DRUG INFORMATION HANDBOOK for NURSING

Including
Assessment, Administration, Monitoring Guidelines and Patient Education

14th Edition

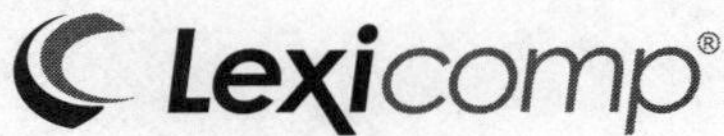

NOTICE

This data is intended to serve the user as a handy reference and not as a complete drug information resource. It does not include information on every therapeutic agent available. The publication covers over 1000 commonly used drugs and is specifically designed to present important aspects of drug data in a more concise format than is typically found in medical literature or product material supplied by manufacturers.

The nature of drug information is that it is constantly evolving because of ongoing research and clinical experience and is often subject to interpretation. While great care has been taken to ensure the accuracy of the information and recommendations presented, the reader is advised that the authors, editors, reviewers, contributors, and publishers cannot be responsible for the continued currency of the information or for any errors, omissions, or the application of this information, or for any consequences arising therefrom. Therefore, the author(s) and/or the publisher shall have no liability to any person or entity with regard to claims, loss, or damage caused, or alleged to be caused, directly or indirectly, by the use of information contained herein. Because of the dynamic nature of drug information, readers are advised that decisions regarding drug therapy must be based on the independent judgment of the clinician, changing information about a drug (eg, as reflected in the literature and manufacturer's most current product information), and changing medical practices. Therefore, this data is designed to be used in conjunction with other necessary information and is not designed to be solely relied upon by any user. The user of this data hereby and forever releases the authors and publishers of this data from any and all liability of any kind that might arise out of the use of this data. The editors are not responsible for any inaccuracy of quotation or for any false or misleading implication that may arise due to the text or formulas as used or due to the quotation of revisions no longer official.

Certain of the authors, editors, and contributors have written this book in their private capacities. No official support or endorsement by any federal or state agency or pharmaceutical company is intended or inferred.

The publishers have made every effort to trace any third party copyright holders, if any, for borrowed material. If they have inadvertently overlooked any, they will be pleased to make the necessary arrangements at the first opportunity.

If you have any suggestions or questions regarding any information presented in this data, please contact our drug information pharmacists at (330) 650-6506. Book revisions are available at our website at http://www.lexi.com/home/revisions/.

This manual was produced using Lexi-Comp's Information Management System™ (LIMS) — A complete publishing service of Lexi-Comp, Inc.

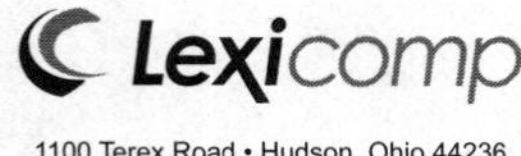

1100 Terex Road • Hudson, Ohio 44236
(330) 650-6506

ISBN 978-1-59195-310-4

TABLE OF CONTENTS

EDITORIAL ADVISORY PANEL

Beth Deen, PharmD, BDNSP
Senior Pediatric Clinical Pharmacy Specialist
Cook Children's Medical Center

Julie A. Dopheide, PharmD, BCPP
Associate Professor of Clinical Pharmacy, Psychiatry and the Behavioral Sciences
Schools of Pharmacy and Medicine
University of Southern California

Teri Dunsworth, PharmD, FCCP, BCPS
Pharmacotherapy Specialist
Lexi-Comp, Inc

Eve Echt, MD
Medical Staff
Department of Radiology
Akron General Medical Center

Michael S. Edwards, PharmD, MBA, BCOP
Chief, Oncology Pharmacy
and *Director, Oncology Pharmacy Residency Program*
Walter Reed Army Medical Center

Vicki L. Ellingrod, PharmD, BCPP
Head, Clinical Pharmacogenomics Laboratory
and *Associate Professor*
Department of Psychiatry
Colleges of Pharmacy and Medicine
University of Michigan

Kelley K. Engle, BSPharm
Medical Science Pharmacist
Lexi-Comp, Inc

Christopher Ensor, PharmD, BCPS (AQ-CV)
Clinical Specialist
Cardiothoracic Transplantation and Mechanical Circulatory Support
The Johns Hopkins Hospital

Erin Fabian, PharmD, RPh
Pharmacotherapy Specialist
Lexi-Comp, Inc

Elizabeth A. Farrington, PharmD, FCCP, FCCM, FPPAG, BCPS
Pharmacist III - Pediatrics
New Hanover Regional Medical Center

Margaret A. Fitzgerald, MS, APRN, BC, NP-C, FAANP
President
Fitzgerald Health Education Associates, Inc.
Family Nurse Practitioner
Greater Lawrence Family Health Center

Lawrence A. Frazee, PharmD, BCPS
Pharmacotherapy Specialist in Internal Medicine
Akron General Medical Center

Matthew A. Fuller, PharmD, BCPS, BCPP, FASHP
Clinical Pharmacy Specialist, Psychiatry
Cleveland Department of Veterans Affairs Medical Center
Associate Clinical Professor of Psychiatry and *Clinical Instructor of Psychology*
Case Western Reserve University
Adjunct Associate Professor of Clinical Pharmacy
University of Toledo

Jason C. Gallagher, PharmD, BCPS
Clinical Pharmacy Specialist, Infectious Diseases
and *Clinical Associate Professor*
Temple University Hospital

Jennifer L. Gardner, PharmD
Neonatal Clinical Pharmacy Specialist
Texas Children's Hospital

Meredith D. Girard, MD, FACP
Medical Staff
Department of Internal Medicine
Summa Health Systems
Assistant Professor Internal Medicine
Northeast Ohio Medical University (NEOMED)

Morton P. Goldman, RPh, PharmD, BCPS, FCCP
Senior Editor
Lexi-Comp, Inc

Julie A. Golembiewski, PharmD
Clinical Associate Professor and *Clinical Pharmacist, Anesthesia/Pain*
Colleges of Pharmacy and Medicine
University of Illinois

Jeffrey P. Gonzales, PharmD, BCPS
Critical Care Clinical Pharmacy Specialist
University of Maryland Medical Center

Roland Grad, MDCM, MSc, CCFP, FCFP
Associate Professor
Department of Family Medicine
McGill University

Larry D. Gray, PhD, ABMM
Director, Clinical Microbiology
TriHealth Laboratories
Bethesda and Good Samaritan Hospitals

Tracy Hagemann, PharmD
Associate Professor
College of Pharmacy
The University of Oklahoma

JoEllen L. Hanigosky, PharmD
Clinical Coordinator
Department of Hematology/Oncology/Bone Marrow Transplant
Children's Hospital of Akron

Martin D. Higbee, PharmD
Associate Professor
Department of Pharmacy Practice and Science
The University of Arizona

EDITORIAL ADVISORY PANEL

Jennifer Fisher Lowe, PharmD, BCOP
Pharmacotherapy Contributor
Lexi-Comp, Inc

Sherry Luedtke, PharmD
Associate Professor
Department of Pharmacy Practice
Texas Tech University HSC School of Pharmacy

Melissa Makii, PharmD, BCPS
Clinical Pharmacy Specialist
Pediatric Oncology
Rainbow Babies & Children's Hospital

Vincent F. Mauro, BS, PharmD, FCCP
Professor of Clinical Pharmacy
and *Adjunct Professor of Medicine*
Colleges of Pharmacy and Medicine
The University of Toledo

Barrie McCombs, MD, FCFP
Medical Information Service Coordinator
The Alberta Rural Physician Action Plan

Christopher McPherson, PharmD
Clinical Pharmacist
Neonatal Intensive Care Unit
St. Louis Children's Hospital

Timothy F. Meiller, DDS, PhD
Professor
Oncology and Diagnostic Sciences
Baltimore College of Dental Surgery
Professor of Oncology
Marlene and Stewart Greenebaum Cancer Center
University of Maryland Medical System

Geralyn M. Meny, MD
Medical Director
American Red Cross, Penn-Jersey Region

Charla E. Miller, RPh, PharmD
Neonatal Clinical Pharmacy Specialist
Wolfson Children's Hospital

Julie Miller, PharmD
Pharmacy Clinical Specialist, Cardiology
Columbus Children's Hospital

Katherine Mills, PharmD
Pharmacotherapy Contributor
Lexi-Comp, Inc

Leah Millstein, MD
Assistant Professor
Division of General Internal Medicine
University of Maryland School of Medicine

Kim Moeller, RN, MSN, OCN, ACNS-BC
Advanced Practice Nurse
Summit Oncology Associates
Akron, Ohio

Kevin M. Mulieri, BS, PharmD
Pediatric Hematology/Oncology Clinical Specialist
Penn State Milton S. Hershey Medical Center
Instructor of Pharmacology
Penn State College of Medicine

Elizabeth A. Neuner, PharmD, BCPS
Infectious Diseases Clinical Specialist
The Cleveland Clinic Foundation

Tom Palma, MS, RPh
Medical Science Pharmacist
Lexi-Comp, Inc

Susie H. Park, PharmD, BCPP
Assistant Professor of Clinical Pharmacy
University of Southern California

Nicole Passerrello, PharmD, BCPS
Pharmacotherapy Specialist
Lexi-Comp, Inc

Alpa Patel, PharmD
Antimicrobial Clinical Pharmacist
University of Louisville Hospital

Gayle Pearson, BSPharm, MSA
Drug Information Pharmacist
Peter Lougheed Centre
Alberta Health Services

James A. Ponto, MS, RPh, BCNP
Chief Nuclear Pharmacist
Department of Radiology
University of Iowa, Hospitals and Clinics
Professor of Clinical Pharmacy
Department of Pharmacy Practice and Science
University of Iowa College of Pharmacy

Amy L. Potts, PharmD, BCPS
Assistant Director
Department of Pharmacy
PGY1 & PGY2 Residency Program Director
Monroe Carell Jr. Children's Hospital at Vanderbilt

James Reissig, PharmD
Assistant Director, Clinical Services
Akron General Medical Center

A.J. (Fred) Remillard, PharmD
Assistant Dean, Research and Graduate Affairs
College of Pharmacy and Nutrition
University of Saskatchewan

Curtis M. Rimmermann, MD, MBA, FACC
Gus P. Karos Chair
Clinical Cardiovascular Medicine
The Cleveland Clinic Foundation

P. David Rogers, PharmD, PhD, FCCP
Director, Clinical and Translational Therapeutics
University of Tennessee College of Pharmacy

Amy Rybarczyk, PharmD, BCPS
Pharmacotherapy Specialist, Internal Medicine
Akron General Medical Center

Jennifer K. Sekeres, PharmD, BCPS
Infectious Diseases Clinical Specialist
The Cleveland Clinic Foundation

EDITORIAL ADVISORY PANEL

DESCRIPTION OF SECTIONS AND FIELDS

Introduction

This and other documents in this section provide guidelines for the use of the handbook including a brief overview of General Nursing Issues (Assessment, Administration, Monitoring, and Patient Education); Patient Factors That Influence Drug Therapy; and Therapeutic Nursing Management of Side Effects.

Individual Drug Monographs

Medications are arranged alphabetically by generic name. Abbreviated monographs contain unique information, commonly for combination formulations.

Monograph Fields

Generic Name	U.S. adopted name.
Pronunciation	Phonetic pronunciation guide.
Brand Names: U.S.	Trade names (manufacturer-specific) found in the United States. The symbol [DSC] appears after trade names that have been recently discontinued.
Index Terms	Other name(s) or accepted abbreviation(s) of the generic drug.
Pharmacologic Category	Unique systematic classification of medications.
Medication Safety Issues	In an effort to promote the safe use of medications, this field is intended to highlight possible sources of medication errors such as sound-alike/look-alike drugs or highly concentrated formulations which require vigilance on the part of healthcare professionals. In addition, medications which have been associated with severe consequences in the event of a medication error are also identified in this field.
Medication Guide Available	Identifies drugs that have an FDA-approved Medication Guide.
Pregnancy Risk Factor	Five categories established by the FDA to indicate the potential of a systemically absorbed drug for causing risk to fetus.
Lactation	Indicates if the drug listed in the monograph is present in breast milk and the manufacturers' recommendation for use while breast-feeding (where recommendation of American Academy of Pediatrics differs, notation is made).
Breast-Feeding Considerations	Information pertinent to or associated with the human use of the drug as it relates to clinical effects on the nursing infant or postpartum woman.
Use	Description of FDA-approved indications of the drug
Unlabeled Use	Information pertaining to non-FDA-approved indications of the drug
Mechanism of Action/Effect	How the drug works in the body to elicit a response
Contraindications	Information pertaining to inappropriate use of the drug as dictated by approved labeling.
Warnings/Precautions	Precautionary considerations, hazardous conditions related to use of the drug, and disease states or patient populations in which the drug should be cautiously used. Boxed warnings, when present, are clearly identified and are adapted from the FDA-approved labeling. Consult the product labeling for the black box warning through the manufacturer's or the FDA website.
Drug Interactions	Agents that, when combined with the drug, may affect therapy; may include the following:
Avoid Concomitant Use	Designates drug combinations which should not be used concomitantly, due to an unacceptable risk:benefit assessment. Frequently, the concurrent use of the agents is explicitly prohibited or contraindicated by the product labeling.
Decreased Effect	Drug combinations that result in a decreased therapeutic effect between the drug listed in the monograph and other drugs or drug classes.
Increased Effect/Toxicity	Drug combinations that result in an increased or toxic therapeutic effect between the drug listed in the monograph and other drugs or drug classes.
Nutritional/Ethanol Interactions	Presents a description of the interaction between the drug listed in the monograph and ethanol, food, or herb/nutraceuticals.
Adverse Reactions	Only side effects >1% are included and are grouped by percentage of incidence (if known)

Pharmacodynamics/Kinetics	May include the following:
Onset of Action	The time after drug administration when therapeutic effect is observed; may also include time for peak therapeutic effect
Duration of Action	Length of therapeutic effect
Product Availability	Provides availability information on products that have been approved by the FDA, but not yet available for use. Estimates for when a product may be available are included, when this information is known. May also provide any unique or critical drug availability issues.
Controlled Substance	The controlled substance classification from the Drug Enforcement Agency (DEA). U.S. schedules are I-V. Schedules vary by country and sometimes state (eg, Massachusetts uses I-VI).
Available Dosage Forms	Information with regard to form, strength, and availability of the drug in the United States. Please consult product labeling for further information.
General Dosage Range	The range of dosing typically used during therapy in children and adults based upon route of administration. The information included is useful for confirming the dose is within the range but should not be used for prescribing purposes. Medications with a variety of indication-specific doses that cannot be encompassed by a range will not have a dose.
Administration	
Oral I.M. I.V. I.V. Detail Inhalation Topical Other	The administration field contains subfields by route regarding issues relative to appropriately giving a medication; includes suggestions on final drug concentrations and/or rates of infusion for parenteral medications and comments regarding the timing of drug administration relative to meals.
Stability	
Reconstitution	Includes comments on solution choice with time or conditions for the mixture to maintain full potency before administration
Storage	Information relating to appropriate storage of the medication prior to opening the manufacturer's original packaging; information is only given if recommendations are for storage at other than room temperature; includes storage requirements for reconstituted products
Nursing Actions	
Physical Assessment	Monitoring guidelines
Patient Education	Suggested items to discuss with the patient or caregiver when taking the medication; may include issues regarding contraception, self-monitoring, precautions, and administration
Dietary Considerations	Includes information on how the medication should be taken relative to meals or food
Related Information	Cross-reference to other pertinent drug information in this handbook

Appendix

The extensive appendix is filled with useful tables and text including conversions, laboratory information, and administration and therapy guidelines.

Alphabetical Index

This is an alphabetical index which provides a quick reference to the monograph section by using the generic names, index terms, and U.S. brand names.

PREGNANCY CATEGORIES

Pregnancy Categories (sometimes referred to as pregnancy risk factors) are a letter system currently required under the *Teratogenic Effects* subsection of the product labeling. The system was initiated in 1979. The categories are required to be part of the package insert for prescription drugs that are systemically absorbed.

The categories are defined as follows:

A Adequate and well-controlled studies in pregnant women have not shown that the drug increases the risk of fetal abnormalities.

B Animal reproduction studies show no evidence of impaired fertility or harm to the fetus; however, no adequate and well-controlled studies have been conducted in pregnant women.
or
Animal reproduction studies have shown adverse events; however, studies in pregnant women have not shown that the drug increases the risk of abnormalities.

C Animal reproduction studies have shown an adverse effect on the fetus. There are no adequate and well-controlled studies in humans and the benefits from the use of the drug in pregnant women may be acceptable, despite its potential risks.
or
Animal reproduction studies have not been conducted.

D Based on human data, the drug can cause fetal harm when administered to pregnant women, but the potential benefits from the use of the drug may be acceptable, despite its potential risks.

X Studies in animals or humans have demonstrated fetal abnormalities (or there is positive evidence of fetal risk based on reports and/or marketing experience) and the risk of using the drug in pregnant women clearly outweighs any possible benefit (for example, safer drugs or other forms of therapy are available).

The categories do not take into consideration nonteratogenic effects (that information is currently presented separately). In 2008, the Food and Drug Administration (FDA) proposed new labeling requirements which would eliminate the use of the pregnancy category system and replace it with scientific data and other information specific to the use of the drug in pregnant women. These proposed changes were suggested because the current category system may be misleading. For instance, some practitioners may believe that risk increases from category A to B to C to D to X, which is not the intent. In addition, practitioners may not be aware that some medications are categorized based on animal data, while others are based on human data. When the new labeling requirements are approved, product labeling will contain pregnancy and lactation subsections, each describing a risk summary, clinical considerations, and section for specific data.

For full descriptions of the current and proposed labeling requirements, refer to the following websites:

Labeling Requirements for Prescription Drugs and/or Insulin (Code of Federal Regulations, Title 21, Volume 4, Revised April 1, 2010). Available at http://www.accessdata.fda.gov/scripts/cdrh/cfdocs/cfCFR/CFRSearch.cfm?fr=201.57

Content and Format of Labeling for Human Prescription Drug and Biological Products; Requirements for Pregnancy and Lactation Labeling (Federal Register, May 29, 2008). Available at http://frwebgate.access.gpo.gov/cgi-bin/getdoc.cgi?dbname=2008_register&docid=fr29my08-33.pdf

GENERAL NURSING ISSUES

ASSESSMENT

Assessment is the *primary* action in the nursing process and it is also a vital part of optimal drug therapy. Assessment activities must precede administering any medication. Appropriate assessment includes not just the particulars of the presenting complaint, but also must include what the patient understands or believes about the problem (eg, etiology and prognosis of complaint, impact of lifestyle habits, etc). Information gathered in primary assessment should serve as a guide to patient education and to identify specific areas that need close monitoring. Generally, assessment starts with a thorough patient history that can include:

- Current complaint: History, observation, laboratory results, other treatments, etc
- Other concurrent conditions: Chronic illnesses
- Past health problems and treatments: Resolved, chronic, treatments effective/noneffective
- Current drugs: Prescription, OTC, home remedies, herbs and herbal medicines
- Past drugs: Reason for taking, effectiveness, adverse effects
- Allergies or adverse effects: Drugs, household products, food products, environmental factors
- Health habits: Caffeine, alcohol, nicotine, street drugs, sleep, activity, nutrition, hydration, sexual activity, pregnant, lactating, use of contraceptives (barrier or oral)
- Physical: Vital signs, weight, height; may include particulars (as necessary) about any body system: pulmonary, cardiac, circulatory, hepatic, renal, gastrointestinal, genitourinary, integument, skeletal, or connective tissues systems
- Psychosocial support: Financial, religious, personal, community

SAFE ADMINISTRATION

Safe administration is grounded in the five "Right" principles: *Right Drug, Right Dose, Right Patient, Right Route, Right Time.*

Right drug: Involves checking drug dispensed with the written prescription. Many drugs have similar names (terbutaline/tolbutamine, calciferol/calcitriol); caution must be used to determine the exact drug prescribed. In addition, a nurse must understand why any particular medication is being prescribed.

Right dose: Requires checking the prescribed dosage, being aware of the "average" or "usual" dosage for that drug, or identifying any particular patient characteristics which may be rational for unusual dosing. Determining the right dose for some medications means titrating dose to monitored physiological parameters determined by hemodynamic or cardiac monitoring, according to kidney or liver function, or calculating dose according to body weight or body surface area.

Right patient: Means identifying each individual patient. Patients in healthcare institutions most generally wear identifying namebands that can be checked prior to administration. When patients are not wearing namebands (eg, at home, in rehabilitation, in outpatient settings), asking patients to identify themselves will reduce medication misadventures.

Right route: Includes consideration of traditional routes (P.O., I.V., I.M., or SubQ, etc). Right route should also include knowledge about whether the dispensed oral drug form can be changed. Can the drug safely be crushed, chewed, dissolved, administered via a nasogastric or any other type of feeding tube. Extended-release formulations should never be crushed, chewed, or dissolved (see Oral Medications That Should Not Be Crushed or Altered on page 1278 in the Appendix). Some intravenous drugs should be administered via a central line because the possibility of peripheral extravasation presents a serious risk for the patient. Some intravenous drugs (eg, ectoposide VP-16, idarubicin, hydroxyzine, ifosfamide, irinotecan, mannitol, mechlorethamine, mitomycin, nafcillin, norepinephrine, phenobarbital, phenylephrine, phenytoin, potassium chloride, vasopressin, etc) are extremely irritating to peripheral veins; this requires their administration via a central line or as dilute solutions at a slow rate given peripherally.

Right time: Necessitates knowledge of a drug's bioavailability; knowing whether the drug should be given at around-the-clock intervals, or whether doses need to be timed in a specific manner. Are there specific dietary considerations? Food will slow the absorption time of many drugs, however, their overall effect will not be affected. Administering medications with food will often reduce the nausea or vomiting that occurs when medications are given on an empty stomach. The drug monographs clearly identify those drugs that must specifically be administered on an empty stomach or should definitely be administered with food. Some monographs include the recommendation for administering in the early part of the day, to reduce night-time sleep interruptions (diuretics).

MONITORING

Nursing actions are found in each monograph and address a wide variety of assessment and monitoring activities. Advanced nurse practitioners may be responsible for both prescribing and monitoring. However, at all times, the nurse responsible for administering the medication or instructing the patient about administration is also responsible for monitoring effectiveness and adverse effects and communicating these details to the prescriber. Some common monitoring responsibilities are described in the following paragraphs.

Assessing patient knowledge/teaching. Specifics regarding the prescribed formulation of the drug and route of administration may require discussing that particular area of concern with a patient (or caregiver) and ensuring that their knowledge is correct and complete. If their knowledge is incomplete or incorrect, then it is vital to teach the patient (or caregiver) the necessary information (eg, correct procedure for using inhalators, instilling ophthalmic medications, inserting a suppository, administering injectable medications, or disposing of needles). Is the patient's knowledge about identifying signs and symptoms of opportunistic infections accurate? Is the patient aware of the precautions necessary with antihypertensives (eg, postural hypotension precautions)? Does the patient understand the rationale for contraception and the difference between oral and barrier forms of contraception? Sometime patients need to be referred to other professionals for advanced education pertaining to their disease and the prescribed drugs (eg, drug monographs for medications used to treat diabetics suggest referring the patient to a diabetic educator).

Monitoring vital signs means more than just identifying normal or abnormal patient responses. It also means communicating any adverse signs or symptoms to the prescriber. When the patient is in danger it may be necessary to discontinue a medication and notify the prescriber. In other instances, it will mean contacting the prescriber for further instructions. Some monitoring is constant, as with emergency drugs; and some is intermittent, as with patient administered medications. Awareness of the need for monitoring, the rationale behind monitoring instructions, and the type of monitoring required is a nursing responsibility.

Monitoring for adverse/toxic response. Known adverse reactions are categorized according to body systems in the Adverse Reactions field. The Physical Assessment section of Nursing Actions also includes reminders about the necessity for monitoring the most threatening or severe of those possible side effects.

Monitoring laboratory test results includes knowing what tests are necessary to monitor drug response and ensuring that ordered tests are done at appropriate times. Communicating laboratory test results to the appropriate prescriber is frequently a nursing responsibility.

Some laboratory tests must be completed prior to administering the first dose of a drug (eg, culture and sensitivity tests, tests that indicate premedication status of liver, kidney, or other systems function). Standard peak and trough serum concentration recommendations are available from most laboratories. Since these may change somewhat among laboratories, it is always best to check with the laboratory that will be completing peak and trough assays to identify their exact timing regulations.

Patient education sections in each drug monograph include the major points that patients need to know about administration safety, including appropriate timing, dietary considerations, drug interaction precautions, and possible actions the patient may take to reduce unpleasant inherent adverse effects (eg, postural hypotension precautions; caution against driving or engaging in hazardous activity because of confusion, dizziness, or impaired judgment; the need to prevent excessive exposure to sunlight because of photosensitivity; and strategies to reduce or prevent nausea and vomiting). See also Therapeutic Nursing Management of Side Effects, found in the Introduction. Adverse effects that should be reported to the prescriber are also identified, including the necessity for informing the prescriber if the patient is pregnant or intends to be pregnant.

Geriatric considerations include information pertinent for that drug in relation to therapy for older patients. In addition to these precautions or information, it is necessary to remember the general effects of aging on drug response, especially the effects that impaired circulation or renal function may have on pharmacokinetics.

PATIENT FACTORS THAT INFLUENCE DRUG THERAPY

Many factors related to an individual patient, or a group of similar patients, can impact the pharmacokinetics of drugs and relate to adverse reactions.

PREGNANCY/LACTATION

The changes that occur during pregnancy may necessitate dosage changes for some drugs. Decreased gastric tract motility, increased blood volume, decreased protein binding sites, and increased glomerular filtration rates may alter the degree of anticipated pharmacotherapeutic response.

Primarily, the concern about drugs during pregnancy is the effect of drugs on the fetus, either teratogenic (causing birth defects) or systemic (causing addiction). Although many drugs cross the placenta, the type of drug, the concentration of that drug, and the gestational age at time of exposure of the fetus are primary determinants of fetal reaction. When prescribing or administering drugs to any childbearing age female, it is vital to ask when her last menstrual period was and, if necessary, to wait for the results of a pregnancy test before starting any drug therapy. Of course, it is best to avoid all drugs during pregnancy, however, in some cases, the physiological context (ie, cardiac output, renal blood flow, etc) may be altered enough to require the use of drugs that are not needed by the same woman when not pregnant.

Most systematically absorbed drugs have been assigned a pregnancy risk factor based on the drugs potential to cause birth defects. This permits an evaluation of the risk:benefit ratio when prescribing or administering drugs becomes necessary. Drugs in the risk factor class "A" are generally considered to be safe for use during pregnancy, class "X" drugs are never safe and are known to be positively teratogenic. See Pregnancy Categories on page 9.

Contraception note: Many drugs will interact with and decrease the effect of oral contraceptives (eg, barbiturates, protease inhibitors, rifampin, and carbamazepine). When a second drug will decrease the effect of oral contraceptives, the patient needs to be educated about the necessity for using a "barrier" (nonhormonal) form of contraception. Barrier contraception (alone or in combination with some form of oral contraception) is often recommended for the patient who must take selected drugs with pregnancy risk factors "D" (idarubicin) or class "X" (isotretinoin).

Because many drugs and substances used by a mother appear in breast milk, care must be taken to evaluate the drug effects on the lactating woman and the infant. Some drugs are identified as being clearly contraindicated during lactation, others may cross into breast milk but adverse side effects on the fetus have not been identified, and for some drugs the administration times should be distanced from nursing time. Nurses should advise lactating women about the effects that drugs may have on the infant.

AGE

All pharmacokinetics (absorption, distribution, metabolism, and excretion) are different in infants, young adults, and elderly patients. Elderly patients may have mildly decreased or severely decreased blood flow to all organs, gastric motility may be slowed, kidney function may be reduced, decreased nutrition may result in decreased albumin, and sedentary lifestyles may have an impact on drug response. Slower gastric motility means that absorption is slowed, resulting in longer time periods to clinical response. Decreased blood flow means that distribution is altered, resulting in decreased response or longer response time. Excretion may be altered with decreased glomerular filtration rates or slower gastric emptying which can result in increased levels of drug remaining in the system.

The ratio between total body water and total body fat also changes with age; older persons have decreased amounts of total body water and higher body fat. This aspect of aging also influences the blood concentration of some drugs. In a person with increased body fat, fat-soluble drugs are distributed to tissues more than to plasma; resulting in a longer response time as the drug must then be redistributed from tissue to plasma. The idiosyncratic response incidence also increases with an aging population. Responses to drugs may be both more exaggerated or diminished with the "usual" doses of some drugs.

In addition, and of major concern with elderly patients, is the incidence of poly-pharmacy; the increased numbers of drugs the patient may be taking. Older patients may have 2, 3, 4, or 5 (or more) chronic conditions for which they are taking medication. In addition, they may be seeing a different prescriber for each of these conditions. Often, it is a nurse who identifies and coordinates the care of these elderly patients, and the nurse must be aware of the possibility for increased incidence of adverse effects.

BODY WEIGHT/BUILD

Most "recommended" dosages of drugs are based on the average size, young or middle aged adult (usually males). Extremely obese or extremely thin patients may be prone to adverse effects as a result of "non-individualized" prescribing. Serum creatinine is a breakdown product of skeletal muscle and its levels in the serum are frequently used to estimate renal function. Decreased muscle mass can result in reduced creatinine from muscle breakdown, leading to a serum creatinine, which is artificially low or appears normal. When dosing is based on estimated creatinine clearance (which is calculated based on the serum creatinine) rather than "actual" creatinine clearance, normal doses may be administered to patients with a diminished capacity for excretion, potentially leading to accumulation and toxicity. This is a particular problem in elderly and/or debilitated patients.

SMOKING, ALCOHOL, NUTRITION, AND HYDRATION

Smoking has a direct impact on liver enzyme activity, blood flow, and the central nervous system. Excessive alcohol intake impacts liver enzymes, renal function, and has an additive effect with most antipsychotic, sedative, or anxiolytic medications, as well as altering responses to many other medications. Nutrition and hydration also play an important part in drug responses and possible adverse reactions. Poor hydration may result in reduced blood flow and excretion. Decreased or prolonged gastric motility can result in slowed excretion and/or prolonged absorption. Poor or inadequate nutrition may result in decreased protein available for binding.

It is vital that a patient's current habits are considered when prescribing, administering, or monitoring drug therapy, but in addition, patients must be aware of the need to inform their professional care provider that they have changed their smoking, alcohol, or dietary patterns. When dosage of theophylline is based on the fact that the patient is a smoker, the theophylline dosage must be adjusted to prevent overdose, if the patient quits smoking. When a patient is on warfarin, drastic increases in the amount of vitamin K intake through increased green leafy vegetables can dramatically alter the dose of warfarin.

OTHER PATIENT FACTORS THAT INFLUENCE DRUG RESPONSE

- Genetic variations
- Differences in circadian patterns
- Disease states
- Psychological temperament

Genetic differences in enzymes may influence the effectiveness of therapy or the incidence of adverse effects (fast acetylators or slow acetylators). The emerging science of pharmacogenomics is devoted to the investigation of these genetic differences in drug response, and offers the hope of truly individualized therapy. Circadian rhythms differ among individuals and have an impact on absorption patterns, hormone secretion, or urinary excretion patterns. Disease states can and do change all aspects of pharmacokinetics. Cirrhosis can impair liver enzyme metabolism rate. Kidney disease will reduce excretion rates for many drugs. Abnormal thyroid function can influence drug metabolism. Diseases which affect blood circulation (eg, hypertension, CHF, Raynaud's phenomena, malignancies, etc) can have an impact on absorption, distribution, and excretion. Diabetes impacts the response to many drugs. Malnutrition, commonly associated with disease, can drastically reduce albumin levels.

See Therapeutic Nursing Management of Side Effects on page 14

THERAPEUTIC NURSING MANAGEMENT OF SIDE EFFECTS

MANAGEMENT OF DRUG-RELATED PROBLEMS

Patients may experience some type of side effect or adverse drug reaction as a result of their drug therapy. The type of effect, the severity, and the frequency of occurrence is dependent on the medication and dose being used, as well as the individual's response to therapy. The following information is presented as helpful tips to assist the patient through these drug-related problems. Pharmacological support may also be required for their management.

Alopecia

- Your hair loss is temporary. Hair usually will begin to grow within 3-6 months of completing drug therapy.
- Your hair may come back with a different texture, color, or thickness.
- Avoid excessive shampooing and hair combing, or harsh hair care products.
- Avoid excessive drying of hair.
- Avoid use of permanents, dyes, or hair sprays.
- Always cover head in cold weather or sunshine.

Anemia

- Observe all bleeding precautions (see Thrombocytopenia).
- Get adequate sleep and rest.
- Be alert for potential for dizziness, fainting, or extreme fatigue.
- Maintain adequate nutrition and hydration.
- Have laboratory tests done as recommended.
- If unusual bleeding occurs, notify prescriber.

Anorexia

- Small frequent meals containing favorite foods may tempt appetite.
- Eat simple foods such as toast, rice, bananas, mashed potatoes, scrambled eggs.
- Eat in a pleasant environment conducive to eating.
- When possible, eat with others.
- Avoid noxious odors when eating.
- Use nutritional supplements high in protein and calories.
- Freezing nutritional supplements sometimes makes them more palatable.
- A small glass of wine (if not contraindicated) may stimulate appetite.
- Mild exercise or short walks may stimulate appetite.
- Request antiemetic medication to reduce nausea or vomiting.

Diarrhea

- Include fiber, high protein foods, and fruits in dietary intake.
- Drink plenty of liquids.
- Buttermilk, yogurt, or boiled milk may be helpful.
- Antidiarrheal agents may be needed. Consult your prescriber.
- Include regular rest periods in your activities.
- Institute skin care regimen to prevent breakdown and promote comfort.

Fluid Retention/Edema

- Elevate legs when sitting.
- Wear support hose.
- Increase physical exercise.
- Maintain adequate hydration; avoiding fluids will not reduce edema.
- Weigh yourself regularly.
- If your prescriber has advised you to limit your salt intake, avoid foods such as ham, bacon, processed meats, and canned foods. Many foods are high in salt content. Read labels carefully.
- Report to prescriber if any of the following occur: Sudden weight gain, decrease in urination, swelling of hands or feed, increase in waist size, wet cough, or difficulty breathing.

Headache

- Lie down.
- Use cool cloth on forehead.
- Avoid caffeine.
- Use mild analgesics. Consult prescriber.

Leukopenia/Neutropenia

- Monitor for signs of infections: Persistent sore throat, fever, chills, fatigue, headache, flu-like symptoms, vaginal discharge, foul-smelling stools.
- Prevent infection. Maintain strict handwashing at all times. Avoid crowds when possible. Avoid exposure to infected persons.
- Avoid exposure to temperature changes.
- Maintain adequate nutrition and hydration.
- Maintain good personal hygiene.
- Avoid injury or skin breaks.
- Avoid vaccinations (unless recommended by healthcare provider).
- Avoid sunburn.

Nausea and Vomiting

- Eat food served cold or at room temperature. Ice chips are sometimes helpful.
- Drink clear liquids in severe cases of nausea. Avoid carbonated beverages.
- Sip liquids slowly.
- Avoid spicy food. Bland foods are easier to digest.
- Rinse mouth with lemon water. Practice good oral hygiene.
- Avoid sweet, fatty, salty foods and foods with strong odors.
- Eat small frequent meals rather than heavy meals.
- Use relaxation techniques and guided imagery.
- Use distractions such as meals, television, reading, games, etc.
- Sleep during intense periods of nausea.
- Chew gum or suck on hard candy or lozenges.
- Eat in an upright (sitting position), rather than semirecumbant.
- Avoid tight constrictive clothing at meal time.
- Use some mild exercise following light meals rather than lying down.
- Request antiemetic medication to reduce nausea or vomiting.

Postural Hypotension

- Use care and rise slowly from sitting or lying position to standing.
- Use care when climbing stairs.
- Initiate ambulation slowly. Get your bearings before you start walking.
- Do not bend over; always squat slowly if you must pick up something from floor.
- Use caution when showering or bathing (use secure handrails).

Stomatitis

- Perform good oral hygiene frequently, especially before and after meals.
- Avoid use of strong or alcoholic commercial mouthwashes.
- Keep lips well lubricated.
- Avoid tobacco or other products that are irritating to the oral mucosa.
- Avoid hot, spicy, excessively salty foods.
- Eat soft foods and drink adequate fluids.
- Request topical or systemic analgesics for painful ulcerations.
- Be alert for and report signs of oral fungal infections.

Thrombocytopenia

- Avoid aspirin and aspirin-containing products.
- Use electric or safety razor and blunt scissors.
- Use soft toothbrush or cotton swabs for oral care. Avoid use of dental floss.
- Avoid use of enemas, cathartics, and suppositories unless approved by prescriber.
- Avoid valsalva maneuvers such as straining at stool.
- Use stool softeners if necessary to prevent constipation. Consult prescriber.
- Avoid blowing nose forcefully.
- Never go barefoot, wear protective foot covering.
- Use care when trimming nails (if necessary).
- Maintain safe environment; arrange furniture to provide safe passageway.
- Maintain adequate lighting in darkened areas to avoid bumping into objects.
- Avoid handling sharp tools or instruments.
- Avoid contact sports or activities that might result in injury.
- Promptly report signs of bleeding; abdominal pain; blood in stool, urine, or vomitus; unusual fatigue; easy bruising; bleeding around gums; or nosebleeds.
- If injection or bloodsticks are necessary, inform healthcare provider that you may have excess bleeding.

Vertigo

- Observe postural hypotension precautions.
- Use caution when driving or using any machinery.
- Avoid sudden position shifts; do not "rush".
- Utilize appropriate supports (eg, cane, walker) to prevent injury.

ALPHABETICAL LISTING OF DRUGS

Abacavir (a BAK a veer)

Brand Names: U.S. Ziagen®

Index Terms Abacavir Sulfate; ABC

Pharmacologic Category Antiretroviral Agent, Reverse Transcriptase Inhibitor (Nucleoside)

Medication Guide Available Yes

Pregnancy Risk Factor C

Lactation Excretion in breast milk unknown/contraindicated

Breast-Feeding Considerations Maternal or infant antiretroviral therapy does not completely eliminate the risk of postnatal HIV transmission. In addition, multiclass-resistant virus has been detected in breast-feeding infants despite maternal therapy. Therefore, in the United States, where formula is accessible, affordable, safe, and sustainable, and the risk of infant mortality due to diarrhea and respiratory infections is low, complete avoidance of breast-feeding by HIV-infected women is recommended to decrease potential transmission of HIV (DHHS [perinatal], 2011).

Use Treatment of HIV infections in combination with other antiretroviral agents

Mechanism of Action/Effect Nucleoside reverse transcriptase inhibitor which interferes with HIV viral RNA-dependent DNA polymerase resulting in inhibition of viral replication

Contraindications Hypersensitivity to abacavir or any component of the formulation (do not rechallenge patients who have experienced hypersensitivity to abacavir regardless of *HLA-B*5701* status); moderate-to-severe hepatic impairment

Warnings/Precautions Abacavir should always be used as a component of a multidrug regimen. **[U.S. Boxed Warning]: Serious and sometimes fatal hypersensitivity reactions have occurred.** Patients testing positive for the presence of the *HLA-B*5701* allele are at an increased risk for hypersensitivity reactions. Screening for *HLA-B*5701* allele status is recommended prior to initiating therapy or reinitiating therapy in patients of unknown status, including patients who previously tolerated therapy. Therapy is **not** recommended in patients testing positive for the *HLA-B*5701* allele. An allergy to abacavir should be reported in the patient's medical record (DHHS, 2011). Reactions usually occur within 9 days of starting abacavir; ~90% occur within 6 weeks. Patients exhibiting symptoms from two or more of the following: Fever, skin rash, constitutional symptoms (malaise, fatigue, aches), respiratory symptoms (eg, pharyngitis, dyspnea, cough), and GI symptoms (eg, abdominal pain, diarrhea, nausea, vomiting) should discontinue therapy immediately and call for medical attention. Abacavir should be permanently discontinued if hypersensitivity cannot be ruled out, even when other diagnoses are possible and regardless of *HLA-B*5701* status. Abacavir SHOULD NOT be restarted because more severe symptoms may occur within hours, including LIFE-THREATENING HYPOTENSION AND DEATH. Fatal hypersensitivity reactions have occurred following the reintroduction of abacavir in patients whose therapy was interrupted (ie, interruption in drug supply, temporary discontinuation while treating other conditions). In some cases, signs of hypersensitivity may have been previously present, but attributed to other medical conditions (eg, acute onset respiratory diseases, gastroenteritis, reactions to other medications). If abacavir is restarted following an interruption in therapy, evaluate the patient for previously unsuspected symptoms of hypersensitivity. To report these events on abacavir hypersensitivity, a registry has been established (1-800-270-0425). A higher incidence of severe hypersensitivity reactions may be associated with a 600 mg once daily dosing regimen.

[U.S. Boxed Warning]: Lactic acidosis and severe hepatomegaly with steatosis (sometimes fatal) have occurred with antiretroviral nucleoside analogues. Female gender, prior liver disease, obesity, and prolonged treatment may increase the risk of hepatotoxicity. May be associated with fat redistribution. Immune reconstitution syndrome may develop; further evaluation and treatment may be required. Use has been associated with an increased risk of myocardial infarction (MI) in observational studies; however, based on a meta-analysis of 26 randomized trials, the FDA has concluded there is not an increased risk. Consider using with caution in patients with risks for coronary heart disease and minimizing modifiable risk factors (eg, hypertension, hyperlipidemia, diabetes mellitus, and smoking) prior to use. Products may contain propylene glycol. Safety and efficacy in children <3 months of age have not been established.

Drug Interactions

Avoid Concomitant Use There are no known interactions where it is recommended to avoid concomitant use.

Decreased Effect

The levels/effects of Abacavir may be decreased by: Protease Inhibitors

Increased Effect/Toxicity

The levels/effects of Abacavir may be increased by: Ganciclovir-Valganciclovir; Ribavirin

Nutritional/Ethanol Interactions Ethanol: Ethanol may increase the risk of toxicity.

Adverse Reactions Hypersensitivity reactions (which may be fatal) occur in ~5% of patients. Symptoms may include anaphylaxis, fever, rash (including erythema multiforme), fatigue, diarrhea, abdominal pain; respiratory symptoms (eg, pharyngitis, dyspnea, cough, adult respiratory distress syndrome, or respiratory failure); headache, malaise, lethargy, myalgia, myolysis, arthralgia, edema, paresthesia, nausea and vomiting, mouth ulcerations, conjunctivitis, lymphadenopathy, hepatic failure, and renal failure.

Note: Rates of adverse reactions were defined during combination therapy with other antiretrovirals (lamivudine and efavirenz **or** lamivudine and zidovudine). Only reactions which occurred at a higher frequency in adults (except where noted) than in the comparator group are noted. Adverse reaction rates attributable to abacavir alone are not available.

>10%:

Central nervous system: Headache (7% to 13%)
Gastrointestinal: Nausea (7% to 19%, children 9%)

1% to 10%:

Central nervous system: Depression (6%), fever/chills (6%, children 9%), anxiety (5%)
Dermatologic: Rash (5% to 6%, children 7%)
Endocrine & metabolic: Triglycerides increased (2% to 6%)
Gastrointestinal: Diarrhea (7%), vomiting (children 9%), amylase increased (2%)
Hematologic: Thrombocytopenia (1%)
Hepatic: AST increased (6%)
Neuromuscular & skeletal: Musculoskeletal pain (5% to 6%)
Miscellaneous: Hypersensitivity reactions (2% to 9%; may include reactions to other components of antiretroviral regimen), infection (ENT 5%)

Available Dosage Forms

Solution, oral:

Ziagen®: 20 mg/mL (240 mL)

Tablet, oral:

Ziagen®: 300 mg

General Dosage Range Dosage adjustment recommended in patients with hepatic impairment

Oral:

Infants and Children ≥3 months to <16 years: 8 mg/kg twice daily (maximum: 300 mg twice daily)

Adolescents ≥16 years and Adults: 600 mg/day in 1-2 divided doses (maximum: 600 mg/day)

Administration

Oral May be administered with or without food.

Stability

Storage Store oral solution and tablets at controlled room temperature of 20°C to 25°C (68°F to 77°F). Oral solution may be refrigerated; do not freeze.

Nursing Actions

Physical Assessment Previous exposure/allergy to abacavir and risk factors for heart disease should be assessed prior to beginning treatment. A medication guide and a warning card (summarizing symptoms of hypersensitivity) are available in each bottle and patients should be provided with this information. Monitor patient closely for any sign of hypersensitivity reaction; can occur within hours or at any time and may be fatal (can also occur at reintroduction with patients who have no history of previous reaction). Assess decrease in infections. Teach patient proper timing of multiple medications and importance of immediately reporting any sign of hypersensitivity or myocardial infarction.

Patient Education You will be provided with a medication guide to help educate you about the medication and a warning card summarizing symptoms of hypersensitivity. This drug will not cure HIV, nor has it been found to reduce transmission of HIV; use appropriate precautions to prevent spread to other persons. This drug is prescribed as one part of a multidrug combination; take exactly as directed for full course of therapy. Maintain adequate hydration, unless instructed to restrict fluids. Avoid alcohol. Frequent blood tests may be required. May cause dizziness, weakness, nausea, and vomiting. Seek immediate emergency care if you experience unusual chest pain, palpitations, or if you suspect you are having a heart attack. Stop drug and report immediately symptoms of hypersensitivity (eg, fever; rash; fatigue, malaise, lethargy; persistent nausea, vomiting, diarrhea, abdominal pain; mouth sores; sore throat, cough, difficulty breathing; headache; swelling of face, mouth or throat; numbness or loss of sensation; pain, tingling, or numbness in toes, feet, muscles or joints; swollen glands; alterations in urinary pattern; swelling of extremities or weight gain). Do not restart without specific instruction by your prescriber.

Dietary Considerations May be taken with or without food.

Abacavir and Lamivudine

(a BAK a veer & la MI vyoo deen)

Brand Names: U.S. Epzicom®

Index Terms Abacavir Sulfate and Lamivudine; Lamivudine and Abacavir

Pharmacologic Category Antiretroviral Agent, Reverse Transcriptase Inhibitor (Nucleoside)

Medication Guide Available Yes

Pregnancy Risk Factor C

Lactation See individual agents.

Use Treatment of HIV infections in combination with other antiretroviral agents

Available Dosage Forms

Tablet:

Epzicom®: Abacavir 600 mg and lamivudine 300 mg

General Dosage Range Oral: *Adults:* One tablet (abacavir 600 mg and lamivudine 300 mg) once daily

Administration

Oral May be administered with or without food.

Nursing Actions

Physical Assessment See individual agents.

Patient Education See individual agents.

Abacavir, Lamivudine, and Zidovudine

(a BAK a veer, la MI vyoo deen, & zye DOE vyoo deen)

Brand Names: U.S. Trizivir®

Index Terms 3TC, Abacavir, and Zidovudine; Azidothymidine, Abacavir, and Lamivudine; AZT, Abacavir, and Lamivudine; Compound S, Abacavir, and Lamivudine; Lamivudine, Abacavir, and Zidovudine; ZDV, Abacavir, and Lamivudine; Zidovudine, Abacavir, and Lamivudine

Pharmacologic Category Antiretroviral Agent, Reverse Transcriptase Inhibitor (Nucleoside)

Medication Guide Available Yes

Pregnancy Risk Factor C

Lactation See individual agents.

Use Treatment of HIV infection (either alone or in combination with other antiretroviral agents) in patients whose regimen would otherwise contain the components of Trizivir®

Available Dosage Forms

Tablet, oral:

Trizivir®: Abacavir 300 mg, lamivudine 150 mg, and zidovudine 300 mg

General Dosage Range Oral: *Adolescents ≥40 kg and Adults:* 1 tablet twice daily

Administration

Oral Administer without regard to food.

Nursing Actions

Physical Assessment See individual agents.

Patient Education See individual agents.

Related Information

Abacavir *on page 18*

LamiVUDine *on page 664*

Zidovudine *on page 1197*

Abatacept (ab a TA sept)

Brand Names: U.S. Orencia®

Index Terms BMS-188667; CTLA-4Ig

Pharmacologic Category Antirheumatic, Disease Modifying; Selective T-Cell Costimulation Blocker

Medication Safety Issues

Sound-alike/look-alike issues:

Orencia® may be confused with Oracea®

Pregnancy Risk Factor C

Lactation Excretion in breast milk unknown/not recommended

Breast-Feeding Considerations Due to the potential for adverse reactions and possible effects on the developing immune system, breast-feeding is not recommended.

Use

Treatment of moderately- to severely-active adult rheumatoid arthritis (RA); may be used as monotherapy or in combination with other DMARDs

Treatment of moderately- to severely-active juvenile idiopathic arthritis (JIA); may be used as monotherapy or in combination with methotrexate

Note: Abatacept should **not** be used in combination with anakinra or TNF-blocking agents

Mechanism of Action/Effect Prevents activation of T cells

Contraindications There are no contraindications listed within the FDA-approved labeling.

Warnings/Precautions Serious and potentially fatal infections (including tuberculosis and sepsis) have been reported, particularly in patients receiving concomitant immunosuppressive therapy. RA patients receiving a concomitant TNF antagonist experienced an even higher rate of serious infection. Caution should be exercised when considering the use of abatacept in any patient with a history of recurrent infections, with conditions that predispose them to infections, or with chronic, latent, or localized infections. Patients who develop a new infection while undergoing treatment should be monitored closely. If a patient develops a serious infection, abatacept should be discontinued. Screen patients for latent tuberculosis infection prior to initiating abatacept; safety in tuberculosis-positive patients has not been established. Treat patients testing positive according to standard therapy prior to initiating abatacept. Adult patients receiving abatacept in combination with TNF-blocking agents had higher rates of infections (including serious infections) than patients on TNF-blocking agents alone. The manufacturer does not recommend concurrent use with anakinra or TNF-blocking agents. Monitor for signs and symptoms of infection when transitioning from TNF-blocking agents to abatacept. Due to the effect of T-cell inhibition on host defenses, abatacept may affect immune responses against infections and malignancies; impact on the development and course of malignancies is not fully defined.

Use caution with chronic obstructive pulmonary disease (COPD), higher incidences of adverse effects (COPD exacerbation, cough, rhonchi, dyspnea) have been observed; monitor closely. Rare cases of hypersensitivity, anaphylaxis, or anaphylactoid reactions have been reported; medications for the treatment of hypersensitivity reactions should be available for immediate use. Patients should be screened for viral hepatitis prior to use; antirheumatic therapy may cause reactivation of hepatitis B. Patients should be brought up to date with all immunizations before initiating therapy. Live vaccines should not be given concurrently or within 3 months of discontinuation of therapy; there is no data available concerning secondary transmission of live vaccines in patients receiving therapy. Powder for injection may contain maltose, which may result in falsely-elevated serum glucose readings on the day of infusion. Higher incidences of infection and malignancy were observed in the elderly; use with caution.

Drug Interactions

Avoid Concomitant Use

Avoid concomitant use of Abatacept with any of the following: Anti-TNF Agents; BCG; Belimumab; Natalizumab; Pimecrolimus; Tacrolimus (Topical); Vaccines (Live)

Decreased Effect

Abatacept may decrease the levels/effects of: BCG; Coccidioidin Skin Test; Sipuleucel-T; Vaccines (Inactivated); Vaccines (Live)

The levels/effects of Abatacept may be decreased by: Echinacea

Increased Effect/Toxicity

Abatacept may increase the levels/effects of: Belimumab; Leflunomide; Natalizumab; Vaccines (Live)

The levels/effects of Abatacept may be increased by: Anti-TNF Agents; Denosumab; Pimecrolimus; Roflumilast; Tacrolimus (Topical); Trastuzumab

Nutritional/Ethanol Interactions Herb/Nutraceutical: Avoid echinacea (has immunostimulant properties; consider therapy modifications).

Adverse Reactions Note: Percentages not always reported; COPD patients experienced a higher frequency of COPD-related adverse reactions (COPD exacerbation, cough, dyspnea, pneumonia, rhonchi)

>10%:

Central nervous system: Headache (≤18%)

Gastrointestinal: Nausea

Respiratory: Nasopharyngitis (12%), upper respiratory tract infection

Miscellaneous: Infection (adults 54%; children 36%), antibody formation (2% to 41%)

1% to 10%:

Cardiovascular: Hypertension (7%)

Central nervous system: Dizziness (9%), fever

Dermatologic: Rash (4%)

Gastrointestinal: Dyspepsia (6%), abdominal pain, diarrhea

Genitourinary: Urinary tract infection (6%)

Local: Injection site reaction (3%)

Neuromuscular & skeletal: Back pain (7%), limb pain (3%)

Respiratory: Cough (8%), bronchitis, pneumonia, rhinitis, sinusitis

Miscellaneous: Infusion-related reactions (≤9%), herpes simplex, immunogenicity (1% to 2%), influenza

Available Dosage Forms

Injection, powder for reconstitution [preservative free]:

Orencia®: 250 mg

Injection, solution [preservative free]:

Orencia®: 125 mg/mL (1 mL)

General Dosage Range

I.V.: Repeat dose at 2 weeks and 4 weeks, then every 4 weeks thereafter

Children ≥6 years and <75 kg: 10 mg/kg/dose

Children ≥6 years and 75-100 kg: 750 mg/dose

Children ≥6 years and >100 kg: 1000 mg/dose

Adults <60 kg: 500 mg/dose

Adults 60-100 kg: 750 mg/dose

Adults >100 kg: 1000 mg/dose

SubQ: *Adults:* 125 mg/dose once weekly

Administration

I.V. Infuse over 30 minutes. Administer through a 0.2-1.2 micron low protein-binding filter

I.V. Detail pH: 7-8

Other SubQ: Allow prefilled syringe to warm to room temperature (for 30-60 minutes) prior to administration. Inject into the front of the thigh (preferred), abdomen (except for 2-inch area around the navel), or the outer area of the upper arms (if administered by a caregiver). Rotate injection sites (≥1 inch apart); do not administer into tender, bruised, red, or hard skin.

Stability

Reconstitution Reconstitute each vial with 10 mL SWFI using the provided silicone-free disposable syringe (discard solutions accidentally reconstituted with siliconized syringe as they may develop translucent particles). Inject SWFI down the side of the vial to avoid foaming. The reconstituted solution contains 25 mg/mL abatacept. Further dilute (using a silicone-free syringe) in 100 mL NS to a final concentration of ≤10 mg/mL. Prior to adding abatacept to the 100 mL bag, the manufacturer recommends withdrawing a volume of NS equal to the abatacept volume required, resulting in a final volume of 100 mL. Mix gently; do not shake.

Storage

Prefilled syringe: Store at 2°C to 8°C (36°F to 46°F); do not freeze. Protect from light.

Powder for injection: Prior to reconstitution, store at 2°C to 8°C (36°F to 46°F); do not freeze. Protect from light. After dilution, may be stored for up to 24 hours at room temperature or refrigerated at 2°C to 8°C (36°F to 46°F). Must be used within 24 hours of reconstitution.

Nursing Actions

Physical Assessment Perform testing for tuberculosis prior to initiating therapy. Assess for infection prior to initiating infusion.

Patient Education You may be more susceptible to infections. Report signs of infection, such as fever, chills, sore throat, and flu-like symptoms. May cause falsely elevated blood glucose readings on day of infusion. You may experience headache, sore throat, and nausea. Report immediately respiratory difficulty including wheezing, hives, dizziness, nausea, flushing, cough, or any signs of infection. Do not receive live vaccines, such as measles, mumps, chickenpox, BCG, or rubella while taking this medication.

Abiraterone Acetate (a bir A ter one AS e tate)

Brand Names: U.S. Zytiga™

Index Terms Abiraterone; CB7630

Pharmacologic Category Antiandrogen; Antineoplastic Agent, Antiandrogen

Pregnancy Risk Factor X

Lactation Excretion in breast milk unknown/not recommended

Use Treatment of metastatic, castration-resistant prostate cancer (in combination with prednisone) in patients previously treated with docetaxel

Available Dosage Forms

Tablet, oral:

Zytiga™: 250 mg

General Dosage Range Dosage adjustment recommended in patients with hepatic impairment or who develop toxicity.

Oral: *Adults:* 1000 mg once daily

Administration

Oral Administer on an empty stomach, at least 1 hour before and 2 hours after food. Swallow tablets whole with water.

Acamprosate (a kam PROE sate)

Brand Names: U.S. Campral®

Index Terms Acamprosate Calcium; Calcium Acetylhomotaurinate

Pharmacologic Category GABA Agonist/Glutamate Antagonist

Pregnancy Risk Factor C

Lactation Excretion in breast milk unknown/use caution

Use Maintenance of alcohol abstinence

Available Dosage Forms

Tablet, delayed release, enteric coated, oral:

Campral®: 333 mg

General Dosage Range Dosage adjustment recommended in patients with renal impairment.

Oral: *Adults:* 666 mg 3 times/day (maximum: 1998 mg/day)

Administration

Oral May be administered without regard to meals (administered with meals during clinical trials to possibly increase compliance). Tablet should be swallowed whole; do not crush or chew.

Nursing Actions

Physical Assessment Can cause depression. Monitor for suicide ideation.

Patient Education Taking this medication helps maintain abstinence only when used as part of a treatment program that includes counseling and support. Swallow tablet whole. Do not chew or crush. Can cause drowsiness. You may experience diarrhea, peripheral edema, insomnia, anxiety, depression, and generalized weakness. Report persistent diarrhea, excessive or sudden weight gain, swelling of extremities, respiratory difficulties, fainting, or thoughts of suicide.

Acarbose (AY car bose)

Brand Names: U.S. Precose®

Pharmacologic Category Antidiabetic Agent, Alpha-Glucosidase Inhibitor

Medication Safety Issues

Sound-alike/look-alike issues:

Precose® may be confused with PreCare®

International issues:

Precose® [U.S., Malaysia] may be confused with Precosa brand name for *Saccharomyces boulardii* [Finland, Sweden]

Pregnancy Risk Factor B

Lactation Excretion in breast milk unknown/not recommended

Breast-Feeding Considerations It is not known if acarbose is found in breast milk; however, low amounts of acarbose are absorbed systemically in adults, which may limit the amount that could distribute into breast milk. Breast-feeding is not recommended by the manufacturer.

Use Adjunct to diet and exercise to lower blood glucose in patients with type 2 diabetes mellitus (noninsulin dependent, NIDDM)

Mechanism of Action/Effect Delays glucose absorption and lowers postprandial hyperglycemia.

Contraindications Hypersensitivity to acarbose or any component of the formulation; patients with diabetic ketoacidosis or cirrhosis; patients with inflammatory bowel disease, colonic ulceration, partial intestinal obstruction, or in patients predisposed to intestinal obstruction; patients who have chronic intestinal diseases associated with marked disorders of digestion or absorption, and in patients who have conditions that may deteriorate as a result of increased gas formation in the intestine

Warnings/Precautions Acarbose given in combination with a sulfonylurea or insulin will cause a further lowering of blood glucose and may increase the hypoglycemic potential of the sulfonylurea or insulin. Treatment-emergent elevations of serum transaminases (AST and/or ALT) occurred in up to 14% of acarbose-treated patients in long-term studies. These serum transaminase elevations appear to be dose related and were asymptomatic, reversible, more common in females, and, in general, were not associated with other evidence of liver dysfunction. Fulminant hepatitis has been reported rarely. It may be necessary to discontinue acarbose and administer insulin if the patient is exposed to stress (ie, fever, trauma, infection, surgery). Use not recommended in patients with significant impairment (S_{cr} >2 mg/dL); use with caution in other patients with renal impairment.

Drug Interactions

Avoid Concomitant Use There are no known interactions where it is recommended to avoid concomitant use.

Decreased Effect

Acarbose may decrease the levels/effects of: Digoxin

The levels/effects of Acarbose may be decreased by: Corticosteroids (Orally Inhaled); Corticosteroids (Systemic); Luteinizing Hormone-Releasing Hormone Analogs; Somatropin; Thiazide Diuretics

Increased Effect/Toxicity

Acarbose may increase the levels/effects of: Hypoglycemic Agents

The levels/effects of Acarbose may be increased by: Herbs (Hypoglycemic Properties); Neomycin; Pegvisomant

Nutritional/Ethanol Interactions Ethanol: Limit ethanol.

Adverse Reactions >10%:

Gastrointestinal: Diarrhea (31%) and abdominal pain (19%) tend to return to pretreatment levels over time; frequency and intensity of flatulence (74%) tend to abate with time

Hepatic: Transaminases increased (≤4%)

Available Dosage Forms

Tablet, oral: 25 mg, 50 mg, 100 mg

Precose®: 25 mg, 50 mg, 100 mg

General Dosage Range Dosage adjustment recommended in patients on concomitant therapy

Oral: *Adults:* Initial: 25 mg 1-3 times/day; Maintenance: 75-300 mg/day in 3 divided doses (maximum: ≤60 kg: 150 mg/day; >60 kg: 300 mg/day)

Administration

Oral Should be **administered with the first bite of each main meal.**

Stability

Storage Store at <25°C (77°F). Protect from moisture.

Nursing Actions

Physical Assessment Teach patient importance of diabetic control.

Patient Education Take this medication with the first bite of each main meal. Do not take other medications with or within 2 hours of this medication unless advised by prescriber. Avoid alcohol. It is important to follow dietary and lifestyle recommendations of prescriber. You will be instructed in signs of hyper-/hypoglycemia. If combining acarbose with other diabetic medication (eg, sulfonylureas, insulin), keep source of glucose in the form of dextrose (NOT table sugar, candy, or cookies) on hand in case hypoglycemia occurs. May cause mild side effects during first weeks of acarbose therapy (eg, bloating, flatulence, diarrhea, abdominal discomfort); these should diminish over time. Report severe or persistent side effects, fever, extended vomiting or flu, or change in color of urine or stool.

Dietary Considerations Take with food (first bite of meal).

Acetaminophen (a seet a MIN oh fen)

Brand Names: U.S. Acephen™ [OTC]; APAP 500 [OTC]; Aspirin Free Anacin® Extra Strength [OTC]; Cetafen® Extra [OTC]; Cetafen® [OTC]; Excedrin® Tension Headache [OTC]; Feverall® [OTC]; Infantaire [OTC]; Little Fevers™ [OTC]; Mapap® Arthritis Pain [OTC]; Mapap® Children's [OTC]; Mapap® Extra Strength [OTC]; Mapap® Infant's [OTC]; Mapap® Junior Rapid Tabs [OTC]; Mapap® [OTC]; Non-Aspirin Pain Reliever [OTC]; Nortemp Children's [OTC]; Ofirmev™; Pain & Fever Children's [OTC]; Pain Eze [OTC]; RapiMed® Children's [OTC]; RapiMed® Junior [OTC]; Silapap Children's [OTC]; Silapap Infant's [OTC]; Triaminic™ Children's Fever Reducer Pain Reliever [OTC]; Tylenol® 8 Hour [OTC]; Tylenol® Arthritis Pain Extended Relief [OTC]; Tylenol® Children's Meltaways [OTC]; Tylenol® Children's [OTC]; Tylenol® Extra Strength [OTC]; Tylenol® Infant's Concentrated [OTC]; Tylenol® Jr. Meltaways [OTC]; Tylenol® [OTC]; Valorin Extra [OTC]; Valorin [OTC]

Index Terms APAP (abbreviation is not recommended); N-Acetyl-P-Aminophenol; Paracetamol

Pharmacologic Category Analgesic, Miscellaneous

Medication Safety Issues

Sound-alike/look-alike issues:

Acephen® may be confused with AcipHex®

FeverALL® may be confused with Fiberall®

Triaminic™ Children's Fever Reducer Pain Reliever may be confused with Triaminic® cough and cold products

Tylenol® may be confused with atenolol, timolol, Tylenol® PM, Tylox®

Other safety concerns:

Duplicate therapy issues: This product contains acetaminophen, which may be a component of combination products. Do not exceed the maximum recommended daily dose of acetaminophen.

The new infant acetaminophen concentration (160 mg/5 mL) is available. All children's liquid acetaminophen products will now be the same 160 mg/5 mL concentration. However, the former infant acetaminophen concentration (80 mg/0.8 mL) may still be available in some pharmacies until supplies run out. Check concentrations closely prior to administering or dispensing (November 2011).

International issues:

Depon [Greece] may be confused with Depen brand name for penicillamine [U.S.]; Depin brand name for nifedipine [India]; Dipen brand name for diltiazem [Greece]

Duorol [Spain] may be confused with Diuril brand name for chlorothiazide [U.S., Canada]

Paralen [Czech Republic] may be confused with Aralen brand name for chloroquine [U.S., Mexico]

Pregnancy Risk Factor C (intravenous)

Lactation Enters breast milk/use caution (AAP rates "compatible"; AAP 2001 update pending)

Breast-Feeding Considerations Low concentrations of acetaminophen are excreted into breast milk and can be detected in the urine of nursing infants. Adverse reactions have generally not been observed; however, a rash caused by acetaminophen exposure was reported in one breast-feeding infant.

Use Treatment of mild-to-moderate pain and fever (analgesic/antipyretic)

I.V.: Additional indication: Management of moderate-to-severe pain when combined with opioid analgesia

Mechanism of Action/Effect Reduces fever by acting on the hypothalamus to cause vasodilatation and sweating

Contraindications Hypersensitivity to acetaminophen or any component of the formulation; severe hepatic impairment or severe active liver disease (Ofirmev™)

Warnings/Precautions Limit dose to <4 g/day. May cause severe hepatotoxicity on acute overdose; in addition, chronic daily dosing in adults has resulted in liver damage in some patients. Use with caution in patients with alcoholic liver disease; consuming ≥3 alcoholic drinks/day may increase the risk of liver damage. Use caution in patients with hepatic impairment or active liver disease. Use of intravenous formulation is contraindicated in patients with severe hepatic impairment or severe active liver disease. Use caution in patients with known G6PD deficiency; rare reports of hemolysis have occurred. Use caution in patients with chronic malnutrition and hypovolemia (intravenous formulation). Use caution in patients with severe renal impairment; consider dosing adjustments. Hypersensitivity and anaphylactic reactions have been reported; discontinue immediately if symptoms of allergic or hypersensitivity reactions occur.

OTC labeling: When used for self-medication, patients should be instructed to contact healthcare provider if used for fever lasting >3 days or for pain lasting >10 days in adults or >5 days in children.

Drug Interactions

Avoid Concomitant Use

Avoid concomitant use of Acetaminophen with any of the following: Pimozide

Decreased Effect

The levels/effects of Acetaminophen may be decreased by: Anticonvulsants (Hydantoin); Barbiturates; CarBAMazepine; Cholestyramine Resin; Cyproterone; Peginterferon Alfa-2b; Tocilizumab

Increased Effect/Toxicity

Acetaminophen may increase the levels/effects of: ARIPiprazole; Busulfan; Dasatinib; Imatinib; Pimozide; Prilocaine; SORAfenib; Vitamin K Antagonists

The levels/effects of Acetaminophen may be increased by: Conivaptan; Dasatinib; Imatinib; Isoniazid; Metyrapone; Probenecid; SORAfenib

Nutritional/Ethanol Interactions

Ethanol: Excessive intake of ethanol may increase the risk of acetaminophen-induced hepatotoxicity. Avoid ethanol or limit to <3 drinks/day.

Food: Rate of absorption may be decreased when given with food.

Herb/Nutraceutical: St John's wort may decrease acetaminophen levels.

Adverse Reactions Oral, Rectal: Frequency not defined:

Dermatologic: Rash

Endocrine & metabolic: May increase chloride, uric acid, glucose; may decrease sodium, bicarbonate, calcium

Hematologic: Anemia; blood dyscrasias (neutropenia, pancytopenia, leukopenia)

Hepatic: Bilirubin increased, alkaline phosphatase increased

Renal: Ammonia increased, nephrotoxicity with chronic overdose, analgesic nephropathy

Miscellaneous: Hypersensitivity reactions (rare)

I.V.:

>10%: Gastrointestinal: Nausea (adults 34%; children ≥5%), vomiting (adults 15%; children ≥5%)

1% to 10%:

Cardiovascular: Edema (peripheral), hypervolemia, hypo/hypertension, tachycardia

Central nervous system: Headache (adults 10%; children ≥1%), insomnia (adults 7%; children ≥1%), agitation (children ≥5%), anxiety, fatigue

Dermatologic: Pruritus (children ≥5%), rash

Endocrine & metabolic: Hypoalbuminemia, hypokalemia, hypomagnesemia, hypophosphatemia

Gastrointestinal: Constipation (children ≥5%), abdominal pain, diarrhea

Hematologic: Anemia

Hepatic: Transaminases increased

Local: Infusion site pain

Neuromuscular & skeletal: Muscle spasms, pain in extremity, trismus

Ocular: Periorbital edema

Renal: Oliguria (children ≥1%)

Respiratory: Atelectasis (children ≥5%), breath sounds abnormal, dyspnea, hypoxia, pleural effusion, pulmonary edema, stridor, wheezing

Pharmacodynamics/Kinetics

Onset of Action

Oral: <1 hour

I.V.: Analgesia: 5-10 minutes; Antipyretic: Within 30 minutes

Peak effect: I.V.: Analgesic: 1 hour

Duration of Action

I.V., Oral: Analgesia: 4-6 hours

I.V.: Antipyretic: ≥6 hours

Available Dosage Forms For available OTC formulations, consult specific product labeling.

General Dosage Range Dosage adjustment recommended in patients with renal impairment

Oral, rectal:

Children 0-3 months: 10-15 mg/kg/dose **or** 40 mg/dose every 4-6 hours as needed (maximum: 2.6 g/day)

Children 4-11 months: 10-15 mg/kg/dose **or** 80 mg/dose every 4-6 hours as needed (maximum: 2.6 g/day)

Children 1-2 years: 10-15 mg/kg/dose **or** 120 mg/dose every 4-6 hours as needed (maximum: 2.6 g/day)

Children 2-3 years: 10-15 mg/kg/dose **or** 160 mg/dose every 4-6 hours as needed (maximum: 2.6 g/day)

Children 4-5 years: 10-15 mg/kg/dose **or** 240 mg/dose every 4-6 hours as needed (maximum: 2.6 g/day)

Children 6-8 years: 10-15 mg/kg/dose **or** 320 mg/dose every 4-6 hours as needed (maximum: 2.6 g/day)

Children 9-10 years: 10-15 mg/kg/dose **or** 400 mg/dose every 4-6 hours as needed (maximum: 2.6 g/day)

Children 11 years: 10-15 mg/kg/dose **or** 480 mg/dose every 4-6 hours as needed (maximum: 2.6 g/day)

Adults: 325-650 mg every 4-6 hours as needed **or** 1000 mg 3-4 times/day as needed (maximum: 4 g/day)

I.V.:

Children 2-12 years: 15 mg/kg every 6 hours **or** 12.5 mg/kg every 4 hours; maximum single dose: 15 mg/kg/dose; maximum daily dose: 75 mg/kg/day (≤3.75 g/day)

Adolescents >12 years and Adults <50 kg: 15 mg/kg every 6 hours **or** 12.5 mg/kg every 4 hours; maximum daily dose: 75 mg/kg/day (≤3.75 g/day)

Adolescents >12 years and Adults ≥50 kg: 650 mg every 4 hours **or** 1000 mg every 6 hours; maximum daily dose: 4 g/day

Administration

Oral Shake suspension well before pouring dose.

I.V. For I.V. infusion only. May administer undiluted over 15 minutes.

Doses <1000 mg (<50 kg): Withdraw appropriate dose from vial and place into separate empty, sterile container prior to administration. Small volume pediatric doses (up to 60 mL) may be placed in a syringe and infused over 15 minutes via syringe pump.

Doses of 1000 mg (≥50 kg): Insert vented I.V. set through vial stopper.

I.V. Detail pH: 5.5

Stability

Reconstitution Injectable solution may be administered directly from the vial without further dilution. For doses <1000 mg, withdraw the appropriate volume and transfer to a separate sterile container (eg, glass bottle, plastic I.V. container, syringe) for administration.

Storage

Injection: Store intact vials at room temperature of 20°C to 25°C (68°F to 77°F); do not refrigerate or freeze. Use within 6 hours of opening vial or transferring to another container. Discard any unused portion; single use vials only.

Oral formulations: Store at controlled room temperature.

Suppositories: Store at <27°C (80°F); do not freeze.

Nursing Actions

Physical Assessment Assess patient for history of liver disease or ethanol abuse (acetaminophen and any ethanol may have adverse liver effects). Ensure adult patients keep daily dose to ≤4 g/day.

Patient Education Oral: Take with food or milk. While using this medication, avoid alcohol and other prescription or OTC medications that contain acetaminophen. Keep dose to below accepted maximum level for specific age group or weight. Encourage patient to report if they took more than maximum dose. This medication will not reduce inflammation; consult prescriber for anti-inflammatory, if needed. Report unusual bleeding (stool, mouth, urine) or bruising, unusual fatigue and weakness, belly pain, yellow eyes or skin, or lack of appetite.

Dietary Considerations Some products may contain phenylalanine and/or sodium.

Acetaminophen and Codeine

(a seet a MIN oh fen & KOE deen)

Brand Names: U.S. Capital® and Codeine; Tylenol® with Codeine No. 3; Tylenol® with Codeine No. 4

Index Terms Codeine and Acetaminophen; Tylenol #2; Tylenol #3; Tylenol Codeine

Pharmacologic Category Analgesic, Opioid

Medication Safety Issues

Sound-alike/look-alike issues:

Tylenol® may be confused with atenolol, timolol, Tylox®

High alert medication:

The Institute for Safe Medication Practices (ISMP) includes this medication among its list of drug classes which have a heightened risk of causing significant patient harm when used in error.

Other safety concerns:

Duplicate therapy issues: This product contains acetaminophen, which may be a component of other combination products. Do not exceed the maximum recommended daily dose of acetaminophen.

T3 is an error-prone abbreviation (mistaken as liothyronine)

International issues:

Codex: Brand name for acetaminophen/codeine [Brazil], but also the brand name for *saccharomyces boulardii* [Italy]

Codex [Brazil] may be confused with Cedax brand name for ceftibuten [U.S. and multiple international markets]

Pregnancy Risk Factor C

Lactation Enters breast milk/use caution

Use Relief of mild-to-moderate pain

Controlled Substance C-III; C-V

Available Dosage Forms

Solution, oral [C-V]: Acetaminophen 120 mg and codeine 12 mg per 5 mL

Suspension, oral [C-V]: Acetaminophen 120 mg and codeine 12 mg per 5 mL

Capital® and Codeine [C-V]: Acetaminophen 120 mg and codeine 12 mg per 5 mL

Tablet [C-III]: Acetaminophen 300 mg and codeine 15 mg; acetaminophen 300 mg and codeine 30 mg; acetaminophen 300 mg and codeine 60 mg

Tylenol® with Codeine No. 3: Acetaminophen 300 mg and codeine 30 mg

Tylenol® with Codeine No. 4: Acetaminophen 300 mg and codeine 60 mg

General Dosage Range Dosage adjustment recommended in patients with renal impairment

Oral:

Acetaminophen:

Children ≤12 years: 10-15 mg/kg/dose every 4-6 hours as needed (maximum: 2.6 g/day)

Children >12 years and Adults: 325-650 mg every 4-6 hours as needed (maximum: 4 g/day)

Codeine:

Children: 0.5-1 mg/kg/dose every 4-6 hours (maximum: 60 mg/dose)

Adults: 15-60 mg/dose every 4-6 hours (maximum: 360 mg/day)

Administration

Oral May be administered with food.

Nursing Actions

Physical Assessment See individual agents.

Patient Education See individual agents.

Related Information

Acetaminophen *on page* 23

Codeine *on page* 268

AcetaZOLAMIDE (a set a ZOLE a mide)

Brand Names: U.S. Diamox® Sequels®

Pharmacologic Category Anticonvulsant, Miscellaneous; Carbonic Anhydrase Inhibitor; Diuretic, Carbonic Anhydrase Inhibitor; Ophthalmic Agent, Antiglaucoma

Medication Safety Issues

International issues:

Diamox [Canada and multiple international markets] may be confused with Diabinese brand name for chlorpropamide [Multiple international markets]; Dobutrex brand name for dobutamine [Multiple international markets]; Trimox brand name for amoxicillin [Brazil]; Zimox brand name for amoxicillin [Italy] and carbidopa/levodopa [Greece]

Pregnancy Risk Factor C

Lactation Enters breast milk/not recommended (AAP rates "compatible"; AAP 2001 update pending)

Use Treatment of glaucoma (chronic simple open-angle, secondary glaucoma, preoperatively in acute angle-closure); drug-induced edema or edema due to congestive heart failure (adjunctive therapy; I.V. and immediate release dosage forms); centrencephalic epilepsies (I.V. and immediate release dosage forms); prevention or amelioration of symptoms associated with acute mountain sickness (immediate and extended release dosage forms)

Unlabeled Use Metabolic alkalosis; respiratory stimulant in stable hypercapnic COPD

Available Dosage Forms

Capsule, extended release, oral: 500 mg

Capsule, sustained release, oral:

Diamox® Sequels®: 500 mg

Injection, powder for reconstitution: 500 mg

Tablet, oral: 125 mg, 250 mg

General Dosage Range Dosage adjustment recommended in patients with renal impairment

I.V.: *Adults:* 250-1000 mg/day

Oral:

Immediate release:

Children: 8-30 mg/kg/day divided in 1-4 doses (maximum: 30 mg/kg/day or 1 g/day)

Adults: 250-1000 mg/day **or** 8-30 mg/kg/day in 1-4 divided doses (maximum: 30 mg/kg/day or 1 g/day) **or** 125-250 mg every 4 hours

Elderly: Initial: 250-500 mg/day

Extended release:

Adults: 500-1000 mg/day

Administration

Oral May be administered with food. May cause an alteration in taste, especially carbonated beverages. Short-acting tablets may be crushed and suspended in cherry or chocolate syrup to disguise the bitter taste of the drug; do not use fruit juices. Alternatively, submerge tablet in 10 mL of hot water and add 10 mL honey or syrup.

I.M. I.M. administration is painful because of the alkaline pH of the drug; use by this route is not recommended.

I.V. I.V.: No specific guidance given by manufacturer, but I.V. push at a rate of up to 500 mg over 3 minutes has been reported in a clinical trial (Mazur, 1999); a study to assess cerebrovascular reserve has used rapid I.V. push of up to 1 g over ≤1 minute (Piepgras, 1990)

I.V. Detail pH: 9.2

Nursing Actions

Physical Assessment Assess allergy history prior to beginning therapy. Monitor for signs of excessive fatigue, malaise, and myalgia. Monitor growth in pediatric patients. Monitor blood glucose levels closely if patients have diabetes.

Patient Education Do not chew or crush long-acting capsule (contents may be sprinkled on soft food). May be administered with food to decrease GI upset. If taking for glaucoma, you will need periodic ophthalmic examinations while taking this medication. Monitor serum glucose closely (may cause altered blood glucose in some patients with diabetes or unusual response to some forms of glucose testing). You may experience increased sensitivity to sunlight, nausea, loss of appetite, or altered taste. Notify your doctor of unusual and persistent nausea, vomiting, diarrhea, sudden change in eyesight, eye pain or irritation, or if seizures are worse or change after starting this medication.

Acetic Acid, Propylene Glycol Diacetate, and Hydrocortisone

(a SEE tik AS id, PRO pa leen GLY kole dye AS e tate, & hye droe KOR ti sone)

Brand Names: U.S. Acetasol® HC; VoSol® HC

Index Terms Acetic Acid, Hydrocortisone, and Propylene Glycol Diacetate; Hydrocortisone, Acetic Acid, and Propylene Glycol Diacetate; Propylene Glycol Diacetate, Acetic Acid, and Hydrocortisone

Pharmacologic Category Otic Agent, Anti-infective

Medication Safety Issues

Sound-alike/look-alike issues:

VoSol® may be confused with Vexol®

Use Treatment of superficial infections of the external auditory canal caused by organisms susceptible to the action of the antimicrobial, complicated by swelling

Available Dosage Forms

Solution, otic [drops]: Acetic acid 2%, propylene glycol diacetate 3%, and hydrocortisone 1% (10 mL)

Acetasol® HC, VoSol® HC: Acetic acid 2%, propylene glycol diacetate 3%, and hydrocortisone 1% (10 mL)

General Dosage Range Otic: *Children ≥3 years and Adults:* Instill 3-5 drops in ear(s) every 4-6 hours

Administration

Other After removing cerumen and debris, solution may be applied by inserting a cotton wick into the ear canal and saturating with the solution. Wick may remain in place for 24 hours and then removed; however, drops should continue to be instilled into ear canal as long as indicated.

Nursing Actions

Physical Assessment See individual agents.

Patient Education See individual agents.

Acyclovir (Systemic) (ay SYE kloe veer)

Brand Names: U.S. Zovirax®

Index Terms Aciclovir; ACV; Acycloguanosine

Pharmacologic Category Antiviral Agent

Medication Safety Issues

Sound-alike/look-alike issues:

Acyclovir may be confused with ganciclovir, Retrovir®, valacyclovir

Zovirax® may be confused with Doribax®, Valtrex®, Zithromax®, Zostrix®, Zyloprim®, Zyvox®

Pregnancy Risk Factor B

Lactation Enters breast milk/use with caution (AAP rates "compatible"; AAP 2001 update pending)

Breast-Feeding Considerations Nursing mothers with herpetic lesions near or on the breast should avoid breast-feeding. Limited data suggest exposure to the nursing infant of ~0.3 mg/kg/day following oral administration of acyclovir to the mother.

Use Treatment of genital herpes simplex virus (HSV) and HSV encephalitis

Unlabeled Use Prevention of HSV reactivation in HIV-positive patients; prevention of HSV reactivation in hematopoietic stem cell transplant (HSCT); prevention of HSV reactivation during periods of neutropenia in patients with cancer; prevention of varicella zoster virus (VZV) reactivation in allogenic HSCT; prevention of CMV reactivation in low-risk allogeneic HSCT; treatment of disseminated HSV or VZV in immunocompromised patients with cancer; empiric treatment of suspected encephalitis in immunocompromised patients with cancer; treatment of initial and prophylaxis of recurrent mucosal and cutaneous herpes simplex (HSV-1 and HSV-2) infections in immunocompromised patients

Mechanism of Action/Effect Inhibits DNA synthesis and viral replication

Contraindications Hypersensitivity to acyclovir, valacyclovir, or any component of the formulation

Warnings/Precautions Use with caution in immunocompromised patients; thrombocytopenic purpura/hemolytic uremic syndrome (TTP/HUS) has been reported. Use caution in the elderly, pre-existing renal disease (may require dosage modification), or in those receiving other nephrotoxic drugs. Renal failure (sometimes fatal) has been reported. Maintain adequate hydration during oral or intravenous therapy. Use I.V. preparation with caution in patients with underlying neurologic abnormalities, serious hepatic or electrolyte abnormalities, or substantial hypoxia.

Varicella-zoster: Treatment should begin within 24 hours of appearance of rash; oral route not recommended for routine use in otherwise healthy children with varicella, but may be effective in patients at increased risk of moderate-to-severe infection (>12 years of age, chronic cutaneous or pulmonary disorders, long-term salicylate therapy, corticosteroid therapy).

Drug Interactions

Avoid Concomitant Use

Avoid concomitant use of Acyclovir (Systemic) with any of the following: Zoster Vaccine

Decreased Effect

Acyclovir (Systemic) may decrease the levels/effects of: Zoster Vaccine

Increased Effect/Toxicity

Acyclovir (Systemic) may increase the levels/effects of: Mycophenolate; Tenofovir; Zidovudine

The levels/effects of Acyclovir (Systemic) may be increased by: Mycophenolate

Nutritional/Ethanol Interactions Food: Does not affect absorption of oral acyclovir.

Adverse Reactions

Oral:

>10%: Central nervous system: Malaise (≤12%)

1% to 10%:

Central nervous system: Headache (≤2%)

Gastrointestinal: Nausea (2% to 5%), vomiting (≤3%), diarrhea (2% to 3%)

Parenteral:

1% to 10%:

Dermatologic: Hives (2%), itching (2%), rash (2%)

Gastrointestinal: Nausea/vomiting (7%)

Hepatic: Liver function tests increased (1% to 2%)

Local: Inflammation at injection site or phlebitis (9%)

Renal: BUN increased (5% to 10%), creatinine increased (5% to 10%), acute renal failure

Available Dosage Forms

Capsule, oral: 200 mg

Zovirax®: 200 mg

Injection, powder for reconstitution: 500 mg, 1000 mg

Injection, solution [preservative free]: 50 mg/mL (10 mL, 20 mL)

Suspension, oral: 200 mg/5 mL (473 mL)

Zovirax®: 200 mg/5 mL (473 mL)

Tablet, oral: 400 mg, 800 mg

Zovirax®: 400 mg, 800 mg

General Dosage Range Dosage adjustment recommended in patients with renal impairment

I.V.:

Children <12 years: 10-20 mg/kg/dose every 8 hours (maximum: 60 mg/kg/day)

Children ≥12 years and Adults: 5-10 mg/kg/dose **or** 500 mg/m²/dose every 8 hours (maximum: 45 mg/kg/day)

Oral:

Children ≥2 years and ≤40 kg: 20 mg/kg/dose 4 times/day (maximum: 800 mg/dose)

Children ≥2 years and >40 kg: 800 mg/dose 4 times/day

Adults: 200-800 mg/dose 3-5 times/day

Administration

Oral May be administered with or without food.

I.V. For I.V. infusion only. Avoid rapid infusion. Infuse over 1 hour to prevent renal damage. Maintain adequate hydration of patient. Check for phlebitis and rotate infusion sites. Avoid I.M. or SubQ administration.

I.V. Detail pH: 10.5-11.6 (reconstituted solution)

Stability

Reconstitution Powder for injection: Reconstitute acyclovir 500 mg powder with SWFI 10 mL; do not use bacteriostatic water containing benzyl alcohol or parabens. For intravenous infusion, dilute in D_5W, D_5NS, $D_5$1/4NS, $D_5$1/2NS, LR, or NS to a final concentration ≤7 mg/mL. Concentrations >10 mg/mL increase the risk of phlebitis.

Storage

Capsule, tablet: Store at controlled room temperature of 15°C to 25°C (59°F to 77°F); protect from moisture.

Injection: Store powder at controlled room temperature of 15°C to 25°C (59°F to 77°F). Reconstituted solutions remain stable for 12 hours at room temperature. Do not refrigerate reconstituted solutions or solutions diluted for infusion as they may precipitate as they may precipitate. Once diluted for infusion, use within 24 hours.

Nursing Actions

Physical Assessment Patient should be adequately hydrated during I.V. therapy and monitored closely during intravenous administration.

Patient Education This is not a cure for herpes, nor will this medication reduce the risk of transmission to others when lesions are present; avoid sexual intercourse when visible lesions are present. Oral doses may be taken with food. Maintain adequate hydration, unless instructed to restrict fluid intake. May cause nausea, vomiting, lightheadedness, dizziness, headache, fever, or muscle pain. Report any change in urination (difficulty urinating, dark colored or concentrated urine), persistent lethargy, acute headache, severe nausea or vomiting, confusion or hallucinations, rash, or respiratory difficulty.

Dietary Considerations May be taken with or without food. Some products may contain sodium.

Related Information

Management of Drug Extravasations *on page 1269*

Acyclovir (Topical) (ay SYE kloe veer)

Brand Names: U.S. Zovirax®

Index Terms Aciclovir; ACV; Acycloguanosine

Pharmacologic Category Antiviral Agent, Topical

Medication Safety Issues

Sound-alike/look-alike issues:

Acyclovir may be confused with ganciclovir, Retrovir®, valacyclovir

Zovirax® may be confused with Doribax®, Valtrex®, Zithromax®, Zostrix®, Zyloprim®, Zyvox®

International issues:

Opthavir [Mexico] may be confused with Optivar brand name for azelastine [U.S.]

Pregnancy Risk Factor B

Use Treatment of herpes labialis (cold sores), mucocutaneous HSV in immunocompromised patients

Available Dosage Forms

Cream, topical:

Zovirax®: 5% (2 g, 5 g)

Ointment, topical:

Zovirax®: 5% (15 g, 30 g)

General Dosage Range Topical:

Children ≥12 years: Cream: Apply 5 times/day

Adults: Cream: Apply 5 times/day; Ointment: 1/2" ribbon for a 4" square surface area 6 times/day

Administration

Topical Not for use in the eye. Apply using a finger cot or rubber glove to avoid transmission to other parts of the body or to other persons.

Nursing Actions

Patient Education Use gloves or finger cot when applying. This is not a cure for herpes, nor will this medication reduce the risk of transmission to others when lesions are present; avoid sexual intercourse when visible lesions are present.

Acyclovir and Hydrocortisone

(ay SYE kloe veer & hye droe KOR ti sone)

Brand Names: U.S. Xerese™

Index Terms Hydrocortisone and Acyclovir; ME-609; Xerclear

Pharmacologic Category Antiviral Agent, Topical; Corticosteroid, Topical

Pregnancy Risk Factor B

Lactation Excretion in breast milk unknown/use caution

Use Treatment of recurrent herpes labialis (cold sores)

General Dosage Range Topical: *Children ≥12 years and Adults:* Apply 5 times/day

Administration

Topical For external use only; not for use in the eye, inside the mouth or nose, or on the genitals. Apply to clean, dry area using a finger cot or rubber glove to avoid transmission to other parts of the body or to other persons. Use sufficient amount to cover the affected area(s), including the outer margin of cold sore; do not rub affected area. Initiate therapy early (ie, during the prodrome or when lesions appear).

Nursing Actions

Physical Assessment See individual agents.

Patient Education See individual agents.

Adalimumab (a da LIM yoo mab)

Brand Names: U.S. Humira®; Humira® Pen

Index Terms Antitumor Necrosis Factor Alpha (Human); D2E7; Human Antitumor Necrosis Factor Alpha

Pharmacologic Category Antirheumatic, Disease Modifying; Gastrointestinal Agent, Miscellaneous; Monoclonal Antibody; Tumor Necrosis Factor (TNF) Blocking Agent

Medication Safety Issues

Sound-alike/look-alike issues:

Humira® may be confused with Humulin®, Humalog®

Humira® Pen may be confused with HumaPen® Memoir®

Medication Guide Available Yes

Pregnancy Risk Factor B

Lactation Excretion in breast milk unknown/not recommended

Breast-Feeding Considerations It is not known whether adalimumab is secreted in human milk. Because many immunoglobulins are secreted in milk and the potential for serious adverse reactions exists, a decision should be made whether to discontinue nursing or discontinue the drug, taking into account the importance of the drug to the mother.

Use

Treatment of active rheumatoid arthritis (moderate-to-severe) and active psoriatic arthritis; may be used alone or in combination with disease-modifying antirheumatic drugs (DMARDs); treatment of ankylosing spondylitis

Treatment of moderately- to severely-active Crohn's disease in patients with inadequate response to conventional treatment, or patients who have lost response to or are intolerant of infliximab

Treatment of moderate-to-severe plaque psoriasis

Treatment of moderately- to severely-active juvenile idiopathic arthritis

Mechanism of Action/Effect Adalimumab decreases signs and symptoms of psoriatic arthritis, rheumatoid arthritis, Crohn's disease, and ankylosing spondylitis; inhibits progression of structural damage in rheumatoid and psoriatic arthritis

Contraindications There are no contraindications listed within the FDA-approved labeling.

Canadian labeling: Additional contraindications (not in U.S. labeling): Hypersensitivity to adalimumab or any component of the formulation; severe infection (eg, sepsis, tuberculosis, opportunistic infection)

Warnings/Precautions [U.S. Boxed Warnings]: Patients should be evaluated for latent tuberculosis infection with a tuberculin skin test prior to therapy. Treatment of latent tuberculosis should be initiated before adalimumab is used. Tuberculosis (disseminated or extrapulmonary) has been reactivated while on adalimumab. Most cases have been reported within the first 8 months of treatment. Doses higher than recommended are associated with an increased risk for tuberculosis reactivation. **Patients with initial negative tuberculin skin tests should receive continued monitoring for tuberculosis throughout treatment; active tuberculosis has developed in this population during treatment.** Rare reactivation of hepatitis B virus (HBV) has occurred in chronic virus carriers; use with caution; evaluate prior to initiation and during treatment.

[U.S. Boxed Warning]: Patients receiving adalimumab are at increased risk for serious infections which may result in hospitalization and/or fatality; infections usually developed in patients receiving concomitant immunosuppressive agents (eg, methotrexate or corticosteroids) and may present as disseminated (rather than local) disease. Active tuberculosis (or reactivation of latent tuberculosis), invasive fungal (including aspergillosis, blastomycosis, candidiasis, coccidioidomycosis, histoplasmosis, and pneumocystosis) and bacterial, viral or other opportunistic infections (including legionellosis and listeriosis) have been reported in patients receiving TNF-blocking agents, including adalimumab. Monitor closely for signs/symptoms of infection. Discontinue for serious infection or sepsis. Consider risks versus benefits prior to use in patients with a history of chronic or recurrent infection. Consider empiric antifungal therapy in patients who are at risk for invasive fungal infection and develop severe systemic illness. Caution should be exercised when considering use in the elderly or in patients with conditions that predispose them to infections (eg, diabetes) or residence/travel from areas of endemic mycoses (blastomycosis, coccidioidomycosis, histoplasmosis), or with latent or localized infections. Do not initiate adalimumab therapy with clinically important active infection. Patients who develop a new infection while undergoing treatment should be monitored closely. **[U.S. Boxed Warning]: Lymphoma and other malignancies have been reported in children and adolescent patients receiving other TNF-blocking agents.** Half the cases are lymphomas (Hodgkin's and non-Hodgkin's) and the other cases are varied, but include malignancies not typically observed in this population. Most patients were receiving concomitant immunosuppressants. **[U.S. Boxed Warning]: Hepatosplenic T-cell lymphoma (HSTCL), a rare T-cell lymphoma, has also been reported primarily in patients with Crohn's disease or ulcerative colitis treated with adalimumab and who received concomitant azathioprine or mercaptopurine; reports occurred predominantly in adolescent and young adult males.** Rare cases of lymphoma have also been reported in association with adalimumab. A higher incidence of nonmelanoma skin cancers was noted in adalimumab treated patients, when compared to the control group. Impact on the development and course of malignancies is not fully defined. May exacerbate pre-existing or recent-onset central or peripheral nervous system demyelinating disorders. Consider discontinuing use in patients who develop peripheral or central nervous system demyelinating disorders during treatment.

May exacerbate pre-existing or recent-onset demyelinating CNS disorders. Worsening and new-onset heart failure (HF) has been reported; use caution in patients with decreased left ventricular function. Use caution in patients with HF. Patients should be brought up to date with all immunizations before initiating therapy. No data are available concerning the effects of adalimumab on vaccination. Live vaccines should not be given concurrently. No data are available concerning secondary transmission of live vaccines in patients receiving adalimumab. Rare cases of pancytopenia (including aplastic anemia) have been reported with TNF-blocking agents; with significant hematologic abnormalities, consider discontinuing therapy. Positive antinuclear antibody titers have been detected in patients (with negative baselines) treated with adalimumab. Rare cases of autoimmune disorder, including lupus-like syndrome, have been reported; monitor and discontinue adalimumab if symptoms develop. May cause hypersensitivity reactions, including anaphylaxis; monitor. Infection and malignancy has been reported at a higher incidence in elderly patients compared to younger adults; use caution in elderly patients. The packaging (needle cover of prefilled syringe) may contain latex. Product may contain polysorbate 80.

Drug Interactions

Avoid Concomitant Use

Avoid concomitant use of Adalimumab with any of the following: Abatacept; Anakinra; BCG; Belimumab; Canakinumab; Certolizumab Pegol; Natalizumab; Pimecrolimus; Rilonacept; Tacrolimus (Topical); Vaccines (Live)

Decreased Effect

Adalimumab may decrease the levels/effects of: BCG; Coccidioidin Skin Test; Sipuleucel-T; Vaccines (Inactivated); Vaccines (Live)

The levels/effects of Adalimumab may be decreased by: Echinacea

Increased Effect/Toxicity

Adalimumab may increase the levels/effects of: Abatacept; Anakinra; Belimumab; Canakinumab; Certolizumab Pegol; Leflunomide; Natalizumab; Rilonacept; Vaccines (Live)

The levels/effects of Adalimumab may be increased by: Abciximab; Denosumab; Pimecrolimus; Roflumilast; Tacrolimus (Topical); Trastuzumab

Nutritional/Ethanol Interactions Herb/nutraceutical: Echinacea may decrease the therapeutic effects of adalimumab; avoid concurrent use.

Adverse Reactions

>10%:

Central nervous system: Headache (12%)
Dermatologic: Rash (6% to 12%)
Local: Injection site reaction (12% to 20%; includes erythema, itching, hemorrhage, pain, swelling)
Neuromuscular & skeletal: CPK increased (15%)
Respiratory: Upper respiratory tract infection (17%), sinusitis (11%)
Miscellaneous: Antibodies to adalimumab (3% to 26%; significance unknown), positive ANA (12%)

5% to 10%:

Cardiovascular: Hypertension (5%)
Endocrine & metabolic: Hyperlipidemia (7%), hypercholesterolemia (6%)
Gastrointestinal: Nausea (9%), abdominal pain (7%)
Genitourinary: Urinary tract infection (8%)
Hepatic: Alkaline phosphatase increased (5%)
Local: Injection site reaction (8%; other than erythema, itching, hemorrhage, pain, swelling)
Neuromuscular & skeletal: Back pain (6%)
Renal: Hematuria (5%)
Miscellaneous: Accidental injury (10%), flu-like syndrome (7%)

1% to 5%:

Cardiovascular: Arrhythmia, atrial fibrillation, chest pain, CHF, coronary artery disorder, heart arrest, MI, palpitation, pericardial effusion, pericarditis, peripheral edema, syncope, tachycardia, thrombosis (leg), vascular disorder
Central nervous system: Confusion, fever, hypertensive encephalopathy, multiple sclerosis, subdural hematoma
Dermatologic: Alopecia, cellulitis, erysipelas
Endocrine & metabolic: Dehydration, menstrual disorder, parathyroid disorder
Gastrointestinal: Diverticulitis, esophagitis, gastroenteritis, gastrointestinal hemorrhage, vomiting
Genitourinary: Cystitis, pelvic pain
Hematologic: Agranulocytosis, granulocytopenia, leukopenia, pancytopenia, paraproteinemia, polycythemia
Hepatic: Cholecystitis, cholelithiasis, hepatic necrosis
Neuromuscular & skeletal: Arthralgia, arthritis, bone fracture, bone necrosis, joint disorder, muscle cramps, myasthenia, pain in extremity, paresthesia, pyogenic arthritis, synovitis, tendon disorder, tremor
Ocular: Cataract
Renal: Kidney calculus, pyelonephritis
Respiratory: Asthma, bronchospasm, dyspnea, lung function decreased, pleural effusion, pneumonia
Miscellaneous: Adenoma, allergic reactions (1%), carcinoma (including breast, gastrointestinal, skin, urogenital), healing abnormality, herpes zoster, ketosis, lupus erythematosus syndrome, lymphoma, melanoma, postsurgical infection, sepsis, tuberculosis (reactivation of latent infection; miliary, lymphatic, peritoneal and pulmonary)

Available Dosage Forms

Injection, solution [preservative free]:

Humira®: 20 mg/0.4 mL (0.4 mL); 40 mg/0.8 mL (0.8 mL)
Humira® Pen: 40 mg/0.8 mL (0.8 mL)

General Dosage Range SubQ:

Children ≥4 years: 15 kg to <30 kg: 20 mg every other week; ≥30 kg: 40 mg every other week

Adults: Initial: 80-160 mg; Maintenance: 40 mg every other week (maximum: 40 mg every week)

Administration

Other For SubQ injection; rotate injection sites. Do not use if solution is discolored. Do not administer to skin which is red, tender, bruised, or hard. Needle cap of the prefilled syringe may contain latex.

Stability

Storage Store under refrigeration at 2°C to 8°C (36°F to 46°F); do not freeze. Protect from light.

Nursing Actions

Physical Assessment Monitor for signs and symptoms of tuberculosis, other infections, enlarged lymph nodes, or skin lesions/eruptions. Assess for liver dysfunction (unusual fatigue, easy bruising or bleeding, jaundice). Monitor PDD at regular intervals during treatment. Teach patient proper injection technique and syringe/needle disposal. Latex-sensitive patients: Needle cap of prefilled syringe contains latex.

Patient Education Inform prescriber of any allergies, history of tuberculosis, or any kind of infection you have. If self-administered, follow directions for injection and needle/syringe disposal exactly. You may be more susceptible to infection. May cause headache or dizziness; if persistent, consult prescriber. Report persistent fever, increased bruising or bleeding, respiratory tract infection, unhealed or infected wounds, urinary tract infection, flu-like symptoms, unexplained weight loss, persistent cough, enlarged lymph nodes, new skin lesions or eruptions, or unusual bump or sore that does not heal. Stop drug and report immediately persistent nausea or abdominal pain; numbness or tingling; problems with vision; weakness in legs; chest pains, respiratory difficulty; weight gain; swelling of extremities; joint pain; skin rash; or redness, swelling, or pain at injection site.

Adapalene (a DAP a leen)

Brand Names: U.S. Differin®

Pharmacologic Category Acne Products; Topical Skin Product, Acne

Pregnancy Risk Factor C

Lactation Excretion in breast milk unknown/use caution

Use Treatment of acne vulgaris

Available Dosage Forms

Cream, topical: 0.1% (45 g)

Differin®: 0.1% (45 g)

Gel, topical: 0.1% (45 g)

Differin®: 0.1% (45 g); 0.3% (45 g)

Lotion, topical:

Differin®: 0.1% (59 mL)

General Dosage Range Topical: *Children >12 years and Adults:* Apply once daily at bedtime

Administration

Topical For external use only. Apply a thin film at night to clean/dry skin; avoid contact with abraded, eczematous, or sunburned skin, mucous membranes, eyes, mouth and angles of the nose. Moisturizers may be used if necessary; avoid alpha hydroxy or glycolic acid-containing products.

Nursing Actions

Patient Education Apply with gloves in thin film at night to thoroughly clean/dry skin; avoid area around eyes or mouth. Do not apply occlusive dressing. Results may take 8-12 weeks to appear. You may experience transient burning or stinging immediately after applying. Report worsening of condition or skin redness, dryness, peeling, or burning that persists between applications. Avoid excessive exposure to sunlight or sunlamps.

Adapalene and Benzoyl Peroxide
(a DAP a leen & BEN zoe il peer OKS ide)

Brand Names: U.S. Epiduo®

Index Terms Benzoyl Peroxide and Adapalene

Pharmacologic Category Acne Products; Topical Skin Product; Topical Skin Product, Acne

Pregnancy Risk Factor C

Lactation Excretion in breast milk unknown/use caution

Use Topical treatment of acne vulgaris

Available Dosage Forms

Gel, topical:

Epiduo®: Adapalene 0.1% and benzoyl peroxide 2.5% (45 g)

General Dosage Range Topical: *Children ≥12 years and Adults:* Apply once daily

Administration

Topical Apply a pea-sized amount for each area of the face (eg, forehead, chin, each cheek). Skin should be clean and dry before applying. For external use only; avoid applying to eyes and mucous membranes.

Nursing Actions

Patient Education See individual agents.

Adefovir (a DEF o veer)

Brand Names: U.S. Hepsera®

Index Terms Adefovir Dipivoxil; Bis-POM PMEA

Pharmacologic Category Antiretroviral Agent, Reverse Transcriptase Inhibitor (Nucleotide)

Pregnancy Risk Factor C

Lactation Excretion in breast milk unknown/not recommended

Use Treatment of chronic hepatitis B with evidence of active viral replication (based on persistent elevation of ALT/AST or histologic evidence), including patients with lamivudine-resistant hepatitis B

Mechanism of Action/Effect Acyclic nucleotide reverse transcriptase inhibitor (adenosine analog) which interferes with HBV viral DNA polymerase resulting in inhibition of viral replication

Contraindications Hypersensitivity to adefovir or any component of the formulation

Warnings/Precautions [U.S. Boxed Warning]: Use with caution in patients with renal dysfunction or in patients at risk of renal toxicity (including concurrent nephrotoxic agents or NSAIDs). Chronic administration may result in nephrotoxicity. Dosage adjustment is required in adult patients with renal dysfunction or in patients who develop renal dysfunction during therapy; no data available for use in children ≥12 years or adolescents with renal impairment. Not recommended as first line therapy of chronic HBV due to weak antiviral activity and high rate of resistance after first year. May be more appropriate as second-line agent in treatment-naïve patients. Combination therapy with lamivudine in nucleoside-naïve patients has not been shown to provide synergistic antiviral effects. In patients with lamivudine-resistant HBV, switching to adefovir monotherapy was associated with a higher risk of adefovir resistance compared to adding adefovir to lamivudine therapy (Lok, 2009).

Calculate creatinine clearance before initiation of therapy. Consider alternative therapy in patients who do not respond to adefovir monotherapy treatment. **[U.S. Boxed Warning]: May cause the development of HIV resistance in patients with unrecognized or untreated HIV infection.** Determine HIV status prior to initiating treatment with adefovir. **[U.S. Boxed Warning]: Fatal cases of lactic acidosis and severe hepatomegaly with steatosis have been reported with the use of nucleoside analogues alone or in combination**

with other antiretrovirals. Female gender, obesity, and prolonged treatment may increase the risk of hepatotoxicity. Treatment should be discontinued in patients with lactic acidosis or signs/symptoms of hepatotoxicity (which may occur without marked transaminase elevations). **[U.S. Boxed Warning]: Acute exacerbations of hepatitis may occur (in up to 25% of patients) when antihepatitis therapy is discontinued.** Exacerbations typically occur within 12 weeks and may be self-limited or resolve upon resuming treatment; risk may be increased with advanced liver disease or cirrhosis. Monitor patients following discontinuation of therapy. Safety and efficacy in children <12 years of age have not been established. Do not use concurrently with tenofovir (Viread®) or any product containing tenofovir (eg, Truvada®, Atripla®, Complera®).

Drug Interactions

Avoid Concomitant Use

Avoid concomitant use of Adefovir with any of the following: Tenofovir

Decreased Effect

Adefovir may decrease the levels/effects of: Tenofovir

Increased Effect/Toxicity

Adefovir may increase the levels/effects of: Tenofovir

The levels/effects of Adefovir may be increased by: Ganciclovir-Valganciclovir; Ribavirin; Tenofovir

Nutritional/Ethanol Interactions

Ethanol: Should be avoided in hepatitis B infection due to potential hepatic toxicity.

Food: Does not have a significant effect on adefovir absorption.

Adverse Reactions

>10%:

Central nervous system: Headache (24% to 25%)

Gastrointestinal: Abdominal pain (15%), diarrhea (up to 13%)

Hepatic: Hepatitis exacerbation (up to 25% within 12 weeks of adefovir discontinuation)

Neuromuscular & skeletal: Weakness (up to 25%)

Renal: Hematuria (grade ≥3: 11%)

1% to 10%:

Dermatologic: Rash, pruritus

Endocrine & metabolic: Hypophosphatemia (<2 mg/dL: 1% and 3% in pre-/post-liver transplant patients, respectively)

Gastrointestinal: Flatulence (up to 8%), dyspepsia (5% to 9%), nausea, vomiting

Neuromuscular & skeletal: Back pain (up to 10%)

Renal: Serum creatinine increased (≥0.5 mg/dL: 2% to 3% in compensated liver disease; incidence may be higher in patients with decompensated cirrhosis or in liver transplant recipients), renal failure

Note: In liver transplant patients with baseline renal dysfunction, frequency of increased serum creatinine has been observed to be as high as 32% to 51% at 48 and 96 weeks post-transplantation, respectively; considering the concomitant use of other potentially nephrotoxic medications, baseline renal insufficiency, and predisposing comorbidities, the role of adefovir in these changes could not be established.

Respiratory: Cough (6% to 8%), rhinitis (up to 5%)

Available Dosage Forms

Tablet, oral:

Hepsera®: 10 mg

General Dosage Range Dosage adjustment recommended in patients with renal impairment

Oral: *Children ≥12 years and Adults:* 10 mg once daily

Administration

Oral May be administered without regard to food.

Stability

Storage Store controlled room temperature of 25°C (77°F).

Nursing Actions

Physical Assessment Assess adherence to regimen. Monitor for lactic acidosis and altered hepatic status on a regular basis throughout therapy.

Patient Education Use appropriate precautions to prevent spread to other persons. You will require frequent blood tests; follow recommended schedule. Maintain adequate hydration, unless instructed to restrict fluid intake. May cause headache, abdominal pain, diarrhea, or weakness. Report unusual bleeding (blood in urine, tarry stools, or easy bruising), unresolved diarrhea, signs of infection (eg, fever, chills, sore throat, burning urination, flu-like symptoms), persistent fatigue, muscle weakness, or changes in urinary pattern.

Dietary Considerations May be taken without regard to food.

Adenosine (a DEN oh seen)

Brand Names: U.S. Adenocard® IV; Adenoscan®

Index Terms 9-Beta-D-Ribofuranosyladenine

Pharmacologic Category Antiarrhythmic Agent, Miscellaneous; Diagnostic Agent

Medication Safety Issues

High alert medication:

The Institute for Safe Medication Practices (ISMP) includes this medication among its list of drugs which have a heightened risk of causing significant patient harm when used in error.

Pregnancy Risk Factor C

Lactation Excretion in breast milk unknown

Use

Adenocard®: Treatment of paroxysmal supraventricular tachycardia (PSVT) including that associated with accessory bypass tracts (Wolff-Parkinson-White syndrome); when clinically advisable, appropriate vagal maneuvers should be attempted prior to adenosine administration; **not effective for conversion of atrial fibrillation, atrial flutter, or ventricular tachycardia**

Adenoscan®: Pharmacologic stress agent used in myocardial perfusion thallium-201 scintigraphy

Unlabeled Use

ACLS/PALS Guidelines (2010): Stable, narrow-complex regular tachycardias; unstable narrow-complex regular tachycardias while preparations are made for synchronized direct-current cardioversion; stable regular monomorphic, wide-complex tachycardia as a therapeutic (if SVT) and diagnostic maneuver

Adenoscan®: Acute vasodilator testing in pulmonary artery hypertension

Available Dosage Forms

Injection, solution [preservative free]: 3 mg/mL (2 mL, 4 mL)

Adenocard® IV: 3 mg/mL (2 mL, 4 mL)

Adenoscan®: 3 mg/mL (20 mL, 30 mL)

General Dosage Range I.V.:

Children <50 kg: Initial: 0.05-0.1 mg/kg/dose (maximum initial dose: 6 mg); repeat: 0.05-0.3 mg/kg/dose (maximum: 0.3 mg/kg/dose or 12 mg/dose)

Children ≥50 kg and Adults: Initial: 6 mg; if not effective, 12 mg may be given; may repeat 12 mg if needed (maximum: 12 mg/dose)

Administration

I.V.

Adenocard®: For rapid bolus I.V. use only; administer I.V. push over 1-2 seconds at a peripheral I.V. site as proximal as possible to trunk (not in lower arm, hand, lower leg, or foot); follow each bolus with a rapid normal saline flush (infants and children ≥5 mL; adults 20 mL). Use of 2 syringes (one with adenosine dose and the other with NS flush) connected to a T-connector or stopcock is recommended. If administered via **central line** in adults, reduce initial dose (ACLS, 2010).

Adenoscan®: For I.V. infusion only via peripheral line

I.V. Detail Do not mix with any other drug in syringe or solution.

Nursing Actions

Physical Assessment Requires use of infusion pump and continuous cardiac and hemodynamic monitoring during infusion. Emergency resuscitation equipment should be immediately available. Monitor for adverse reactions. Adenosine could produce bronchoconstriction in patients with asthma.

Patient Education Adenosine is administered in emergencies; patient education should be appropriate to the situation. May cause facial flushing. Report chest pain or pressure or difficulty breathing immediately.

Adenovirus (Types 4, 7) Vaccine

(ad e noh VYE rus typs for SEV en vak SEEN)

Index Terms Adenovirus Type 4 and Type 7 Vaccine; Adenovirus Vaccine; Adenovirus Vaccine (Types 4 and 7); Type 4 and Type 7 Adenovirus Vaccine

Pharmacologic Category Vaccine, Live (Viral)

Lactation Excretion in breast milk unknown/use caution

Use Prevention of acute febrile respiratory disease caused by adenovirus types 4 and 7 (approved for use in military populations)

Available Dosage Forms

Tablet, enteric coated, oral [combination package]:

Adenovirus type 4 ≥4.5 log_{10} $TCID_{50}$ [contains albumin (human); 100 white tablets]

Adenovirus type 7 ≥4.5 log_{10} $TCID_{50}$ [contains albumin (human); 100 white tablets]

General Dosage Range Oral: *Adolescents ≥17 years and Adults ≤50 years:* One tablet each of type 4 and type 7 as a single vaccine dose

Administration

Oral Oral: Swallow tablets whole, do not chew, crush, or split. Both tablets (type 4 and type 7) are to be taken together as a single dose.

Related Information

Immunization Administration Recommendations *on page 1243*

Aflibercept (a FLIB er sept)

Brand Names: U.S. Eylea™

Index Terms AVE 0005; AVE 005; AVE-0005; VEGF Trap; VEGF Trap-Eye

Pharmacologic Category Ophthalmic Agent; Vascular Endothelial Growth Factor (VEGF) Inhibitor

Pregnancy Risk Factor C

Lactation Excretion in breast milk unknown/not recommended

Use Treatment of neovascular (wet) age-related macular degeneration (AMD)

Available Dosage Forms

Injection, solution, intravitreal [preservative free]:

Eylea™: 40 mg/mL (0.05 mL)

General Dosage Range Intravitreal: *Adults:* 2 mg (0.05 mL) every 4-8 weeks

Administration

Other Ophthalmic: For intravitreal injection only. Remove contents from vial using a 5 micron, 19-gauge 1 1/2 inch filter needle (supplied) attached to a 1 mL syringe (supplied). Discard filter needle and replace with a sterile 30 gauge 1/2 inch needle (supplied) for intravitreal injection procedure (do not use filter needle for intravitreal injection). Depress plunger to expel excess air and medication (plunger tip should align with the 0.05 mL marking on syringe). Adequate anesthesia and a broad-spectrum antimicrobial agent should be administered prior to the procedure.

Nursing Actions

Physical Assessment

Assess allergy history before beginning therapy. Assess visual acuity and intraocular pressure prior to beginning treatment and periodically during treatment. Adequate anesthesia and broad spectrum antibiotic should be administered prior to intravitreous injection. Rare hypersensitivity reactions, including anaphylaxis, can occur within several hours of use; patient should be monitored closely following injection and appropriate emergency equipment should be immediately available. Teach patient/caregiver to report any signs of infection, intraocular discomfort, or visual disturbances.

Patient Education

This treatment will not reverse vision loss, but may decrease further loss. Do not rub eyes or use any ocular products unless recommended by prescriber. You may experience blurred vision, eye pain, infection, or irritation. Notify prescriber immediately of any sign of infection (redness, drainage, eye pain, itching, sensitivity to light, swelling, or change in vision), chest pain, acute headache, or persistent dizziness.

Albendazole (al BEN da zole)

Brand Names: U.S. Albenza®

Pharmacologic Category Anthelmintic

Medication Safety Issues

Sound-alike/look-alike issues:

Albenza® may be confused with Aplenzin™, Relenza®

International issues:

Albenza [U.S.] may be confused with Avanza brand name for mirtazapine [Australia]

Pregnancy Risk Factor C

Lactation Excretion in breast milk unknown/use caution

Use Treatment of parenchymal neurocysticercosis caused by *Taenia solium* and cystic hydatid disease of the liver, lung, and peritoneum caused by *Echinococcus granulosus*

Unlabeled Use Albendazole has activity against *Ascaris lumbricoides* (roundworm); *Ancylostoma caninum*; *Ancylostoma duodenale* and *Necator americanus* (hookworms); cutaneous larva migrans; *Enterobius vermicularis* (pinworm); *Giardia duodenalis* (giardiasis); *Gnathostoma spinigerum*; *Gongylonema* sp; *Mansonella perstans* (filariasis); *Oesophagostomum bifurcum*; *Opisthorchis sinensis* (liver fluke); *Trichinella spiralis* (Trichinellosis); visceral larva migrans (toxocariasis); activity has also been shown against the liver fluke *Clonorchis sinensis*, *Giardia lamblia*, *Cysticercus cellulosae*, and *Echinococcus multilocularis*. Albendazole has also been used for the treatment of intestinal microsporidiosis (*Encephalitozoon intestinalis*), disseminated microsporidiosis (*E. hellem*, *E. cuniculi*, *E. intestinalis*, *Pleistophora* sp, *Trachipleistophora* sp, *Brachiola vesicularum*), and ocular microsporidiosis (*E. hellem*, *E. cuniculi*, *Vittaforma corneae*).

Available Dosage Forms

Tablet, oral:

Albenza®: 200 mg

General Dosage Range Oral:

Children and Adults <60 kg: 15 mg/kg/day in 2 divided doses (maximum: 800 mg/day)

Children and Adults ≥60 kg: 800 mg/day in 2 divided doses (maximum: 800 mg/day)

Administration

Oral Should be administered with a high-fat meal. Administer anticonvulsant and steroid therapy during first week of neurocysticercosis therapy. If patients have difficulty swallowing, tablets may be crushed or chewed, then swallowed with a drink of water.

Nursing Actions

Physical Assessment Monitor laboratory tests for reduction or elimination of ova and parasites. Monitor for elevated LFTs.

Patient Education Laboratory tests may be required; maintain recommended schedule. Take with a high-fat meal. Follow prescriber's suggestions to prevent reinfection. May cause loss of hair (reversible), nausea, vomiting, dizziness, or headaches. Report unusual fever, persistent or unresolved abdominal pain, vomiting, yellowing of skin or eyes, darkening of urine, or light colored stools.

Albumin (al BYOO min)

Brand Names: U.S. Albuked™ 25; Albuked™ 5; Albuminar®-25; Albuminar®-5; AlbuRx® 25; AlbuRx® 5; Albutein®; Buminate; Flexbumin 25%; Human Albumin Grifols® 25%; Kedbumin™; Plasbumin®-25; Plasbumin®-5

Index Terms Albumin (Human); Normal Human Serum Albumin; Normal Serum Albumin (Human); Salt Poor Albumin; SPA

Pharmacologic Category Blood Product Derivative; Plasma Volume Expander, Colloid

Medication Safety Issues

Sound-alike/look-alike issues:

Albutein® may be confused with albuterol

Buminate® may be confused with bumetanide

Pregnancy Risk Factor C

Use Plasma volume expansion and maintenance of cardiac output in the treatment of certain types of shock or impending shock; may be useful for burn patients, ARDS, and cardiopulmonary bypass; other uses considered by some investigators (but not proven) are retroperitoneal surgery, peritonitis, and ascites; unless the condition responsible for hypoproteinemia can be corrected, albumin can provide only symptomatic relief or supportive treatment

Note: Nutritional supplementation is not an appropriate indication.

Unlabeled Use In patients with cirrhosis, administered with diuretics to help facilitate diuresis; large volume paracentesis; volume expansion in dehydrated, mildly hypotensive patients with cirrhosis; to prevent renal impairment and reduce mortality associated with spontaneous bacterial peritonitis (SBP) in patients with cirrhosis

Available Dosage Forms

Injection, solution [preservative free]: 5% [50 mg/mL] (250 mL, 500 mL); 20% [200 mg/mL] (50 mL, 100 mL); 25% [250 mg/mL] (50 mL, 100 mL)

Albuked™ 5: 5% [50 mg/mL] (250 mL)
Albuked™ 25: 25% [250 mg/mL] (50 mL)
Albuminar®-5: 5% [50 mg/mL] (250 mL, 500 mL)
Albuminar®-25: 25% [250 mg/mL] (50 mL, 100 mL)
AlbuRx® 5: 5% [50 mg/mL] (250 mL, 500 mL)
AlbuRx® 25: 25% [250 mg/mL] (50 mL, 100 mL)
Albutein®: 5% [50 mg/mL] (250 mL, 500 mL); 25% [250 mg/mL] (50 mL, 100 mL)
Buminate: 5% [50 mg/mL] (250 mL, 500 mL); 25% [250 mg/mL] (20 mL)
Flexbumin 25%: 25% [250 mg/mL] (50 mL, 100 mL)
Human Albumin Grifols® 25%: 25% [250 mg/mL] (50 mL, 100 mL)
Kedbumin™: 25% [250 mg/mL] (50 mL)
Plasbumin®-5: 5% [50 mg/mL] (50 mL, 250 mL)
Plasbumin®-25: 25% [250 mg/mL] (20 mL, 50 mL, 100 mL)

General Dosage Range I.V.:

Children: 0.5-1 g/kg/dose (10-20 mL/kg/dose) as needed

Adults: 0.5-1 g/kg/dose as needed **or** 25 g/dose may repeat in 15-30 minutes if response inadequate (maximum: 250 g/48 hours)

Administration

I.V. For I.V. administration only. Use within 4 hours after opening vial; discard unused portion. In emergencies, may administer as rapidly as necessary to improve clinical condition. After initial volume replacement:

5%: Do not exceed 2-4 mL/minute in patients with normal plasma volume; 5-10 mL/minute in patients with hypoproteinemia

25%: Do not exceed 1 mL/minute in patients with normal plasma volume; 2-3 mL/minute in patients with hypoproteinemia

I.V. Detail Do not dilute 5% solution. Rapid infusion may cause vascular overload. Albumin 25% may be given undiluted or diluted in normal saline. May give in combination or through the same administration set as saline or carbohydrates. Do not use with ethanol or protein hydrolysates, precipitation may form.

pH: 6.4-7.4

Nursing Actions

Physical Assessment Monitor patient closely for pulmonary edema and cardiac failure (assess vital signs and central venous pressure) during administration. Monitor frequently for hypovolemia or fluid overload. If fever, tachycardia, hypotension, or dyspnea occurs, stop infusion and notify prescriber.

Patient Education This medication can only be administered intravenously. You will be monitored closely during the infusion. Report immediately any pain or bruising at infusion site, acute headache, difficulty breathing, chills, chest pain or tightness, palpitations, or sudden pain.

Albuterol (al BYOO ter ole)

Brand Names: U.S. AccuNeb®; ProAir® HFA; Proventil® HFA; Ventolin® HFA; VoSpire ER®

Index Terms Albuterol Sulfate; Salbutamol; Salbutamol Sulphate

Pharmacologic Category $Beta_2$ Agonist

Medication Safety Issues

Sound-alike/look-alike issues:

Albuterol may be confused with Albutein®, atenolol

Proventil® may be confused with Bentyl®, PriLOSEC®, Prinivil®

Salbutamol may be confused with salmeterol

Ventolin® may be confused with phentolamine, Benylin®, Vantin

Pregnancy Risk Factor C

Lactation Excretion in breast milk unknown/use caution

Use Treatment or prevention of bronchospasm in patients with reversible obstructive airway disease; prevention of exercise-induced bronchospasm

Mechanism of Action/Effect Relaxes bronchial smooth muscle by action on $beta_2$-receptors with little effect on heart rate

Contraindications Hypersensitivity to albuterol or any component of the formulation

Injection formulation (Canadian labeling; product not available in U.S.): Hypersensitivity to albuterol or any component of the formulation; tachyarrhythmias; risk of abortion during first or second trimester

Warnings/Precautions Optimize anti-inflammatory treatment before initiating maintenance treatment with albuterol. Do not use as a component of chronic therapy without an anti-inflammatory agent. Only the mildest forms of asthma (Step 1 and/or exercise-induced) would not require concurrent use based upon asthma guidelines. Patient must be instructed to seek medical attention in cases where acute symptoms are not relieved or a previous level of response is diminished. The need to increase frequency of use may indicate deterioration of asthma, and treatment must not be delayed.

Use caution in patients with cardiovascular disease (arrhythmia or hypertension or HF), convulsive disorders, diabetes, glaucoma, hyperthyroidism, or hypokalemia. Beta-agonists may cause elevation in blood pressure, heart rate, and result in CNS stimulation/excitation. $Beta_2$-agonists may increase risk of arrhythmia, increase serum glucose, or decrease serum potassium.

Immediate hypersensitivity reactions (urticaria, angioedema, rash, bronchospasm) have been reported. Do not exceed recommended dose; serious adverse events, including fatalities, have been associated with excessive use of inhaled sympathomimetics. Rarely, paradoxical bronchospasm may occur with use of inhaled bronchodilating agents; this should be distinguished from inadequate response. All patients should utilize a spacer device or valved holding chamber when using a metered-dose inhaler; in addition, face masks should be used in children <4 years of age.

Drug Interactions

Avoid Concomitant Use

Avoid concomitant use of Albuterol with any of the following: Beta-Blockers (Nonselective); Iobenguane I 123

Decreased Effect

Albuterol may decrease the levels/effects of: Iobenguane I 123

The levels/effects of Albuterol may be decreased by: Alpha-/Beta-Blockers; Beta-Blockers (Beta1 Selective); Beta-Blockers (Nonselective); Betahistine

Increased Effect/Toxicity

Albuterol may increase the levels/effects of: Loop Diuretics; Sympathomimetics; Thiazide Diuretics

The levels/effects of Albuterol may be increased by: Atomoxetine; Cannabinoids; MAO Inhibitors; Tricyclic Antidepressants

Nutritional/Ethanol Interactions

Food: Avoid or limit caffeine (may cause CNS stimulation).

Herb/Nutraceutical: Avoid ephedra, yohimbe (may cause CNS stimulation). Avoid St John's wort (may decrease the levels/effects of albuterol).

Adverse Reactions Incidence of adverse effects is dependent upon age of patient, dose, and route of administration.

Cardiovascular: Angina, atrial fibrillation, arrhythmias, chest discomfort, chest pain, extrasystoles, flushing, hyper-/hypotension, palpitation, supraventricular tachycardia, tachycardia

Central nervous system: CNS stimulation, dizziness, drowsiness, headache, insomnia, irritability, lightheadedness, migraine, nervousness, nightmares, restlessness, seizure

Dermatologic: Angioedema, rash, urticaria

Endocrine & metabolic: Hyperglycemia, hypokalemia, lactic acidosis

Gastrointestinal: Diarrhea, dry mouth, dyspepsia, gastroenteritis, nausea, unusual taste, vomiting

Genitourinary: Micturition difficulty

Local: Injection: Pain, stinging

Neuromuscular & skeletal: Muscle cramps, musculoskeletal pain, tremor, weakness

Otic: Otitis media, vertigo

Respiratory: Asthma exacerbation, bronchospasm, cough, epistaxis, laryngitis, oropharyngeal drying/irritation, oropharyngeal edema, pharyngitis, rhinitis, upper respiratory inflammation, viral respiratory infection

Miscellaneous: Allergic reaction, anaphylaxis, diaphoresis, lymphadenopathy

Pharmacodynamics/Kinetics

Onset of Action Peak effect:

Nebulization/oral inhalation: 0.5-2 hours

CFC-propelled albuterol: 10 minutes

Ventolin® HFA: 25 minutes

Oral: 2-3 hours

Duration of Action Nebulization/oral inhalation: 3-4 hours; Oral: 4-6 hours

Available Dosage Forms

Aerosol, for oral inhalation:

ProAir® HFA: 90 mcg/inhalation (8.5 g)

Proventil® HFA: 90 mcg/inhalation (6.7 g)

Ventolin® HFA: 90 mcg/inhalation (8 g, 18 g)

Solution, for nebulization: 0.083% [2.5 mg/3 mL] (25s, 30s, 60s); 0.5% [100 mg/20 mL] (1s)

Solution, for nebulization [preservative free]: 0.021% [0.63 mg/3 mL] (25s); 0.042% [1.25 mg/3 mL] (25s, 30s); 0.083% [2.5 mg/3 mL] (3 mL, 10s, 24s, 25s, 30s, 60s); 0.5% [2.5 mg/0.5 mL] (10s, 30s)

AccuNeb®: 0.021% [0.63 mg/3 mL] (25s); 0.042% [1.25 mg/3 mL] (25s)

Syrup, oral: 2 mg/5 mL (473 mL, 480 mL)

Tablet, oral: 2 mg, 4 mg

Tablet, extended release, oral: 4 mg, 8 mg

VoSpire ER®: 4 mg, 8 mg

General Dosage Range

Inhalation via metered-dose inhaler (90 mcg/puff): *Children and Adults:* 2 puffs every 4-6 hours **or** 4-8 puffs every 1-4 hours [acute symptoms] **or** 1-2 puffs prior to exercise

Nebulization:

Children <12 years: 0.15-0.3 mg/kg (maximum: 10 mg) every 1-4 hours **or** 0.63-1.25 mg 3-4 times/day **or** 0.5 mg/kg/hour by continuous nebulization

Children ≥12 years: 2.5-10 mg every 1-4 hours **or** 10-15 mg/hour by continuous nebulization

Adults: 2.5-10 mg every 1-4 hours **or** 10-15 mg/hour by continuous nebulization

Oral:

Regular release:

Children 2-6 years: 0.1-0.2 mg/kg/dose 3 times/day (maximum: 12 mg/day)

Children 6-12 years: 2 mg/dose 3-4 times/day (maximum: 24 mg/day)

Children >12 years and Adults: 2-4 mg/dose 3-4 times/day (maximum: 32 mg/day)

Extended release:

Children 6-12 years: 4 mg every 12 hours (maximum: 24 mg/day)

Children >12 years and Adults: 8 mg every 12 hours (maximum: 32 mg/day)

Administration

Oral Do not crush or chew extended release tablets.

I.V. Infusion solution (Canadian labeling; product not available in U.S.): Do not inject undiluted. Reduce concentration by at least 50% before infusing. Administer as a continuous infusion via infusion pump.

Inhalation

Metered-dose inhaler: Shake well before use; prime prior to first use, and whenever inhaler has not been used for >2 weeks or when it has been dropped, by releasing 3-4 test sprays into the air (away from face). HFA inhalers should be cleaned with warm water at least once per week; allow to air dry completely prior to use. A spacer device or valved holding chamber is recommended for use with metered-dose inhalers.

Solution for nebulization: Concentrated solution should be diluted prior to use. Blow-by administration is not recommended, use a mask device if patient unable to hold mouthpiece in mouth for administration.

Stability

Reconstitution Solution for nebulization: To prepare a 2.5 mg dose, dilute 0.5 mL of solution to a total of 3 mL with normal saline; also compatible with cromolyn or ipratropium nebulizer solutions.

Storage

HFA aerosols: Store at 15°C to 25°C (59°F to 77°F).

Ventolin® HFA: Discard when counter reads 000 or 12 months after removal from protective pouch, whichever comes first. Store with mouthpiece down.

Infusion solution (Canadian labeling; product not available in U.S.): Ventolin® I.V.: Store at 15°C to 30°C (59°F to 86°F). Protect from light. After dilution, discard unused portion after 24 hours.

Solution for nebulization (0.5%): Store at 2°C to 25°C (36°F to 77°F).

AccuNeb®: Store at 2°C to 25°C (36°F to 77°F). Do not use if solution changes color or becomes cloudy. Use within 1 week of opening foil pouch.

Syrup: Store at 20°C to 25°C (68°F to 77°F).

Tablet: Store at 20°C to 25°C (68°F to 77°F).

Tablet, extended release: Store at 20°C to 25°C (68°F to 77°F)

Nursing Actions

Physical Assessment Evaluate effectiveness of therapy (relief of airway obstruction). For inpatient care, monitor vital signs and lung sounds prior to and periodically during therapy.

Patient Education Maintain adequate hydration, unless instructed to restrict fluid intake. You may experience nervousness, dizziness, dry mouth, unpleasant taste, or stomach upset. Report unresolved GI upset, dizziness, chest pain or palpitations, nervousness or insomnia, muscle cramping or tremor, or respiratory difficulty.

Self-administered inhalation: Shake canister before using. Sit when using medication. Close eyes when administering albuterol to avoid spraying into eyes. Exhale slowly and completely through nose; inhale deeply through mouth while administering aerosol. Hold breath for 5-10 seconds after inhalation. Wait at least 1 full minute between inhalations. Wash mouthpiece between use. If more than one inhalation medication is used, use albuterol first and wait 5 minutes between medications. Prime inhaler prior to first use, and whenever the inhaler has not been used for more than 2 weeks.

Self-administered nebulizer: Wash hands before and after treatment. Wash and dry nebulizer after each treatment. Twist open the top of one unit-dose vial and squeeze contents into nebulizer reservoir. Connect nebulizer reservoir to the mouthpiece or face mask. Connect nebulizer to compressor. Sit in comfortable, upright position. Place mouthpiece in your mouth or put on face mask and turn on compressor. If face mask is used, avoid leakage around the mask to avoid mist getting into eyes, which may cause vision problems. Breathe calmly and deeply until no more mist is formed in nebulizer (about 5 minutes).

Dietary Considerations Oral forms should be taken with water 1 hour before or 2 hours after meals.

Alcaftadine (al KAF ta deen)

Brand Names: U.S. Lastacaft™

Pharmacologic Category Histamine H_1 Antagonist; Histamine H_1 Antagonist, Second Generation; Mast Cell Stabilizer

Pregnancy Risk Factor B

Lactation Excretion in breast milk unknown/use caution

Use Prevention of itching associated with allergic conjunctivitis

Available Dosage Forms

Solution, ophthalmic:

Lastacaft™: 0.25% (3 mL)

General Dosage Range Ophthalmic: *Children ≥2 years and Adults:* Instill 1 drop into each eye once daily

Administration

Other For topical ophthalmic use only. Contact lenses should be removed prior to application, and may be reinserted 10 minutes after administration. Do not insert contacts if eyes are red. Avoid contaminating the applicator tip with affected eye(s).

Aldesleukin (al des LOO kin)

Brand Names: U.S. Proleukin®

Index Terms IL-2; Interleukin 2; Interleukin-2; Lymphocyte Mitogenic Factor; Recombinant Human Interleukin-2; T-Cell Growth Factor; TCGF; Thymocyte Stimulating Factor

Pharmacologic Category Antineoplastic Agent, Miscellaneous; Biological Response Modulator

Medication Safety Issues

Sound-alike/look-alike issues:

Aldesleukin may be confused with oprelvekin

Proleukin® may be confused with oprelvekin

High alert medication:

The Institute for Safe Medication Practices (ISMP) includes this medication among its list of drug classes which have a heightened risk of causing significant patient harm when used in error.

Pregnancy Risk Factor C

Lactation Excretion in breast milk unknown/not recommended

Use Treatment of metastatic renal cell cancer, metastatic melanoma

Unlabeled Use Treatment of acute myeloid leukemia (AML)

Available Dosage Forms

Injection, powder for reconstitution:

Proleukin®: 22 x 10^6 int. units

General Dosage Range Dosage adjustment recommended in patients who develop toxicities

I.V.: *Adults:* 600,000 int. units/kg every 8 hours (maximum: 14 doses); may repeat after 9 days for a total of 28 doses/course

Administration

I.V. Infuse over 15 minutes. Allow solution to reach room temperature prior to administration. Do not administer with an inline filter. Flush before and after with D_5W, particularly if maintenance I.V. line contains sodium chloride.

Other May be administered by SubQ injection (unlabeled route).

Nursing Actions

Physical Assessment Monitor vital signs; cardiac, respiratory, and CNS status; fluid balance; signs of systemic sepsis; changes in mental status; and laboratory tests daily prior to beginning infusion and for 2 hours following infusion. Closely monitor infusion site for extravasation.

Patient Education Avoid alcohol. Maintain adequate hydration, unless instructed to restrict fluid intake. Can cause hypotension. You will be susceptible to infection. May cause increased sensitivity to sunlight, nausea, vomiting, stomatitis, anorexia, malaise, or weakness. This drug may result in many side effects; you will be monitored and assessed closely during therapy. Report any changes in urination, swelling of extremities, weight gain, unusual bruising or bleeding, chest pain or palpitations, acute dizziness, respiratory difficulty, fever or chills, changes in cognition or mental status, rash, feelings of pain or numbness in extremities, severe or persistent GI upset or diarrhea, vaginal discharge or mouth sores, yellowing of eyes or skin, or changes in color of urine or stool.

Alefacept (a LE fa sept)

Brand Names: U.S. Amevive® [DSC]

Index Terms B 9273; BG 9273; Human LFA-3/IgG (1) Fusion Protein; LFA-3/IgG(1) Fusion Protein, Human

Pharmacologic Category Monoclonal Antibody

Pregnancy Risk Factor B

Lactation Excretion in breast milk unknown/not recommended

Breast-Feeding Considerations It is not known whether alefacept is excreted in breast milk. Since alefacept is an immunosuppressant, and transfer of proteins into breast milk may occur, breast-feeding women are cautioned to discontinue breast-feeding or to discontinue use of the drug while breast-feeding (recommendations per manufacturer).

Use Treatment of moderate-to-severe chronic plaque psoriasis in adults who are candidates for systemic therapy or phototherapy

Mechanism of Action/Effect Alefacept is a monoclonal antibody against a specific receptor on T lymphocytes, and reduces the number of both $CD4^+$ and $CD8^+$ T lymphocytes. It improves symptoms of psoriasis by decreasing the number of activated T lymphocytes, and their production of inflammatory mediators such as interferon gamma.

Contraindications Hypersensitivity to alefacept or any component of the formulation; patients with HIV infection

Warnings/Precautions Hazardous agent - use appropriate precautions for handling and disposal. Has been associated with hypersensitivity reactions; discontinue if anaphylaxis or severe reaction occurs. Alefacept induces a decline in circulating T-lymphocytes ($CD4^+$ and $CD8^+$); $CD4^+$ lymphocyte counts should be monitored every 2 weeks throughout therapy. Do not initiate in pre-existing depression of $CD4^+$ lymphocytes; withhold treatment in any patient who develops a depressed $CD4^+$ lymphocyte count (<250 cells/µL) during treatment and monitor $CD4^+$ lymphocyte counts ▶

weekly; permanently discontinue if CD4+ lymphocyte counts remain <250 cells/µL for 1 month.

Alefacept may increase the risk of malignancies; avoid use in patients with a history of systemic malignancy; use caution in patients at high risk for malignancy. Discontinue if malignancy develops during therapy. Alefacept may increase the risk of infection and may reactivate latent infection; monitor for new infections. Avoid use in patients with clinically important infections or a history of recurrent infections; not recommended for use in patients receiving other immunosuppressant drugs or phototherapy. Discontinue if a serious infection occurs. In postmarketing reports, significant transaminase elevations, as well as rare cases of hepatitis, fatty liver, decompensation of cirrhosis, and acute hepatic failure (a causal relationship not established). Discontinue if signs and symptoms of hepatic injury occur. Safety and efficacy of live or attenuated vaccines have not been evaluated.

Drug Interactions

Avoid Concomitant Use

Avoid concomitant use of Alefacept with any of the following: BCG; Belimumab; Natalizumab; Pimecrolimus; Tacrolimus (Topical); Vaccines (Live)

Decreased Effect

Alefacept may decrease the levels/effects of: BCG; Coccidioidin Skin Test; Sipuleucel-T; Vaccines (Inactivated); Vaccines (Live)

The levels/effects of Alefacept may be decreased by: Echinacea

Increased Effect/Toxicity

Alefacept may increase the levels/effects of: Belimumab; Leflunomide; Natalizumab; Vaccines (Live)

The levels/effects of Alefacept may be increased by: Denosumab; Pimecrolimus; Roflumilast; Tacrolimus (Topical); Trastuzumab

Nutritional/Ethanol Interactions Ethanol: Avoid ethanol (may increase risk of liver toxicity).

Adverse Reactions

≥10%:

Hematologic: Lymphopenia (up to 10% of patients required temporary discontinuation, up to 17% during a second course of therapy)

Local: Injection site reactions (up to 16% of patients; includes pain, inflammation, bleeding, edema, or other reaction)

1% to 10%:

Central nervous system: Chills (6%; primarily during intravenous administration), dizziness (≥2%)

Dermatologic: Pruritus (≥2%)

Gastrointestinal: Nausea (≥2%)

Hepatic: Transaminases increased (2%; AST and ALT ≥3 times ULN)

Neuromuscular & skeletal: Myalgia (≥2%)

Respiratory: Pharyngitis (≥2%), cough (≥2%)

Miscellaneous: Antibodies to alefacept (3%; significance unknown), infection (1% requiring hospitalization), malignancies (1%)

Available Dosage Forms

Injection, powder for reconstitution:

Amevive®: 15 mg

General Dosage Range I.M.: *Adults:* 15 mg once weekly

Administration

I.M. I.M. injections should be administered at least 1 inch from previous administration sites.

Stability

Reconstitution Reconstitute 15 mg vial for I.M. solution with 0.6 mL of SWFI (supplied); reconstituted solution contains 15 mg/0.5 mL of alefacept. Gently swirl to avoid excessive foaming. Do not filter reconstituted solutions.

Storage Store under refrigeration at 2°C to 8°C (36°F to 46°F). Protect from light. Following reconstitution, may be stored for up to 4 hours at 2°C to 8°C (36°F to 46°F). Discard any unused solution within 4 hours of reconstitution.

Nursing Actions

Physical Assessment Monitor closely for the development of malignancies or infections.

Patient Education This medication can only be administered by injection. Report immediately any pain or irritation at injection site; chills; rash; difficulty swallowing or breathing; or feelings of tightness in chest. Avoid alcohol. You will need weekly blood tests while receiving this medication. May cause nausea or muscle pain. Report unusual feelings of fatigue or weakness, signs of infection (eg, cough, runny nose, sore throat, swollen glands, mouth sores, burning on urination, fever, chills), abdominal pain, jaundice, easy bruising, dark urine, or pale stools.

Dietary Considerations Some products may contain sucrose.

Alendronate (a LEN droe nate)

Brand Names: U.S. Fosamax®

Index Terms Alendronate Sodium; Alendronic Acid Monosodium Salt Trihydrate; MK-217

Pharmacologic Category Bisphosphonate Derivative

Medication Safety Issues

Sound-alike/look-alike issues:

Alendronate may be confused with risedronate

Fosamax® may be confused with Flomax®, Fosamax Plus D®, fosinopril, Zithromax®

International issues:

Fosamax [U.S., Canada, and multiple international markets] may be confused with Fisamox brand name for amoxicillin [Australia]

Medication Guide Available Yes

Pregnancy Risk Factor C

Lactation Excretion in breast milk unknown/use caution

Use Treatment and prevention of osteoporosis in postmenopausal females; treatment of osteoporosis in males; Paget's disease of the bone in patients who are symptomatic, at risk for future complications, or with alkaline phosphatase ≥2 times the upper limit of normal; treatment of glucocorticoid-induced osteoporosis in males and females with low bone mineral density who are receiving a daily dosage ≥7.5 mg of prednisone (or equivalent)

Mechanism of Action/Effect A bisphosphonate which inhibits bone resorption via actions on osteoclasts or on osteoclast precursors; decreases the rate of bone resorption, leading to an indirect increase in bone mineral density. In Paget's disease, characterized by disordered resorption and formation of bone, inhibition of resorption leads to an indirect decrease in bone formation; but the newly-formed bone has a more normal architecture.

Contraindications Hypersensitivity to alendronate, other bisphosphonates, or any component of the formulation; hypocalcemia; abnormalities of the esophagus which delay esophageal emptying such as stricture or achalasia; inability to stand or sit upright for at least 30 minutes; oral solution should not be used in patients at risk of aspiration

Warnings/Precautions Use caution in patients with renal impairment (not recommended for use in patients with Cl_{cr} <35 mL/minute); hypocalcemia must be corrected before therapy initiation; ensure adequate calcium and vitamin D intake. May cause irritation to upper gastrointestinal mucosa. Esophagitis, dysphagia, esophageal ulcers, esophageal erosions, and esophageal stricture (rare) have been reported; risk increases in patients unable to comply with dosing instructions. Use with caution in patients with dysphagia, esophageal disease, gastritis, duodenitis, or ulcers (may worsen underlying condition). Discontinue use if new or worsening symptoms develop.

Osteonecrosis of the jaw (ONJ) has been reported in patients receiving bisphosphonates. Risk factors include invasive dental procedures (eg, tooth extraction, dental implants, boney surgery); a diagnosis of cancer, with concomitant chemotherapy or corticosteroids; poor oral hygiene, ill-fitting dentures; and comorbid disorders (anemia, coagulopathy, infection, pre-existing dental disease). Most reported cases occurred after I.V. bisphosphonate therapy; however, cases have been reported following oral therapy. A dental exam and preventative dentistry should be performed prior to placing patients with risk factors on chronic bisphosphonate therapy. The manufacturer's labeling states that discontinuing bisphosphonates in patients requiring invasive dental procedures may reduce the risk of ONJ. However, other experts suggest that there is no evidence that discontinuing therapy reduces the risk of developing ONJ (Assael, 2009). The benefit/risk must be assessed by the treating physician and/or dentist/surgeon prior to any invasive dental procedure. Patients developing ONJ while on bisphosphonates should receive care by an oral surgeon.

Atypical femur fractures have been reported in patients receiving bisphosphonates for treatment/ prevention of osteoporosis. The fractures include subtrochanteric femur (bone just below the hip joint) and diaphyseal femur (long segment of the thigh bone). Some patients experience prodromal pain weeks or months before the fracture occurs. It is unclear if bisphosphonate therapy is the cause for these fractures, although the majority have been reported in patients taking bisphosphonates. Patients receiving long-term (>3-5 years) therapy may be at an increased risk. Discontinue bisphosphonate therapy in patients who develop a femoral shaft fracture.

Severe (and occasionally debilitating) bone, joint, and/or muscle pain have been reported during bisphosphonate treatment. The onset of pain ranged from a single day to several months. Consider discontinuing therapy in patients who experience severe symptoms; symptoms usually resolve upon discontinuation. Some patients experienced recurrence when rechallenged with same drug or another bisphosphonate; avoid use in patients with a history of these symptoms in association with bisphosphonate therapy.

Drug Interactions

Avoid Concomitant Use There are no known interactions where it is recommended to avoid concomitant use.

Decreased Effect

The levels/effects of Alendronate may be decreased by: Antacids; Calcium Salts; Iron Salts; Magnesium Salts; Proton Pump Inhibitors

Increased Effect/Toxicity

Alendronate may increase the levels/effects of: Deferasirox; Phosphate Supplements

The levels/effects of Alendronate may be increased by: Aminoglycosides; Aspirin; Nonsteroidal Anti-Inflammatory Agents

Nutritional/Ethanol Interactions

Ethanol: May increase risk of osteoporosis and gastric irritation. Management: Avoid ethanol.

Food: All food and beverages interfere with absorption. Coadministration with caffeine may reduce alendronate efficacy. Coadministration with dairy products may decrease alendronate absorption. Beverages (especially orange juice and coffee) and food may reduce the absorption of alendronate as much as 60%. Management: Alendronate must be taken with plain water (tablets 6-8 oz; oral solution follow with 2 oz) first thing in the morning and ≥30 minutes before the first food, beverage, or other medication of the day. Do not take with mineral water or with other beverages.

Adverse Reactions Note: Incidence of adverse effects (mostly GI) increases significantly in patients treated for Paget's disease at 40 mg/day.

>10%: Endocrine & metabolic: Hypocalcemia (transient, mild, 18%); hypophosphatemia (transient, mild, 10%)

1% to 10%:

Central nervous system: Headache (up to 3%)

Gastrointestinal: Abdominal pain (1% to 7%), acid reflux (1% to 4%), dyspepsia (1% to 4%), nausea (1% to 4%), flatulence (up to 4%), diarrhea (1% to 3%), gastroesophageal reflux disease (1% to 3%), constipation (up to 3%), esophageal ulcer (up to 2%), abdominal distension (up to 1%), gastritis (up to 1%), vomiting (up to 1%), dysphagia (up to 1%), gastric ulcer (1%), melena (1%)

Neuromuscular & skeletal: Musculoskeletal pain (up to 6%), muscle cramps (up to 1%)

Available Dosage Forms

Tablet, oral: 5 mg, 10 mg, 35 mg, 40 mg, 70 mg

Fosamax®: 10 mg, 70 mg

General Dosage Range Oral: *Adults:* 5-10 mg/day **or** 35-70 mg once weekly (maximum: 70 mg/week) **or** 40 mg once daily [Paget's disease]

Administration

Oral Alendronate must be taken with plain water (tablets 6-8 oz; oral solution follow with 2 oz) first thing in the morning and ≥30 minutes before the first food, beverage, or other medication of the day. Do not take with mineral water or with other beverages. Patients should be instructed to stay upright (not to lie down) for at least 30 minutes **and** until after first food of the day (to reduce esophageal irritation).

Stability

Storage Store tablets and oral solution at room temperature of 15°C to 30°C (59°F to 86°F). Keep in well-closed container.

Nursing Actions

Physical Assessment Monitor for unusual or acute musculoskeletal pain. Monitor blood pressure at the beginning of therapy and periodically during use. Patients at risk for osteonecrosis of the jaw (eg, chemotherapy, corticosteroids, poor oral hygiene) should have dental exams; necessary preventive dentistry should be done before beginning bisphosphonate therapy. Assess ability of patient to comply with administration directions. Teach patient appropriate administration of medication. Instruct patient in lifestyle and dietary changes that will have a beneficial impact.

Patient Education Take first thing in the morning, at least 30 minutes before the first food or beverage of the day. Take tablets with a full 6- to 8-ounce glass of water; follow solution with 2 ounces of water. Wait at least 30 minutes after taking alendronate before eating or drinking anything else. Stay in sitting or standing position for 30 minutes following administration and until after the first food of the day to reduce potential for esophageal irritation. Consult prescriber to determine necessity of lifestyle changes (eg, decreased smoking, decreased alcohol intake). Consult prescriber before having any dental procedures; inform dentist that you are taking this medication. You may experience flatulence, bloating, nausea, acid regurgitation, temporary bone pain, or muscle cramps. Report persistent muscle or bone pain or leg cramps; persistent unresolved GI pain or upset; unusual fever or chills; or pain in mouth, jaws, or teeth.

Dietary Considerations Ensure adequate calcium and vitamin D intake; women and men >50 years of age should consume 1200-1500 mg/day of elemental calcium and 800-1000 int. units/day of vitamin D. Wait at least 30 minutes after taking alendronate before taking any supplement. Alendronate must be taken with plain water first thing in the morning and at least 30 minutes before the first food or beverage of the day. Do not take with mineral water or with other beverages.

Alfuzosin (al FYOO zoe sin)

Brand Names: U.S. Uroxatral®

Index Terms Alfuzosin Hydrochloride

Pharmacologic Category Alpha$_1$ Blocker

Pregnancy Risk Factor B

Use Treatment of the functional symptoms of benign prostatic hyperplasia (BPH)

Unlabeled Use Facilitation of expulsion of ureteral stones

Mechanism of Action/Effect An antagonist of alpha$_1$-adrenoreceptors in the lower urinary tract. Blockade of these adrenoreceptors can cause smooth muscles in the bladder neck and prostate to relax, resulting in an improvement in urine flow rate and a reduction in BPH symptoms.

Contraindications Hypersensitivity to alfuzosin or any component of the formulation; moderate or severe hepatic insufficiency (Child-Pugh class B and C); concurrent use with potent CYP3A4 inhibitors (eg, itraconazole, ketoconazole, ritonavir) or other alpha$_1$-blocking agents

Warnings/Precautions Not intended for use as an antihypertensive drug. May cause significant orthostatic hypotension and syncope, especially with first dose; anticipate a similar effect if therapy is interrupted for a few days, if dosage is rapidly increased, or used with antihypertensives (particularly vasodilators), PDE-5 inhibitors, nitrates or other medications which may result in hypotension. Discontinue if symptoms of angina occur or worsen. Alfuzosin has been shown to prolong the QT interval alone (minimal) and with other drugs with comparable effects on the QT interval (additive); use with caution in patients with known QT prolongation (congenital or acquired). Patients should be cautioned about performing hazardous tasks when starting new therapy or adjusting dosage upward. Discontinue if symptoms of angina occur or worsen. Rule out prostatic carcinoma before beginning therapy. Use caution with severe renal or mild hepatic impairment; contraindicated in moderate-to-severe hepatic impairment. Intraoperative floppy iris syndrome has been observed in cataract surgery patients who were on or were previously treated with alpha$_1$-blockers. Causality has not been established and there appears to be no benefit in discontinuing alpha-blocker therapy prior to surgery. May cause priapism. Contraindicated in patients taking strong CYP3A4 inhibitors or other alpha$_1$-blockers.

Drug Interactions

Avoid Concomitant Use

Avoid concomitant use of Alfuzosin with any of the following: Alpha1-Blockers; CYP3A4 Inhibitors (Strong); Protease Inhibitors; Telaprevir

Decreased Effect

The levels/effects of Alfuzosin may be decreased by: CYP3A4 Inducers (Strong); Deferasirox; Herbs (CYP3A4 Inducers); Tocilizumab

Increased Effect/Toxicity

Alfuzosin may increase the levels/effects of: Alpha1-Blockers; Antihypertensives; Calcium Channel Blockers; Nitroglycerin; QTc-Prolonging Agents

The levels/effects of Alfuzosin may be increased by: Beta-Blockers; CYP3A4 Inhibitors (Moderate); CYP3A4 Inhibitors (Strong); Ivacaftor; MAO Inhibitors; Phosphodiesterase 5 Inhibitors; Protease Inhibitors; Telaprevir

Nutritional/Ethanol Interactions

Food: Food increases the extent of absorption. Management: Administer immediately following a meal at the same time each day.

Herb/Nutraceutical: St John's wort may decrease alfuzosin levels. Management: Avoid St John's wort.

Adverse Reactions 1% to 10%:

Central nervous system: Dizziness (6%), fatigue (3%), headache (3%), pain (1% to 2%)

Gastrointestinal: Abdominal pain (1% to 2%), constipation (1% to 2%), dyspepsia (1% to 2%), nausea (1% to 2%)

Genitourinary: Impotence (1% to 2%)

Respiratory: Upper respiratory tract infection (3%), bronchitis (1% to 2%), pharyngitis (1% to 2%), sinusitis (1% to 2%)

Available Dosage Forms

Tablet, extended release, oral: 10 mg

Uroxatral®: 10 mg

General Dosage Range Oral: *Adults:* 10 mg once daily

Administration

Oral Tablet should be swallowed whole; do not crush or chew. Administer once daily (immediately following a meal); should be taken at the same time each day.

Stability

Storage Store at room temperature of 25°C (77°F); excursions permitted to 15°C to 30°C (59°F to 86°F). Protect from light and moisture.

Nursing Actions

Physical Assessment Assess blood pressure and monitor for hypotension, dizziness, somnolence, and impotence at beginning of therapy and on a regular basis.

Patient Education Take at the same time each day. May cause drowsiness, dizziness, postural hypotension, nausea, or sexual dysfunction (reversible, may resolve with continued use). Report altered CNS status (eg, fatigue), severe dizziness or passing out, or erection that lasts more than 4 hours.

Dietary Considerations Take immediately following a meal at the same time each day.

Aliskiren (a lis KYE ren)

Brand Names: U.S. Tekturna®

Index Terms Aliskiren Hemifumarate; SPP100

Pharmacologic Category Renin Inhibitor

Medication Safety Issues

Sound-alike/look-alike issues:

Tekturna® may be confused with Valturna®

Pregnancy Risk Factor C (1st trimester); D (2nd and 3rd trimesters)

Lactation Excretion in breast milk unknown/not recommended

Use Treatment of hypertension, alone or in combination with other antihypertensive agents

Unlabeled Use Treatment of persistent proteinuria in patients with type 2 diabetes mellitus, hypertension, and nephropathy despite administration of optimized recommended renoprotective therapy (eg, angiotensin II receptor blocker)

Mechanism of Action/Effect Aliskerin is a direct renin inhibitor, resulting in blockade of the conversion of angiotensinogen to angiotensin I. Angiotensin I suppression decreases the formation of angiotensin II (Ang II), resulting in blood pressure reduction.

Contraindications

U.S. labeling: There are no contraindications listed in manufacturer's labeling.

Canada labeling: Hypersensitivity to aliskiren or any component of the formulation; history of angioedema with aliskiren, ACE-inhibitors, or angiotensin receptor blockers; hereditary or idiopathic angioedema. **Note:** To be included with forthcoming changes to the Canadian labeling: Concomitant use with ACE-inhibitors or angiotensin receptor blockers in patients with type 2 diabetes mellitus.

Warnings/Precautions [U.S. Boxed Warning]: Drugs that act on the renin-angiotensin system can cause injury and death to the developing fetus. Discontinue as soon as possible once pregnancy is detected. Since the effect of aliskiren on bradykinin levels is unknown, the risk of kinin-mediated etiologies of angioedema occurring is also unknown. Use with caution in any patient with a history of angioedema (of any etiology) as angioedema, some cases necessitating hospitalization and intubation, has been observed (rarely) with aliskiren use. Discontinue immediately following any signs and symptoms of angioedema; do not readminister. Prolonged frequent monitoring may be required especially if tongue, glottis, or larynx are involved as they are associated with airway obstruction. Patients with a history of airway surgery may have a higher risk of airway obstruction. Early, aggressive, and appropriate management is critical. Hyperkalemia may occur (rarely) during monotherapy; risk may increase in patients with predisposing factors (eg, renal dysfunction, diabetes mellitus or concomitant use with ACE inhibitors, potassium-sparing diuretics, potassium supplements, and/or potassium-containing salts). Symptomatic hypotension may occur (rarely) during the initiation of therapy, particularly in patients with an activated renin-angiotensin system (ie, volume or salt-depleted patients). Use with caution in patients with severe renal impairment; not studied in patients with severe renal impairment (eGFR <30 mL/minute and/or S_{cr} ≥1.7 mg/dL [women]; S_{cr} ≥2 mg/dL [men]), history of dialysis, nephrotic syndrome, or renovascular hypertension. Use with caution or avoid in patients with deteriorating renal function or renal artery stenosis (bilateral or unilateral). Avoid concurrent use with strong inhibitors of P-glycoprotein (eg, cyclosporine, itraconazole).

Drug Interactions

Avoid Concomitant Use

Avoid concomitant use of Aliskiren with any of the following: CycloSPORINE; CycloSPORINE (Systemic); Itraconazole

Decreased Effect

Aliskiren may decrease the levels/effects of: Furosemide

The levels/effects of Aliskiren may be decreased by: Grapefruit Juice; Herbs (Hypertensive Properties); Methylphenidate; Nonsteroidal Anti-Inflammatory Agents; P-glycoprotein/ABCB1 Inducers; Tocilizumab; Yohimbine

Increased Effect/Toxicity

Aliskiren may increase the levels/effects of: Amifostine; Antihypertensives; Hypotensive Agents; RiTUXimab

The levels/effects of Aliskiren may be increased by: Alfuzosin; Atorvastatin; Conivaptan; CycloSPORINE; CycloSPORINE (Systemic); Diazoxide; Herbs (Hypotensive Properties); Itraconazole; Ketoconazole; Ketoconazole (Systemic); MAO Inhibitors; Nonsteroidal Anti-Inflammatory Agents; Pentoxifylline; P-glycoprotein/ABCB1 Inhibitors; Phosphodiesterase 5 Inhibitors; Prostacyclin Analogues; Verapamil

Nutritional/Ethanol Interactions

Food: High-fat meals decrease absorption. Grapefruit juice may decrease the serum concentration of aliskiren. Management: Administer at the same time each day; may take with or without a meal, but consistent administration with regards to meals is recommended. Avoid concomitant use of aliskiren and grapefruit juice.

Herb/Nutraceutical: Some herbal medications may worsen hypertension (eg, licorice); others may increase the antihypertensive effect of aliskiren (eg, shepherd's purse). Management: Avoid bayberry, blue cohosh, cayenne, ephedra, ginger, ginseng (American), kola, licorice, and yohimbe. Avoid black cohosh, California poppy, coleus, golden seal, hawthorn, mistletoe, periwinkle, quinine, and shepherd's purse.

Adverse Reactions 1% to 10%:

Dermatologic: Rash (1%)

Endocrine & metabolic: Hyperkalemia (monotherapy ≤1%; concurrent with ACE inhibitor in patients with diabetes 6%)

Gastrointestinal: Diarrhea (2%)

Hematologic: Creatine kinase increased (>300%: 1%)

Renal: BUN increased (≤7%), serum creatinine increased (≤7%)

Respiratory: Cough (1%)

Pharmacodynamics/Kinetics

Onset of Action Maximum antihypertensive effect: Within 2 weeks

Available Dosage Forms

Tablet, oral:

Tekturna®: 150 mg, 300 mg

General Dosage Range Oral: *Adults:* 150-300 mg once daily (maximum: 300 mg/day)

Administration

Oral Administer at the same time daily; may take with or without a meal, but consistent administration with regards to meals is recommended.

Stability

Storage Store at 25°C (77°F); excursions permitted to 15°C to 30°C (59°F to 86°F). Protect from moisture.

Nursing Actions

Physical Assessment Monitor for angioedema and hypotension at beginning of therapy, when changing dose, and on a regular basis throughout.

Patient Education Take at same time each day; may be taken with meals. This drug does not eliminate the need for diet or exercise regimen. May cause dizziness or hypotension. Report immediately any unusual swelling of eyes, face, lips, mouth, throat, or any difficulty swallowing of breathing; changes in urinary pattern; or palpitations or irregular heartbeat.

Dietary Considerations May be taken with or without food; however, a high-fat meal reduces absorption. Consistent administration with regards to meals is recommended.

Aliskiren, Amlodipine, and Hydrochlorothiazide

(a lis KYE ren, am LOE di peen, & hye droe klor oh THYE a zide)

Brand Names: U.S. Amturnide™

Index Terms Aliskiren, Hydrochlorothiazide, and Amlodipine; Amlodipine Besylate, Aliskiren Hemifumarate, and Hydrochlorothiazide; Amlodipine, Aliskiren, and Hydrochlorothiazide; Amlodipine, Hydrochlorothiazide, and Aliskiren; Hydrochlorothiazide, Aliskiren, and Amlodipine; Hydrochlorothiazide, Amlodipine, and Aliskiren

Pharmacologic Category Antianginal Agent; Calcium Channel Blocker; Calcium Channel Blocker, Dihydropyridine; Diuretic, Thiazide; Renin Inhibitor

Medication Safety Issues

Sound-alike/look-alike issues:

Amturnide™ may be confused with AMILoride

Pregnancy Risk Factor D

Lactation Excretion in breast milk unknown/not recommended

Use Treatment of hypertension (not for initial therapy)

Available Dosage Forms

Tablet, oral:

Amturnide™: Aliskiren 150 mg, amlodipine 5 mg, and hydrochlorothiazide 12.5 mg; Aliskiren 300 mg, amlodipine 5 mg, and hydrochlorothiazide 12.5 mg; Aliskiren 300 mg, amlodipine 5 mg, and hydrochlorothiazide 25 mg; Aliskiren 300 mg, amlodipine 10 mg, and hydrochlorothiazide 12.5 mg; Aliskiren 300 mg, amlodipine 10 mg, and hydrochlorothiazide 25 mg

General Dosage Range Oral: *Adults:* Aliskiren 150-300 mg and Amlodipine 5-10 mg and Hydrochlorothiazide 12.5-25 mg once daily (maximum recommended daily dose: Aliskiren 300 mg; amlodipine 10 mg; hydrochlorothiazide 25 mg)

Administration

Oral Administer at the same time daily. May take with or without a meal, but consistent administration with regard to meals is recommended.

Nursing Actions

Physical Assessment See individual agents.

Patient Education See individual agents.

Aliskiren and Amlodipine

(a lis KYE ren & am LOE di peen)

Brand Names: U.S. Tekamlo™

Index Terms Aliskiren Hemifumarate and Amlodipine Besylate; Amlodipine and Aliskiren

Pharmacologic Category Antianginal Agent; Calcium Channel Blocker; Calcium Channel Blocker, Dihydropyridine; Renin Inhibitor

Pregnancy Risk Factor D

Lactation Excretion in breast milk unknown/not recommended

Use Treatment of hypertension, alone or in combination with other antihypertensive agents, including use as initial therapy in patients likely to need multiple antihypertensives for adequate control

Available Dosage Forms

Tablet, oral:

Tekamlo™: 150/5: Aliskiren 150 mg and amlodipine 5 mg, 300/5: Aliskiren 300 mg and amlodipine 5 mg, 150/10: Aliskiren 150 mg and amlodipine 10 mg, 300/10: Aliskiren 300 mg and amlodipine 10 mg

General Dosage Range Oral: *Adults:* Aliskiren 150-300 mg and amlodipine 5-10 mg once daily (maximum: 300 mg/day [aliskiren]; 10 mg/day [amlodipine])

Administration

Oral Administer at the same time daily. May take with or without a meal, but consistent administration with regards to meals is recommended.

Nursing Actions

Physical Assessment See individual agents.

Patient Education See individual agents.

Aliskiren and Hydrochlorothiazide

(a lis KYE ren & hye droe klor oh THYE a zide)

Brand Names: U.S. Tekturna HCT®

Index Terms Aliskiren Hemifumarate and Hydrochlorothiazide; Hydrochlorothiazide and Aliskiren

Pharmacologic Category Diuretic, Thiazide; Renin Inhibitor

Pregnancy Risk Factor D

Lactation Enters breast milk/not recommended

Use Treatment of hypertension, including use as initial therapy in patients likely to need multiple antihypertensives for adequate control

Available Dosage Forms

Tablet:

Tekturna HCT®: 150/12.5: Aliskiren 150 mg and hydrochlorothiazide 12.5 mg; 150/25: Aliskiren 150 mg and hydrochlorothiazide 25 mg; 300/12.5: Aliskiren 300 mg and hydrochlorothiazide 12.5 mg; 300/25: Aliskiren 300 mg and hydrochlorothiazide 25 mg

General Dosage Range Oral: *Adults:* Aliskiren 150-300 mg and hydrochlorothiazide 12.5-25 mg once daily (maximum: 300 mg/day [aliskiren]; 25 mg/day [hydrochlorothiazide])

Administration

Oral Administer at the same time daily; may take with or without a meal, but consistent administration with regards to meals is recommended.

Nursing Actions

Physical Assessment See individual agents.

Patient Education See individual agents.

Aliskiren and Valsartan
(a lis KYE ren & val SAR tan)

Brand Names: U.S. Valturna®

Index Terms Aliskiren Hemifumarate and Valsartan; Valsartan and Aliskiren

Pharmacologic Category Angiotensin II Receptor Blocker; Renin Inhibitor

Medication Safety Issues

Sound-alike/look-alike issues:

Valturna® may be confused with Tekturna®, valsartan

Pregnancy Risk Factor D

Lactation Excretion in breast milk unknown/not recommended

Use Treatment of hypertension, including use as initial therapy in patients likely to need multiple antihypertensives for adequate control

Available Dosage Forms

Tablet:

Valturna®: 150/160: Aliskiren 150 mg and valsartan 160 mg; 300/320: Aliskiren 300 mg and valsartan 320 mg

General Dosage Range Oral: *Adults:* Aliskiren 150-300 mg and valsartan 160-320 mg once daily (maximum: 300 mg/day [aliskiren]; 320 mg/day [valsartan])

Administration

Oral Administer at the same time daily; may take with or without a meal, but consistent administration with regards to meal is recommended. Avoid taking with high-fat meals.

Nursing Actions

Physical Assessment See individual agents.

Patient Education See individual agents.

Alitretinoin (a li TRET i noyn)

Brand Names: U.S. Panretin®

Pharmacologic Category Antineoplastic Agent, Miscellaneous; Retinoic Acid Derivative

Medication Safety Issues

Sound-alike/look-alike issues:

Panretin® may be confused with pancreatin

High alert medication:

The Institute for Safe Medication Practices (ISMP) includes this medication among its list of drugs which have a heightened risk of causing significant patient harm when used in error.

Pregnancy Risk Factor D

Lactation Excretion in breast milk unknown/not recommended

Use Orphan drug: Topical treatment of cutaneous lesions in AIDS-related Kaposi's sarcoma

Unlabeled Use Cutaneous T-cell lymphomas

Available Dosage Forms

Gel, topical:

Panretin®: 0.1% (60 g)

General Dosage Range Topical: *Adults:* Apply twice daily

Administration

Topical Do not use occlusive dressings.

Nursing Actions

Patient Education For external use only. Avoid use of any product containing DEET, such as insect repellent. Wear protective clothing and/or avoid exposure to direct sun or sunlamps. Wash hands thoroughly before applying. Avoid applying skin products that contain alcohol or harsh chemicals during treatment. Do not apply occlusive dressings. Stop treatment and inform prescriber if rash, skin irritation, redness, scaling, or excessive dryness appears.

Allopurinol (al oh PURE i nole)

Brand Names: U.S. Aloprim®; Zyloprim®

Index Terms Allopurinol Sodium

Pharmacologic Category Antigout Agent; Xanthine Oxidase Inhibitor

Medication Safety Issues

Sound-alike/look-alike issues:

Allopurinol may be confused with Apresoline

Zyloprim® may be confused with ZORprin®, Zovirax®

Pregnancy Risk Factor C

Lactation Enters breast milk/use caution (AAP rates "compatible"; AAP 2001 update pending)

Use

Oral: Management of primary or secondary gout (acute attack, tophi, joint destruction, uric acid lithiasis, and/or nephropathy); management of hyperuricemia associated with cancer treatment for leukemia, lymphoma, or solid tumor malignancies; management of recurrent calcium oxalate calculi (with uric acid excretion >800 mg/day in men and >750 mg/day in women)

I.V.: Management of hyperuricemia associated with cancer treatment for leukemia, lymphoma, or solid tumor malignancies

Mechanism of Action/Effect Allopurinol inhibits xanthine oxidase, the enzyme responsible for the conversion of hypoxanthine to xanthine to uric acid. Allopurinol is metabolized to oxypurinol which is also an inhibitor of xanthine oxidase; allopurinol acts on purine catabolism, reducing the production of uric acid without disrupting the biosynthesis of vital purines.

Contraindications Hypersensitivity to allopurinol or any component of the formulation

Warnings/Precautions Do not use to treat asymptomatic hyperuricemia. Has been associated with a number of hypersensitivity reactions, including severe reactions (vasculitis and Stevens-Johnson syndrome); discontinue at first sign of rash. Reversible hepatotoxicity has been reported; use with caution in patients with pre-existing hepatic impairment. Bone marrow suppression has been reported; use caution with other drugs causing myelosuppression. Caution in renal impairment, dosage adjustments needed. Use with caution in patients taking diuretics concurrently. Risk of skin rash may be increased in patients receiving amoxicillin or ampicillin. The risk of hypersensitivity may be increased in patients receiving thiazides, and possibly ACE inhibitors. Use caution with mercaptopurine or azathioprine; dosage adjustment necessary. Full effect on serum uric acid levels in chronic gout may take several weeks to become evident; gradual titration is recommended.

Drug Interactions

Avoid Concomitant Use

Avoid concomitant use of Allopurinol with any of the following: Didanosine

Decreased Effect

The levels/effects of Allopurinol may be decreased by: Antacids

Increased Effect/Toxicity

Allopurinol may increase the levels/effects of: Amoxicillin; Ampicillin; Anticonvulsants (Hydantoin); AzaTHIOprine; CarBAMazepine; ChlorproPAMIDE; Cyclophosphamide; Didanosine; Mercaptopurine; Theophylline Derivatives; Vitamin K Antagonists

The levels/effects of Allopurinol may be increased by: ACE Inhibitors; Loop Diuretics; Thiazide Diuretics

Nutritional/Ethanol Interactions

Ethanol: May decrease effectiveness.

Iron supplements: Hepatic iron uptake may be increased.

Vitamin C: Large amounts of vitamin C may acidify urine and increase kidney stone formation.

Adverse Reactions

Dermatologic: Rash

Endocrine & metabolic: Gout (acute)

Gastrointestinal: Diarrhea, nausea

Hepatic: Alkaline phosphatase increased, liver enzymes increased

Pharmacodynamics/Kinetics

Onset of Action Peak effect: 1-2 weeks

Available Dosage Forms

Injection, powder for reconstitution: 500 mg (base)

Aloprim®: 500 mg (base)

Tablet, oral: 100 mg, 300 mg

Zyloprim®: 100 mg, 300 mg

General Dosage Range Dosage adjustment recommended in patients with renal impairment

I.V.:

Children: Initial: 200 mg/m^2/day as a single infusion or in equally divided doses at 6-, 8-, or 12-hour intervals

Adults: 200-400 mg/m^2/day as a single infusion or in equally divided doses at 6-, 8-, or 12-hour intervals (maximum: 600 mg/day)

Oral:

Children <6 years: 150 mg/day

Children 6-10 years: 10 mg/kg/day

Children >10 years and Adults: 100-800 mg/day in 1-3 divided doses (maximum: 800 mg/day)

Administration

Oral Do not initiate or discontinue allopurinol during an acute gout attack. Should be administered after meals with plenty of fluid.

I.V. The rate of infusion depends on the volume of the infusion; infuse maximum single daily doses (600 mg/day) over ≥30 minutes. Whenever possible, therapy should be initiated at 24-48 hours before the start of chemotherapy known to cause tumor lysis (including adrenocorticosteroids). I.V. daily dose can be administered as a single infusion or in equally divided doses at 6-, 8-, or 12-hour interval.

Stability

Reconstitution Reconstitute powder for injection with SWFI. Further dilution with NS or D_5W (50-100 mL) to ≤6 mg/mL is recommended.

Storage

Powder for injection: Store at controlled room temperature of 20°C to 25°C (68°F to 77°F). Following preparation, intravenous solutions should be stored at 20°C to 25°C (68°F to 77°F). Do not refrigerate reconstituted and/or diluted product. Must be administered within 10 hours of solution preparation.

Tablet: Store at controlled room temperature of 20°C to 25°C (68°F to 77°F). Protect from moisture and light.

Nursing Actions

Physical Assessment Monitor frequency and severity of gouty attacks.

Patient Education Maintain adequate hydration, unless instructed to restrict fluid intake. Avoid the use of alcohol (especially beer). You may experience drowsiness, nausea, vomiting, heartburn, or hair loss (reversible). Report immediately skin rash or lesions; painful urination or blood in urine or stool; pain or irritation of the eyes; swelling of lips, mouth, or tongue; unusual fatigue; easy bruising or bleeding; yellowing of skin or eyes; any change in color of urine or stool; unresolved nausea or vomiting; or numbness of extremities. Continue medication during gout attacks.

Dietary Considerations Should take oral forms after meals with plenty of fluid. Fluid intake should be administered to yield neutral or slightly alkaline urine and an output of ~2 L (in adults).

Almotriptan (al moh TRIP tan)

Brand Names: U.S. Axert®

Index Terms Almotriptan Malate

Pharmacologic Category Antimigraine Agent; Serotonin 5-$HT_{1B, 1D}$ Receptor Agonist

Medication Safety Issues

Sound-alike/look-alike issues:

Axert® may be confused with Antivert®

Pregnancy Risk Factor C

Lactation Excretion in breast milk unknown/use caution

Use Acute treatment of migraine with or without aura in adults (with a history of migraine) and adolescents (with a history of migraine lasting ≥4 hours when left untreated)

Mechanism of Action/Effect Selective agonist for serotonin receptor in cranial arteries; causes vasoconstriction and relief of migraine.

Contraindications Hypersensitivity to almotriptan or any component of the formulation; hemiplegic or basilar migraine; known or suspected ischemic heart disease (eg, angina pectoris, MI, documented silent ischemia, coronary artery vasospasm, Prinzmetal's variant angina); cerebrovascular syndromes (eg, stroke, transient ischemic attacks); peripheral vascular disease (eg, ischemic bowel disease); uncontrolled hypertension; use within 24 hours of another 5-HT_1 agonist; use within 24 hours of ergotamine derivatives and/or ergotamine-containing medications (eg, dihydroergotamine, ergotamine)

Warnings/Precautions Almotriptan is only indicated for the treatment of acute migraine headache; not indicated for migraine prophylaxis, or the treatment of cluster headaches, hemiplegic migraine, or basilar migraine. If a patient does not respond to the first dose, the diagnosis of acute migraine should be reconsidered.

Almotriptan should not be given to patients with documented ischemic or vasospastic CAD. Patients with risk factors for CAD (eg, hypertension, hypercholesterolemia, smoker, obesity, diabetes, strong family history of CAD, menopause, male >40 years of age) should undergo adequate cardiac evaluation prior to administration; if the cardiac evaluation is "satisfactory," the first dose of almotriptan should be given in the healthcare provider's office (consider ECG monitoring). All patients should undergo periodic evaluation of cardiovascular status during treatment. Cardiac events (coronary artery vasospasm, transient ischemia, myocardial infarction, ventricular tachycardia/fibrillation, cardiac arrest, and death), cerebral/subarachnoid hemorrhage, stroke, peripheral vascular ischemia, and colonic ischemia have been reported with 5-HT_1 agonist administration. Patients who experience sensations of chest pain/pressure/tightness or symptoms suggestive of angina following dosing should be evaluated for coronary artery disease or Prinzmetal's angina before receiving additional doses; if dosing is resumed and similar symptoms recur, monitor with ECG. Significant elevation in blood pressure, including hypertensive crisis, has also been reported on rare occasions following 5-HT_1 agonist administration in patients with and without a history of hypertension.

Transient and permanent blindness and partial vision loss have been reported (rare) with 5-HT_1 agonist administration. Almotriptan contains a sulfonyl group which is structurally different from a sulfonamide. Cross-reactivity in patients with sulfonamide allergy has not been evaluated; however, the manufacturer recommends that caution be exercised in this patient population. Use with caution in liver or renal dysfunction. Symptoms of agitation, confusion, hallucinations, hyper-reflexia, myoclonus, shivering, and tachycardia (serotonin syndrome) may occur with concomitant proserotonergic drugs (ie, SSRIs/SNRIs or triptans) or agents which reduce almotriptan's metabolism. Concurrent use of serotonin precursors (eg, tryptophan) is not recommended. If concomitant administration with SSRIs is warranted, monitor closely, especially at initiation and with dose increases. Efficacy has not been demonstrated in improvement of migraine-associated symptoms (eg, phonophobia, nausea, photophobia) in patients aged 12-17 years (Linder, 2008).

Drug Interactions

Avoid Concomitant Use

Avoid concomitant use of Almotriptan with any of the following: Ergot Derivatives; MAO Inhibitors

Decreased Effect

The levels/effects of Almotriptan may be decreased by: Peginterferon Alfa-2b; Tocilizumab

Increased Effect/Toxicity

Almotriptan may increase the levels/effects of: Ergot Derivatives; Metoclopramide; Serotonin Modulators

The levels/effects of Almotriptan may be increased by: Antipsychotics; CYP3A4 Inhibitors (Strong); Ergot Derivatives; MAO Inhibitors

Adverse Reactions 1% to 10%:

Central nervous system: Somnolence (≤5%), dizziness (≤4%), headache (≤2%)

Gastrointestinal: Nausea (1% to 3%), vomiting (≤2%), xerostomia (1%)

Neuromuscular & skeletal: Paresthesia (≤1%)

Available Dosage Forms

Tablet, oral:

Axert®: 6.25 mg, 12.5 mg

General Dosage Range Dosage adjustment recommended in patients with hepatic or renal impairment and/or on concomitant therapy

Oral: *Children ≥12 years and Adults:* 6.25-12.5 mg in a single dose; may repeat after 2 hours (maximum daily dose: 25 mg)

Administration

Oral Administer without regard to meals.

Stability

Storage Store at 25°C (77°F); excursions permitted to 15°C to 30°C (59°F to 86°F).

Nursing Actions

Physical Assessment Clear diagnosis of migraines and cardiac status should be determined before beginning treatment. Assess risk for coronary artery disease, liver or renal dysfunction, and sulfonamide allergy. Monitor for hypertension and cardiac events. Teach patient proper use (treatment of acute migraine; not prevention of migraine).

Patient Education This drug is to be used to reduce your migraine, not to prevent or reduce the number of attacks. Do not use more than two doses in 24 hours and do not take within 24 hours of any other migraine medication without consulting prescriber. May cause dizziness, fatigue, or drowsiness. Report immediately any chest pain or palpitations, feelings of tightness or pressure in jaw or throat, dizziness, or skin rash.

Dietary Considerations May be taken without regard to meals.

ALPRAZolam (al PRAY zoe lam)

Brand Names: U.S. Alprazolam Intensol™; Niravam™; Xanax XR®; Xanax®

Pharmacologic Category Benzodiazepine

Medication Safety Issues

Sound-alike/look-alike issues:

ALPRAZolam may be confused with alprostadil, LORazepam, triazolam

Xanax® may be confused with Fanapt®, Lanoxin®, Tenex®, Tylox®, Xopenex®, Zantac®, ZyrTEC®

BEERS Criteria medication:

This drug may be inappropriate for use in geriatric patients (high severity risk).

Pregnancy Risk Factor D

Lactation Enters breast milk/not recommended (AAP rates "of concern"; AAP 2001 update pending)

Breast-Feeding Considerations In a study of eight postpartum women, peak concentrations of alprazolam were found in breast milk ~1 hour after the maternal dose and the half-life was ~14 hours. Samples were obtained over 36 hours following a single oral dose of alprazolam 0.5 mg. Metabolites were not detected in breast milk. In this study, the estimated exposure to the breast-feeding infant was ~3% of the weight-adjusted maternal dose. Drowsiness, lethargy, or weight loss in nursing infants have been observed in case reports following maternal use of some benzodiazepines.

Use Treatment of anxiety disorder (GAD); short-term relief of symptoms of anxiety; panic disorder, with or without agoraphobia; anxiety associated with depression

Unlabeled Use Anxiety in children

Mechanism of Action/Effect Binds to stereospecific benzodiazepine receptors on the postsynaptic GABA neuron at several sites within the central nervous system, including the limbic system, reticular formation. Enhancement of the inhibitory effect of GABA on neuronal excitability results by increased neuronal membrane permeability to chloride ions. This shift in chloride ions results in hyperpolarization (a less excitable state) and stabilization.

Contraindications Hypersensitivity to alprazolam or any component of the formulation (cross-sensitivity with other benzodiazepines may exist); narrow-angle glaucoma; concurrent use with ketoconazole or itraconazole

Warnings/Precautions Rebound or withdrawal symptoms, including seizures, may occur following abrupt discontinuation or large decreases in dose (more common in patients receiving >4 mg/day or prolonged treatment); the risk of seizures appears to be greatest 24-72 hours following discontinuation of therapy. Breakthrough anxiety may occur at the end of dosing interval. Use with caution in patients receiving concurrent CYP3A4 inhibitors, moderate or strong CYP3A4 inducers, and major CYP3A4 substrates; consider alternative agents that avoid or lessen the potential for CYP-mediated interactions. Use with caution in renal impairment or predisposition to urate nephropathy; has weak uricosuric properties. Use with caution in elderly; due to increased sensitivity in this age group, smaller doses of benzodiazepines may be safer and as effective. Avoid using doses >2 mg daily of alprazolam (Beers Criteria) Use with caution in or debilitated patients, patients with hepatic disease (including alcoholics) or respiratory disease, or obese patients.

Causes CNS depression (dose related) which may impair physical and mental capabilities. Patients must be cautioned about performing tasks that require mental alertness (eg, operating machinery or driving). Effects with other sedative drugs or ethanol may be potentiated. Benzodiazepines have been associated with falls and traumatic injury and should be used with extreme caution in patients who are at risk of these events.

Use caution in patients with depression, particularly if suicidal risk may be present. Episodes of mania or hypomania have occurred in depressed patients treated with alprazolam. May cause physical or psychological dependence. Acute withdrawal may be precipitated in patients after administration of flumazenil.

Benzodiazepines have been associated with anterograde amnesia. Paradoxical reactions have been reported with benzodiazepines, particularly in adolescent/pediatric or psychiatric patients. Does not have analgesic, antidepressant, or antipsychotic properties.

Drug Interactions

Avoid Concomitant Use

Avoid concomitant use of ALPRAZolam with any of the following: Conivaptan; Indinavir; OLANZapine

Decreased Effect

The levels/effects of ALPRAZolam may be decreased by: CarBAMazepine; CYP3A4 Inducers (Strong); Deferasirox; Rifamycin Derivatives; St Johns Wort; Theophylline Derivatives; Tocilizumab; Yohimbine

Increased Effect/Toxicity

ALPRAZolam may increase the levels/effects of: Alcohol (Ethyl); CloZAPine; CNS Depressants; Methotrimeprazine; Selective Serotonin Reuptake Inhibitors

The levels/effects of ALPRAZolam may be increased by: Antifungal Agents (Azole Derivatives, Systemic); Aprepitant; Boceprevir; Calcium Channel Blockers (Nondihydropyridine); Cimetidine; Conivaptan; Contraceptives (Estrogens); Contraceptives (Progestins); CYP3A4 Inhibitors (Moderate); CYP3A4 Inhibitors (Strong); Dasatinib; Droperidol; Fosaprepitant; Grapefruit Juice; HydrOXYzine; Indinavir; Isoniazid; Ivacaftor; Macrolide Antibiotics; Methotrimeprazine; OLANZapine; Protease Inhibitors; Proton Pump Inhibitors; Selective Serotonin Reuptake Inhibitors; Telaprevir

Nutritional/Ethanol Interactions

Cigarette: Smoking may decrease alprazolam concentrations up to 50%.

Ethanol: Ethanol may increase CNS depression. Management: Avoid ethanol.

Food: Alprazolam serum concentration is unlikely to be increased by grapefruit juice because of alprazolam's high oral bioavailability. The C_{max} of the extended release formulation is increased by 25% when a high-fat meal is given 2 hours before dosing. T_{max} is decreased 33% when food is given immediately prior to dose and increased by 33% when food is given ≥1 hour after dose.

Herb/Nutraceutical: St John's wort may decrease alprazolam levels. Valerian, kava kava, and gotu kola may increase CNS depression. Management: Avoid St John's wort. Avoid valerian, kava kava, and gotu kola.

Adverse Reactions

>10%:

Central nervous system: Abnormal coordination, cognitive disorder, depression, drowsiness, fatigue, irritability, lightheadedness, memory impairment, sedation, somnolence

Endocrine & metabolic: Libido decreased

Gastrointestinal: Appetite increased/decreased, constipation, weight gain/loss, xerostomia

Genitourinary: Micturition difficulty

Neuromuscular & skeletal: Dysarthria

Respiratory: Nasal congestion

1% to 10%:

Cardiovascular: Chest pain, hypotension, palpitation, sinus tachycardia

Central nervous system: Agitation, akathisia, ataxia, attention disturbance, confusion, depersonalization, derealization, disorientation, disinhibition, dizziness, dream abnormalities, fear, hallucination, headache, hypersomnia, hypoesthesia, insomnia, lethargy, malaise, mental impairment, nervousness, nightmares, restlessness, seizure, syncope, talkativeness, vertigo

Dermatologic: Dermatitis, rash

Endocrine & metabolic: Dysmenorrhea, libido increased, menstrual disorders, sexual dysfunction

Gastrointestinal: Abdominal pain, anorexia, diarrhea, dyspepsia, nausea, salivation increased, vomiting

Genitourinary: Incontinence

Hepatic: Bilirubin increased, jaundice, liver enzymes increased

Neuromuscular & skeletal: Arthralgia, back pain, dyskinesia, dystonia, muscle cramps, muscle twitching, myalgia, paresthesia, tremor, weakness

Ocular: Blurred vision

Respiratory: Allergic rhinitis, dyspnea, hyperventilation, upper respiratory infection

Miscellaneous: Diaphoresis

Pharmacodynamics/Kinetics

Onset of Action Immediate release and extended release formulations: 1 hour

Duration of Action Immediate release: 5.1 ± 1.7 hours; Extended release: 11.3 ± 4.2 hours

Controlled Substance C-IV

Available Dosage Forms

Solution, oral:

Alprazolam Intensol™: 1 mg/mL (30 mL)

Tablet, oral: 0.25 mg, 0.5 mg, 1 mg, 2 mg

Xanax®: 0.25 mg, 0.5 mg, 1 mg, 2 mg

Tablet, extended release, oral: 0.5 mg, 1 mg, 2 mg, 3 mg

Xanax XR®: 0.5 mg, 1 mg, 2 mg, 3 mg

Tablet, orally disintegrating, oral: 0.25 mg, 0.5 mg, 1 mg, 2 mg

Niravam™: 0.25 mg, 0.5 mg, 1 mg, 2 mg

General Dosage Range Dosage adjustment recommended in patients with hepatic impairment

Oral:

Immediate release:

Adults: Initial: 0.25-0.5 mg 3 times/day; titrate as needed and tolerated (maximum: 10 mg/day)

Elderly: Initial: 0.25 mg 2-3 times/day; titrate gradually if needed and tolerated

Extended release:

Adults: Initial: 0.5-1 mg once daily; Maintenance: 3-6 mg/day (maximum: 6 mg/day)

Elderly: Initial: 0.5 mg/day; titrate gradually if needed and tolerated

Administration

Oral

Immediate release preparations: Can be administered sublingually if oral administration is not possible; absorption and onset of effect are comparable to oral administration (Scavone,1987; Scavone, 1992)

Extended release tablet: Should be taken once daily in the morning; do not crush, break, or chew.

Orally-disintegrating tablets: Using dry hands, place tablet on top of tongue and allow to disintegrate. If using one-half of tablet, immediately discard remaining half (may not remain stable). Administration with water is not necessary.

Stability

Storage

Immediate release tablets: Store at 20°C to 25°C (68°F to 77°F).

Extended release tablets: Store at 25°C (77°F); excursions permitted to 15°C to 30°C (59°F to 86°F).

Orally-disintegrating tablet: Store at room temperature of 20°C to 25°C (68°F to 77°F). Protect from moisture. Seal bottle tightly and discard any cotton packaged inside bottle.

Nursing Actions

Physical Assessment Assess for signs of CNS depression (sedation, dizziness, confusion, or ataxia). Assess for history of addiction; long-term use can result in dependence, abuse, or tolerance; periodically evaluate need for continued use. For inpatient use, institute safety measures to prevent falls. Taper dosage slowly when discontinuing.

Patient Education Drug may cause physical and/or psychological dependence. Avoid alcohol. You may experience drowsiness, lightheadedness, impaired coordination, dizziness, blurred vision, nausea, vomiting, dry mouth, constipation, altered sexual drive or ability (reversible), or photosensitivity. Report persistent CNS effects (eg, confusion, depression, increased sedation, excitation, headache, agitation, insomnia or nightmares, dizziness, fatigue, impaired coordination, changes in personality, or changes in cognition); changes in urinary pattern; muscle cramping, weakness, tremors, or rigidity; ringing in ears or visual disturbances; chest pain, palpitations, or rapid heartbeat; excessive perspiration; excessive GI symptoms (eg, cramping, constipation, vomiting, anorexia); or worsening of condition.

Dietary Considerations Extended release tablet should be taken once daily in the morning.

Alprostadil (al PROS ta dill)

Brand Names: U.S. Caverject Impulse®; Caverject®; Edex®; Muse®; Prostin VR Pediatric®

Index Terms PGE_1; Prostaglandin E_1

Pharmacologic Category Prostaglandin; Vasodilator

Medication Safety Issues

Sound-alike/look-alike issues:

Alprostadil may be confused with alPRAZolam

Pregnancy Risk Factor X/C (Muse®)

Lactation Not indicated for use in women

Use

Prostin VR Pediatric®: Temporary maintenance of patency of ductus arteriosus in neonates with ductal-dependent congenital heart disease until surgery can be performed. These defects include cyanotic (eg, pulmonary atresia, pulmonary stenosis, tricuspid atresia, Fallot's tetralogy, transposition of the great vessels) and acyanotic (eg, interruption of aortic arch, coarctation of aorta, hypoplastic left ventricle) heart disease.

Caverject®: Treatment of erectile dysfunction of vasculogenic, psychogenic, or neurogenic etiology; adjunct in the diagnosis of erectile dysfunction

Edex®, Muse®: Treatment of erectile dysfunction of vasculogenic, psychogenic, or neurogenic etiology

Unlabeled Use Treatment of pulmonary hypertension in infants and children with congenital heart defects with left-to-right shunts

Available Dosage Forms

Injection, powder for reconstitution:

Caverject Impulse®: 10 mcg, 20 mcg

Caverject®: 20 mcg, 40 mcg

Edex®: 10 mcg, 20 mcg, 40 mcg

Injection, solution: 500 mcg/mL (1 mL)

Prostin VR Pediatric®: 500 mcg/mL (1 mL)

Pellet, urethral:

Muse®: 125 mcg (1s, 6s); 250 mcg (1s, 6s); 500 mcg (1s, 6s); 1000 mcg (1s, 6s)

General Dosage Range

I.V.: *Neonates:* Initial: 0.05-0.1 mcg/kg/minute; Maintenance: 0.01-0.4 mcg/kg/minute

Intracavernous: *Adults:* Initial: 1.25-2.5 mcg; Maintenance: Increase to effective dose no more than 3 times/week with at least 24 hours between doses (maximum: 40 mcg/dose [Edex®]; 60 mcg/dose [Caverject®])

Intraurethral: *Adults:* Initial: 125-250 mcg; Maintenance: As needed (maximum: 2 doses/day)

Administration

I.V. Patent ductus arteriosus (Prostin VR Pediatric®): I.V. continuous infusion into a large vein or alternatively through an umbilical artery catheter placed at the ductal opening; manufacturer recommended maximum concentration for I.V. infusion: 20 mcg/mL

Other Erectile dysfunction: Use a 1/2 inch, 27- to 30-gauge needle. Inject into the dorsolateral aspect of the proximal third of the penis, avoiding visible veins; alternate side of the penis for injections.

Nursing Actions

Physical Assessment Neonate: Monitor closely; apnea has occurred during first hour after administration. **Erectile dysfunction:** After individual dose titration is determined by prescriber, the medication is self-administered. Teach patient appropriate injection technique and syringe/needle disposal.

Patient Education Use no more than 3 times/week, allowing 24 hours between injections. Avoid alcohol. Use alternate sides of penis with each injection. The risk of transmitting blood-borne disease is increased with use of alprostadil injections since a small amount of bleeding at injection site is possible. Stop using and contact prescriber immediately if erections last more than 4 hours, or you experience moderate to severe penile pain. Report penile problems (eg, nodules, new penile pain, rash, bruising, numbness, swelling, signs of infection, abnormal ejaculations); cardiac symptoms (hyper-/hypotension, chest pain, palpitations, irregular heartbeat); flushing, fever, or flu-like symptoms; or respiratory difficulty.

Alteplase (AL te plase)

Brand Names: U.S. Activase®; Cathflo® Activase®

Index Terms Alteplase, Recombinant; Alteplase, Tissue Plasminogen Activator, Recombinant; tPA

Pharmacologic Category Thrombolytic Agent

Medication Safety Issues

Sound-alike/look-alike issues:

Activase® may be confused with Cathflo® Activase®, TNKase®

Alteplase may be confused with Altace®

"tPA" abbreviation should not be used when writing orders for this medication; has been misread as TNKase (tenecteplase)

High alert medication:

The Institute for Safe Medication Practices (ISMP) includes this medication (I.V.) among its list of drugs which have a heightened risk of causing significant patient harm when used in error.

Pregnancy Risk Factor C

Lactation Excretion in breast milk unknown/use caution

Use Management of ST-elevation myocardial infarction (STEMI) for the lysis of thrombi in coronary arteries; management of acute ischemic stroke (AIS); management of acute pulmonary embolism (PE)

Recommended criteria for treatment:

STEMI: Chest pain ≥20 minutes duration, onset of chest pain within 12 hours of treatment (or within prior 12-24 hours in patients with continuing ischemic symptoms), and ST-segment elevation >0.1 mV in at least two contiguous precordial leads or two adjacent limb leads on ECG or new or presumably new left bundle branch block (LBBB)

AIS: Onset of stroke symptoms within 3 hours of treatment

Acute pulmonary embolism: Age ≤75 years: Documented massive PE (defined as acute PE with sustained hypotension [SBP <90 mm Hg for ≤15 minutes or requiring inotropic support], persistent profound bradycardia [HR <40 bpm with signs or symptoms of shock], or pulselessness); alteplase may be considered for submassive PE with clinical evidence of adverse prognosis (eg, new hemodynamic instability, worsening respiratory insufficiency, severe RV dysfunction, or major myocardial necrosis) and low risk of bleeding complications. **Note:** Not recommended for patients with low-risk PE (eg, normotensive, no RV dysfunction, normal biomarkers) or submassive acute PE with minor RV dysfunction, minor myocardial necrosis, and no clinical worsening (Jaff, 2011).

Cathflo® Activase®: Restoration of central venous catheter function

Unlabeled Use Acute ischemic stroke presenting 3-4.5 hours after symptom onset; acute peripheral arterial occlusive disease; pediatric parapneumonic effusion (chest tube instillation)

Mechanism of Action/Effect Dissolves thrombus (clot)

Contraindications Hypersensitivity to alteplase or any component of the formulation

Treatment of STEMI or PE: Active internal bleeding; history of CVA; ischemic stroke within 3 months (Antman, 2004; Jaff, 2011); recent intracranial or intraspinal surgery or trauma; intracranial neoplasm; prior intracranial hemorrhage (Antman, 2004; Jaff, 2011); arteriovenous malformation or aneurysm; known bleeding diathesis; severe uncontrolled hypertension (listed as a relative contraindication in STEMI [Antman, 2004] and PE [Jaff, 2011] guidelines); suspected aortic dissection (Antman, 2004; Jaff, 2011); significant closed head or facial trauma (Antman, 2004; Jaff, 2011) within 3 months with radiographic evidence of bony fracture or brain injury (Jaff, 2011)

Treatment of acute ischemic stroke: Evidence of intracranial hemorrhage or suspicion of subarachnoid hemorrhage on pretreatment evaluation; intracranial or intraspinal surgery within 3 months; stroke or serious head injury within 3 months; history of intracranial hemorrhage; uncontrolled hypertension at time of treatment (eg, >185 mm Hg systolic or >110 mm Hg diastolic); seizure at the onset of stroke; active internal bleeding; intracranial neoplasm; arteriovenous malformation or aneurysm; multilobar cerebral infarction (hypodensity >1/3 cerebral hemisphere; Adams, 2007); clinical presentation suggesting post-MI pericarditis; known bleeding diathesis including but not limited to current use of oral anticoagulants producing an

INR >1.7, an INR >1.7, administration of heparin within 48 hours preceding the onset of stroke with an elevated aPTT at presentation, platelet count <100,000/mm^3.

Additional exclusion criteria within clinical trials:

Presentation <3 hours after initial symptoms (NINDS, 1995): Time of symptom onset unknown, rapidly improving or minor symptoms, major surgery within 2 weeks, GI or urinary tract hemorrhage within 3 weeks, aggressive treatment required to lower blood pressure, glucose level <50 or >400 mg/dL, and arterial puncture at a noncompressible site or lumbar puncture within 1 week.

Presentation 3-4.5 hours after initial symptoms (ECASS-III; Hacke, 2008): Age >80 years, time of symptom onset unknown, rapidly improving or minor symptoms, current use of anticoagulants regardless of INR, glucose level <50 or >400 mg/dL, aggressive intravenous treatment required to lower blood pressure, major surgery or severe trauma within 3 months, baseline National Institutes of Health Stroke Scale (NIHSS) score >25, and history of both stroke and diabetes.

Warnings/Precautions Concurrent heparin anticoagulation may contribute to bleeding. In the treatment of acute ischemic stroke, concurrent use of anticoagulants was not permitted during the initial 24 hours of the <3 hour window trial (NINDS, 1995). Initiation of SubQ heparin (≤10,000 units) or equivalent doses of low molecular weight heparin for prevention of DVT during the first 24 hours of the 3-4.5 hour window trial was permitted and did not increase the incidence of intracerebral hemorrhage (Hacke, 2008). For acute PE, withhold heparin during the 2-hour infusion period. Monitor all potential bleeding sites. Do not use doses >150 mg; associated with increased risk of intracranial hemorrhage. Intramuscular injections and nonessential handling of the patient should be avoided. Venipunctures should be performed carefully and only when necessary. If arterial puncture is necessary, use an upper extremity vessel that can be manually compressed. If serious bleeding occurs, the infusion of alteplase and heparin should be stopped. Avoid aspirin for 24 hours following administration of alteplase; administration within 24 hours increases the risk of hemorrhagic transformation.

For the following conditions, the risk of bleeding is higher with use of thrombolytics and should be weighed against the benefits of therapy: Recent major surgery (eg, CABG, obstetrical delivery, organ biopsy, pregnancy, previous puncture of noncompressible vessels), prolonged CPR with evidence of thoracic trauma, lumbar puncture within 1 week, cerebrovascular disease, recent gastrointestinal or genitourinary bleeding, recent trauma, hypertension (systolic BP >175 mm Hg and/or diastolic BP >110 mm Hg), high likelihood of left heart thrombus (eg, mitral stenosis with atrial fibrillation), acute pericarditis, subacute bacterial endocarditis, hemostatic defects including ones caused by severe renal or hepatic dysfunction, significant hepatic dysfunction, pregnancy, diabetic hemorrhagic retinopathy or other hemorrhagic ophthalmic conditions, septic thrombophlebitis or occluded AV cannula at seriously infected site, advanced age (eg, >75 years), any other condition in which bleeding constitutes a significant hazard or would be particularly difficult to manage because of location. When treating acute MI or pulmonary embolism, use with caution in patients receiving oral anticoagulants. In the treatment of acute ischemic stroke within 3 hours of stroke symptom onset, the current use of oral anticoagulants producing an INR >1.7 is contraindicated.

Coronary thrombolysis may result in reperfusion arrhythmias. Patients who present **within 3 hours** of stroke symptom onset should be treated with alteplase unless contraindications exist. A longer time window (**3-4.5 hours** after symptom onset) has now been formally evaluated and shown to be safe and efficacious for select individuals (del Zoppo, 2009; Hacke, 2008). Treatment of patients with minor neurological deficit or with rapidly improving symptoms is not recommended. Follow standard management for STEMI while infusing alteplase.

Cathflo® Activase®: When used to restore catheter function, use Cathflo® cautiously in those patients with known or suspected catheter infections. Evaluate catheter for other causes of dysfunction before use. Avoid excessive pressure when instilling into catheter.

Drug Interactions

Avoid Concomitant Use There are no known interactions where it is recommended to avoid concomitant use.

Decreased Effect

The levels/effects of Alteplase may be decreased by: Aprotinin; Nitroglycerin

Increased Effect/Toxicity

Alteplase may increase the levels/effects of: Anticoagulants; Drotrecogin Alfa (Activated)

The levels/effects of Alteplase may be increased by: Antiplatelet Agents; Herbs (Anticoagulant/Antiplatelet Properties); Nonsteroidal Anti-Inflammatory Agents; Salicylates

Nutritional/Ethanol Interactions Herb/Nutraceutical: Avoid cat's claw, dong quai, evening primrose, feverfew, red clover, horse chestnut, garlic, green tea, ginseng, ginkgo (all have additional antiplatelet activity).

Adverse Reactions As with all drugs which may affect hemostasis, bleeding is the major adverse effect associated with alteplase. Hemorrhage may occur at virtually any site. Risk is dependent on multiple variables, including the dosage administered, concurrent use of multiple agents which alter hemostasis, and patient predisposition. Rapid lysis of coronary artery thrombi by thrombolytic agents may be associated with reperfusion-related atrial and/or ventricular arrhythmia. **Note:** Lowest rate of bleeding complications expected with dose used to restore catheter function.

1% to 10%:

Cardiovascular: Hypotension

Central nervous system: Fever

Dermatologic: Bruising (1%)

Gastrointestinal: GI hemorrhage (5%), nausea, vomiting

Genitourinary: GU hemorrhage (4%)

Hematologic: Bleeding (0.5% major, 7% minor: GUSTO trial)

Local: Bleeding at catheter puncture site (15.3%, accelerated administration)

Additional cardiovascular events associated **with use in STEMI:** AV block, cardiogenic shock, heart failure, cardiac arrest, recurrent ischemia/infarction, myocardial rupture, electromechanical dissociation, pericardial effusion, pericarditis, mitral regurgitation, cardiac tamponade, thromboembolism, pulmonary edema, asystole, ventricular tachycardia, bradycardia, ruptured intracranial AV malformation, seizure, hemorrhagic bursitis, cholesterol crystal embolization

Additional events associated **with use in pulmonary embolism:** Pulmonary re-embolization, pulmonary edema, pleural effusion, thromboembolism

Additional events associated **with use in stroke:** Cerebral edema, cerebral herniation, seizure, new ischemic stroke

Pharmacodynamics/Kinetics

Duration of Action >50% present in plasma cleared ~5 minutes after infusion terminated, ~80% cleared within 10 minutes

Available Dosage Forms

Injection, powder for reconstitution:

Activase®: 50 mg [29 million int. units], 100 mg [58 million int. units]

Cathflo® Activase®: 2 mg

General Dosage Range

Intracatheter:

Children <30 kg: 110% of the internal lumen volume of the catheter; retain in catheter for 0.5-2 hours; may repeat once (maximum: 2 mg/2 mL/dose)

Children ≥30 kg and Adults: 2 mg (2 mL) retain in catheter for 0.5-2 hours; may repeat once

I.V. infusion: *Adults:* Dosage varies greatly depending on indication

Administration

I.V.

Activase®: ST-elevation MI: Accelerated infusion: Bolus dose may be prepared by one of three methods:

1) Removal of 15 mL reconstituted (1 mg/mL) solution from vial

2) Removal of 15 mL from a port on the infusion line after priming

3) Programming an infusion pump to deliver a 15 mL bolus at the initiation of infusion

Activase®: Acute ischemic stroke: Bolus dose (10% of total dose) may be prepared by one of three methods:

1) Removal of the appropriate volume from reconstituted solution (1 mg/mL)

2) Removal of the appropriate volume from a port on the infusion line after priming

3) Programming an infusion pump to deliver the appropriate volume at the initiation of infusion

Note: Remaining dose for STEMI, AIS, or total dose for acute pulmonary embolism may be administered as follows: Any quantity of drug not to be administered to the patient must be removed from vial(s) prior to administration of remaining dose.

50 mg vial: Either PVC bag or glass vial and infusion set

100 mg vial: Insert spike end of the infusion set through the same puncture site created by transfer device and infuse from vial

If further dilution is desired, may be diluted in equal volume of 0.9% sodium chloride or D_5W to yield a final concentration of 0.5 mg/mL.

I.V. Detail Reconstituted solution should be clear or pale yellow and transparent. Avoid agitation during dilution.

pH: 5-7.3

Other

Cathflo® Activase®: Intracatheter: Instill dose into occluded catheter. Do not force solution into catheter. After a 30-minute dwell time, assess catheter function by attempting to aspirate blood. If catheter is functional, aspirate 4-5 mL of blood in patients ≥10 kg or 3 mL in patients <10 kg to remove Cathflo® Activase® and residual clots. Gently irrigate the catheter with NS. If catheter remains nonfunctional, let Cathflo® Activase® dwell for another 90 minutes (total dwell time: 120 minutes) and reassess function. If catheter function is not restored, a second dose may be instilled.

Pediatric parapneumonic effusion (unlabeled use): Intrapleural: Instill dose into chest tube at time of chest tube placement and clamp drain. After 1 hour dwell time, release clamp and connect chest tube to continuous suction (-20 cm H_2O) (St. Peter, 2009); or instill dose into chest tube after pigtail catheter (chest tube) placement and clamp drain. After 0.75-1 hour dwell time, release clamp and connect chest tube to continuous suction (-20 to -25 cm H_2O) (Hawkins, 2004).

Stability

Reconstitution

Activase®:

50 mg vial: Use accompanying diluent; mix by gentle swirling or slow inversion; do not shake. Vacuum is present in 50 mg vial. Final concentration: 1 mg/mL.

100 mg vial: Use transfer set with accompanying diluent (100 mL vial of sterile water for injection). No vacuum is present in 100 mg vial. Final concentration: 1 mg/mL.

Cathflo® Activase®: Add 2.2 mL SWFI to vial; do not shake. Final concentration: 1 mg/mL.

Storage

Activase®: The lyophilized product may be stored at room temperature (not to exceed 30°C/86°F), or under refrigeration. Once reconstituted, it should be used within 8 hours.

Cathflo® Activase®: Store lyophilized product under refrigeration. The following stability information has also been reported: Intact vials may be stored at room temperature for up to 4 months (Cohen, 2007). Once reconstituted, it should be used within 8 hours.

Nursing Actions

Physical Assessment Monitor vital signs and ECG prior to, during, and after therapy. Report abnormalities to prescriber immediately. Arrhythmias may occur; treatment should be available. Assess infusion site and monitor for hemorrhage during therapy and for 1 hour following therapy. Maintain strict bedrest and monitor regularly for excess bleeding. Use bleeding precautions.

Patient Education This medication can only be administered by infusion; you will be monitored closely during and after treatment. You will have a tendency to bleed easily; use caution to prevent injury. Follow instructions for strict bedrest to reduce the risk of injury. If bleeding occurs, report immediately. Report unusual pain (acute headache, joint pain, chest pain); unusual bruising or bleeding; blood in urine, stool, or vomit; bleeding gums; or change in mentation.

Alvimopan (al VI moe pan)

Brand Names: U.S. Entereg®

Index Terms ADL-2698; LY246736

Pharmacologic Category Gastrointestinal Agent, Miscellaneous; Opioid Antagonist, Peripherally-Acting

Medication Safety Issues

Sound-alike/look-alike issues:

Alvimopan may be confused with almotriptan

Pregnancy Risk Factor B

Lactation Excretion in breast milk unknown/use caution

Use Accelerate the time to upper and lower GI recovery following partial large or small bowel resection surgery with primary anastomosis

Mechanism of Action/Effect An opioid receptor antagonist which blocks opioid binding at the mu receptor; alvimopan has restricted ability to cross the blood-brain barrier at therapeutic doses. It selectively and competitively binds to the GI tract mu opioid receptors and antagonizes the peripheral effects of opioids on gastrointestinal motility and secretion. Does not affect opioid analgesic effects or induce opioid withdrawal symptoms.

Contraindications Patients who have taken therapeutic doses of opioids for more than 7 consecutive days immediately prior to alvimopan

Warnings/Precautions [U.S. Boxed Warning]: For short-term (≤15 doses) hospital use only. Only hospitals that have registered through the ENTEREG Access Support and Education (E.A.S.E.™) Program and met all requirements may use. It will not be dispensed to patients who have been discharged from the hospital. Use not recommended in patients with complete bowel obstruction. Use with caution in patients with hepatic or renal impairment; use not recommended in patients with severe hepatic impairment or ESRD. Use with caution is patients recently exposed to opioids; may be more sensitive to gastrointestinal adverse effects (eg, abdominal pain, diarrhea, nausea and vomiting). Contraindicated in patients who have received therapeutic opioids for >7 consecutive days immediately prior to use. A trend towards an increased incidence of MI was observed in alvimopan (low dose) treated patients compared to placebo in a 12-month study in patients treated with opioids for chronic pain. MI was generally observed more frequently in the initial 1-4 months of treatment. Other studies have not observed this trend and a causal relationship has not been found. Patients of Japanese descent should be monitored closely for gastrointestinal side effects (eg, abdominal pain, cramping, diarrhea) due to possibility of greater drug exposure; discontinue use if side effects occur.

Drug Interactions

Avoid Concomitant Use There are no known interactions where it is recommended to avoid concomitant use.

Decreased Effect There are no known significant interactions involving a decrease in effect.

Increased Effect/Toxicity

The levels/effects of Alvimopan may be increased by: Analgesics (Opioid)

Nutritional/Ethanol Interactions Food: When administered with a high-fat meal, extent and rate of absorption may be reduced (C_{max} and AUC decreased by ~38% and 21%, respectively).

Adverse Reactions 1% to 10%: **Note:** Incidence reported limited to bowel resection patients only.

Endocrine & metabolic: Hypokalemia (10%)

Gastrointestinal: Dyspepsia (7%)

Genitourinary: Urinary retention (3%)
Hematologic: Anemia (5%)
Neuromuscular & skeletal: Back pain (3%)

Available Dosage Forms

Capsule, oral:

Entereg®: 12 mg

General Dosage Range Oral: *Adults:* Initial: 12 mg prior to surgery; Maintenance: 12 mg twice daily (maximum: 15 doses)

Administration

Oral Patient must be hospitalized. Initial dose should be administered 30 minutes to 5 hours prior to surgery. May be administered with or without food.

Stability

Storage Store at 25°C (77°F); excursions permitted to 15°C to 30°C (59°F to 86°F).

Nursing Actions

Physical Assessment For restricted in-hospital use only to improve bowel function.

Patient Education This medication is used to improve bowel function after surgery. Report any gastrointestinal upset, difficulty passing urine, or unusual back pain.

Dietary Considerations Take with or without food; high-fat meals may decrease the rate and extent of absorption

Amantadine (a MAN ta deen)

Index Terms Adamantanamine Hydrochloride; Amantadine Hydrochloride; Symmetrel

Pharmacologic Category Anti-Parkinson's Agent, Dopamine Agonist; Antiviral Agent; Antiviral Agent, Adamantane

Medication Safety Issues

Sound-alike/look-alike issues:

Amantadine may be confused with ranitidine, rimantadine

Symmetrel may be confused with Synthroid®

Pregnancy Risk Factor C

Lactation Enters breast milk/not recommended

Use Prophylaxis and treatment of influenza A viral infection (per manufacturer labeling; also refer to current ACIP guidelines for recommendations during current flu season); treatment of parkinsonism; treatment of drug-induced extrapyramidal symptoms

Available Dosage Forms

Capsule, oral: 100 mg

Capsule, softgel, oral: 100 mg

Solution, oral: 50 mg/5 mL (473 mL)

Syrup, oral: 50 mg/5 mL (10 mL, 473 mL, 480 mL)

Tablet, oral: 100 mg

General Dosage Range Dosage adjustment recommended in patients with renal impairment

Oral:

Children 1-9 years: 4.4-8.8 mg/kg/day in 2 divided doses (maximum: 150 mg/day)

Children ≥10 years and <40 kg: 5 mg/kg/day in 2 divided doses

Children ≥10 years and ≥40 kg: 100 mg twice daily (maximum: 200 mg/day)

Adults: 200-400 mg/day in 2 divided doses (maximum: 400 mg/day)

Elderly: 100-400 mg/day in 2 divided doses (maximum: 400 mg/day)

Nursing Actions

Physical Assessment Recommendations for antiviral susceptibility and effectiveness have changed; amantadine is not recommended for use for the 2011 flu season. Monitor renal function at beginning of therapy and periodically throughout. Assess blood pressure; monitor for signs of fluid retention. When treating Parkinson's disease, taper slowly when discontinuing.

Patient Education Maintain adequate hydration, unless instructed to restrict fluid intake, and void before taking medication. Take last dose of day in the afternoon to reduce incidence of insomnia. May cause dizziness or lightheadedness. Avoid alcohol. You may experience decreased mental alertness or coordination, loss of impulse control (possibly manifested as pathological gambling, libido increases, and/or binge eating), nausea, or dry mouth. Report unusual respiratory difficulty or shortness of breath, change in balance, or changes in mentation (eg, depression, anxiety, irritability, hallucination, slurred speech).

Ambenonium (am be NOE nee um)

Brand Names: U.S. Mytelase®

Index Terms Ambenonium Chloride

Pharmacologic Category Cholinergic Agonist

Lactation Excretion in breast milk unknown/not recommended

Use Treatment of myasthenia gravis

Mechanism of Action/Effect Temporarily improves muscle strength

Contraindications Hypersensitivity to ambenonium or any components of the formulation; concomitant administration with belladonna derivatives, mecamylamine, or other ganglionic-blocking agents

Warnings/Precautions Anticholinergic insensitivity may develop for brief or prolonged periods; reduce or withhold dosages until the patient becomes sensitive again; may require respiratory support. Use with caution in patients with asthma, intestinal obstruction, Parkinson's disease, or urinary tract obstruction. There is a narrow margin between the first appearance of side effects and serious toxic effects; use caution when adjusting dose. Overdose may lead to cholinergic crisis. Temporarily discontinue use if signs of overdose occur (eg, excess gastrointestinal stimulation, excess salivation, miosis, and fasciculations of voluntary muscles). Edrophonium may be used to evaluate the maintenance dose. Avoid use with other cholinergic agents except under strict medical supervision; prior to initiating ambenonium, suspend cholinergic therapy until patient is stabilized. Routine administration of atropine or other belladonna alkaloids with ambenonium is contraindicated.

Drug Interactions

Avoid Concomitant Use There are no known interactions where it is recommended to avoid concomitant use.

Decreased Effect There are no known significant interactions involving a decrease in effect.

Increased Effect/Toxicity

The levels/effects of Ambenonium may be increased by: Acetylcholinesterase Inhibitors; Beta-Blockers

Adverse Reactions Frequency not defined.

Central nervous system: Anxiety, malaise, vertigo

Gastrointestinal: Abdominal cramps, diarrhea, nausea, salivation, vomiting

Genitourinary: Urinary urgency

Neuromuscular & skeletal: Fasciculations, muscle cramps

Ocular: Lacrimation, miosis

Respiratory: Bronchial secretions increased

Miscellaneous: Diaphoresis increased

Available Dosage Forms

Caplet, oral:

Mytelase®: 10 mg

General Dosage Range Oral: *Adults:* Usual dose: 5-25 mg 3-4 times/day; some patients may require as much as 50-75 mg/dose

Administration

Oral Administer 3-4 times/day every 3-4 hours. Medication is usually not required throughout the night.

Stability

Storage Store at controlled room temperature up to 25°C (77°F).

Nursing Actions

Physical Assessment Assess bladder and sphincter adequacy prior to administering medication.

Patient Education This drug will not cure myasthenia gravis, but it may reduce the symptoms. Maintain adequate hydration, unless instructed to restrict fluid intake. May cause dizziness, drowsiness, postural hypotension, vomiting, loss of appetite, or diarrhea. Report persistent abdominal discomfort; significantly increased salivation, sweating, tearing, or urination; flushed skin; chest pain or palpitations; acute headache; unresolved diarrhea; excessive fatigue, insomnia, dizziness, or depression; increased muscle, joint, or body pain; vision changes or blurred vision; or shortness of breath or wheezing.

Ambrisentan (am bri SEN tan)

Brand Names: U.S. Letairis®

Index Terms BSF208075

Pharmacologic Category Endothelin Antagonist; Vasodilator

Medication Guide Available Yes

Pregnancy Risk Factor X

Lactation Excretion in breast milk unknown/not recommended

Use Treatment of pulmonary artery hypertension (PAH) World Health Organization (WHO) Group I to improve exercise ability and decrease the rate of clinical deterioration

Mechanism of Action/Effect Decreases symptoms of pulmonary artery hypertension and slows progression of the disease by causing vasodilation of the pulmonary arteries.

Contraindications Pregnancy

Canadian labeling: Additional contraindications (not in U.S. labeling): Hypersensitivity to ambrisentan or any component of the formulation

Warnings/Precautions [U.S. Boxed Warning]: Use in pregnancy is contraindicated; may cause birth defects. Exclude pregnancy prior to initiation of therapy and monthly thereafter. Two reliable methods of contraception must be used in women of childbearing potential during therapy and for one month after stopping treatment except in patients with tubal ligation or an implanted IUD (Copper T 380A or LNg 20). No other contraceptive measures are required for these patients. A missed menses should be reported to healthcare provider and prompt immediate pregnancy testing. Women should also be educated on the appropriate use of emergency contraception if failure of contraceptive is known or suspected or in the event of unprotected sex.

[U.S. Boxed Warning]: Because of the high likelihood of teratogenic effects, ambrisentan is only available through the LEAP restricted distribution program. Patients, prescribers, and pharmacies must be registered with and meet conditions of LEAP. Call 1-866-664-5327 for more information.

Use caution in patients with low hemoglobin levels. May cause decreases in hemoglobin and hematocrit (monitoring of hemoglobin is recommended. Use not recommended in patients with clinically significant anemia. Development of peripheral edema due to treatment and/or disease state (pulmonary arterial hypertension) may occur; a higher incidence is seen in elderly patients. Sperm count may be reduced in men during treatment (as observed with bosentan). No changes in sperm function or hormone levels have been noted. Fertility issues may require discussion with patient. Increases in serum liver aminotransferases have been reported during postmarketing use; however, in the majority of the cases, alternative causes of hepatotoxicity could be identified. Perform liver enzyme testing only when clinically indicated. Discontinue therapy if signs/symptoms of hepatic injury appear, if serum liver aminotransferases >5 times ULN are observed, or if aminotransferases are increased in the presence of bilirubin >2 times ULN. Hepatotoxicity has been reported with other endothelin receptor antagonists (eg, bosentan); however, ambrisentan may be tried in patients that have experienced asymptomatic increases in liver enzymes caused by another endothelin receptor antagonist after the liver enzymes have returned to normal. Use caution in patients with mild hepatic impairment; use not recommended in patients with moderate-to-severe impairment. There have also been postmarketing reports of fluid retention requiring treatment (eg, diuretics, fluid management, hospitalization). Further evaluation may be necessary to determine cause and appropriate treatment or discontinuation of therapy. Discontinue in any patient with pulmonary edema suggestive of pulmonary veno-occlusive disease (PVOD).

Drug Interactions

Avoid Concomitant Use There are no known interactions where it is recommended to avoid concomitant use.

Decreased Effect

The levels/effects of Ambrisentan may be decreased by: Tocilizumab

Increased Effect/Toxicity

The levels/effects of Ambrisentan may be increased by: Conivaptan; CycloSPORINE; CycloSPORINE (Systemic)

Nutritional/Ethanol Interactions

Food: Grapefruit/grapefruit juice may increase levels/effects of ambrisentan.

Herb/Nutraceutical: Avoid St John's wort (concurrent use may decrease levels/effects of ambrisentan).

Adverse Reactions

>10%:

Cardiovascular: Peripheral edema (17%)

Central nervous system: Headache (15%)

1% to 10%:

Cardiovascular: Palpitation (5%), flushing (4%)

Gastrointestinal: Constipation (4%), abdominal pain (3%)

Hematologic: Hemoglobin decreased (7% to 10%)

Respiratory: Nasal congestion (6%), dyspnea (4%), nasopharyngitis (3%), sinusitis (3%)

Available Dosage Forms

Tablet, oral:

Letairis®: 5 mg, 10 mg

General Dosage Range Dosage adjustment recommended in patients on concomitant therapy.

Oral: *Adults:* Initial: 5 mg once daily (maximum: 10 mg/day)

Administration

Oral Swallow tablet whole. Do not split, crush, or chew tablets. May be administered with or without food.

Stability

Storage Store in original packaging at 25°C (77°F); excursions permitted to 15°C to 30°C (59°F to 86°F).

Nursing Actions

Physical Assessment Assess for symptoms of hepatic problems and fluid retention.

Patient Education Pregnancy must be excluded prior to initiation and monthly thereafter. Two forms of contraception must be used during therapy (except in patients with tubal ligation or an implanted IUD). Avoid grapefruit or grapefruit juice. You may experience headache, nasal congestion, fatigue, or constipation. Report signs of fluid retention (unusual weight gain, swelling of the extremities), shortness of breath, unusual bleeding or bruising, change in color of urine or stool, loss of appetite, abdominal pain, yellowing of skin or eyes, or unusual fatigue.

Dietary Considerations May be taken with or without food. Avoid grapefruit and grapefruit juice.

Amikacin (am i KAY sin)

Index Terms Amikacin Sulfate

Pharmacologic Category Antibiotic, Aminoglycoside

Medication Safety Issues

Sound-alike/look-alike issues:

Amikacin may be confused with Amicar®, anakinra

Amikin® may be confused with Amicar®, Kineret®

Pregnancy Risk Factor D

Lactation Enters breast milk/not recommended

Use Treatment of serious infections (bone infections, respiratory tract infections, endocarditis, and septicemia) due to organisms resistant to gentamicin and tobramycin, including *Pseudomonas*, *Proteus*, *Serratia*, and other gram-negative bacilli; documented infection of mycobacterial organisms susceptible to amikacin

Unlabeled Use Bacterial endophthalmitis

Available Dosage Forms

Injection, solution: 250 mg/mL (2 mL, 4 mL)

General Dosage Range Dosage adjustment recommended in patients with renal impairment

I.M.: *Infants, Children, and Adults:* 5-7.5 mg/kg/dose every 8 hours (maximum: 20 mg/kg/day)

I.V.:

Infants and Children: 5-7.5 mg/kg/dose every 8 hours (maximum: 20 mg/kg/day)

Adults: 5-7.5 mg/kg/dose every 8 hours **or** 15-20 mg/kg as a single daily dose (maximum: 20 mg/kg/day)

Administration

I.M. Administer I.M. injection in large muscle mass. Administer around-the-clock to promote less variation in peak and trough serum levels. Do not mix with other drugs, administer separately.

I.V. Infuse over 30-60 minutes.

Some penicillins (eg, carbenicillin, ticarcillin, and piperacillin) have been shown to inactivate *in vitro*. This has been observed to a greater extent with tobramycin and gentamicin, while amikacin has shown greater stability against inactivation. Concurrent use of these agents may pose a risk of reduced antibacterial efficacy *in vivo*, particularly in the setting of profound renal impairment. However, definitive clinical evidence is lacking. If combination penicillin/aminoglycoside therapy is desired in a patient with renal dysfunction, separation of doses (if feasible), and routine monitoring of aminoglycoside levels, CBC, and clinical response should be considered.

I.V. Detail Administer around-the-clock to promote less variation in peak and trough serum levels. Do not mix with other drugs, administer separately. pH: 3.5-5.5

Other Intrathecal/Intraventricular (unlabeled route): Reserved solely for meningitis due to susceptible gram-negative organisms. Available formulation contains sodium metabisulfite. If possible, consider alternative therapy with gentamicin or tobramycin as both of these agents are available as preservative-free formulations.

Nursing Actions

Physical Assessment Assess allergy history prior to beginning therapy. Monitor for ototoxicity, nephrotoxicity, and neurotoxicity. Hearing and renal status should be assessed before, during, and after therapy.

Patient Education This drug can only be administered by I.V. or I.M. injection. It is important to maintain adequate hydration, unless instructed to restrict fluid intake. Report immediately any change in hearing acuity, ringing or roaring in ears, alteration in balance, vertigo, feeling of fullness in head; pain, tingling, or numbness of any body part; or change in urinary pattern or decrease in urine. Report signs of opportunistic infection (eg, white plaques in mouth, vaginal discharge, unhealed sores, sore throat, unusual fever, chills); persistent diarrhea; or pain, redness, or swelling at injection site.

Related Information

Peak and Trough Guidelines *on page 1276*

AMILoride (a MIL oh ride)

Index Terms Amiloride Hydrochloride

Pharmacologic Category Diuretic, Potassium-Sparing

Medication Safety Issues

Sound-alike/look-alike issues:

AMILoride may be confused with amiodarone, amLODIPine, inamrinone

Pregnancy Risk Factor B

Lactation Excretion in breast milk unknown/not recommended

Use Counteracts potassium loss induced by other diuretics in the treatment of hypertension or edematous conditions including CHF, hepatic cirrhosis, and hypoaldosteronism; usually used in conjunction with more potent diuretics such as thiazides or loop diuretics

Unlabeled Use Cystic fibrosis; reduction of lithium-induced polyuria; pediatric hypertension

Mechanism of Action/Effect Inhibits sodium reabsorption in the distal tubule, cortical collecting tubule, and collecting duct subsequently reducing both potassium and hydrogen excretion resulting in weak natriuretic, diuretic, and antihypertensive activity; increases sodium loss; increases potassium retention; decreases calcium excretion; decreases magnesium loss

Contraindications Hypersensitivity to amiloride or any component of the formulation; presence of elevated serum potassium levels (>5.5 mEq/L); if patient is receiving other potassium-conserving agents (eg, spironolactone, triamterene) or potassium supplementation (medicine, potassium-containing salt substitutes, potassium-rich diet); anuria; acute or chronic renal insufficiency; evidence of diabetic nephropathy. Patients with evidence of renal impairment or diabetes mellitus should not receive this medicine without close, frequent monitoring of serum electrolytes and renal function.

Warnings/Precautions [U.S. Boxed Warning]: Hyperkalemia can occur; patients at risk include those with renal impairment, diabetes, the elderly, and the severely ill. Serum potassium levels must be monitored at frequent intervals especially when dosages are changed or with any illness that may cause renal dysfunction. Excess amounts can lead to profound diuresis with fluid and electrolyte loss; close medical supervision and dose evaluation are required. Watch for and correct electrolyte disturbances; adjust dose to avoid dehydration. In cirrhosis, avoid electrolyte and acid/base imbalances that might lead to hepatic encephalopathy. Use with extreme caution in patients with diabetes mellitus; monitor closely. Discontinue amiloride 3 days prior to glucose tolerance testing. Use with caution in patients who are at risk for metabolic or respiratory acidosis (eg, cardiopulmonary disease, uncontrolled diabetes). Safety and efficacy have not been established in children.

Drug Interactions

Avoid Concomitant Use

Avoid concomitant use of AMILoride with any of the following: CycloSPORINE; CycloSPORINE (Systemic); Tacrolimus; Tacrolimus (Systemic)

Decreased Effect

AMILoride may decrease the levels/effects of: Cardiac Glycosides; QuiNIDine

The levels/effects of AMILoride may be decreased by: Herbs (Hypertensive Properties); Methylphenidate; Nonsteroidal Anti-Inflammatory Agents; Yohimbine

Increased Effect/Toxicity

AMILoride may increase the levels/effects of: ACE Inhibitors; Amifostine; Ammonium Chloride; Antihypertensives; Cardiac Glycosides; CycloSPORINE; CycloSPORINE (Systemic); Dofetilide; Hypotensive Agents; RiTUXimab; Sodium Phosphates; Tacrolimus; Tacrolimus (Systemic)

The levels/effects of AMILoride may be increased by: Alfuzosin; Angiotensin II Receptor Blockers; Diazoxide; Drospirenone; Eplerenone; Herbs (Hypotensive Properties); MAO Inhibitors; Nonsteroidal Anti-Inflammatory Agents; Pentoxifylline; Phosphodiesterase 5 Inhibitors; Potassium Salts; Prostacyclin Analogues; Tolvaptan

Nutritional/Ethanol Interactions Food: Hyperkalemia may result if amiloride is taken with potassium-containing foods.

Adverse Reactions 1% to 10%:

Central nervous system: Headache, fatigue, dizziness

Endocrine & metabolic: Hyperkalemia (up to 10%; risk reduced in patients receiving kaliuretic diuretics), hyperchloremic metabolic acidosis, dehydration, hyponatremia, gynecomastia

Gastrointestinal: Nausea, diarrhea, vomiting, abdominal pain, gas pain, appetite changes, constipation

Genitourinary: Impotence

Neuromuscular & skeletal: Muscle cramps, weakness

Respiratory: Cough, dyspnea

Pharmacodynamics/Kinetics

Onset of Action 2 hours

Duration of Action 24 hours

Available Dosage Forms

Tablet, oral: 5 mg

General Dosage Range Dosage adjustment recommended in patients with renal impairment

Oral:

Adults: 5-10 mg/day in 1-2 divided doses (maximum: 20 mg/day)

Elderly: Initial: 5 mg once daily or every other day

Administration

Oral Administer with food or meals to avoid GI upset.

Nursing Actions

Physical Assessment Monitor electrolytes and fluid status (I & O, weight, blood pressure). Monitor for hyperkalemia.

Patient Education Take early in day with food. Do not increase dietary intake of potassium unless instructed by prescriber. Report muscle cramping or weakness, unresolved nausea or vomiting, palpitations, or respiratory difficulty.

Dietary Considerations Take with food or meals to avoid GI upset. Do not use salt substitutes or low salt milk without checking with healthcare provider.

Amiloride and Hydrochlorothiazide

(a MIL oh ride & hye droe klor oh THYE a zide)

Index Terms Hydrochlorothiazide and Amiloride

Pharmacologic Category Diuretic, Combination

Pregnancy Risk Factor B

Lactation Enters breast milk/contraindicated

Use Potassium-sparing diuretic; antihypertensive

Available Dosage Forms

Tablet: 5/50: Amiloride 5 mg and hydrochlorothiazide 50 mg

General Dosage Range Dosage adjustment recommended in patients with renal impairment

Oral:

Adults: 1-2 tablets (amiloride 5 mg/HCTZ 50 mg per tablet) once daily (maximum: 2 tablets/day)

Elderly: Initial: 1/2 to 1 tablet/day (maximum: 2 tablets/day)

Administration

Oral May administer with food.

Nursing Actions

Physical Assessment See individual agents.

Patient Education See individual agents.

Related Information

AMILoride *on page 59*

Hydrochlorothiazide *on page 570*

Amiodarone

(a MEE oh da rone)

Brand Names: U.S. Cordarone®; Nexterone®; Pacerone®

Index Terms Amiodarone Hydrochloride

Pharmacologic Category Antiarrhythmic Agent, Class III

Medication Safety Issues

Sound-alike/look-alike issues:

Amiodarone may be confused with aMILoride, inamrinone

Cordarone® may be confused with Cardura®, Cordran®

High alert medication:

The Institute for Safe Medication Practices (ISMP) includes this medication among its list of drugs which have a heightened risk of causing significant patient harm when used in error.

BEERS Criteria medication:

This drug may be inappropriate for use in geriatric patients (high severity risk).

Medication Guide Available Yes

Pregnancy Risk Factor D

Lactation Enters breast milk/not recommended (AAP rates "of concern"; AAP 2001 update pending)

Breast-Feeding Considerations Hypothyroidism may occur in nursing infants. Both amiodarone and its active metabolite are excreted in human milk.

Breast-feeding may lead to significant infant exposure and potential toxicity.

Use Management of life-threatening recurrent ventricular fibrillation (VF) or hemodynamically-unstable ventricular tachycardia (VT) refractory to other antiarrhythmic agents or in patients intolerant of other agents used for these conditions

Unlabeled Use

Atrial fibrillation (AF): Pharmacologic conversion of AF to and maintenance of normal sinus rhythm; treatment of AF in patients with heart failure [no accessory pathway] who require heart rate control (ACC/AHA/ESC Practice Guidelines) or in patients with hypertrophic cardiomyopathy (ACCF/AHA Practice Guidelines); prevention of postoperative AF associated with cardiothoracic surgery

Paroxysmal supraventricular tachycardia (SVT) (not initial drug of choice)

Ventricular tachyarrhythmias (ACLS/PALS guidelines): Cardiac arrest with persistent VT or VF if defibrillation, CPR, and vasopressor administration have failed; control of hemodynamically-stable monomorphic VT, polymorphic VT with a normal baseline QT interval, or wide-complex tachycardia of uncertain origin; control of rapid ventricular rate due to accessory pathway conduction in pre-excited atrial arrhythmias (ACLS guidelines) or stable narrow-complex tachycardia (ACLS guidelines)

Adjunct to ICD therapy to suppress symptomatic ventricular tachyarrhythmias in otherwise optimally-treated patients with heart failure (ACC/AHA/ESC Practice Guidelines)

Mechanism of Action/Effect Class III antiarrhythmic agent which inhibits adrenergic stimulation, prolongs the action potential and refractory period in myocardial tissue; decreases AV conduction and sinus node function. Amiodarone shows beta-blocker-like and calcium channel blocker-like effects on SA and AV nodes.

Contraindications Hypersensitivity to amiodarone, iodine, or any component of the formulation; severe sinus-node dysfunction; second- and third-degree heart block (except in patients with a functioning artificial pacemaker); bradycardia causing syncope (except in patients with a functioning artificial pacemaker); cardiogenic shock

Warnings/Precautions [U.S. Boxed Warning]: Only indicated for patients with life-threatening arrhythmias because of risk of toxicity. Alternative therapies should be tried first before using amiodarone. Patients should be hospitalized when amiodarone is initiated. Currently, the 2005 ACLS guidelines recommend I.V. amiodarone as the preferred antiarrhythmic for the treatment of pulseless VT/VF, both life-threatening arrhythmias. In patients with non-life-threatening arrhythmias (eg, atrial fibrillation), amiodarone should be used only if the use of other antiarrhythmics has proven ineffective or are contraindicated.

[U.S. Boxed Warning]: Lung damage (abnormal diffusion capacity) may occur without symptoms. Monitor for pulmonary toxicity. Evaluate new respiratory symptoms; pre-existing pulmonary disease does not increase risk of developing pulmonary toxicity, but if pulmonary toxicity develops then the prognosis is worse. The lowest effective dose should be used as appropriate for the acuity/severity of the arrhythmia being treated. **[U.S. Boxed Warning]: Liver toxicity is common, but usually mild with evidence of increased liver enzymes. Severe liver toxicity can occur and has been fatal in a few cases.**

[U.S. Boxed Warning]: Amiodarone can exacerbate arrhythmias, by making them more difficult to tolerate or reverse; other types of arrhythmias have occurred, including significant heart block, sinus bradycardia new ventricular fibrillation, incessant ventricular tachycardia, increased resistance to cardioversion, and polymorphic ventricular tachycardia associated with QT_c prolongation (torsade de pointes [TdP]). Risk may be increased with concomitant use of other antiarrhythmic agents or drugs that prolong the QT_c interval. Proarrhythmic effects may be prolonged.

Monitor pacing or defibrillation thresholds in patients with implantable cardiac devices (eg, pacemakers, defibrillators). Use very cautiously and with close monitoring in patients with thyroid or liver disease. May cause hyper- or hypothyroidism. Hyperthyroidism may result in thyrotoxicosis and may aggravate or cause breakthrough arrhythmias. If any new signs of arrhythmia appear, hyperthyroidism should be considered. Thyroid function should be monitored prior to treatment and periodically thereafter.

May cause optic neuropathy and/or optic neuritis, usually resulting in visual impairment. Corneal microdeposits occur in a majority of patients, and may cause visual disturbances in some patients (blurred vision, halos); these are not generally considered a reason to discontinue treatment. Corneal refractive laser surgery is generally contraindicated in amiodarone users. Avoid excessive exposure to sunlight; may cause photosensitivity.

Amiodarone is a potent inhibitor of CYP enzymes and transport proteins (including p-glycoprotein), which may lead to increased serum concentrations/toxicity of a number of medications. Particular caution must be used when a drug with QT_c-prolonging potential relies on metabolism via these enzymes, since the effect of elevated concentrations may be additive with the effect of amiodarone. Carefully assess risk:benefit of coadministration of other drugs which may prolong QT_c interval. Patients may still be at risk for amiodarone–related drug interactions after the drug has been discontinued. The pharmacokinetics are complex (due to prolonged duration of action and half-life) and difficult to predict. Correct electrolyte disturbances, especially hypokalemia or hypomagnesemia, prior to use and throughout therapy. Use caution when initiating amiodarone in patients on warfarin. Cases of increased INR with or without bleeding have occurred in patients treated with warfarin; monitor INR closely after initiating amiodarone in these patients.

May cause hypotension and bradycardia (infusion-rate related). Hypotension with rapid administration has been attributed to the emulsifier polysorbate 80. Commercially-prepared premixed solutions do not contain polysorbate 80 and may have a lower incidence of hypotension. Caution in surgical patients; may enhance hemodynamic effect of anesthetics; associated with increased risk of adult respiratory distress syndrome (ARDS) postoperatively. May be inappropriate in the elderly due to a risk of QT_c-interval prolongation, torsade de pointes, and lack of efficacy in the elderly (Beers Criteria). Vials for injection contain benzyl alcohol, which has been associated with "gasping syndrome" in neonates. Commercially-prepared premixed solutions do not contain benzyl alcohol. Commercially-prepared premixed infusion contains the excipient cyclodextrin (sulfobutyl ether beta-cyclodextrin), which may accumulate in patients with renal insufficiency.

Drug Interactions

Avoid Concomitant Use

Avoid concomitant use of Amiodarone with any of the following: Agalsidase Alfa; Agalsidase Beta; Artemether; Conivaptan; Dronedarone; Grapefruit Juice; Lumefantrine; Nilotinib; Pimozide; Propafenone; Protease Inhibitors; QUEtiapine; QuiNINE; Silodosin; Tetrabenazine; Thioridazine; Topotecan; Toremifene; Vandetanib; Vemurafenib; Ziprasidone

Decreased Effect

Amiodarone may decrease the levels/effects of: Agalsidase Alfa; Agalsidase Beta; Clopidogrel; Codeine; Sodium Iodide I131; TraMADol

The levels/effects of Amiodarone may be decreased by: Bile Acid Sequestrants; CYP2C8 Inducers (Strong); CYP3A4 Inducers (Strong); Cyproterone; Deferasirox; Etravirine; Fosphenytoin; Grapefruit Juice; Orlistat; Peginterferon Alfa-2b; P-glycoprotein/ABCB1 Inducers; Phenytoin; Rifamycin Derivatives; Tocilizumab

Increased Effect/Toxicity

Amiodarone may increase the levels/effects of: Antiarrhythmic Agents (Class Ia); ARIPiprazole; Beta-Blockers; Budesonide (Systemic, Oral Inhalation); Cardiac Glycosides; Colchicine; CycloSPORINE; CycloSPORINE (Systemic); CYP2A6 Substrates; CYP2C9 Substrates; CYP2D6 Substrates; CYP3A4 Substrates; Dabigatran Etexilate; Dronedarone; Eplerenone; Everolimus; FentaNYL; Fesoterodine; Flecainide; Fosphenytoin; HMG-CoA Reductase Inhibitors; Lidocaine; Lidocaine (Systemic); Lidocaine (Topical); Loratadine; Lurasidone; P-glycoprotein/ABCB1 Substrates; Phenytoin; Pimecrolimus; Pimozide; Porfimer; Propafenone; Prucalopride; QTc-Prolonging Agents; QuiNINE; Rivaroxaban; Salmeterol; Silodosin; Tetrabenazine; Thioridazine; Topotecan; Toremifene; Vandetanib; Vemurafenib; Vilazodone; Vitamin K Antagonists; Ziprasidone

The levels/effects of Amiodarone may be increased by: Alfuzosin; Artemether; Azithromycin; Azithromycin (Systemic); Boceprevir; Calcium Channel Blockers (Nondihydropyridine); Chloroquine; Cimetidine; Ciprofloxacin; Ciprofloxacin (Systemic); Conivaptan; CYP2C8 Inhibitors (Moderate); CYP2C8 Inhibitors (Strong); CYP3A4 Inhibitors (Moderate); CYP3A4 Inhibitors (Strong); Deferasirox; Eribulin; Fingolimod; Gadobutrol; Grapefruit Juice; Indacaterol; Lidocaine (Topical); Lumefantrine; Nilotinib; P-glycoprotein/ABCB1 Inhibitors; Protease Inhibitors; QUEtiapine; QuiNINE; Telaprevir

Nutritional/Ethanol Interactions

Food: Increases the rate and extent of absorption of amiodarone. Grapefruit juice increases bioavailability of oral amiodarone by 50% and decreases the conversion of amiodarone to N-DEA (active metabolite); altered effects are possible. Management: Take consistently with regard to meals; grapefruit juice should be avoided during therapy.

Herb/Nutraceutical: St John's wort may decrease amiodarone levels or enhance photosensitization. Ephedra may worsen arrythmia. Management: Avoid St John's wort, ephedra and dong quai.

Adverse Reactions In a recent meta-analysis, adult patients taking lower doses of amiodarone (152-330 mg daily for at least 12 months) were more likely to develop thyroid, neurologic, skin, ocular, and bradycardic abnormalities than those taking placebo (Vorperian, 1997). Pulmonary toxicity was similar in both the low-dose amiodarone group and in the placebo group, but there was a trend towards increased toxicity in the amiodarone group. Gastrointestinal and hepatic events were seen to a similar extent in both the low-dose amiodarone group and placebo group. As the frequency of adverse events varies considerably across studies as a function of route and dose, a consolidation of adverse event rates is provided by Goldschlager, 2000.

>10%:

Cardiovascular: Hypotension (I.V. 16%, refractory in rare cases)

Central nervous system (3% to 40%): Abnormal gait/ataxia, dizziness, fatigue, headache, malaise, impaired memory, involuntary movement, insomnia, poor coordination, peripheral neuropathy, sleep disturbances, tremor

Dermatologic: Photosensitivity (10% to 75%)

Endocrine & Metabolic: Hypothyroidism (1% to 22%)

Gastrointestinal: Nausea, vomiting, anorexia, and constipation (10% to 33%)

Hepatic: AST or ALT level >2x normal (15% to 50%)

Ocular: Corneal microdeposits (>90%; causes visual disturbance in <10%)

1% to 10%:

Cardiovascular: CHF (3%), bradycardia (3% to 5%), AV block (5%), conduction abnormalities, SA node dysfunction (1% to 3%), cardiac arrhythmia, flushing, edema. Additional effects associated with I.V. administration include asystole, atrial fibrillation, cardiac arrest, electromechanical dissociation, pulseless electrical activity (PEA), ventricular tachycardia, and cardiogenic shock.

Dermatologic: Slate blue skin discoloration (<10%)

Endocrine & metabolic: Hyperthyroidism (3% to 10%; more common in iodine-deficient regions of the world), libido decreased

Gastrointestinal: Abdominal pain, abnormal salivation, abnormal taste (oral), diarrhea, nausea (I.V.)

Hematologic: Coagulation abnormalities

Hepatic: Hepatitis and cirrhosis (<3%)

Local: Phlebitis (I.V., with concentrations >3 mg/mL)

Ocular: Visual disturbances (2% to 9%), halo vision (<5% occurring especially at night), optic neuritis (1%)

Respiratory: Pulmonary toxicity has been estimated to occur at a frequency between 2% and 7% of patients (some reports indicate a frequency as high as 17%). Toxicity may present as hypersensitivity pneumonitis; pulmonary fibrosis (cough, fever, malaise); pulmonary inflammation; interstitial pneumonitis; or alveolar pneumonitis. ARDS has been reported in up to 2% of patients receiving amiodarone, and postoperatively in patients receiving oral amiodarone.

Miscellaneous: Abnormal smell (oral)

Pharmacodynamics/Kinetics

Onset of Action Oral: 2 days to 3 weeks; I.V.: May be more rapid; Peak effect: 1 week to 5 months

Duration of Action After discontinuing therapy: 7-50 days

Note: Mean onset of effect and duration after discontinuation may be shorter in children than adults

Available Dosage Forms

Infusion, premixed iso-osmotic dextrose solution:

Nexterone®: 150 mg (100 mL); 360 mg (200 mL)

Injection, solution: 50 mg/mL (3 mL, 9 mL, 18 mL)

Tablet, oral: 200 mg, 400 mg

Cordarone®: 200 mg

Pacerone®: 100 mg, 200 mg, 400 mg

General Dosage Range

I.O.: *Children (PALS dosing):* 5 mg/kg (maximum: 300 mg/day); may repeat up to maximum dose of 15 mg/kg/day

I.V.:

Children (PALS dosing): 5 mg/kg (maximum: 300 mg/day); may repeat up to maximum dose of 15 mg/kg/day

Adults: Initial: 150-300 mg bolus **or** 5-7 mg/kg; Maintenance: 1200-1800 mg/day continuous infusion until 10 g total **or** 1 mg/minute infusion for 6 hours, then 0.5 mg/minute infusion for 18 hours (maximum: 2.1 g/day)

Oral: *Adults:* Initial: 600-1600 mg/day until 10 g total; Maintenance: 100-400 mg/day

Administration

Oral Administer consistently with regard to meals. Take in divided doses with meals if GI upset occurs or if taking large daily dose. If GI intolerance occurs with single-dose therapy, use twice daily dosing.

I.V. For infusions >1 hour, use concentrations ≤2 mg/mL unless a central venous catheter is used; commercially-prepared premixed solutions in concentrations of 1.5 mg/mL and 1.8 mg/mL are available. Use only volumetric infusion pump; use of drop counting may lead to underdosage. Administer through an I.V. line located as centrally as possible. For continuous infusions, an in-line filter has been recommended during administration to reduce the incidence of phlebitis. During pulseless VT/VF, administering **undiluted** is preferred (Dager, 2006; Skrifvars, 2004). *The Handbook of Emergency Cardiovascular Care* (Hazinski, 2010) and the 2010 ACLS guidelines do not make any specific recommendations regarding dilution of amiodarone in this setting.

Adjust administration rate to urgency (give more slowly when perfusing arrhythmia present). Slow the infusion rate if hypotension or bradycardia develops. Infusions >2 hours must be administered in a non-PVC container (eg, glass or polyolefin). PVC tubing is recommended for administration regardless of infusion duration. **Note:** I.V. administration at lower flow rates (potentially associated with use in pediatrics) and higher concentrations than recommended may result in leaching of plasticizers (DEHP) from intravenous tubing. DEHP may adversely affect male reproductive tract development. Alternative means of dosing and administration (1 mg/kg aliquots) may need to be considered.

I.V. Detail Incompatible with heparin. Flush with saline prior to and following infusion.

pH: 4.08

Stability

Storage Store undiluted vials and premixed solutions at 20°C to 25°C (68°F to 77°F). Protect from light.

Vials for injection: When admixed in D_5W to a final concentration of 1-6 mg/mL, the solution is stable at room temperature for 24 hours in polyolefin or glass, or for 2 hours in PVC. Infusions >2 hours must be administered in a non-PVC container (eg, glass or polyolefin). Do not use evacuated glass containers; buffer may cause precipitation.

Nursing Actions

Physical Assessment Eye examinations should be performed periodically. Monitor cardiac status closely and assess for CNS changes (ie, abnormal gait/ataxia, dizziness, impaired memory, involuntary movement, poor coordination, peripheral neuropathy, tremor). Monitor for signs of pulmonary toxicity (eg, nonproductive cough, dyspnea, pleuritic pain, weight loss, fever, malaise). **I.V.:** Requires continuous cardiac/hemodynamic monitoring during infusion. Be alert for adverse reactions. **Oral:** Monitor cardiac status prior to treatment and throughout.

Patient Education

I.V.: Emergency use: Patient condition will determine amount of patient education required.

Oral: May be taken with food to reduce GI disturbance, but be consistent. Always take with food or always take without food. Avoid grapefruit juice. Regular blood work, ophthalmic exams, and cardiac assessment will be necessary while taking this medication on a long-term basis. You may experience dizziness, weakness, insomnia, hypotension, nausea, vomiting, loss of appetite, stomach discomfort, abnormal taste, photosensitivity, or decreased libido (reversible). Report persistent dry cough or shortness of breath; chest pain, palpitations, irregular or slow heartbeat; unusual bruising or bleeding; blood in urine or feces (black stool); warmth, swelling, pain in calves; heat or cold intolerance; weight loss or gain; restlessness; hair thinning; changes in menses; sweating; swelling in neck; muscle tremor, weakness, numbness, or changes in gait; fever; malaise; skin rash (bluish-gray color) or irritation; visual disturbances; or changes in urinary patterns.

Dietary Considerations Take consistently with regard to meals. Amiodarone is a potential source of large amounts of inorganic iodine; ~3 mg of inorganic iodine per 100 mg of amiodarone is released into the systemic circulation. Recommended daily allowance for iodine in adults is 150 mcg.

Grapefruit juice is not recommended.

Amitriptyline (a mee TRIP ti leen)

Index Terms Amitriptyline Hydrochloride; Elavil

Pharmacologic Category Antidepressant, Tricyclic (Tertiary Amine)

Medication Safety Issues

Sound-alike/look-alike issues:

Amitriptyline may be confused with aminophylline, imipramine, nortriptyline

Elavil® may be confused with Aldoril®, Eldepryl®, enalapril, Equanil®, Plavix®

BEERS Criteria medication:

This drug may be inappropriate for use in geriatric patients (high severity risk).

Medication Guide Available Yes

Pregnancy Risk Factor C

Lactation Enters breast milk/not recommended (AAP rates "of concern"; AAP 2001 update pending)

Use Relief of symptoms of depression

Unlabeled Use Analgesic for certain chronic and neuropathic pain (including diabetic neuropathy); prophylaxis against migraine headaches; treatment of depressive disorders in children; post-traumatic stress disorder (PTSD)

Available Dosage Forms

Tablet, oral: 10 mg, 25 mg, 50 mg, 75 mg, 100 mg, 150 mg

General Dosage Range Oral:

Adolescents: Initial: 25-50 mg/day; Maintenance: 25-100 mg/day (maximum: 100 mg/day)

Adults: 50-300 mg/day as a single dose at bedtime or in divided doses (maximum: 300 mg/day)

Elderly: Initial: 10-25 mg at bedtime; Maintenance: 25-150 mg/day (maximum: 150 mg/day)

Nursing Actions

Physical Assessment Assess for suicidal tendencies or unusual changes in behavior before beginning therapy and periodically thereafter. Caution patients with diabetes; may increase or decrease serum glucose levels. Taper dosage slowly when discontinuing.

Patient Education It may take several weeks to achieve desired results. Restrict use of alcohol. Maintain adequate hydration, unless instructed to restrict fluid intake. If you have diabetes, monitor glucose levels closely; this medication may alter glucose levels. May cause drowsiness, lightheadedness, impaired coordination, dizziness, blurred vision, constipation, urinary retention, postural hypotension, altered sexual drive or ability (reversible), or photosensitivity. Report persistent CNS effects (eg, nervousness, restlessness, insomnia, headache, agitation, impaired coordination, changes in cognition); suicide ideation; muscle cramping, weakness, tremors, or rigidity; ringing in ears or visual disturbances; chest pain, palpitations, or irregular heartbeat; blurred vision; or worsening of condition.

Related Information

Peak and Trough Guidelines *on page 1276*

AmLODIPine (am LOE di peen)

Brand Names: U.S. Norvasc®

Index Terms Amlodipine Besylate

Pharmacologic Category Antianginal Agent; Calcium Channel Blocker; Calcium Channel Blocker, Dihydropyridine

Medication Safety Issues

Sound-alike/look-alike issues:

AmLODIPine may be confused with aMILoride

Norvasc® may be confused with Navane®, Norvir®, Vascor®

International issues:

Norvasc [U.S., Canada, and multiple international markets] may be confused with Vascor brand name for imidapril [Philippines] and simvastatin [Malaysia, Singapore, and Thailand]

Pregnancy Risk Factor C

Lactation Excretion in breast milk unknown/not recommended

Use Treatment of hypertension; treatment of symptomatic chronic stable angina, vasospastic (Prinzmetal's) angina (confirmed or suspected); prevention of hospitalization due to angina with documented CAD (limited to patients without heart failure or ejection fraction <40%)

Mechanism of Action/Effect Inhibits calcium ion from entering the "slow channels" or select voltage-sensitive areas of vascular smooth muscle and myocardium during depolarization; a peripheral arterial vasodilator that causes a reduction in blood pressure

Contraindications Hypersensitivity to amlodipine or any component of the formulation

Warnings/Precautions Increased angina and/or MI has occurred with initiation or dosage titration of calcium channel blockers. Symptomatic hypotension with or without syncope can rarely occur; blood pressure must be lowered at a rate appropriate for the patient's clinical condition. Use caution in severe aortic stenosis and/or hypertrophic cardiomyopathy with outflow tract obstruction. Use caution in patients with hepatic impairment; may require lower starting dose; titrate slowly with severe hepatic impairment. The most common side effect is peripheral edema; occurs within 2-3 weeks of starting therapy. Reflex tachycardia may occur with use. Peak antihypertensive effect is delayed; dosage titration should occur after 7-14 days on a given dose. Initiate at a lower dose in the elderly.

Drug Interactions

Avoid Concomitant Use

Avoid concomitant use of AmLODIPine with any of the following: Conivaptan; Pimozide

Decreased Effect

AmLODIPine may decrease the levels/effects of: Clopidogrel; QuiNIDine

The levels/effects of AmLODIPine may be decreased by: Barbiturates; Calcium Salts; CarBAMazepine; CYP3A4 Inducers (Strong); Deferasirox; Herbs (CYP3A4 Inducers); Herbs (Hypertensive Properties); Methylphenidate; Nafcillin; Rifamycin Derivatives; Tocilizumab; Yohimbine

Increased Effect/Toxicity

AmLODIPine may increase the levels/effects of: Amifostine; Antihypertensives; ARIPiprazole; Beta-Blockers; Calcium Channel Blockers (Nondihydropyridine); CYP1A2 Substrates; Fosphenytoin; Hypotensive Agents; Magnesium Salts; Neuromuscular-Blocking Agents (Nondepolarizing); Nitroprusside; Phenytoin; Pimozide; QuiNIDine; RiTUXimab; Simvastatin; Tacrolimus; Tacrolimus (Systemic)

The levels/effects of AmLODIPine may be increased by: Alpha1-Blockers; Antifungal Agents (Azole Derivatives, Systemic); Calcium Channel Blockers (Nondihydropyridine); Conivaptan; CycloSPORINE; CycloSPORINE (Systemic); CYP3A4 Inhibitors (Moderate); CYP3A4 Inhibitors (Strong); Dasatinib; Diazoxide; Fluconazole; Grapefruit Juice; Herbs (Hypotensive Properties); Ivacaftor; Macrolide Antibiotics; Magnesium Salts; MAO Inhibitors; Pentoxifylline; Phosphodiesterase 5 Inhibitors; Prostacyclin Analogues; Protease Inhibitors; QuiNIDine

Nutritional/Ethanol Interactions

Food: Grapefruit juice may modestly increase amlodipine levels.

Herb/Nutraceutical: St John's wort may decrease amlodipine levels. Avoid herbs with *hypertensive* properties (bayberry, blue cohosh, cayenne, ephedra, ginger, ginseng [American], kola, licorice). Avoid herbs with *hypotensive* properties (black cohosh, California poppy, coleus, garlic, goldenseal, hawthorn, mistletoe, periwinkle, quinine, shepherd's purse).

Adverse Reactions

>10%: Cardiovascular: Peripheral edema (2% to 15% dose related; HF patients: 27% [Packer, 1996])

1% to 10%:

Cardiovascular: Flushing (1% to 5% dose related), palpitation (1% to 5% dose related)

Central nervous system: Dizziness (1% to 3% dose related), fatigue (5%), somnolence (1% to 2%)

Dermatologic: Rash (1% to 2%), pruritus (1% to 2%)

Endocrine & metabolic: Male sexual dysfunction (1% to 2%)

Gastrointestinal: Nausea (3%), abdominal pain (1% to 2%), dyspepsia (1% to 2%)

Neuromuscular & skeletal: Muscle cramps (1% to 2%), weakness (1% to 2%)

Respiratory: Dyspnea (1% to 2%), pulmonary edema (HF patients: 27% [Packer, 1996])

Pharmacodynamics/Kinetics

Duration of Action Antihypertensive effect: 24 hours

Available Dosage Forms

Tablet, oral: 2.5 mg, 5 mg, 10 mg

Norvasc®: 2.5 mg, 5 mg, 10 mg

General Dosage Range Dosage adjustment recommended in patients with hepatic impairment

Oral:

Children 6-17 years: 2.5-5 mg once daily

Adults: Initial: 5 mg once daily; Maintenance: 2.5-10 mg once daily (maximum: 10 mg/day)

Elderly: 2.5-5 mg once daily

Administration

Oral May be administered without regard to meals.

Stability

Storage Store at room temperature of 15°C to 30°C (59°F to 86°F).

Nursing Actions

Physical Assessment Monitor blood pressure, pulse, frequency and intensity of angina, weight, and peripheral edema.

Patient Education May cause headache or constipation. Report unrelieved headache, severe constipation, peripheral or facial swelling, weight gain, respiratory changes, or worsening of chest pain or pressure.

Dietary Considerations May be taken without regard to meals.

Amlodipine and Atorvastatin

(am LOW di peen & a TORE va sta tin)

Brand Names: U.S. Caduet®

Index Terms Atorvastatin and Amlodipine; Atorvastatin Calcium and Amlodipine Besylate

Pharmacologic Category Antianginal Agent; Antilipemic Agent, HMG-CoA Reductase Inhibitor; Calcium Channel Blocker; Calcium Channel Blocker, Dihydropyridine

Pregnancy Risk Factor X

Lactation Excretion in breast milk unknown/contraindicated

Use For use when treatment with both amlodipine and atorvastatin is appropriate:

Amlodipine: Treatment of hypertension; treatment of chronic stable angina, vasospastic (Prinzmetal's) angina (confirmed or suspected); prevention of hospitalization or to decrease coronary revascularization procedure due to angina with documented CAD (limited to patients without heart failure or ejection fraction <40%)

Atorvastatin: Treatment of dyslipidemias or primary prevention of cardiovascular disease (atherosclerotic) as detailed here:

Primary prevention of cardiovascular disease (high-risk for CVD): To reduce the risk of MI or stroke in patients without evidence of coronary heart disease who have multiple CVD risk factors or type 2 diabetes; also reduces the risk for angina or revascularization procedures in patients with multiple CVD risk factors without evidence of coronary heart disease

Secondary prevention of cardiovascular disease: To reduce the risk of MI, stroke, revascularization procedures, angina, and hospitalization for heart failure

Treatment of dyslipidemias: To reduce elevations in total cholesterol, LDL-C, apolipoprotein B, and triglycerides in patients with elevations of one or more components, and/or to increase low HDL-C as present in heterozygous familial/nonfamilial hypercholesterolemia and mixed dyslipidemia (Fredrickson type IIa and IIb hyperlipidemias); treatment of primary dysbetalipoproteinemia (Fredrickson type III), elevated serum TG levels (Fredrickson type IV), and homozygous familial hypercholesterolemia

Treatment of heterozygous familial hypercholesterolemia (HeFH) in adolescent patients (10-17 years of age, females >1 year postmenarche) having LDL-C ≥190 mg/dL or LDL-C ≥160 mg/dL with positive family history of premature cardiovascular disease (CVD) or with two or more CVD risk factors.

Available Dosage Forms

Tablet, oral: Amlodipine 2.5 mg and atorvastatin 10 mg; Amlodipine 2.5 mg and atorvastatin 20 mg; Amlodipine 2.5 mg and atorvastatin 40 mg; Amlodipine 5 mg and atorvastatin 10 mg; Amlodipine 5 mg and atorvastatin 20 mg; Amlodipine 5 mg and atorvastatin 40 mg; Amlodipine 5 mg and atorvastatin 80 mg; Amlodipine 10 mg and atorvastatin 10 mg; Amlodipine 10 mg and atorvastatin 20 mg; Amlodipine 10 mg and atorvastatin 40 mg; Amlodipine 10 mg and atorvastatin 80 mg

Caduet®:

2.5/10: Amlodipine 2.5 mg and atorvastatin 10 mg; 2.5/20: Amlodipine 2.5 mg and atorvastatin 20 mg; 2.5/40: Amlodipine 2.5 mg and atorvastatin 40 mg

5/10: Amlodipine 5 mg and atorvastatin 10 mg; 5/20: Amlodipine 5 mg and atorvastatin 20 mg; 5/40: Amlodipine 5 mg and atorvastatin 40 mg; 5/80: Amlodipine 5 mg and atorvastatin 80 mg

10/10: Amlodipine 10 mg and atorvastatin 10 mg; 10/20: Amlodipine 10 mg and atorvastatin 20 mg; 10/40: Amlodipine 10 mg and atorvastatin 40 mg; 10/80: Amlodipine 10 mg and atorvastatin 80 mg

General Dosage Range Dosage adjustment recommended in patients on concomitant therapy

Oral:

Children 10-17 years (females >1 year postmenarche): 2.5-5 mg (amlodipine) and 10-20 mg (atorvastatin) once daily (maximum: amlodipine 5 mg/day; atorvastatin 20 mg/day)

Adults: 2.5-10 mg (amlodipine) and 10-80 mg (atorvastatin) once daily (maximum: amlodipine 10 mg/day; atorvastatin 80 mg/day)

Administration

Oral May be administered without regard to meals.

Nursing Actions

Physical Assessment See individual agents.

Patient Education See individual agents.

Amlodipine and Benazepril

(am LOE di peen & ben AY ze pril)

Brand Names: U.S. Lotrel®

Index Terms Benazepril Hydrochloride and Amlodipine Besylate

Pharmacologic Category Angiotensin-Converting Enzyme (ACE) Inhibitor; Antianginal Agent; Calcium Channel Blocker; Calcium Channel Blocker, Dihydropyridine

Pregnancy Risk Factor D

Lactation

Amlodipine: Excretion in breast milk unknown/not recommended

Benazepril: Enters breast milk

Use Treatment of hypertension

Available Dosage Forms

Capsule: 2.5/10: Amlodipine 2.5 mg and benazepril 10 mg; 5/10: Amlodipine 5 mg and benazepril 10 mg; 5/20: Amlodipine 5 mg and benazepril 20 mg; 5/40: Amlodipine 5 mg and benazepril hydrochloride 40 mg; 10/20: Amlodipine 10 mg and benazepril 20 mg; 10/40: Amlodipine 10 mg and benazepril hydrochloride 40 mg

Lotrel®: 2.5/10: Amlodipine 2.5 and benazepril 10 mg; 5/10: Amlodipine 5 mg and benazepril 10 mg; 5/20: Amlodipine 5 mg and benazepril 20 mg; 5/40: Amlodipine 5 mg and benazepril 40 mg; 10/20: Amlodipine 10 mg and benazepril 20 mg; 10/40: Amlodipine 10 mg and benazepril 40 mg

General Dosage Range Dosage adjustment recommended in patients with hepatic impairment

Oral:

Adults: 2.5-10 mg (amlodipine) and 10-40 mg (benazepril) once daily (maximum: amlodipine 10 mg/day; benazepril 80 mg/day)

Elderly: Initial: 2.5 mg/day (based on amlodipine component)

Nursing Actions

Physical Assessment See individual agents.

Patient Education See individual agents.

Related Information

AmLODIPine *on page 65*

Benazepril *on page 122*

Amlodipine and Olmesartan

(am LOE di peen & olme SAR tan)

Brand Names: U.S. Azor™

Index Terms Amlodipine Besylate and Olmesartan Medoxomil; Olmesartan and Amlodipine

Pharmacologic Category Angiotensin II Receptor Blocker; Antianginal Agent; Calcium Channel Blocker; Calcium Channel Blocker, Dihydropyridine

Pregnancy Risk Factor D

Lactation Excretion in breast milk unknown/not recommended

Use Treatment of hypertension, including initial treatment in patients who will require multiple antihypertensives for adequate control

Available Dosage Forms

Tablet:

Azor™: 5/20: Amlodipine 5 mg and olmesartan medoxomil 20 mg; 5/40: Amlodipine 5 mg and olmesartan medoxomil 40 mg; 10/20: Amlodipine 10 mg and olmesartan medoxomil 20 mg; 10/40: Amlodipine 10 mg and olmesartan medoxomil 40 mg

General Dosage Range Oral: *Adults:* Amlodipine 5-10 mg and olmesartan 20-40 mg once daily (maximum: 10 mg/day [amlodipine]; 40 mg/day [olmesartan])

Administration

Oral Administer with or without food.

Nursing Actions

Physical Assessment See individual agents.

Patient Education See individual agents.

Related Information

AmLODIPine *on page 65*

Olmesartan *on page 849*

Amlodipine and Valsartan

(am LOE di peen & val SAR tan)

Brand Names: U.S. Exforge®

Index Terms Amlodipine Besylate and Valsartan; Valsartan and Amlodipine

Pharmacologic Category Angiotensin II Receptor Blocker; Antianginal Agent; Calcium Channel Blocker; Calcium Channel Blocker, Dihydropyridine

Pregnancy Risk Factor D

Lactation Excretion in breast milk unknown/not recommended

Use Treatment of hypertension

Available Dosage Forms

Tablet:

Exforge®: 5/160: Amlodipine 5 mg and valsartan 160 mg; 5/320 mg: Amlodipine 5 mg and valsartan 320 mg; 10/160: Amlodipine 10 mg and valsartan 160 mg; 10/320: Amlodipine 10 mg and valsartan 320 mg

General Dosage Range Oral: *Adults:* Amlodipine 5-10 mg and valsartan 160-320 mg once daily (maximum: 10 mg/day [amlodipine]; 320 mg/day [valsartan])

Administration

Oral Administer with or without food.

Nursing Actions

Physical Assessment See individual agents.

Patient Education See individual agents.

Related Information

AmLODIPine *on page 65*
Valsartan *on page 1161*

Amlodipine, Valsartan, and Hydrochlorothiazide

(am LOE di peen, val SAR tan, & hye droe klor oh THYE a zide)

Brand Names: U.S. Exforge HCT®

Index Terms Amlodipine Besylate, Valsartan, and Hydrochlorothiazide; Amlodipine, Hydrochlorothiazide, and Valsartan; Hydrochlorothiazide, Amlodipine, and Valsartan; Valsartan, Hydrochlorothiazide, and Amlodipine

Pharmacologic Category Angiotensin II Receptor Blocker; Antianginal Agent; Calcium Channel Blocker; Calcium Channel Blocker, Dihydropyridine; Diuretic, Thiazide

Pregnancy Risk Factor D

Lactation Enters breast milk/not recommended

Use Treatment of hypertension (not for initial therapy)

Available Dosage Forms

Tablet, oral:

Exforge HCT®: Amlodipine 5 mg, valsartan 160 mg, and hydrochlorothiazide 12.5 mg; Amlodipine 5 mg, valsartan 160 mg, and hydrochlorothiazide 25 mg; Amlodipine 10 mg, valsartan 160 mg, and hydrochlorothiazide 12.5 mg; Amlodipine 10 mg, valsartan 160 mg, and hydrochlorothiazide 25 mg; Amlodipine 10 mg, valsartan 320 mg, and hydrochlorothiazide 25 mg

General Dosage Range Oral: *Adults:* Amlodipine 5-10 mg and valsartan 160-320 mg and hydrochlorothiazide 12.5-25 mg once daily (maximum: 10 mg/day [amlodipine]; 25 mg/day [hydrochlorothiazide]; 320 mg/day [valsartan])

Administration

Oral Administer with or without food.

Nursing Actions

Physical Assessment See individual agents.

Patient Education See individual agents.

Amoxicillin

(a moks i SIL in)

Brand Names: U.S. Moxatag™

Index Terms *p*-Hydroxyampicillin; Amoxicillin Trihydrate; Amoxil; Amoxycillin

Pharmacologic Category Antibiotic, Penicillin

Medication Safety Issues

Sound-alike/look-alike issues:

Amoxicillin may be confused with amoxapine, Augmentin®

Amoxil may be confused with amoxapine

International issues:

Fisamox [Australia] may be confused with Fosamax brand name for alendronate [U.S., Canada, and multiple international markets] and Vigamox brand name for moxifloxacin [U.S., Canada, and multiple international markets]

Limoxin [Mexico] may be confused with Lanoxin brand name for digoxin [U.S., Canada, and multiple international markets]; Lincocin brand name for lincomycin [U.S., Canada, and multiple international markets]

Zimox: Brand name for amoxicillin [Italy], but also the brand name for carbidopa/levodopa [Greece]

Zimox [Italy] may be confused with Diamox which is the brand name for acetazolamide [Canada and multiple international markets]

Pregnancy Risk Factor B

Lactation Enters breast milk/use caution (AAP rates "compatible"; AAP 2001 update pending)

Breast-Feeding Considerations Very small amounts of amoxicillin are excreted in breast milk. The manufacturer recommends that caution be exercised when administering amoxicillin to nursing women. Nondose-related effects could include modification of bowel flora and allergic sensitization of the infant.

Use Treatment of otitis media, sinusitis, and infections caused by susceptible organisms involving the upper and lower respiratory tract, skin, and urinary tract; prophylaxis of infective endocarditis in patients undergoing surgical or dental procedures; as part of a multidrug regimen for *H. pylori* eradication

Unlabeled Use Postexposure prophylaxis for anthrax exposure with documented susceptible organisms

Mechanism of Action/Effect Interferes with bacterial cell wall synthesis during active multiplication, causing cell wall death and resultant bactericidal activity against susceptible bacteria

Contraindications Hypersensitivity to amoxicillin, penicillin, other beta-lactams, or any component of the formulation

Warnings/Precautions In patients with renal impairment, doses and/or frequency of administration should be modified in response to the degree of renal impairment; in addition, use of certain dosage forms (eg, extended release 775 mg tablet and immediate release 875 mg tablet) should be avoided in patients with Cl_{cr} <30 mL/minute or patients requiring hemodialysis. A high percentage of patients with infectious mononucleosis have developed rash during therapy with amoxicillin; ampicillin-class antibiotics not recommended in these patients. Serious and occasionally severe or fatal hypersensitivity (anaphylactoid) reactions have been reported in patients on penicillin therapy, especially with a history of beta-lactam hypersensitivity, history of sensitivity to multiple allergens, or previous IgE-mediated reactions (eg, anaphylaxis, angioedema, urticaria). Use with caution in asthmatic patients. Prolonged use may result in fungal or bacterial superinfection, including *C. difficile*-associated diarrhea (CDAD) and pseudomembranous colitis; CDAD has been observed >2 months postantibiotic treatment. Chewable tablets contain phenylalanine.

Drug Interactions

Avoid Concomitant Use

Avoid concomitant use of Amoxicillin with any of the following: BCG

Decreased Effect

Amoxicillin may decrease the levels/effects of: BCG; Mycophenolate; Typhoid Vaccine

The levels/effects of Amoxicillin may be decreased by: Fusidic Acid; Tetracycline Derivatives

Increased Effect/Toxicity

Amoxicillin may increase the levels/effects of: Methotrexate; Vitamin K Antagonists

The levels/effects of Amoxicillin may be increased by: Allopurinol; Probenecid

Adverse Reactions Frequency not defined.

Central nervous system: Agitation, anxiety, behavioral changes, confusion, dizziness, headache, hyperactivity (reversible), insomnia, seizure

Dermatologic: Acute exanthematous pustulosis, erythematous maculopapular rash, erythema multiforme, exfoliative dermatitis, hypersensitivity vasculitis, mucocutaneous candidiasis, Stevens-Johnson syndrome, toxic epidermal necrolysis, urticaria

Gastrointestinal: Black hairy tongue, diarrhea, hemorrhagic colitis, nausea, pseudomembranous colitis, tooth discoloration (brown, yellow, or gray; rare), vomiting

Hematologic: Agranulocytosis, anemia, eosinophilia, hemolytic anemia, leukopenia, thrombocytopenia, thrombocytopenia purpura

Hepatic: Acute cytolytic hepatitis, ALT increased, AST increased, cholestatic jaundice, hepatic cholestasis

Renal: Crystalluria

Miscellaneous: Anaphylaxis, serum sickness-like reaction

Available Dosage Forms

Capsule, oral: 250 mg, 500 mg

Powder for suspension, oral: 125 mg/5 mL (80 mL, 100 mL, 150 mL); 200 mg/5 mL (50 mL, 75 mL, 100 mL); 250 mg/5 mL (80 mL, 100 mL, 150 mL); 400 mg/5 mL (50 mL, 75 mL, 100 mL)

Tablet, oral: 500 mg, 875 mg

Tablet, chewable, oral: 125 mg, 200 mg, 250 mg, 400 mg

Tablet, extended release, oral:

Moxatag™: 775 mg

General Dosage Range Dosage adjustment recommended in patients with renal impairment

Oral:

Immediate release:

Infants ≤3 months: 20-30 mg/kg/day divided every 12 hours

Children >3 months and <40 kg: 20-100 mg/kg/day divided every 8-12 hours

Adults: 250-500 mg every 8 hours **or** 500-875 mg twice daily (maximum: 875 mg/dose)

Extended release: *Children ≥12 years and Adults:* 775 mg once daily

Administration

Oral Administer around-the-clock to promote less variation in peak and trough serum levels. The appropriate amount of suspension may be mixed with formula, milk, fruit juice, water, ginger ale, or cold drinks; administer dose immediately after mixing.

Moxatag™ extended release tablet: Administer within 1 hour of finishing a meal.

Some penicillins (eg, carbenicillin, ticarcillin, and piperacillin) have been shown to inactivate aminoglycosides *in vitro*. This has been observed to a greater extent with tobramycin and gentamicin, while amikacin has shown greater stability against inactivation. Concurrent use of these agents may pose a risk of reduced antibacterial efficacy *in vivo*, particularly in the setting of profound renal impairment. However, definitive clinical evidence is lacking. If combination penicillin/aminoglycoside therapy is desired in a patient with renal dysfunction, separation of doses (if feasible), and routine monitoring of aminoglycoside levels, CBC, and clinical response should be considered.

Stability

Storage

Amoxil®: Oral suspension remains stable for 14 days at room temperature or if refrigerated (refrigeration preferred). Unit-dose antibiotic oral syringes are stable at room temperature for at least 72 hours (Tu, 1988).

Moxatag™: Store at 25°C (77°F); excursions permitted to 15°C to 30°C (59°F to 86°F).

Nursing Actions

Physical Assessment Culture and sensitivity report and patient's allergies should be assessed prior to starting therapy. Monitor for opportunistic infection.

Patient Education Multiple daily doses should be taken at equal intervals around-the-clock. May be taken with milk, juice, or food. Maintain adequate hydration, unless instructed to restrict fluid intake. May cause nausea, vomiting, or diarrhea. Report respiratory difficulty; rash, itching, or hives; easy bruising or bleeding; persistent diarrhea; signs of opportunistic infection (eg, unusual sore throat, fever, chills, fatigue, thrush, vaginal discharge); CNS changes (confusion, agitation, dizziness, insomnia); or if condition being treated worsens or does not improve by time prescription is completed.

Dietary Considerations May be taken with food. Some products may contain phenylalanine.

Moxatag™: Take within 1 hour of finishing a meal.

Amoxicillin and Clavulanate

(a moks i SIL in & klav yoo LAN ate)

Brand Names: U.S. Amoclan; Augmentin ES-600® [DSC]; Augmentin XR®; Augmentin®

Index Terms Amoxicillin and Clavulanate Potassium; Amoxicillin and Clavulanic Acid; Clavulanic Acid and Amoxicillin

Pharmacologic Category Antibiotic, Penicillin

Medication Safety Issues

Sound-alike/look-alike issues:

Augmentin® may be confused with amoxicillin, Azulfidine®

Pregnancy Risk Factor B

Lactation Enters breast milk/use caution

Use Treatment of otitis media, sinusitis, and infections caused by susceptible organisms involving the lower respiratory tract, skin and skin structure, and urinary tract; spectrum same as amoxicillin with additional coverage of beta-lactamase producing *B. catarrhalis*, *H. influenzae*, *N. gonorrhoeae*, and *S. aureus* (not MRSA). The expanded coverage of this combination makes it a useful alternative when amoxicillin resistance is present and patients cannot tolerate alternative treatments.

Available Dosage Forms

Powder for suspension, oral: 200: Amoxicillin 200 mg and clavulanate potassium 28.5 mg per 5 mL; 250: Amoxicillin 250 mg and clavulanate potassium 62.5 mg per 5 mL; 400: Amoxicillin 400 mg and clavulanate potassium 57 mg per 5 mL; 600: Amoxicillin 600 mg and clavulanate potassium 42.9 mg per 5 mL

Amoclan:

200: Amoxicillin 200 mg and clavulanate potassium 28.5 mg per 5 mL

400: Amoxicillin 400 mg and clavulanate potassium 57 mg per 5 mL

600: Amoxicillin 600 mg and clavulanate potassium 42.9 mg per 5 mL

Augmentin®:

125: Amoxicillin 125 mg and clavulanate potassium 31.25 mg per 5 mL

250: Amoxicillin 250 mg and clavulanate potassium 62.5 mg per 5 mL

Tablet, oral: 250: Amoxicillin 250 mg and clavulanate potassium 125 mg; 500: Amoxicillin 500 mg and clavulanate potassium 125 mg; 875: Amoxicillin 875 mg and clavulanate potassium 125 mg

Augmentin®:

500: Amoxicillin 500 mg and clavulanate potassium 125 mg

875: Amoxicillin 875 mg and clavulanate potassium 125 mg

Tablet, chewable, oral: 200: Amoxicillin 200 mg and clavulanate potassium 28.5 mg; 400: Amoxicillin 400 mg and clavulanate potassium 57 mg

Tablet, extended release, oral: Amoxicillin 1000 mg and clavulanate acid 62.5 mg

Augmentin XR®: 1000: Amoxicillin 1000 mg and clavulanate acid 62.5 mg

General Dosage Range Dosage adjustment recommended in patients with renal impairment

Oral:

Immediate release:

Infants <3 months: 30 mg/kg/day divided every 12 hours

Children ≥3 months and <40 kg: 25-90 mg/kg/day divided every 12 hours **or** 20-40 mg/kg/day divided every 8 hours

Children >40 kg and Adults: 250-500 mg every 8 hours **or** 875 mg every 12 hours

Extended release: *Children ≥16 years and Adults:* 2000 mg every 12 hours (maximum: 2000 mg/dose)

Administration

Oral Administer around-the-clock to promote less variation in peak and trough serum levels. Administer with food to increase absorption and decrease stomach upset; shake suspension well before use. Extended release tablets should be administered with food.

Some penicillins (eg, carbenicillin, ticarcillin, and piperacillin) have been shown to inactivate aminoglycosides *in vitro*. This has been observed to a greater extent with tobramycin and gentamicin, while amikacin has shown greater stability against inactivation. Concurrent use of these agents may pose a risk of reduced antibacterial efficacy *in vivo*, particularly in the setting of profound renal impairment. However, definitive clinical evidence is lacking. If combination penicillin/aminoglycoside therapy is desired in a patient with renal dysfunction, separation of doses (if feasible), and routine monitoring of aminoglycoside levels, CBC, and clinical response should be considered.

Nursing Actions

Physical Assessment See individual agents.

Patient Education See individual agents.

Related Information

Amoxicillin *on page* 68

Amphotericin B Cholesteryl Sulfate Complex

(am foe TER i sin bee kole LES te ril SUL fate KOM plecks)

Brand Names: U.S. Amphotec®

Index Terms ABCD; Amphotericin B Colloidal Dispersion

Pharmacologic Category Antifungal Agent, Parenteral

Medication Safety Issues

High alert medication:

The Institute for Safe Medication Practices (ISMP) includes this medication among its list of drugs which have a heightened risk of causing significant patient harm when used in error.

Other safety concerns:

Lipid-based amphotericin formulations (Amphotec®) may be confused with conventional formulations (Amphocin®, Fungizone®)

Large overdoses have occurred when conventional formulations were dispensed inadvertently for lipid-based products. Single daily doses of conventional amphotericin formulation never exceed 1.5 mg/kg.

Pregnancy Risk Factor B

Lactation Excretion in breast milk unknown/not recommended

Breast-Feeding Considerations It is not known if amphotericin is excreted into breast milk. Due to its poor oral absorption, systemic exposure to the nursing infant is expected to be decreased; however, because of the potential for toxicity, breast-feeding is not recommended (Mactal-Haaf, 2001).

Use Treatment of invasive aspergillosis in patients who have failed amphotericin B deoxycholate treatment, or who have renal impairment or experience unacceptable toxicity which precludes treatment with amphotericin B deoxycholate in effective doses.

Unlabeled Use Effective in patients with serious *Candida* species infections

Mechanism of Action/Effect Binds to ergosterol altering cell membrane permeability in susceptible fungi and causing leakage of cell components with subsequent cell death

Contraindications Hypersensitivity to amphotericin B or any component of the formulation

Warnings/Precautions Anaphylaxis has been reported with amphotericin B-containing drugs. If severe respiratory distress occurs, the infusion should be immediately discontinued. During the initial dosing, the drug should be administered under close clinical observation. Infusion reactions, sometimes severe, usually subside with continued therapy - manage with decreased rate of infusion and pretreatment with antihistamines/corticosteroids.

Drug Interactions

Avoid Concomitant Use

Avoid concomitant use of Amphotericin B Cholesteryl Sulfate Complex with any of the following: Gallium Nitrate

Decreased Effect

Amphotericin B Cholesteryl Sulfate Complex may decrease the levels/effects of: Saccharomyces boulardii

The levels/effects of Amphotericin B Cholesteryl Sulfate Complex may be decreased by: Antifungal Agents (Azole Derivatives, Systemic)

Increased Effect/Toxicity

Amphotericin B Cholesteryl Sulfate Complex may increase the levels/effects of: Aminoglycosides; Colistimethate; CycloSPORINE; CycloSPORINE (Systemic); Flucytosine; Gallium Nitrate

The levels/effects of Amphotericin B Cholesteryl Sulfate Complex may be increased by: Corticosteroids (Orally Inhaled); Corticosteroids (Systemic)

Adverse Reactions

>10%: Central nervous system: Chills, fever

1% to 10%:

Cardiovascular: Hypotension, tachycardia

Central nervous system: Headache

Dermatologic: Rash

Endocrine & metabolic: Hypokalemia, hypomagnesemia

Gastrointestinal: Nausea, diarrhea, abdominal pain

Hematologic: Thrombocytopenia

Hepatic: LFT change

Neuromuscular & skeletal: Rigors

Renal: Creatinine increased

Respiratory: Dyspnea

Note: Amphotericin B colloidal dispersion has an improved therapeutic index compared to conventional amphotericin B, and has been used safely in patients with amphotericin B-related nephrotoxicity; however, continued decline of renal function has occurred in some patients.

Available Dosage Forms

Injection, powder for reconstitution:

Amphotec®: 50 mg, 100 mg

General Dosage Range I.V.: *Children and Adults:* 3-4 mg/kg/day (maximum: 7.5 mg/kg/day)

Administration

I.V. For a patient who experiences chills, fever, hypotension, nausea, or other nonanaphylactic infusion-related reactions, premedicate with the following drugs 30-60 minutes prior to drug administration: A nonsteroidal (eg, ibuprofen, choline magnesium trisalicylate) with or without diphenhydramine **or** acetaminophen with diphenhydramine **or** hydrocortisone 50-100 mg. If the patient experiences rigors during the infusion, meperidine may be administered. If severe respiratory distress occurs, the infusion should be immediately discontinued.

I.V. Detail Avoid injection faster than 1 mg/kg/hour.

Stability

Reconstitution Reconstitute 50 mg and 100 mg vials with 10 mL and 20 mL of SWI, respectively. The reconstituted vials contain 5 mg/mL of amphotericin B. Shake the vial gently by hand until all solid particles have dissolved. Further dilute amphotericin B colloidal dispersion with D_5W.

Storage Store intact vials under refrigeration. After reconstitution, the solution should be refrigerated at 2°C to 8°C (36°F to 46°F) and used within 24 hours. Concentrations of 0.1-2 mg/mL in D_5W are stable for 14 days at 4°C and 23°C if protected from light, however, due to the occasional formation of subvisual particles, solutions should be used within 48 hours.

Nursing Actions

Physical Assessment Culture and sensitivity and patient history of exposure to amphotericin B should be assessed prior to beginning treatment. Premedication may be ordered to reduce incidence/severity of infusion reaction. Monitor patient closely for infusion related reactions (eg, anaphylaxis, chills, fever, nausea, vomiting, rigors, hypotension, acute respiratory distress); facilities for cardiopulmonary resuscitation should be available.

Patient Education This medication can only be administered by infusion and therapy may last several weeks. You will be monitored closely during and after infusion; report immediately any pain or swelling at infusion site, chills, nausea, chest pain, swelling of face or mouth, difficulty breathing, muscle cramping, acute anxiety, or other infusion reactions. Maintain adequate hydration, unless instructed to restrict fluid intake. May cause postural hypotension, nausea, or vomiting. Report chest pain or palpitations; CNS disturbances; skin rash; unusual chills or fever; persistent nausea, vomiting, or abdominal pain; sore throat; excessive fatigue; swelling of extremities or unusual weight gain; difficulty breathing; pain at infusion site; muscle cramping; or weakness.

Amphotericin B (Conventional)

(am foe TER i sin bee con VEN sha nal)

Index Terms Amphotericin B Deoxycholate; Amphotericin B Desoxycholate; Conventional Amphotericin B

Pharmacologic Category Antifungal Agent, Parenteral

Medication Safety Issues

High alert medication:

The Institute for Safe Medication Practices (ISMP) includes this medication (intrathecal administration) among its list of drugs which have a heightened risk of causing significant patient harm when used in error.

Other safety concerns:

Conventional amphotericin formulations (Amphocin®, Fungizone®) may be confused with lipid-based formulations (AmBisome®, Abelcet®, Amphotec®).

Large overdoses have occurred when conventional formulations were dispensed inadvertently for lipid-based products. Single daily doses of conventional amphotericin formulation never exceed 1.5 mg/kg.

Pregnancy Risk Factor B

Lactation Excretion in breast milk unknown/not recommended

Use Treatment of severe systemic and central nervous system infections caused by susceptible fungi such as *Candida* species, *Histoplasma capsulatum*, *Cryptococcus neoformans*, *Aspergillus* species, *Blastomyces dermatitidis*, *Torulopsis glabrata*, and *Coccidioides immitis*; fungal peritonitis; irrigant for bladder fungal infections; used in fungal infection in patients with bone marrow transplantation, amebic meningoencephalitis, ocular aspergillosis (intraocular injection), candidal cystitis (bladder irrigation), chemoprophylaxis (low-dose I.V.), immunocompromised patients at risk of aspergillosis (intranasal/nebulized), refractory meningitis (intrathecal), coccidioidal arthritis (intra-articular/I.M.).

Low-dose amphotericin B has been administered after bone marrow transplantation to reduce the risk of invasive fungal disease.

Available Dosage Forms

Injection, powder for reconstitution: 50 mg

General Dosage Range Dosage adjustment recommended in patients who develop toxicities

I.V.:

Infants and Children: Test dose: 0.1 mg/kg/dose (maximum: 1 mg); Maintenance: 0.25-1 mg/kg/day given once daily; 1-1.5 mg/kg every other day may be given once therapy is established (maximum: 1.5-4 g cumulative dose)

Adults: Test dose: 1 mg infused; Maintenance: 0.3-1.5 mg/kg/day given once daily; 1-1.5 mg/kg every other day may be given once therapy is established (maximum: 1.5 mg/kg/day)

Administration

I.V. May be infused over 4-6 hours. For a patient who experiences chills, fever, hypotension, nausea, or other nonanaphylactic infusion-related reactions, premedicate with the following drugs 30-60 minutes prior to drug administration: A nonsteroidal (eg, ibuprofen, choline magnesium trisalicylate) ± diphenhydramine **or** acetaminophen with diphenhydramine **or** hydrocortisone. If the patient experiences rigors during the infusion, meperidine may be administered. Bolus infusion of normal saline immediately preceding, or immediately preceding and following amphotericin B may reduce drug-induced nephrotoxicity. Risk of nephrotoxicity increases with amphotericin B doses >1 mg/kg/day. Infusion of admixtures more concentrated than 0.25 mg/mL should be limited to patients absolutely requiring volume contraction.

I.V. Detail Precipitate may form in ionic dialysate solutions.

pH: 5.7 (100 mg/L in D_5W)

Nursing Actions

Physical Assessment Culture and sensitivity and patient history of exposure to amphotericin B should be assessed prior to beginning treatment. Premedication may be ordered to reduce incidence/severity of infusion reaction. Monitor patient closely for infusion-related reactions (eg, anaphylaxis, chills, fever, nausea, vomiting, rigors, hypotension, acute respiratory distress); facilities for cardiopulmonary resuscitation should be available. If acute respiratory distress occurs, stop infusion and notify prescriber.

Patient Education I.V.: You will be monitored closely during and after infusion; report immediately any pain or swelling at infusion site, chills, nausea, chest pain, swelling of face or mouth, difficulty breathing, muscle cramping, acute anxiety, or other infusion reactions. May cause nausea, vomiting, anorexia, generalized muscle or joint pain, or hypotension. Report severe muscle cramping or weakness; chest pain or palpitations; CNS disturbances; skin rash; change in urinary patterns or difficulty voiding; unusual bruising or bleeding; or pain, redness, or swelling at infusion site.

Amphotericin B (Lipid Complex)

(am foe TER i sin bee LIP id KOM pleks)

Brand Names: U.S. Abelcet®

Index Terms ABLC

Pharmacologic Category Antifungal Agent, Parenteral

Medication Safety Issues

High alert medication:

The Institute for Safe Medication Practices (ISMP) includes this medication among its list of drugs which have a heightened risk of causing significant patient harm when used in error.

Other safety concerns:

Lipid-based amphotericin formulations (Abelcet®) may be confused with conventional formulations (Amphocin®, Fungizone®)

Large overdoses have occurred when conventional formulations were dispensed inadvertently for lipid-based products. Single daily doses of conventional amphotericin formulation never exceed 1.5 mg/kg.

Pregnancy Risk Factor B

Lactation Enters breast milk/not recommended

Breast-Feeding Considerations It is not known if amphotericin is excreted into breast milk. Due to its poor oral absorption, systemic exposure to the nursing infant is expected to be decreased; however, because of the potential for toxicity, breast-feeding is not recommended (Mactal-Haaf, 2001).

Use Treatment of aspergillosis or any type of progressive fungal infection in patients who are refractory to or intolerant of conventional amphotericin B therapy

Unlabeled Use Effective in patients with serious *Candida* species infections

Mechanism of Action/Effect Mechanism is like amphotericin - includes binding to ergosterol altering cell membrane permeability in susceptible fungi and causing leakage of cell components with subsequent cell death.

Contraindications Hypersensitivity to amphotericin or any component of the formulation

Warnings/Precautions Anaphylaxis has been reported with amphotericin B-containing drugs. If severe respiratory distress occurs, the infusion should be immediately discontinued. During the initial dosing, the drug should be administered under close clinical observation. Acute reactions (including fever and chills) may occur 1-2 hours after starting an intravenous infusion. These reactions are usually more common with the first few doses and generally diminish with subsequent doses.

Drug Interactions

Avoid Concomitant Use

Avoid concomitant use of Amphotericin B (Lipid Complex) with any of the following: Gallium Nitrate

Decreased Effect

Amphotericin B (Lipid Complex) may decrease the levels/effects of: Saccharomyces boulardii

The levels/effects of Amphotericin B (Lipid Complex) may be decreased by: Antifungal Agents (Azole Derivatives, Systemic)

Increased Effect/Toxicity

Amphotericin B (Lipid Complex) may increase the levels/effects of: Aminoglycosides; Colistimethate; CycloSPORINE; CycloSPORINE (Systemic); Flucytosine; Gallium Nitrate

The levels/effects of Amphotericin B (Lipid Complex) may be increased by: Corticosteroids (Orally Inhaled); Corticosteroids (Systemic)

Adverse Reactions Nephrotoxicity and infusion-related hyperpyrexia, rigor, and chilling are reduced relative to amphotericin deoxycholate.

>10%:

Central nervous system: Chills, fever

Renal: Serum creatinine increased

Miscellaneous: Multiple organ failure

1% to 10%:

Cardiovascular: Hypotension, cardiac arrest

Central nervous system: Headache, pain

Dermatologic: Rash

Endocrine & metabolic: Bilirubinemia, hypokalemia, acidosis

Gastrointestinal: Nausea, vomiting, diarrhea, gastrointestinal hemorrhage, abdominal pain

Renal: Renal failure

Respiratory: Respiratory failure, dyspnea, pneumonia

Available Dosage Forms

Injection, suspension [preservative free]:

Abelcet®: 5 mg/mL (20 mL)

General Dosage Range Dosage adjustment recommended in patients who develop toxicities

I.V.: *Children and Adults:* 2.5-5 mg/kg/day as a single daily dose (maximum: 5 mg/kg/day)

Administration

I.V. For patients who experience nonanaphylactic infusion-related reactions, premedicate 30-60 minutes prior to drug administration with a nonsteroidal anti-inflammatory agent ± diphenhydramine **or** acetaminophen with diphenhydramine **or** hydrocortisone. If the patient experiences rigors during the infusion, meperidine may be administered.

Administer at an infusion rate of 2.5 mg/kg/hour (over 2 hours). Invert infusion container several times prior to administration and every 2 hours during infusion if it exceeds 2 hours.

I.V. Detail Do not use an in-line filter. Flush line with dextrose; normal saline may cause precipitate.

Stability

Reconstitution Shake vial gently to disperse yellow sediment at bottom of container. Dilute with D_5W to 1-2 mg/mL.

Storage Intact vials should be stored at 2°C to 8°C (35°F to 46°F); do not freeze. Protect intact vials from exposure to light. Solutions for infusion are stable for 48 hours under refrigeration and 6 hours at room temperature. Protect from light. Following reconstitution, protect from light.

Nursing Actions

Physical Assessment Patient history of previous exposure to amphotericin B should be assessed before beginning treatment. Premedication may be ordered to reduce incidence/ severity of infusion reaction. Monitor patient closely for infusion related reactions (eg, anaphylaxis, chills, fever, nausea, vomiting, rigors, hypotension, acute respiratory distress); facilities for cardiopulmonary resuscitation should be available. If acute respiratory distress occurs, stop infusion and notify prescriber.

Patient Education This medication can only be administered by infusion and therapy may last several weeks. May cause postural hypotension, nausea, or vomiting. Report chest pain or palpitations; CNS disturbances; skin rash; chills or fever; persistent nausea, vomiting, or abdominal pain; sore throat; excessive fatigue; swelling of extremities or unusual weight gain; respiratory difficulty; pain at infusion site; or muscle cramping or weakness.

Amphotericin B (Liposomal)

(am foe TER i sin bee lye po SO mal)

Brand Names: U.S. AmBisome®

Index Terms L-AmB

Pharmacologic Category Antifungal Agent, Parenteral

Medication Safety Issues

High alert medication:

The Institute for Safe Medication Practices (ISMP) includes this medication among its list of drugs which have a heightened risk of causing significant patient harm when used in error.

Other safety concerns:

Lipid-based amphotericin formulations (AmBisome®) may be confused with conventional formulations (Amphocin®, Fungizone®) or with other lipid-based amphotericin formulations (Abelcet®, Amphotec®)

Large overdoses have occurred when conventional formulations were dispensed inadvertently for lipid-based products. Single daily doses of conventional amphotericin formulation never exceed 1.5 mg/kg.

Pregnancy Risk Factor B

Lactation Excretion in breast milk unknown/not recommended

Breast-Feeding Considerations It is not known if amphotericin is excreted into breast milk. Due to its poor oral absorption, systemic exposure to the nursing infant is expected to be decreased; however, because of the potential for toxicity, breast-feeding is not recommended (Mactal-Haaf, 2001).

Use Empirical therapy for presumed fungal infection in febrile, neutropenic patients; treatment of patients with *Aspergillus* species, *Candida* species, and/or *Cryptococcus* species infections refractory to amphotericin B desoxycholate (conventional amphotericin), or in patients where renal impairment or unacceptable toxicity precludes the use of amphotericin B desoxycholate; treatment of cryptococcal meningitis in HIV-infected patients; treatment of visceral leishmaniasis

Unlabeled Use Treatment of systemic *Histoplasmosis* infection

Mechanism of Action/Effect Amphotericin B, the active ingredient, binds to the sterol component of a cell membrane leading to alterations in cell permeability and cell death. While amphotericin B has a higher affinity for the ergosterol component of the fungal cell membrane, it can also bind to the cholesterol component of the mammalian cell leading to cytotoxicity. AmBisome®, the liposomal preparation of amphotericin B, has been shown to penetrate the cell wall of both extracellular and intracellular forms of susceptible fungi.

Contraindications Hypersensitivity to amphotericin B deoxycholate or any component of the formulation

Warnings/Precautions Patients should be under close clinical observation during initial dosing. As with other amphotericin B-containing products, anaphylaxis has been reported. Facilities for cardiopulmonary resuscitation should be available during administration. Acute infusion reactions (including fever and chills) may occur 1-2 hours after starting infusions; reactions are more common with the first few doses and generally diminish with subsequent doses. Immediately discontinue infusion if severe respiratory distress occurs; the patient should not receive further infusions. Concurrent use of amphotericin B with other nephrotoxic drugs may enhance the potential for drug-induced renal toxicity. Concurrent use with antineoplastic agents may enhance the potential for renal toxicity, bronchospasm or hypotension. Acute pulmonary toxicity has been reported in patients receiving simultaneous leukocyte transfusions and amphotericin B. Safety and efficacy have not been established in patients <1 month of age.

Drug Interactions

Avoid Concomitant Use

Avoid concomitant use of Amphotericin B (Liposomal) with any of the following: Gallium Nitrate

Decreased Effect

Amphotericin B (Liposomal) may decrease the levels/effects of: Saccharomyces boulardii

The levels/effects of Amphotericin B (Liposomal) may be decreased by: Antifungal Agents (Azole Derivatives, Systemic)

Increased Effect/Toxicity

Amphotericin B (Liposomal) may increase the levels/effects of: Aminoglycosides; Colistimethate; CycloSPORINE; CycloSPORINE (Systemic); Flucytosine; Gallium Nitrate

The levels/effects of Amphotericin B (Liposomal) may be increased by: Corticosteroids (Orally Inhaled); Corticosteroids (Systemic)

Adverse Reactions Percentage of adverse reactions is dependent upon population studied and may vary with respect to premedications and underlying illness. Incidence of decreased renal function and infusion-related events are lower than rates observed with amphotericin B deoxycholate.

>10%:

Cardiovascular: Peripheral edema (15%), edema (12% to 14%), tachycardia (9% to 19%), hypotension (7% to 14%), hypertension (8% to 20%), chest pain (8% to 12%), hypervolemia (8% to 12%)

Central nervous system: Chills (29% to 48%), insomnia (17% to 22%), headache (9% to 20%), anxiety (7% to 14%), pain (14%), confusion (9% to 13%)

Dermatologic: Rash (5% to 25%), pruritus (11%)

Endocrine & metabolic: Hypokalemia (31% to 51%), hypomagnesemia (15% to 50%), hyperglycemia (8% to 23%), hypocalcemia (5% to 18%), hyponatremia (9% to 12%)

Gastrointestinal: Nausea (16% to 40%), vomiting (11% to 32%), diarrhea (11% to 30%), abdominal pain (7% to 20%), constipation (15%), anorexia (10% to 14%)

Hematologic: Anemia (27% to 48%), blood transfusion reaction (9% to 18%), leukopenia (15% to 17%), thrombocytopenia (6% to 13%)

Hepatic: Alkaline phosphatase increased (7% to 22%), bilirubinemia (≤18%), ALT increased (15%), AST increased (13%), liver function tests abnormal (not specified) (4% to 13%)

Local: Phlebitis (9% to 11%)

Neuromuscular & skeletal: Weakness (6% to 13%), back pain (12%)

Renal: Nephrotoxicity (14% to 47%), creatinine increased (18% to 40%), BUN increased (7% to 21%), hematuria (14%)

Respiratory: Dyspnea (18% to 23%), lung disorder (14% to 18%), cough (2% to 18%), epistaxis (9% to 15%), pleural effusion (13%), rhinitis (11%)

Miscellaneous: Infusion reactions (4% to 21%), sepsis (7% to 14%), infection (11% to 13%)

2% to 10%:

Cardiovascular: Arrhythmia, atrial fibrillation, bradycardia, cardiac arrest, cardiomegaly, facial swelling, flushing, postural hypotension, valvular heart disease, vascular disorder, vasodilation

Central nervous system: Agitation, abnormal thinking, coma, depression, dysesthesia, dizziness (7% to 9%), hallucinations, malaise, nervousness, seizure, somnolence

Dermatologic: Alopecia, bruising, cellulitis, dry skin, maculopapular rash, petechia, purpura, skin discoloration, skin disorder, skin ulcer, urticaria, vesiculobullous rash

Endocrine & metabolic: Acidosis, fluid overload, hypernatremia (4%), hyperchloremia, hyperkalemia, hypermagnesemia, hyperphosphatemia, hypophosphatemia, hypoproteinemia, lactate dehydrogenase increased, nonprotein nitrogen increased

Gastrointestinal: Abdomen enlarged, amylase increased, dyspepsia, dysphagia, eructation, fecal incontinence, flatulence, gastrointestinal hemorrhage (10%), hematemesis, hemorrhoids, gum/oral hemorrhage, ileus, mucositis, rectal disorder, stomatitis, ulcerative stomatitis, xerostomia

Genitourinary: Vaginal hemorrhage

Hematologic: Coagulation disorder, hemorrhage, prothrombin decreased

Hepatic: Hepatocellular damage, hepatomegaly, veno-occlusive liver disease

Local: Injection site inflammation

Neuromuscular & skeletal: Arthralgia, bone pain, dystonia, myalgia, neck pain, paresthesia, rigors, tremor

Ocular: Conjunctivitis, dry eyes, eye hemorrhage

Renal: Abnormal renal function, acute renal failure, dysuria, renal failure, toxic nephropathy, urinary incontinence

Respiratory: Asthma, atelectasis, dry nose, hemoptysis, hyperventilation, pharyngitis, pneumonia, pulmonary edema, respiratory alkalosis, respiratory insufficiency, respiratory failure, sinusitis, hypoxia (6% to 8%)

Miscellaneous: Allergic reaction, cell-mediated immunological reaction, flu-like syndrome, graft-versus-host disease, herpes simplex, hiccup, procedural complication (8% to 10%), diaphoresis (7%)

Available Dosage Forms

Injection, powder for reconstitution:

AmBisome®: 50 mg

General Dosage Range I.V.: *Children and Adults:* 3-6 mg/kg/day as a single daily dose (maximum: 6 mg/kg/day)

Administration

I.V. Intravenous infusion, over a period of approximately 2 hours. Infusion time may be reduced to approximately 1 hour in patients in whom the treatment is well-tolerated. If the patient experiences discomfort during infusion, the duration of infusion may be increased. Discontinue if severe respiratory distress occurs.

For a patient who experiences chills, fever, hypotension, nausea, or other nonanaphylactic infusion-related reactions, premedicate with the following drugs, 30-60 minutes prior to drug administration: A nonsteroidal (eg, ibuprofen, choline magnesium trisalicylate) ± diphenhydramine **or** acetaminophen with diphenhydramine **or** hydrocortisone. If the patient experiences rigors during the infusion, meperidine may be administered.

I.V. Detail Existing intravenous line should be flushed with D_5W prior to infusion (if not feasible, administer through a separate line). An in-line membrane filter (not less than 1 micron) may be used.

Stability

Reconstitution Reconstitute with 12 mL SWFI to a concentration of 4 mg/mL. The use of any solution other than those recommended, or the presence of a bacteriostatic agent in the solution, may cause precipitation. **Shake the vial vigorously** for 30 seconds, until dispersed into a translucent yellow suspension.

Filtration and dilution: The 5-micron filter should be on the syringe used to remove the reconstituted AmBisome®. Dilute to a final concentration of 1-2 mg/mL (0.2-0.5 mg/mL for infants and small children).

Storage Store intact vials at ≤25°C (≤77°F). Reconstituted vials are stable refrigerated at 2°C to 8°C (36°F to 46°F) for 24 hours. Do not freeze. Manufacturer's labeling states infusion should begin within 6 hours of dilution with D_5W; data on file with Astellas Pharma shows extended formulation stability when admixed in D_5W at 0.2-2 mg/mL (in polyolefin or PVC bags) for up to 11 days when stored refrigerated at 2°C to 8°C (36°F to 46°F).

Nursing Actions

Physical Assessment Culture and sensitivity report and patient's previous exposure to Amphotericin B should be assessed before beginning treatment. Premedication may be ordered to reduce incidence/severity of infusion reaction. Monitor patient closely for infusion-related reactions (eg, anaphylaxis, chills, fever, nausea, vomiting, rigors, hypotension, acute respiratory distress); facilities for cardiopulmonary resuscitation should be available. If acute respiratory distress occurs, stop infusion and notify prescriber.

Patient Education This medication can only be administered by infusion and therapy may last several weeks. You will be monitored closely during and after infusion; report immediately any pain or swelling at infusion site, difficulty breathing or chest pain, chills, nausea, swelling of face or mouth, muscle cramping, acute anxiety, or other infusion reactions. You may experience dizziness, anxiety, confusion, nausea, vomiting, or loss of appetite. Report chest pain or palpitations; CNS disturbances; skin rash; unusual chills or fever; persistent nausea, vomiting, or abdominal pain; sore throat; excessive fatigue; swelling of extremities or unusual weight gain; difficulty breathing; muscle cramping; or weakness.

Ampicillin (am pi SIL in)

Index Terms Aminobenzylpenicillin; Ampicillin Sodium; Ampicillin Trihydrate

Pharmacologic Category Antibiotic, Penicillin

Medication Safety Issues

Sound-alike/look-alike issues:

Ampicillin may be confused with aminophylline

Pregnancy Risk Factor B

Lactation Enters breast milk/use caution

Breast-Feeding Considerations Ampicillin is excreted in breast milk. The manufacturer recommends that caution be exercised when administering ampicillin to nursing women. Due to the low concentrations in human milk, minimal toxicity would be expected in the nursing infant. Non-dose-related effects could include modification of bowel flora and allergic sensitization.

Use Treatment of susceptible bacterial infections (nonbeta-lactamase-producing organisms); treatment or prophylaxis of infective endocarditis; susceptible bacterial infections caused by streptococci, pneumococci, nonpenicillinase-producing staphylococci, *Listeria*, meningococci; some strains of *H. influenzae*, *Salmonella*, *Shigella*, *E. coli*, *Enterobacter*, and *Klebsiella*

Mechanism of Action/Effect Interferes with bacterial cell wall synthesis during active multiplication, causing cell wall death and resultant bactericidal activity against susceptible bacteria

Contraindications Hypersensitivity to ampicillin, any component of the formulation, or other penicillins

Warnings/Precautions Dosage adjustment may be necessary in patients with renal impairment. Serious and occasionally severe or fatal hypersensitivity (anaphylactoid) reactions have been reported in patients on penicillin therapy, especially with a history of beta-lactam hypersensitivity, history of sensitivity to multiple allergens, or previous IgE-mediated reactions (eg, anaphylaxis, angioedema, urticaria). Use with caution in asthmatic patients. High percentage of patients with infectious mononucleosis have developed rash during therapy with ampicillin; ampicillin-class antibiotics not recommended in these patients. Appearance of a rash should be carefully evaluated to differentiate a nonallergic ampicillin rash from a hypersensitivity reaction. Ampicillin rash occurs in 5% to 10% of children receiving ampicillin and is a generalized dull red, maculopapular rash, generally appearing 3-14 days after the start of therapy. It normally begins on the trunk and spreads over most of the body. It may be most intense at pressure areas, elbows, and knees. Prolonged use may result in fungal or bacterial superinfection, including *C. difficile*-associated diarrhea (CDAD) and pseudomembranous colitis; CDAD has been observed >2 months postantibiotic treatment.

Drug Interactions

Avoid Concomitant Use

Avoid concomitant use of Ampicillin with any of the following: BCG

Decreased Effect

Ampicillin may decrease the levels/effects of: Atenolol; BCG; Mycophenolate; Typhoid Vaccine

The levels/effects of Ampicillin may be decreased by: Chloroquine; Fusidic Acid; Lanthanum; Tetracycline Derivatives

Increased Effect/Toxicity

Ampicillin may increase the levels/effects of: Methotrexate; Vitamin K Antagonists

The levels/effects of Ampicillin may be increased by: Allopurinol; Probenecid

Nutritional/Ethanol Interactions Food: Food decreases ampicillin absorption rate; may decrease ampicillin serum concentration. Management: Take at equal intervals around-the-clock, preferably on an empty stomach (1 hour before or 2 hours after meals). Maintain adequate hydration, unless instructed to restrict fluid intake.

Adverse Reactions Frequency not defined.

Central nervous system: Fever, penicillin encephalopathy, seizure

Dermatologic: Erythema multiforme, exfoliative dermatitis, rash, urticaria

Note: Appearance of a rash should be carefully evaluated to differentiate (if possible) nonallergic ampicillin rash from hypersensitivity reaction. Incidence is higher in patients with viral infection, *Salmonella* infection, lymphocytic leukemia, or patients that have hyperuricemia.

Gastrointestinal: Black hairy tongue, diarrhea, enterocolitis, glossitis, nausea, oral candidiasis, pseudomembranous colitis, sore mouth or tongue, stomatitis, vomiting

Hematologic: Agranulocytosis, anemia, hemolytic anemia, eosinophilia, leukopenia, thrombocytopenia purpura

Hepatic: AST increased

Renal: Interstitial nephritis (rare)

Respiratory: Laryngeal stridor

Miscellaneous: Anaphylaxis, serum sickness-like reaction

Available Dosage Forms

Capsule, oral: 250 mg, 500 mg

Injection, powder for reconstitution: 125 mg, 250 mg, 500 mg, 1 g, 2 g, 10 g

Powder for suspension, oral: 125 mg/5 mL (100 mL, 200 mL); 250 mg/5 mL (100 mL, 200 mL)

General Dosage Range Dosage adjustment recommended in patients with renal impairment

I.M., I.V.:

Infants and Children: 100-400 mg/kg/day divided every 6 hours (maximum: 12 g/day)

Adults: 1-2 g every 4-6 hours or 50-250 mg/kg/day in divided doses (maximum: 12 g/day)

Oral:

Infants and Children: 50-100 mg/kg/day divided every 6 hours (maximum: 2-4 g/day)

Adults: 250-500 mg every 6 hours

Administration

Oral Administer around-the-clock to promote less variation in peak and trough serum levels. Administer on an empty stomach (ie, 1 hour prior to, or 2 hours after meals) to increase total absorption.

I.V. Administer around-the-clock to promote less variation in peak and trough serum levels. Administer over 3-5 minutes (125-500 mg) or over 10-15 minutes (1-2 g). More rapid infusion may cause seizures. Ampicillin and gentamicin should not be mixed in the same I.V. tubing.

Some penicillins (eg, carbenicillin, ticarcillin, and piperacillin) have been shown to inactivate aminoglycosides *in vitro*. This has been observed to a greater extent with tobramycin and gentamicin, while amikacin has shown greater stability against inactivation. Concurrent use of these agents may pose a risk of reduced antibacterial efficacy *in vivo*, particularly in the setting of profound renal impairment. However, definitive clinical evidence is lacking. If combination penicillin/aminoglycoside therapy is desired in a patient with renal dysfunction, separation of doses (if feasible), and routine monitoring of aminoglycoside levels, CBC, and clinical response should be considered.

I.V. Detail pH: 8-10 (reconstituted solution)

Stability

Reconstitution I.V.: Minimum volume: Concentration should not exceed 30 mg/mL due to concentration-dependent stability restrictions. Standard diluent: 500 mg/50 mL NS; 1 g/50 mL NS; 2 g/100 mL NS.

Storage

Oral: Oral suspension is stable for 7 days at room temperature or for 14 days under refrigeration.

I.V.:

Solutions for I.M. or direct I.V. should be used within 1 hour. Solutions for I.V. infusion will be inactivated by dextrose at room temperature. If dextrose-containing solutions are to be used, the resultant solution will only be stable for 2 hours versus 8 hours in the 0.9% sodium chloride injection. D_5W has limited stability.

Stability of parenteral admixture in NS at room temperature (25°C) is 8 hours.

Stability of parenteral admixture in NS at refrigeration temperature (4°C) is 2 days.

Nursing Actions

Physical Assessment Allergy history should be assessed prior to starting therapy. Monitor for opportunistic infection (fever, chills, unhealed sores, white plaques in mouth or vagina, purulent vaginal discharge).

Patient Education Take at equal intervals around-the-clock; preferably on an empty stomach (1 hour before or 2 hours after meals). Maintain adequate hydration, unless instructed to restrict fluid intake. May cause nausea, vomiting, or diarrhea. Report immediately any rash; persistent diarrhea; swelling of face, tongue, mouth, or throat; or chest tightness. Report if condition being treated worsens or does not improve by the time prescription is completed.

Dietary Considerations Take on an empty stomach 1 hour before or 2 hours after meals. Some products may contain sodium.

Ampicillin and Sulbactam

(am pi SIL in & SUL bak tam)

Brand Names: U.S. Unasyn®

Index Terms Sulbactam and Ampicillin

Pharmacologic Category Antibiotic, Penicillin

Pregnancy Risk Factor B

Lactation Enters breast milk/use caution

Use Treatment of susceptible bacterial infections involved with skin and skin structure, intra-abdominal infections, gynecological infections; spectrum is that of ampicillin plus organisms producing beta-lactamases such as *S. aureus*, *H. influenzae*, *E. coli*, *Klebsiella*, *Acinetobacter*, *Enterobacter*, and anaerobes

Available Dosage Forms

Injection, powder for reconstitution: 1.5 g [ampicillin 1 g and sulbactam 0.5 g]; 3 g [ampicillin 2 g and sulbactam 1 g]; 15 g [ampicillin 10 g and sulbactam 5 g]

Unasyn®: 1.5 g [ampicillin 1 g and sulbactam 0.5 g]; 3 g [ampicillin 2 g and sulbactam 1 g]; 15 g [ampicillin 10 g and sulbactam 5 g]; 15 g [ampicillin 10 g and sulbactam 5 g

General Dosage Range Dosage adjustment recommended in patients with renal impairment

I.M.: *Adults:* 1-2 g (1.5-3 g Unasyn®) ampicillin every 6 hours (maximum: 8 g ampicillin/day)

I.V.:

Children ≥1 year: 100-400 mg ampicillin/kg/day divided every 6 hours (maximum: 8 g ampicillin/day)

Adults: 1-2 g (1.5-3 g Unasyn®) ampicillin every 6 hours (maximum: 8 g ampicillin/day)

Administration

I.V. Administer around-the-clock to promote less variation in peak and trough serum levels. Administer by slow injection over 10-15 minutes or I.V. over 15-30 minutes. Ampicillin and gentamicin should not be mixed in the same I.V. tubing.

Some penicillins (eg, carbenicillin, ticarcillin, and piperacillin) have been shown to inactivate aminoglycosides *in vitro*. This has been observed to a greater extent with tobramycin and gentamicin, while amikacin has shown greater stability against inactivation. Concurrent use of these agents may pose a risk of reduced antibacterial efficacy *in vivo*, particularly in the setting of profound renal impairment. However, definitive clinical evidence is lacking. If combination penicillin/aminoglycoside therapy is desired in a patient with renal dysfunction, separation of doses (if feasible), and routine monitoring of aminoglycoside levels, CBC, and clinical response should be considered.

I.V. Detail pH: 8-10

Nursing Actions

Physical Assessment See individual agents.

Patient Education See individual agents.

Related Information

Ampicillin *on page* 76

Anastrozole

(an AS troe zole)

Brand Names: U.S. Arimidex®

Index Terms ICI-D1033; ZD1033

Pharmacologic Category Antineoplastic Agent, Aromatase Inhibitor

Medication Safety Issues

Sound-alike/look-alike issues:

Anastrozole may be confused with anagrelide, letrozole

Arimidex® may be confused with Aromasin®

Pregnancy Risk Factor X

Lactation Excretion in breast milk unknown/not recommended

Use First-line treatment of locally-advanced or metastatic breast cancer (hormone receptor-positive or unknown) in postmenopausal women; treatment of advanced breast cancer in postmenopausal women with disease progression following tamoxifen therapy; adjuvant treatment of early hormone receptor-positive breast cancer in postmenopausal women

Unlabeled Use Treatment of recurrent or metastatic endometrial or uterine cancers, treatment of recurrent ovarian cancer

Mechanism of Action/Effect Potent and selective nonsteroidal aromatase inhibitor. By inhibiting aromatase, the conversion of androstenedione to estrone, and testosterone to estradiol, is prevented, thereby decreasing tumor mass or delaying progression in patients with tumors responsive to hormones. Anastrozole causes an 85% decrease in estrone sulfate levels.

Contraindications Hypersensitivity to anastrozole or any component of the formulation; use in women who are or may become pregnant

Warnings/Precautions Hazardous agent - use appropriate precautions for handling and disposal. Use is contraindicated in women who are or may become pregnant. Anastrozole offers no clinical benefit in premenopausal women with breast cancer. Patients with pre-existing ischemic cardiac disease have an increased risk for ischemic cardiovascular events.

Due to decreased circulating estrogen levels, anastrozole is associated with a reduction in bone mineral density (BMD); decreases (from baseline) in total hip and lumbar spine BMD have been reported. Patients with pre-existing osteopenia are at higher risk for developing osteoporosis (Eastell, 2008). When initiating anastrozole treatment, follow available guidelines for bone mineral density management in postmenopausal women with similar fracture risk; concurrent use of bisphosphonates may be useful in patients at risk for fractures.

Elevated total cholesterol levels (contributed to by LDL cholesterol increases) have been reported in patients receiving anastrozole; use with caution in patients with hyperlipidemias; cholesterol levels should be monitored/managed in accordance with current guidelines for patients with LDL elevations. Plasma concentrations in patients with stable hepatic cirrhosis were within the range of concentrations seen in normal subjects across all clinical trials; use has not been studied in patients with severe hepatic impairment. Safety and efficacy in children have not been established.

Drug Interactions

Avoid Concomitant Use

Avoid concomitant use of Anastrozole with any of the following: Estrogen Derivatives; Pimozide

Decreased Effect

The levels/effects of Anastrozole may be decreased by: Estrogen Derivatives; Tamoxifen

Increased Effect/Toxicity

Anastrozole may increase the levels/effects of: ARIPiprazole; Pimozide

Adverse Reactions

>10%:

Cardiovascular: Vasodilatation (25% to 36%), ischemic cardiovascular disease (4%; 17% in patients with pre-existing ischemic heart disease), hypertension (2% to 13%), angina (2%; 12% in patients with pre-existing ischemic heart disease)

Central nervous system: Mood disturbance (19%), fatigue (19%), pain (11% to 17%), headache (9% to 13%), depression (5% to 13%)

Dermatologic: Rash (6% to 11%)

Endocrine & metabolic: Hot flashes (12% to 36%)

Gastrointestinal: Nausea (11% to 19%), vomiting (8% to 13%)

Neuromuscular & skeletal: Weakness (16% to 19%), arthritis (17%), arthralgia (2% to 15%), back pain (10% to 12%), bone pain (6% to 11%), osteoporosis (11%)

Respiratory: Pharyngitis (6% to 14%), cough increased (8% to 11%)

1% to 10%:

Cardiovascular: Peripheral edema (5% to 10%), chest pain (5% to 7%), edema (7%), venous thromboembolic events (2% to 4%), ischemic cerebrovascular events (2%), MI (1%)

Central nervous system: Insomnia (2% to 10%), dizziness (6% to 8%), anxiety (2% to 6%), fever (2% to 5%), malaise (2% to 5%), confusion (2% to 5%), nervousness (2% to 5%), somnolence (2% to 5%), lethargy (1%)

Dermatologic: Alopecia (2% to 5%), pruritus (2% to 5%)

Endocrine & metabolic: Hypercholesterolemia (9%), breast pain (2% to 8%)

Gastrointestinal: Diarrhea (8% to 9%), constipation (7% to 9%), abdominal pain (7% to 9%), weight gain (2% to 9%), anorexia (5% to 7%), xerostomia (6%), dyspepsia (7%), weight loss (2% to 5%)

Genitourinary: Urinary tract infection (2% to 8%), vulvovaginitis (6%), pelvic pain (5%), vaginal bleeding (1% to 5%), vaginitis (4%), vaginal discharge (4%), vaginal hemorrhage (2% to 4%), leukorrhea (2% to 3%), vaginal dryness (2% to 5%)

Hematologic: Anemia (2% to 5%), leukopenia (2% to 5%)

Hepatic: Liver function tests increased (1% to 10%), alkaline phosphatase increased (1% to 10%), gamma GT increased (≤5%)

Local: Thrombophlebitis (2% to 5%)

Neuromuscular & skeletal: Fracture (1% to 10%), arthrosis (7%), paresthesia (5% to 7%), joint disorder (6%), myalgia (2% to 6%), neck pain (2% to 5%), carpal tunnel syndrome (3%), hypertonia (3%)

Ocular: Cataracts (6%)

Respiratory: Dyspnea (8% to 10%), sinusitis (2% to 6%), bronchitis (2% to 5%), rhinitis (2% to 5%)

Miscellaneous: Lymphedema (10%), infection (2% to 9%), flu-like syndrome (2% to 7%), diaphoresis (2% to 5%), cyst (5%), neoplasm (5%), tumor flare (3%)

Pharmacodynamics/Kinetics

Onset of Action Onset of estradiol reduction: 70% reduction after 24 hours; 80% after 2 weeks therapy

Duration of Action Duration of estradiol reduction: 6 days

Available Dosage Forms

Tablet, oral: 1 mg

Arimidex®: 1 mg

General Dosage Range Oral: *Adults:* 1 mg once daily

Administration

Oral May be administered with or without food.

Stability

Storage Store at 20°C to 25°C (68°F to 77°F).

Nursing Actions

Physical Assessment Monitor bone mineral density and cholesterol levels. Monitor for hyperlipidemia, hypotension, CNS changes, thrombophlebitis, and bone pain or fracture at regular intervals during therapy.

Patient Education Maintain adequate hydration, unless instructed to restrict fluid intake. Anastrozole may cause or worsen osteoporosis; discuss ways to decrease this risk with prescriber. You may experience dizziness or fatigue; nausea, vomiting, or loss of appetite; increased pelvic, bone, or tumor pain; hot flashes; rash; or loss of hair. Report chest pain, palpitations, persistent headache, or dizziness; unresolved nausea or vomiting; pain or burning on urination; unusual or persistent nervousness, confusion, or anxiety; flu-like symptoms; or respiratory difficulty.

Dietary Considerations May be taken with or without food.

Anidulafungin (ay nid yoo la FUN jin)

Brand Names: U.S. Eraxis™

Index Terms LY303366

Pharmacologic Category Antifungal Agent, Parenteral; Echinocandin

Pregnancy Risk Factor C

Lactation Excretion in breast milk unknown/use caution

Use Treatment of candidemia and other forms of *Candida* infections (including those of intra-abdominal, peritoneal, and esophageal locus)

Unlabeled Use Treatment of infections due to *Aspergillus* spp.

Mechanism of Action/Effect Noncompetitive inhibitor of 1,3-beta-D-glucan synthase resulting in reduced formation of 1,3-beta-D-glucan, an essential polysaccharide comprising 30% to 60% of *Candida* cell walls (absent in mammalian cells); decreased glucan content leads to osmotic instability and cellular lysis

Contraindications Hypersensitivity to anidulafungin, other echinocandins, or any component of the formulation

Warnings/Precautions Histamine-mediated reactions (eg, urticaria, flushing, hypotension) have been observed; these may be related to infusion rate. Elevated liver function tests, hepatitis, and worsening hepatic failure have been reported. Monitor for progressive hepatic impairment if increased transaminase enzymes noted. Safety and efficacy in pediatric patients, neutropenic patients, or other *Candida* infections (eg, endocarditis, osteomyelitis, meningitis) have not been established.

Drug Interactions

Avoid Concomitant Use There are no known interactions where it is recommended to avoid concomitant use.

Decreased Effect

Anidulafungin may decrease the levels/effects of: Saccharomyces boulardii

Increased Effect/Toxicity There are no known significant interactions involving an increase in effect.

Adverse Reactions 2% to 10%:

Endocrine & metabolic: Hypokalemia (3%)

Gastrointestinal: Diarrhea (3%)

Hepatic: Transaminase increased (<1% to 2%)

Available Dosage Forms

Injection, powder for reconstitution:

Eraxis™: 50 mg, 100 mg

General Dosage Range I.V.: *Adults:* Loading dose: 100-200 mg as a single dose; Maintenance: 50-100 mg daily

Administration

I.V. For intravenous use only; infusion rate should not exceed 1.1 mg/minute

Stability

Reconstitution Aseptically add 15 mL (50 mg vial) or 30 mL (100 mg vial) of sterile water for injection to each vial. Swirl to dissolve; do not shake. Further dilute 50 mg, 100 mg, or 200 mg in 50 mL, 100 mL, or 200 mL, respectively, of D_5W or NS.

Storage Store vials at 2°C to 8°C (36°F to 46°F); do not freeze. The reconstituted solution can be stored for up to 1 hour at 2°C to 8°C (36°F to 46°F) prior to dilution into the infusion solution; do not freeze. If the infusion solution is not used immediately, it should be stored in a refrigerator at 2°C to 8°C (36°F to 46°F) and administered within 24 hours of preparation; do not freeze.

Nursing Actions

Patient Education This medication can only be administered by infusion. Report immediately any pain, burning, or swelling at infusion site, or any signs of allergic reaction (eg, respiratory difficulty or swallowing, back pain, chest tightness, rash, hives, or swelling of lips or mouth). Report diarrhea and muscle cramps or weakness.

Antihemophilic Factor (Human)
(an tee hee moe FIL ik FAK tor HYU man)

Brand Names: U.S. Hemofil M; Koāte®-DVI; Monoclate-P®

Index Terms AHF (Human); Factor VIII (Human)

Pharmacologic Category Antihemophilic Agent; Blood Product Derivative

Medication Safety Issues

Sound-alike/look-alike issues:

Factor VIII may be confused with Factor XIII

Other safety concerns:

Confusion may occur due to the omitting of "Factor VIII" from some product labeling. Review product contents carefully prior to dispensing any antihemophilic factor.

Pregnancy Risk Factor C

Lactation Excretion in breast milk unknown/use caution

Use Prevention and treatment of hemorrhagic episodes in patients with hemophilia A (classic hemophilia); perioperative management of hemophilia A; can be of significant therapeutic value in patients with acquired factor VIII inhibitors not exceeding 10 Bethesda units/mL

Available Dosage Forms

Injection, powder for reconstitution:

Hemofil M: ~250 int. units, ~500 int. units, ~1000 int. units, ~1700 int. units

Koāte®-DVI: ~500 int. units, ~1000 int. units

Monoclate-P®: ~250 int. units, ~500 int. units, ~1000 int. units, ~1500 int. units

General Dosage Range I.V.: *Children and Adults:* Dosage varies greatly depending on indication

Administration

I.V. Over 5-10 minutes (maximum: 10 mL/minute). Infuse Monoclate-P® at 2 mL/minute.

Nursing Actions

Physical Assessment Monitor patient closely during and after infusion for any change in vital signs, cardiac and CNS status, or hypersensitivity reactions (eg, chills, fever, chest pain, respiratory difficulty). Assess results of hematocrit and coagulation studies. Monitor bleeding and coagulation status. Monitor for anemia.

Patient Education This medication can only be given intravenously. Report immediately any sudden-onset headache, rash, chest or back pain, wheezing or respiratory difficulties, hives, itching, low-grade fever, stomach pain, or nausea/vomiting to prescriber. Wear identification indicating that you have a hemophilic condition.

Antihemophilic Factor (Recombinant)

(an tee hee moe FIL ik FAK tor ree KOM be nant)

Brand Names: U.S. Advate; Helixate® FS; Kogenate® FS; Recombinate; Xyntha®; Xyntha® Solofuse™

Index Terms AHF (Recombinant); Factor VIII (Recombinant); rAHF

Pharmacologic Category Antihemophilic Agent

Medication Safety Issues

Sound-alike/look-alike issues:

Factor VIII may be confused with Factor XIII

Other safety concerns:

Confusion may occur due to the omitting of "Factor VIII" from some product labeling. Review product contents carefully prior to dispensing any antihemophilic factor.

Pregnancy Risk Factor C

Lactation Excretion in breast milk unknown/use caution

Use Prevention and treatment of hemorrhagic episodes in patients with hemophilia A (classic hemophilia or congenital factor VIII deficiency); perioperative management of hemophilia A; routine prophylaxis in patients with hemophilia A to prevent bleeding episodes (Advate, Helixate® FS, Kogenate® FS)

Note: Helixate® FS and Kogenate® FS are also approved in children with hemophilia A with no preexisting joint damage to reduce risk of joint damage. In addition, Recombinate can be of therapeutic value in patients with acquired factor VIII inhibitors ≤10 Bethesda units/mL.

Available Dosage Forms

Injection, powder for reconstitution:

Recombinate: 2000 int. units

Injection, powder for reconstitution [preservative free]:

Advate: 250 int. units, 500 int. units, 1000 int. units, 1500 int. units, 2000 int. units, 3000 int. units

Helixate® FS: 250 int. units, 500 int. units, 1000 int. units, 2000 int. units, 3000 int. units

Kogenate® FS: 250 int. units, 500 int. units, 1000 int. units, 2000 int. units, 3000 int. units

Recombinate: 250 int. units, 500 int. units, 1000 int. units, 1500 int. units

Xyntha®: 250 int. units, 500 int. units, 1000 int. units, 2000 int. units

Xyntha® Solofuse™: 1000 int. units, 2000 int. units, 3000 int. units

General Dosage Range I.V.: *Children and Adults:* Dosage varies greatly depending on indication

Administration

I.V. Use administration sets/tubing provided by manufacturer (if provided).

Advate: Infuse over ≤5 minutes (maximum: 10 mL/minute)

Helixate® FS, Kogenate® FS: Infuse over 1-15 minutes; based on patient tolerability

Recombinate reconstituted with 5 mL of SWFI: Infuse at a rate of ≤5 mL/minute (maximum: 5 mL/minute)

Recombinate reconstituted with 10 mL of SWFI: Infuse at a rate of ≤10 mL/minute (maximum: 10 mL/minute)

Xyntha®, Xyntha® Solufuse™: Infuse over several minutes; adjust based on patient comfort. Do not admix or administer in same tubing as other medications.

Nursing Actions

Physical Assessment Monitor patient closely during and after infusion for any change in vital signs, cardiac and CNS status, or hypersensitivity reactions (eg, chills, fever, chest pain, respiratory difficulty). Assess results of hematocrit and coagulation studies. Monitor bleeding and coagulation status. Monitor for anemia.

Patient Education This medication can only be given intravenously. Report immediately to doctor any sudden-onset headache, rash, chest or back pain, wheezing or respiratory difficulties, hives, itching, low-grade fever, change in thinking clearly, change in strength on one side over another, weakness, or significant bleeding or inability to stop bleeding. Wear identification indicating that you have a hemophilic condition.

Antihemophilic Factor/von Willebrand Factor Complex (Human)

(an tee hee moe FIL ik FAK tor von WILL le brand FAK tor KOM plex HYU man)

Brand Names: U.S. Alphanate®; Humate-P®; Wilate®

Index Terms AHF (Human); Factor VIII (Human); Factor VIII Concentrate; FVIII/vWF; von Willebrand Factor/Factor VIII Complex; VWF/FVIII Concentrate; VWF:RCo; vWF:RCof

Pharmacologic Category Antihemophilic Agent; Blood Product Derivative

Medication Safety Issues

Sound-alike/look-alike issues:

Factor VIII may be confused with Factor XIII

Pregnancy Risk Factor C

Lactation Excretion in breast milk unknown/use caution

Use

Factor VIII deficiency: Alphanate®, Humate-P®: Prevention and treatment of hemorrhagic episodes in patients with hemophilia A (classical hemophilia) or acquired factor VIII deficiency (Alphanate® only); **Note:** Wilate® is not approved for use in patients with hemophilia A or acquired factor VIII deficiency

von Willebrand disease (VWD):

Alphanate®: Prophylaxis with surgical and/or invasive procedures in patients with VWD when desmopressin is either ineffective or contraindicated; **Note:** Not indicated for patients with severe VWD undergoing major surgery

Humate-P®: Treatment of spontaneous or trauma-induced bleeding, as well as prevention of excessive bleeding during and after surgery in patients with severe VWD, including mild or moderate disease where use of desmopressin is known or suspected to be inadequate; **Note:** Not indicated for the prophylaxis of spontaneous bleeding episodes

Wilate®: Treatment of spontaneous and trauma-induced bleeding in patients with severe VWD, including mild or moderate disease where use of desmopressin is known or suspected to be inadequate or contraindicated; **Note:** Not indicated for prophylaxis of spontaneous bleeding or prevention of excessive bleeding during and after surgery)

Available Dosage Forms

Injection, powder for reconstitution [human derived]:

Alphanate®:

250 int. units [Factor VIII and VWF:RCo ratio varies by lot]

500 int. units [Factor VIII and VWF:RCo ratio varies by lot]

1000 int. units [Factor VIII and VWF:RCo ratio varies by lot]

1500 int. units [Factor VIII and VWF:RCo ratio varies by lot]

Humate-P®:

FVIII 250 int. units and VWF:RCo 600 int. units

FVIII 500 int. units and VWF:RCo 1200 int. units

FVIII 1000 int. units and VWF:RCo 2400 int. units

Wilate®:

FVIII 500 int. units and VWF:RCo 500 int. units

FVIII 1000 int. units and VWF:RCo 1000 int. units

General Dosage Range I.V.: *Children and Adults:* Dosage varies greatly depending on indication

Administration

I.V.

Alphanate®: Infuse slowly (maximum rate 10 mL/minute)

Humate-P®: Infuse slowly (maximum rate 4 mL/minute)

Wilate®: Infuse slowly at a rate of 2-4 mL/minute

Nursing Actions

Physical Assessment Monitor patient closely during and after infusion for any change in vital signs, cardiac and CNS status, or hypersensitivity reactions (eg, chills, fever, chest pain, respiratory difficulty). Assess results of hematocrit and coagulation studies. Monitor bleeding and coagulation status. Monitor for anemia.

Patient Education This medication can only be given intravenously; administer slowly. Report immediately any sudden-onset headache, rash, chest or back pain, wheezing or respiratory difficulties, hives, itching, low-grade fever, stomach pain, or nausea/vomiting to prescriber. Wear identification indicating that you have a hemophilic condition.

Anti-inhibitor Coagulant Complex

(an TEE in HI bi tor coe AG yoo lant KOM pleks)

Brand Names: U.S. Feiba NF; Feiba VH [DSC]

Index Terms AICC; aPCC; Coagulant Complex Inhibitor

Pharmacologic Category Activated Prothrombin Complex Concentrate (aPCC); Antihemophilic Agent; Blood Product Derivative

Pregnancy Risk Factor C

Use Hemophilia A & B patients with inhibitors who are to undergo surgery or those who are bleeding

Unlabeled Use Acquired hemophilia with factor VIII or inhibitor titers >5 Bethesda units (BU)

Available Dosage Forms

Injection, powder for reconstitution:

Feiba NF: ~500 units, ~1000 units, ~2500 units

General Dosage Range I.V.: *Children and Adults:* 50-100 units/kg every 6-12 hours (maximum: 200 units/kg/day)

Administration

I.V. For I.V. injection or drip infusion only; maximum infusion rate: 2 units/kg/minute. Following reconstitution, complete infusion within 3 hours.

Nursing Actions

Physical Assessment Assess potential for interactions with pharmacological agents patient may be taking that may affect coagulation or platelet function. Monitor patient closely during and after infusion for any change in vital signs, cardiac and CNS status, or hypersensitivity reactions (chills, fever, chest pain, respiratory difficulty). If hypotension develops, the rate of infusion should be slowed and prescriber notified.

Patient Education This medication can only be administered by infusion; you will be monitored during and after infusion. Report immediately any sudden-onset headache, rash, chest or back pain, wheezing or respiratory difficulties, hives, itching, low-grade fever, stomach pain, or nausea/vomiting to prescriber. Wear identification indicating that you have a hemophilic condition.

Antithymocyte Globulin (Equine)

(an te THY moe site GLOB yu lin E kwine)

Brand Names: U.S. Atgam®

Index Terms Antithymocyte Immunoglobulin; ATG; Horse Antihuman Thymocyte Gamma Globulin; Lymphocyte Immune Globulin

Pharmacologic Category Immune Globulin; Immunosuppressant Agent; Polyclonal Antibody

Medication Safety Issues

Sound-alike/look-alike issues:

Antithymocyte globulin equine (Atgam®) may be confused with antithymocyte globulin rabbit (Thymoglobulin®)

Atgam® may be confused with Ativan®

Pregnancy Risk Factor C

Lactation Excretion in breast milk unknown/use caution

Use Prevention and treatment of acute renal allograft rejection; treatment of moderate-to-severe aplastic anemia in patients not considered suitable candidates for bone marrow transplantation

Unlabeled Use Prevention and treatment of other solid organ allograft rejection; prevention or treatment of graft-versus-host disease (GVHD) following allogeneic stem cell transplantation; treatment of myelodysplastic syndrome (MDS)

Available Dosage Forms

Injection, solution:

Atgam®: 50 mg/mL (5 mL)

General Dosage Range I.V.:

Children: Initial: 5-25 mg/kg/day administered daily for 8-14 days; may be followed by administration every other day (maximum: 21 doses in 28 days)

Adults: Initial: 10-20 mg/kg/day administered daily; may be followed by administration every other day (maximum: 21 doses in 28 days)

Administration

I.V. Infuse dose over at least 4 hours. Any severe systemic reaction to the skin test, such as generalized rash, tachycardia, dyspnea, hypotension, or anaphylaxis, should preclude further therapy. Epinephrine and resuscitative equipment should be nearby. Patient may need to be pretreated with an antipyretic, antihistamine, and/or corticosteroid. Mild itching and erythema can be treated with antihistamines. May cause vein irritation (chemical phlebitis) if administered peripherally. Infuse into a vascular shunt, arterial venous fistula, or high-flow central vein through a 0.2-1 micron in-line filter.

First dose: Premedicate with diphenhydramine orally 30 minutes prior to and hydrocortisone I.V. 15 minutes prior to infusion and acetaminophen 2 hours after start of infusion.

Nursing Actions

Physical Assessment Intradermal skin testing and premedication are recommended with the first dose. Treatment for hypersensitivity should be available. Assess for history of previous allergic reactions. Monitor vital signs during infusion and observe for adverse or allergic reactions closely.

Patient Education This medication can only be administered by infusion. You will be closely monitored during the infusion. Ask for assistance if you must get up or change position. Do not have any vaccinations for the next 3 months without consulting prescriber. Immediately report chills; persistent dizziness or nausea; itching or stinging; acute back pain; flank pain; chest pain, tightness, or rapid heartbeat; or respiratory difficulty.

Apomorphine (a poe MOR feen)

Brand Names: U.S. Apokyn®

Index Terms Apomorphine Hydrochloride; Apomorphine Hydrochloride Hemihydrate

Pharmacologic Category Anti-Parkinson's Agent, Dopamine Agonist

Pregnancy Risk Factor C

Lactation Excretion in breast milk unknown/contraindicated

Use Treatment of hypomobility, "off" episodes with Parkinson's disease

Unlabeled Use Treatment of erectile dysfunction

Available Dosage Forms

Injection, solution:

Apokyn®: 10 mg/mL (3 mL)

General Dosage Range Dosage adjustment recommended in patients with renal impairment

SubQ: *Adults:* Initial test dose: 2 mg; Starting dose: 2-3 mg/dose at time of "off" episode; Maintenance dose: 2-6 mg/dose at time of "off" episode (maximum: 20 mg/day; 6 mg/dose; 5 doses/day)

Administration

I.V. Not for I.V. administration.

Other SubQ: Initiate antiemetic 3 days before test dose of apomorphine and continue for 2 months (if patient to be treated) before reassessment. Administer in abdomen, upper arm, or upper leg; change site with each injection. 3 mL cartridges are used with a manual, reusable, multidose injector pen. Injector pen can deliver doses up to 1 mL in 0.02 mL increments. Do not give intravenously; thrombus formation or pulmonary embolism may occur.

Nursing Actions

Physical Assessment Monitor patient closely for 90 minutes following each test dose. Premedication with antiemetic is required prior to each dose. Monitor for orthostatic hypotension, nausea, vomiting, dyskinesias, and excessive sedation or somnolence. Teach patient or caregiver proper injection technique and needle disposal.

Patient Education Follow specific directions for administration with injection pen or syringe and needle disposal. Avoid alcohol. An antiemetic may be prescribed to reduce nausea or vomiting. May cause headache, drowsiness, dizziness, loss of impulse control (possibly manifested as pathological gambling, libido increases, and/or binge eating), postural hypotension, nausea, or vomiting. Report immediately any irregular or rapid heartbeat, chest pain, palpitations, difficulty breathing, or shortness of breath; unusual or sudden sleepiness; unusual muscle or skeletal movements or weakness, tremors, or altered gait; CNS changes (hallucinations, confusion, insomnia, anxiety, or depression); suicide ideation; redness, swelling, or irritation at injection site; changes in the appearance of skin moles; or other unusual skin changes.

Apraclonidine (a pra KLOE ni deen)

Brand Names: U.S. Iopidine®

Index Terms Aplonidine; Apraclonidine Hydrochloride; p-Aminoclonidine

Pharmacologic Category Alpha$_2$ Agonist, Ophthalmic

Medication Safety Issues

Sound-alike/look-alike issues:

Iopidine® may be confused with indapamide, iodine, Lodine®

Pregnancy Risk Factor C

Lactation Excretion in breast milk unknown/use caution

Use Prevention and treatment of postsurgical intraocular pressure (IOP) elevation; short-term, adjunctive therapy in patients who require additional reduction of IOP

Available Dosage Forms

Solution, ophthalmic: 0.5% (5 mL, 10 mL)

Iopidine®: 0.5% (5 mL, 10 mL); 1% (0.1 mL)

General Dosage Range Ophthalmic: *Adults:* 0.5%: Instill 1-2 drops in the affected eye(s) 3 times/day; 1%: Instill 1 drop in operative eye 1 hour prior to and upon completion of surgery

Administration

Other Wait 5 minutes between instillation of other ophthalmic agents to avoid washout of previous dose. After topical instillation, finger pressure should be applied to lacrimal sac to decrease drainage into the nose and throat and minimize possible systemic absorption.

Nursing Actions

Patient Education For use in eyes only. May sting on instillation, do not touch dropper to eye. Visual acuity may be decreased after administration. Night vision may be decreased. Distance vision may be altered.

Aprepitant (ap RE pi tant)

Brand Names: U.S. Emend®

Index Terms L 754030; MK 869

Pharmacologic Category Antiemetic; Substance P/Neurokinin 1 Receptor Antagonist

Medication Safety Issues

Sound-alike/look-alike issues:

Aprepitant may be confused with fosaprepitant

Emend® (aprepitant) oral capsule formulation may be confused with Emend® for injection (fosaprepitant)

Pregnancy Risk Factor B

Lactation Excretion in breast milk unknown/not recommended

Use Prevention of acute and delayed nausea and vomiting associated with moderately- and highly-emetogenic chemotherapy (in combination with other antiemetics); prevention of postoperative nausea and vomiting (PONV)

Mechanism of Action/Effect Prevents acute and delayed vomiting at the substance P/neurokinin 1 (NK$_1$) receptor; augments the antiemetic activity of 5-HT$_3$ receptor antagonists and corticosteroids to inhibit acute and delayed phases of chemotherapy-induced emesis.

Contraindications Hypersensitivity to aprepitant or any component of the formulation; concurrent use with cisapride or pimozide

Warnings/Precautions Use caution with agents primarily metabolized via CYP3A4; aprepitant is a 3A4 inhibitor. Effect on orally administered 3A4 substrates is greater than those administered intravenously. Chronic continuous use is not recommended; however, a single 40 mg aprepitant oral dose is not likely to alter plasma concentrations of CYP3A4 substrates. Use caution with severe hepatic impairment; has not been studied in patients with severe hepatic impairment (Child-Pugh class C). Not studied for treatment of existing nausea and vomiting. Chronic continuous administration is not recommended.

Drug Interactions

Avoid Concomitant Use

Avoid concomitant use of Aprepitant with any of the following: Axitinib; Cisapride; Conivaptan; Pimozide; Tolvaptan

Decreased Effect

Aprepitant may decrease the levels/effects of: ARIPiprazole; Axitinib; Contraceptives (Estrogens); Contraceptives (Progestins); CYP2C9 Substrates; Diclofenac; PARoxetine; Saxagliptin; TOLBUTamide; Warfarin

The levels/effects of Aprepitant may be decreased by: CYP3A4 Inducers (Strong); Cyproterone; Deferasirox; Herbs (CYP3A4 Inducers); PARoxetine; Rifamycin Derivatives; Tocilizumab

Increased Effect/Toxicity

Aprepitant may increase the levels/effects of: ARIPiprazole; Benzodiazepines (metabolized by oxidation); Budesonide (Systemic, Oral Inhalation); Cisapride; Colchicine; Corticosteroids (Systemic); CYP3A4 Substrates; Diltiazem; Eplerenone; Everolimus; FentaNYL; Halofantrine; Ivacaftor; Lurasidone; Pimecrolimus; Pimozide; Propafenone; Ranolazine; Salmeterol; Saxagliptin; Tolvaptan; Vilazodone; Zuclopenthixol

The levels/effects of Aprepitant may be increased by: Antifungal Agents (Azole Derivatives, Systemic); Conivaptan; CYP3A4 Inhibitors (Moderate); CYP3A4 Inhibitors (Strong); Dasatinib; Diltiazem; Ivacaftor

Nutritional/Ethanol Interactions

Food: Aprepitant serum concentration may be increased when taken with grapefruit juice; avoid concurrent use.

Herb/Nutraceutical: Avoid St John's wort (may decrease aprepitant levels).

Adverse Reactions **Note:** Adverse reactions reported as part of a combination chemotherapy regimen or with general anesthesia.

>10%:

Central nervous system: Fatigue (≤18%)

Gastrointestinal: Nausea (6% to 13%), constipation (9% to 10%)

Neuromuscular & skeletal: Weakness (≤18%)

Miscellaneous: Hiccups (11%)

1% to 10%:

Cardiovascular: Hypotension (≤6%), bradycardia (≤4%)

Central nervous system: Dizziness (≤7%)

Endocrine & metabolic: Dehydration (≤6%)

Gastrointestinal: Diarrhea (≤10%), dyspepsia (≤6%), abdominal pain (≤5%), epigastric discomfort (4%), gastritis (4%), stomatitis (3%)

Hepatic: ALT increased (≤6%), AST increased (3%)

Renal: Proteinuria (7%), BUN increased (5%)

Available Dosage Forms

Capsule, oral:

Emend®: 40 mg, 80 mg, 125 mg

Combination package, oral:

Emend®: Capsule: 80 mg (2s) and Capsule: 125 mg (1s)

General Dosage Range Oral: *Adults:* 125 mg on day 1, followed by 80 mg on days 2 and 3 **or** 40 mg within 3 hours prior to induction with anesthesia

Administration

Oral

Chemotherapy induced nausea/vomiting: Administer with or without food. First dose should be given 1 hour prior to antineoplastic therapy; subsequent doses should be given in the morning.

PONV: Administer within 3 hours prior to induction; follow healthcare providers instructions about food/drink restrictions prior to surgery.

Stability

Storage Store at room temperature of 20°C to 25°C (68°F to 77°F).

Nursing Actions

Physical Assessment Monitor for fatigue, weakness, gastrointestinal upset, and dehydration.

Patient Education This medication is intended to prevent or treat nausea/vomiting; it may be prescribed in combination with other medications; follow directions and timing exactly. May by taken with or without food; do not take with grapefruit juice. Report unusual fatigue, weakness, dizziness, disorientation, abdominal discomfort, chest pain, or respiratory distress to prescriber.

Dietary Considerations May be taken with or without food.

Arformoterol (ar for MOE ter ol)

Brand Names: U.S. Brovana®

Index Terms (R,R)-Formoterol L-Tartrate; Arformoterol Tartrate

Pharmacologic Category Beta$_2$-Adrenergic Agonist; Beta$_2$-Adrenergic Agonist, Long-Acting

Medication Guide Available Yes

Pregnancy Risk Factor C

Lactation Excretion in breast milk unknown/use caution

Use Long-term maintenance treatment of bronchoconstriction in chronic obstructive pulmonary disease (COPD), including chronic bronchitis and emphysema

Available Dosage Forms

Solution, for nebulization:

Brovana®: 15 mcg/2 mL (30s, 60s)

General Dosage Range Nebulization: *Adults:* 5 mcg twice daily (maximum: 30 mcg/day)

Administration

Inhalation Nebulization: Remove each vial from individually sealed foil pouch immediately before use. Use with standard jet nebulizer connected to an air compressor, administer with mouthpiece or face mask. Administer vial undiluted and do not mix with other medications in nebulizer.

Nursing Actions

Physical Assessment Teach patient appropriate use and care of nebulizer.

Patient Education This drug is intended for long-term use. Do not mix with other medications in your nebulizer. Maintain adequate hydration, unless instructed to restrict fluid intake. You may experience nervousness, tremor, headache, muscle cramps, trouble sleeping, dizziness, or tiredness. Report rapid heart rate, chest pain, or palpitations; swelling of extremities or weight gain; back or leg pain; increased shortness of breath; or difficulty breathing.

Argatroban (ar GA troh ban)

Pharmacologic Category Anticoagulant, Thrombin Inhibitor

Medication Safety Issues

Sound-alike/look-alike issues:

Argatroban may be confused with Aggrastat®, Orgaran®

High alert medication:

The Institute for Safe Medication Practices (ISMP) includes this medication among its list of drugs which have a heightened risk of causing significant patient harm when used in error.

Pregnancy Risk Factor B

Lactation Excretion in breast milk unknown/not recommended

Use Prophylaxis or treatment of thrombosis in patients with heparin-induced thrombocytopenia (HIT); adjunct to percutaneous coronary intervention (PCI) in patients who have or are at risk of thrombosis associated with HIT

Unlabeled Use To maintain extracorporeal circuit patency (prefilter administration) of continuous renal replacement therapy (CRRT) in critically-ill patients with HIT

Available Dosage Forms

Infusion, premixed in NS: 125 mg (125 mL)

Infusion, premixed in water for injection: 50 mg (50 mL)

Injection, solution: 100 mg/mL (2.5 mL)

General Dosage Range Dosage adjustment recommended in patients with hepatic impairment

I.V.:

Children: Initial dose: 0.75 mcg/kg/minute; dosage may be adjusted in increments of 0.1-0.25 mcg/kg/minute

Adults: Bolus dose: 150-350 mcg/kg during procedure; Infusion: Initial: 2 mcg/kg/minute **or** 25 mcg/kg/minute during procedure; Maintenance: 0.5-10 mcg/kg/minute (maximum: 10 mcg/kg/minute) **or** 25-40 mcg/kg/minute during procedure

Adults (critically-ill): Initial: 0.2 mcg/kg/minute; Maintenance: 0.5-1.3 mcg/kg/minute

Administration

I.V. The 2.5 mL (100 mg/mL) **concentrated** vial **must be diluted to 1 mg/mL** prior to administration. The premixed 50 mL or 125 mL (1 mg/mL) vial requires no further dilution. The premixed 1 mg/mL vial may be inverted for use with an infusion set.

Nursing Actions

Physical Assessment Monitor for abnormal bleeding, GI pain, epistaxis, hematuria, and irritation at infusion site. Observe bleeding precautions.

Patient Education This medication can only be administered by intravenous infusion and you will be monitored with blood tests during therapy. You may have a tendency to bleed easily; use electric razor, brush teeth with soft brush, floss with waxed floss, avoid all scissors or sharp instruments (knives, needles, etc), and avoid injury or bruising. Report stomach cramping or pain, dark or bloody stools, blood in urine, acute headache or confusion, respiratory difficulty, nosebleed, or bleeding from gums.

Aripiprazole (ay ri PIP ray zole)

Brand Names: U.S. Abilify Discmelt®; Abilify®

Index Terms BMS 337039; OPC-14597

Pharmacologic Category Antipsychotic Agent, Atypical

Medication Safety Issues

Sound-alike/look-alike issues:

Abilify® may be confused with Ambien®

ARIPiprazole may be confused with proton pump inhibitors (dexlansoprazole, esomeprazole, lansoprazole, omeprazole, pantoprazole, RABEprazole)

Medication Guide Available Yes

Pregnancy Risk Factor C

Lactation Excretion in breast milk unknown/not recommended

Breast-Feeding Considerations Based on limited data from case reports, small amounts of aripiprazole have been detected in breast milk.

Use

Oral: Acute and maintenance treatment of schizophrenia; acute (manic and mixed episodes) and maintenance treatment of bipolar I disorder as monotherapy or as an adjunct to lithium or valproic acid; adjunctive treatment of major depressive disorder; treatment of irritability associated with autistic disorder

Injection: Agitation associated with schizophrenia or bipolar I disorder

Unlabeled Use Depression with psychotic features; aggression (children); conduct disorder (children); Tourette syndrome (children); psychosis/agitation related to Alzheimer's dementia

Mechanism of Action/Effect Aripiprazole (quinolinone antipsychotic) is a dopamine-serotonin system stabilizer with activity at dopamine and serotonin receptors.

Contraindications Hypersensitivity to aripiprazole or any component of the formulation

Warnings/Precautions [U.S. Boxed Warning]: Elderly patients with dementia-related psychosis treated with antipsychotics are at an increased risk of death compared to placebo. Most deaths appeared to be either cardiovascular (eg, heart failure, sudden death) or infectious (eg, pneumonia) in nature. In addition, an increased incidence of cerebrovascular effects (eg, transient ischemic attack, cerebrovascular accidents) has been reported in studies of placebo-controlled trials of aripiprazole in elderly patients with dementia-related psychosis. Aripiprazole is not approved for the treatment of dementia-related psychosis.

[U.S. Boxed Warning]: Antidepressants increase the risk of suicidal thinking and behavior in children, adolescents, and young adults (18-24 years of age) with major depressive disorder (MDD) and other psychiatric disorders; consider risk prior to prescribing. The possibility of a suicide attempt is inherent in major depression and may persist until remission occurs. Patients treated with antidepressants should be observed for clinical worsening and suicidality, especially during the initial few months of a course of drug therapy, or at times of dose changes, either increases or decreases. Prescriptions should be written for the smallest quantity consistent with good patient care. The patient's family or caregiver should be alerted to monitor patients for the emergence of suicidality and associated behaviors; patients should be instructed to notify their healthcare provider if any of these symptoms or worsening depression or psychosis occur.

Leukopenia, neutropenia, and agranulocytosis (sometimes fatal) have been reported in clinical trials and postmarketing reports with antipsychotic use; presence of risk factors (eg, pre-existing low WBC or history of drug-induced leuko-/neutropenia) should prompt periodic blood count assessment. Discontinue therapy at first signs of blood dyscrasias or if absolute neutrophil count <1000/mm^3.

A medication guide concerning the use of antidepressants should be dispensed with each prescription. **Aripiprazole is not FDA approved for adjunctive treatment of depression in children.**

May cause extrapyramidal symptoms (EPS), including pseudoparkinsonism, acute dystonic reactions, akathisia, and tardive dyskinesia (risk of these reactions is very low relative to typical/conventional antipsychotics, frequencies reported are similar to placebo). Risk of dystonia (and probably other EPS) may be greater with increased doses, use of conventional antipsychotics, males, and younger patients. May be associated with neuroleptic malignant syndrome (NMS).

May be sedating, use with caution in disorders where CNS depression is a feature. May cause orthostatic hypotension (although reported rates are similar to placebo); use caution in patients at risk of this effect or those who would not tolerate transient hypotensive episodes (cerebrovascular disease, cardiovascular disease, or other medications which may predispose).

Use caution in patients with Parkinson's disease; predisposition to seizures; and severe cardiac disease. May alter cardiac conduction; life-threatening arrhythmias have occurred with therapeutic doses of antipsychotics. Esophageal dysmotility and aspiration have been associated with antipsychotic use; use caution in patients at risk of pneumonia (eg, Alzheimer's disease). May alter temperature regulation. Significant weight gain has been observed with antipsychotic therapy; incidence varies with product. Monitor waist circumference and BMI.

Atypical antipsychotics have been associated with development of hyperglycemia; in some cases, may be extreme and associated with ketoacidosis, hyperosmolar coma, or death. Reports of hyperglycemia with aripiprazole therapy have been few and specific risk associated with this agent is not known. Use caution in patients with diabetes or other disorders of glucose regulation; monitor for worsening of glucose control.

Tablets contain lactose; avoid use in patients with galactose intolerance or glucose-galactose malabsorption.

Abilify Discmelt®: Use caution in phenylketonuria; contains phenylalanine.

Drug Interactions

Avoid Concomitant Use

Avoid concomitant use of ARIPiprazole with any of the following: Metoclopramide

Decreased Effect

ARIPiprazole may decrease the levels/effects of: Amphetamines; Anti-Parkinson's Agents (Dopamine Agonist); Quinagolide

The levels/effects of ARIPiprazole may be decreased by: CYP3A4 Inducers; Deferasirox; Lithium formulations; Peginterferon Alfa-2b; Tocilizumab

Increased Effect/Toxicity

ARIPiprazole may increase the levels/effects of: Alcohol (Ethyl); CNS Depressants; Methotrimeprazine; Methylphenidate; Serotonin Modulators

The levels/effects of ARIPiprazole may be increased by: Abiraterone Acetate; Acetylcholinesterase Inhibitors (Central); CYP2D6 Inhibitors (Moderate); CYP2D6 Inhibitors (Strong); CYP2D6 Inhibitors (Weak); CYP3A4 Inhibitors (Moderate); CYP3A4 Inhibitors (Strong); CYP3A4 Inhibitors (Weak); Dasatinib; Droperidol; HydrOXYzine; Ivacaftor; Lithium formulations; Methotrimeprazine; Methylphenidate; Metoclopramide; Tetrabenazine

Nutritional/Ethanol Interactions

Ethanol: May increase CNS depression; monitor for increased effects with coadministration. Caution patients about effects.

Food: Ingestion with a high-fat meal delays time to peak plasma level.

Herb/Nutraceutical: St John's wort may decrease aripiprazole levels. Avoid kava kava, gotu kola, valerian, St John's wort (may increase CNS depression).

Adverse Reactions Unless otherwise noted, frequency of adverse reactions is shown as reported for adult patients receiving oral administration. Spectrum and incidence of adverse effects similar in children; exceptions noted when incidence much higher in children.

>10%:

Central nervous system: Headache (27%; injection 12%), agitation (19%), insomnia (18%), anxiety (17%), EPS (dose related; 5% to 16%; children 6% to 26%), akathisia (dose related; 8% to 13%; injection 2%), sedation (dose related; 5% to 11%; children 8% to 24%; injection 3% to 9%)

Gastrointestinal: Weight gain (2% to 30%; highest frequency in patients with baseline BMI <23 and prolonged use), nausea (15%; injection 9%), constipation (11%), vomiting (11%; children 9% to 14%; injection 3%), dyspepsia (9%)

1% to 10%:

Cardiovascular: Orthostatic hypotension (1% to 4%; injection 1% to 3%), tachycardia (injection 2%), chest pain, hypertension, peripheral edema

Central nervous system: Dizziness (10%; injection 8%), pyrexia (children 5% to 9%), restlessness (5% to 6%), fatigue (dose related; 6%; children 8% to 17%; injection 2%), lethargy (children 2% to 5%), lightheadedness (4%), pain (3%), dystonia (children 1%), hypersomnia (1%), irritability (children 1%), coordination impaired, suicidal ideation

Dermatologic: Rash (children 2%), hyperhidrosis

Endocrine & metabolic: Dysmenorrhea (children 2%)

Gastrointestinal: Salivation increased (dose related; children 4% to 9%), appetite decreased (children 4% to 7%), appetite increased (children 7%), xerostomia (5%), toothache (4%), abdominal discomfort (3%), diarrhea (children 5%), weight loss

Local: Injection site reaction (injection)

Neuromuscular & skeletal: Tremor (dose related; 5% to 6%; children 6% to 10%), extremity pain (4%), stiffness (4%), myalgia (2%), spasm (2%), arthralgia (children 1%), dyskinesia (children 1%), CPK increased, weakness

Ocular: Blurred vision (3%; children 3% to 8%)

Respiratory: Nasopharyngitis (children 6%), pharyngolaryngeal pain (3%), cough (3%), rhinorrhea (children 2%), aspiration pneumonia, dyspnea, nasal congestion

Miscellaneous: Thirst (children 1%)

Pharmacodynamics/Kinetics

Onset of Action Initial: 1-3 weeks

Available Dosage Forms

Injection, solution:

Abilify®: 7.5 mg/mL (1.3 mL)

Solution, oral:

Abilify®: 1 mg/mL (150 mL)

Tablet, oral:

Abilify®: 2 mg, 5 mg, 10 mg, 15 mg, 20 mg, 30 mg

Tablet, orally disintegrating, oral:

Abilify Discmelt®: 10 mg, 15 mg

General Dosage Range Dosage adjustment recommended in patients on concomitant therapy

Oral:

Children 6-9 years: 5-15 mg once daily (maximum: 15 mg/day)

Children ≥10 years: 5-30 mg once daily (maximum: 30 mg/day)

Adults: 10-30 mg once daily (maximum: 30 mg/day)

I.M.: *Adults:* 9.75 mg as a single dose (maximum: 30 mg/day)

Administration

Oral May be administered with or without food. Tablet and oral solution may be interchanged on a mg-per-mg basis, up to 25 mg. Doses using 30 mg tablets should be exchanged for 25 mg oral solution. Orally disintegrating tablets (Abilify Discmelt®) are bioequivalent to the immediate release tablets (Abilify®).

Orally-disintegrating tablet: Remove from foil blister by peeling back (do not push tablet through the foil). Place tablet in mouth immediately upon removal. Tablet dissolves rapidly in saliva and may be swallowed without liquid. If needed, can be taken with liquid. Do not split tablet.

I.M. For I.M. use only; do not administer SubQ or I.V.; inject slowly into deep muscle mass

Stability

Storage

Injection solution: Store at controlled room temperature of 25°C (77°F); excursions permitted to 15°C to 30°C (59°F to 86°F). Protect from light.

Oral solution: Store at controlled room temperature of 25°C (77°F); excursions permitted to 15°C to 30°C (59°F to 86°F). Use within 6 months after opening.

Tablet: Store at controlled room temperature of 25°C (77°F); excursions permitted to 15°C to 30°C (59°F to 86°F).

Nursing Actions

Physical Assessment Assess vital signs, blood pressure, mental status, thoughts of suicide ideation, abnormal involuntary movements, and extrapyramidal symptoms. Weight and waist circumference should be assessed prior to treatment, at 4 weeks, 8 weeks, 12 weeks, and then at quarterly intervals. This drug may alter glucose regulation and control; monitor closely. Monitor for extrapyramidal symptoms prior to and periodically during therapy.

Patient Education Take at the same time of day, without regard to meals. Do not alter dose; it may take some time to achieve desired results. Avoid alcohol. If you have diabetes, monitor blood glucose levels closely prior to treatment and periodically throughout; may cause hyperglycemia. You may be more vulnerable to overheating and dehydration while taking this medication; maintain adequate hydration. May cause headache, dizziness, problems sleeping, anxiety, nausea, vomiting, constipation, or orthostatic hypotension. Report chest pain or palpitations; persistent gastrointestinal effects; tremors; involuntary movements; altered gait; change in vision; change in mental status (especially suicide ideation); or weight gain.

Dietary Considerations May be taken with or without food. Some products may contain phenylalanine.

Armodafinil (ar moe DAF i nil)

Brand Names: U.S. Nuvigil®

Index Terms R-modafinil

Pharmacologic Category Stimulant

Medication Guide Available Yes

Pregnancy Risk Factor C

Lactation Excretion in breast milk unknown/use caution

Use Improve wakefulness in patients with excessive daytime sleepiness associated with narcolepsy and shift work sleep disorder (SWSD); adjunctive therapy for obstructive sleep apnea/hypopnea syndrome (OSAHS)

Mechanism of Action/Effect Armodafinil is a stimulant with effects. The exact mechanism of action of armodafinil is unknown.

Contraindications Hypersensitivity to armodafinil, modafinil, or any component of the formulation

Warnings/Precautions For use following complete evaluation of sleepiness and in conjunction with other standard treatments (eg, CPAP). The degree of sleepiness should be reassessed frequently; some patients may not return to a normal level of wakefulness. Use is not recommended with a history of angina, cardiac ischemia, recent history of myocardial infarction, left ventricular hypertrophy, or patients with mitral valve prolapse who have developed mitral valve prolapse syndrome with previous CNS stimulant use. Blood pressure monitoring may be required in patients on armodafinil. New or additional antihypertensive therapy may be needed.

Serious and life-threatening rashes including Stevens-Johnson syndrome, toxic epidermal necrolysis, and drug rash with eosinophilia and systemic symptoms have been reported with modafinil, the racemate of armodafinil. In clinical trials of modafinil, these rashes were more likely to occur in children; however, in the postmarketing period, serious reactions have occurred in both adults and children. Most cases have been reported within the first 5 weeks of initiating therapy; however, rare cases have occurred after prolonged therapy.

Caution should be exercised when modafinil is given to patients with a history of psychosis; may impair the ability to engage in potentially hazardous activities. Stimulants may unmask tics in individuals with coexisting Tourette's syndrome. Use caution with renal or hepatic impairment (dosage adjustment in hepatic dysfunction is recommended). Use reduced doses in elderly patients. Safety and efficacy in children <17 years of age have not been established.

Drug Interactions

Avoid Concomitant Use

Avoid concomitant use of Armodafinil with any of the following: Axitinib; Clopidogrel; Conivaptan; Iobenguane I 123

Decreased Effect

Armodafinil may decrease the levels/effects of: ARIPiprazole; Axitinib; Clopidogrel; Contraceptives (Estrogens); CycloSPORINE; CycloSPORINE (Systemic); Iobenguane I 123; Saxagliptin

The levels/effects of Armodafinil may be decreased by: CYP3A4 Inducers (Strong); Deferasirox; Herbs (CYP3A4 Inducers); Tocilizumab

Increased Effect/Toxicity

Armodafinil may increase the levels/effects of: Citalopram; CYP2C19 Substrates; Sympathomimetics

The levels/effects of Armodafinil may be increased by: Atomoxetine; Cannabinoids; Conivaptan; CYP3A4 Inhibitors (Moderate); CYP3A4 Inhibitors (Strong); Dasatinib; Ivacaftor; Linezolid

Nutritional/Ethanol Interactions
Ethanol: Avoid or limit ethanol.
Food: Delays absorption, but minimal effects on bioavailability. Food may affect the onset and time course of armodafinil.

Adverse Reactions
>10%: Central nervous system: Headache (14% to 23%; dose-related)
1% to 10%:
Cardiovascular: Palpitation (2%), increased heart rate (1%)
Central nervous system: Dizziness (5%), insomnia (4% to 6%; dose related), anxiety (4%), depression (1% to 3%; dose related), fatigue (2%), agitation (1%), attention disturbance (1%), depressed mood (1%), migraine (1%), nervousness (1%), pain (1%), pyrexia (1%), tremor (1%)
Dermatologic: Rash (1% to 4%; dose related), contact dermatitis (1%), hyperhidrosis (1%)
Gastrointestinal: Nausea (6% to 9%; dose related), xerostomia (2% to 7%; dose related), diarrhea (4%), abdominal pain (2%), dyspepsia (2%), anorexia (1%), appetite decreased (1%), constipation (1%), loose stools (1%), vomiting (1%)
Genitourinary: Polyuria (1%)
Hepatic: GGT increased (1%)
Neuromuscular & skeletal: Paresthesia (1%)
Respiratory: Dyspnea (1%)
Miscellaneous: Flu-like syndrome (1%), thirst (1%)

Controlled Substance C-IV

Available Dosage Forms
Tablet, oral:
Nuvigil®: 50 mg, 150 mg, 250 mg

General Dosage Range Dosage adjustment recommended in patients with hepatic impairment
Oral: *Adults:* 150-250 mg once daily

Administration
Oral May be administered without regard to food.

Stability
Storage Store at 20°C to 25°C (68°F to 77°F).

Nursing Actions
Physical Assessment Monitor blood pressure at the beginning of therapy and periodically throughout.
Patient Education Avoid or limit alcohol. May cause headache, dizziness, dry mouth, or nausea. Report changes in thinking, persistent insomnia or headaches, rash, or chest pain or pressure.

Dietary Considerations Take with or without meals.

Arsenic Trioxide (AR se nik tri OKS id)

Brand Names: U.S. Trisenox®
Index Terms As_2O_3
Pharmacologic Category Antineoplastic Agent, Miscellaneous

Medication Safety Issues
High alert medication:
This medication is in a class the Institute for Safe Medication Practices (ISMP) includes among its list of drugs which have a heightened risk of causing significant patient harm when used in error.

Pregnancy Risk Factor D
Lactation Enters breast milk/not recommended
Use Remission induction and consolidation in patients with relapsed or refractory acute promyelocytic leukemia (APL) characterized by t(15;17) translocation or PML/RAR-alpha gene expression
Unlabeled Use Initial treatment of APL, treatment of myelodysplastic syndrome (MDS)

Available Dosage Forms
Injection, solution [preservative free]:
Trisenox®: 1 mg/mL (10 mL)

General Dosage Range Dosage adjustment recommended for renal impairment.
I.V.: *Children ≥4 years and Adults:* Induction: 0.15 mg/kg/day (maximum: 60 doses); Consolidation: 0.15 mg/kg/day (maximum: 25 doses over a period of up to 5 weeks)

Administration
I.V. I.V. infusion over 1-2 hours. If acute vasomotor reactions occur, infuse over a maximum of 4 hours. Does not require administration via a central venous catheter.
I.V. Detail pH: 7.5-8.5

Nursing Actions
Physical Assessment Monitor cardiac and electrolyte status at beginning of and periodically during therapy.
Patient Education This medication can only be administered by intravenous infusion. Report immediately any redness, swelling, pain, or burning at infusion site. May cause dizziness, fatigue, blurred vision, nausea, vomiting, diarrhea, or decreased appetite. Report immediately unexplained fever; respiratory difficulty; chest pain or palpitations; confusion, lightheadedness, or fainting; unusual joint, back, or muscle pain; or tingling or loss of feeling.

Related Information
Management of Drug Extravasations *on page 1269*

Asenapine (a SEN a peen)

Brand Names: U.S. Saphris®
Pharmacologic Category Antimanic Agent; Antipsychotic Agent, Atypical
Pregnancy Risk Factor C
Lactation Excretion in breast milk unknown/not recommended
Use Acute and maintenance treatment of schizophrenia; treatment of acute mania or mixed

episodes associated with bipolar I disorder (as monotherapy or in combination with lithium or valproate)

Mechanism of Action/Effect Atypical antipsychotic with high affinity for serotonin, dopamine, alpha$_1$- and alpha$_2$-adrenergic receptors, and histamine receptors; no affinity for muscarinic receptors. Results in improvement of psychotic symptoms and reduction of extrapyramidal and antimuscarinic side effects as compared to typical antipsychotics.

Contraindications Hypersensitivity to asenapine or any component of the formulation

Warnings/Precautions [U.S. Boxed Warning]: Elderly patients with dementia-related psychosis treated with atypical antipsychotics are at an increased risk of death compared to placebo. Most deaths appeared to be either cardiovascular (eg, heart failure, sudden death) or infectious (eg, pneumonia) in nature. In addition, an increased incidence of cerebrovascular effects (eg, transient ischemic attack, cerebrovascular accidents) has been reported in studies of placebo-controlled trials of antipsychotics in elderly patients with dementia-related psychosis. Asenapine is not approved for the treatment of dementia-related psychosis.

Leukopenia, neutropenia, and agranulocytosis (sometimes fatal) have been reported in clinical trials and postmarketing reports with antipsychotic use; presence of risk factors (eg, pre-existing low WBC or history of drug-induced leuko/neutropenia) should prompt periodic blood count assessment. Discontinue therapy at first signs of blood dyscrasias or if absolute neutrophil count <1000/mm^3.

May be sedating; use with caution in disorders where CNS depression is a feature. Use with caution in Parkinson's disease. Use with caution in patients at risk of seizures, including those with a history of seizures, head trauma, brain damage, alcoholism, or concurrent therapy with medications which may lower seizure threshold. Use is not recommended in severe hepatic impairment; increased drug concentrations may occur. Esophageal dysmotility and aspiration have been associated with antipsychotic use; use with caution in patients at risk of aspiration pneumonia (ie, Alzheimer's disease). Elevates prolactin levels; use with caution in breast cancer or other prolactin-dependent tumors. May alter temperature regulation.

Use with caution in patients with cardiovascular diseases (eg, heart failure, history of myocardial infarction or ischemia, cerebrovascular disease, conduction abnormalities). May cause orthostatic hypotension; use with caution in patients at risk of this effect (eg, concurrent medication use which may predispose to hypotension/bradycardia or presence of hypovolemia) or in those who would not tolerate transient hypotensive episodes. May result in QT_c prolongation. Risk may be increased by conditions or concomitant medications which cause bradycardia, hypokalemia, and/or hypomagnesemia. Avoid use in combination with QT_c-prolonging drugs and in patients with congenital long QT syndrome or patients with history of cardiac arrhythmia.

May cause extrapyramidal symptoms (EPS), including pseudoparkinsonism, acute dystonic reactions, akathisia, and tardive dyskinesia. Risk of dystonia (and probably other EPS) may be greater with increased doses, use of conventional antipsychotics, males, and younger patients. Risk of neuroleptic malignant syndrome (NMS) may be increased in patients with Parkinson's disease or Lewy body dementia. May cause hyperglycemia; in some cases may be extreme and associated with ketoacidosis, hyperosmolar coma, or death. Use with caution in patients with diabetes or other disorders of glucose regulation; monitor for worsening of glucose control. Significant weight gain has been observed with antipsychotic therapy; incidence varies with product. Monitor waist circumference and BMI. May cause anaphylaxis or hypersensitivity reactions.

The possibility of a suicide attempt is inherent in psychotic illness or bipolar disorder; use caution in high-risk patients during initiation of therapy. Prescriptions should be written for the smallest quantity consistent with good patient care. Use caution in elderly patients.

Drug Interactions

Avoid Concomitant Use

Avoid concomitant use of Asenapine with any of the following: Artemether; Dronedarone; Lumefantrine; Metoclopramide; Nilotinib; Pimozide; QUEtiapine; QuiNINE; Tetrabenazine; Thioridazine; Toremifene; Vandetanib; Vemurafenib; Ziprasidone

Decreased Effect

Asenapine may decrease the levels/effects of: Amphetamines; Anti-Parkinson's Agents (Dopamine Agonist); Quinagolide

The levels/effects of Asenapine may be decreased by: CYP1A2 Inducers (Strong); Cyproterone; Lithium formulations; Peginterferon Alfa-2b; Tocilizumab

Increased Effect/Toxicity

Asenapine may increase the levels/effects of: Alcohol (Ethyl); ARIPiprazole; CNS Depressants; Dronedarone; Methylphenidate; PARoxetine; Pimozide; QTc-Prolonging Agents; QuiNINE; Serotonin Modulators; Tetrabenazine; Thioridazine; Toremifene; Vandetanib; Vemurafenib; Ziprasidone

The levels/effects of Asenapine may be increased by: Abiraterone Acetate; Acetylcholinesterase Inhibitors (Central); Alfuzosin; Artemether; Chloroquine; Ciprofloxacin; Ciprofloxacin (Systemic);

Conivaptan; CYP1A2 Inhibitors (Moderate); CYP1A2 Inhibitors (Strong); Deferasirox; FluvoxaMINE; Gadobutrol; HydrOXYzine; Indacaterol; Lithium formulations; Lumefantrine; MAO Inhibitors; Methylphenidate; Metoclopramide; Nilotinib; QUEtiapine; QuiNINE; Tetrabenazine

Nutritional/Ethanol Interactions Ethanol: May increase CNS depression; monitor for increased effects with coadministration. Caution patients about effects.

Adverse Reactions Actual frequency may be dependent upon dose and/or indication.

>10%:

- Central nervous system: Somnolence (13% to 24%), insomnia (6% to 16%), extrapyramidal symptoms (6% to 12%), headache (12%), akathisia (4% to 11%; dose related), dizziness (3% to 11%)
- Endocrine & metabolic: Hypertriglyceridemia (13% to 15%)

1% to 10%:

- Cardiovascular: Peripheral edema (3%), hypertension (2% to 3%)
- Central nervous system: Hypoesthesia (4% to 7%), fatigue (3% to 4%), anxiety (4%), depression (2%), irritability (1% to 2%)
- Endocrine & metabolic: Cholesterol increased (8% to 9%), glucose increased (5% to 7%), hyperprolactinemia (2% to 3%)
- Gastrointestinal: Constipation (4% to 7%), vomiting (4% to 7%), weight gain (2% to 5%), dyspepsia (3% to 4%), appetite increased (≤4%), salivation increased (≤4%), abnormal taste (3%), toothache (3%), abdominal discomfort (≤3%), xerostomia (1% to 3%)
- Hematologic: Creatine kinase increased (6%)
- Hepatic: Transaminases increased (<1% to 3%)
- Neuromuscular & skeletal: Arthralgia (3%), extremity pain (2%)

Available Dosage Forms

Tablet, sublingual:

Saphris®: 5 mg, 10 mg

General Dosage Range Oral: *Adults:* 5-10 mg twice daily

Administration

Oral Sublingual tablets should be placed under the tongue and allowed to disintegrate. Do not crush, chew, or swallow. Avoid eating or drinking for at least 10 minutes after administration.

Stability

Storage Store at 15°C to 30°C (59°F to 86°F).

Nursing Actions

Physical Assessment Monitor weight prior to treatment and periodically throughout. Be alert to the potential for orthostatic hypotension, especially during the titration phase. Initiate at lower doses and titrate to target dose. Taper dosage slowly when discontinuing.

Patient Education Sublingual tablets should be placed under tongue to dissolve. Avoid eating or drinking for at least 10 minutes. Avoid alcohol. Maintain adequate hydration. If you have diabetes, you may experience increased blood sugars; monitor blood sugars closely. You may experience excess sedation, drowsiness, problems sleeping, restlessness, dizziness, or blurred vision; dry mouth, nausea, or GI upset; postural hypotension; or urinary retention (void before taking medication). Report persistent CNS effects (eg, trembling fingers, altered gait or balance, excessive sedation, seizures, unusual muscle or skeletal movements, anxiety, abnormal thoughts [especially suicide ideation], confusion, personality changes); diaphoresis, chest pain, palpitations, rapid heartbeat, or severe dizziness; respiratory difficulty; or worsening of condition.

Dietary Considerations Avoid eating or drinking for at least 10 minutes after administration.

Asparaginase *(E. coli)*

(a SPEAR a ji nase e ko lye)

Brand Names: U.S. Elspar®

Index Terms *E. coli* Asparaginase; Asparaginase; L-asparaginase (*E. coli*)

Pharmacologic Category Antineoplastic Agent, Miscellaneous; Enzyme

Medication Safety Issues

Sound-alike/look-alike issues:

Asparaginase (*E. coli*) may be confused with asparaginase (*Erwinia*), pegaspargase

Elspar® may be confused with Elaprase®, Erwinaze™, Oncaspar®

High alert medication:

This medication is in a class the Institute for Safe Medication Practices (ISMP) includes among its list of drug classes which have a heightened risk of causing significant patient harm when used in error.

Pregnancy Risk Factor C

Lactation Excretion in breast milk unknown/not recommended

Use Treatment (in combination with other chemotherapy) of acute lymphoblastic leukemia (ALL)

Unlabeled Use Treatment of lymphoblastic lymphoma

Available Dosage Forms

Injection, powder for reconstitution:

Elspar®: 10,000 int. units

General Dosage Range

I.M.: *Children and Adults:* 6000 units/m^2/dose 3 times/week **or** 6000 units/m^2 every ~3 days

I.V.: *Children and Adults:* Dosage varies greatly depending on indication

Intradermal: *Children and Adults:* Test dose: 0.1-0.2 mL of a 20-250 units/mL concentration

Administration

I.M. Doses should be given as a deep intramuscular injection into a large muscle; volumes >2 mL should be divided and administered in 2 separate sites

I.V. Note: I.V. administration greatly increases the risk of allergic reactions and should be avoided if possible.

The following precautions should be taken when administering. Administer in 50-250 mL of D_5W over at least 30-60 minutes. The manufacturer recommends a test dose (0.1 mL of a dilute 20 unit/mL solution) prior to initial administration and when given after an interval of 7 days or more. Institutional policies vary. The skin test site should be observed for at least 1 hour for a wheal or erythema. Note that a negative skin test does not preclude the possibility of an allergic reaction. Desensitization may be performed in patients who have been found to be hypersensitive by the intradermal skin test or who have received previous courses of therapy with the drug. Have epinephrine, diphenhydramine, and hydrocortisone at the bedside. Have a running I.V. in place. A physician should be readily accessible.

I.V. Detail The intradermal skin test is commonly given prior to the initial injection, using a dose of 0.1 mL of 20 units/mL solution (~2 units). The skin test site should be observed for at least 1 hour for a wheal or erythema. Do not infuse through filter.

Gelatinous fiber-like particles may develop on standing. Filtration through a 5-micron filter during administration will remove the particles with no loss of potency.

pH: 7.4; 6.5-8 (active enzyme)

Other Has been administered SubQ in specific protocols

Nursing Actions

Physical Assessment With each dose, monitor patient closely for CNS changes, acute hypersensitivity reaction (may occur in 10% to 35% of patients and may be fatal), hyperglycemia, nausea, or vomiting. In the event of hypersensitivity or hyperglycemia, stop infusion and notify prescriber immediately.

Patient Education This medication can only be given I.M. or I.V. Report immediately any pain or burning at infusion/injection site, rash, chest pain, respiratory difficulty or chest tightness, difficulty swallowing, or sharp back pain. It is vital to maintain adequate hydration, unless instructed to restrict fluid intake, and good nutritional status. May cause acute nausea or vomiting. Report unusual fever or chills, changes in mentation (confusion, agitation, depression, stupor, seizures), yellowing of skin or eyes, unusual bleeding or bruising, unhealed sores, or vaginal discharge.

Asparaginase (*Erwinia*)

(a SPEAR a ji nase er WIN i ah)

Brand Names: U.S. Erwinaze™

Index Terms *Erwinia chrysanthemi*; Asparaginase *Erwinia chrysanthemi*; L-asparaginase (*Erwinia*)

Pharmacologic Category Antineoplastic Agent, Miscellaneous; Enzyme

Medication Safety Issues

Sound-alike/look-alike issues:

Asparaginase *(Erwinia)* may be confused with asparaginase *(E. coli)*, pegaspargase

Erwinaze™ may be confused with Elaprase®, Elspar®, Oncaspar®

High alert medication:

This medication is in a class the Institute for Safe Medication Practices (ISMP) includes among its list of drug classes which have a heightened risk of causing significant patient harm when used in error.

Pregnancy Risk Factor C

Lactation Excretion in breast milk unknown/not recommended

Use Treatment (in combination with other chemotherapy) of acute lymphoblastic leukemia (ALL) in patients with hypersensitivity to *E. coli*-derived asparaginase

Available Dosage Forms

Injection, powder for reconstitution:

Erwinaze™: 10,000 int. units

General Dosage Range

I.M.: *Children and Adults:* 25,000 units/m^2 3 times/week (Mon, Wed, Fri) for 6 doses for each planned pegaspargase dose **or** 25,000 units/m^2 for each planned asparaginase (*E. coli*) dose

Administration

I.M. Volume of each single injection site should be limited to 2 mL; use multiple injections for volumes >2 mL

I.V. *Canadian labeling (additional administration routes not in the U.S. labeling):* May also be administered I.V., although I.M. and SubQ are preferred.

Other *Canadian labeling (additional administration routes not in the U.S. labeling):* May also be administered SubQ, (I.M. and SubQ are the preferred routes).

Nursing Actions

Physical Assessment

With each dose, patient should be monitored closely for acute hypersensitivity reactions, hyperglycemia, pancreatitis, and thrombosis. In event of hypersensitivity or hyperglycemia, infusion should be stopped and prescriber notified immediately.

Patient Education

This medication can only be given I.M. or I.V. Report immediately any pain or burning at infusion/injection site, rash, chest pain, respiratory difficulty or chest tightness, difficulty swallowing, or sharp back pain. May cause nausea or vomiting. Report any signs of bleeding or bruising, trouble breathing, chest pain, severe nausea, vomiting, abdominal pain, severe headaches, or signs of high blood sugar.

Aspirin (AS pir in)

Brand Names: U.S. Ascriptin® Maximum Strength [OTC]; Ascriptin® Regular Strength [OTC]; Aspercin [OTC]; Aspergum® [OTC]; Aspir-low [OTC]; Aspirtab [OTC]; Bayer® Aspirin Extra Strength [OTC]; Bayer® Aspirin Regimen Adult Low Strength [OTC]; Bayer® Aspirin Regimen Children's [OTC]; Bayer® Aspirin Regimen Regular Strength [OTC]; Bayer® Genuine Aspirin [OTC]; Bayer® Plus Extra Strength [OTC]; Bayer® Women's Low Dose Aspirin [OTC]; Buffasal [OTC]; Bufferin® Extra Strength [OTC]; Bufferin® [OTC]; Buffinol [OTC]; Ecotrin® Arthritis Strength [OTC]; Ecotrin® Low Strength [OTC]; Ecotrin® [OTC]; Halfprin® [OTC]; St Joseph® Adult Aspirin [OTC]; Tri-Buffered Aspirin [OTC]

Index Terms Acetylsalicylic Acid; ASA; Baby Aspirin

Pharmacologic Category Antiplatelet Agent; Salicylate

Medication Safety Issues

Sound-alike/look-alike issues:

Aspirin may be confused with Afrin®

Ascriptin® may be confused with Aricept®

Ecotrin® may be confused with Edecrin®, Epogen®

Halfprin® may be confused with Haltran®

ZORprin® may be confused with Zyloprim®

International issues:

Cartia [multiple international markets] may be confused with Cartia XT brand name for diltiazem [U.S.]

Lactation Enters breast milk (AAP recommends use "with caution"; AAP 2001 update pending)

Breast-Feeding Considerations Low amounts of aspirin can be found in breast milk. Milk/plasma ratios ranging from 0.03-0.3 have been reported. Peak levels in breast milk are reported to be at ~9 hours after a dose. Metabolic acidosis was reported in one infant following an aspirin dose of 3.9 g/day in the mother. The WHO considers occasional doses of aspirin to be compatible with breast-feeding, but to avoid long-term therapy and consider monitoring the infant for adverse effects. Other sources suggest avoiding aspirin while breast-feeding due to the theoretical risk of Reye's syndrome.

Use Treatment of mild-to-moderate pain, inflammation, and fever; prevention and treatment of myocardial infarction (MI), acute ischemic stroke, and transient ischemic episodes; management of rheumatoid arthritis, rheumatic fever, osteoarthritis; adjunctive therapy in revascularization procedures (coronary artery bypass graft [CABG], percutaneous transluminal coronary angioplasty [PTCA], carotid endarterectomy), stent implantation

Unlabeled Use Low doses have been used in the prevention of pre-eclampsia, complications associated with autoimmune disorders such as lupus or antiphospholipid syndrome; colorectal cancer; Kawasaki disease; alternative therapy for prevention of thromboembolism associated with atrial fibrillation in patients not candidates for warfarin; pericarditis associated with MI; prosthetic valve thromboprophylaxis; peripheral arterial occlusive disease

Mechanism of Action/Effect Irreversibly inhibits cyclooxygenase-1 and 2 (COX-1 and 2) enzymes, which results in decreased formation of prostaglandin precursors; has antipyretic, analgesic, and anti-inflammatory properties

Contraindications Hypersensitivity to salicylates, other NSAIDs, or any component of the formulation; asthma; rhinitis; nasal polyps; inherited or acquired bleeding disorders (including factor VII and factor IX deficiency); do not use in children (<16 years of age) for viral infections (chickenpox or flu symptoms), with or without fever, due to a potential association with Reye's syndrome; pregnancy (3rd trimester especially)

Warnings/Precautions Use with caution in patients with platelet and bleeding disorders, renal dysfunction, dehydration, erosive gastritis, or peptic ulcer disease. Heavy ethanol use (>3 drinks/day) can increase bleeding risks. Avoid use in severe renal failure or in severe hepatic failure. Low-dose aspirin for cardioprotective effects is associated with a two- to fourfold increase in UGI events (eg, symptomatic or complicated ulcers); risks of these events increase with increasing aspirin dose; during the chronic phase of aspirin dosing, doses >81 mg are not recommended unless indicated (Bhatt, 2008).

Discontinue use if tinnitus or impaired hearing occurs. Caution in mild-to-moderate renal failure (only at high dosages). Patients with sensitivity to tartrazine dyes, nasal polyps, and asthma may have an increased risk of salicylate sensitivity. In the treatment of acute ischemic stroke, avoid aspirin for 24 hours following administration of alteplase; administration within 24 hours increases the risk of hemorrhagic transformation. Concurrent use of aspirin and clopidogrel is not recommended for secondary prevention of ischemic stroke or TIA in patients unable to take oral anticoagulants due to hemorrhagic risk (Furie, 2011). Surgical patients should avoid ASA if possible, for 1-2 weeks prior to surgery, to reduce the risk of excessive bleeding (except in patients with cardiac stents that have not completed their full course of dual antiplatelet therapy [aspirin, clopidogrel]; patient-specific situations need to be discussed with cardiologist; AHA/ACC/SCAI/ACS/ADA Science Advisory provides recommendations). When used concomitantly with ≤325 mg of aspirin, NSAIDs (including selective COX-2 inhibitors) substantially increase the risk of gastrointestinal complications (eg, ulcer); concomitant gastroprotective therapy (eg, proton pump inhibitors) is recommended (Bhatt, 2008).

When used for self-medication (OTC labeling): Children and teenagers who have or are recovering from chickenpox or flu-like symptoms should not use this product. Changes in behavior (along with nausea and vomiting) may be an early sign of Reye's syndrome; patients should be instructed to contact their healthcare provider if these occur.

Drug Interactions

Avoid Concomitant Use

Avoid concomitant use of Aspirin with any of the following: Floctafenine; Influenza Virus Vaccine (Live/Attenuated); Ketorolac; Ketorolac (Nasal); Ketorolac (Systemic)

Decreased Effect

Aspirin may decrease the levels/effects of: ACE Inhibitors; Loop Diuretics; NSAID (Nonselective); Probenecid; Ticagrelor; Tiludronate

The levels/effects of Aspirin may be decreased by: Corticosteroids (Systemic); Nonsteroidal Anti-Inflammatory Agents; NSAID (Nonselective)

Increased Effect/Toxicity

Aspirin may increase the levels/effects of: Alendronate; Anticoagulants; Carbonic Anhydrase Inhibitors; Collagenase (Systemic); Corticosteroids (Systemic); Divalproex; Drotrecogin Alfa (Activated); Heparin; Ibritumomab; Methotrexate; PRALAtrexate; Rivaroxaban; Salicylates; Sulfonylureas; Thrombolytic Agents; Ticagrelor; Tositumomab and Iodine I 131 Tositumomab; Valproic Acid; Varicella Virus-Containing Vaccines; Vitamin K Antagonists

The levels/effects of Aspirin may be increased by: Ammonium Chloride; Antidepressants (Tricyclic, Tertiary Amine); Antiplatelet Agents; Calcium Channel Blockers (Nondihydropyridine); Dasatinib; Floctafenine; Ginkgo Biloba; Glucosamine; Herbs (Anticoagulant/Antiplatelet Properties); Influenza Virus Vaccine (Live/Attenuated); Ketorolac; Ketorolac (Nasal); Ketorolac (Systemic); Loop Diuretics; Nonsteroidal Anti-Inflammatory Agents; NSAID (Nonselective); Omega-3-Acid Ethyl Esters; Pentosan Polysulfate Sodium; Pentoxifylline; Potassium Acid Phosphate; Prostacyclin Analogues; Selective Serotonin Reuptake Inhibitors; Serotonin/Norepinephrine Reuptake Inhibitors; Treprostinil; Vitamin E

Nutritional/Ethanol Interactions

Ethanol: Avoid ethanol (may enhance gastric mucosal damage).

Food: Food may decrease the rate but not the extent of oral absorption.

Folic acid: Hyperexcretion of folate; folic acid deficiency may result, leading to macrocytic anemia.

Iron: With chronic aspirin use and at doses of 3-4 g/day, iron-deficiency anemia may result.

Sodium: Hypernatremia resulting from buffered aspirin solutions or sodium salicylate containing high sodium content. Avoid or use with caution in CHF or any condition where hypernatremia would be detrimental.

Benedictine liqueur, prunes, raisins, tea, and gherkins: Potential salicylate accumulation.

Fresh fruits containing vitamin C: Displace drug from binding sites, resulting in increased urinary excretion of aspirin.

Herb/Nutraceutical: Avoid cat's claw, dong quai, evening primrose, feverfew, garlic, ginger, ginkgo, red clover, horse chestnut, green tea, ginseng (all have additional antiplatelet activity). Limit curry powder, paprika, licorice; may cause salicylate accumulation. These foods contain 6 mg salicylate/100 g. An ordinary American diet contains 10-200 mg/day of salicylate.

Adverse Reactions As with all drugs which may affect hemostasis, bleeding is associated with aspirin. Hemorrhage may occur at virtually any site. Risk is dependent on multiple variables including dosage, concurrent use of multiple agents which alter hemostasis, and patient susceptibility. Many adverse effects of aspirin are dose related, and are rare at low dosages. Other serious reactions are idiosyncratic, related to allergy or individual sensitivity. Accurate estimation of frequencies is not possible. The reactions listed below have been reported for aspirin (frequency not defined).

Cardiovascular: Hypotension, tachycardia, dysrhythmias, edema

Central nervous system: Fatigue, insomnia, nervousness, agitation, confusion, dizziness, headache, lethargy, cerebral edema, hyperthermia, coma

Dermatologic: Rash, angioedema, urticaria

Endocrine & metabolic: Acidosis, hyperkalemia, dehydration, hypoglycemia (children), hyperglycemia, hypernatremia (buffered forms)

Gastrointestinal: Nausea, vomiting, dyspepsia, epigastric discomfort, heartburn, stomach pain, gastrointestinal ulceration (6% to 31%), gastric erosions, gastric erythema, duodenal ulcers

Hematologic: Anemia, disseminated intravascular coagulation (DIC), prothrombin times prolonged, coagulopathy, thrombocytopenia, hemolytic anemia, bleeding, iron deficiency anemia

Hepatic: Hepatotoxicity, transaminases increased, hepatitis (reversible)

Neuromuscular & skeletal: Rhabdomyolysis, weakness, acetabular bone destruction (OA)

Otic: Hearing loss, tinnitus

Renal: Interstitial nephritis, papillary necrosis, proteinuria, renal impairment, renal failure (including cases caused by rhabdomyolysis), BUN increased, serum creatinine increased

Respiratory: Asthma, bronchospasm, dyspnea, laryngeal edema, hyperpnea, tachypnea, respiratory alkalosis, noncardiogenic pulmonary edema

Miscellaneous: Anaphylaxis, prolonged pregnancy and labor, stillbirths, low birth weight, peripartum bleeding, Reye's syndrome

Pharmacodynamics/Kinetics
Duration of Action 4-6 hours
Available Dosage Forms
Caplet, oral: 500 mg
Ascriptin® Maximum Strength [OTC]: 500 mg
Bayer® Aspirin Extra Strength [OTC]: 500 mg
Bayer® Genuine Aspirin [OTC]: 325 mg
Bayer® Plus Extra Strength [OTC]: 500 mg
Bayer® Women's Low Dose Aspirin [OTC]: 81 mg
Caplet, enteric coated, oral:
Bayer® Aspirin Regimen Regular Strength [OTC]: 325 mg
Gum, chewing, oral:
Aspergum® [OTC]: 227 mg (12s)
Suppository, rectal: 300 mg (12s); 600 mg (12s)
Tablet, oral: 325 mg
Ascriptin® Regular Strength [OTC]: 325 mg
Aspercin [OTC]: 325 mg
Aspirtab [OTC]: 325 mg
Bayer® Genuine Aspirin [OTC]: 325 mg
Buffasal [OTC]: 325 mg
Bufferin® [OTC]: 325 mg
Bufferin® Extra Strength [OTC]: 500 mg
Buffinol [OTC]: 324 mg
Tri-Buffered Aspirin [OTC]: 325 mg
Tablet, chewable, oral: 81 mg
Bayer® Aspirin Regimen Children's [OTC]: 81 mg
St Joseph® Adult Aspirin [OTC]: 81 mg
Tablet, enteric coated, oral: 81 mg, 325 mg, 650 mg
Aspir-low [OTC]: 81 mg
Bayer® Aspirin Regimen Adult Low Strength [OTC]: 81 mg
Ecotrin® [OTC]: 325 mg
Ecotrin® Arthritis Strength [OTC]: 500 mg
Ecotrin® Low Strength [OTC]: 81 mg
Halfprin® [OTC]: 81 mg, 162 mg
St Joseph® Adult Aspirin [OTC]: 81 mg
General Dosage Range
Oral:
Children: 10-15 mg/kg/dose every 4-6 hours (maximum: 4 g/day) **or** 60-100 mg/kg/day divided every 4-8 hours **or** 1-20 mg/kg/day as a single dose
Adults: 325-650 mg every 4-6 hours (maximum: 4 g/day) **or** 2.4-5.4 g/day in divided doses **or** 40-325 mg/day as a single dose
Rectal:
Children: 10-15 mg/kg/dose every 4-6 hours (maximum: 4 g/day)
Adults: 300-600 mg every 4-6 hours (maximum: 4 g/day)
Administration
Oral Do not crush enteric coated tablet. Administer with food or a full glass of water to minimize GI distress. For acute myocardial infarction, have patient chew tablet.
Stability
Storage Keep suppositories in refrigerator; do not freeze. Hydrolysis of aspirin occurs upon exposure to water or moist air, resulting in salicylate and acetate, which possess a vinegar-like odor. Do not use if a strong odor is present.
Nursing Actions
Physical Assessment Do not use for persons with allergic reaction to salicylate or other NSAIDs.
Patient Education Take with food or milk. Do not use aspirin with strong vinegar-like odor. While using this medication, avoid alcohol, salicylate-containing foods, other medications containing aspirin or salicylate, or other NSAIDs without consulting prescriber. Maintain adequate hydration, unless instructed to restrict fluid intake. Inform prescribers and dentists that you are taking this medication prior to scheduling any surgery or dental procedure. You may experience nausea, vomiting, gastric discomfort, GI bleeding, ulceration, perforation (can occur with or without pain), or blood in stool. Stop taking aspirin and report ringing in ears, persistent stomach pain, unresolved nausea or vomiting, respiratory difficulty or shortness of breath, unusual bruising or bleeding (mouth, urine, stool), or skin rash.
Dietary Considerations Take with food or large volume of water or milk to minimize GI upset.

Aspirin and Diphenhydramine
(AS pir in & dye fen HYE dra meen)

Brand Names: U.S. Bayer® PM [OTC]
Index Terms ASA and Diphenhydramine; Aspirin and Diphenhydramine Citrate; Diphenhydramine and ASA; Diphenhydramine and Aspirin; Diphenhydramine Citrate and Aspirin
Pharmacologic Category Analgesic, Miscellaneous
Lactation See individual agents.
Use Aid in the relief of insomnia accompanied by minor pain or headache
Available Dosage Forms
Caplet, oral:
Bayer® PM [OTC]: Aspirin 500 mg and diphenhydramine 38.3 mg
General Dosage Range Oral: *Children ≥12 years and Adults:* Two caplets (1000 mg aspirin/77 mg diphenhydramine citrate) at bedtime
Administration
Oral Administer each dose with a full glass of water.
Nursing Actions
Physical Assessment See individual agents.
Patient Education See individual agents.
Related Information
Aspirin *on page 94*
DiphenhydrAMINE (Systemic) *on page 342*

Aspirin and Dipyridamole
(AS pir in & dye peer ID a mole)

Brand Names: U.S. Aggrenox®

Index Terms Aspirin and Extended-Release Dipyridamole; Dipyridamole and Aspirin

Pharmacologic Category Antiplatelet Agent

Medication Safety Issues

Sound-alike/look-alike issues:

Aggrenox® may be confused with Aggrastat®

Pregnancy Risk Factor D

Lactation Enters breast milk/use caution

Breast-Feeding Considerations Both aspirin and dipyridamole are excreted in breast milk.

Use Reduction in the risk of stroke in patients who have had transient ischemia of the brain or ischemic stroke due to thrombosis

Unlabeled Use Hemodialysis graft patency

Mechanism of Action/Effect Antithrombotic action results from additive antiplatelet effects of aspirin and dipyridamole.

Contraindications Hypersensitivity to dipyridamole, aspirin, or any component of the formulation; allergy to NSAIDs; patients with the syndrome of asthma, rhinitis, and nasal polyps; children <16 years of age with viral infections; pregnancy (third trimester; aspirin)

Canadian labeling: Additional contraindications (not in U.S. labeling): Patients with hereditary fructose and/or galactose intolerance

Warnings/Precautions Patients who consume ≥3 alcoholic drinks per day may be at risk of bleeding. Use cautiously use in patients with inherited or acquired bleeding disorders, renal impairment, hypotension, unstable angina, recent MI or hepatic dysfunction. Avoid use in patients with a history of active peptic ulcer disease, severe hepatic failure, or severe renal impairment (Cl_{cr} <10 mL/minute). Monitor for signs and symptoms of GI ulcers and bleeding. Discontinue use if dizziness, tinnitus, or impaired hearing occurs. Discontinue use 24 hours prior to pharmacologic (I.V. dipyridamole) stress testing. Discontinue 1-2 weeks before elective surgical procedures to reduce the risk of bleeding. Use caution in the elderly who are at high risk for adverse events. Dose of aspirin in this combination may not be adequate to prevent for cardiac indications (eg, MI prophylaxis). Avoid use in children due to risk of Reye's syndrome in certain viral illness associated with aspirin component. Formulation may contain lactose and/or sucrose. Use in patients with fructose and/or galactose intolerance is contraindicated in the Canadian labeling.

Drug Interactions

Avoid Concomitant Use

Avoid concomitant use of Aspirin and Dipyridamole with any of the following: Floctafenine; Influenza Virus Vaccine (Live/Attenuated); Ketorolac; Ketorolac (Nasal); Ketorolac (Systemic); Silodosin; Topotecan

Decreased Effect

Aspirin and Dipyridamole may decrease the levels/effects of: ACE Inhibitors; Acetylcholinesterase Inhibitors; Loop Diuretics; NSAID (Nonselective); Probenecid; Ticagrelor; Tiludronate

The levels/effects of Aspirin and Dipyridamole may be decreased by: Corticosteroids (Systemic); Nonsteroidal Anti-Inflammatory Agents; NSAID (Nonselective)

Increased Effect/Toxicity

Aspirin and Dipyridamole may increase the levels/effects of: Adenosine; Alendronate; Anticoagulants; Beta-Blockers; Carbonic Anhydrase Inhibitors; Colchicine; Collagenase (Systemic); Corticosteroids (Systemic); Dabigatran Etexilate; Divalproex; Drotrecogin Alfa (Activated); Everolimus; Heparin; Hypotensive Agents; Ibritumomab; Methotrexate; P-glycoprotein/ABCB1 Substrates; PRALAtrexate; Prucalopride; Regadenoson; Rivaroxaban; Salicylates; Silodosin; Sulfonylureas; Thrombolytic Agents; Ticagrelor; Topotecan; Tositumomab and Iodine I 131 Tositumomab; Valproic Acid; Varicella Virus-Containing Vaccines; Vitamin K Antagonists

The levels/effects of Aspirin and Dipyridamole may be increased by: Ammonium Chloride; Antidepressants (Tricyclic, Tertiary Amine); Antiplatelet Agents; Calcium Channel Blockers (Nondihydropyridine); Dasatinib; Floctafenine; Ginkgo Biloba; Glucosamine; Herbs (Anticoagulant/Antiplatelet Properties); Influenza Virus Vaccine (Live/Attenuated); Ketorolac; Ketorolac (Nasal); Ketorolac (Systemic); Loop Diuretics; Nonsteroidal Anti-Inflammatory Agents; NSAID (Nonselective); Omega-3-Acid Ethyl Esters; Pentosan Polysulfate Sodium; Pentoxifylline; Potassium Acid Phosphate; Prostacyclin Analogues; Selective Serotonin Reuptake Inhibitors; Serotonin/Norepinephrine Reuptake Inhibitors; Treprostinil; Vitamin E

Nutritional/Ethanol Interactions Ethanol: Avoid ethanol (due to GI irritation).

Adverse Reactions

>10%:

Central nervous system: Headache (39%; tolerance usually develops)

Gastrointestinal: Abdominal pain (18%), dyspepsia (18%), nausea (16%), diarrhea (13%)

1% to 10%:

Cardiovascular: Cardiac failure (2%), syncope (1%)

Central nervous system: Fatigue (6%), pain (6%), amnesia (2%), malaise (2%), seizure (2%), confusion (1%), somnolence (1%)

Dermatologic: Purpura (1%)

Gastrointestinal: Vomiting (8%), GI bleeding (4%), melena (2%), rectal bleeding (2%), hemorrhoids (1%), GI hemorrhage (1%), anorexia (1%)

Hematologic: Hemorrhage (3%), anemia (2%)

Neuromuscular & skeletal: Arthralgia (6%), back pain (5%), weakness (2%), arthritis (2%), arthrosis (1%), myalgia (1%)

Respiratory: Cough (2%), epistaxis (2%), upper respiratory tract infection (1%)

Available Dosage Forms

Capsule:

Aggrenox®: Aspirin 25 mg [immediate release] and dipyridamole 200 mg [extended release]

General Dosage Range Oral: *Adults:* 1 capsule (200 mg dipyridamole, 25 mg aspirin) twice daily

Administration

Oral Capsule should be swallowed whole; do not crush or chew. May be administered with or without food.

Stability

Storage Store at 25°C (77°F); excursions permitted to 15°C to 30°C (59°F to 86°F). Protect from excessive moisture.

Nursing Actions

Physical Assessment See individual agents.

Patient Education See individual agents.

Dietary Considerations May be taken with or without food.

Related Information

Aspirin *on page 94*

Dipyridamole *on page 351*

Atenolol (a TEN oh lole)

Brand Names: U.S. Tenormin®

Pharmacologic Category Antianginal Agent; Beta Blocker, Beta-1 Selective

Medication Safety Issues

Sound-alike/look-alike issues:

Atenolol may be confused with albuterol, Altenol®, timolol, Tylenol®

Tenormin® may be confused with Imuran®, Norpramin®, thiamine, Trovan®

Pregnancy Risk Factor D

Lactation Enters breast milk/use caution (AAP recommends "use with caution"; AAP 2001 update pending)

Breast-Feeding Considerations Atenolol is excreted in breast milk and has been detected in the serum and urine of nursing infants. Peak concentrations in breast milk have been reported to occur between 2-8 hours after the maternal dose and in some cases are higher than the peak maternal serum concentration. Although most studies have not reported adverse events in nursing infants, avoiding maternal use while nursing infants with renal dysfunction or infants <44 weeks postconceptual age has been suggested. Beta-blockers with less distribution into breast milk may be preferred. The manufacturer recommends that caution be exercised when administering atenolol to nursing women.

Use Treatment of hypertension, alone or in combination with other agents; management of angina pectoris; secondary prevention postmyocardial infarction

Unlabeled Use Acute ethanol withdrawal (in combination with a benzodiazepine), supraventricular and ventricular arrhythmias, and migraine headache prophylaxis

Mechanism of Action/Effect Competitively blocks response to beta-adrenergic stimulation, selectively blocks beta$_1$-receptors with little or no effect on beta$_2$-receptors except at high doses

Contraindications Hypersensitivity to atenolol or any component of the formulation; sinus bradycardia; sinus node dysfunction; heart block greater than first-degree (except in patients with a functioning artificial pacemaker); cardiogenic shock; uncompensated cardiac failure; pulmonary edema; pregnancy

Warnings/Precautions Consider pre-existing conditions such as sick sinus syndrome before initiating. Administer cautiously in compensated heart failure and monitor for a worsening of the condition (efficacy of atenolol in heart failure has not been established). **[U.S. Boxed Warning]: Beta-blocker therapy should not be withdrawn abruptly (particularly in patients with CAD), but gradually tapered to avoid acute tachycardia, hypertension, and/or ischemia.** Chronic beta-blocker therapy should not be routinely withdrawn prior to major surgery. Beta-blockers should be avoided in patients with bronchospastic disease (asthma). Atenolol, with B$_1$ selectivity, has been used cautiously in bronchospastic disease with close monitoring. May precipitate or aggravate symptoms of arterial insufficiency in patients with PVD and Raynaud's disease; use with caution and monitor for progression of arterial obstruction. Use cautiously in patients with diabetes - may mask hypoglycemic symptoms. May mask signs of hyperthyroidism (eg, tachycardia); use caution if hyperthyroidism is suspected, abrupt withdrawal may precipitate thyroid storm. Alterations in thyroid function tests may be observed. Use cautiously in the renally impaired (dosage adjustment required). Caution in myasthenia gravis or psychiatric disease (may cause CNS depression). Bradycardia may be observed more frequently in elderly patients (>65 years of age); dosage reductions may be necessary. Adequate alpha-blockade is required prior to use of any beta-blocker for patients with untreated pheochromocytoma. May induce or exacerbate psoriasis. Use caution with history of severe anaphylaxis to allergens; patients taking beta-blockers may become more sensitive to repeated challenges. Treatment of anaphylaxis (eg, epinephrine) in patients taking beta-blockers may be ineffective or promote undesirable effects. Use with caution in patients on concurrent digoxin, verapamil, or diltiazem; bradycardia or heart block can occur. Use with caution in patients receiving inhaled anesthetic agents known to depress myocardial contractility.

Drug Interactions

Avoid Concomitant Use

Avoid concomitant use of Atenolol with any of the following: Floctafenine; Methacholine

Decreased Effect

Atenolol may decrease the levels/effects of: Beta2-Agonists; Theophylline Derivatives

The levels/effects of Atenolol may be decreased by: Ampicillin; Herbs (Hypertensive Properties); Methylphenidate; Nonsteroidal Anti-Inflammatory Agents; Yohimbine

Increased Effect/Toxicity

Atenolol may increase the levels/effects of: Alpha-/Beta-Agonists (Direct-Acting); Alpha1-Blockers; Alpha2-Agonists; Amifostine; Antihypertensives; Bupivacaine; Cardiac Glycosides; Cholinergic Agonists; Fingolimod; Hypotensive Agents; Insulin; Lidocaine; Lidocaine (Systemic); Lidocaine (Topical); Mepivacaine; Methacholine; Midodrine; RiTUXimab; Sulfonylureas

The levels/effects of Atenolol may be increased by: Acetylcholinesterase Inhibitors; Amiodarone; Anilidopiperidine Opioids; Calcium Channel Blockers (Dihydropyridine); Calcium Channel Blockers (Nondihydropyridine); Diazoxide; Dipyridamole; Disopyramide; Dronedarone; Floctafenine; Glycopyrrolate; Herbs (Hypotensive Properties); MAO Inhibitors; Pentoxifylline; Phosphodiesterase 5 Inhibitors; Prostacyclin Analogues; Reserpine

Nutritional/Ethanol Interactions

Food: Atenolol serum concentrations may be decreased if taken with food.

Herb/Nutraceutical: Dong quai has estrogenic activity. Ephedra, yohimbe, and ginseng may worsen hypertension. Garlic may have increased antihypertensive effect. Management: Avoid dong quai, ephedra, yohimbe, ginseng, and garlic.

Adverse Reactions 1% to 10%:

Cardiovascular: Persistent bradycardia, hypotension, chest pain, edema, heart failure, second- or third-degree AV block, Raynaud's phenomenon

Central nervous system: Dizziness, fatigue, insomnia, lethargy, confusion, mental impairment, depression, headache, nightmares

Gastrointestinal: Constipation, diarrhea, nausea

Genitourinary: Impotence

Miscellaneous: Cold extremities

Pharmacodynamics/Kinetics

Onset of Action Peak effect: Oral: 2-4 hours

Duration of Action Normal renal function: 12-24 hours

Available Dosage Forms

Tablet, oral: 25 mg, 50 mg, 100 mg

Tenormin®: 25 mg, 50 mg, 100 mg

General Dosage Range Dosage adjustment recommended in patients with renal impairment

Oral:

Children: 0.5-1 mg/kg/dose given daily; range of 0.5-1.5 mg/kg/day (maximum dose: 2 mg/kg/day up to 100 mg/day)

Adults: 25-100 mg/day as a single daily dose (maximum dose: 100 mg/day)

Administration

Oral When administered acutely for cardiac treatment, monitor ECG and blood pressure. May be administered without regard to meals.

Stability

Storage Protect from light.

Nursing Actions

Physical Assessment Monitor blood pressure and heart rate prior to and following first dose and after any change in dosage. Monitor for CHF, edema, new cough, dyspnea, unintentional weight gain, or unresolved fatigue. Advise patients with diabetes to monitor glucose levels closely; beta-blockers may alter glucose tolerance. Taper dosage slowly when discontinuing. Teach patient hypotension precautions to report.

Patient Education Do not stop mediation without prescriber's advice. Take with or without food. Take pulse daily (prior to medication) and follow prescriber's instruction about holding medication. If you have diabetes, monitor serum sugar closely; drug may alter glucose tolerance or mask signs of hypoglycemia. If medication is being tapered, advise patient to limit physical activity to decrease strain on heart. May cause fatigue, dizziness, postural hypotension, alteration in sexual performance (reversible), or constipation. If chest pain or pressure, tightness, or shortness of breath occur, seek medical attention immediately. Report unresolved swelling of extremities, respiratory difficulty or new cough, unresolved fatigue, unusual weight gain, or unresolved constipation.

Dietary Considerations May be taken without regard to meals.

Atenolol and Chlorthalidone

(a TEN oh lole & klor THAL i done)

Brand Names: U.S. Tenoretic®

Index Terms Chlorthalidone and Atenolol

Pharmacologic Category Beta Blocker, Beta-1 Selective; Diuretic, Thiazide

Pregnancy Risk Factor D

Lactation Excretion in breast milk unknown/use caution

Use Treatment of hypertension with a cardioselective beta-blocker and a diuretic

Available Dosage Forms

Tablet, oral: Atenolol 50 mg and chlorthalidone 25 mg; atenolol 100 mg and chlorthalidone 25 mg

Tenoretic®: Atenolol 50 mg and chlorthalidone 25 mg; atenolol 100 mg and chlorthalidone 25 mg

General Dosage Range Dosage adjustment recommended in patients with renal impairment.

Oral: *Adults:* Initial: Atenolol 50 mg and chlorthalidone 25 mg once daily; Maintenance: Atenolol 50-100 mg and chlorthalidone 25 mg once daily (maximum dose: Atenolol 100 mg/day; chlorthalidone 25 mg/day)

Nursing Actions

Physical Assessment See individual agents.

Patient Education See individual agents.

Related Information

Atenolol *on page 98*
Chlorthalidone *on page 228*

Atomoxetine (AT oh mox e teen)

Brand Names: U.S. Strattera®

Index Terms Atomoxetine Hydrochloride; LY139603; Methylphenoxy-Benzene Propanamine; Tomoxetine

Pharmacologic Category Norepinephrine Reuptake Inhibitor, Selective

Medication Safety Issues

Sound-alike/look-alike issues:

Atomoxetine may be confused with atorvastatin

Medication Guide Available Yes

Pregnancy Risk Factor C

Lactation Excretion in breast milk unknown/use caution

Use Treatment of attention deficit/hyperactivity disorder (ADHD)

Mechanism of Action/Effect Selectively inhibits the reuptake of norepinephrine (Ki 4.5nM) with little to no activity at the other neuronal reuptake pumps or receptor sites.

Contraindications Hypersensitivity to atomoxetine or any component of the formulation; use with or within 14 days of MAO inhibitors; narrow-angle glaucoma; current or past history of pheochromocytoma; severe cardiovascular disorders in which the condition would be expected to deteriorate with clinically relevant blood pressure or heart rate increases

Canadian labeling: Additional contraindications (not in U.S. labeling): Symptomatic cardiovascular diseases, moderate-to-severe hypertension; advanced arteriosclerosis; uncontrolled hyperthyroidism

Warnings/Precautions [U.S. Boxed Warning]: Use caution in pediatric patients; may be an increased risk of suicidal ideation. Closely monitor for clinical worsening, suicidality, or unusual changes in behavior; especially during the initial few months of a course of drug therapy, or at times of dose changes, either increases or decreases. The child's family or caregiver should be instructed to closely observe the patient and communicate condition with healthcare provider. New or worsening symptoms of hostility or aggressive behaviors have been associated with atomoxetine, particularly with the initiation of therapy. Use caution in patients with a history of psychotic illness or bipolar disorder; therapy may induce mixed/manic disorder or psychotic symptoms. Atomoxetine is not approved for major depressive disorder. Patients presenting with depressive symptoms should be screened for bipolar disorder. Recommended to be used as part of a comprehensive treatment program for attention deficit disorders. Atomoxetine does not worsen anxiety in patients with existing anxiety disorders or tics related to Tourette's disorder.

Use caution with hepatic disease (dosage adjustments necessary in hepatic impairment). Use may be associated with rare but severe hepatotoxicity; discontinue and do not restart if signs or symptoms of hepatotoxic reaction (eg, jaundice, pruritus, flu-like symptoms) or laboratory evidence of liver disease are noted. Use caution in patients who are poor metabolizers of CYP2D6 metabolized drugs ("poor metabolizers"), bioavailability increases.

Orthostasis can occur; use caution in patients predisposed to hypotension or those with abrupt changes in heart rate or blood pressure. CNS stimulant use has been associated with serious cardiovascular events including sudden death in patients with pre-existing structural cardiac abnormalities or other serious heart problems (sudden death in children and adolescents; sudden death, stroke, and MI in adults). These products should be avoided in patients with known serious structural cardiac abnormalities, cardiomyopathy, serious heart rhythm abnormalities, or other serious cardiac problems that could increase the risk of sudden death that these conditions alone carry. Patients should be carefully evaluated for cardiac disease prior to initiation of therapy. May cause increased heart rate or blood pressure; use caution with hypertension or other cardiovascular disease. Use caution with renal impairment. May cause urinary retention/hesitancy; use caution in patients with history of urinary retention or bladder outlet obstruction. Priapism has been associated with use (rarely). Allergic reactions (including angioneurotic edema, urticaria, and rash) may occur (rare).

Growth should be monitored during treatment. Height and weight gain may be reduced during the first 9-12 months of treatment, but should recover by 3 years of therapy. Safety and efficacy have not been evaluated in pediatric patients <6 years of age.

Drug Interactions

Avoid Concomitant Use

Avoid concomitant use of Atomoxetine with any of the following: Iobenguane I 123; MAO Inhibitors; Pimozide

Decreased Effect

Atomoxetine may decrease the levels/effects of: Iobenguane I 123

The levels/effects of Atomoxetine may be decreased by: Peginterferon Alfa-2b

Increased Effect/Toxicity

Atomoxetine may increase the levels/effects of: ARIPiprazole; Beta2-Agonists; Pimozide; Sympathomimetics

The levels/effects of Atomoxetine may be increased by: Abiraterone Acetate; CYP2D6 Inhibitors (Moderate); CYP2D6 Inhibitors (Strong); Darunavir; MAO Inhibitors

Nutritional/Ethanol Interactions Ethanol: May increase CNS depression; monitor for increased effects with coadministration. Caution patients about effects.

Adverse Reactions Percentages as reported in children and adults; some adverse reactions may be increased in "poor metabolizers" (CYP2D6).

>10%:

Central nervous system: Headache (2% to 19%), insomnia (2% to 15%), somnolence (4% to 11%)

Gastrointestinal: Xerostomia (21%), nausea (7% to 21%), abdominal pain (7% to 18%), appetite decreased (11% to 16%), vomiting (3% to 11%)

1% to 10%:

Cardiovascular: Systolic blood pressure increased (4% to 5%), diastolic pressure increased (≤4%), palpitation (3%), flushing (≥2%), tachycardia (≤2%), orthostatic hypotension (<2%)

Central nervous system: Fatigue/lethargy (6% to 9%), dizziness (5% to 6%), irritability (≤6%), chills (3%), sleep disturbance (3%), mood swings (1% to 2%)

Dermatologic: Hyperhidrosis (4%), rash (2%)

Endocrine & metabolic: Hot flashes (8%), dysmenorrhea (6%), libido decreased (4%), menstruation disturbance (2%), orgasm abnormal (2%)

Gastrointestinal: Constipation (1% to 9%), dyspepsia (4%), anorexia (<3%), weight loss (2% to 3%)

Genitourinary: Erectile disturbance (9%), urinary hesitation/retention (7%), dysuria (3%), ejaculatory disturbance (3%), prostatitis (2%)

Neuromuscular & skeletal: Paresthesia (3% adults; postmarketing observation in children), tremor (2%)

Ocular: Mydriasis (≥2%)

Respiratory: Sinus headache (3%)

Miscellaneous: Jittery feeling (2%)

Available Dosage Forms

Capsule, oral:

Strattera®: 10 mg, 18 mg, 25 mg, 40 mg, 60 mg, 80 mg, 100 mg

General Dosage Range Dosage adjustment recommended in patients with hepatic impairment or on concomitant therapy.

Oral:

Children ≥6 years and ≤70 kg: Initial: 0.5 mg/kg/day in 1-2 divided doses; Maintenance: 0.5-1.4 mg/kg/day in 1-2 divided doses (maximum: 1.4 mg/kg/day **or** 100 mg/day, whichever is less)

Children ≥6 years and >70 kg and Adults: Initial: 40 mg/day in 1-2 divided doses; Maintenance: 40-100 mg/day in 1-2 divided doses (maximum: 100 mg/day)

Administration

Oral May be administered with or without food as a single daily dose in the morning or as two evenly divided doses in morning and late afternoon/early evening. Swallow capsules whole; do not open capsules. If opened accidentally, do not touch eyes; wash hands immediately (product is an ocular irritant).

Stability

Storage Store at room temperature of 25°C (77°F).

Nursing Actions

Physical Assessment Pediatric patients should be screened/monitored for cardiovascular conditions prior to treatment. Monitor growth (height and weight) regularly and for risk of suicide ideation.

Patient Education Take at the same time of day, without regard for meals. You may experience CNS changes; fatigue or lethargy; irritability; sleep disturbances; nausea, vomiting, or decreased appetite; diarrhea; or constipation. Report immediately any chest pain, palpitations, or rapid heartbeat; suicide ideation; or persistent CNS changes (especially any increase in aggression or hostility). Inform prescriber of weight loss, fatigue, dizziness, or palpitations.

Dietary Considerations May be taken with or without food.

Atorvastatin (a TORE va sta tin)

Brand Names: U.S. Lipitor®

Index Terms Atorvastatin Calcium

Pharmacologic Category Antilipemic Agent, HMG-CoA Reductase Inhibitor

Medication Safety Issues

Sound-alike/look-alike issues:

Atorvastatin may be confused with atomoxetine, lovastatin, nystatin, pitavastatin, pravastatin, rosuvastatin, simvastatin

Lipitor® may be confused with labetalol, Levatol®, lisinopril, Loniten®, Lopid®, Mevacor®, Zocor®, ZyrTEC®

Pregnancy Risk Factor X

Lactation Excretion in breast milk unknown/contraindicated

Use Treatment of dyslipidemias or primary prevention of cardiovascular disease (atherosclerotic) as detailed below:

Primary prevention of cardiovascular disease (high-risk for CVD): To reduce the risk of MI or stroke in patients without evidence of heart disease who have multiple CVD risk factors or type 2 diabetes. Treatment reduces the risk for angina or revascularization procedures in patients with multiple risk factors.

Secondary prevention of cardiovascular disease: To reduce the risk of nonfatal MI, nonfatal stroke, revascularization procedures, hospitalization for heart failure, and angina in patients with evidence of coronary heart disease.

Treatment of dyslipidemias: To reduce elevations in total cholesterol (C), LDL-C, apolipoprotein B, and triglycerides in patients with elevations of one or more components, and/or to increase low HDL-C as present in Fredrickson type IIa, IIb, III, and IV hyperlipidemias, heterozygous familial and nonfamilial hypercholesterolemia, and homozygous familial hypercholesterolemia

Treatment of heterozygous familial hypercholesterolemia (HeFH) in adolescent patients (10-17 years of age, females >1 year postmenarche) having LDL-C ≥190 mg/dL or LDL-C ≥160 mg/dL with positive family history of premature cardiovascular disease (CVD) or with two or more CVD risk factors.

Unlabeled Use Secondary prevention in patients who have experienced a noncardioembolic stroke/TIA or following an ACS event regardless of baseline LDL-C using intensive lipid-lowering therapy

Mechanism of Action/Effect Inhibitor of 3-hydroxy-3-methylglutaryl coenzyme A (HMG-CoA) reductase, the rate-limiting enzyme in cholesterol synthesis (reduces the production of mevalonic acid from HMG-CoA); this then results in a compensatory increase in the expression of LDL receptors on hepatocyte membranes and a stimulation of LDL catabolism

Contraindications Hypersensitivity to atorvastatin or any component of the formulation; active liver disease; unexplained persistent elevations of serum transaminases; pregnancy; breast-feeding

Warnings/Precautions Secondary causes of hyperlipidemia should be ruled out prior to therapy. Atorvastatin has not been studied when the primary lipid abnormality is chylomicron elevation (Fredrickson types I and V). Liver function tests must be obtained prior to initiating therapy, repeat if clinically indicated thereafter. May cause hepatic dysfunction. Use with caution in patients who consume large amounts of ethanol or have a history of liver disease; use is contraindicated in patients with active liver disease or unexplained persistent elevations of serum transaminases. Monitoring is recommended. Patients with a history of hemorrhagic stroke may be at increased risk for another hemorrhagic stroke with use.

Rhabdomyolysis with acute renal failure has occurred. Risk is dose related and is increased with concurrent use of lipid-lowering agents which may cause rhabdomyolysis (fibric acid derivatives or niacin at doses ≥1 g/day) or during concurrent use with potent CYP3A4 inhibitors (including amiodarone, clarithromycin, erythromycin, itraconazole, ketoconazole, nefazodone, grapefruit juice in large quantities, verapamil, or protease inhibitors such as indinavir, nelfinavir, or ritonavir). Ensure patient is on the lowest effective atorvastatin dose. If concurrent use of clarithromycin or combination protease inhibitors (eg, lopinavir/ritonavir or ritonavir/saquinavir) is warranted consider dose adjustment of atorvastatin. Do not use with cyclosporine, tipranavir plus ritonavir, or telaprevir. Monitor closely if used with other drugs associated with myopathy. Weigh the risk versus benefit when combining any of these drugs with atorvastatin. Discontinue in any patient in which CPK levels are markedly elevated (>10 times ULN) or if myopathy is suspected/diagnosed. The manufacturer recommends temporary discontinuation for elective major surgery, acute medical or surgical conditions, or in any patient experiencing an acute or serious condition predisposing to renal failure (eg, sepsis, hypotension, trauma, uncontrolled seizures). However, based upon current evidence, HMG-CoA reductase inhibitor therapy should be continued in the perioperative period unless risk outweighs cardioprotective benefit. Use with caution in patients with advanced age, these patients are predisposed to myopathy. Safety and efficacy have not been established in patients <10 years of age or in premenarcheal girls.

Drug Interactions

Avoid Concomitant Use

Avoid concomitant use of Atorvastatin with any of the following: Conivaptan; Pimozide; Red Yeast Rice; Silodosin; Telaprevir; Topotecan

Decreased Effect

Atorvastatin may decrease the levels/effects of: Dabigatran Etexilate; Lanthanum

The levels/effects of Atorvastatin may be decreased by: Antacids; Bexarotene; Bexarotene (Systemic); Bosentan; CYP3A4 Inducers (Strong); Deferasirox; Efavirenz; Etravirine; Fosphenytoin; P-glycoprotein/ABCB1 Inducers; Phenytoin; Rifamycin Derivatives; St Johns Wort; Tocilizumab

Increased Effect/Toxicity

Atorvastatin may increase the levels/effects of: Aliskiren; ARIPiprazole; Colchicine; Dabigatran Etexilate; DAPTOmycin; Digoxin; Diltiazem; Everolimus; Midazolam; P-glycoprotein/ABCB1 Substrates; Pimozide; Prucalopride; Rivaroxaban; Silodosin; Topotecan; Trabectedin; Verapamil

The levels/effects of Atorvastatin may be increased by: Amiodarone; Antifungal Agents (Azole Derivatives, Systemic); Boceprevir; Colchicine; Conivaptan; CycloSPORINE; CycloSPORINE (Systemic); CYP3A4 Inhibitors (Moderate); CYP3A4 Inhibitors (Strong); Cyproterone; Danazol; Dasatinib; Diltiazem; Dronedarone; Eltrombopag; Fenofibrate; Fenofibric Acid; Fluconazole; Fusidic Acid; Gemfibrozil; Grapefruit Juice; Macrolide Antibiotics; Niacin; Niacinamide; P-glycoprotein/ABCB1 Inhibitors; Protease Inhibitors; QuiNINE; Red Yeast Rice; Sildenafil; Telaprevir; Verapamil

Nutritional/Ethanol Interactions

Ethanol: Ethanol may enhance the potential of adverse hepatic effects. Management: Avoid excessive ethanol consumption.

Food: Atorvastatin serum concentrations may be increased by grapefruit juice. Management: Avoid concurrent intake of large quantities of grapefruit juice (>1 quart/day). Red yeast rice contains an estimated 2.4 mg lovastatin per 600 mg rice.

Herb/Nutraceutical: St John's wort may decrease atorvastatin levels.

Adverse Reactions

>10%:

Gastrointestinal: Diarrhea (5% to 14%)

Neuromuscular & skeletal: Arthralgia (4% to 12%)

Respiratory: Nasopharyngitis (4% to 13%)

2% to 10%:

Central nervous system: Insomnia (1% to 5%)

Gastrointestinal: Nausea (4% to 7%), dyspepsia (3% to 6%)

Genitourinary: Urinary tract infection (4% to 8%)

Hepatic: Transaminases increased (2% to 3% with 80 mg/day dosing)

Neuromuscular & skeletal: Limb pain (3% to 9%), myalgia (3% to 8%), muscle spasms (2% to 5%), musculoskeletal pain (2% to 5%)

Respiratory: Pharyngolaryngeal pain (1% to 4%)

Additional class-related events or case reports (not necessarily reported with atorvastatin therapy): Cataracts, cirrhosis, dermatomyositis, eosinophilia, erectile dysfunction, extraocular muscle movement impaired, fulminant hepatic necrosis, gynecomastia, hemolytic anemia, interstitial lung disease, ophthalmoplegia, peripheral nerve palsy, polymyalgia rheumatica, positive ANA, renal failure (secondary to rhabdomyolysis), systemic lupus erythematosus-like syndrome, thyroid dysfunction, tremor, vasculitis, vertigo

Pharmacodynamics/Kinetics

Onset of Action Initial changes: 3-5 days; Maximal reduction in plasma cholesterol and triglycerides: 2 weeks

Available Dosage Forms

Tablet, oral: 10 mg, 20 mg, 40 mg, 80 mg

Lipitor®: 10 mg, 20 mg, 40 mg, 80 mg

General Dosage Range Dosage adjustment recommended in patients on concomitant therapy

Oral:

Children 10-17 years (females >1 year postmenarche): 10-20 mg/day (maximum: 20 mg/day)

Adults: Maintenance: 10-80 mg once daily (maximum: 80 mg/day)

Administration

Oral May be administered with food if desired; may take without regard to time of day.

Stability

Storage Store at controlled room temperature of 20°C to 25°C (68°F to 77°F).

Nursing Actions

Physical Assessment Assess risk potential for interactions with other prescriptions or herbal products patient may be taking that may increase risk of rhabdomyolysis. Monitor CPK prior to initiation and recheck when symptoms are suggestive of myopathy. Assess liver function tests prior to initiation, repeat LFTs if indicated thereafter.

Patient Education May take without regard to food; avoid large intake of grapefruit juice. You will need periodic laboratory evaluation during therapy. This drug does not eliminate the need for prescribed diet or exercise regimen. Avoid excessive alcohol. Report unusual muscle cramping or weakness, yellowing of skin or eyes, easy bruising or bleeding, or unusual fatigue.

Dietary Considerations May take with food if desired; may take without regard to time of day. Before initiation of therapy, patients should be placed on a standard cholesterol-lowering diet for 3-6 months and the diet should be continued during drug therapy. Red yeast rice contains an estimated 2.4 mg lovastatin per 600 mg rice. Atorvastatin serum concentration may be increased when taken with grapefruit juice; avoid concurrent intake of large quantities (>1 quart/day).

Atovaquone (a TOE va kwone)

Brand Names: U.S. Mepron®

Pharmacologic Category Antiprotozoal

Pregnancy Risk Factor C

Lactation Excretion in breast milk unknown/use caution

Use Acute oral treatment of mild-to-moderate *Pneumocystis jirovecii* pneumonia (PCP) in patients who are intolerant to co-trimoxazole; prophylaxis of PCP in patients who are intolerant to co-trimoxazole

Unlabeled Use Treatment of babesiosis; treatment/suppression of *Toxoplasma gondii* encephalitis; primary prophylaxis of HIV-infected persons at high risk for developing *Toxoplasma gondii* encephalitis

Available Dosage Forms

Suspension, oral:

Mepron®: 750 mg/5 mL (5 mL, 210 mL)

General Dosage Range Oral: *Children 13-16 years and Adults:* 1500 mg/day in 1-2 divided doses

Administration

Oral Must be taken administered meals. Shake suspension gently before use. Once opened, the foil pouch can be emptied on a dosing spoon, in a cup, or directly into the mouth.

Nursing Actions

Physical Assessment Monitor for CNS and respiratory changes.

Patient Education Take with high-fat meals. You may experience dizziness or lightheadedness, problems sleeping, rash, weakness, cough, or flu-like symptoms. Report unresolved diarrhea, fever, mouth sores, unresolved headache, abdominal pain, shortness of breath, or vomiting.

Atracurium (a tra KYOO ree um)

Index Terms Atracurium Besylate

Pharmacologic Category Neuromuscular Blocker Agent, Nondepolarizing

Medication Safety Issues

High alert medication:

The Institute for Safe Medication Practices (ISMP) includes this medication among its list of drugs which have a heightened risk of causing significant patient harm when used in error.

Other safety concerns:

United States Pharmacopeia (USP) 2006: The Interdisciplinary Safe Medication Use Expert Committee of the USP has recommended the following:

- Hospitals, clinics, and other practice sites should institute special safeguards in the storage, labeling, and use of these agents and should include these safeguards in staff orientation and competency training.
- Healthcare professionals should be on **high alert** (especially vigilant) whenever a neuromuscular-blocking agent (NMBA) is stocked, ordered, prepared, or administered.

Pregnancy Risk Factor C

Lactation Excretion in breast milk unknown/use caution

Use Adjunct to general anesthesia to facilitate endotracheal intubation and to relax skeletal muscles during surgery; to facilitate mechanical ventilation in ICU patients; does not relieve pain or produce sedation

Mechanism of Action/Effect Blocks neural transmission at the myoneural junction by binding with cholinergic receptor sites

Contraindications Hypersensitivity to atracurium besylate or any component of the formulation

Warnings/Precautions Reduce initial dosage and inject slowly (over 1-2 minutes) in patients in whom substantial histamine release would be potentially hazardous (eg, patients with clinically-important cardiovascular disease). Maintenance of an adequate airway and respiratory support is critical. Certain clinical conditions may result in potentiation or antagonism of neuromuscular blockade:

Potentiation: Electrolyte abnormalities, severe hyponatremia, severe hypocalcemia, severe hypokalemia, hypermagnesemia, neuromuscular diseases, acidosis, acute intermittent porphyria, renal failure, hepatic failure

Antagonism: Alkalosis, hypercalcemia, demyelinating lesions, peripheral neuropathies, diabetes mellitus

Increased sensitivity in patients with myasthenia gravis, Eaton-Lambert syndrome; resistance in burn patients (>30% of body) for period of 5-70 days postinjury; resistance in patients with muscle trauma, denervation, immobilization, infection, chronic treatment with atracurium. Cross-sensitivity with other neuromuscular-blocking agents may occur; use extreme caution in patients with previous anaphylactic reactions. Use caution in the elderly. Bradycardia may be more common with atracurium than with other neuromuscular-blocking agents since it has no clinically-significant effects on heart rate to counteract the bradycardia produced by anesthetics. Should be administered by adequately trained individuals familiar with its use. Some dosage forms may contain benzyl alcohol which has been associated with "gasping syndrome" in neonates.

Drug Interactions

Avoid Concomitant Use

Avoid concomitant use of Atracurium with any of the following: QuiNINE

Decreased Effect

The levels/effects of Atracurium may be decreased by: Acetylcholinesterase Inhibitors; Loop Diuretics

Increased Effect/Toxicity

Atracurium may increase the levels/effects of: Cardiac Glycosides; Corticosteroids (Systemic); OnabotulinumtoxinA; RimabotulinumtoxinB

The levels/effects of Atracurium may be increased by: AbobotulinumtoxinA; Aminoglycosides; Calcium Channel Blockers; Capreomycin; Colistimethate; Inhalational Anesthetics; Ketorolac; Ketorolac (Nasal); Ketorolac (Systemic); Lincosamide Antibiotics; Lithium; Loop Diuretics; Magnesium Salts; Polymyxin B; Procainamide; QuiNIDine; QuiNINE; Spironolactone; Tetracycline Derivatives; Vancomycin

Adverse Reactions Mild, rare, and generally suggestive of histamine release

1% to 10%: Cardiovascular: Flushing

Causes of prolonged neuromuscular blockade: Excessive drug administration; cumulative drug effect, metabolism/excretion decreased (hepatic and/or renal impairment); accumulation of active metabolites; electrolyte imbalance (hypokalemia, hypocalcemia, hypermagnesemia, hypernatremia); hypothermia

Pharmacodynamics/Kinetics

Onset of Action Dose dependent: 2-3 minutes

Duration of Action Recovery begins in 20-35 minutes following initial dose of 0.4-0.5 mg/kg under balanced anesthesia; recovery to 95% of control takes 60-70 minutes

Available Dosage Forms

Injection, solution: 10 mg/mL (10 mL)

Injection, solution [preservative free]: 10 mg/mL (5 mL)

General Dosage Range I.V.:

Children 1 month to 2 years: Initial: 0.3-0.4 mg/kg; Maintenance: Doses as needed to maintain neuromuscular blockade; Infusion: 10-20 mcg/kg/minute

Children >2 years and Adults: Initial: 0.4-0.5 mg/kg; Maintenance: 0.08-1 mg/kg at 15- to 25-minute intervals; Infusion: 5-13 mcg/kg/minute

Administration

I.M. Not for I.M. injection due to tissue irritation.

I.V. May be given undiluted as a bolus injection. Administration via infusion requires the use of an infusion pump. Use infusion solutions within 24 hours of preparation.

I.V. Detail pH: 3.25-3.65 (adjusted)

Stability

Reconstitution Atracurium should not be mixed with alkaline solutions.

Storage Refrigerate intact vials at 2°C to 8°C (36°F to 46°F); protect from freezing. Use vials within 14 days upon removal from the refrigerator to room temperature of 25°C (77°F). Dilutions of 0.2 mg/mL or 0.5 mg/mL in 0.9% sodium chloride, dextrose 5% in water, or 5% dextrose in sodium chloride 0.9% are stable for up to 24 hours at room temperature or under refrigeration.

Nursing Actions

Physical Assessment Ventilatory support must be instituted and maintained until adequate respiratory muscle function and/or airway protection are assured. Other drugs that affect neuromuscular activity may increase/decrease neuromuscular block induced by atracurium. This drug is not an anesthetic or analgesic; pain must be treated with other agents. Continuous monitoring of vital signs, cardiac status, respiratory status, and degree of neuromuscular block (objective assessment with peripheral external nerve stimulator) is mandatory during infusion and until full muscle tone has returned. Safety precautions must be maintained until full muscle tone has returned. It may take longer for return of muscle tone in obese or elderly patients or patients with renal or hepatic disease, myasthenia gravis, myopathy, other neuromuscular disease, dehydration, electrolyte imbalance, or severe acid/base imbalance.

Long-term use: Monitor level of neuromuscular blockade, skeletal muscle movement, and respiratory effort. Reposition patient and provide appropriate skin care, mouth care, and care of patient's eyes every 2-3 hours while sedated. Provide appropriate emotional and sensory support (auditory and environmental).

Patient Education Patient will usually be unconscious prior to administration. Reassurance of constant monitoring and emotional support to reduce fear and anxiety should precede and follow administration. Following return of muscle tone, do not attempt to change position or rise from bed without assistance.

Atropine (A troe peen)

Brand Names: U.S. AtroPen®; Atropine Care™; Isopto® Atropine

Index Terms Atropine Sulfate

Pharmacologic Category Anticholinergic Agent; Anticholinergic Agent, Ophthalmic; Antidote; Antispasmodic Agent, Gastrointestinal; Ophthalmic Agent, Mydriatic

Pregnancy Risk Factor B/C (manufacturer specific)

Lactation Enters breast milk/use caution (AAP rates "compatible"; AAP 2001 update pending)

Breast-Feeding Considerations Trace amounts of atropine are excreted into breast milk. Anticholinergic agents may suppress lactation.

Use

Injection: Preoperative medication to inhibit salivation and secretions; treatment of symptomatic sinus bradycardia, AV block (nodal level); antidote for anticholinesterase poisoning (carbamate insecticides, nerve agents, organophosphate insecticides); adjuvant use with anticholinesterases (eg, edrophonium, neostigmine) to decrease their side effects during reversal of neuromuscular blockade

Note: Use is no longer recommended in the management of asystole or pulseless electrical activity (PEA) (ACLS, 2010).

Ophthalmic: Produce mydriasis and cycloplegia for examination of the retina and optic disc and accurate measurement of refractive errors; produce papillary dilation in inflammatory conditions (eg, uveitis)

Mechanism of Action/Effect Blocks the action of acetylcholine at parasympathetic sites in smooth muscle, secretory glands, and the CNS; increases cardiac output, dries secretions. Atropine reverses the muscarinic effects of cholinergic poisoning due to agents with acetylcholinesterase inhibitor activity by acting as a competitive antagonist of ▶

acetylcholine at muscarinic receptors. The primary goal in cholinergic poisonings is reversal of bronchorrhea and bronchoconstriction. Atropine has no effect on the nicotinic receptors responsible for muscle weakness, fasciculations, and paralysis.

Contraindications Hypersensitivity to atropine or any component of the formulation; narrow-angle glaucoma; adhesions between the iris and lens (ophthalmic product); pyloric stenosis; prostatic hypertrophy

Note: No contraindications exist in the treatment of life-threatening organophosphate or carbamate insecticide or nerve agent poisoning.

Warnings/Precautions Heat prostration may occur in the presence of high environmental temperatures. Psychosis may occur in sensitive individuals or following use of excessive doses. Avoid use if possible in patients with obstructive uropathy or in other conditions resulting in urinary retention; use is contraindicated in patients with prostatic hypertrophy. Avoid use in patients with paralytic ileus, intestinal atony of the elderly or debilitated patient, severe ulcerative colitis, and toxic megacolon complicating ulcerative colitis. Use with caution in patients with autonomic neuropathy, hyperthyroidism, renal or hepatic impairment, myocardial ischemia, HF, tachyarrhythmias (including sinus tachycardia), hypertension, and hiatal hernia associated with reflux esophagitis. Treatment-related blood pressure increases and tachycardia may lead to ischemia, precipitate an MI, or increase arrhythmogenic potential. In heart transplant recipients, atropine will likely be ineffective in treatment of bradycardia due to lack of vagal innervation of the transplanted heart; cholinergic reinnervation may occur over time (years), so atropine may be used cautiously; however, some may experience paradoxical slowing of the heart rate and high-degree AV block upon administration (ACLS, 2010; Bernheim, 2004).

Avoid relying on atropine for effective treatment of type II second-degree or third-degree AV block (with or without a new wide QRS complex). Asystole or bradycardic pulseless electrical activity (PEA): Although no evidence exists for significant detrimental effects, routine use is unlikely to have a therapeutic benefit and is no longer recommended (ACLS, 2010).

AtroPen®: There are no absolute contraindications for the use of atropine in severe organophosphate or carbamate insecticide or nerve agent poisonings; however in mild poisonings, use caution in those patients where the use of atropine would be otherwise contraindicated. Formulation for use by trained personnel only. Clinical symptoms consistent with highly-suspected organophosphate or carbamate insecticides or nerve agent poisoning should be treated with antidote immediately; administration should not be delayed for confirmatory laboratory tests. Signs of atropinization include flushing, mydriasis, tachycardia, and dryness of the mouth or nose. Monitor effects closely when administering subsequent injections as necessary. The presence of these effects is not indicative of the success of therapy; inappropriate use of mydriasis as an indicator of successful treatment has resulted in atropine toxicity. Reversal of bronchial secretions is the preferred indicator of success. Adjunct treatment with a cholinesterase reactivator (eg, pralidoxime) may be required in patients with toxicity secondary to organophosphorus insecticides or nerve agents. Treatment should always include proper evacuation and decontamination procedures; medical personnel should protect themselves from inadvertent contamination. Antidotal administration is intended only for initial management; definitive and more extensive medical care is required following administration. Individuals should not rely solely on antidote for treatment, as other supportive measures (eg, artificial respiration) may still be required. Atropine reverses the muscarinic but not the nicotinic effects associated with anticholinesterase toxicity.

Children and elderly patients may be more sensitive to the anticholinergic effects of atropine; use with caution in children with spastic paralysis.

Drug Interactions

Avoid Concomitant Use There are no known interactions where it is recommended to avoid concomitant use.

Decreased Effect

Atropine may decrease the levels/effects of: Acetylcholinesterase Inhibitors (Central); Secretin

The levels/effects of Atropine may be decreased by: Acetylcholinesterase Inhibitors (Central)

Increased Effect/Toxicity

Atropine may increase the levels/effects of: AbobotulinumtoxinA; Anticholinergics; Cannabinoids; OnabotulinumtoxinA; Potassium Chloride; RimabotulinumtoxinB

The levels/effects of Atropine may be increased by: Pramlintide

Adverse Reactions Severity and frequency of adverse reactions are dose related and vary greatly; listed reactions are limited to significant and/or life-threatening.

Cardiovascular: Arrhythmia, flushing, hypotension, palpitation, tachycardia

Central nervous system: Ataxia, coma, delirium, disorientation, dizziness, drowsiness, excitement, fever, hallucinations, headache, insomnia, nervousness

Dermatologic: Anhidrosis, urticaria, rash, scarlatiniform rash

Gastrointestinal: Bloating, constipation, delayed gastric emptying, loss of taste, nausea, paralytic ileus, vomiting, xerostomia, dry throat, nasal dryness

Genitourinary: Urinary hesitancy, urinary retention

Neuromuscular & skeletal: Weakness
Ocular: Angle-closure glaucoma, blurred vision, cycloplegia, dry eyes, mydriasis, ocular tension increased
Respiratory: Dyspnea, laryngospasm, pulmonary edema
Miscellaneous: Anaphylaxis

Pharmacodynamics/Kinetics

Onset of Action I.M., I.V.: Rapid

Available Dosage Forms

Injection, solution: 0.05 mg/mL (5 mL); 0.1 mg/mL (5 mL, 10 mL); 0.4 mg/mL (1 mL, 20 mL)

AtroPen®: 0.25 mg/0.3 mL (0.3 mL); 0.5 mg/0.7 mL (0.7 mL); 1 mg/0.7 mL (0.7 mL); 2 mg/0.7 mL (0.7 mL)

Injection, solution [preservative free]: 0.4 mg/0.5 mL (0.5 mL); 0.4 mg/mL (1 mL); 1 mg/mL (1 mL)

Ointment, ophthalmic: 1% (3.5 g)

Solution, ophthalmic: 1% (2 mL, 5 mL, 15 mL)

Atropine Care™: 1% (2 mL, 5 mL, 15 mL)

Isopto® Atropine: 1% (5 mL, 15 mL)

General Dosage Range

I.M.; SubQ:

Children ≤5 kg: 0.02 mg/kg/dose every 4-6 hours as needed

Children >5 kg: 0.01-0.02 mg/kg/dose every 4-6 hours as needed (maximum: 0.4 mg/dose; minimum: 0.1 mg/dose)

Adults: 0.4-0.6 mg every 4-6 hours as needed

AtroPen® (I.M.):

Children <6.8 kg: 0.25 mg/dose (maximum: 3 doses)

Children 6.8-18 kg: 0.5 mg/dose (maximum: 3 doses)

Children 18-41 kg: 1 mg/dose (maximum: 3 doses)

Children >41 kg and Adults: 2 mg/dose (maximum: 3 doses)

I.V.: *Children and Adults:* Dosage varies greatly depending on indication

Ophthalmic: *Adults:* Ointment: Apply a small amount in the conjunctival sac up to 3 times/day; Solution (1%): Instill 1-2 drops up to 4 times/day

Administration

I.M. AtroPen®: Administer to the outer thigh. Firmly grasp the autoinjector with the green tip (0.5 mg, 1 mg, and 2 mg autoinjector) or black tip (0.25 mg autoinjector) pointed down; remove the yellow safety release (0.5 mg, 1 mg, and 2 mg autoinjector) or gray safety release (0.25 autoinjector). Jab the green tip at a 90° angle against the outer thigh; may be administered through clothing as long as pockets at the injection site are empty. In thin patients or patients <6.8 kg (15 lb), bunch up the thigh prior to injection. Hold the autoinjector in place for 10 seconds following the injection; remove the autoinjector and massage the injection site. After administration, the needle will be visible; if the needle is not visible, repeat the above steps. After use, bend the needle against a hard surface (needle does not retract) to avoid accidental injury.

I.V. Administer undiluted by rapid I.V. injection; slow injection may result in paradoxical bradycardia. In bradycardia, atropine administration should not delay treatment with external pacing.

I.V. Detail pH: 3-6.5; AtroPen®: pH: 4-5

Other Endotracheal: Dilute in NS or sterile water. Absorption may be greater with sterile water. Stop compressions (if using for cardiac arrest), spray the drug quickly down the tube. Follow immediately with several quick insufflations and continue chest compressions.

Stability

Reconstitution Preparation of bulk atropine solution for mass chemical terrorism: Add atropine sulfate powder to 100 mL NS in polyvinyl chloride bags to yield a final concentration of 1 mg/mL. Stable for 72 hours at 4°C to 8°C (39°F to 46°F); 20°C to 25°C (68°F to 77°F); 32°C to 36°C (90°F to 97°F) (Dix, 2003).

Storage Store injection at controlled room temperature of 15°C to 30°C (59°F to 86°F); avoid freezing. In addition, AtroPen® should be protected from light.

Nursing Actions

Physical Assessment Monitor for tachycardia and hypotension, especially if cardiac problems are present. Ensure patient safety (side rails up, call light within reach), have patient void prior to administration, and ensure adequate hydration. Be alert to the potential of heat prostration in the presence of high temperatures.

Patient Education Maintain adequate hydration, unless instructed to restrict fluid intake. You may experience dizziness, blurred vision, sensitivity to light, dry mouth, nausea, vomiting, orthostatic hypotension, constipation, increased sensitivity to heat and decreased perspiration, or decreased milk supply if breast-feeding. Report hot, dry, flushed skin; blurred vision or vision changes; difficulty swallowing; chest pain, palpitations, or rapid heartbeat; painful or difficult urination; increased confusion, depression, or loss of memory; rapid or difficult respirations; muscle weakness or tremors; or eye pain.

Ophthalmic: Wash hands before using. Sit or lie down, open eye, look at ceiling, and instill prescribed amount of solution. Do not blink for 30 seconds. Close eye, roll eye in all directions, and apply gentle pressure to inner corner of eye for 1-2 minutes. Do not let tip of applicator touch eye; do not contaminate tip of applicator (may cause eye infection, eye damage, or vision loss). Temporary stinging or blurred vision may occur.

Axitinib (ax I ti nib)

Brand Names: U.S. Inlyta®

Index Terms AG-013736; Inlyta®

Pharmacologic Category Antineoplastic Agent, Tyrosine Kinase Inhibitor; Vascular Endothelial Growth Factor (VEGF) Inhibitor

Medication Safety Issues

Sound-alike/look-alike issues:

Axitinib may be confused with gefitinib, imatinib, pazopanib, SORAfenib, SUNItinib, vandetanib, vemurafenib

High alert medication:

This medication is in a class the Institute for Safe Medication Practices (ISMP) includes among its list of drug classes which have a heightened risk of causing significant patient harm when used in error.

Pregnancy Risk Factor D

Lactation Excretion in breast milk unknown/not recommended

Use Treatment of advanced renal cell cancer (RCC) after failure of one prior systemic treatment

Available Dosage Forms

Tablet, oral:

Inlyta®: 1 mg, 5 mg

General Dosage Range Dosage adjustment recommended in patients with hepatic impairment, on concomitant therapy, or who develop toxicities.

Oral: *Adults:* 5 mg every 12 hours; maximum: 10 mg every 12 hours

Administration

Oral Swallow tablet whole with a glass of water. May be taken with or without food. If a dose is missed or vomited, do not make up; resume dosing with the next scheduled dose.

Nursing Actions

Physical Assessment Axitinib is an oral capsule given daily with or without food. Blood pressure needs to be monitored closely even at the start of therapy. Due to altered wound healing, instruct patient to discuss any surgery or procedures with prescriber. Monitor for bleeding, symptoms of hypothyroidism, hyperglycemia, diarrhea, severe abdominal pain, and proper wound healing.

Patient Education Patients should inform prescriber of liver disease, kidney disease, hypertension, thyroid disease, or thrombosis (eg, DVT, PE, CVA, MI). Common side effects include high blood pressure, diarrhea, high blood sugar, weight loss, feeling tired or weak, bleeding problems, and kidney effects. Have patient call prescriber immediately for signs of stroke, heart attack, blood clot, hypothyroidism, severe diarrhea, severe abdominal pain, high blood sugar, or wound that will not heal.

AzaCITIDine (ay za SYE ti deen)

Brand Names: U.S. Vidaza®

Index Terms 5-Azacytidine; 5-AZC; AZA-CR; Azacytidine; Ladakamycin

Pharmacologic Category Antineoplastic Agent, DNA Methylation Inhibitor

Medication Safety Issues

Sound-alike/look-alike issues:

AzaCITIDine may be confused with azaTHIOprine

High alert medication:

This medication is in a class the Institute for Safe Medication Practices (ISMP) includes among its list of drug classes which have a heightened risk of causing significant patient harm when used in error.

Pregnancy Risk Factor D

Lactation Excretion in breast milk unknown/not recommended

Use Treatment of myelodysplastic syndrome (MDS)

Unlabeled Use Treatment of acute myelogenous leukemia (AML)

Available Dosage Forms

Injection, powder for suspension:

Vidaza®: 100 mg

General Dosage Range Dosage adjustment recommended in patients who develop toxicities

I.V., SubQ: *Adults:* 75-100 mg/m^2/day for 7 days/28-day treatment cycle

Administration

I.V. Premedication for nausea and vomiting is recommended. Infuse over 10-40 minutes; infusion must be completed within 1 hour of (vial) reconstitution.

Other SubQ: Premedication for nausea and vomiting is recommended. The manufacturer recommends equally dividing volumes >4 mL into 2 syringes and injecting into 2 separate sites; however, policies for maximum SubQ administration volume may vary by institution; interpatient variations may also apply. Administer subsequent injections at least 1 inch from previous injection sites. Allow refrigerated suspensions to come to room temperature (up to 30 minutes) prior to administration. Resuspend by inverting the syringe 2-3 times and then rolling the syringe between the palms for 30 seconds. If azacitidine suspension comes in contact with the skin, immediately wash with soap and water.

Nursing Actions

Physical Assessment Pretreatment with antiemetic may be ordered to reduce nausea and vomiting. Note specific reconstitution, administration, and storage instructions (I.V. and SubQ stability differs). Monitor patient closely for edema, chest pain, hypotension, CNS changes, gastrointestinal disturbances, and hematologic and hepatic effects.

Patient Education This medication can only be administered by injection or I.V.; report immediately any pain, burning, or swelling at injection/infusion site. Limit oral intake for 4-6 hours before therapy to reduce potential for nausea/vomiting. It is important that you maintain adequate nutrition between treatments and adequate hydration, unless instructed to restrict fluid intake. You may be susceptible to infection. May cause nausea, vomiting, abdominal tenderness, anorexia, mouth sores, or loss of hair (reversible). Report chest pain or palpitations; sore throat, fever, chills, unusual weakness or fatigue; unusual bruising/bleeding; change in color or frequency of urine or stool; itching or burning on urination; difficulty breathing; change in visual acuity; or pain, redness, or swelling at injection site.

AzaTHIOprine (ay za THYE oh preen)

Brand Names: U.S. Azasan®; Imuran®

Index Terms Azathioprine Sodium

Pharmacologic Category Immunosuppressant Agent

Medication Safety Issues

Sound-alike/look-alike issues:

AzaTHIOprine may be confused with azaCITIDine, azidothymidine, azithromycin, Azulfidine®

Imuran® may be confused with Elmiron®, Enduron, Imdur®, Inderal®, Tenormin®

Other safety concerns:

Azathioprine is metabolized to mercaptopurine; concurrent use of these commercially-available products has resulted in profound myelosuppression.

Pregnancy Risk Factor D

Lactation Enters breast milk/not recommended

Breast-Feeding Considerations Due to risk of immunosuppression and serious adverse effects in the nursing infant, breast-feeding is not recommended.

Use Adjunctive therapy in prevention of rejection of kidney transplants; management of active rheumatoid arthritis (RA)

Unlabeled Use Adjunct in prevention of rejection of solid organ (nonrenal) transplants; remission maintenance or reduction of steroid use in Crohn's disease (CD) and in ulcerative colitis (UC); dermatomyositis/polymyositis; erythema multiforme; pemphigus vulgaris, lupus nephritis, chronic refractory immune (idiopathic) thrombocytopenic purpura, relapsed/remitting multiple sclerosis

Mechanism of Action/Effect Antagonizes purine metabolism and may inhibit synthesis of DNA, RNA, and proteins; may also interfere with cellular metabolism and inhibit mitosis; the 6-thioguanine nucleotides appear to mediate the majority of azathioprine's immunosuppressive and toxic effects

Contraindications Hypersensitivity to azathioprine or any component of the formulation; pregnancy (in patients with rheumatoid arthritis); patients with rheumatoid arthritis and a history of treatment with alkylating agents (eg, cyclophosphamide, chlorambucil, melphalan) may have a prohibitive risk of neoplasia with azathioprine treatment

Warnings/Precautions [U.S. Boxed Warning]: Immunosuppressive agents, including azathioprine, are associated with the development of lymphoma and other malignancies, especially of the skin. Hepatosplenic T-Cell Lymphoma (HSTCL), a rare white blood cell cancer that is usually fatal, has predominantly occurred in adolescents and young adults treated for Crohn's disease or ulcerative colitis and receiving TNF blockers (eg, adalimumab, certolizumab pegol, etanercept, golimumab), azathioprine, and/or mercaptopurine. Most cases have occurred in patients treated with a combination of immunosuppressant agents, although there have been reports of HSTCL in patients receiving azathioprine or mercaptopurine monotherapy. Renal transplant patients are also at increased risk for malignancy (eg, skin cancer, lymphoma); limit sun and ultraviolet light exposure and use appropriate sun protection. Dose-related hematologic toxicities (leukopenia, thrombocytopenia, and anemias, including macrocytic anemia, or pancytopenia) may occur; delayed toxicities may also occur. May be more severe with renal transplants undergoing rejection; dosage modification for hematologic toxicity may be necessary. Chronic immunosuppression increases the risk of serious infections; may require dosage reduction. Use with caution in patients with liver disease or renal impairment; monitor hematologic function closely. Azathioprine is metabolized to mercaptopurine; concomitant use may result in profound myelosuppression and should be avoided. Patients with genetic deficiency of thiopurine methyltransferase (TPMT) or concurrent therapy with drugs which may inhibit TPMT may be sensitive to myelosuppressive effects. Patients with intermediate TPMT activity may be at risk for increased myelosuppression; those with low or absent TPMT activity are at risk for developing severe myelotoxicity. TPMT genotyping or phenotyping may assist in identifying patients at risk for developing toxicity. Consider TPMT testing in patients with abnormally low CBC unresponsive to dose reduction. TPMT testing does not substitute for CBC monitoring. Xanthine oxidase inhibitors may increase risk for hematologic toxicity; reduce azathioprine dose when used concurrently with allopurinol; patients with low or absent TPMT activity may require further dose reductions or discontinuation.

Hepatotoxicity (transaminase, bilirubin, and alkaline phosphatase elevations) may occur, usually in renal transplant patients and generally within 6 months of transplant; normally reversible with discontinuation; monitor liver function periodically. Rarely, hepatic sinusoidal obstruction syndrome (SOS; formerly called veno-occlusive disease) has been reported; discontinue if hepatic SOS is suspected. Severe nausea, vomiting, diarrhea, rash, fever, malaise, myalgia, hypotension, and liver enzyme abnormalities may occur within the first several weeks of treatment and are generally reversible upon discontinuation. **[U.S. Boxed Warning]: Should be prescribed by physicians familiar with the risks, including hematologic toxicities and mutagenic potential.** Immune response to vaccines may be diminished. Hazardous agent - use appropriate precautions for handling and disposal.

Drug Interactions

Avoid Concomitant Use

Avoid concomitant use of AzaTHIOprine with any of the following: BCG; Febuxostat; Mercaptopurine; Natalizumab; Pimecrolimus; Tacrolimus (Topical)

Decreased Effect

AzaTHIOprine may decrease the levels/effects of: BCG; Coccidioidin Skin Test; Sipuleucel-T; Vaccines (Inactivated); Vitamin K Antagonists

The levels/effects of AzaTHIOprine may be decreased by: Echinacea

Increased Effect/Toxicity

AzaTHIOprine may increase the levels/effects of: Leflunomide; Mercaptopurine; Natalizumab; Vaccines (Live)

The levels/effects of AzaTHIOprine may be increased by: 5-ASA Derivatives; ACE Inhibitors; Allopurinol; Denosumab; Febuxostat; Pimecrolimus; Ribavirin; Roflumilast; Sulfamethoxazole; Tacrolimus (Topical); Trastuzumab; Trimethoprim

Nutritional/Ethanol Interactions Herb/Nutraceutical: Avoid cat's claw, echinacea (have immunostimulant properties).

Adverse Reactions Frequency not always defined; dependent upon dose, duration, indication, and concomitant therapy.

Central nervous system: Fever, malaise

Gastrointestinal: Nausea/vomiting (RA 12%), diarrhea

Hematologic: Leukopenia (renal transplant >50%; RA 28%), thrombocytopenia

Hepatic: Alkaline phosphatase increased, bilirubin increased, hepatotoxicity, transaminases increased

Neuromuscular & skeletal: Myalgia

Miscellaneous: Infection (renal transplant 20%; RA <1%; includes bacterial, fungal, protozoal, viral), neoplasia (renal transplant 3% [other than lymphoma], 0.5% [lymphoma])

Available Dosage Forms

Injection, powder for reconstitution: 100 mg

Tablet, oral: 50 mg

Azasan®: 75 mg, 100 mg

Imuran®: 50 mg

General Dosage Range Dosage adjustment recommended in patients with renal impairment, on concomitant therapy, or who develop toxicities

I.V.: *Adults:* Transplant immunosuppression: Initial: 3-5 mg/kg/day as a single daily dose; Maintenance: 1-3 mg/kg/day as a single daily dose

Oral: *Adults:*

Transplant immunosuppression: Initial: 3-5 mg/kg/day in 1-2 divided doses; Maintenance: 1-3 mg/kg/day in 1-2 divided doses

Rheumatoid arthritis: Initial: 1 mg/kg/day (50-100 mg) in 1-2 divided doses; Maintenance: 0.5-2.5 mg/kg/day in 1-2 divided doses

Administration

Oral Administering tablets after meals or in divided doses may decrease adverse GI events.

I.V. Can be administered IVP over 5 minutes at a concentration not to exceed 10 mg/mL **or** azathioprine can be further diluted with normal saline, 1/2NS, or D_5W and administered by intermittent infusion usually over 30-60 minutes or by an extended infusion up to 8 hours.

I.V. Detail pH: 9.6

Stability

Reconstitution Powder for injection: Reconstitute each vial with 10 mL sterile water for injection; may further dilute for infusion (in D_5W, 1/2NS, or NS). Use appropriate precautions for handling and disposal.

Storage

Tablet: Store at room temperature of 15°C to 25°C (59°F to 77°F).Protect from light and moisture.

Powder for injection: Store intact vials at room temperature of 15°C to 25°C (59°F to 77°F). Protect from light. Reconstituted solution should be used within 24 hours; solutions diluted in D_5W, 1/2NS, or NS for infusion are stable at room temperature or refrigerated for up to 16 days (Johnson, 1981); however, the manufacturer recommends use within 24 hours of reconstitution.

Nursing Actions

Physical Assessment Monitor for opportunistic infection (eg, fever, mouth and vaginal sores or plaques, unhealed wounds).

Patient Education May take in divided doses or with food if GI upset occurs. You will be susceptible to infection. You may experience nausea, vomiting, loss of appetite. Report abdominal pain and unresolved GI upset (eg, persistent vomiting or diarrhea); unusual fever or chills; bleeding or bruising; sore throat, unhealed sores, or signs of infection; yellowing of skin or eyes; or change in color of urine or stool. For rheumatoid arthritis, response may not occur for up to 3 months. For organ transplant, azathioprine will usually be prescribed with other antirejection medications.

Dietary Considerations May be taken with food.

Azilsartan (ay zil SAR tan)

Brand Names: U.S. edarbi™

Index Terms Azilsartan Medoxomil; AZL-M

Pharmacologic Category Angiotensin II Receptor Blocker

Pregnancy Risk Factor D

Lactation Excretion in breast milk unknown/not recommended

Breast-Feeding Considerations According to the manufacturer, the decision to continue or discontinue breast-feeding during therapy should take into account the risk of exposure to the infant and the benefits of treatment to the mother.

Use Treatment of hypertension; may be used alone or in combination with other antihypertensives

Mechanism of Action/Effect Azilsartan is an angiotensin receptor antagonist which selectively blocks the vasoconstriction and aldosterone-secreting effects of angiotensin II.

Contraindications There are no contraindications listed in manufacturer's labeling.

Warnings/Precautions [U.S. Boxed Warning]: Drugs that act on the renin-angiotensin system can cause injury and death to the developing fetus. Discontinue as soon as possible once pregnancy is detected. Angiotensin II receptor blockers may cause hyperkalemia; avoid potassium supplementation unless specifically required by healthcare provider. Avoid use or use a smaller dose in patients who are volume depleted; correct depletion first. May be associated with deterioration of renal function and/or increases in serum creatinine, particularly in patients with low renal blood flow (eg, renal artery stenosis, heart failure, volume depletion) whose glomerular filtration rate (GFR) is dependent on efferent arteriolar vasoconstriction by angiotensin II. Use with caution in unstented unilateral/bilateral renal artery stenosis. When unstented bilateral renal artery stenosis is present, use is generally avoided due to the elevated risk of deterioration in renal function unless possible benefits outweigh risks. Use with caution in pre-existing renal insufficiency; significant aortic/mitral stenosis. Concurrent use with ACE inhibitors may increase the risk of clinically-significant adverse events (eg, renal dysfunction, hyperkalemia).

Drug Interactions

Avoid Concomitant Use There are no known interactions where it is recommended to avoid concomitant use.

Decreased Effect

The levels/effects of Azilsartan may be decreased by: Herbs (Hypertensive Properties); Methylphenidate; Nonsteroidal Anti-Inflammatory Agents; Rifamycin Derivatives; Yohimbine

Increased Effect/Toxicity

Azilsartan may increase the levels/effects of: ACE Inhibitors; Amifostine; Antihypertensives; Hypotensive Agents; Lithium; Nonsteroidal Anti-Inflammatory Agents; Potassium-Sparing Diuretics; RiTUXimab; Sodium Phosphates

The levels/effects of Azilsartan may be increased by: Alfuzosin; Diazoxide; Eplerenone; Herbs (Hypotensive Properties); MAO Inhibitors; Pentoxifylline; Phosphodiesterase 5 Inhibitors; Potassium Salts; Prostacyclin Analogues; Tolvaptan; Trimethoprim

Nutritional/Ethanol Interactions Herb/Nutraceutical: Avoid ephedra, yohimbe, ginseng (may worsen hypertension). Avoid garlic (may have increased antihypertensive effect).

Adverse Reactions

Cardiovascular: Hypotension, orthostatic hypotension

Central nervous system: Dizziness, fatigue

Gastrointestinal: Diarrhea (2%), nausea

Hematologic: Hemoglobin decreased, hematocrit decreased, leukopenia (rare), RBC decreased, thrombocytopenia (rare)

Neuromuscular & skeletal: Muscle spasm, weakness

Renal: Serum creatinine increased

Respiratory: Cough

Available Dosage Forms

Tablet, oral:

edarbi™: 40 mg, 80 mg

General Dosage Range Oral: *Adults:* 40-80 mg once daily

Administration

Oral Administer without regard to food.

Stability

Storage Store at 25°C (77°F); excursions permitted to 15°C to 30°C (59°F to 86°F). Protect from moisture and light. Dispense and store in original container.

Dietary Considerations May be taken with or without food.

Azithromycin (Systemic) (az ith roe MYE sin)

Brand Names: U.S. Zithromax®; Zithromax® TRI-PAK™; Zithromax® Z-PAK®; Zmax®

Index Terms Azithromycin Dihydrate; Azithromycin Hydrogencitrate; Azithromycin Monohydrate; Z-Pak; Zithromax TRI-PAK™; Zithromax Z-PAK®

Pharmacologic Category Antibiotic, Macrolide

Medication Safety Issues

Sound-alike/look-alike issues:

Azithromycin may be confused with azathioprine, erythromycin

Zithromax® may be confused with Fosamax®, Zinacef®, Zovirax®

Pregnancy Risk Factor B

Lactation Enters breast milk/use caution

Breast-Feeding Considerations Azithromycin is excreted in low amounts into breast milk. The manufacturer recommends that caution be exercised when administering azithromycin to breast-feeding women. Nondose-related effects could include modification of bowel flora.

Use Oral, I.V.: Treatment of acute otitis media due to *H. influenzae*, *M. catarrhalis*, or *S. pneumoniae*; pharyngitis/tonsillitis due to *S. pyogenes*; treatment of mild-to-moderate upper and lower respiratory tract infections, infections of the skin and skin structure, community-acquired pneumonia, pelvic inflammatory disease (PID), sexually-transmitted diseases (urethritis/cervicitis), and genital ulcer disease (chancroid) due to susceptible strains of *Chlamydophila pneumoniae, C. trachomatis, M. catarrhalis, H. influenzae, S. aureus, S. pneumoniae, Mycoplasma genitalium, Mycoplasma pneumoniae*, and *C. psittaci*; acute bacterial exacerbations of chronic obstructive pulmonary disease (COPD) due to *H. influenzae, M. catarrhalis,* or *S. pneumoniae*; acute bacterial sinusitis; prevention, alone or in combination with rifabutin, of MAC in patients with advanced HIV infection; treatment, in combination with ethambutol, of disseminated MAC in patients with advanced HIV infection

Unlabeled Use Prophylaxis of infective endocarditis in patients who are allergic to penicillin and undergoing surgical or dental procedures; pertussis

Mechanism of Action/Effect Inhibits RNA-dependent protein synthesis at the chain elongation step; binds to the 50S ribosomal subunit resulting in blockage of transpeptidation

Contraindications Hypersensitivity to azithromycin, other macrolide (eg, azalide or ketolide) antibiotics, or any component of the formulation; history of cholestatic jaundice/hepatic dysfunction associated with prior azithromycin use

Warnings/Precautions Use with caution in patients with pre-existing liver disease; hepatocellular and/or cholestatic hepatitis, with or without jaundice, hepatic necrosis, failure and death have occurred. Discontinue immediately if symptoms of hepatitis occur (malaise, nausea, vomiting, abdominal colic, fever). Allergic reactions have been reported (rare); reappearance of allergic reaction may occur shortly after discontinuation without further azithromycin exposure. May mask or delay symptoms of incubating gonorrhea or syphilis, so appropriate culture and susceptibility tests should be performed prior to initiating azithromycin. Prolonged use may result in fungal or bacterial superinfection, including *C. difficile*-associated diarrhea (CDAD); CDAD has been observed >2 months postantibiotic treatment. Use caution with renal dysfunction. Prolongation of the QT_c interval has been reported with macrolide antibiotics; use caution in patients at risk of prolonged cardiac repolarization. Use with caution in patients with myasthenia gravis.

Oral suspensions (immediate release and extended release) are not interchangeable.

Drug Interactions

Avoid Concomitant Use

Avoid concomitant use of Azithromycin (Systemic) with any of the following: Artemether; BCG; Dronedarone; Lumefantrine; Nilotinib; Pimozide; QUEtiapine; QuiNINE; Terfenadine; Tetrabenazine; Thioridazine; Toremifene; Vandetanib; Vemurafenib; Ziprasidone

Decreased Effect

Azithromycin (Systemic) may decrease the levels/effects of: BCG; Typhoid Vaccine

The levels/effects of Azithromycin (Systemic) may be decreased by: Tocilizumab

Increased Effect/Toxicity

Azithromycin (Systemic) may increase the levels/effects of: Amiodarone; Cardiac Glycosides; CycloSPORINE; CycloSPORINE (Systemic); Dronedarone; Pimozide; QTc-Prolonging Agents; QuiNINE; Tacrolimus; Tacrolimus (Systemic); Tacrolimus (Topical); Terfenadine; Tetrabenazine; Thioridazine; Toremifene; Vandetanib; Vemurafenib; Vitamin K Antagonists; Ziprasidone

The levels/effects of Azithromycin (Systemic) may be increased by: Alfuzosin; Artemether; Chloroquine; Ciprofloxacin; Ciprofloxacin (Systemic); Conivaptan; Gadobutrol; Indacaterol; Lumefantrine; Nelfinavir; Nilotinib; QUEtiapine; QuiNINE

Nutritional/Ethanol Interactions Food: Rate and extent of GI absorption may be altered depending upon the formulation. Azithromycin suspension, not tablet form, has significantly increased absorption (46%) with food.

Adverse Reactions

>10%: Gastrointestinal: Diarrhea (4% to 9%; high single-dose regimens 12% to 14%), nausea (≤7%; high single-dose regimens 18%)

2% to 10%:

Dermatologic: Pruritus, rash

Gastrointestinal: Abdominal pain, anorexia, cramping, vomiting (especially with high single-dose regimens)

Genitourinary: Vaginitis

Local: (with I.V. administration): Injection site pain, inflammation

Available Dosage Forms

Injection, powder for reconstitution: 500 mg

Zithromax®: 500 mg

Microspheres for suspension, extended release, oral:

Zmax®: 2 g/bottle (60 mL)

Powder for suspension, oral: 100 mg/5 mL (15 mL); 200 mg/5 mL (15 mL, 22.5 mL, 30 mL); 1 g/packet (3s, 10s)

Zithromax®: 100 mg/5 mL (15 mL); 200 mg/5 mL (15 mL, 22.5 mL, 30 mL); 1 g/packet (3s, 10s)

Tablet, oral: 250 mg, 500 mg, 600 mg

Zithromax®: 250 mg, 500 mg, 600 mg

Zithromax® TRI-PAK™: 500 mg

Zithromax® Z-PAK®: 250 mg

General Dosage Range

I.V.: *Adults:* 500 mg as a single daily dose

Oral:

Immediate release:

Children ≥6 months to 2 years: 5-10 mg/kg as a single daily dose (maximum: 500 mg/dose) **or** 30 mg/kg as a single dose (maximum: 1500 mg/dose)

Children ≥2 years: 5-12 mg/kg as single daily dose (maximum: 500 mg/dose) **or** 30 mg/kg as a single dose (maximum: 1500 mg/dose)

Adults: 250-500 mg as a single daily dose **or** 1-2 g as a single dose

Extended release (suspension):

Children ≥6 months and <34 kg: 60 mg/kg as a single dose

Children ≥6 months and ≥34 kg and Adults: 2 g as a single dose

Administration

Oral Immediate release suspension and tablet may be taken without regard to food; extended release suspension should be taken on an empty stomach (at least 1 hour before or 2 hours following a meal), within 12 hours of reconstitution.

I.V. Other medications should not be infused simultaneously through the same I.V. line.

I.V. Detail Infusate concentration and rate of infusion for azithromycin for injection should be either 1 mg/mL over 3 hours or 2 mg/mL over 1 hour.

Stability

Reconstitution Injection (Zithromax®): Prepare initiation solution by adding 4.8 mL of sterile water for injection to the 500 mg vial (resulting concentration: 100 mg/mL). Use of a standard syringe is recommended due to the vacuum in the vial (which may draw additional solution through an automated syringe).

The initial solution should be further diluted to a concentration of 1 mg/mL (500 mL) to 2 mg/mL (250 mL) in 0.9% sodium chloride, 5% dextrose in water, or lactated Ringer's. The diluted solution is stable for 24 hours at or below room temperature (30°C or 86°F) and for 7 days if stored under refrigeration (5°C or 41°F).

Storage

Injection (Zithromax®): Store intact vials of injection at room temperature. Reconstituted solution is stable for 24 hours when stored below 30°C (86°F).

Suspension, immediate release (Zithromax®): Store dry powder below 30°C (86°F). Following reconstitution, store at 5°C to 30°C (41°F to 86°F).

Suspension, extended release (Zmax®): Store dry powder ≤30°C (86°F). Following reconstitution, store at 25°C (77°F); excursions permitted to 15°C to 30°C (59°F to 86°F); do not refrigerate or freeze. Should be consumed within 12 hours following reconstitution.

Tablet (Zithromax®): Store between 15°C to 30°C (59°F to 86°F).

Nursing Actions

Physical Assessment Results of culture and sensitivity tests and patient's allergy history should be assessed prior to beginning therapy. Monitor LFTs and CBC with diff. Instruct patients being treated for STDs about preventing transmission.

Patient Education If administered by infusion, report immediately any redness, swelling, or pain at infusion site. Oral: Take extended release suspension 1 hour before or 2 hours after meals; immediate release suspension and tablets may be taken with or without food; tablet form may be taken with meals to decrease GI effects. Maintain adequate hydration, unless instructed to restrict fluid intake. If taken to treat a sexually-transmitted disease, follow advice of prescriber related to sexual intercourse and preventing transmission. May cause transient abdominal distress, diarrhea, and headache. Report signs of additional infections (eg, sores in mouth or vagina, vaginal discharge, unresolved fever, severe vomiting, or loose or foul-smelling stools).

Dietary Considerations

Some products may contain sodium and/or sucrose.

Oral suspension, immediate release, may be administered with or without food.

Oral suspension, extended release, should be taken on an empty stomach (at least 1 hour before or 2 hours following a meal).

Tablet may be administered with food to decrease GI effects.

Related Information

Compatibility of Drugs *on page 1264*

Aztreonam (AZ tree oh nam)

Brand Names: U.S. Azactam®; Cayston®

Index Terms Azthreonam

Pharmacologic Category Antibiotic, Miscellaneous

Medication Safety Issues

Sound-alike/look-alike issues:

Aztreonam may be confused with azidothymidine

Pregnancy Risk Factor B

Lactation Enters breast milk/not recommended (AAP rates "compatible"; AAP 2001 update pending)

Breast-Feeding Considerations Very small amounts of aztreonam are excreted in breast milk. The poor oral absorption of aztreonam (<1%) may limit adverse effects to the infant. Nondose-related effects could include modification of bowel flora. Maternal use of aztreonam inhalation is not likely to pose a risk to breast-feeding infants.

Use

Injection: Treatment of patients with urinary tract infections, lower respiratory tract infections, septicemia, skin/skin structure infections, intra-abdominal infections, and gynecological infections caused by susceptible gram-negative bacilli

Inhalation: Improve respiratory symptoms in cystic fibrosis (CF) patients with *Pseudomonas aeruginosa*

Mechanism of Action/Effect Monobactam which is active only against gram-negative bacilli; inhibits bacterial cell wall synthesis during active multiplication, causing cell wall destruction

Contraindications Hypersensitivity to aztreonam or any component of the formulation

Warnings/Precautions Rare cross-allergenicity to penicillins and cephalosporins has been reported. Use caution in renal impairment; dosing adjustment required for the injectable formulation. Prolonged use may result in fungal or bacterial superinfection, including *C. difficile*-associated diarrhea (CDAD) and pseudomembranous colitis; CDAD has been observed >2 months postantibiotic treatment. Patients colonized with *Burkholderia cepacia* have not been studied. Safety and efficacy has not been established in patients with FEV_1 <25% or >75% predicted. To reduce the development of resistant bacteria and maintain efficacy reserve use for CF patients with known *Pseudomonas aeruginosa*. Bronchospasm may occur occur following nebulization; administer a bronchodilator prior to treatment.

Drug Interactions

Avoid Concomitant Use

Avoid concomitant use of Aztreonam with any of the following: BCG

Decreased Effect

Aztreonam may decrease the levels/effects of: BCG; Typhoid Vaccine

Increased Effect/Toxicity There are no known significant interactions involving an increase in effect.

Adverse Reactions

Injection: Adults: 1% to 10%:

Dermatologic: Rash

Gastrointestinal: Diarrhea, nausea, vomiting

Local: Thrombophlebitis, pain at injection site

Inhalation:

>10%:

Central nervous system: Pyrexia (13%; more often observed in children)

Respiratory: Cough (54%), nasal congestion (16%), pharyngeal pain (12%), wheezing (16%)

1% to 10%:

Cardiovascular: Chest discomfort (8%)

Dermatologic: Rash (2%)

Gastrointestinal: Abdominal pain (7%), vomiting (6%)

Respiratory: Bronchospasm (3%)

Available Dosage Forms

Infusion, premixed iso-osmotic solution:

Azactam®: 1 g (50 mL); 2 g (50 mL)

Injection, powder for reconstitution: 1 g, 2 g

Azactam®: 1 g, 2 g

Powder for reconstitution, for oral inhalation [preservative free]:

Cayston®: 75 mg

General Dosage Range Dosage adjustment recommended in patients with renal impairment

I.M.:

Children >1 month: 30-50 mg/kg/dose every 6-8 hours (maximum: 8 g/day)

Adults: 500 mg to 1 g every 8-12 hours

I.V.:

Children >1 month: 30-50 mg/kg/dose every 6-8 hours (maximum: 8 g/day)

Adults: 1-2 g every 6-12 hours (maximum: 8 g/day)

Oral inhalation: *Children ≥7 years and Adults:* 75 mg 3 times/day

Administration

I.M. Administer by deep injection into large muscle mass, such as upper outer quadrant of gluteus maximus or the lateral part of the thigh. Doses >1 g should be administered I.V.

I.V. I.V. route is preferred for doses >1 g or in patients with severe life-threatening infections. Administer by slow I.V. push over 3-5 minutes or by intermittent infusion over 20-60 minutes.

I.V. Detail Monitor infusion/injection sites carefully. Administer around-the-clock to promote less variation in peak and trough serum levels.

pH: 4.5-7.5 (aqueous solution)

Inhalation Administer using only an Altera® nebulizer system; **administer alone; do not mix with other nebulizer medications**. Administer a bronchodilator before administration of aztreonam (short-acting: 15 minutes to 4 hours before; long-acting: 30 minutes to 12 hours before). For patients on multiple inhaled therapies, administer bronchodilator first, then mucolytic, and lastly, aztreonam.

To administer Cayston®, pour reconstituted solution into the handset of the nebulizer system, turn unit on. Place the mouthpiece in the patient's mouth and encourage to breath normally through the mouth. Administration time is usually 2-3 minutes. Administer doses ≥4 hours apart.

Stability

Reconstitution

Inhalation: Reconstitute immediately prior to use. Squeeze diluent into opened glass vial. Replace rubber stopper and gently swirl vial until contents have completely dissolved.

I.M.: Reconstitute with at least 3 mL SWFI, sterile bacteriostatic water for injection, NS, or bacteriostatic sodium chloride.

I.V.:

Bolus injection: Reconstitute with 6-10 mL SWFI.

Infusion: Reconstitute to a final concentration ≤2%; the final concentration should not exceed 20 mg/mL.

Storage

Inhalation: Prior to reconstitution, store at 2°C to 8°C (36°F to 46°F). Once removed from refrigeration, aztreonam and the diluent may be stored at room temperature (up to 25°C [77°F]) for ≤28 days. Protect from light. Use immediately after reconstitution.

Injection: Prior to reconstitution, store at room temperature; avoid excessive heat. Reconstituted solutions are colorless to light yellow straw and may turn pink upon standing without affecting potency. Use reconstituted solutions and I.V. solutions (in NS and D_5W) within 48 hours if kept at room temperature (25°C) or 7 days under refrigeration (4°C).

Infusion: Solution for infusion may be frozen at less than -2°C (less than -4°F) for up to 3 months. Thawed solution should be used within 24 hours if thawed at room temperature or within 72 hours if thawed under refrigeration. **Do not refreeze.**

Nursing Actions

Physical Assessment Allergy history should be assessed prior to beginning treatment. I.V.: Infusion site should be monitored closely. Monitor patient closely during first dose for anaphylaxis. Bronchospasm may occur following inhalation administration; a bronchodilator may be ordered prior to treatment.

Patient Education Report immediately any burning, pain, swelling, or redness at infusion or injection site; swelling of mouth or tongue; or chest pain or acute onset of difficulty breathing. May cause nausea or GI distress. Report any respiratory difficulty, coughing, wheezing, persistent diarrhea or vomiting, pain at injection site, unresolved fever, unhealed or new sores in mouth or vagina, or vaginal discharge.

Baclofen (BAK loe fen)

Brand Names: U.S. Gablofen®; Lioresal®

Pharmacologic Category Skeletal Muscle Relaxant

Medication Safety Issues

Sound-alike/look-alike issues:

Baclofen may be confused with Bactroban®

Lioresal® may be confused with lisinopril, Lotensin®

High alert medication:

The Institute for Safe Medication Practices (ISMP) includes this medication (intrathecal administration) among its list of drugs which have a heightened risk of causing significant patient harm when used in error.

Pregnancy Risk Factor C

Lactation Enters breast milk/not recommended

Breast-Feeding Considerations Very small amounts of baclofen were found in the breast milk of a woman 14 days postpartum after oral use. Following a single oral dose of baclofen 20 mg, the total amount of baclofen excreted in breast milk within 26 hours was 22 mcg (Eriksson, 1981). Adverse events were not observed in a nursing infant following maternal use of intrathecal baclofen 200 mcg/day throughout pregnancy and while nursing (Morton, 2009).

Use Treatment of reversible spasticity associated with multiple sclerosis or spinal cord lesions

Orphan drug: Intrathecal: Treatment of intractable spasticity caused by spinal cord injury, multiple sclerosis, and other spinal disease (spinal ischemia or tumor, transverse myelitis, cervical spondylosis, degenerative myelopathy)

Unlabeled Use Intractable hiccups, intractable pain relief, bladder spasticity, trigeminal neuralgia, cerebral palsy, short-term treatment of spasticity in children with cerebral palsy, Huntington's chorea

Mechanism of Action/Effect Inhibits the transmission of both monosynaptic and polysynaptic reflexes at the spinal cord level, possibly by hyperpolarization of primary afferent fiber terminals, with resultant relief of muscle spasticity

Contraindications Hypersensitivity to baclofen or any component of the formulation

Warnings/Precautions Use with caution in patients with seizure disorder or impaired renal function. **[U.S. Boxed Warning]: Avoid abrupt withdrawal of the drug; abrupt withdrawal of intrathecal baclofen has resulted in severe sequelae (hyperpyrexia, obtundation, rebound/exaggerated spasticity, muscle rigidity, and rhabdomyolysis), leading to organ failure and some fatalities.** Risk may be higher in patients with injuries at T-6 or above, history of baclofen withdrawal, or limited ability to communicate. May cause CNS depression, which may impair physical or mental abilities; patients must be cautioned about performing tasks which require mental alertness (eg, operating machinery or driving). Elderly are more sensitive to the effects of baclofen and are more likely to experience adverse CNS effects at higher doses.

Cases (most from pharmacy compounded preparations) of intrathecal mass formation at the implanted catheter tip have been reported; may lead to loss of clinical response, pain or new/worsening neurological effects. Neurosurgical evaluation and/or an appropriate imaging study should be considered if a mass is suspected.

Drug Interactions

Avoid Concomitant Use There are no known interactions where it is recommended to avoid concomitant use.

Decreased Effect There are no known significant interactions involving a decrease in effect.

Increased Effect/Toxicity

Baclofen may increase the levels/effects of: Alcohol (Ethyl); CNS Depressants; Methotrimeprazine; Selective Serotonin Reuptake Inhibitors

The levels/effects of Baclofen may be increased by: Droperidol; HydrOXYzine; Methotrimeprazine

Nutritional/Ethanol Interactions

Ethanol: May increase CNS depression; monitor for increased effects with coadministration. Caution patients about effects.

Herb/Nutraceutical: Avoid valerian, St John's wort, kava kava, gotu kola.

Adverse Reactions

>10%:

Central nervous system: Drowsiness, vertigo, psychiatric disturbances, insomnia, slurred speech, ataxia, hypotonia

Neuromuscular & skeletal: Weakness

1% to 10%:

Cardiovascular: Hypotension

Central nervous system: Fatigue, confusion, headache

Dermatologic: Rash

Gastrointestinal: Nausea, constipation

Genitourinary: Polyuria

Pharmacodynamics/Kinetics

Onset of Action 3-4 days; Peak effect: 5-10 days

Available Dosage Forms

Injection, solution, intrathecal [preservative free]:

Gablofen®: 50 mcg/mL (1 mL); 500 mcg/mL (20 mL); 2000 mcg/mL (20 mL)

Lioresal®: 50 mcg/mL (1 mL); 500 mcg/mL (20 mL); 2000 mcg/mL (5 mL, 20 mL)

Tablet, oral: 10 mg, 20 mg

General Dosage Range

Intrathecal:

Children: Test dose: 25-100 mcg; Initial infusion: Infuse at a 24-hourly rate dosed at twice the test dose

Adults: Test dose: 50-100 mcg; Initial infusion: Infuse at a 24-hourly rate dosed at twice the test dose

Oral:

Adults: Initial: 5 mg 3 times/day; Maintenance: Up to 80 mg/day in 2-3 divided doses

Elderly: Initial: 5 mg 2-3 times/day, increasing gradually as needed

Administration

I.V. Detail pH: 5-7

Other Intrathecal: For screening dosages, dilute with preservative-free sodium chloride to a final concentration of 50 mcg/mL for bolus injection into the subarachnoid space. For maintenance infusions, concentrations of 500-2000 mcg/mL may be used.

Nursing Actions

Physical Assessment Assess cardiovascular and CNS status at beginning of therapy and periodically throughout.

Patient Education Abrupt discontinuation may cause hallucinations. Avoid alcohol use. You may experience transient drowsiness, lethargy, or dizziness. Intrathecal use: Keep scheduled pump refill visits; abrupt interruption can cause serious withdrawal symptoms. Report increased spasticity, itching, numbness, unresolved insomnia, painful urination, change in urinary patterns, constipation, high fever, or persistent confusion.

Basiliximab (ba si LIK si mab)

Brand Names: U.S. Simulect®

Pharmacologic Category Immunosuppressant Agent; Monoclonal Antibody

Pregnancy Risk Factor B

Lactation Excretion in breast milk unknown/not recommended

Breast-Feeding Considerations It is not known whether basiliximab is excreted in human milk. Because many immunoglobulins are secreted in milk and the potential for serious adverse reactions exists, a decision should be made whether to discontinue nursing or discontinue the drug, taking into account the importance of the drug to the mother.

Use Prophylaxis of acute organ rejection in renal transplantation (in combination with cyclosporine and corticosteroids)

Unlabeled Use Treatment of refractory acute graft-versus-host disease (GVHD); prevention of liver or cardiac transplant rejection

Mechanism of Action/Effect Chimeric (murine/human) immunosuppressant monoclonal antibody which blocks the alpha-chain of the interleukin-2 (IL-2) receptor complex; this receptor is expressed on activated T lymphocytes and is a critical pathway for activating cell-mediated allograft rejection

Contraindications Hypersensitivity to basiliximab or any component of the formulation

Warnings/Precautions To be used as a component of an immunosuppressive regimen which includes cyclosporine and corticosteroids. The incidence of lymphoproliferative disorders and/or opportunistic infections may be increased by immunosuppressive therapy. Severe hypersensitivity reactions, occurring within 24 hours, have been reported. Reactions, including anaphylaxis, have occurred both with the initial exposure and/or following re-exposure after several months. Use caution during re-exposure to a subsequent course of therapy in a patient who has previously received basiliximab; patients in whom concomitant immunosuppression was prematurely discontinued due to abandoned transplantation or early graft loss are at increased risk for developing a severe hypersensitivity reaction upon re-exposure. Discontinue permanently if a severe reaction occurs. Medications for the treatment of hypersensitivity reactions should be available for immediate use. Treatment may result in the development of human antimurine antibodies (HAMA); however, limited evidence suggesting the use of muromonab-CD3 or other murine products is not precluded. **[U.S. Boxed Warning]: Should be administered under the supervision of a physician experienced in immunosuppression therapy and organ transplant management.** In renal transplant patients receiving basiliximab plus prednisone, cyclosporine, and mycophenolate, new-onset diabetes, glucose intolerance, and impaired fasting glucose were observed at rates significantly higher than observed in patients receiving prednisone, cyclosporine, and mycophenolate without basiliximab (Aasebo, 2010).

Drug Interactions

Avoid Concomitant Use

Avoid concomitant use of Basiliximab with any of the following: BCG; Belimumab; Natalizumab; Pimecrolimus; Tacrolimus (Topical); Vaccines (Live)

Decreased Effect

Basiliximab may decrease the levels/effects of: BCG; Coccidioidin Skin Test; Sipuleucel-T; Vaccines (Inactivated); Vaccines (Live)

The levels/effects of Basiliximab may be decreased by: Echinacea

Increased Effect/Toxicity

Basiliximab may increase the levels/effects of: Belimumab; Hypoglycemic Agents; Leflunomide; Natalizumab; Vaccines (Live)

The levels/effects of Basiliximab may be increased by: Abciximab; Denosumab; Herbs (Hypoglycemic Properties); Pimecrolimus; Roflumilast; Tacrolimus (Topical); Trastuzumab

Nutritional/Ethanol Interactions Herb/Nutraceutical: Echinacea may diminish the therapeutic effect of basiliximab. Avoid hypoglycemic herbs, including alfalfa, bilberry, bitter melon, burdock, celery, damiana, fenugreek, garcinia, garlic, ginger, ginseng, gymnema, marshmallow, and stinging nettle (may enhance the hypoglycemic effect of basiliximab).

Adverse Reactions Administration of basiliximab did not appear to increase the incidence or severity of adverse effects in clinical trials. Adverse events were reported in 96% of both the placebo and basiliximab groups.

>10%:

Cardiovascular: Hypertension, peripheral edema

Central nervous system: Fever, headache, insomnia, pain

Dermatologic: Acne, wound complications

Endocrine & metabolic: Hypercholesterolemia, hyperglycemia, hyper-/hypokalemia, hyperuricemia, hypophosphatemia

Gastrointestinal: Abdominal pain, constipation, diarrhea, dyspepsia, nausea, vomiting

Genitourinary: Urinary tract infection

Hematologic: Anemia

Neuromuscular & skeletal: Tremor

Respiratory: Dyspnea, infection (upper respiratory)

Miscellaneous: Viral infection

3% to 10%:

Cardiovascular: Abnormal heart sounds, angina, arrhythmia, atrial fibrillation, chest pain, generalized edema, heart failure, hypotension, tachycardia

Central nervous system: Agitation, anxiety, depression, dizziness, fatigue, hypoesthesia, malaise

Dermatologic: Cyst, hypertrichosis, pruritus, rash, skin disorder, skin ulceration

Endocrine & metabolic: Acidosis, dehydration, diabetes mellitus, fluid overload, glucocorticoids increased, hyper-/hypocalcemia, hyperlipemia, hypertriglyceridemia, hypoglycemia, hypomagnesemia, hyponatremia, hypoproteinemia

Gastrointestinal: Abdomen enlarged, esophagitis, flatulence, gastroenteritis, GI hemorrhage, gingival hyperplasia, melena, moniliasis, stomatitis (including ulcerative), weight gain

Genitourinary: Bladder disorder, dysuria, genital edema (male), impotence, ureteral disorder, urinary frequency, urinary retention

Hematologic: Hematoma, hemorrhage, leukopenia, polycythemia, purpura, thrombocytopenia, thrombosis

Neuromuscular & skeletal: Arthralgia, arthropathy, back pain, cramps, fracture, hernia, leg pain, myalgia, neuropathy, paresthesia, rigors, weakness

Ocular: Abnormal vision, cataract, conjunctivitis

Renal: Albuminuria, hematuria, nonprotein nitrogen increased, oliguria, renal function abnormal, renal tubular necrosis

Respiratory: Bronchitis, bronchospasm, cough, pharyngitis, pneumonia, pulmonary edema, sinusitis, rhinitis

Miscellaneous: Accidental trauma, cytomegalovirus (CMV) infection, herpes infection (simplex and zoster), infection, sepsis

Pharmacodynamics/Kinetics

Duration of Action Mean: 36 days (determined by IL-2R alpha saturation)

Available Dosage Forms

Injection, powder for reconstitution:

Simulect®: 10 mg, 20 mg

General Dosage Range I.V.:

Children <35 kg: 10 mg within 2 hours prior to transplant surgery, followed by a second 10 mg dose 4 days after transplantation

Children ≥35 kg and Adults: 20 mg within 2 hours prior to transplant surgery, followed by a second 20 mg dose 4 days after transplantation

Administration

I.V. For intravenous administration only. Infuse as a bolus or I.V. infusion over 20-30 minutes. (Bolus dosing is associated with nausea, vomiting, and local pain at the injection site.) Administer only after assurance that patient will receive renal graft and immunosuppression. For the treatment of acute GVHD (unlabeled use), the dose was diluted in 250 mL NS and administered over 30 minutes (Schmidt-Hieber, 2005).

Stability

Reconstitution Reconstitute with preservative-free sterile water for injection (reconstitute 10 mg vial with 2.5 mL, 20 mg vial with 5 mL). Shake gently to dissolve. May further dilute reconstituted solution with 25 mL (10 mg) or 50 mL (20 mg) 0.9% sodium chloride or dextrose 5% in water. When mixing the solution, gently invert the bag to avoid foaming. Do not shake solutions diluted for infusion.

Storage Store intact vials refrigerated at 2°C to 8°C (36°F to 46°F). Should be used immediately after reconstitution; however, if not used immediately, reconstituted solution may be stored at 2°C to 8°C for up to 24 hours or at room temperature for up to 4 hours. Discard the reconstituted solution if not used within 24 hours.

Nursing Actions

Physical Assessment Monitor infusion site and cardiovascular, respiratory, and renal function during infusion. Allergic reactions, including anaphylaxis, have occurred both with the initial exposure and/or following re-exposure after several months. Treatment of hypersensitivity reactions should be available for immediate use. Monitor closely for opportunistic infection (eg, chills, fever, sore throat, easy bruising or bleeding, mouth sores, unhealed sores).

Patient Education This medication, which may help to reduce transplant rejection, can only be given by infusion. You will be monitored and assessed closely during infusion and thereafter. It is important that you report any changes or problems for evaluation. You will be susceptible to infection. You may experience trouble sleeping or headaches. Report any changes in urination; chest pain or palpitations; dizziness; respiratory difficulty; changes in cognition; rash; feelings of pain or numbness in extremities; weight gain; swelling of extremities; severe GI upset, pain, or diarrhea; unusual back or leg pain or muscle tremors; vision changes; or any sign of infection (eg, chills, fever, sore throat).

Beclomethasone (Oral Inhalation)

(be kloe METH a sone)

Brand Names: U.S. QVAR®

Index Terms Vancenase

Pharmacologic Category Corticosteroid, Inhalant (Oral)

Medication Safety Issues

Sound-alike/look-alike issues:

Vanceril® may be confused with Vancenase

Pregnancy Risk Factor C

Lactation Excretion in breast milk unknown/use caution

Breast-Feeding Considerations Other corticosteroids have been found in breast milk; however, information for beclomethasone is not available.

Use Oral inhalation: Maintenance and prophylactic treatment of asthma; includes those who require corticosteroids and those who may benefit from a dose reduction/elimination of systemically-administered corticosteroids. Not for relief of acute bronchospasm.

Mechanism of Action/Effect Acts at cellular level to prevent or control inflammation

Contraindications Hypersensitivity to beclomethasone or any component of the formulation; status asthmaticus

Warnings/Precautions May cause hypercorticism or suppression of hypothalamic-pituitary-adrenal (HPA) axis, particularly in younger children or in patients receiving high doses for prolonged periods. HPA axis suppression may lead to adrenal crisis. Withdrawal and discontinuation of a corticosteroid should be done slowly and carefully. Particular care is required when patients are transferred from systemic corticosteroids to inhaled products due to possible adrenal insufficiency or withdrawal from steroids, including an increase in allergic symptoms. Patients receiving >20 mg per day of prednisone (or equivalent) may be most susceptible. Fatalities have occurred due to adrenal insufficiency in asthmatic patients during and after transfer from systemic corticosteroids to aerosol steroids; aerosol steroids do **not** provide the systemic steroid needed to treat patients having trauma, surgery, or infections.

Bronchospasm may occur with wheezing after inhalation; if this occurs, stop steroid and treat with a fast-acting bronchodilator. Supplemental steroids (oral or parenteral) may be needed during stress or severe asthma attacks. Not to be used in status asthmaticus or for the relief of acute bronchospasm. Corticosteroid use may cause psychiatric disturbances, including depression, euphoria, insomnia, mood swings, and personality changes. Pre-existing psychiatric conditions may be exacerbated by corticosteroid use. Prolonged use of corticosteroids may also increase the incidence of secondary infection, mask acute infection (including fungal infections), prolong or exacerbate viral infections, or limit response to vaccines. Exposure to chickenpox should be avoided; corticosteroids should not be used to treat ocular herpes simplex. Corticosteroids should not be used for cerebral malaria. Close observation is required in patients with latent tuberculosis and/or TB reactivity; restrict use in active TB (only in conjunction with antituberculosis treatment). Prolonged treatment with corticosteroids has been associated with the development of Kaposi's sarcoma (case reports); if noted, discontinuation of therapy should be considered.

Use with caution in patients with thyroid disease, hepatic impairment, renal impairment, cardiovascular disease, diabetes, glaucoma, cataracts, myasthenia gravis, patients at risk for osteoporosis, patients at risk for seizures, or GI diseases (diverticulitis, peptic ulcer, ulcerative colitis) due to perforation risk. Use caution following acute MI (corticosteroids have been associated with myocardial rupture). Because of the risk of adverse effects, systemic corticosteroids should be used cautiously in the elderly in the smallest possible effective dose for the shortest duration.

Orally-inhaled corticosteroids may cause a reduction in growth velocity in pediatric patients (~1 centimeter per year [range: 0.3-1.8 cm per year] and related to dose and duration of exposure). To minimize the systemic effects of orally-inhaled corticosteroids, each patient should be titrated to the lowest effective dose. Growth should be routinely monitored in pediatric patients. Safety and efficacy have not been established in children <5 years of age. There have been reports of systemic corticosteroid withdrawal symptoms (eg, joint/muscle pain, lassitude, depression) when withdrawing oral inhalation therapy.

Drug Interactions

Avoid Concomitant Use

Avoid concomitant use of Beclomethasone (Oral Inhalation) with any of the following: Aldesleukin; BCG; Natalizumab; Pimecrolimus; Tacrolimus (Topical)

Decreased Effect

Beclomethasone (Oral Inhalation) may decrease the levels/effects of: Aldesleukin; Antidiabetic Agents; BCG; Coccidioidin Skin Test; Corticorelin; Sipuleucel-T; Telaprevir; Vaccines (Inactivated)

The levels/effects of Beclomethasone (Oral Inhalation) may be decreased by: Echinacea

Increased Effect/Toxicity

Beclomethasone (Oral Inhalation) may increase the levels/effects of: Amphotericin B; Deferasirox; Leflunomide; Loop Diuretics; Natalizumab; Thiazide Diuretics

The levels/effects of Beclomethasone (Oral Inhalation) may be increased by: Denosumab; Pimecrolimus; Tacrolimus (Topical); Telaprevir; Trastuzumab

Adverse Reactions Frequency not defined.

Central nervous system: Agitation, depression, dizziness, dysphonia, headache, lightheadedness, mental disturbances

Dermatologic: Acneiform lesions, angioedema, atrophy, bruising, pruritus, purpura, striae, rash, urticaria

Endocrine & metabolic: Cushingoid features, growth velocity reduction in children and adolescents, HPA function suppression, weight gain

Gastrointestinal: Dry/irritated nose, throat and mouth, hoarseness, localized *Candida* or *Aspergillus* infection, loss of smell, loss of taste, nausea, unpleasant smell, unpleasant taste, vomiting

Ocular: Cataracts, glaucoma, intraocular pressure increased

Respiratory: Cough, paradoxical bronchospasm, pharyngitis, sinusitis, wheezing

Miscellaneous: Anaphylactic/anaphylactoid reactions, death (due to adrenal insufficiency, reported during and after transfer from systemic corticosteroids to aerosol in asthmatic patients), immediate and delayed hypersensitivity reactions

Pharmacodynamics/Kinetics

Onset of Action Therapeutic effect: 1-4 weeks

Available Dosage Forms

Aerosol, for oral inhalation:

QVAR®: 40 mcg/inhalation (8.7 g); 80 mcg/inhalation (8.7 g)

General Dosage Range Inhalation:

Children 5-11 years: Initial: 40 mcg twice daily; Maintenance: 80->320 mcg/day in 2 divided doses

Children ≥12 years and Adults: Initial: 40-160 mcg twice daily; Maintenance: 80->480 mcg/day in 2 divided doses

Administration

Inhalation QVAR®: Rinse mouth and throat after use to prevent *Candida* infection. Do not wash or put inhaler in water; mouth piece may be cleaned with a dry tissue or cloth. Prime canister before using.

Stability

Storage Do not store near heat or open flame. Do not puncture canisters. Store at 25°C (77°F); excursions permitted between 15°C to 30°C (59°F to 86°F). Rest QVAR® on concave end of canister with actuator on top.

Nursing Actions

Physical Assessment When changing from systemic steroids to inhalational steroids, taper reduction of systemic medication slowly.

Patient Education It may take 1-4 weeks for you to realize full effects of treatment. Review use of inhaler with prescriber. Keep oral inhaler clean and unobstructed. Always rinse mouth after use of inhaler to prevent infection. If you are also using an inhaled bronchodilator, wait 10 minutes before using this steroid aerosol. Report skin rash, white plaques in mouth, unresolved headache, or worsening of condition or lack of improvement.

Inhalation: Sit when using. Take deep breaths for 3-5 minutes and clear nasal passages before administration. Hold breath for 5-10 seconds after use and wait 1-3 minutes between inhalations. If also using inhaled bronchodilator, use before beclomethasone. Rinse mouth after use to reduce aftertaste and prevent infection.

Belatacept (bel AT a sept)

Brand Names: U.S. Nulojix®

Index Terms BMS-224818; LEA29Y

Pharmacologic Category Selective T-Cell Costimulation Blocker

Medication Guide Available Yes

Pregnancy Risk Factor C

Lactation Excretion in breast milk unknown/not recommended

Breast-Feeding Considerations Due to the potential for adverse reactions and possible effects on the developing immune system, breast-feeding is not recommended.

Use Prophylaxis of organ rejection concomitantly with basiliximab, mycophenolate, and corticosteroids in Epstein-Barr virus (EBV) seropositive kidney transplant recipients

Mechanism of Action/Effect Prevents activation of T cells, a mediator in immunologic rejection associated with kidney transplantation

Contraindications Transplant patients who are Epstein-Barr virus (EBV) seronegative or with unknown EBV status

Warnings/Precautions [U.S. Boxed Warning]: Risk of post-transplant lymphoproliferative disorder (PTLD) is increased, primarily involving the CNS, in patients receiving belatacept compared to patients receiving cyclosporine-based regimens. Degree of immunosuppression is a risk factor for PTLD developing; do not exceed recommended dosing. Patients who are Epstein-Barr virus seronegative (EBV) are at an even higher risk; use is contraindicated in patients without evidence of immunity to EBV. Therapy is only appropriate in patients who are EBV seropositive via evidence of acquired immunity, such as presence of IgG antibodies to viral capsid antigen [VCA] and EBV nuclear antigen [EBNA]. Cytomegalovirus (CMV) infection also increases the risk for PTLD; CMV prophylaxis is recommended for a minimum of 3 months following transplantation. Although CMV disease is a risk for PTLD and CMV seronegative patients are at an increased risk for CMV disease, the clinical role, if any, of determining CMV serology to determine risk of PTLD development has not been determined.

[U.S. Boxed Warning]: Risk for infection is increased. Immunosuppressive therapy may lead to opportunistic infections, sepsis, and/or fatal infections. Tuberculosis (TB) is increased; test patients for latent TB prior to initiation, and treat latent TB infection prior to use. Patients receiving immunosuppressive therapy are at an increased risk of activation of latent viral infections, including John Cunningham virus (JCV) and BK virus infection. Activation of JCV may result in progressive multifocal leukoencephalopathy (PML), a rare and potentially fatal condition affecting the CNS. Symptoms of PML include apathy, ataxia, cognitive deficiencies, confusion, and hemiparesis. Polyoma virus-associated nephropathy (PVAN), primarily from activation of BK virus, may also occur and lead to the deterioration of renal function and/or renal graft loss. Risk factors for the development of PML and PVAN include immunosuppression and treatment with immunosuppressant therapy. The onset of PML or PVAN may warrant a reduction in immunosuppressive therapy; however, in transplant recipients, the risk of reduced immunosuppression and graft rejection should be considered.

[U.S. Boxed Warning]: Risk for malignancy is increased. Malignancy, including skin malignancy and post-transplant lymphoproliferative disease, is associated with the use of immunosuppressants, including belatacept; higher than recommended doses or more frequent dosing is not recommended; patients should be advised to limit their exposure to sunlight/UV light.

[U.S. Boxed Warning]: Therapy is not recommended in liver transplant patients due to increased risk of graft loss and death. [U.S. Boxed Warning]: Should be administered under the supervision of a physician experienced in immunosuppressive therapy. Patients should not be immunized with attenuated or live viral vaccines during or shortly after treatment; safety of immunization following therapy has not been studied. The ENLiST registry has been created to further determine the safety of belatacept, particularly the incidence of PTLD and PML, in EBV seropositive kidney transplant patients. Transplant centers are encouraged to participate (1-800-321-1335).

Drug Interactions

Avoid Concomitant Use

Avoid concomitant use of Belatacept with any of the following: BCG; Belimumab; Natalizumab; Pimecrolimus; Tacrolimus (Topical); Vaccines (Live)

Decreased Effect

Belatacept may decrease the levels/effects of: BCG; Coccidioidin Skin Test; Sipuleucel-T; Vaccines (Inactivated); Vaccines (Live)

The levels/effects of Belatacept may be decreased by: Echinacea

Increased Effect/Toxicity

Belatacept may increase the levels/effects of: Belimumab; Leflunomide; Mycophenolate; Natalizumab; Vaccines (Live)

The levels/effects of Belatacept may be increased by: Denosumab; Pimecrolimus; Roflumilast; Tacrolimus (Topical); Trastuzumab

Adverse Reactions Incidences reported occurred during clinical trials using belatacept compared to a cyclosporine control regimen. All patients also received basiliximab induction, mycophenolate mofetil, and corticosteroids, and were followed up to 3 years.

>10%:

Cardiovascular: Peripheral edema (34%), hypertension (32%), hypotension (18%)

Central nervous system: Fever (28%), headache (21%), insomnia (15%)

Endocrine & metabolic: Hypokalemia (21%), hyperkalemia (20%), hypophosphatemia (19%), dyslipidemia (19%), hyperglycemia (16%), hypocalcemia (13%), hypercholesterolemia (11%)

Gastrointestinal: Diarrhea (39%), constipation (33%), nausea (24%), vomiting (22%), abdominal pain (19%)

Genitourinary: Urinary tract infection (37%), dysuria (11%)

Hematologic: Anemia (45%), leukopenia (20%)

Neuromuscular & skeletal: Arthralgia (17%), back pain (13%)

Renal: Proteinuria (16%; up to 33% 2+ proteinuria at 1 month post-transplant), renal graft dysfunction (25%), hematuria (16%), serum creatinine increased (15%)

Respiratory: Cough (24%), upper respiratory infection (15%), nasopharyngitis (13%), dyspnea (12%)

Miscellaneous: Infection (72% to 82%; serious infection: 24% to 36%), herpes (7% to 14%), CMV (11% to 13%), influenza (11%)

1% to 10%:

Cardiovascular: Arteriovenous fistula thrombosis (<10%), atrial fibrillation (<10%)

Central nervous system: Anxiety (10%), dizziness (9%)

Dermatologic: Alopecia (<10%), hyperhidrosis (<10%), acne (8%)

Endocrine & metabolic: New-onset diabetes (5% to 8%), hypomagnesemia (7%), hyperuricemia (5%)

Gastrointestinal: Stomatitis (<10%), upper abdominal pain (9%)

Genitourinary: Urinary incontinence (<10%)

Hematologic: Hematoma (<10%), neutropenia (<10%)

Neuromuscular & skeletal: Musculoskeletal pain (<10%), tremor (8%)

Renal: Chronic allograft nephropathy (<10%), hydronephrosis (<10%), renal impairment (<10%), renal artery stenosis (<10%), renal tubular necrosis (9%)

Respiratory: Bronchitis (10%)

Miscellaneous: Guillain-Barré syndrome (<10%), lymphocele (<10%), infusion reactions (5%), malignancy (4%), polyoma virus (3% to 4%), antibelatacept antibody development (2%), nonmelanoma skin cancer (2%), tuberculosis (1% to 2%), BK virus-associated nephropathy (1%)

Available Dosage Forms

Injection, powder for reconstitution:

Nulojix®: 250 mg

General Dosage Range I.V.: *Adults:* Initial phase: 10 mg/kg/dose; maintenance phase: 5 mg/kg/dose

Administration

I.V. Administer as an I.V. infusion over 30 minutes using an infusion set with a 0.2-1.2 micron low protein-binding filter. Prior to administration, inspect visually and do not use if solution is discolored or contains particulate matter.

Stability

Reconstitution Reconstitute each vial with 10.5 mL of diluent (SWFI, NS, or D_5W) using the provided silicone-free disposable syringe, and an 18- to 21-gauge needle. Reconstituted using **only** the silicone-free syringe provided (discard if powder is inadvertently mixed using a siliconized syringe, translucent particles may develop). Inject the diluent down the side of the vial to avoid foaming. Rotate the vial and invert with gentle swirling until completely dissolved; do **not** shake vial. The reconstituted solution should be clear to slightly opalescent and colorless to pale yellow. Immediately transfer the reconstituted solution using the same silicone-free syringe to an infusion bag or bottle with NS or D_5W (if NS or D_5W were used to reconstitute, the same fluid should be used to further dilute). The final concentration should range from 2 mg/mL and 10 mg/mL (typical infusion volume is 100 mL). Prior to adding belatacept to the infusion solution, the manufacturer recommends withdrawing a volume equal to the amount of belatacept to be added. Mix gently; do not shake.

Storage Prior to use, store refrigerated at 2°C to 8°C (36°F to 46°F). Protect from light. After dilution, the infusion solution (reconstituted solution must be further diluted immediately) may be stored refrigerated for up to 24 hours, with a maximum of 4 hours of the 24 hours at room temperature, 20°C to 25°C (68°F to 77°F), and room light. Infusion must be completed within 24 hours of reconstitution.

Nursing Actions

Physical Assessment Monitor vital signs as changes in blood pressure can occur. Assess for new-onset or worsening neurological, cognitive, or behavioral signs/symptoms, change in balance or gait, decreased strength, change in vision, and signs or symptoms of infection.

Patient Education Advise patient to avoid sun exposure, tanning beds, sunlamps, and live vaccines. Common side effects include headache, anemia, low white blood cell count, constipation, GI upset, peripheral edema, high blood pressure, loose stools, and cough.

Dietary Considerations Some products may contain sucrose.

Belimumab (be LIM yoo mab)

Brand Names: U.S. Benlysta®

Pharmacologic Category Monoclonal Antibody

Medication Guide Available Yes

Pregnancy Risk Factor C

Lactation Excretion in breast milk unknown/not recommended

Use Treatment of autoantibody-positive (antinuclear antibody [ANA] and/or anti-double-stranded DNA [anti-ds-DNA]) systemic lupus erythematosus (SLE) in addition to standard therapy

Available Dosage Forms

Injection, powder for reconstitution:

Benlysta®: 120 mg, 400 mg

General Dosage Range I.V.: *Adults:* 10 mg/kg every 2 weeks for 3 doses; Maintenance: 10 mg/kg every 4 weeks

Administration

I.V. Administer intravenously over 1 hour through a dedicated I.V. line. Do not give as an I.V. push or bolus. Discontinue infusion for severe hypersensitivity reaction (eg, anaphylaxis, angioedema). The infusion may be slowed or temporarily interrupted for minor reactions. Consider premedicating for prophylaxis against infusion reactions.

Nursing Actions

Patient Education This medication can only be administered by I.V. infusion. Report immediately any pain or irritation at injection site; chills; rash; difficulty swallowing or breathing; or feelings of tightness in chest. Avoid alcohol. May cause nausea, diarrhea, sore throat, and nasal irritation. Report unusual feelings of fatigue or weakness, signs of infection (eg, cough, runny nose, sore throat, swollen glands, mouth sores, burning on urination, fever, chills).

Belladonna and Opium
(bel a DON a & OH pee um)

Index Terms B&O; Opium and Belladonna

Pharmacologic Category Analgesic Combination (Opioid); Antispasmodic Agent, Urinary

Medication Safety Issues

Sound-alike/look-alike issues:

B&O may be confused with beano®

BEERS Criteria medication:

This drug may be inappropriate for use in geriatric patients (high severity risk).

Pregnancy Risk Factor C

Lactation Excretion in breast milk unknown/use caution

Use Relief of moderate-to-severe pain associated with ureteral spasms not responsive to nonopioid analgesics and to space intervals between injections of opiates

Controlled Substance C-II

Available Dosage Forms

Suppository: Belladonna extract 16.2 mg and opium 30 mg; belladonna extract 16.2 mg and opium 60 mg

General Dosage Range Rectal: *Children >12 years and Adults:* 1 suppository 1-2 times/day (maximum: 4 doses/day)

Administration

Other Prior to rectal insertion, the finger and suppository should be moistened. Assist with ambulation.

Nursing Actions

Physical Assessment Monitor blood pressure, CNS and respiratory status, and degree of sedation at beginning of therapy and at regular intervals. May cause physical and/or psychological dependence. For inpatients, implement safety measures (eg, side rails up, call light within reach, instructions to call for assistance) to prevent falls.

Patient Education Drug may cause physical and/or psychological dependence. While using this medication, do not use alcohol. Maintain adequate hydration, unless instructed to restrict fluid intake. May cause hypotension, dizziness, or drowsiness; dry mouth or throat; constipation (if unresolved, consult prescriber about use of stool softeners); photosensitivity; or decreased perspiration. Report chest pain or palpitations, persistent dizziness, changes in mentation, changes in gait, blurred vision, shortness of breath, or respiratory difficulty.

Related Information

Opium Tincture *on page 858*

Benazepril (ben AY ze pril)

Brand Names: U.S. Lotensin®

Index Terms Benazepril Hydrochloride

Pharmacologic Category Angiotensin-Converting Enzyme (ACE) Inhibitor

Medication Safety Issues

Sound-alike/look-alike issues:

Benazepril may be confused with Benadryl®

Lotensin® may be confused with Lioresal®, lovastatin

Pregnancy Risk Factor D

Lactation Enters breast milk

Breast-Feeding Considerations Small amounts of benazepril and benazeprilat are found in breast milk.

Use Treatment of hypertension, either alone or in combination with other antihypertensive agents

Mechanism of Action/Effect Competitive inhibitor of angiotensin-converting enzyme (ACE); prevents conversion of angiotensin I to angiotensin II, a potent vasoconstrictor; results in lower levels of angiotensin II which causes an increase in plasma renin activity and a reduction in aldosterone secretion

Contraindications Hypersensitivity to benazepril or any component of the formulation; patients with a history of angioedema (with or without prior ACE inhibitor therapy)

Warnings/Precautions Anaphylactic reactions may occur rarely with ACE inhibitors. At any time during treatment (especially following first dose) angioedema may occur rarely with ACE inhibitors. It may involve the head and neck (potentially compromising airway) or the intestine (presenting with abdominal pain). African-Americans and patients with idiopathic or hereditary angioedema may be at an increased risk. Prolonged frequent monitoring may be required especially if tongue, glottis, or larynx are involved as they are associated with airway obstruction. Patients with a history of airway surgery may have a higher risk of airway obstruction. Aggressive early and appropriate management is critical. Contraindicated in patients with history of angioedema with or without prior ACE inhibitor therapy. Hypersensitivity reactions may be seen during hemodialysis (eg, CVVHD) with high-flux dialysis membranes (eg, AN69), and rarely, during low density lipoprotein apheresis with dextran sulfate cellulose. Rare cases of anaphylactoid reactions have been reported in patients undergoing sensitization treatment with hymenoptera (bee, wasp) venom while receiving ACE inhibitors.

Symptomatic hypotension with or without syncope can occur with ACE inhibitors (usually with the first several doses); effects are most often observed in volume depleted patients; close monitoring of patient is required especially with initial dosing and dosing increases; blood pressure must be lowered at a rate appropriate for the patient's clinical condition. Initiation of therapy in patients with ischemic heart disease or cerebrovascular disease warrants close observation due to the potential consequences posed by falling blood pressure (eg, MI, stroke). **[U.S. Boxed Warning]: Drugs that act on the renin-angiotensin system can cause injury and death to the developing fetus. Discontinue as soon as possible once pregnancy is detected.** Use with caution in hypertrophic cardiomyopathy with outflow tract obstruction, severe aortic stenosis, or before, during, or immediately after major surgery.

Hyperkalemia may occur with ACE inhibitors; risk factors include renal dysfunction, diabetes mellitus, concomitant use of potassium-sparing diuretics, potassium supplements and/or potassium containing salts. Use cautiously, if at all, with these agents and monitor potassium closely. Cough may occur with ACE inhibitors. Other causes of cough should be considered (eg, pulmonary congestion in patients with heart failure) and excluded prior to discontinuation. Use with caution in patients with diabetes receiving insulin or oral antidiabetic agents; may be at increased risk for episodes of hypoglycemia.

May be associated with deterioration of renal function and/or increases in serum creatinine, particularly in patients with low renal blood flow (eg, renal artery stenosis, heart failure) whose glomerular filtration rate (GFR) is dependent on efferent arteriolar vasoconstriction by angiotensin II; deterioration may result in oliguria, acute renal failure, and progressive azotemia. Small increases in serum creatinine may occur following initiation; consider discontinuation only in patients with progressive and/or significant deterioration in renal function. Use with caution in patients with unstented unilateral/bilateral renal artery stenosis. When unstented bilateral renal artery stenosis is present, use is generally avoided due to the elevated risk of deterioration in renal function unless possible benefits outweigh risks. Concurrent use of angiotensin receptor blockers may increase the risk of clinically-significant adverse events (eg, renal dysfunction, hyperkalemia).

Rare toxicities associated with ACE inhibitors include cholestatic jaundice (which may progress to fulminant hepatic necrosis), agranulocytosis, neutropenia, or leukopenia with myeloid hypoplasia. Patients with collagen vascular diseases (especially with concomitant renal impairment) or renal impairment alone may be at increased risk for hematologic toxicity; periodically monitor CBC with differential in these patients.

Drug Interactions

Avoid Concomitant Use There are no known interactions where it is recommended to avoid concomitant use.

Decreased Effect

Benazepril may decrease the levels/effects of: Hydrochlorothiazide

The levels/effects of Benazepril may be decreased by: Antacids; Aprotinin; Herbs (Hypertensive Properties); Icatibant; Lanthanum; Methylphenidate; Nonsteroidal Anti-Inflammatory Agents; Salicylates; Yohimbine

Increased Effect/Toxicity

Benazepril may increase the levels/effects of: Allopurinol; Amifostine; Antihypertensives; AzaTHIOprine; CycloSPORINE; CycloSPORINE (Systemic); Ferric Gluconate; Gold Sodium Thiomalate; Hypotensive Agents; Iron Dextran Complex; Lithium; Nonsteroidal Anti-Inflammatory Agents; RiTUXimab; Sodium Phosphates

The levels/effects of Benazepril may be increased by: Alfuzosin; Angiotensin II Receptor Blockers; Diazoxide; DPP-IV Inhibitors; Eplerenone; Everolimus; Herbs (Hypotensive Properties); Hydrochlorothiazide; Loop Diuretics; MAO Inhibitors; Pentoxifylline; Phosphodiesterase 5 Inhibitors; Potassium Salts; Potassium-Sparing Diuretics; Prostacyclin Analogues; Sirolimus; Temsirolimus; Thiazide Diuretics; TiZANidine; Tolvaptan; Trimethoprim

Nutritional/Ethanol Interactions

Food: Potassium supplements and/or potassium-containing salts may cause or worsen hyperkalemia. Management: Consult prescriber before consuming a potassium-rich diet, potassium supplements, or salt substitutes.

Herb/Nutraceutical: Some herbal medications may worsen hypertension (eg, licorice); others may increase the antihypertensive effect of benazepril (eg, shepherd's purse). Management: Avoid bayberry, blue cohosh, cayenne, ephedra, ginger, ginseng (American), kola, licorice, and yohimbe. Avoid black cohosh, California poppy, coleus, golden seal, hawthorn, mistletoe, periwinkle, quinine, and shepherd's purse.

Adverse Reactions

1% to 10%:

Cardiovascular: Postural dizziness (2%)

Central nervous system: Headache (6%), dizziness (4%), somnolence (2%)

Renal: Serum creatinine increased (2%), worsening of renal function may occur in patients with bilateral renal artery stenosis or hypovolemia

Respiratory: Cough (1% to 10%)

Eosinophilic pneumonitis, anaphylaxis, renal insufficiency, and renal failure have been reported with other ACE inhibitors. In addition, a syndrome including fever, myalgia, arthralgia, interstitial nephritis, vasculitis, rash, eosinophilia, and elevated ESR has been reported to be associated with ACE inhibitors.

Pharmacodynamics/Kinetics

Onset of Action

Reduction in plasma angiotensin-converting enzyme (ACE) activity: Peak effect: 1-2 hours after 2-20 mg dose

Reduction in blood pressure: Peak effect: Single dose: 2-4 hours; Continuous therapy: 2 weeks

Duration of Action Reduction in plasma angiotensin-converting enzyme (ACE) activity: >90% inhibition for 24 hours after 5-20 mg dose

Available Dosage Forms

Tablet, oral: 5 mg, 10 mg, 20 mg, 40 mg

Lotensin®: 10 mg, 20 mg, 40 mg

General Dosage Range Dosage adjustment recommended in patients with renal impairment

Oral:

Children ≥6 years: Initial: 0.2 mg/kg/day (up to 10 mg/day); Maintenance: 0.1-0.6 mg/kg/day (maximum: 40 mg/day)

Adults: Initial: 5-10 mg/day; Maintenance: 20-80 mg/day in 1-2 divided doses

Stability

Storage Store at ≤30°C (86°F). Protect from moisture.

Nursing Actions

Physical Assessment Blood pressure should be monitored after first doses and periodically throughout.

Patient Education Take first dose at bedtime. Do not take potassium supplements or salt substitutes containing potassium without consulting prescriber. This drug does not eliminate need for diet or exercise regimen as recommended by prescriber. May cause dizziness, fainting, lightheadedness, postural hypotension, nausea, vomiting, abdominal pain, dry mouth, or transient loss of appetite; report if these side effects persist. Report mouth sores; fever or chills; swelling of extremities, face, mouth, or tongue; or respiratory difficulty or unusual cough.

Benazepril and Hydrochlorothiazide

(ben AY ze pril & hye droe klor oh THYE a zide)

Brand Names: U.S. Lotensin HCT®

Index Terms Benazepril Hydrochloride and Hydrochlorothiazide; Hydrochlorothiazide and Benazepril

Pharmacologic Category Angiotensin-Converting Enzyme (ACE) Inhibitor; Diuretic, Thiazide

Pregnancy Risk Factor D

Lactation Enters breast milk/not recommended

Use Treatment of hypertension

Available Dosage Forms

Tablet:

Generics:

5/6.25: Benazepril 5 mg and hydrochlorothiazide 6.25 mg

10/12.5: Benazepril 10 mg and hydrochlorothiazide 12.5 mg

20/12.5: Benazepril 20 mg and hydrochlorothiazide 12.5 mg

20/25: Benazepril 20 mg and hydrochlorothiazide 25 mg

Brands:

Lotensin HCT® 10/12.5: Benazepril 10 mg and hydrochlorothiazide 12.5 mg

Lotensin HCT® 20/12.5: Benazepril 20 mg and hydrochlorothiazide 12.5 mg

Lotensin HCT® 20/25: Benazepril 20 mg and hydrochlorothiazide 25 mg

General Dosage Range Oral: *Adults:* Benazepril 5-20 mg and hydrochlorothiazide 6.25-25 mg daily

Nursing Actions

Physical Assessment See individual agents.

Patient Education See individual agents.

Related Information

Benazepril *on page 122*

Hydrochlorothiazide *on page 570*

Bendamustine (ben da MUS teen)

Brand Names: U.S. Treanda®

Index Terms Bendamustine Hydrochloride; Cytostasan; SDX-105

Pharmacologic Category Antineoplastic Agent; Antineoplastic Agent, Alkylating Agent; Antineoplastic Agent, Alkylating Agent (Nitrogen Mustard)

Medication Safety Issues

Sound-alike/look-alike issues:

Bendamustine may be confused with brentuximab, carmustine, lomustine

High alert medication:

This medication is in a class the Institute for Safe Medication Practices (ISMP) includes among its list of drug classes which have a heightened risk of causing significant patient harm when used in error.

Pregnancy Risk Factor D

Lactation Excretion in breast milk unknown/not recommended

Use Treatment of chronic lymphocytic leukemia (CLL); treatment of progressed indolent B-cell non-Hodgkin's lymphoma (NHL)

Unlabeled Use Treatment of mantle cell lymphoma; salvage therapy for relapsed multiple myeloma; first-line therapy for follicular lymphoma; treatment of Waldenstrom's macroglobulinemia

Available Dosage Forms

Injection, powder for reconstitution:

Treanda®: 25 mg, 100 mg

General Dosage Range Dosage adjustment recommended in patients who develop toxicities

I.V.: *Adults:* 100 mg/m^2 on days 1 and 2 of a 28-day treatment cycle **or** 120 mg/m^2 on days 1 and 2 of a 21-day treatment cycle

Administration

I.V. Infuse over 30 minutes for the treatment of CLL and over 60 minutes for NHL. Prophylactic treatment with allopurinol may be needed in patients at risk for tumor lysis syndrome. Consider premedication with antihistamines, antipyretics, and/or corticosteroids for patients with a previous grade 1 or 2 infusion reaction to bendamustine. Avoid extravasation; monitor I.V. site for redness, swelling, or pain.

I.V. Detail pH: 2.5-3.5

Nursing Actions

Physical Assessment Monitor infusion site closely to avoid extravasation. Monitor infusion reactions, including skin reactions; can occur with first or subsequent cycles and may require premedication or discontinuation.

Patient Education This medication can only be administered by I.V. Report immediately any pain, burning, or swelling at infusion site; sudden onset chest pain; respiratory difficulty; or difficulty swallowing. It is important that you maintain adequate nutrition between treatments and adequate hydration, unless instructed to restrict fluid intake. You will be susceptible to infection. May cause nausea, vomiting, weight loss, or diarrhea. Report immediately chills, fever, skin rash, persistent unusual fatigue, unusual bruising/bleeding, or signs of infection.

Related Information

Management of Drug Extravasations *on page 1269*

Benzonatate (ben ZOE na tate)

Brand Names: U.S. Tessalon®; Zonatuss™

Index Terms Tessalon Perles

Pharmacologic Category Antitussive

Pregnancy Risk Factor C

Lactation Excretion in breast milk unknown/use caution

Use Symptomatic relief of nonproductive cough

Available Dosage Forms

Capsule, oral:

Zonatuss™: 150 mg

Capsule, softgel, oral: 100 mg, 200 mg

Tessalon®: 100 mg, 200 mg

General Dosage Range Oral: *Children >10 years and Adults:* 100-200 mg 3 times/day as needed (maximum: 600 mg/day)

Administration

Oral Swallow capsule whole (do not break. chew, dissolve, cut, or crush).

Nursing Actions

Physical Assessment Assess effectiveness of therapy (relief of cough, lung sounds, and respiratory pattern). Monitor for CNS changes at beginning of therapy and periodically throughout.

Patient Education Do not break or chew capsule. Maintain adequate hydration, unless instructed to restrict fluid intake. You may experience drowsiness, impaired coordination, blurred vision, increased anxiety, upset stomach, or nausea. Report persistent CNS changes (dizziness, sedation, tremor, or agitation), numbness in chest or feeling of chill, visual changes or burning in eyes, numbness of mouth or difficulty swallowing, or lack of improvement or worsening or condition.

Benztropine (BENZ troe peen)

Brand Names: U.S. Cogentin®

Index Terms Benztropine Mesylate

Pharmacologic Category Anti-Parkinson's Agent, Anticholinergic; Anticholinergic Agent

Medication Safety Issues

Sound-alike/look-alike issues:

Benztropine may be confused with bromocriptine

Pregnancy Risk Factor C

Lactation Excretion in breast milk unknown/use caution

Breast-Feeding Considerations It is not known if benztropine is excreted in breast milk. Anticholinergic agents may suppress lactation.

Use Adjunctive treatment of Parkinson's disease; treatment of drug-induced extrapyramidal symptoms (except tardive dyskinesia)

Mechanism of Action/Effect Possesses both anticholinergic and antihistaminic effects. *In vitro* anticholinergic activity approximates that of atropine; *in vivo* it is only about half as active as atropine. Animal data suggest its antihistaminic activity and duration of action approach that of pyrilamine maleate. May also inhibit the reuptake and storage of dopamine, thereby prolonging the action of dopamine.

Contraindications Hypersensitivity to benztropine or any component of the formulation; pyloric or duodenal obstruction, stenosing peptic ulcers; bladder neck obstructions; achalasia; myasthenia gravis; children <3 years of age

Warnings/Precautions Use with caution in older children (dose has not been established). Use with caution in hot weather or during exercise. May cause anhydrosis and hyperthermia, which may be severe. The risk is increased in hot environments, particularly in the elderly, alcoholics, patients with CNS disease, and those with prolonged outdoor exposure.

Elderly patients frequently develop increased sensitivity and require strict dosage regulation - side effects may be more severe in elderly patients with atherosclerotic changes. Use with caution in patients with tachycardia, cardiac arrhythmias, hypertension, hypotension, glaucoma, prostatic hyperplasia (especially in the elderly), any tendency toward urinary retention, liver or kidney disorders, and obstructive disease of the GI or GU tract. When given in large doses or to susceptible patients, may cause weakness and inability to move particular muscle groups.

May be associated with confusion or hallucinations (generally at higher dosages). Intensification of symptoms or toxic psychosis may occur in patients with mental disorders. May cause CNS depression, which may impair physical or mental abilities; patients must be cautioned about performing tasks which require mental alertness (eg, operating machinery or driving). Benztropine does not relieve symptoms of tardive dyskinesia.

Drug Interactions

Avoid Concomitant Use There are no known interactions where it is recommended to avoid concomitant use.

Decreased Effect

Benztropine may decrease the levels/effects of: Acetylcholinesterase Inhibitors (Central); Ioflupane I 123; Secretin

The levels/effects of Benztropine may be decreased by: Acetylcholinesterase Inhibitors (Central); Peginterferon Alfa-2b

Increased Effect/Toxicity

Benztropine may increase the levels/effects of: AbobotulinumtoxinA; Anticholinergics; Cannabinoids; OnabotulinumtoxinA; Potassium Chloride; RimabotulinumtoxinB

The levels/effects of Benztropine may be increased by: Pramlintide

Nutritional/Ethanol Interactions Ethanol: Avoid ethanol (may increase CNS depression).

Adverse Reactions Frequency not defined.

Cardiovascular: Tachycardia

Central nervous system: Confusion, disorientation, memory impairment, toxic psychosis, visual hallucinations

Dermatologic: Rash

Endocrine & metabolic: Heat stroke, hyperthermia

Gastrointestinal: Constipation, dry throat, ileus, nasal dryness, nausea, vomiting, xerostomia

Genitourinary: Urinary retention, dysuria

Ocular: Blurred vision, mydriasis

Miscellaneous: Fever

Pharmacodynamics/Kinetics

Onset of Action Oral: Within 1 hour; Parenteral: Within 15 minutes

Duration of Action 6-48 hours

Available Dosage Forms

Injection, solution: 1 mg/mL

Cogentin®: 1 mg/mL

Tablet, oral: 0.5 mg, 1 mg, 2 mg

General Dosage Range I.M., I.V., Oral: *Adults:* Range: 0.5-8 mg/day

Administration

Oral May be given with or without food.

I.M. May administer I.M. if oral route is unacceptable.

I.V. May administer I.V. if oral route is unacceptable. Manufacturer's labeling states there is no difference in onset of effect after I.V. or I.M. injection and therefore there is usually no need to use the I.V. route. No specific instructions on administering benztropine I.V. are provided in the labeling. The I.V. route has been reported in the literature (slow I.V. push when reported), although specific instructions are lacking (Duncan, 2001; Lydon, 1998; Sachdev, 1993; Schramm, 2002).

I.V. Detail pH: 5-8

Nursing Actions

Physical Assessment Monitor renal function and therapeutic response (eg, Parkinsonian symptoms). Monitor for anticholinergic syndrome (dry mouth and mucous membranes, constipation, epigastric distress, CNS disturbances, paralytic ileus).

Patient Education Take at the same time each day. Do not use alcohol. You may experience drowsiness, dizziness, confusion, blurred vision, increased susceptibility to heat stroke, decreased perspiration, or constipation. Report unresolved nausea, vomiting, or gastric disturbances; rapid or pounding heartbeat, chest pain, or palpitation; respiratory difficulty; CNS changes (hallucination, loss of memory, nervousness, etc); eye pain; prolonged fever; painful or difficult urination; unresolved constipation; increased muscle spasticity or rigidity; skin rash; or significant worsening of condition.

Dietary Considerations Tablet may be taken with or without food.

Benzylpenicilloyl Polylysine
(BEN zil pen i SIL oyl pol i LIE seen)

Brand Names: U.S. Pre-Pen®

Index Terms Benzylpenicilloyl-polylysine; Penicilloyl-polylysine; PPL

Pharmacologic Category Diagnostic Agent

Pregnancy Risk Factor C

Use Adjunct in assessing the risk of administering penicillin (penicillin G or benzylpenicillin) in patients suspected of clinical penicillin hypersensitivity

Unlabeled Use Adjunct in assessment of hypersensitivity to other beta-lactam antibiotics (penicillins and cephalosporins) to determine the safety of penicillin administration in patients with a history of reaction to cephalosporins

Available Dosage Forms

Injection, solution:

Pre-Pen®: 6 x 10^{-5} M (0.25 mL)

General Dosage Range

Intradermal: *Children and Adults:* Inject a volume of skin test solution sufficient to raise a small intradermal bleb ~3 mm in diameter, in duplicate

Puncture test (first step): *Children and Adults:* Apply a small drop of solution to make a single shallow puncture of the epidermis

Administration

Other

Puncture test: Administer initially by puncture technique on the inner volar aspect of the forearm, followed by an intradermal injection only in patients with a negative reaction.

Intradermal: Do **not** administer intradermally to patients with a positive reaction (wheal of 5-15 mm or more in diameter). Administer the intradermal test on the upper, outer arm, below the deltoid muscle in the event a severe hypersensitivity reaction occurs and a tourniquet needs to be applied. During the skin test, immediate treatment with epinephrine should also be available.

Bepotastine
(be poe TAS teen)

Brand Names: U.S. Bepreve®

Index Terms Bepotastine Besilate

Pharmacologic Category Histamine H_1 Antagonist; Histamine H_1 Antagonist, Second Generation; Mast Cell Stabilizer

Pregnancy Risk Factor C

Lactation Excretion in breast milk unknown/use caution

Use Treatment of itching associated with allergic conjunctivitis

Available Dosage Forms

Solution, ophthalmic:

Bepreve®: 1.5% (5 mL, 10 mL)

General Dosage Range Ophthalmic: *Children ≥2 years and Adults:* Instill 1 drop into the affected eye(s) twice daily

Administration

Other For topical ophthalmic use only. Contact lenses should be removed prior to application, may be inserted after 10 minutes. Do not insert contacts if eyes are red. Avoid contaminating the applicator tip with affected eye(s).

Nursing Actions

Patient Education This medication is for external use only. You may experience mild headache or unusual taste after use. Contact prescriber if eye condition worsens or does not improve. Application: Wash hands thoroughly before applying. Remove contact lenses prior to administration and wait 10 minutes before reinserting. Apply this medication in the affected eye(s) as directed by prescriber. Tilt your head back and look up. Pull down lower lid, hold applicator directly over eye, and place 1 drop into lower lid. Close eyes for a minute. Apply gentle pressure with one finger at the corner of eye near the nose. Do not allow dropper to touch eye or any other surface. If you are using another kind of eye medication, wait several minutes before applying other medications.

Besifloxacin
(be si FLOX a sin)

Brand Names: U.S. Besivance™

Index Terms Besifloxacin Hydrochloride; BOL-303224-A; SS734

Pharmacologic Category Antibiotic, Ophthalmic; Antibiotic, Quinolone

Pregnancy Risk Factor C

Lactation Excretion in breast milk unknown/use caution

Use Treatment of bacterial conjunctivitis

Available Dosage Forms

Suspension, ophthalmic:

Besivance™: 0.6% (5 mL)

General Dosage Range Ophthalmic: *Children ≥1 year and Adults:* 1 drop into affected eye(s) 3 times/day (4-12 hours apart)

Administration

Other Ophthalmic: Wash hands before and after instillation. Shake bottle once prior to each administration. Avoid contaminating the applicator tip with affected eye(s).

Nursing Actions

Patient Education Do not wear contact lenses while using this medication. Wash hands before applying; invert bottle and shake once before use. Remove cap and tilt head back; squeeze bottle gently and instill one drop into the affected eye(s). Avoid contaminating the tip; do not touch the tip with fingers or touch the tip to eye. You may experience eye redness or blurred vision. Discontinue immediately and contact prescriber if you experience a rash, pain, or allergic reaction.

Betamethasone (bay ta METH a sone)

Brand Names: U.S. Celestone®; Celestone® Soluspan®; Diprolene®; Diprolene® AF; Luxiq®

Index Terms Betamethasone Dipropionate; Betamethasone Dipropionate, Augmented; Betamethasone Sodium Phosphate; Betamethasone Valerate; Flubenisolone

Pharmacologic Category Corticosteroid, Systemic; Corticosteroid, Topical

Medication Safety Issues

Sound-alike/look-alike issues:

Luxiq® may be confused with Lasix®

International issues:

Beta-Val [U.S.] may be confused with Betanol brand name for metipranolol [Monaco]

Pregnancy Risk Factor C

Lactation Excretion in breast milk unknown/use caution

Breast-Feeding Considerations Corticosteroids are excreted in human milk. The onset of milk secretion after birth may be delayed and the volume of milk produced may be decreased by antenatal betamethasone therapy; this affect was seen when delivery occurred 3-9 days after the betamethasone dose in women between 28 and 34 weeks gestation. Antenatal betamethasone therapy did not affect milk production when birth occurred <3 days or >10 days of treatment. It is not known if systemic absorption following topical administration results in detectable quantities in human milk. Use with caution while breast-feeding; do not apply to nipples.

Use Inflammatory dermatoses such as seborrheic or atopic dermatitis, neurodermatitis, anogenital pruritus, psoriasis, inflammatory phase of xerosis

Unlabeled Use Accelerate fetal lung maturation in patients with preterm labor

Mechanism of Action/Effect Binds to corticosteroid receptors in cell and acts to prevent or control inflammation

Contraindications Hypersensitivity to betamethasone, other corticosteroids, or any component of the formulation; systemic fungal infections; I.M. administration contraindicated in idiopathic thrombocytopenia purpura

Warnings/Precautions Very high potency topical products are not for treatment of rosacea, perioral dermatitis; not for use on face, groin, or axillae; not for use in a diapered area. Avoid concurrent use of other corticosteroids.

May cause hypercorticism or suppression of hypothalamic-pituitary-adrenal (HPA) axis, particularly in younger children or in patients receiving high doses for prolonged periods. HPA axis suppression may lead to adrenal crisis. Withdrawal and discontinuation of a corticosteroid should be done slowly and carefully. Particular care is required when patients are transferred from systemic corticosteroids to inhaled products due to possible adrenal insufficiency or withdrawal from steroids, including an increase in allergic symptoms. Patients receiving >20 mg per day of prednisone (or equivalent) may be most susceptible. Fatalities have occurred due to adrenal insufficiency in asthmatic patients during and after transfer from systemic corticosteroids to aerosol steroids; aerosol steroids do not provide the systemic steroid needed to treat patients having trauma, surgery, or infections. In stressful situations, HPA axis-suppressed patients should receive adequate supplementation with natural glucocorticoids (hydrocortisone or cortisone) rather than betamethasone (due to lack of mineralocorticoid activity).

Topical corticosteroids may be absorbed percutaneously. Absorption of topical corticosteroids may cause manifestations of Cushing's syndrome, hyperglycemia, or glycosuria. Absorption is increased by the use of occlusive dressings, application to denuded skin, or application to large surface areas.

Acute myopathy has been reported with high dose corticosteroids, usually in patients with neuromuscular transmission disorders; may involve ocular and/or respiratory muscles; monitor creatine kinase; recovery may be delayed. Corticosteroid use may cause psychiatric disturbances, including depression, euphoria, insomnia, mood swings, and personality changes. Pre-existing psychiatric conditions may be exacerbated by corticosteroid use. Prolonged use of corticosteroids may also increase the incidence of secondary infection, mask acute infection (including fungal infections), prolong or exacerbate viral infections, or limit response to vaccines. Exposure to chickenpox should be avoided; corticosteroids should not be used to treat ocular herpes simplex. Corticosteroids should not be used for cerebral malaria or viral hepatitis. Close observation is required in patients with latent tuberculosis and/or TB reactivity; restrict use in active TB (only in conjunction with antituberculosis treatment). Prolonged treatment with corticosteroids has been associated with the development of Kaposi's sarcoma (case reports); if noted, discontinuation of therapy should be considered. High-dose corticosteroids should not be used to manage acute head injury.

Use with caution in patients with thyroid disease, hepatic impairment, renal impairment, cardiovascular disease, diabetes, glaucoma, cataracts, myasthenia gravis, patients at risk for osteoporosis, patients at risk for seizures, or GI diseases (diverticulitis, peptic ulcer, ulcerative colitis) due to perforation risk. Use caution following acute MI (corticosteroids have been associated with myocardial rupture). Because of the risk of adverse effects, systemic corticosteroids should be used cautiously in the elderly in the smallest possible effective dose for the shortest duration. Discontinue if skin irritation or contact dermatitis should occur; do not use in patients with decreased skin circulation. Withdraw therapy with gradual tapering of dose.

Topical use in patients ≤12 years of age is not recommended. Children may absorb proportionally larger amounts after topical application and may be more prone to systemic effects. HPA axis suppression, intracranial hypertension, and Cushing's syndrome have been reported in children receiving topical corticosteroids. Prolonged use may affect growth velocity; growth should be routinely monitored in pediatric patients.

Drug Interactions

Avoid Concomitant Use

Avoid concomitant use of Betamethasone with any of the following: Aldesleukin; BCG; Natalizumab; Pimecrolimus; Tacrolimus (Topical)

Decreased Effect

Betamethasone may decrease the levels/effects of: Aldesleukin; Antidiabetic Agents; BCG; Calcitriol; Coccidioidin Skin Test; Corticorelin; Isoniazid; Salicylates; Sipuleucel-T; Telaprevir; Vaccines (Inactivated)

The levels/effects of Betamethasone may be decreased by: Aminoglutethimide; Antacids; Barbiturates; Bile Acid Sequestrants; Echinacea; Mitotane; Primidone; Rifamycin Derivatives

Increased Effect/Toxicity

Betamethasone may increase the levels/effects of: Acetylcholinesterase Inhibitors; Amphotericin B; Deferasirox; Leflunomide; Loop Diuretics; Natalizumab; NSAID (COX-2 Inhibitor); NSAID (Nonselective); Thiazide Diuretics; Vaccines (Live); Warfarin

The levels/effects of Betamethasone may be increased by: Antifungal Agents (Azole Derivatives, Systemic); Aprepitant; Calcium Channel Blockers (Nondihydropyridine); Denosumab; Estrogen Derivatives; Fluconazole; Fosaprepitant; Indacaterol; Macrolide Antibiotics; Neuromuscular-Blocking Agents (Nondepolarizing); Pimecrolimus; Quinolone Antibiotics; Roflumilast; Salicylates; Tacrolimus (Topical); Telaprevir; Trastuzumab

Nutritional/Ethanol Interactions

Ethanol: Avoid ethanol (may enhance gastric mucosal irritation).

Food: Betamethasone interferes with calcium absorption.

Herb/Nutraceutical: Avoid cat's claw, echinacea (have immunostimulant properties).

Adverse Reactions

Systemic:

Cardiovascular: Congestive heart failure, edema, hyper-/hypotension

Central nervous system: Dizziness, headache, insomnia, intracranial pressure increased, lightheadedness, nervousness, pseudotumor cerebri, seizure, vertigo

Dermatologic: Ecchymoses, facial erythema, fragile skin, hirsutism, hyper-/hypopigmentation, perioral dermatitis (oral), petechiae, striae, wound healing impaired

Endocrine & metabolic: Amenorrhea, Cushing's syndrome, diabetes mellitus, growth suppression, hyperglycemia, hypokalemia, menstrual irregularities, pituitary-adrenal axis suppression, protein catabolism, sodium retention, water retention

Local: Injection site reactions (intra-articular use), sterile abscess

Neuromuscular & skeletal: Arthralgia, muscle atrophy, fractures, muscle weakness, myopathy, osteoporosis, necrosis (femoral and humeral heads)

Ocular: Cataracts, glaucoma, intraocular pressure increased

Miscellaneous: Anaphylactoid reaction, diaphoresis, hypersensitivity, secondary infection

Topical:

Dermatologic: Acneiform eruptions, allergic dermatitis, burning, dry skin, erythema, folliculitis, hypertrichosis, irritation, miliaria, pruritus, skin atrophy, striae, vesiculation

Endocrine and metabolic effects have occasionally been reported with topical use.

Available Dosage Forms

Aerosol, foam, topical:
Luxiq®: 0.12% (50 g, 100 g)

Cream, topical: 0.05% (15 g, 45 g, 50 g); 0.1% (15 g, 45 g)
Diprolene® AF: 0.05% (15 g, 50 g)

Gel, topical: 0.05% (15 g, 50 g)

Injection, suspension: Betamethasone sodium phosphate 3 mg and betamethasone acetate 3 mg per 1 mL (5 mL)
Celestone® Soluspan®: Betamethasone sodium phosphate 3 mg and betamethasone acetate 3 mg per 1 mL (5 mL)

Lotion, topical: 0.05% (30 mL, 60 mL); 0.1% (60 mL)
Diprolene®: 0.05% (30 mL, 60 mL)

Ointment, topical: 0.05% (15 g, 45 g, 50 g); 0.1% (15 g, 45 g)
Diprolene®: 0.05% (15 g, 50 g)

Solution, oral:
Celestone®: 0.6 mg/5 mL (118 mL)

General Dosage Range

I.M.:

Children ≤12 years: 0.0175-0.125 mg base/kg/day **or** 0.5-7.5 mg base/m²/day divided every 6-12 hours

Children ≥13 years and Adults: 0.6-9 mg/day divided every 12-24 hours

Intrabursal, intra-articular, intradermal: *Adults:* 0.25-2 mL

Intralesional: *Adults:* Very large joints: 1-2 mL; Large joints: 1 mL; Medium joints: 0.5-1 mL; Small joints: 0.25-0.5 mL

Oral:

Children ≤12 years: 0.0175-0.25 mg/kg/day **or** 0.5-7.5 mg/m²/day divided every 6-8 hours

Children ≥13 years and Adults: 0.6-7.2 mg/day in 2-4 divided doses

Topical: *Children ≥13 years and Adults:* Apply once or twice daily (maximum: 45-50 g/week; 50 mL/week)

Administration

Oral Not for alternate day therapy; once daily doses should be given in the morning. May be administered with food to decrease GI distress.

I.M. Do **not** give injectable sodium phosphate/acetate suspension I.V.

Topical Apply topical sparingly to areas. Not for use on broken skin or in areas of infection. Do not apply to wet skin unless directed; do not cover with occlusive dressing. Do not apply very high potency agents to face, groin, axillae, or diaper area.

Foam: Invert can and dispense a small amount onto a saucer or other cool surface. Do not dispense directly into hands. Pick up small amounts of foam and gently massage into affected areas until foam disappears. Repeat until entire affected scalp area is treated.

Nursing Actions

Physical Assessment Growth should be routinely monitored in pediatric patients. With systemic administration, caution patients with diabetes to monitor glucose levels closely (corticosteroids may alter glucose levels).

Patient Education Take oral medication with or after meals. Avoid alcohol and limit intake of caffeine or stimulants. Prescriber may recommend increased dietary vitamins, minerals, or iron. If you have diabetes, monitor glucose levels closely (antidiabetic medication may need to be adjusted). Inform prescriber if you are experiencing greater-than-normal levels of stress (medication may need adjustment). You may be more susceptible to infection. Some forms of this medication may cause GI upset. Report promptly excessive nervousness or sleep disturbances, signs of infection (eg, sore throat, unhealed injuries), excessive growth of body hair or loss of skin color, vision changes, weight gain, swelling of face or extremities, respiratory difficulty, muscle weakness, change in color of stools (tarry) or persistent abdominal pain, or worsening of condition or failure to improve.

Topical: For external use only. Do not use for eyes, mucous membranes, or open wounds. Before using, wash and dry area gently. Apply in a thin layer (may rub in lightly). Apply light dressing (if necessary) to area being treated. Do not use occlusive dressing unless so advised by prescriber. Avoid prolonged or excessive use around sensitive tissues, genital, or rectal areas. Avoid exposing treated area to direct sunlight. Inform prescriber if condition worsens (redness, swelling, irritation, signs of infection, or open sores) or fails to improve.

Dietary Considerations May be taken with food to decrease GI distress.

Betamethasone and Clotrimazole

(bay ta METH a sone & kloe TRIM a zole)

Brand Names: U.S. Lotrisone®

Index Terms Clotrimazole and Betamethasone

Pharmacologic Category Antifungal Agent, Topical; Corticosteroid, Topical

Medication Safety Issues

Sound-alike/look-alike issues:

Clotrimazole may be confused with co-trimoxazole

Lotrisone® may be confused with Lotrimin®

Pregnancy Risk Factor C

Lactation Excretion in breast milk unknown/use caution

Use Topical treatment of various dermal fungal infections (including tinea pedis, cruris, and corpora in patients ≥17 years of age)

Available Dosage Forms

Cream: Betamethasone 0.05% and clotrimazole 1% (15 g, 45 g)

Lotrisone®: Betamethasone 0.05% and clotrimazole 1% (15 g, 45 g)

Lotion: Betamethasone 0.05% and clotrimazole 1% (30 mL)

Lotrisone®: Betamethasone 0.05% and clotrimazole 1% (30 mL)

General Dosage Range Topical: *Adults:* Apply to affected area twice daily (maximum: 45 g cream/week; 45 mL lotion/week)

Administration

Topical For external use only. Do not use on open wounds. Do not cover with occlusive dressings. Shake lotion well prior to use

Nursing Actions

Physical Assessment See individual agents.

Patient Education See individual agents.

Related Information

Betamethasone *on page 128*

Betaxolol (Systemic) (be TAKS oh lol)

Brand Names: U.S. Kerlone®

Index Terms Betaxolol Hydrochloride

Pharmacologic Category Beta Blocker, Beta-1 Selective

Medication Safety Issues

Sound-alike/look-alike issues:

Betaxolol may be confused with bethanechol, labetalol

Pregnancy Risk Factor C

Lactation Enters breast milk/use caution

Breast-Feeding Considerations Betaxolol is excreted into breast milk in amounts which may have a pharmacologic effect in the nursing infant. The manufacturer recommends that caution be exercised when administering betaxolol to nursing women.

Use Management of hypertension

Unlabeled Use Treatment of coronary artery disease

Mechanism of Action/Effect Competitively blocks $beta_1$-receptors, with little or no effect on $beta_2$-receptors

Contraindications Hypersensitivity to betaxolol or any component of the formulation; sinus bradycardia; heart block greater than first-degree (except in patients with a functioning artificial pacemaker); cardiogenic shock; uncompensated cardiac failure

Warnings/Precautions Consider pre-existing conditions (such as sick sinus syndrome) before initiating. Administer cautiously in compensated heart failure and monitor for a worsening of the condition. Beta-blocker therapy should not be withdrawn abruptly (particularly in patients with CAD), but gradually tapered to avoid acute tachycardia, hypertension, and/or ischemia. Chronic beta-blocker therapy should not be routinely withdrawn prior to major surgery. Use caution with concurrent use of digoxin, verapamil, or diltiazem; bradycardia or heart block can occur. Use with caution in patients receiving inhaled anesthetic agents known to depress myocardial contractility. Bradycardia may be observed more frequently in elderly patients (>65 years of age); dosage reductions may be necessary.

May precipitate or aggravate symptoms of arterial insufficiency in patients with peripheral vascular disease (PVD) and Raynaud's disease; use with caution; monitor for progression of arterial obstruction. In general, beta-blockers should be avoided in patients with bronchospastic disease. Betaxolol, with $beta_1$ selectivity, may be used cautiously in bronchospastic disease with the lowest possible dose (eg, 5-10 mg/day), availability of a bronchodilator, and close monitoring; if dosage increase is indicated, administer in divided doses. Use cautiously in patients with diabetes because it may potentiate and/or mask prominent hypoglycemic symptoms. May mask signs of hyperthyroidism (eg, tachycardia); use caution if hyperthyroidism is suspected, abrupt withdrawal may precipitate thyroid storm. May induce or exacerbate psoriasis. Use with caution in patients with cerebrovascular insufficiency; hypotension and decreased heart rate may reduce cerebral blood flow. Dosage adjustment required in severe renal impairment and in patients on dialysis. Use with caution in patients with myasthenia gravis (may potentiate myasthenia-related muscle weakness, including diplopia and ptosis) or psychiatric disease (may cause CNS depression). Adequate alpha-blockade is required prior to use of any beta-blocker for patients with untreated pheochromocytoma. Use caution with history of severe anaphylaxis to allergens; patients taking beta-blockers may become more sensitive to repeated challenges. Treatment of anaphylaxis (eg, epinephrine) in patients taking beta-blockers may be ineffective or promote undesirable effects.

Drug Interactions

Avoid Concomitant Use

Avoid concomitant use of Betaxolol (Systemic) with any of the following: Floctafenine; Methacholine

Decreased Effect

Betaxolol (Systemic) may decrease the levels/effects of: Beta2-Agonists; Theophylline Derivatives

The levels/effects of Betaxolol (Systemic) may be decreased by: Barbiturates; CYP1A2 Inducers (Strong); Cyproterone; Herbs (Hypertensive Properties); Methylphenidate; Nonsteroidal Anti-Inflammatory Agents; Peginterferon Alfa-2b; Rifamycin Derivatives; Yohimbine

Increased Effect/Toxicity

Betaxolol (Systemic) may increase the levels/effects of: Alpha-/Beta-Agonists (Direct-Acting); Alpha1-Blockers; Alpha2-Agonists; Amifostine; Antihypertensives; Antipsychotic Agents (Phenothiazines); ARIPiprazole; Bupivacaine; Cardiac Glycosides; Cholinergic Agonists; Fingolimod; Hypotensive Agents; Insulin; Lidocaine; Lidocaine (Systemic); Lidocaine (Topical); Mepivacaine; Methacholine; Midodrine; RiTUXimab; Sulfonylureas

The levels/effects of Betaxolol (Systemic) may be increased by: Abiraterone Acetate; Acetylcholinesterase Inhibitors; Aminoquinolines (Antimalarial); Amiodarone; Anilidopiperidine Opioids; Antipsychotic Agents (Phenothiazines); Calcium Channel Blockers (Dihydropyridine); Calcium Channel Blockers (Nondihydropyridine); CYP1A2 Inhibitors (Moderate); CYP1A2 Inhibitors (Strong); Deferasirox; Diazoxide; Dipyridamole; Disopyramide; Dronedarone; Floctafenine; Herbs (Hypotensive Properties); MAO Inhibitors;

Pentoxifylline; Phosphodiesterase 5 Inhibitors; Propafenone; Prostacyclin Analogues; QuiNIDine; Reserpine

Nutritional/Ethanol Interactions Herb/Nutraceutical: Avoid bayberry; blue cohosh, cayenne, ephedra, ginger, ginseng (American), gotu kola, and licorice (may worsen hypertension). Avoid black cohosh, California poppy, coleus, golden seal, hawthorn, mistletoe, periwinkle, quinine, shepherd's purse (may have increased antihypertensive effects).

Adverse Reactions 2% to 10%:

Cardiovascular: Bradycardia (6% to 8%; symptomatic bradycardia: <1% to 2%; dose-dependent), chest pain (2% to 7%), palpitation (2%), edema (≤2%; similar to placebo)

Central nervous system: Fatigue (3% to 10%), insomnia (1% to 5%), lethargy (3%)

Gastrointestinal: Nausea (2% to 6%), dyspepsia (4% to 5%), diarrhea (2%)

Neuromuscular & skeletal: Arthralgia (3% to 5%), paresthesia (2%)

Respiratory: Dyspnea (2%), pharyngitis (2%)

Miscellaneous: Antinuclear antibody positive (5%), cold extremities (2%)

Pharmacodynamics/Kinetics

Onset of Action 1-1.5 hours

Available Dosage Forms

Tablet, oral: 10 mg, 20 mg

Kerlone®: 10 mg, 20 mg

General Dosage Range Dosage adjustment recommended in patients with renal impairment

Oral:

Adults: 5-20 mg/day

Elderly: Initial dose: 5 mg/day

Administration

Oral Absorption is not affected by food.

Stability

Storage Avoid freezing. Store tablets at room temperature of 15°C to 25°C (59°F to 77°F).

Nursing Actions

Physical Assessment Advise patients with diabetes to monitor glucose levels closely; beta-blockers may alter glucose tolerance. Taper dosage slowly when discontinuing.

Patient Education May cause dizziness, fatigue, nausea, or vomiting. If you have diabetes, monitor serum sugar closely; drug may alter glucose tolerance or mask signs of hypoglycemia. Report chest pain, palpitations, or irregular heartbeat; persistent GI upset (eg, nausea, vomiting, diarrhea); unusual cough; respiratory difficulty; swelling or coolness of extremities; or depression.

Bethanechol (be THAN e kole)

Brand Names: U.S. Urecholine®

Index Terms Bethanechol Chloride

Pharmacologic Category Cholinergic Agonist

Medication Safety Issues

Sound-alike/look-alike issues:

Bethanechol may be confused with betaxolol

Pregnancy Risk Factor C

Lactation Excretion in breast milk unknown/not recommended

Use Treatment of acute postoperative and postpartum nonobstructive (functional) urinary retention; treatment of neurogenic atony of the urinary bladder with retention

Unlabeled Use Gastroesophageal reflux

Available Dosage Forms

Tablet, oral: 5 mg, 10 mg, 25 mg, 50 mg

Urecholine®: 5 mg, 10 mg, 25 mg, 50 mg

General Dosage Range Oral: *Adults:* 10-100 mg 2-4 times/day

Administration

Oral Should be administered 1 hour before meals or 2 hours after meals.

Nursing Actions

Physical Assessment Assess bladder and sphincter adequacy prior to administering medication.

Patient Education Take on an empty stomach to avoid nausea or vomiting. Maintain adequate hydration, unless instructed to restrict fluid intake. May cause dizziness, hypotension, vomiting, or loss of appetite. Report persistent abdominal discomfort; significantly increased salivation, sweating, tearing, or urination; flushed skin; chest pain or palpitations; acute headache; unresolved diarrhea; excessive fatigue, insomnia, dizziness, or depression; increased muscle, joint, or body pain; vision changes or blurred vision; or respiratory difficulty or wheezing.

Bevacizumab (be vuh SIZ uh mab)

Brand Names: U.S. Avastin®

Index Terms Anti-VEGF Monoclonal Antibody; Anti-VEGF rhuMAb; rhuMAb-VEGF

Pharmacologic Category Antineoplastic Agent, Monoclonal Antibody; Vascular Endothelial Growth Factor (VEGF) Inhibitor

Medication Safety Issues

Sound-alike/look-alike issues:

Avastin® may be confused with Astelin®

Bevacizumab may be confused with brentuximab, cetuximab, riTUXimab

High alert medication:

This medication is in a class the Institute for Safe Medication Practices (ISMP) includes among its list of drug classes which have a heightened risk of causing significant patient harm when used in error.

International issues:

Avastin [U.S., Canada, and multiple international markets] may be confused with Avaxim, a brand name for hepatitis A vaccine [Canada and multiple international markets]

Pregnancy Risk Factor C

Lactation Excretion in breast milk unknown/not recommended

Use Treatment of metastatic colorectal cancer; treatment of unresectable, locally advanced, recurrent or metastatic nonsquamous, nonsmall cell lung cancer; treatment of progressive glioblastoma; treatment of metastatic renal cell cancer (not an approved use in Canada)

Note: For the treatment of glioblastoma, effectiveness is based on improvement in objective response rate.

Unlabeled Use Treatment of metastatic breast cancer, recurrent cervical cancer, recurrent ovarian cancer, soft tissue sarcomas (angiosarcoma or hemangiopericytoma/solitary fibrous tumor), age-related macular degeneration (AMD)

Available Dosage Forms

Injection, solution [preservative free]:

Avastin®: 25 mg/mL (4 mL, 16 mL)

General Dosage Range I.V.: *Adults:* 5 or 10 mg/kg every 2 weeks **or** 15 mg/kg every 3 weeks

Administration

I.V. I.V. infusion, usually after the other antineoplastic agents. Infuse the initial dose over 90 minutes. The second infusion may be shortened to 60 minutes if the initial infusion is well tolerated. The third and subsequent infusions may be shortened to 30 minutes if the 60-minute infusion is well tolerated. Monitor closely during the infusion for signs/symptoms of an infusion reaction. Some Some institutions use a 10-minute infusion (0.5 mg/kg/minute) for bevacizumab dosed at 5 mg/kg (after tolerance at the 90-, 60-, and 30-minute infusion rates has been established; Reidy, 2007). Do not administer I.V. push.

I.V. Detail pH: 6.2

Other Intravitreal injection (unlabeled use): Adequate local anesthesia and a topical broad-spectrum antimicrobial agent should be administered prior to the procedure; administer topical ophthalmic antibiotics for 3 days after procedure (Avery, 2006; Bashshur, 2006).

Nursing Actions

Physical Assessment Monitor patient closely during infusion for infusion reaction (eg, hypertension, chest pain, wheezing, diaphoresis). If infusion reaction occurs, discontinue and notify prescriber immediately; permanent discontinuation may be necessary. Monitor for gastrointestinal perforation (abdominal pain, constipation, vomiting), heart failure, hypertensive crisis, serious bleeding, and nephrotic syndrome; notify prescriber of serious adverse reactions.

Patient Education This medication can only be administered by infusion; you will be closely monitored during infusion. Report immediately unusual back or abdominal pain; acute headache; difficulty breathing or chest tightness; difficulty swallowing; itching or rash; or redness, swelling, or pain at infusion site. Between treatments, maintain adequate nutrition and hydration, unless instructed to restrict fluid intake. You may experience loss of appetite, nausea, dry mouth, taste changes, loss of hair (will grow back when therapy is completed), or muscle or skeletal pain. Report immediately any unusual bleeding (blood in urine or tarry stool, nose bleeds, vaginal bleeding, bleeding from wound); abdominal pain, vomiting, constipation, or diarrhea; acute headache, dizziness, or confusion; seizure, vision changes, or unusual lethargy; changes in urinary pattern; pain, redness, swelling, or sudden loss of sensation in extremities; skin rash or hives; or unusual infection (fever or chills, cough, sore throat, pain or difficulty passing urine).

Bexarotene (Systemic) (beks AIR oh teen)

Brand Names: U.S. Targretin®

Pharmacologic Category Antineoplastic Agent, Miscellaneous

Medication Safety Issues

High alert medication:

The Institute for Safe Medication Practices (ISMP) includes this medication among its list of drugs which have a heightened risk of causing significant patient harm when used in error.

Pregnancy Risk Factor X

Lactation Excretion in breast milk unknown/not recommended

Breast-Feeding Considerations It is not known if bexarotene is excreted into breast milk. Due to the potential for serious adverse reactions in a nursing infant, the decision to continue or discontinue breast-feeding during therapy should take into account the risk of exposure to the infant and the benefits of treatment to the mother.

Use Treatment of cutaneous manifestations of cutaneous T-cell lymphoma in patients who are refractory to at least one prior systemic therapy

Mechanism of Action/Effect Exact mechanism in is unknown. Acts to inhibit the growth of some tumor cell lines of hematopoietic and squamous cell origin.

Contraindications Hypersensitivity to bexarotene or any component of the formulation; pregnancy

Warnings/Precautions Hazardous agent - use appropriate precautions for handling and disposal. **[U.S. Boxed Warning]: Bexarotene is a retinoid, a drug class associated with birth defects in humans; do not administer during pregnancy.** Pregnancy test needed 1 week before initiation and every month thereafter. Effective contraception must be in place 1 month before initiation, during therapy, and for at least 1 month after discontinuation. Male patients with sexual partners who are pregnant, possibly pregnant, or who could become pregnant, must use condoms during sexual intercourse during treatment and for 1 month after last dose. Induces significant lipid abnormalities in a majority of patients (triglyceride, total cholesterol, and HDL); reversible on discontinuation. Use extreme caution in patients with underlying hypertriglyceridemia. Pancreatitis secondary to hypertriglyceridemia has been reported. Patients with risk factors for pancreatitis (eg, prior pancreatitis, uncontrolled hyperlipidemia, excess ethanol consumption, uncontrolled diabetes, biliary tract disease) should generally not receive bexarotene (oral). Monitor for liver function test abnormalities and discontinue drug if tests are three times the upper limit of normal values for AST, ALT, or bilirubin. Hypothyroidism occurs in about a third of patients. Monitor for signs and symptoms of infection about 4-8 weeks after initiation (leukopenia may occur). Any new visual abnormalities experienced by the patient should be evaluated by an ophthalmologist (cataracts can form, or worsen, especially in the geriatric population). May cause photosensitization. Safety and efficacy are not established in the pediatric population. Use only with extreme caution in patients with hepatic impairment. Limit additional vitamin A intake to <15,000 int. units/day. Use caution with diabetic patients.

Drug Interactions

Avoid Concomitant Use

Avoid concomitant use of Bexarotene (Systemic) with any of the following: Axitinib; Gemfibrozil; Tetracycline Derivatives; Vitamin A

Decreased Effect

Bexarotene (Systemic) may decrease the levels/effects of: ARIPiprazole; Atorvastatin; Axitinib; Contraceptives (Estrogens); Contraceptives (Progestins); PACLitaxel; Saxagliptin

The levels/effects of Bexarotene (Systemic) may be decreased by: Tocilizumab

Increased Effect/Toxicity

Bexarotene (Systemic) may increase the levels/effects of: Porfimer; Vitamin A

The levels/effects of Bexarotene (Systemic) may be increased by: CARBOplatin; Conivaptan; Gemfibrozil; PACLitaxel; Tetracycline Derivatives

Nutritional/Ethanol Interactions

Food: Bioavailability is increased when administered with a fat-containing meal. Serum levels may be increased by grapefruit juice. Management: Administer with food, preferably high-fat meals (peanuts or ice cream). Avoid grapefruit juice.

Herb/Nutraceutical: Dong quai and St John's wort may cause photosensitization. St John's wort may decrease bexarotene levels. Additional vitamin A supplementation may lead to vitamin A toxicity (dry skin, irritation, arthralgias, myalgias, abdominal pain, hepatic changes). Management: Avoid St John's wort and dong quai. Avoid use of vitamin A supplements.

Adverse Reactions First percentage is at a dose of 300 mg/m^2/day; the second percentage is at a dose >300 mg/m^2/day.

>10%:

Cardiovascular: Peripheral edema (13% to 11%)

Central nervous system: Headache (30% to 42%), chills (10% to 13%)

Dermatologic: Rash (17% to 23%), exfoliative dermatitis (10% to 28%)

Endocrine & metabolic: Hyperlipidemia (about 79% in both dosing ranges), hypercholesteremia (32% to 62%), hypothyroidism (29% to 53%)

Hematologic: Leukopenia (17% to 47%)

Neuromuscular & skeletal: Weakness (20% to 45%)

Miscellaneous: Infection (13% to 23%)

<10%:

Cardiovascular: Hemorrhage, hypertension, angina pectoris, right heart failure, tachycardia, cerebrovascular accident

Central nervous system: Fever (5% to 17%), insomnia (5% to 11%), subdural hematoma, syncope, depression, agitation, ataxia, confusion, dizziness, hyperesthesia

Dermatologic: Dry skin (about 10% for both dosing ranges), alopecia (4% to 11%), skin ulceration, acne, skin nodule, maculopapular rash, serous drainage, vesicular bullous rash, cheilitis

Endocrine & metabolic: Hypoproteinemia, hyperglycemia, weight loss/gain, breast pain

Gastrointestinal: Abdominal pain (11% to 4%), nausea (16% to 8%), diarrhea (7% to 42%), vomiting (4% to 13%), anorexia (2% to 23%), constipation, xerostomia, flatulence, colitis, dyspepsia, gastroenteritis, gingivitis, melena, pancreatitis, serum amylase increased

Genitourinary: Albuminuria, hematuria, urinary incontinence, urinary tract infection, urinary urgency, dysuria, kidney function abnormality

Hematologic: Hypochromic anemia (4% to 13%), anemia (6% to 25%), eosinophilia, thrombocythemia, coagulation time increased, lymphocytosis, thrombocytopenia

Hepatic: LDH increase (7% to 13%), hepatic failure

Neuromuscular & skeletal: Back pain (2% to 11%), arthralgia, myalgia, bone pain, myasthenia, arthrosis, neuropathy

Ocular: Dry eyes, conjunctivitis, blepharitis, corneal lesion, visual field defects, keratitis

Otic: Ear pain, otitis externa

Renal: Creatinine increased

Respiratory: Pharyngitis, rhinitis, dyspnea, pleural effusion, bronchitis, cough increased, lung edema, hemoptysis, hypoxia

Miscellaneous: Flu-like syndrome (4% to 13%), bacterial infection (1% to 13%)

Available Dosage Forms

Capsule, oral:

Targretin®: 75 mg

General Dosage Range Oral: *Adults:* 300-400 mg/m² once daily

Administration

Oral Administer capsule following a fat-containing meal.

Stability

Storage Store at 2°C to 25°C (36°F to 77°F). Protect from light.

Nursing Actions

Physical Assessment Monitor pregnancy status, lipid panel, LFTs, thyroid function, and CBC prior to and during therapy. Monitor for CNS or cardiovascular effects, opportunistic infection, visual abnormalities, and hypoglycemia.

Patient Education It is preferable to take capsules after a fat-containing meal. Maintain adequate hydration, unless instructed to restrict fluid intake. Avoid grapefruit juice, St John's wort, or additional vitamin A supplements while using this medication. You may be more susceptible to infection. May cause nausea, vomiting, anorexia, flatulence, constipation, diarrhea, headache, back or muscle pain, or photosensitivity. Report chest pain, rapid heartbeat; unresolved GI effects, headache, back or muscle pain, skin dryness, skin rash or peeling, mucous membrane lesions, altered urinary patterns, flu syndrome or opportunistic infection (eg, weakness, fatigue, white plaques or sores in mouth, vaginal discharge, chills, fever), CNS disturbances (insomnia, dizziness, agitation, confusion, depression), or vision or hearing changes.

Dietary Considerations It is preferable to take the oral capsule following a fat-containing meal. Avoid grapefruit juice.

Bexarotene (Topical) (beks AIR oh teen)

Brand Names: U.S. Targretin®

Pharmacologic Category Antineoplastic Agent, Miscellaneous

Medication Safety Issues

High alert medication:

The Institute for Safe Medication Practices (ISMP) includes this medication among its list of drugs which have a heightened risk of causing significant patient harm when used in error.

Pregnancy Risk Factor X

Lactation Excretion in breast milk unknown/not recommended

Use Treatment of cutaneous lesions in patients with refractory cutaneous T-cell lymphoma (stage 1A and 1B) or who have not tolerated other therapies

Available Dosage Forms

Gel, topical:

Targretin®: 1% (60 g)

General Dosage Range Topical: *Adults:* Initial: Apply once every other day for first week; Maintenance: Apply 1-4 times/day

Administration

Topical Allow gel to dry before covering with clothing. Avoid application to normal skin. Use of occlusive dressings is not recommended.

Nursing Actions

Patient Education Avoid applying to normal skin or mucous membranes. Do not use occlusive dressings.

Bicalutamide (bye ka LOO ta mide)

Brand Names: U.S. Casodex®

Index Terms CDX; ICI-176334

Pharmacologic Category Antineoplastic Agent, Antiandrogen

Medication Safety Issues

Sound-alike/look-alike issues:

Casodex® may be confused with Kapidex [DSC]

International issues:

Casodex [U.S., Canada, and multiple international markets] may be confused with Capadex brand name for propoxyphene/acetaminophen [Australia, New Zealand]

Pregnancy Risk Factor X

Lactation Excretion in breast milk unknown/contraindicated

Use Treatment of metastatic prostate cancer (in combination with an LHRH agonist)

Unlabeled Use Monotherapy for locally-advanced prostate cancer

Available Dosage Forms

Tablet, oral: 50 mg

Casodex®: 50 mg

General Dosage Range Oral: *Adults:* 50 mg once daily

Administration

Oral Dose should be taken at the same time each day with or without food. Treatment for metastatic cancer should be started concomitantly with an LHRH analogue.

Nursing Actions

Physical Assessment Monitor LFTs at baseline and regularly during therapy. Advise patients with diabetes to monitor glucose levels closely (may induce hyperglycemia).

Patient Education Take at the same time each day, with or without food. If you have diabetes, monitor serum glucose closely and notify prescriber of changes (this medication may alter glucose levels). May cause back, breast, or pelvic pain; hot flashes; dizziness, confusion, or drowsiness; nausea or vomiting; constipation; hair loss; impotence; or gynecomastia. Report unusual weight gain or swelling of extremities; easy bruising or bleeding; yellowing of skin or eyes; change in color of urine or stool; unresolved CNS changes (eg, nervousness, chills, insomnia, somnolence); skin rash, redness, or irritation; chest pain or palpitations; respiratory difficulty; urinary retention or inability to void; muscle weakness, tremors, or pain; or persistent gastrointestinal upset.

Bimatoprost (bi MAT oh prost)

Brand Names: U.S. Latisse®; Lumigan®

Pharmacologic Category Ophthalmic Agent, Antiglaucoma; Prostaglandin, Ophthalmic

Pregnancy Risk Factor C

Lactation Excretion in breast milk unknown/use caution

Use Reduction of intraocular pressure (IOP) in patients with open-angle glaucoma or ocular hypertension; hypotrichosis treatment of the eyelashes

Mechanism of Action/Effect Decreases intraocular pressure by increasing outflow of aqueous humor. Increases the percent and duration of hairs in the growth phase, resulting in eyelash growth.

Contraindications

Latisse®: Hypersensitivity to bimatoprost or any component of the formulation

Lumigan®: There are no contraindications listed in the manufacturer's prescribing information.

Warnings/Precautions May cause permanent changes in eye color (increases the amount of brown pigment in the iris), the eyelid skin, and eyelashes. In addition, may increase the length and/or number of eyelashes (may vary between eyes). Use caution in patients with intraocular inflammation, aphakic patients, pseudophakic patients with a torn posterior lens capsule, or patients with risk factors for macular edema. Contains benzalkonium chloride (may be adsorbed by contact lenses). Safety and efficacy have not been determined for use in patients with angle-closure, inflammatory, or neovascular glaucoma. Not recommended for use in pediatrics <16 years of age due to potential concerns regarding long-term use and hyperpigmentation.

Latisse®: Additional warnings: Patients receiving medications to reduce intraocular pressure should consult their healthcare provider prior to using; may interfere with desired reduction of intraocular pressure. Unintentional hair growth may occur on skin that has repeated contact with solution; apply to upper eyelid only, blot away excess.

Drug Interactions

Avoid Concomitant Use There are no known interactions where it is recommended to avoid concomitant use.

Decreased Effect There are no known significant interactions involving a decrease in effect.

Increased Effect/Toxicity

The levels/effects of Bimatoprost may be increased by: Latanoprost

Adverse Reactions Adverse reactions and percentages are for Lumigan® unless noted:

>10%: Ocular: Conjunctival hyperemia (25% to 45%; Latisse®: <4%), growth of eyelashes, ocular pruritus (>10%; Latisse®: <4%)

1% to 10%:

Central nervous system: Headache (1% to 5%)

Dermatologic: Skin hyperpigmentation (Latisse®: <4%), abnormal hair growth

Hepatic: Liver function tests abnormal (1% to 5%)

Neuromuscular & skeletal: Weakness (1% to 5%)

Ocular: Dry eyes (Latisse®: <4%), erythema (eyelid/periorbital region; Latisse® <4%), irritation (Latisse®: <4%), allergic conjunctivitis, asthenopia, blepharitis, burning, cataract, conjunctival edema, conjunctival hemorrhage, discharge, eyelash darkening, foreign body sensation, iris pigmentation increased (may be delayed), pain, photophobia, pigmentation of periocular skin, superficial punctate keratitis, tearing, visual disturbance

Miscellaneous: Infections (10% [primarily colds and upper respiratory tract infections])

Pharmacodynamics/Kinetics

Onset of Action Reduction of IOP: ~4 hours; Peak effect: Maximum reduction of IOP: ~8-12 hours

Available Dosage Forms

Solution, ophthalmic:

Latisse®: 0.03% (3 mL)

Lumigan®: 0.01% (2.5 mL, 5 mL, 7.5 mL); 0.03% (2.5 mL, 5 mL, 7.5 mL)

General Dosage Range

Ophthalmic: *Adults:* Instill 1 drop into affected eye(s) once daily

Ophthalmic, topical: *Adults:* Place 1 drop on applicator and apply evenly along the skin of the upper eyelid at base of eyelashes once daily

Administration

Other

Latisse®: Remove make-up and contact lenses prior to application; ensure face is clean. Apply with the sterile applicator provided only; do not use other brushes or applicators. Use a tissue or cloth to blot any excess solution on the outside of the upper eyelid margin; do not apply to lower eyelash line. Do not reuse applicators; use new applicator for second eye. Applying more than once nightly will not increase eyelash growth; eyelash growth is expected to return to baseline when therapy is discontinued. May reinsert contacts 15 minutes after application.

Lumigan®: May be used with other eye drops to lower intraocular pressure. If using more than one ophthalmic product, wait at least 5 minutes in between application of each medication. Remove contact lenses prior to administration and wait 15 minutes before reinserting.

Stability

Storage Store between 2°C to 25°C (36°F to 77°F).

Nursing Actions

Patient Education For use in eyes only. Wash hands before instilling. Sit or lie down to instill. Open eye, look at ceiling, and instill prescribed amount of solution. Apply gentle pressure to inner corner of eye. Do not let tip of applicator touch eye; do not contaminate tip of applicator (may cause eye infection, eye damage, or vision loss). Contact prescriber concerning continued use of drops if eye infection develops, trauma occurs to the eye, and prior to eye surgery. This product contains benzalkonium chloride which may be adsorbed by contact lenses; remove contacts prior to administration and wait 15 minutes before reinserting. May cause permanent changes in eye color, eyelid, and eyelashes. May also increase the length and/or number of eyelashes. Changes may occur slowly (months to years). May be used with other eye drops to lower intraocular pressure. If using more than one eye drop medicine, wait at least 5 minutes in between application of each medication. Notify prescriber if conjunctivitis or eyelid reactions occur with use of this product.

Bismuth (BIZ muth)

Brand Names: U.S. Bismatrol Maximum Strength [OTC]; Bismatrol [OTC]; Diotame [OTC]; Kao-Tin [OTC]; Kaopectate® Extra Strength [OTC]; Kaopectate® [OTC]; Peptic Relief [OTC]; Pepto Relief [OTC]; Pepto-Bismol® Maximum Strength [OTC]; Pepto-Bismol® [OTC]

Index Terms Bismatrol; Bismuth Subsalicylate; Pink Bismuth

Pharmacologic Category Antidiarrheal

Medication Safety Issues

Sound-alike/look-alike issues:

Kaopectate® may be confused with Kayexalate®

Other safety concerns:

Maalox® Total Relief® is a different formulation than other Maalox® liquid antacid products which contain aluminum hydroxide, magnesium hydroxide, and simethicone.

Canadian formulation of Kaopectate® does not contain bismuth; the active ingredient in the Canadian formulation is attapulgite.

Use Subsalicylate formulation: Symptomatic treatment of mild, nonspecific diarrhea; control of traveler's diarrhea (enterotoxigenic *Escherichia coli*); as part of a multidrug regimen for *H. pylori* eradication to reduce the risk of duodenal ulcer recurrence

Available Dosage Forms For available OTC formulations, consult specific product labeling.

General Dosage Range Oral:

Subsalicylate based on 262 mg/5 mL liquid or 262 mg tablet (diarrhea):

Children 3-6 years: 1/3 tablet **or** 5 mL every 30 minutes to 1 hour as needed (maximum: 8 doses/day)

Children 6-9 years: 2/3 tablet **or** 10 mL every 30 minutes to 1 hour as needed (maximum: 8 doses/day)

Children 9-12 years: 1 tablet **or** 15 mL every 30 minutes to 1 hour as needed (maximum: 8 doses/day)

Subsalicylate based on 262 mg/15 mL liquid or 262 mg tablet:

Children >12 years: Diarrhea: 2 tablets **or** 30 mL every 30 minutes to 1 hour as needed (maximum: 8 doses/day)

Adults:

Diarrhea: 2 tablets **or** 30 mL every 30 minutes to 1 hour as needed (maximum: 8 doses/day)

H. pylori eradication: 524 mg 4 times/day

Administration

Oral Liquids must be shaken prior to use. Chewable tablets should be chewed thoroughly. Nonchewable caplets should be swallowed whole with a full glass of water.

Nursing Actions

Physical Assessment Patient's history with aspirin products should be assessed prior to beginning treatment (contains ASA). Assess other drugs patient may be taking for potential interactions (eg, aspirin products). Monitor for CNS changes, impactions, and tinnitus.

Patient Education Chew tablet well or shake suspension well before using. Maintain adequate fluid intake to prevent dehydration unless instructed to restrict fluid intake. May darken stools and turn tongue black. If diarrhea persists for more than 2 days, consult healthcare provider. If tinnitus (ringing in the ears) occurs, this may indicate toxicity; discontinue use and notify healthcare provider.

Bisoprolol (bis OH proe lol)

Brand Names: U.S. Zebeta®

Index Terms Bisoprolol Fumarate

Pharmacologic Category Beta Blocker, Beta-1 Selective

Medication Safety Issues

Sound-alike/look-alike issues:

Zebeta® may be confused with DiaBeta®, Zetia®

Pregnancy Risk Factor C

Lactation Excretion unknown/use caution

Breast-Feeding Considerations It is not known if bisoprolol is excreted into breast milk. The manufacturer recommends that caution be exercised when administering bisoprolol to nursing women.

Use Treatment of hypertension, alone or in combination with other agents

Unlabeled Use Chronic stable angina, supraventricular arrhythmias, PVCs, heart failure (HF)

Mechanism of Action/Effect Selective inhibitor of $beta_1$-adrenergic receptors; competitively blocks $beta_1$-receptors, with little or no effect on $beta_2$-receptors at doses ≤20 mg

Contraindications Cardiogenic shock; overt cardiac failure; marked sinus bradycardia or heart block greater than first-degree (except in patients with a functioning artificial pacemaker)

Warnings/Precautions Consider pre-existing conditions such as sick sinus syndrome before initiating. Use caution in patients with heart failure; use gradual and careful titration; monitor for symptoms of congestive heart failure. Use with caution in patients with myasthenia gravis, psychiatric disease (may cause CNS depression), bronchospastic disease, undergoing anesthesia; and in those with impaired hepatic function. Bradycardia may be observed more frequently in elderly patients (>65 years of age); dosage reductions may be necessary. Beta-blocker therapy should not be withdrawn abruptly (particularly in patients with CAD), but gradually tapered to avoid acute tachycardia, hypertension, and/or ischemia. Chronic beta-blocker therapy should not be routinely withdrawn prior to major surgery. Can precipitate or aggravate symptoms of arterial insufficiency in patients with PVD and Raynaud's disease; use with caution and monitor for progression of arterial obstruction. Use caution with concurrent use of digoxin, verapamil, or diltiazem; bradycardia or heart block may occur. Use with caution in patients receiving inhaled anesthetic agents known to depress myocardial contractility. Bisoprolol, with beta$_1$-selectivity, may be used cautiously in bronchospastic disease with close monitoring. Use cautiously in patients with diabetes because it can mask prominent hypoglycemic symptoms. May mask signs of hyperthyroidism (eg, tachycardia); use caution if hyperthyroidism is suspected, abrupt withdrawal may precipitate thyroid storm. Dosage adjustment is required in patients with significant hepatic or renal dysfunction. Adequate alpha-blockade is required prior to use of any beta-blocker for patients with untreated pheochromocytoma. May induce or exacerbate psoriasis. Use caution with history of severe anaphylaxis to allergens; patients taking beta-blockers may become more sensitive to repeated challenges. Treatment of anaphylaxis (eg, epinephrine) in patients taking beta-blockers may be ineffective or promote undesirable effects.

Drug Interactions

Avoid Concomitant Use

Avoid concomitant use of Bisoprolol with any of the following: Conivaptan; Floctafenine; Methacholine

Decreased Effect

Bisoprolol may decrease the levels/effects of: Beta2-Agonists; Theophylline Derivatives

The levels/effects of Bisoprolol may be decreased by: Barbiturates; CYP3A4 Inducers (Strong); Deferasirox; Herbs (CYP3A4 Inducers); Herbs (Hypertensive Properties); Methylphenidate; Nonsteroidal Anti-Inflammatory Agents; Peginterferon Alfa-2b; Rifamycin Derivatives; Tocilizumab; Yohimbine

Increased Effect/Toxicity

Bisoprolol may increase the levels/effects of: Alpha-/Beta-Agonists (Direct-Acting); Alpha1-Blockers; Alpha2-Agonists; Amifostine; Antihypertensives; Antipsychotic Agents (Phenothiazines); Bupivacaine; Cardiac Glycosides; Cholinergic Agonists; Fingolimod; Hypotensive Agents; Insulin; Lidocaine; Lidocaine (Systemic); Lidocaine (Topical); Mepivacaine; Methacholine; Midodrine; RiTUXimab; Sulfonylureas

The levels/effects of Bisoprolol may be increased by: Acetylcholinesterase Inhibitors; Aminoquinolines (Antimalarial); Amiodarone; Anilidopiperidine Opioids; Antipsychotic Agents (Phenothiazines); Calcium Channel Blockers (Dihydropyridine); Calcium Channel Blockers (Nondihydropyridine); Conivaptan; CYP3A4 Inhibitors (Moderate); CYP3A4 Inhibitors (Strong); Dasatinib; Diazoxide; Dipyridamole; Disopyramide; Dronedarone; Floctafenine; Herbs (Hypotensive Properties); Ivacaftor; MAO Inhibitors; Pentoxifylline; Phosphodiesterase 5 Inhibitors; Propafenone; Prostacyclin Analogues; QuiNIDine; Reserpine

Nutritional/Ethanol Interactions Herb/Nutraceutical: Avoid dong quai if using for hypertension (has estrogenic activity). Avoid ephedra, yohimbe, ginseng (may worsen hypertension). Avoid garlic (may have increased antihypertensive effect).

Adverse Reactions 1% to 10%:

Cardiovascular: Chest pain (1% to 2%)

Central nervous system: Fatigue (dose related; 6% to 8%), insomnia (2% to 3%), hypoesthesia (1% to 2%)

Gastrointestinal: Diarrhea (dose related; 3% to 4%), nausea (2%), vomiting (1% to 2%)

Neuromuscular & skeletal: Arthralgia, weakness (dose related; ≤2%)

Respiratory: Upper respiratory infection (5%), rhinitis (3% to 4%), sinusitis (dose related; 2%), dyspnea (1% to 2%)

Pharmacodynamics/Kinetics

Onset of Action 1-2 hours

Available Dosage Forms

Tablet, oral: 5 mg, 10 mg

Zebeta®: 5 mg, 10 mg

General Dosage Range Dosage adjustment recommended in patients with renal impairment

Oral: *Adults and Elderly:* Initial: 2.5-5 mg once daily; Maintenance: 2.5-20 mg once daily

Administration

Oral May be administered without regard to meals.

Stability

Storage Store at controlled room temperature 20°C to 25°C (68°F to 77°F). Protect from moisture.

Nursing Actions

Physical Assessment Monitor blood pressure and heart rate prior to and following first dose and with any change in dosage. Taper dosage slowly when discontinuing. Advise patients with diabetes to monitor glucose levels closely; beta-blockers may alter glucose tolerance. Teach patient how to handle orthostatic hypotension.

Patient Education Take with or without food. Take pulse daily (prior to medication) and follow prescriber's instruction about holding medication. If you have diabetes, monitor serum sugar closely; drug may alter glucose tolerance or mask signs of hypoglycemia. May cause fatigue, dizziness, postural hypotension, alteration in sexual performance (reversible), or diarrhea. Report unresolved swelling of extremities, respiratory difficulty or new cough, unresolved fatigue, unusual weight gain, unresolved constipation, or unusual muscle weakness.

Dietary Considerations May be taken without regard to meals.

Bisoprolol and Hydrochlorothiazide

(bis OH proe lol & hye droe klor oh THYE a zide)

Brand Names: U.S. Ziac®

Index Terms Bisoprolol Fumarate and Hydrochlorothiazide; Hydrochlorothiazide and Bisoprolol

Pharmacologic Category Beta Blocker, Beta-1 Selective; Diuretic, Thiazide

Medication Safety Issues

Sound-alike/look-alike issues:

Ziac® may be confused with Tiazac®, Zerit®

Pregnancy Risk Factor C

Lactation Enters breast milk/not recommended

Use Treatment of hypertension

Unlabeled Use Treatment of hypertension in the pediatric patient

Available Dosage Forms

Tablet, oral: 2.5/6.25: Bisoprolol 2.5 mg and hydrochlorothiazide 6.25 mg; 5/6.25: Bisoprolol 5 mg and hydrochlorothiazide 6.25 mg; 10/6.25: Bisoprolol 10 mg and hydrochlorothiazide 6.25 mg

Ziac®: 2.5/6.25: Bisoprolol 2.5 mg and hydrochlorothiazide 6.25 mg; 5/6.25: Bisoprolol 5 mg and hydrochlorothiazide 6.25 mg; 10/6.25: Bisoprolol 10 mg and hydrochlorothiazide 6.25 mg

General Dosage Range Oral: *Adults:* Initial: Bisoprolol 2.5 mg and hydrochlorothiazide 6.25 mg once daily; Maintenance: Bisoprolol 2.5-20 mg and hydrochlorothiazide 6.25-12.5 mg once daily; Maximum dose (manufacturer recommended): Bisoprolol 20 mg and hydrochlorothiazide 12.5 mg once daily

Administration

Oral May be administered without regard to meals.

Nursing Actions

Physical Assessment See individual agents.

Patient Education See individual agents.

Related Information

Bisoprolol *on page 137*

Hydrochlorothiazide *on page 570*

Bleomycin (blee oh MYE sin)

Index Terms Blenoxane; Bleo; Bleomycin Sulfate; BLM

Pharmacologic Category Antineoplastic Agent, Antibiotic

Medication Safety Issues

Sound-alike/look-alike issues:

Bleomycin may be confused with Cleocin®

High alert medication:

This medication is in a class the Institute for Safe Medication Practices (ISMP) includes among its list of drugs which have a heightened risk of causing significant patient harm when used in error.

Pregnancy Risk Factor D

Lactation Excretion in breast milk unknown/not recommended

Breast-Feeding Considerations Due to the potential for serious adverse reactions in the nursing infant, breast-feeding is not recommended.

Use Treatment of squamous cell carcinomas of the head and neck, penis, cervix, or vulva, testicular carcinoma, Hodgkin's lymphoma, and non-Hodgkin's lymphoma; sclerosing agent for malignant pleural effusion

Unlabeled Use Treatment of ovarian germ cell tumors

Mechanism of Action/Effect Inhibits synthesis of DNA; also inhibits (to a lesser degree) RNA and protein synthesis

Contraindications Hypersensitivity to bleomycin or any component of the formulation

Warnings/Precautions Hazardous agent - use appropriate precautions for handling and disposal. **[U.S. Boxed Warning]: Occurrence of pulmonary fibrosis (commonly presenting as pneumonitis; occasionally progressing to pulmonary fibrosis) is the most severe toxicity. Risk is higher in elderly patients or patients receiving >400 units total lifetime dose;** other possible risk factors include smoking and patients with prior radiation therapy or receiving concurrent oxygen. **A severe idiosyncratic reaction consisting of hypotension, mental confusion, fever, chills, and wheezing (similar to anaphylaxis) has been reported in 1% of lymphoma patients treated with bleomycin.** Since these reactions usually occur after the first or second dose, careful monitoring is essential after these doses. Use caution when administering O_2 during surgery to patients who have received bleomycin; the risk of bleomycin-related pulmonary toxicity is increased. Use caution with renal impairment (Cl_{cr} <50 mL/minute), may require dose adjustment. May cause renal or hepatic toxicity. **[U.S. Boxed Warning]: Should be administered under the supervision of an experienced cancer chemotherapy physician**

Drug Interactions

Avoid Concomitant Use

Avoid concomitant use of Bleomycin with any of the following: BCG; Brentuximab Vedotin; Natalizumab; Pimecrolimus; Tacrolimus (Topical); Vaccines (Live)

Decreased Effect

Bleomycin may decrease the levels/effects of: BCG; Cardiac Glycosides; Coccidioidin Skin Test; Sipuleucel-T; Vaccines (Inactivated); Vaccines (Live)

The levels/effects of Bleomycin may be decreased by: Echinacea

Increased Effect/Toxicity

Bleomycin may increase the levels/effects of: Leflunomide; Natalizumab; Vaccines (Live)

The levels/effects of Bleomycin may be increased by: Brentuximab Vedotin; Denosumab; Filgrastim; Gemcitabine; Pimecrolimus; Roflumilast; Sargramostim; Tacrolimus (Topical); Trastuzumab

Adverse Reactions

>10%:

Dermatologic: Pain at the tumor site, phlebitis. About 50% of patients develop erythema, rash, striae, induration, hyperkeratosis, vesiculation, and peeling of the skin, particularly on the palmar and plantar surfaces of the hands and feet. Hyperpigmentation (50%), alopecia, nailbed changes may also occur. These effects appear dose related and reversible with discontinuation.

Gastrointestinal: Stomatitis and mucositis (30%), anorexia, weight loss

Respiratory: Tachypnea, rales, acute or chronic interstitial pneumonitis, and pulmonary fibrosis (5% to 10%); hypoxia and death (1%). Symptoms include cough, dyspnea, and bilateral pulmonary infiltrates. The pathogenesis is not certain, but may be due to damage of pulmonary, vascular, or connective tissue. Response to steroid therapy is variable and somewhat controversial.

Miscellaneous: Acute febrile reactions (25% to 50%)

1% to 10%:

Dermatologic: Skin thickening, diffuse scleroderma, onycholysis, pruritus

Miscellaneous: Anaphylactoid-like reactions (characterized by hypotension, confusion, fever, chills, and wheezing; onset may be immediate or delayed for several hours); idiosyncratic reactions (1% in lymphoma patients)

Available Dosage Forms

Injection, powder for reconstitution: 15 units, 30 units

General Dosage Range Dosage adjustment recommended in patients with renal impairment

I.V.: *Adults:* Dosage varies greatly depending on indication

Intrapleural: *Adults:* 60 units as a single instillation

Administration

I.M. May cause pain at injection site.

I.V. I.V. doses should be administered slowly over 10 minutes.

I.V. Detail pH: 4-6 (reconstituted solution, varies depending on diluent)

Other

Intrapleural: 60 units in 50-100 mL NS; use of topical anesthetics or narcotic analgesia is usually not necessary

SubQ: May cause pain at injection site.

Stability

Reconstitution For I.V. use, reconstitute 15-unit vial with 5 mL with NS and the 30-unit vial with 10 mL NS; for I.M. or SubQ use, reconstitute 15-unit vial with 1-5 mL of SWFI, BWFI, or NS and the 30-unit vial with 2-10 mL of SWFI, BWFI, or NS. For intrapleural use, mix in 50-100 mL of NS. Use appropriate precautions for handling and disposal.

Storage Refrigerate intact vials of powder. Intact vials are stable for up to 4 weeks at room temperature. Solutions reconstituted in NS for are stable for up to 28 days refrigerated and 14 days at room temperature; however, the manufacturer recommends stability of 24 hours in NS at room temperature.

Nursing Actions

Physical Assessment Monitor pulmonary status for fine rales prior to each treatment (may be the first symptom of pulmonary toxicity) and notify physician of any changes. Lymphoma patients should be closely monitored (vital signs every 15 minutes) for 1 hour following test dose before remainder of dose is administered (for first and second dose). Infusion or injection site must be monitored closely to avoid extravasation. Monitor pulmonary, renal, and hepatic function regularly during therapy.

Patient Education This medication can only be administered by injection or infusion; report immediately any redness, burning, pain, or swelling at injection/infusion site. May cause loss of appetite, nausea, or vomiting; mouth sores; fever or chills (will usually resolve); rash, redness, peeling, or increased color of skin; or loss of hair (reversible after cessation of therapy). Report any change in respiratory status; respiratory difficulty; wheezing; air hunger; increased secretions; difficulty expectorating secretions; confusion; unresolved fever or chills; sores in mouth; vaginal itching, burning, or discharge; sudden onset of dizziness; acute headache; or burning, stinging, redness, or swelling at injection site.

Related Information
Management of Drug Extravasations *on page 1269*

Boceprevir (boe SE pre vir)

Brand Names: U.S. Victrelis™

Index Terms SCH503034

Pharmacologic Category Antiviral Agent; Protease Inhibitor

Medication Guide Available Yes

Pregnancy Risk Factor B / X (in combination with ribavirin)

Lactation Excretion in breast milk unknown/not recommended

Breast-Feeding Considerations It is not known if boceprevir or ribavirin are excreted into breast milk. Breast-feeding is not linked to the spread of hepatitis C virus; however, if nipples are cracked or bleeding, breast-feeding is not recommended.

Use Treatment of chronic hepatitis C (CHC) genotype 1 (in combination with peginterferon alfa and ribavirin) in adult patients with compensated liver disease (including cirrhosis) who were previously untreated or have failed prior therapy with peginterferon alfa and ribavirin therapy

Mechanism of Action/Effect Inhibits viral protein synthesis; direct-acting antiviral against the hepatitis C virus

Contraindications Hypersensitivity to boceprevir or any component of the formulation; pregnancy; male partners of pregnant women

Coadministration with CYP 3A4/5 highly-dependent substrates (alfuzosin, cisapride, drospirenone, ergot derivatives, lovastatin, midazolam [oral], pimozide, sildenafil/tadalafil [when used for treatment of pulmonary arterial hypertension], simvastatin, triazolam) or strong CYP 3A4/5 inducers (carbamazepine, phenobarbital, phenytoin, rifampin, St John's wort)

Refer to Peginterferon Alfa and Ribavirin monographs for individual product contraindications.

Canadian labeling: Additional contraindications (not in U.S. labeling): Autoimmune hepatitis, hepatic decompensation (Child-Pugh class B or C)

Warnings/Precautions Avoid pregnancy in female patients and female partners of male patients, during therapy, and for at least 6 months after treatment; two forms of contraception should be used. Safety and efficacy have not been established in patients who have uncompensated cirrhosis, received organ transplants, or been coinfected with hepatitis B or HIV. Monotherapy is not effective for chronic hepatitis C infection. Safety and efficacy have not been established in patients documented to have less than a 2-$\log_{10}$ HCV-RNA decline by treatment week 12 with prior peginterferon alfa and ribavirin therapy. Patients who have less than 0.5-$\log_{10}$ HCV-RNA decline at treatment week 4 with peginterferon alfa and ribavirin when **initiating** boceprevir therapy are predicted to have less than a 2-$\log_{10}$ HCV-RNA decline by treatment week 12. Those poor responders treated with boceprevir will likely not have a sustained virologic response and have a predisposition to viral resistance at treatment failure.

Anemia has been reported with peginterferon alfa and ribavirin; addition of boceprevir is associated with further hemoglobin decreases. With anemia management, average hemoglobin decrease in clinical trials was ~1 g/dL. The addition of boceprevir to peginterferon alfa and ribavirin therapy is also associated with a higher incidence of neutropenia. Dose modifications of peginterferon alfa and ribavirin were needed more often in patients also taking boceprevir. Complete blood counts should be obtained pretreatment and at weeks 4, 8, and 12, as well as other times during treatment. May be severe or life-threatening (rare); discontinuation of therapy may be necessary.

Drug Interactions

Avoid Concomitant Use

Avoid concomitant use of Boceprevir with any of the following: Alfuzosin; Axitinib; CarBAMazepine; Cisapride; Conivaptan; Crizotinib; Dihydroergotamine; Dronedarone; Drospirenone; Efavirenz; Eplerenone; Ergotamine; Everolimus; Fluticasone (Oral Inhalation); Fosphenytoin; Halofantrine; Lapatinib; Lovastatin; Lurasidone; Methylergonovine; Midazolam; Nilotinib; Nisoldipine; PHENobarbital; Phenytoin; Pimozide; Primidone; Ranolazine; Rifabutin; Rifampin; Rivaroxaban; RomiDEPsin; Salmeterol; Sildenafil; Silodosin; Simvastatin; St Johns Wort; Tadalafil; Tamsulosin; Ticagrelor; Tolvaptan; Toremifene; Triazolam

Decreased Effect

Boceprevir may decrease the levels/effects of: Buprenorphine; Contraceptives (Estrogens); Methadone; Prasugrel; Protease Inhibitors; Ritonavir; Ticagrelor; Warfarin

The levels/effects of Boceprevir may be decreased by: CarBAMazepine; CYP3A4 Inducers (Strong); Deferasirox; Efavirenz; Fosphenytoin; PHENobarbital; Phenytoin; Primidone; Protease Inhibitors; Rifabutin; Rifampin; Ritonavir; St Johns Wort; Tocilizumab

Increased Effect/Toxicity

Boceprevir may increase the levels/effects of: Alfuzosin; Almotriptan; Alosetron; ALPRAZolam; Amiodarone; ARIPiprazole; Atorvastatin; Axitinib; Bepridil [Off Market]; Bortezomib; Brentuximab Vedotin; Brinzolamide; Budesonide (Nasal); Budesonide (Systemic, Oral Inhalation); Buprenorphine; Ciclesonide; Cisapride; Colchicine; Conivaptan; Contraceptives (Progestins); Corticosteroids (Orally Inhaled); Crizotinib; CYP3A4 Substrates; Desipramine; Dienogest; Digoxin; Dihydroergotamine; Dronedarone; Drospirenone;

Dutasteride; Efavirenz; Eplerenone; Ergotamine; Everolimus; FentaNYL; Fesoterodine; Flecainide; Fluticasone (Nasal); Fluticasone (Oral Inhalation); GuanFACINE; Halofantrine; Iloperidone; Itraconazole; Ivacaftor; Ixabepilone; Ketoconazole; Ketoconazole (Systemic); Lapatinib; Lovastatin; Lumefantrine; Lurasidone; Maraviroc; Methadone; Methylergonovine; MethylPREDNISolone; Midazolam; Nilotinib; Nisoldipine; Paricalcitol; Pazopanib; Pimecrolimus; Pimozide; Posaconazole; Propafenone; QuiNIDine; Ranolazine; Rifabutin; Rivaroxaban; RomiDEPsin; Ruxolitinib; Salmeterol; Saxagliptin; Sildenafil; Silodosin; Simvastatin; SORAfenib; Tadalafil; Tamsulosin; Ticagrelor; Tolterodine; Tolvaptan; Toremifene; Triazolam; Vardenafil; Vemurafenib; Vilazodone; Voriconazole; Warfarin; Zuclopenthixol

The levels/effects of Boceprevir may be increased by: Itraconazole; Ketoconazole; Ketoconazole (Systemic); Posaconazole; Voriconazole

Adverse Reactions

>10%:

Central nervous system: Fatigue (55% to 58%), chills (33% to 34%), insomnia (30% to 34%), irritability (21% to 22%), dizziness (16% to 19%), headache

Dermatologic: Alopecia (22% to 27%), dry skin (18% to 22%), rash (16% to 17%)

Gastrointestinal: Nausea (43% to 46%), abnormal taste (35% to 44%), appetite decreased (25% to 26%), diarrhea (24% to 25%), vomiting (15% to 20%), xerostomia (11% to 15%)

Hematologic: Anemia (45% to 50%), neutropenia (14% to 31%)

Neuromuscular & skeletal: Arthralgia (19% to 23%), weakness (15% to 21%)

Respiratory: Dyspnea (8% to 11%)

1% to 10%: Hematologic: Thrombocytopenia

Available Dosage Forms

Capsule, oral:

Victrelis™: 200 mg

General Dosage Range Oral: *Adults:* 800 mg 3 times/day

Administration

Oral Administer with food. Doses should be taken approximately every 7-9 hours. Administer concurrently with peginterferon alfa and ribavirin.

Stability

Storage Store refrigerated at 2°C to 8°C (36°F to 46°F). After dispensing, may be stored at room temperature of up to 25°C (77°F) for 3 months; keep container closed tightly; avoid excessive heat.

Dietary Considerations Take with food. The type or timing of a meal is not important as long as dose is taken with food.

Bortezomib (bore TEZ oh mib)

Brand Names: U.S. Velcade®

Index Terms LDP-341; MLN341; PS-341

Pharmacologic Category Antineoplastic Agent; Proteasome Inhibitor

Medication Safety Issues

High alert medication:

This medication is in a class the Institute for Safe Medication Practices (ISMP) includes among its list of drug classes which have a heightened risk of causing significant patient harm when used in error.

Administration issues:

The reconstituted concentrations for I.V. and SubQ administration are different; use caution when calculating the volume for each dose. The manufacturer provides stickers to facilitate identification of the concentration/route for reconstituted vials.

For I.V. or SubQ administration only. Inadvertent intrathecal administration has resulted in death and is contraindicated. Bortezomib should **NOT** be prepared during the preparation of any intrathecal medications and should **NOT** be delivered to the patient at the same time with any medications intended for intrathecal administration.

Pregnancy Risk Factor D

Lactation Excretion in breast milk unknown/not recommended

Use Treatment of multiple myeloma; treatment of relapsed or refractory mantle cell lymphoma

Unlabeled Use Treatment of cutaneous T-Cell lymphomas (mycosis fungoides), peripheral T-cell lymphoma, systemic light-chain amyloidosis, Waldenström's macroglobulinemia

Available Dosage Forms

Injection, powder for reconstitution:

Velcade®: 3.5 mg

General Dosage Range Dosage adjustment recommended in patients with hepatic impairment or who develop toxicities.

I.V., SubQ: *Adults:* Dosage varies greatly depending on indication

Administration

I.V.

Note: The reconstituted concentrations for I.V. and SubQ administration are different; use caution when calculating the volume for each dose. Consider SubQ administration in patients with pre-existing or at high risk for peripheral neuropathy.

Administer via rapid I.V. push (3-5 seconds).

I.V. Detail pH: 2-6.5

Other Note: The reconstituted concentrations for I.V. and SubQ administration are different; use caution when calculating the volume for each dose.

SubQ: Subcutaneous administration of bortezomib 1.3 mg/m^2 days 1, 4, 8, and 11 of a 21-day treatment cycle has been studied in a limited number of patients with relapsed multiple myeloma; doses were administered subcutaneously (concentration of 2.5 mg/mL) into the thigh or abdomen, rotating the injection site with each dose; injections at the same site within a single cycle were avoided (Moreau, 2010; Moreau, 2011). Response rates were similar to I.V. administration; decreased incidence of grade 3 or higher adverse events were observed with SubQ administration. If injection site reaction occurs, the more dilute 1 mg/mL concentration may be used subQ (or I.V. administration of the 1 mg/mL concentration may be considered).

Nursing Actions

Physical Assessment Monitor for peripheral neuropathy, postural hypotension, dehydration, heart failure, and infections. Be alert to the potential for reactivation of herpes.

Patient Education Avoid grapefruit juice, green tea, and ascorbic acid supplements. This medication can be administered intravenously or subcutaneously; you will be monitored during and following infusion. Maintain adequate hydration, unless instructed to restrict fluid intake. If you have diabetes, monitor blood sugars closely; may cause alterations in glycemic control. May cause headache, dizziness, anxiety, sleep disturbances, fever, fatigue, nausea, vomiting, loss of appetite, abnormal taste, constipation, or diarrhea. You may be more susceptible to infection. Report immediately any chest pain, respiratory difficulty, itching, rash, acute headache, throat tightness, pain, redness, or swelling at infusion site. Report swelling in extremities; weight gain; persistent headache; muscle, bone, or back pain; abdominal pain; cramping or loss of sensation or tingling of extremities; unusual bleeding; or changes in vision.

Related Information

Management of Drug Extravasations *on page 1269*

Brentuximab Vedotin

(bren TUX i mab ve DOE tin)

Brand Names: U.S. Adcetris™

Index Terms Anti-CD30 ADC SGN-35; Anti-CD30 Antibody-Drug Conjugate SGN-35; Antibody-Drug Conjugate SGN-35; Brentuximab; SGN-35

Pharmacologic Category Antineoplastic Agent, Monoclonal Antibody

Medication Safety Issues

Sound-alike/look-alike issues:

Brentuximab may be confused with bendamustine, bevacizumab, rituximab

High alert medication:

This medication is in a class the Institute for Safe Medication Practices (ISMP) includes among its list of drug classes which have a heightened risk of causing significant patient harm when used in error.

Pregnancy Risk Factor D

Lactation Excretion in breast milk unknown/not recommended

Use Treatment of Hodgkin lymphoma after failure of at least 2 prior chemotherapy regimens (in patients ineligible for transplant) or after stem cell transplant failure; treatment of systemic anaplastic large cell lymphoma (sALCL) after failure of at least 1 prior chemotherapy regimen

Available Dosage Forms

Injection, powder for reconstitution:

Adcetris™: 50 mg

General Dosage Range Dosage adjustment recommended in patients who develop toxicities.

I.V.: *Adults:* 1.8 mg/kg every 3 weeks (maximum dose: 180 mg)

Administration

I.V. Infuse over 30 minutes. Do not administer as I.V. push or bolus.

I.V. Detail pH: 6.6

Nursing Actions

Physical Assessment Medication is given as an infusion. Inform physician of existing neuropathy or past infusion-related reaction. Monitor for symptoms of new or progressive neuropathy, or symptoms of infection due to neutropenia. Assess patients for changes in mental status or vision or balance problems, which could be symptoms of a rare but fatal encephalopathy (PML, a viral brain infection) and has occurred in patients who have received four or more regimens of chemotherapy.

Patient Education Instruct patients that their immune system may be weakened by this medication, and any symptoms such as cold, fevers, sore throat, rash, or chills should be reported to their doctor. In addition, patients should avoid large crowds and maintain good hand washing when their immune system is decreased. Inform patients that they may experience a hypersensitivity reaction during the infusion or up to 24 hours afterward. Symptoms of this include shortness of breath, chills, cough, itching, nausea, fever, or rash and need to be reported. Common side effects include arthralgias, myalgias, headaches, decreased appetite, nausea, constipation, and diarrhea. Patients need to understand serious side effects to report immediately include decreased urination, muscle weakness, sluggishness, chest pain, hemoptysis or other bleeding, worsening neuropathy, confusion, or changes in thought process, eyesight, or balance. Patients may need to have blood counts monitored to evaluate if they are at risk for bleeding or infections.

Brimonidine (bri MOE ni deen)

Brand Names: U.S. Alphagan® P

Index Terms Brimonidine Tartrate

Pharmacologic Category $Alpha_2$ Agonist, Ophthalmic; Ophthalmic Agent, Antiglaucoma

Medication Safety Issues

Sound-alike/look-alike issues:

Brimonidine may be confused with bromocriptine

Pregnancy Risk Factor B

Lactation Excretion in breast milk unknown/not recommended

Use Lowering of intraocular pressure (IOP) in patients with open-angle glaucoma or ocular hypertension

Available Dosage Forms

Solution, ophthalmic: 0.15% (5 mL, 10 mL, 15 mL); 0.2% (5 mL, 10 mL, 15 mL)

Alphagan® P: 0.1% (5 mL, 10 mL, 15 mL); 0.15% (5 mL, 10 mL, 15 mL)

General Dosage Range Ophthalmic: *Children ≥2 years and Adults:* Instill 1 drop in affected eye(s) 3 times/day

Administration

Other Remove contact lenses prior to administration; wait 15 minutes before reinserting if using products containing benzalkonium chloride. Separate administration of other ophthalmic agents by 5 minutes.

Nursing Actions

Patient Education For use in eyes only. Wash hands before instilling. Remove contacts prior to administration and wait 15 minutes before reinserting. Sit or lie down to instill. Open eye, look at ceiling, and instill prescribed amount of solution. Apply gentle pressure to inner corner of eye. Do not let tip of applicator touch eyes; do not contaminate tip of applicator (may cause eye infection, eye damage, or vision loss). Brimonidine tartrate may cause fatigue or drowsiness in some patients. Avoid engaging in hazardous activities due to potential for decreased mental alertness until response known. Wait at least 15 minutes after instilling brimonidine tartrate before reinserting soft contact lenses.

Brinzolamide (brin ZOH la mide)

Brand Names: U.S. Azopt®

Pharmacologic Category Carbonic Anhydrase Inhibitor; Ophthalmic Agent, Antiglaucoma

Pregnancy Risk Factor C

Lactation Excretion in breast milk unknown/not recommended

Use Treatment of elevated intraocular pressure in patients with ocular hypertension or open-angle glaucoma

Available Dosage Forms

Suspension, ophthalmic:

Azopt®: 1% (10 mL, 15 mL)

General Dosage Range Ophthalmic: *Adults:* Instill 1 drop in affected eye(s) 3 times/day

Administration

Other Remove contact lenses prior to administration; wait 15 minutes before reinserting. If more than one topical ophthalmic drug is being used, administer drugs at least 10 minutes apart. Shake well before use.

Nursing Actions

Patient Education For use in eyes only. Tilt head back, place medication in conjunctival sac, and close eyes. Apply finger pressure at corner of eye for 1 minute following application. Do not let tip of applicator touch eye; do not contaminate tip of applicator (may cause eye infection, eye damage, or vision loss). If using other ophthalmic preparations, administer 10 minutes apart. May cause taste changes, runny nose, or vision changes (blurred vision, dry eye, foreign body sensation, eye discharge, temporary sensitivity to bright light, blurring or stinging). Report skin rash or eye pain.

Bromfenac (BROME fen ak)

Brand Names: U.S. Bromday™

Index Terms Bromfenac Sodium

Pharmacologic Category Nonsteroidal Anti-inflammatory Drug (NSAID), Ophthalmic

Pregnancy Risk Factor C

Lactation Excretion in breast milk unknown/use caution

Use Treatment of postoperative inflammation and reduction in ocular pain following cataract removal

Available Dosage Forms

Solution, ophthalmic: 0.09% (2.5 mL)

Bromday™: 0.09% (1.7 mL)

General Dosage Range Ophthalmic: *Adults:* Bromday™: Instill 1 drop into affected eye(s) once daily

Xibrom®: Instill 1 drop into affected eye(s) twice daily

Administration

Other Remove contact lenses prior to administration and wait 15 minutes before reinserting.

Bromday™: May be used with other eye drops. If using more than 1 ophthalmic product, wait at least 5 minutes between application of each medication.

Nursing Actions

Physical Assessment Assess for intraocular bleeding. Evaluate allergy history with aspirin or other NSAIDs.

Patient Education Do not wear contact lenses while using this medication. Report any abnormal sensation in eye, redness, severe headache, or pain.

Bromocriptine (broe moe KRIP teen)

Brand Names: U.S. Cycloset®; Parlodel®; Parlodel® SnapTabs®

Index Terms Bromocriptine Mesylate; Cycloset®

Pharmacologic Category Anti-Parkinson's Agent, Dopamine Agonist; Antidiabetic Agent, Dopamine Agonist; Ergot Derivative

Medication Safety Issues

Sound-alike/look-alike issues:

Bromocriptine may be confused with benztropine, brimonidine

Cycloset® may be confused with Glyset®

Parlodel® may be confused with pindolol, Provera®

Pregnancy Risk Factor B

Lactation Enters breast milk/contraindicated

Breast-Feeding Considerations A previous indication for prevention of postpartum lactation was withdrawn voluntarily by the manufacturer following reports of serious adverse reactions, including stroke, MI, seizures, and severe hypertension. Use during breast-feeding is specifically contraindicated in the product labeling for Cycloset®. Use in postpartum women with a history of coronary artery disease or other severe cardiovascular conditions is specifically contraindicated in the product labeling for Parlodel® (unless withdrawal of medication is medically contraindicated). Based on the risk/benefit assessment, other treatments should be considered for lactation suppression.

Use Treatment of hyperprolactinemia associated with amenorrhea with or without galactorrhea, infertility, or hypogonadism; treatment of prolactin-secreting adenomas; treatment of acromegaly; treatment of Parkinson's disease

Cycloset®: Management of type 2 diabetes mellitus (noninsulin dependent, NIDDM) as an adjunct to diet and exercise

Unlabeled Use Neuroleptic malignant syndrome

Mechanism of Action/Effect Semisynthetic ergot alkaloid derivative and a dopamine receptor agonist which activates postsynaptic dopamine receptors to decrease prolactin secretion (tuberoinfundibular pathway) and enhance coordinated motor control (nigrostriatal pathways).

In the treatment type 2 diabetes mellitus, bromocriptine's effect on improving glycemic control is unknown; however, when administered during the morning and released into the systemic circulation in a rapid, 'pulse-like' dose, it is believed to affect circadian rhythms thought to play a role in obesity and insulin resistance.

Contraindications Hypersensitivity to bromocriptine, ergot alkaloids, or any component of the formulation

Additional contraindications:

Parlodel®: Uncontrolled hypertension; pregnancy (risk to benefit evaluation must be performed in women who become pregnant during treatment for acromegaly, prolactinoma, or Parkinson's disease - hypertension during treatment should generally result in efforts to withdraw); postpartum women with a history of coronary artery disease or other severe cardiovascular conditions (unless withdrawal of medication is medically contraindicated)

Cycloset®: Syncopal migraine; breast-feeding

Warnings/Precautions Complete evaluation of pituitary function should be completed prior to initiation of treatment of any hyperprolactinemia-associated dysfunction. Use caution in patients with a history of peptic ulcer disease, dementia, or cardiovascular disease (myocardial infarction, arrhythmia). Use with extreme caution or avoid in patients with psychosis. Symptomatic hypotension may occur in a significant number of patients. In addition, hypertension, seizures, MI, and stroke have been rarely associated with bromocriptine therapy. Severe headache or visual changes may precede events. The onset of reactions may be immediate or delayed (often may occur in the second week of therapy). Sudden sleep onset and somnolence have been reported with use, primarily in patients with Parkinson's disease. Patients must be cautioned about performing tasks which require mental alertness.

Use with caution in patients taking strong CYP3A4 inhibitors and/or major CYP3A4 substrates (includes protease inhibitors, azole antifungals, and some macrolide antibiotics); consider alternative agents that avoid or lessen the potential for CYP-mediated interactions. Concurrent antihypertensives or drugs which may alter blood pressure should be used with caution. Concurrent use with levodopa has been associated with an increased risk of hallucinations. Consider dosage reduction and/or discontinuation in patients with hallucinations. Hallucinations may require weeks to months before resolution.

Dopamine agonists have been associated with compulsive behaviors and/or loss of impulse control, which has manifested as pathological gambling, libido increases (hypersexuality), and/or binge eating. Causality has not been established, and controversy exists as to whether this phenomenon is related to the underlying disease, prior behaviors/addictions and/or drug therapy. Dose reduction or discontinuation of therapy has been reported to reverse these behaviors in some, but not all cases. Risk for melanoma development is increased in Parkinson's disease patients; drug causation or factors contributing to risk have not been established. Patients should be monitored closely and periodic skin examinations should be performed.

In the treatment of acromegaly, discontinuation is recommended if tumor expansion occurs during therapy. Digital vasospasm (cold sensitive) may occur in some patients with acromegaly; may require dosage reduction. Patients who receive bromocriptine during and immediately following pregnancy as a continuation of previous therapy (eg, acromegaly) should be closely monitored for cardiovascular effects. Should not be used postpartum in women with coronary artery disease or other cardiovascular disease. Use of bromocriptine to control or prevent lactation or in patients with uncontrolled hypertension is not recommended.

Monitoring and careful evaluation of visual changes during the treatment of hyperprolactinemia is recommended to differentiate between tumor shrinkage and traction on the optic chiasm; rapidly progressing visual field loss requires neurosurgical consultation. Discontinuation of bromocriptine in patients with macroadenomas has been associated with rapid regrowth of tumor and increased prolactin serum levels. Pleural and retroperitoneal fibrosis have been reported with prolonged daily use. Cardiac valvular fibrosis has also been associated with ergot alkaloids.

In the management of type 2 diabetes mellitus, Cycloset® ("quick-release" tablet) should not be interchanged with any other bromocriptine product due to formulation differences and resulting pharmacokinetics. Therapy is not appropriate in patients with diabetic ketoacidosis (DKA) or type 1 diabetes mellitus due to lack of efficacy in these patient populations. There is limited efficacy of use in combination with thiazolidinediones or in combination with insulin. Combination therapy with other hypoglycemic agents may increase risk for hypoglycemic events; dose reduction of concomitant hypoglycemics may be warranted.

Safety and efficacy have not been established in patients with hepatic or renal dysfunction. Safety and effectiveness in patients <11 years of age (for pituitary adenoma) have not been established. Safety has not been established for use >2 years in patients with Parkinson's disease.

Drug Interactions

Avoid Concomitant Use

Avoid concomitant use of Bromocriptine with any of the following: Alpha-/Beta-Agonists; Alpha1-Agonists; Conivaptan; Efavirenz; Itraconazole; Nitroglycerin; Posaconazole; Protease Inhibitors; Serotonin 5-HT1D Receptor Agonists; Voriconazole

Decreased Effect

Bromocriptine may decrease the levels/effects of: Antipsychotics (Typical); Nitroglycerin

The levels/effects of Bromocriptine may be decreased by: Antipsychotics (Atypical); Metoclopramide; Tocilizumab

Increased Effect/Toxicity

Bromocriptine may increase the levels/effects of: Alcohol (Ethyl); Alpha-/Beta-Agonists; Alpha1-Agonists; CycloSPORINE; CycloSPORINE (Systemic); Metoclopramide; Serotonin 5-HT1D Receptor Agonists; Serotonin Modulators

The levels/effects of Bromocriptine may be increased by: Alcohol (Ethyl); Alpha-/Beta-Agonists; Antipsychotics; Antipsychotics (Typical); Conivaptan; CYP3A4 Inhibitors (Moderate); CYP3A4 Inhibitors (Strong); Dasatinib; Efavirenz; Itraconazole; Ivacaftor; Macrolide Antibiotics; MAO Inhibitors; Methylphenidate; Nitroglycerin; Posaconazole; Protease Inhibitors; Serotonin 5-HT1D Receptor Agonists; Voriconazole

Nutritional/Ethanol Interactions

Ethanol: Avoid ethanol (may increase GI side effects or ethanol intolerance).

Herb/Nutraceutical: St John's wort may decrease bromocriptine levels.

Adverse Reactions Note: Frequency of adverse effects may vary by dose and/or indication.

>10%:

- Central nervous system: Dizziness, fatigue, headache
- Gastrointestinal: Constipation, nausea
- Neuromuscular & skeletal: Weakness
- Respiratory: Rhinitis

1% to 10%:

- Cardiovascular: Hypotension (including postural/orthostatic), Raynaud's syndrome exacerbation, syncope
- Central nervous system: Drowsiness, lightheadedness, somnolence
- Endocrine & metabolic: Hypoglycemia (4%; in combination with sulfonylureas or other antidiabetic agents: 7% to 9%)
- Gastrointestinal: Abdominal cramps, anorexia, diarrhea, dyspepsia, GI bleeding, vomiting, xerostomia
- Neuromuscular & skeletal: Digital vasospasm
- Ocular: Amblyopia
- Respiratory: Nasal congestion, sinusitis
- Miscellaneous: Infection, flu-like syndrome

Pharmacodynamics/Kinetics

Onset of Action Parlodel®: Prolactin decreasing effect: 1-2 hours

Available Dosage Forms

Capsule, oral: 5 mg

Parlodel®: 5 mg

Tablet, oral: 2.5 mg

Cycloset®: 0.8 mg

Parlodel® SnapTabs®: 2.5 mg

General Dosage Range Oral:

Children 11-15 years: Initial: 1.25-2.5 mg daily; Maintenance: 2.5-10 mg/day

Children ≥16 years: Initial: 1.25-2.5 mg daily; Maintenance: 2.5-15 mg/day

Adults: Dosage varies greatly depending on indication

Administration

Oral Administer with food to decrease GI distress.

Cycloset®: Administer within 2 hours of waking in the morning.

Stability

Storage Store at or below 25°C (77°F).

Nursing Actions

Physical Assessment Monitor blood pressure at beginning of therapy and periodically during course of treatment.

Patient Education May be prescribed in conjunction with levodopa/carbidopa. Therapeutic effects may take several weeks or months to achieve and you may need frequent monitoring during first weeks of therapy. Take with meals if GI upset occurs. Take at the same time each day. Maintain adequate hydration, unless instructed to restrict fluid intake. Do not use alcohol. Urine or perspiration may appear darker. You may experience drowsiness (can be sudden onset), dizziness, confusion, vision changes, loss of impulse control (possibly manifested as pathological gambling, libido increases, and/or binge eating), orthostatic hypotension, constipation, nasal congestion, nausea, vomiting, loss of appetite, or stomach discomfort. Report unresolved constipation or vomiting; chest pain or irregular heartbeat; acute headache or dizziness; CNS changes (eg, hallucination, loss of memory, seizures, acute headache, nervousness); suicide ideation; painful or difficult urination; increased muscle spasticity, rigidity, or involuntary movements; changes in the appearance of skin moles, skin rash, or other unusual skin changes; or significant worsening of condition.

Dietary Considerations Should be taken with food to decrease GI distress.

Brompheniramine (brome fen IR a meen)

Brand Names: U.S. Bromax [DSC]; LoHist-12 [DSC]

Index Terms Brompheniramine Maleate; Brompheniramine Tannate

Pharmacologic Category Alkylamine Derivative; Histamine H_1 Antagonist; Histamine H_1 Antagonist, First Generation

Pregnancy Risk Factor C

Lactation Excretion in breast milk unknown/not recommended

Use Symptomatic relief of perennial and seasonal allergic rhinitis, vasomotor rhinitis, and other respiratory allergies

General Dosage Range Oral:

Children 6-12 years: LoHist-12: One tablet every 12 hours (maximum: 2 tablets/day)

Children >12 years and Adults:

Bromax: One tablet twice daily

LoHist-12: 1-2 tablets every 12 hours (maximum: 4 tablets/day)

Administration

Oral Extended release tablets are to be swallowed whole; do not crush or chew.

Nursing Actions

Patient Education Follow dosing guidelines closely; measure dosage carefully, especially in pediatric patients. Avoid alcohol. You may experience drowsiness or dizziness. Report persistent sedation, confusion, agitation, blurred vision, or respiratory difficulty.

Budesonide (Systemic, Oral Inhalation) (byoo DES oh nide)

Brand Names: U.S. Entocort® EC; Pulmicort Flexhaler®; Pulmicort Respules®

Pharmacologic Category Corticosteroid, Inhalant (Oral); Corticosteroid, Systemic

Pregnancy Risk Factor C (capsule)/B (inhalation)

Lactation Enters breast milk/use caution

Breast-Feeding Considerations Following use of the powder for oral inhalation, ~0.3% to 1% of the maternal dose was found in breast milk. The maximum concentration appeared within 45 minutes of dosing. Plasma budesonide levels obtained from infants ~90 minutes after breast-feeding (~140 minutes after maternal dose) were below the limit of quantification. Concentrations of budesonide in breast milk are expected to be higher following administration of oral capsules than after an inhaled dose. The use of inhaled corticosteroids is not considered a contraindication to breast-feeding (NAEPP, 2005).

Use

Nebulization: Maintenance and prophylactic treatment of asthma

Oral capsule: Treatment of active Crohn's disease (mild-to-moderate) involving the ileum and/or ascending colon; maintenance of remission (for up to 3 months) of Crohn's disease (mild-to-moderate) involving the ileum and/or ascending colon

Oral inhalation: Maintenance and prophylactic treatment of asthma; includes patients who require oral corticosteroids and those who may benefit from systemic dose reduction/elimination

Mechanism of Action/Effect Anti-inflammatory corticosteroid

Contraindications Hypersensitivity to budesonide or any component of the formulation; primary treatment of status asthmaticus, acute episodes of asthma; not for relief of acute bronchospasm

Canadian labeling: Additional contraindications (not in U.S. labeling): Moderate-to-severe bronchiectasis, pulmonary tuberculosis (active or quiescent), untreated respiratory infection (bacterial, fungal, or viral)

Warnings/Precautions May cause hypercorticism or suppression of hypothalamic-pituitary-adrenal (HPA) axis, particularly in younger children or in patients receiving high doses for prolonged periods. HPA axis suppression may lead to adrenal crisis. Withdrawal and discontinuation of a corticosteroid should be done slowly and carefully. Particular care is required when patients are transferred from systemic corticosteroids to inhaled products due to possible adrenal insufficiency or withdrawal ▶

from steroids, including an increase in allergic symptoms. Patients receiving >20 mg per day of prednisone (or equivalent) may be most susceptible. Fatalities have occurred due to adrenal insufficiency in asthmatic patients during and after transfer from systemic corticosteroids to aerosol steroids; aerosol steroids do not provide the systemic steroid needed to treat patients having trauma, surgery, or infections. Do not use this product to transfer patients directly from oral corticosteroid therapy.

Bronchospasm may occur with wheezing after inhalation; if this occurs stop steroid and treat with a fast-acting bronchodilator (eg, albuterol). Supplemental steroids (oral or parenteral) may be needed during stress or severe asthma attacks. Not to be used in status asthmaticus or for the relief of acute bronchospasm. Acute myopathy has been reported with high-dose corticosteroids, usually in patients with neuromuscular transmission disorders; may involve ocular and/or respiratory muscles; monitor creatine kinase; recovery may be delayed. Corticosteroid use may cause psychiatric disturbances, including depression, euphoria, insomnia, mood swings, and personality changes. Pre-existing psychiatric conditions may be exacerbated by corticosteroid use. Prolonged use of corticosteroids may also increase the incidence of secondary infection, mask acute infection (including fungal infections), prolong or exacerbate viral infections, or limit response to vaccines. Exposure to chickenpox should be avoided; corticosteroids should not be used to treat ocular herpes simplex. Corticosteroids should not be used for cerebral malaria or viral hepatitis. Close observation is required in patients with latent tuberculosis and/or TB reactivity; restrict use in active TB (only in conjunction with antituberculosis treatment). *Candida albicans* infections may occur in the mouth and pharynx; rinsing (and spitting) with water after inhaler use may decrease risk. Prolonged treatment with corticosteroids has been associated with the development of Kaposi's sarcoma (case reports); if noted, discontinuation of therapy should be considered.

Use with caution in patients with thyroid disease, hepatic impairment, renal impairment, cardiovascular disease, diabetes, glaucoma, cataracts, myasthenia gravis, patients at risk for osteoporosis, patients at risk for seizures, or GI diseases (diverticulitis, peptic ulcer, ulcerative colitis) due to perforation risk. Use caution following acute MI (corticosteroids have been associated with myocardial rupture). Because of the risk of adverse effects, systemic corticosteroids should be used cautiously in the elderly in the smallest possible effective dose for the shortest duration.

Orally-inhaled corticosteroids may cause a reduction in growth velocity in pediatric patients (~1 centimeter per year [range: 0.3-1.8 cm per year] and related to dose and duration of exposure). To minimize the systemic effects of orally-inhaled corticosteroids, each patient should be titrated to the lowest effective dose. Growth should be routinely monitored in pediatric patients. Withdraw systemic therapy with gradual tapering of dose. There have been reports of systemic corticosteroid withdrawal symptoms (eg, joint/muscle pain, lassitude, depression) when withdrawing oral inhalation therapy. Pulmicort Flexhaler™ contains lactose; very rare anaphylactic reactions have been reported in patients with severe milk protein allergy.

Drug Interactions

Avoid Concomitant Use

Avoid concomitant use of Budesonide (Systemic, Oral Inhalation) with any of the following: Aldesleukin; BCG; Grapefruit Juice; Natalizumab; Pimecrolimus; Tacrolimus (Topical)

Decreased Effect

Budesonide (Systemic, Oral Inhalation) may decrease the levels/effects of: Aldesleukin; Antidiabetic Agents; BCG; Coccidioidin Skin Test; Corticorelin; Sipuleucel-T; Telaprevir; Vaccines (Inactivated)

The levels/effects of Budesonide (Systemic, Oral Inhalation) may be decreased by: Antacids; Bile Acid Sequestrants; Echinacea; Tocilizumab

Increased Effect/Toxicity

Budesonide (Systemic, Oral Inhalation) may increase the levels/effects of: Amphotericin B; Deferasirox; Leflunomide; Loop Diuretics; Natalizumab; Thiazide Diuretics

The levels/effects of Budesonide (Systemic, Oral Inhalation) may be increased by: CYP3A4 Inhibitors (Moderate); CYP3A4 Inhibitors (Strong); Dasatinib; Denosumab; Grapefruit Juice; Ivacaftor; Pimecrolimus; Tacrolimus (Topical); Telaprevir; Trastuzumab

Nutritional/Ethanol Interactions

Food: Grapefruit juice may double systemic exposure of orally administered budesonide. Administration of capsules with a high-fat meal delays peak concentration, but does not alter the extent of absorption. Management: Avoid grapefruit juice when using oral capsules.

Herb/Nutraceutical: Echinacea may diminish the therapeutic effect of budesonide. Management: Avoid echinacea.

Adverse Reactions Reaction severity varies by dose and duration; not all adverse reactions have been reported with each dosage form.

>10%:

Central nervous system: Headache (≤21%)

Gastrointestinal: Nausea (≤11%)

Respiratory: Respiratory infection, rhinitis

Miscellaneous: Symptoms of HPA axis suppression and/or hypercorticism may occur in >10% of patients following administration of dosage forms which result in higher systemic exposure (ie, oral capsule), but may be less frequent than rates observed with comparator drugs (prednisolone). These symptoms may be rare (<1%) following administration via methods which result in lower exposures (topical).

1% to 10%:

Cardiovascular: Chest pain, edema, flushing, hypertension, palpitation, syncope, tachycardia

Central nervous system: Amnesia, dizziness, dysphonia, emotional lability, fatigue, fever, insomnia, malaise, migraine, nervousness, pain, sleep disorder, somnolence, vertigo

Dermatologic: Acne, alopecia, bruising, contact dermatitis, eczema, hirsutism, pruritus, pustular rash, rash, striae

Endocrine & metabolic: Adrenal insufficiency, hypokalemia, menstrual disorder

Gastrointestinal: Abdominal pain, anorexia, diarrhea, dyspepsia, flatulence, gastroenteritis (including viral), glossitis, intestinal obstruction, oral candidiasis, taste perversion, tongue edema, vomiting, weight gain, xerostomia

Genitourinary: Dysuria, hematuria, nocturia, pyuria

Hematologic: Cervical lymphadenopathy, leukocytosis, purpura

Hepatic: Alkaline phosphatase increased

Neuromuscular & skeletal: Arthralgia, back pain, fracture, hyperkinesis, hypertonia, myalgia, neck pain, paresthesia, weakness

Ocular: Conjunctivitis, eye infection

Otic: Earache, ear infection, external ear infection

Respiratory: Bronchitis, bronchospasm, cough, epistaxis, hoarseness, nasal congestion, nasal irritation, pharyngitis, sinusitis, stridor, throat irritation

Miscellaneous: Abscess, allergic reaction, C-reactive protein increased, erythrocyte sedimentation rate increased, fat distribution (moon face, buffalo hump); flu-like syndrome, herpes simplex, infection, moniliasis, viral infection, voice alteration

Pharmacodynamics/Kinetics

Onset of Action Pulmicort Respules®: 2-8 days; Inhalation: 24 hours

Peak effect: Pulmicort Respules®: 4-6 weeks; Inhalation: 1-2 weeks

Available Dosage Forms

Capsule, enteric coated, oral: 3 mg

Entocort® EC: 3 mg

Powder, for oral inhalation:

Pulmicort Flexhaler®: 90 mcg/inhalation (165 mg); 180 mcg/inhalation (225 mg)

Suspension, for nebulization: 0.25 mg/2 mL (30s); 0.5 mg/2 mL (30s)

Pulmicort Respules®: 0.25 mg/2 mL (30s); 0.5 mg/2 mL (30s); 1 mg/2 mL (30s)

General Dosage Range

Inhalation:

Children ≥6 years: Initial: 180-360 mcg twice daily; Maintenance: 180->800 mcg/day in 2 divided doses

Adults: Initial: 180-720 mcg twice daily; Maintenance: 180->1200 mcg/day in 2 divided doses

Nebulization: *Children 12 months to 8 years:* 0.25-1 mg in 1-2 divided doses

Oral: *Adults:* Initial: 9 mg once daily; Maintenance: 6 mg once daily

Administration

Oral Oral capsule: Capsule should be swallowed whole; do not crush or chew.

Inhalation

Powder for inhalation:

Pulmicort Flexhaler™: Hold inhaler in upright position (mouthpiece up) to load dose. Do not shake prior to use. Unit should be primed prior to first use only. It will not need primed again, even if not used for a long time. Place mouthpiece between lips and inhale forcefully and deeply. Do not exhale through inhaler; do not use a spacer. Dose indicator does not move with every dose, usually only after 5 doses. Discard when dose indicator reads "0". Rinse mouth with water after each use to reduce incidence of candidiasis.

Pulmicort Turbuhaler® [CAN, not available in the U.S.]: Hold inhaler in upright position (mouthpiece up) to load dose. Do not shake inhaler after dose is loaded. Unit should be primed prior to first use. Place mouthpiece between lips and inhale forcefully and deeply; mouthpiece should face up. Do not exhale through inhaler; do not use a spacer. When a red mark appears in the dose indicator window, 20 doses are left. When the red mark reaches the bottom of the window, the inhaler should be discarded. Rinse mouth with water after use to reduce incidence of candidiasis.

Suspension for nebulization: Shake well before using. Use Pulmicort Respules® with jet nebulizer connected to an air compressor; administer with mouthpiece or facemask. Do not use ultrasonic nebulizer. Do not mix with other medications in nebulizer. Rinse mouth following treatments to decrease risk of oral candidiasis (wash face if using face mask).

Stability

Storage

Suspension for nebulization: Store upright at 20°C to 25°C (68°F to 77°F). Protect from light. Do not refrigerate or freeze. Once aluminum package is opened, solution should be used within 2 weeks. Continue to protect from light.

Oral inhaler (Pulmicort Flexhaler™): Store at controlled room temperature of 20°C to 25°C (68°F to 77°F). Protect from moisture.

Nursing Actions

Physical Assessment When changing from systemic steroids to inhalational steroids, taper reduction of systemic medication slowly (may take several months). Growth should be routinely monitored in pediatric patients.

Patient Education May take 1-2 weeks or longer before full effects are seen. Avoid grapefruit juice while taking this medication. May be more susceptible to infection; avoid exposure to chickenpox and measles unless immunity has been established. If exposure to measles or chickenpox occurs, notify your prescriber immediately. Report acute nervousness or inability to sleep; respiratory difficulty, sore throat, hoarseness, bronchitis, or bronchospasms; disturbed menstrual pattern; vision changes; loss of taste or smell perception; or worsening of condition or lack of improvement. Regular eye exams should be considered (risk of cataracts or glaucoma).

Oral capsule: Swallow whole; do not crush or chew capsule.

Inhalation/nebulization: This is not a bronchodilator and will not relieve acute asthma attacks. It may take several days for you to realize full effects of treatment. If you are also using an inhaled bronchodilator, wait 10 minutes before using this steroid aerosol. Take 5-10 deep breaths. Use inhaler on inspiration. Hold breath for 5-10 seconds after inhalation. Allow 1 full minute between inhalations. You may experience dizziness, anxiety, blurred vision, or taste disturbance or aftertaste. Rinse mouth with water following oral treatments to decrease risk of oral candidiasis (wash face if using a face mask).

Dietary Considerations Avoid grapefruit juice when using oral capsules.

Budesonide (Nasal) (byoo DES oh nide)

Brand Names: U.S. Rhinocort Aqua®

Pharmacologic Category Corticosteroid, Nasal

Pregnancy Risk Factor B

Lactation Enters breast milk/use caution

Use Management of symptoms of seasonal or perennial rhinitis

Canadian labeling: Additional use (not in U.S. labeling): Prevention and treatment of nasal polyps

Available Dosage Forms

Suspension, intranasal:

Rhinocort Aqua®: 32 mcg/inhalation (8.6 g)

General Dosage Range Intranasal inhalation: *Children ≥6 years and Adults:* 64 mcg/day as a single 32 mcg spray in each nostril (maximum: 128 mcg/day [children <12 years]; 256 mcg/day [children ≥12 years and adults])

Administration

Inhalation

Powder for nasal inhalation: Rhinocort® Turbuhaler® [CAN, not available in the U.S.]: Hold inhaler in upright position and turn grey grip as far as it will go in one direction and then back to original position. Clicking sound means inhaler is loaded with dose and ready for use. Place nasal adapter into nostril and ensure firm fit. Cover opposite nostril with finger and inhale (sniff) quickly and forcefully. Do not exhale through inhaler. When a red mark appears in the dose indicator window, 20 doses are left. When the red mark reaches the bottom of the window, the inhaler should be discarded

Suspension for nasal inhalation: Shake gently before use. Prime before first use; discard after 120 sprays.

Budesonide and Formoterol
(byoo DES oh nide & for MOH te rol)

Brand Names: U.S. Symbicort®

Index Terms Budesonide and Eformoterol; Eformoterol and Budesonide; Formoterol and Budesonide; Formoterol Fumarate Dihydrate and Budesonide

Pharmacologic Category Beta$_2$ Agonist; Beta$_2$-Adrenergic Agonist, Long-Acting; Corticosteroid, Inhalant (Oral)

Medication Guide Available Yes

Pregnancy Risk Factor C

Lactation

Budesonide: Enters breast milk/use caution

Formoterol: Excretion in breast milk unknown/use caution

Use Treatment of asthma in patients ≥12 years of age where combination therapy is indicated; maintenance treatment of airflow obstruction associated with chronic obstructive pulmonary disease (COPD; including chronic bronchitis and emphysema)

Unlabeled Use Treatment of asthma in children 5-11 years of age where combination therapy is indicated

Mechanism of Action/Effect Formoterol relaxes bronchial smooth muscle by selective action on beta$_2$ receptors with little effect on heart rate. Formoterol has a long-acting effect. Budesonide is a corticosteroid which controls the rate of protein synthesis, depresses the migration of polymorphonuclear leukocytes/fibroblasts, and reverses capillary permeability and lysosomal stabilization at the cellular level to prevent or control inflammation.

Contraindications Hypersensitivity to budesonide, formoterol, or any component of the formulation; need for acute bronchodilation in COPD or asthma (including status asthmaticus)

Canadian labeling: Additional contraindications (not in U.S. labeling): Hypersensitivity to inhaled lactose

Warnings/Precautions [U.S. Boxed Warning]: Long-acting beta$_2$-agonists (LABAs), such as formoterol, increase the risk of asthma-related deaths; budesonide and formoterol should only be used in patients not adequately controlled on a long-term asthma control medication (ie, inhaled corticosteroid) or whose disease severity requires initiation of two maintenance

therapies. In a large, randomized, placebo-controlled U.S. clinical trial (SMART, 2006), salmeterol was associated with an increase in asthma-related deaths (when added to usual asthma therapy); risk is considered a class effect among all LABAs. Data are not available to determine if the addition of an inhaled corticosteroid lessens this increased risk of death associated with LABA use. Assess patients at regular intervals once asthma control is maintained on combination therapy to determine if step-down therapy is appropriate (without loss of asthma control), and the patient can be maintained on an inhaled corticosteroid only. LABAs are not appropriate in patients whose asthma is adequately controlled on low- or medium-dose inhaled corticosteroids. **[U.S. Boxed Warning]: LABAs may increase the risk of asthma-related hospitalization in pediatric and adolescent patients.**

Do **not** use for acute bronchospasm or acute symptomatic COPD. Short-acting beta$_2$-agonist (eg, albuterol) should be used for acute symptoms and symptoms occurring between treatments. Do **not** initiate in patients with significantly worsening or acutely deteriorating asthma or COPD. Increased use and/or ineffectiveness of short-acting beta$_2$-agonists may indicate rapidly deteriorating disease and should prompt re-evaluation of the patient's condition. Patients must be instructed to seek medical attention in cases where acute symptoms are not relieved by short-acting beta-agonist (not formoterol) or a previous level of response is diminished. Medical evaluation must not be delayed. Patients using inhaled, short acting beta$_2$-agonists should be instructed to discontinue routine use of these medications prior to beginning treatment with Symbicort®; short acting agents should be reserved for symptomatic relief of acute symptoms. Data are not available to determine if LABA use increases the risk of death in patients with COPD.

Immediate hypersensitivity reactions (urticaria, angioedema, rash, bronchospasm) have been reported. Do not exceed recommended dose; serious adverse events, including fatalities, have been associated with excessive use of inhaled sympathomimetics. Rarely, paradoxical bronchospasm may occur with use of inhaled bronchodilating agents; this should be distinguished from inadequate response. Pneumonia and other lower respiratory tract infections have been reported in patients with COPD following the use of inhaled corticosteroids; monitor COPD patients closely since pneumonia symptoms may overlap symptoms of exacerbations.

Use caution in patients with cardiovascular disease (arrhythmia or hypertension or HF), seizure disorders, diabetes, hepatic impairment, ocular disease, osteoporosis, thyroid disease, or hypokalemia.

Beta agonists may cause elevation in blood pressure, heart rate, and result in CNS stimulation/excitation. Beta$_2$-agonists may increase risk of arrhythmia, increase serum glucose, or decrease serum potassium. Long-term use may affect bone mineral density in adults. Infections with *Candida albicans* in the mouth and throat (thrush) have been reported with use. Use with caution in patients taking strong CYP3A4 inhibitors (see Drug Interactions); consider alternative agents that avoid or lessen the potential for CYP-mediated interactions.

Budesonide may cause hypercorticism and/or suppression of hypothalamic-pituitary-adrenal (HPA) axis, particularly in younger children or in patients receiving high doses for prolonged periods. Caution is required when patients are transferred from systemic corticosteroids to products with lower systemic bioavailability (ie, inhalation). May lead to possible adrenal insufficiency or withdrawal symptoms, including an increase in allergic symptoms. Patients receiving prolonged therapy ≥20 mg per day of prednisone (or equivalent) may be most susceptible. Aerosol steroids do **not** provide the systemic steroid needed to treat patients having trauma, surgery, or infections.

Orally-inhaled and intranasal corticosteroids may cause a reduction in growth velocity in pediatric patients (~1 centimeter per year [range 0.3-1.8 cm per year] and related to dose and duration of exposure). To minimize the systemic effects of orally-inhaled and intranasal corticosteroids, each patient should be titrated to the lowest effective dose. Growth should be routinely monitored in pediatric patients.

Prolonged use of corticosteroids may also increase the incidence of secondary infection, mask acute infection (including fungal infections), prolong or exacerbate viral infections, or limit response to vaccines. Exposure to chickenpox should be avoided; corticosteroids should not be used to treat ocular herpes simplex. Corticosteroids should not be used for cerebral malaria. Close observation is required in patients with latent tuberculosis and/or TB reactivity restrict use in active TB (only in conjunction with antituberculosis treatment).

Some products available in Canada contain lactose; very rare anaphylactic reactions have been reported in patients with severe milk protein allergy. Withdraw systemic therapy with gradual tapering of dose. There have been reports of systemic corticosteroid withdrawal symptoms (eg, joint/muscle pain, lassitude, depression) when withdrawing oral inhalation therapy.

Drug Interactions

Avoid Concomitant Use

Avoid concomitant use of Budesonide and Formoterol with any of the following: Aldesleukin; BCG; Beta-Blockers (Nonselective); Grapefruit Juice; Iobenguane I 123; Natalizumab; Pimecrolimus; Tacrolimus (Topical)

Decreased Effect

Budesonide and Formoterol may decrease the levels/effects of: Aldesleukin; Antidiabetic Agents; BCG; Coccidioidin Skin Test; Corticorelin; Iobenguane I 123; Sipuleucel-T; Telaprevir; Vaccines (Inactivated)

The levels/effects of Budesonide and Formoterol may be decreased by: Alpha-/Beta-Blockers; Antacids; Beta-Blockers (Beta1 Selective); Beta-Blockers (Nonselective); Betahistine; Bile Acid Sequestrants; Echinacea; Tocilizumab

Increased Effect/Toxicity

Budesonide and Formoterol may increase the levels/effects of: Amphotericin B; Deferasirox; Leflunomide; Loop Diuretics; Natalizumab; Sympathomimetics; Thiazide Diuretics

The levels/effects of Budesonide and Formoterol may be increased by: Atomoxetine; Caffeine; Cannabinoids; CYP3A4 Inhibitors (Moderate); CYP3A4 Inhibitors (Strong); Dasatinib; Denosumab; Grapefruit Juice; Ivacaftor; MAO Inhibitors; Pimecrolimus; Tacrolimus (Topical); Telaprevir; Theophylline Derivatives; Trastuzumab; Tricyclic Antidepressants

Adverse Reactions Note: Percentage of adverse events may be dose related; causation not established. Also see individual agents.

>10%:

- Central nervous system: Headache (7% to 11%)
- Respiratory: Nasopharyngitis (7% to 11%), upper respiratory tract infections (4% to 11%)

1% to 10%:

- Central nervous system: Dizziness (<3%)
- Gastrointestinal: Stomach discomfort (1% to 7%), oral candidiasis (1% to 6%), vomiting (1% to 3%)
- Neuromuscular & skeletal: Back pain (2% to 3%)
- Respiratory: Pharyngolaryngeal pain (6% to 9%), lower respiratory tract infection (3% to 8%), sinusitis (4% to 6%), bronchitis (5%), nasal congestion (3%)
- Miscellaneous: Influenza (2% to 3%)

Pharmacodynamics/Kinetics

Onset of Action Asthma: 15 minutes; maximum benefit: May take ≥2 weeks

Available Dosage Forms

Aerosol for oral inhalation:

Symbicort® 80/4.5: Budesonide 80 mcg and formoterol fumarate dihydrate 4.5 mcg per actuation (6.9 g) [60 metered inhalations]; budesonide 80 mcg and formoterol fumarate dihydrate 4.5 mcg per actuation (10.2 g) [120 metered inhalations]

Symbicort® 160/4.5: Budesonide 160 mcg and formoterol fumarate dihydrate 4.5 mcg per actuation (6 g) [60 metered inhalations]; budesonide 160 mcg and formoterol fumarate dihydrate 4.5 mcg per actuation (10.2 g) [120 metered inhalations]

General Dosage Range Inhalation:

Children 5-11 years: Symbicort® 80/4.5: Two inhalations twice daily (maximum: 4 inhalations/day)

Children ≥12 years: 2 inhalations once or twice daily (maximum: 4 inhalations/day)

Adults: 2 inhalations twice daily (maximum: 4 inhalations/day)

Administration

Inhalation

Symbicort® 80/4.5, Symbicort® 160/4.5: Prior to first use, inhaler must be primed by releasing 2 test sprays into the air; shake well for 5 seconds before each spray. Inhaler must be reprimed if not used for >7 days or if it has been dropped. Shake well for 5 seconds before each use. Discard inhaler after the labeled number of inhalations have been used or within 3 months after removal from foil pouch (do not use the "float test" to determine amount remaining in canister).

Symbicort® Turbuhaler® [CAN; not available in U.S.]:

To "load" inhaler: Turn grip on inhaler as far as it will move in one direction, then turn in opposite direction as far as it will go (inhaler is "loaded" with a dose, indicated by a "click"). Prior to first use, this procedure should be done twice, it does not need to be repeated with subsequent uses even when not used regularly.

Delivery of dose: Instruct patient to place mouthpiece gently between teeth, closing lips around inhaler. Instruct patient to inhale deeply and hold breath held for 5-10 seconds. The amount of drug delivered is small, and the individual will not sense the medication as it is inhaled. Remove mouthpiece prior to exhalation. Patient should not breathe out through the mouthpiece. After use of the inhaler, patient should rinse mouth/oropharynx with water and spit out rinse solution.

Stability

Storage

Symbicort® 80/4.5, Symbicort® 160/4.5: Store at room temperature of 20°C to 25°C (68°F to 77°F) with mouthpiece down. Do not puncture, incinerate, or store near heat or open flame. Discard inhaler after the labeled number of inhalations have been used or within 3 months after removal from foil pouch.

Symbicort® Turbuhaler®: Store at room temperature of 15°C to 30°C. Protect from heat and moisture.

Nursing Actions

Physical Assessment See individual agents.

Patient Education See individual agents.

Related Information

Budesonide (Systemic, Oral Inhalation) *on page 147*

Formoterol *on page 512*

Bumetanide (byoo MET a nide)

Index Terms Bumex

Pharmacologic Category Diuretic, Loop

Medication Safety Issues

Sound-alike/look-alike issues:

Bumetanide may be confused with Buminate®

Bumex® may be confused with Brevibloc®, Buprenex®

International issues:

Bumex [U.S.] may be confused with Permax brand name for pergolide [multiple international markets]

Pregnancy Risk Factor C

Lactation Excretion in breast milk unknown/not recommended

Use Management of edema secondary to heart failure or hepatic or renal disease (including nephrotic syndrome)

Unlabeled Use Treatment of hypertension

Mechanism of Action/Effect Inhibits reabsorption of sodium and chloride in the ascending loop of Henle and proximal renal tubule, causing increased excretion of water, sodium, chloride, magnesium, phosphate, and calcium

Contraindications Hypersensitivity to bumetanide or any component of the formulation; anuria; patients with hepatic coma or in states of severe electrolyte depletion until the condition improves or is corrected

Warnings/Precautions [U.S. Boxed Warning]: Excessive amounts can lead to profound diuresis with fluid and electrolyte loss; close medical supervision and dose evaluation are required. Potassium supplementation and/or use of potassium-sparing diuretics may be necessary to prevent hypokalemia. In cirrhosis, initiate bumetanide therapy with conservative dosing and close monitoring of electrolytes; avoid sudden changes in fluid and electrolyte balance and acid/base status which may lead to hepatic encephalopathy. *In vitro* studies using pooled sera from critically-ill neonates have shown bumetanide to be a potent displacer of bilirubin; avoid use in neonates at risk for kernicterus. Coadministration of antihypertensives may increase the risk of hypotension.

Monitor fluid status and renal function in an attempt to prevent oliguria, azotemia, and reversible increases in BUN and creatinine; close medical supervision of aggressive diuresis required. Bumetanide-induced ototoxicity (usually transient) may occur with rapid I.V. administration, renal impairment, excessive doses, and concurrent use of other ototoxins (eg, aminoglycosides). Asymptomatic hyperuricemia has been reported with use.

Chemical similarities are present among sulfonamides, sulfonylureas, carbonic anhydrase inhibitors, thiazides, and loop diuretics (except ethacrynic acid); the manufacturer's labeling states that bumetanide may be used in patients allergic to furosemide. Use in patients with sulfonylurea allergy is not specifically contraindicated in product labeling; however, a risk of cross-reaction exists in patients with allergy to any of these compounds; avoid use when previous reaction has been severe. Discontinue if signs of hypersensitivity are noted.

Drug Interactions

Avoid Concomitant Use There are no known interactions where it is recommended to avoid concomitant use.

Decreased Effect

Bumetanide may decrease the levels/effects of: Lithium; Neuromuscular-Blocking Agents

The levels/effects of Bumetanide may be decreased by: Bile Acid Sequestrants; Fosphenytoin; Herbs (Hypertensive Properties); Methotrexate; Methylphenidate; Nonsteroidal Anti-Inflammatory Agents; Phenytoin; Probenecid; Salicylates; Yohimbine

Increased Effect/Toxicity

Bumetanide may increase the levels/effects of: ACE Inhibitors; Allopurinol; Amifostine; Aminoglycosides; Antihypertensives; Cardiac Glycosides; CISplatin; Dofetilide; Hypotensive Agents; Lithium; Methotrexate; Neuromuscular-Blocking Agents; RisperiDONE; RiTUXimab; Salicylates; Sodium Phosphates

The levels/effects of Bumetanide may be increased by: Alfuzosin; Beta2-Agonists; Corticosteroids (Orally Inhaled); Corticosteroids (Systemic); CycloSPORINE (Systemic); Diazoxide; Herbs (Hypotensive Properties); Licorice; MAO Inhibitors; Methotrexate; Pentoxifylline; Phosphodiesterase 5 Inhibitors; Probenecid; Prostacyclin Analogues

Nutritional/Ethanol Interactions

Food: Bumetanide serum levels may be decreased if taken with food. It has been recommended that bumetanide be administered without food (Bard, 2004).

Herb/Nutraceutical: Avoid ephedra, yohimbe, ginseng (may worsen hypertension). Avoid dong quai if using for hypertension (has estrogenic activity). Avoid garlic (may have increased antihypertensive effect).

Adverse Reactions

>10%:

Endocrine & metabolic: Hyperuricemia (18%), hypochloremia (15%), hypokalemia (15%)

Renal: Azotemia (11%)

1% to 10%:

Central nervous system: Dizziness (1%)

Endocrine & metabolic: Hyponatremia (9%), hyperglycemia (7%), phosphorus altered (5%), CO_2 content altered (4%), bicarbonate altered (3%), calcium altered (2%)

Neuromuscular & skeletal: Muscle cramps (1%)

Renal: Serum creatinine increased (7%)

Miscellaneous: LDH altered (1%)

Pharmacodynamics/Kinetics

Onset of Action Oral, I.M.: 0.5-1 hour; I.V.: 2-3 minutes

Peak effect: Oral: 1-2 hours; I.V.: 15-30 minutes

Duration of Action 4-6 hours

Available Dosage Forms

Injection, solution: 0.25 mg/mL (2 mL, 4 mL, 5 mL, 10 mL)

Tablet, oral: 0.5 mg, 1 mg, 2 mg

General Dosage Range

I.M., I.V.:

Infants and Children: 0.015-0.1 mg/kg/dose every 6-24 hours (maximum: 10 mg/day)

Adults: 0.5-1 mg/dose; may repeat in 2-3 hours for up to 2 doses (maximum: 10 mg/day)

Oral:

Infants and Children: 0.015-0.1 mg/kg/dose every 6-24 hours (maximum: 10 mg/day)

Adults: 0.5-2 mg 1-2 times/day; may repeat in 4-5 hours for up to 2 doses (maximum: 10 mg/day)

Administration

Oral An alternate-day schedule or a 3-4 daily dosing regimen with rest periods of 1-2 days in between may be the most tolerable and effective regimen for the continued control of edema.

I.V. Administer slowly, over 1-2 minutes.

I.V. Detail pH: 6.8-7.8 (adjusted)

Stability

Storage

I.V.: Store vials at 15°C to 30°C (59°F to 86°F). Infusion solutions should be used within 24 hours after preparation. Light sensitive; discoloration may occur when exposed to light.

Tablet: Store at 15°C to 30°C (59°F to 86°F).

Nursing Actions

Physical Assessment History of allergies and renal, electrolyte, hepatic, and pregnancy status should be assessed prior to beginning treatment. Monitor blood pressure, weight, and fluid status at beginning of therapy and periodically during therapy. Assess therapeutic effectiveness (reduced edema and cardiopulmonary symptoms). Monitor for hypotension, electrolyte imbalance, and ototoxicity.

Patient Education May be taken with food to reduce GI effects. If taking one dose daily, take single dose early in day; if taking twice daily, take last dose early in afternoon to prevent sleep interruptions. Include potassium-rich foods in your daily diet, but do not take supplemental potassium without consulting prescriber. May cause dizziness or weakness. Report palpitations or chest pain, swelling of ankles or feet, weight increase, increased fatigue, muscle cramps, trembling, and any changes in hearing.

Dietary Considerations Administration with food slows the rate and reduces the extent of absorption and may reduce diuretic efficacy (Bard, 2004). May require increased intake of potassium-rich foods.

Bupivacaine (byoo PIV a kane)

Brand Names: U.S. Bupivacaine Spinal; Marcaine®; Marcaine® Spinal; Sensorcaine®; Sensorcaine®-MPF; Sensorcaine®-MPF Spinal

Index Terms Bupivacaine Hydrochloride

Pharmacologic Category Local Anesthetic

Medication Safety Issues

Sound-alike/look-alike issues:

Bupivacaine may be confused with mepivacaine, ropivacaine

Marcaine® may be confused with Narcan®

High alert medication:

The Institute for Safe Medication Practices (ISMP) includes this medication (epidural administration) among its list of drug classes which have a heightened risk of causing significant patient harm when used in error.

Pregnancy Risk Factor C

Lactation Enters breast milk/not recommended

Use Local or regional anesthesia; spinal anesthesia; diagnostic and therapeutic procedures; obstetrical procedures (only 0.25% and 0.5% concentrations)

0.25%: Local infiltration, peripheral nerve block, sympathetic block, caudal or epidural block

0.5%: Peripheral nerve block, caudal and epidural block

0.75% **(not for obstetrical anesthesia)**: Retrobulbar block, epidural block. **Note:** Reserve for surgical procedures where a high degree of muscle relaxation and prolonged effect are necessary

Available Dosage Forms

Injection, solution: 0.25% [2.5 mg/mL] (20 mL, 50 mL); 0.5% [5 mg/mL] (20 mL, 50 mL)

Marcaine®: 0.5% [5 mg/mL] (50 mL)

Sensorcaine®: 0.25% [2.5 mg/mL] (50 mL); 0.5% [5 mg/mL] (50 mL)

Injection, solution [preservative free]: 0.25% [2.5 mg/mL] (10 mL, 20 mL, 30 mL, 50 mL); 0.5% [5 mg/mL] (10 mL, 20 mL, 30 mL); 0.75% [7.5 mg/mL] (10 mL, 20 mL, 30 mL)

Marcaine®: 0.25% [2.5 mg/mL] (10 mL, 30 mL, 50 mL); 0.5% [5 mg/mL] (10 mL, 30 mL); 0.75% [7.5 mg/mL] (10 mL, 30 mL)

Sensorcaine®-MPF: 0.25% [2.5 mg/mL] (10 mL, 30 mL); 0.5% [5 mg/mL] (10 mL, 30 mL); 0.75% [7.5 mg/mL] (10 mL, 30 mL)

Injection, solution, premixed in $D_{8.25}W$ [preservative free]:

Bupivacaine Spinal: 0.75% [7.5 mg/mL] (2 mL)

Marcaine® Spinal: 0.75% [7.5 mg/mL] (2 mL)
Sensorcaine®-MPF Spinal: 0.75% [7.5 mg/mL] (2 mL)

General Dosage Range

Caudal block: *Children >12 years and Adults:* 15-30 mL of 0.25% or 0.5%

Epidural block: *Children >12 years and Adults:* 10-20 mL of 0.25% or 0.5% in 3-5 mL increments **or** 10-20 mL of 0.75% if high degree of muscle relaxation and prolonged effects needed

Infiltration (local): *Children >12 years and Adults:* 0.25% (maximum: 175 mg)

Nerve block: *Children >12 years and Adults:*
Peripheral: 5 mL of 0.25% or 0.5% (maximum: 400 mg/day)
Sympathetic: 20-50 mL of 0.25%

Retrobulbar anesthesia: *Children >12 years and Adults:* 2-4 mL of 0.75%

Spinal: *Adults:* Preservative free solution of 0.75% bupivacaine in 8.25% dextrose:
Cesarean section: 1-1.4 mL
Lower abdominal procedures: 1.6 mL
Lower extremity and perineal procedures: 1 mL
Normal vaginal delivery: 0.8 mL (higher doses may be required in some patients)

Administration

I.V. Detail pH: 4.0-6.5

Other Solutions containing preservatives should not be used for epidural or caudal blocks.

Nursing Actions

Physical Assessment Monitor for return of sensation. Teach patient appropriate interventions to promote safety.

Patient Education This medication is given to reduce sensation in the injected area. You will experience decreased sensation to pain, heat, or cold in the area and/or decreased muscle strength; use necessary caution to reduce incidence of possible injury until full sensation returns. If used in mouth, do not eat or drink until full sensation returns. Immediately report chest pain or palpitations; increased restlessness, anxiety, or dizziness; skeletal or muscle weakness; or respiratory difficulty.

Buprenorphine (byoo pre NOR feen)

Brand Names: U.S. Buprenex®; Butrans®; Subutex® [DSC]

Index Terms Buprenorphine Hydrochloride

Pharmacologic Category Analgesic, Opioid; Analgesic, Opioid Partial Agonist

Medication Safety Issues

Sound-alike/look-alike issues:
Buprenex® may be confused with Brevibloc®, Bumex®

High alert medication:
The Institute for Safe Medication Practices (ISMP) includes this medication among its list of drug classes which have a heightened risk of causing significant patient harm when used in error.

Medication Guide Available Yes

Pregnancy Risk Factor C

Lactation Enters breast milk/not recommended

Use
Injection: Management of moderate-to-severe pain
Sublingual tablet: Treatment of opioid dependence
Transdermal patch: Management of moderate-to-severe chronic pain in patients requiring an around-the-clock opioid analgesic for an extended period of time

Unlabeled Use Injection: Management of opioid withdrawal in heroin-dependent hospitalized patients

Mechanism of Action/Effect Buprenorphine exerts its analgesic effect via high affinity binding to μ opiate receptors in the CNS; displays partial mu agonist and weak kappa antagonist activity

Contraindications Hypersensitivity to buprenorphine or any component of the formulation

Transdermal patch: Additional contraindications: Significant respiratory depression; severe asthma; known or suspected paralytic ileus; management of mild, acute, or intermittent pain; management of pain requiring short-term opioid analgesia; management of postoperative pain

Warnings/Precautions An opioid-containing analgesic regimen should be tailored to each patient's needs and based upon the type of pain being treated (acute versus chronic), the route of administration, degree of tolerance for opioids (naive versus chronic user), age, weight, and medical condition. The optimal analgesic dose varies widely among patients. Doses should be titrated to pain relief/prevention.

May cause CNS depression, which may impair physical or mental abilities. Effects with other sedative drugs or ethanol may be potentiated. Elderly may be more sensitive to CNS depressant and constipating effects. May cause respiratory depression - use caution in patients with respiratory disease or pre-existing respiratory depression. Hypersensitivity reactions, including bronchospasm, angioneurotic edema, and anaphylactic shock, have also been reported. Potential for drug dependency exists, abrupt cessation may precipitate withdrawal. Use caution in elderly, debilitated, pediatric patients, depression or suicidal tendencies. Tolerance, psychological and physical dependence may occur with prolonged use. Partial antagonist activity may precipitate acute narcotic withdrawal in opioid-dependent individuals.

Hepatitis has been reported with buprenorphine use; hepatic events ranged from transient, asymptomatic transaminase elevations to hepatic failure; in many cases, patients had preexisting hepatic dysfunction. Monitor liver function tests in patients at increased risk for hepatotoxicity (eg, history of alcohol abuse, pre-existing hepatic dysfunction, I.V. drug abusers) prior to and during therapy. Use with caution in patients with hepatic impairment; dosage adjustments are recommended in hepatic impairment.

Use with caution in patients with pulmonary or renal function impairment. Also use caution in patients with head injury or increased ICP, biliary tract dysfunction, patients with history of hyperthyroidism, morbid obesity, adrenal insufficiency, prostatic hyperplasia, urinary stricture, CNS depression, toxic psychosis, pancreatitis, alcoholism, delirium tremens, or kyphoscoliosis. May cause hypotension; use with caution in patients with hypovolemia, cardiovascular disease (including acute MI), or drugs which may exaggerate hypotensive effects (including phenothiazines or general anesthetics). May obscure diagnosis or clinical course of patients with acute abdominal conditions. Opioid therapy may lower seizure threshold; use caution in patients with a history of seizure disorders.

Transdermal patch: **[U.S. Boxed Warning]: Do not exceed one 20 mcg/hour transdermal patch due to the risk of QT_c-interval prolongation.** Avoid using in patients with history of long QT syndrome or in patients with predisposing factors increasing the risk of QT abnormalities (eg, concurrent medications such as antiarrhythmics, hypokalemia, unstable heart failure, unstable atrial fibrillation). **[U.S. Boxed Warning]: Healthcare provider should be alert to problems of abuse, misuse, and diversion.**

Sublingual tablets, which are used for induction treatment of opioid dependence, should not be started until effects of withdrawal are evident.

Drug Interactions

Avoid Concomitant Use

Avoid concomitant use of Buprenorphine with any of the following: Atazanavir; Conivaptan; MAO Inhibitors

Decreased Effect

Buprenorphine may decrease the levels/effects of: Analgesics (Opioid); Atazanavir; Pegvisomant

The levels/effects of Buprenorphine may be decreased by: Ammonium Chloride; Boceprevir; CYP3A4 Inducers (Strong); Deferasirox; Efavirenz; Etravirine; Herbs (CYP3A4 Inducers); Mixed Agonist / Antagonist Opioids; Tocilizumab

Increased Effect/Toxicity

Buprenorphine may increase the levels/effects of: Alcohol (Ethyl); Alvimopan; ARIPiprazole; CNS Depressants; Desmopressin; MAO Inhibitors; Selective Serotonin Reuptake Inhibitors; Thiazide Diuretics

The levels/effects of Buprenorphine may be increased by: Amphetamines; Antipsychotic Agents (Phenothiazines); Atazanavir; Boceprevir; Conivaptan; CYP3A4 Inhibitors (Moderate); CYP3A4 Inhibitors (Strong); Dasatinib; Droperidol; HydrOXYzine; Ivacaftor; Succinylcholine

Nutritional/Ethanol Interactions

Ethanol: May increase CNS depression; monitor for increased effects with coadministration. Caution patients about effect.

Herb/Nutraceutical: Avoid valerian, St John's wort, kava kava, gotu kola (may increase CNS depression).

Adverse Reactions

Injection:

>10%: Central nervous system: Sedation

1% to 10%:

Cardiovascular: Hypotension

Central nervous system: Respiratory depression, dizziness, headache

Gastrointestinal: Vomiting, nausea

Ocular: Miosis

Otic: Vertigo

Miscellaneous: Diaphoresis

Tablet:

>10%:

Central nervous system: Headache (30%), pain (24%), insomnia (21% to 25%), anxiety (12%), depression (11%)

Gastrointestinal: Nausea (10% to 14%), abdominal pain (12%), constipation (8% to 11%)

Neuromuscular & skeletal: Back pain (14%), weakness (14%)

Respiratory: Rhinitis (11%)

Miscellaneous: Withdrawal syndrome (19%; placebo 37%), infection (12% to 20%), diaphoresis (12% to 13%)

1% to 10%:

Central nervous system: Chills (6%), nervousness (6%), somnolence (5%), dizziness (4%), fever (3%)

Gastrointestinal: Vomiting (5% to 8%), diarrhea (5%), dyspepsia (3%)

Ocular: Lacrimation (5%)

Respiratory: Cough (4%), pharyngitis (4%)

Miscellaneous: Flu-like syndrome (6%)

Transdermal patch:

>10%:

Central nervous system: Headache (16%), dizziness (16%), somnolence (14%),

Gastrointestinal: Nausea (23%), constipation (14%), vomiting (11%)

Local: Application site pruritus (15%)

1% to 10%:

Cardiovascular: Peripheral edema (7%), chest pain, hypertension

Central nervous system: Fatigue (5%), insomnia (3%), hypoesthesia (2%), anxiety, depression, fever, migraine

Dermatologic: Pruritus (4%), rash (2%)

Gastrointestinal: Xerostomia (7%), diarrhea (3%), abdominal discomfort (2%), anorexia (2%), upper abdominal pain

Genitourinary: Urinary tract infection (3%)

Local: Application site erythema (7%); application site rash (6%), application site irritation

Neuromuscular & skeletal: Pain in extremity (3%), back pain (3%), joint swelling (3%), paresthesia (2%), tremor (2%), muscles spasms, musculoskeletal pain, myalgia, neck pain, weakness

Respiratory: Dyspnea (3%), bronchitis, cough, nasopharyngitis, pharyngolaryngeal pain, sinusitis, upper respiratory tract infection

Miscellaneous: Hyperhydrosis (4%), fall (4%), flu-like syndrome

Pharmacodynamics/Kinetics

Onset of Action Analgesic: I.M: Within 15 minutes; Peak effect: I.M.: ~1 hour; Transdermal patch: Steady state achieved by day 3

Duration of Action I.M.: ≥6 hours

Controlled Substance C-III

Available Dosage Forms

Injection, solution: 0.3 mg/mL (1 mL)

Buprenex®: 0.3 mg/mL (1 mL)

Injection, solution [preservative free]: 0.3 mg/mL (1 mL)

Patch, transdermal:

Butrans®: 5 mcg/hr (4s); 10 mcg/hr (4s); 20 mcg/hr (4s)

Tablet, sublingual: 2 mg, 8 mg

General Dosage Range Dosage adjustment recommended in patients with hepatic impairment.

I.M., I.V.:

Children 2-12 years: 2-6 mcg/kg every 4-6 hours

Children ≥13 years and Adults: Initial: 0.3 mg, may repeat once in 30-60 minutes then every 6-8 hours as needed; Maintenance: 0.15-0.6 mg every 4-8 hours as needed

Elderly: 0.15 mg every 6 hours

Sublingual: *Children ≥16 years and Adults:* Induction: 12-16 mg/day; Maintenance: 12-16 mg/day (target dose: 16 mg/day)

Transdermal: *Adults:* 5-20 mcg/hour applied once every 7 days

Administration

Oral Sublingual: Tablet should be placed under the tongue until dissolved; should not be swallowed. If two or more tablets are needed per dose, all may be placed under the tongue at once, or two at a time. To ensure consistent bioavailability, subsequent doses should always be taken the same way.

I.M. Administer via deep I.M. injection.

I.V. Administer slowly, over at least 2 minutes. Administration over 20-30 minutes preferred when managing opioid withdrawal in heroin-dependent hospitalized patients (Welsh, 2002).

I.V. Detail pH: 3.5-5.5

Other Transdermal patch: Apply to patch to intact, nonirritated skin only. Apply to a hairless or nearly hairless skin site. If hairless site is not available, do not shave skin; hair at application site should be clipped. Prior to application, if the site must be cleaned, clean with clear water and allow to dry completely; do not use soaps, alcohol, lotions or abrasives due to potential for increased skin absorption. Do not use any patch that has been damaged, cut or manipulated in any way. Remove patch from protective pouch immediately before application. Remove the protective backing, and apply the sticky side of the patch to one of eight possible application sites (upper outer arm, upper chest, upper back, or the side of the chest [on either side of the body]). Firmly press patch in place and hold for ~15 seconds. Change patch every 7 days. Rotate patch application sites; wait ≥21 days before reapplying another patch to the same skin site. Avoid exposing application site to external heat sources (eg, heating pad, electric blanket, heat lamp, hot tub). If there is difficulty with patch adhesion, the edges of the system may be taped in place with first-aid tape. If the patch falls off during the 7-day dosing interval, dispose of the patch and apply a new patch to a different skin site.

Stability

Storage

Injection: Protect from excessive heat >40°C (>104°F). Protect from light.

Patch, tablet: Store at room temperature of 25°C (77°F).

Nursing Actions

Physical Assessment Monitor for effectiveness of pain relief. Monitor for possible respiratory depression. Monitor blood pressure, CNS and respiratory status, and degree of sedation prior to treatment and periodically throughout. For inpatients, implement safety measures (eg, side rails up, call light within reach, instructions to call for assistance). Assess patient's physical and/or psychological dependence. Discontinue slowly after prolonged use.

Patient Education Apply transdermal patch to hairless site; if that is impossible, then clip hair; do not shave (as absorption from patch can be increased). Have patient avoid external heat sources (increases absorption from patch). Do not use alcohol, sedatives, tranquilizers, antihistamines, or pain medications without consulting prescriber. May cause dizziness, drowsiness, confusion, or blurred vision. You may experience nausea, vomiting, or constipation. If constipation is unresolved, consult prescriber about use of stool softeners and/or laxatives. Report unresolved nausea or vomiting, severe dizziness, respiratory difficulty or shortness of breath, excessive sedation or unusual weakness, or rapid heartbeat or palpitations.

Take with or without food once daily. May cause hypertension or headache. Report increase or changes in CNS symptoms (confusion, hallucinations, fatigue, aggressive reaction), chest pain or palpitations, dizziness or fainting, difficulty breathing or tightness in chest, or rash.

Buprenorphine and Naloxone

(byoo pre NOR feen & nal OKS one)

Brand Names: U.S. Suboxone®

Index Terms Buprenorphine Hydrochloride and Naloxone Hydrochloride Dihydrate; Naloxone and Buprenorphine; Naloxone Hydrochloride Dihydrate and Buprenorphine Hydrochloride

Pharmacologic Category Analgesic, Opioid; Analgesic, Opioid Partial Agonist

Medication Safety Issues

High alert medication:

The Institute for Safe Medication Practices (ISMP) includes this medication among its list of drug classes which have a heightened risk of causing significant patient harm when used in error.

Medication Guide Available Yes

Pregnancy Risk Factor C

Lactation Buprenorphine: Enters breast milk/not recommended

Use Maintenance treatment for opioid dependence

Mechanism of Action/Effect See individual agents.

Contraindications Hypersensitivity to buprenorphine, naloxone, or any component of the formulation

Warnings/Precautions May cause respiratory depression - use caution in patients with respiratory disease or pre-existing respiratory depression. Potential for drug dependency exists, abrupt cessation may precipitate withdrawal. Hypersensitivity, including bronchospasm, angioneurotic edema, and anaphylactic shock, have been reported. Hepatitis has been reported with buprenorphine use; hepatic events ranged from transient, asymptomatic transaminase elevations to hepatic; in many cases, patients had preexisting hepatic dysfunction. Monitor liver function tests in all patients prior to and during therapy.

Use caution in elderly or debilitated patients. Use with caution in patients with hepatic or pulmonary function impairment. May cause CNS depression, which may impair physical or mental abilities. Patients must be cautioned about performing tasks which require mental alertness (eg, operating machinery or driving). Effects with other sedative drugs or ethanol may be potentiated. May cause orthostatic hypotension; use with caution in patients with hypovolemia, cardiovascular disease (including acute MI), or drugs which may exaggerate hypotension. Elderly may be more sensitive to CNS depressant and constipating effects. Use with caution in patients with head injury or increased ICP, biliary tract dysfunction, pancreatitis, patients with history of ileus or bowel obstruction, hyperthyroidism, adrenal insufficiency, prostatic hyperplasia, urinary stricture, CNS depression, psychosis, alcoholism, delirium tremens, kyphoscoliosis or morbidly obese patients. May obscure diagnosis or clinical course of patients with acute abdominal conditions. Partial antagonist activity of buprenorphine may precipitate acute narcotic withdrawal in opioid-dependent individuals upon rapid discontinuation. Naloxone may precipitate intense withdrawal symptoms in patients addicted to opiates when administered before the opioid effects have subsided, or if misused and administered parenterally by opioid-dependent individuals. Combination product is indicated for maintenance therapy for opioid dependence and should not be used for induction. Buprenorphine/naloxone is not appropriate for pain management; deaths have been reported in opioid-naive patients receiving oral buprenorphine for analgesia. Use caution with switching between formulations; potential for greater bioavailability with sublingual film compared to sublingual tablet; monitor closely for either over- or underdosing when switching patients from one formulation to another. Healthcare provider should be alert to problems of abuse, misuse, and diversion.

Drug Interactions

Avoid Concomitant Use

Avoid concomitant use of Buprenorphine and Naloxone with any of the following: Atazanavir; Conivaptan; MAO Inhibitors

Decreased Effect

Buprenorphine and Naloxone may decrease the levels/effects of: Analgesics (Opioid); Atazanavir; Pegvisomant

The levels/effects of Buprenorphine and Naloxone may be decreased by: Ammonium Chloride; Boceprevir; CYP3A4 Inducers (Strong); Deferasirox; Efavirenz; Etravirine; Herbs (CYP3A4 Inducers); Mixed Agonist / Antagonist Opioids; Tocilizumab

Increased Effect/Toxicity

Buprenorphine and Naloxone may increase the levels/effects of: Alcohol (Ethyl); Alvimopan; ARIPiprazole; CNS Depressants; Desmopressin; MAO Inhibitors; Selective Serotonin Reuptake Inhibitors; Thiazide Diuretics

The levels/effects of Buprenorphine and Naloxone may be increased by: Amphetamines; Antipsychotic Agents (Phenothiazines); Atazanavir; Boceprevir; Conivaptan; CYP3A4 Inhibitors (Moderate); CYP3A4 Inhibitors (Strong); Dasatinib; Droperidol; HydrOXYzine; Ivacaftor; Succinylcholine

Adverse Reactions Also see individual agents.

>10%:

Central nervous system: Headache (36%), pain (22%)

Gastrointestinal: Vomiting (8%), erythema (oral mucosa; film), glossodynia (film), oral hypoesthesia (film)

Miscellaneous: Withdrawal syndrome (25%; placebo 37%), diaphoresis (14%)

1% to 10%:

Cardiovascular: Vasodilation (9%)

Gastrointestinal: Vomiting (7%)

Controlled Substance C-III

Available Dosage Forms

Film, sublingual:

Suboxone®: Buprenorphine 2 mg and naloxone 0.5 mg; buprenorphine 8 mg and naloxone 2 mg

Tablet, sublingual:

Suboxone®: Buprenorphine 2 mg and naloxone 0.5 mg; buprenorphine 8 mg and naloxone 2 mg

General Dosage Range Sublingual: *Children ≥16 years and Adults:* 4-24 mg/day (target dose: 16 mg/day)

Administration

Oral

Sublingual film: Film should be placed under the tongue. Keep under the tongue until film dissolves completely; film should not be chewed, swallowed or moved after placement. If more than one film is needed, the additional film should be placed under the tongue on the opposite side from the first film.

Sublingual tablet: Tablet should be placed under the tongue until dissolved; should not be swallowed. If two or more tablets are needed per dose, all may be placed under the tongue at once, or two at a time. To ensure consistent bioavailability, subsequent doses should always be taken the same way.

Stability

Storage Store at room temperature of 25°C (77°F).

Nursing Actions

Physical Assessment See individual agents.

Patient Education See individual agents.

Dietary Considerations

Ethanol: May increase CNS depression; monitor for increased effects with coadministration. Caution patients about effect.

Herb/Nutraceutical: Avoid valerian, St John's wort, kava kava, gotu kola (may increase CNS depression).

Related Information

Buprenorphine *on page* 155

Naloxone *on page* 808

BuPROPion (byoo PROE pee on)

Brand Names: U.S. Aplenzin™; Budeprion SR®; Budeprion XL®; Buproban®; Wellbutrin SR®; Wellbutrin XL®; Wellbutrin®; Zyban®

Index Terms Bupropion Hydrobromide; Bupropion Hydrochloride

Pharmacologic Category Antidepressant, Dopamine-Reuptake Inhibitor; Smoking Cessation Aid

Medication Safety Issues

Sound-alike/look-alike issues:

Aplenzin™ may be confused with Albenza®, Relenza®

BuPROPion may be confused with busPIRone

Wellbutrin XL® may be confused with Wellbutrin SR®

Zyban® may be confused with Diovan®

Medication Guide Available Yes

Pregnancy Risk Factor C

Lactation Enters breast milk/not recommended (AAP rates "of concern"; AAP 2001 update pending)

Breast-Feeding Considerations Bupropion and its metabolites are excreted into breast milk, although neither bupropion nor its metabolites have been detected in the plasma of breast-fed infants. Adverse events have not been reported in older breast-fed infants; however, a seizure was noted in one 6-month old infant (a causal effect could not be confirmed). Breast-feeding is not recommended by the manufacturer.

Use Treatment of major depressive disorder, including seasonal affective disorder (SAD); adjunct in smoking cessation

Unlabeled Use Attention-deficit/hyperactivity disorder (ADHD); depression associated with bipolar disorder

Mechanism of Action/Effect Antidepressant structurally different from all other marketed antidepressants; like other antidepressants the mechanism of bupropion's activity is not fully understood; relatively weak inhibitor of the neuronal uptake of norepinephrine and dopamine

Contraindications Hypersensitivity to bupropion or any component of the formulation; seizure disorder; history of anorexia/bulimia; use of MAO inhibitors within 14 days; patients undergoing abrupt discontinuation of ethanol or sedatives (including benzodiazepines); patients receiving other dosage forms of bupropion

Warnings/Precautions [U.S. Boxed Warning]: Use in treating psychiatric disorders: Antidepressants increase the risk of suicidal thinking and behavior in children, adolescents, and young adults (18-24 years of age) with major depressive disorder (MDD) and other

psychiatric disorders; consider risk prior to prescribing. Short-term studies did not show an increased risk in patients >24 years of age and showed a decreased risk in patients ≥65 years. All patients must be closely monitored for clinical worsening, suicidality, or unusual changes in behavior, especially during the initiation of therapy (generally first 1-2 months) or following an increase or decrease in dosage. The patient's family or caregiver should be instructed to closely observe the patient and communicate condition with healthcare provider. A medication guide should be dispensed with each prescription. **Bupropion is not FDA approved for use in children.**

[U.S. Boxed Warning]: Use in smoking cessation: Serious neuropsychiatric events, including depression, suicidal thoughts, and suicide, have been reported with use; some cases may have been complicated by symptoms of nicotine withdrawal following smoking cessation. Smoking cessation (with or without treatment) is associated with nicotine withdrawal symptoms and the exacerbation of underlying psychiatric illness; however, some of the behavioral disturbances were reported in treated patients who continued to smoke. These neuropsychiatric symptoms (eg, mood disturbances, psychosis, hostility) have occurred in patients with and without pre-existing psychiatric disease; many cases resolved following therapy discontinuation although in some cases, symptoms persisted. Monitor all patients for behavioral changes and psychiatric symptoms (eg, agitation, depression, suicidal behavior, suicidal ideation); inform patients to discontinue treatment and contact their healthcare provider immediately if they experience any behavioral and/or mood changes.

The possibility of a suicide attempt is inherent in major depression and may persist until remission occurs. Use caution in high-risk patients. Worsening depression and severe abrupt suicidality that are not part of the presenting symptoms may require discontinuation or modification of drug therapy. The patient's family or caregiver should be alerted to monitor patients for the emergence of suicidality and associated behaviors (such as agitation, irritability, hostility, impulsivity, and hypomania) and notify the healthcare provider.

May worsen psychosis in some patients or precipitate a shift to mania or hypomania in patients with bipolar disorder. Patients presenting with depressive symptoms should be screened for bipolar disorder. Monotherapy in patients with bipolar disorder should be avoided. **Bupropion is not FDA approved for bipolar depression.**

The risk of seizures is dose-dependent and increased in patients with a history of seizures, anorexia/bulimia, head trauma, CNS tumor, severe hepatic cirrhosis, abrupt discontinuation of sedative-hypnotics or ethanol, medications which lower seizure threshold (antipsychotics, antidepressants, theophyllines, systemic steroids), stimulants, or hypoglycemic agents. Risk of seizures may also be increased by chewing,crushing, or dividing long-acting products. Risk may be reduced by limiting the daily dose to bupropion hydrochloride ≤450 mg or bupropion hydrobromide 522 mg. Gradually increase dose incrementally to reduce risk. Discontinue and do not restart in patients experiencing a seizure.

May cause CNS stimulation (restlessness, anxiety, insomnia) or anorexia. May increase the risks associated with electroconvulsive therapy. Consider discontinuing, when possible, prior to elective surgery. May cause weight loss; use caution in patients where weight loss is not desirable. The incidence of sexual dysfunction with bupropion is generally lower than with SSRIs.

Use caution in patients with cardiovascular disease, history of hypertension, or coronary artery disease; treatment-emergent hypertension (including some severe cases) has been reported, both with bupropion alone and in combination with nicotine transdermal systems. All children diagnosed with ADHD who may be candidates for stimulant medications should have a thorough cardiovascular assessment to identify risk factors for sudden cardiac death prior to initiation of drug therapy. Use with caution in patients with hepatic or renal dysfunction and in elderly patients; reduced dose and/or frequency may be recommended. Elderly patients may be at greater risk of accumulation during chronic dosing. May cause motor or cognitive impairment in some patients; use with caution if tasks requiring alertness such as operating machinery or driving are undertaken. Arthralgia, myalgia, and fever with rash and other symptoms suggestive of delayed hypersensitivity resembling serum sickness have been reported.

Extended release tablet: Insoluble tablet shell may remain intact and be visible in the stool.

Drug Interactions

Avoid Concomitant Use

Avoid concomitant use of BuPROPion with any of the following: MAO Inhibitors; Methylene Blue; Pimozide; Tamoxifen; Thioridazine

Decreased Effect

BuPROPion may decrease the levels/effects of: Codeine; Iloperidone; Ioflupane I 123; TraMADol

The levels/effects of BuPROPion may be decreased by: CYP2B6 Inducers (Strong); Cyproterone; Efavirenz; Lopinavir; Peginterferon Alfa-2b; Ritonavir; Tocilizumab

Increased Effect/Toxicity

BuPROPion may increase the levels/effects of: Alcohol (Ethyl); ARIPiprazole; Atomoxetine; CYP2D6 Substrates; Fesoterodine; Iloperidone; Methylene Blue; Nebivolol; Pimozide;

Propafenone; Tamoxifen; Tetrabenazine; Thioridazine; Tricyclic Antidepressants

The levels/effects of BuPROPion may be increased by: Alcohol (Ethyl); Conivaptan; CYP2B6 Inhibitors (Moderate); CYP2B6 Inhibitors (Strong); MAO Inhibitors; Quazepam

Nutritional/Ethanol Interactions

Ethanol: May increase CNS depression; monitor for increased effects with coadministration. Caution patients about effects.

Herb/Nutraceutical: Avoid valerian, St John's wort, SAMe, gotu kola, kava kava (may increase CNS depression).

Adverse Reactions Frequencies, when reported, reflect highest incidence reported with sustained release product.

>10%:

Cardiovascular: Tachycardia (11%)

Central nervous system: Headache (25% to 34%), insomnia (11% to 20%), dizziness (6% to 11%)

Gastrointestinal: Xerostomia (17% to 26%), weight loss (14% to 23%), nausea (1% to 18%)

Respiratory: Pharyngitis (3% to 13%)

1% to 10%:

Cardiovascular: Palpitation (2% to 6%), arrhythmias (5%), chest pain (3% to 4%), hypertension (2% to 4%; may be severe), flushing (1% to 4%), hypotension (3%)

Central nervous system: Agitation (2% to 9%), confusion (8%), anxiety (5% to 7%), hostility (6%), nervousness (3% to 5%), sleep disturbance (4%), sensory disturbance (4%), migraine (1% to 4%), abnormal dreams (3%), irritability (2% to 3%), somnolence (2% to 3%), pain (2% to 3%), memory decreased (≤3%), fever (1% to 2%), CNS stimulation (1% to 2%), depression

Dermatologic: Rash (1% to 5%), pruritus (2% to 4%), urticaria (1% to 2%)

Endocrine & metabolic: Menstrual complaints (2% to 5%), hot flashes (1% to 3%), libido decreased (3%)

Gastrointestinal: Constipation (5% to 10%), abdominal pain (2% to 9%), diarrhea (5% to 7%), flatulence (6%), anorexia (3% to 5%), appetite increased (4%), taste perversion (2% to 4%), vomiting (2% to 4%), dyspepsia (3%), dysphagia (≤2%)

Genitourinary: Polyuria (2% to 5%), urinary urgency (≤2%), vaginal hemorrhage (≤2%), UTI (≤1%)

Neuromuscular & skeletal: Tremor (3% to 6%), myalgia (2% to 6%), weakness (2% to 4%), arthralgia (1% to 4%), arthritis (2%), akathisia (≤2%), paresthesia (1% to 2%), twitching (1% to 2%), neck pain

Ocular: Blurred vision (2% to 3%), amblyopia (2%)

Otic: Tinnitus (3% to 6%), auditory disturbance (5%)

Respiratory: Upper respiratory infection (9%), cough increased (1% to 4%), sinusitis (1% to 5%)

Miscellaneous: Infection (8% to 9%), diaphoresis (5% to 6%), allergic reaction (including anaphylaxis, pruritus, urticaria)

Available Dosage Forms

Tablet, oral: 75 mg, 100 mg

Wellbutrin®: 75 mg, 100 mg

Tablet, extended release, oral: 100 mg, 150 mg, 200 mg, 300 mg

Aplenzin™: 174 mg, 348 mg, 522 mg

Budeprion SR®: 100 mg, 150 mg

Budeprion XL®: 300 mg

Buproban®: 150 mg

Wellbutrin XL®: 150 mg, 300 mg

Tablet, sustained release, oral:

Wellbutrin SR®: 100 mg, 150 mg, 200 mg

Zyban®: 150 mg

General Dosage Range Dosage adjustment recommended in patients with hepatic impairment

Oral:

Extended release: *Adults:*

Initial: Hydrochloride salt: 150 mg once daily; Maintenance: 300 mg once daily (maximum: 450 mg/day); Hydrobromide salt: 174-522 mg/day

Immediate release hydrochloride salt:

Adults: Initial: 100 mg twice daily; Maintenance: 100 mg 3 times/day (maximum: 450 mg/day)

Elderly: Initial: 37.5 mg twice daily, increase by 37.5-100 mg every 3-4 days as tolerated

Sustained release hydrochloride salt:

Adults: Initial: 150 mg once daily; Maintenance: 150 mg twice daily (maximum: 400 mg/day)

Elderly: Initial: 100 mg/day, increase by 37.5-100 mg every 3-4 days as tolerated

Administration

Oral May be taken without regard to meals. Zyban® and extended release tablets (hydrochloride and hydrobromide salt formulations) should be swallowed whole; do not crush, chew, or divide. The insoluble shell of the extended-release tablet may remain intact during GI transit and is eliminated in the feces.

Stability

Storage Store at controlled room temperature of 20°C to 25°C (68°F to 77°F).

Aplenzin™, Wellbutrin XL®: Store at 15°C to 30°C (59°F to 86°F).

Nursing Actions

Physical Assessment Perform careful cardiovascular assessment prior to initiating therapy. Monitor blood pressure at beginning of therapy and periodically throughout. Monitor for clinical worsening; neuropsychiatric symptoms, such as changes in behavior, hostility, agitation, and depression; and suicidality, especially at the beginning of therapy or when dose changes occur. Taper dosage slowly when discontinuing.

Patient Education Be aware that bupropion is marketed under different names and should not be taken together; Zyban® is for smoking cessation. Excessive use or abrupt discontinuation of alcohol or sedatives may lower seizure threshold.

Depression: Take in equally divided doses. Do not use alcohol. May cause drowsiness, clouded sensorium, headache, restlessness, agitation, nausea, vomiting, dry mouth, weight loss, constipation, or impotence (reversible). Report persistent CNS effects (eg, agitation, confusion, anxiety, restlessness, insomnia, psychosis, hallucinations, seizures); suicide ideation; muscle weakness or tremor; skin rash or irritation; chest pain or palpitations, abdominal pain or blood in stools; yellowing of skin or eyes; or respiratory difficulty, bronchitis, or unusual cough.

Smoking cessation: May cause dry mouth and insomnia (these may resolve with continued use). Report any respiratory difficulty, unusual cough, dizziness, changes in behavior, agitation, anxiety, suicide ideation, seizures, or muscle tremors.

BusPIRone (byoo SPYE rone)

Index Terms BuSpar; Buspirone Hydrochloride

Pharmacologic Category Antianxiety Agent, Miscellaneous

Medication Safety Issues

Sound-alike/look-alike issues:

BusPIRone may be confused with buPROPion

Pregnancy Risk Factor B

Lactation Excretion in breast milk unknown/not recommended

Use Management of generalized anxiety disorder (GAD)

Unlabeled Use Management of aggression in mental retardation and secondary mental disorders; major depression; potential augmenting agent for antidepressants; premenstrual syndrome

Mechanism of Action/Effect The mechanism of action of buspirone is unknown. Buspirone has a high affinity for serotonin 5-HT_{1A} and 5-HT_2 receptors, without affecting benzodiazepine-GABA receptors. Buspirone has moderate affinity for dopamine D_2 receptors.

Contraindications Hypersensitivity to buspirone or any component of the formulation

Warnings/Precautions Use in severe hepatic or renal impairment is not recommended; does not prevent or treat withdrawal from benzodiazepines. Low potential for cognitive or motor impairment. Use with MAO inhibitors may result in hypertensive reactions. Restlessness syndrome has been reported in small number of patients; monitor for signs of any dopamine-related movement disorders. Buspirone does not exhibit cross-tolerance with benzodiazepines or other sedative/hypnotic agents. If substituting buspirone for any of these agents, gradually withdraw the drug(s) prior to initiating buspirone. Safety and efficacy of buspirone have not been established in children <6 years of age; no long-term safety/efficacy data available in children.

Drug Interactions

Avoid Concomitant Use

Avoid concomitant use of BusPIRone with any of the following: Conivaptan; MAO Inhibitors; Methylene Blue

Decreased Effect

BusPIRone may decrease the levels/effects of: Ioflupane I 123

The levels/effects of BusPIRone may be decreased by: CYP3A4 Inducers (Strong); Deferasirox; Peginterferon Alfa-2b; Rifamycin Derivatives; Tocilizumab; Yohimbine

Increased Effect/Toxicity

BusPIRone may increase the levels/effects of: Alcohol (Ethyl); Antidepressants (Serotonin Reuptake Inhibitor/Antagonist); CNS Depressants; MAO Inhibitors; Methylene Blue; Metoclopramide; Selective Serotonin Reuptake Inhibitors; Serotonin Modulators

The levels/effects of BusPIRone may be increased by: Antifungal Agents (Azole Derivatives, Systemic); Antipsychotics; Calcium Channel Blockers (Nondihydropyridine); Conivaptan; CYP3A4 Inhibitors (Moderate); CYP3A4 Inhibitors (Strong); Dasatinib; Grapefruit Juice; HydrOXYzine; Ivacaftor; Macrolide Antibiotics; Selective Serotonin Reuptake Inhibitors

Nutritional/Ethanol Interactions

Ethanol: Ethanol may increase CNS depression. Management: Monitor for increased effects with coadministration. Caution patients about effects.

Food: Food may decrease the absorption of buspirone, but it may also decrease the first-pass metabolism, thereby increasing the bioavailability of buspirone. Grapefruit juice may cause increased buspirone concentrations. Management: Avoid intake of large quantities of grapefruit juice.

Herb/Nutraceutical: St John's wort may decrease buspirone levels or increase CNS depression. Kava kava, valerian, and gotu kola may increase CNS depression; yohimbe may diminish the therapeutic effect of buspirone. Management: Avoid St John's wort, kava kava, valerian, gotu kola, and yohimbe.

Adverse Reactions

>10%: Central nervous system: Dizziness (12%)

1% to 10%:

Cardiovascular: Chest pain (≥1%)

Central nervous system: Drowsiness (10%), headache (6%), nervousness (5%), lightheadedness (3%), anger/hostility (2%), confusion (2%), excitement (2%), dream disturbance (≥1%)

Dermatologic: Rash (1%)

Gastrointestinal: Nausea (8%), diarrhea (2%)

Neuromuscular & skeletal: Numbness (2%), weakness (2%), musculoskeletal pain (1%), paresthesia (1%), incoordination (1%), tremor (1%)
Ocular: Blurred vision (2%)
Otic: Tinnitus (≥1%)
Respiratory: Nasal congestion (≥1%), sore throat (≥1%)
Miscellaneous: Diaphoresis (1%)

Available Dosage Forms

Tablet, oral: 5 mg, 7.5 mg, 10 mg, 15 mg, 30 mg

General Dosage Range Oral:

Children ≥6 years: Initial: 5 mg daily; Maintenance: Up to 60 mg/day in 2-3 divided doses

Adults: Initial: 7.5 mg twice daily; Maintenance: Up to 60 mg/day in 2 divided doses (target dose: 10-15 mg twice daily)

Elderly: Initial: 5 mg twice daily; Maintenance: 20-30 mg/day (maximum: 60 mg/day)

Stability

Storage Store at USP controlled room temperature of 25°C (77°F). Protect from light.

Nursing Actions

Patient Education May take 2-3 weeks to see full effect; do not discontinue this medicine without consulting prescriber. Avoid large quantities of grapefruit juice. Maintain adequate hydration, unless instructed to restrict fluid intake. You may experience drowsiness, lightheadedness, impaired coordination, dizziness, blurred vision; upset stomach, or nausea. Report persistent vomiting, chest pain or rapid heartbeat, persistent CNS effects (eg, confusion, restlessness, anxiety, insomnia, excitation, headache, dizziness, fatigue, impaired coordination); or worsening of condition.

Dietary Considerations Avoid large quantities of grapefruit juice.

Busulfan (byoo SUL fan)

Brand Names: U.S. Busulfex®; Myleran®

Index Terms Bussulfam; Busulfanum; Busulphan

Pharmacologic Category Antineoplastic Agent, Alkylating Agent

Medication Safety Issues

Sound-alike/look-alike issues:

Myleran® may be confused with Alkeran®, Leukeran®, melphalan, Mylicon®

High alert medication:

This medication is in a class the Institute for Safe Medication Practices (ISMP) includes among its list of drug classes which have a heightened risk of causing significant patient harm when used in error.

Pregnancy Risk Factor D

Lactation Excretion in breast milk unknown/not recommended

Breast-Feeding Considerations According to the manufacturer, the decision to continue or discontinue breast-feeding during therapy should take into account the risk of exposure to the infant and the benefits of treatment to the mother.

Use Palliative treatment of chronic myelogenous leukemia (CML) (oral); conditioning regimen prior to allogeneic hematopoietic progenitor cell transplantation (I.V.) for CML

Unlabeled Use Conditioning regimen prior to hematopoietic stem cell transplant (HSCT) (oral); treatment of polycythemia vera and essential thrombocytosis

Mechanism of Action/Effect Alkylating agent which reacts with the N-7 position of guanosine and interferes with DNA replication and RNA transcription. Interferes with the normal function of DNA by alkylation and cross-linking the strands of DNA.

Contraindications Hypersensitivity to busulfan or any component of the formulation; oral busulfan is contraindicated in patients without a definitive diagnosis of CML

Warnings/Precautions Hazardous agent - use appropriate precautions for handling and disposal. **[U.S. Boxed Warning]: Severe bone marrow suppression is common; reduce dose or discontinue oral busulfan for unusual suppression; may require bone marrow biopsy.** May result in severe neutropenia, thrombocytopenia, anemia, bone marrow failure, and/or pancytopenia; pancytopenia may be prolonged (1 month up to 2 years) and may be reversible. Use with caution in patients with compromised bone marrow reserve (due to prior treatment or radiation therapy). Monitor closely for signs of infection (due to neutropenia) or bleeding (due to thrombocytopenia) Seizures have been reported with use; use caution in patients predisposed to seizures, history of seizures or head trauma; when using as a conditioning regimen for transplant, initiate prophylactic anticonvulsant therapy (eg, phenytoin) prior to treatment. Phenytoin increases busulfan clearance by ≥15%; busulfan kinetics and dosing recommendations for high-dose HSCT conditioning were studied with concomitant phenytoin. If alternate anticonvulsants are used, busulfan clearance may be decreased and dosing should be monitored accordingly.

Bronchopulmonary dysplasia with pulmonary fibrosis ("busulfan lung") is associated with busulfan; onset is delayed with symptoms occurring at an average of 4 years (range: 4 months to 10 years) after treatment; may be fatal. Symptoms generally include a slow onset of cough, dyspnea, and fever (low-grade), although acute symptomatic onset may also occur. Diminished diffusion capacity and decreased pulmonary compliance have been noted with pulmonary function testing. Differential diagnosis should rule out opportunistic pulmonary infection or leukemic pulmonary infiltrates; may require lung biopsy. Discontinue busulfan if toxicity develops. Pulmonary toxicity may be additive if administered with other cytotoxic agents also associated with pulmonary toxicity. Cardiac tamponade as been reported in children with thalassemia treated with high-dose oral busulfan in combination with cyclophosphamide. Busulfan has been causally related to the development of secondary malignancies (tumors and acute leukemias); chromosomal alterations may also occur. Busulfan has been associated with ovarian failure (including failure to achieve puberty).

High busulfan area under the concentration versus time curve (AUC) values (>1500 micromolar•minute) are associated with increased risk of hepatic sinusoidal obstruction syndrome (SOS; formerly called veno-occlusive disease [VOD]) due to conditioning for allogenic HSCT; patients with a history of radiation therapy, prior chemotherapy (≥3 cycles), or prior stem cell transplantation are at increased risk; monitor liver function tests periodically. Oral busulfan doses above 16 mg/kg (based on IBW) and concurrent use with alkylating agents may also increase the risk for hepatic SOS. The solvent in I.V. busulfan, DMA, may impair fertility. DMA may also be associated with hepatotoxicity, hallucinations, somnolence, lethargy, and confusion. **[U.S. Boxed Warning]: Should be administered under the supervision of an experienced cancer chemotherapy physician; for the I.V. formulation, should be experienced in management of HSCT and management of patients with severe pancytopenia; according to the manufacturer, oral busulfan should not be used until CML diagnosis has been established.** Cellular dysplasia in many organs has been observed (in addition to lung dysplasia); giant hyperchromatic nuclei have been noted in adrenal glands, liver, lymph nodes, pancreas, thyroid, and bone marrow. May obscure routine diagnostic cytologic exams (eg, cervical smear).

Drug Interactions

Avoid Concomitant Use

Avoid concomitant use of Busulfan with any of the following: BCG; CloZAPine; Conivaptan; Natalizumab; Pimecrolimus; Tacrolimus (Topical); Vaccines (Live)

Decreased Effect

Busulfan may decrease the levels/effects of: BCG; Coccidioidin Skin Test; Sipuleucel-T; Vaccines (Inactivated); Vaccines (Live); Vitamin K Antagonists

The levels/effects of Busulfan may be decreased by: CYP3A4 Inducers (Strong); Deferasirox; Echinacea; Fosphenytoin; Herbs (CYP3A4 Inducers); Phenytoin; Tocilizumab

Increased Effect/Toxicity

Busulfan may increase the levels/effects of: CloZAPine; Leflunomide; Natalizumab; Vaccines (Live); Vitamin K Antagonists

The levels/effects of Busulfan may be increased by: Acetaminophen; Antifungal Agents (Azole Derivatives, Systemic); Conivaptan; CYP3A4 Inhibitors (Moderate); CYP3A4 Inhibitors (Strong); Dasatinib; Denosumab; Ivacaftor; MetroNIDAZOLE; MetroNIDAZOLE (Systemic); Pimecrolimus; Roflumilast; Tacrolimus (Topical); Trastuzumab

Nutritional/Ethanol Interactions

Ethanol: Avoid ethanol due to GI irritation.

Food: No clear or firm data on the effect of food on busulfan bioavailability.

Herb/Nutraceutical: Avoid St John's wort (may decrease busulfan levels).

Adverse Reactions

I.V.:

>10%:

Cardiovascular: Tachycardia (44%), hypertension (36%; grades 3/4: 7%), edema (28% to 79%), thrombosis (33%), chest pain (26%), vasodilation (25%), hypotension (11%; grades 3/4: 3%)

Central nervous system: Insomnia (84%), fever (80%), anxiety (72% to 75%), headache (69%), chills (46%), pain (44%), dizziness (30%), depression (23%), confusion (11%)

Dermatologic: Rash (57%), pruritus (28%), alopecia (17%)

Endocrine & metabolic: Hypomagnesemia (77%), hyperglycemia (66% to 67%; grades 3/4: 15%), hypokalemia (64%), hypocalcemia (49%), hypophosphatemia (17%)

Gastrointestinal: Vomiting (43% to 100%), nausea (83% to 98%), mucositis/stomatitis (79% to 97%; grades 3/4: 26%), anorexia (85%), diarrhea (84%; grades 3/4: 5%), abdominal pain (72%), dyspepsia (44%), constipation (38%), xerostomia (26%), rectal disorder (25%), abdominal fullness (23%)

Hematologic: Myelosuppression (≤100%), neutropenia (100%; onset: 4 days; median recovery: 13 days [with G-CSF support]), thrombocytopenia (98%; median onset: 5-6 days), lymphopenia (children: 79%), anemia (69%)

Hepatic: Hyperbilirubinemia (49%; grades 3/4: 30%), ALT increased (31%; grades 3/4: 7%), hepatic sinusoidal obstruction syndrome (SOS; veno-occlusive disease) (adults: 8% to 12%; children: 21%), alkaline phosphatase increased (15%), jaundice (12%)

Local: Injection site inflammation (25%), injection site pain (15%)

Neuromuscular & skeletal: Weakness (51%), back pain (23%), myalgia (16%), arthralgia (13%)

Renal: Creatinine increased (21%), oliguria (15%)

Respiratory: Rhinitis (44%), lung disorder (34%), cough (28%), epistaxis (25%), dyspnea (25%), pneumonia (children: 21%), hiccup (18%), pharyngitis (18%)

Miscellaneous: Infection (51%; includes severe bacterial, viral [CMV], and fungal infections), allergic reaction (26%)

1% to 10%:

Cardiovascular: Arrhythmia (5%), cardiomegaly (5%), atrial fibrillation (2%), ECG abnormal (2%), heart block (2%), heart failure (grade 3/4: 2%), pericardial effusion (2%), tamponade (children with thalassemia: 2%), ventricular extrasystoles (2%), hypervolemia

Central nervous system: Lethargy (7%), hallucination (5%), agitation (2%), delirium (2%), encephalopathy (2%), seizure (2%), somnolence (2%), cerebral hemorrhage (1%)

Dermatologic: Vesicular rash (10%), vesiculobullous rash (10%), skin discoloration (8%), maculopapular rash (8%), acne (7%), exfoliative dermatitis (5%), erythema nodosum (2%)

Endocrine & metabolic: Hyponatremia (2%)

Gastrointestinal: Ileus (8%), weight gain (8%), esophagitis (grade 3: 2%), hematemesis (2%), pancreatitis (2%)

Hematologic: Prothrombin time increased (2%)

Hepatic: Hepatomegaly (6%)

Renal: Hematuria (8%), dysuria (7%), hemorrhagic cystitis (grade 3/4: 7%), BUN increased (3%; grades 3/4: 2%)

Respiratory: Asthma (8%), alveolar hemorrhage (5%), hyperventilation (5%), hemoptysis (3%), pleural effusion (3%), sinusitis (3%), atelectasis (2%), hypoxia (2%)

Oral: Frequency not defined:

Dermatologic: Hyperpigmentation of skin (5% to 10%), rash

Endocrine & metabolic: Amenorrhea, ovarian suppression

Gastrointestinal: Xerostomia

Hematologic: Myelosuppression (anemia, leukopenia, thrombocytopenia)

Available Dosage Forms

Injection, solution:

Busulfex®: 6 mg/mL (10 mL)

Tablet, oral:

Myleran®: 2 mg

General Dosage Range

I.V.:

Children ≤12 kg: **HSCT:** 1.1 mg/kg (actual body weight) every 6 hours for 16 doses

Children >12 kg: **HSCT:**0.8 mg/kg (actual body weight) every 6 hours for 16 doses

Adults: **HSCT:** 0.8 mg/kg every 6 hours for 16 doses (use ideal body weight or actual body weight, whichever is lower; use adjusted body weight if obese)

Oral: Dosage adjustment is recommended in patients who experience toxicity:

Children: Induction: 60 mcg/kg/day **or** 1.8 mg/m^2/day; Maintenance: Resume induction dose **or** 1-3 mg/day

Adults: Induction: 60 mcg/kg/day **or** 1.8 mg/m^2/day; usual range: 4-8 mg/day; Maintenance: Resume induction dose **or** 1-3 mg/day

Administration

Oral HSCT only: To facilitate ingestion of high oral doses, may insert multiple tablets into gelatin capsules.

I.V. Intravenous busulfan should be infused over 2 hours via central line. Flush line before and after each infusion with 5 mL D_5W or NS. Do not use polycarbonate syringes or filters for preparation or administration

Stability

Reconstitution Injection: Dilute NS or D_5W. The dilution volume should be ten times the volume of busulfan injection, ensuring that the final concentration of busulfan is 0.5 mg/mL. Always add busulfan to the diluent, and not the diluent to the busulfan. Mix with several inversions. Do not use polycarbonate syringes or filters for preparation or administration.

Storage

Injection: Store intact vials under refrigeration at 2°C to 8°C (36°F to 46°F). Solutions diluted in sodium chloride (NS) injection or dextrose 5% in water (D_5W) for infusion are stable for up to 8 hours at room temperature (25°C [77°F]); the infusion must also be completed within that 8-hour timeframe. Dilution of busulfan injection in NS is stable for up to 12 hours at refrigeration (2°C to 8°C); the infusion must be completed within that 12-hour timeframe.

Tablet: Store at 25°C (77°F); excursions permitted to 15°C to 30°C (59°F to 86°F).

Nursing Actions

Physical Assessment HSCT: Phenytoin or clonazepam may be ordered prophylactically during and for at least 48 hours following completion of busulfan to reduce risk of seizures if patient is predisposed to seizures. Assess CBC with differential, platelet count, and LFTs. Monitor for pulmonary fibrosis or toxicity, adverse hematologic effects, pancytopenia, leukopenia, thrombocytopenia, anemia, and bone marrow suppression during therapy and for several months following therapy.

Patient Education Maintain adequate nutrition and hydration, unless instructed to restrict fluid intake. Avoid excess alcohol and acidic or spicy foods (may increase gastrointestinal irritation). You will be more susceptible to infection. May cause dizziness, insomnia, or confusion; mouth sores; loss of hair or darkening of skin color (reversible when medication is discontinued); nausea, vomiting, or loss of appetite; constipation; diarrhea (consult prescriber if severe or persistent); amenorrhea; sterility; or skin rash. Report palpitations or chest pain, weight gain, CNS changes (anxiety, confusion, depression), unusual cough or difficulty breathing, numbness or tingling of extremities, unusual bruising or bleeding, or pain or changes in urination.

Related Information

Management of Drug Extravasations *on page 1269*

Butalbital, Acetaminophen, and Caffeine (byoo TAL bi tal, a seet a MIN oh fen, & KAF een)

Brand Names: U.S. Alagesic LQ; Anolor 300; Dolgic® Plus; Esgic-Plus™; Esgic®; Fioricet®; Margesic; Orbivan™; Repan®; Zebutal®

Index Terms Acetaminophen, Butalbital, and Caffeine

Pharmacologic Category Barbiturate

Medication Safety Issues

Sound-alike/look-alike issues:

Fioricet® may be confused with Fiorinal®, Florinef®, Lorcet®, Percocet®

Repan® may be confused with Riopan®

Other safety concerns:

Duplicate therapy issues: This product contains acetaminophen, which may be a component of other combination products. Do not exceed the maximum recommended daily dose of acetaminophen.

Pregnancy Risk Factor C

Lactation Enters breast milk/not recommended

Use Relief of the symptomatic complex of tension or muscle contraction headache

Available Dosage Forms

Capsule, oral:

Anolor 300, Esgic®, Margesic: Butalbital 50 mg, acetaminophen 325 mg, and caffeine 40 mg

Esgic-Plus™, Zebutal®: Butalbital 50 mg, acetaminophen 500 mg, and caffeine 40 mg

Orbivan™: Butalbital 50 mg, acetaminophen 300 mg, and caffeine 40 mg

Liquid, oral:

Alagesic LQ: Butalbital 50 mg, acetaminophen 325 mg, and caffeine 40 mg per 15 mL

Tablet, oral: Butalbital 50 mg, acetaminophen 325 mg, and caffeine 40 mg; butalbital 50 mg, acetaminophen 500 mg, and caffeine 40 mg

Dolgic® Plus: Butalbital 50 mg, acetaminophen 750 mg, and caffeine 40 mg

Esgic®, Fioricet®, Repan®: Butalbital 50 mg, acetaminophen 325 mg, and caffeine 40 mg

Esgic-Plus™: Butalbital 50 mg, acetaminophen 500 mg, and caffeine 40 mg

General Dosage Range Oral: *Adults:* 1-2 tablets/capsules or 15-30 mL every 4 hours (maximum: 6 tablets/capsules daily; 180 mL/day)

Nursing Actions

Physical Assessment See individual agents.

Patient Education See individual agents.

Related Information

Acetaminophen *on page 23*

Caffeine *on page 169*

Butalbital, Acetaminophen, Caffeine, and Codeine (byoo TAL bi tal, a seet a MIN oh fen, KAF een, & KOE deen)

Brand Names: U.S. Fioricet® with Codeine

Index Terms Acetaminophen, Caffeine, Codeine, and Butalbital; Caffeine, Acetaminophen, Butalbital, and Codeine; Codeine, Acetaminophen, Butalbital, and Caffeine

Pharmacologic Category Analgesic Combination (Opioid); Barbiturate

Medication Safety Issues

Sound-alike/look-alike issues:

Fioricet® may be confused with Fiorinal®, Florinef®, Lorcet®, Percocet®

Phrenilin may be confused with Phenergan®

High alert medication:

The Institute for Safe Medication Practices (ISMP) includes this medication among its list of drug classes which have a heightened risk of causing significant patient harm when used in error.

Other safety concerns:

Duplicate therapy issues: This product contains acetaminophen, which may be a component of other combination products. Do not exceed the maximum recommended daily dose of acetaminophen.

Pregnancy Risk Factor C (per manufacturer)

Lactation Enters breast milk/not recommended

Use Relief of symptoms of complex tension (muscle contraction) headache

Controlled Substance C-III

Available Dosage Forms

Capsule: Butalbital 50 mg, acetaminophen 325 mg, caffeine 40 mg, and codeine 30 mg

Fioricet® with Codeine: Butalbital 50 mg, acetaminophen 325 mg, caffeine 40 mg, and codeine 30 mg

General Dosage Range Oral: *Adults:* 1-2 capsules every 4 hours (maximum: 6 capsules/day)

Nursing Actions

Physical Assessment See individual agents.

Patient Education See individual agents.

Related Information

Acetaminophen *on page 23*

Caffeine *on page 169*

Codeine *on page 268*

Butalbital and Acetaminophen (byoo TAL bi tal & a seet a MIN oh fen)

Brand Names: U.S. Bupap; Cephadyn; Phrenilin®; Phrenilin® Forte; Promacet; Sedapap®

Index Terms Acetaminophen and Butalbital

Pharmacologic Category Analgesic, Miscellaneous; Barbiturate

Medication Safety Issues

Other safety concerns:

Duplicate therapy issues: This product contains acetaminophen, which may be a component of other combination products. Do not exceed the maximum recommended daily dose of acetaminophen.

Pregnancy Risk Factor C

Lactation Enters breast milk/not recommended

Use Relief of the symptomatic complex of tension or muscle contraction headache

Available Dosage Forms

Tablet:

Phrenilin®: Butalbital 50 mg and acetaminophen 325 mg

Bupap, Cephadyn, Promacet, Sedapap®: Butalbital 50 mg and acetaminophen 650 mg

Capsule:

Phrenilin® Forte: Butalbital 50 mg and acetaminophen 650 mg

General Dosage Range Oral: *Adults:* 1 tablet/capsule every 4 hours as needed (maximum: 6 doses/day) **or** Phrenilin®: 1-2 tablets every 4 hours as needed (maximum: 6 tablets/day)

Nursing Actions

Physical Assessment See individual agents.

Patient Education See individual agents.

Related Information

Acetaminophen *on page 23*

PHENobarbital *on page 909*

Butalbital, Aspirin, and Caffeine

(byoo TAL bi tal, AS pir in, & KAF een)

Brand Names: U.S. Fiorinal®

Index Terms Aspirin, Caffeine, and Butalbital; Butalbital Compound

Pharmacologic Category Barbiturate

Medication Safety Issues

Sound-alike/look-alike issues:

Fiorinal® may be confused with Fioricet®, Florical®, Florinef®

Pregnancy Risk Factor C/D (prolonged use or high doses at term)

Lactation Enters breast milk/use caution due to aspirin content

Use Relief of the symptomatic complex of tension or muscle contraction headache

Controlled Substance C-III

Available Dosage Forms

Capsule: Butalbital 50 mg, aspirin 325 mg, and caffeine 40 mg

Fiorinal®: Butalbital 50 mg, aspirin 325 mg, and caffeine 40 mg

Tablet: Butalbital 50 mg, aspirin 325 mg, and caffeine 40 mg

General Dosage Range Oral: *Adults:* 1-2 tablets/capsules every 4 hours (maximum: 6 tablets/capsules daily)

Nursing Actions

Physical Assessment See individual agents.

Patient Education See individual agents.

Related Information

Aspirin *on page 94*

Caffeine *on page 169*

Butalbital, Aspirin, Caffeine, and Codeine

(byoo TAL bi tal, AS pir in, KAF een, & KOE deen)

Brand Names: U.S. Ascomp® with Codeine; Fiorinal® with Codeine

Index Terms Aspirin, Caffeine, Codeine, and Butalbital; Butalbital Compound and Codeine; Codeine and Butalbital Compound; Codeine, Butalbital, Aspirin, and Caffeine

Pharmacologic Category Analgesic Combination (Opioid); Barbiturate

Medication Safety Issues

Sound-alike/look-alike issues:

Fiorinal® may be confused with Fioricet®, Florical®, Florinef®

High alert medication:

The Institute for Safe Medication Practices (ISMP) includes this medication among its list of drug classes which have a heightened risk of causing significant patient harm when used in error.

Pregnancy Risk Factor C (per manufacturer)

Lactation Enters breast milk/not recommended

Use Relief of symptoms of complex tension (muscle contraction) headache

Controlled Substance C-III

Available Dosage Forms

Capsule: Butalbital 50 mg, aspirin 325 mg, caffeine 40 mg, and codeine 30 mg

Ascomp® with Codeine, Fiorinal® with Codeine: Butalbital 50 mg, aspirin 325 mg, caffeine 40 mg, and codeine 30 mg

General Dosage Range Oral: *Adults:* 1-2 capsules every 4 hours as needed (maximum: 6 capsules/day)

Nursing Actions

Physical Assessment See individual agents.

Patient Education See individual agents.

Related Information

Aspirin *on page 94*

Caffeine *on page 169*

Codeine *on page 268*

Butorphanol

(byoo TOR fa nole)

Index Terms Butorphanol Tartrate; Stadol

Pharmacologic Category Analgesic, Opioid; Analgesic, Opioid Partial Agonist

Medication Safety Issues

Sound-alike/look-alike issues:

Stadol may be confused with Haldol®, sotalol

High alert medication:

The Institute for Safe Medication Practices (ISMP) includes this medication among its list of drug classes which have a heightened risk of causing significant patient harm when used in error.

Pregnancy Risk Factor C

Lactation Enters breast milk (AAP rates "compatible"; AAP 2001 update pending)

Use

Parenteral: Management of moderate-to-severe pain; preoperative medication; supplement to balanced anesthesia; management of pain during labor

Nasal spray: Management of moderate-to-severe pain, including migraine headache pain

Controlled Substance C-IV

Available Dosage Forms

Injection, solution: 1 mg/mL (1 mL); 2 mg/mL (1 mL, 2 mL, 10 mL)

Injection, solution [preservative free]: 1 mg/mL (1 mL); 2 mg/mL (1 mL, 2 mL)

Solution, intranasal: 10 mg/mL (2.5 mL)

General Dosage Range Dosage adjustment recommended in patients with hepatic or renal impairment

I.M.:

Adults: Initial: 2 mg, may repeat every 3-4 hours as needed; Usual range: 1-4 mg every 3-4 hours as needed **or** 2 mg prior to surgery

Elderly: Initial: 1/2 of the recommended dose, repeated dosing generally should be at least 6 hours apart

I.V.:

Adults: Initial: 1 mg, may repeat every 3-4 hours as needed; Usual range: 0.5-2 mg every 3-4 hours as needed **or** 2 mg and/or an incremental dose of 0.5-1 mg (up to 0.06 mg/kg) as supplement to surgery

Elderly: Initial: 1/2 of the recommended dose, repeated dosing generally should be at least 6 hours apart

Intranasal:

Adults: Initial: 1 spray (~1 mg) in 1 nostril, may repeat in 60-90 minutes, then repeat initial dose sequence in 3-4 hours after last dose as needed; may use initial dose of 1 spray in each nostril (2 mg) in patients who will remain recumbent

Elderly: Initial: Should not exceed 1 mg, may repeat after 90-120 minutes

Administration

I.V. Detail pH: 3.0-5.5

Inhalation See Dosing.

Other Intranasal: Consider avoiding simultaneous intranasal migraine sprays; may want to separate by at least 30 minutes

Nursing Actions

Physical Assessment Monitor for effectiveness of pain relief. Monitor blood pressure, CNS and respiratory status, and degree of sedation prior to treatment and periodically throughout. For inpatients, implement safety measures (eg, side rails up, call light within reach, instructions to call for assistance). Assess patient's physical and/or psychological dependence. Discontinue slowly after prolonged use.

Patient Education May cause physical and/or psychological dependence. Do not use alcohol, sedatives, tranquilizers, antihistamines, or pain medications without consulting prescriber. May cause dizziness, drowsiness, confusion, or blurred vision; nausea or vomiting; or loss of appetite. Report unresolved nausea or vomiting; respiratory difficulty or shortness of breath; restlessness, insomnia, euphoria, or nightmares; excessive sedation or unusual weakness; facial flushing, rapid heartbeat, or palpitations; urinary difficulty; or vision changes.

Nasal administration: Do not use more frequently than prescribed. Blow nose prior to administering. Follow instructions on package insert. Insert nozzle of applicator gently into one nostril and exhale. With next breath, squeeze applicator once firmly and quickly once as you breath in. If adequate relief from headache is not achieved within 60-90 minutes, an additional 1 spray may be given. May be repeated in 3-4 hours following last dose, as needed. **Alternatively:** Two sprays may be given, one spray in each nostril, if you are able to remain lying down (in the event of drowsiness or dizziness). Additional doses should not be taken for 3-4 hours. Avoid using simultaneously with other intranasal migraine sprays. Separate by at least 30 minutes.

Related Information

Compatibility of Drugs *on page 1264*

Cabazitaxel (ca baz i TAKS el)

Brand Names: U.S. Jevtana®

Index Terms RPR-116258A; XRP6258

Pharmacologic Category Antineoplastic Agent, Antimicrotubular; Antineoplastic Agent, Taxane Derivative

Medication Safety Issues

High alert medication:

This medication is in a class the Institute for Safe Medication Practices (ISMP) includes among its list of drugs which have a heightened risk of causing significant patient harm when used in error.

Administration issues:

Cabazitaxel requires a two-step dilution process prior to administration.

Pregnancy Risk Factor D

Lactation Excretion in breast milk unknown/not recommended

Use Treatment of hormone-refractory metastatic prostate cancer (in patients previously treated with a docetaxel-containing regimen)

Available Dosage Forms

Injection, solution:

Jevtana®: 40 mg/mL (1.5 mL)

General Dosage Range Dosage adjustment recommended in patients with hepatic impairment or who develop toxicities

I.V.: *Adults:* 25 mg/m^2 once every 3 weeks

Administration

I.V. Infuse over 1 hour using a 0.22 micron inline filter. Do not use polyurethane-containing infusion sets for administration. Allow to reach room temperature prior to infusion. Premedicate with an antihistamine, a corticosteroid, and an H_2 antagonist at least 30 minutes prior to infusion. Observe closely during infusion (for hypersensitivity). Antiemetic prophylaxis (oral or I.V.) is also recommended.

Nursing Actions

Physical Assessment Monitor patient closely for hypersensitivity reaction (rash, erythema, hypotension, bronchospasm); discontinue and notify prescriber. Monitor for hypersensitivity, hypotension, myelosuppression, and GI irritation (including severe diarrhea) prior to, during, and between each infusion.

Patient Education This drug is only administered by intravenous infusion; you will be monitored closely during and following infusions. Immediately report any burning, pain, or swelling at infusion site; any unusual chest pain or tightness, rapid heartbeat, or palpitations; difficulty breathing; difficulty swallowing; or nausea or vomiting during infusion. You will be more susceptible to infection. It is important that you maintain adequate nutrition and fluid intake, unless instructed to restrict fluid intake. May cause fatigue, dizziness, headache, gastrointestinal upset, or loss of hair (will grow back after therapy). Report chest pain, palpitations, or swelling of extremities; difficult breathing; pain or decreased sensation in extremities; or unusual sign of weakness.

Cabergoline (ca BER goe leen)

Pharmacologic Category Ergot Derivative

Pregnancy Risk Factor B

Lactation Excretion in breast milk unknown/not recommended

Use Treatment of hyperprolactinemic disorders, either idiopathic or due to pituitary adenomas

Canadian labeling: Additional use (not in U.S. labeling): Prevention of the onset of physiological lactation in the puerperium when clinically indicated (eg, still born baby or neonatal death, conditions that interfere with suckling, severe acute or chronic mental illness). Note: Not indicated for suppression of established postpartum lactation.

Available Dosage Forms

Tablet, oral: 0.5 mg

General Dosage Range Oral: *Adults:* Initial: 0.25 mg twice weekly; Maintenance: Up to 1 mg twice weekly

Administration

Oral Administer with meals (may increase tolerability).

Caffeine (KAF een)

Brand Names: U.S. Cafcit®; Enerjets [OTC]; No Doz® Maximum Strength [OTC]; Vivarin® [OTC]

Index Terms Caffeine and Sodium Benzoate; Caffeine Citrate; Caffeine Sodium Benzoate; Sodium Benzoate and Caffeine

Pharmacologic Category Stimulant

Pregnancy Risk Factor C

Lactation Enters breast milk/use caution (AAP rates "compatible"; AAP 2001 update pending)

Use

Caffeine citrate: Treatment of idiopathic apnea of prematurity

Caffeine and sodium benzoate: Treatment of acute respiratory depression (not a preferred agent)

Caffeine [OTC labeling]: Restore mental alertness or wakefulness when experiencing fatigue

Unlabeled Use Caffeine and sodium benzoate: Treatment of spinal puncture headache; CNS stimulant; diuretic; augmentation of seizure induction during electroconvulsive therapy (ECT)

Available Dosage Forms

Caplet:

No Doz® Maximum Strength [OTC], Vivarin® [OTC]: 200 mg

Injection, solution [preservative free]: 20 mg/mL (3 mL)

Cafcit®: 20 mg/mL (3 mL)

Lozenge:

Enerjets® [OTC]: 75 mg

Solution, oral [preservative free]: 20 mg/mL (3 mL)

Cafcit®: 20 mg/mL

Tablet: 200 mg

Vivarin® [OTC]: 200 mg

General Dosage Range

I.M. (caffeine and sodium benzoate):

Children: 8 mg/kg every 4 hours as needed

Adults: 250 mg as a single dose; may repeat as needed (maximum: 500 mg/dose; 2500 mg/day)

I.V.:

Neonates (caffeine citrate): Loading dose: 10-20 mg/kg; Maintenance: 5 mg/kg once daily

Children (caffeine and sodium benzoate): 8 mg/kg every 4 hours as needed

Adults (caffeine and sodium benzoate): 250 mg as a single dose; may repeat as needed (maximum: 500 mg/dose; 2500 mg/day) **or** 300-2000 mg (electroconvulsive therapy)

Oral:

Neonates (caffeine citrate): Loading dose: 10-20 mg/kg; Maintenance: 5 mg/kg once daily

Children ≥12 years and Adults: 100-200 mg every 3-4 hours as needed (OTC labeling)

SubQ (caffeine and sodium benzoate): *Children:* 8 mg/kg every 4 hours as needed

Administration

Oral May be administered without regard to feedings or meals. May administer injectable formulation (caffeine citrate) orally.

I.M. Parenteral: **Caffeine and sodium benzoate:** May administer I.M. undiluted

I.V. Parenteral:

Caffeine citrate: Infuse loading dose over at least 30 minutes; maintenance dose may be infused over at least 10 minutes. May administer without dilution or diluted with D_5W to 10 mg caffeine citrate/mL.

Caffeine and sodium benzoate: I.V. as slow direct injection. For spinal headaches, dilute in 1000 mL NS and infuse over 1 hour. Follow with 1000 mL NS; infuse over 1 hour. May administer I.M. undiluted.

Nursing Actions

Patient Education You may experience excitability, flushing, dizziness, insomnia, or agitation. Report excessive excitability or nervousness, chest pain, or respiratory difficulty.

Calcipotriene (kal si POE try een)

Brand Names: U.S. Calcitrene™; Dovonex®

Pharmacologic Category Topical Skin Product; Vitamin D Analog

Pregnancy Risk Factor C

Lactation Excretion in breast milk unknown/use caution

Use Treatment of plaque psoriasis; chronic, moderate-to-severe psoriasis of the scalp

Unlabeled Use Vitiligo

Available Dosage Forms

Cream, topical:

Dovonex®: 0.005% (60 g, 120 g)

Ointment, topical:

Calcitrene™: 0.005% (60 g)

Solution, topical: 0.005% (60 mL)

Dovonex®: 0.005% (60 mL)

General Dosage Range Topical: *Adults:* Cream, solution: Apply a thin film to affected area 2 times/day; Ointment: Apply a thin film to affected area 1-2 times/day

Administration

Topical For external use only.

Cream, ointment: Apply to affected skin; rub in gently and completely. Wash hands thoroughly before and after use.

Solution: Prior to using scalp solution, comb hair to remove debris; apply only to lesions. Rub in gently and completely. Avoid solution spreading or dripping onto forehead. Avoid contact with eyes. Wash hands thoroughly before and after use.

Nursing Actions

Physical Assessment When applied to large areas of skin or for extensive periods of time, monitor for adverse skin or systemic reactions.

Patient Education For external use only. Before using, wash and dry area gently. Wear gloves to apply a thin film to affected area and rub in gently. If dressing is necessary, use a porous dressing. Avoid contact with eyes. Avoid exposing treated area to direct sunlight; sunburn can occur. Report increased swelling, redness, rash, itching, signs of infection, worsening of condition, or lack of healing.

Calcipotriene and Betamethasone

(kal si POE try een & bay ta METH a sone)

Brand Names: U.S. Taclonex Scalp®; Taclonex®

Index Terms Betamethasone Dipropionate and Calcipotriene Hydrate; Calcipotriol and Betamethasone Dipropionate

Pharmacologic Category Corticosteroid, Topical; Vitamin D Analog

Pregnancy Risk Factor C

Lactation Excretion in breast milk unknown/use caution

Use Treatment of psoriasis vulgaris

Unlabeled Use Treatment of corticosteroid-responsive dermatoses

Available Dosage Forms

Ointment, topical:

Taclonex®: Calcipotriene 0.005% and betamethasone 0.064% (60 g, 100 g)

Suspension, topical:

Taclonex Scalp®: Calcipotriene 0.005% and betamethasone 0.064%

General Dosage Range Topical: *Adults:* Apply to affected area once daily (maximum: 100 g/week)

Administration

Topical Wash hands before and after use.

Gel (Xamiol® [CAN]): Shake well before use. Avoid use of occlusive dressings over treated areas.

Ointment: Rub into affected area gently and completely. Do not apply to face, axillae, or groin.

Suspension: Shake well before use. Do not apply within 12 hours of chemical hair treatment. Do not wash hair directly after use.

Nursing Actions

Physical Assessment See individual agents.

Patient Education See individual agents.

Related Information
Betamethasone *on page 128*
Calcipotriene *on page 170*

Calcitonin (kal si TOE nin)

Brand Names: U.S. Fortical®; Miacalcin®
Index Terms Calcitonin (Salmon)
Pharmacologic Category Antidote; Hormone
Medication Safety Issues
Sound-alike/look-alike issues:
Calcitonin may be confused with calcitriol
Miacalcin® may be confused with Micatin®
Administration issues:
Calcitonin nasal spray is administered as a single spray into **one** nostril daily, using alternate nostrils each day.

Pregnancy Risk Factor C
Lactation Excretion in breast milk unknown/not recommended
Use Treatment of Paget's disease of bone (osteitis deformans); adjunctive therapy for hypercalcemia; treatment of osteoporosis in women >5 years postmenopause
Available Dosage Forms
Injection, solution:
Miacalcin®: 200 int. units/mL (2 mL)
Solution, intranasal: 200 int. units/actuation (3.7 mL)
Fortical®: 200 int. units/actuation (3.7 mL)
Miacalcin®: 200 int. units/actuation (3.7 mL)

General Dosage Range
I.M., SubQ: *Adults:* Paget's disease/osteoporosis: 50-100 units every 1-3 days; Hypercalcemia: 4-8 units/kg every 12 hours (maximum: 8 units/kg every 6 hours)
Intranasal: *Adults:* 200 units (1 spray) in one nostril daily

Administration
I.M. Injection solution: May be administered I.M. or SubQ; I.M route is preferred if the injection volume is >2 mL.
Inhalation Nasal spray: Before first use, allow bottle to reach room temperature, then prime pump by releasing at least 5 sprays until full spray is produced. To administer, place nozzle into nostril with head in upright position. Alternate nostrils daily. Do not prime pump before each daily use. Discard after 30 doses.
Other Injection solution: May be administered I.M. or SubQ. SubQ route is preferred for outpatient self-administration unless the injection volume is >2 mL.

Nursing Actions
Physical Assessment Teach patient appropriate administration techniques. Monitor for allergic reaction if calcitonin solution (Miacalcin®) used.
Patient Education If administered by injection, you will be instructed on how to give the injections and dispose of syringes/needles (follow directions exactly). May cause increased warmth and flushing (this should only last about 1 hour after administration; taking drug in evening may minimize these discomforts). Report significant nasal irritation if using nasal spray. Immediately report chest pain, depression, unresolved nausea or constipation, skin rash, palpitations, or respiratory difficulty.

Calcitriol (kal si TRYE ole)

Brand Names: U.S. Calcijex®; Rocaltrol®; Vectical®
Index Terms 1,25 Dihydroxycholecalciferol
Pharmacologic Category Vitamin D Analog
Medication Safety Issues
Sound-alike/look-alike issues:
Calcitriol may be confused with alfacalcidol, Calciferol™, calcitonin, calcium carbonate, captopril, colestipol, paricalcitol, ropinirole
Administration issues:
Dosage is expressed in mcg (micrograms), **not** mg (milligrams); rare cases of acute overdose have been reported

Pregnancy Risk Factor C
Lactation Enters breast milk/not recommended
Use
Oral, injection: Management of hypocalcemia in patients on chronic renal dialysis; management of secondary hyperparathyroidism in patients with chronic kidney disease (CKD); management of hypocalcemia in hypoparathyroidism and pseudohypoparathyroidism
Topical: Management of mild-to-moderate plaque psoriasis

Unlabeled Use Decrease severity of psoriatic lesions in psoriatic vulgaris; vitamin D-dependent rickets
Available Dosage Forms
Capsule, softgel, oral: 0.25 mcg, 0.5 mcg
Rocaltrol®: 0.25 mcg, 0.5 mcg
Injection, solution: 1 mcg/mL (1 mL)
Calcijex®: 1 mcg/mL (1 mL)
Ointment, topical:
Vectical®: 3 mcg/g (100 g)
Solution, oral: 1 mcg/mL (15 mL)
Rocaltrol®: 1 mcg/mL (15 mL)

General Dosage Range Dosage adjustment recommended in patients who develop toxicities
I.V.: *Adults:* 0.5-4 mcg 3 times/week
Oral:
Children: 0.25-0.2 mcg/day **or** 0.01-0.015 mcg/kg/day (maximum: 0.5 mcg/day)
Adults: 0.25 mcg every other day to 2 mcg once daily
Topical: *Adults:* Apply to affected areas twice daily (maximum: 200 g/week)

Administration
Oral May be administered without regard to food. Administer with meals to reduce GI problems.

I.V. May be administered as a bolus dose I.V. through the catheter at the end of hemodialysis.

I.V. Detail pH: 5.9-7.0

Topical Apply externally; not for ophthalmic, oral, or intravaginal use. Do not apply to eyes, lips, or facial skins. Rub in gently so that no medication remains visible. Limit application to only the areas of skin affected by psoriasis.

Nursing Actions

Physical Assessment Provide appropriate nutritional counseling.

Patient Education Maintain recommended diet and calcium supplementation. You may experience nausea, vomiting, loss of appetite, or metallic taste. Report CNS changes, unusual weakness or fatigue, or persistent nausea or vomiting.

Topical: Avoid or limit excessive exposure to sun or phototherapy. Protect skin with sunblock and protective clothing.

Calcium Chloride (KAL see um KLOR ide)

Pharmacologic Category Calcium Salt; Electrolyte Supplement, Parenteral

Medication Safety Issues

Sound-alike/look-alike issues:

Calcium chloride may be confused with calcium gluconate

Administration issues:

Calcium chloride may be confused with calcium gluconate.

Confusion with the different intravenous salt forms of calcium has occurred. There is a three-fold difference in the primary cation concentration between calcium chloride (in which 1g = 13.6 mEq [270 mg] of elemental Ca++) and calcium gluconate (in which 1g = 4.65 mEq [90 mg] of elemental Ca++).

Prescribers should specify which salt form is desired. Dosages should be expressed either as mEq, mg, or grams of the salt form.

Pregnancy Risk Factor C

Use Treatment of acute symptomatic hypocalcemia; cardiac disturbances of hyperkalemia or hypocalcemia; emergent treatment of hypocalcemic tetany; treatment of severe hypermagnesemia

Unlabeled Use Calcium channel blocker overdose; beta-blocker overdose; severe hyperkalemia (K+ >6.5 mEq/L with toxic ECG changes) [ACLS guidelines]; malignant arrhythmias (including cardiac arrest) associated with hypermagnesemia [ACLS guidelines]

Available Dosage Forms

Injection, solution: 10% (10 mL)

Injection, solution [preservative free]: 10% (10 mL)

General Dosage Range I.V.:

Infants and Children: 10-20 mg/kg **or** 35-50 mg/kg every 6-8 hours **or** 32 mg for each 100 mL of citrated blood infused

Adults: 500-1000 mg; repeat as appropriate **or** 20-50 mg/kg/hour **or** 200-500 mg per 500 mL of citrated blood

Administration

I.V. For I.V. administration only; avoid extravasation. Avoid rapid administration (do not exceed 100 mg/minute except in emergency situations). May be given over 2-5 minutes if rapid increase in serum calcium concentration is required. For I.V. infusion, dilute to a maximum concentration of 20 mg/mL and infuse over 1 hour or no greater than 45-90 mg/kg/hour (0.6-1.2 mEq/kg/hour); administration via a central or deep vein is preferred; do not use scalp, small hand or foot veins for I.V. administration since severe necrosis and sloughing may occur. Monitor ECG if calcium is infused faster than 2.5 mEq/minute; **stop the infusion if the patient complains of pain or discomfort.** Warm to body temperature. **Do not infuse calcium chloride in the same I.V. line as phosphate-containing solutions.**

Nursing Actions

Physical Assessment Infusion site should be monitored closely to prevent extravasation.

Patient Education This medication can only be given intravenously. Do not make rapid postural changes while calcium is infusing. Report any feelings of excitation, chest pain, irregular or pounding heartbeat, vomiting, acute headache, or dizziness.

Related Information

Management of Drug Extravasations *on page 1269*

Calcium Gluconate (KAL see um GLOO koe nate)

Brand Names: U.S. Cal-G [OTC]; Cal-GLU™ [OTC]

Pharmacologic Category Calcium Salt; Electrolyte Supplement, Oral; Electrolyte Supplement, Parenteral

Medication Safety Issues

Sound-alike/look-alike issues:

Calcium gluconate may be confused with calcium glubionate

Administration issues:

Calcium gluconate may be confused with calcium chloride.

Confusion with the different intravenous salt forms of calcium has occurred. There is a three-fold difference in the primary cation concentration between calcium gluconate (in which 1g = 4.65 mEq [90 mg] of elemental Ca++) and calcium chloride (in which 1g = 13.6 mEq [270 mg] of elemental Ca++).

Prescribers should specify which salt form is desired. Dosages should be expressed either as mEq, mg, or grams of the salt form.

Pregnancy Risk Factor C

Lactation Enters breast milk

Breast-Feeding Considerations Calcium is excreted in breast milk. The amount of calcium in breast milk is homeostatically regulated and not altered by maternal calcium intake. Calcium requirements are the same in lactating and non-lactating females (IOM, 2011).

Use Treatment and prevention of hypocalcemia; treatment of tetany, cardiac disturbances of hyperkalemia, cardiac resuscitation when epinephrine fails to improve myocardial contractions, hypocalcemia; calcium supplementation; hydrofluoric acid (HF) burns

Unlabeled Use Calcium channel blocker overdose

Mechanism of Action/Effect As dietary supplement, used to prevent or treat negative calcium balance; in osteoporosis, it helps to prevent or decrease the rate of bone loss. The calcium in calcium salts moderates nerve and muscle performance and allows normal cardiac function.

Contraindications Hypersensitivity to calcium gluconate or any component of the formulation; ventricular fibrillation during cardiac resuscitation; digitalis toxicity or suspected digoxin toxicity; hypercalcemia

Warnings/Precautions Injection solution is for I.V. use only; do not inject SubQ or I.M. Avoid too rapid I.V. administration and avoid extravasation. Use with caution in digitalized patients, severe hyperphosphatemia, respiratory failure, or acidosis. May produce cardiac arrest. Hypercalcemia may occur in patients with renal failure; frequent determination of serum calcium is necessary. Use caution with renal disease. Use caution when administering calcium supplements to patients with a history of kidney stones. Solutions may contain aluminum; toxic levels may occur following prolonged administration in premature neonates or patients with renal dysfunction. Oral: Constipation, bloating, and gas are common with oral calcium supplements (especially carbonate salt). Taking calcium (≤500 mg) with food improves absorption. Calcium administration interferes with absorption of some minerals and drugs; use with caution. It is recommended to concomitantly administer vitamin D for optimal calcium absorption.

Drug Interactions

Avoid Concomitant Use

Avoid concomitant use of Calcium Gluconate with any of the following: Calcium Acetate

Decreased Effect

Calcium Gluconate may decrease the levels/effects of: Bisphosphonate Derivatives; Calcium Channel Blockers; Deferiprone; DOBUTamine; Eltrombopag; Estramustine; Phosphate Supplements; Quinolone Antibiotics; Tetracycline Derivatives; Thyroid Products; Trientine

The levels/effects of Calcium Gluconate may be decreased by: Trientine

Increased Effect/Toxicity

Calcium Gluconate may increase the levels/effects of: Calcium Acetate; CefTRIAXone; Vitamin D Analogs

The levels/effects of Calcium Gluconate may be increased by: Thiazide Diuretics

Adverse Reactions Frequency not defined.

I.V.:

Cardiovascular: Arrhythmia, bradycardia, cardiac arrest, hypotension, vasodilation, and syncope may occur following rapid I.V. injection

Central nervous system: Sense of oppression

Gastrointestinal: Chalky taste

Local: Abscess and necrosis following I.M. administration

Neuromuscular & skeletal: Tingling sensation

Miscellaneous: Heat waves

Oral: Gastrointestinal: Constipation

Available Dosage Forms

Capsule, oral:

Cal-G [OTC]: 700 mg

Cal-GLU™ [OTC]: 515 mg

Injection, solution [preservative free]: 10% (10 mL, 50 mL, 100 mL, 200 mL)

Powder, oral: (480 g)

Tablet, oral: 500 mg, 648 mg

General Dosage Range

I.V.: *Children and Adults:* Dosage varies greatly depending on indication

Oral:

Children 1-6 months: Adequate intake: 200 mg/day

Children 7-12 months: Adequate intake: 260 mg/day

Children 1-3 years: RDA: 700 mg/day

Children 4-8 years: RDA: 1000 mg/day

Children 9-18 years: RDA: 1300 mg/day

Children: 200-500 mg/kg/day (calcium gluconate salt containing 0.465 mEq [9.3 mg]/mL elemental calcium) divided every 6 hours

Adults: 500 mg to 2 g 2-4 times/day (calcium gluconate salt containing 0.465 mEq [9.3 mg]/mL elemental calcium)

Adults 19-50 years: RDA: 1000 mg/day

Adults ≥51 years, females: RDA: 1200 mg/day

Adults 51-70 years, males: RDA: 1000 mg/day

Adults >70 years, males: RDA: 1200 mg/day

Administration

I.M. Not for I.M. or SubQ administration

I.V. For I.V. administration only; administer slowly (~1.5 mL calcium gluconate 10% per minute) through a small needle into a large vein in order to avoid too rapid increased in serum calcium and extravasation

Other Not for SubQ administration.

Stability

Storage

Do not refrigerate solutions. IVPB solutions/I.V. infusion solutions are stable for 24 hours at room temperature.

Standard diluent: 1 g/100 mL D_5W or NS; 2 g/100 mL D_5W or NS.

Maximum concentration in parenteral nutrition solutions is variable depending upon concentration and solubility (consult detailed reference).

Nursing Actions

Physical Assessment If administered I.V., monitor ECG, vital signs, and CNS. Observe infusion site closely. Avoid extravasation.

Patient Education Oral: Take with a full glass of water or juice, 1-3 hours after other medications and 1-2 hours before any iron supplements. May cause constipation or dry mouth. Report severe, unresolved GI disturbances and unusual emotional lability (mood swings).

Related Information

Compatibility of Drugs *on page 1264*

Management of Drug Extravasations *on page 1269*

Calcium Phosphate (Tribasic)

(KAL see um FOS fate tri BAY sik)

Brand Names: U.S. Posture® [OTC]

Index Terms Tricalcium Phosphate

Pharmacologic Category Calcium Salt

Use Dietary supplement

Available Dosage Forms For available OTC formulations, consult specific product labeling.

General Dosage Range Oral:

Children 1-6 months: Adequate intake: 200 mg/day

Children 7-12 months: Adequate intake: 260 mg/day

Children 1-3 years: RDA: 700 mg/day

Children 4-8 years: RDA: 1000 mg/day

Children 9-18 years: RDA: 1300 mg/day

Adults: 2 tablets daily

Adults 19-50 years: RDA: 1000 mg/day

Adults ≥51 years, females: RDA: 1200 mg/day

Adults 51-70 years, males: RDA: 1000 mg/day

Adults >70 years, males: RDA: 1200 mg/day

Nursing Actions

Patient Education Take with a full glass of water or juice, 1-3 hours after other medications and 1-2 hours before any iron supplements. May cause constipation or dry mouth. Report severe, unresolved GI disturbances and unusual emotional lability (mood swings).

Candesartan (kan de SAR tan)

Brand Names: U.S. Atacand®

Index Terms Candesartan Cilexetil

Pharmacologic Category Angiotensin II Receptor Blocker; Antihypertensive

Medication Safety Issues

Sound-alike/look-alike issues:

Atacand® may be confused with antacid

Pregnancy Risk Factor C (1st trimester); D (2nd and 3rd trimesters)

Lactation Enters breast milk/contraindicated

Use Alone or in combination with other antihypertensive agents in treating hypertension; treatment of heart failure (NYHA class II-IV)

Mechanism of Action/Effect Blocks the vasoconstrictor and aldosterone-secreting effects of angiotensin II by binding of angiotensin II at the AT1 receptor in many tissues, such as vascular smooth muscle and the adrenal gland. Independent of pathways for angiotensin II synthesis. Does not affect the response to bradykinin; does not bind to block other hormone receptors or ion channels known to be important in cardiovascular regulation.

Contraindications Hypersensitivity to candesartan or any component of the formulation

Warnings/Precautions [U.S. Boxed Warning]: Drugs that act on the renin-angiotensin system can cause injury and death to the developing fetus. Discontinue as soon as possible once pregnancy is detected. May cause hyperkalemia; avoid potassium supplementation unless specifically required by healthcare provider. Avoid use or use a smaller dose in patients who are volume depleted; correct depletion first. May be associated with deterioration of renal function and/or increases in serum creatinine, particularly in patients with low renal blood flow (eg, renal artery stenosis, heart failure) whose glomerular filtration rate (GFR) is dependent on efferent arteriolar vasoconstriction by angiotensin II. Use with caution in unstented unilateral/bilateral renal artery stenosis, pre-existing renal insufficiency, or significant aortic/mitral stenosis. Use with caution in patients with moderate hepatic impairment. Contraindicated with severe hepatic impairment and/or cholestasis. Use caution when initiating in heart failure; may need to adjust dose, and/or concurrent diuretic therapy, because of candesartan-induced hypotension. Hypotension may occur during major surgery and anesthesia; use cautiously before, during, and immediately after such interventions. Although concurrent therapy with an ACE inhibitor may be rational in select patients, concurrent use of ACE inhibitors may increase the risk of clinically-significant adverse events (eg, renal dysfunction, hyperkalemia). Pediatric patients with a GFR <30 mL/minute/1.73m^2 or children <1 year of age should not receive candesartan; has not been evaluated.

Drug Interactions

Avoid Concomitant Use There are no known interactions where it is recommended to avoid concomitant use.

Decreased Effect

The levels/effects of Candesartan may be decreased by: Herbs (Hypertensive Properties);

Methylphenidate; Nonsteroidal Anti-Inflammatory Agents; Yohimbine

Increased Effect/Toxicity

Candesartan may increase the levels/effects of: ACE Inhibitors; Amifostine; Antihypertensives; Hypotensive Agents; Lithium; Nonsteroidal Anti-Inflammatory Agents; Potassium-Sparing Diuretics; RiTUXimab; Sodium Phosphates

The levels/effects of Candesartan may be increased by: Alfuzosin; Diazoxide; Eplerenone; Herbs (Hypotensive Properties); MAO Inhibitors; Pentoxifylline; Phosphodiesterase 5 Inhibitors; Potassium Salts; Prostacyclin Analogues; Tolvaptan; Trimethoprim

Nutritional/Ethanol Interactions

Food: Potassium supplements and/or potassium-containing salts may cause or worsen hyperkalemia. Management: Consult prescriber before consuming a potassium-rich diet, potassium supplements, or salt substitutes.

Herb/Nutraceutical: Dong quai has estrogenic activity. Ephedra, yohimbe, and ginseng may worsen hypertension. Garlic may increase antihypertensive effect of candesartan. Management: Avoid dong quai if using for hypertension. Avoid ephedra, yohimbe, ginseng, and garlic.

Adverse Reactions

Cardiovascular: Angina, hypotension (heart failure 19%), MI, palpitation, tachycardia

Central nervous system: Anxiety, depression, dizziness, drowsiness, fever, headache, lightheadedness, somnolence, vertigo

Dermatologic: Angioedema, rash

Endocrine & metabolic: Hyperglycemia, hyperkalemia (heart failure <1% to 6%), hypertriglyceridemia, hyperuricemia

Gastrointestinal: Dyspepsia, gastroenteritis

Neuromuscular & skeletal: Back pain, CPK increased, myalgia, paresthesia, weakness

Renal: Serum creatinine increased (up to 13% in patients with heart failure with drug discontinuation required in 6%), hematuria

Respiratory: Dyspnea, epistaxis, pharyngitis, rhinitis, upper respiratory tract infection

Miscellaneous: Diaphoresis increased

Pharmacodynamics/Kinetics

Onset of Action 2-3 hours; Peak effect: 6-8 hours

Duration of Action >24 hours

Available Dosage Forms

Tablet, oral:

Atacand®: 4 mg, 8 mg, 16 mg, 32 mg

General Dosage Range Oral:

Children 1 to <6 years: Initial: 0.2 mg/kg/day in 1-2 divided doses; Maintenance: 0.05-0.4 mg/kg/day in 1-2 divided doses (maximum daily dose: 0.4 mg/kg/day)

Children 6 to <17 years: Initial: <50 kg: 4-8 mg/day in 1-2 divided doses; >50 kg: 8-16 mg/day in 1-2 divided doses; Maintenance: 2-32 mg/day in 1-2 divided doses (maximum daily dose: 32 mg/day)

Adults: Initial: 4-16 mg once daily; Maintenance: 4-32 mg/day in 1-2 divided doses

Administration

Oral Administer without regard to meals.

Stability

Storage Store at 25°C (77°F); excursions permitted to 15°C to 30°C (59°F to 86°F).

Nursing Actions

Physical Assessment Assess for potential interactions (eg, increased risk for hypotension, hyperkalemia). Monitor for reduced hypertension. Monitor for tachycardia, CNS changes, hyperglycemia, and hypotension prior to treatment, when changing dose, and throughout therapy.

Patient Education Take with or without food. This drug does not eliminate need for diet or exercise regimen as recommended by prescriber. May cause dizziness, fainting, lightheadedness, postural hypotension, nausea, or vomiting. Report chest pain or palpitations; unusual weight gain or swelling of ankles and hands; persistent fatigue; unusual flu or cold symptoms or dry cough; respiratory difficulty; swelling of eyes, face, or lips; skin rash; muscle pain or weakness; or unusual bleeding (blood in urine).

Candesartan and Hydrochlorothiazide

(kan de SAR tan & hye droe klor oh THYE a zide)

Brand Names: U.S. Atacand HCT®

Index Terms Candesartan Cilexetil and Hydrochlorothiazide; Hydrochlorothiazide and Candesartan

Pharmacologic Category Angiotensin II Receptor Blocker; Diuretic, Thiazide

Pregnancy Risk Factor C/D (2nd and 3rd trimesters)

Lactation Enters breast milk/contraindicated

Use Treatment of hypertension; combination product should not be used for initial therapy

Available Dosage Forms

Tablet:

Atacand HCT®: 16/12.5: Candesartan 16 mg and hydrochlorothiazide 12.5 mg; 32/12.5: Candesartan 32 mg and hydrochlorothiazide 12.5 mg; 32/25: Candesartan 32 mg and hydrochlorothiazide 25 mg

General Dosage Range Oral: *Adults:* Candesartan 16-32 mg/day in 1-2 divided doses and hydrochlorothiazide 12.5-25 mg once daily

Administration

Oral May administer with or without food.

Nursing Actions

Physical Assessment See individual agents.

Patient Education See individual agents.

Related Information

Candesartan *on page 174*

Hydrochlorothiazide *on page 570*

Capecitabine (ka pe SITE a been)

Brand Names: U.S. Xeloda®

Index Terms CAPE

Pharmacologic Category Antineoplastic Agent, Antimetabolite; Antineoplastic Agent, Antimetabolite (Pyrimidine Analog)

Medication Safety Issues

Sound-alike/look-alike issues:

Xeloda® may be confused with Xenical®

High alert medication:

This medication is in a class the Institute for Safe Medication Practices (ISMP) includes among its list of drug classes which have a heightened risk of causing significant patient harm when used in error.

Pregnancy Risk Factor D

Lactation Excretion in breast milk unknown/not recommended

Breast-Feeding Considerations It is not known if the drug is excreted in breast milk. Because of the potential for serious adverse reactions in nursing infants, it is recommended that nursing be discontinued when receiving capecitabine therapy.

Use Treatment of metastatic colorectal cancer; adjuvant therapy of Dukes' C colon cancer; treatment of metastatic breast cancer

Unlabeled Use Treatment of gastric cancer, pancreatic cancer, esophageal cancer, ovarian cancer, metastatic renal cell cancer, neuroendocrine tumors, metastatic CNS lesions

Mechanism of Action/Effect Capecitabine is a prodrug of fluorouracil. It undergoes hydrolysis in the liver and tissues to form fluorouracil. It interferes with DNA (and to a lesser degree RNA) synthesis. Appears to be specific for G_1 and S phases of the cell cycle.

Contraindications Hypersensitivity to capecitabine, fluorouracil, or any component of the formulation; known deficiency of dihydropyrimidine dehydrogenase (DPD); severe renal impairment (Cl_{cr} <30 mL/minute)

Warnings/Precautions Hazardous agent - use appropriate precautions for handling and disposal. Use with caution in patients ≥80 years of age, or with renal or hepatic dysfunction. Patients with baseline moderate renal impairment require dose reduction. Patients with mild-to-moderate renal impairment require careful monitoring and subsequent dose reduction with any grade 2 or higher adverse event. Bone marrow suppression may occur, hematologic toxicity is more common when used in combination therapy; use with caution; dosage adjustments may be required. Canadian labeling recommends that patients with baseline platelets <100,000/mm^3 and/or neutrophils <1500/mm^3 not receive capecitabine therapy and also to withhold for grade 3 or 4 hematologic toxicity during treatment. Use with caution in patients who have received extensive pelvic radiation or alkylating therapy. Use cautiously with warfarin. Rare and unexpected severe toxicity may be attributed to dihydropyrimidine dehydrogenase (DPD) deficiency. Necrotizing enterocolitis (typhlitis) has been reported.

Capecitabine can cause severe diarrhea; median time to first occurrence is 34 days. Subsequent doses should be reduced after grade 3 or 4 diarrhea or recurrence of grade 2 diarrhea. Dehydration may occur rapidly in patients with diarrhea, nausea, vomiting, anorexia, and/or weakness; adequately hydrate prior to treatment initiation. Elderly patients may be a higher risk for dehydration. Note: the Canadian labeling recommends treatment interruption for dehydration requiring I.V. hydration lasting <24 hours and dosage reduction if I.V hydration required for ≥24 hours; correct precipitating factors and ensure rehydration prior to resuming therapy.

Hand-and-foot syndrome is characterized by numbness, dysesthesia/paresthesia, tingling, painless or painful swelling, erythema, desquamation, blistering, and severe pain. If grade 2 or 3 hand-and-foot syndrome occurs, interrupt administration of capecitabine until decreases to grade 1. Following grade 3 hand-and-foot syndrome, decrease subsequent doses of capecitabine. In patients with colorectal cancer, treatment with capecitabine immediately following 6 weeks of fluorouracil/leucovorin (FU/LV) therapy has been associated with an increased incidence of grade ≥3 toxicity, when compared to patients receiving the reverse sequence, capecitabine (two 3-week courses) followed by FU/LV (Hennig, 2008).

There has been cardiotoxicity associated with fluorinated pyrimidine therapy. May be more common in patients with a history of coronary artery disease. **[U.S. Boxed Warning]: Capecitabine may increase the anticoagulant effects of warfarin; monitor closely.**

Safety and efficacy in children <18 years of age have not been established.

Drug Interactions

Avoid Concomitant Use

Avoid concomitant use of Capecitabine with any of the following: BCG; CloZAPine; Natalizumab; Pimecrolimus; Tacrolimus (Topical); Vaccines (Live)

Decreased Effect

Capecitabine may decrease the levels/effects of: BCG; Coccidioidin Skin Test; Sipuleucel-T; Vaccines (Inactivated); Vaccines (Live)

The levels/effects of Capecitabine may be decreased by: Echinacea

Increased Effect/Toxicity

Capecitabine may increase the levels/effects of: Carvedilol; CloZAPine; CYP2C9 Substrates; Diclofenac; Fosphenytoin; Leflunomide; Natalizumab; Phenytoin; Vaccines (Live); Vitamin K Antagonists

The levels/effects of Capecitabine may be increased by: Denosumab; Leucovorin Calcium-Levoleucovorin; Pimecrolimus; Roflumilast; Tacrolimus (Topical); Trastuzumab

Nutritional/Ethanol Interactions Food: Food reduced the rate and extent of absorption of capecitabine.

Adverse Reactions Frequency listed derived from monotherapy trials.

>10%:

Cardiovascular: Edema (9% to 15%)

Central nervous system: Fatigue (16% to 42%), fever (7% to 18%), pain (12%)

Dermatologic: Palmar-plantar erythrodysesthesia (hand-and-foot syndrome) (54% to 60%; grade 3: 11% to 17%; may be dose limiting), dermatitis (27% to 37%)

Gastrointestinal: Diarrhea (47% to 57%; may be dose limiting; grade 3: 12% to 13%; grade 4: 2% to 3%), nausea (34% to 53%), vomiting (15% to 37%), abdominal pain (7% to 35%), stomatitis (22% to 25%), appetite decreased (26%), anorexia (9% to 23%), constipation (9% to 15%)

Hematologic: Lymphopenia (94%; grade 4: 14%), anemia (72% to 80%; grade 4: <1% to 1%), neutropenia (2% to 26%; grade 4: 2%), thrombocytopenia (24%; grade 4: 1%)

Hepatic: Bilirubin increased (22% to 48%; grades 3/4: 11% to 23%)

Neuromuscular & skeletal: Paresthesia (21%)

Ocular: Eye irritation (13% to 15%)

Respiratory: Dyspnea (14%)

5% to 10%:

Cardiovascular: Venous thrombosis (8%), chest pain (6%)

Central nervous system: Headache (5% to 10%), lethargy (10%), dizziness (6% to 8%), insomnia (7% to 8%), mood alteration (5%), depression (5%)

Dermatologic: Nail disorder (7%), rash (7%), skin discoloration (7%), alopecia (6%), erythema (6%)

Endocrine & metabolic: Dehydration (7%)

Gastrointestinal: Motility disorder (10%), oral discomfort (10%), dyspepsia (6% to 8%), upper GI inflammatory disorders (colorectal cancer: 8%), hemorrhage (6%), ileus (6%), taste perversion (colorectal cancer: 6%)

Neuromuscular & skeletal: Back pain (10%), weakness (10%), neuropathy (10%), myalgia (9%), arthralgia (8%), limb pain (6%)

Ocular: Abnormal vision (colorectal cancer: 5%), conjunctivitis (5%)

Respiratory: Cough (7%)

Miscellaneous: Viral infection (colorectal cancer: 5%)

Available Dosage Forms

Tablet, oral:

Xeloda®: 150 mg, 500 mg

General Dosage Range Dosage adjustment recommended in patients with renal impairment or who develop toxicities

Oral: *Adults:* 1250 mg/m^2 twice daily for 2 weeks, every 21 days

Administration

Oral Usually administered in 2 divided doses taken 12 hours apart. Doses should be taken with water within 30 minutes after a meal.

Stability

Storage Store at room temperature of 25°C (77°F); excursions permitted between 15°C and 30°C (59°F and 86°F).

Nursing Actions

Physical Assessment Monitor for adverse reactions periodically during therapy. Teach sexually active female patients the necessity for contraception.

Patient Education Take within 30 minutes after a meal. Maintain adequate hydration, unless instructed to restrict fluid intake. You may be more susceptible to infection. May cause lethargy; dizziness; visual changes; confusion; anxiety; nausea; vomiting; loss of appetite; dry mouth; loss of hair (will grow back when treatment is discontinued); photosensitivity; dry, itchy skin; and dry or irritated eyes (avoid contact lenses). Report persistent or severe diarrhea, vomiting, or abdominal pain; skin rash, redness, tenderness, or peeling (especially hands and feet); respiratory difficulty; chest pain or palpitations; unusual bleeding or bruising; or vision changes.

Dietary Considerations Because current safety and efficacy data are based upon administration with food, it is recommended that capecitabine be administered with food. In all clinical trials, patients were instructed to take with water within 30 minutes after a meal.

Captopril (KAP toe pril)

Index Terms ACE

Pharmacologic Category Angiotensin-Converting Enzyme (ACE) Inhibitor

Medication Safety Issues

Sound-alike/look-alike issues:

Captopril may be confused with calcitriol, Capitrol®, carvedilol

International issues:

Acepril [Great Britain] may be confused with Accupril which is a brand name for quinapril in the U.S.

Acepril: Brand name for captopril [Great Britain], but also the brand name for enalapril [Hungary, Switzerland]; lisinopril [Malaysia]

Pregnancy Risk Factor D

Lactation Enters breast milk/not recommended (AAP rates "compatible"; AAP 2001 update pending)

Breast-Feeding Considerations Captopril is excreted in breast milk. Breast-feeding is not recommended by the manufacturer.

Use Management of hypertension; treatment of heart failure, left ventricular dysfunction after myocardial infarction, diabetic nephropathy

Unlabeled Use To delay the progression of nephropathy and reduce risks of cardiovascular events in hypertensive patients with type 1 or 2 diabetes mellitus; treatment of hypertensive crisis, rheumatoid arthritis; diagnosis of anatomic renal artery stenosis, hypertension secondary to scleroderma renal crisis; diagnosis of aldosteronism, idiopathic edema, Bartter's syndrome, postmyocardial infarction for prevention of ventricular failure; increase circulation in Raynaud's phenomenon, hypertension secondary to Takayasu's disease

Mechanism of Action/Effect Competitive inhibitor of angiotensin-converting enzyme (ACE); prevents conversion of angiotensin I to angiotensin II, a potent vasoconstrictor; results in lower levels of angiotensin II which causes an increase in plasma renin activity and a reduction in aldosterone secretion

Contraindications Hypersensitivity to captopril, any other ACE inhibitor, or any component of the formulation; angioedema related to previous treatment with an ACE inhibitor

Warnings/Precautions Anaphylactic reactions may occur rarely with ACE inhibitors. At any time during treatment (especially following first dose) angioedema may occur rarely with ACE inhibitors; may involve the head and neck (potentially compromising airway) or the intestine (presenting with abdominal pain). African-Americans and patients with idiopathic or hereditary angioedema may be at an increased risk. Prolonged frequent monitoring may be required especially if tongue, glottis, or larynx are involved as they are associated with airway obstruction. Patients with a history of airway surgery may have a higher risk of airway obstruction. Aggressive early and appropriate management is critical. Use in patients with previous angioedema associated with ACE inhibitor therapy is contraindicated. Severe anaphylactoid reactions may be seen during hemodialysis (eg, CVVHD) with high-flux dialysis membranes (eg, AN69), and rarely, during low density lipoprotein apheresis with dextran sulfate cellulose. Rare cases of anaphylactoid reactions have been reported in patients undergoing sensitization treatment with hymenoptera (bee, wasp) venom while receiving ACE inhibitors.

Symptomatic hypotension with or without syncope can occur with ACE inhibitors (usually with the first several doses); effects are most often observed in volume depleted patients; close monitoring of patient is required especially with initial dosing and dosing increases; blood pressure must be lowered at a rate appropriate for the patient's clinical condition. Initiation of therapy in patients with ischemic heart disease or cerebrovascular disease warrants close observation due to the potential consequences posed by falling blood pressure (eg, MI, stroke). Use with caution in hypertrophic cardiomyopathy with outflow tract obstruction, severe aortic stenosis, or before, during, or immediately after major surgery. **[U.S. Boxed Warning]: Drugs that act on the renin-angiotensin system can cause injury and death to the developing fetus. Discontinue as soon as possible once pregnancy is detected.**

Hyperkalemia may occur with ACE inhibitors; risk factors include renal dysfunction, diabetes mellitus, concomitant use of potassium-sparing diuretics, potassium supplements and/or potassium containing salts. Use cautiously, if at all, with these agents and monitor potassium closely. Cough may occur with ACE inhibitors. Other causes of cough should be considered (eg, pulmonary congestion in patients with heart failure) and excluded prior to discontinuation.

May be associated with deterioration of renal function and/or increases in serum creatinine, particularly in patients with low renal blood flow (eg, renal artery stenosis, heart failure) whose glomerular filtration rate (GFR) is dependent on efferent arteriolar vasoconstriction by angiotensin II; deterioration may result in oliguria, acute renal failure, and progressive azotemia. Small increases in serum creatinine may occur following initiation; consider discontinuation only in patients with progressive and/or significant deterioration in renal function. Use with caution in patients with unstented unilateral/bilateral renal artery stenosis. When unstented bilateral renal artery stenosis is present, use is generally avoided due to the elevated risk of deterioration in renal function unless possible benefits outweigh risks. Concurrent use of angiotensin receptor blockers may increase the risk of clinically-significant adverse events (eg, renal dysfunction, hyperkalemia).

Rare toxicities associated with ACE inhibitors include cholestatic jaundice (which may progress to fulminant hepatic necrosis), agranulocytosis, neutropenia, or leukopenia with myeloid hypoplasia. Patients with collagen vascular diseases (especially with concomitant renal impairment) or renal impairment alone may be at increased risk for hematologic toxicity; closely monitor CBC with differential for the first 3 months of therapy and periodically thereafter in these patients.

Drug Interactions

Avoid Concomitant Use There are no known interactions where it is recommended to avoid concomitant use.

Decreased Effect

The levels/effects of Captopril may be decreased by: Antacids; Aprotinin; Herbs (Hypertensive Properties); Icatibant; Lanthanum; Methylphenidate; Nonsteroidal Anti-Inflammatory Agents; Peginterferon Alfa-2b; Salicylates; Yohimbine

Increased Effect/Toxicity

Captopril may increase the levels/effects of: Allopurinol; Amifostine; Antihypertensives; AzaTHIOprine; CycloSPORINE; CycloSPORINE (Systemic); Ferric Gluconate; Gold Sodium Thiomalate; Hypotensive Agents; Iron Dextran Complex; Lithium; Nonsteroidal Anti-Inflammatory Agents; RiTUXimab; Sodium Phosphates

The levels/effects of Captopril may be increased by: Abiraterone Acetate; Alfuzosin; Angiotensin II Receptor Blockers; CYP2D6 Inhibitors (Moderate); CYP2D6 Inhibitors (Strong); Darunavir; Diazoxide; DPP-IV Inhibitors; Eplerenone; Everolimus; Herbs (Hypotensive Properties); Loop Diuretics; MAO Inhibitors; Pentoxifylline; Phosphodiesterase 5 Inhibitors; Potassium Salts; Potassium-Sparing Diuretics; Prostacyclin Analogues; Sirolimus; Temsirolimus; Thiazide Diuretics; TiZANidine; Tolvaptan; Trimethoprim

Nutritional/Ethanol Interactions

Food: Captopril serum concentrations may be decreased if taken with food. Long-term use of captopril may lead to a zinc deficiency which can result in altered taste perception. Potassium supplements and/or potassium-containing salts may cause or worsen hyperkalemia. Management: Take on an empty stomach 1 hour before or 2 hours after meals. Consult prescriber before consuming a potassium-rich diet, potassium supplements, or salt substitutes.

Herb/Nutraceutical: Some herbal medications may worsen hypertension (eg, licorice); others may increase the antihypertensive effect of captopril (eg, shepherd's purse). Management: Avoid bayberry, blue cohosh, cayenne, ephedra, ginger, ginseng (American), kola, yohimbe, and licorice. Avoid black cohosh, california poppy, coleus, golden seal, hawthorn, mistletoe, periwinkle, quinine, and shepherd's purse.

Adverse Reactions

Frequency not defined:

Cardiovascular: Angioedema, cardiac arrest, cerebrovascular insufficiency, rhythm disturbances, orthostatic hypotension, syncope, flushing, pallor, angina, MI, Raynaud's syndrome, CHF

Central nervous system: Ataxia, confusion, depression, nervousness, somnolence

Dermatologic: Bullous pemphigus, erythema multiforme, Stevens-Johnson syndrome, exfoliative dermatitis

Endocrine & metabolic: Alkaline phosphatase increased, bilirubin increased, gynecomastia

Gastrointestinal: Pancreatitis, glossitis, dyspepsia

Genitourinary: Urinary frequency, impotence

Hematologic: Anemia, thrombocytopenia, pancytopenia, agranulocytosis, anemia

Hepatic: Jaundice, hepatitis, hepatic necrosis (rare), cholestasis, hyponatremia (symptomatic), transaminases increased

Neuromuscular & skeletal: Asthenia, myalgia, myasthenia

Ocular: Blurred vision

Renal: Renal insufficiency, renal failure, nephrotic syndrome, polyuria, oliguria

Respiratory: Bronchospasm, eosinophilic pneumonitis, rhinitis

Miscellaneous: Anaphylactoid reactions

1% to 10%:

Cardiovascular: Hypotension (1% to 3%), tachycardia (1%), chest pain (1%), palpitation (1%)

Dermatologic: Rash (maculopapular or urticarial) (4% to 7%), pruritus (2%); in patients with rash, a positive ANA and/or eosinophilia has been noted in 7% to 10%

Endocrine & metabolic: Hyperkalemia (1% to 11%)

Hematologic: Neutropenia may occur in up to 4% of patients with renal insufficiency or collagen-vascular disease

Renal: Proteinuria (1%), serum creatinine increased, worsening of renal function (may occur in patients with bilateral renal artery stenosis or hypovolemia)

Respiratory: Cough (<1% to 2%)

Miscellaneous: Hypersensitivity reactions (rash, pruritus, fever, arthralgia, and eosinophilia) have occurred in 4% to 7% of patients (depending on dose and renal function); dysgeusia - loss of taste or diminished perception (2% to 4%)

Pharmacodynamics/Kinetics

Onset of Action Peak effect: Blood pressure reduction: 1-1.5 hours after dose

Duration of Action Dose related, may require several weeks of therapy before full hypotensive effect

Available Dosage Forms

Tablet, oral: 12.5 mg, 25 mg, 50 mg, 100 mg

General Dosage Range Dosage adjustment recommended in patients with renal impairment

Oral:

Infants: Initial: 0.15-0.3 mg/kg/dose; Maximum: 6 mg/kg/day in 1-4 divided doses

Children: Initial: 0.3-0.5 mg/kg/dose; Maximum: 6 mg/kg/day in 2-4 divided doses

Older Children: Initial: 6.25-12.5 mg every 12-24 hours; Maximum: 6 mg/kg/day

Adolescents: Initial: 12.5-25 mg; Maximum: 450 mg/day

Adults: Initial: 6.25-25 mg 2-3 times/day; Maintenance: 25-450 mg/day in 2-3 divided doses

Administration

Oral Unstable in aqueous solutions; to prepare solution for oral administration, mix prior to administration and use within 10 minutes.

Nursing Actions

Physical Assessment Assess other pharmacological or herbal products patient may be taking that may impact renal function. When beginning therapy, monitor patient closely for anaphylactic reaction or severe angioedema. Monitor renal function tests and blood pressure. Monitor for hypovolemia, angioedema, and postural hypotension when beginning therapy, adjusting dosage, and on a regular basis throughout.

Patient Education Do not use potassium supplement or salt substitutes without consulting prescriber. Take first dose at bedtime. Take all doses on an empty stomach, 1 hour before or 2 hours after meals. This drug does not eliminate need for diet or exercise regimen as recommended by prescriber. May cause dizziness, fainting, lightheadedness, postural hypotension, nausea, vomiting, abdominal pain, dry mouth, or transient loss of appetite. Report immediately swelling or numbness of face, mouth, or throat; unusual chest pain or palpitations; decreased urinary output; fever or chills; swelling of extremities; skin rash; numbness, tingling, or pain in muscles; or respiratory difficulty or unusual cough.

Dietary Considerations Should be taken at least 1 hour before or 2 hours after eating.

Captopril and Hydrochlorothiazide

(KAP toe pril & hye droe klor oh THYE a zide)

Index Terms Hydrochlorothiazide and Captopril

Pharmacologic Category Angiotensin-Converting Enzyme (ACE) Inhibitor; Diuretic, Thiazide

Pregnancy Risk Factor C/D (2nd and 3rd trimesters)

Lactation Enters breast milk/not recommended

Use Management of hypertension

Available Dosage Forms

Tablet: 25/15: Captopril 25 mg and hydrochlorothiazide 15 mg; 25/25: Captopril 25 mg and hydrochlorothiazide 25 mg; 50/15: Captopril 50 mg and hydrochlorothiazide 15 mg; 50/25: Captopril 50 mg and hydrochlorothiazide 25 mg

General Dosage Range Oral: *Adults:* Captopril 25-150 mg and hydrochlorothiazide 15-50 mg once daily

Nursing Actions

Physical Assessment See individual agents.

Patient Education See individual agents.

Related Information

Captopril *on page 177*

Hydrochlorothiazide *on page 570*

CarBAMazepine

(kar ba MAZ e peen)

Brand Names: U.S. Carbatrol®; Epitol®; Equetro®; TEGretol®; TEGretol®-XR

Index Terms CBZ; SPD417

Pharmacologic Category Anticonvulsant, Miscellaneous

Medication Safety Issues

Sound-alike/look-alike issues:

CarBAMazepine may be confused with OXcarbazepine

Epitol® may be confused with Epinal®

TEGretol®, TEGretol®-XR may be confused with Mebaral®, Toprol-XL®, Toradol®, TRENtal®

Medication Guide Available Yes

Pregnancy Risk Factor D

Lactation Enters breast milk/not recommended (AAP rates "compatible"; AAP 2001 update pending)

Breast-Feeding Considerations Carbamazepine and its active epoxide metabolite are found in breast milk. Carbamazepine can also be detected in the serum of nursing infants. Transient hepatic dysfunction has been observed in some case reports. Nursing should be discontinued if adverse events are observed. According to the manufacturer, the decision to continue or discontinue breast-feeding during therapy should take into account the risk of exposure to the infant and the benefits of treatment to the mother. Respiratory depression, seizures, nausea, vomiting, diarrhea, and/or decreased feeding have been observed in neonates exposed to carbamazepine *in utero* and may represent a neonatal withdrawal syndrome.

Use

Carbatrol®, Tegretol®, Tegretol®-XR: Partial seizures with complex symptomatology (psychomotor, temporal lobe), generalized tonic-clonic seizures (grand mal), mixed seizure patterns, trigeminal neuralgia

Equetro®: Acute manic and mixed episodes associated with bipolar 1 disorder

Unlabeled Use Treatment of restless leg syndrome and post-traumatic stress disorders

Mechanism of Action/Effect In addition to anticonvulsant effects, carbamazepine has anticholinergic, antineuralgic, antidiuretic, muscle relaxant, antimanic, antidepressive, and and antiarrhythmic properties; may depress activity in the nucleus ventralis of the thalamus or decrease synaptic transmission or decrease summation of temporal stimulation leading to neural discharge by limiting influx of sodium ions across cell membrane or other unknown mechanisms; stimulates the release of ADH and potentiates its action in promoting reabsorption of water; chemically related to tricyclic antidepressants

Contraindications Hypersensitivity to carbamazepine, tricyclic antidepressants, or any component of the formulation; bone marrow depression; with or within 14 days of MAO inhibitor use; concurrent use of nefazodone

Warnings/Precautions **[U.S. Boxed Warning]: Potentially fatal blood cell abnormalities have been reported.** Patients with a previous history of adverse hematologic reaction to any drug may be at increased risk.

Antiepileptics are associated with an increased risk of suicidal behavior/thoughts with use (regardless of indication); patients should be monitored for signs/symptoms of depression, suicidal tendencies, and other unusual behavior changes during therapy and instructed to inform their healthcare provider immediately if symptoms occur.

Administer carbamazepine with caution to patients with history of cardiac damage, ECG abnormalities (or at risk for ECG abnormalities), hepatic or renal disease. When used to treat bipolar disorder, the smallest effective dose is suggested to reduce the risk for overdose/suicide; high-risk patients should be monitored for suicidal ideations. Prescription should be written for the smallest quantity consistent with good patient care. May activate latent psychosis and/or cause confusion or agitation; elderly patients may be at an increased risk for psychiatric effects. Potentially serious, sometimes fatal multiorgan hypersensitivity reactions have been reported with some antiepileptic drugs; monitor for signs and symptoms of possible disparate manifestations associated with lymphatic, hepatic, renal, and/or hematologic organ systems; gradual discontinuation and conversion to alternate therapy may be required.

Carbamazepine is not effective in absence, myoclonic, or akinetic seizures; exacerbation of certain seizure types have been seen after initiation of carbamazepine therapy in children with mixed seizure disorders. Abrupt discontinuation is not recommended in patients being treated for seizures. Dizziness or drowsiness may occur; caution should be used when performing tasks which require alertness until the effects are known. Effects with other sedative drugs or ethanol may be potentiated. Carbamazepine has a high potential for drug interactions; use caution in patients taking strong CYP3A4 inducers or inhibitors or medications significantly metabolized via CYP1A2, 2B6, 2C9, 2C19, and 3A4. Coadministration of carbamazepine and nefazodone may lead to insufficient plasma levels of nefazodone; combination is contraindicated. Carbamazepine has mild anticholinergic activity; use with caution in patients with increased intraocular pressure, or sensitivity to anticholinergic effects. Severe dermatologic reactions, including toxic epidermal necrolysis and Stevens-Johnson syndrome, although rarely reported, have resulted in fatalities. **[U.S. Boxed Warning]: Use caution and screen for the genetic susceptibility genotype (*HLA-B*1502* allele) in Asian patients. Patients with a positive result should not be started on carbamazepine.** Discontinue if there are any signs of hypersensitivity. Elderly patients may have an increased risk of SIADH-like syndrome.

Administration of the suspension will yield higher peak and lower trough serum levels than an equal dose of the tablet form; consider a lower starting dose given more frequently (same total daily dose) when using the suspension.

Drug Interactions

Avoid Concomitant Use

Avoid concomitant use of CarBAMazepine with any of the following: Axitinib; Boceprevir; Bortezomib; CloZAPine; Conivaptan; Dabigatran Etexilate; Dronedarone; Etravirine; Lurasidone; MAO Inhibitors; Nefazodone; Nilotinib; Praziquantel; Rilpivirine; Roflumilast; SORAfenib; Telaprevir; Ticagrelor; Toremifene; Vandetanib; Voriconazole

Decreased Effect

CarBAMazepine may decrease the levels/effects of: Acetaminophen; ARIPiprazole; Axitinib; Bendamustine; Benzodiazepines (metabolized by oxidation); Boceprevir; Bortezomib; Brentuximab Vedotin; Calcium Channel Blockers (Dihydropyridine); Calcium Channel Blockers (Nondihydropyridine); Caspofungin; CloZAPine; Contraceptives (Estrogens); Contraceptives (Progestins); CycloSPORINE; CycloSPORINE (Systemic); CYP1A2 Substrates; CYP2B6 Substrates; CYP2C19 Substrates; CYP2C8 Substrates; CYP2C9 Substrates; CYP3A4 Substrates; Dabigatran Etexilate; Dasatinib; Diclofenac; Divalproex; Doxycycline; Dronedarone; Etravirine; Exemestane; Felbamate; Flunarizine; Fosphenytoin; Gefitinib; GuanFACINE; Haloperidol; Irinotecan; Ixabepilone; Lacosamide; LamoTRIgine; Linagliptin; Lopinavir; Lurasidone; Maraviroc; Mebendazole; Methadone; MethylPREDNISolone; Nefazodone; Nilotinib; Paliperidone; P-glycoprotein/ABCB1 Substrates; Phenytoin; Praziquantel; Protease Inhibitors; QuiNINE; Rilpivirine; RisperiDONE; Roflumilast; Rufinamide; Selective Serotonin Reuptake Inhibitors; SORAfenib; SUNItinib; Tadalafil; Telaprevir; Temsirolimus; Theophylline Derivatives; Thyroid Products; Ticagrelor; Topiramate; Toremifene; Treprostinil; Tricyclic Antidepressants; Ulipristal; Valproic Acid; Vandetanib; Vecuronium; Vitamin K Antagonists; Voriconazole; Ziprasidone; Zolpidem; Zuclopenthixol

The levels/effects of CarBAMazepine may be decreased by: CYP3A4 Inducers (Strong); Deferasirox; Divalproex; Felbamate; Fosphenytoin; Herbs (CYP3A4 Inducers); Ketorolac; Ketorolac (Nasal); Ketorolac (Systemic); Mefloquine; Methylfolate; Phenytoin; Rufinamide; Theophylline Derivatives; Tocilizumab; Valproic Acid

Increased Effect/Toxicity

CarBAMazepine may increase the levels/effects of: Adenosine; Alcohol (Ethyl); ClomiPRAMINE; CloZAPine; CNS Depressants; Desmopressin; Fosphenytoin; Lithium; MAO Inhibitors; Methotrimeprazine; Phenytoin

The levels/effects of CarBAMazepine may be increased by: Allopurinol; Antifungal Agents (Azole Derivatives, Systemic); Calcium Channel Blockers (Nondihydropyridine); Carbonic

Anhydrase Inhibitors; Cimetidine; Conivaptan; CYP3A4 Inhibitors (Moderate); CYP3A4 Inhibitors (Strong); Danazol; Darunavir; Dasatinib; Droperidol; Fluconazole; Grapefruit Juice; HydrOXYzine; Isoniazid; Ivacaftor; LamoTRIgine; Macrolide Antibiotics; Methotrimeprazine; Nefazodone; Protease Inhibitors; QuiNINE; Selective Serotonin Reuptake Inhibitors; Telaprevir; Thiazide Diuretics; Zolpidem

Nutritional/Ethanol Interactions

Ethanol: Ethanol may increase CNS depression. Management: Avoid concurrent use of ethanol.

Food: Carbamazepine serum levels may be increased if taken with food and/or grapefruit juice. Management Avoid concurrent ingestion of grapefruit juice. Maintain adequate hydration, unless instructed to restrict fluid intake.

Herb/Nutraceutical: Evening primrose may decrease seizure threshold. Valerian, St John's wort, kava kava, and gotu kola may increase CNS depression. Management: Avoid evening primrose. Avoid valerian, St John's wort, kava kava, and gotu kola.

Adverse Reactions Frequency not defined, unless otherwise specified.

Cardiovascular: Arrhythmias, AV block, bradycardia, chest pain (bipolar use), CHF, edema, hyper-/hypotension, lymphadenopathy, syncope, thromboembolism, thrombophlebitis

Central nervous system: Amnesia (bipolar use), anxiety (bipolar use), aseptic meningitis (case report), ataxia (bipolar use 15%), confusion, depression (bipolar use), dizziness (bipolar use 44%), fatigue, headache (bipolar use 22%), sedation, slurred speech, somnolence (bipolar use 32%)

Dermatologic: Alopecia, alterations in skin pigmentation, erythema multiforme, exfoliative dermatitis, photosensitivity reaction, pruritus (bipolar use 8%), purpura, rash, Stevens-Johnson syndrome, toxic epidermal necrolysis, urticaria

Endocrine & metabolic: Chills, fever, hyponatremia, syndrome of inappropriate ADH secretion (SIADH)

Gastrointestinal: Abdominal pain, anorexia, constipation, diarrhea, dyspepsia (bipolar use), gastric distress, nausea (bipolar use 29%), pancreatitis, vomiting (bipolar use 18%), xerostomia (bipolar use)

Genitourinary: Azotemia, impotence, renal failure, urinary frequency, urinary retention

Hematologic: Acute intermittent porphyria, agranulocytosis, aplastic anemia, bone marrow suppression, eosinophilia, leukocytosis, leukopenia, pancytopenia, thrombocytopenia

Hepatic: Abnormal liver function tests, hepatic failure, hepatitis, jaundice

Neuromuscular & skeletal: Back pain, pain (bipolar use 12%), peripheral neuritis, weakness

Ocular: Blurred vision, conjunctivitis, lens opacities, nystagmus

Otic: Hyperacusis, tinnitus

Miscellaneous: Diaphoresis, hypersensitivity (including multiorgan reactions, may include disorders mimicking lymphoma, eosinophilia, hepatosplenomegaly, vasculitis); infection (bipolar use 12%)

Available Dosage Forms

Capsule, extended release, oral: 100 mg, 200 mg, 300 mg

Carbatrol®: 100 mg, 200 mg, 300 mg

Equetro®: 100 mg, 200 mg, 300 mg

Suspension, oral: 100 mg/5 mL (5 mL, 10 mL, 450 mL)

TEGretol®: 100 mg/5 mL (450 mL)

Tablet, oral: 200 mg

Epitol®: 200 mg

TEGretol®: 200 mg

Tablet, chewable, oral: 100 mg

TEGretol®: 100 mg

Tablet, extended release, oral: 200 mg, 400 mg

TEGretol®-XR: 100 mg, 200 mg, 400 mg

General Dosage Range Dosage adjustment recommended in patients with renal impairment.

Oral:

Extended release:

Capsules:

Children <12 years: Receiving ≥400 mg/day of carbamazepine may be converted to extended release capsules (Carbatrol®) using the same total daily dosage divided twice daily

Children 12-15 years: Initial: 400 mg/day; Maintenance: 800-1000 mg/day in 2 divided doses (maximum: 1000 mg/day)

Adolescents >15 years: Initial: 400 mg/day; Maintenance: 800-1200 mg/day in 2 divided doses (maximum: 1200 mg/day)

Adults: Bipolar disorder (Equetro®): Initial: 400 mg/day in 2 divided doses: Maintenance: Adjust by 200 mg daily increments (maximum: 1600 mg/day); Epilepsy: Initial: 400 mg/day; Maintenance: 800-1200 mg/day in 2 divided doses (maximum: 2400 mg/day)

Tablets:

Children 6-12 years: Initial: 200 mg/day; Maintenance: 400-800 mg/day in 2 divided doses (maximum: 1000 mg/day)

Children 12-15 years: Initial: 400 mg/day; Maintenance: 800-1000 mg/day in 2 divided doses (maximum: 1000 mg/day)

Adolescents >15 years and Adults: Initial: 400 mg/day; Maintenance: 800-1200 mg/day in 2 divided doses (maximum: 1200 mg/day)

Immediate release:

Children <6 years: Initial: 10-20 mg/kg/day in 2-3 divided doses (tablets) **or** 4 divided doses (suspension); Maintenance: Up to 35 mg/kg/day in 3-4 divided doses

Children 6-12 years: Initial: 200 mg/day in 2 divided doses (tablets) **or** 4 divided doses (suspension); Maintenance: 400-800 mg/day in 2-4 divided doses (maximum: 1000 mg/day)

Children 12-15 years: Initial: 400 mg/day in 2 divided doses (tablets) **or** 4 divided doses (suspension); Maintenance: 800-1000 mg/day in 3-4 divided doses (maximum: 1000 mg/day)

Adolescents >15 years: Initial: 400 mg/day in 2 divided doses (tablets) **or** 4 divided doses (suspension); Maintenance: 800-1200 mg/day in 3-4 divided doses (maximum: 1200 mg/day)

Adults: Epilepsy: Initial: 400 mg/day in 2 divided doses (tablets) **or** 4 divided doses (suspension); Maintenance: 800-1200 mg/day in 3-4 divided doses (maximum: 2400 mg/day); Trigeminal or glossopharyngeal neuralgia: Initial: 200 mg/day in 2 divided doses; Maintenance: 400-800 mg/day in 2 divided doses (maximum: 1200 mg/day)

Administration

Oral

Suspension: Must be given on a 3-4 times/day schedule versus tablets which can be given 2-4 times/day. Since a given dose of suspension will produce higher peak and lower trough levels than the same dose given as the tablet form, patients given the suspension should be started on lower doses given more frequently (same total daily dose) and increased slowly to avoid unwanted side effects. When carbamazepine suspension has been combined with chlorpromazine or thioridazine solutions, a precipitate forms which may result in loss of effect. Therefore, it is recommended that the carbamazepine suspension dosage form not be administered at the same time with other liquid medicinal agents or diluents. Should be administered with meals.

Extended release capsule (Carbatrol®, Equetro®): Consists of three different types of beads: Immediate release, extended-release, and enteric release. The bead types are combined in a ratio to allow twice daily dosing. May be opened and contents sprinkled over food such as a teaspoon of applesauce; may be administered with or without food; do not crush or chew.

Extended release tablet: Should be inspected for damage. Damaged extended release tablets (without release portal) should not be administered. Should be administered with meals; swallow whole, do not crush or chew.

Nursing Actions

Physical Assessment Monitor therapeutic response (seizure activity, type, duration) at beginning of therapy and periodically throughout. Taper dosage slowly when discontinuing. Observe and teach seizure/safety precautions. Monitor for mental and CNS changes, excessive sedation (especially when initiating or increasing therapy), and suicide ideation.

Patient Education Do not use extended release tablets which have been damaged or crushed. While using this medication, do not use alcohol. Maintain adequate hydration, unless instructed to restrict fluid intake. You may experience drowsiness, dizziness, blurred vision, nausea, vomiting, loss of appetite, or dry mouth. Wear identification of epileptic status and medications. Report CNS changes, suicide ideation, mentation changes, depression, changes in cognition, muscle cramping, weakness, tremors, sore throat, mouth ulcers, swollen glands, fever, jaundice, changes in gait, persistent GI symptoms (cramping, constipation, vomiting, anorexia), rash or skin irritations, unusual bruising or bleeding (mouth, urine, stool), or worsening of seizure activity or loss of seizure control.

Dietary Considerations Drug may cause GI upset, take with large amount of water or food to decrease GI upset. May need to split doses to avoid GI upset.

Related Information

Peak and Trough Guidelines *on page 1276*

Carbidopa and Levodopa

(kar bi DOE pa & lee voe DOE pa)

Brand Names: U.S. Parcopa®; Sinemet®; Sinemet® CR

Index Terms Levodopa and Carbidopa

Pharmacologic Category Anti-Parkinson's Agent, Decarboxylase Inhibitor; Anti-Parkinson's Agent, Dopamine Precursor

Medication Safety Issues

Sound-alike/look-alike issues:

Sinemet® may be confused with Serevent®

International issues:

Zimox: Brand name for carbidopa and levodopa [Greece], but also the brand name for amoxicillin [Italy]

Zimox [Greece] may be confused with Diamox which is a brand name for acetazolamide [Canada and multiple international markets]

Pregnancy Risk Factor C

Lactation Excretion in breast milk unknown/use caution

Use Idiopathic Parkinson's disease; postencephalitic parkinsonism; symptomatic parkinsonism

Duodopa™ intestinal gel: Canadian labeling (not available in U.S.): Treatment of advanced levodopa-responsive Parkinson's disease in which severe motor symptoms are not controlled by other Parkinson's agents

Unlabeled Use Restless leg syndrome

Mechanism of Action/Effect Parkinson's symptoms are due to a lack of striatal dopamine; levodopa circulates in the plasma to the blood-brain-barrier (BBB), where it crosses, to be converted by striatal enzymes to dopamine; carbidopa inhibits the peripheral plasma breakdown of levodopa by inhibiting its decarboxylation, and thereby increases available levodopa at the BBB

Contraindications Hypersensitivity to levodopa, carbidopa, or any component of the formulation; narrow-angle glaucoma; use of MAO inhibitors within prior 14 days (however, may be administered concomitantly with the manufacturer's recommended dose of an MAO inhibitor with selectivity for MAO type B); history of melanoma or undiagnosed skin lesions

Canadian labeling: Additional contraindications: Clinical or laboratory evidence of uncompensated cardiovascular, cerebrovascular, endocrine, renal, hepatic, hematologic or pulmonary disease; when administration of a sympathomimetic amine (eg, epinephrine, norepinephrine or isoproterenol) is contraindicated; intestinal gel therapy in patients with any condition preventing the required placement of a PEG tube for administration.

Warnings/Precautions Use with caution in patients with history of cardiovascular disease (including myocardial infarction and arrhythmias), pulmonary diseases (such as asthma), psychosis, wide-angle glaucoma, peptic ulcer disease, seizure disorder or prone to seizures, and in severe renal and hepatic dysfunction. Use with caution when interpreting plasma/urine catecholamine levels; falsely diagnosed pheochromocytoma has been rarely reported. Severe cases or rhabdomyolysis have been reported. Sudden discontinuation of levodopa may cause a worsening of Parkinson's disease. Elderly may be more sensitive to CNS effects of levodopa. May cause or exacerbate dyskinesias. Patients have reported falling asleep while engaging in activities of daily living; this has been reported to occur without significant warning signs. May cause orthostatic hypotension; Parkinson's disease patients appear to have an impaired capacity to respond to a postural challenge; use with caution in patients at risk of hypotension (such as those receiving antihypertensive drugs) or where transient hypotensive episodes would be poorly tolerated (cardiovascular disease or cerebrovascular disease). Observe patients closely for development of depression with concomitant suicidal tendencies.

Dopamine agonists have been associated with compulsive behaviors and/or loss of impulse control, which has manifested as pathological gambling, libido increases (hypersexuality), and/or binge eating. Causality has not been established, and controversy exists as to whether this phenomenon is related to the underlying disease, prior behaviors/addictions and/or drug therapy. Dose reduction or discontinuation of therapy has been reported to reverse these behaviors in some, but not all cases. Risk for melanoma development is increased in Parkinson's disease patients; drug causation or factors contributing to risk have not been established. Patients should be monitored closely and periodic skin examinations should be performed. Dopaminergic agents have been associated with a syndrome resembling neuroleptic malignant syndrome on abrupt withdrawal or significant dosage reduction after long-term use. Protein in the diet should be distributed throughout the day to avoid fluctuations in levodopa absorption.

Intestinal gel (available in Canada, not available in U.S.): Product should be prescribed only by neurologists experienced in the treatment of Parkinson's disease and who have completed the Duodopa™ Education Program. Response to levodopa/carbidopa intestinal gel therapy should be assessed with a test period (~3 days) of administration via a temporary nasoduodenal tube prior to placement of a percutaneous endoscopic gastrostomy (PEG) tube for permanent access and administration. Sudden deterioration in therapy response with recurring motor symptoms may indicate PEG tube complications (eg, displacement) or obstruction of the infusion device. Tube or infusion device complications may require initiation of oral levodopa/carbidopa therapy until complications are resolved. Discontinue therapy 2-3 hours prior to surgical procedures requiring general anesthesia, if possible. May resume therapy postoperatively when oral fluid intake is permitted.

Drug Interactions

Avoid Concomitant Use There are no known interactions where it is recommended to avoid concomitant use.

Decreased Effect

Carbidopa and Levodopa may decrease the levels/effects of: Antipsychotics (Typical)

The levels/effects of Carbidopa and Levodopa may be decreased by: Antipsychotics (Atypical); Fosphenytoin; Glycopyrrolate; Iron Salts; Methionine; Metoclopramide; Phenytoin; Pyridoxine

Increased Effect/Toxicity

Carbidopa and Levodopa may increase the levels/effects of: MAO Inhibitors

The levels/effects of Carbidopa and Levodopa may be increased by: Antipsychotics (Typical); MAO Inhibitors; Methylphenidate; Sapropterin

Nutritional/Ethanol Interactions

Ethanol: Avoid ethanol (due to CNS depression).

Food: Avoid high protein diets due to potential for impaired levodopa absorption; levodopa competes with certain amino acids for transport across the gut wall or across the blood-brain barrier.

Herb/Nutraceutical: Avoid kava kava (may decrease effects). Pyridoxine (vitamin B_6) in doses >10-25 mg (for levodopa alone) may decrease efficacy. Iron supplements or iron-containing multivitamins may reduce absorption of levodopa.

Adverse Reactions Frequency not defined.

Cardiovascular: Arrhythmia, chest pain, edema, flushing, hypotension, hypertension, MI, orthostatic hypotension, palpitation, phlebitis, syncope

Central nervous system: Agitation, anxiety, ataxia, confusion, delusions, dementia, depression (with or without suicidal tendencies), disorientation, dizziness, dreams abnormal, EPS, euphoria, faintness, falling, fatigue, gait abnormalities, headache, hallucinations, impulse control symptoms, insomnia, malaise, memory impairment, mental acuity decreased, nervousness, neuroleptic malignant syndrome, nightmares, on-off phenomena, paranoid ideation, pathological gambling, psychosis, seizure (causal relationship not established), somnolence

Dermatologic: Alopecia, malignant melanoma, rash

Endocrine & metabolic: Hot flashes, hyperglycemia, hypokalemia, libido increased (including hypersexuality), uric acid increased

Gastrointestinal: Abdominal pain, abdominal distress, anorexia, bruxism, constipation, diarrhea, discoloration of saliva, duodenal ulcer, dyspepsia, dysphagia, flatulence, GI bleeding, heartburn, nausea, sialorrhea, taste alterations, tongue burning sensation, weight gain/loss, vomiting, xerostomia

Genitourinary: Discoloration of urine, glycosuria, urinary frequency, priapism, proteinuria, urinary incontinence, urinary retention, urinary tract infection

Hematologic: Agranulocytosis, anemia, Coombs' test abnormal, hematocrit decreased, hemoglobin decreased, hemolytic anemia, leukopenia

Hepatic: Alkaline phosphatase abnormal, ALT abnormal, AST abnormal, bilirubin abnormal, LDH abnormal

Neuromuscular & skeletal: Back pain, dyskinesias (including choreiform, dystonic and other involuntary movements), leg pain, muscle cramps, muscle twitching, numbness, paresthesia, peripheral neuropathy, shoulder pain, tremor increased, trismus, weakness

Ocular: Blepharospasm, blurred vision, diplopia, Horner's syndrome reactivation, mydriasis, oculogyric crises (may be associated with acute dystonic reactions)

Renal: Difficult urination

Respiratory: Cough, dyspnea, hoarseness, pharyngeal pain, upper respiratory infection

Miscellaneous: Discoloration of sweat, diaphoresis increased, hiccups, hypersensitivity reactions (angioedema, pruritus, urticaria, bullous lesions [including pemphigus-like reactions], Henoch-Schönlein purpura)

Available Dosage Forms

Tablet: 10/100: Carbidopa 10 mg and levodopa 100 mg; 25/100: Carbidopa 25 mg and levodopa 100 mg; 25/250: Carbidopa 25 mg and levodopa 250 mg

Sinemet®:

10/100: Carbidopa 10 mg and levodopa 100 mg

25/100: Carbidopa 25 mg and levodopa 100 mg

25/250: Carbidopa 25 mg and levodopa 250 mg

Tablet, extended release: 25/100: Carbidopa 25 mg and levodopa 100 mg; 50/200: Carbidopa 50 mg and levodopa 200 mg

Tablet, orally disintegrating: 10/100: Carbidopa 10 mg and levodopa 100 mg; 25/100: Carbidopa 25 mg and levodopa 100 mg; 25/250: Carbidopa 25 mg and levodopa 250 mg

Parcopa®:

10/100: Carbidopa 10 mg and levodopa 100 mg [contains phenylalanine 3.4 mg/tablet; mint flavor]

25/100: Carbidopa 25 mg and levodopa 100 mg [contains phenylalanine 3.4 mg/tablet; mint flavor]

25/250: Carbidopa 25 mg and levodopa 250 mg [contains phenylalanine 8.4 mg/tablet; mint flavor]

Tablet, sustained release: 25/100: Carbidopa 25 mg and levodopa 100 mg; 50/200: Carbidopa 50 mg and levodopa 200 mg

Sinemet® CR:

25/100: Carbidopa 25 mg and levodopa 100 mg

50/200: Carbidopa 50 mg and levodopa 200 mg

General Dosage Range Oral: *Adults:* Immediate release: Initial: Carbidopa 25 mg/levodopa 100 mg 3 times/day (maximum: 8 tablets of any strength/day **or** 200 mg of carbidopa and 2000 mg of levodopa); Controlled release: *Adults:* Initial: Carbidopa 50 mg/levodopa 200 mg 2 times/day, at intervals not <6 hours (maximum: 8 tablets/day)

Administration

Oral Tablet formulations: Space doses evenly over the waking hours. Give with meals to decrease GI upset. Controlled release product should not be chewed or crushed. Orally-disintegrating tablets do not require water; the tablet should disintegrate on the tongue's surface before swallowing.

Other Intestinal gel (Canadian labeling; not available in U.S.): Gel is administered directly to the duodenum via a portable infusion pump (CADD-legacy Duodopa™ pump). Administer through a temporary nasoduodenal tube for at least 3 days to evaluate patient response and for dose optimization. Long-term administration requires placement of PEG tube for intestinal infusion. Continuous maintenance dose is infused throughout the day for up to 16 hours.

Stability

Storage

Tablet: Store at 20°C to 25°C (68°F to 77°F); excursions permitted between 15°C to 30°C (59°F to 86°F). Protect from light and moisture.

Intestinal gel (Canadian labeling; not available in U.S.): Store in refrigerator at 2°C to 8°C (36°F to 46°F). Keep in outer carton to protect from light. Cassettes are for single use only and should be discarded daily following infusion (up to 16 hours).

Nursing Actions

Physical Assessment Monitor therapeutic response (eg, activities of daily living, involuntary movements) at beginning of therapy and periodically throughout therapy.

Patient Education Do not crush controlled release form. Duodopa: If successful, trial patient will need PEG tube insertion for long-term treatment. Education will be required for use of portable infusion pump and gel delivery. Make sure to give patient educational materials.

Therapeutic effects may take several weeks or months to achieve and you may need frequent monitoring during first weeks of therapy. Take with meals if GI upset occurs. Do not use alcohol. You may experience drowsiness, dizziness, confusion, vision changes, loss of impulse control (possibly manifested as pathological gambling, libido increases, and/or binge eating), orthostatic hypotension, constipation, dry skin, nausea, vomiting, or loss of appetite. Report unresolved constipation or vomiting, respiratory difficulty, dizziness, CNS changes (hallucination, loss of memory, nervousness, etc), suicide ideation, increased muscle spasticity or rigidity, changes in the appearance of skin moles, skin rash, or significant worsening of condition.

Dietary Considerations Avoid high protein diets (>2 g/kg) which may decrease the efficacy of levodopa via competition with amino acids in crossing the blood-brain barrier. Some products may contain phenylalanine.

CARBOplatin (KAR boe pla tin)

Index Terms CBDCA; Paraplatin

Pharmacologic Category Antineoplastic Agent, Alkylating Agent; Antineoplastic Agent, Platinum Analog

Medication Safety Issues

Sound-alike/look-alike issues:

CARBOplatin may be confused with CISplatin, oxaliplatin

Paraplatin® may be confused with Platinol®

High alert medication:

This medication is in a class the Institute for Safe Medication Practices (ISMP) includes among its list of drugs which have a heightened risk of causing significant patient harm when used in error.

Pregnancy Risk Factor D

Lactation Excretion in breast milk unknown/not recommended

Breast-Feeding Considerations Due to the potential for toxicity in nursing infants, breast-feeding is not recommended.

Use Treatment of advanced ovarian cancer

Unlabeled Use Treatment of bladder cancer, breast cancer (metastatic), central nervous system tumors, cervical cancer (recurrent or metastatic), endometrial cancer, esophageal cancer, head and neck cancer, Hodgkin's lymphoma (relapsed or refractory), malignant pleural mesothelioma, melanoma (advanced or metastatic), merkel cell carcinoma, neuroendocrine tumors (adrenal gland and carcinoid tumors), non-Hodgkin's lymphomas (relapsed or refractory), nonsmall cell lung cancer, prostate cancer, sarcomas (Ewing's sarcoma and osteosarcoma), small-cell lung cancer, testicular cancer, thymic malignancies, unknown primary adenocarcinoma, and as a conditioning regimen prior to hematopoietic stem cell transplantation

Mechanism of Action/Effect Carboplatin is an alkylating agent which covalently binds to DNA; possible cross-linking and interference with the function of DNA

Contraindications History of severe allergic reaction to cisplatin, carboplatin, other platinum-containing formulations, mannitol, or any component of the formulation; should not be used in patients with severe bone marrow depression or significant bleeding

Warnings/Precautions Hazardous agent - use appropriate precautions for handling and disposal. High doses have resulted in severe abnormalities of liver function tests. **[U.S. Boxed Warning]: Bone marrow suppression, which may be severe, is dose related;** reduce dosage in patients with bone marrow suppression; cycles should be delayed until WBC and platelet counts have recovered. Patients who have received prior myelosuppressive therapy and patients with renal dysfunction are at increased risk for bone marrow suppression. Anemia is cumulative.

When calculating the carboplatin dose using the Calvert formula and an estimated glomerular filtration rate (GFR), the laboratory method used to measure serum creatinine may impact dosing. Compared to other methods, standardized isotope dilution mass spectrometry (IDMS) may underestimate serum creatinine values in patients with low creatinine values (eg, ≤0.7 mg/dL) and may overestimate GFR in patients with normal renal function. This may result in higher calculated carboplatin doses and increased toxicities. If using IDMS, the Food and Drug Administration (FDA) recommends that clinicians consider capping estimated GFR at a maximum of 125 mL/minute to avoid potential toxicity.

[U.S. Boxed Warning]: Anaphylactic-like reactions have been reported with carboplatin; may occur within minutes of administration. Epinephrine, corticosteroids and antihistamines have been used to treat symptoms. The risk of allergic reactions (including anaphylaxis) is increased in patients previously exposed to platinum therapy. Skin testing and desensitization protocols have been reported (Confina-Cohen, 2005; Lee, 2004; Markman, 2003). When administered as sequential infusions, taxane derivatives (docetaxel, paclitaxel) should be administered before the platinum derivatives (carboplatin, cisplatin) to limit myelosuppression and to enhance efficacy. Clinically significant hearing loss has been reported to occur in pediatric patients when carboplatin was administered at higher than recommended doses in combination with other ototoxic agents (eg, aminoglycosides). Loss of vision (reversible) has been reported with higher than recommended doses. Peripheral neuropathy occurs infrequently, the incidence of peripheral neuropathy is increased patients >65 years of age and those who have previously received cisplatin treatment. Patients >65 years of age are more likely to develop severe thrombocytopenia. **[U.S. Boxed Warning]: Vomiting may occur;** may be severe in patients who have received prior emetogenic therapy. **[U.S. Boxed Warning]: Should be administered under the supervision of an experienced cancer chemotherapy physician.**

Drug Interactions

Avoid Concomitant Use

Avoid concomitant use of CARBOplatin with any of the following: BCG; CloZAPine; Natalizumab; Pimecrolimus; SORAfenib; Tacrolimus (Topical); Vaccines (Live)

Decreased Effect

CARBOplatin may decrease the levels/effects of: BCG; Coccidioidin Skin Test; Sipuleucel-T; Vaccines (Inactivated); Vaccines (Live)

The levels/effects of CARBOplatin may be decreased by: Echinacea

Increased Effect/Toxicity

CARBOplatin may increase the levels/effects of: Bexarotene; Bexarotene (Systemic); CloZAPine; Leflunomide; Natalizumab; Taxane Derivatives; Topotecan; Vaccines (Live)

The levels/effects of CARBOplatin may be increased by: Aminoglycosides; Denosumab; Pimecrolimus; Roflumilast; SORAfenib; Tacrolimus (Topical); Trastuzumab

Nutritional/Ethanol Interactions Herb/Nutraceutical: Avoid black cohosh, dong quai in estrogen-dependent tumors.

Adverse Reactions Percentages reported with single-agent therapy.

>10%:

Central nervous system: Pain (23%)

Endocrine & metabolic: Hyponatremia (29% to 47%), hypomagnesemia (29% to 43%), hypocalcemia(22% to 31%), hypokalemia (20% to 28%)

Gastrointestinal: Vomiting (65% to 81%), abdominal pain (17%), nausea (without vomiting: 10% to 15%)

Hematologic: Myelosuppression (dose related and dose limiting; nadir at ~21 days; recovery by ~28 days), anemia (71% to 90%; grades 3/4: 21%), leukopenia (85%; grades 3/4: 15% to 26%), neutropenia (67%; grades 3/4: 16% to 21%), thrombocytopenia (62%; grades 3/4: 25% to 35%)

Hepatic: Alkaline phosphatase increased (24% to 37%), AST increased (15% to 19%)

Neuromuscular & skeletal: Weakness (11%)

Renal: Creatinine clearance decreased (27%), BUN increased (14% to 22%)

Miscellaneous: Hypersensitivity/allergic reaction (2% to 16%)

1% to 10%:

Central nervous system: Neurotoxicity (5%)

Dermatologic: Alopecia (2% to 3%)

Gastrointestinal: Constipation (6%), diarrhea (6%), stomatitis/mucositis (1%), taste dysgeusia (1%)

Hematologic: Bleeding (5%), hemorrhagic complications (5%)

Hepatic: Bilirubin increased (5%)

Neuromuscular & skeletal: Peripheral neuropathy (4% to 6%)

Ocular: Visual disturbance (1%)

Otic: Ototoxicity (1%)

Renal: Creatinine increased (6% to 10%)

Miscellaneous: Infection (5%)

Available Dosage Forms

Injection, solution [preservative free]: 10 mg/mL (5 mL, 15 mL, 45 mL, 60 mL)

General Dosage Range Dosage adjustment recommended in renal impairment or who develop toxicities

I.V.: *Adults:* 300-360 mg/m^2 every 4 weeks **or** AUC of 4-6 (using Calvert formula)

Administration

I.V. Usually infused over 15-60 minutes, although some protocols may require infusions up to 24 hours. When administered as sequential infusions, taxane derivatives (docetaxel, paclitaxel) should be administered before platinum derivatives to limit myelosuppression and to enhance efficacy.

Stability

Reconstitution Reconstitute powder to yield a final concentration of 10 mg/mL. Reconstituted carboplatin 10 mg/mL should be further diluted to a final concentration of 0.5-2 mg/mL with D_5W or NS for administration. Use appropriate precautions for handling and disposal.

Storage Store intact vials at room temperature of 25°C (77°F); excursions permitted to 15°C to 30°C (59°F to 86°F). Protect from light. Further dilution to a concentration as low as 0.5 mg/mL is stable at room temperature (25°C) for 8 hours in NS; stable at room temperature or under refrigeration for at least 9 days in D_5W, although the manufacturer states to use within 8 hours due to lack of preservative.

Powder for reconstitution: Reconstituted to a final concentration of 10 mg/mL is stable for 5 days at room temperature (25°C).

Solution for injection: Multidose vials are stable for up to 14 days after opening when stored at room temperature.

Nursing Actions

Physical Assessment Patient allergy history must be assessed prior to therapy. Assess other drugs patient may be taking for potential interactions (especially products that may be ototoxic or nephrotoxic and need for sequencing with taxane derivatives). Assess hematology, electrolytes, and renal and hepatic function tests prior to treatment and on a regular basis during therapy. Monitor for nausea and vomiting (pretreatment with antiemetic may be required), ototoxicity (audiometry may be advisable), bone marrow depression, anemia, bleeding, and peripheral neuropathy.

Patient Education This medicine can only be administered intravenously. Report immediately any redness, burning, pain, or swelling at infusion site. It is important that you maintain adequate nutrition and hydration, unless instructed to restrict fluid intake. You will be susceptible to infection. May cause nausea, vomiting, mouth sores, or loss of hair (reversible). Report chest pain or palpitations; sore throat, fever, chills, unusual fatigue; unusual bruising/bleeding; respiratory difficulty; numbness, pain, or tingling in extremities; muscle cramps or twitching; or change in hearing acuity.

Related Information

Management of Drug Extravasations *on page 1269*

Carboprost Tromethamine

(KAR boe prost tro METH a meen)

Brand Names: U.S. Hemabate®

Index Terms Carboprost; Prostaglandin F_2

Pharmacologic Category Abortifacient; Prostaglandin

Pregnancy Risk Factor C

Lactation Excretion in breast milk unknown

Use Termination of pregnancy; treatment of refractory postpartum uterine bleeding

Unlabeled Use Hemorrhagic cystitis

Available Dosage Forms

Injection, solution:

Hemabate®: 250 mcg/mL (1 mL)

General Dosage Range I.M.: *Adults (females):* Abortion: 250 mcg at 1.5- to 3.5-hour intervals, a 500 mcg dose may be given if uterine response is not adequate after several 250 mcg doses (maximum total dose: 12 mg); Postpartum bleeding: 250 mcg; may repeat if needed (maximum total dose: 2 mg [8 doses])

Administration

I.M. Give deep I.M.; rotate site if repeat injections are required.

I.V. Do not inject I.V.; may result in bronchospasm, hypertension, vomiting, or anaphylaxis.

Nursing Actions

Physical Assessment Note that nausea or vomiting may be significant; premedication with an antiemetic may be considered. Monitor for uterine contractions, hypertension, hemorrhage, respiratory effects, or prolonged or excessively elevated temperature. Report contractions lasting longer than 1 minute or absence of contractions to prescriber. Assess for complete expulsion of uterine contents (fetal tissue).

Patient Education This medication is used to stimulate expulsion of uterine contents (fetal tissue) or stimulate uterine contractions to reduce uterine bleeding. Report increased blood loss, acute abdominal cramping, foul-smelling vaginal discharge, or persistent elevation of temperature. Increased temperature may occur 1-16 hours after therapy and last for several hours.

Carisoprodol (kar eye soe PROE dole)

Brand Names: U.S. Soma®

Index Terms Carisoprodate; Isobamate

Pharmacologic Category Skeletal Muscle Relaxant

Medication Safety Issues

BEERS Criteria medication:

This drug may be inappropriate for use in geriatric patients (high severity risk).

Pregnancy Risk Factor C

Lactation Enters breast milk/use caution

Breast-Feeding Considerations Carisoprodol levels in breast milk may be 2-4 times that of maternal plasma levels. The estimated dose to the infant was reported as 6.9% of the weight adjusted maternal dose in one case report and ~4% of the weight-adjusted maternal dose in another. In both cases, breast milk production was decreased requiring supplemental formula or cessation of breast-feeding. Other than slight sedation reported in one infant, no symptoms of withdrawal or other adverse events were noted in these 2 cases. Effects on long-term development are not known.

Use Short-term (2-3 weeks) treatment of acute musculoskeletal pain

Mechanism of Action/Effect Precise mechanism is not yet clear, but many effects have been ascribed to its central depressant actions. In animals, carisoprodol blocks interneuronal activity and depresses polysynaptic neuron transmission in the spinal cord and reticular formation of the brain. It is also metabolized to meprobamate, which has anxiolytic and sedative effects.

Contraindications Hypersensitivity to carisoprodol, meprobamate, or any component of the formulation; acute intermittent porphyria

Warnings/Precautions Can cause CNS depression, which may impair physical or mental abilities. Patients must be cautioned about performing tasks which require mental alertness (eg, operating machinery or driving); postmarketing reports of motor vehicle accidents have been associated with use. Effects with other CNS-depressant drugs or ethanol may be potentiated. Use with caution in patients with hepatic/renal dysfunction. Tolerance or drug dependence may result from extended use. Limit use to 2-3 weeks; use caution in patients who may be prone to addiction. May precipitate withdrawal after abrupt cessation of prolonged use.

Idiosyncratic reactions and/or severe allergic reactions may occur. Idiosyncratic reactions occur following the initial dose and may include severe weakness, transient quadriplegia, euphoria, or vision loss (temporary). Has been associated (rarely) with seizures in patients with and without seizure history. Carisoprodol should be used with caution in patients who are poor CYP2C19 metabolizers; poor metabolizers have been shown to have a fourfold increase in exposure to carisoprodol and a 50% reduced exposure to the metabolite meprobamate compared to normal metabolizers. This class of medication is poorly tolerated by the elderly due to anticholinergic effects, sedation, and weakness. Efficacy is questionable at dosages tolerated by elderly patients (Beers Criteria).

Drug Interactions

Avoid Concomitant Use There are no known interactions where it is recommended to avoid concomitant use.

Decreased Effect

The levels/effects of Carisoprodol may be decreased by: CYP2C19 Inducers (Strong)

Increased Effect/Toxicity

Carisoprodol may increase the levels/effects of: Alcohol (Ethyl); CNS Depressants; Methotrimeprazine; Selective Serotonin Reuptake Inhibitors

The levels/effects of Carisoprodol may be increased by: CYP2C19 Inhibitors (Moderate); CYP2C19 Inhibitors (Strong); Droperidol; HydrOXYzine; Methotrimeprazine

Nutritional/Ethanol Interactions Ethanol: May increase CNS depression; monitor for increased effects with coadministration. Caution patients about effects.

Adverse Reactions

>10%: Central nervous system: Drowsiness (13% to 17%)

1% to 10%: Central nervous system: Dizziness (7% to 8%), headache (3% to 5%)

Pharmacodynamics/Kinetics

Onset of Action ~30 minutes

Duration of Action 4-6 hours

Controlled Substance C-IV

Available Dosage Forms

Tablet, oral: 350 mg

Soma®: 250 mg, 350 mg

General Dosage Range Oral: *Children ≥16 years and Adults:* 250-350 mg 3 times/day and at bedtime

Administration

Oral Administer with or without food.

Stability

Storage Store at controlled room temperature of 20°C to 25°C (68°F to 77°F).

Nursing Actions

Physical Assessment Monitor for excessive drowsiness at beginning of therapy and periodically throughout. Do not discontinue abruptly; taper dosage slowly (withdrawal symptoms such as abdominal cramping, headache, and insomnia may occur). Teach patient postural hypotension precautions.

Patient Education Do not use alcohol. You may experience drowsiness, dizziness, lightheadedness, nausea, vomiting, cramping, headache, or postural hypotension. Report excessive drowsiness or mental agitation; palpitations, rapid heartbeat, or chest pain; skin rash; muscle cramping or tremors; or respiratory difficulty.

Dietary Considerations May be taken with or without food.

Carisoprodol and Aspirin

(kar eye soe PROE dole & AS pir in)

Index Terms Aspirin and Carisoprodol; Soma Compound

Pharmacologic Category Skeletal Muscle Relaxant

Medication Safety Issues

BEERS Criteria medication:

This drug (carisoprodol) may be inappropriate for use in geriatric patients (high severity risk).

Pregnancy Risk Factor D

Lactation Enters breast milk/not recommended

Use Relief of discomfort associated with acute, painful skeletal muscle conditions

Controlled Substance C-IV

Available Dosage Forms

Tablet: Carisoprodol 200 mg and aspirin 325 mg

General Dosage Range Oral: *Children ≥16 years and Adults:* 1-2 tablets 4 times/day (maximum: 8 tablets/24 hours)

Nursing Actions

Physical Assessment See individual agents.

Patient Education See individual agents.

Related Information

Aspirin *on page 94*

Carisoprodol *on page 188*

Carmustine (kar MUS teen)

Brand Names: U.S. BiCNU®; Gliadel®

Index Terms BCNU; bis(chloroethyl) nitrosourea; bis-chloronitrosourea; Carmustine Polymer Wafer; Carmustinum; WR-139021

Pharmacologic Category Antineoplastic Agent; Antineoplastic Agent, Alkylating Agent; Antineoplastic Agent, Alkylating Agent (Nitrosourea)

Medication Safety Issues

Sound-alike/look-alike issues:

Carmustine may be confused with bendamustine, lomustine

High alert medication:

This medication is in a class the Institute for Safe Medication Practices (ISMP) includes among its list of drug classes which have a heightened risk of causing significant patient harm when used in error.

Pregnancy Risk Factor D

Lactation Excretion in breast milk unknown/not recommended

Breast-Feeding Considerations Due to the potential for serious adverse reactions in the nursing infant, breast-feeding should be discontinued.

Use

Injection: Treatment of brain tumors (glioblastoma, brainstem glioma, medulloblastoma, astrocytoma, ependymoma, and metastatic brain tumors), multiple myeloma, Hodgkin's lymphoma (relapsed or refractory), non-Hodgkin's lymphomas (relapsed or refractory)

Wafer (implant): Adjunct to surgery in patients with recurrent glioblastoma multiforme; adjunct to surgery and radiation in patients with newly-diagnosed high-grade malignant glioma

Unlabeled Use Treatment of mycosis fungoides (topical)

Mechanism of Action/Effect Interferes with the normal function of DNA and RNA by alkylation and cross-linking the strands of DNA and RNA, and by possible protein modification; may also inhibit enzyme processes by carbamylation of amino acids in protein

Contraindications Hypersensitivity to carmustine or any component of the formulation

Warnings/Precautions Hazardous agent - use appropriate precautions for handling and disposal.

[U.S. Boxed Warning]: Injection: Bone marrow suppression (primarily thrombocytopenia and leukopenia) is the major carmustine toxicity; generally is delayed. Monitor blood counts weekly for at least 6 weeks after administration. Myelosuppression is cumulative. When given at the FDA-approved doses, treatment should not be administered less than 6 weeks apart. Consider nadir blood counts from prior dose for dosage adjustment. May cause bleeding (due to thrombocytopenia) or infections (due to neutropenia); monitor closely. Patients must have platelet counts >100,000/mm^3 and leukocytes >4000/mm^3 for a repeat dose. Anemia may occur (less common and less severe than leukopenia or thrombocytopenia). Long-term use is associated with the development of secondary malignancies (acute leukemias and bone marrow dysplasias).

[U.S. Boxed Warnings]: Injection: Dose-related pulmonary toxicity may occur; patients receiving cumulative doses >1400 mg/m^2 are at higher risk. Delayed onset of pulmonary fibrosis (may be fatal) has occurred in children up to 17 years after treatment; this occurred in ages 1-16 for the treatment of intracranial tumors; cumulative doses ranged from 770-1800 mg/m^2 (in combination with cranial radiotherapy). Pulmonary toxicity is characterized by pulmonary infiltrates and/or fibrosis and has been reported from 9 days to 43 months after nitrosourea treatment (including carmustine). Although pulmonary toxicity generally occurs in patients who have received prolonged treatment, pulmonary fibrosis has been reported with cumulative doses <1400 mg/m^2. In addition to high cumulative doses, other risk factors for pulmonary toxicity include history of lung disease and baseline predicted forced vital capacity (FVC) or carbon monoxide diffusing capacity (DL_{CO}) <70%. Baseline and periodic pulmonary function tests are recommended. For high-dose treatment (transplant; unlabeled dose), acute lung injury may occur ~1-3 months post transplant; advise patients to contact their transplant physician for dyspnea, cough, or fever; interstitial pneumonia may be managed with a course of corticosteroids. Children are at higher risk for delayed pulmonary toxicity.

Injection site burning and local tissue reactions, including swelling, pain, erythema, and necrosis have been reported. Monitor infusion site closely for infiltration or injection site reactions. Reversible increases in transaminases, bilirubin and alkaline phosphatase have been reported (rare); monitor liver function tests periodically during treatment. Renal failure, progressive azotemia, and decreased kidney size have been reported in patients who have received large cumulative doses or prolonged treatment (renal toxicity has also been reported in patients who have received lower cumulative doses); monitor renal function tests periodically during treatment. Unlabeled administration (intraarterial intracarotid route) has been associated with ocular toxicity. Consider initiating treatment at the lower end of the dose range in the elderly. Diluent contains ethanol. With wafer implantation, monitor closely for known craniotomy-related complications (seizure, intracranial infection, abnormal wound healing, brain edema); intracerebral mass effect (unresponsive to corticosteroids) has been reported; may lead to brain herniation; avoid communication between the resection cavity and the ventricular system to prevent wafer migration; communications larger than the wafer should be closed prior to implantation; wafer migration may cause obstructive hydrocephalus. **[U.S. Boxed Warning]: Injection: Should be administered under the supervision of an experienced cancer chemotherapy physician.**

Drug Interactions

Avoid Concomitant Use

Avoid concomitant use of Carmustine with any of the following: BCG; CloZAPine; Natalizumab; Pimecrolimus; Tacrolimus (Topical); Vaccines (Live)

Decreased Effect

Carmustine may decrease the levels/effects of: BCG; Cardiac Glycosides; Coccidioidin Skin Test; Sipuleucel-T; Vaccines (Inactivated); Vaccines (Live)

The levels/effects of Carmustine may be decreased by: Echinacea

Increased Effect/Toxicity

Carmustine may increase the levels/effects of: CloZAPine; Leflunomide; Natalizumab; Vaccines (Live)

The levels/effects of Carmustine may be increased by: Cimetidine; Denosumab; Melphalan; Pimecrolimus; Roflumilast; Tacrolimus (Topical); Trastuzumab

Adverse Reactions

I.V.: Frequency not defined:

Cardiovascular: Arrhythmia (with high doses), chest pain, flushing (with rapid infusion), hypotension, tachycardia

Central nervous system: Ataxia, dizziness

Central nervous system: Ethanol intoxication (with high doses), headache

Dermatologic: Hyperpigmentation/skin burning (after skin contact)

Gastrointestinal: Nausea (common; dose related), vomiting (common; dose related), mucositis (with high doses), toxic enterocolitis (with high doses)

Hematologic: Leukopenia (common; onset: 5-6 weeks; recovery: after 1-2 weeks), thrombocytopenia (common: onset:~4 weeks; recovery: after 1-2 weeks), anemia, neutropenic fever, secondary malignancies (acute leukemia, bone marrow dysplasias)

Hepatic: Alkaline phosphatase increased, bilirubin increased, hepatic sinusoidal obstruction syndrome (SOS; veno-occlusive disease; with high doses), transaminases increased

Local: Injection site reactions (burning, erythema, necrosis, pain, swelling)

Ocular: Conjunctival suffusion (with rapid infusion), neuroretinitis

Renal: Kidney size decreased, progressive azotemia, renal failure

Respiratory: Interstitial pneumonitis (with high doses), pulmonary fibrosis, pulmonary hypoplasia, pulmonary infiltrates

Miscellaneous: Allergic reaction, infection (with high doses)

Wafer: ≥4% (percentages reported only where incidence was greater compared to placebo):

Cardiovascular: Deep thrombophlebitis (10%), facial edema (6%), chest pain (5%)

Central nervous system: Brain edema (4% to 23%), confusion (10% to 23%), depression (16%), headache (15%), somnolence (14%), fever (12%), speech disorder (11%), intracranial hypertension (9%), anxiety (7%), facial paralysis (7%), pain (7%), ataxia (6%), hypesthesia (6%), hallucination (5%), seizure (grand mal 5%), meningitis (4%)

Dermatologic: Abnormal wound healing (14% to 16%), rash (5% to 12%)

Endocrine: Diabetes (5%)

Gastrointestinal: Nausea (8% to 22%), vomiting (8% to 21%), constipation (19%), abdominal pain (8%), diarrhea (5%)

Genitourinary: Urinary tract infection (21%)

Hematologic: Hemorrhage (7%)

Local: Abscess (4% to 8%)

Neuromuscular & skeletal: Weakness (22%), back pain (7%)

Available Dosage Forms

Injection, powder for reconstitution:

BiCNU®: 100 mg

Wafer, for implantation:

Gliadel®: 7.7 mg (8s)

General Dosage Range Dosage adjustment recommended in patients with renal impairment or who develop toxicity.

I.V.: *Adults:* 150-200 mg/m^2 every 6-8 weeks **or** 75-100 mg/m^2/day for 2 days every 6-8 weeks

Implantation: *Adults:* 8 wafers placed in the resection cavity (total dose: 61.6 mg)

Administration

I.V. Hazardous agent; use appropriate precautions for handling and disposal. Irritant (alcohol-based diluent). Significant absorption to PVC containers; should be prepared in either glass or polyolefin containers. Infuse over 2 hours (infusions <2 hours may lead to injection site pain or burning); infuse through a free-flowing saline or dextrose infusion, or administer through a central catheter to alleviate venous pain/irritation.

High-dose carmustine (transplant dose; unlabeled use): Infuse over a least 2 hours to avoid excessive flushing, agitation, and hypotension; was infused over 1 hour in some trials (Chopra, 1993). **High-dose carmustine may be fatal if not followed by stem cell rescue.** Monitor vital signs frequently during infusion; patients should be supine during infusion and may require the Trendelenburg position, fluid support, and vasopressor support.

Topical Hazardous agent; use appropriate precautions for handling and disposal. Topical (unlabeled use): Apply solution with brush or gauze pads; ointment and solution should be applied while wearing gloves to involved areas only; avoid contact with eyes or mouth (Zackheim, 2003).

Other Implant: Hazardous agent; use appropriate precautions for handling and disposal; double glove before handling; outer gloves should be discarded as chemotherapy waste after handling wafers. Any wafer or remnant that is removed upon repeat surgery should be discarded as chemotherapy waste. The outer surface of the external foil pouch is not sterile. Open pouch gently; avoid pressure on the wafers to prevent breakage. Wafer that are broken in half may be used, however, wafers broken into more than 2 pieces should be discarded in a biohazard container. Oxidized regenerated cellulose (Surgicel®) may be placed over the wafer to secure; irrigate cavity prior to closure.

Stability

Reconstitution Injection: Reconstitute initially with 3 mL of supplied diluent (dehydrated alcohol injection, USP); then further dilute with SWFI (27 mL), this provides a concentration of 3.3 mg/mL in ethanol 10%; protect from light; further dilute for infusion with D_5W using a non-PVC container.

Storage

Injection: Store intact vials under refrigeration at 2°C to 8°C (36°F to 46°F); provided diluent may be stored in refrigerator or at room temperature; intact vials are stable for 7 days at room temperature. Reconstituted solutions are stable for 24 hours refrigerated (2°C to 8°C) and protected from light. Solutions diluted to a concentration of 0.2 mg/mL in D_5W are stable for 8 hours at room temperature (25°C) in glass or polyolefin containers and protected from light.

Wafer: Store at or below -20°C (-4°F). Unopened foil pouches may be kept at room temperature for up to 6 hours.

Nursing Actions

Physical Assessment An antiemetic may be ordered prior to therapy. I.V.: Monitor infusion site closely to prevent extravasation. Monitor patient closely during and following high-dose BMT infusion; supine position (Trandelenburg position may be necessary), fluid support, and vasopressor support should be available. Assess results of hematology, pulmonary, hepatic, and renal function tests at baseline and periodically during therapy.

Patient Education This medication is usually administered by I.V. Report immediately any pain, burning, or swelling at infusion site; sudden onset chest pain; or difficulty breathing or swallowing. It is important that you maintain adequate nutrition between treatments and adequate hydration, unless instructed to restrict fluid intake. You will be susceptible to infection. May cause nausea, vomiting, anorexia, mouth sores, or hyperpigmentation of skin and loss of hair (reversible). Report immediately any dyspnea, cough, or fever; chest pain or palpitations; sore throat, chills, persistent or unusual fatigue; unusual bruising/bleeding; change in color of urine or stool; change in urinary pattern; change in visual acuity; seizure activity; or CNS changes.

Related Information

Management of Drug Extravasations *on page 1269*

Carvedilol (KAR ve dil ole)

Brand Names: U.S. Coreg CR®; Coreg®

Pharmacologic Category Beta Blocker With Alpha-Blocking Activity

Medication Safety Issues

Sound-alike/look-alike issues:

Carvedilol may be confused with atenolol, captopril, carbidopa, carteolol

Coreg® may be confused with Corgard®, Cortef®, Cozaar®

Pregnancy Risk Factor C

Lactation Excretion in breast milk unknown/not recommended

Breast-Feeding Considerations It is not known if carvedilol is excreted into human milk. The manufacturer suggests that a decision should be made to either discontinue nursing or discontinue the medication.

Use Mild-to-severe heart failure of ischemic or cardiomyopathic origin (usually in addition to standard therapy); left ventricular dysfunction following myocardial infarction (MI) (clinically stable with LVEF ≤40%); management of hypertension

Unlabeled Use Angina pectoris

Mechanism of Action/Effect Nonselective beta-adrenoreceptor and alpha-adrenergic blocking agent, lowers heart rate and blood pressure. Has been shown to lower risk of hospitalization and increase survival in patients with mild to severe heart failure.

Contraindications Serious hypersensitivity to carvedilol or any component of the formulation; decompensated cardiac failure requiring intravenous inotropic therapy; bronchial asthma or related bronchospastic conditions; second- or third-degree AV block, sick sinus syndrome, and severe bradycardia (except in patients with a functioning artificial pacemaker); cardiogenic shock; severe hepatic impairment

Warnings/Precautions Consider pre-existing conditions such as sick sinus syndrome before initiating. Heart failure patients may experience a worsening of renal function (rare); risk factors include ischemic heart disease, diffuse vascular disease, underlying renal dysfunction, and systolic BP <100 mm Hg. Initiate cautiously and monitor for possible deterioration in patient status (eg, symptoms of HF). Worsening heart failure or fluid retention may occur during upward titration; dose reduction or temporary discontinuation may be necessary. Adjustment of other medications (ACE inhibitors and/or diuretics) may also be required. Bradycardia may be observed more frequently in elderly patients (>65 years of age); dosage reductions may be necessary.

Symptomatic hypotension with or without syncope may occur with carvedilol (usually within the first 30 days of therapy); close monitoring of patient is required especially with initial dosing and dosing increases; blood pressure must be lowered at a rate appropriate for the patient's clinical condition. Initiation with a low dose, gradual up-titration, and administration with food may help to decrease the occurrence of hypotension or syncope. Patients should be advised to avoid driving or other hazardous tasks during initiation of therapy due to the risk of syncope. Beta-blocker therapy should not be withdrawn abruptly (particularly in patients with CAD), but gradually tapered to avoid acute tachycardia, hypertension, and/or ischemia. Chronic beta-blocker therapy should not be routinely withdrawn prior to major surgery.

In general, patients with bronchospastic disease should not receive beta-blockers; if used at all, should be used cautiously with close monitoring. May precipitate or aggravate symptoms of arterial insufficiency in patients with PVD and Raynaud's disease; use with caution and monitor for progression of arterial obstruction. Use caution with concurrent use of digoxin, verapamil or diltiazem; bradycardia or heart block can occur. Use with caution in patients receiving inhaled anesthetic agents known to depress myocardial contractility. Use cautiously in patients with diabetes because it can mask prominent hypoglycemic symptoms. In patients with heart failure and diabetes, use of carvedilol may worsen hyperglycemia; may require adjustment of antidiabetic agents. May mask signs of hyperthyroidism (eg, tachycardia); if hyperthyroidism is suspected, carefully manage and monitor; abrupt withdrawal may exacerbate symptoms of hyperthyroidism or precipitate thyroid storm. May induce or exacerbate psoriasis. Use with caution in patients with myasthenia gravis or psychiatric disease (may cause CNS depression). Use with caution in patients with mild-to-moderate hepatic impairment; use is contraindicated in patients with severe impairment. Manufacturer recommends discontinuation of therapy if liver injury occurs (confirmed by laboratory testing). Adequate alpha-blockade is required prior to use of any beta-blocker for patients with untreated pheochromocytoma. Use caution with history of severe anaphylaxis to allergens; patients taking beta-blockers may become more sensitive to repeated challenges. Treatment of anaphylaxis (eg, epinephrine) in patients taking beta-blockers may be ineffective or promote undesirable effects.

Intraoperative floppy iris syndrome has been observed in cataract surgery patients who were on or were previously treated with alpha$_1$-blockers; causality has not been established and there appears to be no benefit in discontinuing alpha-blocker therapy prior to surgery. Instruct patients to inform ophthalmologist of carvedilol use when considering eye surgery.

Drug Interactions

Avoid Concomitant Use

Avoid concomitant use of Carvedilol with any of the following: Beta2-Agonists; Floctafenine; Methacholine; Silodosin; Topotecan

Decreased Effect

Carvedilol may decrease the levels/effects of: Beta2-Agonists; Theophylline Derivatives

The levels/effects of Carvedilol may be decreased by: Barbiturates; Cyproterone; Herbs (Hypertensive Properties); Methylphenidate; Nonsteroidal Anti-Inflammatory Agents; Peginterferon Alfa-2b; P-glycoprotein/ABCB1 Inducers; Rifamycin Derivatives; Tocilizumab; Yohimbine

Increased Effect/Toxicity

Carvedilol may increase the levels/effects of: Alpha-/Beta-Agonists (Direct-Acting); Alpha1-Blockers; Alpha2-Agonists; Amifostine; Antihypertensives; Antipsychotic Agents (Phenothiazines); Bupivacaine; Cardiac Glycosides; Cholinergic Agonists; Colchicine; CycloSPORINE; CycloSPORINE (Systemic); Dabigatran Etexilate; Digoxin; Everolimus; Fingolimod; Hypotensive Agents; Insulin; Lidocaine; Lidocaine (Systemic); Lidocaine (Topical); Mepivacaine; Methacholine; Midodrine; P-glycoprotein/ABCB1 Substrates; Prucalopride; RiTUXimab; Rivaroxaban; Silodosin; Sulfonylureas; Topotecan

The levels/effects of Carvedilol may be increased by: Acetylcholinesterase Inhibitors; Aminoquinolines (Antimalarial); Amiodarone; Anilidopiperidine Opioids; Antipsychotic Agents (Phenothiazines); Calcium Channel Blockers (Dihydropyridine); Calcium Channel Blockers (Nondihydropyridine); Cimetidine; Conivaptan; CYP2C9 Inhibitors (Moderate); CYP2C9 Inhibitors (Strong); CYP2D6 Inhibitors (Moderate); CYP2D6 Inhibitors (Strong); Diazoxide; Dipyridamole; Disopyramide; Dronedarone; Floctafenine; Herbs (Hypotensive Properties); MAO Inhibitors; Pentoxifylline; P-glycoprotein/ABCB1 Inhibitors; Phosphodiesterase 5 Inhibitors; Propafenone; Prostacyclin Analogues; QuiNIDine; Reserpine; Selective Serotonin Reuptake Inhibitors

Nutritional/Ethanol Interactions

Food: Food decreases rate but not extent of absorption. Administration with food minimizes risks of orthostatic hypotension.

Herb/Nutraceutical: Avoid herbs with hypertensive properties (bayberry, blue cohosh, cayenne, ephedra, ginger, ginseng [American], kola, licorice); may diminish the antihypertensive effect of carvedilol. Avoid herbs with hypotensive properties (black cohosh, California poppy, coleus, golden seal, hawthorn, mistletoe, periwinkle, quinine, shepherd's purse); may enhance the hypotensive effect of carvedilol.

Adverse Reactions Note: Frequency ranges include data from hypertension and heart failure trials. Higher rates of adverse reactions have generally been noted in patients with heart failure. However, the frequency of adverse effects associated with placebo is also increased in this population.

>10%:

Cardiovascular: Hypotension (9% to 20%)

Central nervous system: Dizziness (2% to 32%), fatigue (4% to 24%)

Endocrine & metabolic: Hyperglycemia (5% to 12%)

Gastrointestinal: Diarrhea (1% to 12%), weight gain (10% to 12%)

Neuromuscular & skeletal: Weakness (7% to 11%)

1% to 10%:

Cardiovascular: Bradycardia (2% to 10%), syncope (3% to 8%), peripheral edema (1% to 7%), generalized edema (5% to 6%), angina (1% to 6%), dependent edema (≤4%), AV block, cerebrovascular accident, hypertension, hyper-/hypovolemia, postural hypotension, palpitation

Central nervous system: Headache (5% to 8%), depression, fever, hypoesthesia, hypotonia, insomnia, malaise, somnolence, vertigo

Endocrine & metabolic: Hypercholesterolemia (1% to 4%), hypertriglyceridemia (1%), diabetes mellitus, gout, hyperkalemia, hyperuricemia, hypoglycemia, hyponatremia

Gastrointestinal: Nausea (2% to 9%), vomiting (1% to 6%), abdominal pain, melena, periodontitis, weight loss

Genitourinary: Impotence

Hematologic: Anemia, prothrombin decreased, purpura, thrombocytopenia

Hepatic: Alkaline phosphatase increased (1% to 3%), GGT increased, transaminases increased

Neuromuscular & skeletal: Back pain (2% to 7%), arthralgia (1% to 6%), arthritis, muscle cramps, paresthesia

Ocular: Blurred vision (1% to 5%)

Renal: BUN increased (≤6%), nonprotein nitrogen increased (6%), albuminuria, creatinine increased, glycosuria, hematuria, renal insufficiency

Respiratory: Cough (5% to 8%), nasopharyngitis (4%), rales (4%), dyspnea (>3%), pulmonary edema (>3%), rhinitis (2%), nasal congestion (1%), sinus congestion (1%)

Miscellaneous: Injury (3% to 6%), allergy, flu-like syndrome, sudden death

Pharmacodynamics/Kinetics

Onset of Action 1-2 hours; Peak antihypertensive effect: ~1-2 hours

Available Dosage Forms

Capsule, extended release, oral:

Coreg CR®: 10 mg, 20 mg, 40 mg, 80 mg

Tablet, oral: 3.125 mg, 6.25 mg, 12.5 mg, 25 mg

Coreg®: 3.125 mg, 6.25 mg, 12.5 mg, 25 mg

General Dosage Range Oral: *Adults:* Immediate release: Initial: 3.125-6.25 mg twice daily; Maintenance: 6.25-50 mg twice daily (maximum: 50 mg/day [<85 kg]; 100 mg/day [>85 kg]); Extended release: Initial: 10 mg once daily; range: 10-80 mg once daily

Administration

Oral Administer with food to minimize the risk of orthostatic hypotension. Extended release capsules should not be crushed or chewed. Capsules may be opened and sprinkled on applesauce for immediate use.

Stability

Storage

Coreg®: Store at <30°C (<86°F). Protect from moisture.

Coreg CR®: Store at 25°C (77°F); excursions permitted to 15°C to 30°C (59°F to 86°F).

Nursing Actions

Physical Assessment Take blood pressure and heart rate prior to and following first dose and with any change in dosage. Caution patients with diabetes to monitor glucose levels closely (beta-blockers may alter glucose tolerance).

Patient Education Take pulse daily, prior to taking medication; follow prescriber's instruction about holding medication. If you have diabetes, monitor serum glucose closely (drug may alter glucose tolerance or mask signs of hypoglycemia). You may experience fatigue, dizziness, or postural hypotension. Report unresolved swelling of extremities; respiratory difficulty or new cough; unresolved fatigue; or unusual weight gain.

Dietary Considerations Should be taken with food to minimize the risk of orthostatic hypotension.

Caspofungin (kas poe FUN jin)

Brand Names: U.S. Cancidas®

Index Terms Caspofungin Acetate

Pharmacologic Category Antifungal Agent, Parenteral; Echinocandin

Pregnancy Risk Factor C

Lactation Excretion in breast milk unknown/use caution

Use Treatment of invasive *Aspergillus* infections in patients who are refractory or intolerant of other therapy; treatment of candidemia and other *Candida* infections (intra-abdominal abscesses, esophageal, peritonitis, pleural space); empirical treatment for presumed fungal infections in febrile neutropenic patient

Mechanism of Action/Effect Blocks synthesis of a vital component of fungal cell wall, limiting its growth. The cell wall component is unique to specific fungi, limiting any potential for toxicity in mammals.

Contraindications Hypersensitivity to caspofungin or any component of the formulation

Warnings/Precautions Concurrent use of cyclosporine should be limited to patients for whom benefit outweighs risk, due to a high frequency of hepatic transaminase elevations observed during concurrent use. Use caution in hepatic impairment; increased transaminases and rare cases of liver impairment have been reported in pediatric and adult patients. Dosage reduction required in adults with moderate hepatic impairment; safety and efficacy have not been established in children with any degree of hepatic impairment and adults with severe hepatic impairment.

Drug Interactions

Avoid Concomitant Use There are no known interactions where it is recommended to avoid concomitant use.

Decreased Effect

Caspofungin may decrease the levels/effects of: Saccharomyces boulardii; Tacrolimus; Tacrolimus (Systemic)

The levels/effects of Caspofungin may be decreased by: Inducers of Drug Clearance; Rifampin

Increased Effect/Toxicity

The levels/effects of Caspofungin may be increased by: CycloSPORINE; CycloSPORINE (Systemic)

Adverse Reactions

>10%:

Cardiovascular: Hypotension (3% to 20%), peripheral edema (6% to 11%), tachycardia (4% to 11%)

Central nervous system: Fever (6% to 30%), chills (9% to 23%), headache (5% to 15%)

Dermatologic: Rash (4% to 23%)

Endocrine & metabolic: Hypokalemia (5% to 23%)

Gastrointestinal: Diarrhea (6% to 27%), vomiting (6% to 17%), nausea (4% to 15%)

Hematologic: Hemoglobin decreased (18% to 21%), hematocrit decreased (13% to 18%), WBC decreased (12%), anemia (2% to 11%)

Hepatic: Serum alkaline phosphatase increased (9% to 22%), transaminases increased (2% to 18%), bilirubin increased (5% to 13%)

Local: Phlebitis/thrombophlebitis (18%)

Renal: Serum creatinine increased (3% to 11%)

Respiratory: Respiratory failure (2% to 20%), cough (6% to 11%), pneumonia (4% to 11%)

Miscellaneous: Infusion reactions (20% to 35%), septic shock (11% to 14%)

5% to 10%:

Cardiovascular: Hypertension (5% to 6%; children 9% to 10%)

Dermatologic: Erythema (4% to 9%), pruritus (6% to 7%)

Endocrine & metabolic: Hypomagnesemia (7%), hyperglycemia (6%)

Gastrointestinal: Mucosal inflammation (4% to 10%), abdominal pain (4% to 9%)

Hepatic: Albumin decreased (7%)

Local: Infection (1% to 9%, central line)

Renal: Hematuria (10%), blood urea nitrogen increased (4% to 9%)

Respiratory: Dyspnea (9%), pleural effusion (9%), respiratory distress (≤8%), rales (7%)

Miscellaneous: Sepsis (5% to 7%)

Available Dosage Forms

Injection, powder for reconstitution:

Cancidas®: 50 mg, 70 mg

General Dosage Range Dosage adjustment recommended in patients with hepatic impairment or on concomitant therapy

I.V.:

Children 3 months to 17 years: 70 mg/m^2 on day 1, subsequent dosing: 50-70 mg/m^2 once daily (maximum dose: 70 mg/day)

Adults: Initial: 70 mg on day 1; Subsequent dose: 50-70 mg once daily

Administration

I.V. Infuse slowly, over 1 hour

I.V. Detail Monitor during infusion. Isolated cases of possible histamine-related reactions have occurred during clinical trials (rash, flushing, pruritus, facial edema).

Stability

Reconstitution Bring refrigerated vial to room temperature. Reconstitute vials using 0.9% sodium chloride for injection, SWFI, or bacteriostatic water for injection. Mix gently until clear solution is formed; do not use if cloudy or contains particles. Solution should be further diluted with 0.9%, 0.45%, or 0.225% sodium chloride or LR (do not exceed final concentration of 0.5 mg/mL).

Storage Store vials at 2°C to 8°C (36°F to 46°F). Reconstituted solution may be stored at ≤25°C (≤77°F) for 1 hour prior to preparation of infusion solution. Infusion solutions may be stored at ≤25°C (≤77°F) and should be used within 24 hours; up to 48 hours if stored at 2°C to 8°C (36°F to 46°F).

Nursing Actions

Patient Education This medication can only be administered by infusion. Report immediately any pain, burning, or swelling at infusion site or any signs of allergic reaction (eg, respiratory difficulty or swallowing, back pain, chest tightness, rash, hives, swelling of lips or mouth). Report gastrointestinal upset (nausea, vomiting, abdominal pain, diarrhea), swelling of extremities, chest pain or palpations, or unusual cough.

Cefaclor (SEF a klor)

Pharmacologic Category Antibiotic, Cephalosporin (Second Generation)

Medication Safety Issues

Sound-alike/look-alike issues:

Cefaclor may be confused with cephalexin

Pregnancy Risk Factor B

Lactation Enters breast milk/use caution

Breast-Feeding Considerations Small amounts of cefaclor are excreted in breast milk. The manufacturer recommends that caution be exercised when administering cefaclor to nursing women. Nondose-related effects could include modification of bowel flora.

Use Treatment of susceptible bacterial infections including otitis media, lower respiratory tract infections, acute exacerbations of chronic bronchitis, pharyngitis and tonsillitis, urinary tract infections, skin and skin structure infections

Mechanism of Action/Effect Inhibits bacterial cell wall synthesis by binding to one or more of the penicillin-binding proteins (PBPs)

Contraindications Hypersensitivity to cefaclor, any component of the formulation, or other cephalosporins

Warnings/Precautions Modify dosage in patients with severe renal impairment. Prolonged use may result in fungal or bacterial superinfection, including *C. difficile*-associated diarrhea (CDAD) and pseudomembranous colitis; CDAD has been observed >2 months postantibiotic treatment. Use with caution in patients with a history of penicillin allergy, especially IgE-mediated reactions (eg, anaphylaxis, urticaria). Beta-lactamase-negative, ampicillin-resistant (BLNAR) strains of *H. influenzae* should be considered resistant to cefaclor. Extended release tablets are not approved for use in children <16 years of age.

Drug Interactions

Avoid Concomitant Use

Avoid concomitant use of Cefaclor with any of the following: BCG

Decreased Effect

Cefaclor may decrease the levels/effects of: BCG; Typhoid Vaccine

Increased Effect/Toxicity

Cefaclor may increase the levels/effects of: Aminoglycosides

The levels/effects of Cefaclor may be increased by: Probenecid

Nutritional/Ethanol Interactions Food: Cefaclor serum levels may be decreased slightly if taken with food. The bioavailability of cefaclor extended release tablets is decreased 23% and the maximum concentration is decreased 67% when taken on an empty stomach.

Adverse Reactions

1% to 10%:

Dermatologic: Rash (maculopapular, erythematous, or morbilliform) (1% to 2%)

Gastrointestinal: Diarrhea (3%)

Genitourinary: Vaginitis (2%)

Hematologic: Eosinophilia (2%)

Hepatic: Transaminases increased (3%)

Miscellaneous: Moniliasis (2%)

Reactions reported with other cephalosporins: Fever, abdominal pain, superinfection, renal dysfunction, toxic nephropathy, hemorrhage, cholestasis

Available Dosage Forms

Capsule, oral: 250 mg, 500 mg

Powder for suspension, oral: 125 mg/5 mL (75 mL, 150 mL); 250 mg/5 mL (75 mL, 150 mL); 375 mg/5 mL (50 mL, 100 mL)

Tablet, extended release, oral: 500 mg

General Dosage Range Dosage adjustment recommended in patients with renal impairment

Oral:

Children >1 month: 20-40 mg/kg/day divided every 8-12 hours (maximum: 1 g/day)

Adults: 250-500 mg every 8 hours

Administration

Oral Administer around-the-clock to promote less variation in peak and trough serum levels.

Oral suspension: Shake well before using.

Stability

Storage Store at controlled room temperature. Refrigerate suspension after reconstitution. Discard after 14 days. Do not freeze.

Nursing Actions

Physical Assessment Results of culture/sensitivity tests and patient's allergy history should be assessed prior to therapy. Monitor for nephrotoxicity. Hypersensitivity can occur days after therapy is started. Advise patients with diabetes about use of Clinitest®. Teach patient to report hypersensitivity and opportunistic infections.

Patient Education Take at regular intervals around-the-clock, with or without food. Must chill after reconstitution. Do not chew or crush extended release tablets. Maintain adequate hydration, unless instructed to restrict fluid intake. May cause false test results with Clinitest®; use of another type of testing is preferable. May cause diarrhea. Report rash; breathing or swallowing difficulty; persistent diarrhea, nausea, vomiting, or abdominal pain; changes in urinary pattern or pain on urination; opportunistic infection (eg, vaginal itching or drainage, sores in mouth, blood in stool or urine, vaginal itching or drainage, unusual fever or chills); or CNS changes (eg, irritability, agitation, nervousness, insomnia, hallucinations).

Dietary Considerations Capsule and suspension may be taken with or without food.

Cefadroxil (sef a DROKS il)

Index Terms Cefadroxil Monohydrate; Duricef

Pharmacologic Category Antibiotic, Cephalosporin (First Generation)

Pregnancy Risk Factor B

Lactation Enters breast milk (small amounts)/use caution (AAP rates "compatible"; AAP 2001 update pending)

Breast-Feeding Considerations Very small amounts of cefadroxil are excreted in breast milk. The manufacturer recommends that caution be exercised when administering cefadroxil to nursing women. Nondose-related effects could include modification of bowel flora.

Use Treatment of susceptible bacterial infections, including those caused by group A beta-hemolytic *Streptococcus*

Mechanism of Action/Effect Inhibits bacterial cell wall synthesis by binding to one or more of the penicillin-binding proteins (PBPs)

Contraindications Hypersensitivity to cefadroxil, any component of the formulation, or other cephalosporins

Warnings/Precautions Modify dosage in patients with severe renal impairment. Use with caution in patients with a history of penicillin allergy, especially IgE-mediated reactions (eg, anaphylaxis, angioedema, urticaria). Prolonged use may result in fungal or bacterial superinfection, including *C. difficile*-associated diarrhea (CDAD) and pseudomembranous colitis; CDAD has been observed >2 months postantibiotic treatment.

Drug Interactions

Avoid Concomitant Use

Avoid concomitant use of Cefadroxil with any of the following: BCG

Decreased Effect

Cefadroxil may decrease the levels/effects of: BCG; Typhoid Vaccine

Increased Effect/Toxicity

The levels/effects of Cefadroxil may be increased by: Probenecid

Nutritional/Ethanol Interactions Food: Concomitant administration with food, infant formula, or cow's milk does **not** significantly affect absorption.

Adverse Reactions

1% to 10%: Gastrointestinal: Diarrhea

Reactions reported with other cephalosporins: Toxic epidermal necrolysis, abdominal pain, superinfection, renal dysfunction, toxic nephropathy, aplastic anemia, hemolytic anemia, hemorrhage, prothrombin time prolonged, BUN increased, creatinine increased, eosinophilia, pancytopenia, seizure

Available Dosage Forms

Capsule, oral: 500 mg

Powder for suspension, oral: 250 mg/5 mL (50 mL, 100 mL); 500 mg/5 mL (75 mL, 100 mL)

Tablet, oral: 1 g

General Dosage Range Dosage adjustment recommended in patients with renal impairment

Oral:

Children: 30 mg/kg/day in 2 divided doses (maximum: 2 g/day)

Adults: 1-2 g/day in 2 divided doses

Administration

Oral Administer around-the-clock to promote less variation in peak and trough serum levels.

Stability

Reconstitution Refrigerate suspension after reconstitution. Discard after 14 days.

Nursing Actions

Physical Assessment Results of culture/sensitivity tests and patient's allergy history should be assessed prior to therapy. Hypersensitivity can occur several days after therapy is started. Advise patients with diabetes about use of Clinitest®. Teach patient to report hypersensitivity, opportunistic infection, renal dysfunction, and anemia.

Patient Education Take at regular intervals around-the-clock, with or without food. Must be refrigerated for stability purposes. Maintain adequate hydration, unless instructed to restrict fluid intake. May cause false test results with Clinitest®; use of another type of glucose testing is preferable. May cause diarrhea. Report rash; breathing or swallowing difficulty; persistent diarrhea, nausea, vomiting, or abdominal pain; changes in urinary pattern or pain on urination; opportunistic infection (eg, vaginal itching or drainage, sores in mouth, blood in urine or stool, unusual fever or chills); or CNS changes (eg, irritability, agitation, nervousness, insomnia, hallucinations).

Cefazolin (sef A zoe lin)

Index Terms Ancef; Cefazolin Sodium

Pharmacologic Category Antibiotic, Cephalosporin (First Generation)

Medication Safety Issues

Sound-alike/look-alike issues:

CeFAZolin may be confused with cefoTEtan, cefOXitin, cefprozil, cefTAZidime, cefTRIAXone, cephalexin

Pregnancy Risk Factor B

Lactation Enters breast milk (small amounts)/use caution (AAP rates "compatible"; AAP 2001 update pending)

Breast-Feeding Considerations Small amounts of cefazolin are excreted in breast milk. The manufacturer recommends that caution be exercised when administering cefazolin to nursing women. Nondose-related effects could include modification of bowel flora.

Use Treatment of respiratory tract, skin, genital, urinary tract, biliary tract, bone and joint infections, and septicemia due to susceptible gram-positive cocci (except *Enterococcus*); some gram-negative bacilli including *E. coli*, *Proteus*, and *Klebsiella* may be susceptible; surgical prophylaxis

Unlabeled Use Prophylaxis against infective endocarditis

Mechanism of Action/Effect Inhibits bacterial cell wall synthesis by binding to one or more of the penicillin-binding proteins (PBPs)

Contraindications Hypersensitivity to cefazolin sodium, any component of the formulation, or other cephalosporins

Warnings/Precautions Modify dosage in patients with severe renal impairment. Use with caution in patients with a history of penicillin allergy, especially IgE-mediated reactions (eg, anaphylaxis, angioedema, urticaria). Prolonged use may result in fungal or bacterial superinfection, including *C. difficile*-associated diarrhea (CDAD) and pseudomembranous colitis; CDAD has been observed >2 months postantibiotic treatment. May be associated with increased INR, especially in nutritionally-deficient patients, prolonged treatment, hepatic or renal disease. Use with caution in patients with a history of seizure disorder; high levels, particularly in the presence of renal impairment, may increase risk of seizures.

Drug Interactions

Avoid Concomitant Use

Avoid concomitant use of CeFAZolin with any of the following: BCG

Decreased Effect

CeFAZolin may decrease the levels/effects of: BCG; Typhoid Vaccine

Increased Effect/Toxicity

CeFAZolin may increase the levels/effects of: Fosphenytoin; Phenytoin; Vitamin K Antagonists

The levels/effects of CeFAZolin may be increased by: Probenecid

Adverse Reactions Frequency not defined.

Central nervous system: Fever, seizure

Dermatologic: Rash, pruritus, Stevens-Johnson syndrome

Gastrointestinal: Diarrhea, nausea, vomiting, abdominal cramps, anorexia, pseudomembranous colitis, oral candidiasis

Genitourinary: Vaginitis

Hepatic: Transaminases increased, hepatitis

Hematologic: Eosinophilia, neutropenia, leukopenia, thrombocytopenia, thrombocytosis

Local: Pain at injection site, phlebitis

Renal: BUN increased, serum creatinine increased, renal failure

Miscellaneous: Anaphylaxis

Reactions reported with other cephalosporins: Toxic epidermal necrolysis, abdominal pain, cholestasis, superinfection, toxic nephropathy, aplastic anemia, hemolytic anemia, hemorrhage, prothrombin time prolonged, pancytopenia

Available Dosage Forms

Infusion, premixed iso-osmotic dextrose solution: 1 g (50 mL)

Injection, powder for reconstitution: 500 mg, 1 g, 2 g, 10 g, 20 g, 100 g, 300 g

General Dosage Range Dosage adjustment recommended in patients with renal impairment

I.M., I.V.:

Children >1 month: 25-100 mg/kg/day divided every 6-8 hours (maximum: 6 g/day)

Adults: 250 mg to 1.5 g every 6-12 hours (maximum: 12 g/day)

Administration

I.M. Inject deep I.M. into large muscle mass.

I.V. Inject direct I.V. over 5 minutes. Infuse intermittent infusion over 30-60 minutes.

Some penicillins (eg, carbenicillin, ticarcillin, and piperacillin) have been shown to inactivate aminoglycosides *in vitro*. This has been observed to a greater extent with tobramycin and gentamicin, while amikacin has shown greater stability against inactivation. Concurrent use of these agents may pose a risk of reduced antibacterial efficacy *in vivo*, particularly in the setting of profound renal impairment. However, definitive clinical evidence is lacking. If combination penicillin/aminoglycoside therapy is desired in a patient with renal dysfunction, separation of doses (if feasible), and routine monitoring of aminoglycoside levels, CBC, and clinical response should be considered.

I.V. Detail pH: 4.5-6.0

Stability

Reconstitution Dilute 500 mg vial with 2 mL SWFI and 1 g vial with 2.5 mL SWFI; reconstituted solution may be directly injected after further dilution with 5 mL SWFI or further diluted for I.V. administration in 50-100 mL compatible solution; 10 g vial may be diluted with 45 mL to yield 1 g/5 mL or 96 mL to yield 1 g/10 mL.

Storage Store intact vials at room temperature and protect from temperatures exceeding 40°C. Reconstituted solutions of cefazolin are light yellow to yellow. Protection from light is recommended for the powder and for the reconstituted solutions. Reconstituted solutions are stable for 24 hours at room temperature and for 10 days under refrigeration. Stability of parenteral admixture at room temperature (25°C) is 48 hours. Stability of parenteral admixture at refrigeration temperature (4°C) is 14 days.

DUPLEX™: Store at 20°C to 25°C (68°F to 77°F); excursions permitted to 15°C to 30°C (59°F to 86°F) prior to activation. Following activation, stable for 24 hours at room temperature and for 7 days under refrigeration.

Nursing Actions

Physical Assessment Assess results of culture/sensitivity tests and patient's allergy history prior to therapy. Assess anticoagulants patient may be taking for potential interactions. Hypersensitivity can occur several days after therapy is started. Advise patients with diabetes about use of Clinitest®. Teach patient to report hypersensitivity, opportunistic infection, renal dysfunction, and anemia.

Patient Education This medication is administered by injection or infusion. Report immediately any redness, swelling, burning, or pain at injection/infusion site; rash or hives; or respiratory difficulty, chest pain, or difficulty swallowing. Maintain adequate hydration, unless instructed to restrict fluid intake. If you have diabetes, drug may cause false test results with Clinitest® urine glucose monitoring; use of another type of glucose monitoring is preferable. May cause diarrhea. Report rash; breathing or swallowing difficulty; persistent diarrhea, nausea, vomiting, or abdominal pain; changes in urinary pattern or pain on urination; opportunistic infection (eg, vaginal itching or drainage, sores in mouth, blood in stool or urine, unusual fever or chills); or CNS changes (eg, irritability, agitation, nervousness, insomnia, hallucinations).

Dietary Considerations Some products may contain sodium.

Related Information

Compatibility of Drugs *on page 1264*

Cefdinir (SEF di ner)

Brand Names: U.S. Omnicef®

Index Terms CFDN

Pharmacologic Category Antibiotic, Cephalosporin (Third Generation)

Pregnancy Risk Factor B

Lactation Excretion in breast milk unknown

Breast-Feeding Considerations Cefdinir is not detectable in breast milk following a single cefdinir 600 mg dose. It is not known if it would be detectable after multiple doses. If present in breast milk, nondose-related effects could include modification of bowel flora.

Use Treatment of community-acquired pneumonia, acute exacerbations of chronic bronchitis, acute bacterial otitis media, acute maxillary sinusitis, pharyngitis/tonsillitis, and uncomplicated skin and skin structure infections.

Mechanism of Action/Effect Inhibits bacterial cell wall synthesis by binding to one or more of the penicillin-binding proteins (PBPs) which in turn inhibits the final transpeptidation step of peptidoglycan synthesis in bacterial cell walls, thus inhibiting cell wall biosynthesis. Bacteria eventually lyse due to ongoing activity of cell wall autolytic enzymes (autolysins and murein hydrolases) while cell wall assembly is arrested.

Contraindications Hypersensitivity to cefdinir, any component of the formulation, other cephalosporins, or related antibiotics

Warnings/Precautions Administer cautiously to penicillin-sensitive patients, especially IgE-mediated reactions (eg, anaphylaxis, urticaria). Prolonged use may result in fungal or bacterial superinfection, including *C. difficile*-associated diarrhea (CDAD) and pseudomembranous colitis; CDAD has been observed >2 months postantibiotic treatment. Use caution with renal dysfunction (Cl_{cr} <30 mL/minute); dose adjustment may be required.

Drug Interactions

Avoid Concomitant Use

Avoid concomitant use of Cefdinir with any of the following: BCG

Decreased Effect

Cefdinir may decrease the levels/effects of: BCG; Typhoid Vaccine

The levels/effects of Cefdinir may be decreased by: Iron Salts

Increased Effect/Toxicity

Cefdinir may increase the levels/effects of: Aminoglycosides

The levels/effects of Cefdinir may be increased by: Probenecid

Adverse Reactions

>10%: Gastrointestinal: Diarrhea (8% to 15%)

1% to 10%:

Central nervous system: Headache (2%)

Dermatologic: Rash (≤3%)

Endocrine & metabolic: Bicarbonate decreased (≤1%), hyperglycemia (≤1%), hyperphosphatemia (≤1%)

Gastrointestinal: Nausea (≤3%), abdominal pain (≤1%), vomiting (≤1%)

Genitourinary: Vaginal moniliasis (≤4%), urine leukocytes increased (≤2%), urine pH increased (≤1%), urine specific gravity increased (≤1%), vaginitis (≤1%)

Hematologic: Lymphocytes increased (≤2%), eosinophils increased (1%), lymphocytes decreased (1%), platelets increased (≤1%), PMN changes (≤1%), WBC decreased/increased (≤1%)

Hepatic: Alkaline phosphatase increased (≤1%), ALT increased (≤1%)

Renal: Proteinuria (1% to 2%), microhematuria (≤1%), glycosuria (≤1%)

Miscellaneous: GGT increased (≤1%), lactate dehydrogenase increased (≤1%)

Additional reactions reported with other cephalosporins: Agranulocytosis, angioedema, aplastic anemia, asterixis, encephalopathy, hemorrhage, interstitial nephritis, neuromuscular excitability, PT prolonged, seizure, superinfection, and toxic nephropathy

Available Dosage Forms

Capsule, oral: 300 mg

Omnicef®: 300 mg

Powder for suspension, oral: 125 mg/5 mL (60 mL, 100 mL); 250 mg/5 mL (60 mL, 100 mL)

Omnicef®: 125 mg/5 mL (60 mL, 100 mL); 250 mg/5 mL (60 mL, 100 mL)

General Dosage Range Dosage adjustment recommended in patients with renal impairment

Oral:

Children 6 months to 12 years: 14 mg/kg/day in 1-2 divided doses (maximum: 600 mg/day)

Children >12 years and Adults: 600 mg/day in 1-2 divided doses

Administration

Oral Twice daily doses should be given every 12 hours. May be administered with or without food. Manufacturer recommends administering at least 2 hours before or after antacids or iron supplements. Shake suspension well before use.

Stability

Reconstitution Oral suspension should be mixed with 38 mL water for the 60 mL bottle and 63 mL of water for the 100 mL bottle.

Storage Capsules and unmixed powder should be stored at 25°C (77°F); excursions permitted to 15°C to 30°C (59°F to 86°F). Oral suspension should be mixed with 38 mL water for the 60 mL bottle and 63 mL of water for the 100 mL bottle. After mixing, the suspension can be stored at room temperature of 25°C (77°F) for 10 days.

Nursing Actions

Physical Assessment Results of culture/sensitivity tests and patient's allergy history should be assessed prior to therapy. Teach patient to report opportunistic infection and hypersensitivity.

Patient Education Take at regular intervals around-the-clock, with or without food. Chilling oral suspension improves flavor (do not freeze). Maintain adequate hydration, unless instructed to restrict fluid intake. May cause diarrhea, nausea, vomiting, or flatulence. Report rash; breathing or swallowing difficulty; persistent diarrhea, nausea, vomiting, or abdominal pain; changes in urinary pattern or pain on urination; opportunistic infection (eg, vaginal itching or drainage, sores in mouth, blood in stool or urine, unusual fever or chills); or CNS changes (eg, irritability, agitation, nervousness, insomnia, hallucinations).

Cefditoren (sef de TOR en)

Brand Names: U.S. Spectracef®

Index Terms Cefditoren Pivoxil

Pharmacologic Category Antibiotic, Cephalosporin (Third Generation)

Medication Safety Issues

International issues:

Spectracef [U.S., Great Britain, Mexico, Portugal, Spain] may be confused with Spectrocef brand name for cefotaxime [Italy]

Pregnancy Risk Factor B

Lactation Excretion in breast milk unknown/use caution

Breast-Feeding Considerations It is not known whether cefditoren is excreted in human milk. The manufacturer recommends caution when using cefditoren during breast-feeding. Other cephalosporins are considered safe during breast-feeding. If cefditoren reaches the breast milk, the limited oral absorption may minimize the effect on the nursing infant. Nondose-related effects could include modification of bowel flora.

Use Treatment of acute bacterial exacerbation of chronic bronchitis or community-acquired pneumonia (due to susceptible organisms including *Haemophilus influenzae*, *Haemophilus parainfluenzae*, *Streptococcus pneumoniae*-penicillin susceptible only, *Moraxella catarrhalis*); pharyngitis or tonsillitis (*Streptococcus pyogenes*); and uncomplicated skin and skin-structure infections (*Staphylococcus aureus* - not MRSA, *Streptococcus pyogenes*)

Mechanism of Action/Effect Has bactericidal activity against susceptible gram-positive and gram-negative pathogens. Inhibits bacterial cell wall synthesis by binding to one or more of the penicillin-binding proteins (PBPs).

Contraindications Hypersensitivity to cefditoren, any component of the formulation, other cephalosporins, or milk protein; carnitine deficiency

Warnings/Precautions Use with caution in patients with a history of penicillin allergy, especially IgE-mediated reactions (eg, anaphylaxis, urticaria). Prolonged use may result in fungal or bacterial superinfection, including *C. difficile*-associated diarrhea (CDAD) and pseudomembranous colitis; CDAD has been observed >2 months post-antibiotic treatment. Caution in individuals with seizure disorders; high levels, particularly in the presence of renal impairment, may increase risk of seizures. Use caution in patients with renal or hepatic impairment; modify dosage in patients with severe renal impairment. Cefditoren causes renal excretion of carnitine; do not use in patients with carnitine deficiency; not for long-term therapy due to the possible development of carnitine deficiency over time. May prolong prothrombin time; use with caution in patients with a history of bleeding disorder. Cefditoren tablets contain sodium caseinate, which may cause hypersensitivity reactions in patients with milk protein hypersensitivity; this does not affect patients with lactose intolerance.

Drug Interactions

Avoid Concomitant Use There are no known interactions where it is recommended to avoid concomitant use.

Decreased Effect

The levels/effects of Cefditoren may be decreased by: Antacids; H2-Antagonists; Proton Pump Inhibitors

Increased Effect/Toxicity

The levels/effects of Cefditoren may be increased by: Probenecid

Nutritional/Ethanol Interactions Food: Moderate- to high-fat meals increase bioavailability and maximum plasma concentration. Management: Take with meals. Maintain adequate hydration, unless instructed to restrict fluid intake.

Adverse Reactions

>10%: Gastrointestinal: Diarrhea (11% to 15%)

1% to 10%:
Central nervous system: Headache (2% to 3%)
Endocrine & metabolic: Glucose increased (1% to 2%)
Gastrointestinal: Nausea (4% to 6%), abdominal pain (2%), dyspepsia (1% to 2%), vomiting (1%)
Genitourinary: Vaginal moniliasis (3% to 6%)
Hematologic: Hematocrit decreased (2%)
Renal: Hematuria (3%), urinary white blood cells increased (2%)

Reactions reported with other cephalosporins: Anaphylaxis, aplastic anemia, cholestasis, hemorrhage, hemolytic anemia, renal dysfunction, reversible hyperactivity, serum sickness-like reaction, toxic nephropathy

Available Dosage Forms
Tablet, oral: 200 mg, 400 mg
Spectracef®: 200 mg, 400 mg

General Dosage Range Dosage adjustment recommended in patients with renal impairment
Oral: *Children ≥12 years and Adults:* 200-400 mg twice daily

Administration
Oral Administer with meals.

Stability
Storage Store at controlled room temperature of 15°C to 30°C (59°F to 86°F). Protect from light and moisture.

Nursing Actions
Physical Assessment Results of culture/sensitivity tests and patient's allergy history should be assessed prior to therapy. Teach patient to report hypersensitivity, opportunistic infection, gastrointestinal upset, and diarrhea.

Patient Education Take at regular intervals around-the-clock, with food. Maintain adequate hydration, unless instructed to restrict fluid intake. If you have diabetes, monitor glucose levels closely. May cause diarrhea, nausea, or vomiting. Report rash; breathing or swallowing difficulty; persistent diarrhea, nausea, vomiting, or abdominal pain; opportunistic infection (eg, vaginal itching or drainage, sores in mouth, blood in stool or urine, or unusual fever or chills); or CNS changes (eg, irritability, agitation, nervousness, insomnia, hallucinations).

Dietary Considerations Cefditoren should be taken with meals. Plasma carnitine levels are decreased during therapy (39% with 200 mg dosing, 63% with 400 mg dosing); normal concentrations return within 7-10 days after treatment is discontinued.

Cefepime (SEF e pim)

Brand Names: U.S. Maxipime® [DSC]
Index Terms Cefepime Hydrochloride
Pharmacologic Category Antibiotic, Cephalosporin (Fourth Generation)

Medication Safety Issues
Sound-alike/look-alike issues:
Cefepime may be confused with cefixime, cefTAZidime

Pregnancy Risk Factor B

Lactation Enters breast milk/use caution

Breast-Feeding Considerations Small amounts of cefepime are excreted in breast milk. The manufacturer recommends that caution be exercised when administering cefepime to nursing women. Nondose-related effects could include modification of bowel flora.

Use Treatment of uncomplicated and complicated urinary tract infections, including pyelonephritis caused by *Escherichia coli, Klebsiella pneumoniae*, or *Proteus mirabilis*; monotherapy for febrile neutropenia; uncomplicated skin and skin structure infections caused by *Streptococcus pyogenes* or methicillin-susceptible staphylococci; moderate-to-severe pneumonia caused by *Streptococcus pneumoniae, Pseudomonas aeruginosa, Klebsiella pneumoniae*, or *Enterobacter* species; complicated intra-abdominal infections (in combination with metronidazole) caused by *E. coli, P. aeruginosa, K. pneumoniae, Enterobacter* species, or *Bacteroides fragilis* against methicillin-susceptible staphylococci, *Enterobacter* sp, and many other gram-negative bacilli.

Children 2 months to 16 years: Empiric therapy of febrile neutropenia patients, uncomplicated skin/soft tissue infections, pneumonia, and uncomplicated/complicated urinary tract infections, including pyelonephritis.

Unlabeled Use Brain abscess (postneurosurgical prevention); malignant otitis externa; septic lateral/cavernous sinus thrombosis

Mechanism of Action/Effect Inhibits bacterial cell wall synthesis by binding to one or more of the penicillin-binding proteins (PBPs)

Contraindications Hypersensitivity to cefepime, other cephalosporins, penicillins, other beta-lactam antibiotics, or any component of the formulation

Warnings/Precautions Modify dosage in patients with renal impairment (Cl_{cr} ≤60 mL/minute); may increase risk of encephalopathy, myoclonus, and seizures. Use with caution in patients with a history of penicillin or cephalosporin allergy, especially IgE-mediated reactions (eg, anaphylaxis, urticaria). Prolonged use may result in fungal or bacterial superinfection, including *C. difficile*-associated diarrhea (CDAD) and pseudomembranous colitis; CDAD has been observed >2 months postantibiotic treatment. Use with caution in patients with a history of gastrointestinal disease, especially colitis. May be associated with increased INR, especially in nutritionally-deficient patients, prolonged treatment, hepatic or renal disease. Use with caution in patients with a history of seizure disorder; high levels, particularly in the presence of renal impairment, may increase risk of seizures.

Drug Interactions

Avoid Concomitant Use

Avoid concomitant use of Cefepime with any of the following: BCG

Decreased Effect

Cefepime may decrease the levels/effects of: BCG; Typhoid Vaccine

Increased Effect/Toxicity

Cefepime may increase the levels/effects of: Aminoglycosides

The levels/effects of Cefepime may be increased by: Probenecid

Adverse Reactions

>10%: Hematologic: Positive Coombs' test without hemolysis (16%)

1% to 10%:

Central nervous system: Fever (1%), headache (1%)

Dermatologic: Rash (1% to 4%), pruritus (1%)

Endocrine & metabolic: Hypophosphatemia (3%)

Gastrointestinal: Diarrhea (≤3%), nausea (≤2%), vomiting (≤1%)

Hematologic: Eosinophils (2%)

Hepatic: ALT increased (3%), AST increased (2%), PTT abnormal (2%), PT abnormal (1%)

Local: Inflammation, phlebitis, and pain (1%)

Reactions reported with other cephalosporins: Aplastic anemia, erythema multiforme, hemolytic anemia, hemorrhage, pancytopenia, PT prolonged, renal dysfunction, Stevens-Johnson syndrome, superinfection, toxic epidermal necrolysis, toxic nephropathy, vaginitis

Available Dosage Forms

Infusion, premixed iso-osmotic dextrose solution: 1 g (50 mL); 2 g (100 mL)

Injection, powder for reconstitution: 500 mg, 1 g, 2 g

General Dosage Range Dosage adjustment recommended in patients with renal impairment

I.M.:

Children ≥2 months: 50 mg/kg/dose every 12 hours

Adults: 500-1000 mg every 12 hours

I.V.:

Children ≥2 months: 50 mg/kg/dose every 8-12 hours

Adults: 1-2 g every 8-12 hours

Administration

I.M. Inject deep I.M. into large muscle mass.

I.V. Inject direct I.V. over 5 minutes (Garrelts, 1999). Infuse intermittent infusion over 30 minutes.

I.V. Detail pH: 4-6

Stability

Storage

Vials: Store at 20°C to 25°C (68°F to 77°F). Protect from light. After reconstitution, stable in normal saline, D_5W, and a variety of other solutions for 24 hours at room temperature and 7 days refrigerated.

Premixed solution: Store frozen at -20°C (-4°F). Thawed solution is stable for 24 hours at room temperature or 7 days under refrigeration; do not refreeze.

Nursing Actions

Physical Assessment Results of culture/sensitivity tests and patient's allergy history should be assessed prior to therapy. Monitor prothrombin time. Teach patient to report hypersensitivity, nephrotoxicity, and opportunistic infection.

Patient Education This medication is administered by infusion or injection. Report immediately any redness, swelling, burning, or pain at injection/infusion site; itching or hives; chest pain; or difficulty swallowing or breathing. Maintain adequate hydration, unless instructed to restrict fluid intake. May cause diarrhea, nausea, or vomiting. Report rash; breathing or swallowing difficulty; persistent diarrhea, nausea, vomiting, or abdominal pain; changes in urinary pattern or pain on urination; opportunistic infection (eg, vaginal itching or drainage, sores in mouth, blood in stool or urine, unusual fever or chills); or CNS changes (eg, irritability, agitation, nervousness, insomnia, hallucinations).

Cefixime (sef IKS eem)

Brand Names: U.S. Suprax®

Index Terms Cefixime Trihydrate

Pharmacologic Category Antibiotic, Cephalosporin (Third Generation)

Medication Safety Issues

Sound-alike/look-alike issues:

Cefixime may be confused with cefepime

Suprax® may be confused with Sporanox®

International issues:

Cefiton: Brand name for cefixime [Portugal] may be confused with Ceftim brand name for ceftazidime [Portugal]; Ceftime brand name for ceftazidime [Thailand]; Ceftin brand name for cefuroxime [U.S., Canada]

Pregnancy Risk Factor B

Lactation Excretion in breast milk unknown

Breast-Feeding Considerations It is not known if cefixime is excreted in breast milk. The manufacturer recommends that consideration be given to discontinuing nursing temporarily during treatment. Other cephalosporins are considered safe during breast-feeding. If present in breast milk, nondose-related effects could include modification of bowel flora.

Use Treatment of urinary tract infections, otitis media, respiratory infections due to susceptible organisms including *S. pneumoniae* and *S. pyogenes*, *H. influenzae*, and many Enterobacteriaceae; uncomplicated cervical/urethral gonorrhea due to *N. gonorrhoeae*

Mechanism of Action/Effect Inhibits bacterial cell wall synthesis by binding to one or more of the penicillin-binding proteins (PBPs)

Contraindications Hypersensitivity to cefixime, any component of the formulation, or other cephalosporins

Warnings/Precautions Prolonged use may result in fungal or bacterial superinfection, including *C. difficile*-associated diarrhea (CDAD) and pseudomembranous colitis; CDAD has been observed >2 months postantibiotic treatment. Modify dosage in patients with renal impairment. Use with caution in patients with a history of penicillin allergy, especially IgE-mediated reactions (eg, anaphylaxis, urticaria).

Drug Interactions

Avoid Concomitant Use

Avoid concomitant use of Cefixime with any of the following: BCG

Decreased Effect

Cefixime may decrease the levels/effects of: BCG; Typhoid Vaccine

Increased Effect/Toxicity

Cefixime may increase the levels/effects of: Aminoglycosides

The levels/effects of Cefixime may be increased by: Probenecid

Nutritional/Ethanol Interactions Food: Delays cefixime absorption.

Adverse Reactions

>10%: Gastrointestinal: Diarrhea (16%)

2% to 10%: Gastrointestinal: Abdominal pain, nausea, dyspepsia, flatulence, loose stools

Reactions reported with other cephalosporins: Interstitial nephritis, aplastic anemia, hemolytic anemia, hemorrhage, pancytopenia, agranulocytosis, colitis, superinfection

Available Dosage Forms

Powder for suspension, oral:

Suprax®: 100 mg/5 mL (50 mL, 100 mL); 200 mg/5 mL (50 mL, 75 mL)

Tablet, oral:

Suprax®: 400 mg

General Dosage Range Dosage adjustment recommended in patients with renal impairment

Oral:

Children ≥6 months to 12 years and ≤50 kg: 8-20 mg/kg/day divided every 12-24 hours (maximum: 400 mg/day)

Children >12 years or >50 kg and Adults: 400 mg/day divided every 12-24 hours **or** 20-30 mg/kg/day in 2 divided doses

Administration

Oral May be administered with or without food. Administer with food to decrease GI distress. Shake oral suspension well before use.

Stability

Storage After reconstitution, suspension may be stored for 14 days at room temperature or under refrigeration.

Nursing Actions

Physical Assessment Results of culture/sensitivity tests and patient's allergy history should be assessed prior to therapy. Assess prothrombin time. Monitor for anemia, hemorrhage, pancytopenia, agranulocytosis, and colitis during therapy. Teach patient to report hypersensitivity and opportunistic infection.

Patient Education Take at regular intervals around-the-clock, with or without food. Chilling oral suspension improves flavor (do not freeze); shake suspension thoroughly before using. Maintain adequate hydration, unless instructed to restrict fluid intake. May cause nausea, vomiting, or diarrhea. Report rash; breathing or swallowing difficulty; persistent diarrhea, nausea, vomiting, or abdominal pain; changes in urinary pattern or pain on urination; opportunistic infection (eg, vaginal itching or drainage, sores in mouth, blood in stool or urine, unusual fever or chills); or CNS changes (eg, irritability, agitation, nervousness, insomnia, hallucinations).

Dietary Considerations May be taken with food to decrease GI distress.

Cefotaxime (sef oh TAKS eem)

Brand Names: U.S. Claforan®

Index Terms Cefotaxime Sodium

Pharmacologic Category Antibiotic, Cephalosporin (Third Generation)

Medication Safety Issues

Sound-alike/look-alike issues:

Cefotaxime may be confused with cefOXitin, cefuroxime

International issues:

Spectrocef [Italy] may be confused with Spectracef brand name for cefditoren [U.S., Great Britain, Mexico, Portugal, Spain]

Pregnancy Risk Factor B

Lactation Enters breast milk/use caution (AAP rates "compatible"; AAP 2001 update pending)

Breast-Feeding Considerations Very small amounts of cefotaxime are excreted in breast milk. The manufacturer recommends that caution be exercised when administering cefotaxime to nursing women. Nondose-related effects could include modification of bowel flora. The pregnancy-related changes in cefotaxime pharmacokinetics continue into the early postpartum period.

Use Treatment of susceptible organisms in lower respiratory tract, skin and skin structure, bone and joint, urinary tract, intra-abdominal, gynecologic as well as bacteremia/septicemia, and documented or suspected central nervous system infections (eg, meningitis). Active against most gram-negative bacilli (not *Pseudomonas* spp) and gram-positive cocci (not enterococcus). Active against many penicillin-resistant pneumococci.

Mechanism of Action/Effect Inhibits bacterial cell wall synthesis by binding to one or more of the penicillin-binding proteins (PBPs)

Contraindications Hypersensitivity to cefotaxime, any component of the formulation, or other cephalosporins

Warnings/Precautions Modify dosage in patients with severe renal impairment. Prolonged use may result in superinfection. A potentially life-threatening arrhythmia has been reported in patients who received a rapid (<1 minute) bolus injection via central venous catheter. Granulocytopenia and more rarely agranulocytosis may develop during prolonged treatment (>10 days). Minimize tissue inflammation by changing infusion sites when needed. Use with caution in patients with a history of penicillin allergy, especially IgE-mediated reactions (eg, anaphylaxis, urticaria). Prolonged use may result in fungal or bacterial superinfection, including *C. difficile*-associated diarrhea (CDAD) and pseudomembranous colitis; CDAD has been observed >2 months postantibiotic treatment.

Drug Interactions

Avoid Concomitant Use

Avoid concomitant use of Cefotaxime with any of the following: BCG

Decreased Effect

Cefotaxime may decrease the levels/effects of: BCG; Typhoid Vaccine

Increased Effect/Toxicity

Cefotaxime may increase the levels/effects of: Aminoglycosides

The levels/effects of Cefotaxime may be increased by: Probenecid

Adverse Reactions

1% to 10%:

Dermatologic: Pruritus, rash

Gastrointestinal: Colitis, diarrhea, nausea, vomiting

Local: Pain at injection site

Reactions reported with other cephalosporins: Aplastic anemia, hemorrhage, pancytopenia, renal dysfunction, seizure, superinfection, toxic nephropathy.

Available Dosage Forms

Infusion, premixed iso-osmotic solution:

Claforan®: 1 g (50 mL); 2 g (50 mL)

Injection, powder for reconstitution: 500 mg, 1 g, 2 g, 10 g

Claforan®: 500 mg, 1 g, 2 g, 10 g

General Dosage Range Dosage adjustment recommended in patients with hepatic or renal impairment

I.M.:

Infants and Children 1 month to 12 years and <50 kg: 50-200 mg/kg/day in divided doses every 6-8 hours (maximum: 12 g/day)

Children ≥50 kg, Children >12 years, and Adults: 1-2 g every 4-12 hours **or** 0.5-1 g as a single dose

I.V.:

Infants and Children 1 month to 12 years and <50 kg: 50-200 mg/kg/day in divided doses every 6-8 hours (maximum: 12 g/day)

Children ≥50 kg, Children >12 years, and Adults: 1-2 g every 4-12 hours

Administration

I.M. Inject deep I.M. into large muscle mass.

I.V. Inject direct I.V. over at least 3-5 minutes. Infuse intermittent infusion over 30 minutes.

I.V. Detail pH: 5.0-7.5 (injectable solution)

Stability

Reconstitution Reconstituted solution is stable for 12-24 hours at room temperature and 7-10 days when refrigerated and for 13 weeks when frozen. For I.V. infusion in NS or D_5W, solution is stable for 24 hours at room temperature, 5 days when refrigerated, or 13 weeks when frozen in Viaflex® plastic containers. Thawed solutions previously of frozen premixed bags are stable for 24 hours at room temperature or 10 days when refrigerated.

Nursing Actions

Physical Assessment Assess results of culture/sensitivity tests and patient's allergy history prior to therapy. Evaluate CBC with differential. Monitor for diarrhea, nausea/vomiting, and nephrotoxicity regularly during therapy. Teach patient to report hypersensitivity and opportunistic infection.

Patient Education This medication is administered by injection or infusion. Report immediately any redness, swelling, burning, or pain at injection/infusion site; chest pain, palpitations, respiratory difficulty or swallowing; or itching or hives. Maintain adequate hydration, unless instructed to restrict fluid intake. May cause diarrhea, GI distress, or nausea. Report unresolved or persistent diarrhea, opportunistic infection (vaginal itching or drainage, sores in mouth, blood in stool or urine, easy bleeding or bruising, unusual fever or chills), or respiratory difficulty.

Dietary Considerations Some products may contain sodium.

Cefotetan (SEF oh tee tan)

Index Terms Cefotan; Cefotetan Disodium

Pharmacologic Category Antibiotic, Cephalosporin (Second Generation)

Medication Safety Issues

Sound-alike/look-alike issues:

CefoTEtan may be confused with ceFAZolin, cefOXitin, cefTAZidime, Ceftin®, cefTRIAXone

Pregnancy Risk Factor B

Lactation Enters breast milk (small amounts)/use caution

Breast-Feeding Considerations Very small amounts of cefotetan are excreted in human milk. The manufacturer recommends caution when giving cefotetan to a breast-feeding mother. Nondose-related effects could include modification of bowel flora.

Use Surgical prophylaxis; intra-abdominal infections and other mixed infections; respiratory tract, skin and skin structure, bone and joint, urinary tract and gynecologic as well as septicemia; active against gram-negative enteric bacilli including *E. coli*, *Klebsiella*, and *Proteus*; less active against staphylococci and streptococci than first generation cephalosporins, but active against anaerobes including *Bacteroides fragilis*

Mechanism of Action/Effect Inhibits bacterial cell wall synthesis by binding to one or more of the penicillin-binding proteins (PBPs)

Contraindications Hypersensitivity to cefotetan, any component of the formulation, or other cephalosporins; previous cephalosporin-associated hemolytic anemia

Warnings/Precautions Modify dosage in patients with severe renal impairment. Although cefotetan contains the methyltetrazolethiol side chain, bleeding has not been a significant problem. Use with caution in patients with a history of penicillin allergy, especially IgE-mediated reactions (eg, anaphylaxis, urticaria). Cefotetan has been associated with a higher risk of hemolytic anemia relative to other cephalosporins (approximately threefold); monitor carefully during use and consider cephalosporin-associated immune anemia in patients who have received cefotetan within 2-3 weeks (either as treatment or prophylaxis). Prolonged use may result in fungal or bacterial superinfection, including *C. difficile*-associated diarrhea (CDAD) and pseudomembranous colitis; CDAD has been observed >2 months postantibiotic treatment. May be associated with increased INR, especially in nutritionally-deficient patients, prolonged treatment, hepatic or renal disease.

Drug Interactions

Avoid Concomitant Use

Avoid concomitant use of CefoTEtan with any of the following: BCG

Decreased Effect

CefoTEtan may decrease the levels/effects of: BCG; Typhoid Vaccine

Increased Effect/Toxicity

CefoTEtan may increase the levels/effects of: Alcohol (Ethyl); Aminoglycosides; Vitamin K Antagonists

The levels/effects of CefoTEtan may be increased by: Probenecid

Nutritional/Ethanol Interactions Ethanol: Avoid ethanol (may cause a disulfiram-like reaction).

Adverse Reactions

1% to 10%:

Gastrointestinal: Diarrhea (1%)

Hepatic: Transaminases increased (1%)

Miscellaneous: Hypersensitivity reactions (1%)

Reactions reported with other cephalosporins: Seizure, Stevens-Johnson syndrome, toxic epidermal necrolysis, renal dysfunction, toxic nephropathy, cholestasis, aplastic anemia, hemolytic anemia, hemorrhage, pancytopenia, agranulocytosis, colitis, superinfection

Available Dosage Forms

Injection, powder for reconstitution: 1 g, 2 g, 10 g

General Dosage Range Dosage adjustment recommended in patients with renal impairment

I.M.: *Adults:* 1-6 g/day divided every 12 hours **or** 1-2 g every 24 hours **or** 1-2 g prior to surgery

I.V.:

Adolescents: PID: 2 g every 12 hours

Adults: 1-6 g/day divided every 12 hours **or** 1-2 g every 24 hours **or** 1-2 g prior to surgery

Administration

I.M. Inject deep I.M. into large muscle mass.

I.V. Inject direct I.V. over 3-5 minutes. Infuse intermittent infusion over 30 minutes.

I.V. Detail pH: 4.5-6.5 (reconstituted solution)

Stability

Reconstitution Reconstituted solution is stable for 24 hours at room temperature and 96 hours when refrigerated. For I.V. infusion in NS or D_5W solution and after freezing, thawed solution is stable for 24 hours at room temperature or 96 hours when refrigerated. Frozen solution is stable for 12 weeks.

Nursing Actions

Physical Assessment Assess results of culture/sensitivity tests and patient's allergy history prior to therapy. Assess prothrombin time. Advise patients with diabetes about use of Clinitest® (may cause false-positive test). Teach patient to report nephrotoxicity, opportunistic infection, and hypersensitivity reaction.

Patient Education This medication is administered by injection or infusion. Report immediately any redness, swelling, burning, or pain at injection/infusion site, or immediately report any itching, hives, difficulty swallowing, or respiratory difficulty. Maintain adequate hydration, unless instructed to restrict fluid intake. Avoid alcohol during therapy (may cause severe disulfiram-like reactions). May cause false test results with Clinitest®; use of another type of glucose testing is preferable. May cause diarrhea. Report rash; breathing or swallowing difficulty; persistent diarrhea, nausea, vomiting, or abdominal pain; changes in urinary pattern or pain on urination; opportunistic infection (eg, vaginal itching or drainage; sores in mouth; blood in stool or urine; unusual fever or chills); or CNS changes (eg, irritability, agitation, nervousness, insomnia, hallucinations).

Dietary Considerations Some products may contain sodium.

Cefoxitin (se FOKS i tin)

Brand Names: U.S. Mefoxin®

Index Terms Cefoxitin Sodium

Pharmacologic Category Antibiotic, Cephalosporin (Second Generation)

Medication Safety Issues

Sound-alike/look-alike issues:

CefOXitin may be confused with ceFAZolin, cefotaxime, cefoTEtan, cefTAZidime, cefTRIAXone, Cytoxan

Mefoxin® may be confused with Lanoxin®

Pregnancy Risk Factor B

Lactation Enters breast milk/use caution (AAP rates "compatible"; AAP 2001 update pending)

Breast-Feeding Considerations Very small amounts of cefoxitin are excreted in breast milk. The manufacturer recommends that caution be exercised when administering cefoxitin to nursing women. Nondose-related effects could include modification of bowel flora. Cefoxitin pharmacokinetics may be altered immediately postpartum.

Use Less active against staphylococci and streptococci than first generation cephalosporins, but active against anaerobes including *Bacteroides fragilis*; active against gram-negative enteric bacilli including *E. coli*, *Klebsiella*, and *Proteus*; used predominantly for respiratory tract, skin, bone and joint, urinary tract and gynecologic as well as septicemia; surgical prophylaxis; intra-abdominal infections and other mixed infections; indicated for bacterial *Eikenella corrodens* infections

Mechanism of Action/Effect Inhibits bacterial cell wall synthesis by binding to one or more of the penicillin-binding proteins (PBPs)

Contraindications Hypersensitivity to cefoxitin, any component of the formulation, or other cephalosporins

Warnings/Precautions Modify dosage in patients with severe renal impairment. Prolonged use may result in superinfection. Use with caution in patients with a history of penicillin allergy, especially IgE-mediated reactions (eg, anaphylaxis, urticaria). Prolonged use may result in fungal or bacterial superinfection, including *C. difficile*-associated diarrhea (CDAD) and pseudomembranous colitis; CDAD has been observed >2 months postantibiotic treatment.

Drug Interactions

Avoid Concomitant Use

Avoid concomitant use of CefOXitin with any of the following: BCG

Decreased Effect

CefOXitin may decrease the levels/effects of: BCG; Typhoid Vaccine

Increased Effect/Toxicity

CefOXitin may increase the levels/effects of: Aminoglycosides; Vitamin K Antagonists

The levels/effects of CefOXitin may be increased by: Probenecid

Adverse Reactions

1% to 10%: Gastrointestinal: Diarrhea

Reactions reported with other cephalosporins: Agranulocytosis, aplastic anemia, cholestasis, colitis, erythema multiforme, hemolytic anemia, hemorrhage, pancytopenia, renal dysfunction, serum-sickness reactions, seizure, Stevens-Johnson syndrome, superinfection, toxic nephropathy, vaginitis

Available Dosage Forms

Infusion, premixed iso-osmotic dextrose solution:

Mefoxin®: 1 g (50 mL); 2 g (50 mL)

Injection, powder for reconstitution: 1 g, 2 g, 10 g

General Dosage Range Dosage adjustment recommended in patients with renal impairment

I.M.:

Children >3 months: 80-160 mg/kg/day divided every 4-6 hours (maximum: 12 g/day)

Adolescents: 80-160 mg/kg/day divided every 4-6 hours (maximum: 12 g/day) **or** 1-2 g prior to surgery

Adults: 1-2 g every 4-8 hours (maximum: 12 g/day) **or** 1-2 g prior to surgery

I.V.:

Children >3 months: 80-160 mg/kg/day divided every 4-6 hours (maximum: 12 g/day) **or** 30-40 mg/kg prior to surgery

Adolescents: 80-160 mg/kg/day divided every 4-6 hours (maximum: 12 g/day) **or** 1-2 g prior to surgery

Adults: 1-2 g every 4-8 hours (maximum: 12 g/day) **or** 1-2 g prior to surgery

Administration

I.M. Inject deep I.M. into large muscle mass.

I.V. Can be administered IVP over 3-5 minutes at a maximum concentration of 100 mg/mL or I.V. intermittent infusion over 10-60 minutes at a final concentration for I.V. administration not to exceed 40 mg/mL

I.V. Detail pH: 4.2-7.0 (reconstituted solution); 6.5 (frozen premixed solution)

Stability

Reconstitution Reconstitute vials with SWFI, bacteriostatic water for injection, NS, or D_5W. For I.V. infusion, solutions may be further diluted in NS, $D_5 1/4NS$, $D_5 1/2NS$, D_5NS, D_5W, $D_{10}W$, LR, D_5LR, mannitol 10%, or sodium bicarbonate 5%.

Storage Reconstituted solution is stable for 6 hours at room temperature or 7 days when refrigerated; I.V. infusion in NS or D_5W solution is stable for 18 hours at room temperature or 48 hours when refrigerated. Premixed frozen solution, when thawed, is stable for 24 hours at room temperature or 21 days when refrigerated.

Nursing Actions

Physical Assessment Results of culture/sensitivity tests and patient's allergy history should be assessed prior to therapy. Monitor for nephrotoxicity. Evaluate prothrombin time and CBC with differential. Monitor for diarrhea, nausea, vomiting, and nephrotoxicity. Advise patients with diabetes about use of Clinitest®. Teach patient to report hypersensitivity and opportunistic infection.

Patient Education This medication is administered by injection or infusion. Report immediately any redness, swelling, burning, or pain at injection/infusion site; chest pain, palpitations, respiratory difficulty or swallowing; or itching or hives. Maintain adequate hydration, unless instructed to restrict fluid intake. May cause false test results with Clinitest®; use of another type of glucose testing is preferable. May cause diarrhea, GI distress, or nausea. Report rash; breathing or swallowing difficulty; persistent diarrhea, nausea, vomiting, or abdominal pain; changes in urinary pattern or pain on urination; opportunistic infection (eg, vaginal itching or drainage, sores in mouth, blood in stool or urine, unusual fever or chills); or CNS changes (eg, irritability, agitation, nervousness, insomnia, hallucinations).

Dietary Considerations Some products may contain sodium.

Cefpodoxime (sef pode OKS eem)

Index Terms Cefpodoxime Proxetil; Vantin

Pharmacologic Category Antibiotic, Cephalosporin (Third Generation)

Medication Safety Issues

Sound-alike/look-alike issues:

Vantin may be confused with Ventolin®

Pregnancy Risk Factor B

Lactation Enters breast milk (small amounts)/not recommended

Breast-Feeding Considerations Very small amounts of cefpodoxime are excreted in breast milk. Breast-feeding is not recommended by the manufacturer. Other cephalosporins are considered safe during breast-feeding. Nondose-related effects could include modification of bowel flora.

Use Treatment of susceptible acute, community-acquired pneumonia caused by *S. pneumoniae* or nonbeta-lactamase producing *H. influenzae*; acute uncomplicated gonorrhea caused by *N. gonorrhoeae*; uncomplicated skin and skin structure infections caused by *S. aureus* or *S. pyogenes*; acute otitis media caused by *S. pneumoniae*, *H. influenzae*, or *M. catarrhalis*; pharyngitis or tonsillitis; and uncomplicated urinary tract infections caused by *E. coli*, *Klebsiella*, and *Proteus*

Mechanism of Action/Effect Inhibits bacterial cell wall synthesis by binding to one or more of the penicillin-binding proteins (PBPs)

Contraindications Hypersensitivity to cefpodoxime, any component of the formulation, or other cephalosporins

Warnings/Precautions Modify dosage in patients with severe renal impairment. Prolonged use may result in fungal or bacterial superinfection, including *C. difficile*-associated diarrhea (CDAD) and pseudomembranous colitis; CDAD has been observed >2 months postantibiotic treatment. Use with caution in patients with a history of penicillin allergy, especially IgE-mediated reactions (eg, anaphylaxis, urticaria).

Drug Interactions

Avoid Concomitant Use

Avoid concomitant use of Cefpodoxime with any of the following: BCG

Decreased Effect

Cefpodoxime may decrease the levels/effects of: BCG; Typhoid Vaccine

The levels/effects of Cefpodoxime may be decreased by: Antacids; H2-Antagonists

Increased Effect/Toxicity

Cefpodoxime may increase the levels/effects of: Aminoglycosides

The levels/effects of Cefpodoxime may be increased by: Probenecid

Nutritional/Ethanol Interactions Food: Food and/or low gastric pH delays absorption and may increase serum levels. Management: Take with or without food at regular intervals on an around-the-clock schedule to promote less variation in peak and trough serum levels.

Adverse Reactions

>10%:

Dermatologic: Diaper rash (12%)

Gastrointestinal: Diarrhea in infants and toddlers (15%)

1% to 10%:

Central nervous system: Headache (1%)

Dermatologic: Rash (1%)

Gastrointestinal: Diarrhea (7%), nausea (4%), abdominal pain (2%), vomiting (1% to 2%)

Genitourinary: Vaginal infection (3%)

Reactions reported with other cephalosporins: Seizure, Stevens-Johnson syndrome, toxic epidermal necrolysis, erythema multiforme, urticaria, serum-sickness reactions, renal dysfunction, interstitial nephritis toxic nephropathy, cholestasis, aplastic anemia, hemolytic anemia, hemorrhage, pancytopenia, agranulocytosis, colitis, vaginitis, superinfection

Available Dosage Forms

Granules for suspension, oral: 50 mg/5 mL (50 mL, 100 mL); 100 mg/5 mL (50 mL, 100 mL)

Tablet, oral: 100 mg, 200 mg

General Dosage Range Dosage adjustment recommended in patients with renal impairment

Oral:

Children 2 months to 12 years: 10 mg/kg/day divided every 12 hours (maximum: 400 mg/day)

Children ≥12 years and Adults: 100-400 mg every 12 hours **or** 200 mg as a single dose

Administration

Oral Administer around-the-clock to promote less variation in peak and trough serum levels.

Stability

Reconstitution Shake well before using. After mixing, keep suspension in refrigerator. Discard unused portion after 14 days.

Nursing Actions

Physical Assessment Results of culture/sensitivity tests and patient's allergy history should be assessed prior to therapy. Monitor prothrombin time. Monitor for hemolytic anemia, hypoprothrombinemia, and bleeding. Teach patient to report nephrotoxicity, opportunistic infection, and hypersensitivity reaction.

Patient Education Take at regular intervals around-the-clock, with or without food. Shake suspension well before using. Maintain adequate hydration, unless instructed to restrict fluid intake. May cause nausea, vomiting, or diarrhea. Report rash; breathing or swallowing difficulty; persistent diarrhea, nausea, vomiting, or abdominal pain; changes in urinary pattern or pain on urination; opportunistic infection (eg, vaginal itching or drainage, sores in mouth, blood in stool or urine, unusual fever or chills); or CNS changes (eg, irritability, agitation, nervousness, insomnia, hallucinations).

Dietary Considerations May be taken with food.

Cefprozil (sef PROE zil)

Index Terms Cefzil

Pharmacologic Category Antibiotic, Cephalosporin (Second Generation)

Medication Safety Issues

Sound-alike/look-alike issues:

Cefprozil may be confused with ceFAZolin, cefuroxime

Cefzil may be confused with Ceftin®

Pregnancy Risk Factor B

Lactation Enters breast milk/use caution (AAP rates "compatible"; AAP 2001 update pending)

Breast-Feeding Considerations Small amounts of cefprozil are excreted in breast milk. The manufacturer recommends that caution be exercised when administering cefprozil to nursing women. Nondose-related effects could include modification of bowel flora.

Use Treatment of otitis media and infections involving the respiratory tract and skin and skin structure; active against methicillin-sensitive staphylococci, many streptococci, and various gram-negative bacilli including *E. coli*, some *Klebsiella*, *P. mirabilis*, *H. influenzae*, and *Moraxella*.

Mechanism of Action/Effect Inhibits bacterial cell wall synthesis by binding to one or more of the penicillin-binding proteins (PBPs)

Contraindications Hypersensitivity to cefprozil, any component of the formulation, or other cephalosporins

Warnings/Precautions Modify dosage in patients with severe renal impairment. Use with caution in patients with a history of penicillin allergy, especially IgE-mediated reactions (eg, anaphylaxis, urticaria). Prolonged use may result in fungal or bacterial superinfection, including *C. difficile*-associated diarrhea (CDAD) and pseudomembranous colitis; CDAD has been observed >2 months postantibiotic treatment. Some products may contain phenylalanine.

Drug Interactions

Avoid Concomitant Use

Avoid concomitant use of Cefprozil with any of the following: BCG

Decreased Effect

Cefprozil may decrease the levels/effects of: BCG; Typhoid Vaccine

Increased Effect/Toxicity

Cefprozil may increase the levels/effects of: Aminoglycosides

The levels/effects of Cefprozil may be increased by: Probenecid

Nutritional/Ethanol Interactions Food: Food delays cefprozil absorption.

Adverse Reactions

1% to 10%:

Central nervous system: Dizziness (1%)

Dermatologic: Diaper rash (2%)

Gastrointestinal: Diarrhea (3%), nausea (4%), vomiting (1%), abdominal pain (1%)

Genitourinary: Vaginitis, genital pruritus (2%)

Hepatic: Transaminases increased (2%)

Miscellaneous: Superinfection

Reactions reported with other cephalosporins: Seizure, toxic epidermal necrolysis, renal dysfunction, interstitial nephritis, toxic nephropathy, aplastic anemia, hemolytic anemia, hemorrhage, pancytopenia, agranulocytosis, colitis, vaginitis, superinfection

Available Dosage Forms

Powder for suspension, oral: 125 mg/5 mL (50 mL, 75 mL, 100 mL); 250 mg/5 mL (50 mL, 75 mL, 100 mL)

Tablet, oral: 250 mg, 500 mg

General Dosage Range Dosage adjustment recommended in patients with renal impairment

Oral:

Children 6 months to 2 years: 7.5-30 mg/kg/day divided every 12 hours

Children 2-12 years: 7.5-30 mg/kg/day divided every 12 hours **or** 20 mg/kg every 24 hours (maximum: 1 g/day)

Adolescents >12 years and Adults: 250-500 mg every 12 hours **or** 500 mg every 24 hours

Administration

Oral Administer around-the-clock to promote less variation in peak and trough serum levels. Chilling the reconstituted oral suspension improves flavor (do not freeze).

Nursing Actions

Physical Assessment Results of culture/sensitivity tests and patient's allergy history should be assessed prior to therapy. Monitor prothrombin time. Advise patients with diabetes about use of Clinitest® (may cause false-positive test). Teach patient to report opportunistic infection and hypersensitivity reaction.

Patient Education Take at regular intervals around-the-clock, with or without food. Chilling oral suspension improves flavor (do not freeze). Maintain adequate hydration, unless instructed to restrict fluid intake. May cause false test results with Clinitest®; use of another type of glucose testing is preferable. May cause dizziness, nausea, vomiting, or diarrhea. Report rash; breathing or swallowing difficulty; persistent diarrhea, nausea, vomiting, or abdominal pain; changes in urinary pattern or pain on urination; opportunistic infection (eg, vaginal itching or drainage, sores in mouth, blood in stool or urine, unusual fever or chills); or CNS changes (eg, irritability, agitation, nervousness, insomnia, hallucinations).

Dietary Considerations May be taken with food. Oral suspension may contain phenylalanine; consult product labeling.

Ceftaroline Fosamil (sef TAR oh leen FOS a mil)

Brand Names: U.S. Teflaro™

Index Terms PPI-0903; PPI-0903M; T-91825; TAK-599

Pharmacologic Category Antibiotic, Cephalosporin (Fifth Generation)

Pregnancy Risk Factor B

Lactation Excretion in breast milk unknown/use caution

Use Treatment of acute bacterial skin and skin structure infections (ABSSSI) caused by susceptible isolates of *Staphylococcus aureus* (including methicillin-susceptible and -resistant isolates), *Streptococcus pyogenes, Streptococcus agalactiae, Escherichia coli, Klebsiella pneumoniae*, and *Klebsiella oxytoca,* and community-acquired pneumonia (CAP) caused by *Streptococcus pneumoniae* (including cases with concurrent bacteremia), *Staphylococcus aureus* (methicillin-susceptible isolates only), *Haemophilus influenzae, Klebsiella pneumoniae, Klebsiella oxytoca,* and *Escherichia coli*

Mechanism of Action/Effect Inhibits bacterial cell wall synthesis by binding to 1 or more of the penicillin-binding proteins (PBPs)

Contraindications Hypersensitivity to ceftaroline, other cephalosporins, or any component of the formulation

Warnings/Precautions Use with caution in patients with a history of penicillin allergy, especially IgE-mediated reactions (eg, anaphylaxis, angioedema, urticaria). Prolonged use may result in fungal or bacterial superinfection, including *C. difficile*-associated diarrhea (CDAD) and pseudomembranous colitis; CDAD has been observed >2 months postantibiotic treatment. Use with caution in patients with renal impairment (Cl_{cr} ≤50 mL/minute); dosage adjustments recommended.

Drug Interactions

Avoid Concomitant Use

Avoid concomitant use of Ceftaroline Fosamil with any of the following: BCG

Decreased Effect

Ceftaroline Fosamil may decrease the levels/effects of: BCG; Typhoid Vaccine

Increased Effect/Toxicity

The levels/effects of Ceftaroline Fosamil may be increased by: Probenecid

Adverse Reactions

>10%: Hematologic: Positive Coombs' test without hemolysis (~11%)

2% to 10%:

Central nervous system: Headache (3% to 5%), insomnia (3% to 4%)

Dermatologic: Pruritus (3% to 4%), rash (3%)

Endocrine & metabolic: Hypokalemia (2%)

Gastrointestinal: Diarrhea (5%), nausea (4%), constipation (2%), vomiting (2%)

Hepatic: Transaminases increased (2%)

Local: Phlebitis (2%)

Available Dosage Forms

Injection, powder for reconstitution:

Teflaro™: 600 mg

General Dosage Range Dosage adjustment recommended in patients with renal impairment.

I.V.: *Adults:* 600 mg every 12 hours

Administration

I.V. Administer by slow I.V. infusion over 60 minutes.

I.V. Detail pH: 4.8-6.5

Stability

Reconstitution Reconstitute 400 mg or 600 mg vial with 20 mL SWFI; mix gently; reconstituted solution should be further diluted for I.V. administration in 250 mL of a compatible solution (eg, D_5W, NS); use within 6 hours at room temperature or within 24 hours if refrigerated; color of infusion solutions ranges from clear and light to dark yellow depending on concentration and storage conditions.

Storage Store unused vials at 2°C to 8°C (36°F to 46°F); unused vials may be stored at room temperature, up to 25°C (77°F), for ≤7 days.

Ceftazidime (SEF tay zi deem)

Brand Names: U.S. Fortaz®; Tazicef®

Pharmacologic Category Antibiotic, Cephalosporin (Third Generation)

Medication Safety Issues

Sound-alike/look-alike issues:

CefTAZidime may be confused with ceFAZolin, cefepime, cefoTEtan, cefOXitin, cefTRIAXone

Ceptaz® may be confused with Septra®

Tazicef® may be confused with Tazidime®

International issues:

Ceftim [Portugual] and Ceftime [Thailand] brand names for ceftazidime may be confused with Ceftin brand name for cefuroxime [U.S., Canada]; Cefiton brand name for cefixime [Portugal]

Pregnancy Risk Factor B

Lactation Enters breast milk/use caution (AAP rates "compatible"; AAP 2001 update pending)

Breast-Feeding Considerations Very small amounts of ceftazidime are excreted in breast milk. The manufacturer recommends that caution be exercised when administering ceftazidime to nursing women. Ceftazidime in not absorbed when given orally; therefore, any medication that is distributed to human milk should not result in systemic concentrations in the nursing infant. Nondose-related effects could include modification of bowel flora.

Use Treatment of documented susceptible *Pseudomonas aeruginosa* infection and infections due to other susceptible aerobic gram-negative organisms; empiric therapy of a febrile, granulocytopenic patient

Unlabeled Use Bacterial endophthalmitis

Mechanism of Action/Effect Inhibits bacterial cell wall synthesis by binding to one or more of the penicillin-binding proteins (PBPs)

Contraindications Hypersensitivity to ceftazidime, any component of the formulation, or other cephalosporins

Warnings/Precautions Modify dosage in patients with severe renal impairment. Use with caution in patients with a history of penicillin allergy, especially IgE-mediated reactions (eg, anaphylaxis, urticaria). Prolonged use may result in fungal or bacterial superinfection, including *C. difficile*-associated diarrhea (CDAD) and pseudomembranous colitis; CDAD has been observed >2 months post-antibiotic treatment. May be associated with increased INR, especially in nutritionally-deficient patients, prolonged treatment, hepatic or renal disease. Use with caution in patients with a history of seizure disorder; high levels, particularly in the presence of renal impairment, may increase risk of seizures.

Drug Interactions

Avoid Concomitant Use

Avoid concomitant use of CefTAZidime with any of the following: BCG

Decreased Effect

CefTAZidime may decrease the levels/effects of: BCG; Typhoid Vaccine

Increased Effect/Toxicity

CefTAZidime may increase the levels/effects of: Aminoglycosides

The levels/effects of CefTAZidime may be increased by: Probenecid

Adverse Reactions

1% to 10%:

Gastrointestinal: Diarrhea (1%)

Local: Pain at injection site (1%)

Miscellaneous: Hypersensitivity reactions (2%)

Reactions reported with other cephalosporins: Seizure, urticaria, serum-sickness reactions, renal dysfunction, interstitial nephritis, toxic nephropathy, BUN increased, creatinine increased, cholestasis, aplastic anemia, hemolytic anemia, pancytopenia, agranulocytosis, colitis, prolonged PT, hemorrhage, superinfection

Available Dosage Forms

Infusion, premixed iso-osmotic solution:

Fortaz®: 1 g (50 mL); 2 g (50 mL)

Injection, powder for reconstitution: 1 g, 2 g, 6 g

Fortaz®: 500 mg, 1 g, 2 g, 6 g

Tazicef®: 1 g, 2 g, 6 g

General Dosage Range Dosage adjustment recommended in patients with renal impairment

I.M.: *Adults:* 500 mg to 2 g every 8-12 hours

I.V.:

Children 1 month to 12 years: 30-50 mg/kg every 8 hours (maximum: 6 g/day)

Children ≥12 years and Adults: 500 mg to 2 g every 8-12 hours (maximum: 6 g/day)

Administration

I.M. Inject deep I.M. into large mass muscle.

I.V. Ceftazidime can be administered IVP over 3-5 minutes or I.V. intermittent infusion over 15-30 minutes.

I.V. Detail Any carbon dioxide bubbles that may be present in the withdrawn solution should be expelled prior to injection. Administer around-the-clock to promote less variation in peak and trough serum levels.

pH: 5-8 (Fortaz®); 5.0-7.5 (Tazicef®)

Stability

Reconstitution

I.M.: Using SWFI, bacteriostatic water, lidocaine 0.5%, or lidocaine 1%, reconstitute the 500 mg vials with 1.5 mL or the 1 g vials with 3 mL; final concentration of *~280 mg/mL*

I.V.: Using SWFI, reconstitute as follows (**Note:** After reconstitution, may dilute further with a compatible solution to administer via I.V. infusion):

Fortaz®:

~100 mg/mL solution:

500 mg vial: 5.3 mL SWFI (withdraw 5 mL from the reconstituted vial to obtain a 500 mg dose)

1 g vial: 10 mL SWFI (withdraw 10 mL from the reconstituted vial to obtain a 1 g dose)

6 g vial: 56 mL SWFI (withdraw 10 mL from the reconstituted vial to obtain a 1 g dose)

~170 mg/mL solution: 2 g vial: 10 mL SWFI (withdraw 11.5 mL from the reconstituted vial to obtain a 2 g dose)

~200 mg/mL solution: 6 g vial: 26 mL SWFI (withdraw 5 mL from the reconstituted vial to obtain a 1 g dose)

Tazicef®:

~95 mg/mL solution: 1 g vial: 10 mL SWFI (withdraw 10.6 mL from the reconstituted vial to obtain a 1 g dose)

~180 mg/mL solution: 2 g vial: 10 mL SWFI (withdraw 11.2 mL from the reconstituted vial to obtain a 2 g dose)

Fortaz®, Tazicef®: ADD-Vantage® vials: Dilute in 50 or 100 mL of D_5W, NS, or 0.45% sodium chloride in an ADD-Vantage® flexible diluent container only.

Storage

Fortaz®: Store dry vials at 15°C to 30°C (59°F to 86°F). Protect from light. Reconstituted solution and solution further diluted for I.V. infusion are stable for 12 hours at room temperature, for 3 days when refrigerated, or for 12 weeks when frozen at -20°C (-4°F). After freezing, thawed solution in SWFI for I.M. administration is stable for 3 hours at room temperature or for 3 days when refrigerated; thawed solution in NS in a Viaflex® small volume container for I.V. administration is stable for 12 hours at room temperature or for 3 days when refrigerated; and thawed solution in SWFI in the original container is stable for 8 hours at room temperature or for 3 days when refrigerated.

Premixed frozen solution: Store frozen at -20°C (-4°F). Thawed solution is stable for 8 hours at room temperature or for 3 days under refrigeration; do not refreeze.

Fortaz®, Tazicef®: ADD-Vantage® vials: Following dilution, may be stored for up to 12 hours at room temperature or for 3 days under refrigeration. Freezing solutions in the ADD-Vantage® system is not recommended. Joined vials that have not been activated may be used within 14 days.

Tazicef® vials: Store dry vials at 20°C to 25°C (68°F to 77°F). Protect from light. Reconstituted vials and solution further diluted for I.V. infusion are stable for 24 hours at room temperature, for 7 days when refrigerated, or for 12 weeks when frozen at -20°C (-4°F). When thawed, solution is stable for 8 hours at room temperature and 4 days when refrigerated.

Nursing Actions

Physical Assessment Results of culture/sensitivity tests and patient's allergy history should be assessed prior to therapy. Monitor for nephrotoxicity. Assess prothrombin time. Monitor for hemolytic anemia, hypoprothrombinemia, and bleeding. Teach patient to report opportunistic infection and hypersensitivity reaction.

Patient Education This medication is administered by infusion or injection. Report immediately any redness, swelling, burning, or pain at injection/infusion site. Maintain adequate hydration, unless instructed to restrict fluid intake. May cause diarrhea. Report rash; breathing or swallowing difficulty; persistent diarrhea, nausea, vomiting, or abdominal pain; changes in urinary pattern or pain on urination; opportunistic infection (eg, vaginal itching or drainage, sores in mouth, blood in stool or urine, unusual fever or chills); or CNS changes (eg, irritability, agitation, nervousness, insomnia, hallucinations).

Dietary Considerations Some products may contain sodium.

Ceftibuten (sef TYE byoo ten)

Brand Names: U.S. Cedax®

Pharmacologic Category Antibiotic, Cephalosporin (Third Generation)

Medication Safety Issues

Sound-alike/look-alike issues:

Cedax® may be confused with Cidex®

International issues:

Cedax [U.S. and multiple international markets] may be confused with Codex brand name for acetaminophen/codeine [Brazil] and *Saccharomyces boulardii* [Italy]

Pregnancy Risk Factor B

Lactation Excretion in breast milk unknown/use caution

Breast-Feeding Considerations Ceftibuten was not detectable in milk after a single 200 mg dose (limit of detection: 1 mcg/mL). It is not known if it would be detectable after a 400 mg dose or multiple doses. The manufacturer recommends that caution be exercised when administering ceftibuten to nursing women. If ceftibuten does reach the human milk, nondose-related effects could include modification of bowel flora.

Use Treatment of acute exacerbations of chronic bronchitis, acute bacterial otitis media, and pharyngitis/tonsillitis

Mechanism of Action/Effect Inhibits bacterial cell wall synthesis by binding to one or more of the penicillin-binding proteins (PBPs)

Contraindications Hypersensitivity to ceftibuten, any component of the formulation, or other cephalosporins

Warnings/Precautions Modify dosage in patients with moderate-to-severe renal impairment. Prolonged use may result in fungal or bacterial superinfection, including *C. difficile*-associated diarrhea (CDAD) and pseudomembranous colitis; CDAD has been observed >2 months postantibiotic treatment. Use with caution in patients with a history of colitis and other gastrointestinal diseases. Use with caution in patients with a history of penicillin allergy, especially IgE-mediated reactions (eg, anaphylaxis, urticaria). Oral suspension formulation contains sucrose.

Drug Interactions

Avoid Concomitant Use

Avoid concomitant use of Ceftibuten with any of the following: BCG

Decreased Effect

Ceftibuten may decrease the levels/effects of: BCG; Typhoid Vaccine

Increased Effect/Toxicity

Ceftibuten may increase the levels/effects of: Aminoglycosides

The levels/effects of Ceftibuten may be increased by: Probenecid

Adverse Reactions

1% to 10%:

Central nervous system: Headache (≤3%), dizziness (≤1%)

Gastrointestinal: Nausea (≤4%), diarrhea (3% to 4%), dyspepsia (≤2%), loose stools (≤2%), abdominal pain (1% to 2%), vomiting (1% to 2%)

Hematologic: Eosinophils increased (3%), hemoglobin decreased (1% to 2%), platelets increased (≤1%)

Hepatic: ALT increased (≤1%), bilirubin increased (≤1%)

Renal: BUN increased (2% to 4%)

Additional reactions reported with other cephalosporins: Allergic reaction, agranulocytosis, angioedema, aplastic anemia, anaphylaxis, asterixis, cholestasis, drug fever, encephalopathy, erythema multiforme, hemolytic anemia, hemorrhage, interstitial nephritis, neuromuscular excitability, neutropenia, pancytopenia, prolonged PT, renal dysfunction, seizure, superinfection, toxic nephropathy

Available Dosage Forms

Capsule, oral:

Cedax®: 400 mg

Powder for suspension, oral:

Cedax®: 90 mg/5 mL (60 mL, 90 mL, 120 mL); 180 mg/5 mL (30 mL, 60 mL)

General Dosage Range Dosage adjustment recommended in patients with renal impairment

Oral:

Children 6 months to <12 years: 9 mg/kg/day (maximum: 400 mg/day)

Children ≥12 years and Adults: 400 mg once daily

Administration

Oral

Capsule: Administer without regard to food.

Suspension: Administer 2 hours before or 1 hour after meals. Shake well before use.

Stability

Storage Store capsules and powder for suspension at 2°C to 25°C (36°F to 77°F). Reconstituted suspension is stable for 14 days when refrigerated at 2°C to 8°C (36°F to 46°F).

Nursing Actions

Physical Assessment Results of culture/sensitivity tests and patient's allergy history should be assessed prior to therapy. Monitor for nephrotoxicity, hemolytic anemia, hypoprothrombinemia, and bleeding. Teach patient to report opportunistic infection and hypersensitivity reaction.

Patient Education Take at regular intervals around-the-clock. Take capsules with or without food; take suspension 2 hours before or 1 hour after meals. Maintain adequate hydration, unless instructed to restrict fluid intake. May cause headache, dizziness, nausea, vomiting, or diarrhea. Report rash; breathing or swallowing difficulty; persistent diarrhea, nausea, vomiting, or abdominal pain; changes in urinary pattern or pain on urination; opportunistic infection (eg, vaginal itching or drainage, sores in mouth, blood in stool or urine, unusual fever or chills); or CNS changes (eg, irritability, agitation, nervousness, insomnia, hallucinations).

Dietary Considerations

Capsule: Take without regard to food.

Suspension: Take 2 hours before or 1 hour after meals.

CefTRIAXone (sef trye AKS one)

Brand Names: U.S. Rocephin®

Index Terms Ceftriaxone Sodium

Pharmacologic Category Antibiotic, Cephalosporin (Third Generation)

Medication Safety Issues

Sound-alike/look-alike issues:

CefTRIAXone may be confused with CeFAZolin, cefoTEtan, cefOXitin, cefTAZidime, Cetraxal®

Rocephin® may be confused with Roferon®

Pregnancy Risk Factor B

Lactation Enters breast milk/use caution (AAP rates "compatible"; AAP 2001 update pending)

Breast-Feeding Considerations Small amounts of ceftriaxone are excreted in breast milk. The manufacturer recommends that caution be exercised when administering ceftriaxone to nursing women. Nondose-related effects could include modification of bowel flora.

Use Treatment of lower respiratory tract infections, acute bacterial otitis media, skin and skin structure infections, bone and joint infections, intra-abdominal and urinary tract infections, pelvic inflammatory disease (PID), uncomplicated gonorrhea, bacterial septicemia, and meningitis; used in surgical prophylaxis

Unlabeled Use Treatment of chancroid, epididymitis, complicated gonococcal infections; sexually-transmitted diseases (STD); periorbital or buccal cellulitis; salmonellosis or shigellosis; atypical community-acquired pneumonia; epiglottitis, Lyme disease; used in chemoprophylaxis for high-risk contacts (close exposure to patients with invasive meningococcal disease); sexual assault; typhoid fever, Whipple's disease

Mechanism of Action/Effect Inhibits bacterial cell wall synthesis by binding to one or more of the penicillin-binding proteins (PBPs)

Contraindications Hypersensitivity to ceftriaxone sodium, any component of the formulation, or other cephalosporins; **do not use in hyperbilirubinemic neonates**, particularly those who are premature since ceftriaxone is reported to displace bilirubin from albumin binding sites; concomitant use with intravenous calcium-containing solutions/ products in neonates (≤28 days)

Warnings/Precautions Use with caution in patients with a history of penicillin allergy, especially IgE-mediated reactions (eg, anaphylaxis, urticaria). Abnormal gallbladder sonograms have been reported, possibly due to cetriaxone-calcium precipitates; discontinue in patients who develop signs and symptoms of gallbladder disease. Secondary to biliary obstruction, pancreatitis has been reported rarely. Use with caution in patients with a history of GI disease, especially colitis. Severe cases (including some fatalities) of immune-related hemolytic anemia have been reported in patients receiving cephalosporins, including ceftriaxone. Prolonged use may result in fungal or bacterial superinfection, including *C. difficile*-associated diarrhea (CDAD) and pseudomembranous colitis; CDAD has been observed >2 months postantibiotic treatment.

May be associated with increased INR (rarely), especially in nutritionally-deficient patients, prolonged treatment, hepatic or renal disease. No adjustment is generally necessary in patients with renal impairment; use with caution in patients with concurrent hepatic dysfunction and significant renal disease, dosage should not exceed 2 g/day. Ceftriaxone may complex with calcium causing precipitation. Fatal lung and kidney damage associated with calcium-ceftriaxone precipitates has been observed in premature and term neonates. Do not reconstitute, admix, or coadminister with calcium-containing solutions, even via separate infusion lines/sites or at different times in any neonatal patient. Ceftriaxone should not be diluted or administered simultaneously with any calcium-containing solution via a Y-site in any patient. However, ceftriaxone and calcium-containing solution may be administered sequentially of one another for use in patients **other than neonates** if infusion lines are thoroughly flushed, with a compatible fluid, between infusions

Drug Interactions

Avoid Concomitant Use

Avoid concomitant use of CefTRIAXone with any of the following: BCG

Decreased Effect

CefTRIAXone may decrease the levels/effects of: BCG; Typhoid Vaccine

Increased Effect/Toxicity

CefTRIAXone may increase the levels/effects of: Aminoglycosides; Vitamin K Antagonists

The levels/effects of CefTRIAXone may be increased by: Calcium Salts (Intravenous); Probenecid; Ringer's Injection (Lactated)

Adverse Reactions

>10%: Local: Induration (I.M. 5% to 17%), warmth (I.M.), tightness (I.M.)

1% to 10%:

Dermatologic: Rash (2%)

Gastrointestinal: Diarrhea (3%)

Hematologic: Eosinophilia (6%), thrombocytosis (5%), leukopenia (2%)

Hepatic: Transaminases increased (3%)

Local: Tenderness at injection site (I.V. 1%), pain

Renal: BUN increased (1%)

Reactions reported with other cephalosporins: Angioedema, allergic reaction, aplastic anemia, asterixis, cholestasis, encephalopathy, hemorrhage, hepatic dysfunction, hyperactivity (reversible), hypertonia, interstitial nephritis, LDH increased, neuromuscular excitability, pancytopenia, paresthesia, renal dysfunction, superinfection, toxic nephropathy

Available Dosage Forms

Infusion, premixed in D_5W: 1 g (50 mL); 2 g (50 mL)

Injection, powder for reconstitution: 250 mg, 500 mg, 1 g, 2 g, 10 g

Rocephin®: 500 mg, 1 g

General Dosage Range Dosage adjustment recommended in patients with hepatic and renal impairment

I.M.:

Children: 50-100 mg/kg/day divided every 12-24 hours (maximum: 4 g/day) **or** 125 mg or 50 mg/kg as a single dose

Adults: 1-2 g every 12-24 hours **or** 125-250 mg as a single dose

I.V.:

Children: 50-100 mg/kg/day divided every 12-24 hours (maximum: 4 g/day)

Adults: 1-2 g every 12-24 hours

Administration

I.M. Inject deep I.M. into large muscle mass; a concentration of 250 mg/mL or 350 mg/mL is recommended for all vial sizes except the 250 mg size (250 mg/mL is suggested); can be diluted with 1:1 water and 1% lidocaine for I.M. administration.

I.V. Do not reconstitute or coadminister with calcium-containing solutions. Infuse intermittent infusion over 30 minutes.

I.V. Detail pH: 6.6 (premixed infusion solution); 6.7 (1% aqueous solution)

Stability

Reconstitution

I.M. injection: Vials should be reconstituted with appropriate volume of diluent (including D_5W, NS, SWFI, bacteriostatic water, or 1% lidocaine) to make a final concentration of 250 mg/mL or 350 mg/mL.

Volume to add to create a **250 mg/mL** solution:

250 mg vial: 0.9 mL
500 mg vial: 1.8 mL
1 g vial: 3.6 mL
2 g vial: 7.2 mL

Volume to add to create a **350 mg/mL** solution:

500 mg vial: 1.0 mL
1 g vial: 2.1 mL
2 g vial: 4.2 mL

I.V. infusion: Infusion is prepared in two stages: Initial reconstitution of powder, followed by dilution to final infusion solution.

Vials: Reconstitute powder with appropriate I.V. diluent (including SWFI, D_5W, $D_{10}W$, NS) to create an initial solution of ~100 mg/mL. Recommended volume to add:

250 mg vial: 2.4 mL
500 mg vial: 4.8 mL
1 g vial: 9.6 mL
2 g vial: 19.2 mL

Note: After reconstitution of powder, further dilution into a volume of compatible solution (eg, 50-100 mL of D_5W or NS) is recommended.

Piggyback bottle: Reconstitute powder with appropriate I.V. diluent (D_5W or NS) to create a resulting solution of ~100 mg/mL. Recommended initial volume to add:

1 g bottle:10 mL
2 g bottle: 20 mL

Note: After reconstitution, to prepare the final infusion solution, further dilution to 50 mL or 100 mL volumes with the appropriate I.V. diluent (including D_5W or NS) is recommended.

Storage

Powder for injection: Prior to reconstitution, store at room temperature ≤25°C (≤77°F). Protect from light.

Premixed solution (manufacturer premixed): Store at -20°C; once thawed, solutions are stable for 3 days at room temperature of 25°C (77°F) or for 21 days refrigerated at 5°C (41°F). Do not refreeze.

Stability of reconstituted solutions:

10-40 mg/mL: Reconstituted in D_5W, $D_{10}W$, NS, or SWFI: Stable for 2 days at room temperature of 25°C (77°F) or for 10 days when refrigerated at 4°C (39°F). Stable for 26 weeks when frozen at -20°C when reconstituted with D_5W or NS. Once thawed (at room temperature), solutions are stable for 2 days at room temperature of 25°C (77°F) or for 10 days when refrigerated at 4°C (39°F); does not apply to manufacturer's premixed bags. Do not refreeze.

100 mg/mL:

Reconstituted in D_5W, SWFI, or NS: Stable for 2 days at room temperature of 25°C (77°F) or for 10 days when refrigerated at 4°C (39°F).

Reconstituted in lidocaine 1% solution or bacteriostatic water: Stable for 24 hours at room temperature of 25°C (77°F) or for 10 days when refrigerated at 4°C (39°F).

250-350 mg/mL: Reconstituted in D_5W, NS, lidocaine 1% solution, bacteriostatic water, or SWFI: Stable for 24 hours at room temperature of 25°C (77°F) or for 3 days when refrigerated at 4°C (39°F).

Nursing Actions

Physical Assessment Culture/sensitivity tests should be performed and patient's allergy history should be assessed prior to beginning therapy. Monitor prothrombin times.

Patient Education This medication can only be administered by injection or infusion. Report immediately any swelling, pain, burning, or redness at infusion/injection site; back pain; difficulty breathing or swallowing; rapid heartbeat; or chills. Maintain adequate hydration, unless instructed to restrict fluid intake. Report rash; breathing or swallowing difficulty; persistent diarrhea, nausea, vomiting, or abdominal pain; changes in urinary pattern or pain on urination; opportunistic infection (eg, vaginal itching or drainage, sores in mouth, blood in stool or urine, vaginal itching or drainage, unusual fever or chills); or CNS changes (eg, irritability, agitation, nervousness, insomnia, hallucinations).

Dietary Considerations Some products may contain sodium.

Cefuroxime (se fyoor OKS eem)

Brand Names: U.S. Ceftin®; Zinacef®

Index Terms Cefuroxime Axetil; Cefuroxime Sodium

Pharmacologic Category Antibiotic, Cephalosporin (Second Generation)

Medication Safety Issues

Sound-alike/look-alike issues:

Cefuroxime may be confused with cefotaxime, cefprozil, deferoxamine

Ceftin® may be confused with Cefzil®, Cipro®

Zinacef® may be confused with Zithromax®

International issues:

Ceftin [U.S., Canada] may be confused with Cefiton brand name for cefixime [Portugal]; Ceftim brand name for ceftazidime [Portugal]; Ceftime brand name for ceftazidime [Thailand]

Pregnancy Risk Factor B

Lactation Enters breast milk/use caution

Breast-Feeding Considerations Cefuroxime is excreted in breast milk. Manufacturer recommendations vary; caution is recommended if cefuroxime I.V. is given to a nursing woman and it is recommended to consider discontinuing nursing temporarily during treatment following oral cefuroxime. Nondose-related effects could include modification of bowel flora.

Use Treatment of infections caused by staphylococci, group B streptococci, *H. influenzae* (type A and B), *E. coli*, *Enterobacter*, *Salmonella*, and *Klebsiella*; treatment of susceptible infections of the upper and lower respiratory tract, otitis media, urinary tract, uncomplicated skin and soft tissue, bone and joint, sepsis, uncomplicated gonorrhea, and early Lyme disease; surgical prophylaxis

Mechanism of Action/Effect Inhibits bacterial cell wall synthesis by binding to one or more of the penicillin-binding proteins (PBPs)

Contraindications Hypersensitivity to cefuroxime, any component of the formulation, or other cephalosporins

Warnings/Precautions Modify dosage in patients with severe renal impairment. Use with caution in patients with a history of penicillin allergy, especially IgE-mediated reactions (eg, anaphylaxis, urticaria). Prolonged use may result in fungal or bacterial superinfection, including *C. difficile*-associated diarrhea (CDAD) and pseudomembranous colitis; CDAD has been observed >2 months postantibiotic treatment. May be associated with increased INR, especially in nutritionally-deficient patients, prolonged treatment, hepatic or renal disease. Tablets and oral suspension are not bioequivalent (do not substitute on a mg-per-mg basis). Some products may contain phenylalanine.

Drug Interactions

Avoid Concomitant Use

Avoid concomitant use of Cefuroxime with any of the following: BCG

Decreased Effect

Cefuroxime may decrease the levels/effects of: BCG; Typhoid Vaccine

The levels/effects of Cefuroxime may be decreased by: Antacids; H2-Antagonists

Increased Effect/Toxicity

Cefuroxime may increase the levels/effects of: Aminoglycosides

The levels/effects of Cefuroxime may be increased by: Probenecid

Nutritional/Ethanol Interactions Food: Bioavailability is increased with food; cefuroxime serum levels may be increased if taken with food or dairy products.

Adverse Reactions

>10%: Gastrointestinal: Diarrhea (4% to 11%, duration-dependent)

1% to 10%:

Dermatologic: Diaper rash (3%)

Endocrine & metabolic: Alkaline phosphatase increased (2%), lactate dehydrogenase increased (1%)

Gastrointestinal: Nausea/vomiting (3% to 7%)

Genitourinary: Vaginitis (≤5%)

Hematologic: Eosinophilia (7%), hemoglobin and hematocrit decreased (10%)

Hepatic: Transaminases increased (2% to 4%)

Local: Thrombophlebitis (2%)

Reactions reported with other cephalosporins: Agranulocytosis, aplastic anemia, asterixis, encephalopathy, hemorrhage, neuromuscular excitability, serum-sickness reactions, superinfection, toxic nephropathy

Available Dosage Forms

Infusion, premixed iso-osmotic solution:

Zinacef®: 750 mg (50 mL); 1.5 g (50 mL)

Injection, powder for reconstitution: 750 mg, 1.5 g, 7.5 g, 75 g

Zinacef®: 750 mg, 1.5 g, 7.5 g

Powder for suspension, oral: 125 mg/5 mL (100 mL); 250 mg/5 mL (50 mL, 100 mL)

Ceftin®: 125 mg/5 mL (100 mL); 250 mg/5 mL (50 mL, 100 mL)

Tablet, oral: 250 mg, 500 mg

Ceftin®: 250 mg, 500 mg

General Dosage Range Dosage adjustment recommended in patients with renal impairment

I.M., I.V.:

Children 3 months to 12 years: 75-150 mg/kg/day divided every 8 hours (maximum: 6 g/day)

Adolescents >12 years and Adults: 750 mg to 1.5 g every 6-8 hours (maximum: 6 g/day) **or** 1.5 g as a single dose

Oral:

Children 3 months to 12 years: 20-30 mg/kg/day in 2 divided doses **or** 125-250 mg every 12 hours (maximum: 1 g/day)

Adolescents >12 years and Adults: 125-500 mg every 12 hours **or** 1 g as a single dose

Administration

Oral Administer with food. Shake well before use.

I.M. Inject deep I.M. into large muscle mass.

I.V. Inject direct I.V. over 3-5 minutes. Infuse intermittent infusion over 15-30 minutes.

I.V. Detail pH: 6.0-8.5 (vials); 5.0-7.5 (frozen premixed solution)

Stability

Storage

Injection: Reconstituted solution is stable for 24 hours at room temperature and 48 hours when refrigerated. I.V. infusion in NS or D_5W solution is stable for 24 hours at room temperature, 7 days when refrigerated, or 26 weeks when frozen. After freezing, thawed solution is stable for 24 hours at room temperature or 21 days when refrigerated.

Oral suspension: Prior to reconstitution, store at 2°C to 30°C (36°F to 86°F). Reconstituted suspension is stable for 10 days at 2°C to 8°C (36°F to 46°F).

Tablet: Store at 15°C to 30°C (59°F to 86°F).

Nursing Actions

Physical Assessment Results of culture/sensitivity tests and patient's allergy history should be assessed prior to therapy. Monitor for nephrotoxicity. Assess prothrombin times. Monitor for hemolytic anemia, hypoprothrombinemia, and bleeding. Advise patients with diabetes about use of Clinitest® (may cause false-positive test). Teach patient to report opportunistic infection and hypersensitivity reaction.

Patient Education If administered by injection or infusion, report immediately any swelling, redness, or pain at injection/infusion site; respiratory difficulty or swallowing; chest pain; or rash. Oral tablets or suspension should be taken at regular intervals around-the-clock, with food. Shake well before using oral suspension. Maintain adequate hydration, unless instructed to restrict fluid intake. May cause false test results with Clinitest®; use of another type of glucose testing is preferable. Report rash; breathing or swallowing difficulty; persistent diarrhea, nausea, vomiting, or abdominal pain; changes in urinary pattern or pain on urination; opportunistic infection (eg, vaginal itching or drainage, sores in mouth, blood in stool or urine, unusual fever or chills); or CNS changes (eg, irritability, agitation, nervousness, insomnia, hallucinations).

Dietary Considerations Some products may contain phenylalanine and/or sodium.

Oral suspension: May be taken with food.

Celecoxib (se le KOKS ib)

Brand Names: U.S. CeleBREX®

Pharmacologic Category Nonsteroidal Anti-inflammatory Drug (NSAID), COX-2 Selective

Medication Safety Issues

Sound-alike/look-alike issues:

CeleBREX® may be confused with CeleXA®, Cerebyx®, Cervarix®, Clarinex®

Medication Guide Available Yes

Pregnancy Risk Factor C (prior to 30 weeks gestation)/D (≥30 weeks gestation)

Lactation Enters breast milk/use caution

Breast-Feeding Considerations Small amounts of celecoxib are found in breast milk. The manufacturer recommends that caution be exercised when administering celecoxib to nursing women.

Use Relief of the signs and symptoms of osteoarthritis, ankylosing spondylitis, juvenile idiopathic arthritis (JIA), and rheumatoid arthritis; management of acute pain; treatment of primary dysmenorrhea

Mechanism of Action/Effect Inhibits prostaglandin synthesis by decreasing the activity of the enzyme, cyclooxygenase-2 (COX-2), which results in decreased formation of prostaglandin precursors; has antipyretic, analgesic, and anti-inflammatory properties. Celecoxib does not inhibit cyclooxygenase-1 (COX-1) at therapeutic concentrations.

Contraindications Hypersensitivity to celecoxib, sulfonamides, aspirin, other NSAIDs, or any component of the formulation; perioperative pain in the setting of coronary artery bypass graft (CABG) surgery

Canadian labeling: Additional contraindications (not in U.S. labeling): Pregnancy (third trimester); women who are breast-feeding; severe, uncontrolled heart failure; active gastrointestinal ulcer (gastric, duodenal, peptic) or bleeding; inflammatory bowel disease; cerebrovascular bleeding; severe liver impairment or active hepatic disease; severe renal impairment (Cl_{cr} <30 mL/minute) or deteriorating renal disease; known hyperkalemia; use in children

Warnings/Precautions [U.S. Boxed Warning]: NSAIDs are associated with an increased risk of serious (and potentially fatal) adverse cardiovascular thrombotic events, including MI and stroke. Risk may be increased with duration of use or pre-existing cardiovascular risk factors or disease. Carefully evaluate individual cardiovascular risk profiles prior to prescribing. New-onset or exacerbation of hypertension may occur (NSAIDS may impair response to thiazide or loop diuretics); may contribute to cardiovascular events; monitor blood pressure; use with caution in patients with hypertension. May cause sodium and fluid retention; use with caution in patients with edema, cerebrovascular disease, or ischemic heart disease. Avoid use in heart failure. Long-term cardiovascular risk in children has not been evaluated.

[U.S. Boxed Warning]: Celecoxib is contraindicated for treatment of perioperative pain in the setting of coronary artery bypass graft (CABG) surgery. Risk of MI and stroke may be increased with use following CABG surgery.

[U.S. Boxed Warning]: NSAIDs may increase risk of serious gastrointestinal ulceration, bleeding, and perforation (may be fatal). These events may occur at any time during therapy and without warning. Use caution with a history of GI disease (bleeding or ulcers), concurrent therapy with aspirin, anticoagulants and/or corticosteroids, smoking, use of alcohol, the elderly or debilitated patients. When used concomitantly with ≤325 mg of aspirin, a substantial increase in the risk of gastrointestinal complications (eg, ulcer) occurs; concomitant gastroprotective therapy (eg, proton pump inhibitors) is recommended (Bhatt, 2008).

Use the lowest effective dose for the shortest duration of time, consistent with individual patient goals, to reduce risk of cardiovascular or GI adverse events. Alternate therapies should be considered for patients at high risk.

NSAIDs may cause serious skin adverse events including exfoliative dermatitis, Stevens-Johnson syndrome (SJS), and toxic epidermal necrolysis (TEN); may occur without warning and in patients without prior known sulfa allergy. Anaphylactoid reactions may occur, even without prior exposure; patients with "aspirin triad" (bronchial asthma, aspirin intolerance, rhinitis) may be at increased risk. Do not use in patients who experience bronchospasm, asthma, rhinitis, or urticaria with NSAID or aspirin therapy. Use with caution in other forms of asthma.

Use with caution in patients with decreased hepatic (dosage adjustments are recommended for moderate hepatic impairment; not recommended for patients with severe hepatic impairment) or renal function. Transaminase elevations have been reported with use; closely monitor patients with any abnormal LFT. Severe hepatic reactions (eg, fulminant hepatitis, liver failure) have occurred with NSAID use, rarely; discontinue if signs or symptoms of liver disease develop, if systemic manifestations occur, or with persistent or worsening abnormal hepatic function tests. NSAID use may compromise existing renal function; dose-dependent decreases in prostaglandin synthesis may result from NSAID use, causing a reduction in renal blood flow which may cause renal decompensation (usually reversible). Patients with impaired renal function, dehydration, heart failure, liver dysfunction, those taking diuretics, ACE inhibitors, angiotensin II receptor blockers, and the elderly are at greater risk for renal toxicity. Rehydrate patient before starting therapy; monitor renal function closely. Not recommended for use in patients with advanced renal disease or severe renal insufficiency; discontinue use with persistent or worsening abnormal renal function tests. Long-term NSAID use may result in renal papillary necrosis. Should not be considered a treatment or replacement of corticosteroid-dependent diseases.

Anaphylactoid reactions may occur, even with no prior exposure to celecoxib. Use with caution in patients with known or suspected deficiency of cytochrome P450 isoenzyme 2C9; poor metabolizers may have higher plasma levels due to reduced metabolism; consider reduced initial doses. Alternate therapies should be considered in patients with JIA who are poor metabolizers of CYP2C9.

Anemia may occur with use; monitor hemoglobin or hematocrit in patients on long-term treatment. Celecoxib does not affect PT, PTT or platelet counts; does not inhibit platelet aggregation at approved doses.

When used for juvenile idiopathic arthritis (JIA), celecoxib is not FDA-approved in children <2 years of age or in children <10 kg. Use caution with systemic onset JIA (may be at risk for disseminated intravascular coagulation). Safety and efficacy have not been established for use in children for indications other than JIA.

Drug Interactions

Avoid Concomitant Use

Avoid concomitant use of Celecoxib with any of the following: Floctafenine; Ketorolac; Ketorolac (Nasal); Ketorolac (Systemic); Thioridazine

Decreased Effect

Celecoxib may decrease the levels/effects of: ACE Inhibitors; Aliskiren; Angiotensin II Receptor Blockers; Antiplatelet Agents; Beta-Blockers; Codeine; Eplerenone; HydrALAZINE; Loop Diuretics; Potassium-Sparing Diuretics; Selective Serotonin Reuptake Inhibitors; Thiazide Diuretics; TraMADol

The levels/effects of Celecoxib may be decreased by: Bile Acid Sequestrants; CYP2C9 Inducers (Strong); Peginterferon Alfa-2b; Tocilizumab

Increased Effect/Toxicity

Celecoxib may increase the levels/effects of: Aliskiren; Aminoglycosides; Anticoagulants; Antiplatelet Agents; ARIPiprazole; Bisphosphonate Derivatives; CycloSPORINE; CycloSPORINE (Systemic); CYP2C8 Substrates; CYP2D6 Substrates; Deferasirox; Desmopressin; Digoxin; Eplerenone; Fesoterodine; Haloperidol; Lithium; Methotrexate; Nebivolol; Nonsteroidal Anti-Inflammatory Agents; Porfimer; Potassium-Sparing Diuretics; PRALAtrexate; Prilocaine; Quinolone Antibiotics; Tamoxifen; Thioridazine; Thrombolytic Agents; Vancomycin; Vitamin K Antagonists

The levels/effects of Celecoxib may be increased by: ACE Inhibitors; Angiotensin II Receptor Blockers; Antidepressants (Tricyclic, Tertiary Amine); Conivaptan; Corticosteroids (Systemic); CycloSPORINE; CycloSPORINE (Systemic); CYP2C9 Inhibitors (Moderate); CYP2C9 Inhibitors (Strong); Floctafenine; Herbs (Anticoagulant/Antiplatelet Properties); Ketorolac; Ketorolac (Nasal); Ketorolac (Systemic); Probenecid; Propafenone; Selective Serotonin Reuptake Inhibitors; Sodium Phosphates; Treprostinil

Nutritional/Ethanol Interactions

Ethanol: Avoid ethanol (increased GI irritation).

Food: Peak concentrations are delayed and AUC is increased by 10% to 20% when taken with a high-fat meal.

Herb/Nutraceutical: Avoid concomitant use with herbs possessing anticoagulation/antiplatelet properties, including alfalfa, anise, bilberry, bladderwrack, bromelain, cat's claw, celery, chamomile, coleus, cordyceps, dong quai, evening primrose, fenugreek, feverfew, garlic, ginger, ginkgo biloba, ginseng (American, Panax, Siberian), grapeseed, green tea, guggul, horse chestnuts, horseradish, licorice, prickly ash, red clover, reishi, SAMe (S-adenosylmethionine), sweet clover, turmeric, white willow.

Adverse Reactions

≥2%

- Cardiovascular: Peripheral edema
- Central nervous system: Dizziness, fever, headache, insomnia
- Dermatologic: Rash
- Gastrointestinal: Abdominal pain, diarrhea, dyspepsia, flatulence, nausea, vomiting
- Neuromuscular & skeletal: Arthralgia, back pain
- Respiratory: Cough, nasopharyngitis, pharyngitis, rhinitis, sinusitis, upper respiratory tract infection

0.1% to 1.9%:

- Cardiovascular: Angina, aortic valve incompetence, chest pain, coronary artery disorder, edema, facial edema, hypertension (aggravated), MI, palpitation, sinus bradycardia, tachycardia, ventricular hypertrophy
- Central nervous system: Anxiety, depression, fatigue, hypoesthesia, migraine, nervousness, pain, somnolence, vertigo
- Dermatologic: Alopecia, bruising, cellulitis, dermatitis, dry skin, photosensitivity, pruritus, rash (erythematous), rash (maculopapular), urticaria
- Endocrine & metabolic: Hot flashes, hypercholesterolemia, hyperglycemia, hypokalemia, ovarian cyst, testosterone decreased
- Gastrointestinal: Anorexia, appetite increased, constipation, diverticulitis, dysphagia, eructation, esophagitis, gastritis, gastroenteritis, gastroesophageal reflux, gastrointestinal ulcer, hemorrhoids, hiatal hernia, melena, stomatitis, tenesmus, weight gain, xerostomia
- Genitourinary: Cystitis, dysuria, urinary frequency
- Hematologic: Anemia, thrombocythemia
- Hepatic: Alkaline phosphatase increased, transaminases increased
- Neuromuscular & skeletal: Arthrosis, CPK increased, hypertonia, leg cramps, myalgia, paresthesia, synovitis, tendonitis
- Ocular: Conjunctival hemorrhage, vitreous floaters
- Otic: Deafness, labyrinthitis, tinnitus
- Renal: Albuminuria, BUN increased, creatinine increased, hematuria, nonprotein nitrogen increased, renal calculi
- Respiratory: Bronchitis, bronchospasm, dyspnea, epistaxis, laryngitis, pneumonia
- Miscellaneous: Allergic reactions, allergy aggravated, cyst, diaphoresis, flu-like syndrome

Available Dosage Forms

Capsule, oral:

CeleBREX®: 50 mg, 100 mg, 200 mg, 400 mg

General Dosage Range Dosage adjustment recommended in patients with hepatic impairment

Oral:

Children ≥2 years and ≥10 kg to ≤25 kg: 50 mg twice daily

Children ≥2 years and >25 kg: 100 mg twice daily

Adults: 100-400 mg/day in 1-2 divided doses

Administration

Oral May be administered without regard to meals. Capsules may be swallowed whole or the entire contents emptied onto a teaspoon of cool or room temperature applesauce. The contents of the capsules sprinkled onto applesauce may be stored under refrigeration for up to 6 hours.

Stability

Storage Store at 25°C (77°F); excursions permitted to 15°C to 30°C (59°F to 86°F).

Nursing Actions

Physical Assessment Assess allergy history (aspirin, NSAIDs, salicylates). Monitor blood pressure at the beginning of therapy and periodically during use. Monitor effectiveness of therapy (pain, range of motion, mobility, ADL function, inflammation).

Patient Education May be taken with food to reduce GI upset. Avoid alcohol. You may experience dizziness, confusion, blurred vision, anorexia, nausea, vomiting, taste disturbance, or gastric distress; GI bleeding, ulceration, or perforation can occur with or without pain. Stop taking medication and report immediately stomach pain or cramping, unusual bleeding or bruising (blood in vomitus, stool, or urine), chest pain, shortness of breath, weakness of extremities, or slurring of speech. Report skin rash, unusual fatigue, flu-like symptoms, jaundice, weakness, sudden weight gain or edema, changes in hearing (ringing in ears) or vision, changes in urination pattern, or respiratory difficulty.

Dietary Considerations May be taken without regard to meals.

Cephalexin (sef a LEKS in)

Brand Names: U.S. Keflex®

Index Terms Cephalexin Monohydrate

Pharmacologic Category Antibiotic, Cephalosporin (First Generation)

Medication Safety Issues

Sound-alike/look-alike issues:

Cephalexin may be confused with cefaclor, ceFAZolin, ciprofloxacin

Keflex® may be confused with Keppra®, Valtrex®

Pregnancy Risk Factor B

Lactation Enters breast milk (small amounts)/use caution

Breast-Feeding Considerations Small amounts of cephalexin are excreted in breast milk. The manufacturer recommends that caution be exercised when administering cephalexin to nursing women. Maximum milk concentration occurs ~4 hours after a single oral dose and gradually disappears by 8 hours after administration. Nondose-related effects could include modification of bowel flora.

Use Treatment of susceptible bacterial infections including respiratory tract infections, otitis media, skin and skin structure infections, bone infections, and genitourinary tract infections, including acute prostatitis; alternative therapy for acute infective endocarditis prophylaxis

Mechanism of Action/Effect Inhibits bacterial cell wall synthesis by binding to one or more of the penicillin-binding proteins (PBPs)

Contraindications Hypersensitivity to cephalexin, any component of the formulation, or other cephalosporins

Warnings/Precautions Modify dosage in patients with severe renal impairment. Use with caution in patients with a history of penicillin allergy, especially IgE-mediated reactions (eg, anaphylaxis, urticaria). Prolonged use may result in fungal or bacterial superinfection, including *C. difficile*-associated diarrhea (CDAD) and pseudomembranous colitis; CDAD has been observed >2 months postantibiotic treatment. May be associated with increased INR, especially in nutritionally-deficient patients, prolonged treatment, hepatic or renal disease.

Drug Interactions

Avoid Concomitant Use

Avoid concomitant use of Cephalexin with any of the following: BCG

Decreased Effect

Cephalexin may decrease the levels/effects of: BCG; Typhoid Vaccine

The levels/effects of Cephalexin may be decreased by: Zinc Salts

Increased Effect/Toxicity

Cephalexin may increase the levels/effects of: MetFORMIN

The levels/effects of Cephalexin may be increased by: Probenecid

Nutritional/Ethanol Interactions Food: Peak antibiotic serum concentration is lowered and delayed, but total drug absorbed is not affected. Cephalexin serum levels may be decreased if taken with food.

Adverse Reactions Frequency not defined.

Central nervous system: Agitation, confusion, dizziness, fatigue, hallucinations, headache

Dermatologic: Angioedema, erythema multiforme (rare), rash, Stevens-Johnson syndrome (rare), toxic epidermal necrolysis (rare), urticaria

Gastrointestinal: Abdominal pain, diarrhea, dyspepsia, gastritis, nausea (rare), pseudomembranous colitis, vomiting (rare)

Genitourinary: Genital pruritus, genital moniliasis, vaginitis, vaginal discharge

Hematologic: Eosinophilia, hemolytic anemia, neutropenia, thrombocytopenia

Hepatic: ALT increased, AST increased, cholestatic jaundice (rare), transient hepatitis (rare)

Neuromuscular & skeletal: Arthralgia, arthritis, joint disorder

Renal: Interstitial nephritis (rare)

Miscellaneous: Allergic reactions, anaphylaxis

Available Dosage Forms

Capsule, oral: 250 mg, 500 mg

Keflex®: 250 mg, 500 mg, 750 mg

Powder for suspension, oral: 125 mg/5 mL (100 mL, 200 mL); 250 mg/5 mL (100 mL, 200 mL)

Tablet, oral: 250 mg, 500 mg

General Dosage Range Dosage adjustment recommended in patients with renal impairment

Oral:

Children >1-15 years: 25-100 mg/kg/day divided every 6-12 hours (maximum: 4 g/day) **or** 50 mg/kg prior to procedure (maximum: 2 g)

Adolescents >15 years: 25-100 mg/kg/day divided every 6-12 hours (maximum: 4 g/day) **or** 50 mg/kg prior to procedure (maximum: 2 g) **or** 500 mg every 12 hours

Adults: 250-1000 mg every 6 hours **or** 500 mg every 12 hours (maximum: 4 g/day) **or** 2 g prior to procedure

Administration

Oral Take without regard to food. If GI distress, take with food. Give around-the-clock to promote less variation in peak and trough serum levels.

Stability

Storage

Capsule: Store at 15°C to 30°C (59°F to 86°F).

Powder for oral suspension: Refrigerate suspension after reconstitution; discard after 14 days.

Nursing Actions

Physical Assessment Assess results of culture/sensitivity tests and patient's allergy history prior to therapy. Monitor for nephrotoxicity. Advise patients with diabetes about use of Clinitest® (may cause false-positive test). Teach patient to report opportunistic infection and hypersensitivity reaction.

Patient Education Take at regular intervals around-the-clock, with or without food. Maintain adequate hydration, unless instructed to restrict fluid intake. May cause false test results with Clinitest®; use of another type of glucose testing is preferable. May cause diarrhea. Report rash; breathing or swallowing difficulty; persistent diarrhea, nausea, vomiting, or abdominal pain; changes in urinary pattern or pain on urination;

opportunistic infection (eg, vaginal itching or drainage, sores in mouth, blood in stool or urine, unusual fever or chills); or CNS changes (eg, irritability, agitation, nervousness, insomnia, hallucinations).

Dietary Considerations Take without regard to food. If GI distress, take with food.

Certolizumab Pegol (cer to LIZ u mab PEG ol)

Brand Names: U.S. Cimzia®

Index Terms CDP870

Pharmacologic Category Antirheumatic, Disease Modifying; Gastrointestinal Agent, Miscellaneous; Tumor Necrosis Factor (TNF) Blocking Agent

Medication Guide Available Yes

Pregnancy Risk Factor B

Lactation Excretion in breast milk unknown/not recommended

Use Treatment of moderately- to severely-active Crohn's disease in patients who have inadequate response to conventional therapy; moderately- to severely-active rheumatoid arthritis (as monotherapy or in combination with nonbiological disease-modifying antirheumatic drugs [DMARDS])

Mechanism of Action/Effect Elevated levels of TNF-alpha have a role in the inflammatory process associated with Crohn's disease and in joint destruction associated with rheumatoid arthritis. Certolizumab pegol binds to and selectively neutralizes human TNF-alpha activity, inhibiting the role of TNF-alpha as a mediator in the inflammatory process.

Contraindications There are no contraindications listed within the manufacturer's labeling.

Warnings/Precautions [U.S. Boxed Warning]: Patients receiving certolizumab are at increased risk for serious infections which may result in hospitalization and/or fatality; infections usually developed in patients receiving concomitant immunosuppressive agents (eg, methotrexate or corticosteroids) and may present as disseminated (rather than local) disease. Active tuberculosis (or reactivation of latent tuberculosis), invasive fungal (including aspergillosis, blastomycosis, candidiasis, coccidioidomycosis, histoplasmosis, and pneumocystosis) and bacterial, viral or other opportunistic infections (including legionellosis and listeriosis) have been reported in patients receiving TNF-blocking agents, including certolizumab. Monitor closely for signs/symptoms of infection. Discontinue for serious infection or sepsis. Consider risks versus benefits prior to use in patients with a history of chronic or recurrent infection. Consider empiric antifungal therapy in patients who are at risk for invasive fungal infection and develop severe systemic illness. Caution should be exercised when considering use in the elderly or in patients with conditions that predispose them to infections (eg, diabetes) or residence/travel from areas of endemic mycoses (blastomycosis, coccidioidomycosis, histoplasmosis), or with latent or localized infections. Do not initiate certolizumab therapy with clinically important active infection. Patients who develop a new infection while undergoing treatment should be monitored closely. **[U.S. Boxed Warning]: Lymphoma and other malignancies have been reported in children and adolescent patients receiving other TNF-blocking agents.** Use of TNF blockers may affect defenses against malignancies; impact on the development and course of malignancies is not fully defined. Lymphoma has been noted in clinical trials. Chronic immunosuppressant therapy use may be a predisposing factor for malignancy development; rheumatoid arthritis alone has been previously associated with an increased rate of lymphoma.

Tuberculosis has been reported with certolizumab treatment. **[U.S. Boxed Warnings]: Patients should be evaluated for tuberculosis risk factors and for latent tuberculosis infection (with a tuberculin skin test) prior to therapy. Treatment of latent tuberculosis should be initiated before use. Patients with initial negative tuberculin skin tests should receive continued monitoring for tuberculosis throughout treatment;** active tuberculosis has developed in this population during treatment. Use with caution in patients who have resided in regions where tuberculosis is endemic. If appropriate, antituberculosis therapy should be considered (prior to certolizumab treatment) in patients with several or with highly significant risk factors for tuberculosis development.

Rare reactivation of hepatitis B virus (HBV) has occurred in chronic virus carriers; use with caution; evaluate prior to initiation and during treatment.

Hypersensitivity reactions, including angioedema, dyspnea, rash, serum sickness and urticaria have been reported (rarely) with treatment; discontinue and do not resume therapy if hypersensitivity occurs. Use with caution in patients who have experienced hypersensitivity with other TNF blockers. Use with caution in heart failure patients; worsening heart failure and new onset heart failure have been reported with TNF blockers, including certolizumab pegol; monitor closely. Rare cases of pancytopenia and other significant cytopenias, including aplastic anemia and have been reported with TNF-blocking agents. Leukopenia and thrombocytopenia have occurred with certolizumab; use with caution in patients with underlying hematologic disorders; consider discontinuing therapy with significant hematologic abnormalities. Autoantibody formation may develop; rarely resulting in autoimmune disorder, including lupus-like syndrome; monitor and discontinue if symptoms develop. A small number of patients (8%) develop antibodies to certolizumab during therapy.

Antibody-positive patients may have an increased incidence of adverse events (including injection site pain/erythema, abdominal pain and erythema nodosum). Use with caution in patients with pre-existing or recent-onset CNS demyelinating disorders; rare cases of optic neuritis, seizure, peripheral neuropathy, and demyelinating disease (new onset or exacerbation) have been reported.

The manufacturer does not recommend concurrent use with anakinra or other tumor necrosis factor (TNF) blocking agents due to the risk of serious infections. Do not use in combination with biologic DMARDS. Patients should be up to date with all immunizations before initiating therapy; live vaccines should not be given concurrently. There is no data available concerning the effects of therapy on vaccination or secondary transmission of live vaccines in patients receiving therapy. Use has not been studied in patients with renal impairment; however, the pharmacokinetics of the pegylated (polyethylene glycol) component may be dependent on renal function. Use with caution in the elderly, may be at higher risk for infections.

Drug Interactions

Avoid Concomitant Use

Avoid concomitant use of Certolizumab Pegol with any of the following: Abatacept; Anakinra; Anti-TNF Agents; BCG; Canakinumab; Natalizumab; Pimecrolimus; Rilonacept; RiTUXimab; Tacrolimus (Topical); Vaccines (Live)

Decreased Effect

Certolizumab Pegol may decrease the levels/effects of: BCG; Coccidioidin Skin Test; Sipuleucel-T; Vaccines (Inactivated); Vaccines (Live)

The levels/effects of Certolizumab Pegol may be decreased by: Echinacea; Pegloticase

Increased Effect/Toxicity

Certolizumab Pegol may increase the levels/effects of: Abatacept; Anakinra; Canakinumab; Leflunomide; Natalizumab; Rilonacept; Vaccines (Live)

The levels/effects of Certolizumab Pegol may be increased by: Anti-TNF Agents; Denosumab; Pimecrolimus; RiTUXimab; Roflumilast; Tacrolimus (Topical); Trastuzumab

Nutritional/Ethanol Interactions Herb/Nutraceutical: Echinacea may decrease the therapeutic effects of certolizumab; avoid concurrent use.

Adverse Reactions

>10%:

Central nervous system: Headache (5% to 18%)

Gastrointestinal: Nausea (≤11%)

Respiratory: Upper respiratory infection (6% to 20%), nasopharyngitis (4% to 13%)

Miscellaneous: Infection (14% to 38%; serious: 3%)

1% to 10%:

Cardiovascular: Hypertension (≤5%)

Central nervous system: Dizziness (≤6%), fever (≤5%), fatigue (≤3%)

Dermatologic: Rash (9%)

Gastrointestinal: Abdominal pain (≤6%), vomiting (5%)

Genitourinary: Urinary tract infection (≤8%)

Local: Injection site reactions (includes bleeding, burning, erythema, inflammation, pain, rash: ≤7%; incidence higher with placebo)

Neuromuscular & skeletal: Arthralgia (6% to 7%), back pain (≤4%)

Respiratory: Cough (≤6%), bronchitis (≤3%), pharyngitis (≤3%)

Miscellaneous: Antibody formation (7% to 8%), positive ANA (≤4%)

Available Dosage Forms

Injection, powder for reconstitution [preservative free]:

Cimzia®: 200 mg

Injection, solution [preservative free]:

Cimzia®: 200 mg/mL (1 mL)

General Dosage Range SubQ: Adults: Initial: 400 mg, repeat dose 2 and 4 weeks after initial dose; Maintenance: 400 mg every 4 weeks **or** 200 mg every other week

Administration

Other SubQ: Bring to room temperature prior to administration. Total dose requires 2 vials **or** 2 prefilled syringes. After reconstitution (of vials), draw each vial into separate syringes (using 20-gauge needles).

Administer each syringe subcutaneously (using provided 23-gauge needle) to separate sites on abdomen or thigh. Rotate injections sites; do not administer to areas where skin is tender, bruised, red, or hard.

Stability

Reconstitution Vials: Allow to reach room temperature prior to reconstitution. Using aseptic technique, reconstitute each vial with 1 mL sterile water for injection (provided) to a concentration of ~200 mg/mL; the manufacturer recommends using a 20-gauge needle (provided). Gently swirl to facilitate wetting of powder; do not shake. Allow vials to set undisturbed (may take up to 30 minutes) until fully reconstituted. Reconstituted solutions should not contain visible particles or gels in the solution.

Storage Prior to reconstitution, store refrigerated at 2°C to 8°C (36°F to 46°F); do not freeze. Bring to room temperature prior to administration.

Prefilled syringe: Protect from light.

Vials: Reconstituted vials may be retained at room temperature for ≤2 hours or refrigerated (do not freeze) for ≤24 hours prior to administration.

Nursing Actions

Physical Assessment Perform tuberculin skin test prior to initiating therapy. Monitor for signs of tuberculosis and other infections throughout therapy. Do not initiate therapy if active infection is present. Assess results of PPD at regular intervals during treatment. Teach patient proper injection technique and syringe/needle disposal.

Patient Education Inform prescriber of allergies, history of tuberculosis, or any kind of infection you have. If self-administered, follow directions for injection and needle/syringe disposal exactly. You may be more susceptible to infection. May cause headache, nausea, or dizziness. Report persistent fever; respiratory tract infection; infected wounds; urinary tract infection; flu-like symptoms; signs of fluid retention (unusual weight gain, swelling of the extremities); shortness of breath; or redness, swelling, or pain at injection site.

Cetirizine (se TI ra zeen)

Brand Names: U.S. All Day Allergy [OTC]; ZyrTEC® Allergy [OTC]; ZyrTEC® Children's Allergy [OTC]; ZyrTEC® Children's Hives Relief [OTC]

Index Terms Cetirizine Hydrochloride; P-071; UCB-P071

Pharmacologic Category Histamine H_1 Antagonist; Histamine H_1 Antagonist, Second Generation; Piperazine Derivative

Medication Safety Issues

Sound-alike/look-alike issues:

ZyrTEC® may be confused with Lipitor®, Serax, Xanax®, Zantac®, Zerit®, Zocor®, ZyPREXA®, ZyrTEC-D®

ZyrTEC® (cetirizine) may be confused with ZyrTEC® Itchy Eye (ketotifen)

Breast-Feeding Considerations Cetirizine is excreted into breast milk.

Use Perennial and seasonal allergic rhinitis and other allergic symptoms including urticaria; chronic idiopathic urticaria

Mechanism of Action/Effect Competes with histamine for H_1-receptor sites on effector cells in the GI tract, blood vessels, and respiratory tract

Contraindications Hypersensitivity to cetirizine, hydroxyzine, or any component of the formulation

Warnings/Precautions Cetirizine should be used cautiously in patients with hepatic or renal dysfunction; dosage adjustment recommended. Use with caution in the elderly; may be more sensitive to adverse effects. May cause drowsiness; use caution performing tasks which require alertness (eg, operating machinery or driving). Effects may be potentiated when used with other sedative drugs or ethanol.

Drug Interactions

Avoid Concomitant Use There are no known interactions where it is recommended to avoid concomitant use.

Decreased Effect

Cetirizine may decrease the levels/effects of: Acetylcholinesterase Inhibitors (Central); Benzylpenicilloyl Polylysine; Betahistine

The levels/effects of Cetirizine may be decreased by: Acetylcholinesterase Inhibitors (Central); Amphetamines; P-glycoprotein/ABCB1 Inducers; Tocilizumab

Increased Effect/Toxicity

Cetirizine may increase the levels/effects of: Alcohol (Ethyl); Anticholinergics; CNS Depressants; Methotrimeprazine; Selective Serotonin Reuptake Inhibitors

The levels/effects of Cetirizine may be increased by: Conivaptan; Droperidol; HydrOXYzine; Methotrimeprazine; P-glycoprotein/ABCB1 Inhibitors; Pramlintide

Nutritional/Ethanol Interactions Ethanol: May increase CNS depression; monitor for increased effects with coadministration. Caution patients about effects.

Adverse Reactions

>10%: Central nervous system: Headache (children 11% to 14%, placebo 12%), somnolence (adults 14%, children 2% to 4%)

2% to 10%:

Central nervous system: Insomnia (children 9%, adults <2%), fatigue (adults 6%), malaise (4%), dizziness (adults 2%)

Gastrointestinal: Abdominal pain (children 4% to 6%), dry mouth (adults 5%), diarrhea (children 2% to 3%), nausea (children 2% to 3%, placebo 2%), vomiting (children 2% to 3%)

Respiratory: Epistaxis (children 2% to 4%, placebo 3%), pharyngitis (children 3% to 6%, placebo 3%), bronchospasm (children 2% to 3%, placebo 2%)

Pharmacodynamics/Kinetics

Onset of Action Suppression of skin wheal and flare: 0.7 hours (Simons, 1999)

Duration of Action Suppression of skin wheal and flare: ≥24 hours (Simons, 1999)

Available Dosage Forms

Capsule, liquid gel, oral:

ZyrTEC® Allergy [OTC]: 10 mg

Solution, oral: 5 mg/5 mL (5 mL)

Syrup, oral: 5 mg/5 mL (5 mL, 118 mL, 120 mL, 473 mL, 480 mL)

ZyrTEC® Children's Allergy [OTC]: 5 mg/5 mL (118 mL)

ZyrTEC® Children's Hives Relief [OTC]: 5 mg/5 mL (118 mL)

Tablet, oral: 5 mg, 10 mg

All Day Allergy [OTC]: 10 mg

ZyrTEC® Allergy [OTC]: 10 mg

Tablet, chewable, oral: 5 mg, 10 mg

All Day Allergy [OTC]: 5 mg

ZyrTEC® Children's Allergy [OTC]: 5 mg, 10 mg

General Dosage Range Dosage adjustment recommended in patients with hepatic or renal impairment

Oral:

Children 6-12 months: 2.5 mg once daily

Children 12 months to <2 years: 2.5 mg once or twice daily

Children 2-5 years: 2.5-5 mg/day in 1-2 divided doses

Children ≥6 years and Adults: 5-10 mg once daily

Elderly: Initial: 5 mg once daily

Administration

Oral May be administered with or without food.

Stability

Storage Store at room temperature.

Syrup: Store at room temperature of 15°C to 30°C (59°F to 86°F), or under refrigeration at 2°C to 8°C (36°F to 46°F).

Nursing Actions

Patient Education Avoid use of alcohol. You may experience drowsiness, dizziness, or dry mouth. Report persistent sedation, confusion, agitation, persistent nausea or vomiting, blurred vision, or lack of improvement or worsening of condition.

Dietary Considerations May be taken with or without food.

Cetuximab (se TUK see mab)

Brand Names: U.S. Erbitux®

Index Terms C225; IMC-C225; MOAB C225

Pharmacologic Category Antineoplastic Agent, Monoclonal Antibody; Epidermal Growth Factor Receptor (EGFR) Inhibitor

Medication Safety Issues

Sound-alike/look-alike issues:

Cetuximab may be confused with bevacizumab

Pregnancy Risk Factor C

Lactation Excretion in breast milk is unknown/not recommended

Breast-Feeding Considerations According to the manufacturer, the decision to continue or discontinue breast-feeding during therapy should take into account the risk of exposure to the infant and the benefits of treatment to the mother. If breast-feeding is interrupted for cetuximab treatment, based on the half-life, breast-feeding should not be resumed for at least 60 days following the last cetuximab dose.

Use Treatment of EGFR-expressing metastatic colorectal cancer (as a single agent or in combination with irinotecan); treatment of squamous cell cancer of the head and neck (as a single agent for recurrent or metastatic disease after platinum-based chemotherapy failure; in combination with radiation therapy as initial treatment of locally or regionally advanced disease; in combination with platinum and fluorouracil-based chemotherapy as first-line treatment of locoregional or metastatic disease)

Note: Subset analyses (retrospective) in metastatic colorectal cancer trials have not shown a benefit with EGFR inhibitor treatment in patients whose tumors have codon 12 or 13 *KRAS* mutations; use is not recommended in these patients.

Unlabeled Use Treatment of EGFR-expressing advanced nonsmall cell lung cancer (NSCLC)

Mechanism of Action/Effect EGFR inhibitor; inhibits cell growth, induces apoptosis and decreases matrix metalloproteinase and vascular endothelial growth factor production.

Contraindications There are no contraindications listed in the manufacturer's labeling

Warnings/Precautions [U.S. Boxed Warning]: Serious infusion reactions have been reported in ~3% of patients; fatal outcome has been reported rarely; interrupt infusion promptly and permanently discontinue for serious infusion reactions. Reactions have included airway obstruction (bronchospasm, stridor, hoarseness), hypotension, loss of consciousness, shock, MI, and/or cardiac arrest. Approximately 90% of reactions occur with the first infusion despite the use of prophylactic antihistamines. Immediate treatment for anaphylactic/anaphylactoid reactions should be available during administration. The manufacturer recommends monitoring patients for at least 1 hour following completion of infusion, or longer if a reaction occurs. Mild-to-moderate infusion reactions are managed by slowing the infusion rate (by 50%) and administering antihistamines. Patients with pre-existing IgE antibody against cetuximab (specific for galactose-α-1,3-galactose) are reported to have a higher incidence of severe hypersensitivity reaction. Severe hypersensitivity reaction has been reported more frequently in patients living in the middle south area of the United States, including North Carolina and Tennessee (Chung, 2008; O'Neil, 2007).

[U.S. Boxed Warning]: In patients with squamous cell head and neck cancer, cardiopulmonary arrest and/or sudden death has occurred in 2% of patients receiving radiation therapy in combination with cetuximab and in 3% of patients receiving combination chemotherapy (platinum and fluorouracil-based) with cetuximab. Closely monitor serum electrolytes (magnesium, potassium, calcium) during and after cetuximab treatment (monitor for at least 8 weeks after treatment). Use caution with history of coronary artery disease, HF, and arrhythmias; fatalities have been reported. Interstitial lung disease (ILD) has been reported; use caution with pre-existing lung disease; interrupt treatment for acute onset or worsening of pulmonary symptoms; permanently discontinue with confirmed ILD.

Acneiform rash has been reported in 76% to 88% of patients (severe in 1% to 17%), usually developing within the first 2 weeks of therapy; may require dose modification; generally resolved after discontinuation in most patients, although persisted beyond 28 days in some patients; monitor for dermatologic toxicity and corresponding infections. Acneiform rash should be treated with topical and/or oral antibiotics; topical corticosteroids are not recommended. Other dermatologic toxicities, including dry skin, fissures, hypertrichosis, paronychial inflammation, and skin infections have been reported; related ocular toxicities (blepharitis, conjunctivitis, keratitis, ulcerative keratitis with decreased visual acuity) may also occur. Sunlight may exacerbate skin reactions (limit sun exposure). Hypomagnesemia is common (may be severe); the onset of electrolyte disturbance may occur within days to months after initiation of treatment; monitor magnesium, calcium, and potassium during treatment and for at least 8 weeks after completion; may require electrolyte replacement. Non-neutralizing anticetuximab antibodies were detected in 5% of evaluable patients. Safety has not been established when used in combination with radiation therapy **and** cisplatin; fatalities and serious cardiotoxicity, pneumonia or other adverse events have been observed. Patients with colorectal cancer with tumors with a codon 12 or 13 *KRAS* mutation are unlikely to benefit from EGFR inhibitor therapy and should not receive cetuximab treatment. In trials for colorectal cancer, evidence of EGFR expression was required, although the response rate did not correlate with either the percentage of cells positive for EGFR or the intensity of expression. EGFR expression has been detected in nearly all patients with head and neck cancer, therefore laboratory evidence of EGFR expression is not necessary for head and neck cancers.

Drug Interactions

Avoid Concomitant Use There are no known interactions where it is recommended to avoid concomitant use.

Decreased Effect There are no known significant interactions involving a decrease in effect.

Increased Effect/Toxicity There are no known significant interactions involving an increase in effect.

Adverse Reactions Except where noted, percentages reported for studies with cetuximab monotherapy.

>10%:

Central nervous system: Fatigue (89%), pain (51%), headache (33%), fever (30%), insomnia (30%), confusion (15%), anxiety (14%), chills/rigors (13%), depression (13%)

Dermatologic: Acneiform rash (all studies: 76% to 88%; grades 3/4: 1% to 17%; onset: ≤14 days), rash (89%), dry skin (49%), pruritus (40%), nail changes (21%)

Endocrine & metabolic: Hypomagnesemia (all studies: 55%; grades 3/4: 6% to 17%)

Gastrointestinal: Abdominal pain (59%), constipation (46%), diarrhea (39%), vomiting (37%), stomatitis (25%), xerostomia (11%)

Neuromuscular & skeletal: Bone pain (15%)

Respiratory: Dyspnea (48%), cough (29%)

Miscellaneous: Infection (all studies: 13% to 35%), infusion reaction (all studies: 15% to 21%; grades 3/4: 2% to 5%; 90% of severe reactions occurred with first infusion)

1% to 10%:

Cardiovascular: Cardiopulmonary arrest (2%; with radiation therapy; 3% with platinum/fluorouracil-based chemotherapy)

Renal: Renal failure (all studies: 1%)

Miscellaneous: Sepsis (all studies: 1% to 4%)

Available Dosage Forms

Injection, solution [preservative free]:

Erbitux®: 2 mg/mL (50 mL, 100 mL)

General Dosage Range Dosage adjustment recommended in patients who develop toxicities

I.V.: *Adults:* Loading dose: 400 mg/m^2; Maintenance: 250 mg/m^2 weekly

Administration

I.V. I.V. infusion; loading dose over 2 hours, weekly maintenance dose over 1 hour. Do not administer as I.V. push or bolus. Do not shake or dilute. Administer via infusion pump or syringe pump. Following the infusion, an observation period (1 hour) is recommended; longer observation time (following an infusion reaction) may be required. Premedication with an H_1 antagonist prior to the initial dose is recommended. The maximum infusion rate is 10 mg/minute. Administer through a low protein-binding 0.22 micrometer in-line filter. Use 0.9% NaCl to flush line at the end of infusion.

For biweekly administration (unlabeled frequency and dose), the initial dose was infused over 120 minutes and subsequent doses infused over 60 minutes (Pfeiffer, 2007).

I.V. Detail pH: 7-7.4; may contain a small amount of visible white, amorphous cetuximab particles

Stability

Reconstitution Reconstitution is not required. Appropriate dose should be added to empty sterile container; do not shake or dilute.

Storage Store unopened vials refrigerated at 2°C to 8°C (36°F to 46°F); do not freeze. Preparations in infusion containers are stable for up to 12 hours refrigerated at 2°C to 8°C (36°F to 46°F) and up to 8 hours at room temperature of 20°C to 25°C (68°F to 77°F).

Nursing Actions

Physical Assessment Premedication with antihistamines may be prescribed. Monitor patient closely for airway obstruction, hives, and hypotension during and for at least 1 hour following infusion. Treatment for anaphylactic reactions should be available. In case of severe infusion reaction, stop infusion and notify prescriber. Instruct patient to report skin reactions, cough, dyspnea, gastrointestinal upset, and opportunistic infection. Monitor for skin reactions and signs of dermatologic toxicities. Monitor electrolytes up to 8 weeks after treatments.

Patient Education This medication can only be administered by infusion and you will be closely monitored during each infusion. The first infusion takes longer to infuse. Report immediately unusual chest tightness; difficulty breathing or swallowing; itching or skin rash; back pain or acute headache; or redness, swelling, or pain at infusion site. Maintain adequate nutrition and hydration, unless instructed to restrict fluid intake. Patient may experience feelings of weakness or fatigue, nausea, vomiting, loss of appetite, diarrhea, headache, back pain, acne from rash, skin dryness, or loss of hair or nails (may grow back after therapy). Report immediately chest pain, irregular heartbeat, or palpitations; difficulty breathing; persistent gastrointestinal disturbances (pain, constipation, diarrhea, vomiting); CNS changes (depression or insomnia); skin rash, dryness, or cracking; or any signs of infection. Instruct patients to avoid direct sunlight, including tanning booths. Wear sunscreen and protective clothing while receiving this medication and up to 2 months after treatment is complete.

Cevimeline (se vi ME leen)

Brand Names: U.S. Evoxac®

Index Terms Cevimeline Hydrochloride

Pharmacologic Category Cholinergic Agonist

Medication Safety Issues

Sound-alike/look-alike issues:

Cevimeline may be confused with Savella®

Evoxac® may be confused with Eurax®

Pregnancy Risk Factor C

Lactation Excretion in breast milk unknown/not recommended

Use Treatment of symptoms of dry mouth in patients with Sjögren's syndrome

Available Dosage Forms

Capsule, oral:

Evoxac®: 30 mg

General Dosage Range Oral: *Adults:* 30 mg 3 times/day

Administration

Oral Administer with or without food.

Nursing Actions

Patient Education Take with or without food. You may experience decreased visual acuity, GI distress, nausea, diarrhea, or headache. Report unresolved diarrhea; abdominal pain; flatulence; anorexia; excessive salivation or sweating; unresolved respiratory distress; runny nose; cold or flu symptoms; joint, bone, or muscle weakness, pain, tremor, or cramping; chest pain or palpitations; swelling of extremities; or weight gain.

Chenodiol (kee noe DYE ole)

Brand Names: U.S. Chenodal™

Index Terms CDCA; Chenodeoxycholic Acid

Pharmacologic Category Bile Acid

Pregnancy Risk Factor X

Lactation Excretion in breast milk unknown/use caution

Use Oral dissolution of radiolucent cholesterol gallstones in selected patients as an alternative to surgery

Unlabeled Use Cerebrotendinous xanthomatosis (CTX)

Available Dosage Forms

Tablet, oral:

Chenodal™: 250 mg

General Dosage Range Oral: *Adults:* Initial: 250 mg twice daily; Maintenance: 13-16 mg/kg/day in 2 divided doses

Nursing Actions

Patient Education Medication may need to be taken for 24 months before dissolution will occur. Blood studies and x-rays studies will be necessary during therapy. Report persistent diarrhea and gallstone attacks (abdominal pain, nausea and vomiting, yellowing of skin or eyes).

Chloral Hydrate (KLOR al HYE drate)

Brand Names: U.S. Somnote®

Index Terms Chloral; Hydrated Chloral; Trichloroacetaldehyde Monohydrate

Pharmacologic Category Hypnotic, Nonbenzodiazepine

Medication Safety Issues

High alert medication:

The Institute for Safe Medication Practices (ISMP) includes this medication among its list of drugs which have a heightened risk of causing significant patient harm when used in error.

Pregnancy Risk Factor C

Lactation Enters breast milk/not recommended

Use Short-term sedative and hypnotic (<2 weeks); sedative/hypnotic for diagnostic procedures; sedative prior to EEG evaluations

Controlled Substance C-IV

Available Dosage Forms

Capsule, oral:

Somnote®: 500 mg

Syrup, oral: 500 mg/5 mL (5 mL, 473 mL, 480 mL)

General Dosage Range Oral:

Children: Dosage varies greatly depending on indication

Adults: 250 mg 3 times/day **or** 500-1000 mg at bedtime or prior to procedure (maximum: 2 g/day)

Elderly: Hypnotic (oral): Initial: 250 mg at bedtime

Administration

Oral Chilling the syrup may help to mask unpleasant taste. Do not crush capsule (contains drug in liquid form). Gastric irritation may be minimized by diluting dose in water or other oral liquid.

Other Rectal administration: May administer chloral hydrate syrup rectally.

Nursing Actions

Physical Assessment For short-term use. Assess for history of addiction; long-term use can result in dependence, abuse, or tolerance. Monitor for excessive sedation. For inpatient use, institute safety measures (side rails, night light, call bell, assistance with ambulation) to prevent falls.

Patient Education Drug may cause physical and/or psychological dependence. While using this medication, do not use alcohol. You may experience drowsiness, dizziness, blurred vision, nausea, vomiting, unpleasant taste, or diarrhea. Report skin rash, CNS changes (confusion, depression, increased sedation, excitation, headache, insomnia, or nightmares), unresolved GI distress, chest pain or palpitations, or ineffectiveness of medication.

Chlorambucil (klor AM byoo sil)

Brand Names: U.S. Leukeran®

Index Terms CB-1348; Chlorambucilum; Chloraminophene; Chlorbutinum; WR-139013

Pharmacologic Category Antineoplastic Agent, Alkylating Agent

Medication Safety Issues

Sound-alike/look-alike issues:

Chlorambucil may be confused with Chloromycetin®

Leukeran® may be confused with Alkeran®, leucovorin, Leukine®, Myleran®

High alert medication:

This medication is in a class the Institute for Safe Medication Practices (ISMP) includes among its list of drug classes which have a heightened risk of causing significant patient harm when used in error.

Pregnancy Risk Factor D

Lactation Excretion in breast milk unknown/not recommended

Use Management of chronic lymphocytic leukemia (CLL), Hodgkin lymphoma, non-Hodgkin's lymphomas (NHL)

Unlabeled Use Treatment of nephrotic syndrome (steroid sensitive) in children, treatment of Waldenström's macroglobulinemia

Available Dosage Forms

Tablet, oral:

Leukeran®: 2 mg

General Dosage Range Dosage adjustment recommended in patients with hepatic impairment or who develop toxicities

Oral: *Adults:* 0.1-0.2 mg/kg/day for 3-6 weeks **or** 0.4 mg/kg intermittently, biweekly, or monthly (may increase by 0.1 mg/kg/dose)

Administration

Oral Usually administered as a single dose; preferably on an empty stomach.

Nursing Actions

Physical Assessment Monitor for hematologic myelosuppression, hypersensitivity rash, drug fever, seizures, gastrointestinal upset, and hepatotoxicity. Teach sexually-active female patients necessity for contraception.

Patient Education Maintain adequate hydration, unless instructed to restrict fluid intake. Avoid alcohol and acidic, spicy, or hot foods. May cause menstrual irregularities and/or sterility. You will be more susceptible to infection. May cause nausea, vomiting, or mouth sores. Report CNS changes (agitation, confusion, hallucinations, seizures); easy bruising or bleeding; unusual rash; persistent nausea, vomiting, or mouth sores; yellowing of skin or dark urine; or respiratory difficulty.

ChlordiazePOXIDE (klor dye az e POKS ide)

Index Terms Librium; Methaminodiazepoxide Hydrochloride

Pharmacologic Category Benzodiazepine

Medication Safety Issues

Sound-alike/look-alike issues:

ChlordiazePOXIDE may be confused with chlorproMAZINE

Librium may be confused with Librax®

BEERS Criteria medication:

This drug may be inappropriate for use in geriatric patients (high severity risk).

Lactation Enters breast milk

Use Management of anxiety disorder or for the short-term relief of symptoms of anxiety; withdrawal symptoms of acute alcoholism; preoperative apprehension and anxiety

Controlled Substance C-IV

Available Dosage Forms

Capsule, oral: 5 mg, 10 mg, 25 mg

General Dosage Range Dosage adjustment recommended in patients with renal or hepatic impairment.

Oral:

Children ≥6 years: 10-30 mg/day in 2-4 divided doses

Adults: 15-100 mg/day in 3-4 divided doses

Elderly: 10-20 mg/day in 2-4 divided doses

Administration

Oral Administer in divided doses.

Nursing Actions

Physical Assessment Assess for signs of CNS depression (sedation, dizziness, confusion, or ataxia). Assess for history of addiction; long-term use can result in dependence, abuse, or tolerance; periodically evaluate need for continued use. For inpatient use, institute safety measures to prevent falls. Taper dosage slowly when discontinuing.

Patient Education Drug may cause physical and/or psychological dependence. Do not use alcohol. Maintain adequate hydration, unless instructed to restrict fluid intake. You may experience drowsiness, lightheadedness, impaired coordination, dizziness, blurred vision, dry mouth, constipation, or altered sexual drive or ability (reversible).

Report persistent CNS effects (eg, euphoria, confusion, increased sedation, depression); chest pain, palpitations, or rapid heartbeat; muscle cramping, weakness, tremors, rigidity, or altered gait; or worsening of condition.

Related Information

Management of Drug Extravasations *on page 1269*

Chloroquine (KLOR oh kwin)

Brand Names: U.S. Aralen®

Index Terms Chloroquine Phosphate

Pharmacologic Category Aminoquinoline (Antimalarial)

Medication Safety Issues

International issues:

Aralen [U.S., Mexico] may be confused with Paralen brand name for acetaminophen [Czech Republic]

Lactation Enters breast milk/not recommended (AAP considers "compatible"; AAP 2001 update pending)

Use Suppression/chemoprophylaxis or treatment of acute malaria due to susceptible *Plasmodium malariae, P. vivax, P. ovale, P. falciparum*; extraintestinal amebiasis

Unlabeled Use Rheumatoid arthritis; discoid lupus erythematosus

Available Dosage Forms

Tablet, oral: 250 mg, 500 mg

Aralen®: 500 mg

General Dosage Range Dosage adjustment recommended in patients with renal impairment

Oral: *Children and Adults:* Dosage varies greatly depending on indication

Administration

Oral May be taken with meals to decrease GI upset. Chloroquine phosphate tablets have also been mixed with chocolate syrup or enclosed in gelatin capsules to mask the bitter taste.

Nursing Actions

Physical Assessment Assess results of CBC and monitor for retinopathy, hearing loss, or myopathy regularly. Teach patient to report anemia, muscle weakness, or visual or auditory changes.

Patient Education It is important to complete full course of therapy. May be taken with meals to decrease GI upset and bitter aftertaste. Avoid excessive alcohol when taking this medication. You should have regular ophthalmic exams (every 4-6 months) if using this medication over extended periods. May cause skin discoloration (blue/black), hair bleaching, or skin rash. If you have psoriasis, may cause exacerbation. May cause headache, nausea, vomiting, loss of appetite, or increased sensitivity to sunlight. Report vision changes, any change in hearing acuity or ringing in ears, rash or itching, persistent diarrhea or GI disturbances, chest pain or palpitations, CNS changes, unusual fatigue, or easy bruising or bleeding.

ChlorproMAZINE (klor PROE ma zeen)

Index Terms Chlorpromazine Hydrochloride; CPZ; Thorazine

Pharmacologic Category Antimanic Agent; Antipsychotic Agent, Typical, Phenothiazine

Medication Safety Issues

Sound-alike/look-alike issues:

ChlorproMAZINE may be confused with chlordiazePOXIDE, chlorproPAMIDE, clomiPRAMINE, prochlorperazine, promethazine

Thorazine may be confused with thiamine, thioridazine

Lactation Enters breast milk/not recommended (AAP rates "of concern"; AAP 2001 update pending)

Use Management of psychotic disorders (control of mania, treatment of schizophrenia); control of nausea and vomiting; relief of restlessness and apprehension before surgery; acute intermittent porphyria; adjunct in the treatment of tetanus; intractable hiccups; combativeness and/or explosive hyperexcitable behavior in children 1-12 years of age and in short-term treatment of hyperactive children

Unlabeled Use Behavioral symptoms associated with dementia (elderly); psychosis/agitation related to Alzheimer's dementia

Available Dosage Forms

Injection, solution: 25 mg/mL (1 mL, 2 mL)

Tablet, oral: 10 mg, 25 mg, 50 mg, 100 mg, 200 mg

General Dosage Range

I.M., I.V.:

Children ≥6 months: 0.5-1 mg/kg every 6-8 hours (maximum: <5 years [<22.7 kg]: 40 mg/day; 5-12 years [22.7-45.5 kg]: 75 mg/day)

Adults: Initial: 25 mg; may repeat (25-50 mg) in 1-4 hours; Usual dose: 300-800 mg/day (maximum: 400 mg every 4-6 hours)

Oral:

Children ≥6 months: 0.5-1 mg/ kg every 4-6 hours as needed

Adults: Dosage varies greatly depending on indication

Administration

I.V. Do not administer SubQ (tissue damage and irritation may occur); for direct I.V. injection: Dilute with normal saline to a maximum concentration of 1 mg/mL, administer slow I.V. at a rate not to exceed 0.5 mg/minute in children and 1 mg/minute in adults. For treatment of intractable hiccups the manufacturer recommends diluting 25-50 mg of chlorpromazine in 500-1000 ml of normal saline. To reduce the risk of hypotension, patients receiving I.V. chlorpromazine must remain lying down during and for 30 minutes after the injection.

Note: Avoid skin contact with solution; may cause contact dermatitis.

Nursing Actions

Physical Assessment Review ophthalmic exam results. Monitor mental status, mood, affect, and gait. Monitor for suicide ideation, depression, excess sedation, extrapyramidal symptoms, and CNS changes at beginning of therapy and periodically throughout. I.V./I.M.: Significant hypotension may occur. Initiate at lower doses and taper dosage slowly when discontinuing.

Patient Education Avoid alcohol. Maintain adequate hydration, unless instructed to restrict fluid intake. You may experience excess drowsiness, lightheadedness, dizziness, blurred vision, dry mouth, upset stomach, nausea, vomiting, anorexia, constipation, postural hypotension, urinary retention, ejaculatory dysfunction (reversible), decreased perspiration, or photosensitivity. Report persistent CNS effects (trembling fingers, altered gait or balance, excessive sedation, seizures, unusual movements, anxiety, suicide ideation, abnormal thoughts, confusion, personality changes); chest pain, palpitations, rapid heartbeat, or severe dizziness; unresolved urinary retention or changes in urinary pattern; altered menstrual pattern, change in libido, swelling or pain in breasts (male or female); vision changes, skin rash, irritation, or changes in color of skin (gray-blue); or worsening of condition.

Chlorthalidone (klor THAL i done)

Brand Names: U.S. Thalitone®

Index Terms Hygroton

Pharmacologic Category Diuretic, Thiazide

Pregnancy Risk Factor B

Lactation Enters breast milk/not recommended (AAP rates "compatible"; AAP 2001 update pending)

Use Management of mild-to-moderate hypertension when used alone or in combination with other agents; treatment of edema associated with heart failure or nephrotic syndrome. Recent studies have found chlorthalidone effective in the treatment of isolated systolic hypertension in the elderly.

Unlabeled Use Pediatric hypertension

Available Dosage Forms

Tablet, oral: 25 mg, 50 mg

Thalitone®: 15 mg

General Dosage Range Oral:

Adults: 12.5-100 mg/day **or** 100 mg 3 times/week (maximum: 200 mg/day)

Elderly: Initial: 12.5-25 mg/day or every other day

Nursing Actions

Physical Assessment Allergy history should be assessed prior to beginning therapy. Monitor blood pressure, fluid status, and electrolyte balance regularly during long-term therapy. Caution patients with diabetes to monitor glucose levels; may reduce effect of oral hypoglycemics.

Patient Education Take once-daily dose in morning or last of daily doses early in the day to avoid night-time disturbances. You may need to make dietary changes (eg, your prescriber may recommend a potassium supplement or foods high in potassium; do not increase your potassium intake unless recommended to do so). If using oral hypoglycemics, monitor glucose levels closely (this medication may reduce effect of oral hypoglycemics). May cause sensitivity to sunlight, anorexia, or GI distress. Report muscle twitching or cramps; nausea or vomiting; confusion; numbness of extremities; loss of appetite or GI distress; severe rash, redness, or itching of skin; chest pain or palpitations; respiratory difficulty; or unusual weight loss.

Chlorzoxazone (klor ZOKS a zone)

Brand Names: U.S. Lorzone™; Parafon Forte® DSC

Pharmacologic Category Skeletal Muscle Relaxant

Medication Safety Issues

BEERS Criteria medication:

This drug may be inappropriate for use in geriatric patients (high severity risk).

Lactation Excretion in breast milk unknown

Use Symptomatic treatment of muscle spasm and pain associated with acute musculoskeletal conditions

Mechanism of Action/Effect Acts on the spinal cord and subcortical levels by depressing polysynaptic reflexes

Contraindications Hypersensitivity to chlorzoxazone or any component of the formulation; impaired liver function

Warnings/Precautions This class of medication is poorly tolerated by the elderly due to anticholinergic effects, sedation, and weakness. Efficacy is questionable at dosages tolerated by elderly patients (Beers Criteria).

Drug Interactions

Avoid Concomitant Use

Avoid concomitant use of Chlorzoxazone with any of the following: Pimozide

Decreased Effect

The levels/effects of Chlorzoxazone may be decreased by: Cyproterone; Peginterferon Alfa-2b; Tocilizumab

Increased Effect/Toxicity

Chlorzoxazone may increase the levels/effects of: Alcohol (Ethyl); ARIPiprazole; CNS Depressants; Methotrimeprazine; Pimozide; Selective Serotonin Reuptake Inhibitors

The levels/effects of Chlorzoxazone may be increased by: Conivaptan; Disulfiram; Droperidol; HydrOXYzine; Isoniazid; Methotrimeprazine

Nutritional/Ethanol Interactions Ethanol: May increase CNS depression; monitor for increased effects with coadministration. Caution patients about effects.

Adverse Reactions Frequency not defined.

Central nervous system: Dizziness, drowsiness lightheadedness, paradoxical stimulation, malaise

Dermatologic: Rash, petechiae, ecchymoses (rare), angioneurotic edema

Gastrointestinal: Nausea, vomiting, stomach cramps

Genitourinary: Urine discoloration

Hepatic: Liver dysfunction

Miscellaneous: Anaphylaxis (very rare)

Pharmacodynamics/Kinetics

Onset of Action ~1 hour

Duration of Action 6-12 hours

Available Dosage Forms

Caplet, oral:

Parafon Forte® DSC: 500 mg

Tablet, oral: 500 mg

Lorzone™: 375 mg, 750 mg

General Dosage Range Oral:

Children: 20 mg/kg/day **or** 600 mg/m^2/day in 3-4 divided doses

Adults: 250-750 mg 3-4 times/day

Elderly: Initial: 250 mg 2-4 times/day

Nursing Actions

Physical Assessment Monitor for effectiveness and CNS sedation.

Patient Education Take with food. Do not use alcohol. You may experience drowsiness, dizziness, lightheadedness, or postural hypotension. Report excessive drowsiness.

Cholestyramine Resin

(koe LES teer a meen REZ in)

Brand Names: U.S. Prevalite®; Questran®; Questran® Light

Pharmacologic Category Antilipemic Agent, Bile Acid Sequestrant

Pregnancy Risk Factor C

Lactation Does not enter breast milk/use caution

Use Adjunct in the management of primary hypercholesterolemia; pruritus associated with elevated levels of bile acids; regression of arteriolosclerosis

Unlabeled Use Diarrhea associated with excess fecal bile acids (Westergaard, 2007); may be used to enhance elimination of digoxin when non-life-threatening toxicity occurs (Henderson, 1988)

Available Dosage Forms

Powder for suspension, oral: Cholestyramine resin 4 g/5 g of powder (210 g); Cholestyramine resin 4 g/5.7 g of powder (239.4 g); Cholestyramine resin 4 g/9 g of powder (378 g); Cholestyramine resin 4 g/5 g packet (60s); Cholestyramine resin 4 g/5.7 g packet (60s); Cholestyramine resin 4 g/9 g packet (60s)

Prevalite®: Cholestyramine resin 4 g/5.5 g of powder (231 g); Cholestyramine resin 4 g/5.5 g packet (42s, 60s)

Questran®: Cholestyramine resin 4 g/9 g of powder (378 g); Cholestyramine resin 4 g/9 g packet (60s)

Questran® Light: Cholestyramine resin 4 g/5 g of powder (210 g); Cholestyramine resin 4 g/5 g packet (60s)

General Dosage Range Oral: *Adults:* 4-24 g/day in 1-6 divided doses

Administration

Oral Mix powder with 60-180 mL water or other noncarbonated liquid prior to administration and mix well; may also be taken with highly fluid soups, applesauce or crushed pineapple; not to be taken in dry form. Suspension should not be sipped or held in mouth for prolonged periods (may cause tooth discoloration or enamel decay). Administration at mealtime is recommended. Twice-daily dosing is recommended, but may be administered in 1-6 doses/day.

Nursing Actions

Physical Assessment Monitor GI effects and nutritional status periodically throughout therapy.

Patient Education Take once or twice a day as directed. Do not take the powder in its dry form; mix with fluid. Cholestyramine may lower absorption of many medications; check proper administration times. Ongoing medical follow-up and laboratory tests may be required. You may experience GI effects (these should resolve after continued use), nausea and vomiting, or constipation. Report unusual stomach cramping, pain or blood in stool, or unresolved nausea, vomiting, or constipation.

Choline Magnesium Trisalicylate

(KOE leen mag NEE zhum trye sa LIS i late)

Index Terms Tricosal; Trilisate

Pharmacologic Category Salicylate

Pregnancy Risk Factor C/D (3rd trimester)

Lactation Enters breast milk/use caution

Use Management of osteoarthritis, rheumatoid arthritis, and other arthritis; acute painful shoulder

Available Dosage Forms

Liquid, oral: 500 mg/5 mL (240 mL)

General Dosage Range Oral:

Children <37 kg: 50 mg/kg/day in 2 divided doses

Children ≥37 kg: 2250 mg/day in divided doses

Adults: 500 mg to 1.5 g 2-3 times/day **or** 3 g at bedtime

Elderly: 750 mg 3 times/day

Administration

Oral Liquid may be mixed with fruit juice just before drinking. Do not administer with antacids. Take with a full glass of water and remain in an upright position for 15-30 minutes after administration.

Nursing Actions

Physical Assessment Do not use for persons with allergic reaction to salicylates or other NSAIDs. Monitor for effectiveness of pain relief.

Patient Education Take with food or milk. While using this medication, do not use alcohol. You may experience nausea, vomiting, or gastric discomfort; GI bleeding, ulceration, or perforation can occur with or without pain. Report ringing in ears, persistent stomach pain, unresolved nausea or vomiting, respiratory difficulty or shortness of breath, unusual bruising or bleeding (mouth, urine, stool), or skin rash.

Chorionic Gonadotropin (Human)

(kor ee ON ik goe NAD oh troe pin HYU man)

Brand Names: U.S. Novarel®; Pregnyl®

Index Terms CG; hCG

Pharmacologic Category Gonadotropin; Ovulation Stimulator

Pregnancy Risk Factor X

Lactation Excretion in breast milk unknown/use caution

Use Induces ovulation and pregnancy in anovulatory, infertile females; treatment of hypogonadotropic hypogonadism, prepubertal cryptorchidism; spermatogenesis induction with follitropin alfa

Available Dosage Forms

Injection, powder for reconstitution: 10,000 units

Novarel®: 10,000 units

Pregnyl®: 10,000 units

General Dosage Range I.M.:

Children: Dosage varies greatly depending on indication

Adults (females): 5000-10,000 units 1 day following last dose of menotropins

Adults (males): 1000-2000 units 2-3 times/week

Administration

I.M. I.M. administration only

Nursing Actions

Physical Assessment If self-administered, teach patient appropriate injection technique and syringe/needle disposal.

Patient Education This medication can only be administered by injection. If self-administered, follow instruction for reconstitution, injection, and needle disposal. May cause headache, depression, irritability, or restlessness. Contact prescriber if symptoms are severe or do not resolve with use. Contact prescriber if breasts swell; if you experience swelling of legs or feet; or if there is pain, redness, or swelling at injection site.

Chorionic Gonadotropin (Recombinant)

(kor ee ON ik goe NAD oh troe pin ree KOM be nant)

Brand Names: U.S. Ovidrel®

Index Terms Choriogonadotropin Alfa; r-hCG

Pharmacologic Category Gonadotropin; Ovulation Stimulator

Pregnancy Risk Factor X

Lactation Excretion in breast milk unknown/use caution

Use As part of an assisted reproductive technology (ART) program, induces ovulation in infertile females who have been pretreated with follicle stimulating hormones (FSH); induces ovulation and pregnancy in infertile females when the cause of infertility is functional

Mechanism of Action/Effect Luteinizing hormone analogue produced by recombinant DNA techniques; stimulates late follicular maturation and intitates rupture of the ovarian follicle once follicular development has occurred

Contraindications Hypersensitivity to hCG preparations or any component of the formulation; primary ovarian failure; uncontrolled thyroid or adrenal dysfunction; uncontrolled organic intracranial lesion (ie, pituitary tumor); abnormal uterine bleeding, ovarian cyst or enlargement of undetermined origin; sex hormone dependent tumors; pregnancy

Warnings/Precautions Ovarian enlargement may occur; may be accompanied by abdominal distention or abdominal pain and generally regresses without treatment within 2-3 weeks. If ovaries are abnormally enlarged on the last day of treatment, withhold hCG to reduce the risk of ovarian hyperstimulation syndrome (OHSS). OHSS is characterized by severe ovarian enlargement, abdominal pain/distention, nausea, vomiting, diarrhea, dyspnea, and oliguria, and may be accompanied by ascites, pleural effusion, hypovolemia, electrolyte imbalance, hemoperitoneum, and thromboembolic events. If severe hyperstimulation occurs, stop treatment and hospitalize patient. This syndrome develops rapidly with 24 hours to several days and generally occurs during the 7-10 days immediately following treatment.

Arterial thromboembolic events have been reported in association with and separate from OHSS. These medications should only be used by healthcare providers who are thoroughly familiar with infertility problems and their management. Multiple births may result from the use of these medications; advise patients of the potential risk of multiple births before starting the treatment. Safety and efficacy have not been established in the elderly or in children.

Drug Interactions

Avoid Concomitant Use There are no known interactions where it is recommended to avoid concomitant use.

Decreased Effect There are no known significant interactions involving a decrease in effect.

Increased Effect/Toxicity There are no known significant interactions involving an increase in effect.

Adverse Reactions

2% to 10%:

Endocrine & metabolic: Ovarian cyst (3%), ovarian hyperstimulation (<2% to 3%)

Gastrointestinal: Abdominal pain (3% to 4%), nausea (3%), vomiting (3%)

Local: Injection site: Pain (8%), bruising (3% to 5%), reaction (<2% to 3%), inflammation (<2% to 2%)

Miscellaneous: Postoperative pain (5%)

<2%:

Cardiovascular: Cardiac arrhythmia, heart murmur

Central nervous system: Dizziness, emotional lability, fever, headache, insomnia, malaise

Dermatologic: Pruritus, rash

Endocrine & metabolic: Breast pain, hot flashes, hyperglycemia, intermenstrual bleeding, vaginal hemorrhage

Gastrointestinal: Abdominal enlargement, diarrhea, flatulence

Genitourinary: Cervical carcinoma, cervical lesion, dysuria, genital herpes, genital moniliasis, leukorrhea, urinary incontinence, urinary tract infection, vaginal discomfort, vaginal hemorrhage, vaginitis

Hematologic: Leukocytosis

Neuromuscular & skeletal: Back pain, paresthesia

Renal: Albuminuria

Respiratory: Cough, pharyngitis, upper respiratory tract infection

Miscellaneous: Ectopic pregnancy, hiccups

In addition, the following have been reported with menotropin therapy: Adnexal torsion, hemoperitoneum, mild-to-moderate ovarian enlargement, pulmonary and vascular complications. Ovarian neoplasms have also been reported (rare) with multiple drug regimens used for ovarian induction (relationship not established).

Available Dosage Forms

Injection, solution:

Ovidrel®: 257.5 mcg/0.515 mL (0.515 mL)

General Dosage Range SubQ: *Adults (females):* 250 mcg given 1 day following last dose of follicle stimulating agent

Administration

Other For SubQ use only; inject into stomach area.

Stability

Storage Prefilled syringe: Prior to dispensing, store at 2°C to 8°C (36°F to 46°F). Patient may store at 25°C (77°F) for up to 30 days. Protect from light.

Nursing Actions

Physical Assessment For use only under the supervision/direction of an infertility prescriber. If self-administered, teach patient proper storage, reconstitution, injection technique, and needle/syringe disposal.

Patient Education Note that there is a risk of multiple births associated with treatment. This drug must be administered exactly as scheduled (1 day following last dose of follicle stimulating agent); maintain a calendar of treatment days. Keep all ultrasound and laboratory appointments as instructed by prescriber. Avoid strenuous exercise, especially those with pelvic involvement. You may experience nausea, vomiting, GI upset, or hot flashes; if persistent consult prescriber. Report immediately any persistent abdominal pain, vomiting, or acute pelvic pain; chest pain or palpitations; or shortness of breath.

Ciclesonide (Oral Inhalation)

(sye KLES oh nide)

Brand Names: U.S. Alvesco®

Pharmacologic Category Corticosteroid, Inhalant (Oral)

Pregnancy Risk Factor C

Lactation Excretion in breast milk unknown/use caution

Breast-Feeding Considerations Systemic corticosteroids are excreted in human milk. It is not known if sufficient quantities of ciclesonide are absorbed following oral inhalation to produce detectable amounts in breast milk; however, oral absorption is limited (<1%). The use of inhaled corticosteroids is not considered a contraindication to breast-feeding (NAEPP, 2005).

Use Prophylactic management of bronchial asthma

Mechanism of Action/Effect Ciclesonide is a nonhalogenated, glucocorticoid prodrug that is hydrolyzed to the pharmacologically active metabolite des-ciclesonide following administration. Des-ciclesonide has a high affinity for the glucocorticoid receptor and exhibits anti-inflammatory activity. The mechanism of action for corticosteroids is believed to be a combination of three important properties − anti-inflammatory activity, immunosuppressive properties, and antiproliferative actions.

Contraindications Hypersensitivity to ciclesonide or any component of the formulation; primary treatment of acute asthma or status asthmaticus; moderate-to-severe bronchiectasis

Canadian labeling: Additional contraindications (not in U.S. labeling): Untreated fungal, bacterial, or tuberculosis infections of the respiratory tract; moderate-to-severe bronchiectasis

Warnings/Precautions May cause hypercorticism or suppression of hypothalamic-pituitary-adrenal (HPA) axis, particularly in younger children or in patients receiving high doses for prolonged periods. HPA axis suppression may lead to adrenal crisis. Withdrawal and discontinuation of a corticosteroid should be done slowly and carefully. Particular care is required when patients are transferred from systemic corticosteroids to inhaled products due to possible adrenal insufficiency or withdrawal from steroids, including an increase in allergic symptoms. Patients receiving >20 mg per day of prednisone (or equivalent) may be most susceptible. Fatalities have occurred due to adrenal insufficiency in asthmatic patients during and after transfer from systemic corticosteroids to aerosol steroids; aerosol steroids do **not** provide the systemic steroid needed to treat patients having trauma, surgery, or infections.

Bronchospasm may occur with wheezing after inhalation; if this occurs stop steroid and treat with a fast-acting bronchodilator. Supplemental steroids (oral or parenteral) may be needed during stress or severe asthma attacks. Not to be used in status asthmaticus or for the relief of acute bronchospasm. Oropharyngeal thrush due to candida albicans infection may occur with use. Prolonged use of corticosteroids may also increase the incidence of secondary infection, mask acute infection (including fungal infections), prolong or exacerbate viral infections, or limit response to vaccines. Exposure to chickenpox and measles should be avoided; corticosteroids should not be used to treat ocular herpes simplex. Close observation is required in patients with latent tuberculosis and/or TB reactivity; restrict use in active TB (only in conjunction with antituberculosis treatment). Use in patients with TB is contraindicated in the Canadian labeling. Prolonged treatment with corticosteroids has been associated with the development of Kaposi's sarcoma (case reports); if noted, discontinuation of therapy should be considered.

Use with caution in patients with thyroid disease, severe hepatic impairment, glaucoma, cataracts, patients at risk for osteoporosis, and patients at risk for seizures.

Orally inhaled corticosteroids may cause a reduction in growth velocity in pediatric patients (~1 cm per year [range: 0.3-1.8 cm per year] and related to dose and duration of exposure). To minimize the systemic effects of orally inhaled corticosteroids, each patient should be titrated to the lowest effective dose. Growth should be routinely monitored in pediatric patients.

Drug Interactions

Avoid Concomitant Use

Avoid concomitant use of Ciclesonide (Oral Inhalation) with any of the following: Aldesleukin

Decreased Effect

Ciclesonide (Oral Inhalation) may decrease the levels/effects of: Aldesleukin; Corticorelin; Telaprevir

The levels/effects of Ciclesonide (Oral Inhalation) may be decreased by: Tocilizumab

Increased Effect/Toxicity

Ciclesonide (Oral Inhalation) may increase the levels/effects of: Deferasirox

The levels/effects of Ciclesonide (Oral Inhalation) may be increased by: CYP3A4 Inhibitors (Moderate); Dasatinib; Ivacaftor; Telaprevir

Adverse Reactions

>10%:

Central nervous system: Headache (≤11%)

Respiratory: Nasopharyngitis (≤11%)

1% to 10%:

Cardiovascular: Facial edema (≥3%)

Central nervous system: Dizziness (≥3%), fatigue (≥3%), dysphonia (1%)

Dermatologic: Urticaria (≥3%)

Gastrointestinal: Gastroenteritis (≥3%), oral candidiasis (≥3%)

Neuromuscular & skeletal: Arthralgia (≤4%), musculoskeletal chest pain (≥3%), back pain (≥3%), extremity pain (≥3%)

Ocular: Conjunctivitis (≥3%)

Otic: Ear pain (2%)

Respiratory: Upper respiratory infection (≤9%), epistaxis (≤8%), nasal congestion (≤6%), sinusitis (≤6%), pharyngolaryngeal pain (≤ 5%), hoarseness (≥3%), pneumonia (≥3%), paradoxical bronchospasm (2%)

Miscellaneous: Influenza (≥3%)

Available Dosage Forms

Aerosol, for oral inhalation:

Alvesco®: 80 mcg/inhalation (6.1 g); 160 mcg/inhalation (6.1 g)

General Dosage Range Oral inhalation: *Children ≥12 years and Adults:* 100-800 mcg/day (1-2 puffs once or twice daily) (maximum: 640 mcg/day)

Administration

Inhalation Remove mouthpiece cover, place inhaler in mouth, close lips around mouthpiece, and inhale slowly and deeply. Press down on top of inhaler after slow inhalation has begun. Remove inhaler while holding breath for approximately 10 seconds. Breathe out slowly and replace mouthpiece on inhaler. Do not wash or place inhaler in water. Clean mouthpiece using a dry cloth or tissue once weekly. Discard after the "discard by" date or after labeled number of doses has been used, even if container is not completely empty.

Shaking is not necessary since drug is formulated as a solution aerosol. Prime inhaler prior to initial use or if not in use for ≥1 week by releasing 3 puffs into the air.

Stability

Storage Store at 15°C to 30°C (59°F to 86°F); do not freeze.

Nursing Actions

Physical Assessment Growth should be monitored periodically with long-term use in children. Do not discontinue abruptly after long-term use.

Patient Education Not intended for treatment of acute asthma attacks. You may be susceptible to infections. Avoid exposure to chickenpox or measles. Report persistent headache, nosebleeds, fungal infection in the mouth, bad taste, sore throat or tongue, worsening of condition, or lack of improvement.

Ciclesonide (Nasal) (sye KLES oh nide)

Brand Names: U.S. Omnaris™

Index Terms Zetonna

Pharmacologic Category Corticosteroid, Nasal

Pregnancy Risk Factor C

Lactation Excretion in breast milk unknown/use caution

Use Management of seasonal and perennial allergic rhinitis

Product Availability Zetonna™ nasal aerosol: FDA approved January 2012; availability is currently undetermined. Consult prescribing information for additional information.

Available Dosage Forms

Suspension, intranasal:

Omnaris™: 50 mcg/inhalation (12.5 g)

General Dosage Range Intranasal: *Children ≥6 years and Adults:* 2 sprays (50 mcg/spray) per nostril once daily (maximum: 200 mcg/day)

Administration

Other Intranasal: Shake bottle gently before using. Prime pump prior to first use (press 8 times until fine mist appears) or if spray has not been used in 4 consecutive days (press 1 time or until a fine mist appears). Blow nose to clear nostrils. Insert applicator into nostril, keeping bottle upright, and close off the other nostril. Breathe in through nose. While inhaling, press pump to release spray. Avoid spraying directly onto the nasal septum. Nasal applicator may be removed and rinsed with warm water to clean. Discard after the "discard by" date or after labeled number of doses has been used, even if bottle is not completely empty.

Cidofovir (si DOF o veer)

Brand Names: U.S. Vistide®

Pharmacologic Category Antiviral Agent

Pregnancy Risk Factor C

Lactation Excretion in breast milk unknown/contraindicated

Breast-Feeding Considerations The CDC recommends **not** to breast-feed if diagnosed with HIV to avoid postnatal transmission of the virus.

Use Treatment of cytomegalovirus (CMV) retinitis in patients with acquired immunodeficiency syndrome (AIDS). **Note:** Should be administered with probenecid.

Mechanism of Action/Effect Nucleotide analog that selectively inhibits viral DNA polymerase, suppressing viral DNA synthesis

Contraindications Hypersensitivity to cidofovir; history of clinically-severe hypersensitivity to probenecid or other sulfa-containing medications; serum creatinine >1.5 mg/dL; Cl_{cr} <55 mL/minute; urine protein ≥100 mg/dL (≥2+ proteinuria); use with or within 7 days of nephrotoxic agents; direct intraocular injection

Warnings/Precautions Hazardous agent - use appropriate precautions for handling and disposal. **[U.S. Boxed Warning]: Dose-dependent nephrotoxicity requires dose adjustment or discontinuation if changes in renal function occur during therapy (eg, proteinuria, glycosuria, decreased serum phosphate, uric acid or bicarbonate, and elevated creatinine). Neutropenia has been reported;** monitor counts during therapy. Cases of ocular hypotony have also occurred; monitor intraocular pressure. Monitor for signs of metabolic acidosis. Safety and efficacy have not been established in children or the elderly. Administration must be accompanied by oral probenecid and intravenous saline prehydration. **[U.S. Boxed Warning]: Indicated only for CMV retinitis treatment in HIV patients; possibly carcinogenic and teratogenic based on animal data. May cause hypospermia.**

Drug Interactions

Avoid Concomitant Use There are no known interactions where it is recommended to avoid concomitant use.

Decreased Effect There are no known significant interactions involving a decrease in effect.

Increased Effect/Toxicity There are no known significant interactions involving an increase in effect.

Adverse Reactions

>10%:

Central nervous system: Chills, fever, headache, pain

Dermatologic: Alopecia, rash

Gastrointestinal: Nausea, vomiting, diarrhea, anorexia

Hematologic: Anemia, neutropenia

Neuromuscular & skeletal: Weakness

Ocular: Intraocular pressure decreased, iritis, ocular hypotony, uveitis

Renal: Creatinine increased, proteinuria, renal toxicity

Respiratory: Cough, dyspnea

Miscellaneous: Infection, oral moniliasis, serum bicarbonate decreased

1% to 10%:

Renal: Fanconi syndrome

Respiratory: Pneumonia

Frequency not defined (limited to important or life-threatening reactions):

Cardiovascular: Cardiomyopathy, cardiovascular disorder, CHF, edema, postural hypotension, shock, syncope, tachycardia

Central nervous system: Agitation, amnesia, anxiety, confusion, convulsion, dizziness, hallucinations, insomnia, malaise, vertigo

Dermatologic: Photosensitivity reaction, skin discoloration, urticaria

Endocrine & metabolic: Adrenal cortex insufficiency

Gastrointestinal: Abdominal pain, aphthous stomatitis, colitis, constipation, dysphagia, fecal incontinence, gastritis, GI hemorrhage, gingivitis, melena, proctitis, splenomegaly, stomatitis, tongue discoloration

Genitourinary: Urinary incontinence

Hematologic: Hypochromic anemia, leukocytosis, leukopenia, lymphadenopathy, lymphoma-like reaction, pancytopenia, thrombocytopenia, thrombocytopenic purpura

Hepatic: Hepatomegaly, hepatosplenomegaly, jaundice, liver function tests abnormal, liver damage, liver necrosis

Local: Injection site reaction

Neuromuscular & skeletal: Tremor

Ocular: Amblyopia, blindness, cataract, conjunctivitis, corneal lesion, diplopia, vision abnormal

Otic: Hearing loss

Miscellaneous: Allergic reaction, sepsis

Available Dosage Forms

Injection, solution [preservative free]:

Vistide®: 75 mg/mL (5 mL)

General Dosage Range Dosage adjustment recommended in patients with renal impairment

I.V.: *Adults:* Induction: 5 mg/kg once weekly for 2 consecutive weeks; Maintenance: 5 mg/kg once every 2 weeks

Administration

I.V. For I.V. infusion only. Infuse over 1 hour. Hydrate with 1 L of 0.9% NS I.V. prior to cidofovir infusion. A second liter may be administered over a 1- to 3-hour period immediately following infusion, if tolerated.

I.V. Detail pH: 6.7-7.6

Stability

Reconstitution Dilute dose in NS 100 mL prior to infusion.

Storage Store at controlled room temperature 20°C to 25°C (68°F to 77°F). Store admixtures under refrigeration for ≤24 hours. Cidofovir infusion admixture should be administered within 24 hours of preparation at room temperature or refrigerated. Admixtures should be allowed to equilibrate to room temperature prior to use.

Nursing Actions

Physical Assessment Administration must be accompanied by oral probenecid and intravenous saline prehydration. Pretreatment with probenecid and both pre- and post-treatment hydration may be ordered. Monitor infusion site closely to avoid extravasation. Monitor for CNS changes, anemia, renal status, and visual acuity. Instruct patient to report any changes in vision or eye pain.

Patient Education This drug can only be administered I.V. Report immediately any pain, stinging, or swelling at infusion site. You may be more susceptible to infection. May cause hair loss (reversible), headache, anxiety, confusion, diarrhea, nausea, heartburn, vomiting, constipation, or postural hypotension. Report severe unresolved vomiting, constipation, or diarrhea; chills, fever, signs of infection; respiratory difficulty or unusual coughing; palpitations, chest pain, or syncope; CNS changes (eg, hallucinations, depression, excessive sedation, amnesia, seizures, insomnia); or vision changes.

Cilostazol (sil OH sta zol)

Brand Names: U.S. Pletal®

Index Terms OPC-13013

Pharmacologic Category Antiplatelet Agent; Phosphodiesterase Enzyme Inhibitor

Medication Safety Issues

Sound-alike/look-alike issues:

Pletal® may be confused with Plendil®

Pregnancy Risk Factor C

Lactation Excretion in breast milk unknown/not recommended

Breast-Feeding Considerations It is not known whether cilostazol is excreted in human milk. Because of the potential risk to nursing infants, a decision to discontinue the drug or discontinue nursing should be made.

Use Symptomatic management of peripheral vascular disease, primarily intermittent claudication

Unlabeled Use Adjunct with aspirin and clopidogrel for prevention of stent thrombosis and restenosis after coronary stent placement

Mechanism of Action/Effect Cilostazol and its metabolites are inhibitors of phosphodiesterase III. As a result, cyclic AMP is increased leading to reversible inhibition of platelet aggregation, vasodilation, and inhibition of vascular smooth muscle cell proliferation.

Contraindications Hypersensitivity to cilostazol or any component of the formulation; heart failure (HF) of any severity; hemostatic disorders or active bleeding

Warnings/Precautions [U.S. Boxed Warning]: The use of this drug is contraindicated in patients with heart failure. Use with caution in severe underlying heart disease. Use with caution in patients receiving other platelet aggregation inhibitors or in patients with thrombocytopenia. Discontinue therapy if thrombocytopenia or leukopenia occur; progression to agranulocytosis (reversible) has been reported when cilostazol was not immediately stopped. When cilostazol and clopidogrel are used concurrently, manufacturer recommends checking bleeding times. Withhold for at least 4-6 half-lives prior to elective surgical procedures. Use with caution in patients receiving CYP3A4 inhibitors (eg, ketoconazole or erythromycin) or CYP2C19 inhibitors (eg, omeprazole). If concurrent use is warranted, consider dosage adjustment of cilostazol. Use caution in moderate-to-severe hepatic impairment. Use cautiously in severe renal impairment (Cl_{cr} <25 mL/minute).

Drug Interactions

Avoid Concomitant Use

Avoid concomitant use of Cilostazol with any of the following: Conivaptan

Decreased Effect

The levels/effects of Cilostazol may be decreased by: CYP3A4 Inducers (Strong); Cyproterone; Deferasirox; Herbs (CYP3A4 Inducers); Nonsteroidal Anti-Inflammatory Agents; Peginterferon Alfa-2b; Tocilizumab

Increased Effect/Toxicity

Cilostazol may increase the levels/effects of: Anticoagulants; Antiplatelet Agents; Collagenase (Systemic); Drotrecogin Alfa (Activated); Ibritumomab; Rivaroxaban; Salicylates; Thrombolytic Agents; Tositumomab and Iodine I 131 Tositumomab

The levels/effects of Cilostazol may be increased by: Antifungal Agents (Azole Derivatives, Systemic); Conivaptan; CYP2C19 Inhibitors (Moderate); CYP2C19 Inhibitors (Strong); CYP3A4 Inhibitors (Moderate); CYP3A4 Inhibitors (Strong); Dasatinib; Esomeprazole; Glucosamine; Herbs (Anticoagulant/Antiplatelet Properties); Ivacaftor; Macrolide Antibiotics; Nonsteroidal Anti-Inflammatory Agents; Omega-3-Acid Ethyl Esters; Omeprazole; Pentosan Polysulfate Sodium; Pentoxifylline; Prostacyclin Analogues; Vitamin E

Nutritional/Ethanol Interactions

Food: Taking cilostazol with a high-fat meal may increase peak concentration by 90%. Grapefruit juice may increase serum levels of cilostazol and enhance toxic effects. Management: Administer cilostazol on an empty stomach 30 minutes before or 2 hours after meals. Avoid concurrent ingestion of grapefruit juice.

Herb/Nutraceutical: St John's wort may decrease the levels/effects of cilostazol. Other herbs/nutraceuticals have additional antiplatelet activity. Management: Avoid alfalfa, anise, bilberry, bladderwrack, bromelain, cat's claw, chamomile, coleus, cordyceps, dong quai, evening primrose oil, fenugreek, feverfew, garlic, ginger, ginkgo biloba, ginseng (American), ginseng (Panax), ginseng (Siberian), grapeseed, green tea, guggul, horse chestnut seed, horseradish, licorice, prickly ash, red clover, reishi, SAMe (S-adenosylmethionine), St John's wort, sweet clover, turmeric, and white willow.

Adverse Reactions

>10%:

Central nervous system: Headache (27% to 34%)

Gastrointestinal: Abnormal stools (12% to 15%), diarrhea (12% to 19%)

Respiratory: Rhinitis (7% to 12%)

Miscellaneous: Infection (10% to 14%)

2% to 10%:

Cardiovascular: Peripheral edema (7% to 9%), palpitation (5% to 10%), tachycardia (4%)

Central nervous system: Dizziness (9% to 10%), vertigo (up to 3%)

Gastrointestinal: Dyspepsia (6%), nausea (6% to 7%), abdominal pain (4% to 5%), flatulence (2% to 3%)

Neuromuscular & skeletal: Back pain (6% to 7%), myalgia (2% to 3%)

Respiratory: Pharyngitis (7% to 10%), cough (3% to 4%)

Pharmacodynamics/Kinetics

Onset of Action 2-4 weeks; may require up to 12 weeks

Available Dosage Forms

Tablet, oral: 50 mg, 100 mg

Pletal®: 50 mg, 100 mg

General Dosage Range Dosage adjustment recommended in patients on concomitant therapy

Oral: *Adults:* 100 mg twice daily

Administration

Oral Administer cilostazol 30 minutes before or 2 hours after meals.

Stability

Storage Store at 25°C (77°F); excursions permitted to 15°C to 30°C (59°F to 86°F).

Nursing Actions

Patient Education Take on empty stomach (30 minutes before or 2 hours after meals). Inform prescribers and dentists that you are taking this medication prior to scheduling any surgery or dental procedure. You may experience nervousness, dizziness, fatigue, nausea, vomiting, flatulence, or postural hypotension. Report chest pain, palpitations, unusual heartbeat, swelling of extremities, unusual bleeding, unresolved GI upset or pain, dizziness, nervousness, sleeplessness, fatigue, muscle cramping or tremor, or unusual cough.

Dietary Considerations It is best to take cilostazol 30 minutes before or 2 hours after meals.

Cimetidine (sye MET i deen)

Brand Names: U.S. Tagamet HB 200® [OTC]

Pharmacologic Category Histamine H_2 Antagonist

Medication Safety Issues

Sound-alike/look-alike issues:

Cimetidine may be confused with simethicone

BEERS Criteria medication:

This drug may be inappropriate for use in geriatric patients (low severity risk).

Pregnancy Risk Factor B

Lactation Enters breast milk/not recommended (AAP rates "compatible"; AAP 2001 update pending)

Use Short-term treatment of active duodenal ulcers and benign gastric ulcers; maintenance therapy of duodenal ulcer; treatment of gastric hypersecretory states; treatment of gastroesophageal reflux disease (GERD)

OTC labeling: Prevention or relief of heartburn, acid indigestion, or sour stomach

Unlabeled Use Part of a multidrug regimen for *H. pylori* eradication to reduce the risk of duodenal ulcer recurrence

Available Dosage Forms

Solution, oral: 300 mg/5 mL (237 mL, 240 mL, 250 mL, 473 mL, 480 mL)

Tablet, oral: 200 mg, 300 mg, 400 mg, 800 mg

Tagamet HB 200® [OTC]: 200 mg

General Dosage Range Dosage adjustment recommended in patients with renal impaiment

Oral:

Children <12 years: 20-40 mg/kg/day divided every 6 hours

Children ≥12 years: 20-40 mg/kg/day divided every 6 hours **or** 200 mg 1-2 times/day [OTC]

Adults: 300-600 mg 4 times/day **or** 400-800 mg 1-2 times/day **or** 200 mg 1-2 times/day [OTC]

Administration

Oral Administer with meals so that the drug's peak effect occurs at the proper time (peak inhibition of gastric acid secretion occurs at 1 and 3 hours after dosing in fasting subjects and approximately 2 hours in nonfasting subjects. This correlates well with the time food is no longer in the stomach offering a buffering effect). Stagger doses of antacids with cimetidine.

Nursing Actions

Physical Assessment Monitor for CNS changes, agitation, and gastric bleeding regularly during therapy.

Patient Education Take with meals. Avoid excess alcohol. May cause headache, dizziness, agitation, nausea, vomiting, or diarrhea. Report chest pain or palpitations; CNS changes (confusion, agitation); persistent diarrhea, nausea, vomiting, or heartburn; black tarry stools or coffee ground-like emesis; rash; unusual bleeding or bruising; sore throat; or fever; or unexplained weight loss.

Cinacalcet (sin a KAL cet)

Brand Names: U.S. Sensipar®

Index Terms AMG 073; Cinacalcet Hydrochloride

Pharmacologic Category Calcimimetic

Pregnancy Risk Factor C

Lactation Excretion in breast milk unknown/not recommended

Use Treatment of secondary hyperparathyroidism in patients with chronic kidney disease (CKD) on dialysis; treatment of hypercalcemia in patients with parathyroid carcinoma; treatment of severe hypercalcemia in patients with primary hyperparathyroidism who are unable to undergo parathyroidectomy

Available Dosage Forms

Tablet, oral:

Sensipar®: 30 mg, 60 mg, 90 mg

General Dosage Range Dosage adjustment recommended in patients on concomitant therapy or who develop toxicities

Oral: *Adults:* Initial: 30 mg once or twice daily; Maintenance: Increase dose incrementally every 2-4 weeks to normalize calcium levels or maintain iPTH level (maximum: 360 mg/day [parathyroid cancer, primary hyperparathyroidism]; 180 mg/day [secondary hyperparathyroidism])

Administration

Oral Administer with food or shortly after a meal. Do not break or divide tablet; should be taken whole.

Nursing Actions

Physical Assessment Monitor for hypocalcemia (paresthesias, myalgia, cramping, tetany, seizures) at beginning of therapy and regularly thereafter.

Patient Education Take with food; do not break, chew, or crush tablet (swallow whole). You may experience dizziness, nausea, vomiting, loss of appetite, or diarrhea. Report any muscle cramping, twitches, tremors, or spasms; chest pain or palpitations; or unresolved gastrointestinal disturbance.

Ciprofloxacin (Systemic)

(sip roe FLOKS a sin)

Brand Names: U.S. Cipro®; Cipro® I.V.; Cipro® XR

Index Terms Ciprofloxacin Hydrochloride

Pharmacologic Category Antibiotic, Quinolone

Medication Safety Issues

Sound-alike/look-alike issues:

Ciprofloxacin may be confused with cephalexin

Cipro® may be confused with Ceftin®

Medication Guide Available Yes

Pregnancy Risk Factor C

Lactation Enters breast milk/not recommended (AAP rates "compatible"; AAP 2001 update pending)

Breast-Feeding Considerations Ciprofloxacin is excreted in breast milk. Breast-feeding is not recommended by the manufacturer. Due to the low concentrations in human milk, minimal toxicity would be expected in the nursing infant and infant serum levels were undetectable in one report. Nondose-related effects could include modification of bowel flora. There has been a single case report of perforated pseudomembranous colitis in a breast-feeding infant whose mother was taking ciprofloxacin.

Use

Children: Complicated urinary tract infections and pyelonephritis due to *E. coli*. **Note:** Although effective, ciprofloxacin is not the drug of first choice in children.

Children and Adults: To reduce incidence or progression of disease following exposure to aerolized *Bacillus anthracis*.

Adults: Treatment of the following infections when caused by susceptible bacteria: Urinary tract infections; acute uncomplicated cystitis in females; chronic bacterial prostatitis; lower respiratory tract infections (including acute exacerbations of chronic bronchitis); acute sinusitis; skin and skin structure infections; bone and joint infections; complicated intra-abdominal infections (in combination with metronidazole); infectious diarrhea; typhoid fever due to *Salmonella typhi* (eradication of chronic typhoid carrier state has not been proven); uncomplicated cervical and urethra gonorrhea (due to *N. gonorrhoeae*); nosocomial pneumonia; empirical therapy for febrile neutropenic patients (in combination with piperacillin)

Note: As of April 2007, the CDC no longer recommends the use of fluoroquinolones for the treatment of gonococcal disease.

Unlabeled Use Acute pulmonary exacerbations in cystic fibrosis (children); cutaneous/gastrointestinal/oropharyngeal anthrax (treatment, children and adults); disseminated gonococcal infection (adults); chancroid (adults); prophylaxis to *Neisseria meningitidis* following close contact with an infected person; empirical therapy (oral) for febrile neutropenia in low-risk cancer patients; HACEK group endocarditis; infectious diarrhea (children); periodontitis

Mechanism of Action/Effect Inhibits DNA-gyrase in susceptible organisms; inhibits relaxation of supercoiled DNA and promotes breakage of double-stranded DNA

Contraindications Hypersensitivity to ciprofloxacin, any component of the formulation, or other quinolones; concurrent administration of tizanidine

Warnings/Precautions [U.S. Boxed Warning]: There have been reports of tendon inflammation and/or rupture with quinolone antibiotics; risk may be increased with concurrent corticosteroids, organ transplant recipients, and in patients >60 years of age. Rupture of the Achilles tendon sometimes requiring surgical repair has been reported most frequently; but other tendon sites (eg, rotator cuff, biceps) have also been reported. Strenuous physical activity, rheumatoid arthritis, and renal impairment may be an independent risk factor for tendonitis. Discontinue at first sign of tendon inflammation or pain. May occur even after discontinuation of therapy. Use with caution in patients with rheumatoid arthritis; may increase risk of tendon rupture. CNS effects may occur (tremor, restlessness, confusion, and very rarely hallucinations, increased intracranial pressure [including pseudotumor cerebri] or seizures). Use with caution in patients with known or suspected CNS disorder. Potential for seizures, although very rare, may be increased with concomitant NSAID therapy. Use with caution in individuals at risk of seizures. Fluoroquinolones may prolong QT_c interval; avoid use in patients with a history of QT_c prolongation, uncorrected hypokalemia, hypomagnesemia, or concurrent administration of other medications known to prolong the QT interval (including Class Ia and Class III antiarrhythmics, cisapride, erythromycin, antipsychotics, and tricyclic antidepressants). Prolonged use may result in fungal or bacterial superinfection, including *C. difficile*-associated diarrhea (CDAD) and pseudomembranous colitis; CDAD has been observed >2 months postantibiotic treatment. Rarely crystalluria has occurred; urine alkalinity may increase the risk. Ensure adequate hydration during therapy. Adverse effects, including those related to joints and/or surrounding tissues, are increased in pediatric patients and therefore, ciprofloxacin should not be considered as drug of choice in children (exception is anthrax treatment). Rare cases of peripheral neuropathy may occur.

Fluoroquinolones have been associated with the development of serious, and sometimes fatal, hypoglycemia, most often in elderly diabetics but also in patients without diabetes. This occurred most frequently with gatifloxacin (no longer available systemically), but may occur at a lower frequency with other quinolones.

Severe hypersensitivity reactions, including anaphylaxis, have occurred with quinolone therapy. Reactions may present as typical allergic symptoms after a single dose, or may manifest as severe idiosyncratic dermatologic, vascular, pulmonary, renal, hepatic, and/or hematologic events, usually after multiple doses. Prompt discontinuation of drug should occur if skin rash or other symptoms arise. **[U.S. Boxed Warning]: Quinolones may exacerbate myasthenia gravis; avoid use (rare, potentially life-threatening weakness of respiratory muscles may occur).** Use caution in renal impairment. Avoid excessive sunlight and take precautions to limit exposure (eg, loose fitting clothing, sunscreen); may cause moderate-to-severe phototoxicity reactions. Discontinue use if photosensitivity occurs. Since ciprofloxacin is ineffective in the treatment of syphilis and may mask symptoms, all patients should be tested for syphilis at the time of gonorrheal diagnosis and 3 months later. Hemolytic reactions may (rarely) occur with quinolone use in patients with latent or actual G6PD deficiency.

Ciprofloxacin is a potent inhibitor of CYP1A2. Coadministration of drugs which depend on this pathway may lead to substantial increases in serum concentrations and adverse effects.

Drug Interactions

Avoid Concomitant Use

Avoid concomitant use of Ciprofloxacin (Systemic) with any of the following: BCG; TiZANidine

Decreased Effect

Ciprofloxacin (Systemic) may decrease the levels/effects of: BCG; Fosphenytoin; Mycophenolate; Phenytoin; Sulfonylureas; Typhoid Vaccine

The levels/effects of Ciprofloxacin (Systemic) may be decreased by: Antacids; Calcium Salts; Didanosine; Iron Salts; Lanthanum; Magnesium

Salts; P-glycoprotein/ABCB1 Inducers; Quinapril; Sevelamer; Sucralfate; Zinc Salts

Increased Effect/Toxicity

Ciprofloxacin (Systemic) may increase the levels/effects of: ARIPiprazole; Bendamustine; Caffeine; Corticosteroids (Systemic); CYP1A2 Substrates; Erlotinib; Methotrexate; Pentoxifylline; Porfimer; QTc-Prolonging Agents; ROPINIRole; Ropivacaine; Sulfonylureas; Theophylline Derivatives; TiZANidine; Varenicline; Vitamin K Antagonists

The levels/effects of Ciprofloxacin (Systemic) may be increased by: Insulin; Nonsteroidal Anti-Inflammatory Agents; P-glycoprotein/ABCB1 Inhibitors; Probenecid

Nutritional/Ethanol Interactions

Food: Food decreases rate, but not extent, of absorption. Ciprofloxacin serum levels may be decreased if taken with divalent or trivalent cations. Ciprofloxacin may increase serum caffeine levels if taken concurrently. Rarely, crystalluria may occur. Enteral feedings may decrease plasma concentrations of ciprofloxacin probably by >30% inhibition of absorption. Management: May administer with food to minimize GI upset. Avoid or take ciprofloxacin 2 hours before or 6 hours after antacids, dairy products, or calcium-fortified juices alone or in a meal containing >800 mg calcium, oral multivitamins, or mineral supplements containing divalent and/or trivalent cations. Restrict caffeine intake if excessive cardiac or CNS stimulation occurs. Ensure adequate hydration during therapy. Ciprofloxacin should not be administered with enteral feedings. The feeding would need to be discontinued for 1-2 hours prior to and after ciprofloxacin administration. Nasogastric administration produces a greater loss of ciprofloxacin bioavailability than does nasoduodenal administration.

Herb/Nutraceutical: Dong quai and St John's wort may also cause photosensitization. Management: Avoid dong quai and St John's wort.

Adverse Reactions 1% to 10%:

Central nervous system: Neurologic events (children 2%, includes dizziness, insomnia, nervousness, somnolence); fever (children 2%); headache (I.V. administration); restlessness (I.V. administration)

Dermatologic: Rash (children 2%, adults 1%)

Gastrointestinal: Nausea (3%); diarrhea (children 5%, adults 2%); vomiting (children 5%, adults 1%); abdominal pain (children 3%, adults <1%); dyspepsia (children 3%)

Hepatic: ALT increased, AST increased (adults 1%)

Local: Injection site reactions (I.V. administration)

Respiratory: Rhinitis (children 3%)

Available Dosage Forms

Infusion, premixed in D_5W: 200 mg (100 mL); 400 mg (200 mL)

Cipro® I.V.: 200 mg (100 mL); 400 mg (200 mL)

Infusion, premixed in D_5W [preservative free]: 200 mg (100 mL); 400 mg (200 mL)

Injection, solution: 10 mg/mL (20 mL, 40 mL, 120 mL)

Injection, solution [preservative free]: 10 mg/mL (20 mL, 40 mL)

Microcapsules for suspension, oral:

Cipro®: 250 mg/5 mL (100 mL); 500 mg/5 mL (100 mL)

Tablet, oral: 100 mg, 250 mg, 500 mg, 750 mg

Cipro®: 250 mg, 500 mg

Tablet, extended release, oral: 500 mg, 1000 mg

Cipro® XR: 500 mg, 1000 mg

General Dosage Range Dosage adjustment recommended in patients with renal impairment

I.V.:

Children: 20-30 mg/kg/day divided every 12 hours (maximum: 800 mg/day)

Adults: 200-400 mg every 8-12 hours

Oral:

Extended release: *Adults:* 500-1000 mg every 24 hours

Immediate release:

Children: 20-30 mg/kg/day in 2 divided doses (maximum: 1.5 g/day)

Adults: 250-750 mg every 12 hours or 250 mg to 1 g as a single dose

Administration

Oral May administer with food to minimize GI upset; avoid antacid use; maintain proper hydration and urine output. Administer immediate release ciprofloxacin and Cipro® XR at least 2 hours before or 6 hours after antacids or other products containing calcium, iron, or zinc (including dairy products or calcium-fortified juices). Separate oral administration from drugs which may impair absorption (see Drug Interactions).

Oral suspension: Should not be administered through feeding tubes (suspension is oil-based and adheres to the feeding tube). Patients should avoid chewing on the microcapsules.

Nasogastric/orogastric tube: Crush immediate-release tablet and mix with water. Flush feeding tube before and after administration. Hold tube feedings at least 1 hour before and 2 hours after administration.

Tablet, extended release: Do not crush, split, or chew. May be administered with meals containing dairy products (calcium content <800 mg), but not with dairy products alone.

I.V. Administer by slow I.V. infusion over 60 minutes into a large vein.

I.V. Detail Administer slowly to reduce the risk of venous irritation (burning, pain, erythema, and swelling).

pH: 3.3-3.9 (vials); 3.5-4.6 (PVC bags)

Stability

Reconstitution Injection, vial: May be diluted with NS, D_5W, SWFI, $D_{10}W$, $D_5$1/4NS, $D_5$1/2NS, LR.

Storage

Injection:

Premixed infusion: Store between 5°C to 25°C (41°F to 77°F); avoid freezing. Protect from light.

Vial: Store between 5°C to 30°C (41°F to 86°F); avoid freezing. Protect from light. Diluted solutions of 0.5-2 mg/mL are stable for up to 14 days refrigerated or at room temperature.

Microcapsules for oral suspension: Prior to reconstitution, store below 25°C (77°F). Protect from freezing. Following reconstitution, store below 30°C (86°F) for up to 14 days. Protect from freezing.

Tablet:

Immediate release: Store below 30°C (86°F).

Extended release: Store at room temperature of 15°C to 30°C (59°F to 86°F).

Nursing Actions

Physical Assessment Results of culture and sensitivity tests should be assessed prior to beginning therapy. I.V.: See Administration specifics. Monitor for hypersensitivity reactions (severe reactions, including anaphylaxis, have occurred with quinolone therapy), persistent diarrhea (*C. difficile*-associated colitis can occur post-treatment), and changes in CNS.

Patient Education Infusion: Report immediately any redness, swelling, or pain at infusion site; any swelling of mouth, lips, tongue, or throat; chest pain or tightness; respiratory difficulty; back pain; sudden itching; or skin rash. Oral: Take exactly according to specific instructions (eg, timing with meals, dairy products, antacids or products containing calcium, iron or zinc differs with each formulation). Do not crush, split, or chew extended release tablets or chew on microcapsules in oral suspension. Maintain adequate hydration, unless instructed to restrict fluid intake. You may experience nausea, vomiting, anorexia, or increased sensitivity to sunlight. If tendon inflammation or pain occurs or if you experience signs of an allergic reaction (eg, itching, skin rash, respiratory difficulty, facial edema or difficulty swallowing, loss of consciousness, tingling, chest pain, palpitations), discontinue use and contact prescriber immediately. Report persistent GI disturbances, CNS changes (eg, excessive sleepiness, agitation, tremors), vision changes, respiratory difficulty, signs of opportunistic infection (eg, sore throat, chills, fever, burning, itching on urination, vaginal discharge, white plaques in mouth), persistent diarrhea, or worsening of condition.

Dietary Considerations Food: Drug may cause GI upset; take without regard to meals (manufacturer prefers that immediate release tablet is taken 2 hours after meals). Extended release tablet may be taken with meals that contain dairy products (calcium content <800 mg), but not with dairy products alone.

Dairy products, calcium-fortified juices, oral multivitamins, and mineral supplements: Absorption of ciprofloxacin is decreased by divalent and trivalent cations. The manufacturer states that the usual dietary intake of calcium (including meals which include dairy products) has not been shown to interfere with ciprofloxacin absorption. Immediate release ciprofloxacin and Cipro® XR may be taken 2 hours before or 6 hours after any of these products.

Caffeine: Patients consuming regular large quantities of caffeinated beverages may need to restrict caffeine intake if excessive cardiac or CNS stimulation occurs.

Related Information

Compatibility of Drugs *on page 1264*

Ciprofloxacin (Ophthalmic)

(sip roe FLOKS a sin)

Brand Names: U.S. Ciloxan®

Index Terms Ciprofloxacin Hydrochloride

Pharmacologic Category Antibiotic, Ophthalmic; Antibiotic, Quinolone

Medication Safety Issues

Sound-alike/look-alike issues:

Ciprofloxacin may be confused with cephalexin

Ciloxan® may be confused with Cytoxan

Pregnancy Risk Factor C

Lactation Use caution (AAP rates "compatible"; AAP 2001 update pending)

Use Treatment of superficial ocular infections (corneal ulcers, conjunctivitis) due to susceptible strains

Available Dosage Forms

Ointment, ophthalmic:

Ciloxan®: 3.33 mg/g (3.5 g)

Solution, ophthalmic: 3.5 mg/mL (2.5 mL, 5 mL, 10 mL)

Ciloxan®: 3.5 mg/mL (5 mL)

General Dosage Range Ophthalmic:

Ointment: *Children >2 years and Adults:* Apply a 1/2" ribbon into the conjunctival sac 3 times/day for the first 2 days, followed by a 1/2" ribbon applied twice daily

Solution: *Children >1 year and Adults:* Conjunctivitis: Instill 1-2 drops in eye(s) every 2 hours while awake for 2 days, then 1-2 drops every 4 hours while awake; Corneal ulcer: Instill 2 drops into affected eye every 15 minutes for the first 6 hours, then 2 drops every 30 minutes for the remainder of the first day; on day 2 instill 2 drops into the affected eye hourly; on days 3-14 instill 2 drops every 4 hours

Administration

Other For topical ophthalmic use only; avoid touching tip of applicator to eye or other surfaces.

Nursing Actions

Patient Education Wash hands prior to instilling eye medication. Do not touch dropper to eye or any other surface. Do not wear contact lenses while using this medication (check with prescriber before using again). Tilt head back, look upward, and pull lower eyelid down to make a pouch. Drop prescribed number of drops directly into eye. Close eye, place one finger at corner of eye near nose, and apply gentle pressure. Do not blink or rub eye. If also using ointment, use drops before ointment. May cause temporary stinging or burning. Report persistent eye discomfort, itching, redness, unusual tearing, feeling as if something is in your eye, blurred vision, eye pain, worsening vision, a bad taste in your mouth, sensitivity to light, skin rash, difficulty breathing, or worsening of symptoms.

Ciprofloxacin (Otic) (sip roe FLOKS a sin)

Brand Names: U.S. Cetraxal®

Index Terms Ciprofloxacin Hydrochloride

Pharmacologic Category Antibiotic, Otic; Antibiotic, Quinolone

Medication Safety Issues

Sound-alike/look-alike issues:

Cetraxal® may be confused with cefTRIAXone

Ciprofloxacin may be confused with cephalexin

Pregnancy Risk Factor C

Lactation Not recommended (AAP rates "compatible"; AAP 2001 update pending)

Use Treatment of acute otitis externa due to susceptible strains of *Pseudomonas aeruginosa* or *Staphylococcus aureus*

Available Dosage Forms

Solution, otic [preservative free]:

Cetraxal®: 0.5 mg/0.25 mL (14s)

General Dosage Range Otic: *Children ≥1 year and Adults:* 0.5 mg (0.25 mL) every 12 hours

Administration

Other For otic use only. Prior to use, warm solution by holding container in hands for at least 1 minute. Patient should lie down with affected ear upward and medication instilled. Patients should remain in the position for at least 1 minute to allow penetration of solution.

Nursing Actions

Patient Education Store containers in foil pouch until immediately prior to use. Wash hands prior to instilling medication. Warm container by holding in hands for at least 1 minute before instilling (cold solution may cause dizziness). Lie with affected ear upward and then instill solution. Remain in this position for 1 minute. Repeat for opposite ear if necessary. Report increased pain, headache, rash, or if condition does not improve after one week.

Ciprofloxacin and Dexamethasone

(sip roe FLOKS a sin & deks a METH a sone)

Brand Names: U.S. Ciprodex®

Index Terms Ciprofloxacin Hydrochloride and Dexamethasone; Dexamethasone and Ciprofloxacin

Pharmacologic Category Antibiotic, Otic; Antibiotic/Corticosteroid, Otic; Corticosteroid, Otic

Pregnancy Risk Factor C

Lactation Excretion in breast milk unknown/not recommended

Use Treatment of acute otitis media in pediatric patients with tympanostomy tubes or acute otitis externa in children and adults

Available Dosage Forms

Suspension, otic:

Ciprodex®: Ciprofloxacin 0.3% and dexamethasone 0.1% (7.5 mL)

General Dosage Range Otic: *Children and Adults:* Instill 4 drops into affected ear(s) twice daily

Administration

Other Otic: Prior to instillation, bottle should be warmed in hands for 1-2 minutes. Shake suspension well immediately before using. Patient should lie with affected ear upward and remain in this position for 60 seconds following application. Drops should be instilled directly into tympanostomy tube (if present) and tragus should be pumped 5 times to facilitate penetration into the middle ear.

Nursing Actions

Physical Assessment See individual agents.

Patient Education See individual agents.

Related Information

Ciprofloxacin (Otic) *on page 240*

Ciprofloxacin and Hydrocortisone

(sip roe FLOKS a sin & hye droe KOR ti sone)

Brand Names: U.S. Cipro® HC

Index Terms Ciprofloxacin Hydrochloride and Hydrocortisone; Hydrocortisone and Ciprofloxacin

Pharmacologic Category Antibiotic/Corticosteroid, Otic

Pregnancy Risk Factor C

Use Treatment of acute otitis externa, sometimes known as "swimmer's ear"

Available Dosage Forms

Suspension, otic:

Cipro® HC: Ciprofloxacin 0.2% and hydrocortisone 1% (10 mL)

General Dosage Range Otic: *Children >1 year and Adults:* 3 drops into affected ear(s) twice daily

Nursing Actions

Physical Assessment See individual agents.

Patient Education See individual agents.

Related Information

Ciprofloxacin (Otic) *on page 240*

Cisapride (SIS a pride)

Brand Names: U.S. Propulsid®

Pharmacologic Category Gastrointestinal Agent, Prokinetic

Medication Safety Issues

Sound-alike/look-alike issues:

Propulsid® may be confused with propranolol

Medication Guide Available Yes

Pregnancy Risk Factor C

Lactation Enters breast milk/use caution (AAP rates "compatible"; AAP 2001 update pending)

Use Treatment of nocturnal symptoms of gastroesophageal reflux disease (GERD); has demonstrated effectiveness for gastroparesis, refractory constipation, and nonulcer dyspepsia

General Dosage Range

Oral:

Children: 0.15-0.3 mg/kg 3-4 times/day (maximum: 10 mg/dose)

Adults: Initial: 5-10 mg 4 times/day, may increase to 20 mg 4 times/day if needed

Nursing Actions

Physical Assessment Cardiac status must be evaluated prior to therapy (12-lead ECG). Monitor ECG, electrolyte balance, and renal function. Monitor for tachycardia, fatigue, diarrhea, and other abdominal symptoms.

Patient Education Take before meals. Avoid alcohol and grapefruit juice. May cause increased sedation, headache, and anxiety. Immediately report rapid heartbeat, palpitations, chest pain, or tightness. Report severe abdominal pain, prolonged diarrhea, weight loss, and extreme fatigue.

Cisatracurium (sis a tra KYOO ree um)

Brand Names: U.S. Nimbex®

Index Terms Cisatracurium Besylate

Pharmacologic Category Neuromuscular Blocker Agent, Nondepolarizing

Medication Safety Issues

Sound-alike/look-alike issues:

Nimbex® may be confused with Revex®

High alert medication:

The Institute for Safe Medication Practices (ISMP) includes this medication among its list of drugs which have a heightened risk of causing significant patient harm when used in error.

Other safety concerns:

United States Pharmacopeia (USP) 2006: The Interdisciplinary Safe Medication Use Expert Committee of the USP has recommended the following:

- Hospitals, clinics, and other practice sites should institute special safeguards in the storage, labeling, and use of these agents and should include these safeguards in staff orientation and competency training.
- Healthcare professionals should be on high alert (especially vigilant) whenever a neuromuscular-blocking agent (NMBA) is stocked, ordered, prepared, or administered.

Pregnancy Risk Factor B

Lactation Excretion in breast milk unknown/use caution

Use Adjunct to general anesthesia to facilitate endotracheal intubation and to relax skeletal muscles during surgery; to facilitate mechanical ventilation in ICU patients; does not relieve pain or produce sedation

Mechanism of Action/Effect Blocks neural transmission at the myoneural junction by binding with cholinergic receptor sites

Contraindications Hypersensitivity to cisatracurium besylate or any component of the formulation

Warnings/Precautions Maintenance of an adequate airway and respiratory support is critical; certain clinical conditions may result in potentiation or antagonism of neuromuscular blockade:

Potentiation: Electrolyte abnormalities, severe hyponatremia, severe hypocalcemia, severe hypokalemia, hypermagnesemia, neuromuscular diseases, acidosis, acute intermittent porphyria, renal failure, hepatic failure

Antagonism: Alkalosis, hypercalcemia, demyelinating lesions, peripheral neuropathies, diabetes mellitus

Increased sensitivity in patients with myasthenia gravis, Eaton-Lambert syndrome; resistance in burn patients (>30% of body) for period of 5-70 days postinjury; resistance in patients with muscle trauma, denervation, immobilization, infection. Cross-sensitivity with other neuromuscular-blocking agents may occur; use extreme caution in patients with previous anaphylactic reactions. Bradycardia may be more common with cisatracurium than with other neuromuscular blocking agents since it has no clinically significant effects on heart rate to counteract the bradycardia produced by anesthetics. Use caution in the elderly. Should be administered by adequately trained individuals familiar with its use. Some dosage forms may contain benzyl alcohol which has been associated with "gasping syndrome" in neonates.

Drug Interactions

Avoid Concomitant Use

Avoid concomitant use of Cisatracurium with any of the following: QuiNINE

Decreased Effect

The levels/effects of Cisatracurium may be decreased by: Acetylcholinesterase Inhibitors; Loop Diuretics

Increased Effect/Toxicity

Cisatracurium may increase the levels/effects of: Cardiac Glycosides; Corticosteroids (Systemic); OnabotulinumtoxinA; RimabotulinumtoxinB

The levels/effects of Cisatracurium may be increased by: AbobotulinumtoxinA; Aminoglycosides; Calcium Channel Blockers; Capreomycin; Colistimethate; Inhalational Anesthetics; Ketorolac; Ketorolac (Nasal); Ketorolac (Systemic); Lincosamide Antibiotics; Lithium; Loop Diuretics; Magnesium Salts; Polymyxin B; Procainamide;

QuiNIDine; QuiNINE; Spironolactone; Tetracycline Derivatives; Vancomycin

Pharmacodynamics/Kinetics

Onset of Action I.V.: 2-3 minutes; Peak effect: 3-5 minutes

Duration of Action Recovery begins in 20-35 minutes when anesthesia is balanced; recovery is attained in 90% of patients in 25-93 minutes

Available Dosage Forms

Injection, solution:

Nimbex®: 2 mg/mL (5 mL, 10 mL); 10 mg/mL (20 mL)

General Dosage Range I.V.:

Children 1-23 months: Intubating dose: 0.15 mg/kg

Children 2-12 years: Intubating dose: 0.1-0.15 mg/kg over 5-15 seconds; Infusion: Initial: 3 mcg/kg/minute; Maintenance: 1-2 mcg/kg/minute (surgery) **or** 0.5-10 mcg/kg/minute (ICU)

Children >12 years: Infusion: Initial: 3 mcg/kg/minute; Maintenance: 1-2 mcg/kg/minute (surgery) **or** 0.5-10 mcg/kg/minute (ICU)

Adults: Intubating dose: 0.1-0.2 mg/kg; Infusion: Initial: 3 mcg/kg/minute; Maintenance: 1-2 mcg/kg/minute (surgery) **or** 0.5-10 mcg/kg/minute (ICU)

Administration

I.M. Not for I.M. injection, too much tissue irritation.

I.V. Administer I.V. only. The use of a peripheral nerve stimulator will permit the most advantageous use of cisatracurium, minimize the possibility of overdosage or underdosage and assist in the evaluation of recovery.

Give undiluted as a bolus injection. Continuous administration requires the use of an infusion pump.

Stability

Storage Refrigerate intact vials at 2°C to 8°C (36°F to 46°F). Use vials within 21 days upon removal from the refrigerator to room temperature (25°C to 77°F). Per the manufacturer, dilutions of 0.1-0.2 mg/mL in 0.9% sodium chloride (NS) or dextrose 5% in water (D_5W) are stable for up to 24 hours at room temperature or under refrigeration and in D_5LR for up to 24 hours in the refrigerator. *Additional stability data:* Dilutions of 0.1, 2, and 5 mg/mL in D_5W or NS are stable in the refrigerator for up to 30 days; at room temperature (23ºC), dilutions of 0.1 and 2 mg/mL began exhibiting substantial drug loss between 7-14 days; dilutions of 5 mg/mL in D_5W or NS are stable for up to 30 days at room temperature (23ºC) (Xu, 1998). Usual concentration: 0.1-0.4 mg/mL.

Nursing Actions

Physical Assessment Ventilatory support must be instituted and maintained until adequate respiratory muscle function and/or airway protection are assured. This drug is not an anesthetic or analgesic; pain must be treated with other agents. Continuous monitoring of vital signs, cardiac status, respiratory status, and degree of neuromuscular block (objective assessment with peripheral external nerve stimulator) is mandatory during infusion and until full muscle tone has returned. **Note:** It may take longer for return of muscle tone in obese or elderly patients or patients with renal or hepatic disease, myasthenia gravis, myopathy, other neuromuscular disease, dehydration, electrolyte imbalance, or severe acid/base imbalance.

Long-term use: Monitor level of neuromuscular blockade, skeletal muscle movement, and respiratory effort. Reposition patient and provide appropriate skin care, mouth care, and care of patient's eyes every 2-3 hours while sedated. Provide appropriate emotional and sensory support (auditory and environmental).

Patient Education Patient will usually be unconscious prior to administration. Reassurance of constant monitoring and emotional support to reduce fear and anxiety should precede and follow administration. Following return of muscle tone, do not attempt to change position or rise from bed without assistance.

Related Information

Compatibility of Drugs *on page 1264*

CISplatin (SIS pla tin)

Index Terms CDDP; Platinol; Platinol-AQ

Pharmacologic Category Antineoplastic Agent, Alkylating Agent; Antineoplastic Agent, Platinum Analog

Medication Safety Issues

Sound-alike/look-alike issues:

CISplatin may be confused with CARBOplatin, oxaliplatin

High alert medication:

This medication is in a class the Institute for Safe Medication Practices (ISMP) includes among its list of drugs which have a heightened risk of causing significant patient harm when used in error.

Administration issues:

Doses >100 mg/m^2 once every 3-4 weeks are rarely used and should be verified with the prescriber.

Pregnancy Risk Factor D

Lactation Enters breast milk/not recommended

Use Treatment of advanced bladder cancer, metastatic testicular cancer, and metastatic ovarian cancer

Unlabeled Use Treatment of head and neck cancer, breast cancer, gastric cancer, esophageal cancer, cervical cancer, prostate cancer, nonsmall cell lung cancer, small cell lung cancer; Hodgkin's and non-Hodgkin's lymphoma; neuroblastoma; sarcomas, myeloma, melanoma, mesothelioma, hepatoblastoma, and osteosarcoma

Mechanism of Action/Effect Inhibits DNA synthesis

Contraindications Hypersensitivity to cisplatin, other platinum-containing compounds, or any component of the formulation (anaphylactic-like reactions have been reported); pre-existing renal impairment; myelosuppression; hearing impairment

Warnings/Precautions Hazardous agent - use appropriate precautions for handling and disposal. **[U.S. Boxed Warning]: Doses >100 mg/m^2 once every 3-4 weeks are rarely used and should be verified with the prescriber.** Patients should receive adequate hydration, with or without diuretics, prior to and for 24 hours after cisplatin administration. Reduce dosage in renal impairment. **[U.S. Boxed Warning]: Cumulative renal toxicity may be severe.** Elderly patients may be more susceptible to nephrotoxicity and peripheral neuropathy; select dose cautiously and monitor closely. **[U.S. Boxed Warnings]: Dose-related toxicities include myelosuppression, nausea, and vomiting. Ototoxicity, especially pronounced in children, is manifested by tinnitus or loss of high frequency hearing and occasionally, deafness.** Severe and possibly irreversible neuropathies may occur with higher than recommended doses or more frequent regimen. Serum electrolytes, particularly magnesium and potassium, should be monitored and replaced as needed during and after cisplatin therapy. When administered as sequential infusions, taxane derivatives (docetaxel, paclitaxel) should be administered before platinum derivatives (carboplatin, cisplatin). **[U.S. Boxed Warnings]: Anaphylactic-like reactions have been reported; may be managed with epinephrine, corticosteroids, and/or antihistamines. Should be administered under the supervision of an experienced cancer chemotherapy physician.**

Drug Interactions

Avoid Concomitant Use

Avoid concomitant use of CISplatin with any of the following: BCG; CloZAPine; Natalizumab; Pimecrolimus; Tacrolimus (Topical); Vaccines (Live)

Decreased Effect

CISplatin may decrease the levels/effects of: BCG; Coccidioidin Skin Test; Fosphenytoin; Phenytoin; Sipuleucel-T; Vaccines (Inactivated); Vaccines (Live)

The levels/effects of CISplatin may be decreased by: Echinacea

Increased Effect/Toxicity

CISplatin may increase the levels/effects of: Aminoglycosides; CloZAPine; Leflunomide; Natalizumab; Taxane Derivatives; Topotecan; Vaccines (Live); Vinorelbine

The levels/effects of CISplatin may be increased by: Denosumab; Loop Diuretics; Pimecrolimus; Roflumilast; Tacrolimus (Topical); Trastuzumab

Nutritional/Ethanol Interactions Herb/Nutraceutical: Avoid black cohosh, dong quai in estrogen-dependent tumors.

Adverse Reactions

>10%:

Central nervous system: Neurotoxicity: Peripheral neuropathy is dose- and duration-dependent.

Gastrointestinal: Nausea and vomiting (76% to 100%)

Hematologic: Myelosuppression (25% to 30%; nadir: day 18-23; recovery: by day 39; mild with moderate doses, mild-to-moderate with high-dose therapy)

Hepatic: Liver enzymes increased

Renal: Nephrotoxicity (acute renal failure and chronic renal insufficiency)

Otic: Ototoxicity (10% to 30%; manifested as high frequency hearing loss; ototoxicity is especially pronounced in children)

1% to 10%: Local: Tissue irritation

Available Dosage Forms

Injection, solution [preservative free]: 1 mg/mL (50 mL, 100 mL, 200 mL)

General Dosage Range Dosage adjustment recommended in patients with renal impairment

I.V.: *Adults:* 50-70 mg/m^2 every 3-4 weeks **or** 75-100 mg/m^2/day every 4 weeks **or** 20 mg/m^2/day for 5 days every 3 weeks

Administration

I.V. Irritant. Perform pretreatment hydration (see General Dosage Range).

I.V.: Rate of administration has varied from a 15- to 120-minute infusion, 1 mg/minute infusion, 6- to 8-hour infusion, 24-hour infusion, or per protocol.

I.V. Detail pH: 3.5-5.5 (reconstituted solution); 3.7-6.0 (aqueous injection)

Stability

Reconstitution The infusion solution should have a final sodium chloride concentration ≥0.2%.

Storage Store intact vials at room temperature 15°C to 25°C (59°F to 77°F). Protect from light. Do not refrigerate solution as a precipitate may form. Further dilution **stability is dependent on the chloride ion concentration** and should be mixed in solutions of NS (at least 0.3% NaCl). After initial entry into the vial, solution is stable for 28 days protected from light or for at least 7 days under fluorescent room light at room temperature. Further dilutions in NS, D_5/0.45% NaCl or D_5/NS to a concentration of 0.05-2 mg/mL are stable for 72 hours at 4°C to 25°C. The infusion solution should have a final sodium chloride concentration ≥0.2%.

Nursing Actions

Physical Assessment Verify any dose exceeding 100 mg/m^2 per course. Assess potential for interactions with other drugs patient may be taking (especially ototoxins or nephrotoxins). Patient should be vigorously hydrated prior to and for 24 hours following infusion. Evaluate any changes in auditory status prior to each treatment and regularly during therapy. Cisplatin is emetogenic; antiemetic should be administered prior to each treatment and as needed between infusions. Infusion site must be monitored closely to reduce potential for extravasation. Anaphylaxis-like reaction is possible; emergency medication should be readily available. Monitor for acute or chronic renal failure; peripheral neuropathy and ototoxicity may be irreversible. Teach patient importance of adequate hydration.

Patient Education This medication can only be administered by I.V. Report immediately any burning, pain, itching, or redness at infusion site; difficulty breathing or swallowing; swelling of mouth or throat; or chest pain or palpitations. It is important that you maintain adequate hydration, unless instructed to restrict fluid intake, and adequate nutrition. May cause severe nausea or vomiting that can be delayed for up to 48 hours after infusion and last for 1 week (consult prescriber for appropriate antiemetic medication). May cause mouth sores or loss of hair (reversible). You will be susceptible to infection. Report promptly any pain, tingling, loss of sensation, or cramping in extremities; ringing in ears or change in hearing; difficulty breathing or swallowing; fever or chills; unusual fatigue; or unusual bruising/ bleeding.

Dietary Considerations Some products may contain sodium.

Related Information

Management of Drug Extravasations *on page 1269*

Citalopram (sye TAL oh pram)

Brand Names: U.S. CeleXA®

Index Terms Citalopram Hydrobromide; Nitalapram

Pharmacologic Category Antidepressant, Selective Serotonin Reuptake Inhibitor

Medication Safety Issues

Sound-alike/look-alike issues:

CeleXA® may be confused with CeleBREX®, Cerebyx®, Ranexa™, ZyPREXA®

Medication Guide Available Yes

Pregnancy Risk Factor C

Lactation Enters breast milk/consider risk:benefit

Breast-Feeding Considerations Citalopram and its metabolites are excreted in human milk. According to the manufacturer, the decision to continue or discontinue breast-feeding during therapy should take into account the risk of exposure to the infant and the benefits of treatment to the mother. Excessive somnolence, decreased feeding, colic, irritability, restlessness, and weight loss have been reported in breast-fed infants. The long-term effects on development and behavior have not been studied; therefore, citalopram should be prescribed to a mother who is breast-feeding only when the benefits outweigh the potential risks.

Use Treatment of depression

Unlabeled Use Smoking cessation; ethanol abuse; obsessive-compulsive disorder (OCD) in children; diabetic neuropathy

Mechanism of Action/Effect A bicyclic phthalane derivative, citalopram selectively inhibits serotonin reuptake in the presynaptic neurons thus increasing serotonergic activity in the brain.

Contraindications Hypersensitivity to citalopram or any component of the formulation; concomitant use with MAO inhibitors or within 2 weeks of discontinuing MAO inhibitors; concomitant use with pimozide; patients with congenital long QT syndrome

Warnings/Precautions [U.S. Boxed Warning]: Antidepressants increase the risk of suicidal thinking and behavior in children, adolescents, and young adults (18-24 years of age) with major depressive disorder (MDD) and other psychiatric disorders; consider risk prior to prescribing. Short-term studies did not show an increased risk in patients >24 years of age and showed a decreased risk in patients ≥65 years. Closely monitor patients for clinical worsening, suicidality, or unusual changes in behavior, particularly during the initial 1-2 months of therapy or during periods of dosage adjustments (increases or decreases); the patient's family or caregiver should be instructed to closely observe the patient and communicate condition with healthcare provider. A medication guide concerning the use of antidepressants should be dispensed with each prescription. **Citalopram is not FDA approved for use in children.**

The possibility of a suicide attempt is inherent in major depression and may persist until remission occurs. Use caution in high-risk patients. Worsening depression and severe abrupt suicidality that are not part of the presenting symptoms may require discontinuation or modification of drug therapy. The patient's family or caregiver should be alerted to monitor patients for the emergence of suicidality and associated behaviors (such as agitation, irritability, hostility, impulsivity, and hypomania) and call healthcare provider.

May worsen psychosis in some patients or precipitate a shift to mania or hypomania in patients with bipolar disorder. Patients presenting with depressive symptoms should be screened for bipolar disorder. Monotherapy in patients with bipolar disorder should be avoided. **Citalopram is not FDA approved for the treatment of bipolar depression.**

Serotonin syndrome and neuroleptic malignant syndrome (NMS)-like reactions have occurred with serotonin/norepinephrine reuptake inhibitors (SNRIs) and selective serotonin reuptake inhibitors (SSRIs) when used alone, and particularly when used in combination with serotonergic agents (eg, triptans) or antidopaminergic agents (eg, antipsychotics). Concurrent use with MAO inhibitors is contraindicated. May increase the risks associated with electroconvulsive therapy. Has a low potential to impair cognitive or motor performance; caution operating hazardous machinery or driving.

May result in QT_c prolongation. Risk may be increased by conditions or concomitant medications which cause bradycardia, heart failure, hypokalemia, and/or hypomagnesemia; ECG monitoring is recommended. Avoid doses >40 mg/day. Use is contraindicated in patients with congenital long QT syndrome. Use with caution in patients with hepatic or renal dysfunction, in elderly patients, concomitant CNS depressants, and pregnancy (high doses of citalopram have been associated with teratogenicity in animals). Use with caution in patients with a previous seizure disorder or condition predisposing to seizures such as brain damage or alcoholism. Use caution with concomitant use of aspirin, NSAIDs, warfarin, or other drugs that affect coagulation; the risk of bleeding may be potentiated. May cause hyponatremia/SIADH (elderly at increased risk); volume depletion and diuretics may increase risk. May cause or exacerbate sexual dysfunction. Upon discontinuation of citalopram therapy, gradually taper dose. If intolerable symptoms occur following a decrease in dosage or upon discontinuation of therapy, then resuming the previous dose with a more gradual taper should be considered.

Drug Interactions

Avoid Concomitant Use

Avoid concomitant use of Citalopram with any of the following: Artemether; Conivaptan; Dronedarone; Iobenguane I 123; Lumefantrine; MAO Inhibitors; Methylene Blue; Nilotinib; Pimozide; QUEtiapine; QuiNINE; Tetrabenazine; Thioridazine; Toremifene; Tryptophan; Vandetanib; Vemurafenib; Ziprasidone

Decreased Effect

Citalopram may decrease the levels/effects of: Iobenguane I 123; Ioflupane I 123

The levels/effects of Citalopram may be decreased by: CarBAMazepine; CYP2C19 Inducers (Strong); CYP3A4 Inducers (Strong); Cyproheptadine; Deferasirox; NSAID (COX-2 Inhibitor); NSAID (Nonselective); Peginterferon Alfa-2b; Tocilizumab

Increased Effect/Toxicity

Citalopram may increase the levels/effects of: Alpha-/Beta-Blockers; Anticoagulants; Antidepressants (Serotonin Reuptake Inhibitor/Antagonist); Antiplatelet Agents; Aspirin; BusPIRone; CarBAMazepine; CloZAPine; Collagenase (Systemic); Desmopressin; Dextromethorphan; Dronedarone; Drotrecogin Alfa (Activated); Ibritumomab; Lithium; Methadone; Methylene Blue; Metoclopramide; Mexiletine; NSAID (COX-2 Inhibitor); NSAID (Nonselective); Pimozide; QTc-Prolonging Agents; QuiNINE; RisperiDONE; Rivaroxaban; Salicylates; Serotonin Modulators; Tetrabenazine; Thioridazine; Thrombolytic Agents; Toremifene; Tositumomab and Iodine I 131 Tositumomab; TraMADol; Tricyclic Antidepressants; Vandetanib; Vemurafenib; Vitamin K Antagonists; Ziprasidone

The levels/effects of Citalopram may be increased by: Alcohol (Ethyl); Alfuzosin; Analgesics (Opioid); Antipsychotics; Artemether; BusPIRone; Chloroquine; Cimetidine; Ciprofloxacin; Ciprofloxacin (Systemic); CNS Depressants; Conivaptan; CYP2C19 Inhibitors (Moderate); CYP2C19 Inhibitors (Strong); CYP3A4 Inhibitors (Moderate); CYP3A4 Inhibitors (Strong); Fluconazole; Gadobutrol; Glucosamine; Herbs (Anticoagulant/Antiplatelet Properties); Indacaterol; Ivacaftor; Linezolid; Lumefantrine; Macrolide Antibiotics; MAO Inhibitors; Metoclopramide; Nilotinib; Omega-3-Acid Ethyl Esters; Pentosan Polysulfate Sodium; Pentoxifylline; Prostacyclin Analogues; QUEtiapine; QuiNINE; TraMADol; Tryptophan; Vitamin E

Nutritional/Ethanol Interactions

Ethanol: May increase CNS depression; monitor for increased effects with coadministration. Caution patients about effects.

Herb/Nutraceutical: Avoid valerian, St John's wort, SAMe, kava kava, and gotu kola (may increase CNS depression).

Adverse Reactions

>10%:

Central nervous system: Somnolence (18%; dose related), insomnia (15%; dose related)

Gastrointestinal: Nausea (21%), xerostomia (20%)

Miscellaneous: Diaphoresis (11%; dose related)

1% to 10%:

Cardiovascular: Postural hypotension, tachycardia

Central nervous system: Fatigue (5%; dose related), anorexia (4%), anxiety (4%), agitation (3%), fever (2%), yawning (2%; dose related), amnesia, apathy, concentration impaired, confusion, depression, migraine, suicide attempt

Dermatologic: Rash, pruritus

Endocrine & metabolic: Libido decreased (1% to 4%), dysmenorrhea (3%), amenorrhea, sexual dysfunction

Gastrointestinal: Diarrhea (8%), dyspepsia (5%), vomiting (4%), abdominal pain (3%), flatulence, salivation increased, taste perversion, weight gain/loss

Genitourinary: Ejaculation disorder (6%), impotence (3%; dose related), polyuria
Neuromuscular & skeletal: Tremor (8%), arthralgia (2%), myalgia (2%), paresthesia
Ocular: Abnormal accommodation
Respiratory: Rhinitis (5%), upper respiratory tract infection (5%), sinusitis (3%), cough

Pharmacodynamics/Kinetics

Onset of Action Depression: The onset of action is within a week; however, individual response varies greatly and full response may not be seen until 8-12 weeks after initiation of treatment.

Available Dosage Forms

Solution, oral: 10 mg/5 mL (240 mL)
Tablet, oral: 10 mg, 20 mg, 40 mg
CeleXA®: 10 mg, 20 mg, 40 mg

General Dosage Range Dosage adjustment recommended in patients with hepatic impairment

Oral: *Adults:* Initial: 20 mg/day; Maintenance: 20-40 mg/day

Administration

Oral May be administered without regard to food.

Stability

Storage Store at 20°C to 25°C (68°F to 77°F); excursions permitted to 15°C to 30°C (59°F to 86°F). Protect from light.

Nursing Actions

Physical Assessment Assess mental status for depression, signs of clinical worsening, suicide ideation, anxiety, social functioning, mania, or panic attack. Teach patient hypotensive precautions. Taper dosage slowly when discontinuing.

Patient Education It may take up to 3 weeks to see therapeutic effects from this medication. May be taken with or without food. Avoid alcohol. You may experience sexual dysfunction (reversible). May cause dizziness, anxiety, blurred vision, nausea, or dry mouth. Report confusion or impaired concentration, suicide ideation, severe headache, palpitations, rash, insomnia or nightmares, changes in personality, muscle weakness or tremors, altered gait pattern, signs and symptoms of respiratory infection, or excessive perspiration.

Dietary Considerations May be taken without regard to food.

Cladribine (KLA dri been)

Brand Names: U.S. Leustatin®

Index Terms 2-CdA; 2-Chlorodeoxyadenosine

Pharmacologic Category Antineoplastic Agent, Antimetabolite; Antineoplastic Agent, Antimetabolite (Purine Analog)

Medication Safety Issues

Sound-alike/look-alike issues:

Cladribine may be confused with clevidipine, clofarabine, fludarabine
Leustatin® may be confused with lovastatin

High alert medication:

This medication is in a class the Institute for Safe Medication Practices (ISMP) includes among its list of drug classes which have a heightened risk of causing significant patient harm when used in error.

Pregnancy Risk Factor D

Lactation Excretion in breast milk unknown/not recommended

Use Treatment of hairy cell leukemia

Unlabeled Use Treatment of acute myeloid leukemia (AML), chronic lymphocytic leukemia (CLL), non-Hodgkin's lymphomas (mantle cell), Waldenström's macroglobulinemia, refractory Langerhans cell histiocytosis

Available Dosage Forms

Injection, solution [preservative free]: 1 mg/mL (10 mL)
Leustatin®: 1 mg/mL (10 mL)

General Dosage Range Dosage adjustment recommended in patients with renal impairment

I.V.: *Adults:* Continuous infusion: 0.09 mg/kg/day for 7 days

Administration

I.V. Administer as a continuous infusion; may also be administered over 30 minutes or over 2 hours (unlabeled administration rates) depending on indication and/or protocol.

Other May also be administered subcutaneously (unlabeled administration route; Laszlo, 2010)

Nursing Actions

Physical Assessment Monitor for myelosuppression, cardiac changes, and renal failure regularly during therapy and following therapy (patients should be considered immunosuppressed for up to 1 year after cladribine therapy).

Patient Education This drug can only be administered by infusion. It is important to maintain adequate nutrition and hydration during therapy. You will be more susceptible to infection during therapy and for up to 1 year following therapy. May cause nausea, vomiting, muscle weakness or pain, or mouth sores. Report immediately rash, unusual excessive fatigue, and/or signs of infection. Report rapid heartbeat or palpitations; unusual bruising or bleeding; persistent GI disturbances; diarrhea or constipation; yellowing of eyes or skin; change in color of urine or stool; swelling, warmth, or pain in extremities; or difficult respirations.

Related Information

Management of Drug Extravasations *on page 1269*

Clarithromycin (kla RITH roe mye sin)

Brand Names: U.S. Biaxin®; Biaxin® XL

Pharmacologic Category Antibiotic, Macrolide

Medication Safety Issues

Sound-alike/look-alike issues:

Clarithromycin may be confused with Claritin®, clindamycin, erythromycin

Pregnancy Risk Factor C

Lactation Excretion in breast milk unknown/use caution

Breast-Feeding Considerations It is not known if clarithromycin is excreted in human breast milk. The manufacturer recommends that caution be exercised when administering clarithromycin to breast-feeding women.

Other macrolides are considered compatible with breast-feeding and clarithromycin is used therapeutically in infants. Nondose-related effects could include modification of bowel flora.

Use

Children:

Acute otitis media (*H. influenzae, M. catarrhalis*, or *S. pneumoniae*)

Community-acquired pneumonia due to susceptible *Mycoplasma pneumoniae, S. pneumoniae*, or *Chlamydia pneumoniae* (TWAR)

Pharyngitis/tonsillitis due to susceptible *S. pyogenes*, acute maxillary sinusitis due to susceptible *H. influenzae, S. pneumoniae*, or *Moraxella catarrhalis*, uncomplicated skin/skin structure infections due to susceptible *S. aureus, S. pyogenes,* and mycobacterial infections

Prevention of disseminated mycobacterial infections due to MAC disease in patients with advanced HIV infection

Adults:

Pharyngitis/tonsillitis due to susceptible *S. pyogenes*

Acute maxillary sinusitis due to susceptible *H. influenzae, M. catarrhalis,* or *S. pneumoniae*

Acute exacerbation of chronic bronchitis due to susceptible *H. influenzae, H. parainfluenzae, M. catarrhalis*, or *S. pneumoniae*

Community-acquired pneumonia due to susceptible *H. influenzae, H. parainfluenzae, Mycoplasma pneumoniae, S. pneumoniae,* or *Chlamydia pneumoniae* (TWAR), *Moraxella catarrhalis*

Uncomplicated skin/skin structure infections due to susceptible *S. aureus, S. pyogenes*

Disseminated mycobacterial infections due to *M. avium* or *M. intracellulare*

Prevention of disseminated mycobacterial infections due to *M. avium* complex (MAC) disease (eg, patients with advanced HIV infection)

Duodenal ulcer disease due to *H. pylori* in regimens with other drugs including amoxicillin and lansoprazole or omeprazole, ranitidine bismuth citrate, bismuth subsalicylate, tetracycline, and/ or an H_2 antagonist

Unlabeled Use Pertussis (CDC guidelines); alternate antibiotic for prophylaxis of infective endocarditis in patients who are allergic to penicillin and undergoing surgical or dental procedures (ACC/ AHA guidelines)

Mechanism of Action/Effect Exerts its antibacterial action by binding to 50S ribosomal subunit resulting in inhibition of protein synthesis. The 14-OH metabolite of clarithromycin is twice as active as the parent compound against some organisms.

Contraindications Hypersensitivity to clarithromycin, erythromycin, or any macrolide antibiotic; use with ergot derivatives, pimozide, cisapride, astemizole, terfenadine, colchicine (if patient has concomitant renal or hepatic impairment); history of cholestatic jaundice or hepatic dysfunction with prior clarithromycin use

Warnings/Precautions Dosage adjustment required with severe renal impairment; decreased dosage or prolonged dosing interval may be appropriate. May cause hepatotoxicity (elevated liver function tests, hepatitis, jaundice, hepatic failure); use caution with preexisting hepatic disease or hepatotoxic medications. Use with caution in patients with myasthenia gravis. Colchicine toxicity (including fatalities) has been reported with concomitant use; concomitant use is contraindicated in patients with renal or hepatic impairment. Prolonged use may result in fungal or bacterial superinfection, including *C. difficile*-associated diarrhea (CDAD) and pseudomembranous colitis; CDAD has been observed >2 months postantibiotic treatment. Macrolides (including clarithromycin) have been associated with rare QT prolongation and ventricular arrhythmias, including torsade de pointes. Use caution in patients with coronary artery disease. Avoid use of extended release tablets (Biaxin® XL) in patients with known stricture/narrowing of the GI tract.

Drug Interactions

Avoid Concomitant Use

Avoid concomitant use of Clarithromycin with any of the following: Alfuzosin; Artemether; Axitinib; BCG; Cisapride; Conivaptan; Crizotinib; Dihydroergotamine; Disopyramide; Dronedarone; Eplerenone; Ergotamine; Everolimus; Fluticasone (Oral Inhalation); Halofantrine; Lapatinib; Lovastatin; Lumefantrine; Lurasidone; Nilotinib; Nisoldipine; Pimozide; QUEtiapine; QuiNINE; Ranolazine; Rivaroxaban; RomiDEPsin; Salmeterol; Silodosin; Simvastatin; Tamsulosin; Terfenadine; Tetrabenazine; Thioridazine; Ticagrelor; Tolvaptan; Topotecan; Toremifene; Vandetanib; Vemurafenib; Ziprasidone

Decreased Effect

Clarithromycin may decrease the levels/effects of: BCG; Clopidogrel; Prasugrel; Ticagrelor; Typhoid Vaccine; Zidovudine

The levels/effects of Clarithromycin may be decreased by: CYP3A4 Inducers (Strong); Deferasirox; Etravirine; Herbs (CYP3A4 Inducers); Protease Inhibitors; Tocilizumab

Increased Effect/Toxicity

Clarithromycin may increase the levels/effects of: Alfentanil; Alfuzosin; Almotriptan; Alosetron; Antifungal Agents (Azole Derivatives, Systemic); Antineoplastic Agents (Vinca Alkaloids); ARIPiprazole; Axitinib; Benzodiazepines (metabolized by oxidation); Bortezomib; Brentuximab Vedotin; Brinzolamide; Budesonide (Nasal); Budesonide (Systemic, Oral Inhalation); BusPIRone; Calcium Channel Blockers; CarBAMazepine; Cardiac Glycosides; Ciclesonide; Cilostazol; Cisapride; CloZAPine; Colchicine; Conivaptan; Corticosteroids (Orally Inhaled); Corticosteroids (Systemic); Crizotinib; CycloSPORINE; CycloSPORINE (Systemic); CYP3A4 Inducers (Strong); CYP3A4 Substrates; Dabigatran Etexilate; Dienogest; Dihydroergotamine; Disopyramide; Dronedarone; Dutasteride; Eletriptan; Eplerenone; Ergot Derivatives; Ergotamine; Everolimus; FentaNYL; Fesoterodine; Fluticasone (Nasal); Fluticasone (Oral Inhalation); GlipiZIDE; GlyBURIDE; GuanFACINE; Halofantrine; HMG-CoA Reductase Inhibitors; Iloperidone; Ivacaftor; Ixabepilone; Lapatinib; Lovastatin; Lumefantrine; Lurasidone; Maraviroc; MethylPREDNISolone; Nilotinib; Nisoldipine; Paricalcitol; Pazopanib; P-glycoprotein/ABCB1 Substrates; Pimecrolimus; Pimozide; Propafenone; Protease Inhibitors; Prucalopride; QTc-Prolonging Agents; QuiNIDine; QuiNINE; Ranolazine; Repaglinide; Rifamycin Derivatives; Rivaroxaban; RomiDEPsin; Ruxolitinib; Salmeterol; Saxagliptin; Selective Serotonin Reuptake Inhibitors; Sildenafil; Silodosin; Simvastatin; Sirolimus; SORAfenib; Tacrolimus; Tacrolimus (Systemic); Tacrolimus (Topical); Tadalafil; Tamsulosin; Telaprevir; Temsirolimus; Terfenadine; Tetrabenazine; Theophylline Derivatives; Thioridazine; Ticagrelor; Tolterodine; Tolvaptan; Topotecan; Toremifene; Vandetanib; Vardenafil; Vemurafenib; Vilazodone; Vitamin K Antagonists; Zidovudine; Ziprasidone; Zopiclone; Zuclopenthixol

The levels/effects of Clarithromycin may be increased by: Alfuzosin; Antifungal Agents (Azole Derivatives, Systemic); Artemether; Chloroquine; Ciprofloxacin; Ciprofloxacin (Systemic); CYP3A4 Inducers (Strong); CYP3A4 Inhibitors (Moderate); CYP3A4 Inhibitors (Strong); Gadobutrol; Indacaterol; Lumefantrine; Nilotinib; Protease Inhibitors; QUEtiapine; QuiNINE; Telaprevir

Nutritional/Ethanol Interactions

Food: Immediate release: Food delays rate, but not extent of absorption; Extended release: Food increases clarithromycin AUC by ~30% relative to fasting conditions.

Herb/Nutraceutical: St John's wort may decrease clarithromycin levels.

Adverse Reactions 1% to 10%:

Central nervous system: Headache (adults and children 2%)

Dermatologic: Rash (children 3%)

Gastrointestinal: Abnormal taste (adults 3% to 7%), diarrhea (adults 3% to 6%; children 6%), vomiting (children 6%), nausea (adults 3%), abdominal pain (adults 2%; children 3%), dyspepsia (adults 2%)

Hepatic: Prothrombin time increased (adults 1%)

Renal: BUN increased (4%)

Available Dosage Forms

Granules for suspension, oral: 125 mg/5 mL (50 mL, 100 mL); 250 mg/5 mL (50 mL, 100 mL)

Biaxin®: 125 mg/5 mL (50 mL, 100 mL); 250 mg/5 mL (50 mL, 100 mL)

Tablet, oral: 250 mg, 500 mg

Biaxin®: 250 mg, 500 mg

Tablet, extended release, oral: 500 mg

Biaxin® XL: 500 mg

General Dosage Range Dosage adjustment recommended in patients with renal impairment

Oral:

Extended release: *Adults:* 1000 mg once daily

Immediate release:

Children: 15 mg/kg/day divided every 12 hours (maximum: 1 g/day) **or** 15 mg/kg prior to procedure (maximum: 500 mg)

Adults: 250-500 mg every 8-12 hours **or** 500 mg prior to procedure

Administration

Oral Clarithromycin immediate release tablets and oral suspension may be administered with or without meals. Give every 12 hours rather than twice daily to avoid peak and trough variation. Shake suspension well before each use.

Extended release tablets: Should be given with food. Do not crush or chew extended release tablet.

Stability

Storage

Immediate release 250 mg tablets and granules for oral suspension: Store at controlled room temperature of 15°C to 30°C (59°F to 86°F). Reconstituted oral suspension should not be refrigerated because it might gel; microencapsulated particles of clarithromycin in suspension are stable for 14 days when stored at room temperature. Protect tablets from light.

Immediate release 500 mg tablets and Biaxin® XL: Store at controlled room temperature of 20°C to 25°C (68°F to 77°F); excursions permitted to 15°C to 30°C (59°F to 86°F).

Nursing Actions

Physical Assessment Results of culture and sensitivity tests and patient's allergy history should be evaluated prior to therapy.

Patient Education Tables and suspension may be taken with or without meals or milk. Extended release formulation (XL) should be taken with meals; do not break or chew extended release tablets. Maintain adequate hydration, unless instructed to restrict fluid intake. May cause nausea, heartburn, abnormal taste, diarrhea, headaches, or abdominal pain. Report rapid heartbeat or palpitations, persistent fever or chills, easy bruising or bleeding, joint pain, severe persistent diarrhea, skin rash, sores in mouth, or foul-smelling urine.

Dietary Considerations Clarithromycin immediate release tablets and oral suspension may be given with or without meals, and may be taken with milk. Extended release tablets should be taken with food.

Clevidipine (klev ID i peen)

Brand Names: U.S. Cleviprex®

Index Terms Clevidipine Butyrate

Pharmacologic Category Calcium Channel Blocker; Calcium Channel Blocker, Dihydropyridine

Medication Safety Issues

Sound-alike/look-alike issues:

Clevidipine may be confused with cladribine, clofarabine, clomiPRAMINE

Cleviprex® may be confused with Claravis™

Pregnancy Risk Factor C

Lactation Excretion in breast milk unknown/not recommended

Use Management of hypertension

Mechanism of Action/Effect Dihydropyridine calcium channel blocker with potent arterial vasodilating activity. Inhibits calcium ion influx in arterial smooth muscle, producing a decrease in mean arterial pressure (MAP) by reducing systemic vascular resistance.

Contraindications Hypersensitivity to clevidipine or any component of the formulation (soybeans, soy products, eggs, egg products); hypertriglyceridemia or complications of hypertriglyceridemia (eg, acute pancreatitis); lipoid nephrosis; severe aortic stenosis

Warnings/Precautions Symptomatic hypotension with or without syncope and reflex tachycardia may rarely occur. Blood pressure must be lowered at a rate appropriate for the patient's clinical condition; dosage reductions may be necessary. Treatment of clevidipine-induced tachycardia with beta-blockers is **not** recommended. After prolonged use, discontinuation may cause rebound hypertension; monitor closely for ≥8 hours after discontinuation. Use with caution in patients with heart failure (may worsen symptoms). Clevidipine is formulated within a 20% fat emulsion (0.2 g/mL); hypertriglyceridemia is an expected side effect with high-dose or extended treatment periods; median infusion duration in clinical trials was approximately 6.5 hours (Aronson, 2008). Patients who develop hypertriglyceridemia (eg, >500 mg/dL) are at risk of developing pancreatitis. A reduction in the quantity of concurrently administered lipids may be necessary. Use is contraindicated in patients with hypertriglyceridemia or complications associated with hypertriglyceridemia (eg, acute pancreatitis) and lipoid nephrosis. Withdrawal from concomitant beta-blocker therapy should be done gradually. Initiate therapy at the low end of the dosage range in the elderly, with careful upward titration if needed. Use within 12 hours of puncturing vial; maintain aseptic technique while handling.

Drug Interactions

Avoid Concomitant Use There are no known interactions where it is recommended to avoid concomitant use.

Decreased Effect

Clevidipine may decrease the levels/effects of: QuiNIDine

The levels/effects of Clevidipine may be decreased by: Calcium Salts; Herbs (Hypertensive Properties); Methylphenidate; Yohimbine

Increased Effect/Toxicity

Clevidipine may increase the levels/effects of: Amifostine; Antihypertensives; Beta-Blockers; Calcium Channel Blockers (Nondihydropyridine); Hypotensive Agents; Magnesium Salts; Neuromuscular-Blocking Agents (Nondepolarizing); Nitroprusside; QuiNIDine; RiTUXimab

The levels/effects of Clevidipine may be increased by: Alpha1-Blockers; Calcium Channel Blockers (Nondihydropyridine); Diazoxide; Herbs (Hypotensive Properties); Magnesium Salts; MAO Inhibitors; Pentoxifylline; Phosphodiesterase 5 Inhibitors; Prostacyclin Analogues; QuiNIDine

Nutritional/Ethanol Interactions Herb/Nutraceutical: Avoid bayberry, blue cohosh, cayenne, ephedra, ginger, ginseng (American), kola, licorice (may worsen hypertension). Avoid black cohosh, California poppy, coleus, golden seal, hawthorn, mistletoe, periwinkle, quinine, shepherd's purse (may have increased antihypertensive effect).

Adverse Reactions

>10%:

Cardiovascular: Atrial fibrillation (21%)

Central nervous system: Fever (19%), insomnia (12%)

Gastrointestinal: Nausea (5% to 21%)

1% to 10%:

Central nervous system: Headache (6%)

Gastrointestinal: Vomiting (3%)

Hematologic: Postprocedural hemorrhage (3%)

Renal: Acute renal failure (9%)

Respiratory: Pneumonia (3%), respiratory failure (3%)

Pharmacodynamics/Kinetics

Onset of Action 2-4 minutes after start of infusion

Duration of Action I.V.: 5-15 minutes

Available Dosage Forms

Injection, emulsion:

Cleviprex®: 0.5 mg/mL (50 mL, 100 mL)

General Dosage Range I.V.: *Adults:* Initial: 1-2 mg/hour; Usual maintenance: 4-6 mg/hour; Maximum: 21 mg/hour (1000 mL/24 hours)

Administration

I.V. I.V.: Maintain aseptic technique. Do not use if contamination is suspected. Do not dilute. Invert vial gently several times to ensure uniformity of emulsion prior to administration. Administer as a slow continuous infusion via central or peripheral line, using infusion device allowing for calibrated infusion rates. Use within 12 hours of puncturing vial; discard any tubing and unused portion, including that currently being infused.

I.V. Detail pH: 6.0-8.0

Stability

Storage Store in refrigerator at 2°C to 8°C (36°F to 46°F). Unopened vials are stable for 2 months at room temperature. Vials are stable for 12 hours once opened. Protect from light during storage. Do not freeze.

Nursing Actions

Physical Assessment Assess allergy history prior to treatment (soybeans or soy products, eggs or egg products). Monitor cardiac status and blood pressure closely during therapy and for a minimum of 8 hours after discontinuation (rebound hypertension may occur). Caution patient to call for assistance when rising or changing position until response to drug is known.

Patient Education This medication can only be administered by infusion. Report immediately any pain, burning, or swelling at infusion site or any signs of allergic reaction (eg, respiratory difficulty or swallowing, back pain, chest tightness, rash, hives, swelling of lips or mouth). Ask for assistance when rising or changing position until response to drug is known. Report chest pain or palpitations, headache, dizziness, nausea, vomiting, or difficulty breathing.

Dietary Considerations Clevidipine is formulated in an oil-in-water emulsion containing 200 mg/mL of lipid (2 kcal/mL). If on parenteral nutrition, may need to adjust the amount of lipid infused. Emulsion contains soybean oil, egg yolk phospholipids, and glycerin.

Clidinium and Chlordiazepoxide

(kli DI nee um & klor dye az e POKS ide)

Brand Names: U.S. Librax®

Index Terms Chlordiazepoxide and Clidinium

Pharmacologic Category Antispasmodic Agent, Gastrointestinal; Benzodiazepine

Medication Safety Issues

Sound-alike/look-alike issues:

Librax® may be confused with Librium

BEERS Criteria medication:

This drug may be inappropriate for use in geriatric patients (high severity risk).

Pregnancy Risk Factor D

Lactation Enters breast milk/contraindicated

Use Adjunct treatment of peptic ulcer; treatment of irritable bowel syndrome

Available Dosage Forms

Capsule: Clidinium 2.5 mg and chlordiazepoxide 5 mg

Librax®: Clidinium 2.5 mg and chlordiazepoxide 5 mg

General Dosage Range Oral: *Adults:* 1-2 capsules 3-4 times/day

Administration

Oral Administer before meals. **Caution:** Do not abruptly discontinue after prolonged use; taper dose gradually.

Nursing Actions

Physical Assessment See individual agents.

Patient Education See individual agents.

Related Information

ChlordiazePOXIDE *on page 226*

Clindamycin (Systemic) (klin da MYE sin)

Brand Names: U.S. Cleocin HCl®; Cleocin Pediatric®; Cleocin Phosphate®

Index Terms Clindamycin Hydrochloride; Clindamycin Palmitate

Pharmacologic Category Antibiotic, Lincosamide

Medication Safety Issues

Sound-alike/look-alike issues:

Cleocin® may be confused with bleomycin, Clinoril®, Cubicin®, Lincocin®

Clindamycin may be confused with clarithromycin, Claritin®, vancomycin

Pregnancy Risk Factor B

Lactation Enters breast milk/not recommended (AAP rates "compatible"; AAP 2001 update pending)

Breast-Feeding Considerations Small amounts of clindamycin transfer to human milk. The manufacturer does not recommend the use of clindamycin during breast-feeding. Nondose-related effects could include modification of bowel flora. One case of bloody stools in an infant occurred after a mother received clindamycin while breast-feeding; however, a casual relationship was not confirmed.

Use Treatment of susceptible bacterial infections, mainly those caused by anaerobes, streptococci, pneumococci, and staphylococci; pelvic inflammatory disease (I.V.)

Unlabeled Use May be useful in PCP; alternate treatment for toxoplasmosis; bacterial vaginosis (oral); alternate treatment for MRSA infections; alternate antibiotic for prophylaxis of infective endocarditis in patients who are allergic to penicillin and undergoing surgical or dental procedures (ACC/AHA guidelines); treatment of severe or uncomplicated malaria; treatment of babesiosis

Mechanism of Action/Effect Reversibly binds to 50S ribosomal subunits preventing peptide bond formation thus inhibiting bacterial protein synthesis; bacteriostatic or bactericidal depending on drug concentration, infection site, and organism

Contraindications Hypersensitivity to clindamycin, lincomycin, or any component of the formulation

Warnings/Precautions Dosage adjustment may be necessary in patients with severe hepatic dysfunction. **[U.S. Boxed Warning]: Can cause severe and possibly fatal colitis.** Prolonged use may result in fungal or bacterial superinfection, including *C. difficile*-associated diarrhea (CDAD) and pseudomembranous colitis; CDAD has been observed >2 months postantibiotic treatment. Use with caution in patients with a history of gastrointestinal disease. Discontinue drug if significant diarrhea, abdominal cramps, or passage of blood and mucus occurs. Some dosage forms contain benzyl alcohol or tartrazine. Use caution in atopic patients. Not appropriate for use in the treatment of meningitis due to inadequate penetration into the CSF.

Drug Interactions

Avoid Concomitant Use

Avoid concomitant use of Clindamycin (Systemic) with any of the following: BCG; Erythromycin; Erythromycin (Systemic)

Decreased Effect

Clindamycin (Systemic) may decrease the levels/effects of: BCG; Erythromycin (Systemic); Typhoid Vaccine

The levels/effects of Clindamycin (Systemic) may be decreased by: Erythromycin; Kaolin

Increased Effect/Toxicity

Clindamycin (Systemic) may increase the levels/effects of: Neuromuscular-Blocking Agents

Nutritional/Ethanol Interactions

Food: Peak concentrations may be delayed with food.

Herb/Nutraceutical: St John's wort may decrease clindamycin levels.

Adverse Reactions Frequency not defined.

Cardiovascular: Cardiac arrest (rare; I.V. administration), hypotension (rare; I.V. administration)

Dermatologic: Erythema multiforme (rare), exfoliative dermatitis (rare), pruritus, rash, Stevens-Johnson syndrome (rare), urticaria

Gastrointestinal: Abdominal pain, diarrhea, esophagitis, nausea, pseudomembranous colitis, vomiting

Genitourinary: Vaginitis

Hematologic: Agranulocytosis, eosinophilia (transient), neutropenia (transient), thrombocytopenia

Hepatic: Jaundice, liver function test abnormalities

Local: Induration/pain/sterile abscess (I.M.), thrombophlebitis (I.V.)

Neuromuscular & skeletal: Polyarthritis (rare)

Renal: Renal dysfunction (rare)

Miscellaneous: Anaphylactoid reactions (rare)

Available Dosage Forms

Capsule, oral: 75 mg, 150 mg, 300 mg

Cleocin HCl®: 75 mg, 150 mg, 300 mg

Granules for solution, oral: 75 mg/5 mL (100 mL)

Cleocin Pediatric®: 75 mg/5 mL (100 mL)

Infusion, premixed in D_5W:

Cleocin Phosphate®: 300 mg (50 mL); 600 mg (50 mL); 900 mg (50 mL)

Injection, solution: 150 mg/mL (2 mL, 4 mL, 6 mL, 60 mL)

Cleocin Phosphate®: 150 mg/mL (2 mL, 4 mL, 6 mL, 60 mL)

General Dosage Range

I.M., I.V.:

Children >1 month: 20-40 mg/kg/day in 3-4 divided doses

Adults: 1.2-2.7 g/day in 2-4 divided doses (maximum: 4.8 g/day)

Oral:

Children: 8-20 mg/kg/day as hydrochloride or 8-25 mg/kg/day as palmitate in 3-4 divided doses (minimum dose of palmitate: 37.5 mg 3 times/day)

Adults: 150-450 mg every 6-8 hours (maximum: 1.8 g/day)

Administration

Oral Administer oral dosage form with a full glass of water to minimize esophageal ulceration. Give around-the-clock to promote less variation in peak and trough serum levels.

I.M. Deep I.M. sites, rotate sites. Do not exceed 600 mg in a single injection.

I.V. Never administer as bolus; administer by I.V. intermittent infusion over at least 10-60 minutes, at a rate **not** to exceed 30 mg/minute (do not exceed 1200 mg/hour). Final concentration for administration should not exceed 18 mg/mL.

I.V. Detail pH: 6.0-6.3 (usual); 5.5-7.0 (range)

Stability

Storage

Capsule: Store at room temperature of 20°C to 25°C (68°F to 77°F).

I.V.: Infusion solution in NS or D_5W solution is stable for 16 days at room temperature, 32 days refrigerated, or 8 weeks frozen. Prior to use, store vials and premixed bags at controlled room temperature 20°C to 25°C (68°F to 77°F). After initial use, discard any unused portion of vial after 24 hours.

Oral solution: Do not refrigerate reconstituted oral solution (it will thicken). Following reconstitution, oral solution is stable for 2 weeks at room temperature of 20°C to 25°C (68°F to 77°F).

Nursing Actions

Physical Assessment Previous allergy history should be assessed prior to beginning therapy. Monitor cardiac status and blood pressure and keep patient recumbent after infusion until blood pressure is stabilized.

Patient Education

I.M., I.V.: Report any burning, pain, swelling, or redness at infusion or injection site.

Oral: Take each dose with a full glass of water. You may experience nausea or vomiting. Report dizziness; persistent GI effects (pain, diarrhea, vomiting); skin redness, rash, or burning; fever; chills; unusual bruising or bleeding; signs of infection; excessive fatigue; yellowing of eyes or skin; change in color of urine or blackened stool; swelling, warmth, or pain in extremities; difficult respirations; bloody or fatty stool (do not take antidiarrheal without consulting prescriber); or lack of improvement or worsening of condition.

Dietary Considerations May be taken with food.

Related Information

Compatibility of Drugs *on page 1264*

Clindamycin (Topical) (klin da MYE sin)

Brand Names: U.S. Cleocin T®; Cleocin®; Cleocin® Vaginal Ovule; Clindagel®; ClindaMax®; ClindaReach® [DSC]; Clindesse®; Evoclin®

Index Terms Clindamycin Phosphate

Pharmacologic Category Antibiotic, Lincosamide; Topical Skin Product, Acne

Medication Safety Issues

Sound-alike/look-alike issues:

Cleocin® may be confused with bleomycin, Clinoril®, Cubicin®, Lincocin®

Clindamycin may be confused with clarithromycin, Claritin®, vancomycin

Pregnancy Risk Factor B

Lactation Enters breast milk/not recommended (AAP rates "compatible"; AAP 2001 update pending)

Use Treatment of bacterial vaginosis (vaginal cream, vaginal suppository); topically in treatment of severe acne

Available Dosage Forms

Aerosol, foam, topical: 1% (50 g, 100 g)

Evoclin®: 1% (50 g, 100 g)

Cream, vaginal: 2% (40 g)

Cleocin®: 2% (40 g)

Clindesse®: 2% (5 g)

Gel, topical: 1% (30 g, 60 g)

Cleocin T®: 1% (30 g, 60 g)

Clindagel®: 1% (40 mL, 75 mL)

ClindaMax®: 1% (30 g, 60 g)

Lotion, topical: 1% (60 mL)

Cleocin T®: 1% (60 mL)

ClindaMax®: 1% (60 mL)

Pledget, topical: 1% (60s, 69s)

Cleocin T®: 1% (60s)

Solution, topical: 1% (30 mL, 60 mL)

Cleocin T®: 1% (30 mL, 60 mL)

Suppository, vaginal:

Cleocin® Vaginal Ovule: 100 mg (3s)

General Dosage Range

Intravaginal: *Adults:* Insert 1 ovule or applicatorful once daily **or** 1 applicatorful as a single dose (Clindesse®)

Topical: *Children ≥12 years and Adults:* Apply once or twice daily

Administration

Topical

Foam: Dispense directly into cap or onto a cool surface; do not dispense directly into hands or face (foam will melt on contact with warm skin). Apply in small amounts to face using fingertips and gently massage into affected areas until foam disappears. Avoid contact with eyes.

Gel: Avoid contact with eyes.

Lotion: Shake well immediately before using.

Solution or pledget: Avoid contact with eyes, mouth or other mucous membranes; solution/pledget contains an alcohol base and if inadvertent contact with mucous membranes occurs, rinse with liberal amounts of water. Remove pledget from foil immediately before use; discard after single use. May use more than one pledget for each application to cover area.

Other Intravaginal:

Cream: Insertion with the applicator should be as far as possible into the vagina without causing discomfort.

Ovule: The foil should be removed; if the applicator is used for insertion, it should be washed for additional use.

Nursing Actions

Patient Education

Topical, foam: Wash hands thoroughly or wear gloves. Do not dispense directly onto hands or face (foam will begin to melt on contact with warm skin). Dispense an amount that will cover the affected area directly into the cap or onto a cool surface. If can seems warm or foam seems runny, run can under cold water. Pick up small amounts of foam with fingertips and gently massage into affected areas until foam disappears. Wash hands thoroughly. Wait 30 minutes before shaving or applying make-up.

Topical gel, lotion, or solution: Wash hands thoroughly before applying or wear gloves. Apply thin film of gel, lotion, or solution to affected area. May apply porous dressing. Wash hands thoroughly. Wait 30 minutes before shaving or applying make-up. Report persistent burning, swelling, itching, excessive dryness, or worsening of condition.

Vaginal: Wash hands before using. At bedtime: If using applicator, gently insert full applicator into vagina and expel cream. Wash applicator with soap and water following use. If using suppository, insert high into vagina. Remain lying down for 30 minutes following administration. Avoid intercourse during therapy. Report dizziness, nausea, vomiting, stomach cramps, headache, or lack of improvement or worsening of condition.

Clindamycin and Benzoyl Peroxide

(klin da MYE sin & BEN zoe il peer OKS ide)

Brand Names: U.S. Acanya®; BenzaClin®; Duac®; Duac® CS [DSC]

Index Terms Benzoyl Peroxide and Clindamycin; Clindamycin Phosphate and Benzoyl Peroxide

Pharmacologic Category Acne Products; Topical Skin Product; Topical Skin Product, Acne

Pregnancy Risk Factor C

Lactation Excretion in breast milk unknown/not recommended

Use Topical treatment of acne vulgaris

Available Dosage Forms

Gel, topical: Clindamycin 1% and benzoyl peroxide 5% (50 g)

Acanya®: Clindamycin 1.2% and benzoyl peroxide 2.5% (50 g)

BenzaClin®: Clindamycin 1% and benzoyl peroxide 5% (25 g, 35 g, 50 g)

Duac®: Clindamycin 1.2% and benzoyl peroxide 5% (45 g)

General Dosage Range Topical: *Children ≥12 years and Adults:* Apply once daily (Acanya®, Duac® CS) **or** twice daily (BenzaClin®) to affected areas

Administration

Topical Skin should be clean and dry before applying. For external use only; avoid applying to inside nose, mouth, eyes, and mucous membranes.

Nursing Actions

Physical Assessment See individual agents.

Patient Education See individual agents.

Related Information

Clindamycin (Topical) *on page 252*

Clindamycin and Tretinoin

(klin da MYE sin & TRET i noyn)

Brand Names: U.S. Veltin™; Ziana®

Index Terms Clindamycin Phosphate and Tretinoin; Tretinoin and Clindamycin; Veltin™

Pharmacologic Category Acne Products; Retinoic Acid Derivative; Topical Skin Product; Topical Skin Product, Acne

Pregnancy Risk Factor C

Lactation Excretion in breast milk unknown/use caution

Use Treatment of acne vulgaris

Available Dosage Forms

Gel, topical:

Veltin™: Clindamycin phosphate 1.2% and tretinoin 0.025% (30 g, 60 g)

Ziana®: Clindamycin phosphate 1.2% and tretinoin 0.025% (30 g, 60 g)

General Dosage Range Topical: *Children ≥12 years and Adults:* Apply pea-size amount to entire face once daily at bedtime

Administration

Topical At bedtime, clean face with a mild soap and pat dry before applying medication. A pea-size amount should be applied to one fingertip and then dotted on chin, cheeks, nose, and forehead. Gently rub over entire face or entire affected area while avoiding eyes, mouth, angles of nose, and mucous membranes.

Nursing Actions

Physical Assessment See individual agents.

Patient Education See individual agents.

Clobazam (KLOE ba zam)

Brand Names: U.S. Onfi™

Pharmacologic Category Benzodiazepine

Medication Safety Issues

Sound-alike/look-alike issues:

Clobazam may be confused with clonazePAM

Medication Guide Available Yes

Lactation Enters breast milk/not recommended

Use Adjunctive treatment of seizures associated with Lennox-Gastaut syndrome

Canadian labeling: Adjunctive treatment of epilepsy

Unlabeled Use Catamenial epilepsy; epilepsy (monotherapy)

Controlled Substance C-IV

Available Dosage Forms

Tablet, oral:

Onfi™: 5 mg, 10 mg, 20 mg

General Dosage Range Dosage adjustment recommended in patients with hepatic impairment or CYP2C19 poor metabolizers.

Oral: *Children ≥2 years and Adults:* Initial: 5-10 mg/day; Maintenance: Up to 40 mg/day

Administration

Oral May be administered with or without food. Tablets can be crushed and mixed in applesauce.

Nursing Actions

Physical Assessment Evaluate tolerance of medication including CNS depression (ability to function without excessive sedation or coordination impairment). For inpatient use, institute safety measures to prevent falls.

Patient Education Drug may cause physical and/or psychological dependence. While using this medication, do not use alcohol. You may experience drowsiness, dizziness, blurred vision, or constipation. Wear identification that you are taking an antiepileptic medication. Report excessive drowsiness, dizziness, fatigue, or impaired coordination; CNS changes (confusion, depression, increased sedation, excitation, headache, agitation, insomnia, or nightmares) or changes in cognition; respiratory difficulty or shortness of breath; mood changes; worsening of seizure activity; or loss of seizure control.

ClomiPHENE (KLOE mi feen)

Brand Names: U.S. Clomid®; Serophene®

Index Terms Clomiphene Citrate

Pharmacologic Category Ovulation Stimulator; Selective Estrogen Receptor Modulator (SERM)

Medication Safety Issues

Sound-alike/look-alike issues:

ClomiPHENE may be confused with clomiPRAMINE, clonidine

Clomid® may be confused with clonidine

Serophene® may be confused with Sarafem®

Pregnancy Risk Factor X

Lactation Excretion in breast milk unknown/use caution

Breast-Feeding Considerations Clomiphene may decrease lactation.

Use Treatment of ovulatory failure in patients desiring pregnancy

Mechanism of Action/Effect Clomiphene is a racemic mixture consisting of zuclomiphene (~38%) and enclomiphene (~62%) each with distinct pharmacologic properties. Zuclomiphene is more potent in inducing ovulation. Ovulation occurs by stimulating the release of pituitary gonadotropins, causing growth of the ovarian follicle followed by follicular rupture.

Contraindications Hypersensitivity to clomiphene citrate or any of its components; liver disease; abnormal uterine bleeding; enlargement or development of ovarian cyst (not due to polycystic ovarian syndrome); uncontrolled thyroid or adrenal dysfunction; presence of an organic intracranial lesion such as pituitary tumor; pregnancy

Warnings/Precautions Ovarian enlargement may occur with use; may be accompanied by abdominal distention or abdominal pain and generally regresses without treatment within 2-3 weeks. Do not continue dosing until ovaries are of normal size. Ovarian hyperstimulation syndrome (OHSS) is characterized by severe ovarian enlargement, abdominal pain/distention, nausea, vomiting, diarrhea, dyspnea, and oliguria, and may be accompanied by ascites, pleural effusion, hypovolemia, electrolyte imbalance, hemoperitoneum, and thromboembolic events. If severe hyperstimulation occurs, stop treatment and hospitalize patient. This syndrome develops rapidly within 24 hours to several days and generally occurs during the 7-10 days immediately following treatment. Use with caution in patients unusually sensitive to pituitary gonadotropins (eg, PCOS). To minimize risks, use only at the lowest effective dose. Blurring or other visual symptoms can occur; patients with visual disturbances should discontinue therapy and have an eye exam. Multiple births may result from the use of these medications; advise patient of the potential risk of multiple births before starting the treatment.

Drug Interactions

Avoid Concomitant Use There are no known interactions where it is recommended to avoid concomitant use.

Decreased Effect There are no known significant interactions involving a decrease in effect.

Increased Effect/Toxicity There are no known significant interactions involving an increase in effect.

Adverse Reactions

>10%: Endocrine & metabolic: Ovarian enlargement (14%)

1% to 10%:

Central nervous system: Headache (1%)

Endocrine & metabolic: Hot flashes (10%), breast discomfort (2%), abnormal uterine bleeding (1%)

Gastrointestinal: Distention/bloating/discomfort (6%), nausea (2%), vomiting (2%)

Ocular: Visual symptoms (2%, includes blurring of vision, diplopia, floaters, lights, phosphenes, photophobia, scotomata, waves)

Pharmacodynamics/Kinetics

Onset of Action Ovulation: 5-10 days following course of treatment

Duration of Action Effects are cumulative; ovulation may occur in the cycle following the last treatment

Available Dosage Forms

Tablet, oral: 50 mg

Clomid®: 50 mg

Serophene®: 50 mg

General Dosage Range Oral: *Adults (females):* First course: 50 mg/day for 5 days; Second course (if needed): 100 mg/day for 5 days

Administration

Oral The total daily dose should be taken at one time to maximize effectiveness.

Stability

Storage Store at room temperature of 15°C to 30°C (59°F to 86°F). Protect from light, heat, and excessive humidity.

Nursing Actions

Physical Assessment Teach patient proper use (eg, measuring basal body temperature and timing of intercourse).

Patient Education There may be a risk of multiple pregnancies with therapy. Follow recommended schedule of dosing exactly. May cause hot flashes. Report sudden abdominal discomfort, bloating or pain, nausea, or vomiting.

ClomiPRAMINE (kloe MI pra meen)

Brand Names: U.S. Anafranil®

Index Terms Clomipramine Hydrochloride

Pharmacologic Category Antidepressant, Tricyclic (Tertiary Amine)

Medication Safety Issues

Sound-alike/look-alike issues:

ClomiPRAMINE may be confused with chlorproMAZINE, clevidipine, clomiPHENE, desipramine, Norpramin®

Anafranil® may be confused with alfentanil, enalapril, nafarelin

Medication Guide Available Yes

Pregnancy Risk Factor C

Lactation Enters breast milk/not recommended (AAP rates "of concern"; AAP 2001 update pending)

Breast-Feeding Considerations Based on information from three mother-infant pairs, following maternal use of clomipramine 75-150 mg/day, the estimated exposure to the breast-feeding infant would be 0.4% to 4% of the weight-adjusted maternal dose. Adverse events have not been reported in nursing infants (information from seven cases). Infants should be monitored for signs of adverse events; routine monitoring of infant serum concentrations is not recommended.

Use Treatment of obsessive-compulsive disorder (OCD)

Unlabeled Use Depression, panic attacks, chronic pain

Mechanism of Action/Effect Clomipramine appears to affect serotonin uptake while its active metabolite, desmethylclomipramine, affects norepinephrine uptake

Contraindications Hypersensitivity to clomipramine, other tricyclic agents, or any component of the formulation; use of MAO inhibitors within 14 days; use in a patient during the acute recovery phase of MI

Warnings/Precautions [U.S. Boxed Warning]: Antidepressants increase the risk of suicidal thinking and behavior in children, adolescents, and young adults (18-24 years of age) with major depressive disorder (MDD) and other psychiatric disorders; consider risk prior to prescribing. Short-term studies did not show an increased risk in patients >24 years of age and showed a decreased risk in patients ≥65 years. Closely monitor for clinical worsening, suicidality, or unusual changes in behavior; the patient's family or caregiver should be instructed to closely observe the patient and communicate condition with healthcare provider. A medication guide should be dispensed with each prescription. **Clomipramine is FDA approved for the treatment of OCD in children ≥10 years of age.**

The possibility of a suicide attempt is inherent in major depression and may persist until remission occurs. Monitor for worsening of depression or suicidality, especially during initiation of therapy (generally first 1-2 months) or with dose increases or decreases. Use caution in high-risk patients. Worsening depression and severe abrupt suicidality that are not part of the presenting symptoms may require discontinuation or modification of drug therapy. The patient's family or caregiver should be alerted to monitor patients for the emergence of suicidality and associated behaviors (such as agitation, irritability, hostility, impulsivity, and hypomania) and notify the healthcare provider.

May worsen psychosis in some patients or precipitate a shift to mania or hypomania in patients with bipolar disorder. Patients presenting with depressive symptoms should be screened for bipolar disorder. Monotherapy in patients with bipolar disorder should be avoided. **Clomipramine is not FDA approved for bipolar depression.**

TCAs may rarely cause bone marrow suppression; monitor for any signs of infection and obtain CBC if symptoms (eg, fever, sore throat) evident. May cause seizures (relationship to dose and/or duration of therapy) - do not exceed maximum doses. Use caution in patients with a previous seizure disorder or condition predisposing to seizures such as brain damage, alcoholism, or concurrent therapy with other drugs which lower the seizure threshold. May increase the risks associated with electroconvulsive therapy. Has been associated with a high incidence of sexual dysfunction. Weight gain may occur. Hyperpyrexia has been observed with TCAs in combination with anticholinergics and/or neuroleptics, particularly during hot weather.

The degree of sedation, anticholinergic effects, and conduction abnormalities are high relative to other antidepressants. Clomipramine often causes drowsiness/sedation, resulting in impaired performance of tasks requiring alertness (eg, operating machinery or driving). Sedative effects may be additive with other CNS depressants and/or ethanol. The risk of orthostasis is moderate to high relative to other antidepressants. Use with caution in patients with a history of cardiovascular disease (including previous MI, stroke, tachycardia, or conduction abnormalities). Use with caution in patients with urinary retention, benign prostatic hyperplasia, narrow-angle glaucoma, xerostomia, visual problems, constipation, or a history of bowel obstruction.

Consider discontinuing, when possible, prior to elective surgery. Therapy should not be abruptly discontinued in patients receiving high doses for prolonged periods. Use with caution in hyperthyroid patients or those receiving thyroid supplementation. Use with caution in patients with hepatic or renal dysfunction and in elderly patients.

Drug Interactions

Avoid Concomitant Use

Avoid concomitant use of ClomiPRAMINE with any of the following: Artemether; Dronedarone; Iobenguane I 123; Lumefantrine; MAO Inhibitors; Methylene Blue; Nilotinib; Pimozide; QUEtiapine; QuiNINE; Tetrabenazine; Thioridazine; Toremifene; Vandetanib; Vemurafenib; Ziprasidone

Decreased Effect

ClomiPRAMINE may decrease the levels/effects of: Acetylcholinesterase Inhibitors (Central); Alpha2-Agonists; Codeine; Iobenguane I 123

The levels/effects of ClomiPRAMINE may be decreased by: Acetylcholinesterase Inhibitors (Central); Barbiturates; CYP1A2 Inducers (Strong); CYP2C19 Inducers (Strong); Cyproterone; Peginterferon Alfa-2b; St Johns Wort; Tocilizumab

Increased Effect/Toxicity

ClomiPRAMINE may increase the levels/effects of: Alpha-/Beta-Agonists (Direct-Acting); Alpha1-Agonists; Amphetamines; Anticholinergics; Aspirin; Beta2-Agonists; CYP2D6 Substrates; Desmopressin; Dronedarone; Fesoterodine; Methylene Blue; Metoclopramide; Milnacipran; Nebivolol; NSAID (COX-2 Inhibitor); NSAID (Nonselective); Pimozide; QTc-Prolonging Agents; QuiNIDine; QuiNINE; Serotonin Modulators; Sodium Phosphates; Sulfonylureas; Tamoxifen; Tetrabenazine; Thioridazine; Toremifene; TraMADol; Vandetanib; Vemurafenib; Vitamin K Antagonists; Yohimbine; Ziprasidone

The levels/effects of ClomiPRAMINE may be increased by: Abiraterone Acetate; Alfuzosin; Altretamine; Antipsychotics; Artemether; BuPROPion; CarBAMazepine; Chloroquine; Cimetidine; Cinacalcet; Ciprofloxacin; Ciprofloxacin (Systemic); Conivaptan; CYP1A2 Inhibitors (Moderate); CYP1A2 Inhibitors (Strong); CYP2C19 Inhibitors (Moderate); CYP2C19 Inhibitors (Strong); CYP2D6 Inhibitors (Moderate); CYP2D6 Inhibitors (Strong); Deferasirox; Dexmethylphenidate; Divalproex; DULoxetine; Gadobutrol; Grapefruit Juice; Indacaterol; Linezolid; Lithium; Lumefantrine; MAO Inhibitors; Methylphenidate; Metoclopramide; Nilotinib; Pramlintide; Protease Inhibitors; QUEtiapine; QuiNIDine; QuiNINE; Selective Serotonin Reuptake Inhibitors; Terbinafine; Terbinafine (Systemic); Valproic Acid

Nutritional/Ethanol Interactions

Ethanol: Ethanol may increase CNS depression. Management: Avoid ethanol.

Food: Serum concentrations/toxicity may be increased by grapefruit juice. Management: Avoid grapefruit juice.

Herb/Nutraceutical: St John's wort may increase the metabolism of clomipramine. Clomipramine may increase the serum concentration of yohimbe. Avoid valerian, St John's wort, SAMe, kava kava, and yohimbe.

Adverse Reactions Data shown for children reflects both children and adolescents studied in clinical trials.

>10%:

Central nervous system: Dizziness (54%), somnolence (54%), drowsiness, headache (52%; children 28%), fatigue (39%), insomnia (25%; children 11%), malaise, nervousness (18%; children 4%)

Endocrine & metabolic: Libido changes (21%), hot flushes (5%)

Gastrointestinal: Xerostomia (84%, children 63%) constipation (47%; children 22%), nausea (33%; children 9%), dyspepsia (22%; children 13%), weight gain (18%; children 2%), diarrhea (13%; children 7%), anorexia (12%; children 22%), abdominal pain (11%), appetite increased (11%)

Genitourinary: Ejaculation failure (42%), impotence (20%), micturition disorder (14%; children 4%)

Neuromuscular & skeletal: Tremor (54%), myoclonus (13%; children 2%), myalgia (13%)

Ocular: Abnormal vision (18%; children 7%)

Respiratory: Pharyngitis (14%), rhinitis (12%)

Miscellaneous: Diaphoresis increased (29%; children 9%)

1% to 10%:

Cardiovascular: Flushing (8%), postural hypotension (6%), palpitation (4%), tachycardia (4%; children 2%), chest pain (4%), edema (2%)

Central nervous system: Anxiety (9%), memory impairment (9%), twitching (7%), depression (5%), concentration impaired (5%), fever (4%), hypertonia (4%), abnormal dreaming (3%), agitation (3%), confusion (3%), migraine (3%), pain (3%), psychosomatic disorder (3%), speech disorder (3%), yawning (3%), aggressiveness (children 2%), chills (2%), depersonalization (2%), emotional lability (2%), irritability (2%), panic reaction (1%)

Dermatologic: Rash (8%), pruritus (6%), purpura (3%), dermatitis (2%), acne (2%), dry skin (2%), urticaria (1%)

Endocrine & metabolic: Amenorrhea (1%), breast enlargement (2%), breast pain (1%), hot flashes (5%), lactation (nonpuerperal) (4%)

Gastrointestinal: Taste disturbance (8%), vomiting (7%), flatulence (6%), dental caries and teeth grinding (5%), dysphagia (2%), esophagitis (1%)

Genitourinary: UTI (2% to 6%), micturition frequency (5%), dysuria (2%), leucorrhea (2%), vaginitis (2%), urinary retention (2%)

Neuromuscular & skeletal: Paresthesia (9%), back pain (6%), arthralgia (3%), paresis (children 2%), weakness (1%)

Ocular: Lacrimation abnormal (3%), mydriasis (2%), conjunctivitis (1%)

Otic: Tinnitus (6%)

Respiratory: Sinusitis (6%), coughing (6%), bronchospasm (2%; children 7%), epistaxis (2%)

Available Dosage Forms

Capsule, oral: 25 mg, 50 mg, 75 mg

Anafranil®: 25 mg, 50 mg, 75 mg

General Dosage Range Oral:

Children ≥10 years: Initial: 25 mg/day; Maintenance: Up to 3 mg/kg/day (maximum: 200 mg/day)

Adults: Initial: 25 mg/day; Maintenance: Up to 250 mg/day

Administration

Oral During titration, may divide doses and administer with meals to decrease gastrointestinal side effects. After titration, may administer total daily dose at bedtime to decrease daytime sedation.

Nursing Actions

Physical Assessment If history of cardiac problems, monitor cardiac status closely. Be alert to the potential of new or increased seizure activity. Observe for clinical worsening, suicidality, or unusual behavior changes, especially during the initial few months of therapy or during dosage changes. Instruct family or caregiver to observe the patient's behavior closely and communicate any changes to prescriber. Taper dosage slowly when discontinuing.

Patient Education Take multiple dose medication with meals to reduce side effects. Take single daily dose at bedtime to reduce daytime sedation. The effect of this drug may take several weeks to appear. Do not use alcohol. May cause weight gain, dizziness, drowsiness, headache, seizures, dry mouth or unpleasant aftertaste, constipation, or orthostatic hypotension. Report unresolved constipation or GI upset, unusual muscle weakness, palpitations, or persistent CNS disturbances (hallucinations, suicidality, seizures, delirium, insomnia, or impaired gait).

ClonazePAM (kloe NA ze pam)

Brand Names: U.S. KlonoPIN®

Pharmacologic Category Benzodiazepine

Medication Safety Issues

Sound-alike/look-alike issues:

ClonazePAM may be confused with clobazam, cloNIDine, clorazepate, cloZAPine, LORazepam

KlonoPIN® may be confused with cloNIDine, clorazepate, cloZAPine, LORazepam

Medication Guide Available Yes

Pregnancy Risk Factor D

Lactation Enters breast milk/not recommended

Breast-Feeding Considerations Clonazepam enters breast milk. Drowsiness, lethargy, or weight loss in nursing infants have been observed in case reports following maternal use of some benzodiazepines.

Use Alone or as an adjunct in the treatment of petit mal variant (Lennox-Gastaut), akinetic, and myoclonic seizures; petit mal (absence) seizures unresponsive to succimides; panic disorder with or without agoraphobia

Unlabeled Use Restless legs syndrome; neuralgia; multifocal tic disorder; parkinsonian dysarthria; bipolar disorder; adjunct therapy for schizophrenia; burning mouth syndrome

Mechanism of Action/Effect The exact mechanism is unknown, but believed to be related to its ability to enhance the activity of GABA; suppresses the spike-and-wave discharge in absence seizures by depressing nerve transmission in the motor cortex

Contraindications Hypersensitivity to clonazepam or any component of the formulation (cross-sensitivity with other benzodiazepines may exist); significant liver disease; narrow-angle glaucoma; pregnancy

Warnings/Precautions Antiepileptics are associated with an increased risk of suicidal behavior/thoughts with use (regardless of indication); patients should be monitored for signs/symptoms of depression, suicidal tendencies, and other unusual behavior changes during therapy and instructed to inform their healthcare provider immediately if symptoms occur.

Use with caution in elderly or debilitated patients, patients with hepatic disease (including alcoholics), or renal impairment. Use with caution in patients with respiratory disease or impaired gag reflex or ability to protect the airway from secretions (salivation may be increased). Worsening of seizures may occur when added to patients with multiple seizure types. Concurrent use with valproic acid may result in absence status. Monitoring of CBC and liver function tests has been recommended during prolonged therapy.

Causes CNS depression (dose related) resulting in sedation, dizziness, confusion, or ataxia which may impair physical and mental capabilities. Patients must be cautioned about performing tasks which require mental alertness (eg, operating machinery or driving). Use with caution in patients receiving other CNS depressants or psychoactive agents. Effects with other sedative drugs or ethanol may be potentiated. Benzodiazepines have been associated with falls and traumatic injury and should be used with extreme caution in patients who are at risk of these events (especially the elderly).

Use caution in patients with depression, particularly if suicidal risk may be present. Use with caution in patients with a history of drug dependence. Benzodiazepines have been associated with dependence and acute withdrawal symptoms, including seizures, on discontinuation or reduction in dose. Acute withdrawal, including seizures, may be precipitated in patients after administration of flumazenil to patients receiving long-term benzodiazepine therapy.

Benzodiazepines have been associated with anterograde amnesia. Paradoxical reactions, including hyperactive or aggressive behavior, have been reported with benzodiazepines, particularly in adolescent/pediatric or psychiatric patients. Does not have analgesic, antidepressant, or antipsychotic properties.

Drug Interactions

Avoid Concomitant Use

Avoid concomitant use of ClonazePAM with any of the following: Conivaptan; OLANZapine

Decreased Effect

The levels/effects of ClonazePAM may be decreased by: CarBAMazepine; CYP3A4 Inducers (Strong); Deferasirox; Rifamycin Derivatives; St Johns Wort; Theophylline Derivatives; Tocilizumab; Yohimbine

Increased Effect/Toxicity

ClonazePAM may increase the levels/effects of: Alcohol (Ethyl); CloZAPine; CNS Depressants; Fosphenytoin; Methotrimeprazine; Phenytoin; Selective Serotonin Reuptake Inhibitors

The levels/effects of ClonazePAM may be increased by: Antifungal Agents (Azole Derivatives, Systemic); Aprepitant; Calcium Channel Blockers (Nondihydropyridine); Cimetidine; Conivaptan; Contraceptives (Estrogens); Contraceptives (Progestins); CYP3A4 Inhibitors (Moderate); CYP3A4 Inhibitors (Strong); Dasatinib; Droperidol; Fosaprepitant; Grapefruit Juice; HydrOXYzine; Isoniazid; Ivacaftor; Macrolide Antibiotics; Methotrimeprazine; OLANZapine; Proton Pump Inhibitors; Selective Serotonin Reuptake Inhibitors

Nutritional/Ethanol Interactions

Ethanol: May increase CNS depression; monitor for increased effects with coadministration. Caution patients about effects.

Food: Clonazepam serum concentration is unlikely to be increased by grapefruit juice because of clonazepam's high oral bioavailability.

Herb/Nutraceutical: St John's wort may decrease clonazepam levels. Avoid valerian, St John's wort, kava kava, gotu kola (may increase CNS depression).

Adverse Reactions Reactions reported in patients with seizure and/or panic disorder. Frequency not always defined.

Cardiovascular: Edema (ankle or facial), palpitation

Central nervous system: Amnesia, ataxia (seizure disorder ~30%; panic disorder 5%), behavior problems (seizure disorder ~25%), coma, confusion, depression, dizziness, drowsiness (seizure disorder ~50%), emotional lability, fatigue, fever, hallucinations, headache, hypotonia, hysteria, insomnia, intellectual ability reduced, memory disturbance, nervousness; paradoxical reactions (including aggressive behavior, agitation, anxiety, excitability, hostility, irritability, nervousness, nightmares, sleep disturbance, vivid dreams); psychosis, slurred speech, somnolence (panic disorder 37%), suicidal attempt, suicide ideation, vertigo

Dermatologic: Hair loss, hirsutism, skin rash

Endocrine & metabolic: Dysmenorrhea, libido increased/decreased

Gastrointestinal: Abdominal pain, anorexia, appetite increased/decreased, coated tongue, constipation, dehydration, diarrhea, gastritis, gum soreness, nausea, weight changes (loss/gain), xerostomia

Genitourinary: Colpitis, dysuria, ejaculation delayed, enuresis, impotence, micturition frequency, nocturia, urinary retention, urinary tract infection

Hematologic: Anemia, eosinophilia, leukopenia, thrombocytopenia

Hepatic: Alkaline phosphatase increased (transient), hepatomegaly, serum transaminases increased (transient)

Neuromuscular & skeletal: Choreiform movements, coordination abnormal, dysarthria, muscle pain, muscle weakness, myalgia, tremor

Ocular: Blurred vision, eye movements abnormal, diplopia, nystagmus

Respiratory: Chest congestion, cough, bronchitis, hypersecretions, pharyngitis, respiratory depression, respiratory tract infection, rhinitis, rhinorrhea, shortness of breath, sinusitis

Miscellaneous: Allergic reaction, aphonia, dysdiadochokinesis, encopresis, "glassy-eyed" appearance, hemiparesis, lymphadenopathy

Pharmacodynamics/Kinetics

Onset of Action 20-60 minutes

Duration of Action Infants and young children: 6-8 hours; Adults: ≤12 hours

Controlled Substance C-IV

Available Dosage Forms

Tablet, oral: 0.5 mg, 1 mg, 2 mg

KlonoPIN®: 0.5 mg, 1 mg, 2 mg

Tablet, orally disintegrating, oral: 0.125 mg, 0.25 mg, 0.5 mg, 1 mg, 2 mg

General Dosage Range Oral:

Children <10 years or <30 kg: Initial: 0.01-0.03 mg/kg/day in 2-3 divided doses (maximum: 0.05 mg/kg/day); Maintenance: 0.1-0.2 mg/kg/day in 3 divided doses (maximum: 0.2 mg/kg/day)

Children ≥10 years or ≥30 kg and Adults: Panic disorders: Initial: 0.25 mg twice daily; Maintenance: 1-4 mg/day in 2 divided doses; Seizure disorders: Initial: Up to 1.5 mg/day in 3 divided doses; Maintenance: 0.05-2 mg/kg/day (maximum: 20 mg/day)

Administration

Oral Orally-disintegrating tablet: Open pouch and peel back foil on the blister; do not push tablet through foil. Use dry hands to remove tablet and place in mouth. May be swallowed with or without water. Use immediately after removing from package.

Nursing Actions

Physical Assessment Assess for signs of CNS depression (sedation, dizziness, confusion, or ataxia). Assess history of addiction; long-term use can result in dependence, abuse, or tolerance; periodically evaluate need for continued use. For inpatient use, institute safety measures to prevent falls. Taper dosage slowly when discontinuing. Teach patient seizure precautions (if administered for seizures).

Patient Education Drug may cause physical and/or psychological dependence. While using this medication, do not use alcohol. You may experience drowsiness, dizziness, blurred vision, nausea, vomiting, loss of appetite, dry mouth, or constipation. If medication is used to control seizures, wear identification that you are taking an antiepileptic medication. Report excessive drowsiness, dizziness, fatigue, or impaired coordination; CNS changes (confusion, depression, increased sedation, excitation, headache, agitation, insomnia, or nightmares) or changes in cognition; respiratory difficulty or shortness of breath; changes in urinary pattern; changes in sexual activity; muscle cramping, weakness, tremors, or rigidity; ringing in ears or visual disturbances; excessive perspiration; excessive GI symptoms (cramping, constipation, vomiting, anorexia); or worsening of seizure activity or loss of seizure control.

CloNIDine (KLON i deen)

Brand Names: U.S. Catapres-TTS®-1; Catapres-TTS®-2; Catapres-TTS®-3; Catapres®; Duraclon®; Kapvay™; Nexiclon™ XR

Index Terms Clonidine Hydrochloride

Pharmacologic Category $Alpha_2$-Adrenergic Agonist

Medication Safety Issues

Sound-alike/look-alike issues:

CloNIDine may be confused with Clomid®, clomiPHENE, clonazePAM, cloZAPine, KlonoPIN®, quiNIDine

Catapres® may be confused with Cataflam®, Combipres

High alert medication:

The Institute for Safe Medication Practices (ISMP) includes this medication (epidural administration) among its list of drug classes which have a heightened risk of causing significant patient harm when used in error.

BEERS Criteria medication:

This drug may be inappropriate for use in geriatric patients (low severity risk).

Administration issues:

Use caution when interpreting dosing information. Pediatric dose for epidural infusion expressed as mcg/kg/**hour**.

Other safety concerns:

Transdermal patch may contain conducting metal (eg, aluminum); remove patch prior to MRI. Errors have occurred when the inactive, optional adhesive cover has been applied instead of the active clonidine-containing patch.

Pregnancy Risk Factor C

Lactation Enters breast milk/not recommended

Breast-Feeding Considerations Enters breast milk with concentrations approximately twice maternal serum concentrations

Use

Oral:

Immediate release: Management of hypertension (monotherapy or as adjunctive therapy)

Extended release:

Kapvay™: Treatment of attention-deficit/hyperactivity disorder (ADHD) (monotherapy or as adjunctive therapy)

Nexiclon™ XR: Management of hypertension (monotherapy or as adjunctive therapy)

Epidural (Duraclon®): For continuous epidural administration as adjunctive therapy with opioids for treatment of severe cancer pain in patients tolerant to or unresponsive to opioids alone; epidural clonidine is generally more effective for neuropathic pain and less effective (or possibly ineffective) for somatic or visceral pain

Transdermal patch: Management of hypertension (monotherapy or as adjunctive therapy)

Unlabeled Use Heroin or nicotine withdrawal; severe pain; dysmenorrhea; vasomotor symptoms associated with menopause; ethanol dependence; prophylaxis of migraines; glaucoma; diabetes-associated diarrhea; impulse control disorder, clozapine-induced sialorrhea; aid in the diagnosis of growth hormone deficiency; attention-deficit/hyperactivity disorder (ADHD) and associated insomnia in children; Tourette's syndrome in children; aggression associated with conduct disorder

Mechanism of Action/Effect Stimulates $alpha_2$-adrenoceptors in the brain stem, thus activating an inhibitory neuron, resulting in reduced sympathetic outflow from the CNS, producing a decrease in peripheral resistance, renal vascular resistance, heart rate, and blood pressure; epidural clonidine may produce pain relief at spinal presynaptic and postjunctional $alpha_2$-adrenoceptors by preventing pain signal transmission; pain relief occurs only for the body regions innervated by the spinal segments where analgesic concentrations of clonidine exist; in the treatment of ADHD, the mechanism of action is unknown.

Contraindications Hypersensitivity to clonidine hydrochloride or any component of the formulation

Epidural administration: Injection site infection; concurrent anticoagulant therapy; bleeding diathesis; administration above the C4 dermatome

Warnings/Precautions May cause CNS depression, which may impair physical or mental abilities; patients must be cautioned about performing tasks which require mental alertness (eg, operating machinery or driving). Sedating effects may be potentiated when used with other CNS-depressant drugs or ethanol. Use with caution in patients with severe coronary insufficiency; conduction disturbances; recent MI, CVA, or chronic renal insufficiency. May cause dose dependent reductions in heart rate; use with caution in patients with preexisting bradycardia or those predisposed to developing bradycardia. Caution in sinus node dysfunction. Use with caution in patients concurrently receiving agents known to reduce SA node function and/or AV nodal conduction (eg, digoxin, diltiazem, metoprolol, verapamil). May cause significant xerostomia. Clonidine may cause eye dryness in patients who wear contact lenses.

[U.S. Boxed Warning]: Must dilute concentrated epidural injectable (500 mcg/mL) solution prior to use. Epidural clonidine is not recommended for perioperative, obstetrical, or postpartum pain due to risk of hemodynamic instability. Clonidine injection should be administered via a continuous epidural infusion device. Monitor closely for catheter-related infection such as meningitis or epidural abscess. Epidural clonidine is not recommended for use in patients with severe cardiovascular disease or hemodynamic instability; may lead to cardiovascular instability (hypotension, bradycardia). Symptomatic hypotension may occur with use; in all patients, use epidural clonidine with caution due to the potential for severe hypotension especially in women and those of low body weight. Most hypotensive episodes occur within the first 4 days of initiation; however, episodes may occur throughout the duration of therapy.

Gradual withdrawal is needed (taper oral immediate release or epidural dose gradually over 2-4 days to avoid rebound hypertension) if drug needs to be stopped. Patients should be instructed about abrupt discontinuation (causes rapid increase in BP and symptoms of sympathetic overactivity). In patients on both a beta-blocker and clonidine where withdrawal of clonidine is necessary, withdraw the beta-blocker first and several days before clonidine withdrawal, then slowly decrease clonidine. In children and adolescents, extended release formulation (Kapvay™) should be tapered in decrements of no more than 0.1 mg every 3-7 days. Discontinue oral immediate release formulations within 4 hours of surgery then restart as soon as possible afterwards. Discontinue oral extended release formulations up to 28 hours prior to surgery, then restart the following day.

Oral formulations of clonidine (immediate release versus extended release) are not interchangeable on a mg:mg basis due to different pharmacokinetic profiles. This includes commercially available oral suspension (Nexiclon™ XR) which is an extended release preparation and should not be used interchangeably with any extemporaneously prepared clonidine oral suspension.

Transdermal patch may contain conducting metal (eg, aluminum); remove patch prior to MRI. Due to the potential for altered electrical conductivity, remove transdermal patch before cardioversion or defibrillation. Localized contact sensitization to the transdermal system has been reported; in these patients, allergic reactions (eg, generalized rash, urticaria, angioedema) have also occurred following subsequent substitution of oral therapy.

Clonidine may be inappropriate for use in the elderly due to CNS adverse events and orthostatic hypotension (Beers Criteria). In pediatric patients, epidural clonidine should be reserved for cancer patients with severe intractable pain, unresponsive to other analgesics or epidural or spinal opioids. Use oral formulations with caution in pediatric patients since children commonly have gastrointestinal illnesses with vomiting and are susceptible to hypertensive episodes due to abrupt inability to take oral medication.

Drug Interactions

Avoid Concomitant Use

Avoid concomitant use of CloNIDine with any of the following: Iobenguane I 123

Decreased Effect

CloNIDine may decrease the levels/effects of: Iobenguane I 123

The levels/effects of CloNIDine may be decreased by: Antidepressants (Alpha2-Antagonist); Herbs (Hypertensive Properties); Serotonin/Norepinephrine Reuptake Inhibitors; Tricyclic Antidepressants; Yohimbine

Increased Effect/Toxicity

CloNIDine may increase the levels/effects of: Amifostine; Antihypertensives; Hypotensive Agents; RiTUXimab

The levels/effects of CloNIDine may be increased by: Alfuzosin; Beta-Blockers; Diazoxide; Herbs (Hypotensive Properties); MAO Inhibitors; Methylphenidate; Pentoxifylline; Phosphodiesterase 5 Inhibitors; Prostacyclin Analogues

Nutritional/Ethanol Interactions

Ethanol: Avoid ethanol (may increase CNS depression). *In vitro* studies have shown high concentrations of alcohol may increase the rate of release of Nexiclon™ XR.

Herb/Nutraceutical: Avoid dong quai if using for hypertension (has estrogenic activity). Avoid ephedra, yohimbe, ginseng (may worsen hypertension). Avoid valerian, St John's wort, kava kava, gotu kola (may increase CNS depression).

Adverse Reactions Frequency not always defined.

Oral, Transdermal: Incidence of adverse events may be less with transdermal compared to oral due to the lower peak/trough ratio.

Cardiovascular: Bradycardia (≤4%), palpitation (1%), tachycardia (1%), arrhythmia, atrioventricular block, chest pain, CHF, ECG abnormalities, flushing, orthostatic hypotension, pallor, Raynaud's phenomenon, syncope

Central nervous system: Drowsiness (12% to 38%), headache (1% to 29%), fatigue (4% to 16%), dizziness (2% to 16%), sedation (3% to 10%), insomnia (≤6%), lethargy (3%), nervousness (1% to 3%), mental depression (1%), aggression, agitation, anxiety, behavioral changes, CVA, delirium, delusional perception, fever, hallucinations (visual and auditory), irritability, malaise, nightmares, restlessness, vivid dreams

Dermatologic: Transient localized skin reactions characterized by pruritus and erythema (transdermal 15% to 50%), contact dermatitis (transdermal 8% to 34%), vesiculation (transdermal 7%), allergic contact sensitization (transdermal 5%), hyperpigmentation (transdermal 5%), burning (transdermal 3%), edema (3%), excoriation (transdermal 3%) blanching (transdermal 1%), generalized macular rash (1%), papules (transdermal 1%), throbbing (transdermal 1%), alopecia, angioedema, hives, localized hypopigmentation (transdermal), rash, urticaria

Endocrine & metabolic: Sexual dysfunction (3%), gynecomastia (1%), creatine phosphokinase increased (transient; oral), hyperglycemia (transient; oral), libido decreased

Gastrointestinal: Xerostomia (≤40%), constipation (2% to 10%), anorexia (1%), taste perversion (1%), weight gain (<1%), abdominal pain (oral), diarrhea, nausea, parotid gland pain (oral), parotitis (oral), pseudo-obstruction (oral), throat pain, vomiting

Genitourinary: Erectile dysfunction (2% to 3%), nocturia (1%), dysuria, enuresis, urinary retention

Hematologic: Thrombocytopenia (oral)

Hepatic: Liver function test (mild transient abnormalities; ≤1%), hepatitis

Neuromuscular & skeletal: Weakness (10%), arthralgia (1%), myalgia (1%), leg cramps (<1%), numbness (localized, transdermal), pain in extremities, paresthesia, tremor

Ocular: Accommodation disorder, blurred vision, burning eyes, dry eyes, lacrimation decreased, lacrimation increased

Otic: Ear pain, otitis media

Renal: Pollakiuria

Respiratory: Asthma, epistaxis, nasal congestion, nasal dryness, nasopharyngitis, respiratory tract infection, rhinorrhea

Miscellaneous: Withdrawal syndrome (1%), flu-like syndrome, thirst

Epidural: Note: The following adverse events occurred more often than placebo in cancer patients with intractable pain being treated with concurrent epidural morphine.

>10%:

Cardiovascular: Hypotension (45%), postural hypotension (32%)

Central nervous system: Confusion (13%), dizziness (13%)

Gastrointestinal: Xerostomia (13%)

1% to 10%:

Cardiovascular: Chest pain (5%)

Central nervous system: Hallucinations (5%)

Gastrointestinal: Nausea/vomiting (8%)

Otic: Tinnitus (5%)

Miscellaneous: Diaphoresis (5%)

Pharmacodynamics/Kinetics

Onset of Action Oral: 0.5-1 hour; Transdermal: Initial application: 2-3 days

Duration of Action 6-10 hours

Available Dosage Forms

Injection, solution [preservative free]: 100 mcg/mL (10 mL); 500 mcg/mL (10 mL)

Duraclon®: 100 mcg/mL (10 mL); 500 mcg/mL (10 mL)

Patch, transdermal: 0.1 mg/24 hours (4s); 0.2 mg/24 hours (4s); 0.3 mg/24 hours (4s)

Catapres-TTS®-1: 0.1 mg/24 hours (4s)

Catapres-TTS®-2: 0.2 mg/24 hours (4s)

Catapres-TTS®-3: 0.3 mg/24 hours (4s)

Suspension, extended release, oral:

Nexiclon™ XR: 0.09 mg/mL (118 mL)

Tablet, oral: 0.1 mg, 0.2 mg, 0.3 mg

Catapres®: 0.1 mg, 0.2 mg, 0.3 mg

Tablet, extended release, oral:

Kapvay™: 0.1 mg

Nexiclon™ XR: 0.17 mg

General Dosage Range Note: Dosing is expressed as the salt (clonidine hydrochloride) unless otherwise noted.

Epidural:

Children: Initial: 0.5 mcg/kg/**hour**

Adults: Initial: 30 mcg/hour; Maintenance: Up to 40 mcg/hour

Oral, immediate release:

Adults: Initial: 0.1 mg twice daily; Maintenance: 0.1-0.8 mg/day in 2 divided doses (maximum: 2.4 mg/day)

Elderly: Initial: 0.1 mg once daily

Oral, extended release:

Children ≥6 years: (Kapvay™): Initial: 0.1 mg at bedtime; maximum: 0.4 mg/day [ADHD use]

Adults (Nexiclon™ XR): Initial: 0.17 mg clonidine base once daily at bedtime; maintenance: 0.17-0.52 mg/day clonidine base once daily (maximum: 0.52 mg/day clonidine base) [antihypertensive]

Transdermal: *Adults:* Initial: 0.1 mg/24 hour patch applied once every 7 days; Maintenance: 0.1-0.3 mg/24 hour patch applied once every 7 days (maximum: 0.6 mg/24 hours)

Administration

Oral May be taken with or without food. Do not discontinue clonidine abruptly. If needed, gradually reduce dose over 2-4 days to avoid rebound hypertension.

Extended release products:

Kapvay™: Swallow whole; do not crush, split, or chew.

Nexiclon™ XR: Tablets may be split. Shake suspension well before use.

Topical Transdermal patch: Patches should be applied weekly at a consistent time to a clean, hairless area of the upper outer arm or chest. Rotate patch sites weekly. Redness under patch may be reduced if a topical corticosteroid spray is applied to the area before placement of the patch.

Other Epidural: Specialized techniques are required for continuous epidural administration; administration via this route should only be performed by qualified individuals familiar with the techniques of epidural administration and patient management problems associated with this route. Familiarization of the epidural infusion device is essential. Do not discontinue clonidine abruptly; if needed, gradually reduce dose over 2-4 days to avoid withdrawal symptoms.

Stability

Reconstitution Epidural formulation: Prior to administration, the 500 mcg/mL concentration must be diluted in 0.9% sodium chloride for injection (preservative-free) to a final concentration of 100 mcg/mL.

Storage

Epidural formulation: Store at 25°C (77°F); excursions permitted to 15°C to 30°C (59°F to 86°F). **Preservative free;** discard unused portion.

Oral suspension, tablets: Store at 25°C (77°F); excursions permitted to 15°C to 30°C (59°F to 86°F). Protect from light.

Transdermal patches: Store below 30°C (86°F).

Nursing Actions

Physical Assessment Assess potential for interactions with other medications that may cause additive hypotension, bradycardia, or CNS depression. Monitor blood pressure and mental status throughout. Advise patients using oral hypoglycemic agents or insulin to check glucose levels closely; clonidine may decrease the symptoms of hypoglycemia. When discontinuing, monitor blood pressure and taper dose gradually (over 1 week for oral, 2-4 days for epidural).

Patient Education Take at bedtime. If using patch, check daily for correct placement; rotate patch sites weekly. Remove patch while having MRI scan; can cause burns. Do not skip doses or discontinue without consulting prescriber (this drug must be discontinued on a specific schedule to prevent serious adverse effects). This medication may cause drowsiness, dizziness, fatigue, insomnia, decreased libido or sexual function (will resolve when drug is discontinued), postural hypotension, constipation, dry mouth, or nausea. Report chest pain, palpitations, or change in heartbeat; changes in urinary pattern; persistent nervousness, depression, lethargy, insomnia, or nightmares; sudden weight gain; unusual or persistent swelling of ankles, feet, or extremities; or skin reaction to transdermal patch.

Clopidogrel (kloh PID oh grel)

Brand Names: U.S. Plavix®

Index Terms Clopidogrel Bisulfate

Pharmacologic Category Antiplatelet Agent; Antiplatelet Agent, Thienopyridine

Medication Safety Issues

Sound-alike/look-alike issues:

Plavix® may be confused with Elavil®, Paxil®, Pradax™ (Canada), Pradaxa®

Medication Guide Available Yes

Pregnancy Risk Factor B

Lactation Excretion in breast milk unknown/not recommended

Use Reduces rate of atherothrombotic events (myocardial infarction, stroke, vascular deaths) in patients with recent MI or stroke, or established peripheral arterial disease; reduces rate of atherothrombotic events in patients with unstable angina (UA) or non-ST-segment elevation (NSTEMI) managed medically or with percutaneous coronary intervention (PCI) (with or without stent) or CABG; reduces rate of death and atherothrombotic events in patients with ST-segment elevation MI (STEMI) managed medically

Canadian labeling: Additional use (not in U.S. labeling): Prevention of atherothrombotic and thromboembolic events, including stroke, in patients with atrial fibrillation with at least 1 risk factor for vascular events who are not suitable for treatment with an anticoagulant and are at a low risk for bleeding.

Unlabeled Use In patients with allergy or major gastrointestinal intolerance to aspirin, initial treatment of acute coronary syndromes (ACS) or prevention of coronary artery bypass graft closure (saphenous vein); stable coronary artery disease (in combination with aspirin)

Mechanism of Action/Effect Irreversibly blocks platelet aggregation; platelets blocked by clopidogrel are affected for the remainder of their lifespan (~7-10 days).

Contraindications Hypersensitivity to clopidogrel or any component of the formulation; active pathological bleeding such as peptic ulcer or intracranial hemorrhage

Canadian labeling: Additional contraindications (not in U.S. labeling): Significant liver impairment or cholestatic jaundice

Warnings/Precautions [U.S. Boxed Warning]: Patients with one or more copies of the variant *CYP2C19*2* and/or *CYP2C19*3* alleles (and potentially other reduced-function variants) may have reduced conversion of clopidogrel to its active thiol metabolite. Lower active metabolite exposure may result in reduced platelet inhibition and, thus, a higher rate of cardiovascular events following MI or stent thrombosis following PCI. Although evidence is insufficient to recommend routine genetic testing, tests are available to determine CYP2C19 genotype and may be used to determine therapeutic strategy; alternative treatment or treatment strategies may be considered if patient is identified as a CYP2C19 poor metabolizer. Genetic testing may be considered prior to initiating clopidogrel in patients at moderate or high risk for poor outcomes (eg, PCI in patients with extensive and/or very complex disease). The optimal dose for CYP2C19 poor metabolizers has yet to be determined. After initiation of clopidogrel, functional testing (eg, VerifyNow® P2Y12 assay) may also be done to determine clopidogrel responsiveness (Holmes, 2010).

Use with caution in patients who may be at risk of increased bleeding, including patients with PUD, trauma, or surgery. In patients with coronary stents, premature interruption of therapy may result in stent thrombosis with subsequent fatal and nonfatal MI. Duration of therapy, in general, is determined by the type of stent placed (bare metal or drug eluting) and whether an ACS event was ongoing at the time of placement. Consider discontinuing 5 days before elective surgery (except in patients with cardiac stents that have not completed their full course of dual antiplatelet therapy; patient-specific situations need to be discussed with cardiologist; AHA/ACC/SCAI/ACS/ADA Science Advisory provides recommendations). Discontinue at least 5 days before elective CABG; when urgent CABG is necessary, the ACCF/AHA CABG guidelines recommend discontinuation for at least 24 hours prior to surgery (Hillis, 2011).

Because of structural similarities, cross-reactivity is possible among the thienopyridines (clopidogrel, prasugrel, and ticlopidine); use with caution or avoid in patients with previous thienopyridine hypersensitivity. Use of clopidogrel is contraindicated in patients with hypersensitivity to clopidogrel, although desensitization may be considered for mild-to-moderate hypersensitivity.

Use caution in concurrent treatment with anticoagulants (eg, heparin, warfarin) or other antiplatelet drugs; bleeding risk is increased. Concurrent use with drugs known to inhibit CYP2C19 (eg, proton pump inhibitors) may reduce levels of active metabolite and subsequently reduce clinical efficacy and increase the risk of cardiovascular events; if possible, avoid concurrent use of moderate-to-strong CYP2C19 inhibitors. In patients requiring antacid therapy, consider use of an acid-reducing agent lacking (eg, ranitidine) or with less CYP2C19 inhibition. According to the manufacturer, if a PPI is necessary, the use of pantoprazole, a weak CYP2C19 inhibitor, is recommended since it has been shown to have less of an effect on the pharmacologic activity of clopidogrel; lansoprazole exhibits the most potent CYP2C19 inhibition (Li, 2004). Others have recommended the continued use of PPIs, regardless of the degree of inhibition, in patients with multiple risk factors for GI bleeding who are also receiving clopidogrel since no evidence has established clinically meaningful differences in outcome; however, a clinically-significant interaction cannot be excluded in those who are poor metabolizers of clopidogrel. Staggering PPIs with clopidogrel is not recommended until further evidence is available (Abraham, 2010). Concurrent use of aspirin and clopidogrel is not recommended for secondary prevention of ischemic stroke or TIA in patients unable to take oral anticoagulants due to hemorrhagic risk (Furie, 2011).

Use with caution in patients with severe liver or renal disease (experience is limited). Cases of TTP (usually occurring within the first 2 weeks of therapy), resulting in some fatalities, have been reported; urgent plasmapheresis is required. Use in patients with severe hepatic impairment or cholestatic jaundice is contraindicated in the Canadian labeling. Cases of TTP (usually occurring within the first 2 weeks of therapy), resulting in some fatalities, have been reported; urgent plasmapheresis is required.

Assess bleeding risk carefully prior to initiating therapy in patients with atrial fibrillation (Canadian labeling; not an approved use in U.S. labeling); in clinical trials, a significant increase in major bleeding events (including intracranial hemorrhage and fatal bleeding events) were observed in patients receiving clopidogrel plus aspirin versus aspirin alone. Vitamin K antagonist (VKA) therapy (in suitable patients) has demonstrated a greater benefit in stroke reduction than aspirin (with or without clopidogrel).

Drug Interactions

Avoid Concomitant Use

Avoid concomitant use of Clopidogrel with any of the following: CYP2C19 Inhibitors (Moderate); CYP2C19 Inhibitors (Strong); Omeprazole

Decreased Effect

The levels/effects of Clopidogrel may be decreased by: Amiodarone; Calcium Channel Blockers; CYP2C19 Inhibitors (Moderate); CYP2C19 Inhibitors (Strong); Dexlansoprazole; Esomeprazole; Lansoprazole; Macrolide Antibiotics; Nonsteroidal Anti-Inflammatory Agents; Omeprazole; Pantoprazole; RABEprazole; Tocilizumab

Increased Effect/Toxicity

Clopidogrel may increase the levels/effects of: Anticoagulants; Antiplatelet Agents; Collagenase (Systemic); CYP2B6 Substrates; Drotrecogin Alfa (Activated); Ibritumomab; Rivaroxaban; Salicylates; Thrombolytic Agents; Tositumomab and Iodine I 131 Tositumomab; Warfarin

The levels/effects of Clopidogrel may be increased by: Conivaptan; Dasatinib;

Glucosamine; Herbs (Anticoagulant/Antiplatelet Properties); Nonsteroidal Anti-Inflammatory Agents; Omega-3-Acid Ethyl Esters; Pentosan Polysulfate Sodium; Pentoxifylline; Prostacyclin Analogues; Rifamycin Derivatives; Vitamin E

Nutritional/Ethanol Interactions Herb/Nutraceutical: Avoid alfalfa, anise, bilberry, bladderwrack, bromelain, cat's claw, chamomile, coleus, cordyceps, dong quai, evening primrose oil, fenugreek, feverfew, garlic, ginger, ginkgo biloba, ginseng (American), ginseng (Panax), ginseng (Siberian), grape seed, green tea, guggul, horse chestnut seed, horseradish, licorice, prickly ash, red clover, reishi, SAMe (S-adenosylmethionine), sweet clover, turmeric, white willow (all have additional antiplatelet activity).

Adverse Reactions As with all drugs which may affect hemostasis, bleeding is associated with clopidogrel. Hemorrhage may occur at virtually any site. Risk is dependent on multiple variables, including the concurrent use of multiple agents which alter hemostasis and patient susceptibility.

3% to 10%:

- Dermatologic: Rash (4%), pruritus (3%)
- Hematologic: Bleeding (major 4%; minor 5%), purpura/bruising (5%), epistaxis (3%)

1% to 3%:

- Gastrointestinal: GI hemorrhage (2%)
- Hematologic: Hematoma

Pharmacodynamics/Kinetics

Onset of Action

Onset of action: Inhibition of platelet aggregation (IPA): Dose-dependent:

300-600 mg loading dose: Detected within 2 hours

50-100 mg/day: Detected by the second day of treatment

Peak effect: Time to maximal IPA: Dose-dependent: **Note:** Degree of IPA based on adenosine diphosphate (ADP) concentration used during light aggregometry:

300-600 mg loading dose:

ADP 5 micromole/L: 20% to 30% IPA at 6 hours post administration (Montelescot, 2006)

ADP 20 micromole/L: 30% to 37% IPA at 6 hours post administration (Montelescot, 2006)

50-100 mg/day: ADP 5 micromole/L: 50% to 60% IPA at 5-7 days (Herbert, 1993)

Available Dosage Forms

Tablet, oral:

Plavix®: 75 mg, 300 mg

General Dosage Range Oral: *Adults:* Loading dose: 300 mg (maximum: 600 mg); Maintenance: 75 mg once daily

Administration

Oral May be administered without regard to meals.

Stability

Storage Store at 25°C (77°F); excursions permitted to 15°C to 30°C (59°F to 86°F).

Nursing Actions

Physical Assessment Because of the effect on platelets, there is an increased risk of bleeding. Clopidogrel is contraindicated and should be discontinued 5-10 days before surgery given potential for bleeding; assess risk of temporarily discontinuing clopidogrel in patients with recently placed cardiac stents. Review patients' medications, as omeprazole and other proton pump inhibitors may decrease clopidogrel's effectiveness. Monitor for enhanced bleeding effects if used concurrently with warfarin. Inform patients to call for help immediately if there is concern for a new heart attack or stroke.

Patient Education Patients should inform their prescriber if they have a history of hemophilia, GI bleed, stroke, CVA, or taking warfarin. Patients need to be informed that they may bruise or bleed easily. Patients should inform their prescriber if they develop bloody or black stools, gum or nose bleeding, unusual menstrual or heavy periods, or coughing or vomiting blood. In addition, patients need to call for help immediately if they develop symptoms of stroke or heart attack. Symptoms include chest or jaw pain, shortness of breath, sweating or weakness, slurred speech, sudden vision changes, or confusion. Due to potential bleeding risks, prescribers need to discuss with the patient's cardiologist the risk vs benefit of clopidogrel in the face of surgery.

Dietary Considerations May be taken without regard to meals.

Clorazepate (klor AZ e pate)

Brand Names: U.S. Tranxene® T-Tab®

Index Terms Clorazepate Dipotassium; Tranxene T-Tab

Pharmacologic Category Benzodiazepine

Medication Safety Issues

Sound-alike/look-alike issues:

Clorazepate may be confused with clofibrate, clonazepam, KlonoPIN®

BEERS Criteria medication:

This drug may be inappropriate for use in geriatric patients (high severity risk).

Medication Guide Available Yes

Lactation Enters breast milk/not recommended

Use Treatment of generalized anxiety disorder; management of ethanol withdrawal; adjunct anticonvulsant in management of partial seizures

Controlled Substance C-IV

Available Dosage Forms

Tablet, oral: 3.75 mg, 7.5 mg, 15 mg

Tranxene® T-Tab®: 3.75 mg, 7.5 mg, 15 mg

General Dosage Range Oral:

Children 9-12 years: Initial: 3.75-7.5 mg twice daily; Maintenance: Up to 60 mg/day in 2-3 divided doses

Children >12 years: Initial: Up to 7.5 mg 2-3 times/day; Maintenance: Up to 90 mg/day

Adults: Initial: 7.5-15 mg 2-4 times/day; Maintenance: Up to 90 mg/day

Elderly: Anxiety: 7.5 mg 1-2 times/day

Nursing Actions

Physical Assessment Assess for signs of CNS depression (sedation, dizziness, confusion, ataxia, potential for suicide ideation). Assess for history of addiction; long-term use can result in dependence, abuse, or tolerance; periodically evaluate need for continued use. For inpatient use, institute safety measures to prevent falls. Taper dosage slowly when discontinuing.

Patient Education Drug may cause physical and/or psychological dependence. Do not use alcohol. You may experience drowsiness, lightheadedness, impaired coordination, dizziness, blurred vision, nausea, vomiting, dry mouth, constipation, altered sexual drive or ability (reversible), or photosensitivity. Report persistent CNS effects (eg, confusion, depression, suicide ideation, increased sedation, excitation, headache, agitation, insomnia or nightmares, dizziness, fatigue, impaired coordination, changes in personality, or changes in cognition); changes in urinary pattern; muscle cramping, weakness, tremors, or rigidity; ringing in ears or visual disturbances; chest pain, palpitations, or rapid heartbeat; excessive perspiration; excessive GI symptoms (cramping, constipation, vomiting, anorexia); or worsening of condition.

Clotrimazole (Oral) (kloe TRIM a zole)

Index Terms Mycelex

Pharmacologic Category Antifungal Agent, Oral Nonabsorbed

Medication Safety Issues

Sound-alike/look-alike issues:

Clotrimazole may be confused with co-trimoxazole

Mycelex may be confused with Myoflex®

International issues:

Cloderm: Brand name for clotrimazole [Germany], but also brand name for alclomethasone [Indonesia]; clobetasol [China, India, Malaysia, Singapore, Thailand]; clocortolone [U.S., Canada]

Canesten [multiple international markets] may be confused with Canesten Bifonazol Comp brand name for bifonazole/urea [Austria]; Canesten Extra brand name for bifonazole [China, Germany]; Canesten Extra Nagelset brand name for bifonazole/urea [Denmark]; Canesten Fluconazole brand name for fluconazole [New Zealand]; Canesten Oasis brand name for sodium citrate [Great Britain]; Canesten Once Daily brand name for bifonazole [Australia]; Canesten Oral brand name for fluconazole [United Kingdom]; Cenestin brand name for estrogens (conjugated A/synthetic) [U.S., Canada]

Mycelex: Brand name for clotrimazole [U.S.] may be confused with Mucolex brand name for bromhexine [Malaysia]; carbocisteine [Thailand]

Pregnancy Risk Factor C

Lactation Excretion in breast milk unknown

Use Treatment of susceptible fungal infections, including oropharyngeal candidiasis; limited data suggest that clotrimazole troches may be effective for prophylaxis against oropharyngeal candidiasis in neutropenic patients

Available Dosage Forms

Troche, oral: 10 mg

General Dosage Range Oral: *Children >3 years and Adults:* Prophylaxis: 10 mg 3 times/day; Treatment: 10 mg 5 times/day

Administration

Oral Troche: Allow to dissolve slowly over 15-30 minutes.

Nursing Actions

Patient Education Do not swallow oral medication whole; allow to dissolve slowly in mouth. You may experience nausea or vomiting. Report signs of opportunistic infection (eg, white plaques in mouth, fever, chills, perianal itching, vaginal itching or discharge, fatigue, unhealed wounds or sores).

Clozapine (KLOE za peen)

Brand Names: U.S. Clozaril®; FazaClo®

Pharmacologic Category Antipsychotic Agent, Atypical

Medication Safety Issues

Sound-alike/look-alike issues:

CloZAPine may be confused with clonazePAM, cloNIDine, KlonoPIN®

Clozaril® may be confused with Clinoril®, Colazal®

Pregnancy Risk Factor B

Lactation Enters breast milk/not recommended (AAP rates "of concern"; AAP 2001 update pending)

Breast-Feeding Considerations Clozapine was found to accumulate in breast milk in concentrations higher than the maternal plasma.

Use Treatment-refractory schizophrenia; to reduce risk of recurrent suicidal behavior in schizophrenia or schizoaffective disorder

Unlabeled Use Schizoaffective disorder, bipolar disorder, childhood psychosis, severe obsessive-compulsive disorder; psychosis/agitation related to Alzheimer's dementia

Mechanism of Action/Effect Clozapine (dibenzodiazepine antipsychotic) exhibits weak antagonism of D_1, D_2, D_3, and D_5 dopamine receptor subtypes, but shows high affinity for D_4; in addition, it blocks the serotonin ($5HT_2$), alpha-adrenergic, histamine H_1, and cholinergic receptors

Contraindications Hypersensitivity to clozapine or any component of the formulation; history of agranulocytosis or severe granulocytopenia with clozapine; uncontrolled epilepsy, severe central nervous system depression or comatose state; paralytic ileus; myeloproliferative disorders or use with other agents which have a well-known risk of agranulocytosis or bone marrow suppression

Canadian labeling: Additional contraindications (not in U.S. labeling): Active hepatic disease associated with nausea, anorexia, or jaundice; progressive hepatic disease or hepatic failure; severe renal impairment; severe cardiac disease (eg, myocarditis); patients unable to undergo blood testing

Warnings/Precautions [U.S. Boxed Warning]: Elderly patients with dementia-related psychosis treated with antipsychotics are at an increased risk of death compared to placebo. Most deaths appeared to be either cardiovascular (eg, heart failure, sudden death) or infectious (eg, pneumonia) in nature. Clozapine is not approved for the treatment of dementia-related psychosis.

[U.S. Boxed Warning]: Significant risk of agranulocytosis, potentially life-threatening. Therapy should not be initiated in patients with WBC <3500 cells/mm^3 or ANC <2000 cells/mm^3 or history of myeloproliferative disorder. WBC testing should occur periodically on an on-going basis (see prescribing information for monitoring details) to ensure that acceptable WBC/ANC counts are maintained. Initial episodes of moderate leukopenia or granulopoietic suppression confer up to a 12-fold increased risk for subsequent episodes of agranulocytosis. WBCs must be monitored weekly for at least 4 weeks after therapy discontinuation or until WBC is ≥3500/mm^3 and ANC is ≥2000/mm^3. Use with caution in patients receiving other marrow suppressive agents. Eosinophilia has been reported to occur with clozapine. Interrupt therapy for eosinophil count >4000/mm^3. May resume therapy when eosinophil count <3000/mm^3. (**Note:** The Canadian labeling recommends discontinuing therapy for eosinophil count >3000/mm^3; may resume therapy when eosinophil count <1000/mm^3). Due to the significant risk of agranulocytosis, it is strongly recommended that a patient must fail at least two trials of other primary medications for the treatment of schizophrenia (of adequate dose and duration) before initiating therapy with clozapine.

Cognitive and/or motor impairment (sedation) is common with clozapine, resulting in impaired performance of tasks requiring alertness (eg, operating machinery or driving); use caution in patients receiving general anesthesia. **[U.S. Boxed Warning]: Seizures have been associated with clozapine use in a dose-dependent manner;** use with caution in patients at risk of seizures, including those with a history of seizures, head trauma, brain damage, alcoholism, or concurrent therapy with medications which may lower seizure threshold. Benign transient temperature elevation (>100.4°F) may occur; peaking within the first 3 weeks of treatment. Rule out infection, agranulocytosis, and neuroleptic malignant syndrome (NMS) in patients presenting with fever. However, clozapine may also be associated with severe febrile reactions, including neuroleptic malignant syndrome (NMS). Clozapine's potential for extrapyramidal symptoms (including tardive dyskinesia) appears to be extremely low. Risk of dystonia (and probably other EPS) may be greater with increased doses, use of conventional antipsychotics, males, and younger patients.

Deep vein thrombosis, myocarditis, pericarditis, pericardial effusion, cardiomyopathy, and HF have also been associated with clozapine. **[U.S. Boxed Warning]: Fatalities due to myocarditis have been reported; highest risk in the first month of therapy, however, later cases also reported.** Myocarditis or cardiomyopathy should be considered in patients who present with signs/symptoms of heart failure (dyspnea, fatigue, orthopnea, paroxysmal nocturnal dyspnea, peripheral edema), chest pain, palpitations, new electrocardiographic abnormalities (arrhythmias, ST-T wave abnormalities), or unexplained fever. Patients with tachycardia during the first month of therapy should be closely monitored for other signs of myocarditis. Discontinue clozapine if myocarditis is suspected; do not rechallenge in patients with clozapine-related myocarditis. The reported rate of myocarditis in clozapine-treated patients appears to be 17-322 times greater than in the general population. Clozapine should be discontinued in patients with confirmed cardiomyopathy unless benefit clearly outweighs risk. Rare cases of thromboembolism, including pulmonary embolism and stroke resulting in fatalities, have been associated with clozapine.

An increased incidence of cerebrovascular effects (eg, transient ischemic attack, stroke), including fatalities, has been reported in placebo-controlled trials of atypical antipsychotics in elderly patients with dementia-related psychosis.

May cause anticholinergic effects; use with caution in patients with urinary retention, benign prostatic hyperplasia, narrow-angle glaucoma, xerostomia, visual problems, constipation, or history of bowel obstruction. May cause hyperglycemia; in some cases may be extreme and associated with ketoacidosis, hyperosmolar coma, or death. Use with caution in patients with diabetes or other disorders of glucose regulation; monitor for worsening of glucose control. Antipsychotic use has been associated with esophageal dysmotility and aspiration; use with caution in patients at risk of pneumonia (eg, Alzheimer's disease). Use with caution in patients with hepatic disease or impairment; monitor hepatic function regularly. Hepatitis has been reported as a consequence of therapy. Discontinuation of therapy may be necessary with significant elevations in liver function tests; may reinitiate with close monitoring and if values return to normal. Use with caution in patients with renal disease.

Use caution with cardiovascular or pulmonary disease; gradually increase dose. **[U.S. Boxed Warning]: May cause orthostatic hypotension (with or without syncope);** generally occurs more frequently with initial titration and in association with rapid dose increases; use with caution in patients at risk of hypotension or in patients where transient hypotensive episodes would be poorly tolerated (cardiovascular disease or cerebrovascular disease). Concurrent use with benzodiazepines may increase the risk of severe cardiopulmonary reactions. May cause tachycardia (including sustained); sustained tachycardia is not limited to a reflex response to orthostatic hypotension, and is present in all positions.

The possibility of a suicide attempt is inherent in psychotic illness or bipolar disorder; use caution in high-risk patients during initiation of therapy. Prescriptions should be written for the smallest quantity consistent with good patient care.

Medication should not be stopped abruptly; taper off over 1-2 weeks. If conditions warrant abrupt discontinuation (leukopenia, myocarditis, cardiomyopathy), monitor patient for psychosis and cholinergic rebound (headache, nausea, vomiting, diarrhea). Significant weight gain has been observed with antipsychotic therapy; incidence varies with product. Monitor waist circumference and BMI. Elderly patients are more susceptible to adverse effects (including agranulocytosis, cardiovascular, anticholinergic, and tardive dyskinesia). Clozapine levels may be lower in patients who smoke. Smoking cessation may cause toxicity in a patient stabilized on clozapine. Monitor change in smoking. FazaClo® oral disintegrating tablets contain phenylalanine.

Drug Interactions

Avoid Concomitant Use

Avoid concomitant use of CloZAPine with any of the following: Artemether; Dronedarone; Lumefantrine; Metoclopramide; Myelosuppressive Agents; Nilotinib; Pimozide; QUEtiapine; QuiNINE; Tetrabenazine; Thioridazine; Toremifene; Vandetanib; Vemurafenib; Ziprasidone

Decreased Effect

CloZAPine may decrease the levels/effects of: Amphetamines; Anti-Parkinson's Agents (Dopamine Agonist); Codeine; Quinagolide

The levels/effects of CloZAPine may be decreased by: CarBAMazepine; CYP1A2 Inducers (Strong); Cyproterone; Fosphenytoin; Lithium formulations; Omeprazole; Phenytoin; Tocilizumab

Increased Effect/Toxicity

CloZAPine may increase the levels/effects of: Alcohol (Ethyl); Anticholinergics; ARIPiprazole; CNS Depressants; CYP2D6 Substrates; Dronedarone; Fesoterodine; Methylphenidate; Nebivolol; Pimozide; QTc-Prolonging Agents; QuiNINE; Serotonin Modulators; Tamoxifen; Tetrabenazine; Thioridazine; Toremifene; Vandetanib; Vemurafenib; Ziprasidone

The levels/effects of CloZAPine may be increased by: Abiraterone Acetate; Acetylcholinesterase Inhibitors (Central); Alfuzosin; Artemether; Benzodiazepines; Chloroquine; Cimetidine; Ciprofloxacin; Ciprofloxacin (Systemic); Conivaptan; CYP1A2 Inhibitors (Moderate); CYP1A2 Inhibitors (Strong); Deferasirox; Gadobutrol; HydrOXYzine; Indacaterol; Lithium formulations; Lumefantrine; Macrolide Antibiotics; MAO Inhibitors; Methylphenidate; Metoclopramide; Myelosuppressive Agents; Nefazodone; Nilotinib; Omeprazole; Pramlintide; QUEtiapine; QuiNINE; Selective Serotonin Reuptake Inhibitors; Tetrabenazine

Nutritional/Ethanol Interactions

Ethanol: May increase CNS depression; monitor for increased effects with coadministration. Caution patients about effects.

Herb/Nutraceutical: St John's wort may decrease clozapine levels. Avoid kava kava, gotu kola, valerian, St John's wort (may increase CNS depression).

Adverse Reactions

>10%:

Cardiovascular: Tachycardia (25%)

Central nervous system: Drowsiness (39% to 46%), dizziness (19% to 27%), insomnia (2% to 20%)

Gastrointestinal: Sialorrhea (31% to 48%), weight gain (4% to 31%), constipation (14% to 25%), nausea/vomiting (3% to 17%)

1% to 10%:

Cardiovascular: Hypotension (9%), syncope (6%), hypertension (4%), angina (1%), ECG changes (1%)

Central nervous system: Headache (7%), agitation (4%), akinesia (4%), nightmares (4%), restlessness (4%), akathisia (3%), confusion (3%), seizure (3%), anxiety (1%), ataxia (1%), depression (1%), lethargy (1%), myoclonic jerks (1%), slurred speech (1%)

Dermatologic: Rash (2%)

Gastrointestinal: Abdominal discomfort/heartburn (4% to 14%), xerostomia (6%), diarrhea (2%), anorexia (1%), throat discomfort (1%)

Genitourinary: Urinary abnormalities (eg, abnormal ejaculation, retention, urgency, incontinence; 1% to 2%)

Hematologic: Agranulocytosis (1%), eosinophilia (1%), leukocytosis, leukopenia

Hepatic: Liver function tests abnormal (1%)

Neuromuscular & skeletal: Tremor (6%), hypokinesia (4%), rigidity (3%), hyperkinesia (1%), weakness (1%), pain (1%), spasm (1%)

Ocular: Visual disturbances (5%)

Respiratory: Dyspnea (1%), nasal congestion (1%)
Miscellaneous: Diaphoresis (6%), tongue numbness (1%)

Available Dosage Forms

Tablet, oral: 25 mg, 50 mg, 100 mg, 200 mg
Clozaril®: 25 mg, 100 mg

Tablet, orally disintegrating, oral:
FazaClo®: 12.5 mg, 25 mg, 100 mg, 150 mg, 200 mg

General Dosage Range Dosage adjustment recommended in patients who develop toxicities

Oral: *Adults:* Initial: 12.5 mg once or twice daily; Maintenance: 12.5-900 mg/day (maximum: 900 mg/day)

Administration

Oral May be taken without regard to food. Total daily dose may be divided into uneven doses with larger dose administered at bedtime.

Canadian labeling: Maintenance dosing ≤200 mg/day may be administered as single dose in the evening.

Orally-disintegrating tablet: Should be removed from foil blister by peeling apart (do not push tablet through the foil). Remove immediately prior to use. Place tablet in mouth and allow to dissolve; swallow with saliva. If dosing requires splitting tablet, throw unused portion away.

Stability

Storage Store at ≤30°C (86°F).
FazaClo®: Store at 25°C (77°F); excursions permitted to 15°C to 30°C (59°F to 86°F). Protect from moisture; do not remove from package until ready to use.

Nursing Actions

Physical Assessment Initiate at lower doses and taper dosage slowly when discontinuing. Instruct patients with diabetes to monitor blood glucose levels frequently; may cause hyperglycemia. Be alert to the potential for cardiac abnormalities. Monitor weight prior to treatment and at least monthly. Review ophthalmic exam and monitor mental status, mood, and affect prior to treatment and periodically throughout. Monitor for orthostatic hypotension, ECG changes, and anticholinergic and extrapyramidal symptoms.

Patient Education Avoid alcohol. Maintain adequate hydration. If you have diabetes, monitor blood glucose levels frequently. You may experience headache, excess drowsiness, dizziness, or blurred vision; constipation; dry mouth, nausea, or vomiting; or postural hypotension. You may be prone to infections; report fever, sore throat, or other possible signs of infection. Report persistent CNS effects (insomnia, depression, altered consciousness); palpitations, rapid heartbeat, or severe dizziness; vision changes; hypersalivation, tearing, or sweating; seizures; chest pain or shortness of breath; excessive fatigue; or worsening of condition.

Dietary Considerations May be taken without regard to food. Some products may contain phenylalanine.

Codeine (KOE deen)

Index Terms Codeine Phosphate; Codeine Sulfate; Methylmorphine

Pharmacologic Category Analgesic, Opioid; Antitussive

Medication Safety Issues

Sound-alike/look-alike issues:
Codeine may be confused with Cardene®, Cordran®, iodine, Lodine

High alert medication:
The Institute for Safe Medication Practices (ISMP) includes this medication among its list of drug classes which have a heightened risk of causing significant patient harm when used in error.

Pregnancy Risk Factor C

Lactation Enters breast milk/use caution (AAP rates "compatible"; AAP 2001 update pending)

Use Treatment of mild-to-moderate pain

Unlabeled Use Short-term relief of coughing in select patients

Controlled Substance C-II

Available Dosage Forms

Powder, for prescription compounding: USP: 100% (10 g, 25 g)

Tablet, oral: 15 mg, 30 mg, 60 mg

General Dosage Range Dosage adjustment recommended in patients with renal and hepatic impairment

Oral: *Adults:* Initial: 15-60 mg every 4 hours as needed; maximum total daily dose: 360 mg/day

Administration

Oral May administer without regard to meals. Take with food or milk to decrease adverse GI effects.

Controlled release tablets: Codeine Contin® (Canadian availability; not available in U.S.): Tablets should be swallowed whole; do not chew, dissolve, or crush. All strengths may be halved, **except** the 50 mg tablets; half tablets should also be swallowed intact.

Nursing Actions

Physical Assessment Monitor for effectiveness of pain relief. Monitor blood pressure, CNS and respiratory status, and degree of sedation prior to treatment and periodically throughout. May cause physical and/or psychological dependence. For inpatients, implement safety measures (eg, side rails up, call light within reach, instructions to call for assistance). Assess patient's physical and/or psychological dependence. Discontinue slowly after prolonged use.

Patient Education May cause physical and/or psychological dependence. Do not use alcohol, sedatives, tranquilizers, antihistamines, or pain medications without consulting prescriber.

Maintain adequate hydration, unless instructed to restrict fluid intake. May cause dizziness, drowsiness, confusion, agitation, impaired coordination, or blurred vision; nausea or vomiting; loss of appetite; or constipation (if unresolved, consult prescriber about use of stool softeners). Report confusion, insomnia, excessive nervousness, excessive sedation or drowsiness, or shakiness; acute GI upset; respiratory difficulty or shortness of breath; facial flushing, rapid heartbeat, or palpitations; urinary difficulty; unusual muscle weakness; or vision changes.

Colchicine (KOL chi seen)

Brand Names: U.S. Colcrys®

Pharmacologic Category Antigout Agent

Medication Safety Issues

Sound-alike/look-alike issues:

Colchicine may be confused with Cortrosyn®

Medication Guide Available Yes

Pregnancy Risk Factor C

Lactation Enters breast milk/use caution (AAP rates "compatible"; AAP 2001 update pending)

Breast-Feeding Considerations Colchicine enters breast milk; exclusively breast-fed infants are expected to receive <10% of the weight-adjusted maternal dose (limited data).

Use Prevention and treatment of acute gout flares; treatment of familial Mediterranean fever (FMF)

Unlabeled Use Primary biliary cirrhosis; pericarditis

Mechanism of Action/Effect Reduces the deposition of urate crystals that perpetuates the inflammatory response

Contraindications Concomitant use of a P-glycoprotein (P-gp) or strong CYP3A4 inhibitor in presence of renal or hepatic impairment

Canadian labeling: Additional contraindications (not in U.S. labeling): Hypersensitivity to colchicine; serious gastrointestinal, hepatic, renal, and cardiac disease

Warnings/Precautions Hazardous agent - use appropriate precautions for handling and disposal. Myelosuppression (eg, thrombocytopenia, leukopenia, granulocytopenia, pancytopenia) and aplastic anemia have been reported in patients receiving therapeutic doses. Neuromuscular toxicity (including rhabdomyolysis) has been reported in patients receiving therapeutic doses; patients with renal dysfunction and elderly patients are at increased risk. Concomitant use of cyclosporine, diltiazem, verapamil, fibrates, and statins may increase the risk of myopathy. Clearance is decreased in renal or hepatic impairment; monitor closely for adverse effects/toxicity. Dosage adjustments may be required depending on degree of impairment or indication, and may be affected by the use of concurrent medication (CYP3A4 or P-gp inhibitors). Concurrent use of P-gp or strong CYP3A4 inhibitors is contraindicated in renal impairment; fatal toxicity has been reported. Colchicine does not have analgesic activity and should not be used to treat pain from other causes. Colchicine requires dosage adjustment when used concurrently with protease inhibitor regimens. Colchicine does not have analgesic activity and should not be used to treat pain from other causes. Canadian labeling does not include recommendations for use in children.

Drug Interactions

Avoid Concomitant Use

Avoid concomitant use of Colchicine with any of the following: Axitinib

Decreased Effect

Colchicine may decrease the levels/effects of: ARIPiprazole; Axitinib; Cyanocobalamin; Saxagliptin

The levels/effects of Colchicine may be decreased by: P-glycoprotein/ABCB1 Inducers; Tocilizumab

Increased Effect/Toxicity

Colchicine may increase the levels/effects of: HMG-CoA Reductase Inhibitors

The levels/effects of Colchicine may be increased by: CYP3A4 Inhibitors (Moderate); CYP3A4 Inhibitors (Strong); Dasatinib; Digoxin; Fibric Acid Derivatives; P-glycoprotein/ABCB1 Inhibitors; Telaprevir

Nutritional/Ethanol Interactions

Ethanol: Management: Avoid ethanol.

Food: Grapefruit juice may increase colchicine serum concentrations. Management: Administer orally with water and maintain adequate fluid intake. Dose adjustment may be required based on indication if ingesting grapefruit juice. Avoid grapefruit juice with hepatic or renal impairment.

Herb/Nutraceutical: Cyanocobalamin (vitamin B_{12}) absorption may be decreased by colchicine and result in macrocytic anemia or neurologic dysfunction. Management: Consider supplementing with vitamin B_{12}.

Adverse Reactions

>10%: Gastrointestinal: Gastrointestinal disorders including abdominal pain, cramping, nausea, vomiting (up to 26%), diarrhea (up to 23%)

1% to 10%: Respiratory: Pharyngolaryngeal pain (3%)

Pharmacodynamics/Kinetics

Onset of Action Oral: Pain relief: ~18-24 hours

Available Dosage Forms

Tablet, oral: 0.6 mg

Colcrys®: 0.6 mg

General Dosage Range Dosage adjustment recommended in patients with renal impairment or on concomitant therapy

Oral:

Children 4-6 years: 0.3-1.8 mg/day in 1-2 divided doses

Children 6-12 years: 0.9-1.8 mg/day in 1-2 divided doses

Children 12-16 years: 1.2-2.4 mg/day in 1-2 divided doses

Children >16 years and Adults: 0.6-2.4 mg/day in 1-2 divided doses **or** Initial: 1.2 mg; repeat with 0.6 mg in 1 hour (maximum total therapy: 1.8 mg)

Administration

Oral Administer orally with water and maintain adequate fluid intake. May be administered without regard to meals.

Stability

Storage Store at 20°C to 25°C (68°F to 77°F). Protect from light.

Nursing Actions

Patient Education Consult prescriber about a low-purine diet. Maintain adequate hydration, unless instructed to restrict fluid intake. Avoid grapefruit and grapefruit juice. You may experience diarrhea, nausea, vomiting, anorexia, or hair loss (reversible). Stop medication and report to prescriber if severe vomiting, watery or bloody diarrhea, or abdominal pain occurs. Report muscle tremors or weakness, numbness or tingling in fingers or toes, fatigue, numbness or tingling in fingers or toes, easy bruising or bleeding, yellowing of eyes or skin, or pale stool or dark urine.

Dietary Considerations May be taken without regard to meals. May need to supplement with vitamin B_{12}. Avoid grapefruit juice.

Colchicine and Probenecid

(KOL chi seen & proe BEN e sid)

Index Terms ColBenemid; Probenecid and Colchicine

Pharmacologic Category Anti-inflammatory Agent; Antigout Agent; Uricosuric Agent

Use Treatment of chronic gouty arthritis when complicated by frequent, recurrent acute attacks of gout

Available Dosage Forms

Tablet: Colchicine 0.5 mg and probenecid 0.5 g

General Dosage Range Dosage adjustment recommended in patients with renal impairment

Oral: *Adults:* Initial: One tablet daily; Maintenance: 1 tablet twice daily

Administration

Oral Do not initiate therapy until acute attack has subsided.

Nursing Actions

Physical Assessment See individual agents.

Patient Education See individual agents.

Related Information

Colchicine *on page 269*

Probenecid *on page 952*

Colesevelam (koh le SEV a lam)

Brand Names: U.S. Welchol®

Pharmacologic Category Antilipemic Agent, Bile Acid Sequestrant

Pregnancy Risk Factor B

Lactation Does not enter breast milk/use caution

Use Management of elevated LDL in primary hypercholesterolemia (Fredrickson type IIa) when used alone or in combination with an HMG-CoA reductase inhibitor; management of heterozygous familial hypercholesterolemia (heFH) in adolescent patients (males and postmenarcheal females 10-17 years of age) when used alone or in combination with an HMG-CoA reductase inhibitor, in patients who after an adequate trial of dietary therapy have LDL-C ≥190 mg/dL or LDL-C ≥160 mg/dL with positive family history of premature cardiovascular disease (CVD) or with two or more CVD risk factors; improve glycemic control in type 2 diabetes mellitus (noninsulin dependent, NIDDM) in conjunction with diet, exercise, and insulin or oral antidiabetic agents

Available Dosage Forms

Granules for suspension, oral:

Welchol®: 3.75 g/packet (30s)

Tablet, oral:

Welchol®: 625 mg

General Dosage Range Oral: *Children 10-17 years (males and postmenarchal females) and Adults:* 3.75 g/day in 1-2 divided doses

Administration

Oral Educate the patient on dietary guidelines.

Tablets: Administer with meal(s) and a liquid. Due to tablet size, it is recommended that any patient who has trouble swallowing tablets should use the oral suspension form.

Granules for oral suspension: Administer with meal(s). Empty 1 packet into a glass; add 1/2-1 cup (4-8 ounces) of water, fruit juice, or a diet soft drink and mix well. Powder is not to be taken in dry form (to avoid GI distress).

Nursing Actions

Physical Assessment Many other medications should not be administered with colesevelam.

Patient Education Many other medications should be taken 1 hour before or 4 hours after colesevelam. You may experience constipation. Report persistent GI upset, skeletal or muscle pain or weakness, or respiratory difficulties.

Colestipol (koe LES ti pole)

Brand Names: U.S. Colestid®; Colestid® Flavored

Index Terms Colestipol Hydrochloride

Pharmacologic Category Antilipemic Agent, Bile Acid Sequestrant

Medication Safety Issues

Sound-alike/look-alike issues:

Colestipol may be confused with calcitriol

Lactation Does not enter breast milk/use caution

Use Adjunct in management of primary hypercholesterolemia

Unlabeled Use Diarrhea associated with excess fecal bile acids (Westergaard, 2007); relief of pruritus associated with elevated levels of bile acids (Datta, 1963; Scaldaferri, 2011)

Available Dosage Forms

Granules for suspension, oral: 5 g/scoop (500 g); 5 g/packet (30s, 90s)

Colestid®: 5 g/scoop (300 g, 500 g); 5 g/packet (30s, 90s)

Colestid® Flavored: 5 g/scoop (450 g); 5 g/packet (60s)

Tablet, oral: 1 g

Colestid®: 1 g

General Dosage Range Oral: *Adults:* Granules: Initial: 5 g 1-2 times/day; Maintenance: 5-30 g/day once or in divided doses; Tablets: Initial: 2 g 1-2 times/day; Maintenance: 2-16 g/day once or in divided doses

Administration

Oral Other drugs should be administered at least 1 hour before or 4 hours after colestipol.

Granules: Do not administer in dry form (to avoid GI distress). Dry granules should be added to at least 90 mL of liquid and stirred until completely mixed; may be mixed with any beverage or added to soups, cereal, or pulpy fruits. Rinse glass with a small amount of liquid to ensure all medication is taken.

Tablets: Administer tablets 1 at a time, swallowed whole, with plenty of liquid. Do not cut, crush, or chew tablets.

Nursing Actions

Physical Assessment Monitor bowel function. Be alert to potential for constipation or hemorrhoid problems.

Patient Education Take granules with 3-4 oz of water or fruit juice. Rinse glass with small amount of water to ensure full dose is taken. Take tablets one at a time. Other medications should be taken 1 hour before or 4 hours after colestipol. You may experience constipation, drowsiness, or dizziness. Report acute gastric pain, tarry stools, or respiratory difficulty.

Crizotinib (kriz OH ti nib)

Brand Names: U.S. Xalkori®

Index Terms C-Met/Hepatocyte Growth Factor Receptor Tyrosine Kinase Inhibitor PF-02341066; C-Met/HGFR Tyrosine Kinase Inhibitor PF-02341066; MET Tyrosine Kinase Inhibitor PF-02341066; PF-02341066

Pharmacologic Category Antineoplastic Agent, Anaplastic Lymphoma Kinase Inhibitor; Antineoplastic Agent, Tyrosine Kinase Inhibitor

Medication Safety Issues

Sound-alike/look-alike issues:

Crizotinib may be confused with erlotinib, gefitinib

High alert medication:

This medication is in a class the Institute for Safe Medication Practices (ISMP) includes among its list of drug classes which have a heightened risk of causing significant patient harm when used in error.

Pregnancy Risk Factor D

Lactation Excretion in breast milk unknown/not recommended

Use Treatment of locally advanced or metastatic nonsmall cell lung cancer (NSCLC) that is anaplastic lymphoma kinase positive (as detected by an FDA-approved test)

Available Dosage Forms

Capsule, oral:

Xalkori®: 200 mg, 250 mg

General Dosage Range Dosage adjustment recommended in patients who develop toxicities.

Oral: *Adults:* 250 mg twice daily

Administration

Oral Swallow capsules whole (do not crush, dissolve, or open capsules). May be administered with or without food. If a dose is missed, take as soon as remembered unless it is <6 hours prior to the next scheduled dose (skip the dose if <6 hours before the next dose); do not take 2 doses at the same time to make up for a missed dose.

Nursing Actions

Physical Assessment Monitor electrolytes (potassium, magnesium), especially in patients with heart disease, vision, and ECG for QT prolongation. Patients may need ophthalmic evaluation in case of visual changes. Monitor for pulmonary symptoms.

Patient Education Visual changes can happen in the first 1-2 weeks. Inform your doctor if you notice changes or see floaters. Use caution with driving or operating heavy machinery due to vision changes or dizziness. Nausea, vomiting, diarrhea, and constipation are less serious side effects. Side effects that are more serious include fainting, fast heart rate, unusual bleeding or bruising, fever, chills, and body aches. Side effects that require immediate attention include hives; difficulty breathing; swelling of the face, lips, throat, or tongue; passing out; fast heartbeat; or sudden change in eye sight.

Cromolyn (Systemic, Oral Inhalation) (KROE moe lin)

Brand Names: U.S. Gastrocrom®

Index Terms Cromoglycic Acid; Cromolyn Sodium; Disodium Cromoglycate; DSCG

Pharmacologic Category Mast Cell Stabilizer

Pregnancy Risk Factor B

Lactation Excretion in breast milk unknown/use caution

Breast-Feeding Considerations No data available on whether cromolyn enters into breast milk or clinical effects on the infant. Use of cromolyn is not considered a contraindication to breast-feeding.

Use

Inhalation: May be used as an adjunct in the prophylaxis of allergic disorders, including asthma; prevention of exercise-induced bronchospasm

Oral: Systemic mastocytosis

Unlabeled Use Oral: Food allergy, treatment of inflammatory bowel disease

Mechanism of Action/Effect Prevents the mast cell release of histamine, leukotrienes, and slow-reacting substance of anaphylaxis

Contraindications Hypersensitivity to cromolyn or any component of the formulation; acute asthma attacks

Warnings/Precautions Severe anaphylactic reactions may occur rarely; cromolyn is a prophylactic drug with no benefit for acute situations; caution should be used when withdrawing the drug or tapering the dose as symptoms may reoccur; use with caution in patients with a history of cardiac arrhythmias. Dosage of oral product should be decreased with hepatic or renal dysfunction.

Drug Interactions

Avoid Concomitant Use There are no known interactions where it is recommended to avoid concomitant use.

Decreased Effect There are no known significant interactions involving a decrease in effect.

Increased Effect/Toxicity There are no known significant interactions involving an increase in effect.

Adverse Reactions Frequency not defined.

Cardiovascular: Angioedema, chest pain, edema, flushing, palpitation, premature ventricular contractions, tachycardia

Central nervous system: Anxiety, behavior changes, convulsions, depression, dizziness, fatigue, hallucinations, headache, irritability, insomnia, lethargy, migraine, nervousness, hypoesthesia, postprandial lightheadedness, psychosis

Dermatologic: Erythema, photosensitivity, pruritus, purpura, rash, urticaria

Gastrointestinal: Abdominal pain, constipation, diarrhea, dyspepsia, dysphagia, esophagospasm, flatulence, glossitis, nausea, stomatitis, vomiting

Genitourinary: Dysuria, urinary frequency

Hematologic: Neutropenia, pancytopenia, polycythemia

Hepatic: Liver function test abnormal

Local: Burning

Neuromuscular & skeletal: Arthralgia, leg stiffness, leg weakness, myalgia, paresthesia

Otic: Tinnitus

Respiratory: Dyspnea, pharyngitis

Miscellaneous: Lupus erythematosus

Pharmacodynamics/Kinetics

Onset of Action Response to treatment: Oral: May occur within 2-6 weeks

Available Dosage Forms

Solution, for nebulization: 20 mg/2 mL (60s, 120s)

Solution, oral:

Gastrocrom®: 100 mg/5 mL (96s)

General Dosage Range

Inhalation: Nebulization: *Children ≥2 years and Adults:* Initial: 20 mg 4 times/day; Maintenance: 20 mg 3-4 times/day **or** 20 mg prior to exercise or allergen exposure

Oral:

Children 2-12 years: 100 mg 4 times/day (maximum: 40 mg/kg/day)

Children >12 years and Adults: 200 mg 4 times/day (maximum: 40 mg/kg/day)

Administration

Oral Oral solution: Open ampul and squeeze contents into glass of water; stir well. Administer at least 30 minutes before meals and at bedtime.

Stability

Storage Store at room temperature of 15°C to 30°C (59°F to 86°F). Protect from light. Do not use oral solution if solution becomes discolored or forms a precipitate.

Nursing Actions

Physical Assessment This is prophylactic therapy, not to be used for acute situations.

Patient Education

Oral: Take at least 30 minutes before meals. You may experience dizziness, nervousness, diarrhea, headache, or muscle pain. Report persistent insomnia; skin rash; abdominal pain or difficulty swallowing; unusual cough, bronchospasm, or respiratory difficulty; or if condition worsens or fails to improve.

Nebulizer: Prepare nebulizer according to package instructions. Clear as much mucus as possible before use. Rinse mouth following each use to reduce unpleasant aftertaste. Report if symptoms worsen or condition fails to improve.

Dietary Considerations Oral: Should be taken at least 30 minutes before meals.

Cyanocobalamin (sye an oh koe BAL a min)

Brand Names: U.S. CaloMist™ [DSC]; Ener-B® [OTC]; Nascobal®; Twelve Resin-K [OTC]

Index Terms Vitamin B_{12}

Pharmacologic Category Vitamin, Water Soluble

Pregnancy Risk Factor A/C (dose exceeding RDA recommendation); C (intranasal)

Lactation Enters breast milk/compatible

Use Treatment of pernicious anemia; vitamin B_{12} deficiency due to dietary deficiencies or malabsorption diseases, inadequate secretion of intrinsic factor, and inadequate utilization of B_{12} (eg, during neoplastic treatment); increased B_{12} requirements due to pregnancy, thyrotoxicosis, hemorrhage, malignancy, liver or kidney disease

CaloMist™: Maintenance of vitamin B_{12} concentrations after initial correction in patients with B_{12} deficiency without CNS involvement

Available Dosage Forms

Injection, solution: 1000 mcg/mL (1 mL, 10 mL, 30 mL)

Lozenge, oral: 50 mcg (100s); 100 mcg (100s); 250 mcg (100s, 250s); 500 mcg (100s, 250s)

Lozenge, sublingual: 500 mcg (100s)

Solution, intranasal:

Nascobal®: 500 mcg/spray (2.3 mL)

Tablet, for buccal application/oral/sublingual: Twelve Resin-K [OTC]: 1000 mcg

Tablet, oral: 50 mcg, 100 mcg, 250 mcg, 500 mcg, 1000 mcg

Ener-B® [OTC]: 100 mcg, 500 mcg, 1000 mcg

Tablet, sublingual: 1000 mcg, 2500 mcg, 5000 mcg

Tablet, timed release, oral: 1000 mcg

Ener-B® [OTC]: 1500 mcg

General Dosage Range

I.M., SubQ: *Children and Adults:* Dosage varies greatly depending on indication

Intranasal: *Adults:* Nascobal®: 500 mcg in one nostril once weekly; CaloMist™: Maintenance therapy (following correction of vitamin B_{12} deficiency): 50-100 mcg/day

Oral: *Adults:* 250-2000 mcg/day

Administration

Oral Not recommended due to variable absorption; however, oral therapy of 1000-2000 mcg/day has been effective for anemia if I.M./SubQ routes refused or not tolerated.

I.M. I.M. or deep SubQ are preferred routes of administration.

I.V. Not recommended

I.V. Detail pH: 4.5-7.0

Other Intranasal: Nasal spray:

Nascobal®: Prior to initial dose, activate (prime) spray nozzle by pumping unit quickly and firmly until first appearance of spray, then prime twice more. The unit must be reprimed once immediately before each subsequent use. Administer 1 hour before or after ingestion of hot foods/ liquids.

CaloMist™: Prime unit by spraying 7 times. If ≥5 days since use, reprime with 2 sprays. Separate from other intranasal medications by several hours.

Nursing Actions

Physical Assessment Provide patient appropriate nutritional counseling.

Patient Education Pernicious anemia may require treatment for life. Report skin rash, muscle cramps, or weakness.

Cyclobenzaprine (sye kloe BEN za preen)

Brand Names: U.S. Amrix®; Fexmid®; Flexeril®

Index Terms Cyclobenzaprine Hydrochloride

Pharmacologic Category Skeletal Muscle Relaxant

Medication Safety Issues

Sound-alike/look-alike issues:

Cyclobenzaprine may be confused with cycloSERINE, cyproheptadine

Flexeril® may be confused with Floxin®

BEERS Criteria medication:

This drug may be inappropriate for use in geriatric patients (high severity risk).

International issues:

Flexin: Brand name for cyclobenzaprine [Chile], but also the brand name for diclofenac [Argentina] and orphenadrine [Israel]

Flexin [Chile] may be confused with Floxin brand name for flunarizine [Thailand], norfloxacin [South Africa], ofloxacin [U.S., Canada], and perfloxacin [Philippines]; Fluoxine brand name for fluoxetine [Thailand]

Pregnancy Risk Factor B

Lactation Excretion in breast milk unknown/use caution

Use Treatment of muscle spasm associated with acute, painful musculoskeletal conditions

Unlabeled Use Treatment of muscle spasm associated with acute temporomandibular joint pain (TMJ)

Mechanism of Action/Effect Centrally-acting skeletal muscle relaxant pharmacologically related to tricyclic antidepressants; reduces tonic somatic motor activity influencing both alpha and gamma motor neurons

Contraindications Hypersensitivity to cyclobenzaprine or any component of the formulation; during or within 14 days of MAO inhibitors; hyperthyroidism; congestive heart failure; arrhythmias; heart block or conduction disturbances; acute recovery phase of MI

Warnings/Precautions May cause CNS depression, which may impair physical or mental abilities; patients must be cautioned about performing tasks which require mental alertness (eg, operating machinery or driving). Cyclobenzaprine shares the toxic potentials of the tricyclic antidepressants (including arrhythmias, tachycardia, and conduction time prolongation) and the usual precautions of tricyclic antidepressant therapy should be observed; use with caution in patients with urinary hesitancy or retention, angle-closure glaucoma or increased intraocular pressure, hepatic impairment, or in the elderly. This class of medication is poorly tolerated by the elderly due to anticholinergic effects, sedation, and weakness; efficacy is questionable at dosages tolerated by elderly patients (Beers Criteria). Extended release capsules not recommended for use in mild-to-severe hepatic impairment or in the elderly. Do not use concomitantly or within 14 days after MAO inhibitors; combination may cause hypertensive crisis, severe convulsions. Effects may be potentiated when used with other CNS depressants or ethanol.

Drug Interactions

Avoid Concomitant Use

Avoid concomitant use of Cyclobenzaprine with any of the following: MAO Inhibitors

Decreased Effect

Cyclobenzaprine may decrease the levels/effects of: Acetylcholinesterase Inhibitors (Central)

The levels/effects of Cyclobenzaprine may be decreased by: Acetylcholinesterase Inhibitors (Central); Cyproterone; Peginterferon Alfa-2b; Tocilizumab

Increased Effect/Toxicity

Cyclobenzaprine may increase the levels/effects of: Alcohol (Ethyl); Anticholinergics; CNS Depressants; MAO Inhibitors; Metoclopramide; Serotonin Modulators

The levels/effects of Cyclobenzaprine may be increased by: Abiraterone Acetate; Antipsychotics; Conivaptan; CYP1A2 Inhibitors (Moderate); CYP1A2 Inhibitors (Strong); Deferasirox; HydrOXYzine; Pramlintide

Nutritional/Ethanol Interactions

Ethanol: May increase CNS depression; monitor for increased effects with coadministration. Caution patients about effects.

Food: Food increases bioavailability (peak plasma concentrations increased by 35% and area under the curve by 20%) of the extended release capsule.

Herb/Nutraceutical: Avoid valerian, kava kava, gotu kola (may increase CNS depression).

Adverse Reactions

>10%:

Central nervous system: Drowsiness (29% to 39%), dizziness (1% to 11%)

Gastrointestinal: Xerostomia (21% to 32%)

1% to 10%:

Central nervous system: Fatigue (1% to 6%), headache (1% to 5%), confusion (1% to 3%), irritability (1% to 3%), mental acuity decreased (1% to 3%), nervousness (1% to 3%), somnolence (1% to 2%)

Gastrointestinal: Dyspepsia (≤4%), abdominal pain (1% to 3%), constipation (1% to 3%), diarrhea (1% to 3%), gastric regurgitation (1% to 3%), nausea (1% to 3%), unpleasant taste (1% to 3%)

Neuromuscular & skeletal: Weakness (1% to 3%)

Ocular: Blurred vision (1% to 3%)

Respiratory: Pharyngitis (1% to 3%), upper respiratory infection (1% to 3%)

Available Dosage Forms

Capsule, extended release, oral: 15 mg, 30 mg

Amrix®: 15 mg, 30 mg

Tablet, oral: 5 mg, 10 mg

Fexmid®: 7.5 mg

Flexeril®: 5 mg, 10 mg

General Dosage Range Dosage adjustment recommended in patients with hepatic impairment

Oral capsule, extended release: *Adults:* Usual: 15 mg once daily (maximum: 30 mg once daily)

Oral tablet, immediate release:

Children ≥15 years and Adults: Initial: 5 mg 3 times/day; Maintenance: 5-10 mg 3 times/day

Elderly: Initial: 5 mg

Administration

Oral Extended release capsules: Administer at the same time each day. Do not crush or chew.

Stability

Storage

Amrix®, Flexeril®: Store at 25°C (77°F); excursions permitted to 15°C to 30°C (59°F to 86°F).

Fexmid®: Store at 20°C to 25°C (68°F to 77°F).

Nursing Actions

Physical Assessment May cause significant CNS depression. Caution patients about sedation.

Patient Education Do not use alcohol. You may experience drowsiness, dizziness, lightheadedness, or urinary retention. Report excessive drowsiness or skin rash.

Cyclophosphamide (sye kloe FOS fa mide)

Index Terms CPM; CTX; CYT; Cytoxan; Neosar

Pharmacologic Category Antineoplastic Agent, Alkylating Agent

Medication Safety Issues

Sound-alike/look-alike issues:

Cyclophosphamide may be confused with cycloSPORINE, ifosfamide

Cytoxan may be confused with cefOXitin, Ciloxan®, cytarabine, CytoGam®, Cytosar®, Cytosar-U, Cytotec®

High alert medication:

This medication is in a class the Institute for Safe Medication Practices (ISMP) includes among its list of drugs which have a heightened risk of causing significant patient harm when used in error.

Pregnancy Risk Factor D

Lactation Enters breast milk/not recommended

Breast-Feeding Considerations Due to the potential for adverse effects and tumorigenicity, cyclophosphamide is not recommended in breast-feeding women.

Use

Oncology-related uses: Treatment of Hodgkin's lymphoma, non-Hodgkin's lymphoma (including Burkitt's lymphoma), chronic lymphocytic leukemia (CLL), chronic myelocytic leukemia (CML), acute myelocytic leukemia (AML), acute lymphocytic leukemia (ALL), mycosis fungoides, multiple myeloma, neuroblastoma, retinoblastoma; breast cancer; ovarian adenocarcinoma

Nononcology uses: Treatment of refractory nephrotic syndrome in children

Unlabeled Use

Oncology-related uses: Ewing's sarcoma, rhabdomyosarcoma, Wilms tumor, ovarian germ cell tumors, small cell lung cancer, testicular cancer, pheochromocytoma, bone marrow transplantation conditioning regimen

Nononcology uses: Severe rheumatoid disorders, Wegener's granulomatosis, myasthenia gravis, multiple sclerosis, systemic lupus erythematosus, lupus nephritis, autoimmune hemolytic anemia, idiopathic thrombocytic purpura (ITP), and antibody-induced pure red cell aplasia; juvenile idiopathic arthritis (JIA)

Mechanism of Action/Effect Interferes with the normal function of DNA by alkylation and cross-linking the strands of DNA, and by possible protein modification; cyclophosphamide also possesses potent immunosuppressive activity; note that cyclophosphamide must be metabolized to its active form in the liver

Contraindications Hypersensitivity to cyclophosphamide or any component of the formulation; severely depressed bone marrow function

Warnings/Precautions Hazardous agent - use appropriate precautions for handling and disposal. Dosage adjustment may be needed for renal or hepatic failure. Hemorrhagic cystitis may occur; increased hydration and frequent voiding is recommended. Immunosuppression may occur; monitor for infections. May cause cardiotoxicity (HF, usually with higher doses); may potentiate the cardiotoxicity of anthracyclines. May impair fertility; interferes with oogenesis and spermatogenesis. Secondary malignancies (usually delayed) have been reported

Drug Interactions

Avoid Concomitant Use

Avoid concomitant use of Cyclophosphamide with any of the following: BCG; Belimumab; CloZAPine; Etanercept; Natalizumab; Pimecrolimus; Pimozide; Tacrolimus (Topical); Vaccines (Live)

Decreased Effect

Cyclophosphamide may decrease the levels/effects of: BCG; Cardiac Glycosides; Coccidioidin Skin Test; Sipuleucel-T; Vaccines (Inactivated); Vaccines (Live); Vitamin K Antagonists

The levels/effects of Cyclophosphamide may be decreased by: CYP2B6 Inducers (Strong); Echinacea; Tocilizumab

Increased Effect/Toxicity

Cyclophosphamide may increase the levels/effects of: ARIPiprazole; CloZAPine; Leflunomide; Natalizumab; Pimozide; Succinylcholine; Vaccines (Live); Vitamin K Antagonists

The levels/effects of Cyclophosphamide may be increased by: Allopurinol; Belimumab; Conivaptan; CYP2B6 Inhibitors (Moderate); CYP2B6 Inhibitors (Strong); Denosumab; Etanercept; Pentostatin; Pimecrolimus; Quazepam; Roflumilast; Tacrolimus (Topical); Trastuzumab

Nutritional/Ethanol Interactions Herb/Nutraceutical: Avoid black cohosh, dong quai in estrogen-dependent tumors.

Adverse Reactions

>10%:

Dermatologic: Alopecia (40% to 60%) but hair will usually regrow although it may be a different color and/or texture. Hair loss usually begins 3-6 weeks after the start of therapy.

Endocrine & metabolic: Fertility: May cause sterility; interferes with oogenesis and spermatogenesis; may be irreversible in some patients; gonadal suppression (amenorrhea)

Gastrointestinal: Nausea and vomiting (usually beginning 6-10 hours after administration; severe with high-dose therapy); anorexia, diarrhea, mucositis, and stomatitis are also seen

Genitourinary: Severe, potentially fatal, acute hemorrhagic cystitis or urinary fibrosis (7% to 40%)

Hematologic: Anemia, leukopenia (dose-related; recovery: 7-10 days after cessation), thrombocytopenia

1% to 10%:

Cardiovascular: Facial flushing

Central nervous system: Headache

Dermatologic: Skin rash

Respiratory: Nasal congestion occurs when I.V. doses are administered too rapidly; patients experience runny eyes, rhinorrhea, sinus congestion, and sneezing during or immediately after the infusion.

Available Dosage Forms

Injection, powder for reconstitution: 500 mg, 1 g, 2 g

Tablet, oral: 25 mg, 50 mg

General Dosage Range Dosage adjustment recommended in patients with hepatic or renal impairment

I.V.: *Children and Adults:* Dosage varies greatly depending on indication

Oral: *Children and Adults:* 1-5 mg/kg/day

Administration

Oral Tablets are not scored and should not be cut or crushed. To minimize the risk of bladder irritation, do not administer tablets at bedtime.

I.V. IVPB or continuous intravenous infusion; I.V. infusions may be administered over 1-24 hours. Doses >500 mg to approximately 2 g may be administered over 20-30 minutes.

To minimize bladder toxicity, increase normal fluid intake during and for 1-2 days after cyclophosphamide dose. Most adult patients will require a fluid intake of at least 2 L/day. High-dose regimens should be accompanied by vigorous hydration with or without mesna therapy.

I.V. Detail Slow IVP in doses ≤1 g. High-dose regimens should be accompanied by vigorous hydration with or without mesna therapy.

BMT only: Approaches to reduction of hemorrhagic cystitis include infusion of 0.9% NaCl 3 L/m²/24 hours, infusion of 0.9% NaCl 3 L/m²/24 hours with continuous 0.9% NaCl bladder irrigation 300-1000 mL/hour, and infusion of 0.9% NaCl 1.5-3 L/m²/24 hours with intravenous mesna. Hydration should begin at least 4 hours before cyclophosphamide and continue at least 24 hours after completion of cyclophosphamide. The dose of daily mesna used should equal the daily dose of cyclophosphamide. Mesna can be administered as a continuous 24-hour intravenous infusion or be given in divided doses every 4 hours. Mesna should begin at the start of treatment, and continue at least 24 hours following the last dose of cyclophosphamide.

pH: 3-9 (reconstituted solution)

Stability

Reconstitution Reconstitute vials with SWI, NS, or D_5W to a concentration of 20 mg/mL.

Storage Store intact vials of powder at room temperature of 15°C to 30°C (59°F to 86°F). Reconstituted solutions are stable for 24 hours at room temperature and 6 days under refrigeration 2°C to 8°C (36°F to 46°F). Further dilutions in D_5W or NS are stable for 24 hours at room temperature (25°C) and 6 days at refrigeration.

Nursing Actions

Physical Assessment Assess other drugs patient may be taking that may increase or prolong nephrotoxicity and cardiotoxicity. Note infusion specifics in Administration, including recommendations for pre- and posthydration. Monitor infusion site to prevent extravasation. Monitor hemorrhagic cystitis, leukopenia, and renal tubular necrosis prior to each infusion and regularly during therapy. Teach patient importance of adequate hydration.

Patient Education Take during or after meals; do not take at night. Maintain adequate hydration unless instructed to restrict fluid intake and void frequently to reduce incidence of bladder irritation. You will be more susceptible to infection. May cause loss of hair (reversible, although regrowth hair may be different color or texture), infertility or amenorrhea, nausea or vomiting, headache, nasal congestion or cold symptoms, or mouth sores. Report any difficulty or pain with urination; chest pain, rapid heartbeat, or palpitations; easy bruising or bleeding; unusual rash; persistent nausea or vomiting; swelling of extremities; respiratory difficulty; or unusual fatigue.

Dietary Considerations Tablets should be administered during or after meals.

Related Information

Management of Drug Extravasations *on page 1269*

CycloSPORINE (Systemic)

(SYE kloe spor een)

Brand Names: U.S. Gengraf®; Neoral®; SandIMMUNE®

Index Terms CsA; CyA; Cyclosporin A

Pharmacologic Category Calcineurin Inhibitor; Immunosuppressant Agent

Medication Safety Issues

Sound-alike/look-alike issues:

CycloSPORINE may be confused with cyclophosphamide, Cyklokapron®, cycloSERINE

CycloSPORINE modified (Neoral®, Gengraf®) may be confused with cycloSPORINE non-modified (SandIMMUNE®)

Gengraf® may be confused with Prograf®

Neoral® may be confused with Neurontin®, Nizoral®

SandIMMUNE® may be confused with SandoSTATIN®

Pregnancy Risk Factor C

Lactation Enters breast milk/not recommended

Use Prophylaxis of organ rejection in kidney, liver, and heart transplants, has been used with azathioprine and/or corticosteroids; severe, active rheumatoid arthritis (RA) not responsive to methotrexate alone; severe, recalcitrant plaque psoriasis in nonimmunocompromised adults unresponsive to or unable to tolerate other systemic therapy

Unlabeled Use Allogenic stem cell transplants for prevention and treatment of graft-versus-host disease; also used in some cases of severe autoimmune disease (eg, SLE) that are resistant to corticosteroids and other therapy; focal segmental glomerulosclerosis; severe ulcerative colitis

Mechanism of Action/Effect Inhibits T-lymphocytes and lymphokine production and release in a reversible manner.

Contraindications Hypersensitivity to cyclosporine or any component of the formulation. I.V. cyclosporine is contraindicated in hypersensitivity to polyoxyethylated castor oil (Cremophor® EL).

Rheumatoid arthritis and psoriasis: Abnormal renal function, uncontrolled hypertension, malignancies. Concomitant treatment with PUVA or UVB therapy, methotrexate, other immunosuppressive agents, coal tar, or radiation therapy are also contraindications for use in patients with psoriasis.

Warnings/Precautions Hazardous agent - use appropriate precautions for handling and disposal. **[U.S. Boxed Warning]: Renal impairment, including structural kidney damage has occurred (when used at high doses); monitor renal function closely.** Elevations in serum creatinine and BUN generally respond to dosage reductions. Use caution with other potentially nephrotoxic drugs (eg, acyclovir, aminoglycoside antibiotics, amphotericin B, ciprofloxacin). **[U.S. Boxed Warning]: Increased risk of lymphomas and other malignancies, particularly those of the skin;** risk is related to intensity/duration of therapy and the use of >1 immunosuppressive agent; all patients should avoid excessive sun/UV light exposure. **[U.S. Boxed Warning]: Increased risk of infection; fatal infections have been reported.** Latent viral infections may be activated (including BK virus which is associated with nephropathy) and result in serious adverse effects. **[U.S. Boxed Warning]: May cause hypertension.** Use caution when changing dosage forms. **[U.S. Boxed Warning]: Cyclosporine (modified) has increased bioavailability as compared to cyclosporine (non-modified) and cannot be used interchangeably without close monitoring.** Monitor cyclosporine concentrations closely following the addition, modification, or deletion of other medications; live, attenuated vaccines may be less effective; use should be avoided. Increased hepatic enzymes and bilirubin have occurred (when used at high doses); improvement usually seen with dosage reduction.

Transplant patients: To be used initially with corticosteroids. May cause significant hyperkalemia and hyperuricemia, seizures (particularly if used with high dose corticosteroids), and encephalopathy. Other neurotoxic events (eg, optic disc edema including papilledema and visual impairment) have been reported rarely. Make dose adjustments based on cyclosporine blood concentrations. **[U.S. Boxed Warning]: Adjustment of dose should only be made under the direct supervision of an experienced physician.** Anaphylaxis has been reported with I.V. use; reserve for patients who cannot take oral form. **[U.S. Boxed Warning]: Risk of skin cancer may be increased in transplant patients.** Due to the increased risk for nephrotoxicity in renal transplantation, avoid using standard doses of cyclosporine in combination with everolimus; reduced cyclosporine doses are recommended; monitor cyclosporine concentrations closely. Cyclosporine and everolimus combination therapy may increase the risk for proteinuria. Cyclosporine combined with either everolimus or sirolimus may increase the risk for thrombotic microangiopathy/thrombotic thrombocytopenic purpura/hemolytic uremic syndrome (TMA/TTP/HUS).

Psoriasis: Patients should avoid excessive sun exposure; safety and efficacy in children <18 years of age have not been established. **[U.S. Boxed Warning]: Risk of skin cancer may be increased with a history of PUVA and possibly methotrexate or other immunosuppressants, UVB, coal tar, or radiation.**

Rheumatoid arthritis: Safety and efficacy for use in juvenile idiopathic arthritis (JIA) have not been established. If receiving other immunosuppressive agents, radiation or UV therapy, concurrent use of cyclosporine is not recommended.

Products may contain corn oil, ethanol, or propylene glycol; injection also contains Cremophor® EL (polyoxyethylated castor oil), which has been associated with rare anaphylactic reactions.

Drug Interactions

Avoid Concomitant Use

Avoid concomitant use of CycloSPORINE (Systemic) with any of the following: Aliskiren; BCG; Bosentan; Conivaptan; Crizotinib; Dronedarone; Eplerenone; Natalizumab; Pimecrolimus; Pimozide; Pitavastatin; Potassium-Sparing Diuretics; Silodosin; Sitaxentan; Tacrolimus; Tacrolimus (Systemic); Tacrolimus (Topical); Topotecan; Vaccines (Live)

Decreased Effect

CycloSPORINE (Systemic) may decrease the levels/effects of: BCG; Coccidioidin Skin Test; GlyBURIDE; Mycophenolate; Sipuleucel-T; Vaccines (Inactivated); Vaccines (Live)

The levels/effects of CycloSPORINE (Systemic) may be decreased by: Armodafinil; Ascorbic Acid; Barbiturates; Bosentan; CarBAMazepine; Colesevelam; CYP3A4 Inducers (Strong); Deferasirox; Dexamethasone; Dexamethasone (Systemic); Echinacea; Efavirenz; Fibric Acid Derivatives; Fosphenytoin; Griseofulvin; Imipenem; MethylPREDNISolone; Modafinil; Nafcillin; Orlistat; P-glycoprotein/ABCB1 Inducers; Phenytoin; PrednisoLONE; PrednisoLONE (Systemic); PredniSONE; Rifamycin Derivatives; Somatostatin Analogs; St Johns Wort; Sulfinpyrazone [Off Market]; Sulfonamide Derivatives; Terbinafine; Tocilizumab; Vitamin E

Increased Effect/Toxicity

CycloSPORINE (Systemic) may increase the levels/effects of: Aliskiren; Ambrisentan; ARIPiprazole; Bosentan; Budesonide (Systemic, Oral Inhalation); Calcium Channel Blockers (Dihydropyridine); Calcium Channel Blockers (Nondihydropyridine); Cardiac Glycosides; Caspofungin; Colchicine; CYP3A4 Substrates; Dabigatran Etexilate; Dexamethasone; Dexamethasone (Systemic); DOXOrubicin; Dronedarone; Etoposide; Etoposide Phosphate; Everolimus; Ezetimibe; FentaNYL; Fibric Acid Derivatives; Halofantrine; HMG-CoA Reductase Inhibitors; Imipenem; Leflunomide; Loop Diuretics; Lurasidone; Methotrexate; MethylPREDNISolone; Minoxidil; Minoxidil (Systemic); Minoxidil (Topical); Natalizumab; Nonsteroidal Anti-Inflammatory Agents; P-glycoprotein/ABCB1 Substrates; Pimozide; Pitavastatin; PrednisoLONE; PrednisoLONE (Systemic); PredniSONE; Propafenone; Protease Inhibitors; Prucalopride; Repaglinide; Rivaroxaban; Salmeterol; Silodosin; Sirolimus;

Sitaxentan; Tacrolimus; Tacrolimus (Systemic); Tacrolimus (Topical); Topotecan; Vaccines (Live); Vilazodone; Zuclopenthixol

The levels/effects of CycloSPORINE (Systemic) may be increased by: ACE Inhibitors; AcetaZOLAMIDE; Aminoglycosides; Amiodarone; Amphotericin B; Androgens; Antifungal Agents (Azole Derivatives, Systemic); Bromocriptine; Calcium Channel Blockers (Nondihydropyridine); Carvedilol; Chloramphenicol; Conivaptan; Crizotinib; CYP3A4 Inhibitors (Moderate); CYP3A4 Inhibitors (Strong); Dasatinib; Denosumab; Dexamethasone; Dexamethasone (Systemic); Eplerenone; Ezetimibe; Fluconazole; GlyBURIDE; Grapefruit Juice; Imatinib; Imipenem; Macrolide Antibiotics; Melphalan; Methotrexate; MethylPREDNISolone; Metoclopramide; MetroNIDAZOLE; MetroNIDAZOLE (Systemic); Nonsteroidal Anti-Inflammatory Agents; Norfloxacin; Omeprazole; P-glycoprotein/ABCB1 Inhibitors; Pimecrolimus; Potassium-Sparing Diuretics; PrednisoLONE; PrednisoLONE (Systemic); PredniSONE; Protease Inhibitors; Pyrazinamide; Quinupristin; Roflumilast; Sirolimus; Sulfonamide Derivatives; Tacrolimus; Tacrolimus (Systemic); Tacrolimus (Topical); Telaprevir; Temsirolimus; Trastuzumab

Nutritional/Ethanol Interactions

Food: Grapefruit juice increases cyclosporine serum concentrations. Management: Avoid grapefruit juice.

Herb/Nutraceutical: St John's wort may increase the metabolism of and decrease plasma levels of cyclosporine; organ rejection and graft loss have been reported. Cat's claw and echinacea have immunostimulant properties. Management: Avoid St John's wort, cat's claw, and echinacea.

Adverse Reactions Adverse reactions reported with systemic use, including rheumatoid arthritis, psoriasis, and transplantation (kidney, liver, and heart). Percentages noted include the highest frequency regardless of indication/dosage. Frequencies may vary for specific conditions or formulation.

>10%:

Cardiovascular: Hypertension (8% to 53%), edema (5% to 14%)

Central nervous system: Headache (2% to 25%)

Dermatologic: Hirsutism (21% to 45%), hypertrichosis (5% to 19%)

Endocrine & metabolic: Triglycerides increased (15%), female reproductive disorder (9% to 11%)

Gastrointestinal: Nausea (23%), diarrhea (3% to 13%), gum hyperplasia (2% to 16%), abdominal discomfort (<1% to 15%), dyspepsia (2% to 12%)

Neuromuscular & skeletal: Tremor (7% to 55%), paresthesia (1% to 11%), leg cramps/muscle contractions (2% to 12%)

Renal: Renal dysfunction/nephropathy (10% to 38%), creatinine increased (16% to ≥50%)

Respiratory: Upper respiratory infection (1% to 14%)

Miscellaneous: Infection (3% to 25%)

Kidney, liver, and heart transplant only (≤2% unless otherwise noted):

Cardiovascular: Flushes (<1% to 4%), MI

Central nervous system: Convulsions (1% to 5%), anxiety, confusion, fever, lethargy

Dermatologic: Acne (1% to 6%), brittle fingernails, hair breaking, pruritus

Endocrine & metabolic: Gynecomastia (<1% to 4%), hyperglycemia

Gastrointestinal: Nausea (2% to 10%), vomiting (2% to 10%), diarrhea (3% to 8%), abdominal discomfort (<1% to 7%), cramps (0% to 4%), anorexia, constipation, gastritis, mouth sores, pancreatitis, swallowing difficulty, upper GI bleed, weight loss

Hematologic: Leukopenia (<1% to 6%), anemia, thrombocytopenia

Hepatic: Hepatotoxicity (<1% to 7%)

Neuromuscular & skeletal: Paresthesia (1% to 3%), joint pain, muscle pain, tingling, weakness

Ocular: Conjunctivitis, visual disturbance

Otic: Hearing loss, tinnitus

Renal: Hematuria

Respiratory: Sinusitis (<1% to 7%)

Miscellaneous: Lymphoma (<1% to 6%), allergic reactions, hiccups, night sweats

Rheumatoid arthritis only (1% to <3% unless otherwise noted):

Cardiovascular: Hypertension (8%), edema (5%), chest pain (4%), arrhythmia (2%), abnormal heart sounds, cardiac failure, MI, peripheral ischemia

Central nervous system: Dizziness (8%), pain (6%), insomnia (4%), depression (3%), migraine (2%), anxiety, hypoesthesia, emotional lability, impaired concentration, malaise, nervousness, paranoia, somnolence, vertigo

Dermatologic: Purpura (3%), abnormal pigmentation, angioedema, cellulitis, dermatitis, dry skin, eczema, folliculitis, nail disorder, pruritus, skin disorder, urticaria

Endocrine & metabolic: Menstrual disorder (3%), breast fibroadenosis, breast pain, diabetes mellitus, goiter, hot flashes, hyperkalemia, hyperuricemia, hypoglycemia, libido increased/decreased

Gastrointestinal: Vomiting (9%), flatulence (5%), gingivitis (4%), gum hyperplasia (2%), constipation, dry mouth, dysphagia, enanthema, eructation, esophagitis, gastric ulcer, gastritis, gastroenteritis, gingival bleeding, glossitis, peptic ulcer, salivary gland enlargement, taste perversion, tongue disorder, gum hyperplasia, weight loss/gain

Genitourinary: Leukorrhea (1%), abnormal urine, micturition urgency, nocturia, polyuria, pyelonephritis, urinary incontinence, uterine hemorrhage

Hematologic: Anemia, leukopenia

Hepatic: Bilirubinemia

Neuromuscular & skeletal: Paresthesia (8%), tremor (8%), leg cramps/muscle contractions (2%), arthralgia, bone fracture, joint dislocation, myalgia, neuropathy, stiffness, synovial cyst, tendon disorder, weakness

Ocular: Abnormal vision, cataract, conjunctivitis, eye pain

Otic: Tinnitus, deafness, vestibular disorder

Renal: BUN increased, hematuria, renal abscess

Respiratory: Cough (5%), dyspnea (5%), sinusitis (4%), abnormal chest sounds, bronchospasm, epistaxis

Miscellaneous: Infection (9%), abscess, allergy, bacterial infection, carcinoma, fungal infection, herpes simplex, herpes zoster, lymphadenopathy, moniliasis, diaphoresis increased, tonsillitis, viral infection

Psoriasis only (1% to <3% unless otherwise noted):

Cardiovascular: Chest pain, flushes

Central nervous system: Psychiatric events (4% to 5%), pain (3% to 4%), dizziness, fever, insomnia, nervousness, vertigo

Dermatologic: Hypertrichosis (5% to 7%), acne, dry skin, folliculitis, keratosis, pruritus, rash, skin malignancies

Endocrine & metabolic: Hot flashes

Gastrointestinal: Nausea (5% to 6%), diarrhea (5% to 6%), gum hyperplasia (4% to 6%), abdominal discomfort (3% to 6%), dyspepsia (2% to 3%), abdominal distention, appetite increased, constipation, gingival bleeding

Genitourinary: Micturition increased

Hematologic: Bleeding disorder, clotting disorder, platelet disorder, red blood cell disorder

Hepatic: Hyperbilirubinemia

Neuromuscular & skeletal: Paresthesia (5% to 7%), arthralgia (1% to 6%)

Ocular: Abnormal vision

Respiratory: Bronchospasm (5%), cough (5%), dyspnea (5%), rhinitis (5%), respiratory infection

Miscellaneous: Flu-like syndrome (8% to 10%)

Available Dosage Forms

Capsule, oral: 100 mg

Gengraf®: 25 mg, 100 mg

Capsule, softgel, oral: 25 mg, 50 mg, 100 mg

Neoral®: 25 mg, 100 mg

SandIMMUNE®: 25 mg, 100 mg

Injection, solution: 50 mg/mL (5 mL)

SandIMMUNE®: 50 mg/mL (5 mL)

Solution, oral: 100 mg/mL (50 mL)

Gengraf®: 100 mg/mL (50 mL)

Neoral®: 100 mg/mL (50 mL)

SandIMMUNE®: 100 mg/mL (50 mL)

General Dosage Range Dosage adjustment recommended in patients with renal impairment

I.V. (non-modified): *Children and Adults:* Initial dose: 5-6 mg/kg/day or one-third of the oral dose as a single dose; Maintenance: 3-7.5 mg/kg/day in 2-3 divided doses or give as continuous infusion over 24 hours

Oral:

Modified:

Children and Adults: Transplant: Heart: 7 ± 3 mg/kg/day in 2 divided doses; Liver: 8 ± 4 mg/kg/day in 2 divided doses; Renal: 9 ± 3 mg/kg/day in 2 divided doses

Adults: Initial: 2.5 mg/kg/day in 2 divided doses; Maintenance: Up to 4 mg/kg/day

Non-modified: *Children and Adults:* Initial: 10-14 mg/kg/day for 1-2 weeks; Maintenance: Taper by 5% per week to 3-10 mg/kg/day

Administration

Oral Oral solution: Do not administer liquid from plastic or styrofoam cup. May dilute Neoral® oral solution with orange juice or apple juice. May dilute Sandimmune® oral solution with milk, chocolate milk, or orange juice. Avoid changing diluents frequently. Mix thoroughly and drink at once. Use syringe provided to measure dose. Mix in a glass container and rinse container with more diluent to ensure total dose is taken. Do not rinse syringe before or after use (may cause dose variation).

Combination therapy with renal transplantation:

Everolimus: Administer cyclosporine at the same time as everolimus

Sirolimus: Administer cyclosporine 4 hours prior to sirolimus

I.V. The manufacturer recommends that following dilution, intravenous admixture be administered over 2-6 hours. However, many transplant centers administer as divided doses (2-3 doses/day) or as a 24-hour continuous infusion. Patients should be under continuous observation for at least the first 30 minutes of the infusion, and should be monitored frequently thereafter. To minimize leaching of DEHP, non-PVC sets should be used for administration.

I.V. Detail Anaphylaxis has been reported with I.V. use; reserve for patients who cannot take oral form. Patients should be under continuous observation for at least the first 30 minutes of the infusion, and should be monitored frequently thereafter. Maintain patent airway; other supportive measures and agents for treating anaphylaxis should be present when I.V. drug is given. Discard solution after 24 hours.

Stability

Reconstitution Injection: To minimize leaching of DEHP, non-PVC containers and sets should be used for preparation and administration.

Sandimmune® injection: Injection should be further diluted (1 mL [50 mg] of concentrate in 20-100 mL of D_5W or NS) for administration by intravenous infusion.

Storage

Capsule: Store at controlled room temperature.

Injection: Store at controlled room temperature; do not refrigerate. Ampuls and vials should be protected from light. Stability of injection of parenteral admixture at room temperature (25°C) is 6 hours in PVC; 12-24 hours in Excel®, PAB® containers, or glass.

Oral solution: Store at controlled room temperature; do not refrigerate. Use within 2 months after opening; should be mixed in glass containers.

Nursing Actions

Physical Assessment Monitor kidney and hepatic function closely. Monitor blood pressure and assess for signs of fluid retention periodically. Monitor for infection (eg, fever, mouth, and vaginal sores or plaques, unhealed wounds). I.V: Monitor closely for first 30 minutes of infusion and frequently thereafter to assess for CNS changes or hypertension.

Patient Education Oral: Take dose at the same time each day. You will be susceptible to infection. Avoid excessive exposure to sun. Practice good oral hygiene to reduce gum inflammation; see a dentist regularly during treatment. Report severe headache; mouth sores or swollen gums; signs of infection; persistent nausea, vomiting, or diarrhea; or change in urination. Increase in blood pressure or damage to the kidney is possible. Your prescriber will need to monitor you closely. Do not change one brand of cyclosporine for another; any changes must be done by your prescriber. If you are taking this medication for psoriasis, your risk of cancer may be increased when taking additional medications.

Oral solution: Dilute Neoral® with orange juice or apple juice. Dilute Sandimmune® with milk, chocolate milk, or orange juice. Mix thoroughly and drink at once. Mix in a glass container (do not use plastic or styrofoam) and rinse container with more juice/milk to ensure total dose is taken.

Dietary Considerations Administer this medication consistently with relation to time of day and meals. Avoid grapefruit juice with oral cyclosporine use.

Related Information

Peak and Trough Guidelines *on page 1276*

CycloSPORINE (Ophthalmic)

(SYE kloe spor een)

Brand Names: U.S. Restasis®

Index Terms CsA; CyA; Cyclosporin A

Pharmacologic Category Immunosuppressant Agent

Medication Safety Issues

Sound-alike/look-alike issues:

CycloSPORINE may be confused with cyclophosphamide, Cyklokapron®, cycloSERINE

Pregnancy Risk Factor C

Lactation Excretion unknown/use caution

Use Increase tear production when suppressed tear production is presumed to be due to keratoconjunctivitis sicca-associated ocular inflammation (in patients not already using topical anti-inflammatory drugs or punctal plugs)

Available Dosage Forms

Emulsion, ophthalmic [preservative free]:

Restasis®: 0.05% (0.4 mL)

General Dosage Range Ophthalmic (Restasis®): *Children ≥16 years and Adults:* Instill 1 drop in each eye every 12 hours

Administration

Other Prior to use, invert vial several times to obtain a uniform emulsion. Remove contact lenses prior to instillation of drops; may be reinserted 15 minutes after administration. May be used with artificial tears; allow 15 minute interval between products.

Cyproheptadine (si proe HEP ta deen)

Index Terms Cyproheptadine Hydrochloride; Periactin

Pharmacologic Category Histamine H_1 Antagonist; Histamine H_1 Antagonist, First Generation; Piperidine Derivative

Medication Safety Issues

Sound-alike/look-alike issues:

Cyproheptadine may be confused with cyclobenzaprine

Periactin may be confused with Percodan®, Persantine®

International issues:

Periactin brand name for cyproheptadine [U.S., multiple international markets] may be confused with Perative brand name for an enteral nutrition preparation [multiple international markets] and brand name for ketoconazole [Argentina]

BEERS Criteria medication:

This drug may be inappropriate for use in geriatric patients (high severity risk).

Pregnancy Risk Factor B

Lactation Excretion in breast milk unknown/contraindicated

Use Perennial and seasonal allergic rhinitis and other allergic symptoms including urticaria

Unlabeled Use Migraine headache prophylaxis, pruritus, spasticity associated with spinal cord damage

Available Dosage Forms

Syrup, oral: 2 mg/5 mL (473 mL, 480 mL)

Tablet, oral: 4 mg

General Dosage Range

Oral:

Children 2-6 years: 2 mg every 8-12 hours (not to exceed 12 mg/day)

Children 7-14 years: 4 mg every 8-12 hours (not to exceed 16 mg/day)

Adults: 4-20 mg/day divided every 8 hours (not to exceed 0.5 mg/kg/day)

Nursing Actions

Physical Assessment Monitor weight periodically. Monitor for excess anticholinergic effects at beginning of therapy and periodically throughout.

Patient Education Avoid use of alcohol. You may experience drowsiness, dizziness, dry mouth, nausea, or abdominal pain. Report persistent sedation, confusion, agitation, blurred vision, respiratory difficulty, or lack of improvement or worsening of condition.

Cyproterone (sye PROE ter one)

Index Terms Cyproterone Acetate; SH 714

Pharmacologic Category Antiandrogen

Use Palliative treatment of advanced prostate cancer

Product Availability Not available in U.S.

General Dosage Range

I.M.: *Adults (males):* 300 mg (3 mL) once weekly **or** every 2 weeks

Oral: *Adults (males):* 100-300 mg/day in 2-3 divided doses

Administration

Oral Administer tablets at the same time each day, after meals and with liquids. Tablets may be divided into equal halves.

I.M. Administer I.M. injections slowly and avoid intravascular injection which can lead to pulmonary microembolism.

Cytarabine (Conventional)

(sye TARE a been con VEN sha nal)

Index Terms Ara-C; Arabinosylcytosine; Conventional Cytarabine; Cytarabine; Cytarabine Hydrochloride; Cytosar-U; Cytosine Arabinosine Hydrochloride

Pharmacologic Category Antineoplastic Agent, Antimetabolite; Antineoplastic Agent, Antimetabolite (Pyrimidine Analog)

Medication Safety Issues

Sound-alike/look-alike issues:

Cytarabine may be confused with clofarabine, Cytosar®, Cytoxan, vidarabine

Cytarabine (conventional) may be confused with cytarabine liposomal

Cytosar-U may be confused with cytarabine, Cytovene®, Cytoxan, Neosar

High alert medication:

This medication is in a class the Institute for Safe Medication Practices (ISMP) includes among its list of drugs classes which have a heightened risk of causing significant patient harm when used in error.

Administration issues:

Intrathecal medication safety: The American Society of Clinical Oncology (ASCO)/Oncology Nursing Society (ONS) chemotherapy administration safety standards (Jacobson, 2009) encourage the following safety measures for intrathecal chemotherapy:

- Intrathecal medication should not be prepared during the preparation of any other agents
- After preparation, store in an isolated location or container clearly marked with a label identifying as "intrathecal" use only
- Delivery to the patient should only be with other medications also intended for administration into the central nervous system

Pregnancy Risk Factor D

Lactation Excretion in breast milk unknown/not recommended

Breast-Feeding Considerations Due to the potential for serious adverse reactions in the nursing infant, breast-feeding is not recommended.

Use Remission induction in acute myeloid leukemia (AML), treatment of acute lymphocytic leukemia (ALL) and chronic myelocytic leukemia (CML; blast phase); prophylaxis and treatment of meningeal leukemia

Unlabeled Use AML consolidation treatment, AML salvage treatment; acute promyelocytic leukemia (APL) consolidation treatment; treatment of primary central nervous system (CNS) lymphoma; treatment of chronic lymphocytic leukemia (CLL); treatment of relapsed or refractory Hodgkin lymphoma; treatment of non-Hodgkin's lymphomas (NHL)

Mechanism of Action/Effect Inhibition of DNA synthesis in S Phase of cell division; degree of its cytotoxicity correlates linearly with its incorporation into DNA, therefore, incorporation into the DNA is responsible for drug activity and toxicity

Contraindications Hypersensitivity to cytarabine or any component of the formulation

Warnings/Precautions Hazardous agent - use appropriate precautions for handling and disposal. **[U.S. Boxed Warning]: Myelosuppression (leukopenia, thrombocytopenia and anemia) is the major toxicity of cytarabine.** Use with caution in patients with prior drug-induced bone marrow suppression. Monitor blood counts frequently; once blasts are no longer apparent in the peripheral blood, bone marrow should be monitored frequently. Monitor for signs of infection or neutropenic fever due to neutropenia or bleeding due to thrombocytopenia.

High-dose regimens are associated with CNS, gastrointestinal, ocular (reversible corneal toxicity and hemorrhagic conjunctivitis; prophylaxis with ophthalmic corticosteroid drops is recommended), pulmonary toxicities and cardiomyopathy. Neurotoxicity associated with high-dose treatment may present as acute cerebellar toxicity (with or without cerebral impairment), personality changes, or may be severe with seizure and/or coma; may be delayed, occurring up to 3-8 days after treatment has begun. Risk factors for neurotoxicity include cumulative cytarabine dose, prior CNS disease and renal impairment; high-dose therapy (>18 g/m^2 per cycle) and age >50 years also increase the risk for cerebellar toxicity (Herzig, 1987). Tumor lysis syndrome and subsequent hyperuricemia may occur with high dose cytarabine; monitor, consider allopurinol and hydrate accordingly. There have been case reports of fatal cardiomyopathy when high dose cytarabine was used in combination with cyclophosphamide as a preparation regimen for transplantation.

Use with caution in patients with impaired renal and hepatic function; may be at higher risk for CNS toxicities; dosage adjustments may be necessary. A sudden respiratory arrest syndrome is characterized by fever, myalgia, bone pain, chest pain, maculopapular rash, conjunctivitis, and malaise, and may occur 6-12 hours following administration; may be managed with corticosteroids. Anaphylaxis resulting in acute cardiopulmonary arrest has been reported (rare). There have been reports of acute pancreatitis in patients receiving continuous infusion and in patients previously treated with L-asparaginase. **[U.S. Boxed Warning]: Should be administered under the supervision of an experienced cancer chemotherapy physician. Due to the potential toxicities, induction treatment with cytarabine should be in a facility with sufficient laboratory and supportive resources.** Some products may contain benzyl alcohol; do not use products containing benzyl alcohol or products reconstituted with bacteriostatic diluent intrathecally or for high-dose cytarabine regimens. When used for intrathecal administration, should not be prepared during the preparation of any other agents; after preparation, store intrathecal medications in an isolated location or container clearly marked with a label identifying as "intrathecal" use only; delivery of intrathecal medications to the patient should only be with other medications also intended for administration into the central nervous system (Jacobson, 2009).

Drug Interactions

Avoid Concomitant Use

Avoid concomitant use of Cytarabine (Conventional) with any of the following: BCG; CloZAPine; Natalizumab; Pimecrolimus; Tacrolimus (Topical); Vaccines (Live)

Decreased Effect

Cytarabine (Conventional) may decrease the levels/effects of: BCG; Cardiac Glycosides; Coccidioidin Skin Test; Flucytosine; Sipuleucel-T; Vaccines (Inactivated); Vaccines (Live)

The levels/effects of Cytarabine (Conventional) may be decreased by: Echinacea

Increased Effect/Toxicity

Cytarabine (Conventional) may increase the levels/effects of: CloZAPine; Leflunomide; Natalizumab; Vaccines (Live)

The levels/effects of Cytarabine (Conventional) may be increased by: Denosumab; Pimecrolimus; Roflumilast; Tacrolimus (Topical); Trastuzumab

Adverse Reactions

Frequent:

Central nervous system: Fever

Dermatologic: Rash

Gastrointestinal: Anal inflammation, anal ulceration, anorexia, diarrhea, mucositis, nausea, vomiting

Hematologic: Myelosuppression, neutropenia (onset: 1-7 days; nadir [biphasic]: 7-9 days and at 15-24 days; recovery [biphasic]: 9-12 days and at 24-34 days), thrombocytopenia (onset: 5 days; nadir: 12-15 days; recovery 15-25 days), anemia, bleeding, leukopenia, megaloblastosis, reticulocytes decreased

Hepatic: Hepatic dysfunction, transaminases increased (acute)

Local: Thrombophlebitis

Less frequent:

Cardiovascular: Chest pain, pericarditis

Central nervous system: Dizziness, headache, neural toxicity, neuritis

Dermatologic: Alopecia, pruritus, skin freckling, skin ulceration, urticaria

Gastrointestinal: Abdominal pain, bowel necrosis, esophageal ulceration, esophagitis, pancreatitis, sore throat

Genitourinary: Urinary retention

Hepatic: Jaundice

Local: Injection site cellulitis

Ocular: Conjunctivitis

Renal: Renal dysfunction

Respiratory: Dyspnea

Miscellaneous: Allergic edema, anaphylaxis, sepsis

Infrequent and/or case reports: Acute respiratory distress syndrome, amylase increased, angina, aseptic meningitis, cardiopulmonary arrest (acute), cerebral dysfunction, cytarabine syndrome (bone pain, chest pain, conjunctivitis, fever, maculopapular rash, malaise, myalgia); exanthematous pustulosis, hepatic sinusoidal obstruction syndrome (SOS; veno-occlussive disease), hyperuricemia, injection site inflammation (SubQ injection), injection site pain (SubQ injection), interstitial pneumonitis, lipase increased, paralysis (intrathecal and I.V. combination therapy), reversible posterior leukoencephalopathy syndrome (RPLS), rhabdomyolysis, toxic megacolon

Adverse events associated with high-dose cytarabine (CNS, gastrointestinal, ocular, and pulmonary toxicities are more common with high-dose regimens):

Cardiovascular: Cardiomegaly, cardiomyopathy (in combination with cyclophosphamide)

Central nervous system: Cerebellar toxicity, coma, neurotoxicity (up to 55% in patients with renal impairment), personality change, somnolence

Dermatologic: Alopecia (complete), desquamation, rash (severe)

Gastrointestinal: Gastrointestinal ulcer, pancreatitis, peritonitis, pneumatosis cystoides intestinalis

Hepatic: Hyperbilirubinemia, liver abscess, liver damage, necrotizing colitis

Neuromuscular & skeletal: Peripheral neuropathy (motor and sensory)

Ocular: Corneal toxicity, hemorrhagic conjunctivitis

Respiratory: Pulmonary edema, syndrome of sudden respiratory distress

Miscellaneous: Sepsis

Adverse events associated with intrathecal cytarabine administration:

Central nervous system: Accessory nerve paralysis, fever, necrotizing leukoencephalopathy (with concurrent cranial irradiation, I.T. methotrexate, and I.T. hydrocortisone), neurotoxicity, paraplegia

Gastrointestinal: Dysphagia, nausea, vomiting

Ocular: Blindness (with concurrent systemic chemotherapy and cranial irradiation), diplopia

Respiratory: Cough, hoarseness

Miscellaneous: Aphonia

Available Dosage Forms

Injection, powder for reconstitution: 100 mg, 500 mg, 1 g, 2 g

Injection, solution: 20 mg/mL (25 mL); 100 mg/mL (20 mL)

Injection, solution [preservative free]: 20 mg/mL (5 mL, 50 mL); 100 mg/mL (20 mL)

General Dosage Range Dosage adjustment recommended in patients with hepatic or renal impairment

I.V.: *Children and Adults:* AML Induction: 100-200 mg/m²/day for 7 days

Administration

I.V. Infuse standard dose therapy for AML (100-200 mg/m²/day) as a continuous infusion. Infuse high-dose therapy (unlabeled) over 1-3 hours (usually). Other rates have been used, refer to specific reference.

Other

I.T.: Intrathecal doses should be administered as soon as possible after preparation.

May also be administered SubQ.

Stability

Reconstitution Use appropriate precautions for handling and disposal. **Note:** Solutions containing bacteriostatic agents may be used for SubQ and standard-dose (100-200 mg/m²) I.V. cytarabine preparations, but should not be used for the preparation of either intrathecal doses or high-dose I.V. therapies.

I.V.:

Powder for reconstitution: Reconstitute with bacteriostatic water for injection (for standard-dose).

For I.V. infusion: Further dilute in 250-1000 mL 0.9% NaCl or D_5W.

Intrathecal: Powder for reconstitution: Reconstitute with preservative free sodium chloride 0.9%; may further dilute to preferred final volume (volume generally based on institution or practitioner preference; may be up to 12 mL) with Elliott's B solution, sodium chloride 0.9% or lactated Ringer's. Intrathecal medications should not be prepared during the preparation of any other agents.

Triple intrathecal therapy (TIT): Cytarabine 30-50 mg with hydrocortisone sodium succinate 15-25 mg and methotrexate 12 mg; compatible together for up to 24 hours in a syringe; however, should be administered administer as soon as possible after preparation because intrathecal preparations are preservative free

Storage Store intact vials of powder for injection at room temperature of 20°C to 25°C (68°F to 77°F); store intact vials of solution at room temperature of 15°C to 30°C (59°F to 86°F).

I.V.:

Powder for reconstitution: Reconstituted solutions should be stored at room temperature and used within 48 hours.

For I.V. infusion: Solutions for I.V. infusion diluted in D_5W or NS are stable for 7 days at room temperature, although the manufacturer recommends administration as soon as possible after preparation.

Intrathecal: Administer as soon as possible after preparation. After preparation, store intrathecal medications in an isolated location or container clearly marked with a label identifying as "intrathecal" use only.

Nursing Actions

Physical Assessment To be administered under the supervision of an experienced cancer chemotherapy physician. Ocular pain and conjunctivitis reactions may be reduced with ophthalmic corticosteroid premedication. Monitor patient closely throughout treatment, especially with high-dose regimens, for adverse gastrointestinal and pulmonary response, CNS toxicities, and cardiomyopathy.

Patient Education This drug is administered by infusion or injection. Report immediately any redness, swelling, burning, or pain at injection/infusion site; sudden difficulty breathing or swallowing; chest pain; or chills. Maintain adequate hydration. You will be more susceptible to infection. May cause nausea, vomiting, loss of appetite, diarrhea, mouth sores, dizziness, headache, confusion, or brittle or dry hair or loss of hair (may reverse after treatment). Report immediately any signs of respiratory distress, chest pain or palpitations, CNS changes, change in gait, skin rash or ulceration, unusual bruising or bleeding, persistent GI upset, yellowing of eyes or skin, change in color of urine, pain on urination, blackened stool, pain passing stool, pain or numbness in joints or muscles, blurred vision, or change in visual acuity.

Cytomegalovirus Immune Globulin (Intravenous-Human)

(sye toe meg a low VYE rus i MYUN GLOB yoo lin in tra VEE nus HYU man)

Brand Names: U.S. CytoGam®

Index Terms CMV-IGIV

Pharmacologic Category Blood Product Derivative; Immune Globulin

Medication Safety Issues

Sound-alike/look-alike issues:

CytoGam® may be confused with Cytoxan, Gamimune® N

Pregnancy Risk Factor C

Lactation Excretion in breast milk unknown

Use Prophylaxis of cytomegalovirus (CMV) disease associated with kidney, lung, liver, pancreas, and heart transplants; concomitant use with ganciclovir should be considered in organ transplants (other than kidney) from CMV seropositive donors to CMV seronegative recipients

Unlabeled Use Adjunct therapy in the treatment of CMV disease in immunocompromised patients

Available Dosage Forms

Injection, solution [preservative free]:

CytoGam®: 50 mg (± 10 mg)/mL (50 mL)

General Dosage Range I.V.: *Adults:* Initial: 150 mg/kg with 72 hours of transplant; 2-, 4-, 6- and 8 weeks after transplant: 100 mg/kg (kidney) **or** 150 mg/kg (liver, lung, pancreas, heart); 12 and 16 weeks after transplant: 50 mg/kg (kidney) **or** 100 mg/kg (liver, lung, pancreas, heart)

Administration

I.V. For I.V. use only. Administer as separate infusion. Infuse beginning at 15 mg/kg/hour, then increase to 30 mg/kg/hour after 30 minutes if no untoward reactions. May titrate up to 60 mg/kg/hour. Do not administer faster than 75 mL/hour. Begin infusion within 6 hours of entering vial, complete infusion within 12 hours.

I.V. Detail Administer through an I.V. line containing an in-line filter (pore size 15 micron) using an infusion pump. Do not mix with other infusions; do not use if turbid. Begin infusion within 6 hours of entering vial, complete infusion within 12 hours.

Infuse at 15 mg/kg/hour. If no adverse reactions occur within 30 minutes, may increase rate to 30 mg/kg/hour. If no adverse reactions occur within the second 30 minutes, may increase rate to 60 mg/kg/hour; maximum rate of infusion: 75 mL/hour. When infusing subsequent doses, may decrease titration interval from 30 minutes to 15 minutes. If patient develops nausea, back pain, or flushing during infusion, slow the rate or temporarily stop the infusion. Discontinue if blood pressure drops or in case of anaphylactic reaction.

Nursing Actions

Physical Assessment Assess for history of previous allergic reactions. Monitor vital signs during infusion and observe for adverse or allergic reactions.

Patient Education This medication can only be administered by infusion. You will be monitored closely during the infusion. You may experience nausea. Do not have any vaccinations for the next 3 months without consulting prescriber. Immediately report chills, muscle cramping, low back pain, chest pain or tightness, or respiratory difficulty.

Related Information

Immunization Administration Recommendations *on page 1243*

Dacarbazine (da KAR ba zeen)

Index Terms DIC; Dimethyl Triazeno Imidazole Carboxamide; DTIC; DTIC-Dome; Imidazole Carboxamide; Imidazole Carboxamide Dimethyltriazene; WR-139007

Pharmacologic Category Antineoplastic Agent, Alkylating Agent (Triazene)

Medication Safety Issues

Sound-alike/look-alike issues:

Dacarbazine may be confused with procarbazine

High alert medication:

This medication is in a class the Institute for Safe Medication Practices (ISMP) includes among its list of drugs which have a heightened risk of causing significant patient harm when used in error.

Pregnancy Risk Factor C

Lactation Excretion in breast milk unknown/not recommended

Use Treatment of malignant melanoma, Hodgkin's disease

Unlabeled Use Treatment of soft-tissue sarcomas, islet cell tumors, pheochromocytoma, medullary carcinoma of the thyroid

Available Dosage Forms

Injection, powder for reconstitution: 100 mg, 200 mg

General Dosage Range Dosage adjustment recommended in patients with renal impairment

I.V.:

Children: 375 mg/m^2 on days 1 and 15, repeat every 28 days

Adults: 375 mg/m^2 days 1 and 15 every 4 weeks **or** 250 mg/m^2 days 1-5 every 3 weeks

Administration

I.V. Irritant. Infuse over 30-60 minutes; may also be administered as a continuous infusion (unlabeled administration rate) depending on the protocol

I.V. Detail Rapid infusion may cause severe venous irritation.

Extravasation management: Local pain, burning sensation, and irritation at the injection site may be relieved by local application of hot packs. If extravasation occurs, apply cold packs. Protect exposed tissue from light following extravasation.

pH: 3-4

Nursing Actions

Physical Assessment Antiemetic premedication may be ordered (emetic potential is moderately high). Monitor patient closely for anaphylactic reaction; emergency treatment should be available. Monitor infusion site closely; extravasation can cause severe cellulitis or tissue necrosis.

Patient Education This drug can only be given by infusion. Report immediately any pain, burning, or swelling at infusion site; chest pain; or difficulty breathing or swallowing. Limit oral intake for 4-6 hours before infusion. Maintain adequate nutrition and hydration, unless instructed to restrict fluid intake. You will be more susceptible to infection. May cause nausea, vomiting, loss of appetite, hair loss (reversible), headache, fever, sinus congestion, or muscle aches. Report immediately any numbness in extremities or change in gait, respiratory distress or respiratory difficulty, change in urinary pattern, rash, easy bruising or bleeding, yellowing of eyes or skin, change in color of urine, or blackened stool.

Related Information

Management of Drug Extravasations *on page 1269*

DACTINomycin (dak ti noe MYE sin)

Brand Names: U.S. Cosmegen®

Index Terms ACT-D; Actinomycin; Actinomycin CI; Actinomycin D; DACT

Pharmacologic Category Antineoplastic Agent, Antibiotic

Medication Safety Issues

Sound-alike/look-alike issues:

DACTINomycin may be confused with Dacogen®, DAPTOmycin, DAUNOrubicin

Actinomycin may be confused with achromycin

High alert medication:

This medication is in a class the Institute for Safe Medication Practices (ISMP) includes among its list of drug classes which have a heightened risk of causing significant patient harm when used in error.

Pregnancy Risk Factor D

Lactation Excretion in breast milk unknown/not recommended

Use Treatment of Wilms' tumor, childhood rhabdomyosarcoma, Ewing's sarcoma, metastatic testicular tumors (nonseminomatous), gestational trophoblastic neoplasm; regional perfusion (palliative or adjunctive) of locally recurrent or locoregional solid tumors (sarcomas, carcinomas and adenocarcinomas)

Unlabeled Use Treatment of ovarian cancer (germ cell or stromal tumors), osteosarcoma, soft tissue sarcoma (other than rhabdomyosarcoma)

Available Dosage Forms

Injection, powder for reconstitution: 0.5 mg

Cosmegen®: 0.5 mg

General Dosage Range

I.V.:

Children >6 months: 15 mcg/kg/day **or** 400-600 mcg/m^2/day for 5 days every 3-6 weeks

Adults: 12-15 mcg/kg/day **or** 400-600 mcg/m^2/day for 5 days every 3-6 weeks **or** 1000 mcg/m^2 on day 1 **or** 500 mcg/dose days 1 and 2

Regional perfusion: *Adults:* Lower extremity or pelvis: 50 mcg/kg; Upper extremity: 35 mcg/kg

Administration

I.V. Slow I.V. push or infuse over 10-15 minutes. Avoid extravasation. Do not filter with cellulose ester membrane filters. Do not administer I.M. or SubQ.

I.V. Detail pH: 5.5-7.0 (reconstituted solution)

Nursing Actions

Physical Assessment Monitor infusion site closely; extravasation can cause severe cellulitis or tissue necrosis. Monitor laboratory tests and patient response on a regular basis throughout (toxic effects may be delayed 2-4 days following a course of treatment and may take 1-2 weeks to reach maximum severity).

Patient Education This drug is given by infusion and you will be closely monitored. Report immediately any pain, burning, or swelling at infusion site; sudden chest pain, difficulty breathing or swallowing, or chills. Between infusions, maintain adequate nutrition and hydration. You will be more susceptible to infection. May cause fatigue or malaise, nausea, vomiting, loss of appetite, diarrhea, or hair loss (reversible). Report unresolved nausea, vomiting, diarrhea, or abdominal pain; difficulty swallowing; or rash.

Related Information

Management of Drug Extravasations *on page 1269*

Dalfampridine (dal FAM pri deen)

Brand Names: U.S. Ampyra™

Index Terms 4-aminopyridine; 4-AP; EL-970; Fampridine-SR

Pharmacologic Category Potassium Channel Blocker

Medication Safety Issues

Sound-alike/look-alike issues:

Ampyra™ may be confused with anakinra

Dalfampridine may be confused with delavirdine, desipramine

Medication Guide Available Yes

Pregnancy Risk Factor C

Lactation Excretion in breast milk unknown/not recommended

Use Treatment to improve walking in multiple sclerosis (MS) patients

Available Dosage Forms

Tablet, extended release, oral:

Ampyra™: 10 mg

General Dosage Range Oral: Extended release: *Adults:* 10 mg every 12 hours

Administration

Oral May be administered with or without food. Do not chew, crush, dissolve, or divide tablet.

Nursing Actions

Physical Assessment If seizures occur, discontinue medication.

Patient Education Take with or without food. Discontinue and consult prescriber if you experience a seizure. You may experience dizziness or headache. Report any sign of urinary tract infection (change in urinary pattern or pain on urination), relapse of multiple sclerosis, persistent headache or dizziness, unusual muscle weakness, or difficulty with balance.

Dalteparin (dal TE pa rin)

Brand Names: U.S. Fragmin®

Index Terms Dalteparin Sodium

Pharmacologic Category Low Molecular Weight Heparin

Medication Safety Issues

High alert medication:

The Institute for Safe Medication Practices (ISMP) includes this medication among its list of drugs which have a heightened risk of causing significant patient harm when used in error.

National Patient Safety Goals:

The Joint Commission (TJC) requires healthcare organizations that provide anticoagulant therapy to have a process in place to reduce the risk of anticoagulant-associated patient harm. Patients receiving anticoagulants should receive individualized care through a defined process that includes standardized ordering, dispensing, administration, monitoring and education. This does not apply to routine short-term use of anticoagulants for prevention of venous thromboembolism when the expectation is that the patient's laboratory values will remain within or close to normal values (NPSG.03.05.01).

Pregnancy Risk Factor B

Lactation Enters breast milk/use caution

Breast-Feeding Considerations In lactating women receiving prophylactic doses of dalteparin, small amounts of anti-xa activity was noted in breast milk. The milk/plasma ratio was <0.025 to 0.224. Oral absorption of low molecular weight heparin is extremely low.

Use Prevention of deep vein thrombosis (DVT) which may lead to pulmonary embolism, in patients requiring abdominal surgery who are at risk for thromboembolism complications (eg, patients >40 years of age, obesity, patients with malignancy, history of DVT or pulmonary embolism, and surgical procedures requiring general anesthesia and lasting >30 minutes); prevention of DVT in patients undergoing hip-replacement surgery; patients immobile during an acute illness; prevention of ischemic complications in patients with unstable angina or non-Q-wave myocardial infarction on concurrent aspirin therapy; in patients with cancer, extended treatment (6 months) of acute symptomatic venous thromboembolism (DVT and/or PE) to reduce the recurrence of venous thromboembolism

Unlabeled Use Active treatment of deep vein thrombosis (noncancer patients)

Mechanism of Action/Effect Low molecular weight heparin analog; the commercial product contains 3% to 15% heparin; has been shown to inhibit both factor Xa and factor IIa (thrombin), however, the antithrombotic effect of dalteparin is characterized by a higher ratio of antifactor Xa to antifactor IIa activity (ratio = 4)

Contraindications Hypersensitivity to dalteparin or any component of the formulation; history of heparin-induced thrombocytopenia (HIT) or HIT with thrombosis; hypersensitivity to heparin or pork products; patients with active major bleeding; patients with unstable angina, non-Q-wave MI, or acute venous thromboembolism undergoing epidural/neuraxial anesthesia

Warnings/Precautions [U.S. Boxed Warning]: Spinal or epidural hematomas, including subsequent paralysis, may occur with recent or anticipated neuraxial anesthesia (epidural or spinal) or spinal puncture in patients anticoagulated with LMWH or heparinoids. Consider risk versus benefit prior to spinal procedures; risk is increased by the use of concomitant agents which may alter hemostasis, the use of indwelling epidural catheters for analgesia, a history of spinal deformity or spinal surgery, as well as traumatic or repeated epidural or spinal punctures. Use of dalteparin is contraindicated in patients undergoing epidural/neuraxial anesthesia. Patient should be observed closely for bleeding if enoxaparin is administered during or immediately following diagnostic lumbar puncture, epidural anesthesia, or spinal anesthesia.

Use with caution in patients with pre-existing thrombocytopenia, recent childbirth, subacute bacterial endocarditis, peptic ulcer disease, pericarditis or pericardial effusion, liver or renal function impairment, recent lumbar puncture, vasculitis, concurrent use of aspirin (increased bleeding risk), previous hypersensitivity to heparin, heparin-associated thrombocytopenia. Monitor platelet count closely. Rare cases of thrombocytopenia (some with thrombosis) have occurred. Consider discontinuation of dalteparin in any patient developing significant thrombocytopenia related to initiation of dalteparin especially when associated with a positive *in vitro* test for antiplatelet antibodies. Use caution in patients with congenital or drug-induced thrombocytopenia or platelet defects. Cancer patients with thrombocytopenia may require dose adjustments for treatment of acute venous thromboembolism. In patients with a history of heparin-induced thrombocytopenia (HIT) or HIT with thrombosis, dalteparin is contraindicated.

Monitor patient closely for signs or symptoms of bleeding. Certain patients are at increased risk of bleeding. Risk factors include bacterial endocarditis; congenital or acquired bleeding disorders; active ulcerative or angiodysplastic GI diseases; severe uncontrolled hypertension; hemorrhagic stroke; or use shortly after brain, spinal, or ophthalmology surgery; in patients treated concomitantly with platelet inhibitors; recent GI bleeding; thrombocytopenia or platelet defects; severe liver disease; hypertensive or diabetic retinopathy; or in patients undergoing invasive procedures.

Use with caution in patients with severe renal impairment; accumulation may occur with repeated dosing increasing the risk for bleeding. Multidose vials contain benzyl alcohol and should not be used in pregnant women. In neonates, large amounts of benzyl alcohol (>100 mg/kg/day) have been associated with fatal toxicity (gasping syndrome). Heparin can cause hyperkalemia by affecting aldosterone. Similar reactions could occur with dalteparin. Monitor for hyperkalemia. Do **not** administer intramuscularly. Not to be used interchangeably (unit for unit) with heparin or any other low molecular weight heparins.

There is no consensus for adjusting/correcting the weight-based dosage of LMWH for patients who are morbidly obese (BMI ≥40 kg/m^2). For patients undergoing inpatient bariatric surgery, the American College of Chest Physicians Practice Guidelines suggest using a higher thromboprophylaxis dose of LMWH for obese patients (Geerts, 2008).

Drug Interactions

Avoid Concomitant Use

Avoid concomitant use of Dalteparin with any of the following: Rivaroxaban

Decreased Effect There are no known significant interactions involving a decrease in effect.

Increased Effect/Toxicity

Dalteparin may increase the levels/effects of: Anticoagulants; Collagenase (Systemic); Deferasirox; Drotrecogin Alfa (Activated); Ibritumomab; Rivaroxaban; Tositumomab and Iodine I 131 Tositumomab

The levels/effects of Dalteparin may be increased by: 5-ASA Derivatives; Antiplatelet Agents; Dasatinib; Herbs (Anticoagulant/Antiplatelet Properties); Nonsteroidal Anti-Inflammatory Agents; Pentosan Polysulfate Sodium; Pentoxifylline; Prostacyclin Analogues; Salicylates; Thrombolytic Agents

Nutritional/Ethanol Interactions Herb/Nutraceutical: Alfalfa, anise, bilberry, bladderwrack, bromelain, cat's claw, celery, chamomile, coleus, cordyceps, dong quai, evening primrose oil, fenugreek, feverfew, garlic, ginger, ginkgo biloba, ginseng (American), ginseng (panax), ginseng (Siberian), grapeseed, green tea, guggul, horse chestnut seed, horseradish, licorice, prickly ash, red clover, reishi, SAMe (s-adenosylmethionine), sweet clover, turmeric, white willow (all have additional antiplatelet/anticoagulant activity)

Adverse Reactions Note: As with all anticoagulants, bleeding is the major adverse effect of dalteparin. Hemorrhage may occur at virtually any site. Risk is dependent on multiple variables.

>10%: Hematologic: Bleeding (3% to 14%), thrombocytopenia (including heparin-induced thrombocytopenia), <1%; cancer clinical trials: ~11%)

1% to 10%:

Hematologic: Major bleeding (up to 6%), wound hematoma (up to 3%)

Hepatic: AST >3 times upper limit of normal (5% to 9%), ALT >3 times upper limit of normal (4% to 10%)

Local: Pain at injection site (up to 12%), injection site hematoma (up to 7%)

Pharmacodynamics/Kinetics

Onset of Action Anti-Xa activity: Within 1-2 hours

Duration of Action >12 hours

Available Dosage Forms

Injection, solution:

Fragmin®: 25,000 anti-Xa int. units/mL (3.8 mL)

Injection, solution [preservative free]:

Fragmin®: 10,000 anti-Xa int. units/mL (1 mL); 2500 anti-Xa int. units/0.2 mL (0.2 mL); 5000 anti-Xa int. units/0.2 mL (0.2 mL); 7500 anti-Xa int. units/0.3 mL (0.3 mL); 12,500 anti-Xa int. units/0.5 mL (0.5 mL); 15,000 anti-Xa int. units/0.6 mL (0.6 mL); 18,000 anti-Xa int. units/0.72 mL (0.72 mL)

General Dosage Range SubQ: *Adults:* Prophylaxis: 2500-5000 int. units daily; Treatment: 120 int. units/kg every 12 hours (maximum: 10,000 int. units/dose) **or** ~150-200 int. units/kg (maximum: 18,000 int. units/dose) once daily

Administration

Other For deep SubQ injection **only**. May be injected in a U-shape to the area surrounding the navel, the upper outer side of the thigh, or the upper outer quadrangle of the buttock. Use thumb and forefinger to lift a fold of skin when injecting dalteparin to the navel area or thigh. Insert needle at a 45- to 90-degree angle. The entire length of needle should be inserted. Do not expel air bubble from fixed-dose syringe prior to injection. Air bubble (and extra solution, if applicable) may be expelled from graduated syringes. In order to minimize bruising, do not rub injection site.

To convert from I.V. unfractionated heparin (UFH) infusion to SubQ dalteparin (Nutescu, 2007): Calculate specific dose for dalteparin based on indication, discontinue UFH and begin dalteparin within 1 hour

To convert from SubQ dalteparin to I.V. UFH infusion (Nutescu, 2007): Discontinue dalteparin; calculate specific dose for I.V. UFH infusion based on indication; omit heparin bolus/ loading dose

Converting from SubQ dalteparin dosed every 12 hours: Start I.V. UFH infusion 10-11 hours after last dose of dalteparin

Converting from SubQ dalteparin dosed every 24 hours: Start I.V. UFH infusion 22-23 hours after last dose of dalteparin

Stability

Storage Store at temperatures of 20°C to 25°C (68°F to 77°F). Multidose vials may be stored for up to 2 weeks at room temperature after entering.

Nursing Actions

Physical Assessment Bleeding precautions should be observed. Teach patient about bleeding precautions.

Patient Education This drug can only be administered by injection. You may have a tendency to bleed easily while taking this drug. Report unusual fever; unusual bleeding or bruising (bleeding gums, nosebleed, blood in urine, dark stool); pain in joints or back; severe headache or confusion; skin rash; redness, swelling, or pain at injection site; or severe dizziness.

Danazol (DA na zole)

Index Terms Danocrine

Pharmacologic Category Androgen

Medication Safety Issues

Sound-alike/look-alike issues:

Danazol may be confused with Dantrium®

Pregnancy Risk Factor X

Lactation Enters breast milk/contraindicated

Use Treatment of endometriosis, fibrocystic breast disease, and hereditary angioedema

Available Dosage Forms

Capsule, oral: 50 mg, 100 mg, 200 mg

General Dosage Range Oral:

Adults (females): 100-800 mg/day in 2 divided doses

Adults (females/males): Hereditary angioedema: Initial: 200 mg 2-3 times/day; after favorable response decrease dosage by 50% or less

Nursing Actions

Physical Assessment Monitor for hypertension, increased LDL, CNS changes, jaundice, and hematuria. Caution patients with diabetes to monitor glucose levels closely; may enhance the glucose-lowering effect of hypoglycemic agents. Teach patient good self-breast exam technique.

Patient Education Therapy may take up to several months depending on purpose for therapy. If you have diabetes, monitor serum glucose closely and notify prescriber of changes; this medication can alter hypoglycemic requirements. Consult prescriber for appropriate self-breast-exam technique. May cause headache, sleeplessness, anxiety, acne, growth of body hair, deepening of voice, loss of libido, impotence, or menstrual irregularity (usually reversible). Report changes in menstrual pattern, deepening of voice or unusual growth of body hair, persistent penile erections, fluid retention (eg, swelling of ankles, feet, or hands, respiratory difficulty, or sudden weight gain), change in color of urine or stool, yellowing of eyes or skin, or unusual bruising or bleeding.

Dantrolene (DAN troe leen)

Brand Names: U.S. Dantrium®; Revonto™

Index Terms Dantrolene Sodium

Pharmacologic Category Skeletal Muscle Relaxant

Medication Safety Issues

Sound-alike/look-alike issues:

Dantrium® may be confused with danazol, Daraprim®

Revonto™ may be confused with Revatio®

Pregnancy Risk Factor C

Lactation Enters breast milk/not recommended

Use Treatment of spasticity associated with upper motor neuron disorders (eg, spinal cord injury, stroke, cerebral palsy, or multiple sclerosis); management of malignant hyperthermia; prevention of malignant hyperthermia in susceptible individuals (preoperative/postoperative administration)

Unlabeled Use Neuroleptic malignant syndrome (NMS)

Available Dosage Forms

Capsule, oral: 25 mg, 50 mg, 100 mg

Dantrium®: 25 mg, 50 mg, 100 mg

Injection, powder for reconstitution:

Dantrium®: 20 mg

Revonto™: 20 mg

General Dosage Range

I.V.: *Children and Adults:* 1-2.5 mg/kg; may repeat up to cumulative dose of 10 mg/kg **or** 2.5 mg/kg as a single dose

Oral:

Children: 4-8 mg/kg/day in 4 divided doses **or** 0.5-2 mg/kg/dose 1-3 times/day (maximum: 400 mg/day)

Adults: 4-8 mg/kg/day in 4 divided doses **or** 25-100 mg 1-3 times/day (maximum: 400 mg/day)

Administration

I.V. Therapeutic or emergency dose can be administered with rapid continuous I.V. push. Follow-up doses should be administered over 2-3 minutes.

I.V. Detail pH ~9.5 (after reconstitution)

Nursing Actions

Physical Assessment I.V.: Monitor vital signs, cardiac function, respiratory status, and I.V. site (extravasation very irritating to tissues) frequently during infusion.

Patient Education Do not use alcohol. You may experience drowsiness, dizziness, lightheadedness, nausea, vomiting, or diarrhea.

Related Information

Management of Drug Extravasations *on page 1269*

Darbepoetin Alfa (dar be POE e tin AL fa)

Brand Names: U.S. Aranesp®; Aranesp® SingleJect®

Index Terms Erythropoiesis-Stimulating Agent (ESA); Erythropoiesis-Stimulating Protein; NESP; Novel Erythropoiesis-Stimulating Protein

Pharmacologic Category Colony Stimulating Factor; Growth Factor; Recombinant Human Erythropoietin

Medication Safety Issues

Sound-alike/look-alike issues:

Aranesp® may be confused with Aralast, Aricept®

Darbepoetin alfa may be confused with dalteparin, epoetin alfa, epoetin beta

Medication Guide Available Yes

Pregnancy Risk Factor C

Lactation Excretion in breast milk unknown/use caution

Use Treatment of anemia due to concurrent myelosuppressive chemotherapy in patients with cancer (nonmyeloid malignancies) receiving chemotherapy (palliative intent) for a planned minimum of 2 additional months of chemotherapy; treatment of anemia due to chronic kidney disease (including patients on dialysis and not on dialysis)

Note: Darbepoetin is **not** indicated for use under the following conditions:

- Cancer patients receiving hormonal therapy, therapeutic biologic products, or radiation therapy unless also receiving concurrent myelosuppressive chemotherapy
- Cancer patients receiving myelosuppressive chemotherapy when the expected outcome is curative
- As a substitute for RBC transfusion in patients requiring immediate correction of anemia

Note: In clinical trials, darbepoetin has not demonstrated improved quality of life, fatigue, or well-being.

Unlabeled Use Treatment of symptomatic anemia in myelodysplastic syndrome (MDS)

Mechanism of Action/Effect Stimulates production of red blood cells within the bone marrow. There is a dose response relationship with this effect. This results in an increase in red blood cell counts followed by a rise in hematocrit and hemoglobin levels. When administered SubQ or I.V., darbepoetin's half-life is ~3 times that of epoetin alfa.

Contraindications Hypersensitivity to darbepoetin or any component of the formulation; uncontrolled hypertension; pure red cell aplasia (due to darbepoetin or other erythropoietin protein drugs)

Warnings/Precautions [U.S. Boxed Warning]: Erythropoiesis-stimulating agents (ESAs) increased the risk of serious cardiovascular events, thromboembolic events, stroke, and/or tumor progression in clinical studies when administered to target hemoglobin levels >11 g/dL (and provide no additional benefit); a rapid rise in hemoglobin (>1 g/dL over 2 weeks) may also contribute to these risks. **[U.S. Boxed Warning]: A shortened overall survival and/or increased risk of tumor progression or recurrence has been reported in studies with breast, cervical, head and neck, lymphoid, and non-small cell lung cancer patients.** It is of note that in these studies, patients received ESAs to a target hemoglobin of ≥12 g/dL; although risk has not been excluded when dosed to achieve a target hemoglobin of <12 g/dL. **[U.S. Boxed Warnings]: To decrease these risks, and risk of cardio- and thrombovascular events, use ESAs in cancer patients only for the treatment of anemia related to concurrent myelosuppressive chemotherapy and use the lowest dose needed to avoid red blood cell transfusions. Discontinue ESA following completion of the chemotherapy course. ESAs are <u>not</u> indicated for patients receiving myelosuppressive therapy when the anticipated outcome is curative.** A dosage modification is appropriate if hemoglobin levels rise >1 g/dL per 2-week time period during treatment (Rizzo, 2010). Use of ESAs has been associated with an increased risk of venous thromboembolism (VTE) without a reduction in transfusions in patients >65 years of age with cancer (Hershman, 2009). Improved anemia symptoms, quality of life, fatigue, or well-being have not been demonstrated in controlled clinical trials. **[U.S. Boxed Warning]: Because of the risks of decreased survival and increased risk of tumor growth or progression, all healthcare providers and hospitals are required to enroll and comply with the ESA APPRISE (Assisting Providers and Cancer Patients with Risk Information for the Safe use of ESAs) Oncology Program prior to prescribing or dispensing ESAs to cancer patients.** Prescribers and patients will have to provide written documentation of discussed risks prior to each course.

[U.S. Boxed Warning]: An increased risk of death, serious cardiovascular events, and stroke was reported in patients with chronic kidney disease (CKD) administered ESAs to target hemoglobin levels ≥11 g/dL; use the lowest dose sufficient to reduce the need for RBC transfusions. An optimal target hemoglobin level, dose or dosing strategy to reduce these risks has not been identified in clinical trials. Hemoglobin rising >1 g/dL in a 2-week period may contribute to the risk (dosage reduction recommended). CKD patients who exhibit an inadequate hemoglobin response to ESA therapy may be at a higher risk for cardiovascular events and mortality compared to other patients. ESA therapy may reduce dialysis efficacy (due to increase in red blood cells and decrease in plasma volume); adjustments in dialysis parameters may be needed. Patients treated with epoetin may require increased heparinization during dialysis to prevent clotting of the extracorporeal circuit. CKD patients not requiring dialysis may have a better response to darbepoetin and may require lower doses. An increased risk of DVT has been observed in patients treated with epoetin undergoing surgical orthopedic procedures. Darbepoetin is **not** approved for reduction in allogeneic red blood cell transfusions in patients scheduled for surgical procedures. The risk for seizures is increased with darbepoetin use in patients with CKD; use with caution in patients with a history of seizures. Monitor closely for neurologic symptoms during the first several months of therapy. Use with caution in patients with hypertension; hypertensive encephalopathy has been reported. Use is contraindicated in patients with uncontrolled hypertension. If hypertension is difficult to control, reduce or hold darbepoetin alfa. Due to the delayed onset of erythropoiesis, darbepoetin alfa is **not** recommended for acute correction of severe anemia or as a substitute for emergency transfusion. Consider discontinuing in patients who receive a renal transplant.

Prior to treatment, correct or exclude deficiencies of iron, vitamin B_{12}, and/or folate, as well as other factors which may impair erythropoiesis (inflammatory conditions, infections, bleeding). Prior to and during therapy, iron stores must be evaluated. Supplemental iron is recommended if serum ferritin <100 mcg/L or serum transferrin saturation <20%; most patients with CKD will require iron supplementation. Poor response should prompt evaluation of these potential factors, as well as possible malignant processes and hematologic disease (thalassemia, refractory anemia, myelodysplastic disorder), occult blood loss, hemolysis, osteitis fibrosa cystic, and/or bone marrow fibrosis. Severe anemia and pure red cell aplasia (PRCA) with associated neutralizing antibodies to erythropoietin has been reported, predominantly in patients with CKD receiving SubQ darbepoetin (the I.V. route is preferred for hemodialysis patients). Cases have also been reported in patients with hepatitis C who were receiving ESAs, interferon, and ribavirin. Patients with a sudden loss of response to darbepoetin (with severe anemia and a low reticulocyte count) should be evaluated for PRCA with associated neutralizing antibodies to erythropoietin; discontinue treatment (permanently) in patients with PRCA secondary to neutralizing antibodies to erythropoietin. Antibodies may cross-react; do not switch to another ESA in patients who develop antibody-mediated anemia.

Potentially serious allergic reactions have been reported (rarely). Discontinue immediately (and permanently) in patients who experience serious allergic/anaphylactic reactions. Some products may contain albumin and the packaging of some formulations may contain latex.

Drug Interactions

Avoid Concomitant Use There are no known interactions where it is recommended to avoid concomitant use.

Decreased Effect There are no known significant interactions involving a decrease in effect.

Increased Effect/Toxicity There are no known significant interactions involving an increase in effect.

Nutritional/Ethanol Interactions Ethanol: Should be avoided due to adverse effects on erythropoiesis.

Adverse Reactions

>10%:

Cardiovascular: Hypertension (31%), peripheral edema (17%), edema (6% to 13%)

Gastrointestinal: Abdominal pain (10% to 13%)

Respiratory: Dyspnea (17%), cough (12%)

1% to 10%:

Cardiovascular: Angina, fluid overload, hypotension, MI, thromboembolic events

Central nervous system: Cerebrovascular disorder

Dermatologic: Rash/erythema

Local: AV graft thrombosis, vascular access complications

Respiratory: Pulmonary embolism

Pharmacodynamics/Kinetics

Onset of Action Increased hemoglobin levels not generally observed until 2-6 weeks after initiating treatment

Available Dosage Forms

Injection, solution [preservative free]:

Aranesp®: 25 mcg/mL (1 mL); 40 mcg/mL (1 mL); 60 mcg/mL (1 mL); 100 mcg/mL (1 mL); 150 mcg/0.75 mL (0.75 mL); 200 mcg/mL (1 mL); 300 mcg/mL (1 mL)

Aranesp® SingleJect®: 25 mcg/0.42 mL (0.42 mL); 40 mcg/0.4 mL (0.4 mL); 60 mcg/0.3 mL (0.3 mL); 100 mcg/0.5 mL (0.5 mL); 150 mcg/0.3 mL (0.3 mL); 200 mcg/0.4 mL (0.4 mL); 300 mcg/0.6 mL (0.6 mL); 500 mcg/mL (1 mL)

General Dosage Range

I.V.:

Children 1-18 years: 6.25-200 mcg/week

Adults: 0.45 mcg/kg once weekly **or** every 4 weeks **or** 0.75 mcg/kg once every 2 weeks **or** 6.25-200 mcg/week

SubQ:

Children 1-18 years: 6.25-200 mcg/week

Adults: 0.45-4.5 mcg/kg/week **or** 0.45 mcg/kg every 4 weeks **or** 0.75 mcg/kg once every 2 weeks **or** 500 mcg once every 3 weeks **or** 6.25-200 mcg/week

Administration

I.V. May be administered by I.V. injection. The I.V. route is recommended in hemodialysis patients. Do not shake; vigorous shaking may denature darbepoetin alfa, rendering it biologically inactive. Do not dilute or administer in conjunction with other drug solutions. Discard any unused portion of the vial; do not pool unused portions.

Other May be administered SubQ.

Stability

Storage Store at 2°C to 8°C (36°F to 46°F); do not freeze. Do not shake. Protect from light. Store in original carton until use. The following stability information has also been reported: May be stored at room temperature for up to 7 days (Cohen, 2007).

Nursing Actions

Physical Assessment Monitor blood pressure closely during therapy. If administered by intravenous infusion, lines should be monitored closely for possible clotting. Monitor for hyper-/hypotension, edema, thrombosis, stroke, TIA, and anemia. Teach patient proper SubQ injection technique and syringe/needle disposal. Evaluate history of hypertension or seizures and potential risk for thromboembolism prior to beginning therapy. Assess blood chemistries, hemoglobin/hematocrit, serum ferritin, and transferrin saturation prior to and on a regular basis during therapy.

Patient Education If self-administered, follow exact directions for injection and needle disposal. You will require frequent blood tests to determine appropriate dosage and reduce potential for severe adverse effects; maintaining laboratory testing schedule is vital. You may experience fever, headache, trouble sleeping, itching, skin pain, nausea, vomiting, diarrhea, heartburn, or upper respiratory congestion. Report onset of severe headache, unusual dizziness, or blurred vision; sudden and rapid weight gain; numbness or weakness, especially on one side of the body; severe headaches; confusion; chest pain or irregular heartbeat; leg pain and tenderness; muscular tremors or seizure activity; or difficulty breathing.

Dietary Considerations Supplemental iron intake may be required in patients with low iron stores.

Darifenacin (dar i FEN a sin)

Brand Names: U.S. Enablex®

Index Terms Darifenacin Hydrobromide; UK-88,525

Pharmacologic Category Anticholinergic Agent

Pregnancy Risk Factor C

Lactation Excretion in breast milk unknown/use caution

Breast-Feeding Considerations Although human data are not available, darifenacin is excreted in the breast milk in animals.

Use Management of symptoms of bladder overactivity (urge incontinence, urgency, and frequency)

Mechanism of Action/Effect Blocks muscarinic/cholinergic receptors (M3 subtype) on the smooth muscle of the urinary bladder to limit bladder contractions, reducing the symptoms of bladder irritability/overactivity (urge incontinence, urgency and frequency).

Contraindications Hypersensitivity to darifenacin or any component of the formulation; uncontrolled narrow-angle glaucoma; urinary retention, paralytic ileus, GI or GU obstruction

Warnings/Precautions May cause drowsiness and/or blurred vision, which may impair physical or mental abilities; patients must be cautioned about performing tasks which require mental alertness (eg, operating machinery or driving). May occur in the presence of increased environmental temperature; use caution in hot weather and/or exercise. Use with caution with hepatic impairment; dosage limitation is required in moderate hepatic impairment (Child-Pugh class B). Not recommended for use in severe hepatic impairment (Child-Pugh class C). Use with caution in patients with clinically-significant bladder outlet obstruction or prostatic hyperplasia (nonobstructive). Use caution in patients with decreased GI motility, constipation, hiatal hernia, reflux esophagitis, and ulcerative colitis. Use caution in patients with myasthenia gravis. In patients with controlled narrow-angle glaucoma, darifenacin should be used with extreme caution and only when the potential benefit outweighs risks of treatment. Use with caution in patients taking strong CYP3A4 inhibitors (see Drug Interactions); dosage limitation of darifenacin is required.

Drug Interactions

Avoid Concomitant Use

Avoid concomitant use of Darifenacin with any of the following: Conivaptan; Pimozide; Thioridazine

Decreased Effect

Darifenacin may decrease the levels/effects of: Acetylcholinesterase Inhibitors (Central); Codeine; Secretin; TraMADol

The levels/effects of Darifenacin may be decreased by: Acetylcholinesterase Inhibitors (Central); CYP3A4 Inducers (Strong); Deferasirox; Herbs (CYP3A4 Inducers); Peginterferon Alfa-2b; Tocilizumab

Increased Effect/Toxicity

Darifenacin may increase the levels/effects of: AbobotulinumtoxinA; Anticholinergics; ARIPiprazole; Cannabinoids; CYP2D6 Substrates; Fesoterodine; Nebivolol; OnabotulinumtoxinA; Pimozide; Potassium Chloride; RimabotulinumtoxinB; Tamoxifen; Thioridazine

The levels/effects of Darifenacin may be increased by: Conivaptan; CYP3A4 Inhibitors (Moderate); CYP3A4 Inhibitors (Strong); Dasatinib; Ivacaftor; Pramlintide; Propafenone

Nutritional/Ethanol Interactions Herb/Nutraceutical: Darifenacin serum concentration may be decreased by St John's wort (avoid concurrent use.)

Adverse Reactions

>10%: Gastrointestinal: Xerostomia (19% to 35%), constipation (15% to 21%)

1% to 10%:

Cardiovascular: Hypertension (≥1%), peripheral edema (≥1%)

Central nervous system: Headache (7%), dizziness (<2%), pain (≥1%)

Dermatological: Dry skin (≥1%), pruritus (≥1%), rash (≥1%)

Gastrointestinal: Dyspepsia (3% to 8%), abdominal pain (2% to 4%), nausea (2% to 4%), vomiting (≥1%), weight gain (≥1%)

Genitourinary: Urinary tract infection (4% to 5%), vaginitis (≥1%), urinary retention (acute)

Neuromuscular & skeletal: Weakness (<3%), arthralgia (≥1%), back pain (≥1%)

Ocular: Dry eyes (2%), abnormal vision (≥1%)

Respiratory: Bronchitis (≥1%), pharyngitis (≥1%), rhinitis (≥1%), sinusitis (≥1%)

Miscellaneous: Flu-like syndrome (1% to 3%)

Available Dosage Forms

Tablet, extended release, oral:

Enablex®: 7.5 mg, 15 mg

General Dosage Range Dosage adjustment recommended in patients with hepatic impairment or on concomitant therapy

Oral: *Adults:* Initial: 7.5 mg once daily; Maintenance: 7.5-15 mg once daily

Administration

Oral Tablet should be taken with liquid and swallowed whole; do not chew, crush, or split tablet. May be taken without regard to food.

Stability

Storage Store at 25°C (77°F); excursions permitted to 15°C to 30°C (59°F to 86°F). Protect from light.

Nursing Actions

Patient Education Swallow tablet whole. May cause headache, dizziness, nervousness, sleepiness, abdominal discomfort, diarrhea, constipation, dry mouth, nausea, or vomiting. Report back pain, muscle spasms, alteration in gait, or numbness of extremities; unresolved or persistent constipation, diarrhea, or vomiting; symptoms of upper respiratory infection or flu; or difficulty urinating, pain on urination, or abdominal pain.

Dietary Considerations May be taken without regard to meals, with or without food.

Darunavir (dar OO na veer)

Brand Names: U.S. Prezista®

Index Terms Darunavir Ethanolate; TMC-114

Pharmacologic Category Antiretroviral Agent, Protease Inhibitor

Pregnancy Risk Factor C

Lactation Excretion in breast milk unknown/not recommended

Breast-Feeding Considerations Maternal or infant antiretroviral therapy does not completely eliminate the risk of postnatal HIV transmission. In addition, multiclass-resistant virus has been detected in breast-feeding infants despite maternal therapy. Therefore, in the United States, where formula is accessible, affordable, safe, and sustainable, and the risk of infant mortality due to diarrhea and respiratory infections is low, complete avoidance of breast-feeding by HIV-infected women is recommended to decrease potential transmission of HIV (DHHS [perinatal], 2011).

Use Treatment of HIV-1 infections in combination with ritonavir and other antiretroviral agents

Mechanism of Action/Effect Blocks the site of HIV-1 protease activity, resulting in the formation of immature, noninfectious viral particles.

Contraindications Coadministration with medications highly dependent upon CYP3A4 for clearance and for which increased levels are associated with serious and/or life-threatening events (includes alfuzosin, cisapride, ergot alkaloids [eg, dihydroergotamine, ergonovine, ergotamine, methylergonovine], lovastatin, midazolam [oral], pimozide, rifampin, sildenafil (when used for pulmonary artery hypertension [eg, Revatio®]), simvastatin, St John's wort, triazolam

Canadian labeling: Additional contraindications: Hypersensitivity to darunavir or any component of the formulation; coadministration with amiodarone, lidocaine (systemic), quinidine; severe (Child-Pugh class C) hepatic impairment

Warnings/Precautions Coadministration with ritonavir is required (DHHS, 2011). Use with caution in patients taking strong CYP3A4 inhibitors, moderate or strong CYP3A4 inducers and major CYP3A4 substrates (see Drug Interactions); consider alternative agents that avoid or lessen the potential for CYP-mediated interactions. Do not coadminister colchicine in patient with renal or hepatic impairment; avoid concurrent use with salmeterol.

Use with caution in patients with hepatic impairment, including active chronic hepatitis; consider interruption or discontinuation with worsening hepatic function. Not recommended in severe hepatic impairment (contraindicated in Canadian labeling). Infrequent cases of drug-induced hepatitis (including acute and cytolytic) have been reported. Liver injury has been reported with use (including some fatalities), though generally in patients on multiple medications, with advanced HIV disease, hepatitis B/C coinfection, and/or immune reconstitution syndrome. Monitor patients closely; consider interrupting or discontinuing therapy if signs/symptoms of liver impairment occur.

May cause fat redistribution (buffalo hump, increased abdominal girth, breast engorgement, facial atrophy). Immune reconstitution syndrome, including inflammatory responses to indolent infections, has been associated with antiretroviral therapy; additional evaluation and treatment may be required. May increase cholesterol and/or triglycerides. Pancreatitis has been observed with use. Risk for pancreatitis may be increased in patients with elevated triglycerides, advanced HIV disease, or history of pancreatitis. Protease inhibitors have been associated with glucose dysregulation; use caution in patients with diabetes. Use with caution in patients with sulfonamide allergy (contains sulfa moiety) or hemophilia. Protease inhibitors have been associated with a variety of hypersensitivity events (some severe), including rash, anaphylaxis (rare), angioedema, bronchospasm, erythema multiforme, Stevens-Johnson syndrome (rare), and/or toxic epidermal necrolysis. Discontinue treatment if severe skin reactions develop. Severe skin reactions may be accompanied by fever, malaise, fatigue, arthralgias, hepatitis, oral lesion, blisters, conjunctivitis, and/or eosinophilia. Mild-to-moderate rash may occur early in treatment and resolve with continued therapy. Treatment history and resistance data should guide use of darunavir with ritonavir.

Drug Interactions

Avoid Concomitant Use

Avoid concomitant use of Darunavir with any of the following: Alfuzosin; Amiodarone; Axitinib; Cisapride; Conivaptan; Crizotinib; Dronedarone; Eplerenone; Ergot Derivatives; Everolimus; Fluticasone (Oral Inhalation); Fosphenytoin; Halofantrine; Lapatinib; Lopinavir; Lovastatin; Lurasidone; Midazolam; Nilotinib; Nisoldipine; PHENobarbital; Phenytoin; Pimozide; QuiNIDine; Ranolazine; Rifampin; Rivaroxaban; RomiDEPsin; Salmeterol; Saquinavir; Silodosin; Simvastatin; St Johns Wort; Tamsulosin; Telaprevir; Ticagrelor; Tolvaptan; Topotecan; Toremifene; Triazolam; Voriconazole

Decreased Effect

Darunavir may decrease the levels/effects of: Abacavir; Boceprevir; Clarithromycin; Contraceptives (Estrogens); Delavirdine; Didanosine; Divalproex; Etravirine; Meperidine; Methadone; Norethindrone; PARoxetine; Prasugrel; Sertraline; Telaprevir; Theophylline Derivatives; Ticagrelor; Valproic Acid; Voriconazole; Warfarin; Zidovudine

The levels/effects of Darunavir may be decreased by: Boceprevir; CarBAMazepine; CYP3A4 Inducers (Strong); Deferasirox; Efavirenz; Fosphenytoin; Garlic; Lopinavir; PHENobarbital; Phenytoin; Rifampin; Saquinavir; St Johns Wort; Telaprevir; Tenofovir; Tocilizumab

Increased Effect/Toxicity

Darunavir may increase the levels/effects of: Alfuzosin; Almotriptan; Alosetron; ALPRAZolam; Amiodarone; Antifungal Agents (Azole Derivatives, Systemic); ARIPiprazole; Axitinib; Bortezomib; Brentuximab Vedotin; Brinzolamide; Budesonide (Nasal); Budesonide (Systemic, Oral Inhalation); Calcium Channel Blockers (Dihydropyridine); Calcium Channel Blockers (Nondihydropyridine); CarBAMazepine; Ciclesonide; Cisapride; Clarithromycin; Colchicine; Conivaptan; Corticosteroids (Orally Inhaled); Crizotinib; CycloSPORINE; CycloSPORINE (Systemic); CYP2D6 Substrates; CYP3A4 Substrates; Dabigatran Etexilate; Dienogest; Digoxin; Dronedarone; Dutasteride; Efavirenz; Enfuvirtide; Eplerenone; Ergot Derivatives; Everolimus; FentaNYL; Fesoterodine; Fluticasone (Nasal); Fluticasone (Oral Inhalation); Fusidic Acid; GuanFACINE; Halofantrine; HMG-CoA Reductase Inhibitors; Iloperidone; Ivacaftor; Ixabepilone; Lapatinib; Lidocaine; Lidocaine (Systemic); Lidocaine (Topical); Lovastatin; Lumefantrine; Lurasidone; Maraviroc; Meperidine; MethylPREDNISolone; Midazolam; Nefazodone; Nilotinib; Nisoldipine; Paricalcitol; Pazopanib; P-glycoprotein/ABCB1 Substrates; Pimecrolimus; Pimozide; Propafenone; Protease Inhibitors; Prucalopride; QuiNIDine; Ranolazine; Rifabutin; Rilpivirine; Rivaroxaban; RomiDEPsin; Ruxolitinib; Salmeterol; Saxagliptin; Sildenafil; Silodosin; Simvastatin; Sirolimus; SORAfenib; Tacrolimus; Tacrolimus (Systemic); Tacrolimus (Topical); Tadalafil; Tamsulosin; Temsirolimus; Tenofovir;

Ticagrelor; Tolterodine; Tolvaptan; Topotecan; Toremifene; TraZODone; Triazolam; Tricyclic Antidepressants; Vardenafil; Vemurafenib; Vilazodone; Zuclopenthixol

The levels/effects of Darunavir may be increased by: Antifungal Agents (Azole Derivatives, Systemic); Clarithromycin; CycloSPORINE; CycloSPORINE (Systemic); CYP3A4 Inhibitors (Moderate); CYP3A4 Inhibitors (Strong); Dasatinib; Delavirdine; Efavirenz; Enfuvirtide; Etravirine; Fusidic Acid; Rifabutin

Nutritional/Ethanol Interactions

Food: Absorption and bioavailability are increased when administered with food. Management: Take with meals.

Herb/Nutraceutical: St John's wort may decrease the plasma levels of darunavir. Garlic may decrease the serum concentration of darunavir. Management: Taking St John's wort concomitantly with darunavir is contraindicated. Use of garlic supplements with darunavir is not recommended.

Adverse Reactions As a class, protease inhibitors potentially cause dyslipidemias which includes elevated cholesterol and triglycerides and a redistribution of body fat centrally to cause increased abdominal girth, buffalo hump, facial atrophy, and breast enlargement. These agents also cause hyperglycemia. Frequency of adverse events is reported for darunavir/ritonavir. See also Ritonavir monograph.

>10%:

Endocrine & metabolic: Hypercholesterolemia (grade 2: 16% to 25%; grade 3: 1% to 10%), LDL increased (grade 2: 14%; grade 3: 5% to 8%)

Gastrointestinal: Vomiting (children 13% to 14%; adults 2% to 5%), diarrhea (children 11% to 19%; adults 8% to 14%)

2% to 10%:

Central nervous system: Headache (children 9%; adults 3% to 6%), fatigue (children 3%; adults ≤2%)

Dermatologic: Rash (children 5% to 10%; adults 6% to 7%)

Endocrine & metabolic: Hyperglycemia (grade 2: 7% to 10%; grade 3: ≤1%; grade 4: <1%), triglycerides increased (grade 2: 3% to 10%; grade 3: 1% to 7%; grade 4: ≤3%), diabetes mellitus (2%)

Gastrointestinal: Abdominal pain (children 10%; adults 5% to 6%), nausea (3% to 7%), amylase increased (grade 2: 5% to 6%; grade 3: 3% to 7%), lipase increased (grade 2: 2% to 3%; grade 3: ≤2%; grade 4: <1%), abdominal distention (2%), anorexia (2%), dyspepsia (2%)

Hepatic: ALT increased (grade 2: 7%, grade 3: 2% to 3%; grade 4: ≤1%), AST increased (grade 2: 6%; grade 3: 2% to 4%; grade 4: <1%), alkaline phosphatase (grade 2: ≤2%; grade 3: <1%)

Neuromuscular & skeletal: Weakness (≤3%)

Product Availability Prezista® 100 mg/mL oral suspension: FDA approved December 2011; availability expected in the second quarter of 2012

Available Dosage Forms

Tablet, oral:

Prezista®: 75 mg, 150 mg, 400 mg, 600 mg

General Dosage Range Dosage adjustment recommended in patients on concomitant therapy or who develop toxicities.

Oral:

Children ≥6 years and ≥20 kg to <30 kg: Darunavir: 375 mg twice daily; Ritonavir: 50 mg twice daily

Children ≥6 years and ≥30 kg to <40 kg: Darunavir: 450 mg twice daily; Ritonavir: 60 mg twice daily

Children ≥6 years and ≥40 kg: Darunavir: 600 mg twice daily; Ritonavir: 100 mg twice daily

Adults: Darunavir: 600 mg twice daily; Ritonavir: 100 mg twice daily **or** Darunavir: 800 mg once daily; Ritonavir: 100 mg once daily

Administration

Oral Coadministration with ritonavir and food is required (bioavailability is increased).

Stability

Storage Store at 25°C (77°F); excursions permitted to 15°C to 30°C (59°F to 86°F).

Nursing Actions

Physical Assessment Monitor for adherence to regimen. Monitor for hypersensitivity reaction, gastrointestinal disturbance (nausea, vomiting, diarrhea) that can lead to dehydration and weight loss, hyperlipidemia, and redistribution of body fat. Caution patients with diabetes to monitor glucose levels closely; protease inhibitors may cause alterations in glucose regulation or new onset diabetes. Teach patient proper timing of multiple medications.

Patient Education This drug will not cure HIV, nor has it been found to reduce transmission of HIV; use appropriate precautions to prevent spread to other persons. This drug is prescribed as one part of a multidrug combination; take exactly as directed for full course of therapy. Take with food. Maintain adequate nutrition and hydration, unless instructed to restrict fluid intake. Frequent blood tests may be required. You may be advised to check your glucose levels; this drug can cause hyperglycemia. May cause body changes due to redistribution of body fat, facial atrophy, or breast enlargement (normal effects of drug); nausea or vomiting; diarrhea; or headache. Inform prescriber if you experience signs of hypersensitivity (rash, difficulty swallowing or breathing, swelling of mouth or tongue); unresolved persistent vomiting, diarrhea, or abdominal pain; respiratory difficulty or chest pain; unusual bleeding or bruising; or dark-colored urine or light stool.

Dietary Considerations Absorption increased with food. Take with meals.

DAUNOrubicin (Conventional)

(daw noe ROO bi sin con VEN sha nal)

Brand Names: U.S. Cerubidine®

Index Terms Conventional Daunomycin; Daunomycin; DAUNOrubicin Hydrochloride; Rubidomycin Hydrochloride

Pharmacologic Category Antineoplastic Agent, Anthracycline

Medication Safety Issues

Sound-alike/look-alike issues:

DAUNOrubicin may be confused with DACTINOmycin, DOXOrubicin, DOXOrubicin liposomal, epirubicin, IDArubicin, valrubicin

Conventional formulation (Cerubidine®, DAUNOrubicin hydrochloride) may be confused with the liposomal formulation (DaunoXome®)

High alert medication:

The Institute for Safe Medication Practices (ISMP) includes this medication among its list of drug classes which have a heightened risk of causing significant patient harm when used in error.

Pregnancy Risk Factor D

Lactation Excretion in breast milk unknown/not recommended

Use Treatment of acute lymphocytic leukemia (ALL) and acute myeloid leukemia (AML)

Mechanism of Action/Effect Inhibition of DNA and RNA synthesis by intercalation between DNA base pairs and by steric obstruction. Daunomycin intercalates at points of local uncoiling of the double helix. Although the exact mechanism is unclear, it appears that direct binding to DNA (intercalation) and inhibition of DNA repair (topoisomerase II inhibition) result in blockade of DNA and RNA synthesis and fragmentation of DNA.

Contraindications Hypersensitivity to daunorubicin or any component of the formulation

Warnings/Precautions Hazardous agent - use appropriate precautions for handling and disposal. Use with caution in patients who have received radiation therapy; reduce dosage in patients who are receiving radiation therapy simultaneously. **[U.S. Boxed Warnings]: Use caution with renal impairment or in the presence of hepatic dysfunction; dosage reduction is recommended. Potent vesicant; if extravasation occurs, severe local tissue damage leading to ulceration and necrosis, and pain may occur. For I.V. administration only. Severe bone marrow suppression may occur. [U.S. Boxed Warning]: May cause cumulative, dose-related myocardial toxicity (concurrent or delayed).** Total cumulative dose should take into account previous or concomitant treatment with cardiotoxic agents or irradiation of chest. The incidence of irreversible myocardial toxicity increases as the total cumulative (lifetime) dosages approach:

550 mg/m^2 in adults

400 mg/m^2 in adults receiving chest radiation

300 mg/m^2 in children >2 years of age

10 mg/kg in children <2 years of age

Although the risk increases with cumulative dose, irreversible cardiotoxicity may occur at any dose level. Patients with pre-existing heart disease, hypertension, concurrent administration of other antineoplastic agents, prior or concurrent chest irradiation, advanced age; and infants and children are at increased risk. Monitor left ventricular (LV) function (baseline and periodic) with ECHO or MUGA scan; monitor ECG.

Secondary leukemias may occur when used with combination chemotherapy or radiation therapy. **[U.S. Boxed Warning]: Should be administered under the supervision of an experienced cancer chemotherapy physician.**

Drug Interactions

Avoid Concomitant Use

Avoid concomitant use of DAUNOrubicin (Conventional) with any of the following: BCG; CloZAPine; Natalizumab; Pimecrolimus; Tacrolimus (Topical); Vaccines (Live)

Decreased Effect

DAUNOrubicin (Conventional) may decrease the levels/effects of: BCG; Cardiac Glycosides; Coccidioidin Skin Test; Sipuleucel-T; Vaccines (Inactivated); Vaccines (Live)

The levels/effects of DAUNOrubicin (Conventional) may be decreased by: Cardiac Glycosides; Echinacea; P-glycoprotein/ABCB1 Inducers

Increased Effect/Toxicity

DAUNOrubicin (Conventional) may increase the levels/effects of: CloZAPine; Leflunomide; Natalizumab; Vaccines (Live)

The levels/effects of DAUNOrubicin (Conventional) may be increased by: Bevacizumab; Denosumab; P-glycoprotein/ABCB1 Inhibitors; Pimecrolimus; Roflumilast; Tacrolimus (Topical); Taxane Derivatives; Trastuzumab

Nutritional/Ethanol Interactions Ethanol: Avoid ethanol (due to GI irritation).

Adverse Reactions

>10%:

Cardiovascular: Transient ECG abnormalities (supraventricular tachycardia, S-T wave changes, atrial or ventricular extrasystoles); generally asymptomatic and self-limiting. CHF, dose related, may be delayed for 7-8 years after treatment.

Dermatologic: Alopecia(reversible), radiation recall
Gastrointestinal: Mild nausea or vomiting, stomatitis
Genitourinary: Discoloration of urine (red)
Hematologic: Myelosuppression (onset: 7 days; nadir: 10-14 days; recovery: 21-28 days), primarily leukopenia; thrombocytopenia and anemia

1% to 10%:
Dermatologic: Skin "flare" at injection site; discoloration of saliva, sweat, or tears
Endocrine & metabolic: Hyperuricemia
Gastrointestinal: Abdominal pain, GI ulceration, diarrhea

Available Dosage Forms

Injection, powder for reconstitution: 20 mg
Cerubidine®: 20 mg

Injection, solution [preservative free]: 5 mg/mL (4 mL, 10 mL)

General Dosage Range Dosage adjustment recommended in patients with hepatic or renal impairment

I.V.:
Children <2 years or BSA <0.5 m²: 1 mg/kg/dose per protocol with frequency dependent on regimen employed (maximum cumulative dose: 10 mg/kg)
Children ≥2 years and BSA ≥0.5 m²: 25 mg/m² on day 1 every week for 4 cycles **or** 30-60 mg/m²/day for 3 days (maximum cumulative dose: 300 mg/m²)
Adults <60 years: 30-60 mg/m²/day for 2-3 days (maximum cumulative dose: 550 mg/m²; 400 mg/m² with chest irradiation)
Adults ≥60 years: 30 mg/m²/day for 2-3 days (maximum cumulative dose: 550 mg/m²; 400 mg/m² with chest irradiation)

Administration

I.V. Vesicant. **Never** administer I.M. or SubQ. Administer as slow I.V. push over 1-5 minutes into the tubing of a rapidly infusing I.V. solution of D_5W or NS or dilute in 100 mL of D_5W or NS and infuse over 15-30 minutes.

I.V. Detail Avoid extravasation, can cause severe tissue damage. Flush with 5-10 mL of I.V. solution before and after drug administration.

pH: 4.5-6.5

Stability

Reconstitution Dilute vials of powder for injection with 4 mL SWFI for a final concentration of 5 mg/mL. May further dilute in 100 mL D_5W or NS.

Storage Store intact vials of powder for injection at room temperature of 15°C to 30°C (59°F to 86°F); intact vials of solution for injection should be refrigerated at 2°C to 8°C (36°F to 46°F). Protect from light. Reconstituted solution is stable for 4 days at 15°C to 25°C. Further dilution in D_5W, LR, or NS is stable at room temperature (25°C) for up to 4 weeks if protected from light.

Nursing Actions

Physical Assessment Monitor infusion site closely; extravasation can cause severe cellulitis or tissue necrosis (if drug is infiltrated, apply ice to the area, elevate the limb, and consult institutional policy immediately). Monitor for hypertension, tachycardia, cough, dyspnea, and gastrointestinal upset prior to each infusion and throughout therapy.

Patient Education This medication can only be administered I.V. Report immediately any swelling, pain, burning, or redness at infusion site. Avoid alcohol. It is important to maintain adequate nutrition and hydration, unless instructed to restrict fluid intake. You will be more susceptible to infection. May cause nausea or vomiting, diarrhea, loss of hair (reversible), or red-pink urine (normal). Report immediately chest pain, swelling of extremities, respiratory difficulty, palpitations, or rapid heartbeat. Report unresolved nausea, vomiting, or diarrhea; alterations in urinary pattern (increased or decreased); opportunistic infection (eg, fever, chills, unusual bruising or bleeding fatigue, purulent vaginal discharge, unhealed mouth sores); abdominal pain or blood in stools; excessive fatigue; or yellowing of eyes or skin.

Related Information

Management of Drug Extravasations *on page 1269*

Decitabine (de SYE ta been)

Brand Names: U.S. Dacogen®

Index Terms 5-Aza-2'-deoxycytidine; 5-Aza-dCyd; Deoxyazacytidine; Dezocitidine

Pharmacologic Category Antineoplastic Agent, DNA Methylation Inhibitor

Medication Safety Issues

Sound-alike/look-alike issues:
Dacogen® may be confused with DACTINomycin

High alert medication:
This medication is in a class the Institute for Safe Medication Practices (ISMP) includes among its list of drug classes which have a heightened risk of causing significant patient harm when used in error.

Pregnancy Risk Factor D

Lactation Excretion in breast milk unknown/not recommended

Breast-Feeding Considerations Due to the potential for serious adverse reactions in the nursing infant, breast-feeding is not recommended.

Use Treatment of myelodysplastic syndrome (MDS)

Unlabeled Use Treatment of acute myelogenous leukemia (AML), sickle cell anemia

Mechanism of Action/Effect Hypomethylating agent

Contraindications There are no contraindications listed within the manufacturer's labeling.

Warnings/Precautions Hazardous agent - use appropriate precautions for handling and disposal. The dose-limiting toxicity is bone marrow suppression; worsening neutropenia is common in first two treatment cycles and may not correlate with progression of underlying MDS; may require dosage adjustment (after the first cycle), growth factor support and/or antimicrobial agents; monitor for infection. Not studied in hepatic and renal disease; use caution.

Drug Interactions

Avoid Concomitant Use

Avoid concomitant use of Decitabine with any of the following: CloZAPine

Decreased Effect There are no known significant interactions involving a decrease in effect.

Increased Effect/Toxicity

Decitabine may increase the levels/effects of: CloZAPine

Adverse Reactions

>10%:

Cardiovascular: Peripheral edema (25% to 27%), pallor (23%), edema (5% to 18%), cardiac murmur (16%), hypotension (6% to 11%)

Central nervous system: Fever (6% to 53%), fatigue (46%), headache (23% to 28%), insomnia (14% to 28%), dizziness (18% to 21%), chills (16%), pain (5% to 13%), confusion (8% to 12%), lethargy (12%), anxiety (9% to 11%), hypoesthesia (11%)

Dermatologic: Petechiae (12% to 39%), bruising (9% to 22%), rash (11% to 19%), erythema (5% to 14%), cellulitis (9% to 12%), lesions (5% to 11%), pruritus (9% to 11%)

Endocrine & metabolic: Hyperglycemia (6% to 33%), hypoalbuminemia (7% to 24%), hypomagnesemia (5% to 24%), hypokalemia (12% to 22%), hyperkalemia (13%), hyponatremia (19%)

Gastrointestinal: Nausea (40% to 42%), constipation (30% to 35%), diarrhea (28% to 34%), vomiting (16% to 25%), anorexia/appetite decreased (8% to 23%), abdominal pain (5% to 14%), oral mucosal petechiae (13%), stomatitis (11% to 12%), dyspepsia (10% to 12%)

Hematologic: Neutropenia (38% to 90%; grades 3/4: 37% to 87%; recovery 28-50 days), thrombocytopenia (27% to 89%; grades 3/4: 24% to 85%), anemia (31% to 82%; grades 3/4: 22%), febrile neutropenia (20% to 29%; grades 3/4: 23%), leukopenia (6% to 28%; grades 3/4: 22%), lymphadenopathy (12%)

Hepatic: Hyperbilirubinemia (6% to 14%), alkaline phosphatase increased (11%)

Local: Tenderness (11%)

Neuromuscular & skeletal: Rigors (22%), arthralgia (17% to 20%), limb pain (18% to 19%), back pain (17% to 18%), weakness (15%)

Respiratory: Cough (27% to 40%), dyspnea (29%), pneumonia (20% to 22%), pharyngitis (16%), lung crackles (14%), epistaxis (13%)

5% to 10%:

Cardiovascular: Tachycardia (8%), chest pain/discomfort (6% to 7%), facial edema (6%), hypertension (6%), heart failure (5%)

Central nervous system: Depression (9%), malaise (5%)

Dermatologic: Alopecia (8%), dry skin (8%), urticaria (6%)

Endocrine & metabolic: Hyperuricemia (10%), LDH increased (8%), bicarbonate increased (6%), dehydration (6% to 8%), hypochloremia (6%), bicarbonate decreased (5%), hypoproteinemia (5%)

Gastrointestinal: Mucosal inflammation (9%), weight loss (9%), gingival bleeding (8%), hemorrhoids (8%), loose stools (7%), tongue ulceration (7%), dysphagia (5% to 6%), oral candidiasis (6%), toothache (6%), abdominal distension (5%), gastroesophageal reflux (5%), glossodynia (5%), lip ulceration (5%), oral pain (5%), tooth abscess (5%)

Genitourinary: Urinary tract infection (7%), dysuria (6%), polyuria (5%)

Hematologic: Bacteremia (5% to 8%), hematoma (5%), pancytopenia (5%), thrombocythemia (5%)

Hepatic: Ascites (10%), AST increased (10%), hypobilirubinemia (5%)

Local: Catheter infection (8%), catheter site erythema (5%), catheter site pain (5%), injection site swelling (5%)

Neuromuscular & skeletal: Myalgia (5% to 9%), falling (8%), chest wall pain (7%), muscle spasm (7%), bone pain (6%), musculoskeletal pain/discomfort (5% to 6%), crepitation (5%)

Ocular: Blurred vision (6%)

Otic: Ear pain (6%)

Respiratory: Breath sounds abnormal (5% to 10%), hypoxia (10%), upper respiratory tract infection (10%), pharyngolaryngeal pain (8%), rales (8%), pulmonary edema (6%), sinusitis (5% to 6%), pleural effusion (5%), postnasal drip (5%), sinus congestion (5%)

Miscellaneous: Candidal infection (10%), staphylococcal infection (7%), transfusion reaction (7%), night sweats (5%)

Available Dosage Forms

Injection, powder for reconstitution:

Dacogen®: 50 mg

General Dosage Range Dosage adjustment recommended in patients who develop toxicities

I.V.: *Adults:* 15 mg/m^2 every 8 hours for 3 days every 6 weeks **or** 20 mg/m^2 daily for 5 days every 28 days

Administration

I.V. Infuse over 1-3 hours. Premedication with antiemetics is recommended.

I.V. Detail pH: 6.7-7.3

Stability

Reconstitution Vials should be reconstituted with 10 mL SWFI to a concentration of 5 mg/mL. Immediately further dilute with 50-250 mL NS, D_5W, or lactated Ringer's to a final concentration of 0.1-1 mg/mL. Use appropriate precautions for handling and disposal. Solutions not administered within 15 minutes of preparation should be prepared with cold (2°C to 8°C [36°F to 46°F]) infusion solutions.

Storage Store vials at 25°C (77°F); excursions permitted to 15°C to 30°C (59°F to 86°F). Solutions diluted for infusion may be stored for up to 7 hours under refrigeration at 2°C to 8°C (36°F to 46°F) if prepared with cold infusion fluids.

Nursing Actions

Physical Assessment Premedication with antiemetic may be ordered. Monitor for worsening neutropenia, thrombocytopenia, anemia, pulmonary edema, gastrointestinal disturbance, CNS changes, hyperglycemia, and infection prior to each cycle and periodically as indicated during therapy. Advise patients with diabetes to monitor serum glucose closely (may cause hyperglycemia).

Patient Education This medication can only be administered by intravenous infusion. Report immediately any redness, swelling, pain, or burning at infusion site, or any adverse response during infusion (eg, respiratory difficulty, facial edema, pain, restlessness, tremor, wheezing). Maintain adequate nutrition and hydration, unless instructed to restrict fluid intake. You may be more susceptible to infection. If you have diabetes, you should monitor serum glucose closely; may cause hyperglycemia. May cause lethargy, dizziness, visual changes, confusion, anxiety, nausea, vomiting, loss of appetite, dry mouth, mouth sores, loss of hair (may grow back when treatment is discontinued), diarrhea, or constipation. Report respiratory difficulty; chest pain or palpitations; unusual bleeding, bruising, or rash; or any sign of urinary tract infection (itching or burning) or opportunistic infection (eg, sore throat, fever, chills, fatigue, thrush, vaginal discharge, diarrhea).

Deferasirox (de FER a sir ox)

Brand Names: U.S. Exjade®

Index Terms ICL670

Pharmacologic Category Chelating Agent

Medication Safety Issues

Sound-alike/look-alike issues:

Deferasirox may be confused with deferiprone, deferoxamine

Pregnancy Risk Factor C

Lactation Excretion in breast milk unknown/not recommended

Use Treatment of chronic iron overload due to blood transfusions (transfusional hemosiderosis)

Available Dosage Forms

Tablet for suspension, oral:

Exjade®: 125 mg, 250 mg, 500 mg

General Dosage Range Dosage adjustment recommended in patients with renal or hepatic impairment or on concomitant therapy

Oral: *Children ≥2 years and Adults:* Initial: 20 mg/kg once daily; Maintenance: 20-30 mg/kg once daily (maximum dose: 40 mg/kg/day)

Administration

Oral Do not chew or swallow whole tablets. Completely disperse tablets in water, orange juice, or apple juice (use 3.5 ounces for total doses <1 g; 7 ounces for doses ≥1 g); stir to form a fine suspension and drink entire contents. Rinse remaining residue with more fluid; drink. Administer at same time each day on an empty stomach, 30 minutes before food. Do not take simultaneously with aluminum-containing antacids.

Nursing Actions

Physical Assessment Assess hearing and vision prior to initiating therapy and periodically during treatment. Observe for skin rash. Mild-to-moderate rashes will usually resolve spontaneously. Assess for signs of liver dysfunction (eg, unusual fatigue, easy bruising or bleeding, jaundice), gastrointestinal bleeding (blood in vomitus or stool), and renal dysfunction (eg, unusual weight gain, swelling of extremities, decrease in urine output).

Patient Education Take on an empty stomach at least 30 minutes prior to eating. Do not chew tablets or swallow whole. Disperse in water, orange juice, or apple juice and drink immediately. Any residue remaining should be resuspended in a small volume of liquid and swallowed. Do not take with antacids. Maintain adequate hydration, unless instructed to restrict fluid intake. You may experience a fever, headache, abdominal pain, nausea, diarrhea, cough, sore throat, or dizziness. Report severe rashes, changes in vision or hearing, weight gain, swelling of extremities, decrease in urine output, shortness of breath, unusual bleeding or bruising, blood in vomitus or stool, change in color of urine or stool, yellowing of skin or eyes, or unusual fatigue.

Deferiprone (de FER i prone)

Brand Names: U.S. Ferriprox®

Index Terms APO-066; Ferriprox®

Pharmacologic Category Chelating Agent

Medication Safety Issues

Sound-alike/look-alike issues:

Deferiprone may be confused with deferoxamine, deferasirox

Pregnancy Risk Factor D

Lactation Excretion in breast milk unknown/not recommended

Use Treatment of transfusional iron overload due to thalassemia syndromes with inadequate response to other chelation therapy

Available Dosage Forms

Tablet, oral:

Ferriprox®: 500 mg

General Dosage Range Oral: *Adults:* 25-33 mg/kg 3 times/day (maximum: 99 mg/kg/day)

Administration

Oral Administer in the morning, at mid day and in the evening. Administration with food may decrease nausea.

Nursing Actions

Physical Assessment

Assess allergy history prior to beginning therapy. May monitor bloodwork for neutropenia or increased ALT or AST.

Patient Education

Take it with or without food. May take with food if it causes stomach upset. Common side effects are nausea, vomiting, belly or joint pain, change in color of urine to red or brown. Low white blood cell count or infections may rarely occur. Call prescriber for signs or symptoms of infection (fever over 100.5°F (38°C), chills, sore throat, ear or sinus pain, cough, sputum, dysuria, mouth sores, or wound that won't heal), dizziness or syncope, rapid heartbeat, seizures, dark urine, yellow skin or eyes, feeling very tired or weak, or severe abdominal pain.

Deferoxamine (de fer OKS a meen)

Brand Names: U.S. Desferal®

Index Terms Deferoxamine Mesylate; Desferrioxamine; DFM

Pharmacologic Category Antidote; Chelating Agent

Medication Safety Issues

Sound-alike/look-alike issues:

Deferoxamine may be confused with cefuroxime, deferasirox, deferiprone

Desferal® may be confused with desflurane, Desyrel®, Dexferrum®

International issues:

Desferal [U.S., Canada, and multiple international markets] may be confused with Deseril brand name for methysergide [Australia, Belgium, Great Britain, Netherlands]; Disophrol brand name for dexbrompheniramine and pseudoephedrine [Czech Republic, Poland, Turkey]

Pregnancy Risk Factor C

Lactation Excretion in breast milk unknown/use caution

Use Adjunct in the treatment of acute iron intoxication; treatment of chronic iron overload secondary to multiple transfusions

Canadian labeling (unlabeled use in the U.S.): Diagnosis of aluminum overload; treatment of chronic aluminum overload in patients with end-stage renal failure undergoing maintenance dialysis

Unlabeled Use Diagnosis or treatment of aluminum induced toxicity associated with chronic kidney disease (CKD)

Available Dosage Forms

Injection, powder for reconstitution: 500 mg, 2 g

Desferal®: 500 mg, 2 g

General Dosage Range Dosage adjustment recommended in patients with renal impairment

I.M.: *Adults:* Initial: 1000 mg, followed by 500 mg every 4 hours for 2 doses; Maintenance: 500 mg every 4-12 hours **or** 500-1000 mg once daily (maximum: 6000 mg/day)

I.V.:

Children ≥3 years: 20-40 mg/kg/day 5-7 days per week; dose should not exceed 40 mg/kg/day until growth has ceased

Adults: Initial: 1000 mg, followed by 500 mg every 4 hours for 2 doses; Maintenance: 500 mg every 4-12 hours (maximum: 6000 mg/day) **or** 40-50 mg/kg/day (maximum: 60 mg/kg/day) 5-7 days per week

SubQ:

Children ≥3 years: 20-40 mg/kg/day (maximum: 1000-2000 mg/day)

Adults: 1000-2000 mg/day **or** 20-40 mg/kg/day

Administration

I.M. I.M. administration may be used for patients with acute iron toxicity that do not exhibit severe symptoms (per the manufacturer); may also be used in the treatment of chronic iron toxicity.

I.V. Urticaria, flushing of the skin, hypotension, and shock have occurred following rapid I.V. administration; limiting infusion rate to 15mg/kg/hour may help avoid infusion-related adverse effects.

Acute iron toxicity: The manufacturer states that the I.M. route is preferred; however, the I.V. route is generally preferred in patients with severe toxicity (ie, patients in shock). For the first 1000 mg, infuse at 15 mg/kg/hour. Subsequent doses may be given over 4-12 hours at a rate not to exceed 125 mg/hour.

Chronic iron overload: Administer over 8-12 hours for 5-7 days per week; rate not to exceed 15 mg/kg/hour. In patients with poor compliance, deferoxamine may be administered on the same day of blood transfusion, either prior to or following transfusion; do not administer concurrently with transfusion. Longer infusion times (24 hours) and I.V. administration may be required in patients with severe cardiac iron deposition (Brittenham, 2011).

Diagnosis or treatment of aluminum-induced toxicity with CKD: Administer dose over 1 hour during the last hour of dialysis (K/DOQI guidelines, 2003).

Other SubQ: When administered for chronic iron overload, administration over 8-12 hours using a portable infusion pump is generally recommended; however, longer infusion times (24 hours) may also be used. Topical anesthetic or glucocorticoid creams may be used for induration or erythema (Brittenham, 2011).

Nursing Actions

Physical Assessment Infuse slowly and monitor infusion site. Monitor for acute reactions; urticaria, hypotension, and shock can occur following rapid I.V. administration. With chronic therapy, perform ophthalmologic exam (fundoscopy, slit-lamp exam) and audiometry. Teach patient proper injection technique and syringe/needle disposal. Monitor for adverse cardiac, respiratory, or CNS symptoms and teach patient importance of reporting adverse symptoms.

Patient Education You will be monitored closely for effects of this medication and frequent blood or urine tests may be necessary. Your urine may show a reddish discoloration. Report chest pain; rapid heartbeat; headache; pain, swelling, or irritation at infusion site; skin rash; changes or loss of hearing or vision; or acute abdominal or leg cramps.

Degarelix (deg a REL ix)

Brand Names: U.S. Firmagon®

Index Terms Degarelix Acetate; FE200486

Pharmacologic Category Antineoplastic Agent, Gonadotropin-Releasing Hormone Antagonist; Gonadotropin Releasing Hormone Antagonist

Medication Safety Issues

Sound-alike/look-alike issues:

Degarelix may be confused with cetrorelix, ganirelix

Pregnancy Risk Factor X

Lactation Excretion in breast milk unknown/not recommended

Use Treatment of advanced prostate cancer

Available Dosage Forms

Injection, powder for reconstitution:

Firmagon®: 80 mg, 120 mg

General Dosage Range SubQ: *Adults:* Loading dose: 240 mg; Maintenance dose: 80 mg every 28 days

Administration

I.V. Not for I.V. use.

Other Not for I.V. use. Administer SubQ in the abdominal area by grasping skin and elevating SubQ tissue; insert the needle deeply at an angle not ≤45 degrees. Avoid pressure exposed areas (eg, waistband, belt, or near ribs); rotate injection site. Inject loading dose as two 3 mL injections (40 mg/mL); maintenance dose should be administered as a single 4 mL injection (20 mg/mL); begin maintenance dose 28 days after initial loading dose.

Nursing Actions

Physical Assessment Monitor PSA and serum testosterone levels, LFTs, electrolytes, and bone density on a regular basis during therapy. Supplemental calcium and vitamin D may be ordered to reduce risk of osteoporosis due to androgen deprivation.

Patient Education This drug can only be administered by injection in abdominal area at regularly scheduled intervals. It is important that you maintain adequate nutrition and fluid intake; dietary supplements of calcium or vitamins may be recommended. You may experience hot flashes, dizziness, headache, insomnia, fatigue, nausea, diarrhea, or constipation. Report any injection site reaction (pain, redness, swelling), acute headache, signs of urinary tract infection (pain, itching, change in urinary pattern), or persistent back or muscle pain or weakness.

Delavirdine (de la VIR deen)

Brand Names: U.S. Rescriptor®

Index Terms DLV; U-90152S

Pharmacologic Category Antiretroviral Agent, Reverse Transcriptase Inhibitor (Non-nucleoside)

Medication Safety Issues

Sound-alike/look-alike issues:

Delavirdine may be confused with dalfampridine

Pregnancy Risk Factor C

Lactation Excretion in breast milk unknown/contraindicated

Breast-Feeding Considerations Maternal or infant antiretroviral therapy does not completely eliminate the risk of postnatal HIV transmission. In addition, multiclass-resistant virus has been detected in breast-feeding infants despite maternal therapy. Therefore, in the United States, where formula is accessible, affordable, safe, and sustainable, and the risk of infant mortality due to diarrhea and respiratory infections is low, complete avoidance of breast-feeding by HIV-infected women is recommended to decrease potential transmission of HIV (DHHS [perinatal], 2011).

Use Treatment of HIV-1 infection in combination with at least two additional antiretroviral agents

Mechanism of Action/Effect Delavirdine binds directly to reverse transcriptase, blocking RNA-dependent and DNA-dependent DNA polymerase activities

Contraindications Hypersensitivity to delavirdine or any component of the formulation; concurrent use of alprazolam, astemizole, cisapride, ergot alkaloids, midazolam, pimozide, rifampin, terfenadine, or triazolam

Warnings/Precautions Use with caution in patients with hepatic or renal dysfunction; due to rapid emergence of resistance, delavirdine should not be used as monotherapy or as a component of an initial antiretroviral regimen; cross-resistance may be conferred to other non-nucleoside reverse transcriptase inhibitors, although potential for cross-resistance with protease inhibitors is low. Long-term effects of delavirdine are not known. May cause redistribution of fat (eg, buffalo hump, peripheral wasting with increased abdominal girth, cushingoid appearance). Immune reconstitution syndrome may develop resulting in the occurrence of an inflammatory response to an indolent or residual opportunistic infection; further evaluation and treatment may be required. Safety and efficacy have not been established in children. Rash, which occurs frequently, may require discontinuation of therapy; usually occurs within 1-3 weeks and lasts <2 weeks. Most patients may resume therapy following a treatment interruption. Use with caution in patients taking strong CYP3A4 inhibitors, moderate or strong CYP3A4 inducers and major CYP3A4 substrates (see Drug Interactions); consider alternative agents that avoid or lessen the potential for CYP-mediated interactions.

Drug Interactions

Avoid Concomitant Use

Avoid concomitant use of Delavirdine with any of the following: Alfuzosin; Astemizole; Axitinib; Clopidogrel; Conivaptan; Crizotinib; Dronedarone; Eplerenone; Etravirine; Everolimus; Fluticasone (Oral Inhalation); Fosamprenavir; Fosphenytoin; H2-Antagonists; Halofantrine; Lapatinib; Lovastatin; Lurasidone; Nilotinib; Nisoldipine; Phenytoin; Pimozide; Proton Pump Inhibitors; Ranolazine; Rilpivirine; Rivaroxaban; RomiDEPsin; Salmeterol; Silodosin; Simvastatin; St Johns Wort; Tamoxifen; Tamsulosin; Terfenadine; Thioridazine; Ticagrelor; Tolvaptan; Toremifene

Decreased Effect

Delavirdine may decrease the levels/effects of: Clopidogrel; Codeine; Etravirine; Prasugrel; Rilpivirine; Ticagrelor; TraMADol

The levels/effects of Delavirdine may be decreased by: Antacids; CYP3A4 Inducers (Strong); Deferasirox; Fosamprenavir; Fosphenytoin; H2-Antagonists; Peginterferon Alfa-2b; Phenytoin; Protease Inhibitors; Proton Pump Inhibitors; Rifamycin Derivatives; St Johns Wort; Tocilizumab

Increased Effect/Toxicity

Delavirdine may increase the levels/effects of: Alfuzosin; Almotriptan; Alosetron; ARIPiprazole; Astemizole; Atomoxetine; Axitinib; Bortezomib; Brentuximab Vedotin; Brinzolamide; Budesonide (Nasal); Budesonide (Systemic, Oral Inhalation); Carvedilol; Ciclesonide; Citalopram; Colchicine; Conivaptan; Corticosteroids (Orally Inhaled); Crizotinib; CYP2C19 Substrates; CYP2C9 Substrates; CYP2D6 Substrates; CYP3A4 Substrates; Diclofenac; Dienogest; Dronedarone; Dutasteride; Eplerenone; Etravirine; Everolimus; FentaNYL; Fesoterodine; Fluticasone (Nasal); Fluticasone (Oral Inhalation); Fosamprenavir; Fosphenytoin; GuanFACINE; Halofantrine; Iloperidone; Ivacaftor; Ixabepilone; Lapatinib; Lovastatin; Lumefantrine; Lurasidone; Maraviroc; MethylPREDNISolone; Nebivolol; Nilotinib; Nisoldipine; PACLitaxel; Paricalcitol; Pazopanib; Phenytoin; Pimecrolimus; Pimozide; Propafenone; Protease Inhibitors; Ranolazine; Rifamycin Derivatives; Rilpivirine; Rivaroxaban; RomiDEPsin; Ruxolitinib; Salmeterol; Saxagliptin; Sildenafil; Silodosin; Simvastatin; SORAfenib; Tadalafil; Tamoxifen; Tamsulosin; Terfenadine; Tetrabenazine; Thioridazine; Ticagrelor; Tolterodine; Tolvaptan; Toremifene; Vardenafil; Vemurafenib; Vilazodone; Zuclopenthixol

Nutritional/Ethanol Interactions Herb/Nutraceutical: Delavirdine serum concentration may be decreased by St John's wort; avoid concurrent use.

Adverse Reactions

Frequency of adverse reactions reported from occurrence in clinical trials with delavirdine when used as part of combination antiretroviral therapy.

>10%:

Central nervous system: Headache (19% to 20%), depressive symptoms (10% to 15%), fever (4% to 12%)

Dermatologic: Rash (16% to 32%)

Gastrointestinal: Nausea (20% to 25%), vomiting (3% to 11%)

1% to 10%:

Central nervous system: Anxiety (6% to 8%)

Endocrine & metabolic: Transaminases increased (2% to 5%), amylase increased (3%), bilirubin increased (2%)

Gastrointestinal: Diarrhea, vomiting, abdominal pain (4% to 6%)

Hematologic: Prothrombin time increased (2%), hemoglobin decreased (1% to 3%)

Respiratory: Bronchitis (6% to 8%)

Frequency not defined (limited to important or life threatening): Abscess, adenopathy, alkaline phosphatase increased, allergic reaction, angioedema, anorexia, arrhythmia, bloody stool, bone pain, bruising, cardiac insufficiency, cardiac rate abnormal, cardiomyopathy, chest congestion, cognitive impairment, colitis, confusion, conjunctivitis, dermal leukocytoclastic vasculitis, desquamation, diverticulitis, dyspnea, emotional lability, eosinophilia, erythema multiforme, fecal incontinence, fungal dermatitis, gamma glutamyl transpeptidase increased, gastroenteritis, gastrointestinal bleeding, granulocytosis, gum hemorrhage, hallucination, hematuria, hepatomegaly, hyperglycemia, hyperkalemia, hypertension, hypertriglyceridemia, hyperuricemia, hypocalcemia, hyponatremia, hypophosphatemia, infection, jaundice, kidney pain, leukopenia, lipase increased, menstrual irregularities, moniliasis (oral/vaginal), pancreatitis, pancytopenia, paralysis, peripheral vascular disorder, pneumonia, postural hypotension, purpura, redistribution of body ▶

fat, renal calculi, serum creatinine increased, spleen disorder, Stevens-Johnson syndrome, tetany, thrombocytopenia, urinary tract infection, vertigo

Available Dosage Forms

Tablet, oral:

Rescriptor®: 100 mg, 200 mg

General Dosage Range Oral: *Children ≥16 years and Adults:* 400 mg 3 times/day

Administration

Oral Patients with achlorhydria should take the drug with an acidic beverage. Antacids and delavirdine should be separated by 1 hour. A dispersion of delavirdine may be prepared by adding four 100 mg tablets to at least 3 oz of water. Allow to stand for a few minutes and stir until uniform dispersion. Drink immediately. Rinse glass and mouth, then swallow the rinse to ensure total dose administered. The 200 mg tablets should be taken intact.

Stability

Storage Store at 20°C to 25°C (68°F to 77°F). Protect from humidity.

Nursing Actions

Physical Assessment Monitor for rash and gastrointestinal upset. Teach patient proper timing of multiple medications.

Patient Education You will be provided with a list of specific medications that should not be used during therapy. This drug will not cure HIV, nor has it been found to reduce transmission of HIV; use appropriate precautions to prevent spread to other persons. This drug is prescribed as one part of a multidrug combination; take exactly as directed for full course of therapy. May be taken with or without food. Take 200 mg tablets intact (do not chew or dissolve). You may mix four 100 mg tablets in 3-5 oz of water; allow to stand a few minutes and stir; drink immediately; rinse glass and mouth (swallow rinse solution) following ingestion to ensure total dose administered. Maintain adequate hydration, unless instructed to restrict fluid intake. Frequent blood tests may be required. May cause nausea or vomiting; consult prescriber if symptoms persist. Report skin rash, muscle weakness, persistent headache, depression, fatigue, or gastrointestinal upset.

Dietary Considerations May be taken without regard to meals.

Demeclocycline (dem e kloe SYE kleen)

Index Terms Declomycin; Demeclocycline Hydrochloride; Demethylchlortetracycline

Pharmacologic Category Antibiotic, Tetracycline Derivative

Pregnancy Risk Factor D

Lactation Enters breast milk/not recommended

Use Treatment of susceptible bacterial infections (acne, gonorrhea, pertussis, and urinary tract infections) caused by both gram-negative and gram-positive organisms

Unlabeled Use Treatment of chronic syndrome of inappropriate secretion of antidiuretic hormone (SIADH)

Available Dosage Forms

Tablet, oral: 150 mg, 300 mg

General Dosage Range Oral:

Children ≥8 years: 8-12 mg/kg/day divided every 6-12 hours

Adults: 600 mg/day in 2 or 4 divided doses

Administration

Oral Administer 1 hour before or 2 hours after food or milk with plenty of fluid.

Nursing Actions

Physical Assessment Results of culture and sensitivity tests and patient's allergy history should be assessed prior to beginning therapy. Monitor for rash, anaphylactic reactions, anemia, and CNS changes. Advise patients with diabetes about use of Clinitest®.

Patient Education Take on an empty stomach (1 hour before or 2 hours after meals with plenty of fluid). Take at regularly scheduled intervals around-the-clock. Avoid antacids, iron, and dairy products within 2 hours of taking demeclocycline. May cause photosensitivity, dizziness, lightheadedness, nausea, vomiting, or diarrhea. Report rash or intense itching, yellowing of skin or eyes, change in color of urine or stools, fever or chills, dark urine or pale stools, vaginal itching or discharge, foul-smelling stools, excessive thirst or urination, acute headache, unresolved or persistent diarrhea, or respiratory difficulty.

Denileukin Diftitox (de ni LOO kin DIF ti toks)

Brand Names: U.S. ONTAK®

Index Terms DAB389 Interleukin-2; DAB_{389}IL-2; DABIL2

Pharmacologic Category Antineoplastic Agent, Miscellaneous

Medication Safety Issues

High alert medication:

The Institute for Safe Medication Practices (ISMP) includes this medication among its list of drug classes which have a heightened risk of causing significant patient harm when used in error.

Lactation Excretion in breast milk unknown/not recommended

Use Treatment of persistent or recurrent cutaneous T-cell lymphoma (CTCL) whose malignant cells express the CD25 component of the IL-2 receptor

Unlabeled Use Treatment of CTCL types mycosis fungoides (MF) and Sézary syndrome (SS); peripheral T-cell lymphoma (second-line treatment)

Available Dosage Forms

Injection, solution:

ONTAK®: 150 mcg/mL (2 mL)

General Dosage Range Dosage adjustment recommended in patients who develop toxicities

I.V.: *Adults:* 9 or 18 mcg/kg/day days 1-5 every 21 days

Administration

I.V. For I.V. use only. Infuse over 30-60 minutes. Should **not** be given as a rapid I.V. bolus. Discontinue or reduce infusion rate for infusion related reactions; discontinue for severe infusion reaction. Do not administer through an in-line filter. Premedicate with an antihistamine and acetaminophen; consider corticosteroid premedication.

I.V. Detail pH: 6.9-7.2

Nursing Actions

Physical Assessment Premedication may be ordered. Monitor patient closely for acute hypersensitivity reaction during and for 24-48 hours following infusion (resuscitation equipment should be immediately available during infusion). If serious infusion reaction occurs, discontinue immediately and notify prescriber. Following infusion, patient should be monitored or taught to monitor for delayed vascular leak syndrome (eg, hypotension, edema, hypoalbuminemia), gastrointestinal effects, fever, pain, and respiratory infection. Teach patient to report signs of infection.

Patient Education This medication can only be administered via intravenous infusion. During infusion, report immediately any chills; chest pain, respiratory difficulty, or tightness in throat; or redness, swelling, pain, or burning at infusion site. Maintain adequate hydration, unless instructed to restrict fluids. You may be more susceptible to infection. May cause nausea, vomiting, anorexia, flatulence, constipation, diarrhea, headache, back or muscle pain, dizziness, weakness, or confusion. Report unresolved GI effects; headache or back or muscle pain; skin dryness, rash, or sores; altered urinary patterns; flu syndrome or infection (eg, weakness, fatigue, white plaques or sores in mouth, vaginal discharge, chills, fever); CNS disturbances (insomnia, dizziness, agitation, confusion, depression); unusual bleeding or bruising; blood in urine or stool; or swelling of extremities.

Denosumab (den OH sue mab)

Brand Names: U.S. Prolia®; Xgeva™

Index Terms AMG-162

Pharmacologic Category Bone-Modifying Agent; Monoclonal Antibody

Medication Safety Issues

Other safety concerns:

Duplicate therapy issues: Prolia® contains denosumab, which is the same ingredient contained in Xgeva™; patients receiving Xgeva™ should not be treated with Prolia®

Medication Guide Available Yes

Pregnancy Risk Factor C

Lactation Excretion unknown/not recommended

Breast-Feeding Considerations According to the manufacturer, the decision to continue or discontinue breast-feeding during therapy should take into account the risk of exposure to the infant and the benefits of treatment to the mother. In animal studies, mammary gland development was impaired following exposure to denosumab during pregnancy, resulting in impaired lactation postpartum.

Use Treatment of osteoporosis in postmenopausal women at high risk for fracture; treatment of bone loss in men receiving androgen deprivation therapy (ADT) for nonmetastatic prostate cancer; treatment of bone loss in women receiving aromatase inhibitor (AI) therapy for breast cancer; prevention of skeletal-related events (eg, fracture, spinal cord compression, bone pain requiring surgery/radiation therapy) in patients with bone metastases from solid tumors

Unlabeled Use Treatment of bone destruction caused by rheumatoid arthritis

Mechanism of Action/Effect Denosumab is a monoclonal antibody which causes decreased bone resorption and increased bone mass.

Contraindications

Prolia®: Pre-existing hypocalcemia

Xgeva™: There are no contraindications listed in the manufacturer's labeling.

Warnings/Precautions Denosumab may cause or exacerbate hypocalcemia. Monitor calcium levels; correct pre-existing hypocalcemia prior to therapy. Use caution in patients with a history of hypoparathyroidism, thyroid surgery, parathyroid surgery, malabsorption syndromes, excision of small intestine, severe renal impairment/dialysis or other conditions which would predispose the patient to hypocalcemia; monitor calcium, phosphorus, and magnesium closely during therapy. Ensure adequate calcium and vitamin D intake; supplement with calcium and vitamin D; magnesium supplementation may also be necessary. Incidence of infections may be increased, including serious skin infections, abdominal, urinary, ear, or periodontal infections. Endocarditis has also been reported following use. Patients should be advised to contact healthcare provider if signs or symptoms of severe infection or cellulitis develop. Use with caution in patients with impaired immune systems or using concomitant immunosuppressive therapy; may be at increased risk for serious infections. Evaluate the need for continued treatment with serious infection. Osteonecrosis of the jaw (ONJ) has been reported in patients receiving denosumab. ONJ may manifest as jaw pain, osteomyelitis, osteitis, bone erosion, tooth/periodontal infection, toothache, gingival ulceration/erosion. Risk factors include invasive dental procedures (eg, tooth extraction, dental implants, boney surgery); a diagnosis of cancer, concomitant chemotherapy or corticosteroids, poor oral hygiene, ill-fitting dentures; and comorbid disorders (anemia, coagulopathy, infection, pre-existing dental disease). Patients should maintain good oral hygiene during treatment. A dental exam and preventative dentistry should be performed prior to therapy. The benefit/risk must be assessed by the treating physician and/or dentist/surgeon prior to any invasive dental procedure; avoid invasive procedures in patients with bone metastases receiving therapy for prevention of skeletal-related events. Patients developing ONJ while on denosumab therapy should receive care by a dentist or oral surgeon; extensive dental surgery to treat ONJ may exacerbate ONJ; evaluate individually and consider discontinuing if extensive dental surgery is necessary.

Postmenopausal osteoporosis: For use in women at high risk for fracture which is defined as a history of osteoporotic fracture or multiple risk factors for fracture. May also be used in women who failed or did not tolerate other therapies.

Bone metastases: Denosumab is not indicated for the prevention of skeletal-related events in patients with multiple myeloma. In trials of with multiple myeloma patients, denosumab was noninferior to zoledronic acid in delaying time to first skeletal-related event and mortality was increased in a subset of the denosumab-treated group.

Denosumab therapy results in significant suppression of bone turnover; the long term effects of treatment are not known but may contribute to adverse outcomes such as ONJ, atypical fractures, or delayed fracture healing; monitor. Use with caution in patients with renal impairment (Cl_{cr} <30 mL/minute) or patients on dialysis; risk of hypocalcemia is increased. Dose adjustment is not needed. Dermatitis, eczema, and rash (which are not necessarily specific to the injection site) have been reported; consider discontinuing if severe symptoms occur. Packaging may contain natural latex rubber. May impair bone growth in children with open growth plates or inhibit eruption of dentition. Do not administer Prolia® and Xgeva™ to the same patient for different indications.

Drug Interactions

Avoid Concomitant Use There are no known interactions where it is recommended to avoid concomitant use.

Decreased Effect There are no known significant interactions involving a decrease in effect.

Increased Effect/Toxicity

Denosumab may increase the levels/effects of: Immunosuppressants

Nutritional/Ethanol Interactions Ethanol: Avoid ethanol (may increase risk of osteoporosis).

Adverse Reactions A postmarketing safety program for Prolia® is available to collect information on adverse events; more information is available at http://www.proliasafety.com. To report adverse events for either Prolia® or Xgeva™, prescribers may also call Amgen at 800-772-6436 or FDA at 800-332-1088.

>10%:

Central nervous system: Fatigue (Xgeva™: 45%), headache (Xgeva™: 13%)

Dermatologic: Dermatitis (11%), eczema (11%), rash (3% to 11%)

Endocrine & metabolic: Hypophosphatemia (Xgeva™: 32%; grade 3: 15%), hypocalcemia (2%; Xgeva™: 18%; grade 3: 3%)

Gastrointestinal: Nausea (Xgeva™: 31%), diarrhea (Xgeva™: 20%)

Neuromuscular & skeletal: Weakness (Xgeva™: 45%), arthralgia (14%), limb pain (10% to 12%), back pain (12%)

Respiratory: Dyspnea (Xgeva™: 21%), cough (Xgeva™: 15%)

1% to 10%:

Cardiovascular: Peripheral edema (5%), angina (3%)

Endocrine & metabolic: Hypercholesterolemia (7%)

Gastrointestinal: Flatulence (2%)

Neuromuscular & skeletal: Musculoskeletal pain (6%), sciatica (5%), bone pain (4%), myalgia (3%), osteonecrosis of the jaw (ONJ; ≤2%)

Ocular: Cataracts (≤5%)

Respiratory: Upper respiratory tract infection (5%)

Miscellaneous: New malignancies (5%), infections (nonfatal, serious; 4%)

Pharmacodynamics/Kinetics

Onset of Action Decreases markers of bone resorption by ~85% within 3 days; maximal reductions observed within 1 month

Duration of Action Markers of bone resorption return to baseline within 12 months of discontinuing therapy

Available Dosage Forms

Injection, solution [preservative free]:

Prolia®: 60 mg/mL (1 mL)

Xgeva™: 70 mg/mL (1.7 mL)

General Dosage Range SubQ: *Adults:* Prolia®: 60 mg every 6 months; Xgeva™: 120 mg every 4 weeks

Administration

Other SubQ: Prior to administration, bring to room temperature in original container (allow to stand ~15-30 minutes); do not warm by any other method. Solution may contain trace amounts of translucent to white protein particles; do not use if cloudy, discolored (normal solution should be clear and colorless to pale yellow), or contains excessive particles or foreign matter. Avoid vigorous shaking. Administer via SubQ injection in the upper arm, upper thigh, or abdomen.

Prolia®: If a dose is missed, administer as soon as possible, then continue dosing every 6 months from the date of the last injection.

Stability

Storage Prior to use, store in original carton under refrigeration, 2°C to 8°C (36°F to 46°F). Do not freeze. Prior to use, bring to room temperature of 25°C (77°F) in original container (usually takes 15-30 minutes); do not use any other methods for warming. Use within 14 days once at room temperature. Protect from direct heat and light; do not expose to temperatures >25°C (77°F). Avoid vigorous shaking.

Nursing Actions

Physical Assessment Denosumab is given as an injection, subcutaneously, once every 6 months. Serious reactions can include hypocalcemia. Obtain lab results prior to administering drug and correct calcium, especially if creatinine clearance is <30 mL/minute. Instruct patient that drug should be taken along with vitamin D and calcium. There is a risk for osteonecrosis of the jaw, which requires a baseline dental exam prior to administering this drug.

Patient Education Patients should be instructed to take calcium along with vitamin D daily while receiving denosumab. Inform patients of symptoms of hypocalcemia, such as muscle spasms, cramps, or changes in mental status, including confusion or unusual fatigue. Other side effects include numbness or tingling of the mouth, fingers, or toes; fast or slow heartbeat; jaw pain or swelling; gum infection; or loose teeth. Due to the potential risk of osteonecrosis of the jaw, inform patients of need for good oral hygiene, which includes brushing and flossing. A dental exam and repair of dentures should be complete prior to beginning treatment. Patients should inform their prescriber of history of gum disease, anemia, blood clots, or thyroid or parathyroid disease. It may be difficult to tell skin changes from a serious reaction; therefore, notify prescriber of skin changes, such as redness, blistering, or peeling at injection site.

Dietary Considerations Ensure adequate calcium and vitamin D intake to prevent or treat hypocalcemia. Calcium 1000 mg/day and vitamin D ≥400 units/day is recommended in product labeling (Prolia®).

Women and men >50 years of age should consume elemental calcium 1200-1500 mg/day and vitamin D 800-1000 int. units/day (National Osteoporosis Foundation Guidelines, 2010).

Desipramine (des IP ra meen)

Brand Names: U.S. Norpramin®

Index Terms Desipramine Hydrochloride; Desmethylimipramine Hydrochloride

Pharmacologic Category Antidepressant, Tricyclic (Secondary Amine)

Medication Safety Issues

Sound-alike/look-alike issues:

Desipramine may be confused with clomiPRAMINE, dalfampridine, diphenhydrAMINE, disopyramide, imipramine, nortriptyline

Norpramin® may be confused with clomiPRAMINE, imipramine, Normodyne®, Norpace®, nortriptyline, Tenormin®

International issues:

Norpramin: Brand name for desipramine [U.S., Canada], but also the brand name for enalapril/hydrochlorothiazide [Portugal]; omeprazole [Spain]

Medication Guide Available Yes

Lactation Enters breast milk (AAP rates "of concern"; AAP 2001 update pending)

Use Treatment of depression

Unlabeled Use Analgesic adjunct in chronic pain; peripheral neuropathies (including diabetic neuropathy); attention-deficit/hyperactivity disorder (ADHD); depression in children ≤12 years of age

Available Dosage Forms

Tablet, oral: 10 mg, 25 mg, 50 mg, 75 mg, 100 mg, 150 mg

Norpramin®: 10 mg, 25 mg, 50 mg, 75 mg, 100 mg, 150 mg

General Dosage Range Oral:

Adolescents: 25-100 mg/day in single or divided doses (maximum: 150 mg/day)

Adults: 100-200 mg/day in single or divided doses (maximum: 300 mg/day)

Elderly: 25-100 mg/day in single or divided doses (maximum: 150 mg/day)

Nursing Actions

Physical Assessment Monitor CNS status. Assess cardiac and seizure history prior to initiating therapy. Assess for suicidal tendencies before beginning therapy, during initiation of therapy, or following an increase or decrease of dosage. Caution patients with diabetes to monitor glucose levels closely; may increase or decrease serum glucose levels. Taper dose slowly when discontinuing.

Patient Education It may take 2-3 weeks to achieve desired results. Avoid alcohol. Maintain adequate hydration, unless instructed to restrict fluid intake. May cause drowsiness, lightheadedness, impaired coordination, dizziness, blurred vision, loss of appetite or disturbed taste, constipation, urinary retention, postural hypotension, altered sexual drive or ability (reversible), or photosensitivity. Report chest pain, palpitations, or rapid heartbeat; persistent adverse CNS effects (eg, suicide ideation, nervousness, restlessness, insomnia, anxiety, excitation, headache, agitation, impaired coordination, changes in cognition); muscle cramping, weakness, tremors, or rigidity; seizures; blurred vision or eye pain; breast enlargement or swelling; yellowing of skin or eyes; or worsening of condition.

Related Information

Peak and Trough Guidelines *on page 1276*

Desirudin (des i ROO din)

Brand Names: U.S. Iprivask®

Index Terms CGP-39393; Desulfato-Hirudin; Desulfatohirudin; Desulphatohirudin; r-Hirudin; Recombinant Desulfatohirudin; Recombinant Hirudin

Pharmacologic Category Anticoagulant, Thrombin Inhibitor

Medication Safety Issues

High alert medication:

The Institute for Safe Medication Practices (ISMP) includes this medication among its list of drugs which have a heightened risk of causing significant patient harm when used in error.

Pregnancy Risk Factor C

Lactation Excretion in breast milk unknown/use caution

Use Prophylaxis of deep vein thrombosis (DVT) in patients undergoing surgery for hip replacement

Mechanism of Action/Effect Desirudin is a direct, highly selective thrombin inhibitor. Reversibly binds to the active thrombin site of free and clot-associated thrombin. Inhibits fibrin formation, activation of coagulation factors V, VII, and XIII, and thrombin-induced platelet aggregation resulting in a dose-dependent prolongation of the activated partial thromboplastin time (aPTT).

Contraindications Hypersensitivity to natural or recombinant hirudins; active bleeding and/or irreversible coagulation disorders

Warnings/Precautions [U.S. Boxed Warning]: Patients with recent or anticipated neuraxial anesthesia (epidural or spinal anesthesia) are at risk of epidural or spinal hematoma and subsequent paralysis. Consider risk versus benefit prior to neuraxial anesthesia; risk is increased by concomitant agents which may alter hemostasis, as well as traumatic or repeated epidural or spinal puncture. Patient should be observed closely for bleeding and signs and symptoms of neurological impairment if therapy is administered during or immediately following diagnostic lumbar puncture, epidural anesthesia, or spinal anesthesia.

Allergic and hypersensitivity reactions, including anaphylaxis and fatal anaphylactoid reactions have been reported with other hirudin derivatives. Exercise caution when re-exposing patients (anaphylaxis has been reported). Monitor patient closely for signs or symptoms of bleeding. Certain patients are at increased risk of bleeding. Risk factors include bacterial endocarditis; congenital or acquired bleeding disorders; active ulcerative or angiodysplastic GI diseases; severe uncontrolled hypertension; history of hemorrhagic stroke; use shortly after brain, spinal, or ophthalmology surgery; patients treated concomitantly with platelet inhibitors; recent GI bleeding; thrombocytopenia or platelet defects; renal impairment; hepatic impairment; hypertensive or diabetic retinopathy; or in patients undergoing invasive procedures. Do not administer with other agents that increase the risk of hemorrhage unless coadministration cannot be avoided. Discontinue if bleeding occurs. Contraindicated with active bleeding and/or irreversible coagulation disorders.

Do **not** administer intramuscularly (I.M.). Do not use interchangeably (unit-for-unit) with other hirudins. Use with caution in patients with moderate-to-severe renal dysfunction (Cl_{cr} <60 mL/minute/1.73 m^2); dosage reduction is necessary; monitor aPTT and renal function daily. The American College of Chest Physicians recommends against the use of desirudin in patients with Cl_{cr} <30 mL/minute (Hirsh, 2008). Use with caution in the elderly; elimination half-life prolonged in patients >75 years of age.

Drug Interactions

Avoid Concomitant Use

Avoid concomitant use of Desirudin with any of the following: Rivaroxaban

Decreased Effect There are no known significant interactions involving a decrease in effect.

Increased Effect/Toxicity

Desirudin may increase the levels/effects of: Anticoagulants; Collagenase (Systemic); Deferasirox; Ibritumomab; Rivaroxaban; Tositumomab and Iodine I 131 Tositumomab

The levels/effects of Desirudin may be increased by: Antiplatelet Agents; Dasatinib; Herbs (Anticoagulant/Antiplatelet Properties); Nonsteroidal Anti-Inflammatory Agents; Pentosan Polysulfate Sodium; Prostacyclin Analogues; Salicylates; Thrombolytic Agents

Nutritional/Ethanol Interactions Herb/Nutraceutical: Avoid alfalfa, anise, bilberry, bladderwrack, bromelain, cat's claw, celery, coleus, cordyceps, dong quai, evening primrose oil, fenugreek, feverfew, garlic, ginger, ginkgo biloba, ginseng (American/Panax/Siberian), grapeseed, green tea, guggul, horse chestnut seed, horseradish, licorice, prickly ash, red clover, reishi, sweet clover, turmeric, white willow (all possess anticoagulant or antiplatelet activity and as such, may enhance the anticoagulant effects of desirudin).

Adverse Reactions As with all anticoagulants, bleeding is the major adverse effect. Hemorrhage may occur at any site.

2% to 10%:

Gastrointestinal: Nausea (2%)

Hematologic: Hematoma (6%), hemorrhage (major, <1% to 3%; may include cases of intracranial, retroperitoneal, intraocular, intraspinal, or prosthetic joint hemorrhage), anemia (3%)

Local: Injection site mass (4%), deep thrombophlebitis (2%)

Miscellaneous: Wound secretion (4%)

Available Dosage Forms

Injection, powder for reconstitution [preservative free]:

Iprivask®: 15 mg

General Dosage Range Dosage adjustment recommended in patients with renal impairment

SubQ: *Adults:* 15 mg every 12 hours

Administration

I.M. Do **not** administer I.M.

Other For SubQ administration only. Administration should be alternated between the left and right anterolateral and left and right posterolateral thigh or abdominal wall. Insert needle into a skin fold held between the thumb and forefinger; the skin fold should be held throughout the injection. Do not rub injection site. Do not mix with other injections or infusions. Administer according to recommended regimen.

Stability

Reconstitution Attach enclosed vial adapter to vial containing desirudin. Remove syringe cap and attach provided syringe containing diluent to adapter on vial. Slowly push plunger down to transfer entire contents of syringe into vial. Do not remove syringe from vial adapter. Gently swirl solution; round tablet in vial will dissolve within 10 seconds. Resultant solution concentration is 31.5 mg/mL (15.75 mg/0.5 mL provides a 15 mg dose). Turn vial upside down; withdraw appropriate dose amount back into syringe. Remove syringe from vial. Attach enclosed Eclipse™ needle (or any needle appropriate for subcutaneous administration); pull pink lever down and uncap needle; ready for injection. After injection, flip up pink lever to cover needle until it snaps into place; dispose of syringe appropriately.

Storage Store at 25°C (77°F); excursions permitted to 15°C to 30°C (59°F to 86°F). Protect from light. Following reconstitution, solution may be stored at room temperature for up to 24 hours. Discard unused solution after 24 hours.

Nursing Actions

Physical Assessment Monitor patient closely for anaphylactic reaction; treatment for anaphylactic reactions should be available. Bleeding precautions should be observed and patient monitored for signs or symptoms of bleeding (discontinue if bleeding occurs). Monitor for hypersensitivity reaction and bleeding regularly during therapy. Teach patient bleeding precautions.

Patient Education This drug can only be administered by SubQ injection. Report immediately any pain, swelling, burning, or bleeding at injection site; chest pain or difficulty breathing; or swelling of mouth or throat. You may have a tendency to bleed easily; brush teeth with soft brush, floss with waxed floss, use electric razor, avoid scissors or anything sharp, and use caution to prevent falls or injury.

Desloratadine (des lor AT a deen)

Brand Names: U.S. Clarinex®

Pharmacologic Category Histamine H_1 Antagonist; Histamine H_1 Antagonist, Second Generation; Piperidine Derivative

Medication Safety Issues

Sound-alike/look-alike issues:

Clarinex® may be confused with Celebrex®

Pregnancy Risk Factor C

Lactation Enters breast milk/not recommended

Breast-Feeding Considerations Desloratadine is excreted into breast milk. According to the manufacturer, the decision to continue or discontinue breast-feeding during therapy should take into account the risk of exposure to the infant and the benefits of treatment to the mother.

Use Relief of nasal and non-nasal symptoms of seasonal allergic rhinitis (SAR) and perennial allergic rhinitis (PAR); treatment of chronic idiopathic urticaria (CIU)

Mechanism of Action/Effect Desloratadine is a long-acting antihistamine with selective H_1 receptor antagonistic activity.

Contraindications Hypersensitivity to desloratadine, loratadine, or any component of the formulation

Warnings/Precautions Dose should be adjusted in patients with liver or renal impairment. Use with caution in patients known to be slow metabolizers of desloratadine (incidence of side effects may be increased). Some products may contain phenylalanine. Safety and efficacy have not been established for children <6 months of age.

Drug Interactions

Avoid Concomitant Use There are no known interactions where it is recommended to avoid concomitant use.

Decreased Effect

Desloratadine may decrease the levels/effects of: Acetylcholinesterase Inhibitors (Central); Benzylpenicilloyl Polylysine; Betahistine

The levels/effects of Desloratadine may be decreased by: Acetylcholinesterase Inhibitors (Central); Amphetamines; P-glycoprotein/ABCB1 Inducers

Increased Effect/Toxicity

Desloratadine may increase the levels/effects of: Alcohol (Ethyl); Anticholinergics; CNS Depressants; Methotrimeprazine; Selective Serotonin Reuptake Inhibitors

The levels/effects of Desloratadine may be increased by: Droperidol; HydrOXYzine; Methotrimeprazine; P-glycoprotein/ABCB1 Inhibitors; Pramlintide

Nutritional/Ethanol Interactions

Ethanol: May increase CNS depression; monitor for increased effects with coadministration. Caution patients about effects.

Food: Does not affect bioavailability.

Adverse Reactions

>10%: Central nervous system: Headache (14%)

1% to 10%:
Central nervous system: Fatigue (2% to 5%), somnolence (2%), dizziness (4%)
Endocrine & metabolic: Dysmenorrhea (2%)
Gastrointestinal: Xerostomia (3%), nausea (5%), dyspepsia (3%)
Neuromuscular & skeletal: Myalgia (2% to 3%)
Respiratory: Pharyngitis (3% to 4%)

Pharmacodynamics/Kinetics

Onset of Action Within 1 hour

Duration of Action 24 hours

Available Dosage Forms

Syrup, oral:
Clarinex®: 0.5 mg/mL (480 mL)

Tablet, oral:
Clarinex®: 5 mg

Tablet, orally disintegrating, oral:
Clarinex®: 2.5 mg, 5 mg

General Dosage Range Dosage adjustment recommended in adult patients with hepatic or renal impairment

Oral:
Children 6-11 months: 1 mg once daily
Children 1-5 years: 1.25 mg once daily
Children 6-11 years: 2.5 mg once daily
Children ≥12 years and Adults: 5 mg once daily

Administration

Oral May be taken with or without food.

RediTabs® should be placed on the tongue; tablet will disintegrate immediately. May be taken with or without water.

Syrup: A commercially-available measuring dropper or syringe calibrated to deliver 2 mL or 2.5 mL should be used to administer age-appropriate doses in children.

Stability

Storage Syrup, tablet, orally-disintegrating tablet: Store at 25°C (77°F); excursions permitted between 15°C to 30°C (59°F to 86°F). Protect from moisture and excessive heat (85°F). Use orally-disintegrating tablet immediately after opening blister package. Syrup should be protected from light.

Nursing Actions

Patient Education Avoid use of alcohol. You may experience headache, drowsiness, dizziness, dry mouth, dry throat, or nausea. Report rapid heartbeat, shortness of breath, or skin rash.

Dietary Considerations May be taken with or without food. Some products may contain phenylalanine.

Desmopressin (des moe PRES in)

Brand Names: U.S. DDAVP®; Stimate®

Index Terms 1-Deamino-8-D-Arginine Vasopressin; Desmopressin Acetate

Pharmacologic Category Antihemophilic Agent; Hemostatic Agent; Vasopressin Analog, Synthetic

Pregnancy Risk Factor B

Lactation Excretion in breast milk unknown/use caution

Use

Injection: Treatment of diabetes insipidus; maintenance of hemostasis and control of bleeding in hemophilia A with factor VIII coagulant activity levels >5% and mild-to-moderate classic von Willebrand's disease (type 1) with factor VIII coagulant activity levels >5%

Nasal solutions (DDAVP® Nasal Spray and DDAVP® Rhinal Tube): Treatment of central diabetes insipidus

Nasal spray (Stimate®): Maintenance of hemostasis and control of bleeding in hemophilia A with factor VIII coagulant activity levels >5% and mild-to-moderate classic von Willebrand's disease (type 1) with factor VIII coagulant activity levels >5%

Tablet: Treatment of central diabetes insipidus, temporary polyuria and polydipsia following pituitary surgery or head trauma, primary nocturnal enuresis

Unlabeled Use Uremic bleeding associated with acute or chronic renal failure; prevention of surgical bleeding in patients with uremia

Mechanism of Action/Effect Enhances reabsorption of water in the kidneys by increasing permeability of the collecting ducts; raises plasma levels of von Willebrand factor and factor VIII

Contraindications Hypersensitivity to desmopressin or any component of the formulation; hyponatremia or a history of hyponatremia; moderate-to-severe renal impairment (Cl_{cr}<50 mL/minute)

Canadian labeling: Additional contraindications (not in U.S. labeling): Type 2B or platelet-type (pseudo) von Willebrand's disease (injection, intranasal, oral, sublingual); known hyponatremia, habitual or psychogenic polydipsia, cardiac insufficiency or other conditions requiring diuretic therapy (intranasal, sublingual); nephrosis, severe hepatic dysfunction (sublingual); primary nocturnal enuresis (intranasal)

Warnings/Precautions Allergic reactions and anaphylaxis have been reported rarely with both the I.V. and intranasal formulations. Fluid intake should be adjusted downward in the elderly and very young patients to decrease the possibility of water intoxication and hyponatremia. Use may rarely lead to extreme decreases in plasma osmolality, resulting in seizures, coma, and death. Use caution with cystic fibrosis, heart failure, renal dysfunction, polydipsia (habitual or psychogenic [contraindicated in Canadian labeling]), or other conditions associated with fluid and electrolyte imbalance due to potential hyponatremia. Use caution with coronary artery insufficiency or hypertensive cardiovascular disease; may increase or decrease blood pressure leading to changes in heart rate. Consider switching from nasal to intravenous solution if changes in the nasal mucosa (scarring, edema) occur leading to unreliable absorption. Use caution in patients predisposed to thrombus formation; thrombotic events (acute cerebrovascular thrombosis, acute myocardial infarction) have occurred (rare).

Desmopressin (intranasal and I.V.), when used for hemostasis in hemophilia, is not for use in hemophilia B, type 2B von Willebrand disease, severe classic von Willebrand disease (type 1), or in patients with factor VIII antibodies. In general, desmopressin is also not recommended for use in patients with ≤5% factor VIII activity level, although it may be considered in selected patients with activity levels between 2% and 5%.

Consider switching from nasal to intravenous administration if changes in the nasal mucosa (scarring, edema) occur leading to unreliable absorption. Consider alternative rout of administration (I.V. or intranasal) with inadequate therapeutic response at maximum recommended oral doses. Therapy should be interrupted if patient experiences an acute illness (eg, fever, recurrent vomiting or diarrhea), vigorous exercise, or any condition associated with an increase in water consumption. Some patients may demonstrate a change in response after long-term therapy (>6 months) characterized as decreased response or a shorter duration of response.

Drug Interactions

Avoid Concomitant Use There are no known interactions where it is recommended to avoid concomitant use.

Decreased Effect

The levels/effects of Desmopressin may be decreased by: Demeclocycline; Lithium

Increased Effect/Toxicity

Desmopressin may increase the levels/effects of: Lithium

The levels/effects of Desmopressin may be increased by: Analgesics (Opioid); CarBAMazepine; ChlorproMAZINE; LamoTRIgine; Nonsteroidal Anti-Inflammatory Agents; Selective Serotonin Reuptake Inhibitors; Tricyclic Antidepressants

Nutritional/Ethanol Interactions Ethanol: Avoid ethanol (may decrease antidiuretic effect).

Adverse Reactions Frequency may not be defined (may be dose or route related).

Cardiovascular: Blood pressure increased/decreased (I.V.), facial flushing

Central nervous system: Headache (2% to 5%), dizziness (intranasal; ≤3%), chills (intranasal; 2%)

Dermatologic: Rash

Endocrine & metabolic: Hyponatremia, water intoxication

Gastrointestinal: Abdominal pain (intranasal; 2%), gastrointestinal disorder (intranasal; ≤2%), nausea (intranasal; ≤2%), abdominal cramps, sore throat

Hepatic: Transient increases in liver transaminases (associated primarily with tablets)

Local: Injection: Burning pain, erythema, and swelling at the injection site

Neuromuscular & Skeletal: Weakness (intranasal; ≤2%)

Ocular: Conjunctivitis (intranasal; ≤2%), eye edema (intranasal; ≤2%), lacrimation disorder (intranasal; ≤2%)

Respiratory: Rhinitis (intranasal; 3% to 8%), epistaxis (intranasal; ≤3%), nostril pain (intranasal; ≤2%), cough, nasal congestion, upper respiratory infection

Pharmacodynamics/Kinetics

Onset of Action

Intranasal: Antidiuretic: 15-30 minutes; Increased factor VIII and von Willebrand factor (vWF) activity (dose related): 30 minutes

Peak effect: Antidiuretic: 1 hour; Increased factor VIII and vWF activity: 1.5 hours

I.V. infusion: Increased factor VIII and vWF activity: 30 minutes (dose related)

Peak effect: 1.5-2 hours

Oral tablet: Antidiuretic: ~1 hour

Peak effect: 4-7 hours

Duration of Action Intranasal, I.V. infusion, Oral tablet: ~6-14 hours

Available Dosage Forms

Injection, solution: 4 mcg/mL (1 mL, 10 mL)

DDAVP®: 4 mcg/mL (1 mL, 10 mL)

Solution, intranasal: 0.1 mg/mL (2.5 mL, 5 mL)

DDAVP®: 0.1 mg/mL (2.5 mL, 5 mL)

Stimate®: 1.5 mg/mL (2.5 mL)

Tablet, oral: 0.1 mg, 0.2 mg

DDAVP®: 0.1 mg, 0.2 mg

General Dosage Range

I.V.:

Infants and Children ≥3 months: 0.3 mcg/kg as a single dose, may repeat dose if needed

Adults: 2-4 mcg/day in 2 divided doses **or** one-tenth (1/10) of the intranasal maintenance dose **or** 0.3 mcg/kg as a single dose

Intranasal:

Infants 3-11 months: Initial: 5 mcg/day (0.05 mL/day) in 1-2 divided doses; Maintenance: 5-30 mcg/day (0.05-0.3 mL/day) in 1-2 divided doses

Children 12 months to 12 years: Initial: 5 mcg/day (0.05 mL/day) in 1-2 divided doses; Maintenance: 5-30 mcg/day (0.05-0.3 mL/day) in 1-2 divided doses **or** 150 mcg (1 spray of high concentration) as a single dose

Children >12 years and Adults <50 kg: 10-40 mcg/day (0.1-0.4 mL) in 1-3 divided doses **or** 150 mcg (1 spray of high concentration spray) as a single dose

Children >12 years and Adults ≥50 kg: 10-40 mcg/day in 1-3 divided doses **or** 300 mcg (1 spray each nostril of high concentration spray) as a single dose

Oral:

Children 4-5 years: Initial: 0.05 mg twice daily; Maintenance: 0.1-1.2 mg/day in 2-3 divided doses

Children ≥6 years: Initial: 0.05 mg twice daily **or** 0.2 mg at bedtime; Maintenance: 0.1-1.2 mg/day in 2-3 divided doses **or** 0.2-0.6 mg at bedtime

Adults: 0.2-0.6 mg at bedtime **or** 0.1-1.2 mg/day in 2-3 divided doses

SubQ: *Adults:* 2-4 mcg/day in 2 divided doses **or** one-tenth (1/10) of the intranasal maintenance dose

Administration

I.M. Central diabetes insipidus: Withdraw dose from ampul into appropriate syringe size (eg, insulin syringe). Further dilution is not required. Administer as direct injection.

I.V.

I.V. push: Central diabetes insipidus: Withdraw dose from ampul into appropriate syringe size (eg, insulin syringe). Further dilution is not required. Administer as direct injection.

I.V. infusion:

Hemophilia A, von Willebrand disease (type 1), and prevention of surgical bleeding in patients with uremia (unlabeled) (Mannucci, 1983): Infuse over 15-30 minutes

Acute uremic bleeding (unlabeled) (Watson, 1984): May infuse over 10 minutes

Other

Intranasal:

DDAVP®: Nasal pump spray: Delivers 0.1 mL (10 mcg); for doses <10 mcg or for other doses which are not multiples, use rhinal tube. DDAVP® Nasal spray delivers fifty 10 mcg doses. For 10 mcg dose, administer in one nostril. Any solution remaining after 50 doses should be discarded. Pump must be primed prior to first use.

DDAVP® Rhinal tube: Insert top of dropper into tube (arrow marked end) in downward position. Squeeze dropper until solution reaches desired calibration mark. Disconnect dropper. Grasp the tube 3/4 inch from the end and insert tube into nostril until the fingertips reach the nostril. Place opposite end of tube into the mouth (holding breath). Tilt head back and blow with a strong, short puff into the nostril (for very young patients, an adult should blow solution into the child's nose). Reseal dropper after use.

SubQ: Central diabetes insipidus: Withdraw dose from ampul into appropriate syringe size (eg, insulin syringe). Further dilution is not required. Administer as direct injection.

Stability

Reconstitution DDAVP®: Dilute solution for injection in 10-50 mL NS for I.V. infusion (10 mL for children ≤10 kg: 50 mL for adults and children >10 kg).

Storage

DDAVP®:

Nasal spray: Store at controlled room temperature of 20°C to 25°C (68°F to 77°F). Keep nasal spray in upright position.

Rhinal Tube solution: Store refrigerated at 2°C to 8°C (36°F to 46°F). May store at controlled room temperature of 20°C to 25°C (68°F to 77°F) for up to 3 weeks.

Solution for injection: Store refrigerated at 2°C to 8°C (36°F to 46°F).

Tablet: Store at controlled room temperature of 20°C to 25°C (68°F to 77°F).

DDAVP® Melt (CAN; not available in U.S.): Store at 15°C to 25°C (59°F to 77°F) in original container. Protect from moisture.

Stimate® nasal spray: Store refrigerated at 2°C to 8°C (36°F to 46°F). May store at controlled room temperature of 22°C (72°F) for up to 3 weeks.

Nursing Actions

Physical Assessment Monitor for thromboembolism, hyponatremia, and water intoxication regularly throughout therapy.

Patient Education Avoid alcohol; may decrease effect of medication. Avoid overhydration; follow prescriber instructions for fluid intake. Report increased weight or swelling of extremities; excessive thirst; unresolved headache; chest pain or palpitation; respiratory difficulty; acute heartburn, nausea, vomiting, or abdominal cramping; CNS changes (agitation, chills, coma, dizziness, insomnia, confusion); or rash. If using intranasal product, inspect nasal membranes regularly and report swelling, redness, irritation, or increased nasal congestion.

Desvenlafaxine (des ven la FAX een)

Brand Names: U.S. Pristiq®

Index Terms O-desmethylvenlafaxine; ODV

Pharmacologic Category Antidepressant, Serotonin/Norepinephrine Reuptake Inhibitor

Medication Guide Available Yes

Pregnancy Risk Factor C

Lactation Enters breast milk/not recommended

Breast-Feeding Considerations Desvenlafaxine is excreted in human milk and can be detected in the serum of nursing infants. The manufacturer recommends breast-feeding during therapy only if the expected benefits to the mother outweigh any potential risk to the infant.

Use Treatment of major depressive disorder

Mechanism of Action/Effect Desvenlafaxine is a serotonin and norepinephrine reuptake inhibitor.

Contraindications Hypersensitivity to desvenlafaxine, venlafaxine or any component of the formulation; use of MAO inhibitors within 14 days; should not initiate MAO inhibitor within 7 days of discontinuing desvenlafaxine

Warnings/Precautions [U.S. Boxed Warning]: Antidepressants increase the risk of suicidal thinking and behavior in children, adolescents, and young adults (18-24 years of age) with major depressive disorder (MDD) and other psychiatric disorders; consider risk prior to prescribing. Short-term studies did not show an increased risk in patients >24 years of age and showed a decreased risk in patients ≥65 years. Closely monitor for clinical worsening, suicidality, or unusual changes in behavior; the patient's family or caregiver should be instructed to closely observe the patient and communicate condition with healthcare provider. A medication guide should be dispensed with each prescription. **Desvenlafaxine is not FDA approved for use in children.**

The possibility of a suicide attempt is inherent in major depression and may persist until remission occurs. Monitor for worsening of depression or suicidality, especially during initiation of therapy (generally first 1-2 months) or with dose increases or decreases. Use caution in high-risk patients. Worsening depression and severe abrupt suicidality that are not part of the presenting symptoms may require discontinuation or modification of drug therapy. The patient's family or caregiver should be alerted to monitor patients for the emergence of suicidality and associated behaviors (such as agitation, irritability, hostility, impulsivity, and hypomania) and call healthcare provider.

May worsen psychosis in some patients or precipitate a shift to mania or hypomania in patients with bipolar disorder. Patients presenting with depressive symptoms should be screened for bipolar disorder. Monotherapy in patients with bipolar disorder should be avoided. **Desvenlafaxine is not FDA approved for the treatment of bipolar depression.**

Serotonin syndrome and neuroleptic malignant syndrome (NMS)-like reactions have occurred with serotonin/norepinephrine reuptake inhibitors (SNRIs) and selective serotonin reuptake inhibitors (SSRIs) when used alone, and particularly when used in combination with serotonergic agents (eg, triptans) or antidopaminergic agents (eg, antipsychotics). Concurrent use with MAO inhibitors is contraindicated. Do not begin desvenlafaxine within 14 days of terminating MAO-I therapy; do not initiate MAO-I treatment within 7 days of discontinuing desvenlafaxine. May cause sustained increase in blood pressure or heart rate; dose related. Control pre-existing hypertension prior to initiation of desvenlafaxine. Use caution in patients with recent history of MI, unstable heart disease, or cerebrovascular disease; may cause increases in serum lipids (cholesterol, LDL, triglycerides). Use caution in patients with renal impairment; dose reduction required in severe renal impairment. Use caution in patients with hepatic impairment; clearance is decreased and average AUC is increased; dosage adjustment is recommended. May cause hyponatremia/SIADH (elderly at increased risk); volume depletion (diuretics may increase risk).

Interstitial lung disease and eosinophilic pneumonia have been rarely reported with venlafaxine (the parent drug of desvenlafaxine); may present as progressive dyspnea, cough, and/or chest pain. Prompt evaluation and possible discontinuation of therapy may be necessary. Use cautiously in patients with a history of seizures. The risks of cognitive or motor impairment are low. May cause or exacerbate sexual dysfunction. May impair platelet aggregation, resulting in bleeding.

Abrupt discontinuation or dosage reduction after extended (≥6 weeks) therapy may lead to agitation, dysphoria, nervousness, anxiety, and other symptoms; discontinuation symptoms may also occur when switching from another antidepressant. When discontinuing therapy or switching antidepressants, dosage should be tapered gradually over at least a 2-week period. If intolerable symptoms occur following a decrease in dosage or upon discontinuation of therapy, then resuming the previous dose with a more gradual taper should be considered. Use caution in patients with increased intraocular pressure or at risk of acute narrow-angle glaucoma.

Drug Interactions

Avoid Concomitant Use

Avoid concomitant use of Desvenlafaxine with any of the following: Axitinib; Iobenguane I 123; MAO Inhibitors; Methylene Blue

Decreased Effect

Desvenlafaxine may decrease the levels/effects of: Alpha2-Agonists; Axitinib; Iobenguane I 123; Ioflupane I 123; Saxagliptin

The levels/effects of Desvenlafaxine may be decreased by: Tocilizumab

Increased Effect/Toxicity

Desvenlafaxine may increase the levels/effects of: Alpha-/Beta-Agonists; Aspirin; Methylene Blue; Metoclopramide; NSAID (Nonselective); Serotonin Modulators; Vitamin K Antagonists

The levels/effects of Desvenlafaxine may be increased by: Alcohol (Ethyl); Antipsychotics; Linezolid; MAO Inhibitors

Nutritional/Ethanol Interactions

Ethanol: May increase CNS depression; monitor for increased effects with coadministration. Caution patients about effects.

Herb/Nutraceutical: Avoid St John's wort (may increase risk of serotonin syndrome and/or excessive sedation).

Adverse Reactions Reported for 50-100 mg/day.

>10%:

Central nervous system: Dizziness (10% to 13%), insomnia (9% to 12%)

Gastrointestinal: Nausea (22% to 26%), xerostomia (11% to 17%), diarrhea (9% to 11%)
Miscellaneous: Diaphoresis (10% to 11%)
1% to 10%:
Cardiovascular: Palpitation (≤3%), orthostatic hypotension (<2%; elderly 8%), syncope (<2%), hypertension (dose related; ≤1% of patients taking 50-100 mg daily had sustained diastolic BP ≥90 mm Hg)
Central nervous system: Somnolence (≤9%), fatigue (7%), anxiety (3% to 5%), abnormal dreams (2% to 3%), irritability (2%), vertigo (1% to 2%), feeling jittery (≤2%), depersonalization (<2%), extrapyramidal symptoms (<2%), hypomania (<2%), seizures (<2%), concentration decreased (≤1%)
Dermatologic: Rash (1%)
Endocrine & metabolic: Libido decreased (males 4% to 5%), cholesterol (increased by ≥50 mg/dL and ≥261 mg/dL: 3% to 4%), anorgasmia (females 1%; males ≤3%), hot flushes (1%), low density lipoprotein cholesterol (increased by ≥50 mg/dL and ≥190 mg/dL: ≤1%), sexual dysfunction (males ≤1%)
Gastrointestinal: Constipation (9%), anorexia (5% to 8%), vomiting (≤4%), weight loss (≤2%), weight gain (<2%)
Genitourinary: Urinary hesitancy (≤1%)
Hepatic: Liver function tests abnormal (<2%)
Neuromuscular & skeletal: Tremor (≤3%), paresthesia (2%), weakness (≤2%), stiffness (<2%)
Ocular: Blurred vision (3% to 4%), mydriasis (2%)
Otic: Tinnitus (≤2%)
Renal: Proteinuria (6% to 8%)
Respiratory: Epistaxis (<2%)
Miscellaneous: Ejaculation retarded (1% to 5%), erectile dysfunction (3% to 6%), bruxism (<2%), hypersensitivity reaction (<2%), yawning (1%), ejaculation failure (≤1%)
Class-wide adverse effects: Gastrointestinal hemorrhage, hallucinations, photosensitivity

Available Dosage Forms

Tablet, extended release, oral:
Pristiq®: 50 mg, 100 mg

General Dosage Range Dosage adjustment recommended in patients with hepatic or renal impairment

Oral: *Adults:* Initial: 50 mg once daily

Administration

Oral May be taken with or without food. Swallow tablet whole; do not crush, chew, break, or dissolve. When discontinuing therapy, extend dosing interval to taper.

Nursing Actions

Physical Assessment Observe for clinical worsening, suicidality, or unusual behavior changes; especially during the initial few months of therapy or during dosage changes. Monitor vital signs at the beginning and periodically throughout therapy. Taper dosage slowly when discontinuing.

Patient Education It may take 2-3 weeks to achieve desired results. Extended release capsules should be swallowed whole; do not crush or chew. Avoid alcohol. Maintain adequate hydration, unless instructed to restrict fluid intake. You may experience excess drowsiness or insomnia, lightheadedness, dizziness, blurred vision, headache, nausea, vomiting, anorexia, dry mouth, constipation, diarrhea, postural hypotension, urinary retention, or sexual dysfunction (reversible). Report persistent CNS effects (eg, insomnia, restlessness, fatigue, anxiety, abnormal thoughts, suicide ideation, confusion, personality changes, impaired cognitive function), muscle cramping or tremors, chest pain, palpitations, rapid heartbeat, unusual bleeding or bruising, or worsening of condition.

Dietary Considerations May be taken with or without food.

Dexamethasone (Systemic)

(deks a METH a sone)

Brand Names: U.S. Baycadron™; Dexamethasone Intensol™; DexPak® 10 Day TaperPak®; DexPak® 13 Day TaperPak®; DexPak® 6 Day TaperPak®

Index Terms Decadron; Dexamethasone Sodium Phosphate

Pharmacologic Category Anti-inflammatory Agent; Antiemetic; Corticosteroid, Systemic

Medication Safety Issues

Sound-alike/look-alike issues:

Dexamethasone may be confused with desoximetasone, dextroamphetamine
Decadron® may be confused with Percodan®

Pregnancy Risk Factor C

Lactation Excretion in breast milk unknown/use caution

Breast-Feeding Considerations Corticosteroids are excreted in human milk; information specific to dexamethasone has not been located.

Use Primarily as an anti-inflammatory or immunosuppressant agent in the treatment of a variety of diseases including those of allergic, dermatologic, endocrine, hematologic, inflammatory, neoplastic, nervous system, renal, respiratory, rheumatic, and autoimmune origin; may be used in management of cerebral edema, chronic swelling, as a diagnostic agent, diagnosis of Cushing's syndrome, antiemetic

Unlabeled Use Dexamethasone suppression test as an indicator of depression and/or risk of suicide; prevention and treatment of acute mountain sickness and high altitude cerebral edema; accelerate fetal lung maturation in patients with preterm labor

Mechanism of Action/Effect Decreases inflammation by suppression of neutrophil migration, decreased production of inflammatory mediators, and reversal of increased capillary permeability; suppresses normal immune response.

Dexamethasone's mechanism of antiemetic activity is unknown.

Contraindications Hypersensitivity to dexamethasone or any component of the formulation; systemic fungal infections, cerebral malaria

Warnings/Precautions Use with caution in patients with thyroid disease, hepatic impairment, renal impairment, cardiovascular disease, diabetes, glaucoma, cataracts, myasthenia gravis, patients at risk for osteoporosis, patients at risk for seizures, or GI diseases (diverticulitis, peptic ulcer, ulcerative colitis) due to perforation risk. Use caution following acute MI (corticosteroids have been associated with myocardial rupture). Because of the risk of adverse effects, systemic corticosteroids should be used cautiously in the elderly in the smallest possible effective dose for the shortest duration. May affect growth velocity; growth should be routinely monitored in pediatric patients. Withdraw therapy with gradual tapering of dose.

May cause hypercorticism or suppression of hypothalamic-pituitary-adrenal (HPA) axis, particularly in younger children or in patients receiving high doses for prolonged periods. HPA axis suppression may lead to adrenal crisis. Withdrawal and discontinuation of a corticosteroid should be done slowly and carefully. Particular care is required when patients are transferred from systemic corticosteroids to inhaled products due to possible adrenal insufficiency or withdrawal from steroids, including an increase in allergic symptoms. Patients receiving >20 mg per day of prednisone (or equivalent) may be most susceptible. Fatalities have occurred due to adrenal insufficiency in asthmatic patients during and after transfer from systemic corticosteroids to aerosol steroids; aerosol steroids do not provide the systemic steroid needed to treat patients having trauma, surgery, or infections. Dexamethasone does not provide adequate mineralocorticoid activity in adrenal insufficiency (may be employed as a single dose while cortisol assays are performed). The lowest possible dose should be used during treatment; discontinuation and/or dose reductions should be gradual.

Acute myopathy has been reported with high dose corticosteroids, usually in patients with neuromuscular transmission disorders; may involve ocular and/or respiratory muscles; monitor creatine kinase; recovery may be delayed. Corticosteroid use may cause psychiatric disturbances, including depression, euphoria, insomnia, mood swings, and personality changes. Pre-existing psychiatric conditions may be exacerbated by corticosteroid use. Prolonged use of corticosteroids may also increase the incidence of secondary infection, mask acute infection (including fungal infections), prolong or exacerbate viral infections, or limit response to vaccines. Exposure to chickenpox should be avoided; corticosteroids should not be used to treat ocular herpes simplex. Corticosteroids should not be used for cerebral malaria or viral hepatitis. Close observation is required in patients with latent tuberculosis and/or TB reactivity; restrict use in active TB (only in conjunction with antituberculosis treatment). Prolonged treatment with corticosteroids has been associated with the development of Kaposi's sarcoma (case reports); if noted, discontinuation of therapy should be considered. High-dose corticosteroids should not be used to manage acute head injury.

Drug Interactions

Avoid Concomitant Use

Avoid concomitant use of Dexamethasone (Systemic) with any of the following: Aldesleukin; Axitinib; BCG; Conivaptan; Dabigatran Etexilate; Lurasidone; Natalizumab; Nisoldipine; Pimecrolimus; Praziquantel; Rilpivirine; SORAfenib; Tacrolimus (Topical); Ticagrelor; Toremifene

Decreased Effect

Dexamethasone (Systemic) may decrease the levels/effects of: Aldesleukin; Antidiabetic Agents; ARIPiprazole; Axitinib; BCG; Boceprevir; Brentuximab Vedotin; Calcitriol; Caspofungin; Coccidioidin Skin Test; Corticorelin; CycloSPORINE; CycloSPORINE (Systemic); CYP3A4 Substrates; Dabigatran Etexilate; Dasatinib; Exemestane; Gefitinib; GuanFACINE; Isoniazid; Ixabepilone; Linagliptin; Lurasidone; Maraviroc; NIFEdipine; Nisoldipine; P-glycoprotein/ABCB1 Substrates; Praziquantel; Rilpivirine; Salicylates; Sipuleucel-T; SORAfenib; Tadalafil; Telaprevir; Ticagrelor; Toremifene; Ulipristal; Vaccines (Inactivated); Zuclopenthixol

The levels/effects of Dexamethasone (Systemic) may be decreased by: Aminoglutethimide; Antacids; Barbiturates; Bile Acid Sequestrants; CYP3A4 Inducers (Strong); Echinacea; Mitotane; P-glycoprotein/ABCB1 Inducers; Primidone; Rifamycin Derivatives; Tocilizumab

Increased Effect/Toxicity

Dexamethasone (Systemic) may increase the levels/effects of: Acetylcholinesterase Inhibitors; Amphotericin B; CycloSPORINE; CycloSPORINE (Systemic); Deferasirox; Leflunomide; Lenalidomide; Loop Diuretics; Natalizumab; NSAID (COX-2 Inhibitor); NSAID (Nonselective); Thalidomide; Thiazide Diuretics; Vaccines (Live); Warfarin

The levels/effects of Dexamethasone (Systemic) may be increased by: Antifungal Agents (Azole Derivatives, Systemic); Aprepitant; Asparaginase (E. coli); Asparaginase (Erwinia); Calcium Channel Blockers (Nondihydropyridine); Conivaptan; CycloSPORINE; CycloSPORINE (Systemic); CYP3A4 Inhibitors (Moderate); CYP3A4 Inhibitors (Strong); Dasatinib; Denosumab; Estrogen

Derivatives; Fluconazole; Fosaprepitant; Indacaterol; Macrolide Antibiotics; Neuromuscular-Blocking Agents (Nondepolarizing); P-glycoprotein/ABCB1 Inhibitors; Pimecrolimus; Quinolone Antibiotics; Roflumilast; Salicylates; Tacrolimus (Topical); Telaprevir; Trastuzumab

Nutritional/Ethanol Interactions

Ethanol: Avoid ethanol (may enhance gastric mucosal irritation).

Food: Dexamethasone interferes with calcium absorption. Limit caffeine.

Herb/Nutraceutical: Avoid cat's claw, echinacea (have immunostimulant properties).

Adverse Reactions Frequency not defined.

Cardiovascular: Arrhythmia, bradycardia, cardiac arrest, cardiomyopathy, CHF, circulatory collapse, edema, hypertension, myocardial rupture (post-MI), syncope, thromboembolism, vasculitis

Central nervous system: Depression, emotional instability, euphoria, headache, intracranial pressure increased, insomnia, malaise, mood swings, neuritis, personality changes, pseudotumor cerebri (usually following discontinuation), psychic disorders, seizure, vertigo

Dermatologic: Acne, allergic dermatitis, alopecia, angioedema, bruising, dry skin, erythema, fragile skin, hirsutism, hyper-/hypopigmentation, hypertrichosis, perianal pruritus (following I.V. injection), petechiae, rash, skin atrophy, skin test reaction impaired, striae, urticaria, wound healing impaired

Endocrine & metabolic: Adrenal suppression, carbohydrate tolerance decreased, Cushing's syndrome, diabetes mellitus, glucose intolerance decreased, growth suppression (children), hyperglycemia, hypokalemic alkalosis, menstrual irregularities, negative nitrogen balance, pituitary-adrenal axis suppression, protein catabolism, sodium retention

Gastrointestinal: Abdominal distention, appetite increased, gastrointestinal hemorrhage, gastrointestinal perforation, nausea, pancreatitis, peptic ulcer, ulcerative esophagitis, weight gain

Genitourinary: Altered (increased or decreased) spermatogenesis

Hepatic: Hepatomegaly, transaminases increased

Local: Postinjection flare (intra-articular use), thrombophlebitis

Neuromuscular & skeletal: Arthropathy, aseptic necrosis (femoral and humoral heads), fractures, muscle mass loss, myopathy (particularly in conjunction with neuromuscular disease or neuromuscular-blocking agents), neuropathy, osteoporosis, parasthesia, tendon rupture, vertebral compression fractures, weakness

Ocular: Cataracts, exophthalmos, glaucoma, intraocular pressure increased

Renal: Glucosuria

Respiratory: Pulmonary edema

Miscellaneous: Abnormal fat deposition, anaphylactoid reaction, anaphylaxis, avascular necrosis, diaphoresis, hiccups, hypersensitivity, impaired wound healing, infections, Kaposi's sarcoma, moon face, secondary malignancy

Pharmacodynamics/Kinetics

Onset of Action Acetate: Prompt

Duration of Action Metabolic effect: 72 hours; acetate is a long-acting repository preparation

Available Dosage Forms

Elixir, oral: 0.5 mg/5 mL (237 mL)
Baycadron™: 0.5 mg/5 mL (237 mL)

Injection, solution: 4 mg/mL (1 mL, 5 mL, 30 mL); 10 mg/mL (1 mL, 10 mL)

Injection, solution [preservative free]: 10 mg/mL (1 mL)

Solution, oral: 0.5 mg/5 mL (240 mL, 500 mL)
Dexamethasone Intensol™: 1 mg/mL (30 mL)

Tablet, oral: 0.5 mg, 0.75 mg, 1 mg, 1.5 mg, 2 mg, 4 mg, 6 mg
DexPak® 6 Day TaperPak®: 1.5 mg
DexPak® 10 Day TaperPak®: 1.5 mg
DexPak® 13 Day TaperPak®: 1.5 mg

General Dosage Range

I.M.:

Children: 0.03-2 mg/kg/day or 0.6-10 mg/m^2/day divided every 6-12 hours

Adults: 0.75-9 mg/day or 0.03-2 mg/kg/day or 0.6-0.75 mg/m^2/day in divided doses every 6-12 hours **or** 4 mg every 4-6 hours

I.V.:

Children: 0.03-2 mg/kg/day or 0.6-10 mg/m^2/day divided every 6-12 hours **or** 10 mg/m^2/dose every 12-24 hours on days of chemotherapy

Adults: Dosage varies greatly depending on indication

Intra-articular, intralesional, or soft tissue:

Adults: 0.4-6 mg/day

Oral:

Children: 0.03-2 mg/kg/day or 0.6-10 mg/m^2/day divided every 6-12 hours

Adults: Dosage varies greatly depending on indication

Administration

Oral Administer oral formulation with meals to decrease GI upset. **Note:** Oral administration of dexamethasone for croup may be prepared using a parenteral dexamethasone formulation and mixing it with an oral flavored syrup. (Bjornson, 2004)

I.V. Administer as a 5-10 minute bolus; rapid injection is associated with a high incidence of perineal discomfort.

I.V. Detail pH: 7.0-8.5

Topical Topical formulation is for external use. Do not use on open wounds.

Stability

Reconstitution Injection should be diluted in 50-100 mL NS or D_5W.

Storage Injection solution: Store at room temperature; protect from light and freezing.

Stability of injection of parenteral admixture at room temperature (25°C): 24 hours.

Stability of injection of parenteral admixture at refrigeration temperature (4°C): 2 days; protect from light and freezing.

Nursing Actions

Physical Assessment Caution patients with diabetes to monitor glucose levels closely (corticosteroids may alter glucose levels).

Patient Education Oral: Take with or after meals as this may cause stomach upset. Other side effects may include weight gain, mood changes, change in body fat, or weak bones with long term use. Avoid alcohol and limit intake of caffeine or stimulants. Prescriber may recommend increased dietary vitamins, minerals, or iron. If you have diabetes, monitor glucose levels closely (antidiabetic medication may need to be adjusted). Inform prescriber if you are experiencing greater-than-normal levels of stress (medication may need adjustment). You may be more susceptible to infection. Report promptly excessive nervousness or sleep disturbances, signs of infection (eg, sore throat, unhealed injuries), excessive growth of body hair or loss of skin color, vision changes (change in eyesight, eye pain, or irritation), swelling of face or extremities, respiratory difficulty, muscle weakness, tarry stool, persistent abdominal pain, or worsening of condition or failure to improve.

Dietary Considerations May be taken with meals to decrease GI upset. May need diet with increased potassium, pyridoxine, vitamin C, vitamin D, folate, calcium, and phosphorus.

Dexamethasone (Ophthalmic)

(deks a METH a sone)

Brand Names: U.S. Maxidex®; Ozurdex®

Index Terms Dexamethasone Sodium Phosphate

Pharmacologic Category Anti-inflammatory Agent, Ophthalmic; Corticosteroid, Ophthalmic

Medication Safety Issues

Sound-alike/look-alike issues:

Dexamethasone may be confused with desoximetasone, dextroamphetamine

Maxidex® may be confused with Maxzide®

Pregnancy Risk Factor C

Lactation Excretion in breast milk unknown/use caution

Use Management of steroid responsive inflammatory conditions such as allergic conjunctivitis, iritis, or cyclitis; symptomatic treatment of corneal injury from chemical, radiation, or thermal burns, or penetration of foreign bodies

Ophthalmic intravitreal implant (Ozurdex®): Treatment of macular edema following branch retinal vein occlusion (BRVO) or central retinal vein occlusion (CRVO); treatment of noninfective uveitis

Available Dosage Forms

Implant, intravitreal:

Ozurdex®: 0.7 mg (1s)

Solution, ophthalmic: 0.1% (5 mL)

Suspension, ophthalmic:

Maxidex®: 0.1% (5 mL)

General Dosage Range

Intravitreal: *Adults:* 0.7 mg implant in affected eye

Ophthalmic:

Children: Instill 1-2 drops into conjunctival sac every hour during the day and every other hour during the night; gradually reduce dose to 2-4 times/day

Adults:

Solution: Instill 1-2 drops into conjunctival sac every hour during the day and every other hour during the night; gradually reduce dose to every 3-4 hours, then to 3-4 times/day

Suspension: Instill 1-2 drops up to 4-6 times/day or hourly in severe cases

Administration

Other

Ophthalmic solution, suspension: Remove soft contact lenses prior to using solutions containing benzalkonium chloride. Do not touch tip of container to eye.

Ophthalmic implant (intravitreal injection): Ozurdex®: Administer under controlled aseptic conditions (eg, sterile gloves, sterile drape, sterile eyelid speculum). Adequate anesthesia and a broad-spectrum bactericidal agent should be administered prior to injection. In the sterile field, open foil pouch, remove applicator, and pull the safety tab straight off of the applicator (do not twist or flex the tab). If administration is required in the second eye, a new applicator should be used and the sterile field, syringe, gloves, drapes, and eyelid speculum should be changed.

Nursing Actions

Physical Assessment Monitor intraocular pressure if used >10 days.

Patient Education For use in eyes only. Wash hands before using. Lie down or tilt your head back and look upward. Put drops of suspension or solution inside lower eyelid. Close eye and roll eyeball in all directions. Do not blink for 1/2 minute. Apply gentle pressure to inner corner of eye for 30 seconds. Do not use any other eye preparation for at least 10 minutes. Do not let tip of applicator touch eye; do not contaminate tip of applicator (may cause eye infection, eye damage, or vision loss). You may be more sensitive to bright light. Inform prescriber if condition worsens, fails to improve, or if you experience eye pain or disturbances of vision.

Dexchlorpheniramine

(deks klor fen EER a meen)

Index Terms Dexchlorpheniramine Maleate

Pharmacologic Category Alkylamine Derivative; Histamine H_1 Antagonist; Histamine H_1 Antagonist, First Generation

Medication Safety Issues

BEERS Criteria medication:

This drug may be inappropriate for use in geriatric patients (high severity risk).

Pregnancy Risk Factor B

Lactation Excretion in breast milk unknown/not recommended

Use Perennial and seasonal allergic rhinitis and other allergic symptoms including urticaria

Available Dosage Forms

Syrup, oral: 2 mg/5 mL (473 mL)

General Dosage Range Oral:

Regular release:

Children 2-5 years: 0.5 mg every 4-6 hours

Children 6-11 years: 1 mg every 4-6 hours

Adults: 2 mg every 4-6 hours

Timed release:

Children 6-11 years: 4 mg at bedtime

Adults: 4-6 mg at bedtime **or** every 8-10 hours

Administration

Oral May be administered without regard to meals.

Nursing Actions

Patient Education Avoid use of alcohol. You may experience drowsiness, dizziness, dry mouth, nausea, or abdominal pain. Report persistent sedation, confusion, agitation, blurred vision, respiratory difficulty, lack of improvement, or worsening of condition.

Dexlansoprazole (deks lan SOE pra zole)

Brand Names: U.S. Dexilant™

Index Terms Kapidex; TAK-390MR

Pharmacologic Category Proton Pump Inhibitor; Substituted Benzimidazole

Medication Safety Issues

Sound-alike/look-alike issues:

Dexlansoprazole may be confused with aripiprazole, lansoprazole

Kapidex [DSC] may be confused with Casodex®, Kadian®

International issues:

Kapidex [DSC] may be confused with Capadex which is a brand name for propoxyphene/acetaminophen combination product [Australia, New Zealand]

Pregnancy Risk Factor B

Lactation Excretion in breast milk unknown/not recommended

Use Short-term (4 weeks) treatment of heartburn associated with nonerosive GERD; short-term (up to 8 weeks) treatment of all grades of erosive esophagitis; to maintain healing of erosive esophagitis for up to 6 months

Mechanism of Action/Effect A proton pump inhibitor which decreases acid secretion in gastric parietal cells

Contraindications Hypersensitivity to dexlansoprazole or any component of the formulation

Warnings/Precautions Use of proton pump inhibitors (PPIs) may increase the risk of gastrointestinal infections (eg, *Salmonella, Campylobacter*). Relief of symptoms does not preclude the presence of a gastric malignancy. Atrophic gastritis (by biopsy) has been noted with long-term omeprazole therapy; this may also occur with dexlansoprazole. No occurrences of enterochromaffin-like (ECL) cell carcinoids, dysplasia, or neoplasia, such as those seen in rodent studies, have been reported in humans. Patients with moderate hepatic impairment (Child-Pugh class B) may require dosage reductions; no studies have been conducted in patients with severe hepatic impairment.

PPIs may diminish the therapeutic effect of clopidogrel, thought to be due to reduced formation of the active metabolite of clopidogrel. The manufacturer of clopidogrel recommends either avoidance of omeprazole or use of a PPI with less potent CYP2C19 inhibition (eg, pantoprazole). Lansoprazole exhibits the most potent CYP2C19 inhibition; given the potency of CYP2C19 inhibitory activity, avoidance of dexlansoprazole would appear prudent. Others have recommended the continued use of PPIs, regardless of the degree of inhibition, in patients with a history of GI bleeding or multiple risk factors for GI bleeding who are also receiving clopidogrel since no evidence has established clinically meaningful differences in outcome; however, a clinically-significant interaction cannot be excluded in those who are poor metabolizers of clopidogrel (Abraham, 2010; Levine, 2011).

Increased incidence of osteoporosis-related bone fractures of the hip, spine, or wrist may occur with PPI therapy. Patients on high-dose (multiple daily doses) or long-term therapy (≥1 year) should be monitored. Use the lowest effective dose for the shortest duration of time, use vitamin D and calcium supplementation, and follow appropriate guidelines to reduce risk of fractures in patients at risk.

Hypomagnesemia, reported rarely, usually with prolonged PPI use of >3 months (most cases >1 year of therapy); may be symptomatic or asymptomatic; severe cases may cause tetany, seizures, and cardiac arrhythmias. Consider obtaining serum magnesium concentrations prior to beginning long-term therapy, especially if taking concomitant digoxin, diuretics, or other drugs known to cause hypomagnesemia; and periodically thereafter. Hypomagnesemia may be corrected by magnesium supplementation, although discontinuation of dexlansoprazole may be necessary; magnesium levels typically return to normal within 1 week of stopping.

Drug Interactions

Avoid Concomitant Use

Avoid concomitant use of Dexlansoprazole with any of the following: Delavirdine; Erlotinib; Nelfinavir; Posaconazole; Rilpivirine

Decreased Effect

Dexlansoprazole may decrease the levels/effects of: Atazanavir; Bisphosphonate Derivatives; Cefditoren; Clopidogrel; Dabigatran Etexilate; Dasatinib; Delavirdine; Erlotinib; Gefitinib; Indinavir; Iron Salts; Itraconazole; Ketoconazole; Ketoconazole (Systemic); Mesalamine; Mycophenolate; Nelfinavir; Posaconazole; Rilpivirine; Vismodegib

The levels/effects of Dexlansoprazole may be decreased by: Tipranavir

Increased Effect/Toxicity

Dexlansoprazole may increase the levels/effects of: Amphetamines; Benzodiazepines (metabolized by oxidation); Dexmethylphenidate; Methotrexate; Methylphenidate; Raltegravir; Saquinavir; Tacrolimus; Tacrolimus (Systemic); Voriconazole

The levels/effects of Dexlansoprazole may be increased by: Fluconazole; Ketoconazole; Ketoconazole (Systemic)

Nutritional/Ethanol Interactions Ethanol: Avoid ethanol (may cause gastric mucosal irritation).

Adverse Reactions 2% to 10%:

Gastrointestinal: Diarrhea (5%), abdominal pain (4%), nausea (3%), flatulence (1% to 3%), vomiting (1% to 2%)

Respiratory: Upper respiratory tract infection (2% to 3%)

Available Dosage Forms

Capsule, delayed release, oral:

Dexilant™: 30 mg, 60 mg

General Dosage Range Dosage adjustment recommended in patients with hepatic impairment

Oral: *Adults:* 30-60 mg once daily

Administration

Oral May be administered without regard to meals; some patients may benefit from premeal administration if symptoms do not adequately respond to post-meal dosing. Capsules should be swallowed whole; alternatively, patients who are unable to swallow capsules may open the capsule, sprinkle the intact granules onto 1 tablespoon of applesauce, and swallow intact granules immediately.

Stability

Storage Store at 25°C (77°F); excursions permitted to 15°C to 30°C (59°F to 86°F).

Nursing Actions

Patient Education Do not crush or chew capsules. Capsule may be opened and contents added to applesauce. Avoid alcohol. You may experience stomach pain, diarrhea, nausea and/or vomiting, or gas. Report persistent abdominal pain, unresolved severe diarrhea, or persistent vomiting.

Dietary Considerations May be taken without regard to meals; some patients may benefit from premeal administration if symptoms do not adequately respond to post-meal dosing.

Dexmethylphenidate (dex meth il FEN i date)

Brand Names: U.S. Focalin XR®; Focalin®

Index Terms Dexmethylphenidate Hydrochloride

Pharmacologic Category Central Nervous System Stimulant

Medication Safety Issues

Sound-alike/look-alike issues:

Dexmethylphenidate may be confused with methadone

Focalin® may be confused with Folotyn®

Medication Guide Available Yes

Pregnancy Risk Factor C

Lactation Excretion in breast milk unknown/use caution

Breast-Feeding Considerations It is not known if dexmethylphenidate is excreted into breast milk. Dexmethylphenidate is the more active *d-threo*-enantiomer of racemic methylphenidate, and methylphenidate is excreted into breast milk. Refer to Methylphenidate monograph for additional information.

Use Treatment of attention-deficit/hyperactivity disorder (ADHD)

Mechanism of Action/Effect CNS stimulant

Contraindications Hypersensitivity to dexmethylphenidate, methylphenidate, or any component of the formulation; marked anxiety, tension, and agitation; glaucoma; motor tics, family history or diagnosis of Tourette's syndrome; use with or within 14 days following MAO inhibitor therapy

Warnings/Precautions CNS stimulant use has been associated with serious cardiovascular events including sudden death in patients with pre-existing structural cardiac abnormalities or other serious heart problems (sudden death in children and adolescents; sudden death, stroke, and MI in adults). These products should be avoided in patients with known serious structural cardiac abnormalities, cardiomyopathy, serious heart rhythm abnormalities, or other serious cardiac problems that could increase the risk of sudden death that these conditions alone carry. Patients should be carefully evaluated for cardiac disease prior to initiation of therapy. Use of stimulants can cause an increase in blood pressure (average 2-4 mm Hg) and increases in heart rate (average 3-6 bpm), although some patients may have larger than average increases. Use caution with hypertension, hyperthyroidism, or other cardiovascular conditions that might be exacerbated by increases in blood pressure or heart rate.

Has demonstrated value as part of a comprehensive treatment program for ADHD. Use with caution in patients with bipolar disorder (may induce mixed/manic episode). May exacerbate symptoms of behavior and thought disorder in psychotic patients; new onset psychosis or mania may occur with stimulant use; observe for symptoms of aggression and/or hostility. Use caution with seizure disorders (may reduce seizure threshold). Use caution in patients with history of ethanol or drug abuse. May exacerbate symptoms of behavior and thought disorder in psychotic patients. **[U.S. Boxed Warning]: Potential for drug dependency exists - avoid abrupt discontinuation in patients who have received for prolonged periods.** Visual disturbances have been reported (rare). Stimulant use has been associated with growth suppression. Growth should be monitored during treatment.

Drug Interactions

Avoid Concomitant Use

Avoid concomitant use of Dexmethylphenidate with any of the following: Iobenguane I 123; MAO Inhibitors

Decreased Effect

Dexmethylphenidate may decrease the levels/effects of: Iobenguane I 123; Ioflupane I 123

Increased Effect/Toxicity

Dexmethylphenidate may increase the levels/effects of: Fosphenytoin; PHENobarbital; Phenytoin; Primidone; Sympathomimetics; Tricyclic Antidepressants; Vitamin K Antagonists

The levels/effects of Dexmethylphenidate may be increased by: Antacids; Atomoxetine; Cannabinoids; H2-Antagonists; MAO Inhibitors; Proton Pump Inhibitors

Nutritional/Ethanol Interactions

Ethanol: Avoid ethanol (may cause CNS depression).

Food: High-fat meal may increase time to peak concentration.

Herb/Nutraceutical: Avoid ephedra (may cause hypertension or arrhythmias) and yohimbe (also has CNS stimulatory activity).

Adverse Reactions Actual frequency may be dependent upon dose and/or formulation.

>10%:

Central nervous system: Headache (25% to 39%), insomnia (children 5% to 17%), restlessness (adults 12%), anxiety (5% to 11%)

Gastrointestinal: Appetite decreased (children 30%), xerostomia (adults 7% to 20%), abdominal pain (children 15%)

1% to 10%:

Central nervous system: Dizziness (adults 6%), fever (children 5%), irritability (children ≤5%), depression (children ≤3%), mood swings (children ≤3%)

Dermatologic: Pruritus (children ≤3%)

Gastrointestinal: Nausea (children 9%), dyspepsia (5% to 9%), vomiting (children 2% to 9%), anorexia (children 5% to 7%), pharyngolaryngeal pain (adults 4% to 7%)

Respiratory: Nasal congestion (children ≤5%)

Frequency not defined: Ocular: Accommodation difficulties, blurred vision

Also refer to Methylphenidate for adverse effects seen with other methylphenidate products.

Pharmacodynamics/Kinetics

Onset of Action Extended release: ≥0.5 hours

Duration of Action Extended release: 12 hours

Controlled Substance C-II

Available Dosage Forms

Capsule, extended release, oral:

Focalin XR®: 5 mg, 10 mg, 15 mg, 20 mg, 25 mg, 30 mg, 35 mg, 40 mg

Tablet, oral: 2.5 mg, 5 mg, 10 mg

Focalin®: 2.5 mg, 5 mg, 10 mg

General Dosage Range Oral:

Extended release:

Children ≥6 years: Initial: 5 mg once daily; Maintenance: Up to 30 mg/day

Adults: Initial: 10 mg once daily; Maintenance: Up to 40 mg/day

Immediate release: *Children ≥6 years and Adults:* Initial: 2.5 mg twice daily; Maintenance: Up to 20 mg/day in 2 divided doses (at least 4 hours apart)

Administration

Oral

Capsule: Should be administered once daily in the morning; do not crush or chew. Capsules may be opened and contents sprinkled over a spoonful of applesauce; consume immediately; do not store for future use.

Tablet: Should be administered at least 4 hours apart; may be taken with or without food.

Stability

Storage Store at 25°C (77°F); excursions permitted to 15°C to 30°C (59°F to 86°F). Protect from light and moisture.

Nursing Actions

Physical Assessment Perform careful cardiovascular assessment prior to initiating therapy. Monitor vital signs at beginning of therapy and periodically throughout. In children, monitor growth pattern. If growth/weight gain is not as expected, may need to discontinue medication. Taper dosage when discontinuing from long-term therapy.

Patient Education Response may take some time. You may experience decreased appetite or weight loss, restlessness, impaired judgment, headache, dry mouth, or dizziness. Report unresolved rapid heartbeat, chest pain, difficulty breathing, excessive agitation, nervousness, insomnia, tremors, dizziness, or skin rash.

Dietary Considerations May be taken without regard to meals.

Dexrazoxane (deks ray ZOKS ane)

Brand Names: U.S. Totect®; Zinecard®

Index Terms ICRF-187

Pharmacologic Category Antidote; Cardioprotectant

Medication Safety Issues

Sound-alike/look-alike issues:

Zinecard® may be confused with Gemzar®

Pregnancy Risk Factor C (Zinecard®) / D (Totect®)

Lactation Excretion in breast milk unknown/not recommended

Use

Zinecard®: Reduction of the incidence and severity of cardiomyopathy associated with doxorubicin administration in women with metastatic breast cancer who have received a cumulative doxorubicin dose of 300 mg/m^2 and who would benefit from continuing therapy with doxorubicin. (Not recommended for use with initial doxorubicin therapy.)

Totect®: Treatment of anthracycline-induced extravasation.

Unlabeled Use Reduction of the incidence and severity of cardiomyopathy associated with doxorubicin administration (cumulative doses >300 mg/m^2) in patients with malignancies other than metastatic breast cancer who would benefit from continuing therapy with doxorubicin; reduction of the incidence and severity of cardiomyopathy associated with continued epirubicin administration for advanced breast cancer

Available Dosage Forms

Injection, powder for reconstitution: 250 mg, 500 mg

Totect®: 500 mg

Zinecard®: 250 mg, 500 mg

General Dosage Range Dosage adjustment recommended in patients with renal impairment

I.V.: *Adults:* A 10:1 ratio of dexrazoxane:doxorubicin (500 mg/m^2 dexrazoxane: 50 mg/m^2 doxorubicin) **or** 1000 mg/m^2 on days 1 and 2 (maximum dose: 2000 mg), followed by 500 mg/m^2 on day 3 (maximum dose: 1000 mg)

Administration

I.V.

Prevention of doxorubicin cardiomyopathy: Administer by slow I.V. push or rapid (5-15 minutes) I.V. infusion. Administer doxorubicin within 30 minutes after beginning the infusion with dexrazoxane.

Treatment of anthracycline extravasation: Administer I.V. over 1-2 hours; begin infusion as soon as possible, within 6 hours of extravasation. Infusion solution should be at room temperature prior to administration. Infuse in a large vein in an area remote from the extravasation. If extravasation is also being managed with cooling, withhold cooling beginning 15 minutes before dexrazoxane infusion; continue withholding cooling until 15 minutes after infusion is completed. Day 2 and 3 doses should be administered at approximately the same time (± 3 hours) as the dose on day 1. For I.V. administration; **not** for local infiltration into extravasation

Nursing Actions

Physical Assessment Monitor cardiac function closely. Assess infusion site frequently. Avoid extravasation.

Patient Education This I.V. medication is given to reduce incidence of cardiac complications with doxorubicin. Report promptly any pain at infusion site. You will be more susceptible to infections. Report shortness of breath, chest discomfort, unusual bleeding, fever, or swelling of extremities.

Related Information

Management of Drug Extravasations *on page 1269*

Dextroamphetamine (deks troe am FET a meen)

Brand Names: U.S. Dexedrine® Spansule®; ProCentra®

Index Terms Dextroamphetamine Sulfate

Pharmacologic Category Stimulant

Medication Safety Issues

Sound-alike/look-alike issues:

Dexedrine® may be confused with dextran, Excedrin®

Dextroamphetamine may be confused with dexamethasone

BEERS Criteria medication:

This drug may be inappropriate for use in geriatric patients (high severity risk).

Medication Guide Available Yes

Pregnancy Risk Factor C

Lactation Enters breast milk/not recommended

Use Narcolepsy; attention-deficit/hyperactivity disorder (ADHD)

Unlabeled Use Depression

Controlled Substance C-II

Available Dosage Forms

Capsule, extended release, oral: 5 mg, 10 mg, 15 mg

Capsule, sustained release, oral:

Dexedrine® Spansule®: 5 mg, 10 mg, 15 mg

Solution, oral:

ProCentra®: 5 mg/5 mL (480 mL)

Tablet, oral: 5 mg, 10 mg

General Dosage Range Oral:

Children 3-5 years: Initial: 2.5 mg once daily; Maintenance: 0.1-0.5 mg/kg once daily (maximum: 40 mg/day)

Children 6-12 years: Initial: 5 mg once or twice daily; Maintenance: 5-20 mg (0.1-0.5 mg/kg) once daily (maximum: 40 mg [ADHD]: 60 mg [narcolepsy])

Children >12 years: Initial: 5-10 mg/day in 1-2 divided doses; Maximum: Up to 40 mg/day [ADHD] or 60 mg/day [narcolepsy]

Adults: Initial: 10 mg once daily; Maximum: Up to 60 mg/day

Administration

Oral Administer initial dose upon awakening; do not administer doses late in the evening due to potential for insomnia.

Immediate release tablets and oral solution: If needed, 1-2 additional doses may be administered at intervals of 4-6 hours.

Extended release or sustained release capsules: Do not crush sustained release drug products. Formulations may be used for once-daily administration, if appropriate.

Nursing Actions

Physical Assessment Assess for history of suicidal tendencies. Monitor blood pressure and vital signs at start of therapy, when changing dosage, and at regular intervals throughout. Monitor serum glucose closely in patients with diabetes and monitor weight closely; weight loss may occur. Taper dosage slowly when discontinuing.

Patient Education Take early in day to avoid sleep disturbance, 30 minutes before meals. Avoid alcohol or caffeine. You may experience restlessness, impaired judgment, dry mouth, nausea or vomiting, constipation, or diarrhea. Patients with diabetes need to monitor serum glucose closely. Report chest pain, palpitations, difficulty breathing, fainting, extreme fatigue or depression, CNS changes (aggressiveness, restlessness, euphoria, sleep disturbances), or weight loss.

Dextroamphetamine and Amphetamine

(deks troe am FET a meen & am FET a meen)

Brand Names: U.S. Adderall XR®; Adderall®

Index Terms Amphetamine and Dextroamphetamine

Pharmacologic Category Stimulant

Medication Safety Issues

Sound-alike/look-alike issues:

Adderall® may be confused with Inderal®

BEERS Criteria medication:

This drug may be inappropriate for use in geriatric patients (high severity risk).

Medication Guide Available Yes

Pregnancy Risk Factor C

Lactation Enters breast milk/contraindicated

Use Attention-deficit/hyperactivity disorder (ADHD); narcolepsy

Mechanism of Action/Effect Amphetamines release catecholamines from storage sites in the nerve terminals.

Contraindications Hypersensitivity to dextroamphetamine, amphetamine, or any component of the formulation; advanced arteriosclerosis; symptomatic cardiovascular disease; moderate-to-severe hypertension; hyperthyroidism; hypersensitivity or idiosyncrasy to the sympathomimetic amines; glaucoma; agitated states; patients with a history of drug abuse; with or within 14 days following MAO inhibitor (hypertensive crisis)

Warnings/Precautions [U.S. Boxed Warning]: Use has been associated with serious cardiovascular events including sudden death in patients with pre-existing structural cardiac abnormalities or other serious heart problems (sudden death in children and adolescents; sudden death, stroke and MI in adults. These products should be avoided in the patients with known serious structural cardiac abnormalities, cardiomyopathy, serious heart rhythm abnormalities, or other serious cardiac problems that could increase the risk of sudden death that these conditions alone carry. Patients should be carefully evaluated for cardiac disease prior to initiation of therapy. Use with caution in patients with hypertension and other cardiovascular conditions that might be exacerbated by increases in blood pressure or heart rate. Amphetamines may impair the ability to engage in potentially hazardous activities. May cause visual disturbances.

Use with caution in patients with psychiatric or seizure disorders. May exacerbate symptoms of behavior and thought disorder in psychotic patients. Stimulants may unmask tics in individuals with coexisting Tourette's syndrome. **[U.S. Boxed Warning]: Potential for drug dependency exists; prolonged use may lead to drug dependency.** Use is contraindicated in patients with history of ethanol or drug abuse. Prescriptions should be written for the smallest quantity consistent with good patient care to minimize possibility of overdose. Abrupt discontinuation following high doses or for prolonged periods may result in symptoms for withdrawal.

May be inappropriate for use in the elderly due to CNS stimulant adverse effects (Beers Criteria). Safety and efficacy have not been established in children <3 years of age. Appetite suppression may occur; monitor weight during therapy, particularly in children. Use of stimulants has been associated with suppression of growth; monitor growth rate during treatment.

Drug Interactions

Avoid Concomitant Use

Avoid concomitant use of Dextroamphetamine and Amphetamine with any of the following: Iobenguane I 123; MAO Inhibitors

Decreased Effect

Dextroamphetamine and Amphetamine may decrease the levels/effects of: Antihistamines; Ethosuximide; Iobenguane I 123; Ioflupane I 123; PHENobarbital; Phenytoin

The levels/effects of Dextroamphetamine and Amphetamine may be decreased by: Ammonium Chloride; Antipsychotics; Gastrointestinal Acidifying Agents; Lithium; Methenamine; Peginterferon Alfa-2b

Increased Effect/Toxicity

Dextroamphetamine and Amphetamine may increase the levels/effects of: Analgesics (Opioid); Sympathomimetics

The levels/effects of Dextroamphetamine and Amphetamine may be increased by: Alkalinizing Agents; Antacids; Atomoxetine; Cannabinoids; Carbonic Anhydrase Inhibitors; MAO Inhibitors; Proton Pump Inhibitors; Tricyclic Antidepressants

Nutritional/Ethanol Interactions

Ethanol: Ethanol use may increase CNS depression. Potential for drug dependency may increase with prolonged use. Management: Avoid ethanol. Use is contraindicated for patients with history of ethanol or drug abuse.

Food: Dextroamphetamine serum levels may be altered if taken with acidic food, juices, or vitamin C. Management: Avoid caffeine. Take 30 minutes before meals.

Herb/Nutraceutical: Ephedra may cause hypertension or arrhythmias. Management: Avoid ephedra.

Adverse Reactions

As reported with Adderall XR®:

>10%:

Central nervous system: Insomnia (12% to 27%), headache (up to 26% in adults)

Gastrointestinal: Appetite decreased (22% to 36%), abdominal pain (11% to 14%), dry mouth (2% to 35%), weight loss (4% to 11%)

1% to 10%:

Cardiovascular: Tachycardia (up to 6% in adults), palpitation (2% to 4%)

Central nervous system: Emotional lability (2% to 9%), agitation (up to 8% in adults), anxiety (8%), dizziness (2% to 7%), nervousness (6%), fever (5%), somnolence (2% to 4%)

Dermatologic: Photosensitization (2% to 4%)

Endocrine & metabolic: Dysmenorrhea (2% to 4%), impotence (2% to 4%), libido decreased (2% to 4%)

Gastrointestinal: Nausea (2% to 8%), vomiting (2% to 7%), diarrhea (2% to 6%), constipation (2% to 4%), dyspepsia (2% to 4%)

Genitourinary: Urinary tract infection (5%)

Neuromuscular & skeletal: Twitching (2% to 4%), weakness (2% to 6%)

Respiratory: Dyspnea (2% to 4%)

Miscellaneous: Diaphoresis (2% to 4%), infection (2% to 4%), speech disorder (2% to 4%)

Adverse reactions reported with other amphetamines include: Adverse reactions reported with other amphetamines include: Anaphylaxis, angioedema, anorexia, cardiomyopathy, depression, dyskinesia, dysphoria, euphoria, exacerbation of motor and phonic tics, exacerbation of Tourette's syndrome, hypertension, MI, overstimulation, psychosis, rash, restlessness, seizure, stroke, taste disturbance, tremor, urticaria

Pharmacodynamics/Kinetics

Onset of Action 30-60 minutes

Duration of Action 4-6 hours

Controlled Substance C-II

Available Dosage Forms

Capsule, extended release, oral:

5 mg [dextroamphetamine sulfate 1.25 mg, dextroamphetamine saccharate 1.25 mg, amphetamine aspartate monohydrate 1.25 mg, amphetamine sulfate 1.25 mg]

10 mg [dextroamphetamine sulfate 2.5 mg, dextroamphetamine saccharate 2.5 mg, amphetamine aspartate monohydrate 2.5 mg, amphetamine sulfate 2.5 mg]

15 mg [dextroamphetamine sulfate 3.75 mg, dextroamphetamine saccharate 3.75 mg, amphetamine aspartate monohydrate 3.75 mg, amphetamine sulfate 3.75 mg]

20 mg [dextroamphetamine sulfate 5 mg, dextroamphetamine saccharate 5 mg, amphetamine aspartate monohydrate 5 mg, amphetamine sulfate 5 mg]

25 mg [dextroamphetamine sulfate 6.25 mg, dextroamphetamine saccharate 6.25 mg, amphetamine aspartate monohydrate 6.25 mg, amphetamine sulfate 6.25 mg]

30 mg [dextroamphetamine sulfate 7.5 mg, dextroamphetamine saccharate 7.5 mg, amphetamine aspartate monohydrate 7.5 mg, amphetamine sulfate 7.5 mg]

Adderall XR®:

5 mg [dextroamphetamine 1.25 mg, dextroamphetamine saccharate 1.25 mg, amphetamine aspartate monohydrate 1.25 mg, amphetamine sulfate 1.25 mg]

10 mg [dextroamphetamine sulfate 2.5 mg, dextroamphetamine saccharate 2.5 mg, amphetamine aspartate monohydrate 2.5 mg, amphetamine sulfate 2.5 mg]

15 mg [dextroamphetamine sulfate 3.75 mg, dextroamphetamine saccharate 3.75 mg, amphetamine aspartate monohydrate 3.75 mg, amphetamine sulfate 3.75 mg]

20 mg [dextroamphetamine sulfate 5 mg, dextroamphetamine saccharate 5 mg, amphetamine aspartate monohydrate 5 mg, amphetamine sulfate 5 mg]

25 mg [dextroamphetamine sulfate 6.25 mg, dextroamphetamine saccharate 6.25 mg, amphetamine aspartate monohydrate 6.25 mg, amphetamine sulfate 6.25 mg]

30 mg [dextroamphetamine sulfate 7.5 mg, dextroamphetamine saccharate 7.5 mg, amphetamine aspartate monohydrate 7.5 mg, amphetamine sulfate 7.5 mg]

Tablet, oral: 5 mg, 7.5 mg, 10 mg, 12.5 mg, 15 mg, 20 mg, 30 mg
- 5 mg [dextroamphetamine sulfate 1.25 mg, dextroamphetamine saccharate 1.25 mg, amphetamine aspartate monohydrate 1.25 mg, amphetamine sulfate 1.25 mg]
- 7.5 mg [dextroamphetamine sulfate 1.875 mg, dextroamphetamine saccharate 1.875 mg, amphetamine aspartate monohydrate 1.875 mg, amphetamine sulfate 1.875 mg]
- 10 mg [dextroamphetamine sulfate 2.5 mg, dextroamphetamine saccharate 2.5 mg, amphetamine aspartate monohydrate 2.5 mg, amphetamine sulfate 2.5 mg]
- 12.5 mg [dextroamphetamine sulfate 3.125 mg, dextroamphetamine saccharate 3.125 mg, amphetamine aspartate monohydrate 3.125 mg, amphetamine sulfate 3.125 mg]
- 15 mg [dextroamphetamine sulfate 3.75 mg, dextroamphetamine saccharate 3.75 mg, amphetamine aspartate monohydrate 3.75 mg, amphetamine sulfate 3.75 mg]
- 20 mg [dextroamphetamine sulfate 5 mg, dextroamphetamine saccharate 5 mg, amphetamine aspartate monohydrate 5 mg, amphetamine sulfate 5 mg]
- 30 mg [dextroamphetamine sulfate 7.5 mg, dextroamphetamine saccharate 7.5 mg, amphetamine aspartate monohydrate 7.5 mg, amphetamine sulfate 7.5 mg]

Adderall®:
- 5 mg [dextroamphetamine sulfate 1.25 mg, dextroamphetamine saccharate 1.25 mg, amphetamine aspartate monohydrate 1.25 mg, amphetamine sulfate 1.25 mg]
- 7.5 mg [dextroamphetamine sulfate 1.875 mg, dextroamphetamine saccharate 1.875 mg, amphetamine aspartate monohydrate 1.875 mg, amphetamine sulfate 1.875 mg]
- 10 mg [dextroamphetamine sulfate 2.5 mg, dextroamphetamine saccharate 2.5 mg, amphetamine aspartate monohydrate 2.5 mg, amphetamine sulfate 2.5 mg]
- 12.5 mg [dextroamphetamine sulfate 3.125 mg, dextroamphetamine saccharate 3.125 mg, amphetamine aspartate monohydrate 3.125 mg, amphetamine sulfate 3.125 mg]
- 15 mg [dextroamphetamine sulfate 3.75 mg, dextroamphetamine saccharate 3.75 mg, amphetamine aspartate monohydrate 3.75 mg, amphetamine sulfate 3.75 mg]
- 20 mg [dextroamphetamine sulfate 5 mg, dextroamphetamine saccharate 5 mg, amphetamine aspartate monohydrate 5 mg, amphetamine sulfate 5 mg]
- 30 mg [dextroamphetamine sulfate 7.5 mg, dextroamphetamine saccharate 7.5 mg, amphetamine aspartate monohydrate 7.5 mg, amphetamine sulfate 7.5 mg]

General Dosage Range Oral:

Extended release:

Children 6-12 years: Initial: 5-10 mg once daily; Maintenance: Up to 30 mg/day

Adolescents 13-17 years: Initial: 10 mg once daily; Maintenance: 10-20 mg once daily (maximum: 60 mg/day)

Adults: 20 mg once daily (maximum: 60 mg/day)

Immediate release:

Children 3-5 years: Initial: 2.5 mg once daily; Maintenance: Up to 40 mg/day in 1-3 divided doses

Children 6-12 years: Initial: 5 mg once or twice daily; Maintenance: Up to 40 mg/day [ADHD] or 60 mg/day [narcolepsy] in 1-3 divided doses

Children >12 years and Adults: Initial: 5-10 mg in 1-2 divided doses; Maintenance: Up to 40 mg/day [ADHD] or 60 mg/day [narcolepsy] in 1-3 divided doses

Administration

Oral

Adderall®: To avoid insomnia, last daily dose should be administered no less than 6 hours before retiring.

Adderall XR®: Should be given by noon. Capsule may be swallowed whole or it may be opened and the contents sprinkled on applesauce. Applesauce should be consumed immediately without chewing. Do not divide the contents of the capsule.

Stability

Storage Store at controlled room temperature of 15°C to 30°C (59°F to 86°F). Protect from light.

Nursing Actions

Physical Assessment See individual agents.

Patient Education See individual agents.

Related Information

Dextroamphetamine *on page 319*

Dextromethorphan and Chlorpheniramine

(deks troe meth OR fan & klor fen IR a meen)

Brand Names: U.S. Coricidin® HBP Cough & Cold [OTC]; Dimetapp® Children's Long Acting Cough Plus Cold [OTC]; Robitussin® Children's Cough & Cold Long-Acting [OTC]; Robitussin® Cough & Cold Long-Acting [OTC] [DSC]; Scot-Tussin® DM Maximum Strength [OTC]; Triaminic® Children's Softchews® Cough & Runny Nose [OTC]

Index Terms Chlorpheniramine and Dextromethorphan; Chlorpheniramine Maleate and Dextromethorphan Hydrobromide; Dextromethorphan Hydrobromide and Chlorpheniramine Maleate

Pharmacologic Category Alkylamine Derivative; Antitussive; Histamine H_1 Antagonist; Histamine H_1 Antagonist, First Generation

Use Symptomatic relief of runny nose, sneezing, itchy/watery eyes, cough, and other upper respiratory symptoms associated with hay fever, common cold, or upper respiratory allergies

Available Dosage Forms

Syrup:

Dimetapp® Children's Long Acting Cough Plus Cold [OTC]: Dextromethorphan 7.5 mg and chlorpheniramine 1 mg per 5 mL (118 mL)

Robitussin® Children's Cough and Cold Long-Acting [OTC]: Dextromethorphan 15 mg and chlorpheniramine 2 mg per 5 mL (118 mL)

Scot-Tussin® DM Maximum Strength [OTC]: Dextromethorphan 15 mg and chlorpheniramine 2 mg per 5 mL (118 mL)

Tablet:

Coricidin® HBP Cough and Cold [OTC]: Dextromethorphan 30 mg and chlorpheniramine 4 mg

Tablet, softchew:

Triaminic® Children's Softchews® Cough & Runny Nose [OTC]: Dextromethorphan 5 mg and chlorpheniramine 1 mg

General Dosage Range Oral:

Children 6-11 years: Dextromethorphan 10-15 mg and chlorpheniramine 2 mg every 4-6 hours as needed (maximum: 60 mg dextromethorphan and 10 mg chlorpheniramine/24 hours)

Children ≥12 years and Adults: Dextromethorphan 30 mg and chlorpheniramine 4 mg every 6 hours as needed (maximum: 120 mg dextromethorphan and 16 mg chlorpheniramine/24 hours)

Administration

Oral Triaminic® Children's Softchews® Cough & Runny Nose: Dissolve in mouth or chew prior to swallowing.

Dextromethorphan and Quinidine

(deks troe meth OR fan & KWIN i deen)

Brand Names: U.S. Nuedexta™

Index Terms Dextromethorphan Hydrobromide and Quinidine Sulfate; Quinidine and Dextromethorphan

Pharmacologic Category N-Methyl-D-Aspartate Receptor Antagonist

Pregnancy Risk Factor C

Lactation Use caution

Use Treatment of pseudobulbar affect (PBA)

Available Dosage Forms

Capsule, oral:

Nuedexta™: Dextromethorphan hydrobromide 20 mg and quinidine sulfate 10 mg

General Dosage Range

Oral: *Adults:* Initial: Once capsule once daily for 7 days; Maintenance: One capsule twice daily

Administration

Oral May be administered with or without food. Administer twice-daily doses every 12 hours.

Nursing Actions

Physical Assessment See individual agents.

Patient Education See individual agents.

Diazepam (dye AZ e pam)

Brand Names: U.S. Diastat®; Diastat® AcuDial™; Diazepam Intensol™; Valium®

Pharmacologic Category Benzodiazepine

Medication Safety Issues

Sound-alike/look-alike issues:

Diazepam may be confused with diazoxide, diltiazem, Ditropan, LORazepam

Valium® may be confused with Valcyte®

BEERS Criteria medication:

This drug may be inappropriate for use in geriatric patients (high severity risk).

Pregnancy Risk Factor D

Lactation Enters breast milk/not recommended (AAP rates "of concern"; AAP 2001 update pending)

Breast-Feeding Considerations Diazepam and N-desmethyldiazepam can be found in breast milk; the oxazepam metabolite has also been detected in the urine of a nursing infant. Drowsiness, lethargy, or weight loss in nursing infants have been observed in case reports following maternal use of some benzodiazepines, including diazepam.

Use Management of anxiety disorders, ethanol withdrawal symptoms; skeletal muscle relaxant; treatment of convulsive disorders; preoperative or preprocedural sedation and amnesia

Rectal gel: Management of selected, refractory epilepsy patients on stable regimens of antiepileptic drugs requiring intermittent use of diazepam to control episodes of increased seizure activity

Unlabeled Use Panic disorders; short-term treatment of spasticity in children with cerebral palsy; sedation for mechanically-ventilated patients in the intensive care unit

Mechanism of Action/Effect Binds to stereospecific benzodiazepine receptors on the postsynaptic GABA neuron at several sites within the central nervous system, including the limbic system, reticular formation. Enhancement of the inhibitory effect of GABA on neuronal excitability results by increased neuronal membrane permeability to chloride ions. This shift in chloride ions results in hyperpolarization (a less excitable state) and stabilization.

Contraindications Hypersensitivity to diazepam or any component of the formulation (cross-sensitivity with other benzodiazepines may exist); myasthenia gravis; severe respiratory insufficiency; severe hepatic insufficiency; sleep apnea syndrome; acute narrow-angle glaucoma; not for use in children <6 months of age (oral)

Warnings/Precautions Withdrawal has also been associated with an increase in the seizure frequency. Use with caution with drugs which may decrease diazepam metabolism. Use with caution in debilitated patients, obese patients, patients with hepatic disease (including alcoholics), or renal impairment. Active metabolites with extended half-lives may lead to delayed accumulation and adverse effects. Use with caution in patients with respiratory disease or impaired gag reflex.

Acute hypotension, muscle weakness, apnea, and cardiac arrest have occurred with parenteral administration. Acute effects may be more prevalent in patients receiving concurrent barbiturates, narcotics, or ethanol. Appropriate resuscitative equipment and qualified personnel should be available during administration and monitoring. Avoid use of the injection in patients with shock, coma, or acute ethanol intoxication. Intra-arterial injection or extravasation of the parenteral formulation should be avoided. Parenteral formulation contains propylene glycol, which has been associated with toxicity when administered in high dosages. Administration of rectal gel should only be performed by individuals trained to recognize characteristic seizure activity and monitor response.

Causes CNS depression (dose-related) resulting in sedation, dizziness, confusion, or ataxia which may impair physical and mental capabilities. Patients must be cautioned about performing tasks which require mental alertness (eg, operating machinery or driving). Use with caution in patients receiving other CNS depressants or psychoactive agents. Effects with other sedative drugs or ethanol may be potentiated. The dosage of narcotics should be reduced by approximately 1/3 when diazepam is added. Benzodiazepines have been associated with falls and traumatic injury and should be used with extreme caution in patients who are at risk of these events (especially the elderly). Benzodiazepines with long half-lives may produce prolonged sedation and increase the risk of falls and fracture. Short- or intermediate-acting benzodiazepines are preferred in elderly patients (Beers Criteria).

Use with caution in patients taking strong CYP3A4 inhibitors, moderate or strong CYP3A4 and CYP2C19 inducers and major CYP3A4 substrates.

Use caution in patients with depression or anxiety associated with depression, particularly if suicidal risk may be present. Use with caution in patients with a history of drug dependence. Benzodiazepines have been associated with dependence and acute withdrawal symptoms on discontinuation or reduction in dose. Acute withdrawal, including seizures, may be precipitated in patients after administration of flumazenil to patients receiving long-term benzodiazepine therapy.

Diazepam has been associated with anterograde amnesia. Psychiatric and paradoxical reactions, including hyperactive or aggressive behavior, have been reported with benzodiazepines, particularly in adolescent/pediatric or elderly patients. Does not have analgesic, antidepressant, or antipsychotic properties.

Rectal gel: Safety and efficacy have not been established in children <2 years of age.

Oral: Safety and efficacy have not been established in children <6 months of age.

Injection: Safety and efficacy have not been established in children <30 days of age. Solution for injection may contain sodium benzoate, benzyl alcohol, or benzoic acid. Large amounts have been associated with "gasping syndrome" in neonates.

Drug Interactions

Avoid Concomitant Use

Avoid concomitant use of Diazepam with any of the following: Conivaptan; OLANZapine; Pimozide

Decreased Effect

The levels/effects of Diazepam may be decreased by: CarBAMazepine; CYP2C19 Inducers (Strong); CYP3A4 Inducers (Strong); Cyproterone; Deferasirox; Rifamycin Derivatives; St Johns Wort; Theophylline Derivatives; Tocilizumab; Yohimbine

Increased Effect/Toxicity

Diazepam may increase the levels/effects of: Alcohol (Ethyl); ARIPiprazole; CloZAPine; CNS Depressants; Fosphenytoin; Methotrimeprazine; Phenytoin; Pimozide; Selective Serotonin Reuptake Inhibitors

The levels/effects of Diazepam may be increased by: Antifungal Agents (Azole Derivatives, Systemic); Aprepitant; Calcium Channel Blockers (Nondihydropyridine); Cimetidine; Conivaptan; Contraceptives (Estrogens); Contraceptives (Progestins); CYP2C19 Inhibitors (Moderate); CYP2C19 Inhibitors (Strong); CYP3A4 Inhibitors (Moderate); CYP3A4 Inhibitors (Strong); Dasatinib; Disulfiram; Droperidol; Fosamprenavir; Fosaprepitant; Grapefruit Juice; HydrOXYzine; Isoniazid; Ivacaftor; Macrolide Antibiotics; Methotrimeprazine; OLANZapine; Proton Pump Inhibitors; Ritonavir; Saquinavir; Selective Serotonin Reuptake Inhibitors

Nutritional/Ethanol Interactions

Ethanol: Ethanol may increase CNS depression. Potential for drug dependency exists. Management: Avoid ethanol.

Food: Diazepam serum concentrations may be increased if taken with food. Grapefruit juice may increase diazepam serum concentrations. Management: Avoid concurrent use of grapefruit juice. Maintain adequate hydration, unless instructed to restrict fluid intake.

Herb/Nutraceutical: St John's wort may decrease diazepam levels. Yohimbe may decrease the effectiveness of diazepam. Kava kava, valerian, and gotu kola may increase CNS depression. Avoid St John's wort, yohimbe, kava kava, valerian, and gotu kola.

Adverse Reactions Frequency not defined. Adverse reactions may vary by route of administration.

Cardiovascular: Hypotension, vasodilatation

Central nervous system: Amnesia, ataxia, confusion, depression, drowsiness, fatigue, headache, slurred speech, paradoxical reactions (eg, aggressiveness, agitation, anxiety, delusions, hallucinations, inappropriate behavior, increased muscle spasms, insomnia, irritability, psychoses, rage, restlessness, sleep disturbances, stimulation), vertigo

Dermatologic: Rash

Endocrine & metabolic: Libido changes

Gastrointestinal: Constipation, diarrhea, nausea, salivation changes (dry mouth or hypersalivation)

Genitourinary: Incontinence, urinary retention

Hepatic: Jaundice

Local: Phlebitis, pain with injection

Neuromuscular & skeletal: Dysarthria, tremor, weakness

Ocular: Blurred vision, diplopia

Respiratory: Apnea, asthma, respiratory rate decreased

Pharmacodynamics/Kinetics

Onset of Action I.V.: Status epilepticus: Almost immediate

Duration of Action I.V.: Status epilepticus: 20-30 minutes

Controlled Substance C-IV

Available Dosage Forms

Gel, rectal: 10 mg (2 mL); 20 mg (4 mL); 5 mg/mL (0.5 mL)

Diastat®: 5 mg/mL (0.5 mL)

Diastat® AcuDial™: 10 mg (2 mL); 20 mg (4 mL)

Injection, solution: 5 mg/mL (2 mL, 10 mL)

Solution, oral: 5 mg/5 mL (5 mL, 500 mL)

Diazepam Intensol™: 5 mg/mL (30 mL)

Tablet, oral: 2 mg, 5 mg, 10 mg

Valium®: 2 mg, 5 mg, 10 mg

General Dosage Range

I.M.: *Children >30 days and Adults:* Dosage varies greatly depending on indication

I.V.: *Children >30 days and Adults:* Dosage varies greatly depending on indication

Oral:

Children: 0.12-1 mg/kg/day divided every 6-8 hours **or** 0.2-0.3 mg/kg (maximum: 10 mg) prior to procedures

Adolescents: 0.12-0.8 mg/kg/day divided every 6-8 hours **or** 10 mg prior to procedures

Adults: Dosage varies greatly depending on indication

Rectal:

Gel:

Children 2-5 years: Initial: 0.5 mg/kg (maximum dose: 20 mg); may repeat in 4-12 hours if needed

Children 6-11 years: Initial: 0.3 mg/kg (maximum dose: 20 mg); may repeat in 4-12 hours if needed

Children ≥12 years and Adults: Initial: 0.2 mg/kg (maximum dose: 20 mg); may repeat in 4-12 hours if needed

Administration

Oral Intensol™ should be diluted before use.

I.V. Continuous infusion is not recommended because of precipitation in I.V. fluids and absorption of drug into infusion bags and tubing. In children, do not exceed 1-2 mg/minute IVP; in adults 5 mg/minute.

I.V. Detail pH: 6.2-6.9

Other Rectal gel: Prior to administration, confirm that prescribed dose is visible and correct, and that the green "ready" band is visible. Patient should be positioned on side (facing person responsible for monitoring), with top leg bent forward. Insert rectal tip (lubricated) into rectum and push in plunger gently over 3 seconds. Remove tip of rectal syringe after 3 additional seconds. Buttocks should be held together for 3 seconds after removal. Dispose of syringe appropriately.

Stability

Reconstitution Per manufacturer, do not mix I.V. product with other medications.

Storage

Injection: Store at 20° to 25°C (68° to 77°F); excursions permitted to 15°C to 30°C (59°F to 86°F). Protect from light. Potency is retained for up to 3 months when kept at room temperature. Most stable at pH 4-8; hydrolysis occurs at pH <3.

Rectal gel: Store at 25°C (77°F); excursion permitted to 15°C to 30°C (59°F to 86°F).

Tablet: Store at 15°C to 30°C (59°F to 86°F).

Nursing Actions

Physical Assessment Assess for history of addiction; long-term use can result in dependence, abuse, or tolerance; periodically evaluate need for continued use. Monitor blood pressure and CNS status. For inpatient use, institute safety measures to prevent falls. Taper dosage slowly when discontinuing. Teach patient seizure precautions (if administered for seizures).

Patient Education Drug may cause physical and/or psychological dependence. While using this medication, do not use alcohol. Maintain adequate hydration, unless instructed to restrict fluid intake. You may experience drowsiness, dizziness, blurred vision, nausea, vomiting, loss of appetite, dry mouth, or constipation. If medication is used to control seizures, wear identification that you are taking an antiepileptic medication. Report CNS changes (confusion, depression, excitation, insomnia, dizziness, fatigue, or impaired coordination) or changes in cognition, respiratory difficulty, or worsening of seizure activity or loss of seizure control.

Related Information
Management of Drug Extravasations *on page 1269*

Diclofenac (Systemic) (dye KLOE fen ak)

Brand Names: U.S. Cambia™; Cataflam®; Voltaren®-XR; Zipsor™

Index Terms Diclofenac Potassium; Diclofenac Sodium; Voltaren

Pharmacologic Category Nonsteroidal Anti-inflammatory Drug (NSAID); Nonsteroidal Anti-inflammatory Drug (NSAID), Oral

Medication Safety Issues

Sound-alike/look-alike issues:

Diclofenac may be confused with Diflucan®

Cataflam® may be confused with Catapres®

Voltaren may be confused with traMADol, Ultram®, Verelan®

International issues:

Diclofenac may be confused with Duphalac brand name for lactulose [multiple international markets]

Flexin: Brand name for diclofenac [Argentina], but also the brand name for cyclobenzaprine [Chile] and orphenadrine [Israel]

Flexin [Argentina] may be confused with Floxin brand name for flunarizine [Thailand], norfloxacin [South Africa], ofloxacin [U.S., Canada], and perfloxacin [Philippines]

Medication Guide Available Yes

Pregnancy Risk Factor C (oral)/D (≥30 weeks gestation [oral])

Lactation Excreted in breast milk/not recommended

Breast-Feeding Considerations Low concentrations of diclofenac can be found in breast milk. Breast-feeding is not recommended by the manufacturer. Use while breast-feeding is contraindicated in Canadian labeling.

Use

Capsule: Relief of mild-to-moderate acute pain

Immediate-release tablet: Relief of mild-to-moderate pain; primary dysmenorrhea; acute and chronic treatment of rheumatoid arthritis, osteoarthritis

Delayed-release tablet: Acute and chronic treatment of rheumatoid arthritis, osteoarthritis, ankylosing spondylitis

Extended-release tablet: Chronic treatment of osteoarthritis, rheumatoid arthritis

Oral solution: Treatment of acute migraine with or without aura

Suppository (CAN; not available in U.S.): Symptomatic treatment of rheumatoid arthritis and osteoarthritis (including degenerative joint disease of hip)

Unlabeled Use Juvenile idiopathic arthritis (JIA)

Mechanism of Action/Effect Reversibly inhibits cyclooxygenase-1 and 2 (COX-1 and 2) enzymes, which results in decreased formation of prostaglandin precursors; has antipyretic, analgesic, and anti-inflammatory properties

Contraindications Hypersensitivity to diclofenac or any component of the formulation; hypersensitivity to bovine protein (capsule formulation only); patients who exhibit asthma, urticaria, or other allergic-type reactions after taking aspirin or other NSAIDs; perioperative pain in the setting of coronary artery bypass graft (CABG) surgery

Canadian labeling: Additional contraindications (not in U.S. labeling): Uncontrolled heart failure, active gastric/duodenal/peptic ulcer; active GI bleed or perforation; regional ulcer, gastritis, or ulcerative colitis; cerebrovascular bleeding or other bleeding disorders; inflammatory bowel disease; severe hepatic impairment; active hepatic disease; severe renal impairment (Cl_{cr} <30 mL/minute) or deteriorating renal disease; known hyperkalemia; patients <16 years of age; breast-feeding; pregnancy (third trimester); use of diclofenac suppository if recent history of bleeding or inflammatory lesions of rectum/anus

Warnings/Precautions [U.S. Boxed Warning]: NSAIDs are associated with an increased risk of adverse cardiovascular thrombotic events, including MI and stroke. Risk may be increased with duration of use or pre-existing cardiovascular risk factors or disease. Carefully evaluate individual cardiovascular risk profiles prior to prescribing. May cause new-onset hypertension or worsening of existing hypertension. Monitor blood pressure closely. Use caution with fluid retention. Avoid use in heart failure. Concurrent administration of ibuprofen, and potentially other nonselective NSAIDs, may interfere with aspirin's cardioprotective effect. **[U.S. Boxed Warning]: Use is contraindicated for treatment of perioperative pain in the setting of coronary artery bypass graft (CABG) surgery.** Risk of MI and stroke may be increased with use following CABG surgery.

NSAID use may compromise existing renal function; dose-dependent decreases in prostaglandin synthesis may result from NSAID use, reducing renal blood flow which may cause renal decompensation. NSAID use may increase the risk for hyperkalemia. Patients with impaired renal function, dehydration, heart failure, liver dysfunction, those taking diuretics and ACEI, and the elderly are at greater risk of renal toxicity and hyperkalemia. Rehydrate patient before starting therapy; monitor renal function closely. Not recommended for use in patients with advanced renal disease. Long-term NSAID use may result in renal papillary necrosis while persistent urinary symptoms (eg, dysuria, bladder pain), cystitis, or hematuria may occur anytime after initiating NSAID therapy. Discontinue therapy with symptom onset and evaluate for origin.

[U.S. Boxed Warning]: NSAIDs may increase risk of gastrointestinal irritation, inflammation, ulceration, bleeding, and perforation. These events may occur at any time during therapy and without warning. Use caution with a history of GI disease (bleeding or ulcers), concurrent therapy with aspirin, anticoagulants and/or corticosteroids, smoking, use of alcohol, the elderly or debilitated patients. When used concomitantly with ≤325 mg of aspirin, a substantial increase in the risk of gastrointestinal complications (eg, ulcer) occurs; concomitant gastroprotective therapy (eg, proton pump inhibitors) is recommended (Bhatt, 2008).

Use the lowest effective dose for the shortest duration of time, consistent with individual patient goals, to reduce risk of cardiovascular or GI adverse events. Alternate therapies should be considered for patients at high risk.

NSAIDs may cause photosensitivity or serious skin adverse events including exfoliative dermatitis, Stevens-Johnson syndrome (SJS), and toxic epidermal necrolysis (TEN); discontinue use at first sign of skin rash or hypersensitivity. Anaphylactoid reactions may occur, even without prior exposure; patients with "aspirin triad" (bronchial asthma, aspirin intolerance, rhinitis) may be at increased risk. Do not use in patients who experience bronchospasm, asthma, rhinitis, or urticaria with NSAID or aspirin therapy. Use caution in other forms of asthma. Platelet adhesion and aggregation may be decreased; may prolong bleeding time; patients with coagulation disorders or who are receiving anticoagulants should be monitored closely. Anemia may occur; patients on long-term NSAID therapy should be monitored for anemia. Rarely, NSAID use may cause severe blood dyscrasias (eg, agranulocytosis, aplastic anemia, thrombocytopenia).

Use with caution in patients with impaired hepatic function. Closely monitor patients with any abnormal LFT. Diclofenac can cause transaminase elevations; initiate monitoring 4-8 weeks into therapy. Rarely, severe hepatic reactions (eg, fulminant hepatitis, liver failure) have occurred; discontinue all formulations if signs or symptoms of liver disease develop, or if systemic manifestations occur. Use with caution in hepatic porphyria (may trigger attack).

NSAIDS may cause drowsiness, dizziness, blurred vision, and other neurologic effects which may impair physical or mental abilities; patients must be cautioned about performing tasks which require mental alertness (eg, operating machinery or driving). Discontinue use with blurred or diminished vision and perform ophthalmologic exam. Monitor vision with long-term therapy. The elderly are at increased risk for adverse effects (especially peptic ulceration, CNS effects, and renal toxicity) from NSAIDs even at low doses. May increase the risk of aseptic meningitis, especially in patients with systemic lupus erythematosus (SLE) and mixed connective tissue disorders.

Withhold for at least 4-6 half-lives prior to surgical or dental procedures. Safety and efficacy have not been established in children.

Capsule: Contains gelatin; use is contraindicated in patients with history of hypersensitivity to bovine protein.

Oral solution: Only indicated for the acute treatment of migraine; not indicated for migraine prophylaxis or cluster headache. Not bioequivalent to other forms of diclofenac (even same dose); do not interchange products. Contains phenylalanine.

Drug Interactions

Avoid Concomitant Use

Avoid concomitant use of Diclofenac (Systemic) with any of the following: Floctafenine; Ketorolac; Ketorolac (Nasal); Ketorolac (Systemic); Pimozide

Decreased Effect

Diclofenac (Systemic) may decrease the levels/effects of: ACE Inhibitors; Aliskiren; Angiotensin II Receptor Blockers; Antiplatelet Agents; Beta-Blockers; Eplerenone; HydrALAZINE; Loop Diuretics; Potassium-Sparing Diuretics; Salicylates; Selective Serotonin Reuptake Inhibitors; Thiazide Diuretics

The levels/effects of Diclofenac (Systemic) may be decreased by: Bile Acid Sequestrants; Cyproterone; Nonsteroidal Anti-Inflammatory Agents; Peginterferon Alfa-2b; Salicylates; Tocilizumab

Increased Effect/Toxicity

Diclofenac (Systemic) may increase the levels/effects of: Aliskiren; Aminoglycosides; Anticoagulants; Antiplatelet Agents; ARIPiprazole; Bisphosphonate Derivatives; Collagenase (Systemic); CycloSPORINE; CycloSPORINE (Systemic); Deferasirox; Desmopressin; Digoxin; Drotrecogin Alfa (Activated); Eplerenone; Haloperidol; Ibritumomab; Lithium; Methotrexate; Nonsteroidal Anti-Inflammatory Agents; PEMEtrexed; Pimozide; Porfimer; Potassium-Sparing Diuretics; PRALAtrexate; Quinolone Antibiotics; Rivaroxaban; Salicylates; Thrombolytic Agents; Tositumomab and Iodine I 131 Tositumomab; Vancomycin; Vitamin K Antagonists

The levels/effects of Diclofenac (Systemic) may be increased by: ACE Inhibitors; Angiotensin II Receptor Blockers; Antidepressants (Tricyclic, Tertiary Amine); Conivaptan; Corticosteroids (Systemic); CycloSPORINE; CycloSPORINE (Systemic); Dasatinib; Floctafenine; Glucosamine; Herbs (Anticoagulant/Antiplatelet Properties); Ketorolac; Ketorolac (Nasal); Ketorolac (Systemic); Nonsteroidal Anti-Inflammatory Agents; Omega-3-Acid Ethyl Esters; Pentosan Polysulfate Sodium; Pentoxifylline; Probenecid; Prostacyclin Analogues; Selective Serotonin

Reuptake Inhibitors; Serotonin/Norepinephrine Reuptake Inhibitors; Sodium Phosphates; Treprostinil; Vitamin E; Voriconazole

Nutritional/Ethanol Interactions

Ethanol: Avoid ethanol (may enhance gastric mucosal irritation).

Herb/Nutraceutical: Avoid alfalfa, anise, bilberry, bladderwrack, bromelain, cat's claw, celery, chamomile, coleus, cordyceps, dong quai, evening primrose, fenugreek, feverfew, garlic, ginger, ginkgo biloba, grapeseed, green tea, ginseng (Siberian), guggul, horse chestnut, horseradish, licorice, prickly ash, red clover, reishi, SAMe (s-adenosylmethionine), sweet clover, turmeric, white willow (all have additional antiplatelet activity).

Adverse Reactions

Oral:

1% to 10%:

Cardiovascular: Edema

Central nervous system: Dizziness, headache

Dermatologic: Pruritus, rash

Endocrine & metabolic: Fluid retention

Gastrointestinal: Abdominal distension, abdominal pain, constipation, diarrhea, dyspepsia, flatulence, GI perforation, heartburn, nausea, peptic ulcer/GI bleed, vomiting

Hematologic: Anemia, bleeding time increased

Hepatic: Liver enzyme abnormalities (>3 x ULN; ≤4%)

Otic: Tinnitus

Renal: Renal function abnormal

Miscellaneous: Diaphoresis increased

Rectal suppository (CAN; not available in U.S.): Also refer to adverse reactions associated with oral formulations.

Pharmacodynamics/Kinetics

Onset of Action

Cataflam® (potassium salt) is more rapid than the sodium salt because it dissolves in the stomach instead of the duodenum

Suppository: more rapid onset, but slower rate of absorption when compared to enteric coated tablet

Available Dosage Forms

Capsule, liquid filled, oral:

Zipsor™: 25 mg

Powder for solution, oral:

Cambia™: 50 mg/packet (1s)

Tablet, oral: 50 mg

Cataflam®: 50 mg

Tablet, delayed release, enteric coated, oral: 25 mg, 50 mg, 75 mg

Tablet, extended release, oral: 100 mg

Voltaren®-XR: 100 mg

General Dosage Range Oral:

Immediate release capsule: *Adults:* 100 mg/day in 4 divided doses

Immediate release tablet: *Adults:* 100-200 mg/day in 2-4 divided doses

Delayed release tablet: *Adults:* 100-200 mg/day in 2-5 divided doses

Extended release tablet: *Adults:* 100-200 mg/day

Oral solution: *Adults:* 50 mg once

Administration

Oral Do not crush delayed or extended release tablets. Administer with food or milk to avoid gastric distress. Take with full glass of water to enhance absorption.

Oral solution: Empty contents of packet into 1-2 ounces (30-60 mL) of water (do not use other liquids), mix well and administer immediately; food may reduce effectiveness.

Other Rectal suppository: Remove entire plastic wrapping prior to inserting rectally.

Stability

Storage

Capsule, oral solution: Store at 25°C (77°F); excursions permitted to 15°C to 30°C (59°F to 86°F). Protect from moisture.

Suppository (CAN; not available in U.S.): Store at 15°C to 30°C (59°F to 86°F); protect from heat.

Tablet: Store below 30°C (86°F). Protect from moisture; store in tight container.

Nursing Actions

Physical Assessment Monitor blood pressure at the beginning of therapy and periodically during use. Schedule ophthalmic evaluations for patients who develop eye complaints during long-term NSAID therapy.

Patient Education Do not crush or chew tablets. Take with 8 oz of water, along with food or milk products to reduce GI distress. Avoid alcohol. You may experience dizziness, nervousness, headache, nausea, vomiting, dry mouth, heartburn, or constipation; GI bleeding, ulceration, or perforation can occur with or without pain; discontinue medication and contact prescriber if persistent abdominal pain or cramping or blood in stool occurs. Report chest pain or palpitations; respiratory difficulty; bruising/bleeding or blood in urine, stool, mouth, or vomitus; unusual fatigue; skin rash or itching; jaundice, unusual weight gain, or swelling of extremities; change in vision or ringing in ears.

Dietary Considerations Oral formulations may be taken with food to decrease GI distress. Food may reduce effectiveness of oral solution. Some products may contain phenylalanine.

Diclofenac potassium = Cataflam®; potassium content: 5.8 mg (0.15 mEq) per 50 mg tablet

Diclofenac (Topical) (dye KLOE fen ak)

Brand Names: U.S. Flector®; Pennsaid®; Solaraze®; Voltaren® Gel

Index Terms Diclofenac Diethylamine [CAN]; Diclofenac Epolamine; Diclofenac Sodium

Pharmacologic Category Nonsteroidal Anti-inflammatory Drug (NSAID); Nonsteroidal Anti-inflammatory Drug (NSAID), Topical

Medication Safety Issues

Sound-alike/look-alike issues:

Diclofenac may be confused with Diflucan®

Voltaren® may be confused with traMADol, Ultram®, Verelan®

Other safety concerns:

Transdermal patch (Flector®) contains conducting metal (eg, aluminum); remove patch prior to MRI.

International issues:

Diclofenac may be confused with Duphalac brand name for lactulose [multiple international markets]

Flexin: Brand name for diclofenac [Argentina], but also the brand name for cyclobenzaprine [Chile] and orphenadrine [Israel]

Flexin [Argentina] may be confused with Floxin brand name for flunarizine [Thailand], norfloxacin [South Africa], ofloxacin [U.S., Canada], and perfloxacin [Philippines]

Medication Guide Available Yes

Pregnancy Risk Factor B (topical gel 3%) / C (topical gel 1%, topical solution, topical patch) / D (topical solution ≥30 weeks gestation)

Lactation Not recommended

Use

Topical gel 1%: Relief of osteoarthritis pain in joints amenable to topical therapy (eg, ankle, elbow, foot, hand, knee, wrist)

Canadian labeling (not in U.S. labeling): Relief of pain associated with acute, localized joint/ muscle injuries (eg, sports injuries, strains) in patients ≥16 years of age

Topical gel 3%: Actinic keratosis (AK) in conjunction with sun avoidance

Topical patch: Acute pain due to minor strains, sprains, and contusions

Topical solution: Relief of osteoarthritis pain of the knee

Available Dosage Forms

Gel, topical:

Solaraze®: 3% (100 g)

Voltaren® Gel: 1% (100 g)

Patch, transdermal:

Flector®: 1.3% (30s)

Solution, topical:

Pennsaid®: 1.5% (150 mL)

General Dosage Range Topical: *Adults:*

1% gel: Apply 2-4 g to affected joint 4 times/day (maximum: 16 g/day single joint of lower extremity, 8 g/day single joint of upper extremity); Maximum total body dose of 1% gel should not exceed 32 g per day.

3% gel: Apply to lesion area twice daily

Patch: Apply 1 patch twice daily

Solution: Apply 40 drops to each affected knee 4 times/day

Administration

Topical

Topical gel: Do not cover with occlusive dressings or apply sunscreens, cosmetics, lotions, moisturizers, insect repellents or other topical medications to affected area. Do not wash area for 1 hour following application. Wash hands immediately after application (unless hands are treated joint). Avoid sunlight to exposure areas.

1% formulation: Apply gel to affected area or joint and rub into skin gently, making sure to apply to entire affected area or joint.

3% formulation: Apply to lesion with gel and smooth into skin gently.

Topical solution: Apply to clean, dry, intact skin; do not apply to eyes, mucous membranes, or open wounds. Wash hands before and after use. Apply 10 drops at a time either directly onto knee **or** into hand then onto knee (helps avoid spillage). Repeat procedure until total dose applied. Spread evenly around knee (front, back, sides). Allow knee to dry before applying clothing. Do not shower or bathe for at least 30 minutes after applying. Do not apply heat or occlusive dressing to treated knee; protect treated knee from sunlight. Cosmetics, insect repellant, lotion, moisturizer, sunscreens, or other topical medication may be applied to treated knee once solution has dried.

Transdermal patch: Apply to intact, nondamaged skin. Remove transparent liner prior to applying to skin. Wash hands after applying as well as after removal of patch. May tape down edges of patch, if peeling occurs. Should not be worn while bathing or showering. Fold used patches so the adhesive side sticks to itself; dispose of used patches out of reach of children and pets.

Nursing Actions

Patient Education

Gel: This preparation is for topical use only. Use at regular intervals. Wash hands before and after use. Gently apply enough of the gel to cover the lesion. Do not wrap skin where applied in airtight or occlusive dressing. Advise prescriber if you are using any other skin preparations. Avoid direct sunlight and sunlamps while using this medication. You may experience dry skin, itching, peeling, swelling, or tingling at site of application. If severe skin reaction develops, stop applications and notify your prescriber at once.

Transdermal patch: Remove patch prior to MRI. Do not wear during bathing or showering. Apply to clear, healthy skin, avoiding eyes and mucous membranes.

Diclofenac and Misoprostol

(dye KLOE fen ak & mye soe PROST ole)

Brand Names: U.S. Arthrotec®

Index Terms Misoprostol and Diclofenac

Pharmacologic Category Nonsteroidal Anti-inflammatory Drug (NSAID), Oral; Prostaglandin

Medication Guide Available Yes

Pregnancy Risk Factor X

Lactation Enters breast milk/use caution

Use Treatment of osteoarthritis and rheumatoid arthritis in patients at high risk for NSAID-induced gastric and duodenal ulceration

Available Dosage Forms

Tablet:

Arthrotec® 50: Diclofenac 50 mg and misoprostol 200 mcg

Arthrotec® 75: Diclofenac 75 mg and misoprostol 200 mcg

General Dosage Range Oral: *Adults:* Arthrotec® 50: One tablet 2-4 times/day; Arthrotec® 75: One tablet twice daily

Administration

Oral Incidence of diarrhea may be lessened by having patient take dose right after meals and avoiding magnesium containing antacids. Tablets should not be crushed or chewed. Therapy is usually begun on the second or third day of the next normal menstrual period in women of child bearing potential.

Nursing Actions

Physical Assessment See individual agents.

Patient Education See individual agents.

Related Information

Diclofenac (Systemic) *on page 326*

Misoprostol *on page 783*

Dicloxacillin (dye kloks a SIL in)

Index Terms Dicloxacillin Sodium

Pharmacologic Category Antibiotic, Penicillin

Pregnancy Risk Factor B

Lactation Excretion in breast milk unknown/use caution

Use Treatment of systemic infections such as pneumonia, skin and soft tissue infections, and osteomyelitis caused by penicillinase-producing staphylococci

Available Dosage Forms

Capsule, oral: 250 mg, 500 mg

General Dosage Range Oral:

Children <40 kg: 12.5-100 mg/kg/day divided every 6 hours

Children >40 kg: 125-250 mg every 6 hours

Adults: 125-1000 mg every 6-8 hours

Administration

Oral Administer 1 hour before or 2 hours after meals. Administer around-the-clock to promote less variation in peak and trough serum levels.

Nursing Actions

Physical Assessment Assess allergy history prior to beginning therapy.

Patient Education Take medication with a large glass of water 1 hour before or 2 hours after meals. Take at regular intervals around-the-clock. May cause some gastric distress and diarrhea. Report fever, vaginal itching, persistent diarrhea, sores in the mouth, loose foul-smelling stools, yellowing of skin or eyes, or change in color of urine or stool.

Didanosine (dye DAN oh seen)

Brand Names: U.S. Videx®; Videx® EC

Index Terms ddI; Dideoxyinosine

Pharmacologic Category Antiretroviral Agent, Reverse Transcriptase Inhibitor (Nucleoside)

Medication Safety Issues

Sound-alike/look-alike issues:

Videx® may be confused with Lidex®

Medication Guide Available Yes

Pregnancy Risk Factor B

Lactation Excretion in breast milk unknown/contraindicated

Breast-Feeding Considerations Maternal or infant antiretroviral therapy does not completely eliminate the risk of postnatal HIV transmission. In addition, multiclass-resistant virus has been detected in breast-feeding infants despite maternal therapy. Therefore, in the United States, where formula is accessible, affordable, safe, and sustainable, and the risk of infant mortality due to diarrhea and respiratory infections is low, complete avoidance of breast-feeding by HIV-infected women is recommended to decrease potential transmission of HIV (DHHS [perinatal], 2011).

Use Treatment of HIV infection; always to be used in combination with at least two other antiretroviral agents

Mechanism of Action/Effect Didanosine, a purine nucleoside (adenosine) analog and the deamination product of dideoxyadenosine (ddA), inhibits HIV replication *in vitro* in both T cells and monocytes. Didanosine is converted within the cell to the mono-, di-, and triphosphates of ddA. These ddA triphosphates act as substrate and inhibitor of HIV reverse transcriptase substrate and inhibitor of HIV reverse transcriptase thereby blocking viral DNA synthesis and suppressing HIV replication.

Contraindications Concurrent administration with allopurinol or ribavirin

Warnings/Precautions [U.S. Boxed Warning]: Pancreatitis (sometimes fatal) has been reported; incidence is dose related. Risk factors for developing pancreatitis may include a previous history of the condition, concurrent cytomegalovirus or *Mycobacterium avium-intracellulare* infection, renal impairment, advanced age, and concomitant use of stavudine, pentamidine, or hydroxyurea. Discontinue didanosine if clinical signs of pancreatitis occur. **[U.S. Boxed Warning]: Lactic acidosis, symptomatic hyperlactatemia, and severe hepatomegaly with steatosis (sometimes fatal) have occurred with antiretroviral nucleoside analogues, including didanosine.** Hepatotoxicity may occur even in the absence of marked transaminase elevations; suspend therapy in any patient developing clinical/laboratory findings which suggest hepatotoxicity. Hepatotoxicity and hepatic failure (including fatal cases) have been reported in HIV patients receiving combination drug therapy with didanosine and stavudine or hydroxyurea, or didanosine, stavudine, and hydroxyurea; avoid these combinations. Not currently recommended in combination with tenofovir due to failure and resistance. Noncirrhotic portal hypertension may develop within months to years of starting didanosine therapy. Signs may include elevated liver enzymes, esophageal varices, hematemesis, ascites, and splenomegaly. Noncirrhotic portal hypertension may lead to liver failure and/or death. Discontinue use in patients with evidence of this condition. Pregnant women may be at increased risk of lactic acidosis and liver damage. Use with caution in patients with hepatic impairment; safety and efficacy have not been established in patients with significant hepatic disease. Patients on combination antiretroviral therapy with hepatic impairment may be at increased risk of potentially severe and fatal hepatic toxicity; consider interruption or discontinuation of therapy if hepatic impairment worsens.

Peripheral neuropathy occurs in ~20% of patients receiving the drug. If symptomatic, discontinue therapy; after resolution of symptoms, reinitiation of therapy at a reduced dose may be tolerated. Permanently discontinue if neuropathy recurs. Retinal changes (including retinal depigmentation) and optic neuritis have been reported in adults and children using didanosine. Patients should undergo retinal examination every 6-12 months. Use caution in renal impairment; dose reduction recommended for Cl_{cr} <60 mL/minute. May cause redistribution of fat (eg, buffalo hump, peripheral wasting with increased abdominal girth, cushingoid appearance). Patients may develop immune reconstitution syndrome resulting in the occurrence of an inflammatory response to an indolent or residual opportunistic infection; further evaluation and treatment may be required. Didanosine delayed release capsules are indicated for once-daily use.

Drug Interactions

Avoid Concomitant Use

Avoid concomitant use of Didanosine with any of the following: Alcohol (Ethyl); Allopurinol; Febuxostat; Hydroxyurea; Ribavirin; Tenofovir

Decreased Effect

Didanosine may decrease the levels/effects of: Antifungal Agents (Azole Derivatives, Systemic); Atazanavir; Indinavir; Quinolone Antibiotics; Rilpivirine

The levels/effects of Didanosine may be decreased by: Atazanavir; Darunavir; Lopinavir; Methadone; Rilpivirine; Tenofovir; Tipranavir

Increased Effect/Toxicity

Didanosine may increase the levels/effects of: Hydroxyurea

The levels/effects of Didanosine may be increased by: Alcohol (Ethyl); Allopurinol; Febuxostat; Ganciclovir-Valganciclovir; Hydroxyurea; Ribavirin; Stavudine; Tenofovir

Nutritional/Ethanol Interactions

Ethanol: Ethanol increases risk of pancreatitis. Management: Avoid ethanol.

Food: Food decreases AUC and C_{max}; serum levels may be decreased by 55%. Management: Administer on an empty stomach at least 30 minutes before or 2 hours after eating depending on dosage form.

Adverse Reactions As reported in monotherapy studies; risk of toxicity may increase when combined with other agents.

>10%:

Gastrointestinal: Diarrhea (19% to 28%), amylase increased (15% to 17%), abdominal pain (7% to 13%)

Neuromuscular & skeletal: Peripheral neuropathy (17% to 20%)

1% to 10%:

Dermatologic: Rash/pruritus (7% to 9%)

Endocrine & metabolic: Uric acid increased (2% to 3%)

Gastrointestinal: Pancreatitis (1% to 7% dose dependent); patients >65 years of age had a higher frequency of pancreatitis than younger patients patients (10% vs 5% in younger patients)

Hepatic: AST increased (7% to 9%), ALT increased (6% to 9%), alkaline phosphatase increased (1% to 4%)

Available Dosage Forms

Capsule, delayed release, enteric coated beadlets, oral: 125 mg, 200 mg, 250 mg, 400 mg

Videx® EC: 125 mg, 200 mg, 250 mg, 400 mg

Capsule, delayed release, enteric coated pellets, oral: 200 mg, 250 mg, 400 mg

Powder for solution, oral:

Videx®: 2 g/bottle, 4 g/bottle

General Dosage Range Dosage adjustment recommended in patients with renal impairment

Oral:

Delayed release:

Children ≥6 years and 20 kg to <25 kg: 200 mg once daily

Children ≥6 years and 25 kg to <60 kg and Adults <60 kg: 250 mg once daily

Children and Adults ≥60 kg: 400 mg once daily

Pediatric powder for oral solution (Videx®):

Infants 2 weeks to 8 months: 100 mg/m² twice daily

Children >8 months to 18 years: 120 mg/m² twice daily

Adolescents and Adults <60 kg: 125 mg twice daily **or** 250 mg once daily

Adolescents and Adults ≥60 kg: 200 mg twice daily **or** 400 mg once daily

Administration

Oral Pediatric powder for oral solution: Administer on an empty stomach at least 30 minutes before or 2 hours after eating. Prior to dispensing, the powder should be mixed with purified water USP to an initial concentration of 20 mg/mL and then further diluted with an appropriate antacid suspension to a final mixture of 10 mg/mL. Shake well prior to use.

Videx® EC: Administer on an empty stomach at least 1 hour before or 2 hours after eating; swallow capsule whole.

Stability

Reconstitution Videx® pediatric powder: Add 100 mL or 200 mL purified water, USP to the 2 g or 4 g container, respectively, to achieve a 20 mg/mL solution. Immediately mix the resulting solution with an equal volume of Mylanta® Maximum Strength (or equivalent) to achieve a final concentration of 10 mg/mL.

Storage Delayed release capsules should be stored in tightly closed bottles at controlled room temperature of 25°C (77°F). Unreconstituted powder should be stored at 15°C to 30°C (59°F to 86°F). Reconstituted pediatric solution is stable for 30 days if refrigerated.

Nursing Actions

Physical Assessment Monitor for hepatotoxicity, peripheral neuropathy, gastrointestinal pain, and vision changes regularly during therapy. Teach patient proper timing of multiple medications.

Patient Education This drug will not cure HIV, nor has it been found to reduce transmission of HIV; use appropriate precautions to prevent spread to other persons. This drug is prescribed as one part of a multidrug combination; take exactly as directed for full course of therapy. Do not break or chew delayed release capsules. Maintain adequate hydration, unless instructed to restrict fluid intake. Frequent blood tests may be required. You may be advised to have a retinal exam periodically. May cause nausea, vomiting, diarrhea, or changes in body fat (increased in upper back, neck, breast, and around trunk; decreased in legs, arms, and face). Report immediately any loss of sensation, numbness, or tingling in fingers, toes, or feet; persistent unresolved abdominal distress (pain, nausea, vomiting, diarrhea); changes in vision; or signs of infection (burning on urination, perineal itching, white plaques in mouth, unhealed sores, persistent sore throat, cough).

Dietary Considerations Take on an empty stomach; administer at least 30 minutes before or 2 hours after eating

Dienogest (dye EN oh jest)

Pharmacologic Category Antiandrogen

Medication Safety Issues

Sound-alike/look-alike issues:

Visanne® may be confused with Vyvanse®

Lactation Excretion in breast milk unknown/contraindicated

Breast-Feeding Considerations It is not known whether dienogest is excreted into human breast milk. The risk of thromboembolism may be increased immediately postpartum.

Use Management of pelvic pain associated with endometriosis

Mechanism of Action/Effect Dienogest is a steroid with antiandrogen properties that lacks androgen, mineralcorticoid or glucocorticoid activity. Decreases estradiol production and thus suppresses estradiol's trophic effects on eutopic and ectopic endometrium. Inhibits cellular proliferation via direct antiproliferative, immunologic, and antiangiogenic effects.

Contraindications Hypersensitivity to dienogest or any component of the formulation; undiagnosed abnormal vaginal bleeding; active venous thromboembolic disorder; history of or current arterial and cardiovascular disease (eg, MI, CVA); diabetes mellitus with vascular involvement; history of or current severe hepatic disease where liver function tests remain abnormal; history of or current hepatic neoplasia (benign or malignant); known or suspected sex-hormone-dependent malignancy; ocular lesions due to ophthalmic vascular disease, such as partial or complete vision loss or defect in visual fields; current or history of migraine with focal aura; breast-feeding; known or suspected pregnancy

Warnings/Precautions Use is associated with irregular menstrual bleeding (eg amenorrhea, infrequent or frequent bleeding, prolonged bleeding) and may be aggravated in some women (eg, those with fibroids). Bleeding patterns generally show a reduced intensity over time. If bleeding irregularities continue with prolonged use, appropriate diagnostic measures should be taken to rule out endometrial pathology (eg, endometrial sampling, pelvic ultrasound). Consider discontinuation of therapy with prolonged heavy bleeding. Pretreatment menstrual bleeding patterns return within 2 months of therapy discontinuation. The use of combination hormonal contraceptives has been associated with a slight increase in the frequency of breast cancer however studies are not consistent. Data is insufficient to determine if progestin only contraceptives also increase this risk. Routine breast examinations are recommended during therapy. Persistent ovarian cysts which are often asymptomatic may occur during therapy. Use is associated with a moderate decrease in endogenous estrogen levels; in a small study, a reduction in mean bone mineral density was not observed 6 months after initiating therapy though long term data are not available.

Use with caution in women with diabetes. Use with caution in patients with depression; discontinue use with onset of clinically relevant depression or with aggravation of pre-existing depression. Use is contraindicated in patients with a history of or current severe hepatic disease. Patients with a prior history of cholestatic jaundice during pregnancy or due to the use of sex steroids should discontinue use of dienogest if cholestatic jaundice reoccurs during therapy. Rare cases of benign and malignant hepatic tumors have been reported with use.

Progestin-only therapy has been associated with a slight but non-significant increase risk of VTE in some studies; discontinue therapy promptly with suspicion or symptoms of a thrombotic event. Discontinue use in patients with prolonged immobilization and at least 4 weeks prior to elective surgery; may resume therapy 2 weeks after complete remobilization. The risk of stroke may be increased in women with hypertension. Discontinue if clinically significant hypertension develops during therapy. The risk of cardiovascular side effects is increased in women who smoke cigarettes. Women should be advised not to smoke.

Progestin use has been associated with retinal vascular lesions; discontinue pending examination in case of sudden vision loss, complete loss of vision, sudden onset of proptosis, diplopia, or migraine. Chloasma may occur occasionally; women with a history of chloasma should avoid sun or ultraviolet radiation exposure during therapy. Patients with a prior history of pruritus during pregnancy or due to use of sex steroids should discontinue dienogest therapy if pruritus reoccurs during therapy. Not indicated for use prior to menarche or in the geriatric population. Not intended for use as a contraceptive.

Drug Interactions

Avoid Concomitant Use

Avoid concomitant use of Dienogest with any of the following: CYP3A4 Inducers (Strong); Griseofulvin

Decreased Effect

Dienogest may decrease the levels/effects of: Vitamin K Antagonists

The levels/effects of Dienogest may be decreased by: Acitretin; Aminoglutethimide; Aprepitant; Artemether; Barbiturates; Bexarotene; Bexarotene (Systemic); Bile Acid Sequestrants; Bosentan; CarBAMazepine; Clobazam; CYP3A4 Inducers (Strong); Deferasirox; Felbamate; Fosaprepitant; Fosphenytoin; Griseofulvin; LamoTRIgine; Mycophenolate; Nevirapine; OXcarbazepine; Phenytoin; Prucalopride; Retinoic Acid Derivatives; Rifamycin Derivatives; St Johns Wort; Telaprevir; Tocilizumab; Topiramate

Increased Effect/Toxicity

Dienogest may increase the levels/effects of: Benzodiazepines (metabolized by oxidation); Selegiline; Tranexamic Acid; Voriconazole

The levels/effects of Dienogest may be increased by: Boceprevir; CYP3A4 Inhibitors (Strong); Herbs (Progestogenic Properties); Voriconazole

Nutritional/Ethanol Interactions Herb/Nutraceutical: St John's wort may induce dienogest hepatic metabolism and decrease its systemic exposure.

Adverse Reactions 1% to 10%:

Central nervous system: Headache (7%), depression (3%), sleep disturbance (2%), irritability (1%), migraine (1%), nervousness (1%)

Dermatologic: Acne (2%), alopecia (1%)

Endocrine & metabolic: Breast discomfort (5%), ovarian cyst (3%), libido decreased (2%)

Gastrointestinal: Nausea (4%), weight gain (4%), abdominal pain (2%)

Genitourinary: Vaginal bleeding (1%)

Neuromuscular & skeletal: Weakness (2%)

Product Availability Not available in the U.S.

General Dosage Range Oral: *Adult females:* 2 mg once daily

Administration

Oral Administer without regard to meals. If a dose is not absorbed due to vomiting and/or diarrhea within 3-4 hours of administration, repeat dose.

Stability

Storage Store in original packaging at 15°C to 30°C (59°F to 86°F).

Nursing Actions

Physical Assessment

Monitor for possible side effects such as headache, depression, breast soreness, nausea, vomiting, and weight gain. If patient immobilized or having surgery, be sure to notify their prescriber or have them call their prescriber to discuss as medication should be temporarily stopped.

Patient Education

Take with or without food. May need to repeat dose if vomiting soon after taking. May cause headache, depression, breast soreness, nausea/vomiting, and weight gain. Report to prescriber if blood pressure increases, occurrence of ankle swelling or pain, depression, dark urine or yellow skin, or acute change in eyesight.

Diethylpropion (dye eth il PROE pee on)

Index Terms Amfepramone; Diethylpropion Hydrochloride

Pharmacologic Category Anorexiant; Sympathomimetic

Medication Safety Issues

BEERS Criteria medication:

This drug may be inappropriate for use in geriatric patients (high severity risk).

Pregnancy Risk Factor B

Lactation Enters breast milk/use caution

Use Short-term (few weeks) adjunct in the management of exogenous obesity

Pharmacotherapy for weight loss is recommended only for obese patients with a body mass index ≥30 kg/m², or ≥27 kg/m² in the presence of other risk factors such as hypertension, diabetes, and/or dyslipidemia or a high waist circumference; therapy should be used in conjunction with a comprehensive weight management program.

Controlled Substance C-IV

Available Dosage Forms

Tablet, oral: 25 mg

Tablet, controlled release, oral: 75 mg

General Dosage Range Oral:

Controlled release: *Children >16 years and Adults:* 75 mg at midmorning

Immediate release: *Children >16 years and Adults:* 25 mg 3 times/day

Administration

Oral Dose should not be administered in evening or at bedtime.

Tablet: Administer 1 hour before meals.

Tablet, controlled release: Do not crush tablet; administer at midmorning.

Nursing Actions

Physical Assessment Assess for history of psychopathology, homicidal or suicidal tendencies, or addiction; long-term use can result in dependence, abuse, or tolerance. Periodically evaluate the need for continued use. Monitor blood pressure and vital signs prior to treatment, when changing dosage, and at regular intervals during therapy. Monitor serum glucose closely in patients with diabetes (amphetamines may alter antidiabetic requirements). Taper dosage slowly when discontinuing.

Patient Education Drug may cause physical and/ or psychological dependence. Do not crush or chew extended release tablets. Take early in day to avoid sleep disturbance, 1 hour before meals. Avoid alcohol, caffeine, or OTC medications that act as stimulants. You may experience restlessness, euphoria, or impaired judgment; dry mouth; nausea or vomiting; constipation; diarrhea; or altered libido (reversible). Patients with diabetes need to monitor serum glucose closely (may alter antidiabetic medication requirements). Report chest pain, palpitations, or irregular heartbeat; muscle weakness or tremors; extreme fatigue or depression; CNS changes (aggressiveness, restlessness, euphoria, sleep disturbances); severe abdominal distress or cramping; changes in sexual activity; changes in urinary pattern; or blurred vision.

Difenoxin and Atropine

(dye fen OKS in & A troe peen)

Brand Names: U.S. Motofen®

Index Terms Atropine and Difenoxin

Pharmacologic Category Antidiarrheal

Pregnancy Risk Factor C

Lactation Enters breast milk/contraindicated

Use Treatment of diarrhea

Controlled Substance C-IV

Available Dosage Forms

Tablet, oral:

Motofen®: Difenoxin 1 mg and atropine 0.025 mg

General Dosage Range Oral: *Adults:* 2 tablets (each tablet contains difenoxin hydrochloride 1 mg and atropine sulfate 0.025 mg) initially, then 1 tablet after each loose stool (maximum: 8 tablets/ day)

Nursing Actions

Physical Assessment See individual agents.

Patient Education See individual agents.

Related Information

Atropine *on page 105*

Difluprednate (dye floo PRED nate)

Brand Names: U.S. Durezol®

Pharmacologic Category Corticosteroid, Ophthalmic

Medication Safety Issues

Sound-alike/look-alike issues:

Durezol® may be confused with Durasal™

Pregnancy Risk Factor C

Lactation Excretion in breast milk unknown/use caution

Use Treatment of inflammation and pain following ocular surgery

Available Dosage Forms

Emulsion, ophthalmic:

Durezol®: 0.05% (5 mL)

General Dosage Range Ophthalmic: *Adults:* Instill 1 drop in affected eye(s) 2-4 times/day

Nursing Actions

Patient Education Do not allow dropper to touch any surface of the eye to avoid contamination. If pain in eye, redness, or itching becomes aggravated, contact prescriber. Do not wear contact lens while using this medication.

Digoxin (di JOKS in)

Brand Names: U.S. Lanoxin®

Index Terms Digitalis

Pharmacologic Category Antiarrhythmic Agent, Miscellaneous; Cardiac Glycoside

Medication Safety Issues

Sound-alike/look-alike issues:

Digoxin may be confused with Desoxyn®, doxepin

Lanoxin® may be confused with Lasix®, levothyroxine, Levoxyl®, Levsinex®, Lomotil®, Mefoxin®, naloxone, Xanax®

High alert medication:

The Institute for Safe Medication Practices (ISMP) includes this medication among its list of drugs which have a heightened risk of causing significant patient harm when used in error.

BEERS Criteria medication:

This drug may be inappropriate for use in geriatric patients (low severity risk).

International issues:

Lanoxin [U.S., Canada, and multiple international markets] may be confused with Limoxin brand name for ambroxol [Indonesia] and amoxicillin [Mexico]

Pregnancy Risk Factor C

Lactation Enters breast milk/use caution (AAP rates "compatible"; AAP 2001 update pending)

Breast-Feeding Considerations Digoxin is excreted into breast milk and similar concentrations are found within mother's serum and milk. The manufacturer recommends that caution be used in nursing women.

Use Treatment of mild-to-moderate (or stage C as recommended by the ACCF/AHA) heart failure (HF); atrial fibrillation (rate-control)

Note: In treatment of atrial fibrillation (AF), use is not considered first-line unless AF coexistent with heart failure or in sedentary patients (Fuster, 2006).

Unlabeled Use Fetal tachycardia with or without hydrops; to slow ventricular rate in supraventricular tachyarrhythmias such as supraventricular tachycardia (SVT) excluding atrioventricular reciprocating tachycardia (AVRT)

Mechanism of Action/Effect

Heart failure: Inhibition of the sodium/potassium ATPase pump in myocardial cells results in a transient increase of intracellular sodium, which in turn promotes calcium influx via the sodium-calcium exchange pump leading to increased contractility.

Supraventricular arrhythmias: Direct suppression of the AV node conduction to increase effective refractory period and decrease conduction velocity - positive inotropic effect, enhanced vagal tone, and decreased ventricular rate to fast atrial arrhythmias. Atrial fibrillation may decrease sensitivity and increase tolerance to higher serum digoxin concentrations.

Contraindications Hypersensitivity to digoxin (rare) or other forms of digitalis, or any component of the formulation; ventricular fibrillation

Warnings/Precautions Watch for proarrhythmic effects (especially with digoxin toxicity). Withdrawal in clinically stable patients with HF may lead to recurrence of HF symptoms. During an episode of atrial fibrillation or flutter in patients with an accessory bypass tract (eg, Wolff-Parkinson-White syndrome), use has been associated with increased anterograde conduction down the accessory pathway leading to ventricular fibrillation; avoid use in such patients. Avoid use in patients with second- or third-degree heart block (except in patients with a functioning artificial pacemaker); incomplete AV block (eg, Stokes-Adams attack) may progress to complete block with digoxin administration. HF patients with preserved left ventricular function including patients with restrictive cardiomyopathy, constrictive pericarditis, and amyloid heart disease may be susceptible to digoxin toxicity; avoid use unless used to control ventricular response with atrial fibrillation. Digoxin should not be used in patients with low EF, sinus rhythm, and no HF symptoms since the risk of harm may be greater than clinical benefit. Avoid use in patients with hypertrophic cardiomyopathy (HCM) and outflow tract obstruction unless used to control ventricular response with atrial fibrillation; outflow obstruction may worsen due to the positive inotropic effects of digoxin.

Use with caution in patients with hyperthyroidism, hypothyroidism, recent acute MI (within 6 months), sinus nodal disease (eg, sick sinus syndrome). Reduce dose with renal impairment and when amiodarone, propafenone, quinidine, or verapamil are added to a patient on digoxin; use with caution in patients taking strong inducers or inhibitors of P-glycoprotein (eg, cyclosporine). Avoid rapid I.V. administration of calcium in digitalized patients; may produce serious arrhythmias.

Atrial arrhythmias associated with hypermetabolic states are very difficult to treat; treat underlying condition first; if digoxin is used, ensure digoxin toxicity does not occur. Patients with beri beri heart disease may fail to adequately respond to digoxin therapy; treat underlying thiamine deficiency concomitantly. Correct electrolyte disturbances, especially hypokalemia or hypomagnesemia, prior to use and throughout therapy; toxicity may occur despite therapeutic digoxin concentrations. Hypercalcemia may increase the risk of digoxin toxicity; maintain normocalcemia. It is not necessary to routinely reduce or hold digoxin therapy prior to elective electrical cardioversion for atrial fibrillation; however, exclusion of digoxin toxicity (eg, clinical and ECG signs) is necessary prior to cardioversion. If signs of digoxin excess exist, withhold digoxin and delay cardioversion until toxicity subsides; usually >24 hours. Use with caution in the elderly; may develop exaggerated serum/tissue concentrations due to age-related alterations in clearance and pharmacodynamics differences; dosage reduction may be necessary; in general, avoid doses >0.125 mg/day (Beers Criteria).

Drug Interactions

Avoid Concomitant Use There are no known interactions where it is recommended to avoid concomitant use.

Decreased Effect

Digoxin may decrease the levels/effects of: Antineoplastic Agents (Anthracycline, Systemic)

The levels/effects of Digoxin may be decreased by: 5-ASA Derivatives; Acarbose; Aminoglycosides; Antineoplastic Agents; Antineoplastic Agents (Anthracycline, Systemic); Bile Acid ▶

Sequestrants; Kaolin; PenicillAMINE; P-glycoprotein/ABCB1 Inducers; Potassium-Sparing Diuretics; St Johns Wort; Sucralfate; Tocilizumab

Increased Effect/Toxicity

Digoxin may increase the levels/effects of: Adenosine; Colchicine; Dronedarone; Midodrine

The levels/effects of Digoxin may be increased by: Aminoquinolines (Antimalarial); Amiodarone; Antithyroid Agents; Atorvastatin; Beta-Blockers; Boceprevir; Calcium Channel Blockers (Nondihydropyridine); Calcium Polystyrene Sulfonate; Carvedilol; Conivaptan; CycloSPORINE; CycloSPORINE (Systemic); Dronedarone; Etravirine; Glycopyrrolate; Itraconazole; Loop Diuretics; Macrolide Antibiotics; Milnacipran; Nefazodone; Neuromuscular-Blocking Agents; NIFEdipine; Nonsteroidal Anti-Inflammatory Agents; Paricalcitol; P-glycoprotein/ABCB1 Inhibitors; Posaconazole; Potassium-Sparing Diuretics; Propafenone; Protease Inhibitors; QuiNIDine; QuiNINE; Ranolazine; Reserpine; SitaGLIPtin; Sodium Polystyrene Sulfonate; Spironolactone; Telaprevir; Telmisartan; Ticagrelor; Tolvaptan; Vitamin D Analogs

Nutritional/Ethanol Interactions

Food: Digoxin peak serum concentrations may be decreased if taken with food. Meals containing increased fiber (bran) or foods high in pectin may decrease oral absorption of digoxin.

Herb/Nutraceutical: Avoid ephedra (risk of cardiac stimulation). Avoid natural licorice (causes sodium and water retention and increases potassium loss).

Adverse Reactions Incidence not always reported.

Cardiovascular: Accelerated junctional rhythm, asystole, atrial tachycardia with or without block, AV dissociation, first-, second- (Wenckebach), or third-degree heart block, facial edema, PR prolongation, PVCs (especially bigeminy or trigeminy), ST segment depression, ventricular tachycardia or ventricular fibrillation

Central nervous system: Dizziness (6%), mental disturbances (5%), headache (4%), apathy, anxiety, confusion, delirium, depression, fever, hallucinations

Dermatologic: Rash (erythematous, maculopapular [most common], papular, scarlatiniform, vesicular or bullous), pruritus, urticaria, angioneurotic edema

Gastrointestinal: Nausea (4%), vomiting (2%), diarrhea (4%), abdominal pain, anorexia

Neuromuscular & skeletal: Weakness

Ocular: Visual disturbances (blurred or yellow vision)

Respiratory: Laryngeal edema

Children are more likely to experience cardiac arrhythmia as a sign of excessive dosing. The most common are conduction disturbances or tachyarrhythmia (atrial tachycardia with or without block) and junctional tachycardia. Ventricular tachyarrhythmias are less common. In infants, sinus bradycardia may be a sign of digoxin toxicity. Any arrhythmia seen in a child on digoxin should be considered as digoxin toxicity. The gastrointestinal and central nervous system symptoms are not frequently seen in children.

Pharmacodynamics/Kinetics

Onset of Action

Heart rate control: Oral: 1-2 hours; I.V.: 5-60 minutes

Peak effect: Heart rate control: Oral: 2-8 hours; I.V.: 1-6 hours; **Note:** In patients with atrial fibrillation, median time to ventricular rate control in one study was 6 hours (range: 3-15 hours) (Siu, 2009)

Duration of Action Adults: 3-4 days

Available Dosage Forms

Injection, solution: 250 mcg/mL (1 mL, 2 mL)

Lanoxin®: 100 mcg/mL (1 mL); 250 mcg/mL (2 mL)

Solution, oral: 50 mcg/mL (2.5 mL, 5 mL, 60 mL)

Tablet, oral: 125 mcg, 250 mcg

Lanoxin®: 125 mcg, 250 mcg

General Dosage Range Dosage adjustment recommended in patients with renal impairment

I.M., I.V.:

Preterm infants: Digitalizing dose: 15-25 mcg/kg; Maintenance: 4-6 mcg/kg/day in divided doses every 12 hours

Full-term infants: Digitalizing dose: 20-30 mcg/kg; Maintenance: 5-8 mcg/kg/day in divided doses every 12 hours

Children 1 month to 2 years: Digitalizing dose: 30-50 mcg/kg; Maintenance: 7.5-12 mcg/kg/day in divided doses every 12 hours

Children 2-5 years: Digitalizing dose: 25-35 mcg/kg; Maintenance: 6-9 mcg/kg/day in divided doses every 12 hours

Children 5-10 years: Digitalizing dose: 15-30 mcg/kg; Maintenance: 4-8 mcg/kg/day in divided doses every 12 hours

Children >10 years: Digitalizing dose: 8-12 mcg/kg; Maintenance: 2-3 mcg/kg once daily

Adults: Digitalizing dose: 0.5-1 mg; Maintenance: 0.1-0.4 mg once daily

Oral:

Preterm infants: Digitalizing dose: 20-30 mcg/kg; Maintenance: 5-7.5 mcg/kg/day in divided doses every 12 hours

Full-term infants: Digitalizing dose: 25-35 mcg/kg; Maintenance: 6-10 mcg/kg/day in divided doses every 12 hours

Children 1 month to 2 years: Digitalizing dose: 35-60 mcg/kg; Maintenance: 10-15 mcg/kg/day in divided doses every 12 hours

Children 2-5 years: Digitalizing dose: 30-40 mcg/kg; Maintenance: 7.5-10 mcg/kg/day in divided doses every 12 hours

Children 5-10 years: Digitalizing dose: 20-35 mcg/kg; Maintenance: 5-10 mcg/kg/day in divided doses every 12 hours

Children >10 years: Digitalizing dose: 10-15 mcg/kg; Maintenance: 2.5-5 mcg/kg once daily

Adults: Digitalizing dose: 0.75-1.5 mg; Maintenance: 0.125-0.5 mg once daily

Administration

I.M. I.V. route preferred. If I.M. injection necessary, administer by deep injection followed by massage at the injection site. Inject no more than 2 mL per injection site. May cause intense pain.

I.V. May be administered undiluted or diluted fourfold in D_5W, NS, or SWFI for direct injection. Less than fourfold dilution may lead to drug precipitation. Inject slowly over ≥5 minutes

I.V. Detail pH: 6.8-7.2

Stability

Storage Store at 25°C (77°F); excursions permitted to 15°C to 30°C (59°F to 86°F). Protect elixir, injection, and tablets from light.

Nursing Actions

Physical Assessment Monitor laboratory tests when beginning or changing dosage, especially with I.V. administration. I.V.: Monitor ECG continuously. Oral: Monitor apical pulse before administering any dose. Teach patient to report noncardiac signs of toxicity (eg, anorexia, blurred vision, "yellow" vision, confusion).

Patient Education Maintain adequate dietary intake of potassium (do not increase without consulting prescriber). Adequate dietary potassium will reduce risk of digoxin toxicity. Take pulse at the same time each day; hold medication as directed by prescriber. Notify prescriber of acute changes in pulse. Report loss of appetite, nausea, vomiting, persistent diarrhea, swelling of extremities, palpitations, "yellowing" or blurred vision, mental confusion or depression, or unusual fatigue.

Dietary Considerations Maintain adequate amounts of potassium in diet to decrease risk of hypokalemia (hypokalemia may increase risk of digoxin toxicity).

Related Information

Management of Drug Extravasations *on page 1269*

Peak and Trough Guidelines *on page 1276*

Digoxin Immune Fab (di JOKS in i MYUN fab)

Brand Names: U.S. DigiFab®

Index Terms Antidigoxin Fab Fragments, Ovine

Pharmacologic Category Antidote

Pregnancy Risk Factor C

Lactation Excretion in breast milk unknown/use caution

Use Treatment of life-threatening or potentially life-threatening digoxin intoxication, including:

- acute digoxin ingestion (ie, >10 mg in adults; >0.1 mg/kg or >4 mg in children; ingestions resulting in serum concentrations >10 ng/mL)
- chronic ingestions leading to steady-state digoxin concentrations >6 ng/mL in adults or >4 ng/mL in children
- manifestations of digoxin toxicity due to overdose (eg, life-threatening ventricular arrhythmias, progressive bradycardia, second- or third-degree heart block not responsive to atropine, serum potassium >5.5 mEq/L in adults or >6 mEq/L in children)

Available Dosage Forms

Injection, powder for reconstitution:
DigiFab®: 40 mg

General Dosage Range I.V.:

Acute ingestion of known amount: *Children and Adults:* Digoxin Immune Fab Dose (vials) = Total body load (mg) / (0.5)

Based on steady-state digoxin concentration:

Infants and Children ≤20 kg: Digoxin Immune Fab Dose (mg) = [(serum digoxin concentration [ng/mL] x weight [kg]) / 100] x (digoxin immune Fab amount per vial [mg/vial])

Note: Digoxin immune Fab amount per vial: 40 mg/vial.

Children >20 kg and Adults: Digoxin Immune Fab Dose (vials) = (serum digoxin concentration [ng/mL] x weight [kg]) / 100

Amount ingested and blood level unknown:

Children ≤20 kg: Acute toxicity: 20 vials total in 2 divided doses; Chronic toxicity: 1 vial may be sufficient

Children >20 kg and Adults: Acute toxicity: 20 vials total in 2 divided doses; Chronic toxicity: 6 vials

Administration

I.V. I.V. infusion over at least 30 minutes is preferred. May also be given by bolus injection if cardiac arrest is imminent (infusion-related reaction may occur). Small doses (eg, those required in infants or small children) may be administered using a tuberculin syringe as undiluted digoxin immune Fab or diluted with NS to a concentration of 1 mg/mL digoxin immune Fab. Stopping the infusion and restarting at a slower rate may help if an infusion-related reaction occurs.

Nursing Actions

Physical Assessment Assess allergy history prior to administration. Monitor lab values, cardiac status, vital signs, and blood pressure during and following infusion. Monitor for signs of reoccurrence of cardiac toxicity.

Patient Education Immediately report dizziness, palpitations, cramping, respiratory difficulty, rash, or itching.

Dihydrocodeine, Aspirin, and Caffeine (dye hye droe KOE deen, AS pir in, & KAF een)

Brand Names: U.S. Synalgos®-DC

Index Terms Dihydrocodeine Compound

Pharmacologic Category Analgesic, Opioid

Medication Safety Issues

Sound-alike/look-alike issues:

Synalgos®-DC may be confused with Synagis®

High alert medication:

The Institute for Safe Medication Practices (ISMP) includes this medication among its list of drug classes which have a heightened risk of causing significant patient harm when used in error.

Pregnancy Risk Factor B/D (prolonged use or high doses at term)

Lactation Excretion in breast milk unknown/use caution

Use Management of mild-to-moderate pain that requires relaxation

Controlled Substance C-III

Available Dosage Forms

Capsule, oral:

Synalgos®-DC: Dihydrocodeine 16 mg, aspirin 356.4 mg, and caffeine 30 mg

General Dosage Range Oral: *Adults:* 1-2 capsules every 4-6 hours as needed

Nursing Actions

Physical Assessment See individual agents.

Patient Education See individual agents.

Related Information

Aspirin *on page 94*

Caffeine *on page 169*

Dihydroergotamine (dye hye droe er GOT a meen)

Brand Names: U.S. D.H.E. 45®; Migranal®

Index Terms DHE; Dihydroergotamine Mesylate

Pharmacologic Category Antimigraine Agent; Ergot Derivative

Pregnancy Risk Factor X

Lactation Enters breast milk/contraindicated

Use Treatment of migraine headache with or without aura; injection also indicated for treatment of cluster headaches

Unlabeled Use Adjunct for DVT prophylaxis for hip surgery, for orthostatic hypotension, xerostomia secondary to antidepressant use, and pelvic congestion with pain

Available Dosage Forms

Injection, solution: 1 mg/mL (1 mL)

D.H.E. 45®: 1 mg/mL (1 mL)

Solution, intranasal:

Migranal®: 4 mg/mL (1 mL)

General Dosage Range

I.M., SubQ: *Adults:* 1 mg initially, may repeat hourly up to 3 mg total (maximum: 6 mg/week)

I.V.: *Adults:* 1 mg initially, may repeat hourly up to 2 mg total (maximum: 6 mg/week)

Intranasal: *Adults:* 1 spray (0.5 mg) in each nostril initially, may repeat after 15 minutes up to 4 sprays total (maximum: 6 sprays/24 hours; 8 sprays/week)

Administration

I.M. May administer by intramuscular injection.

I.V. Administer slowly over 2-3 minutes (Raskin protocol)

Other

Intranasal: Prior to administration of nasal spray, the nasal spray applicator must be primed (pumped 4 times); in order to let the drug be absorbed through the skin in the nose, patients should not inhale deeply through the nose while spraying or immediately after spraying; for best results, treatment should be initiated at the first symptom or sign of an attack; however, nasal spray can be used at any stage of a migraine attack

SubQ: May administer by subcutaneous injection.

Nursing Actions

Physical Assessment Monitor for hypertension and cardiac events. Teach patient proper use (treatment of acute migraine). Teach patient proper storage, administration, injection technique, and syringe/needle disposal.

Patient Education Take this drug as rapidly as possible when first headache symptoms occur. May cause drowsiness or feelings of numbness or tingling of fingers, toes, or face. Report heart palpitations, severe nausea or vomiting, and severe numbness of fingers or toes.

Diltiazem (dil TYE a zem)

Brand Names: U.S. Cardizem®; Cardizem® CD; Cardizem® LA; Cartia XT®; Dilacor XR®; Dilt-CD; Dilt-XR; Diltia XT®; Diltzac; Matzim™ LA; Taztia XT®; Tiazac®

Index Terms Diltiazem Hydrochloride

Pharmacologic Category Antianginal Agent; Antiarrhythmic Agent, Class IV; Calcium Channel Blocker; Calcium Channel Blocker, Nondihydropyridine

Medication Safety Issues

Sound-alike/look-alike issues:

Cardizem® may be confused with Cardene®, Cardene SR®, Cardizem CD®, Cardizem SR®, cortisone

Cartia XT® may be confused with Procardia XL®

Diltiazem may be confused with Calan®, diazepam, Dilantin®

Tiazac® may be confused with Tigan®, Tiazac® XC [CAN], Ziac®

High alert medication:

The Institute for Safe Medication Practices (ISMP) includes this medication (I.V. formulation) among its list of drug classes which have a heightened risk of causing significant patient harm when used in error.

Administration issues:

Significant differences exist between oral and I.V. dosing. Use caution when converting from one route of administration to another.

International issues:

Cardizem [U.S., Canada, and multiple international markets] may be confused with Cardem brand name for celiprolol [Spain]

Cartia XT [U.S.] may be confused with Cartia brand name for aspirin [multiple international markets]

Dilacor XR [U.S.] may be confused with Dilacor brand name for verapamil [Brazil]

Dipen [Greece] may be confused with Depen brand name for penicillamine [U.S.]; Depin brand name for nifedipine [India]; Depon brand name for acetaminophen [Greece]

Tiazac: Brand name for diltiazem [U.S, Canada], but also the brand name for pioglitazone [Chile]

Pregnancy Risk Factor C

Lactation Enters breast milk/not recommended (AAP considers "compatible"; AAP 2001 update pending)

Breast-Feeding Considerations Diltiazem is excreted into breastmilk in concentrations similar to those in the maternal plasma.

Use

Oral: Essential hypertension; chronic stable angina or angina from coronary artery spasm

Injection: Control of rapid ventricular rate in patients with atrial fibrillation or atrial flutter; conversion of paroxysmal supraventricular tachycardia (PSVT)

Unlabeled Use

ACLS guidelines: Injection: Stable narrow-complex tachycardia uncontrolled or unconverted by adenosine or vagal maneuvers or if SVT is recurrent

Pediatric hypertension

Mechanism of Action/Effect Nondihydropyridine calcium channel blocker which inhibits calcium ion from entering the "slow channels" or select voltage-sensitive areas of vascular smooth muscle and myocardium during depolarization, producing a relaxation of coronary vascular smooth muscle and coronary vasodilation; increases myocardial oxygen delivery in patients with vasospastic angina

Contraindications

Oral: Hypersensitivity to diltiazem or any component of the formulation; sick sinus syndrome (except in patients with a functioning artificial pacemaker); second- or third-degree AV block (except in patients with a functioning artificial pacemaker); severe hypotension (systolic <90 mm Hg); acute MI and pulmonary congestion

Intravenous (I.V.): Hypersensitivity to diltiazem or any component of the formulation; sick sinus syndrome (except in patients with a functioning artificial pacemaker); second- or third-degree AV block (except in patients with a functioning artificial pacemaker); severe hypotension (systolic <90 mm Hg); cardiogenic shock; administration concomitantly or within a few hours of the administration of I.V. beta-blockers; atrial fibrillation or flutter associated with accessory bypass tract (eg, Wolff-Parkinson-White syndrome); ventricular tachycardia (with wide-complex tachycardia, must determine whether origin is supraventricular or ventricular)

Canadian labeling: Additional contraindications (not in U.S. labeling): I.V. and Oral: Pregnancy; use in women of childbearing potential

Warnings/Precautions Can cause first-, second-, and third-degree AV block or sinus bradycardia and risk increases with agents known to slow cardiac conduction. The most common side effect is peripheral edema; occurs within 2-3 weeks of starting therapy. Symptomatic hypotension with or without syncope can rarely occur; blood pressure must be lowered at a rate appropriate for the patient's clinical condition. Use caution when using diltiazem together with a beta-blocker; may result in conduction disturbances, hypotension, and worsened LV function. Simultaneous administration of I.V. diltiazem and an I.V. beta-blocker or administration within a few hours of each other may result in asystole and is contraindicated. Use with other agents known to either reduce SA node function and/or AV nodal conduction (eg, digoxin) or reduce sympathetic outflow (eg, clonidine) may increase the risk of serious bradycardia. Use caution in left ventricular dysfunction (may exacerbate condition). Avoid use of diltiazem in patients with heart failure and reduced ejection fraction (Hunt, 2009). Use with caution with hypertrophic obstructive cardiomyopathy; routine use is currently not recommended due to insufficient evidence (Maron, 2003). Use with caution in hepatic or renal dysfunction. Transient dermatologic reactions have been observed with use; if reaction persists, discontinue. May (rarely) progress to erythema multiforme or exfoliative dermatitis.

Drug Interactions

Avoid Concomitant Use

Avoid concomitant use of Diltiazem with any of the following: Conivaptan; Pimozide; Tolvaptan

Decreased Effect

Diltiazem may decrease the levels/effects of: Clopidogrel

The levels/effects of Diltiazem may be decreased by: Barbiturates; Calcium Salts; CarBAMazepine; Colestipol; CYP3A4 Inducers (Strong); Deferasirox; Herbs (Hypertensive Properties); Methylphenidate; Nafcillin; Peginterferon Alfa-2b; P-glycoprotein/ABCB1 Inducers; Rifamycin Derivatives; Tocilizumab; Yohimbine

Increased Effect/Toxicity

Diltiazem may increase the levels/effects of: Alfentanil; Amifostine; Amiodarone; Antihypertensives; Aprepitant; ARIPiprazole; Atorvastatin;

Benzodiazepines (metabolized by oxidation); Beta-Blockers; Budesonide (Systemic, Oral Inhalation); BusPIRone; Calcium Channel Blockers (Dihydropyridine); CarBAMazepine; Cardiac Glycosides; Colchicine; Corticosteroids (Systemic); CycloSPORINE; CycloSPORINE (Systemic); CYP3A4 Substrates; Dronedarone; Eletriptan; Eplerenone; Everolimus; Fingolimod; Fosaprepitant; Fosphenytoin; Halofantrine; Hypotensive Agents; Lithium; Lovastatin; Lurasidone; Magnesium Salts; Midodrine; Neuromuscular-Blocking Agents (Nondepolarizing); Nitroprusside; Phenytoin; Pimecrolimus; Pimozide; Propafenone; QuiNIDine; Ranolazine; Red Yeast Rice; RiTUXimab; Rivaroxaban; Salicylates; Salmeterol; Saxagliptin; Simvastatin; Tacrolimus; Tacrolimus (Systemic); Tacrolimus (Topical); Tolvaptan; Vilazodone; Zuclopenthixol

The levels/effects of Diltiazem may be increased by: Alpha1-Blockers; Anilidopiperidine Opioids; Antifungal Agents (Azole Derivatives, Systemic); Aprepitant; Atorvastatin; Calcium Channel Blockers (Dihydropyridine); Cimetidine; Conivaptan; CycloSPORINE; CycloSPORINE (Systemic); CYP3A4 Inhibitors (Moderate); CYP3A4 Inhibitors (Strong); Dasatinib; Diazoxide; Dronedarone; Fluconazole; Fosaprepitant; Grapefruit Juice; Herbs (Hypotensive Properties); Lovastatin; Macrolide Antibiotics; Magnesium Salts; MAO Inhibitors; Pentoxifylline; P-glycoprotein/ABCB1 Inhibitors; Phosphodiesterase 5 Inhibitors; Prostacyclin Analogues; Protease Inhibitors; Simvastatin

Nutritional/Ethanol Interactions

Ethanol: Ethanol may increase risk of hypotension or vasodilation. Management: Avoid ethanol.

Food: Diltiazem serum levels may be elevated if taken with food. Serum concentrations were not altered by grapefruit juice in small clinical trials.

Herb/Nutraceutical: St John's wort may decrease diltiazem levels. Some herbal medications may worsen hypertension (eg, licorice); others may increase the antihypertensive effect of diltiazem (eg, shepherd's purse). Management: Avoid St John's wort, bayberry, blue cohosh, cayenne, ephedra, ginger, ginseng (American), kola, licorice, and yohimbe. Avoid black cohosh, California poppy, coleus, golden seal, hawthorn, mistletoe, periwinkle, quinine, and shepherd's purse.

Adverse Reactions Note: Frequencies represent ranges for various dosage forms. Patients with impaired ventricular function and/or conduction abnormalities may have higher incidence of adverse reactions.

>10%:

Cardiovascular: Edema (2% to 15%)

Central nervous system: Headache (5% to 12%)

2% to 10%:

Cardiovascular: AV block (first degree 2% to 8%), edema (lower limb 2% to 8%), pain (6%), bradycardia (2% to 6%), hypotension (<2% to 4%), vasodilation (2% to 3%), extrasystoles (2%), flushing (1% to 2%), palpitation (1% to 2%)

Central nervous system: Dizziness (3% to 10%), nervousness (2%)

Dermatologic: Rash (1% to 4%)

Endocrine & metabolic: Gout (1% to 2%)

Gastrointestinal: Dyspepsia (1% to 6%), constipation (<2% to 4%), vomiting (2%), diarrhea (1% to 2%)

Local: Injection site reactions: Burning, itching (4%)

Neuromuscular & skeletal: Weakness (1% to 4%), myalgia (2%)

Respiratory: Rhinitis (<2% to 10%), pharyngitis (2% to 6%), dyspnea (1% to 6%), bronchitis (1% to 4%), cough (≤3), sinus congestion (1% to 2%)

Pharmacodynamics/Kinetics

Onset of Action Oral: Immediate release tablet: 30-60 minutes; I.V.: 3 minutes

Duration of Action I.V.: Bolus: 1-3 hours; Continuous infusion (after discontinuation): 0.5-10 hours

Available Dosage Forms

Capsule, extended release, oral: 60 mg, 90 mg, 120 mg, 180 mg, 240 mg, 300 mg, 360 mg, 420 mg

Cardizem® CD: 120 mg, 180 mg, 240 mg, 300 mg, 360 mg

Cartia XT®: 120 mg, 180 mg, 240 mg, 300 mg

Dilacor XR®: 240 mg

Dilt-CD: 120 mg, 180 mg, 240 mg, 300 mg

Dilt-XR: 120 mg, 180 mg, 240 mg

Diltia XT®: 120 mg, 180 mg, 240 mg

Diltzac: 120 mg, 180 mg, 240 mg, 300 mg, 360 mg

Taztia XT®: 120 mg, 180 mg, 240 mg, 300 mg, 360 mg

Tiazac®: 120 mg, 180 mg, 240 mg, 300 mg, 360 mg, 420 mg

Injection, powder for reconstitution: 100 mg

Injection, solution: 5 mg/mL (5 mL, 10 mL, 25 mL)

Tablet, oral: 30 mg, 60 mg, 90 mg, 120 mg

Cardizem®: 30 mg, 60 mg, 90 mg, 120 mg

Tablet, extended release, oral:

Cardizem® LA: 120 mg, 180 mg, 240 mg, 300 mg, 360 mg, 420 mg

Matzim™ LA: 180 mg, 240 mg, 300 mg, 360 mg, 420 mg

General Dosage Range

I.V.: *Adults:* Bolus: 0.25 mg/kg, may repeat 0.35 mg/kg after 15 minutes; Infusion: 5-15 mg/hour

Oral:

Extended release: *Adults:* Initial: 120-240 mg once daily **or** 60-120 mg twice daily; Maintenance: 120-540 mg once daily **or** 240-360 mg/day in 2 divided doses

Immediate release: *Adults:* Initial: 30 mg 4 times/day; Maintenance: 120-320 mg/day in divided doses

Administration

Oral

Immediate release tablet (Cardizem®): Administer before meals and at bedtime.

Long acting dosage forms: Do not open, chew, or crush; swallow whole.

Cardizem® CD, Cardizem® LA, Cartia XT®, Dilt-CD,Matzim™ LA: May be administered without regards to meals.

Dilacor XR®, Dilt-XR, Diltia XT®: Administer on an empty stomach.

Taztia XT™, Tiazac®: Capsules may be opened and sprinkled on a spoonful of applesauce. Applesauce should not be hot and should be swallowed without chewing, followed by drinking a glass of water.

Tiazac® XC [CAN; not available in U.S.]: Administer at bedtime

I.V. Bolus doses given over 2 minutes with continuous ECG and blood pressure monitoring. Continuous infusion should be via infusion pump.

I.V. Detail Response to bolus may require several minutes to reach maximum. Response may persist for several hours after infusion is discontinued.

pH: 3.7-4.1

Stability

Storage

Capsule, tablet: Store at room temperature. Protect from light.

Solution for injection: Store in refrigerator at 2°C to 8°C (36°F to 46°F); do not freeze. May be stored at room temperature for up to 1 month. Following dilution to ≤1 mg/mL with $D_5$1/2NS, D_5W, or NS, solution is stable for 24 hours at room temperature or under refrigeration.

Nursing Actions

Physical Assessment Assess potential for interactions with other agents that may cause increased risk of bradycardia, conduction delays, or decreased cardiac output. I.V. requires use of infusion pump and continuous cardiac and hemodynamic monitoring. Monitor therapeutic effectiveness according to use (hypertension, angina, atrial fib/flutter, or PSVT).

Patient Education Oral: Do not crush or chew extended release form. Avoid or limit alcohol and caffeine. May cause dizziness or lightheadedness, nausea, vomiting, or constipation. Report chest pain, palpitations, or irregular heartbeat; persistent diarrhea; unusual cough or respiratory difficulty; swelling of extremities; muscle tremors or weakness; confusion or acute lethargy; or skin rash.

Dinoprostone (dye noe PROST one)

Brand Names: U.S. Cervidil®; Prepidil®; Prostin E2®

Index Terms PGE_2; Prostaglandin E_2

Pharmacologic Category Abortifacient; Prostaglandin

Medication Safety Issues

International issues:

Cervidil brand name for dinoprostone [U.S., Canada, Australia, New Zealand], but also the brand name for gemeprost [Italy]

Pregnancy Risk Factor C

Lactation Excretion in breast milk unknown

Use

Endocervical gel: Promote cervical ripening in patients at or near term in whom there is a medical or obstetrical indication for the induction of labor

Suppositories: Terminate pregnancy from 12th through 20th week of gestation; evacuate uterus in cases of missed abortion or intrauterine fetal death up to 28 weeks of gestation; manage benign hydatidiform mole (nonmetastatic gestational trophoblastic disease)

Vaginal insert: Initiation and/or continuation of cervical ripening in patients at or near term in whom there is a medical or obstetrical indication for the induction of labor

Available Dosage Forms

Gel, endocervical:

Prepidil®: 0.5 mg/3 g (3 g)

Insert, vaginal:

Cervidil®: 10 mg (1s)

Suppository, vaginal:

Prostin E2®: 20 mg (5s)

General Dosage Range

Endocervical: *Children (females of reproductive age) and Adults (females):* 0.5 mg; may repeat every 6 hours if needed. Maximum cumulative dose: 1.5 mg/24 hours

Intravaginal: *Children (females of reproductive age) and Adults (females):* Insert: 10 mg; remove at onset of active labor or after 12 hours; Suppository: 20 mg every 3-5 hours until abortion occurs

Administration

Other

Endocervical gel: Bring to room temperature just prior to use. Do not force the warming process (eg, water bath, microwave). Avoid contact with skin while handling; wash hands thoroughly with soap and water after administration. For cervical ripening, patient should be supine in the dorsal position. The appropriate catheter length should be based on degree of effacement; 20 mm for no effacement; 10 mm if 50% effaced. Patient should remain supine for 15-30 minutes following administration. The manufacturer recommends waiting 6-12 hours after dinoprostone gel administration before initiating oxytocin.

Vaginal insert: One vaginal insert is placed transversely in the posterior fornix of the vagina immediately after removal from its foil package. Patients should remain in the recumbent position for 2 hours after insertion, but thereafter may be ambulatory. Do not use without retrieval system. Product does not need warmed prior to use. A water miscible lubricant may be used to facilitate insertion (avoid excessive use of lubricant). Ensure complete removal of system at completion of therapy. The manufacturer recommends waiting ≥30 minutes after removing the dinoprostone vaginal insert before initiating oxytocin.

Vaginal suppository: Insert high into vagina after removal from its foil package. Bring to room temperature just prior to use. Patient should remain supine for 10 minutes following insertion.

Nursing Actions

Physical Assessment Monitor temperature closely. Monitor uterine tone and vaginal discharge closely throughout procedure and postprocedure. Monitor abortion for completeness (other measures may be necessary if incomplete).

Patient Education Nausea and vomiting, cramping or uterine pain, or fever may occur. Report acute pain, respiratory difficulty, or skin rash. Closely monitor for vaginal discharge for several days. Report heavy vaginal bleeding, itching, malodorous or bloody discharge, or severe cramping.

DiphenhydrAMINE (Systemic)

(dye fen HYE dra meen)

Brand Names: U.S. Aler-Cap [OTC]; Aler-Dryl [OTC]; Aler-Tab [OTC]; AllerMax® [OTC]; Altaryl [OTC]; Anti-Hist [OTC]; Banophen™ [OTC]; Benadryl® Allergy Quick Dissolve [OTC]; Benadryl® Allergy [OTC]; Benadryl® Children's Allergy FastMelt® [OTC]; Benadryl® Children's Allergy Perfect Measure™ [OTC]; Benadryl® Children's Allergy [OTC]; Benadryl® Children's Dye Free Allergy [OTC]; Benadryl® Dye-Free Allergy [OTC]; Compoz® [OTC]; Diphen [OTC]; Diphenhist® [OTC]; Geri-Dryl; Histaprin [OTC]; Nytol® Quick Caps [OTC]; Nytol® Quick Gels [OTC]; PediaCare® Children's Allergy [OTC]; PediaCare® Children's NightTime Cough [OTC]; Siladryl Allergy [OTC]; Silphen [OTC]; Simply Sleep® [OTC]; Sleep-ettes D [OTC]; Sleep-Tabs [OTC]; Sleepinal® [OTC]; Sominex® Maximum Strength [OTC]; Sominex® [OTC]; Theraflu® Thin Strips® Multi Symptom [OTC]; Triaminic Thin Strips® Children's Cough & Runny Nose [OTC]; Twilite® [OTC]; Unisom® SleepGels® Maximum Strength [OTC]; Unisom® SleepMelts™ [OTC]

Index Terms Diphenhydramine Citrate; Diphenhydramine Hydrochloride; Diphenhydramine Tannate

Pharmacologic Category Ethanolamine Derivative; Histamine H_1 Antagonist; Histamine H_1 Antagonist, First Generation

Medication Safety Issues

Sound-alike/look-alike issues:

DiphenhydrAMINE may be confused with desipramine, dicyclomine, dimenhyDRINATE

Benadryl® may be confused with benazepril, Bentyl®, Benylin®, Caladryl®

BEERS Criteria medication:

This drug may be inappropriate for use in geriatric patients (high severity risk).

International issues:

Sominex brand name for diphenhydramine [U.S., Canada], but also the brand name for promethazine [Great Britain]; valerian [Chile]

Pregnancy Risk Factor B

Lactation Enters breast milk/contraindicated

Breast-Feeding Considerations Infants may be more sensitive to the effects of antihistamines. Use while breast-feeding is contraindicated by the manufacturer.

Use Symptomatic relief of allergic symptoms caused by histamine release including nasal allergies and allergic dermatosis; adjunct to epinephrine in the treatment of anaphylaxis; nighttime sleep aid; prevention or treatment of motion sickness; antitussive; management of Parkinsonian syndrome including drug-induced extrapyramidal symptoms

Mechanism of Action/Effect Competes with histamine for H_1-receptor sites on effector cells in the gastrointestinal tract, blood vessels, and respiratory tract; anticholinergic and sedative effects are also seen

Contraindications Hypersensitivity to diphenhydramine or any component of the formulation; acute asthma; neonates or premature infants; breast-feeding; use as a local anesthetic (injection)

Warnings/Precautions Causes sedation, caution must be used in performing tasks which require alertness (eg, operating machinery or driving). Sedative effects of CNS depressants or ethanol are potentiated. Should not be used as a hypnotic in the elderly; may cause excessive sedation and confusion; may be inappropriate in this age group when used as an antihistamine due to potent anticholinergic effects (nonanticholinergic antihistamines preferred); when used for emergency allergic reactions, use the smallest effective dose (Beers Criteria). Antihistamines may cause excitation in young children. Use with caution in patients with angle-closure glaucoma, pyloroduodenal obstruction (including stenotic peptic ulcer), urinary tract obstruction (including bladder neck obstruction and symptomatic prostatic hyperplasia), asthma, hyperthyroidism, increased intraocular pressure, and cardiovascular disease (including hypertension and tachycardia). Some preparations contain soy protein; avoid use in patients with soy protein or peanut allergies. Some products may contain phenylalanine.

Self-medication (OTC use): Do not use with other products containing diphenhydramine, even ones used on the skin. Oral products are not for OTC use in children <6 years of age.

Drug Interactions

Avoid Concomitant Use

Avoid concomitant use of DiphenhydrAMINE (Systemic) with any of the following: Thioridazine

Decreased Effect

DiphenhydrAMINE (Systemic) may decrease the levels/effects of: Acetylcholinesterase Inhibitors (Central); Benzylpenicilloyl Polylysine; Betahistine; Codeine; TraMADol

The levels/effects of DiphenhydrAMINE (Systemic) may be decreased by: Acetylcholinesterase Inhibitors (Central); Amphetamines

Increased Effect/Toxicity

DiphenhydrAMINE (Systemic) may increase the levels/effects of: Alcohol (Ethyl); Anticholinergics; ARIPiprazole; CNS Depressants; CYP2D6 Substrates; Fesoterodine; Methotrimeprazine; Nebivolol; Selective Serotonin Reuptake Inhibitors; Tamoxifen; Thioridazine

The levels/effects of DiphenhydrAMINE (Systemic) may be increased by: Droperidol; HydrOXYzine; Methotrimeprazine; Pramlintide; Propafenone

Nutritional/Ethanol Interactions

Ethanol: May increase CNS depression; monitor for increased effects with coadministration. Caution patients about effects.

Herb/Nutraceutical: Avoid valerian, St John's wort, kava kava, gotu kola (may increase CNS depression).

Adverse Reactions Frequency not defined.

Cardiovascular: Chest tightness, extrasystoles, hypotension, palpitation, tachycardia

Central nervous system: Chills, confusion, convulsion, disturbed coordination, dizziness, euphoria, excitation, fatigue, headache, insomnia, irritability, nervousness, paradoxical excitement, restlessness, sedation, sleepiness, vertigo

Endocrine & metabolic: Menstrual irregularities (early menses)

Gastrointestinal: Anorexia, constipation, diarrhea, dry mucous membranes, epigastric distress, nausea, throat tightness, vomiting, xerostomia

Genitourinary: Difficult urination, urinary frequency, urinary retention

Hematologic: Agranulocytosis, hemolytic anemia, thrombocytopenia

Neuromuscular & skeletal: Neuritis, paresthesia, tremor

Ocular: Blurred vision, diplopia

Otic: Labyrinthitis (acute), tinnitus

Respiratory: Nasal stuffiness, thickening of bronchial secretions, wheezing

Miscellaneous: Anaphylactic shock, diaphoresis

Pharmacodynamics/Kinetics

Duration of Action

Histamine-induced wheel suppression: ≤10 hours (Simons, 1990)

Histamine-induced flare suppression: ≤12 hours (Simons, 1990)

Available Dosage Forms

Caplet, oral:

Aler-Dryl [OTC]: 50 mg
AllerMax® [OTC]: 50 mg
Anti-Hist [OTC]: 25 mg
Compoz® [OTC]: 50 mg
Histaprin [OTC]: 25 mg
Nytol® Quick Caps [OTC]: 25 mg
Simply Sleep® [OTC]: 25 mg
Sleep-ettes D [OTC]: 50 mg
Sominex® Maximum Strength [OTC]: 50 mg
Twilite® [OTC]: 50 mg

Capsule, oral: 25 mg, 50 mg

Aler-Cap [OTC]: 25 mg
Banophen™ [OTC]: 25 mg
Benadryl® Allergy [OTC]: 25 mg
Diphen [OTC]: 25 mg
Diphenhist® [OTC]: 25 mg
Sleepinal® [OTC]: 50 mg

Capsule, liquid gel, oral: 25 mg

Capsule, softgel, oral:

Benadryl® Dye-Free Allergy [OTC]: 25 mg
Compoz® [OTC]: 50 mg
Nytol® Quick Gels [OTC]: 50 mg
Unisom® SleepGels® Maximum Strength [OTC]: 50 mg

Captab, oral:

Diphenhist® [OTC]: 25 mg

Elixir, oral:

Altaryl [OTC]: 12.5 mg/5 mL (480 mL, 3840 mL)
Banophen™ [OTC]: 12.5 mg/5 mL (120 mL, 480 mL)

Injection, solution: 50 mg/mL (1 mL, 10 mL)

Injection, solution [preservative free]: 50 mg/mL (1 mL)

Liquid, oral:

AllerMax® [OTC]: 12.5 mg/5 mL (120 mL)
Benadryl® Children's Allergy [OTC]: 12.5 mg/5 mL (118 mL, 236 mL)
Benadryl® Children's Allergy Perfect Measure™ [OTC]: 12.5 mg/5 mL (5 mL)
Benadryl® Children's Dye Free Allergy [OTC]: 12.5 mg/5 mL (118 mL)
Siladryl Allergy [OTC]: 12.5 mg/5 mL (118 mL, 237 mL, 473 mL)

Solution, oral: 12.5 mg/5 mL (5 mL, 10 mL, 20 mL)

Diphenhist® [OTC]: 12.5 mg/5 mL (120 mL, 480 mL)

Strip, orally disintegrating, oral:

Benadryl® Allergy Quick Dissolve [OTC]: 25 mg (10s)

Theraflu® Thin Strips® Multi Symptom [OTC]: 25 mg (12s, 24s)
Triaminic Thin Strips® Children's Cough & Runny Nose [OTC]: 12.5 mg (14s)

Syrup, oral:
PediaCare® Children's Allergy [OTC]: 12.5 mg/5 mL (118 mL)
PediaCare® Children's NightTime Cough [OTC]: 12.5 mg/5 mL (118 mL)
Silphen [OTC]: 12.5 mg/5 mL (118 mL, 237 mL, 473 mL)

Tablet, oral: 25 mg, 50 mg
Aler-Tab [OTC]: 25 mg
Banophen™ [OTC]: 25 mg
Benadryl® Allergy [OTC]: 25 mg
Geri-Dryl: 25 mg
Sleep-Tabs [OTC]: 25 mg
Sominex® [OTC]: 25 mg

Tablet, orally dissolving, oral:
Benadryl® Children's Allergy FastMelt® [OTC]: 12.5 mg
Unisom® SleepMelts™ [OTC]: 25 mg

General Dosage Range

I.M., I.V.:
Children: 5 mg/kg/day **or** 150 mg/m²/day in divided every 6-8 hours (maximum: 300 mg/day)
Adults: 10-100 per dose (maximum: 400 mg/day)
Elderly: Initial: 25 mg 2-3 times/day

Oral:
Children 2 to <6 years: 5 mg/kg/day **or** 150 mg/m²/day in divided every 6-8 hours (maximum: 300 mg/day) **or** 6.25 mg every 4-6 hours (maximum: 37.5 mg/day)
Children 6 to <12 years: 5 mg/kg/day **or** 150 mg/m²/day in divided every 6-8 hours (maximum: 300 mg/day) **or** 12.5-25 mg every 4-6 hours (maximum: 150 mg/day)
Children ≥12 years: 5 mg/kg/day **or** 150 mg/m²/day in divided doses every 6-8 hours **or** 25-50 mg every 4-6 hours (maximum: 300 mg/day) **or** 50 mg at bedtime
Adults: 25-50 mg every 4-6 hours (maximum: 400 mg/day) **or** 50 mg at bedtime
Elderly: Initial: 25 mg 2-3 times/day

Administration

Oral When used to prevent motion sickness, first dose should be given 30 minutes prior to exposure.

I.V. Injection solution: For I.V. or I.M. administration only. Local necrosis may result with SubQ or intradermal use. For I.V. administration, inject at a rate ≤25 mg/minute.

I.V. Detail pH: 5-6

Stability

Storage Injection: Store at room temperature of 15°C to 30°C (59°F to 86°F); protect from freezing. Protect from light.

Nursing Actions

Physical Assessment Monitor for excess anticholinergic effects at beginning of therapy and periodically throughout.

Patient Education Avoid use of alcohol. You may experience drowsiness, dizziness, dry mouth, nausea, or vomiting. Report persistent sedation, confusion, agitation, blurred vision, respiratory difficulty, lack of improvement, or worsening of condition.

Dietary Considerations Some products may contain sodium and/or phenylalanine.

DiphenhydrAMINE (Topical)

(dye fen HYE dra meen)

Brand Names: U.S. Banophen™ Anti-Itch [OTC]; Benadryl® Extra Strength Itch Stopping [OTC]; Benadryl® Itch Relief Extra Strength [OTC]; Benadryl® Itch Stopping Extra Strength [OTC]; Benadryl® Itch Stopping [OTC]; Dermamycin® [OTC]; Diphenhist® [OTC] [DSC]

Index Terms Diphenhydramine Hydrochloride

Pharmacologic Category Ethanolamine Derivative; Histamine H_1 Antagonist; Histamine H_1 Antagonist, First Generation; Topical Skin Product

Medication Safety Issues

Sound-alike/look-alike issues:
DiphenhydrAMINE may be confused with desipramine, dicyclomine, dimenhyDRINATE
Benadryl® may be confused with benazepril, Bentyl®, Benylin®, Caladryl®

Administration issues:
Institute for Safe Medication Practices (ISMP) has reported cases of patients mistakenly *swallowing* Benadryl® Itch Stopping [OTC] gel intended for topical application. Unclear labeling and similar packaging of the topical gel in containers resembling an oral liquid are factors believed to be contributing to the administration errors. The topical gel contains camphor which can be toxic if swallowed. ISMP has requested the manufacturer to make the necessary changes to prevent further confusion.

Use Topically for relief of pain and itching associated with insect bites, minor cuts and burns, or rashes due to poison ivy, poison oak, and poison sumac

Available Dosage Forms

Cream, topical: 2% (30 g)
Banophen™ Anti-Itch [OTC]: 2% (28.4 g)
Benadryl® Itch Stopping [OTC]: 1% (14.2 g, 28.3 g)
Benadryl® Itch Stopping Extra Strength [OTC]: 2% (14.2 g, 28.3 g)
Dermamycin® [OTC]: 2% (28 g)

Gel, topical:
Benadryl® Extra Strength Itch Stopping [OTC]: 2% (120 mL)

Liquid, topical:
Benadryl® Itch Relief Extra Strength [OTC]: 2% (14 mL)
Benadryl® Itch Stopping Extra Strength [OTC]: 2% (59 mL)
Dermamycin® [OTC]: 2% (60 mL)

General Dosage Range Topical: *Children ≥2 years and Adults:* Apply 1% or 2% up to 3-4 times/day

Diphenhydramine and Phenylephrine (dye fen HYE dra meen & fen il EF rin)

Brand Names: U.S. Aldex® CT; Benadryl-D® Allergy & Sinus [OTC]; Benadryl-D® Children's Allergy & Sinus [OTC]; Dimetapp® Children's Nighttime Cold & Congestion [OTC]; Robitussin® Night Time Cough & Cold [OTC] [DSC]; Triaminic® Children's Night Time Cold & Cough [OTC]; Triaminic® Children's Thin Strips® Night Time Cold & Cough [OTC]

Index Terms Diphenhydramine Hydrochloride and Phenylephrine Hydrochloride; Diphenhydramine Tannate and Phenylephrine Tannate; Phenylephrine and Diphenhydramine; Phenylephrine Hydrochloride and Diphenhydramine Hydrochloride; Phenylephrine Tannate and Diphenhydramine Tannate

Pharmacologic Category Alpha-Adrenergic Agonist; Decongestant; Ethanolamine Derivative; Histamine H_1 Antagonist; Histamine H_1 Antagonist, First Generation

Pregnancy Risk Factor C

Lactation Excretion in breast milk unknown/contraindicated

Use Temporary relief of symptoms of allergic rhinitis, sinusitis, and other upper respiratory conditions, including sinus/nasal congestion, sneezing, stuffy/runny nose, itchy/watery eyes, and cough

Available Dosage Forms

Liquid, oral:

Benadryl-D® Children's Allergy & Sinus [OTC]: Diphenhydramine 12.5 mg and phenylephrine 5 mg per 5 mL (118 mL)

Strip, orally disintegrating:

Triaminic® Children's Thin Strips® Night Time Cold & Cough [OTC]: Diphenhydramine 12.5 mg and phenylephrine 5 mg

Syrup, oral:

Dimetapp® Children's Nighttime Cold and Congestion [OTC]: Diphenhydramine 6.25 mg and phenylephrine 2.5 mg per 5 mL (120 mL)

Triaminic® Children's Night Time Cold & Cough [OTC]: Diphenhydramine 6.25 mg and phenylephrine 2.5 mg per 5 mL (118 mL)

Tablet, oral:

Benadryl-D® Allergy & Sinus [OTC]: Diphenhydramine 25 mg and phenylephrine 10 mg

Tablet, chewable, oral:

Aldex® CT: Diphenhydramine 12.5 mg and phenylephrine 5 mg

General Dosage Range Oral:

Children 6-11 years: Aldex® CT: 1/2 to 1 tablet every 6 hours; OTC labeling: 5-10 mL or 1 strip every 4 hours as needed (maximum: 6 doses/24 hours)

Children ≥12 years and Adults: Aldex® CT: 1-2 tablets every 6 hours; OTC labeling: 10-20 mL every 4 hours as needed or 1 tablet every 4 hours as needed (maximum: 6 doses/24 hours)

Nursing Actions

Physical Assessment See individual agents.

Patient Education See individual agents.

Diphenoxylate and Atropine (dye fen OKS i late & A troe peen)

Brand Names: U.S. Lomotil®

Index Terms Atropine and Diphenoxylate

Pharmacologic Category Antidiarrheal

Medication Safety Issues

Sound-alike/look-alike issues:

Lomotil® may be confused with LaMICtal®, LamISIL®, lamoTRIgine, Lanoxin®, Lasix®

International issues:

Lomotil [U.S., Canada, and multiple international markets] may be confused with Ludiomil brand name for maprotiline [multiple international markets]

Lomotil: Brand name for diphenoxylate [U.S., Canada, and multiple international markets], but also the brand name for loperamide [Mexico, Philippines]

Pregnancy Risk Factor C

Lactation Enters breast milk/use caution

Use Treatment of diarrhea

Controlled Substance C-V

Available Dosage Forms

Solution, oral: Diphenoxylate 2.5 mg and atropine 0.025 mg per 5 mL

Tablet, oral: Diphenoxylate 2.5 mg and atropine 0.025 mg

General Dosage Range Oral:

Children 2-12 years: Initial: Diphenoxylate 0.3-0.4 mg/kg/day in 4 divided doses (maximum: 10 mg/day); Maintenance: Reduce as needed, may be as low as 25% of the initial daily dose

Adults: Initial: Diphenoxylate 5 mg 4 times/day (maximum: 20 mg/day); Maintenance: Reduce as needed, may be as low as 5 mg/day

Administration

Oral If there is no response within 48 hours of continuous therapy, this medication is unlikely to be effective and should be discontinued; if chronic diarrhea is not improved symptomatically within 10 days at maximum dosage, control is unlikely with further use. Use of the liquid preparation is recommended in children <13 years of age; use plastic dropper provided when measuring liquid.

Nursing Actions

Physical Assessment See individual agents.

Patient Education See individual agents.

Related Information

Atropine *on page 105*

Diphtheria and Tetanus Toxoids, Acellular Pertussis, and Poliovirus Vaccine

(dif THEER ee a & TET a nus TOKS oyds, ay CEL yoo lar per TUS sis & POE lee oh VYE rus vak SEEN)

Brand Names: U.S. Kinrix®

Index Terms Diphtheria and Tetanus Toxoids and Acellular Pertussis Adsorbed, and Inactivated Poliovirus Vaccine Combined; Diphtheria, Tetanus Toxoids, Acellular Pertussis (DTaP); DTaP-IPV; Poliovirus, Inactivated (IPV)

Pharmacologic Category Vaccine, Inactivated (Bacterial); Vaccine, Inactivated (Viral)

Pregnancy Risk Factor C

Use Active immunization against diphtheria, tetanus, pertussis, and poliomyelitis, used as the 5th dose in the DTaP series and the 4th dose in the IPV series

The Advisory Committee on Immunization Practices (ACIP) recommends routine vaccination for use as the fifth dose in the DTaP series and the fourth dose in the IPV series in children who received DTaP (Infanrix®) and/or DTaP-Hepatitis B-IPV (Pediarix®) as the first 3 doses and DTaP (Infanrix®) as the fourth dose. Whenever feasible, the same manufacturer should be used to provide the pertussis component; however, vaccination should not be deferred if a specific brand is not known or is not available.

Available Dosage Forms

Injection, suspension [preservative free]:

Kinrix®: Diphtheria toxoid 25 Lf, tetanus toxoid 10 Lf, acellular pertussis antigens [inactivated pertussis toxin 25 mcg, filamentous hemagglutinin 25 mcg, pertactin 8 mcg], type 1 poliovirus 40 D-antigen units, type 2 poliovirus 8 D-antigen units, and type 3 poliovirus 32 D-antigen units per 0.5 mL (0.5 mL)

General Dosage Range I.M.: *Children 4-6 years:* 0.5 mL

Administration

I.M. For I.M. use only; do not administer intradermally, I.V., or SubQ. Shake well prior to use; do not use unless a homogeneous, turbid, white suspension forms. Discard if the suspension is discolored or if there are cracks in the vial or syringe. Administer in the deltoid muscle of the upper arm. Do not administer additional vaccines or immunoglobulins at the same site, or using the same syringe.

For patients at risk of hemorrhage following intramuscular injection, the ACIP recommends "it should be administered intramuscularly if, in the opinion of the physician familiar with the patients bleeding risk, the vaccine can be administered by this route with reasonable safety. If the patient receives antihemophilia or other similar therapy, intramuscular vaccination can be scheduled shortly after such therapy is administered. A fine needle (23 gauge or smaller) can be used for the vaccination and firm pressure applied to the site (without rubbing) for at least 2 minutes. The patient should be instructed concerning the risk of hematoma from the injection." Patients on anticoagulant therapy should be considered to have the same bleeding risks and treated as those with clotting factor disorders (CDC, 2011).

Simultaneous administration of vaccines helps ensure the patients will be fully vaccinated by the appropriate age. Simultaneous administration of vaccines is defined as administering >1 vaccine on the same day at different anatomic sites. The use of licensed combination vaccines is generally preferred over separate injections of the equivalent components. Separate vaccines should not be combined in the same syringe unless indicated by product specific labeling. Separate needles and syringes should be used for each injection. The ACIP prefers each dose of a specific vaccine in a series come from the same manufacturer when possible. Adolescents and adults should be vaccinated while seated or lying down. In general, preterm infants should be vaccinated at the same chronological age as full-term infants (CDC, 2011).

Antipyretics have not been shown to prevent febrile seizures. Antipyretics may be used to treat fever or discomfort following vaccination (CDC, 2011). One study reported that routine prophylactic administration of acetaminophen to prevent fever prior to vaccination decreased the immune response of some vaccines; the clinical significance of this reduction in immune response has not been established (Prymula, 2009).

Nursing Actions

Physical Assessment Treatment for anaphylactic reactions should be immediately available during vaccine use. For I.M. use only. U.S. federal law requires entry into the patient's medical record.

Patient Education Notify prescriber immediately of any acute reaction to vaccination (eg, difficulty breathing or swallowing, chest pain or palpitations, acute headache, rash, seizures, high fever). Follow directions for care of injection site; report persistent redness, swelling, or signs of infection at injection site. May cause drowsiness or loss of appetite; if these persist beyond 1-2 days or become severe, consult prescriber.

Related Information

Immunization Administration Recommendations *on page 1243*

Immunization Recommendations *on page 1248*

Diphtheria and Tetanus Toxoids, Acellular Pertussis, Hepatitis B (Recombinant), Poliovirus (Inactivated), and *Haemophilus influenzae* B Conjugate (Adsorbed) Vaccine

(dif THEER ee a & TET a nus TOKS oyds, ay CEL yoo lar per TUS sis, hep a TYE tis bee ree KOM be nant, POE lee oh VYE rus in ak ti VAY ted, & hem OF fi lus in floo EN za bee KON joo gate ad SORBED vak SEEN)

Index Terms Diphtheria and Tetanus Toxoids and Acellular Pertussis, Hepatitis B (Recombinant), Inactivated Poliovirus Vaccine, and *Haemophilus influenzae* Type B Combined; DTaP-HepB-IPV-Hib

Pharmacologic Category Vaccine, Inactivated (Bacterial, Viral)

Medication Safety Issues

Sound-alike/look-alike issues:

Infanrix Hexa™ may be confused with Infanrix®

Use Active primary immunization against diphtheria, tetanus, pertussis, hepatitis B, poliomyelitis and disease caused by *Haemophilus influenzae* type b in infants and children 6 weeks to 2 years of age; booster immunization (at 18 months) in infants who previously received a full primary vaccination course of each component of the vaccine

Product Availability Not available in U.S.

General Dosage Range I.M.: *Children 6 weeks to 2 years:* Primary immunization: 0.5 mL every 8 weeks for a total of 3 doses; booster dose: 0.5 mL

Administration

I.M. Administer by I.M. injection only, preferably in the anterolateral aspects of the thigh or the deltoid muscle of the upper arm. Do not administer intravenously or subcutaneously. Do not inject into the gluteal area (suboptimal hepatitis B immune response) or areas where major nerve trunks may be located. Fractional dosing (use of reduced volume) is not recommended. If more than one vaccine is to be given by IM injection use separate limbs. Rotate injection sites when completing vaccination series.

Acetaminophen may be used when needed to provide comfort; however, routine prophylactic administration of acetaminophen to prevent fever due to vaccine use is not recommended. There is evidence of a decreased immune response to some vaccines associated with acetaminophen administration; the clinical significance of this reduction in immune response has not been established.

Nursing Actions

Physical Assessment See individual agents.

Patient Education See individual agents.

Diphtheria and Tetanus Toxoids, Acellular Pertussis, Poliovirus and *Haemophilus* b Conjugate Vaccine

(dif THEER ee a & TET a nus TOKS oyds ay CEL yoo lar per TUS sis POE lee oh VYE rus & hem OF fi lus bee KON joo gate vak SEEN)

Brand Names: U.S. Pentacel®

Index Terms *Haemophilus* B Conjugate (Hib); *Haemophilus* B Polysaccharide; Diphtheria Toxoid; Diphtheria, Tetanus Toxoids, Acellular Pertussis (DTaP); DTaP-IPV/Hib; Pertussis, Acellular (Adsorbed); Poliovirus, Inactivated (IPV); Tetanus Toxoid

Pharmacologic Category Vaccine, Inactivated (Bacterial); Vaccine, Inactivated (Viral)

Medication Safety Issues

Administration issues:

Pentacel® is supplied in two vials, one containing DTaP-IPV liquid and one containing Hib powder, which must be mixed together in order to administer the recommended vaccine components.

Pregnancy Risk Factor C

Use Active immunization against diphtheria, tetanus, pertussis, poliomyelitis, and invasive disease caused by *H. influenzae* type b in children 6 weeks through 4 years of age

Advisory Committee on Immunization Practices (ACIP) recommends that Pentacel® (DTaP-IPV/Hib) may be used to provide the recommended DTaP, IPV, and Hib immunization in children <5 years of age. Whenever feasible, the same manufacturer should be used to provide the pertussis component; however, vaccination should not be deferred if a specific brand is not known or is not available. The Hib component in Pentacel® contains a tetanus toxoid conjugate. A Hib vaccine containing the PRP-OMP conjugate (PedvaxHIB®) may provide a more rapid seroconversion following the first dose and may be preferable to use in certain populations (eg, American Indian or Alaska Native children).

Available Dosage Forms

Injection, suspension:

Pentacel®: Diphtheria toxoid 15 Lf, tetanus toxoid 5 Lf, acellular pertussis antigens, poliovirus, and *Haemophilus* b capsular polysaccharide 10 mcg per 0.5 mL (0.5 mL)

General Dosage Range I.M.: *Children 6 weeks to ≤4 years:* 0.5 mL

Administration

I.M. For I.M. administration only. Do not administer I.V. or SubQ. Administer in the anterolateral aspect of thigh in children <1 year of age or deltoid muscle of upper arm in older children. Do not administer to gluteal area or areas near a major nerve trunk. Do not administer additional vaccines or immunoglobulins at the same site or using the same syringe.

For patients at risk of hemorrhage following intramuscular injection, the ACIP recommends: "It should be administered intramuscularly if, in the opinion of the physician familiar with the patient's bleeding risk, the vaccine can be administered by this route with reasonable safety. If the patient receives antihemophilia or other similar therapy, intramuscular vaccination can be scheduled shortly after such therapy is administered. A fine needle (23-gauge or smaller) can be used for the vaccination and firm pressure applied to the site (without rubbing) for at least 2 minutes. The patient should be instructed concerning the risk of hematoma from the injection." Patients on anticoagulant therapy should be considered to have the same bleeding risks and treated as those with clotting factor disorders (CDC, 2011).

Simultaneous administration of vaccines helps ensure the patients will be fully vaccinated by the appropriate age. Simultaneous administration of vaccines is defined as administering >1 vaccine on the same day at different anatomic sites. The use of licensed combination vaccines is generally preferred over separate injections of the equivalent components. Separate vaccines should not be combined in the same syringe unless indicated by product specific labeling. Separate needles and syringes should be used for each injection. The ACIP prefers each dose of a specific vaccine in a series come from the same manufacturer when possible. Adolescents and adults should be vaccinated while seated or lying down. In general, preterm infants should be vaccinated at the same chronological age as full-term infants (CDC, 2011).

Antipyretics have not been shown to prevent febrile seizures. Antipyretics may be used to treat fever or discomfort following vaccination (CDC, 2011). One study reported that routine prophylactic administration of acetaminophen to prevent fever prior to vaccination decreased the immune response of some vaccines; the clinical significance of this reduction in immune response has not been established (Prymula, 2009).

Nursing Actions

Physical Assessment U.S. federal law requires entry into the patient's medical record.

Related Information

Immunization Administration Recommendations *on page 1243*

Immunization Recommendations *on page 1248*

Diphtheria and Tetanus Toxoids, and Acellular Pertussis Vaccine

(dif THEER ee a & TET a nus TOKS oyds & ay CEL yoo lar per TUS sis vak SEEN)

Brand Names: U.S. Adacel®; Boostrix®; Daptacel®; Infanrix®

Index Terms DTaP; Tdap; Tetanus Toxoid, Reduced Diphtheria Toxoid, and Acellular Pertussis, Adsorbed; Tripedia

Pharmacologic Category Vaccine, Inactivated (Bacterial)

Medication Safety Issues

Sound-alike/look-alike issues:

Adacel® (Tdap) may be confused with Daptacel® (DTaP)

Tdap (Adacel®, Boostrix®) may be confused with DTaP (Daptacel®, Infanrix®, Tripedia)

Administration issues:

Carefully review product labeling to prevent inadvertent administration of Tdap when DTaP is indicated. Tdap contains lower amounts of diphtheria toxoid and some pertussis antigens than DTaP.

Tdap is not indicated for use in children <10 years of age

DTaP is not indicated for use in persons ≥7 years of age

Guidelines are available in case of inadvertent administration of these products; refer to ACIP recommendations, February 2006 available at http://www.cdc.gov/mmwr/preview/mmwrhtml/rr55e223a1.htm

Other safety concerns:

DTaP: Diphtheria and tetanus toxoids and acellular pertussis vaccine

DTP: Diphtheria and tetanus toxoids and pertussis vaccine (unspecified pertussis antigens)

DTwP: Diphtheria and tetanus toxoids and whole-cell pertussis vaccine (no longer available on U.S. market)

Tdap: Tetanus toxoid, reduced diphtheria toxoid, and acellular pertussis vaccine

Pregnancy Risk Factor C

Lactation Excretion in breast milk unknown/use caution

Use

Daptacel®, Infanrix® (DTaP): Active immunization against diphtheria, tetanus, and pertussis from age 6 weeks through 6 years of age (prior to seventh birthday)

Adacel®, Boostrix® (Tdap): Active booster immunization against diphtheria, tetanus, and pertussis

The Advisory Committee on Immunization Practices (ACIP) recommends routine vaccination for the following:

Children 6 weeks to <7 years (DTaP):

- For primary immunization against diphtheria, tetanus and pertussis
- Pediatric patients who are wounded in bombings or similar mass casualty events and who have penetrating injuries or nonintact skin exposure, and have an uncertain vaccination history should receive a tetanus booster with DTaP (if no contraindications exist) (CDC, 57 [RR6], 2008)

Children 7-10 years (Tdap):

- Children not fully vaccinated against pertussis should receive a single dose of Tdap (if no contraindications exist) (CDC, 60[1], 2011)
- Children never vaccinated against diphtheria, tetanus, or pertussis, or whose vaccination status is not known should receive a series of three vaccinations containing tetanus and diphtheria toxoids and the first dose should be with Tdap (CDC, 60[1], 2011)

Adolescents 11-18 years (Tdap):

- A single dose of Tdap as a booster dose in adolescents who have completed the recommended childhood DTaP vaccination series (preferred age of administration is 11-12 years) (CDC, 60[1], 2011)

Adolescents ≥11 years and Adults (Tdap):

- Persons wounded in bombings or similar mass casualty events and who cannot confirm receipt of a tetanus booster within the previous 5 years and who have penetrating injuries or nonintact skin exposure should receive a single dose of Tdap (CDC, 57 [RR6] 2008)

Adults 19-64 years (Tdap): A single dose of Tdap should be given to replace a single dose of the 10-year Td booster in patients who have not previously received Tdap or for whom vaccine status is not known, and as soon as feasible to all:

- Pregnant (>20 weeks gestation) or postpartum women (CDC, 57[RR4], 2008; CDC, 60[41], 2011; CDC, 61[4], 2012)
- Close contacts of children <12 months of age; Tdap should ideally be administered at least 2 weeks prior to beginning close contact (CDC, 55 [RR17], 2006; CDC, 60[41], 2011; CDC, 61 [4], 2012)
- Healthcare providers with direct patient contact (CDC, 55[RR17], 2006; CDC, 61[4], 2012)

Adults ≥65 years who have not previously received Tdap:

- All adults ≥65 years may receive a single dose of Tdap in place of a dose of Td (CDC, 60[1], 2011; CDC, 60[41], 2011)
- Adults ≥65 years who anticipate close contact with children <12 months of age should receive a single dose of Tdap in place a of a dose of Td (CDC, 60[1], 2011; CDC, 60[41], 2011)

Note: Tdap is currently recommended for a single dose only (all age groups) (CDC, 60[1], 2011)

Available Dosage Forms

Injection, suspension [Tdap, booster formulation]:

Adacel®: Diphtheria 2 Lf units, tetanus 5 Lf units, and acellular pertussis antigens per 0.5 mL (0.5 mL)

Boostrix®: Diphtheria 2.5 Lf units, tetanus 5 Lf units, and acellular pertussis antigens per 0.5 mL (0.5 mL)

Injection, suspension [DTaP, active immunization formulation]:

Daptacel®: Diphtheria 15 Lf units, tetanus 5 Lf units, and acellular pertussis antigens per 0.5 mL (0.5 mL)

Infanrix®: Diphtheria 25 Lf units, tetanus 10 Lf units, and acellular pertussis antigens per 0.5 mL (0.5 mL) [preservative free]

General Dosage Range I.M.:

Children 6 weeks to <7 years: Primary immunization: 0.5 mL per dose, total of 5 doses

Children ≥10 years and Adults: Booster immunization: 0.5 mL as a single dose

Administration

I.M. Shake suspension well.

Adacel®, Boostrix®: Administer only I.M. in deltoid muscle of upper arm.

Daptacel®, Infanrix®: Administer only I.M. in anterolateral aspect of thigh or deltoid muscle of upper arm.

If feasible, the same brand of DTaP should be used for all doses in the series (CDC, 60 [2], 2011).

For patients at risk of hemorrhage following intramuscular injection, the ACIP recommends "it should be administered intramuscularly if, in the opinion of the physician familiar with the patients bleeding risk, the vaccine can be administered by this route with reasonable safety. If the patient receives antihemophilia or other similar therapy, intramuscular vaccination can be scheduled shortly after such therapy is administered. A fine needle (23 gauge or smaller) can be used for the vaccination and firm pressure applied to the site (without rubbing) for at least 2 minutes. The patient should be instructed concerning the risk of hematoma from the injection." Patients on anticoagulant therapy should be considered to have the same bleeding risks and treated as those with clotting factor disorders (CDC, 60[2], 2011).

Simultaneous administration of vaccines helps ensure the patients will be fully vaccinated by the appropriate age. Simultaneous administration of vaccines is defined as administering >1 vaccine on the same day at different anatomic sites. The use of licensed combination vaccines is generally preferred over separate injections of the equivalent components. Separate vaccines should not be combined in the same syringe unless indicated by product specific labeling. Separate needles and syringes should be used for each injection. The ACIP prefers each dose of a specific vaccine in a series come from the same manufacturer when possible. Adolescents and adults should be vaccinated while seated or lying down. In general, preterm infants should be vaccinated at the same chronological age as full-term infants (CDC, 60[2], 2011).

Antipyretics have not been shown to prevent febrile seizures. Antipyretics may be used to treat fever or discomfort following vaccination (CDC, 2011). One study reported that routine prophylactic administration of acetaminophen to prevent fever prior to vaccination decreased the immune response of some vaccines; the clinical significance of this reduction in immune response has not been established (Prymula, 2009).

Nursing Actions

Physical Assessment U.S. federal law requires entry into the patient's medical record.

Related Information

Immunization Administration Recommendations *on page 1243*

Immunization Recommendations *on page 1248*

Diphtheria, Tetanus Toxoids, Acellular Pertussis, Hepatitis B (Recombinant), and Poliovirus (Inactivated) Vaccine

(dif THEER ee a, TET a nus TOKS oyds, ay CEL yoo lar per TUS sis, hep a TYE tis bee ree KOM be nant, & POE lee oh VYE rus in ak ti VAY ted vak SEEN)

Brand Names: U.S. Pediarix®

Index Terms Diphtheria and Tetanus Toxoids and Acellular Pertussis Adsorbed, Hepatitis B (Recombinant) and Inactivated Poliovirus Vaccine Combined; Diphtheria, Tetanus Toxoids, Acellular Pertussis, Hepatitis B (Recombinant), and Poliovirus Vaccine; DTaP-HepB-IPV

Pharmacologic Category Vaccine, Inactivated (Bacterial); Vaccine, Inactivated (Viral)

Pregnancy Risk Factor C

Use Combination vaccine for the active immunization against diphtheria, tetanus, pertussis, hepatitis B virus (all known subtypes), and poliomyelitis (caused by poliovirus types 1, 2, and 3)

The Advisory Committee on Immunization Practices (ACIP) recommends Pediarix® for the following:

- Primary vaccination for DTaP, Hep B, and IPV in children at 2, 4, and 6 months of age.
- To complete the primary vaccination series in children who have received DTaP (Infanrix®) and who are scheduled to receive the other components of the vaccine. Whenever feasible, the same manufacturer should be used to provide the pertussis component; however, vaccination should not be deferred if a specific brand is not known or is not available. HepB and IPV from different manufacturers are interchangeable.

Available Dosage Forms

Injection, suspension [preservative free]:

Pediarix®: Diphtheria toxoid 25 Lf, tetanus toxoid 10 Lf, acellular pertussis antigens per 0.5 mL (0.5 mL)

General Dosage Range I.M.: *Children 6 weeks to <7 years:* 0.5 mL/dose for a total of 3 doses

Administration

I.M. For I.M. use only; do not administer I.V., SubQ, or intradermally. Shake well prior to use; do not use unless a homogeneous, turbid, white suspension forms. Administer in the anterolateral aspects of the thigh or the deltoid muscle of the upper arm. Do not inject in the gluteal area (suboptimal hepatitis B immune response) or where there may be a major nerve trunk. Do not administer additional vaccines or immunoglobulins at the same site, or using the same syringe.

For patients at risk of hemorrhage following intramuscular injection, the ACIP recommends "it should be administered intramuscularly if, in the opinion of the physician familiar with the patients bleeding risk, the vaccine can be administered by this route with reasonable safety. If the patient receives antihemophilia or other similar therapy, intramuscular vaccination can be scheduled shortly after such therapy is administered. A fine needle (23 gauge or smaller) can be used for the vaccination and firm pressure applied to the site (without rubbing) for at least 2 minutes. The patient should be instructed concerning the risk of hematoma from the injection." Patients on anticoagulant therapy should be considered to have the same bleeding risks and treated as those with clotting factor disorders (CDC, 2011).

Simultaneous administration of vaccines helps ensure the patients will be fully vaccinated by the appropriate age. Simultaneous administration of vaccines is defined as administering >1 vaccine on the same day at different anatomic sites. The use of licensed combination vaccines is generally preferred over separate injections of the equivalent components. Separate vaccines should not be combined in the same syringe unless indicated by product specific labeling. Separate needles and syringes should be used for each injection. The ACIP prefers each dose of a specific vaccine in a series come from the same manufacturer when possible. Adolescents and adults should be vaccinated while seated or lying down. In general, preterm infants should be vaccinated at the same chronological age as full-term infants (CDC, 2011).

Antipyretics have not been shown to prevent febrile seizures. Antipyretics may be used to treat fever or discomfort following vaccination (CDC, 2011). One study reported that routine prophylactic administration of acetaminophen to prevent fever prior to vaccination decreased the immune response of some vaccines; the clinical significance of this reduction in immune response has not been established (Prymula, 2009).

Nursing Actions

Physical Assessment Children who are moderately-to-severely ill should not get this vaccination until they have recovered. Assess any hypersensitivity history prior to administering. Treatment for anaphylactic/anaphylactoid reaction should be available. Antipyretics should be administered at time of and for 24 hours following vaccination to patients at high-risk for seizures. U.S. federal law requires entry into the patient's medical record.

Patient Education Inform prescriber of all previous allergic reactions. Three doses will be required for effective immunity; consult prescriber for appropriate schedule of vaccinations. May cause increased sleeping, restlessness, fussiness, decreased appetite, or fever. Use antipyretic if directed by prescriber. May cause some redness, pain, or swelling at injection site; consult prescriber if excessive or persistent. Notify prescriber immediately of any severe reactions (eg, fever >105°F within 48 hours, inconsolable crying that occurs within 48 hours and lasts 3 hours, seizures that occur within 3 days).

Related Information

Immunization Administration Recommendations *on page 1243*

Immunization Recommendations *on page 1248*

Dipyridamole (dye peer ID a mole)

Brand Names: U.S. Persantine®

Pharmacologic Category Antiplatelet Agent; Vasodilator

Medication Safety Issues

Sound-alike/look-alike issues:

Dipyridamole may be confused with disopyramide

Persantine® may be confused with Periactin

International issues:

Persantine [U.S., Canada, Belgium, Denmark, France] may be confused with Permitil brand name for sildenafil [Argentina]

BEERS Criteria medication:

This drug may be inappropriate for use in geriatric patients (low severity risk).

Pregnancy Risk Factor B

Lactation Enters breast milk/use caution

Use

Oral: Used with warfarin to decrease thrombosis in patients after artificial heart valve replacement

I.V.: Diagnostic agent in CAD

Unlabeled Use Stroke prevention (in combination with aspirin)

Available Dosage Forms

Injection, solution: 5 mg/mL (2 mL, 10 mL)

Tablet, oral: 25 mg, 50 mg, 75 mg

Persantine®: 25 mg, 50 mg, 75 mg

General Dosage Range

I.V.: *Adults:* 0.14 mg/kg/minute for 4 minutes (maximum: 60 mg)

Oral: *Children ≥12 years and Adults:* 75-100 mg 4 times/day

Administration

Oral Administer with water 1 hour before meals.

I.V. I.V.: Infuse diluted solution over 4 minutes.

Nursing Actions

Physical Assessment Observe bleeding precautions. Oral: Monitor blood pressure on a regular basis. I.V.: Continuous ECG and blood pressure monitoring necessary during infusion.

Patient Education Take tablet with water 1 hour before meals. Inform prescribers and dentists that you are taking this medication prior to scheduling any surgery or dental procedure. You may experience mild headache, transient diarrhea, or temporary dizziness. You may have a tendency to bleed easily. Report chest pain, redness around mouth, acute abdominal cramping or severe diarrhea, acute and persistent headache or dizziness, rash, respiratory difficulty, or swelling of extremities.

Disulfiram (dye SUL fi ram)

Brand Names: U.S. Antabuse®

Pharmacologic Category Aldehyde Dehydrogenase Inhibitor

Medication Safety Issues

Sound-alike/look-alike issues:

Disulfiram may be confused with Diflucan®

Lactation Excretion in breast milk unknown/not recommended

Use Management of chronic alcoholism

Available Dosage Forms

Tablet, oral: 250 mg, 500 mg

Antabuse®: 250 mg, 500 mg

General Dosage Range Oral: *Adults:* Initial: 500 mg once daily; Maintenance: 125-500 mg once daily (maximum: 500 mg/day)

Administration

Oral Administration of any medications containing alcohol, including topicals, is contraindicated. Do not administer disulfiram if ethanol has been consumed within the prior 12 hours.

Nursing Actions

Physical Assessment Do not administer until the patient has abstained from ethanol for 12 hours. Monitor laboratory tests and for CNS changes (eg, sedation, restlessness, peripheral neuropathy, and optic or retrobulbar neuritis) prior to treatment and periodically. Advise patient about disulfiram reaction if alcohol is ingested.

Patient Education Tablets can be crushed or mixed with water or juice. Metallic aftertaste may occur; this will go away. Do not drink any alcohol, including products containing alcohol (such as cough and cold syrups or some mouthwashes), or use alcohol-containing skin products while taking this medication and for at least 3 days (preferably 14 days) after stopping this medication. Drowsiness, tiredness, or visual changes may occur. Notify prescriber of any weakness, nausea, vomiting, decreased appetite, yellowing of skin or eyes, dark-colored urine, or numbness of fingers or feet.

Divalproex (dye VAL proe ex)

Brand Names: U.S. Depakote®; Depakote® ER; Depakote® Sprinkle

Index Terms Divalproex Sodium; Valproate Semisodium; Valproic Acid Derivative

Pharmacologic Category Anticonvulsant, Miscellaneous; Antimanic Agent; Histone Deacetylase Inhibitor

Medication Safety Issues

Sound-alike/look-alike issues:

Depakote® may be confused with Depakene®, Depakote® ER, Senokot®

Depakote® ER may be confused with divalproex enteric coated

Pregnancy Risk Factor D

Lactation Enters breast milk/not recommended (AAP considers "compatible"; AAP 2001 update pending)

Breast-Feeding Considerations Breast milk concentrations of valproic acid have been reported as 1% to 10% of maternal concentration. The weight-adjusted dose to the infant has been calculated to be ~4%.

Use Monotherapy and adjunctive therapy in the treatment of patients with complex partial seizures; monotherapy and adjunctive therapy of simple and complex absence seizures; adjunctive therapy in patients with multiple seizure types that include absence seizures

Depakote®, Depakote® ER: Mania associated with bipolar disorder; migraine prophylaxis

Unlabeled Use Diabetic neuropathy

Mechanism of Action/Effect Causes increased availability of gamma-aminobutyric acid (GABA), an inhibitory neurotransmitter, to brain neurons or may enhance the action of GABA or mimic its action at postsynaptic receptor sites

Contraindications Hypersensitivity to divalproex, derivatives, or any component of the formulation; hepatic disease or significant impairment; urea cycle disorders

Warnings/Precautions [U.S. Boxed Warning]: Hepatic failure resulting in fatalities has occurred in patients; children <2 years of age are at considerable risk. Other risk factors include organic brain disease, mental retardation with severe seizure disorders, congenital metabolic disorders, and patients on multiple anticonvulsants. Hepatotoxicity has usually been reported within 6 months of therapy initiation. Monitor patients closely for appearance of malaise, weakness, facial edema, anorexia, jaundice, and vomiting; discontinue immediately with signs/symptom of significant or suspected impairment. Liver function tests should be performed at baseline and at regular intervals after initiation of therapy, especially within the first 6 months. Hepatic dysfunction may progress despite discontinuing treatment. Should only be used as monotherapy in children <2 years of age and patients at high risk for hepatotoxicity. Contraindicated with severe impairment.

[U.S. Boxed Warning]: Cases of life-threatening pancreatitis, occurring at the start of therapy or following years of use, have been reported in adults and children. Some cases have been hemorrhagic with rapid progression of initial symptoms to death. Promptly evaluate symptoms of abdominal pain, nausea, vomiting, and/or anorexia; should generally be discontinued if pancreatitis is diagnosed.

[U.S. Boxed Warning]: May cause teratogenic effects such as neural tube defects (eg, spina bifida). Use in women of childbearing potential requires that benefits of use in mother be weighed against the potential risk to fetus, especially when used for conditions not associated with permanent injury or risk of death (eg, migraine).

May cause severe thrombocytopenia, inhibition of platelet aggregation, and bleeding. Tremors may indicate overdosage; use with caution in patients receiving other anticonvulsants. Hypersensitivity reactions affecting multiple organs have been reported in association with divalproex use; may include dermatologic and/or hematologic changes (eosinophilia, neutropenia, thrombocytopenia) or symptoms of organ dysfunction.

Hyperammonemia and/or encephalopathy, sometimes fatal, have been reported following the initiation of divalproex therapy and may be present with normal transaminase levels. Ammonia levels should be measured in patients who develop unexplained lethargy and vomiting, changes in mental status, or in patients who present with hypothermia (unintentional drop in core body temperature to <35°C/95°F). Discontinue therapy if ammonia levels are increased and evaluate for possible urea cycle disorder (UCD); contraindicated in patients with UCD. Evaluation of UCD should be considered for the following patients prior to the start of therapy: History of unexplained encephalopathy or coma; encephalopathy associated with protein load; pregnancy or postpartum encephalopathy; unexplained mental retardation; history of elevated plasma ammonia or glutamine; history of cyclical vomiting and lethargy; episodic extreme irritability, ataxia; low BUN or protein avoidance; family history of UCD or unexplained infant deaths (particularly male); or signs or symptoms of UCD (hyperammonemia, encephalopathy, respiratory alkalosis). Hypothermia has been reported with divalproex therapy; may or may not be associated with hyperammonemia; may also occur with concomitant topiramate therapy.

In vitro studies have suggested divalproex stimulates the replication of HIV and CMV viruses under experimental conditions. The clinical consequence of this is unknown, but should be considered when monitoring affected patients.

Antiepileptics are associated with an increased risk of suicidal behavior/thoughts with use (regardless of indication); patients should be monitored for signs/symptoms of depression, suicidal tendencies, and other unusual behavior changes during therapy and instructed to inform their healthcare provider immediately if symptoms occur.

Anticonvulsants should not be discontinued abruptly because of the possibility of increasing seizure frequency; divalproex should be withdrawn gradually to minimize the potential of increased seizure frequency, unless safety concerns require a more rapid withdrawal. Concomitant use with carbapenem antibiotics may reduce valproic acid levels to subtherapeutic levels; monitor levels frequently and consider alternate therapy if levels drop significantly or lack of seizure control occurs. Concomitant use with clonazepam may induce absence status. Patients treated for bipolar disorder should be monitored closely for clinical worsening or suicidality; prescriptions should be written for the smallest quantity consistent with good patient care.

CNS depression may occur with divalproex use. Patients must be cautioned about performing tasks which require mental alertness (operating machinery or driving). Effects with other sedative drugs or ethanol may be potentiated. Use with caution in the elderly.

Drug Interactions

Avoid Concomitant Use There are no known interactions where it is recommended to avoid concomitant use.

Decreased Effect

Divalproex may decrease the levels/effects of: CarBAMazepine; Fosphenytoin; OXcarbazepine; Phenytoin

The levels/effects of Divalproex may be decreased by: Barbiturates; CarBAMazepine; Carbapenems; Cyproterone; Ethosuximide; Fosphenytoin; Methylfolate; Phenytoin; Primidone; Protease Inhibitors; Rifampin

Increased Effect/Toxicity

Divalproex may increase the levels/effects of: Barbiturates; Ethosuximide; LamoTRIgine; LORazepam; Paliperidone; Primidone; RisperiDONE; Rufinamide; Temozolomide; Topiramate; Tricyclic Antidepressants; Vorinostat; Zidovudine

The levels/effects of Divalproex may be increased by: ChlorproMAZINE; Felbamate; GuanFACINE; Salicylates

Nutritional/Ethanol Interactions

Ethanol: Avoid ethanol (may increase CNS depression).

Food: Food may delay but does not affect the extent of absorption. Valproic acid serum concentrations may be decreased if taken with food. Milk has no effect on absorption.

Herb/Nutraceutical: Avoid evening primrose (seizure threshold decreased).

Adverse Reactions

>10%:

Central nervous system: Headache (≤31%), somnolence (≤30%), dizziness (12% to 25%), insomnia (>1% to 15%), nervousness (>1% to 11%), pain (1% to 11%)

Dermatologic: Alopecia (>1% to 24%)

Gastrointestinal: Nausea (15% to 48%), vomiting (7% to 27%), diarrhea (7% to 23%), abdominal pain (7% to 23%), dyspepsia (7% to 23%), anorexia (>1% to 12%)

Hematologic: Thrombocytopenia (1% to 24%; dose related)

Neuromuscular & skeletal: Tremor (≤57%), weakness (6% to 27%)

Ocular: Diplopia (>1% to 16%), amblyopia/blurred vision (≤12%)

Miscellaneous: Infection (≤20%), flu-like syndrome (12%)

1% to 10%:

Cardiovascular: Peripheral edema (>1% to 8%), chest pain (>1% to <5%), edema (>1% to <5%), facial edema (>1% to <5%), hypertension (>1% to <5%), hypotension (>1% to <5%), palpitation (>1% to <5%), postural hypotension (>1% to <5%), tachycardia (>1% to <5%), vasodilation (>1% to <5%), arrhythmia

Central nervous system: Ataxia (>1% to 8%), amnesia (>1% to 7%), emotional lability (>1% to 6%), fever (>1% to 6%), abnormal thinking (≤6%), depression (>1% to 5%), abnormal dreams (>1% to <5%), agitation (>1% to <5%), anxiety (>1% to <5%), catatonia (>1% to <5%), chills (>1% to <5%), confusion (>1% to <5%), coordination abnormal (>1% to <5%), hallucination (>1% to <5%), malaise (>1% to <5%), personality disorder (>1% to <5%), speech disorder (>1% to <5%), tardive dyskinesia (>1% to <5%), vertigo (>1% to <5%), euphoria (1%), hypoesthesia (1%)

Dermatologic: Rash (>1% to 6%), bruising (>1% to 5%), discoid lupus erythematosus (>1% to <5%), dry skin (>1% to <5%), furunculosis (>1% to <5%), petechia (>1% to <5%), pruritus (>1% to <5), seborrhea (>1% to <5%)

Endocrine & metabolic: Amenorrhea (>1% to <5%), dysmenorrhea (>1% to <5%), metrorrhagia (>1% to <5%), hypoproteinemia

Gastrointestinal: Weight gain (4% to 9%), weight loss (6%), appetite increased (≤6%), constipation (>1% to 5%), xerostomia (>1% to 5%), eructation (>1% to <5%), fecal incontinence (>1% to <5%), flatulence (>1% to <5%), gastroenteritis (>1% to <5%), glossitis (>1% to <5%), hematemesis (>1% to <5%), pancreatitis (>1% to <5%), periodontal abscess (>1% to <5%), stomatitis (>1% to <5%), taste perversion (>1% to <5%), dysphagia, gum hemorrhage, mouth ulceration

Genitourinary: Cystitis (>1% to 5%), dysuria (>1% to 5%), urinary frequency (>1% to <5%), urinary incontinence (>1% to <5%), vaginal hemorrhage (>1% to 5%), vaginitis (>1% to <5%)

Hepatic: ALT increased (>1% to <5%), AST increased (>1% to <5%)

Local: Injection site pain (3%), injection site reaction (2%), injection site inflammation (1%)

Neuromuscular & skeletal: Back pain (≤8%), abnormal gait (>1% to <5%), arthralgia (>1% to <5%), arthrosis (>1% to <5%), dysarthria (>1% to <5%), hypertonia (>1% to <5%), hypokinesia (>1% to <5%), leg cramps (>1% to <5%), myalgia (>1% to <5%), myasthenia (>1% to <5%), neck pain (>1% to <5%), neck rigidity (>1% to <5%), paresthesia (>1% to <5%), reflex increased (>1% to <5%), twitching (>1% to <5%)

Ocular: Nystagmus (1% to 8%), dry eyes (>1% to 5%), eye pain (>1% to 5%), abnormal vision (>1% to <5%), conjunctivitis (>1% to <5%)

Otic: Tinnitus (1% to 7%), ear pain (>1% to 5%), deafness (>1% to <5%), otitis media (>1% to <5%)

Respiratory: Pharyngitis (2% to 8%), bronchitis (5%), rhinitis (>1% to 5%), dyspnea (1% to 5%), cough (>1% to <5%), epistaxis (>1% to <5%), pneumonia (>1% to <5%), sinusitis (>1% to <5%)

Miscellaneous: Diaphoresis (1%), hiccups

Available Dosage Forms

Capsule, sprinkle, oral: 125 mg

Depakote® Sprinkle: 125 mg

Tablet, delayed release, oral: 125 mg, 250 mg, 500 mg

Depakote®: 125 mg, 250 mg, 500 mg

Tablet, extended release, oral: 250 mg, 500 mg

Depakote® ER: 250 mg, 500 mg

General Dosage Range Dosage adjustment recommended in patients with hepatic impairment

Oral:

Children and Adults: Simple and complex absence seizures: Initial: 15 mg/kg/day; Maintenance: Up to 60 mg/kg/day

Children ≥10 years and Adults: Complex partial seizures: Initial: 10-15 mg/kg/day in 1-3 divided doses; Maintenance: Up to 60 mg/kg/day

Children ≥16 years and Adults: Migraine prophylaxis: Depakote® ER: 500-1000 mg once daily; Depakote® 250 mg twice daily (maximum: 1000 mg/day)

Adults: Mania: Depakote®: Initial: 750 mg/day in divided doses; Depakote® ER: Initial: 25 mg/kg/day given once daily; Maintenance: Up to 60 mg/kg/day

Administration

Oral

Depakote® ER: Swallow whole; do not crush or chew. Patients who need dose adjustments smaller than 500 mg/day for migraine prophylaxis should be changed to Depakote® delayed release tablets.

Depakote® Sprinkle capsules may be swallowed whole or open capsule and sprinkle on small amount (1 teaspoonful) of soft food and use immediately (do not store or chew).

Stability

Storage

Depakote® tablet: Store below 30°C (86°F).

Depakote® Sprinkles: Store below 25°C (77°F).

Depakote® ER: Store at controlled room temperature of 25°C (77°F).

Nursing Actions

Physical Assessment Educate patients about accident prevention with a seizure disorder.

Patient Education Oral: Do not crush or chew capsule or enteric-coated pill. While using this medication, do not use alcohol. Maintain adequate hydration, unless instructed to restrict fluid intake. You may experience nervousness, decreased appetite, insomnia, headache, sleepiness, dizziness, visual changes, and hair loss. Report suicide ideation or depression; alterations in menstrual cycle; abdominal cramps, unresolved diarrhea, vomiting, or constipation; skin rash; tremors; unusual bruising or bleeding; blood in urine, stool, or vomitus; malaise; weakness; facial swelling; yellowing of skin or eyes; persistent abdominal pain; excessive sedation; change in mental status; extreme lethargy; or restlessness.

Dietary Considerations Divalproex may cause GI upset; take with large amount of water or food to decrease GI upset. May need to split doses to avoid GI upset.

Depakote® Sprinkle capsule contents may be mixed with semisolid food (eg, applesauce or pudding) in patients having difficulty swallowing; particles should be swallowed and not chewed.

DOBUTamine (doe BYOO ta meen)

Index Terms Dobutamine Hydrochloride

Pharmacologic Category Adrenergic Agonist Agent

Medication Safety Issues

Sound-alike/look-alike issues:

DOBUTamine may be confused with DOPamine

High alert medication:

The Institute for Safe Medication Practices (ISMP) includes this medication among its list of drugs which have a heightened risk of causing significant patient harm when used in error.

Pregnancy Risk Factor B

Lactation Excretion in breast milk unknown/use caution

Use Short-term management of patients with cardiac decompensation

Unlabeled Use Positive inotropic agent for use in myocardial dysfunction related to sepsis; stress echocardiography

Mechanism of Action/Effect Stimulates $beta_1$-adrenergic receptors, causing increased contractility and heart rate, with little effect on $beta_2$- or alpha-receptors

Contraindications Hypersensitivity to dobutamine or sulfites (some contain sodium metabisulfate), or any component of the formulation; idiopathic hypertrophic subaortic stenosis (IHSS)

Warnings/Precautions May increase heart rate. Patients with atrial fibrillation may experience an increase in ventricular response. An increase in blood pressure is more common, but occasionally a patient may become hypotensive. May exacerbate ventricular ectopy. If needed, correct hypovolemia first to optimize hemodynamics. Ineffective therapeutically in the presence of mechanical obstruction such as severe aortic stenosis. Use caution post-MI (can increase myocardial oxygen demand). Use cautiously in the elderly starting at lower end of the dosage range. Use with extreme caution in patients taking MAO inhibitors. Dobutamine in combination with stress echo may be used diagnostically. Product may contain sodium sulfite.

Drug Interactions

Avoid Concomitant Use

Avoid concomitant use of DOBUTamine with any of the following: Iobenguane I 123

Decreased Effect

DOBUTamine may decrease the levels/effects of: Iobenguane I 123

The levels/effects of DOBUTamine may be decreased by: Calcium Salts

Increased Effect/Toxicity

DOBUTamine may increase the levels/effects of: Sympathomimetics

The levels/effects of DOBUTamine may be increased by: Atomoxetine; Cannabinoids; COMT Inhibitors; Linezolid

Adverse Reactions Incidence of adverse events is not always reported.

Cardiovascular: Increased heart rate, increased blood pressure, increased ventricular ectopic activity, hypotension, premature ventricular beats (5%, dose related), anginal pain (1% to 3%), nonspecific chest pain (1% to 3%), palpitation (1% to 3%)

Central nervous system: Fever (1% to 3%), headache (1% to 3%), paresthesia

Endocrine & metabolic: Slight decrease in serum potassium

Gastrointestinal: Nausea (1% to 3%)

Hematologic: Thrombocytopenia (isolated cases)

Local: Phlebitis, local inflammatory changes and pain from infiltration, cutaneous necrosis (isolated cases)

Neuromuscular & skeletal: Mild leg cramps

Respiratory: Dyspnea (1% to 3%)

Pharmacodynamics/Kinetics

Onset of Action I.V.: 1-10 minutes; Peak effect: 10-20 minutes

Available Dosage Forms

Infusion, premixed in D_5W: 1 mg/mL (250 mL, 500 mL); 2 mg/mL (250 mL); 4 mg/mL (250 mL)

Injection, solution: 12.5 mg/mL (20 mL, 40 mL)

General Dosage Range I.V.: *Children and Adults:* 2.5-20 mcg/kg/minute (maximum: 40 mcg/kg/minute)

Administration

I.V. Always administer via infusion device; administer into large vein.

I.V. Detail pH: 2.5-5.5

Stability

Reconstitution Remix solution every 24 hours. Pink discoloration of solution indicates slight oxidation but **no** significant loss of potency.

Standard adult diluent: 250 mg/500 mL D_5W; 500 mg/500 mL D_5W.

Storage Store reconstituted solution under refrigeration for 48 hours or 6 hours at room temperature. Stability of parenteral admixture at room temperature (25°C) is 48 hours; at refrigeration (4°C) stability is 7 days.

Nursing Actions

Physical Assessment Infusion pump and frequent cardiac monitoring are required.

Patient Education When administered in emergencies, patient education should be appropriate to the situation. If patient is aware, instruct to promptly report chest pain, palpitations, rapid heartbeat, headache, nervousness or restlessness, nausea or vomiting, or respiratory difficulty.

Related Information

Compatibility of Drugs *on page 1264*

Docetaxel (doe se TAKS el)

Brand Names: U.S. Docefrez™; Taxotere®

Index Terms Docefrez™; RP-6976

Pharmacologic Category Antineoplastic Agent, Antimicrotubular; Antineoplastic Agent, Natural Source (Plant) Derivative; Antineoplastic Agent, Taxane Derivative

Medication Safety Issues

Sound-alike/look-alike issues:

DOCEtaxel may confused with PACLitaxel

Taxotere® may be confused with Taxol®

High alert medication:

This medication is in a class the Institute for Safe Medication Practices (ISMP) includes among its list of drug classes which have a heightened risk of causing significant patient harm when used in error.

Administration issues:

Multiple concentrations: Docetaxel is available as a one-vial formulation at concentrations of 10 mg/mL (generic formulation) and 20 mg/mL (concentrate; Taxotere®), and as a lyophilized powder (Docefrez™) which is reconstituted (with provided diluent) to 20 mg/0.8 mL (20 mg vial) or 24 mg/mL (80 mg vial). Docetaxel was previously available as a two-vial formulation (a concentrated docetaxel solution vial and a diluent vial) resulting in a reconstituted concentration of 10 mg/mL. The two-vial formulation has been discontinued by the manufacturer. Admixture errors have occurred due to the availability of various docetaxel concentrations.

Pregnancy Risk Factor D

Lactation Excretion in breast milk unknown/not recommended

Use Treatment of breast cancer (locally advanced/metastatic or adjuvant treatment of operable node-positive); locally-advanced or metastatic nonsmall cell lung cancer (NSCLC); hormone refractory, metastatic prostate cancer; advanced gastric adenocarcinoma; locally-advanced squamous cell head and neck cancer

Unlabeled Use Treatment of bladder cancer (metastatic), ovarian cancer, cervical cancer (relapsed), esophageal cancer, small cell lung cancer (relapsed), soft tissue sarcoma, Ewing's sarcoma, osteosarcoma, and unknown-primary adenocarcinoma

Available Dosage Forms

Injection, powder for reconstitution:

Docefrez™: 20 mg, 80 mg

Injection, solution: 10 mg/mL (2 mL, 8 mL, 16 mL)

Taxotere®: 20 mg/mL (1 mL, 4 mL)

General Dosage Range Dosage adjustment recommended in patients with hepatic impairment, on concomitant therapy, or who develop toxicities.

I.V.: *Adults:* 60-100 mg/m^2 every 3 weeks

Administration

I.V. Administer I.V. infusion over 1-hour through nonsorbing polyethylene lined (non-DEHP) tubing; in-line filter is not necessary (the use of a filter during administration is not recommended by the manufacturer). Infusion should be completed within 4 hours of final preparation. **Note:** Premedication with corticosteroids for 3 days, beginning the day before docetaxel administration, is recommended to prevent hypersensitivity reactions and fluid retention.

Nursing Actions

Physical Assessment Severe hypersensitivity reactions have been reported; premedication with dexamethasone may be advisable. Assess vital signs and weight prior to administration and monitor patient continuously during infusion (dosing adjustment may be necessary). Monitor for neutropenia, severe fluid retention, pleural effusion, and opportunistic infections prior to each infusion and on a regular basis.

Patient Education This medication can only be administered by infusion; report immediately any pain, burning, swelling, or redness at infusion site, difficulty breathing or swallowing, chest pain, or sudden chills. It is important to maintain adequate nutrition and hydration, unless instructed to restrict fluid intake. Ensure premedication prior to administration to prevent hypersensitivity. You will be more susceptible to infection. May cause nausea or vomiting, loss of hair (reversible), or diarrhea. Report immediately swelling of extremities, respiratory difficulty, unusual weight gain, abdominal distention, chest pain, palpitations, fever, chills, unusual bruising or bleeding, signs of infection, excessive fatigue, or rash.

Related Information

Management of Drug Extravasations *on page 1269*

Dofetilide (doe FET il ide)

Brand Names: U.S. Tikosyn®

Pharmacologic Category Antiarrhythmic Agent, Class III

Medication Guide Available Yes

Pregnancy Risk Factor C

Lactation Excretion in breast milk unknown/not recommended

Use Maintenance of normal sinus rhythm in patients with chronic atrial fibrillation/atrial flutter of longer than 1-week duration who have been converted to normal sinus rhythm; conversion of atrial fibrillation and atrial flutter to normal sinus rhythm

Unlabeled Use Alternative antiarrhythmic for the treatment of atrial fibrillation in patients with hypertrophic cardiomyopathy (HCM)

Available Dosage Forms

Capsule, oral:

Tikosyn®: 125 mcg, 250 mcg, 500 mcg

General Dosage Range Dosage adjustment recommended in patients with renal impairment

Oral: *Adults:* Initial: 500 mcg twice daily; Maintenance: 125-500 mcg twice daily **or** 125 mcg once daily

Administration

Oral Swallow capsules whole, do not chew or crush; Do not use damaged or opened capsules.

Nursing Actions

Physical Assessment Must be initiated or reinitiated by a cardiologist in a setting with continuous ECG monitoring for a period of time at beginning or adjustment of therapy. Monitor for signs of electrolyte imbalance (muscle weakness, spasms, twitching, numbness, lethargy, irregular heartbeat, and seizures).

Patient Education Do not open capsules. If you miss a dose, take your normal amount at the next scheduled time. You will need regular cardiac checkups and blood tests when taking this medication. You may experience headache, dizziness, difficulty sleeping, abdominal pain, diarrhea, or nausea. Inform prescriber immediately if you experience fainting, severe GI discomfort or diarrhea, chest palpitations, irregular heartbeat, chest pain, increased thirst, respiratory difficulty, skin rash, back pain, or alteration in muscle strength or gait.

Dolasetron (dol A se tron)

Brand Names: U.S. Anzemet®

Index Terms Dolasetron Mesylate; MDL 73,147EF

Pharmacologic Category Antiemetic; Selective 5-HT_3 Receptor Antagonist

Medication Safety Issues

Sound-alike/look-alike issues:

Anzemet® may be confused with Aldomet, Antivert®, Avandamet®

Dolasetron may be confused with granisetron, ondansetron, palonosetron

Pregnancy Risk Factor B

Lactation Excretion in breast milk unknown/use caution

Use

U.S. labeling:

Injection: Prevention and treatment of postoperative nausea and vomiting

Oral: Prevention of nausea and vomiting associated with emetogenic cancer chemotherapy (initial and repeat courses); prevention of postoperative nausea and vomiting

Canadian labeling: Oral: Prevention of nausea and vomiting associated with emetogenic cancer chemotherapy (initial and repeat courses)

Available Dosage Forms

Injection, solution:

Anzemet®: 20 mg/mL (0.625 mL, 5 mL, 25 mL)

Tablet, oral:

Anzemet®: 50 mg, 100 mg

General Dosage Range

I.V.:

Children 2-16 years: 0.35 mg/kg as a single dose (maximum: 12.5 mg)

Adults: 12.5 mg or 100 mg as a single dose

Oral:

Children 2-16 years: 1.2-1.8 mg/kg as a single dose (maximum: 100 mg/dose)

Adults: 100 mg as single dose

Administration

Oral When unable to administer in tablet form, dolasetron injection may be diluted in apple or apple-grape juice and taken orally; this dilution is stable for 2 hours at room temperature.

I.V. I.V. injection may be given either undiluted IVP over 30 seconds or diluted in 50 mL of compatible fluid and infused over 15 minutes. Flush line before and after dolasetron administration.

I.V. Detail pH: 3.2-3.8

Nursing Actions

Physical Assessment Allergy history to selective 5-HT_3 receptor antagonists should be assessed prior to administering. Assess other drugs patient may be taking that may prolong QT interval. I.V.: Follow infusion specifics. Oral and I.V. doses have different schedules and should not be administered on "PRN" basis.

Patient Education This drug is given to reduce the incidence of nausea and vomiting. If this medication is given by intravenous infusion you will be monitored during infusion. Report immediately any chest pain, respiratory difficulty, or pain or itching at infusion site. You may experience headache, drowsiness, or dizziness. Report chest pain or palpitations, persistent headache, excessive drowsiness, fever, constipation, or diarrhea.

Donepezil (doh NEP e zil)

Brand Names: U.S. Aricept®; Aricept® ODT

Index Terms E2020

Pharmacologic Category Acetylcholinesterase Inhibitor (Central)

Medication Safety Issues

Sound-alike/look-alike issues:

Aricept® may be confused with AcipHex®, Ascriptin®, and Azilect®

Pregnancy Risk Factor C

Lactation Excretion in breast milk unknown/not recommended

Use Treatment of mild, moderate, or severe dementia of the Alzheimer's type

Unlabeled Use Behavioral syndromes in dementia; mild-to-moderate dementia associated with Parkinson's disease; Lewy body dementia

Mechanism of Action/Effect Alzheimer's disease is characterized by cholinergic deficiency in the cortex and basal forebrain, which contributes to cognitive deficits. Donepezil reversibly and noncompetitively inhibits centrally-active acetylcholinesterase, the enzyme responsible for hydrolysis of acetylcholine. This appears to result in increased concentrations of acetylcholine available for synaptic transmission in the central nervous system.

Contraindications Hypersensitivity to donepezil, piperidine derivatives, or any component of the formulation

Warnings/Precautions Cholinesterase inhibitors may have vagotonic effects which may cause bradycardia and/or heart block with or without a history of cardiac disease; syncopal episodes have been associated with donepezil. Alzheimer's treatment guidelines consider bradycardia to be a relative contraindication for use of centrally-active cholinesterase inhibitors. Use with caution with sick sinus syndrome or other supraventricular cardiac conduction abnormalities, COPD, or asthma. Use with caution in patients with a history of seizure disorder; cholinomimetics may potentially cause generalized seizures, although seizure activity may also result from Alzheimer's disease. Use with caution in patients at risk of ulcer disease (eg, previous history or NSAID use), or in patients with bladder outlet obstruction. May cause dose-related diarrhea, nausea, and/or vomiting, which usually resolves in 1-3 weeks. May cause anorexia and/or weight loss (dose-related). May exaggerate neuromuscular blockade effects of depolarizing neuromuscular-blocking agents (eg, succinylcholine).

Drug Interactions

Avoid Concomitant Use There are no known interactions where it is recommended to avoid concomitant use.

Decreased Effect

Donepezil may decrease the levels/effects of: Anticholinergics; Neuromuscular-Blocking Agents (Nondepolarizing)

The levels/effects of Donepezil may be decreased by: Anticholinergics; Dipyridamole; Peginterferon Alfa-2b; Tocilizumab

Increased Effect/Toxicity

Donepezil may increase the levels/effects of: Antipsychotics; Beta-Blockers; Cholinergic Agonists; Succinylcholine

The levels/effects of Donepezil may be increased by: Conivaptan; Corticosteroids (Systemic)

Nutritional/Ethanol Interactions Herb/Nutraceutical: St John's wort may decrease donepezil levels. Ginkgo biloba may increase adverse effects/toxicity of acetylcholinesterase inhibitors.

Adverse Reactions

>10%:

Central nervous system: Insomnia (2% to 14%)

Gastrointestinal: Nausea (3% to 19%; dose related), diarrhea (5% to 15%; dose related)

Miscellaneous: Accident (7% to 13%), infection (11%)

1% to 10%:

Cardiovascular: Hypertension (3%), chest pain (2%), hemorrhage (2%), syncope (2%), hypotension, atrial fibrillation, bradycardia, ECG abnormal, edema, heart failure, hot flashes, peripheral edema, vasodilation

Central nervous system: Headache (3% to 10%), pain (3% to 9%), fatigue (1% to 8%), dizziness (2% to 8%), abnormal dreams (3%), hostility (3%), nervousness (1% to 3%), hallucinations (3%), depression (2% to 3%), confusion (2%), emotional lability (2%), personality disorder (2%), fever (2%), somnolence (2%), abnormal crying, aggression, agitation, anxiety, aphasia, delusions, irritability, restlessness, seizure, vertigo

Dermatologic: Bruising (4% to 5%), eczema (3%), pruritus, rash, skin ulcer, urticaria

Endocrine & metabolic: Dehydration (1% to 2%), hyperlipemia (2%), libido increased

Gastrointestinal: Anorexia (2% to 8%), vomiting (3% to 9%; dose related), weight loss (3% to 5%; dose related), abdominal pain, bloating, constipation, dyspepsia, epigastric pain, fecal incontinence, gastroenteritis, GI bleeding, toothache

Genitourinary: Urinary frequency (2%), urinary incontinence (1% to 3%), cystitis, hematuria, glycosuria, nocturia, UTI

Hematologic: Contusion (≤2%), anemia

Hepatic: Alkaline phosphatase increased

Neuromuscular & skeletal: Muscle cramps (3% to 8%), back pain (3%), CPK increased (3%), arthritis (1% to 2%), ataxia, bone fracture, gait abnormal, lactate dehydrogenase increased, paresthesia, tremor, weakness (1% to 2%)

Ocular: Blurred vision, cataract, eye irritation

Respiratory: Bronchitis, cough increased, dyspnea, pharyngitis, pneumonia, sore throat

Miscellaneous: Diaphoresis, fungal infection, flu symptoms, wandering

Available Dosage Forms

Tablet, oral: 5 mg, 10 mg

Aricept®: 5 mg, 10 mg, 23 mg

Tablet, orally disintegrating, oral: 5 mg, 10 mg

Aricept® ODT: 5 mg, 10 mg

General Dosage Range Oral: *Adults:* 5 mg once daily; Maintenance: 5-23 mg once daily

Administration

Oral Administer at bedtime without regard to food.

Aricept® 5 mg or 10 mg tablet: Swallow whole with water; do not split or crush per manufacturer's labeling. However, data available from the manufacturer showed that bioavailability was not affected by disintegration or dissolution when administered as a solution compared to a tablet during a bioequivalence study (data on file, Eisai Inc).

Aricept® 23 mg tablet: Swallow whole with water; do **NOT** crush or chew due to an increased rate of absorption. The 23 mg strength is provided in a unique film-coated formulation different from the 5 mg or 10 mg tablet strengths, which results in an altered pharmacokinetic profile.

Aricept® ODT: Allow tablet to dissolve completely on tongue and follow with water.

Stability

Storage Store at 15°C to 30°C (59°F to 86°F).

Nursing Actions

Physical Assessment Assess bladder adequacy prior to treatment. Monitor for cholinergic crisis (DUMBELS - **d**iarrhea, **u**rination, **m**iosis, **b**ronchospasm/**b**radycardia, **e**xcitability, **l**acrimation, and **s**alivation/excessive **s**weating). Monitor pulse.

Patient Education This medication will not cure the disease, but may help reduce symptoms. May cause dizziness, sedation, or hypotension; vomiting or loss of appetite; or diarrhea. Report persistent abdominal discomfort; significantly increased salivation, sweating, tearing, or urination; flushed skin; chest pain or palpitations; acute headache; unresolved diarrhea; excessive fatigue, insomnia, dizziness, or depression; increased muscle, joint, or body pain; vision changes or blurred vision; or shortness of breath or wheezing.

Dietary Considerations May take with or without food.

DOPamine (DOE pa meen)

Index Terms Dopamine Hydrochloride; Intropin

Pharmacologic Category Adrenergic Agonist Agent

Medication Safety Issues

Sound-alike/look-alike issues:

DOPamine may be confused with DOBUTamine, Dopram®

High alert medication:

The Institute for Safe Medication Practices (ISMP) includes this medication among its list of drugs which have a heightened risk of causing significant patient harm when used in error.

Pregnancy Risk Factor C

Lactation Excretion in breast milk unknown/use caution

Use Adjunct in the treatment of shock (eg, MI, open heart surgery, renal failure, cardiac decompensation) which persists after adequate fluid volume replacement

Unlabeled Use Symptomatic bradycardia or heart block unresponsive to atropine or pacing

Mechanism of Action/Effect Stimulates both adrenergic and dopaminergic receptors, lower doses are mainly dopaminergic stimulating and produce renal and mesenteric vasodilation, higher doses also are both dopaminergic and $beta_1$-adrenergic stimulating and produce cardiac stimulation and renal vasodilation; large doses stimulate alpha-adrenergic receptors

Contraindications Hypersensitivity to sulfites (commercial preparation contains sodium bisulfite); pheochromocytoma; ventricular fibrillation

Warnings/Precautions Use with caution in patients with cardiovascular disease or cardiac arrhythmias or patients with occlusive vascular disease. Correct hypovolemia and electrolytes when used in hemodynamic support. May cause increases in HR and arrhythmia. Use with caution in post-MI patients. Use with extreme caution in patients taking MAO inhibitors. Avoid extravasation; infuse into a large vein if possible. Avoid infusion into leg veins. Watch I.V. site closely. **[U.S. Boxed Warning]: If extravasation occurs, infiltrate the area with diluted phentolamine (5-10 mg in 10-15 mL of saline) with a fine hypodermic needle. Phentolamine should be administered as soon as possible after extravasation is noted.** Product may contain sodium metabisulfite.

Drug Interactions

Avoid Concomitant Use

Avoid concomitant use of DOPamine with any of the following: Inhalational Anesthetics; Iobenguane I 123; Lurasidone

Decreased Effect

DOPamine may decrease the levels/effects of: Iobenguane I 123

Increased Effect/Toxicity

DOPamine may increase the levels/effects of: Lurasidone; Sympathomimetics

The levels/effects of DOPamine may be increased by: Atomoxetine; Cannabinoids; COMT Inhibitors; Inhalational Anesthetics; Linezolid

Adverse Reactions Frequency not defined.

Cardiovascular: Ectopic beats, tachycardia, anginal pain, palpitation, hypotension, vasoconstriction

Central nervous system: Headache

Gastrointestinal: Nausea and vomiting

Respiratory: Dyspnea

Pharmacodynamics/Kinetics

Onset of Action Adults: 5 minutes

Duration of Action Adults: <10 minutes

Available Dosage Forms

Infusion, premixed in D_5W: 0.8 mg/mL (250 mL, 500 mL); 1.6 mg/mL (250 mL, 500 mL); 3.2 mg/mL (250 mL)

Injection, solution: 40 mg/mL (5 mL, 10 mL); 80 mg/mL (5 mL, 10 mL); 160 mg/mL (5 mL)

General Dosage Range I.V.:

Children: 1-20 mcg/kg/minute (maximum: 50 mcg/kg/minute)

Adults: 1-50 mcg/kg/minute

Administration

I.V. Vesicant. **Must be diluted prior to use.** Do not discontinue suddenly - sudden discontinuation may lead to marked hypotension.

I.V. Detail Monitor continuously for free flow. Administration into an umbilical arterial catheter is not recommended; central line administration.

Extravasation management: Due to short half-life, withdrawal of drug is often only necessary treatment. Use phentolamine as antidote. Mix 5 mg with 9 mL of NS; inject a small amount of this dilution into extravasated area. Blanching should reverse immediately. Monitor site. If blanching should recur, additional injections of phentolamine may be needed.

pH: 3.3-3.6

Stability

Storage Protect from light. Solutions that are darker than slightly yellow should not be used.

Nursing Actions

Physical Assessment Infusion pump and continuous cardiac and hemodynamic monitoring are required for inpatient therapy. Assess I.V. site frequently. Monitor cardiac status and renal function. Monitor for peripheral ischemia.

Patient Education When administered in emergencies, patient education should be appropriate to the situation. If patient is aware, instruct to promptly report chest pain, palpitations, rapid heartbeat, headache, nervousness or restlessness, nausea or vomiting, or respiratory difficulty.

Related Information

Compatibility of Drugs *on page 1264*

Management of Drug Extravasations *on page 1269*

Doripenem (dore i PEN em)

Brand Names: U.S. Doribax®

Index Terms S-4661

Pharmacologic Category Antibiotic, Carbapenem

Medication Safety Issues

Sound-alike/look-alike issues:

Doripenem may be confused with ertapenem

Doribax® may be confused with Zovirax®

Pregnancy Risk Factor B

Lactation Excretion in breast milk unknown/use caution

Breast-Feeding Considerations It is not known if doripenem is excreted into breast milk. The manufacturer recommends that caution be exercised when administering doripenem to nursing women.

Use Treatment of complicated intra-abdominal infections and complicated urinary tract infections (including pyelonephritis) due to susceptible aerobic gram-positive, aerobic gram-negative (including *Pseudomonas aeruginosa*), and anaerobic bacteria

Canadian labeling: Additional use (not in U.S. labeling): Treatment of healthcare-associated pneumonia (including ventilator-associated pneumonia)

Unlabeled Use

Treatment of intravascular catheter-related bloodstream infection due to extended-spectrum β-lactamase (ESBL)-producing *Escherichia coli* and *Klebsiella* spp

Mechanism of Action/Effect Inhibits cell wall synthesis in susceptible bacteria

Contraindications Known serious hypersensitivity to doripenem or other carbapenems (eg, ertapenem, imipenem, meropenem); anaphylactic reactions to beta-lactam antibiotics

Warnings/Precautions Serious hypersensitivity reactions, including anaphylaxis, and skin reactions have been reported in patients receiving beta-lactams. Use may result in fungal or bacterial superinfection, including *C. difficile*-associated diarrhea (CDAD) and pseudomembranous colitis; CDAD has been observed >2 months postantibiotic treatment. Not indicated for the treatment of pneumonia including ventilator-associated pneumonia; decreased efficacy and increased mortality associated with use. Use with caution in patients with renal impairment; dosage adjustment required in patients with moderate-to-severe renal dysfunction. Carbapenems have been associated with CNS adverse effects, including confusional states and seizures (myoclonic); use caution with CNS disorders (eg, brain lesions and history of seizures) and adjust dose in renal impairment to avoid drug accumulation, which may increase seizure risk. May decrease divalproex sodium/valproic acid concentrations leading to breakthrough seizures; concomitant use not recommended. Administer via intravenous infusion only. Per manufacturer's labeling, investigational experience of doripenem via inhalation resulted in pneumonitis.

Drug Interactions

Avoid Concomitant Use

Avoid concomitant use of Doripenem with any of the following: BCG; Probenecid

Decreased Effect

Doripenem may decrease the levels/effects of: BCG; Divalproex; Typhoid Vaccine; Valproic Acid

Increased Effect/Toxicity

The levels/effects of Doripenem may be increased by: Probenecid

Adverse Reactions

>10%:

Central nervous system: Headache (4% to 16%)

Gastrointestinal: Nausea (4% to 12%), diarrhea (6% to 11%)

1% to 10%:

Dermatologic: Rash (1% to 5%; includes allergic/bullous dermatitis, erythema, macular/papular eruptions, urticaria, and erythema multiforme), pruritus (≤3%)

Gastrointestinal: Oral candidiasis (1%)

Hematologic: Anemia (2% to 10%)

Hepatic: Transaminases increased (1% to 2%)

Local: Phlebitis (4% to 8%)

Renal: Renal impairment/failure (≤1%)

Miscellaneous: Vulvomycotic infection (1% to 2%)

Available Dosage Forms

Injection, powder for reconstitution:

Doribax®: 250 mg, 500 mg

General Dosage Range Dosage adjustment recommended in patients with renal impairment

I.V.: *Adults:* 500 mg every 8 hours

Administration

I.V. Infuse intravenously over 1 hour. Use of 4-hour infusion has been shown to increase %T>MIC. **Note:** The Canadian labeling recommends a 4-hour infusion in late-onset ventilator-associated pneumonia (>5 days ventilation [not an approved indication in the U.S. labeling])

Stability

Reconstitution Reconstitute 250 mg vial with 10 mL of SWFI or NS; further dilute for infusion with 50 mL or 100 mL of NS or D_5W. Shake gently until clear. Reconstitute 500 mg vial with 10 mL of SWFI or NS; further dilute for infusion with 100 mL of NS or D_5W. Shake gently until clear. Reconstituted vial may be stored for up to 1 hour prior to preparation of infusion solution. To prepare a 250 mg dose using a 500 mg vial, reconstitute the 500 mg vial with 10 mL of SWFI or NS and further dilute with 100 mL of compatible solution as above, but remove and discard 55 mL from the infusion bag to leave the remaining solution containing the 250 mg dose.

Storage Store dry powder vials at 15°C to 30°C (59°F to 86°F). Stability of solution when diluted in NS is 12 hours at room temperature or 72 hours under refrigeration; stability in D_5W is 4 hours at room temperature and 24 hours under refrigeration.

Nursing Actions

Physical Assessment Results of culture and sensitivity tests and patient history of previous allergies should be assessed prior to beginning treatment. Monitor closely for adverse reactions.

Patient Education This medication can only be administered intravenously. Report warmth, swelling, or irritation at infusion site; difficulty breathing; facial swelling; or acute anxiety. Maintain adequate nutrition and hydration, unless instructed to restrict fluid intake. Report prolonged GI effects (diarrhea, nausea), skin rash, or excessive or persistent fatigue or weakness.

Dornase Alfa (DOOR nase AL fa)

Brand Names: U.S. Pulmozyme®

Index Terms Recombinant Human Deoxyribonuclease; rhDNase

Pharmacologic Category Enzyme; Mucolytic Agent

Pregnancy Risk Factor B

Lactation Excretion in breast milk unknown/use caution

Use Management of cystic fibrosis patients to reduce the frequency of respiratory infections that require parenteral antibiotics in patients with FVC ≥40% of predicted; in conjunction with standard therapies, to improve pulmonary function in patients with cystic fibrosis

Available Dosage Forms

Solution, for nebulization [preservative free]:

Pulmozyme®: 2.5 mg/2.5 mL (30s)

General Dosage Range Inhalation: *Children ≥3 months and Adults:* 2.5 mg once daily

Nursing Actions

Physical Assessment Teach patient appropriate use of nebulizer.

Patient Education Inform prescriber of any allergies you have. Report skin rash, respiratory difficulty, wheezing, or cough. Self-administered nebulizer: Do not combine with any other medications in the nebulizer. Wash hands before and after treatment. Wash and dry nebulizer after each treatment. Twist open the top of one unit dose vial and squeeze contents into nebulizer reservoir. Connect nebulizer reservoir to the mouthpiece or face mask. Connect nebulizer to compressor. Sit in comfortable, upright position. Put on face mask and turn on compressor. Avoid leakage around the mask to avoid mist getting into eyes. Breathe calmly and deeply until no more mist is formed in nebulizer (about 5 minutes).

Dorzolamide (dor ZOLE a mide)

Brand Names: U.S. Trusopt®

Index Terms Dorzolamide Hydrochloride

Pharmacologic Category Carbonic Anhydrase Inhibitor; Ophthalmic Agent, Antiglaucoma

Pregnancy Risk Factor C

Lactation Excretion in breast milk unknown/not recommended

Use Treatment of elevated intraocular pressure in patients with ocular hypertension or open-angle glaucoma

Available Dosage Forms

Solution, ophthalmic: 2% (10 mL)

Trusopt®: 2% (10 mL)

General Dosage Range Ophthalmic: *Children and Adults:* Instill 1 drop into affected eye(s) 3 times/day

Administration

Other If more than one topical ophthalmic drug is being used, administer the drugs at least 10 minutes apart. Remove contact lens prior to administration and wait 15 minutes before reinserting. Instruct patients to avoid allowing the tip of the dispensing container to contact the eye or surrounding structures. Ocular solutions can become contaminated by common bacteria known to cause ocular infections. Serious damage to the eye and subsequent loss of vision may occur from using contaminated solutions.

Nursing Actions

Patient Education For use in eyes only. If serious or unusual reactions or signs of hypersensitivity occur, contact ophthalmologist. If any ocular reactions occur, particularly conjunctivitis and lid reactions, notify prescriber. Avoid allowing the tip of the dispensing container to contact the eye or surrounding structures. Take out contact lenses before using medicine. Lenses can be replaced 15 minutes after medicine is given.

Doxazosin (doks AY zoe sin)

Brand Names: U.S. Cardura®; Cardura® XL

Index Terms Doxazosin Mesylate

Pharmacologic Category Alpha$_1$ Blocker

Medication Safety Issues

Sound-alike/look-alike issues:

Doxazosin may be confused with doxapram, doxepin, DOXOrubicin

Cardura® may be confused with Cardene®, Cordarone®, Cordran®, Coumadin®, K-Dur®, Ridaura®

BEERS Criteria medication:

This drug may be inappropriate for use in geriatric patients (low severity risk).

Pregnancy Risk Factor C

Lactation Excretion in breast milk unknown/use caution

Breast-Feeding Considerations The extended release formulation is not indicated for use in women.

Use

Immediate release formulation: Treatment of hypertension as monotherapy or in conjunction with diuretics, ACE inhibitors, beta-blockers, or calcium antagonists

Immediate release and extended release formulations: Treatment of urinary outflow obstruction and/or obstructive and irritative symptoms associated with benign prostatic hyperplasia (BPH)

Unlabeled Use Pediatric hypertension

Mechanism of Action/Effect

Hypertension: Competitively inhibits postsynaptic alpha$_1$-adrenergic receptors which results in vasodilation of veins and arterioles and a decrease in total peripheral resistance and blood pressure; ~50% as potent on a weight by weight basis as prazosin.

BPH: Competitively inhibits postsynaptic alpha$_1$-adrenergic receptors in prostatic stromal and bladder neck tissues. This reduces the sympathetic tone-induced urethral stricture causing BPH symptoms.

Contraindications Hypersensitivity to quinazolines (prazosin, terazosin), doxazosin, or any component of the formulation

Warnings/Precautions Can cause significant orthostatic hypotension and syncope, especially with first dose; anticipate a similar effect if therapy is interrupted for a few days, if dosage is rapidly increased, or if another antihypertensive drug (particularly vasodilators) or a PDE-5 inhibitor is introduced. Discontinue if symptoms of angina occur or worsen. Patients should be cautioned about performing hazardous tasks when starting new therapy or adjusting dosage upward. Prostate cancer should be ruled out before starting for BPH. Use with caution in mild-to-moderate hepatic impairment; not recommended in severe dysfunction. Intraoperative floppy iris syndrome has been observed in cataract surgery patients who were on or were previously treated with alpha$_1$-blockers. Causality has not been established and there appears to be no benefit in discontinuing alpha-blocker therapy prior to surgery. May be inappropriate in the elderly due to potential for dry mouth, hypotension, and urinary problems (Beers Criteria).

The extended release formulation consists of drug within a nondeformable matrix; following drug release/absorption, the matrix/shell is expelled in the stool. The use of nondeformable products in patients with known stricture/narrowing of the GI tract has been associated with symptoms of obstruction. Use caution in patients with increased GI retention (eg, chronic constipation) as doxazosin exposure may be increased. Extended release formulation is not indicated for use in women or for the treatment of hypertension.

Drug Interactions

Avoid Concomitant Use

Avoid concomitant use of Doxazosin with any of the following: Alpha1-Blockers

Decreased Effect

The levels/effects of Doxazosin may be decreased by: Herbs (Hypertensive Properties); Methylphenidate; Yohimbine

Increased Effect/Toxicity

Doxazosin may increase the levels/effects of: Alpha1-Blockers; Amifostine; Antihypertensives; Calcium Channel Blockers; Hypotensive Agents; RiTUXimab

The levels/effects of Doxazosin may be increased by: Beta-Blockers; Diazoxide; Herbs (Hypotensive Properties); MAO Inhibitors; Pentoxifylline; Phosphodiesterase 5 Inhibitors; Prostacyclin Analogues

Nutritional/Ethanol Interactions Herb/Nutraceutical: Avoid dong quai if using for hypertension (has estrogenic activity). Avoid ephedra, yohimbe, ginseng (may worsen hypertension). Avoid saw palmetto when used for BPH (due to limited experience with this combination). Avoid garlic (may have increased antihypertensive effect).

Adverse Reactions Note: Type and frequency of adverse reactions reflect combined data from BPH and hypertension trials and immediate release and extended release products.

>10%: Central nervous system: Dizziness (5% to 19%), headache (5% to 14%)

1% to 10%:

Cardiovascular: Orthostatic hypotension (dose related; 0.3% up to 2%), edema (3% to 4%), hypotension (1% to 2%), palpitation (1% to 2%),

chest pain (1% to 2%), arrhythmia (1%), syncope (2%), flushing (1%)
Central nervous system: Fatigue (8% to 12%), somnolence (1% to 5%), nervousness (2%), pain (2%), vertigo (2% to 4%), insomnia (1%), anxiety (1%), paresthesia (1%), movement disorder (1%), ataxia (1%), hypertonia (1%), depression (1%)
Dermatologic: Rash (1%), pruritus (1%)
Endocrine & metabolic: Sexual dysfunction (2%)
Gastrointestinal: Abdominal pain (2%), diarrhea (2%), dyspepsia (1% to 2%), nausea (1% to 3%), xerostomia (1% to 2%), constipation (1%), flatulence (1%)
Genitourinary: Urinary tract infection (1%), impotence (1%), polyuria (2%), incontinence (1%)
Neuromuscular & skeletal: Back pain (2% to 3%), weakness (1% to 7%), arthritis (1%), muscle weakness (1%), myalgia (≤1%), muscle cramps (1%)
Ocular: Abnormal vision (1% to 2%), conjunctivitis (1%)
Otic: Tinnitus (1%)
Respiratory: Respiratory tract infection (5%), rhinitis (3%), dyspnea (1% to 3%), respiratory disorder (1%), epistaxis (1%)
Miscellaneous: Diaphoresis increased (1%), flu-like syndrome (1%)

Pharmacodynamics/Kinetics

Duration of Action >24 hours

Available Dosage Forms

Tablet, oral: 1 mg, 2 mg, 4 mg, 8 mg
Cardura®: 1 mg, 2 mg, 4 mg, 8 mg

Tablet, extended release, oral:
Cardura® XL: 4 mg, 8 mg

General Dosage Range Oral:
Extended release: *Adults:* Initial: 4 mg once daily; Maintenance: 4-8 mg/day (maximum: 8 mg/day)
Immediate release:
Adults: Initial: 1-4 mg once daily; Maintenance: 4-8 mg/day (maximum: 8 mg/day [BPH]; 16 mg/day [Hypertension])
Elderly: Initial: 0.5 mg once daily

Administration

Oral Cardura® XL: Tablets should be swallowed whole; do not crush, chew, or divide. Administer with morning meal.

Stability

Storage Store at 25°C (77°F); excursions permitted to 15°C to 30°C (59°F to 86°F).

Nursing Actions

Physical Assessment Assess blood pressure and monitor for hypotension, CNS changes, and urinary retention prior to treatment and on a regular basis. When discontinuing, monitor blood pressure and taper dose slowly over 1 week or more.

Patient Education Do not crush or chew extended release forms, swallow whole. Tablet shell may be visible in the stool. Follow recommended diet and exercise program. May cause drowsiness, dizziness, postural hypotension, or nausea. Report increased nervousness or depression; sudden weight gain; unusual or persistent swelling of ankles, feet, or extremities; palpitations or rapid heartbeat; or muscle weakness, fatigue, or pain.

Dietary Considerations Cardura® XL: Take with morning meal.

Doxepin (Systemic) (DOKS e pin)

Brand Names: U.S. Silenor®

Index Terms Doxepin Hydrochloride

Pharmacologic Category Antidepressant, Tricyclic (Tertiary Amine)

Medication Safety Issues

Sound-alike/look-alike issues:
Doxepin may be confused with digoxin, doxapram, doxazosin, Doxidan®, doxycycline
SINEquan® may be confused with saquinavir, SEROquel®, Singulair®, Zonegran®

BEERS Criteria medication:
This drug may be inappropriate for use in geriatric patients (high severity risk).

International issues:
Doxal [Finland] may be confused with Doxil brand name for doxorubicin (liposomal) [U.S., Israel]
Doxal brand name for doxepin [Finland] but also brand name for pyridoxine/thiamine [Brazil]

Medication Guide Available Yes

Pregnancy Risk Factor C

Lactation Enters breast milk/use caution (AAP rates "of concern"; AAP 2001 update pending)

Use Depression; treatment of insomnia (with difficulty of sleep maintenance)

Unlabeled Use Analgesic for certain chronic and neuropathic pain; anxiety

Available Dosage Forms

Capsule, oral: 10 mg, 25 mg, 50 mg, 75 mg, 100 mg, 150 mg

Solution, oral: 10 mg/mL (118 mL, 120 mL)

Tablet, oral:
Silenor®: 3 mg, 6 mg

General Dosage Range Dosage adjustment recommended for oral route in patients with hepatic impairment

Oral:
Adults: Initial: 25-150 mg/day in 2-3 divided doses; Maintenance: Up to 300 mg/day in single (≤150 mg) or divided doses; 3-6 mg once daily prior to bedtime (insomnia)
Elderly: Initial: 10-25 mg at bedtime; Maintenance: Up to 75 mg at bedtime

Administration

Oral Do not mix oral concentrate with carbonated beverages (physically incompatible).
Silenor®: Administer within 30 minutes prior to bedtime; do not take within 3 hours of food

Nursing Actions

Physical Assessment Monitor CNS status. Be alert for signs of clinical worsening, suicidal ideation, or other changes in behavior. Taper dosage slowly when discontinuing.

Patient Education It may take several weeks to achieve desired results. Avoid alcohol. Maintain adequate hydration, unless instructed to restrict fluid intake. You may experience drowsiness, lightheadedness, impaired coordination, dizziness, blurred vision, constipation, urinary retention, postural hypotension, altered sexual drive or ability (reversible), or photosensitivity. Report persistent CNS effects (eg, nervousness, restlessness, insomnia, anxiety, excitation, suicide ideation, headache, agitation, impaired coordination, changes in cognition); muscle cramping, weakness, tremors, or rigidity; chest pain, palpitations, or irregular heartbeat; blurred vision or eye pain; yellowing of skin or eyes; or worsening of condition.

Doxepin (Topical) (DOKS e pin)

Brand Names: U.S. Prudoxin™; Zonalon®

Index Terms Doxepin Hydrochloride

Pharmacologic Category Topical Skin Product

Medication Safety Issues

Sound-alike/look-alike issues:

Doxepin may be confused with digoxin, doxapram, doxazosin, Doxidan®, doxycycline

Zonalon® may be confused with Zone-A®

International issues:

Doxal [Finland] may be confused with Doxil brand name for doxorubicin (liposomal) [U.S., Israel]

Doxal brand name for doxepin [Finland] but also brand name for pyridoxine/thiamine [Brazil]

Pregnancy Risk Factor B

Lactation Enters breast milk/not recommended (AAP rates "of concern"; AAP 2001 update pending)

Use Short-term (<8 days) management of moderate pruritus in adults with atopic dermatitis or lichen simplex chronicus

Unlabeled Use Cream: Treatment of burning mouth syndrome and neuropathic pain

Available Dosage Forms

Cream, topical:

Prudoxin™: 5% (45 g)

Zonalon®: 5% (30 g, 45 g)

General Dosage Range

Dental: *Adults:* Apply 3-4 times/day

Topical: *Adults:* Apply a thin film 4 times/day (maximum total therapy: 8 days)

Administration

Topical Apply thin film to affected area; use of occlusive dressings is not recommended.

Nursing Actions

Patient Education Apply in thin layer; do not overuse. Report increased skin irritation, worsening of condition, or lack of improvement.

Doxercalciferol (doks er kal si fe FEER ole)

Brand Names: U.S. Hectorol®

Index Terms 1α-Hydroxyergocalciferol

Pharmacologic Category Vitamin D Analog

Pregnancy Risk Factor B

Lactation Excretion in breast milk unknown/not recommended

Use Treatment of secondary hyperparathyroidism in patients with chronic kidney disease

Available Dosage Forms

Capsule, softgel, oral:

Hectorol®: 0.5 mcg, 1 mcg, 2.5 mcg

Injection, solution:

Hectorol®: 2 mcg/mL (1 mL, 2 mL)

General Dosage Range

I.V.: *Adults:* Initial: 4 mcg 3 times/week after dialysis; Maintenance: Up to 18 mcg/week

Oral:

Adults (dialysis patients): Initial: 10 mcg 3 times/week at dialysis; Maintenance: Up to 60 mcg/week

Adults (predialysis patients): Initial: 1 mcg/day; Maintenance: Up to 3.5 mcg/day

Nursing Actions

Physical Assessment Provide appropriate nutritional counseling.

Patient Education Stop other vitamin D products. Report headache, dizziness, weakness, sleepiness, severe nausea, vomiting, dry mouth, loss of appetite, constipation, metallic taste, muscle and/or bone pain, malaise, and difficulty thinking or concentrating. Follow diet and calcium supplements as directed by prescriber.

DOXOrubicin (doks oh ROO bi sin)

Brand Names: U.S. Adriamycin®

Index Terms ADR (error-prone abbreviation); Adria; Conventional Doxorubicin; Doxorubicin Hydrochloride; Hydroxydaunomycin Hydrochloride; Hydroxyldaunorubicin Hydrochloride

Pharmacologic Category Antineoplastic Agent, Anthracycline

Medication Safety Issues

Sound-alike/look-alike issues:

DOXOrubicin may be confused with DACTINomycin, DAUNOrubicin, DAUNOrubicin liposomal, doxapram, doxazosin, DOXOrubicin liposomal, epirubicin, IDArubicin, valrubicin

Adriamycin PFS® may be confused with achromycin, Aredia®, Idamycin®

Conventional formulation (Adriamycin PFS®, Adriamycin RDF®) may be confused with the liposomal formulation (Doxil®)

High alert medication:

The Institute for Safe Medication Practices (ISMP) includes this medication among its list of drug classes which have a heightened risk of causing significant patient harm when used in error.

Administration issues:

Use caution when selecting product for preparation and dispensing; indications, dosages and adverse event profiles differ between conventional DOXOrubicin hydrochloride solution and DOXOrubicin liposomal. Both formulations are the same concentration. As a result, serious errors have occurred.

Other safety concerns:

ADR is an error-prone abbreviation

International issues:

Doxil® may be confused with Doxal® which is a brand name for doxepin in Finland, a brand name for doxycycline in Austria, and a brand name for pyridoxine/thiamine combination in Brazil

Rubex, a discontinued brand name for DOXOrubicin in the U.S, is a brand name for ascorbic acid in Ireland

Pregnancy Risk Factor D

Lactation Enters breast milk/not recommended

Breast-Feeding Considerations Doxorubicin and its metabolites are found in breast milk. Due to the potential for serious adverse reactions in the nursing infant, breast-feeding should be discontinued during treatment.

Use Treatment of acute lymphocytic leukemia (ALL), acute myeloid leukemia (AML), Hodgkin's disease, malignant lymphoma, soft tissue and bone sarcomas, thyroid cancer, small cell lung cancer, breast cancer, gastric cancer, ovarian cancer, bladder cancer, neuroblastoma, and Wilms' tumor

Unlabeled Use Treatment of multiple myeloma, endometrial carcinoma, uterine sarcoma, head and neck cancer, liver cancer, kidney cancer

Mechanism of Action/Effect Inhibits DNA and RNA synthesis, active throughout cell cycle, results in cell death.

Contraindications Hypersensitivity to doxorubicin, any component of the formulation, or to other anthracyclines or anthracenediones; recent MI, severe myocardial insufficiency, severe arrhythmia; previous therapy with high cumulative doses of doxorubicin, daunorubicin, idarubicin, or other anthracycline and anthracenediones; baseline neutrophil count <1500/mm^3; severe hepatic impairment

Warnings/Precautions Hazardous agent - use appropriate precautions for handling and disposal. **[U.S. Boxed Warning]: May cause cumulative, dose-related, myocardial toxicity (early or delayed).** Cardiotoxicity is dose-limiting. Total cumulative dose should take into account previous or concomitant treatment with cardiotoxic agents or irradiation of chest. The incidence of irreversible myocardial toxicity increases as the total cumulative (lifetime) dosages approach 450-500 mg/m^2. Although the risk increases with cumulative dose, irreversible cardiotoxicity may occur at any dose level. Patients with pre-existing heart disease, hypertension, concurrent administration of other antineoplastic agents, prior or concurrent chest irradiation, advanced age; and infants and children are at increased risk. Alternative administration schedules (weekly or continuous infusions) have are associated with less cardiotoxicity Baseline and periodic monitoring of ECG and LVEF (with either ECHO or MUGA scan) is recommended. **[U.S. Boxed Warnings]: Reduce dose in patients with impaired hepatic function; dose-limiting severe myelosuppression (primarily leukopenia and neutropenia) may occur. Secondary acute myelogenous leukemia and myelodysplastic syndrome have been reported following treatment.** May cause tumor lysis syndrome and hyperuricemia (in patients with rapidly growing tumors).

Children are at increased risk for developing delayed cardiotoxicity; follow-up cardiac function monitoring is recommended. Doxorubicin may contribute to prepubertal growth failure in children; may also contribute to gonadal impairment (usually temporary). Radiation recall pneumonitis has been reported in children receiving concomitant dactinomycin and doxorubicin. **[U.S. Boxed Warnings]: For I.V. administration only. Potent vesicant; if extravasation occurs, severe local tissue damage leading to ulceration, necrosis, and pain may occur. Should be administered under the supervision of an experienced cancer chemotherapy physician.** Use caution when selecting product for preparation and dispensing; indications, dosages and adverse event profiles differ between conventional doxorubicin hydrochloride solution and doxorubicin liposomal. Both formulations are the same concentration. As a result, serious errors have occurred.

Drug Interactions

Avoid Concomitant Use

Avoid concomitant use of DOXOrubicin with any of the following: BCG; CloZAPine; Conivaptan; Dabigatran Etexilate; Natalizumab; Pimecrolimus; Pimozide; Tacrolimus (Topical); Vaccines (Live)

Decreased Effect

DOXOrubicin may decrease the levels/effects of: BCG; Cardiac Glycosides; Coccidioidin Skin Test; Dabigatran Etexilate; Linagliptin; P-glycoprotein/ABCB1 Substrates; Sipuleucel-T; Stavudine; Vaccines (Inactivated); Vaccines (Live); Vitamin K Antagonists; Zidovudine

The levels/effects of DOXOrubicin may be decreased by: Cardiac Glycosides; CYP3A4 Inducers (Strong); Deferasirox; Echinacea; Peginterferon Alfa-2b; P-glycoprotein/ABCB1 Inducers; Tocilizumab

Increased Effect/Toxicity

DOXOrubicin may increase the levels/effects of: ARIPiprazole; CloZAPine; CYP2B6 Substrates; Leflunomide; Natalizumab; Pimozide; Vaccines (Live); Vitamin K Antagonists; Zidovudine

The levels/effects of DOXOrubicin may be increased by: Bevacizumab; Conivaptan; CycloSPORINE; CycloSPORINE (Systemic); CYP2D6 Inhibitors (Moderate); CYP2D6 Inhibitors (Strong); CYP3A4 Inhibitors (Moderate); CYP3A4 Inhibitors (Strong); Dasatinib; Denosumab; P-glycoprotein/ABCB1 Inhibitors; Pimecrolimus; Roflumilast; SORAfenib; Tacrolimus (Topical); Taxane Derivatives; Trastuzumab

Nutritional/Ethanol Interactions Herb/Nutraceutical: Avoid St John's wort (may decrease doxorubicin levels). Avoid black cohosh, dong quai in estrogen-dependent tumors.

Adverse Reactions Frequency not defined.

Cardiovascular:

Acute cardiotoxicity: Atrioventricular block, bradycardia, bundle branch block, ECG abnormalities, extrasystoles (atrial or ventricular), sinus tachycardia, ST-T wave changes, supraventricular tachycardia, tachyarrhythmia, ventricular tachycardia

Delayed cardiotoxicity: LVEF decreased, CHF (manifestations include ascites, cardiomegaly, dyspnea, edema, gallop rhythm, hepatomegaly, oliguria, pleural effusion, pulmonary edema, tachycardia); myocarditis, pericarditis

Central nervous system: Malaise

Dermatologic: Alopecia, itching, photosensitivity, radiation recall, rash; discoloration of saliva, sweat, or tears

Endocrine & metabolic: Amenorrhea, dehydration, infertility (may be temporary), hyperuricemia

Gastrointestinal: Abdominal pain, anorexia, colon necrosis, diarrhea, GI ulceration, mucositis, nausea, vomiting

Genitourinary: Discoloration of urine

Hematologic: Leukopenia/neutropenia (75%; nadir: 10-14 days; recovery: by day 21); thrombocytopenia and anemia

Local: Skin "flare" at injection site, urticaria

Neuromuscular & skeletal: Weakness

Available Dosage Forms

Injection, powder for reconstitution: 10 mg, 50 mg

Adriamycin®: 10 mg, 20 mg, 50 mg

Injection, solution [preservative free]: 2 mg/mL (5 mL, 10 mL, 25 mL, 75 mL, 100 mL)

Adriamycin®: 2 mg/mL (5 mL, 10 mL, 25 mL, 100 mL)

General Dosage Range

Dosage adjustment recommended in patients with hepatic impairment or who develop toxicities

I.V.: *Children and Adults:* Dosage varies greatly depending on indication

Administration

I.V. Vesicant. Administer I.V. push over at least 3-5 minutes or by continuous infusion (infusion via central venous line recommended).

I.V. Detail May be further diluted in either NS of D_5W for I.V. administration. Avoid extravasation associated with severe ulceration and soft tissue necrosis. Flush with 5-10 mL of I.V. solution before and after drug administration. Incompatible with heparin. Monitor for local erythematous streaking along vein and/or facial flushing (may indicate rapid infusion rate).

pH: 3.8-6.5 (lyophilized doxorubicin HCl reconstituted with sodium chloride 0.9%); 2.5-4.5 (adjusted solution)

Stability

Reconstitution Reconstitute lyophilized powder with NS to a final concentration of 2 mg/mL (may further dilute in 50-1000 mL D_5W or NS for infusion). Unstable in solutions with a pH <3 or >7.

Storage Store intact vials of solution under refrigeration at 2°C to 8°C. Protected from light. Store intact vials of lyophilized powder at room temperature (15°C to 30°C). Reconstituted vials are stable for 7 days at room temperature (25°C) and 15 days under refrigeration (5°C) when protected from light. Infusions are stable for 48 hours at room temperature (25°C) when protected from light. Solutions diluted in 50-1000 mL D_5W or NS are stable for 48 hours at room temperature (25°C) when protected from light.

Nursing Actions

Physical Assessment Premedication with antiemetic may be ordered (especially with larger doses). Monitor infusion site closely; extravasation can cause sloughing or tissue necrosis (do not apply heat or sodium bicarbonate). Teach patient importance of adequate hydration.

Patient Education This medication can only be administered intravenously. Report immediately any swelling, pain, burning, or redness at infusion site. Maintain adequate nutrition. You will be more susceptible to infection. May cause nausea or vomiting, diarrhea, loss of hair (reversible), or darker yellow urine (normal). Report immediately chest pain, swelling of extremities, respiratory difficulty, palpitations, or rapid heartbeat. Report unresolved nausea, vomiting, or diarrhea; alterations in urinary pattern (increased or decreased); opportunistic infection (fever, chills, unusual bruising or bleeding fatigue, purulent vaginal discharge, unhealed mouth sores); abdominal pain or blood in stools; excessive fatigue; or yellowing of eyes or skin.

Related Information

Management of Drug Extravasations *on page 1269*

DOXOrubicin (Liposomal)

(doks oh ROO bi sin lye po SO mal)

Brand Names: U.S. Doxil®

Index Terms DOXOrubicin Hydrochloride (Liposomal); DOXOrubicin Hydrochloride Liposome; Lipodox; Liposomal DOXOrubicin; Pegylated DOXOrubicin Liposomal; Pegylated Liposomal DOXOrubicin

Pharmacologic Category Antineoplastic Agent, Anthracycline

Medication Safety Issues

Sound-alike/look-alike issues:

DOXOrubicin liposomal may be confused with DACTINomycin, DAUNOrubicin, DAUNOrubicin liposomal, doxapram, doxazosin, DOXOrubicin, epirubicin, IDArubicin, valrubicin

DOXOrubicin liposomal may be confused with DAUNOrubicin liposomal

Doxil® may be confused with Doxy 100™, Paxil®

Liposomal formulation (Doxil®) may be confused with the conventional formulation (Adriamycin PFS®, Adriamycin RDF®)

High alert medication:

This medication is in a class the Institute for Safe Medication Practices (ISMP) includes among its list of drug classes which have a heightened risk of causing significant patient harm when used in error.

Administration issues:

Use caution when selecting product for preparation and dispensing; indications, dosages and adverse event profiles differ between conventional DOXOrubicin hydrochloride solution and DOXOrubicin liposomal. Both formulations are the same concentration. As a result, serious errors have occurred. Liposomal formulation of doxorubicin should NOT be substituted for doxorubicin hydrochloride on a mg-per-mg basis.

International issues:

Doxil [U.S., Israel] may be confused with Doxal brand name for doxepin [Finland} and pyridoxine/thiamine [Brazil]

Pregnancy Risk Factor D

Lactation Excretion in breast milk unknown/contraindicated

Breast-Feeding Considerations Due to the potential for serious adverse reactions in the nursing infant, breast-feeding is contraindicated.

Use Treatment of ovarian cancer (progressive or recurrent), multiple myeloma (after failure of at least 1 prior therapy), and AIDS-related Kaposi's sarcoma (after failure of or intolerance to prior systemic therapy)

Unlabeled Use Treatment of metastatic breast cancer, Hodgkin's lymphoma, cutaneous T-cell lymphomas (mycosis fungoides and Sézary syndrome), advanced soft tissue sarcomas; advanced or metastatic uterine sarcoma

Mechanism of Action/Effect Inhibits DNA and RNA synthesis of susceptible bacteria, active throughout cell cycle, results in cell death

Contraindications Hypersensitivity to doxorubicin liposomal, conventional doxorubicin, or any component of the formulation; breast-feeding

Warnings/Precautions Hazardous agent - use appropriate precautions for handling and disposal.

[U.S. Boxed Warning]: Doxorubicin may cause cumulative, dose-related myocardial toxicity (concurrent or delayed). Doxorubicin liposomal should be used with caution in patients with high cumulative doses of any anthracycline. Total cumulative dose should also account for previous or concomitant treatment with other cardiotoxic agents or irradiation of chest. The incidence of irreversible myocardial toxicity increases as the total cumulative (lifetime) dosages approach 450-550 mg/m^2; or 400 mg/m^2 in patients who have received prior mediastinal radiation therapy or concurrent therapy with other cardiotoxic agents (eg, cyclophosphamide). Although the risk increases with cumulative dose, irreversible cardiotoxicity may occur with anthracycline treatment at any dose level. Patients with pre-existing heart disease, hypertension, concurrent administration of other antineoplastic agents, prior or concurrent chest irradiation, and advanced age are at increased risk. Evaluate left ventricular ejection fraction (LVEF) prior to treatment and periodically during treatment. The onset of symptoms of anthracycline-induced HF and/or cardiomyopathy may be delayed.

[U.S. Boxed Warning]: Acute infusion reactions may occur, some may be serious/life-threatening, including fatal allergic/anaphylactoid-like reactions. Infusion reactions typically occur with the first infusion and may include flushing, dyspnea, facial swelling, headache, chills, back pain, hypotension, and/or tightness of chest/throat. Reactions usually resolve with termination of infusion, or in some cases, slowing the infusion rate. Medication for the treatment of reactions should be readily available in the event of severe reactions. Infuse doxorubicin liposomal at 1 mg/minute initially to minimize risk of infusion reaction.

[U.S. Boxed Warning]: Use with caution in patients with hepatic impairment; dosage reduction is recommended. Use in patients with hepatic impairment has not been adequately studied; dosing adjustment recommendations in multiple myeloma patients with hepatic impairment is not available. **[U.S. Boxed Warning]: Severe myelosuppression may occur.** Palmar-plantar erythrodysesthesia (hand-foot syndrome) has been reported in up to 51% of patients with ovarian cancer, 19% of patients with multiple myeloma, and ~3% in patients with Kaposi's sarcoma. May occur early in treatment, but is usually seen after 2-3 treatment cycles. Dosage modification may be required. In severe cases, treatment discontinuation may be required. **[U.S. Boxed Warning]: Liposomal formulations of doxorubicin should NOT be substituted for conventional doxorubicin hydrochloride on a mg-per-mg basis.**

Doxorubicin may potentiate the toxicity of cyclophosphamide (hemorrhagic cystitis) and mercaptopurine (hepatotoxicity). Radiation recall reaction has been reported with doxorubicin liposomal treatment after radiation therapy. Radiation-induced toxicity (to the myocardium, mucosa, skin, and liver) may be increased by doxorubicin.

Drug Interactions

Avoid Concomitant Use

Avoid concomitant use of DOXOrubicin (Liposomal) with any of the following: BCG; CloZAPine; Conivaptan; Natalizumab; Pimecrolimus; Tacrolimus (Topical); Vaccines (Live)

Decreased Effect

DOXOrubicin (Liposomal) may decrease the levels/effects of: BCG; Cardiac Glycosides; Coccidioidin Skin Test; Sipuleucel-T; Stavudine; Vaccines (Inactivated); Vaccines (Live); Zidovudine

The levels/effects of DOXOrubicin (Liposomal) may be decreased by: Cardiac Glycosides; CYP3A4 Inducers (Strong); Deferasirox; Echinacea; Herbs (CYP3A4 Inducers); Peginterferon Alfa-2b; Tocilizumab

Increased Effect/Toxicity

DOXOrubicin (Liposomal) may increase the levels/effects of: CloZAPine; CYP2B6 Substrates; Leflunomide; Natalizumab; Vaccines (Live); Zidovudine

The levels/effects of DOXOrubicin (Liposomal) may be increased by: Abiraterone Acetate; Bevacizumab; Conivaptan; CYP2D6 Inhibitors (Moderate); CYP2D6 Inhibitors (Strong); CYP3A4 Inhibitors (Moderate); CYP3A4 Inhibitors (Strong); Darunavir; Dasatinib; Denosumab; Ivacaftor; Pimecrolimus; Roflumilast; Tacrolimus (Topical); Taxane Derivatives; Trastuzumab

Nutritional/Ethanol Interactions

Ethanol: Avoid ethanol (due to GI irritation).

Herb/Nutraceutical: St John's wort may decrease doxorubicin levels.

Adverse Reactions

>10%:

Cardiovascular: Peripheral edema (≤11%)

Central nervous system: Fever (8% to 21%), headache (≤11%), pain (≤21%)

Dermatologic: Palmar-plantar erythrodysesthesia/hand-foot syndrome (≤51% in ovarian cancer [grades 3/4: 24%]; 3% in Kaposi's sarcoma), rash (≤29% in ovarian cancer, ≤5% in Kaposi's sarcoma), alopecia (9% to 19%)

Gastrointestinal: Nausea (17% to 46%), stomatitis (5% to 41%), vomiting (8% to 33%), constipation (≤30%), diarrhea (5% to 21%), anorexia (≤20%), mucositis (≤14%), dyspepsia (≤12%), intestinal obstruction (≤11%)

Hematologic: Myelosuppression (onset: 7 days; nadir: 10-14 days; recovery: 21-28 days), thrombocytopenia (13% to 65%; grades 3/4: 1%), neutropenia (12% to 62%; grade 4: 4%), leukopenia (36%), anemia (6% to 74%; grade 4: <1%)

Neuromuscular & skeletal: Weakness (7% to 40%), back pain (≤12%)

Respiratory: Pharyngitis (≤16%), dyspnea (≤15%)

Miscellaneous: Infection (≤12%)

1% to 10%:

Cardiovascular: Cardiac arrest, chest pain, deep thrombophlebitis, edema, hypotension, pallor, tachycardia, vasodilation

Central nervous system: Agitation, anxiety, chills, confusion, depression, dizziness, emotional lability, insomnia, somnolence, vertigo

Dermatologic: Acne, bruising, dry skin (6%), exfoliative dermatitis, fungal dermatitis, furunculosis, maculopapular rash, pruritus, skin discoloration, vesiculobullous rash

Endocrine & metabolic: Dehydration, hypercalcemia, hyperglycemia, hypokalemia, hyponatremia

Gastrointestinal: Abdomen enlarged, anorexia, ascites, cachexia, dyspepsia, dysphagia, esophagitis, flatulence, gingivitis, glossitis, ileus, mouth ulceration, oral moniliasis, rectal bleeding, taste perversion, weight loss, xerostomia

Genitourinary: Cystitis, dysuria, leukorrhea, pelvic pain, polyuria, urinary incontinence, urinary tract infection, urinary urgency, vaginal bleeding, vaginal moniliasis

Hematologic: Hemolysis, prothrombin time increased

Hepatic: ALT increased, alkaline phosphatase increased, hyperbilirubinemia

Local: Thrombophlebitis

Neuromuscular & skeletal: Arthralgia, hypertonia, myalgia, neuralgia, neuritis (peripheral), neuropathy, paresthesia (≤10%), pathological fracture

Ocular: Conjunctivitis, dry eyes, retinitis

Otic: Ear pain

Renal: Albuminuria, hematuria

Respiratory: Apnea, cough (≤10%), epistaxis, pleural effusion, pneumonia, rhinitis, sinusitis

Miscellaneous: Allergic reaction; infusion-related reactions (7%; includes bronchospasm, chest tightness, chills, dyspnea, facial edema, flushing, headache, herpes simplex/zoster, hypotension, pruritus); moniliasis, diaphoresis

Available Dosage Forms

Injection, solution:

Doxil®: 2 mg/mL (10 mL, 25 mL)

General Dosage Range Dosage adjustment recommended in patients with hepatic impairment or who develop toxicities

I.V.: *Adults:* 20-30 mg/m^2 every 3 weeks **or** 50 mg/m^2 every 4 weeks

Administration

I.V. Irritant; avoid extravasation. Administer IVPB over 60 minutes; manufacturer recommends administering at initial rate of 1 mg/minute to minimize risk of infusion reactions until the absence of a reaction has been established, then increase the infusion rate for completion over 1 hour. Do **NOT** administer undiluted, as a bolus injection, or I.M. or SubQ.

Do **NOT** infuse with in-line filters. Avoid extravasation (irritant), monitor site; extravasation may occur without stinging or burning. Flush with 5-10 mL of D_5W solution before and after drug administration (do not rapidly flush through the I.V. line), incompatible with heparin flushes. Monitor for local erythematous streaking along vein and/or facial flushing (may indicate rapid infusion rate).

Stability

Reconstitution Doses of doxorubicin liposomal ≤90 mg must be diluted in 250 mL of D_5W prior to administration. Doses >90 mg should be diluted in 500 mL D_5W. Solution is not a clear, but has a red, translucent appearance due to the liposomal dispersion. Use appropriate precautions for handling and disposal.

Storage Store intact vials of solution under refrigeration at 2°C to 8°C (36°F to 46°F); avoid freezing. Prolonged freezing may adversely affect liposomal drug products, however, short-term freezing (<1 month) does not appear to have a deleterious effect. Diluted doxorubicin hydrochloride liposome injection may be refrigerated at 2°C to 8°C (36°F to 46°F); administer within 24 hours. **Do not infuse with in-line filters.**

Nursing Actions

Physical Assessment Radiation recall may be experienced with this drug, noted by a reddened, burned appearance over the area radiated. Note and be aware of past cumulative doxorubicin dose, as patients can develop cardiotoxicity. Obtain MUGA scan or ECHO prior to doxorubicin (liposomal) therapy to evaluate for ejection fraction. Verify drug is mixed in D_5W solution. If patient is at home and needs help with ADLs, thorough instruction on handling body fluids should be reviewed. This drug has a potential for hypersensitivity reactions and patients should be prescribed Benadryl® as a premedication. Monitor closely throughout infusion for HSR, as these have the potential to be fatal.

Patient Education Instruct patients to inform prescriber if they have received past chemotherapy, especially doxorubicin, or radiation therapy, or if they have liver or heart disease. Inform patients to monitor for symptoms of infection, fever, chills, cough, sore throat, and painful urination. Teach patients symptoms of hypersensitivity reactions, which includes shortness of breath, flushing, chest tightness, or back pain. Patients' families or caregivers should understand the importance of wearing gloves and protecting themselves from blood or body fluids at home. Urine may be reddened or discolored during the first urination after medication is received. Patients should be cautioned against wearing tight, constrictive clothing or clothing that causes friction, as this can potentiate palmar-plantar erythematous areas. Patients will lose their hair about 10 days to 2 weeks after this drug has been initiated.

Related Information

Management of Drug Extravasations *on page 1269*

Doxycycline (doks i SYE kleen)

Brand Names: U.S. Adoxa®; Adoxa® Pak™ 1/150 [DSC]; Adoxa® Pak™ 1/75 [DSC]; Alodox™; Doryx®; Doxy 100™; Monodox®; Ocudox™; Oracea®; Oraxyl™; Periostat®; Vibramycin®

Index Terms Doxycycline Calcium; Doxycycline Hyclate; Doxycycline Monohydrate

Pharmacologic Category Antibiotic, Tetracycline Derivative

Medication Safety Issues

Sound-alike/look-alike issues:

Doxycycline may be confused with dicyclomine, doxepin, doxylamine

Doxy100™ may be confused with Doxil®

Monodox® may be confused with Maalox®

Oracea® may be confused with Orencia®

Vibramycin® may be confused with vancomycin, Vibativ™

Pregnancy Risk Factor D

Lactation Enters breast milk/not recommended

Breast-Feeding Considerations Tetracyclines, including doxycycline, are excreted in breast milk and therefore, breast-feeding is not recommended by the manufacturer.

Doxycycline is less bound to the calcium in maternal milk which may lead to increased absorption compared to other tetracyclines. Only minimal amounts of doxycycline are excreted in human milk and the relative amount of tooth staining has been reported to be lower when compared to other tetracycline analogs. Nondose-related effects could include modification of bowel flora.

Use Principally in the treatment of infections caused by susceptible *Rickettsia*, *Chlamydia*, and *Mycoplasma*; alternative to mefloquine for malaria prophylaxis; treatment for syphilis, uncomplicated *Neisseria gonorrhoeae*, *Listeria*, *Actinomyces israelii*, and *Clostridium* infections in penicillin-allergic patients; used for community-acquired pneumonia and other common infections due to susceptible organisms; anthrax due to *Bacillus anthracis,* including inhalational anthrax (postexposure); treatment of infections caused by uncommon susceptible gram-negative and gram-positive organisms including *Borrelia recurrentis*, *Ureaplasma urealyticum*, *Haemophilus ducreyi*, *Yersinia pestis*, *Francisella tularensis*, *Vibrio cholerae*, *Campylobacter fetus*, *Brucella* spp, *Bartonella bacilliformis*, and *Klebsiella granulomatis,* Q fever, Lyme disease; treatment of inflammatory lesions associated with rosacea; intestinal amebiasis; severe acne

Unlabeled Use Sclerosing agent for pleural effusion injection; vancomycin-resistant enterococci (VRE); alternate treatment for MRSA infections; treatment of periodontitis (refractory); localized juvenile periodontitis (LJP)

Mechanism of Action/Effect Inhibits protein synthesis by binding with the 30S and possibly the 50S ribosomal subunit(s) of susceptible bacteria; may also cause alterations in the cytoplasmic membrane

Doxycycline inhibits collagenase *in vitro* and has been shown to inhibit collagenase in the gingival crevicular fluid in adults with periodontitis

Contraindications Hypersensitivity to doxycycline, tetracycline or any component of the formulation; children <8 years of age (except in treatment of anthrax exposure and tickborne rickettsial disease)

Warnings/Precautions Photosensitivity reaction may occur with this drug; avoid prolonged exposure to sunlight or tanning equipment. Antianabolic effects of tetracyclines can increase BUN (dose-related). Autoimmune syndromes have been reported. Hepatotoxicity rarely occurs; if symptomatic, conduct LFT and discontinue drug. Pseudotumor cerebri has been (rarely) reported with tetracycline use; usually resolves with discontinuation. Prolonged use may result in fungal or bacterial superinfection, including *C. difficile*-associated diarrhea (CDAD) and pseudomembranous colitis; CDAD has been observed >2 months postantibiotic treatment. May cause tissue hyperpigmentation, enamel hypoplasia, or permanent tooth discoloration; use of tetracyclines should be avoided during tooth development (children <8 years of age) unless other drugs are not likely to be effective or are contraindicated. However, recommended in treatment of anthrax exposure and tickborne rickettsial diseases. Do not use during pregnancy. In addition to affecting tooth development, tetracycline use has been associated with retardation of skeletal development and reduced bone growth.

Additional specific warnings: Oracea®: Should not be used for the treatment or prophylaxis of bacterial infections, since the lower dose of drug per capsule may be subefficacious and promote resistance. Syrup contains sodium metabisulfite. Effectiveness of products intended for use in periodontitis has not been established in patients with coexistent oral candidiasis; use with caution in patients with a history or predisposition to oral candidiasis.

Drug Interactions

Avoid Concomitant Use

Avoid concomitant use of Doxycycline with any of the following: BCG; Pimozide; Retinoic Acid Derivatives

Decreased Effect

Doxycycline may decrease the levels/effects of: BCG; Penicillins; Typhoid Vaccine

The levels/effects of Doxycycline may be decreased by: Antacids; Barbiturates; Bile Acid Sequestrants; Bismuth; Bismuth Subsalicylate; Calcium Salts; CarBAMazepine; Fosphenytoin; Iron Salts; Lanthanum; Magnesium Salts; Phenytoin; Quinapril; Sucralfate

Increased Effect/Toxicity

Doxycycline may increase the levels/effects of: ARIPiprazole; Neuromuscular-Blocking Agents; Pimozide; Porfimer; Retinoic Acid Derivatives; Vitamin K Antagonists

Nutritional/Ethanol Interactions

Ethanol: Chronic ethanol ingestion may reduce the serum concentration of doxycycline.

Food: Doxycycline serum levels may be slightly decreased if taken with food or milk. Administration with iron or calcium may decrease doxycycline absorption. May decrease absorption of calcium, iron, magnesium, zinc, and amino acids.

Herb/Nutraceutical: St John's wort may decrease doxycycline levels. Avoid dong quai, St John's wort (may also cause photosensitization).

Adverse Reactions Frequency not defined.

Cardiovascular: Intracranial hypertension, pericarditis

Dermatologic: Angioneurotic edema, erythema multiforme, exfoliative dermatitis (rare), photosensitivity, rash, skin hyperpigmentation, Stevens-Johnson syndrome, toxic epidermal necrolysis, urticaria

Endocrine & metabolic: Brown/black discoloration of thyroid gland (no dysfunction reported), hypoglycemia

Gastrointestinal: Anorexia, diarrhea, dysphagia, enterocolitis, esophagitis (rare), esophageal ulcerations (rare), glossitis, inflammatory lesions in anogenital region, nausea, oral (mucosal) pigmentation, pseudomembranous colitis, tooth discoloration (children), vomiting

Hematologic: Eosinophilia, hemolytic anemia, neutropenia, thrombocytopenia

Hepatic: Hepatotoxicity (rare)

Renal: BUN increased (dose related)

Miscellaneous: Anaphylactoid purpura, anaphylaxis, bulging fontanels (infants), serum sickness, SLE exacerbation

Note: Adverse effects in clinical trials occurring at a frequency more than 1% greater than placebo:

Periostat®: Diarrhea, dyspepsia, joint pain, menstrual cramp, nausea, dyspepsia, pain

Oracea®: Abdominal distention, abdominal pain, anxiety, AST increased, back pain, fungal infection, hyperglycemia, influenza, LDH increased, nasal congestion, nasopharyngitis, pain, sinus headache, sinusitis, xerostomia

Available Dosage Forms

Capsule, oral: 50 mg, 100 mg, 150 mg

Adoxa®: 150 mg

Monodox®: 50 mg, 75 mg, 100 mg

Ocudox™: 50 mg

Oracea®: 40 mg [30 mg (immediate release) and 10 mg (delayed release)]

Oraxyl™: 20 mg

Vibramycin®: 100 mg

Injection, powder for reconstitution: 100 mg

Doxy 100™: 100 mg

Powder for suspension, oral:

Vibramycin®: 25 mg/5 mL (60 mL)

Syrup, oral:

Vibramycin®: 50 mg/5 mL (473 mL)

Tablet, oral: 20 mg, 50 mg, 75 mg, 100 mg, 150 mg

Alodox™: 20 mg

Periostat®: 20 mg

Tablet, delayed release coated beads, oral: 75 mg, 100 mg

Tablet, delayed release coated pellets, oral: Doryx®: 150 mg

General Dosage Range

I.V.:

Children ≤8 years: 2.2 mg/kg every 12 hours

Children >8 years and ≤45 kg: 2-5 mg/kg/day in 1-2 divided doses (maximum: 200 mg/day)

Children >8 years and >45 kg and Adults: 100-200 mg/day in 1-2 divided doses

Oral:

Children ≤8 years: 2.2 mg/kg every 12 hours

Children >8 years and ≤45 kg: 2-5 mg/kg/day in 1-2 divided doses (maximum: 200 mg/day)

Children >8 years and >45 kg: 100-200 mg/day in 1-2 divided doses

Adults: 100-200 mg/day in 1-2 divided doses **or** 300 mg as a single dose **or** 40 mg/day in 1-2 divided doses

Administration

Oral Oral administration is preferable unless patient has significant nausea and vomiting; I.V. and oral routes are bioequivalent. May give with meals to decrease GI upset. Capsule and tablet: Administer with at least 8 ounces of water and have patient sit up for at least 30 minutes after taking to reduce the risk of esophageal irritation and ulceration.

Oracea®: Take on an empty stomach 1 hour before or 2 hours after meals.

Doryx®: May be administered by carefully breaking up the tablet and sprinkling tablet contents on a spoonful of cold applesauce. The delayed release pellets must not be crushed or damaged when breaking up tablet. Should be administered immediately after preparation and without chewing.

I.V. Infuse slowly, usually over 1-4 hours. Avoid extravasation. Oral administration is preferable unless patient has significant nausea and vomiting; I.V. and oral routes are bioequivalent.

I.V. Detail Avoid extravasation. Very irritating to vein; use central line if possible.

pH: 1.8-3.3 (reconstituted solution)

Other Intrapleural (unlabeled route): Add to 100 mL NS and instill into chest tube (Porcel, 2006)

Stability

Reconstitution I.V. infusion: Following reconstitution with sterile water for injection, dilute to a final concentration of 0.1-1 mg/mL using a compatible solution.

Storage

Capsule, tablet: Store at controlled room temperature of 25°C (77°F); excursions permitted to 15°C to 30°C (59°F to 86°F). Protect from light.

I.V. infusion: Protect from light. Stability varies based on solution.

Nursing Actions

Physical Assessment Results of culture and sensitivity test and patient's allergy history should be assessed prior to beginning therapy. I.V.: Infusion site may be closely monitored; extravasation can be very irritating to veins (use of central line is preferable). Teach patient importance of adequate hydration and photosensitivity precautions.

Patient Education If administered by infusion, report immediately any acute back pain, difficulty breathing or swallowing, chest tightness, pain, redness, or swelling at infusion site. Oral: Medication may be taken with food if gastric irritation occurs. Avoid alcohol and maintain adequate hydration, unless instructed to restrict fluid intake. Patient may be sensitive to sunlight. May cause nausea, vomiting, or diarrhea. Do not take antidiarrheal medication without instruction from prescriber. Report skin rash or itching; easy bruising or bleeding; yellowing of skin or eyes; pale stool or dark urine; unhealed mouth sores; vaginal itching or discharge; persistent diarrhea; and fever, chills, or unusual cough. Inform prescriber if you think you are pregnant.

Dietary Considerations

Tetracyclines (in general): Take with food if gastric irritation occurs. While administration with food may decrease GI absorption of doxycycline by up to 20%, administration on an empty stomach is not recommended due to GI intolerance. Of currently available tetracyclines, doxycycline has the least affinity for calcium.

Oracea®: Take on an empty stomach 1 hour before or 2 hours after meals.

Some products may contain sodium.

Dronabinol (droe NAB i nol)

Index Terms Delta-9 THC; Delta-9-tetrahydro-cannabinol; Tetrahydrocannabinol; THC

Pharmacologic Category Antiemetic; Appetite Stimulant

Medication Safety Issues

Sound-alike/look-alike issues:

Dronabinol may be confused with droperidol

Pregnancy Risk Factor C

Lactation Enters breast milk/not recommended

Use Chemotherapy-associated nausea and vomiting refractory to other antiemetic(s); AIDS-related anorexia

Unlabeled Use Cancer-related anorexia

Controlled Substance C-III

Available Dosage Forms

Capsule, soft gelatin, oral: 2.5 mg, 5 mg, 10 mg

General Dosage Range Oral:

Children: Initial: 5 mg/m^2 as a single dose; Maintenance: 5 mg/m^2/dose every 2-4 hours for a total of 4-6 doses/day (maximum: 15 mg/m^2/dose)

Adults: Initial: 5 mg/m^2 as a single dose; Maintenance: 5 mg/m^2/dose every 2-4 hours for a total of 4-6 doses/day (maximum: 15 mg/m^2/dose) **or** Initial: 2.5 mg twice daily; Maintenance: Titrate up to 20 mg/day in 2 divided doses

Nursing Actions

Physical Assessment Monitor for CNS changes, psychotic reactions; this drug is the psychoactive substance in marijuana.

Patient Education Avoid alcohol. May cause psychotic reaction, impaired coordination or judgment, faintness, dizziness, drowsiness, clumsiness, unsteadiness, or muscular weakness. Report excessive or persistent CNS changes (euphoria, anxiety, depression, memory lapse, bizarre thought patterns, excitability, inability to control thoughts or behavior, fainting), respiratory difficulties, and rapid heartbeat.

Dronedarone (droe NE da rone)

Brand Names: U.S. Multaq®

Index Terms Dronedarone Hydrochloride; SR33589

Pharmacologic Category Antiarrhythmic Agent, Class III

Medication Guide Available Yes

Pregnancy Risk Factor X

Lactation Excretion in breast milk unknown/contraindicated

Breast-Feeding Considerations It is not known whether dronedarone is secreted in human milk. Because the potential for serious adverse reactions exists, a decision should be made whether to discontinue nursing or discontinue the drug, taking into account the importance of the drug to the mother.

Use To reduce the risk of hospitalization for atrial fibrillation (AF) in patients in sinus rhythm with a history of paroxysmal or persistent AF

Unlabeled Use Alternative antiarrhythmic for the treatment of atrial fibrillation in patients with hypertrophic cardiomyopathy (HCM)

Mechanism of Action/Effect A noniodinated antiarrhythmic agent structurally related to amiodarone exhibiting properties of all 4 antiarrhythmic classes. Dronedarone prolongs the action potential and refractory period in myocardial tissue, and slows heart rate through inhibition of calcium channels and beta$_1$-receptors.

Contraindications Permanent atrial fibrillation (patients in whom sinus rhythm will not or cannot be restored);symptomatic heart failure (HF with recent decompensation requiring hospitalization or NYHA Class IV symptoms; second- or third-degree heart block or sick sinus syndrome (except in patients with a functioning artificial pacemaker); bradycardia <50 bpm; concomitant use of strong CYP3A4 inhibitors (eg, ketoconazole, itraconazole, voriconazole, cyclosporine, telithromycin, clarithromycin, nefazodone, or ritonavir); concomitant use of drugs or herbal products known to prolong the QT interval increasing the risk for torsade de pointes (eg, phenothiazine antipsychotics, tricyclic antidepressants, certain oral macrolide antibiotics, or class I and III antiarrhythmics); QT$_c$ (Bazett) interval ≥500 msec or PR interval >280 msec; liver toxicity related to previous amiodarone use; severe hepatic impairment; pregnancy; breast-feeding

Canadian labeling: Additional contraindications (not in U.S. labeling): Hypersensitivity to dronedarone or any component of the formulation; permanent atrial fibrillation of any duration where sinus rhythm cannot be restored and further attempts to restore it are no longer considered; history of or current heart failure regardless of NYHA class; left ventricular systolic dysfunction; sinus node dysfunction; atrial conduction defects; complete or distal bundle branch block, unstable hemodynamic conditions; hepatic or pulmonary toxicity related to prior amiodarone use

Warnings/Precautions [U.S. Boxed Warning]: The risk of death is doubled when used in patients with symptomatic heart failure with recent decompensation requiring hospitalization or NYHA Class IV symptoms; use is contraindicated in these patients. New-onset or worsening HF symptoms have been observed in postmarketing studies. If patient develops new or worsening HF symptoms (eg, weight gain, dependent edema, or increasing shortness of breath) requiring hospitalization while on therapy, discontinue dronedarone. Canadian labeling contraindicates use of dronedarone in patients with a history of or current heart failure, regardless of NYHA class.

[U.S. Boxed Warning]: Use in patients with permanent atrial fibrillation doubles the risk of death, stroke and hospitalization for heart failure. Use is contraindicated in patients with AF who will not or can not be converted to normal sinus rhythm. Monitor ECG at least every 3 months. Cardiovert patients who are in AF (if clinically indicated) or discontinue dronedarone. Initiate appropriate antithrombotic therapy prior to starting dronedarone.

Dronedarone induces a moderate prolongation of the QT interval (average ~10 msec); much greater effects have been observed. Use in patients with QT_c (Bazett) interval ≥500 msec is contraindicated; discontinue use of dronedarone if this occurs during therapy. Following initiation, dronedarone may produce a slight increase in serum creatinine (~0.1 mg/dL) due to inhibition of tubular secretion; glomerular filtration rate is not affected; effect is reversible upon discontinuation. Interstitial lung disease (including pulmonary fibrosis and pneumonitis) has been reported with use. Evaluate patients with onset of dyspnea or nonproductive cough for pulmonary toxicity. Canadian labeling recommends discontinuing therapy with confirmed pulmonary toxicity.

Severe liver injury, including acute liver failure leading to liver transplant, has been rarely reported. If liver injury is suspected, discontinue therapy and evaluate liver enzymes/bilirubin. Appropriate treatment should be started and therapy should not be reinitiated if liver injury is confirmed. Advise patients to report any signs or symptoms of hepatic injury (unusual fatigue, jaundice, nausea, vomiting, abdominal pain, and/or fever). Consider periodic monitoring of serum liver enzymes and bilirubin, especially during the first 6 months of therapy. Use with caution in patients with mild-to-moderate hepatic impairment; use is contraindicated in severe hepatic impairment.

Chronic administration of antiarrhythmic drugs may affect defibrillation or pacing thresholds; assess when initiating dronedarone and during therapy. Correct electrolyte disturbances, especially hypokalemia or hypomagnesemia, prior to use and throughout therapy. Dronedarone is a moderate inhibitor of CYP3A4 and CYP2D6 enzymes and has potential to inhibit p-glycoprotein, which may lead to increased serum concentrations/toxicity of a number of medications. Use caution when initiating dronedarone in patients on warfarin. Cases of increased INR with or without bleeding have occurred in patients treated with warfarin; monitor INR closely after initiating dronedarone in these patients. Women of childbearing potential should use effective contraceptive methods during treatment. Initiate appropriate antithrombotic therapy prior to starting dronedarone.

Drug Interactions

Avoid Concomitant Use

Avoid concomitant use of Dronedarone with any of the following: Artemether; CycloSPORINE; CycloSPORINE (Systemic); CYP3A4 Inducers (Strong); CYP3A4 Inhibitors (Strong); Grapefruit Juice; Lumefantrine; Nilotinib; Pimozide; QTc-Prolonging Agents; QUEtiapine; QuiNINE; Silodosin; St Johns Wort; Tetrabenazine; Thioridazine; Topotecan; Toremifene; Vandetanib; Vemurafenib; Ziprasidone

Decreased Effect

Dronedarone may decrease the levels/effects of: Codeine; TraMADol

The levels/effects of Dronedarone may be decreased by: CYP3A4 Inducers (Strong); Deferasirox; St Johns Wort; Tocilizumab

Increased Effect/Toxicity

Dronedarone may increase the levels/effects of: ARIPiprazole; Atorvastatin; Beta-Blockers; Budesonide (Systemic, Oral Inhalation); Calcium Channel Blockers (Nondihydropyridine); Colchicine; CYP2D6 Substrates; CYP3A4 Substrates; Dabigatran Etexilate; Digoxin; DOCEtaxel; Eplerenone; Everolimus; FentaNYL; Fesoterodine; Ivacaftor; Lidocaine (Topical); Lovastatin; Lurasidone; P-glycoprotein/ABCB1 Substrates; Pimecrolimus; Pimozide; Prucalopride; QTc-Prolonging Agents; QuiNINE; Red Yeast Rice; Rivaroxaban; Salmeterol; Silodosin; Simvastatin; Tamoxifen; Tetrabenazine; Thioridazine; Topotecan; Toremifene; Vandetanib; Vemurafenib; Vilazodone; Vitamin K Antagonists; Ziprasidone

The levels/effects of Dronedarone may be increased by: Alfuzosin; Artemether; Calcium Channel Blockers (Nondihydropyridine); Chloroquine; Ciprofloxacin; Ciprofloxacin (Systemic); CycloSPORINE; CycloSPORINE (Systemic); CYP3A4 Inhibitors (Moderate); CYP3A4 Inhibitors (Strong); Digoxin; Eribulin; Fingolimod; Gadobutrol; Grapefruit Juice; Indacaterol; Ivacaftor; Lidocaine (Topical); Lumefantrine; Nilotinib; QTc-Prolonging Agents; QUEtiapine; QuiNINE

Nutritional/Ethanol Interactions

Food: Food increases the rate and extent of absorption of dronedarone; bioavailability is increased 11% with a high-fat meal. Grapefruit juice increases bioavailability of dronedarone threefold; altered effects are possible. Management: Take with food. Grapefruit/grapefruit juice should be avoided during therapy.

Herb/Nutraceutical: St John's wort may decrease dronedarone levels; ephedra may worsen arrhythmia. Management: Avoid St John's wort, ephedra, and dong quai.

Adverse Reactions

>10%:

Cardiovascular: QT_c (Bazett) prolongation (28% [placebo: 19%]; defined as >450 msec in males or >470 msec in females)

Renal: Serum creatinine increased ≥10% (51%; occurred 5 days after initiation)

1% to 10%:

Cardiovascular: Bradycardia (3%)

Dermatologic: Allergic dermatitis (≤5%), dermatitis (≤5%), eczema (≤5%), pruritus (≤5%), rash (≤5%; described as generalized, macular, maculopapular, erythematous)

Gastrointestinal: Diarrhea (9%), nausea (5%), abdominal pain (4%), dyspepsia (2%), vomiting (2%)

Neuromuscular & skeletal: Weakness (7%)

Available Dosage Forms

Tablet, oral:

Multaq®: 400 mg

General Dosage Range Oral: *Adults:* 400 mg twice daily

Administration

Oral Administer with morning and evening meal.

Stability

Storage Store at 25°C (77°F); excursions permitted to 15°C to 30°C (59°F to 86°F).

Nursing Actions

Patient Education Take with food. Avoid grapefruit juice. You may experience diarrhea, nausea, or weakness. Report weight gain, swelling of extremities, or shortness of breath.

Dietary Considerations Take with a meal. Grapefruit juice is not recommended.

Droperidol (droe PER i dole)

Index Terms Dehydrobenzperidol

Pharmacologic Category Antiemetic; Antipsychotic Agent, Typical

Medication Safety Issues

Sound-alike/look-alike issues:

Droperidol may be confused with dronabinol

Pregnancy Risk Factor C

Lactation Excretion in breast milk unknown/use caution

Use Prevention and/or treatment of nausea and vomiting from surgical and diagnostic procedures

Available Dosage Forms

Injection, solution: 2.5 mg/mL (2 mL)

Injection, solution [preservative free]: 2.5 mg/mL (2 mL)

General Dosage Range I.M., I.V.:

Children 2-12 years: Maximum: 0.1 mg/kg; additional doses may be repeated

Adults: Maximum initial dose: 2.5 mg; additional doses of 1.25 mg may be administered

Administration

I.V. According to the manufacturer, I.V. push administration should be slow. For I.V. infusion, dilute in 50-100 mL NS or D_5W. May also administer I.M.

I.V. Detail pH: 3.0-3.8

Nursing Actions

Physical Assessment Monitor vital signs and cardiac and respiratory status on a frequent basis and especially immediately following administration and for several hours afterward. Monitor for extrapyramidal symptoms for 24-48 hours after therapy. Monitor for orthostatic hypotension until the patient is stable.

Patient Education This drug may cause you to feel very sleepy; do not attempt to get up without assistance. May cause dizziness or constipation. Immediately report any respiratory difficulty, confusion, or palpitations.

Drospirenone and Estradiol (droh SPYE re none & es tra DYE ole)

Brand Names: U.S. Angeliq®

Index Terms E2 and DRSP; Estradiol and Drospirenone

Pharmacologic Category Estrogen and Progestin Combination

Lactation Enters breast milk/not recommended

Use Treatment of moderate-to-severe vasomotor symptoms associated with menopause; treatment of vulvar and vaginal atrophy associated with menopause

Product Availability Angeliq® (drospirenone 0.25 mg and estradiol 0.5 mg) tablets: FDA approved March 2012; anticipated availability currently undetermined

Available Dosage Forms

Tablet:

Angeliq®: Drospirenone 0.5 mg and estradiol 1 mg

General Dosage Range Oral: *Adults (females):* 1 tablet daily

Nursing Actions

Physical Assessment See individual agents.

Patient Education See individual agents.

DULoxetine (doo LOX e teen)

Brand Names: U.S. Cymbalta®

Index Terms (+)-(*S*)-*N*-Methyl-γ-(1-naphthyloxy)-2-thiophenepropylamine Hydrochloride; Duloxetine Hydrochloride; LY248686

Pharmacologic Category Antidepressant, Serotonin/Norepinephrine Reuptake Inhibitor

Medication Safety Issues

Sound-alike/look-alike issues:

Cymbalta® may be confused with Symbyax®

DULoxetine may be confused with FLUoxetine

Medication Guide Available Yes

Pregnancy Risk Factor C

Lactation Enters breast milk/not recommended

Breast-Feeding Considerations Duloxetine is excreted in human milk and has been detected in the serum of a nursing infant. Breast-feeding is not recommended by the manufacturer. The long-term effects on neurobehavior have not been studied, thus one should prescribe duloxetine to a mother who is breast-feeding only when the benefits outweigh the potential risks.

Use Acute and maintenance treatment of major depressive disorder (MDD); treatment of generalized anxiety disorder (GAD); management of diabetic peripheral neuropathic pain (DPNP); management of fibromyalgia (FM); chronic musculoskeletal pain (eg, chronic low back pain, osteoarthritis)

Unlabeled Use Treatment of stress incontinence

Mechanism of Action/Effect Inhibits reuptake of both norepinephrine and serotonin (SNRI); improves symptoms of depression and chronic pain

Contraindications Concomitant use or within 2 weeks of MAO inhibitors; uncontrolled narrow-angle glaucoma

Note: MAO inhibitor therapy must be stopped for 14 days before duloxetine is initiated. Treatment with MAO inhibitors should not be initiated until 5 days after the discontinuation of duloxetine.

Canadian labeling: Additional contraindications (not in U.S. labeling): Hypersensitivity to duloxetine or any component of the formulation; hepatic impairment; severe renal impairment (eg, Cl_{cr} <30 mL/minute) or end-stage renal disease (ESRD); concomitant use with thioridazine or with CYP1A2 inhibitors

Warnings/Precautions [U.S. Boxed Warning]: Antidepressants increase the risk of suicidal thinking and behavior in children, adolescents, and young adults (18-24 years of age) with major depressive disorder (MDD) and other psychiatric disorders; consider risk prior to prescribing. Short-term studies did not show an increased risk in patients >24 years of age and showed a decreased risk in patients ≥65 years. Closely monitor for clinical worsening, suicidality, or unusual changes in behavior; the patient's family or caregiver should be instructed to closely observe the patient and communicate condition with healthcare provider. A medication guide concerning the use of antidepressants in children and teenagers should be dispensed with each prescription. **Duloxetine is not FDA approved for use in children.**

The possibility of a suicide attempt is inherent in major depression and may persist until remission occurs. Patients treated with antidepressants should be observed for clinical worsening and suicidality, especially during the initial (generally first 1-2 months) few months of a course of drug therapy, or at times of dose changes, either increases or decreases. Use caution in high-risk patients. Worsening depression and severe abrupt suicidality that are not part of the presenting symptoms may require discontinuation or modification of drug therapy. The patient's family or caregiver should be alerted to monitor patients for the emergence of suicidality and associated behaviors (such as agitation, irritability, hostility, impulsivity, and hypomania) and call healthcare provider.

May worsen psychosis in some patients or precipitate a shift to mania or hypomania in patients with bipolar disorder. Patients presenting with depressive symptoms should be screened for bipolar disorder. Monotherapy in patients with bipolar disorder should be avoided. **Duloxetine is not FDA approved for the treatment of bipolar depression.**

May cause orthostatic hypotension/syncope at therapeutic doses especially within the first week of therapy and after dose increases. Monitor blood pressure with initiation of therapy, dose increases (especially in patients receiving >60 mg/day), or with concomitant use of vasodilators, CYP2D6 inhibitors/substrates, or CYP1A2 inhibitors. Use caution in patients with hypertension. May increase blood pressure. Rare cases of hypertensive crisis have been reported in patients with pre-existing hypertension; evaluate blood pressure prior to initiating therapy and periodically thereafter; consider dose reduction or gradual discontinuation of therapy in individuals with sustained hypertension during therapy.

Modest increases in serum glucose and hemoglobin A_{1c} (Hb A_{1c}) levels have been observed in some diabetic patients receiving duloxetine therapy for diabetic peripheral neuropathic pain (DPNP). Duloxetine may cause increased urinary resistance; advise patient to report symptoms of urinary hesitation/difficulty. Has a low potential to impair cognitive or motor performance. Use caution with a previous seizure disorder or condition predisposing to seizures such as brain damage or alcoholism. Avoid use in patients with substantial ethanol intake, evidence of chronic liver disease, or hepatic impairment (contraindicated in Canadian labeling). Rare cases of hepatic failure (including fatalities) have been reported with use. Hepatitis with abdominal pain, hepatomegaly, elevated transaminase levels >20 times the upper limit of normal (ULN) with and without jaundice have all been observed. Discontinue therapy with the presentation of jaundice or other signs of hepatic dysfunction and do not reinitiate therapy unless another source or cause is identified. Use caution in patients with impaired gastric motility (eg, some diabetics) may affect stability of the capsule's enteric coating.

May cause hyponatremia/SIADH (elderly at increased risk); volume depletion (diuretics may increase risk). Use with caution in patients with controlled narrow angle glaucoma. May cause or exacerbate sexual dysfunction. Use caution with renal impairment (contraindicated in Canadian labeling for severe renal impairment or ESRD). Use caution with concomitant CNS depressants. May impair platelet aggregation; use caution with concomitant use of NSAIDs, ASA, or other drugs that affect coagulation; the risk of bleeding may be potentiated.

Serotonin syndrome and neuroleptic malignant syndrome (NMS)-like reactions have occurred with serotonin/norepinephrine reuptake inhibitors (SNRIs) and selective serotonin reuptake inhibitors (SSRIs) when used alone, and particularly when used in combination with serotonergic agents (eg, triptans) or antidopaminergic agents (eg, antipsychotics). Concurrent use with MAO inhibitors is contraindicated. Use caution during concurrent therapy with triptans and drugs which lower the seizure threshold; concurrent use of serotonin precursors (eg, tryptophan) is not recommended. To discontinue therapy with duloxetine, gradually taper dose. If intolerable symptoms occur following a decrease in dosage or upon discontinuation of therapy, then resuming the previous dose with a more gradual taper should be considered. May increase the risks associated with electroconvulsive therapy. Consider discontinuing, when possible, prior to elective surgery. Formulation contains sucrose; patients with fructose intolerance, glucose-galactose malabsorption, or sucrase-isomaltase deficiency should avoid use.

Drug Interactions

Avoid Concomitant Use

Avoid concomitant use of DULoxetine with any of the following: Iobenguane I 123; MAO Inhibitors; Methylene Blue

Decreased Effect

DULoxetine may decrease the levels/effects of: Alpha2-Agonists; Codeine; Iobenguane I 123; Ioflupane I 123

The levels/effects of DULoxetine may be decreased by: CYP1A2 Inducers (Strong); Cyproterone; Peginterferon Alfa-2b

Increased Effect/Toxicity

DULoxetine may increase the levels/effects of: Alpha-/Beta-Agonists; Aspirin; CYP2D6 Substrates; Fesoterodine; Methylene Blue; Metoclopramide; Nebivolol; NSAID (Nonselective); Serotonin Modulators; Tamoxifen; Tricyclic Antidepressants

The levels/effects of DULoxetine may be increased by: Abiraterone Acetate; Alcohol (Ethyl); Antipsychotics; CYP1A2 Inhibitors (Moderate); CYP1A2 Inhibitors (Strong); CYP2D6 Inhibitors (Moderate); CYP2D6 Inhibitors (Strong); Darunavir; Deferasirox; FluvoxaMINE; Linezolid; MAO Inhibitors; PARoxetine; Propafenone

Nutritional/Ethanol Interactions

Ethanol: Ethanol may increase hepatotoxic potential of duloxetine and increase CNS depression. Management: Avoid ethanol.

Herb/Nutraceutical: Some herbal medications may increase CNS depression. Management: Avoid valerian, St John's wort, SAMe, kava kava, and gotu kola.

Adverse Reactions

>10%:

Central nervous system: Headache (13% to 14%), somnolence (10% to 12%; dose related), fatigue (10 to 11%)

Gastrointestinal: Nausea (23% to 25%), xerostomia (11% to 15%; dose related)

1% to 10%:

Cardiovascular: Palpitation (1% to 2%)

Central nervous system: Dizziness (10%), insomnia (10%; dose related), agitation (3% to 5%), anxiety (3%), dreams abnormal (1% to 2%), yawning (1% to 2%), hypoesthesia (≥1%), lethargy (≥1%), vertigo (≥1%), chills (1%), sleep disorder (1%)

Dermatologic: Hyperhydrosis (6% to 7%)

Endocrine & metabolic: Libido decreased (2% to 4%), hot flushes (1% to 3%), orgasm abnormality (1% to 3%)

Gastrointestinal: Constipation (10%; dose related), diarrhea (9% to 10%), appetite decreased (7% to 9%; dose related), abdominal pain (4% to 6%), vomiting (3% to 5%), dyspepsia (2%), weight loss (2%), flatulence (≥1%), taste abnormal (≥1%), weight gain (≥1%)

Genitourinary: Erectile dysfunction (4% to 5%), ejaculation delayed (3%; dose related), ejaculatory dysfunction (2%)

Hepatic: ALT >3x ULN (1%)

Neuromuscular & skeletal: Muscle spasms (3%), tremor (2% to 3%; dose related), musculoskeletal pain (≥1%), paresthesia (≥1%), rigors (≥1%)

Ocular: Blurred vision (1% to 3%)

Respiratory: Nasopharyngitis (5%), cough (3%)

Miscellaneous: Influenza (3%)

Available Dosage Forms

Capsule, delayed release, enteric coated pellets, oral:

Cymbalta®: 20 mg, 30 mg, 60 mg

General Dosage Range Oral:

Adults: 30-60 mg/day in 1-2 divided doses (maximum: 120 mg/day)

Elderly: Initial: 20 mg 1-2 times/day

Administration

Oral Capsule should be swallowed whole; do not crush or chew. Although the manufacturer does not recommend opening the capsule to facilitate administration; the contents of capsule may be sprinkled on applesauce or in apple juice and swallowed (without chewing) immediately. Do not sprinkle contents on chocolate pudding (Wells, 2008). Administer without regard to meals.

Stability

Storage Store at 25°C (77°F); excursions permitted to 15°C to 30°C (59°F to 86°F)

Nursing Actions

Physical Assessment Monitor blood pressure (can cause elevation or orthostatic hypotension) at the beginning of treatment and periodically throughout. Monitor for worsening of depression and suicide ideation. Taper dosage slowly when discontinuing. Do not discontinue abruptly.

Patient Education Swallow capsule whole; do not open or crush. It may take 2-3 weeks to achieve desired results. Maintain adequate hydration, unless instructed to restrict fluid intake. Avoid alcohol use. If you have diabetes, monitor blood glucose levels closely. May cause increase in glycemic levels. Can cause drowsiness, dizziness, fatigue, or insomnia. You may experience headache, nausea, diarrhea, constipation, appetite decrease, or xerostomia. Report persistent insomnia, dizziness, headache, suicide ideation, worsening of anxiety, panic attacks, agitation, irritability, akathisia, hostility, hypomania, and mania.

Dietary Considerations May be taken without regard to meals.

Dutasteride (doo TAS teer ide)

Brand Names: U.S. Avodart®

Pharmacologic Category 5 Alpha-Reductase Inhibitor

Pregnancy Risk Factor X

Lactation Excretion in breast milk unknown/contraindicated in women of childbearing potential

Use Treatment of symptomatic benign prostatic hyperplasia (BPH) as monotherapy or combination therapy with tamsulosin

Unlabeled Use Treatment of male pattern baldness

Mechanism of Action/Effect Inhibits the conversion of testosterone to dihydrotestosterone (DHT) via 5α-reductase DHT stimulates prostatic cell hyperplasia.

Contraindications Hypersensitivity to dutasteride, other 5α-reductase inhibitors (eg, finasteride), or any component of the formulation; children; women of childbearing potential; pregnancy

Warnings/Precautions Hazardous agent - use appropriate precautions for handling and disposal. Pregnant women or women trying to conceive should not handle the product; active ingredient can be absorbed through the skin and may negatively impact fetal development. Urological diseases, including prostate cancer, and/or obstructive uropathy should be ruled out before initiating. Avoid donating blood during or for 6 months following treatment due to risk of administration to a pregnant female transfusion recipient. Use caution in hepatic impairment and with concurrent use of potent, chronic CYP3A4 inhibitors. Reduces PSA by ~50% within 3-6 months of use; if following serial PSAs, re-establish a new baseline ≥3 months after treatment initiation and monitor PSA periodically thereafter. If interpreting an isolated PSA value in a patient treated for ≥3 months, then double the PSA value for comparison to a normal PSA value in an untreated man. Failure to demonstrate a meaningful PSA decrease (<50%) or a PSA increase while on this medication may be associated with an increased risk for prostate cancer (NCCN Prostate Cancer Early Detection Guidelines, v.1.2011). Patients on a 5-alpha-reductase inhibitor (5-ARI) with any increase in PSA levels, even if within normal limits, should be evaluated; may indicate presence of prostate cancer. When compared to placebo, 5-ARIs have been shown to reduce the overall incidence of prostate cancer, although an increase in the incidence of high-grade prostate cancers has been observed; 5-ARIs are not FDA-approved for the prevention of prostate cancer.

Drug Interactions

Avoid Concomitant Use There are no known interactions where it is recommended to avoid concomitant use.

Decreased Effect

The levels/effects of Dutasteride may be decreased by: Tocilizumab

Increased Effect/Toxicity

The levels/effects of Dutasteride may be increased by: CYP3A4 Inhibitors (Strong)

Nutritional/Ethanol Interactions

Ethanol: No effect or interaction noted.

Food: Maximum serum concentrations reduced by 10% to 15% when taken with food; not clinically significant.

Herb/Nutraceutical: St John's wort may decrease dutasteride levels. Avoid saw palmetto (concurrent use has not been adequately studied).

Adverse Reactions

1% to 10%: Endocrine & metabolic: Impotence (1% to 5%), libido decreased (≤3%), ejaculation disorders (≤1%), gynecomastia (including breast tenderness, breast enlargement; ≤1%)

Note: Frequency of adverse events (except gynecomastia) tends to decrease with continued use (>6 months).

Available Dosage Forms

Capsule, softgel, oral:

Avodart®: 0.5 mg

General Dosage Range Oral: *Adults (males):* 0.5 mg once daily

Administration

Oral May be administered without regard to meals. Capsule should be swallowed whole; do not chew or open; contact with opened capsule can cause oropharyngeal irritation. Should not be touched or handled by women who are pregnant or are of childbearing age.

Stability

Storage Store at controlled room temperature of 25°C (77°F); excursions permitted to 15°C to 30°C (59°F to 86°F).

Dietary Considerations May be taken without regard to meals.

Dutasteride and Tamsulosin

(doo TAS teer ide & tam SOO loe sin)

Brand Names: U.S. Jalyn™

Index Terms Tamsulosin and Dutasteride; Tamsulosin Hydrochloride and Dutasteride

Pharmacologic Category 5 Alpha-Reductase Inhibitor; $Alpha_1$ Blocker

Pregnancy Risk Factor X

Lactation Excretion in breast milk unknown/not indicated for use in women

Use Treatment of symptomatic benign prostatic hyperplasia (BPH)

Available Dosage Forms

Capsule, oral:

Jalyn™: Dutasteride 0.5 mg and tamsulosin hydrochloride 0.4 mg

General Dosage Range Oral: *Adults (males):* 1 capsule (0.5 mg dutasteride/0.4 mg tamsulosin) once daily

Administration

Oral Administer 30 minutes after the same meal each day. Capsules should be swallowed whole; do not crush, chew, or open. Oropharyngeal contact with capsule contents may result in irritation of the mucosa.

Nursing Actions

Physical Assessment See individual agents.

Patient Education See individual agents.

Edrophonium

(ed roe FOE nee um)

Brand Names: U.S. Enlon®

Index Terms Edrophonium Chloride

Pharmacologic Category Acetylcholinesterase Inhibitor; Antidote; Diagnostic Agent

Lactation Excretion in breast milk unknown

Use Diagnosis of myasthenia gravis; differentiation of cholinergic crises from myasthenia crises; reversal of nondepolarizing neuromuscular blockers

Available Dosage Forms

Injection, solution:

Enlon®: 10 mg/mL (15 mL)

General Dosage Range

I.M.:

Infants: 0.5-1 mg

Children ≤34 kg: 1 mg

Children >34 kg: 5 mg

Adults: 10 mg, followed by 2 mg if no response

I.V.:

Infants: 0.1 mg, followed by 0.4 mg if no response (maximum total dose: 0.5 mg)

Children ≤34 kg: 0.04 mg/kg as single dose or followed by 0.16 mg/kg if no response **or** 1 mg, followed by 1mg every 30-45 seconds if no response (maximum total dose: 5 mg)

Children >34 kg: 0.04 mg/kg as single dose or followed by 0.16 mg/kg if no response **or** 2 mg, followed by 1 mg every 30-45 seconds if no response (maximum total dose: 10 mg)

Adults: 2 mg test dose, followed by 8 mg if no response **or** 1-10 mg as a single dose **or** 10 mg every 5-10 minutes up to 40 mg **or** 1 mg; may repeat after 1 minute

Administration

I.V. Detail pH: 5.4

Nursing Actions

Physical Assessment Administration of edrophonium for MG diagnosis is supervised by a neurologist and use as a neuromuscular blocking agent is supervised by an anesthesiologist. Nursing responsibilities include careful monitoring of the patient during and following procedure for cholinergic crisis; keep atropine at hand for antidote. Ascertain that patients receiving the medication for MG testing will have been advised by their neurologist about drug effects. Patient should never be left alone until all drug effects and the possibility of cholinergic crisis have passed.

Efavirenz

(e FAV e renz)

Brand Names: U.S. Sustiva®

Pharmacologic Category Antiretroviral Agent, Reverse Transcriptase Inhibitor (Non-nucleoside)

Pregnancy Risk Factor D

Lactation Enters breast milk/contraindicated

Breast-Feeding Considerations Efavirenz is excreted into breast milk. Although breast-feeding is not recommended, plasma concentrations of efavirenz in nursing infants have been reported as ~13% of maternal plasma concentrations.

Maternal or infant antiretroviral therapy does not completely eliminate the risk of postnatal HIV transmission. In addition, multiclass-resistant virus has been detected in breast-feeding infants despite maternal therapy. Therefore, in the United States, where formula is accessible, affordable, safe, and sustainable, and the risk of infant mortality due to diarrhea and respiratory infections is low, complete avoidance of breast-feeding by HIV-infected women is recommended to decrease potential transmission of HIV (DHHS [perinatal], 2011).

Use Treatment of HIV-1 infections in combination with at least two other antiretroviral agents

Mechanism of Action/Effect As a non-nucleoside reverse transcriptase inhibitor, efavirenz has activity against HIV-1 by binding to reverse transcriptase. It consequently blocks the RNA-dependent and DNA-dependent DNA polymerase activities including HIV-1 replication. It does not require intracellular phosphorylation for antiviral activity.

Contraindications Hypersensitivity to efavirenz or any component of the formulation; concurrent use of bepridil, cisapride, midazolam, pimozide, triazolam, voriconazole (with standard [eg, unadjusted] voriconazole and efavirenz doses), or ergot alkaloids (includes dihydroergotamine, ergotamine, ergonovine, methylergonovine)

Warnings/Precautions Do not use as single-agent therapy; avoid pregnancy; women of child-bearing potential should undergo pregnancy testing prior to initiation of therapy; use caution with other agents metabolized by cytochrome P450 isoenzyme 3A4 (see Contraindications); use caution with history of mental illness/drug abuse (predisposition to psychological reactions); may cause CNS and psychiatric symptoms, which include impaired concentration, dizziness or drowsiness (avoid potentially hazardous tasks such as driving or operating machinery if these effects are noted); CNS effects may be potentiated when used with other sedative drugs or ethanol. Serious psychiatric side effects have been associated with efavirenz, including severe depression, suicide, paranoia, and mania. May cause mild-to-moderate maculopapular rash; usually occurs within 2 weeks of starting therapy; discontinue if severe rash (involving blistering, desquamation, mucosal involvement, or fever) develops. Children are more susceptible.

Caution in patients with known or suspected hepatitis B or C infection (monitoring of liver function is recommended) or Child-Pugh class A hepatic impairment; not recommended in Child-Pugh class B or C hepatic impairment. Persistent elevations of serum transaminases >5 times the upper limit of normal should prompt evaluation - benefit of continued therapy should be weighed against possible risk of hepatotoxicity. Increases in total cholesterol and triglycerides have been reported; screening should be done prior to therapy and periodically throughout treatment. May cause redistribution of fat (eg, buffalo hump, peripheral wasting with increased abdominal girth, cushingoid appearance). Patients may develop immune reconstitution syndrome resulting in the occurrence of an inflammatory response to an indolent or residual opportunistic infection; further evaluation and treatment may be required. Use with caution in patients with a history of seizure disorder; seizures have been associated with use.

Drug Interactions

Avoid Concomitant Use

Avoid concomitant use of Efavirenz with any of the following: Axitinib; Bepridil [Off Market]; Boceprevir; Bortezomib; Cisapride; Clopidogrel; Crizotinib; Dienogest; Dronedarone; Ergot Derivatives; Etravirine; Lapatinib; Lurasidone; Midazolam; Nevirapine; Nilotinib; Nisoldipine; Pazopanib; Pimozide; Posaconazole; Praziquantel; Ranolazine; Rilpivirine; Rivaroxaban; Roflumilast; RomiDEPsin; SORAfenib; St Johns Wort; Ticagrelor; Tolvaptan; Toremifene; Triazolam; Vandetanib

Decreased Effect

Efavirenz may decrease the levels/effects of: ARIPiprazole; Atazanavir; Atorvastatin; Axitinib; Boceprevir; Bortezomib; Brentuximab Vedotin; Buprenorphine; BuPROPion; Caspofungin; Clarithromycin; Clopidogrel; Crizotinib; CycloSPORINE; CycloSPORINE (Systemic); CYP3A4 Substrates; Darunavir; Dasatinib; Dienogest; Dronedarone; Etonogestrel; Etravirine; Everolimus; Exemestane; Gefitinib; GuanFACINE; Imatinib; Itraconazole; Ixabepilone; Lapatinib; Linagliptin; Lopinavir; Lovastatin; Lurasidone; Maraviroc; Methadone; NIFEdipine; Nilotinib; Nisoldipine; Norgestimate; Pazopanib; Posaconazole; Pravastatin; Praziquantel; Protease Inhibitors; Raltegravir; Ranolazine; Rifabutin; Rilpivirine; Rivaroxaban; Roflumilast; RomiDEPsin; Saxagliptin; Sertraline; Simvastatin; Sirolimus; SORAfenib; SUNItinib; Tacrolimus; Tacrolimus (Systemic); Tadalafil; Telaprevir; Ticagrelor; Tolvaptan; Toremifene; Ulipristal; Vandetanib; Vemurafenib; Vitamin K Antagonists; Voriconazole; Zuclopenthixol

The levels/effects of Efavirenz may be decreased by: CYP2B6 Inducers (Strong); CYP3A4 Inducers (Strong); Deferasirox; Fosphenytoin; Nevirapine; Phenytoin; Rifabutin; Rifampin; St Johns Wort; Telaprevir; Tocilizumab

Increased Effect/Toxicity

Efavirenz may increase the levels/effects of: Alcohol (Ethyl); ARIPiprazole; Bepridil [Off Market]; Budesonide (Systemic, Oral Inhalation); Carvedilol; Cisapride; Citalopram; Clarithromycin; CNS Depressants; Colchicine; CYP2C19 Substrates; CYP2C9 Substrates; CYP3A4 Substrates; Eplerenone; Ergot Derivatives; Etravirine; FentaNYL; Fosphenytoin; Halofantrine; Ivacaftor; Lurasidone; Methotrimeprazine; Midazolam; Nevirapine; PACLitaxel; Phenytoin; Pimecrolimus; Pimozide; Propafenone; Protease Inhibitors; Ranolazine; Rilpivirine; Salmeterol; Saxagliptin; Selective Serotonin Reuptake Inhibitors; Tolvaptan; Triazolam; Vilazodone; Vitamin K Antagonists; Zuclopenthixol

The levels/effects of Efavirenz may be increased by: Boceprevir; Clarithromycin; Conivaptan; CYP2B6 Inhibitors (Moderate); CYP2B6 Inhibitors (Strong); Darunavir; Droperidol; HydrOXYzine; Methotrimeprazine; Nevirapine; Quazepam; Voriconazole

Nutritional/Ethanol Interactions

Ethanol: Ethanol may increase hepatotoxic potential of efavirenz and increase CNS depression. Management: Limit or avoid ethanol.

Food: High-fat meals increase the absorption of efavirenz. CNS effects are possible. ▶

Management: Avoid high-fat meals. Administer at or before bedtime on an empty stomach.

Herb/Nutraceutical: St John's wort may decrease efavirenz serum levels. Management: Avoid concurrent use.

Adverse Reactions Unless otherwise noted, frequency of adverse events is as reported in adults receiving combination antiretroviral therapy.

>10%:

Central nervous system: Dizziness (2% to 28%; children 16%), fever (children 21%), depression (up to 19%; severe: 1% to 2%), insomnia (up to 16%), anxiety (2% to 13%), pain (1% to 13%; children 14%), headache (2% to 8%; children 11%)

Dermatologic: Rash (5% to 26%, grade 3/4: <1%; children up to 46%, grade 3/4: 2% to 4%)

Endocrine & metabolic: HDL increased (25% to 35%), total cholesterol increased (20% to 40%), triglycerides increased (≥751 mg/dL: 6% to 11%)

Gastrointestinal: Diarrhea (3% to 14%; children: up to 39%), nausea (2% to 12%; children 12%), vomiting (3% to 6%; children 12%)

Respiratory: Cough (children 16%)

1% to 10%:

Central nervous system: Impaired concentration (up to 8%), somnolence (up to 7%), fatigue (up to 8%), abnormal dreams (1% to 6%), nervousness (2% to 7%), hallucinations (1%)

Dermatologic: Pruritus (up to 9%)

Endocrine & metabolic: Hyperglycemia (>250 mg/dL: 2% to 5%)

Gastrointestinal: Dyspepsia (up to 4%), abdominal pain (2% to 3%), anorexia (up to 2%), amylase increased (grade 3/4: up to 6%)

Hematologic: Neutropenia (grade 3/4: 2% to 10%)

Hepatic: Transaminases increased (grade 3/4: 2% to 8%, incidence higher with hepatitis B and/or C coinfection)

Available Dosage Forms

Capsule, oral:

Sustiva®: 50 mg, 200 mg

Tablet, oral:

Sustiva®: 600 mg

General Dosage Range Dosage adjustment recommended in patients on concomitant therapy

Oral:

Children ≥3 years and 10 kg to <15 kg: 200 mg once daily

Children ≥3 years and 15 kg to <20 kg: 250 mg once daily

Children ≥3 years and 20 kg to <25 kg: 300 mg once daily

Children ≥3 years and 25 kg to <32.5 kg: 350 mg once daily

Children ≥3 years and 32.5 kg to <40 kg: 400 mg once daily

Children ≥3 years and ≥40 kg and Adults: 600 mg once daily

Administration

Oral Administer on an empty stomach. Dosing at or before bedtime is recommended to limit central nervous system effects (DHHS, 2011). Tablets should not be broken. Some clinicians recommend opening capsules and adding to liquid or food for patients that cannot swallow capsules; however, no pharmacokinetic data are available and this is not recommended (DHHS [pediatric], 2010).

Stability

Storage Store at controlled room temperature of 25°C (77°F); excursion permitted to 15°C to 30°C (59°F to 86°F).

Nursing Actions

Physical Assessment Assess adherence with regimen and progression of disease. Monitor for CNS changes, rash, and gastrointestinal upset. Teach patient proper timing of multiple medications.

Patient Education This drug will not cure HIV, nor has it been found to reduce transmission of HIV; use appropriate precautions to prevent spread to other persons. This medication will be prescribed with a combination of other medications; time these medications as directed by prescriber. Take on an empty stomach. Maintain adequate hydration, unless instructed to restrict fluid intake. Frequent blood tests may be required. You may be advised to check your glucose levels; this drug can cause hyperglycemia. May cause dizziness, insomnia, impaired concentration, nausea, vomiting, abdominal pain, or diarrhea. May cause changes in body fat, increased fat in upper back and neck and around trunk, and loss of fat from extremities and face. Report immediately any CNS changes (depression, anxiety, suicide ideation, abnormal dreams, hallucinations, nervousness, impaired concentration), rash, or persistent gastrointestinal upset.

Dietary Considerations Should be taken on an empty stomach.

Efavirenz, Emtricitabine, and Tenofovir

(e FAV e renz, em trye SYE ta been, & te NOE fo veer)

Brand Names: U.S. Atripla®

Index Terms Emtricitabine, Efavirenz, and Tenofovir; FTC, TDF, and EFV; Tenofovir Disoproxil Fumarate, Efavirenz, and Emtricitabine

Pharmacologic Category Antiretroviral Agent, Reverse Transcriptase Inhibitor (Non-nucleoside); Antiretroviral Agent, Reverse Transcriptase Inhibitor (Nucleoside); Antiretroviral Agent, Reverse Transcriptase Inhibitor (Nucleotide)

Pregnancy Risk Factor D

Lactation See individual agents.

Breast-Feeding Considerations See individual agents.

Use Treatment of HIV infection

Mechanism of Action/Effect See individual agents.

Contraindications History of clinically-significant hypersensitivity (eg, Stevens-Johnson syndrome, erythema multiforme, or toxic skin reactions) to efavirenz, concurrent use of bepridil, cisapride, midazolam, triazolam, voriconazole, ergot alkaloids (includes dihydroergotamine, ergotamine, ergonovine, methylergonovine), St John's wort, pimozide

Warnings/Precautions [U.S. Boxed Warning]: Lactic acidosis and severe hepatomegaly with steatosis have been reported with nucleoside analogues, including fatal cases. Not recommended in patients with moderate or severe hepatic impairment (Child-Pugh class B, C). Use caution in patients with mild hepatic impairment (Child-Pugh class A), HBV or HCV coinfection, elevated transaminases or use of concomitant hepatotoxic drugs. Use caution in hepatic impairment. Use with caution in patients with risk factors for liver disease (risk may be increased in obese patients or prolonged exposure) and suspend treatment in any patient who develops clinical or laboratory findings suggestive of lactic acidosis or hepatotoxicity (transaminase elevation may/may not accompany hepatomegaly and steatosis). Persistent elevations of serum transaminases >5 times the upper limit of normal should prompt evaluation - benefit of continued therapy should be weighed against possible risk of hepatotoxicity. May cause redistribution of fat (eg, buffalo hump, peripheral wasting with increased abdominal girth, cushingoid appearance).

[U.S. Boxed Warning]: Safety and efficacy during coinfection of HIV and HBV have not been established; acute, severe exacerbations of HBV have been reported following discontinuation of antiretroviral therapy. All patients with HIV should be tested for HBV prior to initiation of treatment. Caution in patients with known or suspected hepatitis B or C infection (monitoring of liver function is recommended). In HBV coinfected patients, monitor hepatic function closely for several months following discontinuation.

Avoid pregnancy; women of childbearing potential should undergo pregnancy testing prior to initiation of therapy. Use with caution in patients taking strong CYP3A4 inhibitors, moderate or strong CYP3A4 inducers and major CYP3A4 substrates (see Drug Interactions); consider alternative agents that avoid or lessen the potential for CYP-mediated interactions. Immune reconstitution syndrome may develop resulting in the occurrence of an inflammatory response to an indolent or residual opportunistic infection; further evaluation and treatment may be required. Discontinue if severe rash (involving blistering, desquamation, mucosal involvement or fever) develops. Do not use concurrently with adefovir or lamivudine (or lamivudine-combination products). To avoid duplicate therapy, do not use concurrently with efavirenz emtricitabine, tenofovir, or any combination of these drugs.

Use caution with history of mental illness/drug abuse (predisposition to psychological reactions); may cause CNS and psychiatric symptoms, which include impaired concentration, dizziness or drowsiness (avoid potentially hazardous tasks such as driving or operating machinery if these effects are noted); serious psychiatric side effects have been associated with efavirenz, including severe depression, suicidal ideation, paranoia, and mania. Seizures have been associated with efavirenz use; use caution in patients with a history of seizure disorder.

May cause osteomalacia (which may contribute to fractures) and/or renal toxicity (acute renal failure and/or Fanconi syndrome); avoid use with concurrent or recent nephrotoxic therapy; monitor renal function and possible bone abnormalities during therapy. Product is a fixed-dose combination and is not appropriate for use in renal impairment (Cl_{cr} <50 mL/minute).

Use has been associated with decreases in bone mineral density. Consider monitoring of bone density in patients at risk for osteopenia or with a history of pathologic fractures; consider calcium and vitamin D supplementation. Fixed dose combination product; safety and efficacy have not been established in pediatric patients <18 years of age. In children <40 kg, the dose of efavirenz would be excessive.

Drug Interactions

Avoid Concomitant Use

Avoid concomitant use of Efavirenz, Emtricitabine, and Tenofovir with any of the following: Adefovir; Axitinib; Bepridil [Off Market]; Boceprevir; Bortezomib; Cisapride; Clopidogrel; Crizotinib; Didanosine; Dienogest; Dronedarone; Ergot Derivatives; Etravirine; LamiVUDine; Lapatinib; Lurasidone; Midazolam; Nevirapine; Nilotinib; Nisoldipine; Pazopanib; Pimozide; Posaconazole; Praziquantel; Ranolazine; Rilpivirine; Rivaroxaban; Roflumilast; RomiDEPsin; SORAfenib; St Johns Wort; Ticagrelor; Tolvaptan; Toremifene; Triazolam; Vandetanib

Decreased Effect

Efavirenz, Emtricitabine, and Tenofovir may decrease the levels/effects of: ARIPiprazole; Atazanavir; Atorvastatin; Axitinib; Boceprevir; Bortezomib; Brentuximab Vedotin; Buprenorphine; BuPROPion; Caspofungin; Clarithromycin; Clopidogrel; Crizotinib; CycloSPORINE; CycloSPORINE (Systemic); CYP3A4 Substrates; Darunavir; Dasatinib; Didanosine; Dienogest; Dronedarone; Etonogestrel; Etravirine; Everolimus; Exemestane; Gefitinib; GuanFACINE; Imatinib; Itraconazole; Ixabepilone; Lapatinib; Linagliptin; Lopinavir;

Lovastatin; Lurasidone; Maraviroc; Methadone; NIFEdipine; Nilotinib; Nisoldipine; Norgestimate; Pazopanib; Posaconazole; Pravastatin; Praziquantel; Protease Inhibitors; Raltegravir; Ranolazine; Rifabutin; Rilpivirine; Rivaroxaban; Roflumilast; RomiDEPsin; Saxagliptin; Sertraline; Simvastatin; Sirolimus; SORAfenib; SUNItinib; Tacrolimus; Tacrolimus (Systemic); Tadalafil; Telaprevir; Ticagrelor; Tolvaptan; Toremifene; Ulipristal; Vandetanib; Vemurafenib; Vitamin K Antagonists; Voriconazole; Zuclopenthixol

The levels/effects of Efavirenz, Emtricitabine, and Tenofovir may be decreased by: Adefovir; CYP2B6 Inducers (Strong); CYP3A4 Inducers (Strong); Deferasirox; Fosphenytoin; Nevirapine; Phenytoin; Rifabutin; Rifampin; St Johns Wort; Telaprevir; Tocilizumab

Increased Effect/Toxicity

Efavirenz, Emtricitabine, and Tenofovir may increase the levels/effects of: Adefovir; Alcohol (Ethyl); ARIPiprazole; Bepridil [Off Market]; Budesonide (Systemic, Oral Inhalation); Carvedilol; Cisapride; Citalopram; Clarithromycin; CNS Depressants; Colchicine; CYP2C19 Substrates; CYP2C9 Substrates; CYP3A4 Substrates; Didanosine; Eplerenone; Ergot Derivatives; Etravirine; FentaNYL; Fosphenytoin; Ganciclovir-Valganciclovir; Halofantrine; Ivacaftor; Lurasidone; Methotrimeprazine; Midazolam; Nevirapine; PACLitaxel; Phenytoin; Pimecrolimus; Pimozide; Propafenone; Protease Inhibitors; Ranolazine; Rilpivirine; Salmeterol; Saxagliptin; Selective Serotonin Reuptake Inhibitors; Tolvaptan; Triazolam; Vilazodone; Vitamin K Antagonists; Zuclopenthixol

The levels/effects of Efavirenz, Emtricitabine, and Tenofovir may be increased by: Acyclovir-Valacyclovir; Adefovir; Atazanavir; Boceprevir; Clarithromycin; Conivaptan; CYP2B6 Inhibitors (Moderate); CYP2B6 Inhibitors (Strong); Darunavir; Droperidol; Ganciclovir-Valganciclovir; HydrOXYzine; LamiVUDine; Lopinavir; Methotrimeprazine; Nevirapine; Protease Inhibitors; Quazepam; Ribavirin; Telaprevir; Voriconazole

Nutritional/Ethanol Interactions

Ethanol: Ethanol may increase hepatotoxic potential of efavirenz. Ethanol may also increase CNS depression; monitor for increased effects with coadministration. Caution patients about effects.

Food: Avoid high-fat meals (increase the absorption of efavirenz). Food decreases peak plasma concentrations of emtricitabine, but does not alter the extent of absorption or overall systemic exposure. Fatty meals may increase the bioavailability of tenofovir.

Herb/Nutraceutical: St John's wort may decrease efavirenz serum levels. Concurrent use is contraindicated.

Adverse Reactions The complete adverse reaction profile of combination therapy has not been established. **See individual agents.** The following adverse effects were noted in clinical trials with combination therapy:

>10%: Endocrine & metabolic: Hypercholesterolemia (22%)

1% to 10%:

- Central nervous system: Depression (9%), fatigue (9%), dizziness (8%), headache (6%), anxiety (5%), insomnia (5%), somnolence (4%), abnormal dreams
- Dermatologic: Rash (7%)
- Endocrine & metabolic: Triglycerides increased (4%), hyperglycemia (2%)
- Gastrointestinal: Nausea (9%), diarrhea (9%), serum amylase increased (8%), vomiting (2%)
- Hematologic: Neutropenia (3%)
- Hepatic: AST increased (3%), ALT increased (2%), alkaline phosphatase increased (1%)
- Neuromuscular & skeletal: Creatine increased (9%)
- Renal: Hematuria (3%)
- Respiratory: Sinusitis (8%), upper respiratory infection (8%), nasopharyngitis (5%)

Available Dosage Forms

Tablet:

Atripla®: Efavirenz 600 mg, emtricitabine 200 mg, and tenofovir disoproxil fumarate 300 mg

General Dosage Range Oral: *Adults:* 1 tablet (efavirenz 600 mg/emtricitabine 200 mg/tenofovir 300 mg) once daily

Administration

Oral Should be taken on an empty stomach, normally at bedtime to increase gastrointestinal tolerance and decrease nervous system manifestations.

Stability

Storage Store at 25°C (77°F); excursions permitted between 15°C to 30°C (59°F to 86°F). Dispense only in original container.

Nursing Actions

Physical Assessment See individual agents.

Patient Education See individual agents.

Dietary Considerations Should be taken on an empty stomach. In patients with history of bone fracture or osteopenia, consider calcium and vitamin D supplementation.

Eletriptan (el e TRIP tan)

Brand Names: U.S. Relpax®

Index Terms Eletriptan Hydrobromide

Pharmacologic Category Antimigraine Agent; Serotonin 5-$HT_{1B, 1D}$ Receptor Agonist

Pregnancy Risk Factor C

Lactation Enters breast milk/use caution

Breast-Feeding Considerations Eight women were given a single dose of eletriptan 80 mg. The amount of drug detected in breast milk over 24 hours was ~0.02% of the maternal dose and the milk-to-plasma ratio was variable. The presence of the active metabolite was not measured.

Use Acute treatment of migraine, with or without aura

Mechanism of Action/Effect Selective agonist for serotonin receptor in cranial arteries; causes vasoconstriction and relief of migraine

Contraindications Hypersensitivity to eletriptan or any component of the formulation; ischemic heart disease (angina pectoris, history of myocardial infarction, or proven silent ischemia) or in patients with symptoms consistent with ischemic heart disease, coronary artery vasospasm, or Prinzmetal's angina; cerebrovascular syndromes (including strokes, transient ischemic attacks); peripheral vascular syndromes (including ischemic bowel disease); uncontrolled hypertension; use within 24 hours of ergotamine derivatives; use within 24 hours of another 5-HT_1 agonist; management of hemiplegic or basilar migraine; severe hepatic impairment

Warnings/Precautions Only indicated for treatment of acute migraine; not indicated for migraine prophylaxis, or for the treatment of cluster headache, hemiplegic or basilar migraine. If a patient does not respond to the first dose, the diagnosis of migraine should be reconsidered. Do not give to patients with risk factors for CAD until a cardiovascular evaluation has been performed; if evaluation is satisfactory, the healthcare provider should administer the first dose (consider ECG monitoring) and cardiovascular status should be periodically evaluated. Cardiac events (coronary artery vasospasm, transient ischemia, MI, ventricular tachycardia/fibrillation, cardiac arrest, and death), cerebral/subarachnoid hemorrhage, stroke, peripheral vascular ischemia, and colonic ischemia have been reported with 5-HT_1 agonist administration. Patients who experience sensations of chest pain/pressure/tightness or symptoms suggestive of angina following dosing should be evaluated for coronary artery disease or Prinzmetal's angina before receiving additional doses; if dosing is resumed and similar symptoms recur, monitor with ECG. Significant elevation in blood pressure, including hypertensive crisis, has also been reported on rare occasions in patients with and without a history of hypertension. Use with caution with mild-to-moderate hepatic impairment. Symptoms of agitation, confusion, hallucinations, hyperreflexia, myoclonus, shivering, and tachycardia (serotonin syndrome) may occur with concomitant proserotonergic drugs (ie, SSRIs/SNRIs or triptans) or agents which reduce eletriptan's metabolism. Concurrent use of serotonin precursors (eg, tryptophan) is not recommended. If concomitant administration with SSRIs is warranted, monitor closely, especially at initiation and with dose increases. Use not recommended within 72 hours in patients taking strong CYP3A4 inhibitors.

Drug Interactions

Avoid Concomitant Use

Avoid concomitant use of Eletriptan with any of the following: Conivaptan; Ergot Derivatives

Decreased Effect

The levels/effects of Eletriptan may be decreased by: Tocilizumab

Increased Effect/Toxicity

Eletriptan may increase the levels/effects of: Ergot Derivatives; Metoclopramide; Serotonin Modulators

The levels/effects of Eletriptan may be increased by: Antifungal Agents (Azole Derivatives, Systemic); Antipsychotics; Calcium Channel Blockers (Nondihydropyridine); Conivaptan; CYP3A4 Inhibitors (Moderate); CYP3A4 Inhibitors (Strong); Dasatinib; Ergot Derivatives; Fluconazole; Ivacaftor; Macrolide Antibiotics

Nutritional/Ethanol Interactions Food: High-fat meal increases bioavailability.

Adverse Reactions 1% to 10%:

Cardiovascular: Chest pain/tightness (1% to 4%; placebo 1%), palpitation

Central nervous system: Dizziness (3% to 7%; placebo 3%), somnolence (3% to 7%; placebo 4%), headache (3% to 4%; placebo 3%), chills, pain, vertigo

Gastrointestinal: Nausea (4% to 8%; placebo 5%), xerostomia (2% to 4%, placebo 2%), dysphagia (1% to 2%), abdominal pain/discomfort (1% to 2%; placebo 1%), dyspepsia (1% to 2%; placebo 1%)

Neuromuscular & skeletal: Weakness (4% to 10%), paresthesia (3% to 4%), back pain, hypertonia, hypoesthesia

Respiratory: Pharyngitis

Miscellaneous: Diaphoresis

Available Dosage Forms

Tablet, oral:

Relpax®: 20 mg, 40 mg

General Dosage Range Oral: *Adults:* 20-40 mg as a single dose, may repeat (maximum: 80 mg/day)

Stability

Storage Store at 25°C (77°F); excursions permitted to 15°C to 30°C (59°F to 86°F).

Nursing Actions

Physical Assessment Monitor for hypertension and cardiac events. Teach patient proper use (treatment of acute migraine).

Patient Education This drug is to be used to reduce your migraine, not to prevent the number of attacks. Do not crush, break, or chew tablet. If headache improves but returns, dose may be repeated after 2 hours. Do not exceed two doses in 24 hours. May cause dizziness, drowsiness, nausea, vomiting, or abdominal pain. Report immediately any chest pain, tightness, or palpitations; muscle weakness or tremors; back pain; respiratory difficulty; changes in CNS (abnormal thought processes, depression, insomnia, confusion, agitation); swelling of eyelids, face, lips, or throat; rash; or hives.

Eltrombopag (el TROM boe pag)

Brand Names: U.S. Promacta®

Index Terms Eltrombopag Olamine; Revolade®; SB-497115; SB-497115-GR

Pharmacologic Category Colony Stimulating Factor; Thrombopoietic Agent

Medication Guide Available Yes

Pregnancy Risk Factor C

Lactation Excretion in breast milk unknown/not recommended

Breast-Feeding Considerations Due to the potential for serious adverse effects in the nursing infant, breast-feeding is not recommended.

Use Treatment of thrombocytopenia in patients with chronic immune (idiopathic) thrombocytopenic purpura (ITP) at risk for bleeding who have had insufficient response to corticosteroids, immune globulin, or splenectomy

Mechanism of Action/Effect Thrombopoietin (TPO) nonpeptide agonist which increases platelet counts by binding to and activating the human TPO receptor.

Contraindications There are no contraindications listed within the manufacturer's labeling.

Warnings/Precautions [U.S. Boxed Warning]: May cause hepatotoxicity; obtain ALT, AST, and bilirubin prior to treatment initiation, every 2 weeks during adjustment phase, then monthly (after stable dose established); obtain fractionation for elevated bilirubin levels. Repeat abnormal liver function tests within 3-5 days; if confirmed abnormal, monitor weekly until resolves, stabilizes, or returns to baseline. Discontinue treatment for ALT levels ≥3 times the upper limit of normal (ULN) and which are progressive, or persistent (≥4 weeks), or accompanied by increased direct bilirubin, or accompanied by clinical signs of liver injury or evidence of hepatic decompensation. Reinitiation is not recommended; hepatotoxicity usually recurred with retreatment after therapy interruption; however, if the benefit of treatment outweighs the hepatotoxicity risk, initiate carefully, and monitor liver function tests weekly during the dose adjustment phase; permanently discontinue if hepatotoxicity recurs with rechallenge. Use with caution in patients with pre-existing hepatic impairment (clearance may be reduced); dosage reductions are recommended in patients with hepatic dysfunction; monitor closely.

May increase the risk for bone marrow reticulin formation or progression; collagen fibrosis (not associated with cytopenias) was observed in clinical trials. In an extension study, myelofibrosis (≤grade 1) was observed in a majority of bone marrow biopsies performed after 1 year of treatment. Monitor peripheral blood smear for cellular morphologic abnormalities; analyze CBC monthly; discontinue treatment with onset of new or worsening abnormalities (eg, teardrop and nucleated RBC, immature WBC) or cytopenias and consider bone marrow biopsy (with staining for fibrosis).

Thromboembolism may occur with excess increases in platelet levels. Use with caution in patients with known risk factors for thromboembolism (eg, Factor V Leiden, ATIII deficiency, antiphospholipid syndrome, chronic liver disease). Portal venous thrombosis was reported in a study of non-ITP patients with chronic liver disease (not an FDA-approved indication) receiving eltrombopag 75 mg once daily for 14 days as a preparative regimen prior to invasive procedures to reduce platelet transfusions. Stimulation of cell surface thrombopoietin (TPO) receptors may increase the risk for hematologic malignancies.

Cataract formation or worsening was observed in clinical trials. Monitor regularly for signs and symptoms of cataracts; obtain ophthalmic exam at baseline and during therapy. Use with caution in patients at risk for cataracts (eg, advanced age, long-term glucocorticoid use). Allow at least 4 hours between dosing of eltrombopag and antacids, minerals (eg, iron, calcium, aluminum, magnesium, selenium, zinc), or foods high in calcium; may reduce eltrombopag levels. Patients of East-Asian ethnicity (eg, Chinese, Japanese, Korean, Taiwanese) may have greater drug exposure (compared to non-East Asians); therapy should be initiated with lower starting doses. Use with caution in renal impairment (any degree) and monitor closely; initial dosage adjustment is not necessary.

Indicated only when the degree of thrombocytopenia and clinical conditions increase the risk for bleeding; use the lowest dose necessary to achieve and maintain platelet count ≥50,000/mm³. Do not use to normalize platelet counts. Discontinue if platelet count does not respond to a level to avoid clinically important bleeding after 4 weeks at the maximum recommended dose.

Drug Interactions

Avoid Concomitant Use There are no known interactions where it is recommended to avoid concomitant use.

Decreased Effect

The levels/effects of Eltrombopag may be decreased by: Aluminum Hydroxide; Calcium Salts; Cyproterone; Iron Salts; Magnesium Salts; Selenium; Sucralfate; Zinc Salts

Increased Effect/Toxicity

Eltrombopag may increase the levels/effects of: CYP2C8 Substrates; Deferiprone; OATP1B1/SLCO1B1 Substrates; Rosuvastatin

Nutritional/Ethanol Interactions Food: Food, especially dairy products, may decrease the absorption of eltrombopag. Management: Take on an empty stomach at least 1 hour before or 2 hours after a meal. Separate intake from antacids, foods high in calcium, or minerals (eg, iron, calcium, aluminum, magnesium, selenium, zinc) by at least 4 hours.

Adverse Reactions

>10%: Hepatic: Liver function tests abnormal (11%)

1% to 10%:

Central nervous system: Headache (10%), fatigue (4%)

Dermatologic: Rash (3%), alopecia (2%)

Gastrointestinal: Diarrhea (9%), nausea (4% to 9%), vomiting (6%), xerostomia (2%)

Genitourinary: Urinary tract infection (5%)

Hematologic: Myelofibrosis (Extension study: Grade ≤1: 93%; grade 2: 7%), rebound thrombocytopenia (8%)

Hepatic: Hyperbilirubinemia (6%), ALT increased (5% to 6%), AST increased (4%), alkaline phosphatase increased (2%)

Neuromuscular & skeletal: Myalgia (5%), back pain (3%), paresthesia (3%)

Ocular: Cataract (4% to 7%)

Respiratory: Upper respiratory infection (7%), oropharyngeal pain (4%), pharyngitis (4%)

Miscellaneous: Influenza (3%)

Pharmacodynamics/Kinetics

Onset of Action Platelet count increase: Within 1-2 weeks; Peak platelet count increase: 14-16 days

Duration of Action Platelets return to baseline: 1-2 weeks after last dose

Product Availability

Promacta® 12.5 mg tablets (new strength): FDA approved December 2011; expected availability currently unknown.

Product labeling for Promacta® has also been updated to include dosage adjustment recommendations utilizing the new 12.5 mg strength.

Available Dosage Forms

Tablet, oral:

Promacta®: 25 mg, 50 mg, 75 mg

General Dosage Range Dosage adjustment recommended in patients with hepatic impairment, of East-Asian ethnicity, or who develop toxicities

Oral: *Adults:* 50 mg once daily (maximum: 75 mg/day)

Administration

Oral Administer on an empty stomach, 1 hour before or 2 hours after a meal. Do not administer concurrently with antacids, foods high in calcium, or minerals (eg, iron, calcium, aluminum, magnesium, selenium, zinc); separate by at least 4 hours. Do not administer more than one dose within 24 hours.

Stability

Storage Store at room temperature of 25°C (77°F); excursions permitted to 15°C to 30°C (59°F to 86°F).

Nursing Actions

Patient Education Take on an empty stomach, 1 hour before or 2 hours after a meal and at least 4 hours before or after any dairy products or multivitamins with minerals. You will require frequent blood tests to determine appropriate dosage and to reduce potential for severe adverse effects; maintaining laboratory testing schedule is vital. May cause nausea; vomiting; loss of appetite; or muscle, joint, back, or limb pain. Report new or persistent fatigue, yellowing of skin or eyes, unusual or increased bruising or bleeding, or change in vision.

Dietary Considerations Take on an empty stomach (1 hour before or 2 hours after a meal). Food, especially dairy products, may decrease the absorption of eltrombopag; allow at least 4 hours between dosing of eltrombopag and polyvalent cation intake (eg, dairy products, calcium-rich foods, multivitamins with minerals).

Emtricitabine (em trye SYE ta been)

Brand Names: U.S. Emtriva®

Index Terms BW524W91; Coviracil; FTC

Pharmacologic Category Antiretroviral Agent, Reverse Transcriptase Inhibitor (Nucleoside)

Pregnancy Risk Factor B

Lactation Excretion in breast milk unknown/contraindicated

Breast-Feeding Considerations Maternal or infant antiretroviral therapy does not completely eliminate the risk of postnatal HIV transmission. In addition, multiclass-resistant virus has been detected in breast-feeding infants despite maternal therapy. Therefore, in the United States, where formula is accessible, affordable, safe, and sustainable, and the risk of infant mortality due to diarrhea and respiratory infections is low, complete avoidance of breast-feeding by HIV-infected women is recommended to decrease potential transmission of HIV (DHHS [perinatal], 2011).

Use Treatment of HIV infection in combination with at least two other antiretroviral agents

Mechanism of Action/Effect Nucleoside reverse transcriptase inhibitor which interferes with viral RNA-dependent DNA synthesis, resulting in inhibition of viral replication.

Contraindications Hypersensitivity to emtricitabine or any component of the formulation

Warnings/Precautions [U.S. Boxed Warning]: Lactic acidosis, severe hepatomegaly with steatosis, and hepatic failure have occurred rarely with emtricitabine (similar to other nucleoside analogues). Some cases have been fatal; stop treatment if lactic acidosis or hepatotoxicity occur. Prior liver disease, obesity, extended duration of therapy, and female gender may represent risk factors for severe hepatic reactions. Testing for hepatitis B is recommended prior to the initiation of therapy; **[U.S. Boxed Warnings]: Hepatitis B may be exacerbated following discontinuation of emtricitabine; not indicated for treatment of chronic hepatitis B; safety and efficacy in HIV/HBV coinfected patients not established.** May be associated with fat redistribution (buffalo hump, increased abdominal girth, breast engorgement, facial atrophy, and dyslipidemia). Immune reconstitution syndrome may develop resulting in the occurrence of an inflammatory response to an indolent or residual opportunistic infection; further evaluation and treatment may be required. Use caution in patients with renal impairment (dosage adjustment required).

Drug Interactions

Avoid Concomitant Use

Avoid concomitant use of Emtricitabine with any of the following: LamiVUDine

Decreased Effect There are no known significant interactions involving a decrease in effect.

Increased Effect/Toxicity

The levels/effects of Emtricitabine may be increased by: Ganciclovir-Valganciclovir; LamiVUDine; Ribavirin

Nutritional/Ethanol Interactions Food: Food decreases peak plasma concentrations, but does not alter the extent of absorption or overall systemic exposure.

Adverse Reactions Clinical trials were conducted in patients receiving other antiretroviral agents, and it is not possible to correlate frequency of adverse events with emtricitabine alone. The range of frequencies of adverse events is generally comparable to comparator groups, with the exception of hyperpigmentation, which occurred more frequently in patients receiving emtricitabine. Unless otherwise noted, percentages are as reported in adults.

>10%:

Central nervous system: Dizziness (4% to 25%), headache (6% to 22%), fever (children 18%), insomnia (5% to 16%), abnormal dreams (2% to 11%)

Dermatologic: Hyperpigmentation (children 32%; adults 2% to 4%; primarily of palms and/or soles but may include tongue, arms, lip and nails; generally mild and nonprogressive without associated local reactions such as pruritus or rash); rash (17% to 30%; includes pruritus, maculopapular rash, vesiculobullous rash, pustular rash, and allergic reaction)

Gastrointestinal: Diarrhea (children 20%; adults 9% to 23%), vomiting (children 23%; adults 9%), nausea (13% to 18%), abdominal pain (8% to 14%), gastroenteritis (children 11%)

Neuromuscular & skeletal: Weakness (12% to 16%), CPK increased (grades 3/4: 11% to 12%)

Otic: Otitis media (children 23%)

Respiratory: Cough (children 28%; adults 14%), rhinitis (children 20%; adults 12% to 18%), pneumonia (children 15%)

Miscellaneous: Infection (children 44%)

1% to 10%:

Central nervous system: Depression (6% to 9%), neuropathy/neuritis (4%)

Endocrine & metabolic: Serum triglycerides increased (grades 3/4: 4% to 10%), disordered glucose homeostasis (grades 3/4: 2% to 3%), serum amylase increased (grades 3/4: children 9%; adults 2% to 5%), serum lipase increased (grades 3/4: ≤1%)

Gastrointestinal: Dyspepsia (4% to 8%), serum amylase increased (grades 3/4: 8%)

Genitourinary: Hematuria (grades 3/4: 3%)

Hematologic: Anemia (children: 7%), neutropenia (grades 3/4: children 2%; adults 5%)

Hepatic: Transaminases increased (grades 3/4: 2% to 6%), alkaline phosphatase increased (>550 units/L: 1%), bilirubin increased (grades 3/4: 1%)

Neuromuscular & skeletal: Creatinine kinase increased (grades 3/4: 9%), myalgia (4% to 6%), paresthesia (5% to 6%), arthralgia (3% to 5%)

Respiratory: Upper respiratory tract infection (8%), sinusitis (8%), pharyngitis (5%)

Available Dosage Forms

Capsule, oral:

Emtriva®: 200 mg

Solution, oral:

Emtriva®: 10 mg/mL (170 mL)

General Dosage Range Dosage adjustment recommended in patients with renal impairment

Oral:

Capsule: *Children 3 months to 17 years and >33 kg and Adults:* 200 mg once daily

Solution:

Children <3 months: 3 mg/kg/day

Children 3 months to 17 years: 6 mg/kg once daily (maximum: 240 mg/day)

Adults: 240 mg once daily

Administration

Oral May be administered with or without food.

Stability

Storage Store capsules at 15°C to 30°C (59°F to 86°F). Solution should be stored under refrigeration at 2°C to 8°C (36°F to 46°F). Once dispensed, may be stored at 15°C to 30°C (59°F to 86°F) if used within 3 months.

Nursing Actions

Physical Assessment Assess viral load and CD4 count. Monitor for lactic acidosis periodically during therapy. Teach patient proper timing of multiple medications.

Patient Education This drug will not cure HIV, nor has it been found to reduce transmission of HIV. Use appropriate precautions to prevent spread to other people. This drug is prescribed as one part of a multidrug combination; time multiple medications exactly as directed for full course of therapy. Take with or without food. Maintain adequate hydration, unless instructed to restrict fluid intake. Frequent blood tests may be required. May cause hyperpigmentation of hands, soles, or lips (normal). May cause headache, dizziness, insomnia, nausea, vomiting, abdominal pain, and diarrhea. Report persistent fast or rapid heartbeat, weakness or tiredness, muscle pain, respiratory difficulty, gastrointestinal upset, rash, diarrhea, signs of infection (burning on urination, perineal itching, white plaques in mouth, unhealed sores, persistent sore throat, or cough), yellowing of skin or eyes, dark urine, or light stool.

Dietary Considerations May be taken with or without food.

Emtricitabine and Tenofovir

(em trye SYE ta been & te NOE fo veer)

Brand Names: U.S. Truvada®

Index Terms Tenofovir and Emtricitabine

Pharmacologic Category Antiretroviral Agent, Reverse Transcriptase Inhibitor (Nucleoside); Antiretroviral Agent, Reverse Transcriptase Inhibitor (Nucleotide)

Pregnancy Risk Factor B

Lactation See individual agents.

Breast-Feeding Considerations See individual agents.

Use Treatment of HIV infection in combination with other antiretroviral agents

Unlabeled Use Treatment of hepatitis B in patients with antiviral-resistant HBV or coinfection with HIV; pre-exposure prophylaxis (PrEP) for prevention of HIV infection in men who have sex with men who are at high risk for acquiring HIV

Mechanism of Action/Effect Inhibits the production of new HIV virus by blocking the viral enzyme responsible for making DNA from viral RNA.

Contraindications There are no contraindications listed within the FDA-approved labeling.

Warnings/Precautions Not recommended as a component of a triple nucleoside regimen.

[U.S. Boxed Warning]: Lactic acidosis and severe hepatomegaly with steatosis have been reported with nucleoside and nucleotide analogues (eg, tenofovir), including fatal cases. Use with caution in patients with risk factors for liver disease (risk may be increased in obese patients or prolonged exposure) and suspend treatment in any patient who develops clinical or laboratory findings suggestive of lactic acidosis (transaminase elevation may/may not accompany hepatomegaly and steatosis). Use caution in hepatic impairment; no dosage adjustment is required; limited studies indicate the pharmacokinetics of tenofovir are not altered in hepatic dysfunction.

Use caution in moderate renal impairment (Cl_{cr} <50 mL/minute); dosage adjustment required. Calculate creatinine clearance prior to initiation in all patients; monitor renal function during therapy (including recalculation of creatinine clearance and serum phosphorus) in patients at risk for renal impairment, including those with previous renal decline on adefovir. May cause osteomalacia and/or renal toxicity; avoid use in patients with Cl_{cr} <30 mL/minute or concurrent therapy with other nephrotoxic drugs; monitor for possible bone abnormalities during therapy. All patients with HIV should be tested for HBV prior to initiation of treatment.

[U.S. Boxed Warning]: Safety and efficacy during coinfection of HIV and HBV have not been established; acute, severe exacerbations of HBV have been reported following discontinuation of antiretroviral therapy. In HBV coinfected patients, monitor hepatic function closely for several months following discontinuation. May cause redistribution of fat (eg, buffalo hump, peripheral wasting with increased abdominal girth, cushingoid appearance). Immune reconstitution syndrome may develop resulting in the occurrence of an inflammatory response to an indolent or residual opportunistic infection; further evaluation and treatment may be required. Do not use concurrently with adefovir, emtricitabine, tenofovir, lamivudine, or lamivudine-combination products.

Drug Interactions

Avoid Concomitant Use

Avoid concomitant use of Emtricitabine and Tenofovir with any of the following: Adefovir; Didanosine; LamiVUDine

Decreased Effect

Emtricitabine and Tenofovir may decrease the levels/effects of: Atazanavir; Didanosine; Protease Inhibitors

The levels/effects of Emtricitabine and Tenofovir may be decreased by: Adefovir

Increased Effect/Toxicity

Emtricitabine and Tenofovir may increase the levels/effects of: Adefovir; Didanosine; Ganciclovir-Valganciclovir

The levels/effects of Emtricitabine and Tenofovir may be increased by: Acyclovir-Valacyclovir; Adefovir; Atazanavir; Ganciclovir-Valganciclovir; LamiVUDine; Lopinavir; Protease Inhibitors; Ribavirin; Telaprevir

Nutritional/Ethanol Interactions Food: Food decreases peak plasma concentrations, but does not alter the extent of absorption or overall systemic exposure.

Adverse Reactions The adverse reaction profile of combination therapy has not been established. See individual agents.

Available Dosage Forms

Tablet:

Truvada®: Emtricitabine 200 mg and tenofovir 300 mg

General Dosage Range Dosage adjustment recommended in patients with renal impairment

Oral: *Children ≥12 (and >35 kg) and Adults:* 1 tablet (emtricitabine 200 mg and tenofovir 300 mg) once daily

Administration

Oral May be administered with or without food.

Stability

Storage Store tablets at 25°C (77°F); excursions permitted to 15°C to 30°C (59°F to 86°F).

Nursing Actions

Physical Assessment See individual agents.

Patient Education See individual agents.

Dietary Considerations May be taken without regard to meals. Consider calcium and vitamin D supplementation in patients with history of bone fracture or osteopenia.

Emtricitabine, Rilpivirine, and Tenofovir

(em trye SYE ta been, ril pi VIR een, & te NOE fo veer)

Brand Names: U.S. Complera™

Index Terms FTC/RPV/TDF; Rilpivirine, Emtricitabine, and Tenofovir; Tenofovir Disoproxil Fumarate, Rilpivirine, and Emtricitabine; Tenofovir, Emtricitabine, and Rilpivirine

Pharmacologic Category Antiretroviral Agent, Reverse Transcriptase Inhibitor (Non-nucleoside); Antiretroviral Agent, Reverse Transcriptase Inhibitor (Nucleoside); Antiretroviral Agent, Reverse Transcriptase Inhibitor (Nucleotide)

Pregnancy Risk Factor B

Lactation See individual agents.

Use Treatment of human immunodeficiency virus type 1 (HIV 1) infection in antiretroviral treatment-naive adult patients

Available Dosage Forms

Tablet, oral:

Complera™: Emtricitabine 200 mg, rilpivirine 25 mg, and tenofovir 300 mg

General Dosage Range Oral: *Adults:* One tablet once daily

Administration

Oral Administer with a meal (preferably high fat).

Nursing Actions

Physical Assessment See individual agents.

Patient Education See individual agents.

Enalapril (e NAL a pril)

Brand Names: U.S. Vasotec®

Index Terms Enalapril Maleate

Pharmacologic Category Angiotensin-Converting Enzyme (ACE) Inhibitor

Medication Safety Issues

Sound-alike/look-alike issues:

Enalapril may be confused with Anafranil®, Elavil®, Eldepryl®, ramipril

Administration issues:

Significant differences exist between oral and I.V. dosing. Use caution when converting from one route of administration to another.

International issues:

Acepril [Hungary, Switzerland] may be confused with Accupril which is a brand name for quinapril [U.S., Canada, multiple international markets]

Acepril: Brand name for enalapril [Hungary, Switzerland], but also brand name for captopril [Great Britain]; lisinopril [Malaysia]

Pregnancy Risk Factor D

Lactation Enters breast milk/not recommended (AAP rates "compatible"; AAP 2001 update pending)

Breast-Feeding Considerations Enalapril and enalaprilat are excreted in breast milk. Breast-feeding is not recommended by the manufacturer.

Use Treatment of hypertension; treatment of symptomatic heart failure; treatment of asymptomatic left ventricular dysfunction

Unlabeled Use To delay the progression of nephropathy and reduce risks of cardiovascular events in hypertensive patients with type 1 or 2 diabetes mellitus; hypertensive crisis, diabetic nephropathy, hypertension secondary to scleroderma renal crisis, diagnosis of aldosteronism, idiopathic edema, Bartter's syndrome, postmyocardial infarction for prevention of ventricular failure

Mechanism of Action/Effect Competitive inhibitor of angiotensin-converting enzyme (ACE); prevents conversion of angiotensin I to angiotensin II, a potent vasoconstrictor; results in lower levels of angiotensin II which causes an increase in plasma renin activity and a reduction in aldosterone secretion

Contraindications Hypersensitivity to enalapril or enalaprilat; angioedema related to previous treatment with an ACE inhibitor; patients with idiopathic or hereditary angioedema

Warnings/Precautions Anaphylactic reactions may occur rarely with ACE inhibitors. At any time during treatment (especially following first dose) angioedema may occur rarely with ACE inhibitors; it may involve the head and neck (potentially compromising airway) or the intestine (presenting with abdominal pain). African-Americans may be at an increased risk. Prolonged frequent monitoring may be required especially if tongue, glottis, or larynx are involved as they are associated with airway obstruction. Patients with a history of airway surgery may have a higher risk of airway obstruction. Aggressive early and appropriate management is critical. Use in patients with idiopathic or hereditary angioedema or previous angioedema associated with ACE inhibitor therapy is contraindicated. Severe anaphylactoid reactions may be seen during hemodialysis (eg, CVVHD) with high-flux dialysis membranes (eg, AN69), and rarely, during low density lipoprotein apheresis with dextran sulfate cellulose. Rare cases of anaphylactoid reactions have been reported in patients undergoing sensitization treatment with hymenoptera (bee, wasp) venom while receiving ACE inhibitors.

Symptomatic hypotension with or without syncope can occur with ACE inhibitors (usually with the first several doses); effects are most often observed in volume depleted patients; correct volume depletion prior to initiation; close monitoring of patient is required especially with initial dosing and dosing increases; blood pressure must be lowered at a rate appropriate for the patient's clinical condition. Initiation of therapy in patients with ischemic heart disease or cerebrovascular disease warrants close observation due to the potential consequences posed by falling blood pressure (eg, MI, stroke). Use with caution in hypertrophic cardiomyopathy with outflow tract obstruction, severe aortic stenosis, or before, during, or immediately after major surgery. **[U.S. Boxed Warning]: Drugs that act on the renin-angiotensin system can cause injury and death to the developing fetus. Discontinue as soon as possible once pregnancy is detected.**

Hyperkalemia may occur with ACE inhibitors; risk factors include renal dysfunction, diabetes mellitus, concomitant use of potassium-sparing diuretics, potassium supplements, and/or potassium-containing salts. Use cautiously, if at all, with these agents and monitor potassium closely. Cough may occur with ACE inhibitors. Other causes of cough should be considered (eg, pulmonary congestion in patients with heart failure) and excluded prior to discontinuation.

May be associated with deterioration of renal function and/or increases in serum creatinine, particularly in patients with low renal blood flow (eg, renal artery stenosis, heart failure) whose glomerular filtration rate (GFR) is dependent on efferent arteriolar vasoconstriction by angiotensin II; deterioration may result in oliguria, acute renal failure, and progressive azotemia. Small increases in serum creatinine may occur following initiation; consider discontinuation only in patients with progressive and/or significant deterioration in renal function. Use with caution in patients with unstented unilateral/bilateral renal artery stenosis. When unstented bilateral renal artery stenosis is present, use is generally avoided due to the elevated risk of deterioration in renal function unless possible benefits outweigh risks. Concurrent use of angiotensin receptor blockers may increase the risk of clinically-significant adverse events (eg, renal dysfunction, hyperkalemia).

Rare toxicities associated with ACE inhibitors include cholestatic jaundice (which may progress to fulminant hepatic necrosis), agranulocytosis, neutropenia or leukopenia with myeloid hypoplasia. Patients with collagen vascular diseases (especially with concomitant renal impairment) or renal impairment alone may be at increased risk for hematologic toxicity; periodically monitor CBC with differential in these patients.

Drug Interactions

Avoid Concomitant Use There are no known interactions where it is recommended to avoid concomitant use.

Decreased Effect

The levels/effects of Enalapril may be decreased by: Antacids; Aprotinin; Herbs (Hypertensive Properties); Icatibant; Lanthanum; Methylphenidate; Nonsteroidal Anti-Inflammatory Agents; Salicylates; Yohimbine

Increased Effect/Toxicity

Enalapril may increase the levels/effects of: Allopurinol; Amifostine; Antihypertensives; AzaTHIOprine; CycloSPORINE; CycloSPORINE (Systemic); Ferric Gluconate; Gold Sodium Thiomalate; Hypotensive Agents; Iron Dextran Complex; Lithium; Nonsteroidal Anti-Inflammatory Agents; RiTUXimab; Sodium Phosphates

The levels/effects of Enalapril may be increased by: Alfuzosin; Angiotensin II Receptor Blockers; Diazoxide; DPP-IV Inhibitors; Eplerenone; Everolimus; Herbs (Hypotensive Properties); Loop Diuretics; MAO Inhibitors; Pentoxifylline; Phosphodiesterase 5 Inhibitors; Potassium Salts; Potassium-Sparing Diuretics; Prostacyclin Analogues; Sirolimus; Temsirolimus; Thiazide Diuretics; TiZANidine; Tolvaptan; Trimethoprim

Nutritional/Ethanol Interactions

Food: Potassium supplements and/or potassium-containing salts may cause or worsen hyperkalemia. Management: Consult prescriber before consuming a potassium-rich diet, potassium supplements, or salt substitutes.

Herb/Nutraceutical: Some herbal medications may worsen hypertension (eg, licorice); others may increase the antihypertensive effect of enalapril (eg, shepherd's purse). Management: Avoid bayberry, blue cohosh, cayenne, ephedra, ginger, ginseng (American), kola, licorice, and yohimbe. Avoid black cohosh, California poppy, coleus, golden seal, hawthorn, mistletoe, periwinkle, quinine, and shepherd's purse.

Adverse Reactions Note: Frequency ranges include data from hypertension and heart failure trials. Higher rates of adverse reactions have generally been noted in patients with CHF. However, the frequency of adverse effects associated with placebo is also increased in this population.

1% to 10%:

Cardiovascular: Hypotension (1% to 7%), chest pain (2%), syncope (≤2%), orthostasis (2%), orthostatic hypotension (2%)

Central nervous system: Headache (2% to 5%), dizziness (4% to 8%), fatigue (2% to 3%)

Dermatologic: Rash (2%)

Gastrointestinal: Abnormal taste, abdominal pain, vomiting, nausea, diarrhea, anorexia, constipation

Neuromuscular & skeletal: Weakness

Renal: Serum creatinine increased (≤20%), worsening of renal function (in patients with bilateral renal artery stenosis or hypovolemia)

Respiratory (1% to 2%): Bronchitis, cough, dyspnea

Pharmacodynamics/Kinetics

Onset of Action ~1 hour; Peak effect: 4-6 hours

Duration of Action 12-24 hours

Available Dosage Forms

Tablet, oral: 2.5 mg, 5 mg, 10 mg, 20 mg

Vasotec®: 2.5 mg, 5 mg, 10 mg, 20 mg

General Dosage Range Dosage adjustment recommended in patients with renal impairment.

Oral:

Children 1 month to 17 years: Initial: 0.08 mg/kg/day (up to 5 mg) in 1-2 divided doses; Maintenance: Up to 0.58 mg/kg (40 mg)

Adults: Initial: 2.5-5 mg/day in 1-2 divided doses; Maintenance: 2.5-40 mg/day in 1-2 divided doses

Nursing Actions

Physical Assessment Assess potential for interactions with other pharmacological agents or herbal products that may impact fluid balance or cardiac status. Monitor blood pressure closely with first dose or change in dose. Monitor laboratory tests closely during first 3 months and regularly thereafter. Monitor for anaphylactic reaction, hypovolemia, angioedema, and postural hypotension.

Patient Education Do not use potassium supplement or salt substitutes without consulting prescriber. Take first dose at bedtime. This drug does not eliminate need for diet or exercise regimen as recommended by prescriber. May cause dizziness, fainting, lightheadedness, postural hypotension, nausea, vomiting, abdominal pain, dry mouth, or transient loss of appetite. Report persistent nausea and vomiting; chest pain or palpitations; mouth sores; fever or chills; swelling of extremities, face, mouth, or tongue; skin rash; numbness, tingling, or pain in muscles; or respiratory difficulty or unusual cough.

Dietary Considerations Limit salt substitutes or potassium-rich diet.

Enalapril and Hydrochlorothiazide

(e NAL a pril & hye droe klor oh THYE a zide)

Brand Names: U.S. Vaseretic®

Index Terms Enalapril Maleate and Hydrochlorothiazide; Hydrochlorothiazide and Enalapril

Pharmacologic Category Angiotensin-Converting Enzyme (ACE) Inhibitor; Diuretic, Thiazide

Medication Safety Issues

International issues:

Norpramin: Brand name for enalapril/hydrochlorothiazide [Portugal], but also the brand name for desipramine [U.S., Canada]; omeprazole [Spain]

Pregnancy Risk Factor D

Lactation Enters breast milk/not recommended

Use Treatment of hypertension

Available Dosage Forms

Tablet: 5/12.5: Enalapril 5 mg and hydrochlorothiazide 12.5 mg; 10/25: Enalapril 10 mg and hydrochlorothiazide 25 mg

Vaseretic®: 10/25: enalapril 10 mg and hydrochlorothiazide 25 mg

General Dosage Range Oral: *Adults:* Enalapril 5-10 mg and hydrochlorothiazide 12.5-25 mg once daily (maximum: 40 mg/day [enalapril]; 50 mg/day [hydrochlorothiazide])

Nursing Actions

Physical Assessment See individual agents.

Patient Education See individual agents.

Related Information

Enalapril *on page 388*

Hydrochlorothiazide *on page 570*

Enalaprilat (en AL a pril at)

Pharmacologic Category Angiotensin-Converting Enzyme (ACE) Inhibitor

Medication Safety Issues

Administration issues:

Significant differences exist between oral and I.V. dosing. Use caution when converting from one route of administration to another.

Pregnancy Risk Factor C (1st trimester); D (2nd and 3rd trimesters)

Lactation Enters breast milk/not recommended (AAP rates "compatible"; AAP 2001 update pending)

Breast-Feeding Considerations Enalapril and enalaprilat are excreted in breast milk. Breast-feeding is not recommended by the manufacturer.

Use Treatment of hypertension when oral therapy is not practical

Unlabeled Use Severe congestive heart failure in infants, acute cardiogenic pulmonary edema

Mechanism of Action/Effect Competitive inhibitor of angiotensin-converting enzyme (ACE); prevents conversion of angiotensin I to angiotensin II, a potent vasoconstrictor; results in lower levels of angiotensin II which causes an increase in plasma renin activity and a reduction in aldosterone secretion

Contraindications Hypersensitivity to enalapril or enalaprilat; angioedema related to previous treatment with an ACE inhibitor; patients with idiopathic or hereditary angioedema

Warnings/Precautions Anaphylactic reactions may occur rarely with ACE inhibitors. At any time during treatment (especially following first dose) angioedema may occur rarely with ACE inhibitors; it may involve the head and neck (potentially compromising airway) or the intestine (presenting with abdominal pain). African-Americans may be at an increased risk. Prolonged frequent monitoring may be required especially if tongue, glottis, or larynx are involved as they are associated with airway obstruction. Patients with a history of airway surgery may have a higher risk of airway obstruction. Aggressive early and appropriate management is critical. Use in patients with idiopathic or hereditary angioedema or previous angioedema associated with ACE inhibitor therapy is contraindicated. Severe anaphylactoid reactions may be seen during hemodialysis (eg, CVVHD) with high-flux dialysis membranes (eg, AN69), and rarely, during low density lipoprotein apheresis with dextran sulfate cellulose. Rare cases of anaphylactoid reactions have been reported in patients undergoing sensitization treatment with hymenoptera (bee, wasp) venom while receiving ACE inhibitors.

Symptomatic hypotension with or without syncope can occur with ACE inhibitors (usually with the first several doses); effects are most often observed in volume-depleted patients; correct volume depletion prior to initiation; close monitoring of patient is required especially with initial dosing and dosing increases; blood pressure must be lowered at a rate appropriate for the patient's clinical condition. Initiation of therapy in patients with ischemic heart disease or cerebrovascular disease warrants close observation due to the potential consequences posed by falling blood pressure (eg, MI, stroke). Use with caution in hypertrophic cardiomyopathy with outflow tract obstruction, severe aortic stenosis, or before, during, or immediately after major surgery. **[U.S. Boxed Warning]: Based on human data, ACEIs can cause injury and death to the developing fetus when used in the second and third trimesters. ACEIs should be discontinued as soon as possible once pregnancy is detected.** Injection contains benzyl alcohol which has been associated with "gasping syndrome" in neonates.

Hyperkalemia may occur with ACE inhibitors; risk factors include renal dysfunction, diabetes mellitus, concomitant use of potassium-sparing diuretics, potassium supplements, and/or potassium-containing salts. Use cautiously, if at all, with these agents and monitor potassium closely. Cough may occur with ACE inhibitors. Other causes of cough should be considered (eg, pulmonary congestion in patients with heart failure) and excluded prior to discontinuation.

May be associated with deterioration of renal function and/or increases in serum creatinine, particularly in patients with low renal blood flow (eg, renal artery stenosis, heart failure) whose glomerular filtration rate (GFR) is dependent on efferent arteriolar vasoconstriction by angiotensin II; deterioration may result in oliguria, acute renal failure, and progressive azotemia. Small increases in serum creatinine may occur following initiation; consider discontinuation only in patients with progressive and/or significant deterioration in renal function. Use with caution in patients with unstented unilateral/bilateral renal artery stenosis. When unstented bilateral renal artery stenosis is present, use is generally avoided due to the elevated risk of deterioration in renal function unless possible benefits outweigh risks. Concurrent use of angiotensin receptor blockers may increase the risk of clinically-significant adverse events (eg, renal dysfunction, hyperkalemia).

Rare toxicities associated with ACE inhibitors include cholestatic jaundice (which may progress to fulminant hepatic necrosis), agranulocytosis, neutropenia, or leukopenia with myeloid hypoplasia. Patients with collagen vascular diseases (especially with concomitant renal impairment) or renal impairment alone may be at increased risk for hematologic toxicity; periodically monitor CBC with differential in these patients.

Drug Interactions

Avoid Concomitant Use There are no known interactions where it is recommended to avoid concomitant use.

Decreased Effect

The levels/effects of Enalaprilat may be decreased by: Aprotinin; Herbs (Hypertensive Properties); Icatibant; Methylphenidate; Nonsteroidal Anti-Inflammatory Agents; Salicylates; Yohimbine

Increased Effect/Toxicity

Enalaprilat may increase the levels/effects of: Allopurinol; Amifostine; Antihypertensives; AzaTHIOprine; CycloSPORINE; CycloSPORINE (Systemic); Ferric Gluconate; Gold Sodium Thiomalate; Hypotensive Agents; Iron Dextran Complex; Lithium; Nonsteroidal Anti-Inflammatory Agents; RiTUXimab; Sodium Phosphates

The levels/effects of Enalaprilat may be increased by: Alfuzosin; Angiotensin II Receptor Blockers; Diazoxide; DPP-IV Inhibitors; Eplerenone; Everolimus; Herbs (Hypotensive Properties); Loop ▶

Diuretics; MAO Inhibitors; Pentoxifylline; Phosphodiesterase 5 Inhibitors; Potassium Salts; Potassium-Sparing Diuretics; Prostacyclin Analogues; Sirolimus; Temsirolimus; Thiazide Diuretics; TiZANidine; Tolvaptan; Trimethoprim

Nutritional/Ethanol Interactions Herb/Nutraceutical: Avoid bayberry, blue cohosh, cayenne, ephedra, ginger, ginseng (American), kola, licorice (may worsen hypertension). Avoid black cohosh, California poppy, coleus, golden seal, hawthorn, mistletoe, periwinkle, quinine, shepherd's purse (may have increased antihypertensive effect).

Adverse Reactions Note: Since enalapril is converted to enalaprilat, adverse reactions associated with enalapril may also occur with enalaprilat (also refer to Enalapril monograph). Frequency ranges include data from hypertension and heart failure trials. Higher rates of adverse reactions have generally been noted in patients with CHF. However, the frequency of adverse effects associated with placebo is also increased in this population.

1% to 10%:

Cardiovascular: Hypotension (2% to 5%)

Central nervous system: Headache (3%)

Gastrointestinal: Nausea (1%)

Pharmacodynamics/Kinetics

Onset of Action I.V.: ≤15 minutes; Peak effect: I.V.: 1-4 hours

Duration of Action I.V.: ~6 hours

Available Dosage Forms

Injection, solution: 1.25 mg/mL (1 mL, 2 mL)

General Dosage Range Dosage adjustment recommended in patients with renal impairment.

I.V.: *Adults:* 0.625-5 mg every 6 hours

Administration

I.V. Administer direct IVP over at least 5 minutes or dilute in up to 50 mL of a compatible solution and infuse; discontinue diuretic, if possible, for 2-3 days before beginning enalaprilat therapy.

Stability

Storage Enalaprilat is a clear, colorless solution which should be stored at <30°C (86°F). I.V. is stable for 24 hours at room temperature in D_5W, NS, D_5NS, or D_5LR.

Nursing Actions

Physical Assessment Assess potential for interactions with other pharmacological agents or herbal products that may impact fluid balance or cardiac status. Monitor blood pressure closely with first dose or change in dose. Monitor laboratory tests closely during first 3 months and regularly thereafter. Monitor for anaphylactic reaction, hypovolemia, angioedema, and postural hypotension.

Patient Education Do not use potassium supplement or salt substitutes without consulting prescriber. This drug does not eliminate need for diet or exercise regimen as recommended by prescriber. May cause dizziness, fainting, lightheadedness, postural hypotension, nausea, vomiting, abdominal pain, dry mouth, or transient loss of appetite. Report persistent nausea and vomiting; chest pain or palpitations; mouth sores; fever or chills; swelling of extremities, face, mouth, or tongue; skin rash; numbness, tingling, or pain in muscles; or respiratory difficulty or unusual cough.

Dietary Considerations Limit salt substitutes or potassium-rich diet.

Enfuvirtide (en FYOO vir tide)

Brand Names: U.S. Fuzeon®

Index Terms T-20

Pharmacologic Category Antiretroviral Agent, Fusion Protein Inhibitor

Pregnancy Risk Factor B

Lactation Excretion in breast milk unknown/contraindicated

Breast-Feeding Considerations Maternal or infant antiretroviral therapy does not completely eliminate the risk of postnatal HIV transmission. In addition, multiclass-resistant virus has been detected in breast-feeding infants despite maternal therapy. Therefore, in the United States, where formula is accessible, affordable, safe, and sustainable, and the risk of infant mortality due to diarrhea and respiratory infections is low, complete avoidance of breast-feeding by HIV-infected women is recommended to decrease potential transmission of HIV (DHHS [perinatal], 2011).

Use Treatment of HIV-1 infection in combination with other antiretroviral agents in treatment-experienced patients with evidence of HIV-1 replication despite ongoing antiretroviral therapy

Mechanism of Action/Effect Inhibits the fusion of HIV-1 virus with CD4 cells

Contraindications Hypersensitivity to enfuvirtide or any component of the formulation

Warnings/Precautions Use is not recommended in antiretroviral therapy-naive patients (DHHS, 2011). Monitor closely for signs/symptoms of pneumonia; associated with an increased incidence during clinical trials, particularly in patients with a low CD4 cell count, high initial viral load, I.V. drug use, smoking, or a history of lung disease. May cause hypersensitivity reactions (symptoms may include rash, fever, nausea, vomiting, hypotension, and elevated transaminases). In addition, local injection site reactions are common. An inflammatory response to indolent or residual opportunistic infections (immune reconstitution syndrome) has occurred with antiretroviral therapy; further investigation is warranted. Administration using a needle-free device has been associated with nerve pain (including neuralgia and/or paresthesia lasting up to 6 months), bruising, and hematomas when administered at sites where large nerves are close to the skin; only administer medication in recommended sites and use caution in patients with coagulation disorders (eg, hemophilia) or receiving anticoagulants. Safety and efficacy have not been established in children <6 years of age.

Drug Interactions

Avoid Concomitant Use There are no known interactions where it is recommended to avoid concomitant use.

Decreased Effect There are no known significant interactions involving a decrease in effect.

Increased Effect/Toxicity

Enfuvirtide may increase the levels/effects of: Protease Inhibitors

The levels/effects of Enfuvirtide may be increased by: Protease Inhibitors

Adverse Reactions

>10%:

Gastrointestinal: Diarrhea (32%), nausea (23%)

Local: Injection site infection (children 11%), injection site reactions (98%; may include pain, erythema, induration, pruritus, ecchymosis, nodule or cyst formation)

1% to 10%:

Dermatologic: Folliculitis (2%)

Gastrointestinal: Weight loss (7%), abdominal pain (4%), appetite decreased (3%), pancreatitis (3%), anorexia (2%), xerostomia (2%)

Hematologic: Eosinophilia (2% to 9%)

Hepatic: Transaminases increased (4%, grade 4: 1%)

Local: Injection site infection (adults 2%)

Neuromuscular & skeletal: CPK increased (3% to 7%), limb pain (3%), myalgia (3%)

Ocular: Conjunctivitis (2%)

Respiratory: Sinusitis (6%), cough (4%), bacterial pneumonia (3%)

Miscellaneous: Infections (4% to 6%), herpes simplex (4%), flu-like syndrome (2%)

Available Dosage Forms

Injection, powder for reconstitution [preservative free]:

Fuzeon®: 108 mg

General Dosage Range Dosage adjustment recommended in patients with renal impairment

SubQ:

Children 6-16 years: 2 mg/kg twice daily (maximum: 90 mg/dose)

Adolescents ≥16 years and Adults: 90 mg twice daily

Administration

Other Inject subcutaneously into upper arm, abdomen, or anterior thigh. Do not inject into moles, the navel, over a blood vessel or skin abnormalities such as scar tissue, surgical scars, bruises, or tattoos. In addition, do not inject in or near sites where large nerves are close to the skin including the elbow, knee, groin, or buttocks. Rotate injection site, give injections at a site different from the preceding injection site; do not inject into any site where an injection site reaction is evident. Bioequivalence was found to be similar in a study comparing standard administration using a needle versus a needle-free device.

Stability

Reconstitution Reconstitute with 1.1 mL SWFI; tap vial for 10 seconds and roll gently to ensure contact with diluent; then allow to stand until solution is completed; may require up to 45 minutes to form solution (108 mg/1.2 mL).

Storage Store powder at 15°C to 30°C (59°F to 86°F). Reconstituted solutions should be refrigerated and must be used within 24 hours.

Nursing Actions

Physical Assessment Monitor for pneumonia, neuropathy, and CNS changes on a regular basis throughout therapy. Teach patient or caregiver proper use (eg, reconstitution, injection procedure, needle/syringe disposal, and proper timing of mediations). Teach patient to report hypersensitivity reaction and injection site infection.

Patient Education This drug will not cure HIV, nor has it been found to reduce transmission of HIV; use appropriate precautions to prevent spread to other persons. This drug is prescribed as one part of a multidrug combination; take exactly as directed for full course of therapy. This drug can only be administered by injection; follow exact injection instructions that come with your medication. Do not mix any other medications in the same syringe. Inject into the upper arm, abdomen, or anterior thigh; do not inject in the same area you did the time before and do not inject around the naval, into scar tissues, a bruise, a mole, or where there is an injection site reaction. Make sure you have an adequate supply of medications on hand; do not allow supply to run out. Do not miss or skip a dose; if you miss a dose, take the missed dose as soon as you can and take the next dose as scheduled. If it is close to the time for the next dose, wait and take the next dose as regularly scheduled. Do not take two doses at the same time. May cause injection site reactions, such as itching, swelling, redness, pain, hardened skin, or bumps. May cause insomnia, anorexia, or constipation. Notify prescriber immediately if you experience a hypersensitivity reaction (rash, fever, nausea, vomiting, hypotension, blood in urine) or injection site becomes infected (red, painful, swollen, drainage). Report CNS disturbances (depression, anxiety), weakness, loss of feeling, muscle pain, respiratory infections, difficulty breathing, flu-like symptoms, unusual cough, fever, alteration in urinary pattern, or swelling of legs or feet.

Enoxaparin (ee noks a PA rin)

Brand Names: U.S. Lovenox®

Index Terms Enoxaparin Sodium

Pharmacologic Category Low Molecular Weight Heparin

Medication Safety Issues

Sound-alike/look-alike issues:

Lovenox® may be confused with Lasix®, Levaquin®, Lotronex®, Protonix®

High alert medication:

The Institute for Safe Medication Practices (ISMP) includes this medication among its list of drugs which have a heightened risk of causing significant patient harm when used in error.

National Patient Safety Goals:

The Joint Commission (TJC) requires healthcare organizations that provide anticoagulant therapy to have a process in place to reduce the risk of anticoagulant-associated patient harm. Patients receiving anticoagulants should receive individualized care through a defined process that includes standardized ordering, dispensing, administration, monitoring and education. This does not apply to routine short-term use of anticoagulants for prevention of venous thromboembolism when the expectation is that the patient's laboratory values will remain within or close to normal values (NPSG.03.05.01).

Pregnancy Risk Factor B

Lactation Excretion in breast milk unknown/use caution

Breast-Feeding Considerations This drug has a high molecular weight that would minimize excretion in breast milk and is inactivated by the GI tract which further reduces the risk to the infant.

Use

Acute coronary syndromes: Unstable angina (UA), non-ST-elevation (NSTEMI), and ST-elevation myocardial infarction (STEMI)

DVT prophylaxis: Following hip or knee replacement surgery, abdominal surgery, or in medical patients with severely-restricted mobility during acute illness who are at risk for thromboembolic complications

DVT treatment (acute): Inpatient treatment (patients with and without pulmonary embolism) and outpatient treatment (patients without pulmonary embolism)

Note: High-risk patients include those with one or more of the following risk factors: >40 years of age, obesity, general anesthesia lasting >30 minutes, malignancy, history of deep vein thrombosis or pulmonary embolism

Unlabeled Use Prophylaxis and treatment of thromboembolism in children; anticoagulant bridge therapy during temporary interruption of vitamin K antagonist therapy in patients at high risk for thromboembolism; DVT prophylaxis following moderate-risk general surgery, major gynecologic surgery and following higher-risk general surgery for cancer; management of venous thromboembolism (VTE) during pregnancy; anticoagulant used during percutaneous coronary intervention (PCI)

Mechanism of Action/Effect Low molecular weight heparin that blocks factor Xa and IIa to prevent thrombus and clot formation

Contraindications Hypersensitivity to enoxaparin, heparin, or any component of the formulation; thrombocytopenia associated with a positive *in vitro* test for antiplatelet antibodies in the presence of enoxaparin; hypersensitivity to pork products; active major bleeding; not for I.M. use

Warnings/Precautions **[U.S. Boxed Warning]: Spinal or epidural hematomas, including subsequent paralysis, may occur with recent or anticipated neuraxial anesthesia (epidural or spinal anesthesia) or spinal puncture in patients anticoagulated with LMWH or heparinoids.** Consider risk versus benefit prior to spinal procedures; risk is increased by the use of concomitant agents which may alter hemostasis, the use of indwelling epidural catheters for analgesia, a history of spinal deformity or spinal surgery, as well as a history of traumatic or repeated epidural or spinal punctures. Patient should be observed closely for bleeding and signs and symptoms of neurological impairment if therapy is administered during or immediately following diagnostic lumbar puncture, epidural anesthesia, or spinal anesthesia.

Do not administer intramuscularly. Not recommended for thromboprophylaxis in patients with prosthetic heart valves (especially pregnant women). Not to be used interchangeably (unit for unit) with heparin or any other low molecular weight heparins. Use caution in patients with history of heparin-induced thrombocytopenia. Monitor patient closely for signs or symptoms of bleeding. Certain patients are at increased risk of bleeding. Risk factors include bacterial endocarditis; congenital or acquired bleeding disorders; active ulcerative or angiodysplastic GI diseases; severe uncontrolled hypertension; history of hemorrhagic stroke; use shortly after brain, spinal, or ophthalmic surgery; patients treated concomitantly with platelet inhibitors; recent GI bleeding; thrombocytopenia or platelet defects; severe liver disease; hypertensive or diabetic retinopathy; or in patients undergoing invasive procedures. Monitor platelet count closely. Rare cases of thrombocytopenia have occurred. Discontinue therapy and consider alternative treatment if platelets are <100,000/mm^3 and/or thrombosis develops. Rare cases of thrombocytopenia with thrombosis have occurred. Use caution in patients with congenital or drug-induced thrombocytopenia or platelet defects. Risk of bleeding may be increased in women <45 kg and in men <57 kg. Use caution in patients with renal failure; dosage adjustment needed if Cl_{cr} <30 mL/minute. Use with caution in the elderly (delayed elimination may occur); dosage alteration/adjustment may be required (eg, omission of I.V. bolus in acute STEMI in patients ≥75 years of age). Monitor for hyperkalemia; can cause hyperkalemia possibly by suppressing aldosterone production. Multiple-dose vials contain benzyl alcohol (use caution in pregnant women). In neonates, large amounts of benzyl alcohol (>100 mg/kg/day) have been associated with fatal toxicity (gasping syndrome).

There is no consensus for adjusting/correcting the weight-based dosage of LMWH for patients who are morbidly obese (BMI ≥40 kg/m²). For patients undergoing inpatient bariatric surgery, the American College of Chest Physicians Practice Guidelines suggest using a higher thromboprophylaxis dose of LMWH for obese patients (Geerts, 2008).

Drug Interactions

Avoid Concomitant Use

Avoid concomitant use of Enoxaparin with any of the following: Rivaroxaban

Decreased Effect There are no known significant interactions involving a decrease in effect.

Increased Effect/Toxicity

Enoxaparin may increase the levels/effects of: Anticoagulants; Collagenase (Systemic); Deferasirox; Drotrecogin Alfa (Activated); Ibritumomab; Rivaroxaban; Tositumomab and Iodine I 131 Tositumomab

The levels/effects of Enoxaparin may be increased by: 5-ASA Derivatives; Antiplatelet Agents; Dasatinib; Herbs (Anticoagulant/Antiplatelet Properties); Nonsteroidal Anti-Inflammatory Agents; Pentosan Polysulfate Sodium; Pentoxifylline; Prostacyclin Analogues; Salicylates; Thrombolytic Agents

Nutritional/Ethanol Interactions Herb/Nutraceutical: Avoid cat's claw, dong quai, evening primrose, feverfew, garlic, ginger, ginkgo, red clover, horse chestnut, green tea, ginseng (all have additional antiplatelet activity).

Adverse Reactions As with all anticoagulants, bleeding is the major adverse effect of enoxaparin. Hemorrhage may occur at virtually any site. Risk is dependent on multiple variables. At the recommended doses, single injections of enoxaparin do not significantly influence platelet aggregation or affect global clotting time (ie, PT or aPTT).

1% to 10%:

Central nervous system: Fever (5% to 8%), confusion, pain

Dermatologic: Erythema, bruising

Gastrointestinal: Nausea (3%), diarrhea

Hematologic: Hemorrhage (major, <1% to 4%; includes cases of intracranial, retroperitoneal, or intraocular hemorrhage; incidence varies with indication/population), thrombocytopenia (moderate 1%; severe 0.1% - see **"Note"** below), anemia (<2%)

Hepatic: ALT increased, AST increased

Local: Injection site hematoma (9%), local reactions (irritation, pain, ecchymosis, erythema)

Renal: Hematuria (<2%)

Note: Thrombocytopenia with thrombosis: Cases of heparin-induced thrombocytopenia (some complicated by organ infarction, limb ischemia, or death) have been reported.

Pharmacodynamics/Kinetics

Onset of Action Peak effect: SubQ: Antifactor Xa and antithrombin (antifactor IIa): 3-5 hours

Duration of Action 40 mg dose: Antifactor Xa activity: ~12 hours

Available Dosage Forms

Injection, solution:

Lovenox®: 100 mg/mL (3 mL)

Injection, solution [preservative free]: 30 mg/0.3 mL (0.3 mL); 40 mg/0.4 mL (0.4 mL); 60 mg/0.6 mL (0.6 mL); 80 mg/0.8 mL (0.8 mL); 100 mg/mL (1 mL); 120 mg/0.8 mL (0.8 mL); 150 mg/mL (1 mL)

Lovenox®: 30 mg/0.3 mL (0.3 mL); 40 mg/0.4 mL (0.4 mL); 60 mg/0.6 mL (0.6 mL); 80 mg/0.8 mL (0.8 mL); 100 mg/mL (1 mL); 120 mg/0.8 mL (0.8 mL); 150 mg/mL (1 mL)

General Dosage Range Dosage adjustment recommended in patients with renal impairment

SubQ: *Adults:* Prophylaxis: 30 mg every 12 hours **or** 40 mg once daily; Treatment: 1 mg/kg every 12 hours **or** 1.5 mg/kg once daily

STEMI indication only:

<75 years: 30 mg I.V. bolus plus 1 mg/kg SubQ every 12 hours

≥75 years: 0.75 mg/kg SubQ every 12 hours

Administration

I.M. Do **not** administer I.M.

I.V. May be administered I.V. as part of treatment for ST-elevation myocardial infarction (STEMI) only in patients <75 years of age or during PCI. The manufacturer recommends using the multiple-dose vial to prepare I.V. doses. Do not mix or coadminister with other medications.

I.V. Detail pH: 5.5-7.5

Other Should be administered by deep SubQ injection to the left or right anterolateral and left or right posterolateral abdominal wall. To avoid loss of drug from the 30 mg and 40 mg syringes, do not expel the air bubble from the syringe prior to injection. In order to minimize bruising, do not rub injection site. An automatic injector (Lovenox EasyInjector™) is available with the 30 mg and 40 mg syringes to aid the patient with self-injections. **Note:** Enoxaparin is available in 100 mg/mL and 150 mg/mL concentrations.

To convert from I.V. unfractionated heparin (UFH) infusion to SubQ enoxaparin (Nutescu, 2007): Calculate specific dose for enoxaparin based on indication, discontinue UFH and begin enoxaparin within 1 hour.

To convert from SubQ enoxaparin to I.V. UFH infusion (Nutescu, 2007): Discontinue enoxaparin, calculate specific dose for I.V. UFH infusion based on indication, omit heparin bolus/loading dose:

Converting from SubQ enoxaparin dosed every 12 hours: Start I.V. UFH infusion 10-11 hours after last dose of enoxaparin

Converting from SubQ enoxaparin dosed every 24 hours: Start I.V. UFH infusion 22-23 hours after last dose of enoxaparin

Stability

Storage Store at 25°C (77°F); excursions permitted to 15°C to 30°C (59°F to 86°F); do not freeze.

Nursing Actions

Physical Assessment Use caution in presence or history of conditions that increase risk of bleeding. Monitor for bleeding. Teach patient about bleeding precautions.

Patient Education This drug can only be administered by injection. If self-administered, follow exact directions for injection and needle disposal. You may have a tendency to bleed easily while taking this drug. Report unusual bleeding or bruising (bleeding gums, nosebleed, blood in urine, dark stool); pain in joints or back; redness, swelling, burning, or pain at injection site; severe headache or confusion; or any rash.

Entacapone (en TA ka pone)

Brand Names: U.S. Comtan®

Pharmacologic Category Anti-Parkinson's Agent, COMT Inhibitor

Pregnancy Risk Factor C

Lactation Excretion in breast milk unknown/use caution

Use Adjunct to levodopa/carbidopa therapy in patients with idiopathic Parkinson's disease who experience "wearing-off" symptoms at the end of a dosing interval

Mechanism of Action/Effect Entacapone inhibits COMT peripherally and alters the pharmacokinetics of levodopa so serum levels of levodopa become more sustained when used with levodopa/carbidopa combinations.

Contraindications Hypersensitivity to entacapone or any of component of the formulation

Warnings/Precautions May cause orthostatic hypotension and syncope; Parkinson's disease patients appear to have an impaired capacity to respond to a postural challenge; use with caution in patients at risk of hypotension (such as those receiving antihypertensive drugs) or where transient hypotensive episodes would be poorly tolerated (cardiovascular disease or cerebrovascular disease). Parkinson's patients being treated with dopaminergic agonists ordinarily require careful monitoring for signs and symptoms of postural hypotension, especially during dose escalation, and should be informed of this risk. May cause hallucinations, which may improve with reduction in levodopa therapy. Use with caution in patients with pre-existing dyskinesias; exacerbation of pre-existing dyskinesia and severe rhabdomyolysis has been reported. Levodopa dosage reduction may be required, particularly in patients with levodopa dosages >600 mg daily or with moderate-to-severe dyskinesia prior to initiation. Entacapone, in conjunction with other drug therapy that alters brain biogenic amine concentrations (eg, MAO inhibitors, SSRIs), has been associated with a syndrome resembling neuroleptic malignant syndrome (hyperpyrexia and confusion - some fatal) on abrupt withdrawal or dosage reduction. Concomitant use of entacapone and nonselective MAO inhibitors should be avoided. Selegiline is a selective MAO type B inhibitor (when given orally at ≤10 mg/day) and can be taken with entacapone.

Dopaminergic agents have been associated with compulsive behaviors and/or loss of impulse control, which has manifested as pathological gambling, libido increases (hypersexuality), and/or binge eating. Causality has not been established, and controversy exists as to whether this phenomenon is related to the underlying disease, prior behaviors/addictions and/or drug therapy. Dose reduction or discontinuation of therapy has been reported to reverse these behaviors in some, but not all cases. Risk for melanoma development is increased in Parkinson's disease patients; drug causation or factors contributing to risk have not been established. Patients should be monitored closely and periodic skin examinations should be performed. Dopaminergic agents from the ergot class have also been associated with fibrotic complications, such as retroperitoneal fibrosis, pulmonary infiltrates or effusion and pleural thickening. It is unknown whether non-ergot, pro-dopaminergic agents like entacapone confer this risk. Use caution in patients with hepatic impairment or severe renal impairment. Do not withdraw therapy abruptly. Discoloration of urine, saliva, or sweat to dark colors (red, brown, black) may be observed during therapy. Use with caution in patients with lower gastrointestinal disease or an increased risk of dehydration; has been associated with delayed development of diarrhea (usual onset after 4-12 weeks). Diarrhea may be a sign of drug-induced colitis. Discontinue use with prolonged diarrhea.

Drug Interactions

Avoid Concomitant Use

Avoid concomitant use of Entacapone with any of the following: Pimozide

Decreased Effect There are no known significant interactions involving a decrease in effect.

Increased Effect/Toxicity

Entacapone may increase the levels/effects of: Alcohol (Ethyl); ARIPiprazole; CNS Depressants; COMT Substrates; MAO Inhibitors;

Methotrimeprazine; Pimozide; Selective Serotonin Reuptake Inhibitors

The levels/effects of Entacapone may be increased by: Droperidol; HydrOXYzine; Methotrimeprazine

Nutritional/Ethanol Interactions

Ethanol: May increase CNS depression; monitor for increased effects with coadministration. Caution patients about effects.

Food: Entacapone has been reported to chelate iron and decreasing serum iron levels were noted in clinical trials; however, clinically significant anemia has not been observed.

Adverse Reactions

>10%:

Gastrointestinal: Nausea (14%)

Neuromuscular & skeletal: Dyskinesia (25%), placebo (15%)

1% to 10%:

Cardiovascular: Orthostatic hypotension (4%), syncope (1%)

Central nervous system: Dizziness (8%), fatigue (6%), hallucinations (4%), anxiety (2%), somnolence (2%), agitation (1%)

Dermatologic: Purpura (2%)

Gastrointestinal: Diarrhea (10%), abdominal pain (8%), constipation (6%), vomiting (4%), dry mouth (3%), dyspepsia (2%), flatulence (2%), gastritis (1%), taste perversion (1%)

Genitourinary: Brown-orange urine discoloration (10%)

Neuromuscular & skeletal: Hyperkinesia (10%), hypokinesia (9%), back pain (4%), weakness (2%)

Respiratory: Dyspnea (3%)

Miscellaneous: Diaphoresis increased (2%), bacterial infection (1%)

Pharmacodynamics/Kinetics

Onset of Action Rapid; Peak effect: 1 hour

Available Dosage Forms

Tablet, oral:

Comtan®: 200 mg

General Dosage Range Oral: *Adults:* 200 mg with each dose of levodopa/carbidopa (maximum: 1600 mg/day)

Administration

Oral Always administer in association with levodopa/carbidopa; can be combined with both the immediate and sustained release formulations of levodopa/carbidopa. May be administered without regard to meals. Should not be abruptly withdrawn from patient's therapy due to significant worsening of symptoms.

Nursing Actions

Physical Assessment Monitor for postural hypotension, increased dyskinesias, and CNS changes (hallucinations, compulsive behaviors). Dose should be tapered slowly when discontinued. Teach patient proper timing of multiple medications.

Patient Education This drug is prescribed as one part of a multidrug combination; take exactly as directed for full course of therapy. Avoid alcohol. Periodic laboratory tests and skin exams may be required. May cause dizziness, fatigue, sleepiness, postural hypotension, unusual taste, nausea, vomiting, flatulence, upset stomach, or brown- or orange-colored urine (normal). Report any CNS changes (unusual compulsiveness, increased libido, binge eating), any new or increased abnormal skeletal movements or weakness, persistent gastrointestinal problems, hallucinations, changes in the appearance of skin moles, or other unusual skin changes.

Dietary Considerations May be taken without regard to meals.

Epinastine (ep i NAS teen)

Brand Names: U.S. Elestat®

Index Terms Epinastine Hydrochloride

Pharmacologic Category Histamine H_1 Antagonist; Histamine H_1 Antagonist, Second Generation

Pregnancy Risk Factor C

Lactation Excretion in breast milk unknown/use caution

Use Treatment of allergic conjunctivitis

Available Dosage Forms

Solution, ophthalmic: 0.05% (5 mL)

Elestat®: 0.05% (5 mL)

General Dosage Range Ophthalmic: *Children ≥2 years and Adults:* Instill 1 drop into each eye twice daily

Administration

Other For ophthalmic use only; avoid touching tip of applicator to eye or other surfaces. Contact lenses should be removed prior to application, may be reinserted after 10 minutes. Do not wear contact lenses if eyes are red.

Nursing Actions

Physical Assessment For ophthalmic use only.

Patient Education For ophthalmic use only. Do not wear contact lenses if eyes are red. May cause headache. Wash hands before using. Remove contact lenses before application (may be reinserted after 10 minutes). Gently pull lower eyelid forward and instill prescribed amount in lower eyelid. Avoid touching tip of dropper to eye. Close eye and roll eyeball in all directions. May cause blurred vision, temporary stinging, or burning sensation.

EPINEPHrine (Systemic, Oral Inhalation) (ep i NEF rin)

Brand Names: U.S. Adrenalin®; EpiPen 2-Pak®; EpiPen Jr 2-Pak®; EpiPen® Jr. [DSC]; EpiPen® [DSC]; Primatene® Mist [OTC] [DSC]; S2® [OTC]; Twinject®

Index Terms Adrenaline; Epinephrine Bitartrate; Epinephrine Hydrochloride; Racemic Epinephrine; Racepinephrine

Pharmacologic Category Alpha/Beta Agonist

Medication Safety Issues

Sound-alike/look-alike issues:

EPINEPHrine may be confused with ePHEDrine

Epifrin® may be confused with ephedrine, EpiPen®

High alert medication:

The Institute for Safe Medication Practices (ISMP) includes this medication among its list of drugs which have a heightened risk of causing significant patient harm when used in error.

Administration issues:

Medication errors have occurred due to confusion with epinephrine products expressed as ratio strengths (eg, 1:1000 vs 1:10,000).

Epinephrine 1:1000 = 1 mg/mL and is most commonly used I.M.

Epinephrine 1:10,000 = 0.1 mg/mL and is used I.V.

Medication errors have occurred when topical epinephrine 1 mg/mL (1:1000) has been inadvertently injected. Vials of injectable and topical epinephrine look very similar. Epinephrine should always be appropriately labeled with the intended administration.

International issues:

EpiPen [U.S., Canada, and multiple international markets] may be confused with Epigen brand name for glycyrrhizinic acid [Argentina, Mexico, Russia] and Epopen brand name for epoetin alfa [Spain]

Pregnancy Risk Factor C

Lactation Excretion in breast milk unknown

Use Treatment of bronchospasms, bronchial asthma, viral croup, anaphylactic reactions, cardiac arrest; added to local anesthetics to decrease systemic absorption of intraspinal and local anesthetics and increase duration of action; decrease superficial hemorrhage

Unlabeled Use ACLS guidelines: Ventricular fibrillation (VF) or pulseless ventricular tachycardia (VT) unresponsive to initial defibrillatory shocks; pulseless electrical activity; asystole; hypotension/shock unresponsive to volume resuscitation; symptomatic bradycardia unresponsive to atropine or pacing; inotropic support

Mechanism of Action/Effect Stimulates alpha-, beta$_1$-, and beta$_2$-adrenergic receptors resulting in relaxation of smooth muscle of the bronchial tree, cardiac stimulation (increasing myocardial oxygen consumption), and dilation of skeletal muscle vasculature; small doses can cause vasodilation via beta$_2$-vascular receptors; large doses may produce constriction of skeletal and vascular smooth muscle

Contraindications There are no absolute contraindications to the use of injectable epinephrine (including EpiPen®, EpiPen® Jr, and Twinject®) in a life-threatening situation.

Oral inhalation: Concurrent use or within 2 weeks of MAO inhibitors

Injectable solution: Per the manufacturer, contraindicated in narrow-angle glaucoma; shock; during general anesthesia with halogenated hydrocarbons or cyclopropane (currently not available in U.S.); individuals with organic brain damage; with local anesthesia of the digits; during labor; heart failure; coronary insufficiency

Warnings/Precautions Use with caution in elderly patients, patients with diabetes mellitus, cardiovascular diseases (eg, coronary artery disease, hypertension), thyroid disease, cerebrovascular disease, Parkinson's disease, or patients taking tricyclic antidepressants. Some products contain sulfites as preservatives; the presence of sulfites in some products (eg, EpiPen® and Twinject®) should not deter administration during a serious allergic or other emergency situation even if the patient is sulfite-sensitive. Accidental injection into digits, hands, or feet may result in local reactions, including injection site pallor, coldness and hypoesthesia or injury, resulting in bruising, bleeding, discoloration, erythema or skeletal injury; patient should seek immediate medical attention if this occurs. Rapid I.V. administration may cause death from cerebrovascular hemorrhage or cardiac arrhythmias; however, rapid I.V. administration during pulseless arrest is necessary.

Oral inhalation: Use with caution in patients with prostate enlargement or urinary retention; may cause temporary worsening of symptoms.

Self medication (OTC use): Oral inhalation: Prior to self-medication, patients should contact healthcare provider. The product should only be used in persons with a diagnosis of asthma. If symptoms are not relieved in 20 minutes or become worse do not continue to use the product - seek immediate medical assistance. The product should not be used more frequently or at higher doses than recommended unless directed by a healthcare provider. This product should not be used in patients who have required hospitalization for asthma or if a patient is taking prescription medication for asthma. Do not use if you have taken a MAO inhibitor (certain drugs used for depression, Parkinson's disease, or other conditions) within 2 weeks.

Drug Interactions

Avoid Concomitant Use

Avoid concomitant use of EPINEPHrine (Systemic, Oral Inhalation) with any of the following: Ergot Derivatives; Iobenguane I 123; Lurasidone

Decreased Effect

EPINEPHrine (Systemic, Oral Inhalation) may decrease the levels/effects of: Benzylpenicilloyl Polylysine; Iobenguane I 123

The levels/effects of EPINEPHrine (Systemic, Oral Inhalation) may be decreased by: Spironolactone

Increased Effect/Toxicity

EPINEPHrine (Systemic, Oral Inhalation) may increase the levels/effects of: Bromocriptine; Lurasidone; Sympathomimetics

The levels/effects of EPINEPHrine (Systemic, Oral Inhalation) may be increased by: Antacids; Atomoxetine; Beta-Blockers; Cannabinoids; Carbonic Anhydrase Inhibitors; COMT Inhibitors; Ergot Derivatives; Inhalational Anesthetics; MAO Inhibitors; Serotonin/Norepinephrine Reuptake Inhibitors; Tricyclic Antidepressants

Nutritional/Ethanol Interactions Herb/Nutraceutical: Avoid ephedra, yohimbe (may cause CNS stimulation).

Adverse Reactions Frequency not defined.

Cardiovascular: Angina, cardiac arrhythmia, chest pain, flushing, hypertension, pallor, palpitation, sudden death, tachycardia (parenteral), vasoconstriction, ventricular ectopy

Central nervous system: Anxiety (transient), apprehensiveness, cerebral hemorrhage, dizziness, headache, insomnia, lightheadedness, nervousness, restlessness

Gastrointestinal: Dry throat, loss of appetite, nausea, vomiting, xerostomia

Genitourinary: Acute urinary retention in patients with bladder outflow obstruction

Neuromuscular & skeletal: Tremor, weakness

Ocular: Allergic lid reaction, burning, eye pain, ocular irritation, precipitation of or exacerbation of narrow-angle glaucoma, transient stinging

Respiratory: Dyspnea, pulmonary edema

Miscellaneous: Diaphoresis

Pharmacodynamics/Kinetics

Onset of Action Bronchodilation: SubQ: ~5-10 minutes; Inhalation: ~1 minute

Available Dosage Forms

Injection, solution: 0.1 mg/mL (10 mL); 1 mg/mL (1 mL, 30 mL)

Adrenalin®: 1 mg/mL (1 mL, 30 mL)

EpiPen 2-Pak®: 0.3 mg/0.3 mL (2 mL)

EpiPen Jr 2-Pak®: 0.15 mg/0.3 mL (2 mL)

Twinject®: 0.15 mg/0.15 mL (1.1 mL); 0.3 mg/0.3 mL (1.1 mL)

Injection, solution [preservative free]: 1 mg/mL (1 mL)

Solution, for oral inhalation [preservative free]: S2® [OTC]: 2.25% (0.5 mL)

General Dosage Range

I.M.:

Adults: 0.3-0.5 mg (**1:1000** [1 mg/mL] solution) every 15-20 minutes

EpiPen® Jr., Twinject®: *Children 15-29 kg:* 0.15 mg as single dose; may repeat if needed

EpiPen®, Twinject®: *Children ≥30 kg and Adults:* 0.3 mg as single dose; may repeat if needed

Inhalation: *Children ≥4 years and Adults:* 1 inhalation; may repeat once after 1 minute, then do not use again for at least 3 hours

I.V. (**1:10,000** [0.1 mg/mL] solution):

Children: 0.01 mg/kg kg (maximum single dose: 1 mg) every 3-5 minutes as needed **or** 0.1-1 mcg/kg/minute as a continuous infusion **or** 0.01 mg/kg every 20 minutes (hypersensitivity reaction)

Adults: 1 mg every 3-5 minutes (up to 0.2 mg/kg) **or** 1-10 mcg/minute as a continuous infusion

Nebulization (S2® Racepinephrine, OTC):

Children <4 years: Jet nebulizer: 0.05 mL/kg (maximum dose: 0.5 mL) diluted in 3 mL NS up to every 2 hours

Children ≥4 years and Adults:

Hand-bulb nebulizer: Add 0.5 mL (~10 drops) to nebulizer; 1-3 inhalations up to every 3 hours if needed

Jet nebulizer: Add 0.5 mL (~10 drops) to nebulizer and dilute with 3 mL of NS. Administer over ~15 minutes every 3-4 hours as needed.

SubQ:

Children: 0.01 mg/kg (**1:1000** [1 mg/mL] solution) every 20 minutes for 3 doses or as condition requires (maximum: 0.3 mg/dose)

Adults: 0.3-0.5 mg (**1:1000** [1 mg/mL] solution) every 15-20 minutes for 3 doses or as condition requires

EpiPen® Jr, Twinject®: *Children 15-29 kg:* 0.15 mg as single dose; may repeat if needed

EpiPen®, Twinject®: *Children ≥30 kg and Adults:* 0.3 mg as single dose; may repeat if needed

Administration

I.M. I.M. administration into the buttocks should be avoided. I.M. administration in the anterolateral aspect of the middle third of the thigh is preferred in the setting of anaphylaxis (ACLS guidelines, 2010; Kemp, 2008). EpiPen®, EpiPen® Jr, and Twinject® Auto-Injectors should only be injected into the anterolateral aspect of the thigh, through clothing if necessary.

Note: EpiPen® and EpiPen® Jr Auto-Injectors contain a single, fixed-dose of epinephrine. Twinject® Auto-Injectors contain two doses; the first fixed-dose is available for auto-injection; the second dose is available for manual injection following partial disassembly of device.

I.V. When administering as a continuous infusion, central line administration is preferred. I.V. infusions require an infusion pump.

I.V. Detail Extravasation management: Use phentolamine as antidote. Mix 5 mg phentolamine with 9 mL of NS. Inject a small amount of this dilution into extravasated area. Blanching should reverse immediately. Monitor site. If blanching should recur, additional injections of phentolamine may be needed.

pH: 2.5-5.0

Inhalation S2®: If using jet nebulizer: Administer over ~15 minutes; must be diluted. If using hand-held rubber bulb nebulizer, dilution is not required.

Other

Endotracheal: Dilute in NS or sterile water. Absorption may be greater with sterile water (Naganobu, 2000). Stop compressions, spray drug quickly down tube. Follow immediately with several quick insufflations and continue chest compressions. May cause false-negative reading with exhaled CO_2 detectors; use second method to confirm tube placement if CO_2 is not detected (Neumar, 2010).

Subcutaneous: SubQ administration results in slower absorption and is less reliable. I.M. administration into the buttocks should be avoided. I.M. administration in the anterolateral aspect of the middle third of the thigh is preferred in the setting of anaphylaxis (ACLS guidelines, 2010; Kemp, 2008). EpiPen®, EpiPen® Jr, and Twinject® Auto-Injectors should only be injected into the anterolateral aspect of the thigh, through clothing if necessary.

Note: EpiPen® and EpiPen® Jr Auto-Injectors contain a single, fixed-dose of epinephrine. Twinject® Auto-Injectors contain two doses; the first fixed-dose is available for auto-injection; the second dose is available for manual injection following partial disassembly of device.

Stability

Reconstitution

S2®: Dilution not required when administered via hand-bulb nebulizer; dilute with NS 3-5 mL if using jet nebulizer.

Standard I.V. diluent: 1 mg/250 mL NS.

Preparation of adult I.V. infusion: Dilute 1 mg in 250 mL of D_5W or NS (4 mcg/mL).

Storage Epinephrine is sensitive to light and air. Protection from light is recommended. Oxidation turns drug pink, then a brown color. **Solutions should not be used if they are discolored or contain a precipitate.**

Adrenalin®: Store between 15°C to 25°C (59°F to 77°F); do not freeze. Protect from light. The 1:1000 solution should be discarded 30 days after initial use.

EpiPen® and EpiPen® Jr: Store at 25°C (77°F); excursions permitted to 15°C to 30°C (59°F to 86°F); do not freeze or refrigerate. Protect from light by storing in carrier tube provided.

Twinject®: Store between 20°C to 25°C (68°F to 77°F); excursions permitted to 15°C to 30°C (59°F to 86°F); do not freeze or refrigerate. Protect from light.

Primatene® Mist: Store between 20°C to 25°C (68°F to 77°F).

S2®: Store between 2°C to 20°C (36°F to 68°F). Protect from light.

Stability of injection of parenteral admixture at room temperature (25°C) or refrigeration (4°C) is 24 hours.

Nursing Actions

Physical Assessment Monitor for hypertension, CNS excitability, urinary retention, and dysrhythmias. I.V. (cardiovascular therapy): Central line with infusion pump and continuous cardiac/hemodynamic monitoring is necessary.

Patient Education Avoid other stimulants to avoid serious overdose reactions. You may experience dizziness, blurred vision, restlessness, or difficulty urinating. Report excessive nervousness or excitation, inability to sleep, facial flushing, pounding heartbeat, muscle tremors or weakness, chest pain or palpitations, or increased sweating.

Aerosol: Use aerosol or nebulizer as per instructions. Clear as much mucus as possible before use. Rinse mouth following each use. If more than one inhalation is necessary, wait 1 minute between inhalations. May cause restlessness or nervousness. Report persistent nervousness, restlessness, sleeplessness, palpitations, tachycardia, chest pain, muscle tremors, dizziness, flushing, or if breathing difficulty persists.

Related Information

Management of Drug Extravasations *on page 1269*

EPINEPHrine (Nasal) (ep i NEF rin)

Brand Names: U.S. Adrenalin®

Index Terms Adrenaline; Epinephrine Hydrochloride

Pharmacologic Category Alpha/Beta Agonist

Medication Safety Issues

Sound-alike/look-alike issues:

EPINEPHrine may be confused with ePHEDrine

Use Treatment of nasal congestion

Available Dosage Forms

Solution, intranasal:

Adrenalin®: 1 mg/mL (30 mL)

General Dosage Range Intranasal: *Children ≥6 years and Adults:* Apply **1:1000** (1 mg/mL) solution locally as drops, spray, or with sterile swab

Nursing Actions

Physical Assessment Monitor for hypertension, CNS excitability, urinary retention, dysrhythmias, and respiratory depression.

Patient Education Avoid other stimulants to avoid serious overdose reactions. You may experience dizziness, blurred vision, restlessness, or difficulty urinating. Report excessive nervousness or excitation, inability to sleep, facial flushing, pounding heartbeat, muscle tremors or weakness, chest pain or palpitations, or increased sweating.

Epirubicin (ep i ROO bi sin)

Brand Names: U.S. Ellence®

Index Terms Epidoxorubicin; Epirubicin Hydrochloride; Pidorubicin; Pidorubicin Hydrochloride

Pharmacologic Category Antineoplastic Agent, Anthracycline

Medication Safety Issues

Sound-alike/look-alike issues:

Epirubicin may be confused with DOXOrubicin, DAUNOrubicin, eribulin, idarubicin

International issues:

Ellence [U.S.] may be confused with Elase brand name for dornase alfa [Chile, France, Malaysia]

High alert medication:

This drug is in a class the Institute for Safe Medication Practices (ISMP) includes among its list of drug classes which have a heightened risk of causing significant patient harm when used in error.

Pregnancy Risk Factor D

Lactation Excretion in breast milk unknown/not recommended

Breast-Feeding Considerations Excretion in human breast milk is unknown, however, other anthracyclines are excreted. According to the manufacturers, the decision to continue or discontinue breast-feeding during therapy should take into account the risk of exposure to the infant and the benefits of treatment to the mother.

Use Adjuvant therapy component for primary breast cancer

Unlabeled Use Treatment of esophageal cancer, gastric cancer, soft tissue sarcoma, uterine sarcoma

Mechanism of Action/Effect Epirubicin is an anthracycline agent which inhibits DNA and RNA synthesis throughout the cell cycle.

Contraindications Hypersensitivity to epirubicin or any component of the formulation, other anthracyclines, or anthracenediones; previous anthracycline treatment up to maximum cumulative dose; severe myocardial insufficiency, severe arrhythmias; recent myocardial infarction

Warnings/Precautions Hazardous agent - use appropriate precautions for handling and disposal.

[U.S. Boxed Warning]: Myocardial toxicity, including heart failure (HF) may occur, particularly in patients who have received prior anthracyclines, prior or concomitant radiotherapy to the mediastinal/pericardial area, who have pre-existing cardiac disease (active or dormant), or with concomitant cardiotoxic medications. Cardiotoxicity may be concurrent or delayed (months to years after treatment). The risk of HF is ~0.9% at a cumulative dose of 550 mg/m², ~1.6% at a cumulative dose of 700 mg/m², and ~3.3% at a cumulative dose of 900 mg/m². Cardiotoxicity may also occur at lower cumulative doses or without risk factors. The risk of delayed cardiotoxicity increases more steeply with cumulative doses >900 mg/m² and this dose should be exceeded only with extreme caution. Acute toxicity, primarily sinus tachycardia and/or ECG abnormalities, including arrhythmia, and delayed toxicity, including decreased left ventricular ejection fraction (LVEF) and HF, have been described. Delayed toxicity usually develops late in the course of therapy or within 2-3 months after completion. Toxicity may be additive with other anthracyclines or anthracenediones, and may be increased in pediatric patients. Regular monitoring of LVEF and discontinuation at the first sign of impairment is recommended especially in patients with cardiac risk factors or impaired cardiac function. Discontinue treatment with signs of decreased LVEF. The half life of other cardiotoxic agents must be considered in sequential therapy; avoid epirubicin for up to 24 weeks after completing trastuzumab treatment.

[U.S. Boxed Warning]: May cause severe myelosuppression; neutropenia is the dose-limiting toxicity; severe thrombocytopenia or anemia may occur; obtain baseline and periodic blood counts. Patients should recover from myelosuppression due to prior chemotherapy treatment before beginning treatments. Thrombophlebitis and thromboembolic phenomena (including pulmonary embolism) have occurred.

[U.S. Boxed Warning]: Reduce dosage in patients with mild-to-moderate hepatic impairment (not recommended in severe hepatic impairment; predominantly hepatically eliminated) and in patients with serum creatinine >5 mg/dL (has not been studied in patients on dialysis); monitor hepatic and renal function at baseline and during treatment. May cause tumor lysis syndrome (TLS), although generally generally does not occur in patients with breast cancer; if TLS risk is suspected, consider monitoring serum uric acid, potassium, calcium, phosphate, and serum creatinine after initial administration; hydration and allopurinol prophylaxis may minimize potential TLS complications. Radiation recall (inflammatory) has been reported; epirubicin may have radiosensitizing activity. **[U.S. Boxed Warning]: Treatment with anthracyclines (including epirubicin) may increase the risk of secondary acute myelogenous leukemia (AML). AML is more common when given in combination with other antineoplastic agents, in patients who have received multiple courses of previous chemotherapy, or with escalated cumulative anthracycline doses (>720 mg/m² for epirubicin). In breast cancer**

patients, the risk for treatment-related AML or myelodysplastic syndrome (MDS) was estimated at 0.3% at 3 years, 0.5% at 5 years, and 0.6% at 8 years after treatment. The latency period for secondary leukemias may be short (1-3 years).

[U.S. Boxed Warning]: For I.V. administration only, severe local tissue damage and necrosis will result if extravasation occurs (vesicant); not for I.M. or SubQ use. Injection in to a small vein or repeated administration in the same vein may result in venous sclerosis. Women ≥70 years of age should be closely monitored for toxicity. **[U.S. Boxed Warning]: Should be administered under the supervision of an experienced cancer chemotherapy physician.** Epirubicin is emetogenic; consider prophylactic antiemetics prior to administration. Patients should recover from acute toxicities (stomatitis, myelosuppression, infections) prior to initiating treatment. Assess baseline labs (blood counts, bilirubin, ALT, AST, serum creatinine) and cardiac function (with LVEF). Prophylactic antibiotics should be administered with the CDF-120 regimen. Patients should not be immunized with live viral vaccines during or shortly after treatment. Inactivated vaccines may be administered (response may be diminished).

Drug Interactions

Avoid Concomitant Use

Avoid concomitant use of Epirubicin with any of the following: BCG; Cimetidine; CloZAPine; Natalizumab; Pimecrolimus; Tacrolimus (Topical); Vaccines (Live)

Decreased Effect

Epirubicin may decrease the levels/effects of: BCG; Cardiac Glycosides; Coccidioidin Skin Test; Sipuleucel-T; Vaccines (Inactivated); Vaccines (Live)

The levels/effects of Epirubicin may be decreased by: Cardiac Glycosides; Echinacea

Increased Effect/Toxicity

Epirubicin may increase the levels/effects of: CloZAPine; Leflunomide; Natalizumab; Vaccines (Live)

The levels/effects of Epirubicin may be increased by: Bevacizumab; Cimetidine; Denosumab; Pimecrolimus; Roflumilast; Tacrolimus (Topical); Taxane Derivatives; Trastuzumab

Nutritional/Ethanol Interactions

Ethanol: Avoid ethanol (due to GI irritation).

Herb/Nutraceutical: Avoid black cohosh, dong quai in estrogen-dependent tumors.

Adverse Reactions Percentages reported as part of combination chemotherapy regimens.

>10%:

Central nervous system: Lethargy (1% to 46%)

Dermatologic: Alopecia (70% to 96%)

Endocrine & metabolic: Amenorrhea (69% to 72%), hot flashes (5% to 39%)

Gastrointestinal: Nausea/vomiting (83% to 92%; grades 3/4: 22% to 25%), mucositis (9% to 59%; grades 3/4: ≤9%), diarrhea (7% to 25%)

Hematologic: Leukopenia (50% to 80%; grades 3/4: 2% to 59%), neutropenia (54% to 80%; grades 3/4: 11% to 67%; nadir: 10-14 days; recovery: by day 21), anemia (13% to 72%; grades 3/4: ≤6%), thrombocytopenia (5% to 49%; grades 3/4: ≤5%)

Local: Injection site reactions (3% to 20%; grades 3/4: <1%)

Ocular: Conjunctivitis (1% to 15%)

Miscellaneous: Infection (15% to 22%; grades 3/4: ≤2%)

1% to 10%:

Cardiovascular: LVEF decreased (asymptomatic; delayed: 1% to 2%), HF (0.4% to 1.5%)

Central nervous system: Fever (1% to 5%)

Dermatologic: Rash (1% to 9%), skin changes (1% to 5%)

Gastrointestinal: Anorexia (2% to 3%)

Hematologic: Neutropenic fever (grades 3/4: ≤6%)

Available Dosage Forms

Injection, powder for reconstitution: 50 mg

Injection, solution [preservative free]: 2 mg/mL (5 mL, 25 mL, 75 mL, 100 mL)

Ellence®: 2 mg/mL (25 mL, 100 mL)

General Dosage Range Dosage adjustment recommended in patients with hepatic or renal impairment or who develop toxicities

I.V.: *Adults:* 100 mg/m^2 on day 1 every 3 weeks **or** 60 mg/m^2 on days 1 and 8 every 4 weeks

Administration

I.V. Infuse over 15-20 minutes or slow I.V. push; if lower doses due to dose reduction are administered, may reduce infusion time proportionally. Do not infuse over <3 minutes. Infuse into a free-flowing I.V. solution. Avoid the use of veins over joints or in extremities with compromised venous or lymphatic drainage. Monitor infusion site; avoid extravasation.

Stability

Reconstitution Use appropriate precautions for handling and disposal. Reconstitute lyophilized powder with SWFI (25 mL for the 50 mg vial or 100 mL for the 200 mg vial) to a final concentration of 2 mg/mL.

Storage Protect from light.

Solution: Store intact vials refrigerated at 2°C to 8°C (36°F to 46°F); do not freeze. Product may "gel" at refrigerated temperatures; will return to slightly viscous solution after 2-4 hours at room temperature (15°C to 30°C). Discard unused solution from single dose vials within 24 hours of entry.

Lyophilized powder: Store at room temperature of 25°C (77°F); excursions permitted to 15°C to 30°C (59°F to 86°F). Reconstituted solutions are stable for 24 hours when stored at 2°C to 8°C (36°F to 46°F) or at room temperature.

Nursing Actions

Physical Assessment Note specific infusion instructions. Premedication with an antiemetic may be ordered (emetogenic). Monitor infusion site closely to prevent extravasation; severe local tissue necrosis will result if extravasation occurs. Monitor for acute nausea and vomiting, anemia, cardiotoxicity, infection, and bleeding. Teach patient importance of adequate hydration.

Patient Education This medication can only be administered by infusion. Report immediately any swelling, pain, burning, or redness at infusion site, sudden difficulty breathing or swallowing, chest pain, or chills. Maintain adequate nutrition and hydration, unless instructed to restrict fluid intake. You will be more susceptible to infection. May cause nausea or vomiting; if severe, contact prescriber for antiemetic. May cause diarrhea, loss of hair (reversible), hyperpigmentation of skin or nails, mouth sores, or changes in menstrual cycle (consult prescriber). Report chest pain, swelling of extremities, palpitations, or rapid heartbeat; respiratory difficulty or unusual cough; pain, redness, unusual warmth in extremities; unresolved nausea, vomiting, or diarrhea; alterations in urinary pattern (increased or decreased); opportunistic infection (fever, chills, unusual bruising or bleeding, fatigue, purulent vaginal discharge, unhealed mouth sores); skin rash; abdominal pain; or blood in urine or stool.

Related Information

Management of Drug Extravasations *on page 1269*

Eplerenone (e PLER en one)

Brand Names: U.S. Inspra™

Pharmacologic Category Diuretic, Potassium-Sparing; Selective Aldosterone Blocker

Medication Safety Issues

Sound-alike/look-alike issues:

Inspra™ may be confused with Spiriva®

Pregnancy Risk Factor B

Lactation Excretion in breast milk unknown/not recommended

Use Treatment of hypertension (may be used alone or in combination with other antihypertensive agents); treatment of heart failure (HF) following acute MI

Mechanism of Action/Effect Aldosterone increases blood pressure primarily by inducing sodium reabsorption. Eplerenone reduces blood pressure by blocking aldosterone binding at mineralocorticoid receptors found in the kidney, heart, blood vessels and brain.

Contraindications Serum potassium >5.5 mEq/L at initiation; Cl_{cr} ≤30 mL/minute; concomitant use of strong CYP3A4 inhibitors (see Drug Interactions for details)

The following additional contraindications apply to patients with hypertension: Type 2 diabetes mellitus (noninsulin dependent, NIDDM) with microalbuminuria; serum creatinine >2.0 mg/dL in males or >1.8 mg/dL in females; Cl_{cr} <50 mL/minute; concomitant use with potassium supplements or potassium-sparing diuretics

Warnings/Precautions Dosage adjustment needed for patients on moderate CYP3A4 inhibitors. Monitor closely for hyperkalemia; increases in serum potassium were dose related during clinical trials and rates of hyperkalemia also increased with declining renal function. Safety and efficacy have not been established in patients with severe hepatic impairment. Use with caution in HF patients post-MI with diabetes (especially if patient has proteinuria); risk of hyperkalemia is increased. Risk of hyperkalemia is increased with declining renal function. Use with caution in patients with mild renal impairment; contraindicated with moderate-severe impairment (HTN: Cl_{cr} <50 mL/minute; other indications: Cl_{cr} ≤30 mL/minute).

Drug Interactions

Avoid Concomitant Use

Avoid concomitant use of Eplerenone with any of the following: CycloSPORINE; CycloSPORINE (Systemic); CYP3A4 Inhibitors (Strong); Itraconazole; Ketoconazole; Ketoconazole (Systemic); Posaconazole; Tacrolimus; Tacrolimus (Systemic); Voriconazole

Decreased Effect

The levels/effects of Eplerenone may be decreased by: CYP3A4 Inducers (Strong); Deferasirox; Herbs (CYP3A4 Inducers); Herbs (Hypertensive Properties); Methylphenidate; Nonsteroidal Anti-Inflammatory Agents; Tocilizumab; Yohimbine

Increased Effect/Toxicity

Eplerenone may increase the levels/effects of: ACE Inhibitors; Amifostine; Angiotensin II Receptor Blockers; Antihypertensives; CycloSPORINE; CycloSPORINE (Systemic); Hypotensive Agents; Potassium Salts; Potassium-Sparing Diuretics; RiTUXimab; Tacrolimus; Tacrolimus (Systemic)

The levels/effects of Eplerenone may be increased by: Alfuzosin; Calcium Channel Blockers (Nondihydropyridine); CYP3A4 Inhibitors (Moderate); CYP3A4 Inhibitors (Strong); Dasatinib; Diazoxide; Fluconazole; Herbs (Hypotensive Properties); Itraconazole; Ivacaftor; Ketoconazole; Ketoconazole (Systemic); Macrolide Antibiotics; MAO Inhibitors; Nitrofurantoin; Nonsteroidal Anti-Inflammatory Agents; Pentoxifylline; Phosphodiesterase 5 Inhibitors; Posaconazole; Prostacyclin Analogues; Protease Inhibitors; Trimethoprim; Voriconazole

Nutritional/Ethanol Interactions

Food: Grapefruit juice increases eplerenone AUC ~25%.

Herb/Nutraceutical: St John's wort may decrease levels of eplerenone. Avoid black cohosh, California poppy, coleus, golden seal, hawthorn, mistletoe, periwinkle, quinine, shepherd's purse (may have increased antihypertensive effect). Avoid bayberry, blue cohosh, cayenne, ephedra, ginger, ginseng (American), kola, licorice (may diminish the antihypertensive effect).

Adverse Reactions

>10%: Endocrine & metabolic: Hyperkalemia ([HF post-MI: K >5.5 mEq/L: 16%; K ≥6 mEq/L: 6%] [HTN: K >5.5 mEq/L at doses ≤100 mg: ≤1%; doses >100 mg: 9%]), hypertriglyceridemia (1% to 15%, dose related)

1% to 10%:

- Central nervous system: Dizziness (3%), fatigue (2%)
- Endocrine & metabolic: Hyponatremia (2%, dose related), breast pain (males <1% to 1%), gynecomastia (males <1% to 1%), hypercholesterolemia (<1% to 1%)
- Gastrointestinal: Diarrhea (2%), abdominal pain (1%)
- Genitourinary: Abnormal vaginal bleeding (<1% to 2%)
- Renal: Creatinine increased (HF post-MI: 6%), albuminuria (1%)
- Respiratory: Cough (2%)
- Miscellaneous: Flu-like syndrome (2%)

Available Dosage Forms

Tablet, oral: 25 mg, 50 mg

Inspra™: 25 mg, 50 mg

General Dosage Range Dosage adjustment recommended in patients on concomitant therapy or based on potassium concentrations

Oral: *Adults:* Initial: 25-50 mg once daily; Maintenance: 50 mg once or twice daily (maximum: 100 mg/day)

Administration

Oral May be administered with or without food.

Stability

Storage Store at controlled room temperature of 25°C (77°F).

Nursing Actions

Physical Assessment Monitor potassium levels, blood pressure, and renal function prior to and periodically during therapy. Monitor for hypotension and hyperkalemia at beginning of and at regular intervals during therapy.

Patient Education Take at the same time of day, without regard for meals. It may take up to 4 weeks to achieve desired results. Do not use potassium supplement or salt substitutes without consulting prescriber. This drug does not eliminate need for diet or exercise regimen as recommended by prescriber. May cause dizziness, high triglyceride levels, and increased potassium levels. Report muscle weakness, diarrhea, and abdominal pain.

Dietary Considerations May be taken with or without food. Do not use salt substitutes containing potassium.

Epoetin Alfa (e POE e tin AL fa)

Brand Names: U.S. Epogen®; Procrit®

Index Terms *r*HuEPO; *r*HuEPO-α; EPO; Erythropoiesis-Stimulating Agent (ESA); Erythropoietin

Pharmacologic Category Colony Stimulating Factor; Growth Factor; Recombinant Human Erythropoietin

Medication Safety Issues

Sound-alike/look-alike issues:

Epoetin alfa may be confused with darbepoetin alfa, epoetin beta

Epogen® may be confused with Neupogen®

International issues:

Epopen [Spain] may be confused with EpiPen brand name for epinephrine [U.S., Canada, and multiple international markets]

Medication Guide Available Yes

Pregnancy Risk Factor C

Lactation Excretion in breast milk unknown/use caution

Breast-Feeding Considerations When administered enterally to neonates (mixed with human milk or infant formula), *r*HuEPO-α did not significantly increase serum EPO concentrations. If passage via breast milk does occur, risk to a nursing infant appears low. Avoid the use of multidose vials in nursing women (due to the benzyl alcohol content).

Use Treatment of anemia due to concurrent myelosuppressive chemotherapy in patients with cancer (nonmyeloid malignancies) receiving chemotherapy (palliative intent) for a planned minimum of 2 additional months of chemotherapy; treatment of anemia due to chronic kidney disease (including patients on dialysis and not on dialysis) to decrease the need for RBC transfusion; treatment of anemia associated with HIV (zidovudine) therapy when endogenous erythropoietin levels ≤500 mUnits/mL; reduction of allogeneic RBC transfusion for elective, noncardiac, nonvascular surgery when perioperative hemoglobin is >10 to ≤13 g/dL and there is a high risk for blood loss

Note: Epoetin is **not** indicated for use under the following conditions:

- Cancer patients receiving hormonal therapy, therapeutic biologic products, or radiation therapy unless also receiving concurrent myelosuppressive chemotherapy
- Cancer patients receiving myelosuppressive chemotherapy when the expected outcome is curative
- Surgery patients who are willing to donate autologous blood
- Surgery patients undergoing cardiac or vascular surgery

- As a substitute for RBC transfusion in patients requiring immediate correction of anemia

Note: In clinical trials (and one meta-analysis), epoetin has not demonstrated improved quality of life, fatigue, or well-being.

Unlabeled Use Treatment of symptomatic anemia in myelodysplastic syndrome (MDS)

Mechanism of Action/Effect Induces red blood cell production in the bone marrow to be released into the blood stream where they mature to erythrocytes; results in rise in hematocrit and hemoglobin levels

Contraindications Hypersensitivity to epoetin or any component of the formulation; uncontrolled hypertension; pure red cell aplasia (due to epoetin or other epoetin protein drugs); multidose vials contain benzyl alcohol and are contraindicated in neonates, infants, pregnant women, and nursing women

Warnings/Precautions [U.S. Boxed Warning]: Erythropoiesis-stimulating agents (ESAs) increased the risk of serious cardiovascular events, thromboembolic events, stroke, mortality, and/or tumor progression in clinical studies when administered to target hemoglobin levels >11 g/dL (and provide no additional benefit); a rapid rise in hemoglobin (>1 g/dL over 2 weeks) may also contribute to these risks. **[U.S. Boxed Warning]: A shortened overall survival and/or increased risk of tumor progression or recurrence has been reported in studies with breast, cervical, head and neck, lymphoid, and non-small cell lung cancer patients.** It is of note that in these studies, patients received ESAs to a target hemoglobin of ≥12 g/dL; although risk has not been excluded when dosed to achieve a target hemoglobin of <12 g/dL. **[U.S. Boxed Warnings]: To decrease these risks, and risk of cardio- and thrombovascular events, use the lowest dose needed to avoid red blood cell transfusions. Use ESAs in cancer patients only for the treatment of anemia related to concurrent myelosuppressive chemotherapy; discontinue ESA following completion of the chemotherapy course. ESAs are not indicated for patients receiving myelosuppressive therapy when the anticipated outcome is curative.** A dosage modification is appropriate if hemoglobin levels rise >1 g/dL per 2-week time period during treatment (Rizzo, 2010). Use of ESAs has been associated with an increased risk of venous thromboembolism (VTE) without a reduction in transfusions in patients with cancer (Hershman, 2009). Improved anemia symptoms, quality of life, fatigue, or well-being have not been demonstrated in controlled clinical trials. **[U.S. Boxed Warning]: Because of the risks of decreased survival and increased risk of tumor growth or progression, all healthcare providers and hospitals are required to enroll and comply with the ESA APPRISE (Assisting Providers and Cancer Patients with Risk Information for the Safe use of ESAs) Oncology Program prior to prescribing or dispensing ESAs to cancer patients.** Prescribers and patients will have to provide written documentation of discussed risks prior to each epoetin course.

[U.S. Boxed Warning]: An increased risk of death, serious cardiovascular events, and stroke was reported in chronic kidney disease (CKD) patients administered ESAs to target hemoglobin levels ≥11 g/dL; use the lowest dose sufficient to reduce the need for RBC transfusions. An optimal target hemoglobin level, dose or dosing strategy to reduce these risks has not been identified in clinical trials. Hemoglobin rising >1 g/dL in a 2-week period may contribute to the risk (dosage reduction recommended). Chronic kidney disease patients who exhibit an inadequate hemoglobin response to ESA therapy may be at a higher risk for cardiovascular events and mortality compared to other patients. ESA therapy may reduce dialysis efficacy (due to increase in red blood cells and decrease in plasma volume); adjustments in dialysis parameters may be needed. Patients treated with epoetin may require increased heparinization during dialysis to prevent clotting of the extracorporeal circuit. **[U.S. Boxed Warning]: DVT prophylaxis is recommended in perisurgery patients due to the risk of DVT.** Increased mortality was also observed in patients undergoing coronary artery bypass surgery who received epoetin alfa; these deaths were associated with thrombotic events. Epoetin is **not** approved for reduction of red blood cell transfusion in patients undergoing cardiac or vascular surgery and is **not** indicated for surgical patients willing to donate autologous blood.

Use with caution in patients with hypertension (contraindicated in uncontrolled hypertension) or with a history of seizures; hypertensive encephalopathy and seizures have been reported. If hypertension is difficult to control, reduce or hold epoetin alfa. An excessive rate of rise of hemoglobin is associated with hypertension or exacerbation of hypertension; decrease the epoetin dose if the hemoglobin increase exceeds 1 g/dL in any 2-week period. Blood pressure should be controlled prior to start of therapy and monitored closely throughout treatment. The risk for seizures is increased with epoetin use in patients with CKD; monitor closely for neurologic symptoms during the first several months of therapy. Due to the delayed onset of erythropoiesis, epoetin alfa is **not** recommended for acute correction of severe anemia or as a substitute for emergency transfusion.

Prior to treatment, correct or exclude deficiencies of iron, vitamin B_{12}, and/or folate, as well as other factors which may impair erythropoiesis (inflammatory conditions, infections). Prior to and periodically ▶

during therapy, iron stores must be evaluated. Supplemental iron is recommended if serum ferritin <100 mcg/L or serum transferrin saturation <20%; most patients with chronic kidney disease will require iron supplementation. Poor response should prompt evaluation of these potential factors, as well as possible malignant processes and hematologic disease (thalassemia, refractory anemia, myelodysplastic disorder), occult blood loss, hemolysis, ostetis fibrosa cystic, and/or bone marrow fibrosis. Severe anemia and pure red cell aplasia (PRCA) with associated neutralizing antibodies to erythropoietin has been reported, predominantly in patients with CKD receiving SubQ epoetin (the I.V. route is preferred for hemodialysis patients). Cases have also been reported in patients with hepatitis C who were receiving ESAs, interferon, and ribavirin. Patients with a sudden loss of response to epoetin alfa (with severe anemia and a low reticulocyte count) should be evaluated for PRCA with associated neutralizing antibodies to erythropoietin; discontinue treatment (permanently) in patients with PRCA secondary to neutralizing antibodies to epoetin.

Potentially serious allergic reactions have been reported (rarely). Discontinue immediately (and permanently) in patients who experience serious allergic/anaphylactic reactions. Some products may contain albumin. Multidose vials contain benzyl alcohol; do not use in premature infants.

Drug Interactions

Avoid Concomitant Use There are no known interactions where it is recommended to avoid concomitant use.

Decreased Effect There are no known significant interactions involving a decrease in effect.

Increased Effect/Toxicity There are no known significant interactions involving an increase in effect.

Adverse Reactions

>10%:

- Cardiovascular: Hypertension (3% to 28%)
- Central nervous system: Fever (10% to 42%), headache (5% to 18%)
- Dermatologic: Pruritus (12% to 21%), rash (2% to 19%)
- Gastrointestinal: Nausea (35% to 56%), vomiting (12% to 28%)
- Local: Injection site reaction (7% to 13%)
- Neuromuscular & skeletal: Arthralgia (10% to 16%)
- Respiratory: Cough (4% to 26%)

1% to 10%:

- Cardiovascular: Deep vein thrombosis, edema, thrombosis
- Central nervous system: Chills, depression, dizziness, insomnia
- Dermatologic: Urticaria
- Endocrine & metabolic: Hyperglycemia, hypokalemia
- Gastrointestinal: Dysphagia, stomatitis, weight loss
- Hematologic: Leukopenia
- Local: Clotted vascular access
- Neuromuscular & skeletal: Bone pain, muscle spasm, myalgia
- Respiratory: Pulmonary embolism, respiratory congestion, upper respiratory infection

Pharmacodynamics/Kinetics

Onset of Action Several days; Peak effect: Hemoglobin level: 2-6 weeks

Available Dosage Forms

Injection, solution:

Epogen®: 10,000 units/mL (2 mL); 20,000 units/mL (1 mL)

Procrit®: 10,000 units/mL (2 mL); 20,000 units/mL (1 mL)

Injection, solution [preservative free]:

Epogen®: 2000 units/mL (1 mL); 3000 units/mL (1 mL); 4000 units/mL (1 mL); 10,000 units/mL (1 mL)

Procrit®: 2000 units/mL (1 mL); 3000 units/mL (1 mL); 4000 units/mL (1 mL); 10,000 units/mL (1 mL); 40,000 units/mL (1 mL)

General Dosage Range I.V., SubQ: Children and Adults: Dosage varies greatly depending on indication

Administration

I.V. Patients with CKD on hemodialysis: I.V. route preferred; it may be administered into the venous line at the end of the dialysis procedure

Note: SubQ administration is the preferred route in other patient populations.

I.V. Detail pH: 6.6-7.2 (single dose vial); 5.8-6.4 (multidose vial)

Other SubQ: SubQ is the preferred route of administration **except** in patients with CKD on hemodialysis; 1:1 dilution with bacteriostatic NS (containing benzyl alcohol) acts as a local anesthetic to reduce pain at the injection site

Stability

Reconstitution Prior to SubQ administration, preservative free solutions may be mixed with bacteriostatic NS containing benzyl alcohol 0.9% in a 1:1 ratio.

Storage Vials should be stored at 2°C to 8°C (36°F to 46°F); **do not freeze or shake**. Protect from light.

Single-dose 1 mL vial contains no preservative: Use one dose per vial. Do not re-enter vial; discard unused portions.

Single-dose vials (except 40,000 units/mL vial) are stable for 2 weeks at room temperature (Cohen, 2007). Single-dose 40,000 units/mL vial is stable for 1 week at room temperature.

Multidose 1 mL or 2 mL vial contains preservative. Store at 2°C to 8°C after initial entry and between doses. Discard 21 days after initial entry.

Multidose vials (with preservative) are stable for 1 week at room temperature (Cohen, 2007).

Prefilled syringes containing the 20,000 units/mL formulation with preservative are stable for 6 weeks refrigerated (2°C to 8°C) (Naughton, 2003).

Dilutions of 1:10 and 1:20 (1 part epoetin:19 parts sodium chloride) are stable for 18 hours at room temperature (Ohls, 1996).

Prior to SubQ administration, preservative free solutions may be mixed with bacteriostatic NS containing benzyl alcohol 0.9% in a 1:1 ratio (Corbo, 1992).

Dilutions of 1:10 in $D_{10}W$ with human albumin 0.05% or 0.1% are stable for 24 hours.

Nursing Actions

Physical Assessment Evaluate history of hypertension or seizures and potential risk for thromboembolism prior to beginning therapy. Blood pressure should be monitored closely and controlled during therapy. If administered by intravenous infusion, lines should be monitored closely for possible clotting. Assess blood chemistries, hemoglobin/hematocrit, serum ferritin, and transferrin saturation prior to and on a regular basis during therapy; dosage adjustment and iron supplements may be necessary. Monitor for hypertension, thrombotic events, edema, and anemia. Serious allergic or anaphylactic reactions may require discontinuation of treatment. Teach patient proper SubQ injection technique and syringe/needle disposal.

Patient Education If self-administered, follow exact directions for injection and needle disposal. You will require frequent blood tests to determine appropriate dosage and reduce potential for severe adverse effects; maintaining laboratory testing schedule is vital. Report skin rash; difficulty swallowing; onset of severe headache, unusual dizziness, or blurred vision; chest pain; muscular tremors or seizure activity; or difficulty breathing.

Epoprostenol (e poe PROST en ole)

Brand Names: U.S. Flolan®; Veletri®

Index Terms Epoprostenol Sodium; PGI_2; PGX; Prostacyclin

Pharmacologic Category Prostacyclin; Prostaglandin; Vasodilator

Medication Safety Issues

High alert medication:

The Institute for Safe Medication Practices (ISMP) includes this medication among its list of drugs which have a heightened risk of causing significant patient harm when used in error.

Pregnancy Risk Factor B

Lactation Excretion in breast milk unknown/use caution

Use Treatment of pulmonary arterial hypertension (PAH) (WHO Group I) in patients with NYHA Class III or IV symptoms to improve exercise capacity

Unlabeled Use Acute vasodilator testing in pulmonary arterial hypertension (PAH)

Inhalation: Intraoperative treatment of pulmonary hypertension in patients undergoing cardiac surgery with cardiopulmonary bypass; post-cardiothoracic surgery pulmonary hypertension, right ventricular dysfunction, or refractory hypoxemia

Available Dosage Forms

Injection, powder for reconstitution: 0.5 mg, 1.5 mg

Flolan®: 0.5 mg, 1.5 mg

Veletri®: 1.5 mg

General Dosage Range I.V.: *Adults:* Initial: 1-2 ng/kg/minute; increase dose in increments of 1-2 ng/kg/minute every 15 minutes until response

Administration

I.V. The ambulatory infusion pump should be small and lightweight, be able to adjust infusion rates in 2 ng/kg/minute increments, have occlusion, end of infusion, and low battery alarms, have ± 6% accuracy of the programmed rate, and have positive continuous or pulsatile pressure with intervals ≤3 minutes between pulses. The reservoir should be made of polyvinyl chloride, polypropylene, or glass. Immediate access to back up pump, infusion sets and medication is essential to prevent treatment interruptions.

I.V. Detail When given on an ongoing basis, must be infused through a central venous catheter. Peripheral infusion may be used temporarily until central line is established. Infuse using an infusion pump. Avoid abrupt withdrawal (including interruptions in delivery) or sudden large reductions in dosing.

pH: 10.2-10.8

Inhalation Inhalation is an unlabeled route of administration.

Intraoperative administration: Administer via jet nebulizer connected to the inspiratory limb of the ventilator near the endotracheal tube with a bypass oxygen flow of 8 L/minute to achieve administration of a high proportion of small particles (Fattouch, 2006; Hache, 2003).

Post-cardiothoracic surgery: May also be administered via jet nebulizer connected to the inspiratory limb of the ventilator near the endotracheal tube or via face mask with a Venturi attachment for aerosolization with a bypass oxygen flow of 2-3 L/minute (De Wet, 2004). **Note:** Glycine buffer diluent may cause ventilator valve malfunction; it has been recommended that filters be changed on the ventilator every 2 hours; may also use a ventilator heating coil (De Wet, 2004).

Nursing Actions

Physical Assessment Monitor patient's ability to manage a central venous catheter in the home setting. Review with patient the importance of infection control practices for the management of a central venous catheter. **Institutional:** Continuous pulmonary and hemodynamic arterial monitoring, protimes. **Home therapy:** Avoid sudden rate reduction or abrupt withdrawal or interruption of therapy. When adjustment in rate is made, monitor blood pressure (standing and supine) and pulse for several hours to ensure tolerance to new rate. Monitor for bleeding. Monitor vital signs daily. Monitor for improved pulmonary function (decreased exertional dyspnea, fatigue, syncope, chest pain) and improved quality of life. Be alert for any infusion pump malfunction.

Patient Education Therapy on this drug will probably be long-term. You may experience mild headache, nausea, vomiting, diarrhea, weight loss, nervousness, dizziness, or muscular pains. Report immediately any signs or symptoms of acute or severe headache; back pain; increased difficult breathing; flushing; fever or chills; any unusual bleeding or bruising; chest pain; palpitations; difficulty breathing; increased pain, irritation, or pus formed at I.V. site; or any onset of unresolved diarrhea.

Eprosartan (ep roe SAR tan)

Brand Names: U.S. Teveten®

Pharmacologic Category Angiotensin II Receptor Blocker

Pregnancy Risk Factor D

Lactation Not recommended

Use Treatment of hypertension; may be used alone or in combination with other antihypertensives

Mechanism of Action/Effect Eprosartan is an angiotensin receptor antagonist which blocks the vasoconstriction and aldosterone-secreting effects of angiotensin II.

Contraindications Hypersensitivity to eprosartan or any component of the formulation

Warnings/Precautions [U.S. Boxed Warning]: Drugs that act on the renin-angiotensin system can cause injury and death to the developing fetus. Discontinue as soon as possible once pregnancy is detected. May cause hyperkalemia; avoid potassium supplementation unless specifically required by healthcare provider. Avoid use or use a smaller dose in patients who are volume depleted; correct depletion first. May be associated with deterioration of renal function and/or increases in serum creatinine, particularly in patients with low renal blood flow (eg, renal artery stenosis, heart failure) whose glomerular filtration rate (GFR) is dependent on efferent arteriolar vasoconstriction by angiotensin II. Use with caution in unstented unilateral/bilateral renal artery stenosis. When unstented bilateral renal artery stenosis is present, use is generally avoided due to the elevated risk of deterioration in renal function unless possible benefits outweigh risks. Use with caution in pre-existing renal insufficiency; significant aortic/mitral stenosis. Concurrent use of ACE inhibitors may increase the risk of clinically-significant adverse events (eg, renal dysfunction, hyperkalemia).

Drug Interactions

Avoid Concomitant Use There are no known interactions where it is recommended to avoid concomitant use.

Decreased Effect

The levels/effects of Eprosartan may be decreased by: Herbs (Hypertensive Properties); Methylphenidate; Nonsteroidal Anti-Inflammatory Agents; Yohimbine

Increased Effect/Toxicity

Eprosartan may increase the levels/effects of: ACE Inhibitors; Amifostine; Antihypertensives; Hypotensive Agents; Lithium; Nonsteroidal Anti-Inflammatory Agents; Potassium-Sparing Diuretics; RiTUXimab; Sodium Phosphates

The levels/effects of Eprosartan may be increased by: Alfuzosin; Diazoxide; Eplerenone; Herbs (Hypotensive Properties); MAO Inhibitors; Pentoxifylline; Phosphodiesterase 5 Inhibitors; Potassium Salts; Prostacyclin Analogues; Tolvaptan; Trimethoprim

Nutritional/Ethanol Interactions Herb/Nutraceutical: Dong quai has estrogenic activity. Some herbal medications may worsen hypertension (eg, ephedra); garlic may have additional antihypertensive effects. Management: Avoid dong quai if using for hypertension. Avoid ephedra, yohimbe, ginseng, and garlic.

Adverse Reactions 1% to 10%:

Central nervous system: Fatigue (2%), depression (1%)

Endocrine & metabolic: Hypertriglyceridemia (1%)

Gastrointestinal: Abdominal pain (2%)

Genitourinary: Urinary tract infection (1%)

Respiratory: Upper respiratory tract infection (8%), rhinitis (4%), pharyngitis (4%), cough (4%)

Miscellaneous: Viral infection (2%), injury (2%)

Available Dosage Forms

Tablet, oral: 600 mg

Teveten®: 400 mg, 600 mg

General Dosage Range Oral: *Adults:* Initial: 400-600 mg once daily; Maintenance: 400-800 mg/day in 1-2 divided doses

Nursing Actions

Physical Assessment Monitor for hypotension on a regular basis during therapy.

Patient Education This drug does not eliminate need for diet or exercise regimen as recommended by prescriber. May cause dizziness, fainting, lightheadedness, or postural hypotension. Report chest pain or palpitations; respiratory infection or cold symptoms; unusual cough; swelling of face, tongue, lips, or extremities; changes in urinary pattern; or extreme fatigue.

Eprosartan and Hydrochlorothiazide

(ep roe SAR tan & hye droe klor oh THYE a zide)

Brand Names: U.S. Teveten® HCT

Index Terms Eprosartan Mesylate and Hydrochlorothiazide; Hydrochlorothiazide and Eprosartan

Pharmacologic Category Angiotensin II Receptor Blocker; Diuretic, Thiazide

Pregnancy Risk Factor D

Lactation Enters breast milk/not recommended

Use Treatment of hypertension (not indicated for initial treatment)

Available Dosage Forms

Tablet:

Teveten® HCT: 600 mg/12.5 mg: Eprosartan 600 mg and hydrochlorothiazide 12.5 mg; 600 mg/25 mg: Eprosartan 600 mg and hydrochlorothiazide 25 mg

General Dosage Range Oral: *Adults:* Eprosartan 600 mg and hydrochlorothiazide 12.5-25 mg once daily

Administration

Oral May be administered without regard to meals.

Nursing Actions

Physical Assessment See individual agents.

Patient Education See individual agents.

Related Information

Eprosartan *on page 408*

Hydrochlorothiazide *on page 570*

Eptifibatide

(ep TIF i ba tide)

Brand Names: U.S. Integrilin®

Index Terms Intrifiban

Pharmacologic Category Antiplatelet Agent, Glycoprotein IIb/IIIa Inhibitor

Medication Safety Issues

High alert medication:

The Institute for Safe Medication Practices (ISMP) includes this medication among its list of drugs which have a heightened risk of causing significant patient harm when used in error.

Pregnancy Risk Factor B

Lactation Excretion in breast milk unknown/use caution

Use Treatment of patients with acute coronary syndrome (unstable angina/non-ST-segment elevation myocardial infarction [UA/NSTEMI]), including patients who are to be managed medically and those undergoing percutaneous coronary intervention (PCI including angioplasty, intracoronary stenting)

Unlabeled Use To support PCI during ST-elevation myocardial infarction (administered at the time of primary PCI); elective PCI for stable ischemic heart disease (in combination with unfractionated heparin)

Mechanism of Action/Effect Eptifibatide is a glycoprotein IIb/IIIa receptor antagonist that reversibly blocks platelet aggregation and prevents thrombosis.

Contraindications Hypersensitivity to eptifibatide or any component of the product; active abnormal bleeding within the previous 30 days or a history of bleeding diathesis; history of stroke within 30 days or a history of hemorrhagic stroke; severe hypertension (systolic blood pressure >200 mm Hg or diastolic blood pressure >110 mm Hg) not adequately controlled on antihypertensive therapy; major surgery within the preceding 6 weeks; current or planned administration of another parenteral GP IIb/IIIa inhibitor; dependency on hemodialysis

Canadian labeling: Additional contraindications (not in U.S. labeling): PT >1.2 times control or INR ≥2.0; known history of intracranial disease (eg, neoplasm, arteriovenous malformation, aneurysm); severe renal impairment (Cl_{cr} <30 mL/minute); thrombocytopenia (<100,000 cells/mm^3); clinically significant liver disease

Warnings/Precautions Bleeding is the most common complication. Most major bleeding occurs at the arterial access site where the cardiac catheterization was done. When bleeding can not be controlled with pressure, discontinue infusion and heparin. Patients <70 kg may be at greater risk for major and minor bleeding. Discontinue ≥2-4 hours prior to coronary artery bypass graft surgery (Hillis, 2011). Use caution in patients with hemorrhagic retinopathy or with other drugs that affect hemostasis. Use with extreme caution in patients with platelet counts <100,000/mm^3 (contraindicated in the Canadian labeling). If platelet count decreases to <100,000/mm^3 during therapy, discontinue eptifibatide and heparin if administered concurrently.

Concurrent use with thrombolytics has not been established as safe and is generally not recommended (Goodman, 2008). Minimize invasive procedures, including arterial and venous punctures, I.M. injections, and nasogastric tube insertion. Prior to sheath removal, the aPTT or ACT should be checked (do not remove unless aPTT is <45 seconds or the ACT <150 seconds). Use caution in renal dysfunction (estimated Cl_{cr} <50 mL/minute, using Cockcroft-Gault equation); dosage adjustment required. Use is contraindicated in patients dependent upon hemodialysis.

Drug Interactions

Avoid Concomitant Use There are no known interactions where it is recommended to avoid concomitant use.

Decreased Effect

The levels/effects of Eptifibatide may be decreased by: Nonsteroidal Anti-Inflammatory Agents

Increased Effect/Toxicity

Eptifibatide may increase the levels/effects of: Anticoagulants; Antiplatelet Agents; Collagenase

(Systemic); Drotrecogin Alfa (Activated); Ibritumomab; Rivaroxaban; Salicylates; Thrombolytic Agents; Tositumomab and Iodine I 131 Tositumomab

The levels/effects of Eptifibatide may be increased by: Dasatinib; Glucosamine; Herbs (Anticoagulant/Antiplatelet Properties); Nonsteroidal Anti-Inflammatory Agents; Omega-3-Acid Ethyl Esters; Pentosan Polysulfate Sodium; Pentoxifylline; Prostacyclin Analogues; Vitamin E

Nutritional/Ethanol Interactions Herb/Nutraceutical: Avoid alfalfa, anise, bilberry, bladderwrack, bromelain, cat's claw, celery, coleus, cordyceps, dong quai, evening primrose oil, fenugreek, feverfew, garlic, ginger, ginkgo biloba, ginseng (American), ginseng (Panax), ginseng (Siberian), grapeseed, green tea, guggul, horse chestnut seed, horseradish, licorice, prickly ash, red clover, reishi, same (s-adenosylmethionine), sweet clover, turmeric, and white willow (all have additional antiplatelet activity).

Adverse Reactions Bleeding is the major drug-related adverse effect. Access site is often primary source of bleeding complications. Incidence of bleeding is also related to heparin intensity. Patients weighing <70 kg may have an increased risk of major bleeding.

>10%: Hematologic: Bleeding (major: 1% to 11%; minor: 3% to 14%; transfusion required: 2% to 13%)

1% to 10%:

Cardiovascular: Hypotension (up to 7%)
Hematologic: Thrombocytopenia (1% to 3%)
Local: Injection site reaction

Pharmacodynamics/Kinetics

Onset of Action Within 1 hour

Duration of Action Platelet function restored ~4 hours following discontinuation

Available Dosage Forms

Injection, solution:

Integrilin®: 0.75 mg/mL (100 mL); 2 mg/mL (10 mL, 100 mL)

General Dosage Range Dosage adjustment recommended in patients with renal impairment

I.V.: *Adults:* Bolus: 180 mcg/kg (maximum: 22.6 mg), repeat once for PCI; Infusion: 2 mcg/kg/minute (maximum: 15 mg/hour)

Administration

I.V. Do not shake vial. Administer bolus doses by I.V. push over 1-2 minutes. Begin continuous infusion immediately following bolus administration; administer directly from the 100 mL vial.

I.V. Detail Visually inspect for discoloration or particulate matter prior to administration. The bolus dose should be withdrawn from the 10 mL vial into a syringe. The 100 mL vial should be spiked with a vented infusion set.

Stability

Storage Vials should be stored refrigerated at 2°C to 8°C (36°F to 46°F). Vials can be kept at room temperature for 2 months, after which they must be discarded. Protect from light until administration. Do not use beyond the expiration date. Discard any unused portion left in the vial.

Nursing Actions

Physical Assessment Monitor vital signs prior to, during, and after therapy. Assess infusion insertion site during and after therapy (every 15 minutes or as institutional policy). Observe and teach patient bleeding precautions. Monitor closely for signs of excessive bleeding (CNS changes; blood in urine, stool, or vomitus; unusual bruising or bleeding).

Patient Education This medication can only be administered intravenously. You will have a tendency to bleed easily while medication is being administered. Report unusual bruising or bleeding (eg, blood in urine, stool, or vomitus; bleeding gums), dizziness or vision changes, or back pain.

Ergocalciferol (er goe kal SIF e role)

Brand Names: U.S. Calciferol™ [OTC]; Drisdol®; Drisdol® [OTC]

Index Terms Activated Ergosterol; D2; Viosterol; Vitamin D2

Pharmacologic Category Vitamin D Analog

Medication Safety Issues

Sound-alike/look-alike issues:

Calciferol™ may be confused with calcitriol
Drisdol® may be confused with Drysol™
Ergocalciferol may be confused with alfacalcidol, cholecalciferol

Administration issues:

Liquid vitamin D preparations have the potential for dosing errors when administered to infants. Droppers should be clearly marked to easily provide 400 international units. For products intended for infants, the FDA recommends that accompanying droppers deliver no more than 400 international units per dose.

Pregnancy Risk Factor C (manufacturer); A/C (dose exceeding RDA recommendation; per expert analysis)

Lactation Enters breast milk/use caution

Use Treatment of refractory rickets, hypophosphatemia, hypoparathyroidism; dietary supplement

Unlabeled Use Prevention and treatment of vitamin D deficiency in patients with chronic kidney disease (CKD); osteoporosis prevention

Available Dosage Forms

Capsule, oral: 50,000 int. units

Drisdol®: 50,000 int. units

Capsule, softgel, oral: 50,000 int. units, 50,000 units

Solution, oral: 8000 int. units/mL (60 mL)

Calciferol™ [OTC]: 8000 int. units/mL (60 mL)
Drisdol® [OTC]: 8000 int. units/mL (60 mL)

Tablet, oral: 400 int. units

General Dosage Range Oral:
Children 0-12 months: Adequate intake: 400 int. units/day
Children 1 year to Adults ≤70 years: RDA: 600 int. units/day
Elderly >70 years: RDA: 800 int. units/day

Nursing Actions

Physical Assessment Provide patient appropriate nutritional counseling.

Patient Education Your prescriber may recommend a special diet. You may experience nausea, vomiting, or metallic taste. Report weakness, unresolved nausea or vomiting, or CNS irritability.

Ergonovine (er goe NOE veen)

Index Terms Ergometrine Maleate; Ergonovine Maleate

Pharmacologic Category Ergot Derivative

Lactation Enters breast milk/contraindicated

Use Prevention and treatment of postpartum and postabortion hemorrhage caused by uterine atony

Unlabeled Use Diagnostically to identify Prinzmetal's angina

Product Availability Not available in the U.S.

General Dosage Range I.M., I.V.: *Adults:* 0.2 mg, may repeat in 2-4 hours if needed, up to maximum of 5 total doses

Administration

I.M. May be administered by I.M injection.

I.V. I.V. use should be limited to patients with severe uterine bleeding or other life-threatening emergency situations. I.V. doses should be administered over a period of not <1 minute.

Nursing Actions

Physical Assessment Blood pressure should be monitored, especially with I.V. use. For postpartum use, monitor character and amount of vaginal bleeding. Monitor patient response, including ergotamine toxicity (eg, headache, ringing in ears, nausea and vomiting, diarrhea, numbness or coldness of extremities, confusion, hallucinations, dyspnea, chest pain, convulsions). When used to test for Prinzmetal's angina during coronary arteriography, emergency equipment, including nitroglycerin, must be on hand. When used at any time other than postpartum, determine that patient is not pregnant.

Patient Education For angina diagnosis, cardiologist will instruct patient about what to expect. For postpartum hemorrhage (an emergency situation), patient needs to know why the drug is being given and what side effects she might experience (eg, mild nausea and vomiting, dizziness, headache, ringing ears) and be instructed to report respiratory difficulty, acute headache, numbness or cold feeling in extremities, or severe abdominal cramping.

Eribulin (er i BUE lin)

Brand Names: U.S. Halaven™

Index Terms B1939; E7389; ER-086526; Eribulin Mesylate; Halichondrin B Analog

Pharmacologic Category Antineoplastic Agent, Antimicrotubular

Medication Safety Issues

Sound-alike/look-alike issues:
Eribulin may be confused with epirubicin, erlotinib

High alert medication:
This medication is in a class the Institute for Safe Medication Practices (ISMP) includes among its list of drug classes which have a heightened risk of causing significant patient harm when used in error.

Pregnancy Risk Factor D

Lactation Excretion in breast milk unknown/not recommended

Use Treatment of metastatic breast cancer in patients who have received at least 2 prior chemotherapy regimens

Available Dosage Forms

Injection, solution:
Halaven™: 0.5 mg/mL (2 mL)

General Dosage Range Dosage adjustment recommended in patients with renal or hepatic impairment or who develop toxicities

I.V.: *Adults:* 1.4 mg/m^2/dose days 1 and 8 every 3 weeks

Administration

I.V. Infuse over 2-5 minutes. May be administered undiluted or diluted in 100 mL normal saline.

Erlotinib (er LOE tye nib)

Brand Names: U.S. Tarceva®

Index Terms CP358774; Erlotinib Hydrochloride; OSI-774

Pharmacologic Category Antineoplastic Agent, Tyrosine Kinase Inhibitor; Epidermal Growth Factor Receptor (EGFR) Inhibitor

Medication Safety Issues

Sound-alike/look-alike issues:
Erlotinib may be confused with crizotinib, eribulin, gefitinib, imatinib, SUNItinib, vandetanib

High alert medication:
This medication is in a class the Institute for Safe Medication Practices (ISMP) includes among its list of drug classes which have a heightened risk of causing significant patient harm when used in error.

Pregnancy Risk Factor D

Lactation Excretion in breast milk unknown/not recommended

Use Treatment of locally advanced or metastatic nonsmall cell lung cancer (NSCLC) refractory to at least 1 prior chemotherapy regimen (as monotherapy); maintenance treatment of locally advanced or metastatic NCSLC which has not progressed after 4-6 cycles of first line platinum-based chemotherapy; locally advanced, unresectable or metastatic pancreatic cancer (first-line therapy in combination with gemcitabine)

Unlabeled Use First-line treatment of NSCLC with known EGFR mutation; treatment of head and neck cancer

Mechanism of Action/Effect Inhibits the intracellular phosphorylation of tyrosine kinase associated with epidermal growth factor receptor (EGFR) which is located on both normal and cancer cells causing cell death.

Contraindications There are no contraindications listed within the FDA-approved manufacturer's labeling.

Canadian labeling: Hypersensitivity to erlotinib or any component of the formulation

Warnings/Precautions Hazardous agent - use appropriate precautions for handling and disposal. Rare, sometimes fatal, pulmonary toxicity, including interstitial lung disease (acute respiratory distress syndrome, interstitial pneumonia, obliterative bronchiolitis, pneumonitis, pulmonary fibrosis, and pulmonary infiltrates) has occurred; symptoms may begin within 5 days to more than 9 months after treatment initiation (median: 39 days). Interrupt therapy for unexplained pulmonary symptoms (dyspnea, cough, and fever); discontinue for confirmed ILD.

Liver enzyme elevations have been reported. Hepatic failure and hepatorenal syndrome have also been reported, particularly in patients with baseline hepatic impairment. Monitor liver function; patients with any hepatic impairment (total bilirubin >ULN; Child-Pugh class A, B, or C) should be closely monitored, including those with hepatic disease due to tumor burden; use with extreme caution in patients with total bilirubin >3 times ULN. Dosage reduction, interruption or discontinuation may be recommended for changes in hepatic function. Acute renal failure and renal insufficiency (with/without hypokalemia) have been reported; use with caution in patients with or at risk for renal impairment. Monitor closely for dehydration; monitor renal function and electrolytes in patients at risk for dehydration. Gastrointestinal perforation has been reported with use; risk for perforation is increased with concurrent anti-angiogenic agents, corticosteroids, NSAIDs, and/or taxane based-therapy, and patients with history of peptic ulcers or diverticular disease; permanently discontinue in patients who develop perforation.

Bullous, blistering, or exfoliating skin conditions, some suggestive of Stevens-Johnson or toxic epidermal necrolysis (TEN) have been reported with use. Generalized or severe acneiform, erythematous or maculopapular rash may occur. Skin rash may correlate with treatment response and prolonged survival (Saif, 2008); management of skin rashes that are not serious should include alcohol-free lotions, topical antibiotics, or topical corticosteroids, or if necessary, oral antibiotics and systemic corticosteroids; avoid sunlight. Reduce dose or temporarily interrupt treatment for severe skin reactions; interrupt or discontinue treatment for bullous, blistering or exfoliative skin toxicity. Corneal perforation and ulceration have been reported with use; abnormal eyelash growth, keratoconjunctivitis sicca, or keratitis have also been reported and are known risk factors for corneal ulceration/perforation. Interrupt or discontinue treatment in patients presenting with eye pain or other acute or worsening ocular symptoms.

Use caution with cardiovascular disease; MI, CVA, and microangiopathic hemolytic anemia with thrombocytopenia have been noted in patients receiving concomitant erlotinib and gemcitabine. Elevated INR and bleeding events have been reported; use caution with concomitant anticoagulant therapy. Erlotinib levels may be lower in patients who smoke; advise patients to stop smoking. Smokers treated with 300 mg/day exhibited steady-state erlotinib levels comparable to former- and never-smokers receiving 150 mg/day (Hughes, 2009). Concurrent use with CYP3A4 inhibitors and moderate or strong CYP3A4 inducers may affect erlotinib levels; consider alternative agents to CYP3A4 inducers to avoid the potential for CYP-mediated interactions; use with caution in patients taking strong CYP3A4 inhibitors. Consider erlotinib dosage modification if concurrent use with CYP3A4 inhibitors/inducers cannot be avoided. In patients with NSCLC, EGFR mutations, specifically exon 19 deletions and exon 21 mutation (L858R), are associated with better response to erlotinib (Riely, 2006); erlotinib treatment is not recommended in patients with *K-ras* mutations; they are not likely to benefit from erlotinib treatment (Eberhard, 2005; Miller, 2008). Concurrent erlotinib plus platinum-based chemotherapy is not recommended for first line treatment of locally advanced or metastatic NSCLC due to a lack of clinical benefit. Product may contain lactose; avoid use in patients with Lapp lactase deficiency, glucose-galactose malabsorption, or glucose intolerance. Safety and efficacy have not been established in children.

Drug Interactions

Avoid Concomitant Use

Avoid concomitant use of Erlotinib with any of the following: Conivaptan; Proton Pump Inhibitors

Decreased Effect

Erlotinib may decrease the levels/effects of: Cardiac Glycosides; Vitamin K Antagonists

The levels/effects of Erlotinib may be decreased by: Antacids; CYP3A4 Inducers (Strong); Cyproterone; Deferasirox; H2-Antagonists; Herbs (CYP3A4 Inducers); Proton Pump Inhibitors; Rifampin; Tocilizumab

Increased Effect/Toxicity

Erlotinib may increase the levels/effects of: Vitamin K Antagonists

The levels/effects of Erlotinib may be increased by: Antifungal Agents (Azole Derivatives, Systemic); Ciprofloxacin; Ciprofloxacin (Systemic); Conivaptan; CYP3A4 Inhibitors (Moderate); CYP3A4 Inhibitors (Strong); Dasatinib; FluvoxaMINE; Ivacaftor

Nutritional/Ethanol Interactions

Food: Erlotinib bioavailability is increased with food. Grapefruit or grapefruit juice may decrease metabolism and increase erlotinib plasma concentrations. Management: Take on an empty stomach at least 1 hour before or 2 hours after the ingestion of food. Avoid grapefruit and grapefruit juice. Maintain adequate nutrition and hydration, unless instructed to restrict fluid intake.

Herb/Nutraceutical: St John's wort may increase metabolism and decrease erlotinib concentrations. Management: Avoid St John's wort.

Adverse Reactions

Adverse reactions reported with monotherapy:

>10%:

Central nervous system: Fatigue (9% to 52%)

Dermatologic: Rash (49% to 75%; grade 3: 6% to 8%; grade 4: <1%; median onset: 8 days), pruritus (7% to 13%), dry skin (4% to 12%)

Gastrointestinal: Diarrhea (20% to 54%; grade 3: 2% to 6%; grade 4: <1%; median onset: 12 days), anorexia (9% to 52%), nausea (33%), vomiting (23%), stomatitis (17%), abdominal pain (11%)

Ocular: Conjunctivitis (12%), keratoconjunctivitis sicca (12%)

Respiratory: Dyspnea (41%), cough (33%)

Miscellaneous: Infection (24%)

1% to 10%:

Dermatologic: Acne (6%), dermatitis acneiform (5%), paronychia (4%)

Gastrointestinal: Weight loss (4%)

Hepatic: ALT increased (grade 2: 2% to 4%; grade 3: 1%), hyperbilirubinemia (grade 2: 4%; grade 3: <1%)

Respiratory: Pneumonitis/pulmonary infiltrate (3%), pulmonary fibrosis (3%)

Adverse reactions reported with combination (erlotinib plus gemcitabine) therapy:

Cardiovascular: Edema (37%), thrombotic events (grades 3/4: 11%), deep venous thrombosis (4%), cerebrovascular accident (2%; including cerebral hemorrhage), MI/myocardial ischemia (2%), arrhythmia, syncope

Central nervous system: Fatigue (79%), fever (36%), depression (19%), dizziness (15%), headache (15%), anxiety (13%)

Dermatologic: Rash (69%), alopecia (14%)

Gastrointestinal: Nausea (60%), anorexia (52%), diarrhea (48%), abdominal pain (46%), vomiting (42%), weight loss (39%), stomatitis (22%), dyspepsia (17%), flatulence (13%), ileus, pancreatitis

Hematologic: Hemolytic anemia, microangiopathic hemolytic anemia with thrombocytopenia (1%)

Hepatic: ALT increased (grade 2: 31%, grade 3: 13%, grade 4: <1%), AST increased (grade 2: 24%, grade 3: 10%, grade 4 <1%), hyperbilirubinemia (grade 2: 17%, grade 3: 10%, grade 4: <1%)

Neuromuscular & skeletal: Bone pain (25%), myalgia (21%), neuropathy (13%), rigors (12%)

Renal: Renal insufficiency

Respiratory: Dyspnea (24%), cough (16%), interstitial lung disease (ILD)-like events (3%)

Miscellaneous: Infection (39%)

Available Dosage Forms

Tablet, oral:

Tarceva®: 25 mg, 100 mg, 150 mg

General Dosage Range Dosage adjustment recommended in patients with hepatic impairment, on concomitant therapy, who smoke, or who develop toxicities

Oral: *Adults:* 100-150 mg/day

Administration

Oral The manufacturer recommends administration on an empty stomach (at least 1 hour before or 2 hours after the ingestion of food).

For patients unable to swallow whole, tablets may be dissolved in 100 mL water and administered orally or via feeding tube (silicone-based); to ensure full dose is received, rinse container with 40 mL water, administer residue and repeat rinse (data on file, Genentech; Siu, 2007; Soulieres, 2004).

Stability

Storage Store at room temperature of 25°C (77°F); excursions permitted to 15°C and 30°C (59°F and 86°F).

Nursing Actions

Physical Assessment Monitor for gastrointestinal perforation, diarrhea, ocular reactions, severe skin reactions, and interstitial lung disease; notify prescriber if any occur.

Patient Education Take 1 hour before or 2 hours after food, and avoid grapefruit or grapefruit juice. If unable to swallow whole, tablets may be dissolved in 100 mL of water; rinse residue in container with 40 mL of water to assure full dose. If you are a smoker, inform prescriber if you stop smoking. Maintain adequate nutrition and hydration, unless instructed to restrict fluid intake. May cause fatigue, rash or dry skin, loss of hair (may grow back when treatment is completed), nausea, or anorexia. Report any persistent skin rash, blisters, or skin eruptions; persistent or severe gastrointestinal changes, including diarrhea, abdominal pain, nausea, or vomiting; eye pain or visual changes; difficulty breathing or unusual cough or fever; or signs of infection.

Dietary Considerations Take this medicine an empty stomach, 1 hour before or 2 hours after a meal. Avoid grapefruit juice.

Ertapenem (er ta PEN em)

Brand Names: U.S. INVanz®

Index Terms Ertapenem Sodium; L-749,345; MK0826

Pharmacologic Category Antibiotic, Carbapenem

Medication Safety Issues

Sound-alike/look-alike issues:

Ertapenem may be confused with doripenem, imipenem, meropenem

INVanz® may be confused with AVINza®, I.V. vancomycin

Pregnancy Risk Factor B

Lactation Enters breast milk/use caution

Breast-Feeding Considerations Ertapenem is excreted in breast milk. The low concentrations in milk and low oral bioavailability suggest minimal exposure risk to the infant. Although the manufacturer recommends that caution be exercised when administering ertapenem to nursing women, most penicillins and carbapenems are safe for use in breast-feeding. Nondose-related effects could include modification of bowel flora.

Use Treatment of the following moderate-to-severe infections: Complicated intra-abdominal infections, complicated skin and skin structure infections (including diabetic foot infections without osteomyelitis, animal and human bites), complicated UTI (including pyelonephritis), acute pelvic infections (including postpartum endomyometritis, septic abortion, postsurgical gynecologic infections), and community-acquired pneumonia. Prophylaxis of surgical site infection following elective colorectal surgery. Antibacterial coverage includes aerobic gram-positive organisms, aerobic gram-negative organisms, and anaerobic organisms.

Note: Methicillin-resistant *Staphylococcus aureus, Enterococcus* spp, penicillin-resistant strains of *Streptococcus pneumoniae, Acinetobacter*, and *Pseudomonas aeruginosa*, are **resistant** to ertapenem while most extended-spectrum β-lactamase (ESBL)-producing bacteria remain sensitive to ertapenem.

Unlabeled Use Treatment of intravenous catheter-related bloodstream infection

Mechanism of Action/Effect Inhibits cell wall biosynthesis; cell wall assembly is arrested and the bacteria eventually lyse.

Contraindications Hypersensitivity to ertapenem, other carbapenems (eg, doripenem, imipenem, meropenem), or any component of the formulation; anaphylactic reactions to beta-lactam antibiotics. If using intramuscularly, known hypersensitivity to local anesthetics of the amide type (lidocaine is the diluent).

Warnings/Precautions Use caution with renal impairment. Dosage adjustment required in patients with moderate-to-severe renal dysfunction; elderly patients often require lower doses (based upon renal function). Prolonged use may result in fungal or bacterial superinfection, including *C. difficile*-associated diarrhea (CDAD) and pseudomembranous colitis; CDAD has been observed >2 months postantibiotic treatment. Has been associated with CNS adverse effects, including confusional states and seizures; use caution with CNS disorders (eg, brain lesions, history of seizures, or renal impairment). Serious hypersensitivity reactions, including anaphylaxis, have been reported (some without a history of previous allergic reactions to beta-lactams). Doses for I.M. administration are mixed with lidocaine; consult Lidocaine (Systemic) on page 694 information for associated Warnings/Precautions. May decrease divalproex sodium/valproic acid concentrations leading to breakthrough seizures; concomitant use not recommended. Safety and efficacy have not been established in children <3 months of age.

Drug Interactions

Avoid Concomitant Use

Avoid concomitant use of Ertapenem with any of the following: BCG

Decreased Effect

Ertapenem may decrease the levels/effects of: BCG; Divalproex; Typhoid Vaccine; Valproic Acid

Increased Effect/Toxicity

The levels/effects of Ertapenem may be increased by: Probenecid

Adverse Reactions Note: Percentages reported in adults.

1% to 10%:

Cardiovascular: Edema (3%), chest pain (1% to 2%), hypertension (1% to 2%), hypotension (1% to 2%), tachycardia (1% to 2%)

Central nervous system: Headache (6% to 7%); altered mental status (eg, agitation, confusion, disorientation, mental acuity decreased, somnolence, stupor) (3% to 5%); fever (2% to 5%), insomnia (3%), dizziness (2%), fatigue (1%), anxiety (1%)

Dermatologic: Rash (2% to 3%), pruritus (1% to 2%), erythema (1% to 2%)

Endocrine & metabolic: Hypokalemia (2%), hyperglycemia (1% to 2%), hyperkalemia (≤1%)

Gastrointestinal: Diarrhea (9% to 10%), nausea (6% to 9%), abdominal pain (4%), vomiting (4%), constipation (3% to 4%), acid regurgitation (1% to 2%), dyspepsia (1%), oral candidiasis (≤1%)

Genitourinary: Urine WBCs increased (2% to 3%), urine RBCs increased (1% to 3%), vaginitis (1% to 3%)

Hematologic: Thrombocytosis (4% to 7%), hematocrit/hemoglobin decreased (3% to 5%), eosinophils increased (1% to 2%), leukopenia (1% to 2%), neutrophils decreased (1% to 2%), thrombocytopenia (1%), prothrombin time increased (≤1%)

Hepatic: Hepatic enzyme increased (7% to 9%), alkaline phosphatase increase (4% to 7%), albumin decreased (1% to 2%), bilirubin (total) increased (1% to 2%)

Local: Infused vein complications (5% to 7%), phlebitis/thrombophlebitis (2%), extravasation (1% to 2%)

Neuromuscular & skeletal: Weakness (1%), leg pain (≤1%)

Renal: Serum creatinine increased (1%)

Respiratory: Dyspnea (1% to 3%), cough (1% to 2%), pharyngitis (1%), rales/rhonchi (1%), respiratory distress (≤1%)

Available Dosage Forms

Injection, powder for reconstitution:

INVanz®: 1 g

General Dosage Range Dosage adjustment recommended in patients with renal impairment

I.M., I.V.:

Children 3 months to 12 years: 15 mg/kg twice daily (maximum: 1 g/day)

Adolescents ≥13 years and Adults: 1 g once daily or as single dose

Administration

I.M. Avoid injection into a blood vessel. Make sure patient does not have an allergy to lidocaine or another anesthetic of the amide type. Administer by deep I.M. injection into a large muscle mass (eg, gluteal muscle or lateral part of the thigh). Do not administer I.M. preparation or drug reconstituted for I.M. administration intravenously.

I.V. Infuse over 30 minutes

I.V. Detail pH 7.5

Stability

Reconstitution

I.M.: Reconstitute 1 g vial with 3.2 mL of 1% lidocaine HCl injection (without epinephrine). Shake well.

I.V.: Reconstitute 1 g vial with 10 mL of sterile water for injection, 0.9% sodium chloride injection, or bacteriostatic water for injection. Shake well. For adults, transfer dose to 50 mL of 0.9% sodium chloride injection; for children, dilute dose with NS to a final concentration ≤20 mg/mL.

Storage Before reconstitution store at ≤25°C (77°F).

I.M.: Use within 1 hour after preparation.

I.V.: Reconstituted I.V. solution may be stored at room temperature and must be used within 6 hours **or** refrigerated, stored for up to 24 hours and used within 4 hours after removal from refrigerator. Do not freeze.

Nursing Actions

Physical Assessment Results of culture and sensitivity tests and patient history of previous allergies should be assessed prior to beginning treatment. Monitor closely for adverse reactions, especially CNS adverse effects (history of seizures, head injuries, or other CNS events increases risk).

Patient Education This medication can only be administered intravenously or by intramuscular injections; report warmth, swelling, or irritation at infusion or injection site. Maintain adequate hydration, unless instructed to restrict fluid intake, and nutrition. Report unresolved nausea or vomiting. Report immediately any CNS changes (eg, dizziness, disorientation, headaches, confusion, or seizures). Report prolonged GI effects, persistent diarrhea, vomiting, or abdominal pain; change in respirations or respiratory difficulty; chest pain or palpitations; skin rash; foul-smelling vaginal discharge; or white plaques in mouth.

Dietary Considerations Some products may contain sodium.

Erythromycin (Systemic) (er ith roe MYE sin)

Brand Names: U.S. E.E.S.®; Ery-Tab®; EryPed®; Erythro-RX; Erythrocin®; Erythrocin® Lactobionate-I.V.; PCE®

Index Terms Erythromycin Base; Erythromycin Ethylsuccinate; Erythromycin Lactobionate; Erythromycin Stearate

Pharmacologic Category Antibiotic, Macrolide

Medication Safety Issues

Sound-alike/look-alike issues:

Erythromycin may be confused with azithromycin, clarithromycin

Eryc® may be confused with Emcyt®, Ery-Tab®

Pregnancy Risk Factor B

Lactation Enters breast milk/use caution (AAP considers "compatible"; AAP 2001 update pending)

Breast-Feeding Considerations Erythromycin is excreted in breast milk; therefore, the manufacturer recommends that caution be exercised when administering erythromycin to breast-feeding women.

Due to the low concentrations in human milk, minimal toxicity would be expected in the nursing infant. One case report and a cohort study raise the possibility for a connection with pyloric stenosis in neonates exposed to erythromycin via breast milk and an alternative antibiotic may be preferred for breast-feeding mothers of infants in this age group. Nondose-related effects could include modification of bowel flora.

Use Treatment of susceptible bacterial infections including *S. pyogenes*, some *S. pneumoniae*, some *S. aureus*, *M. pneumoniae*, *Legionella pneumophila*, diphtheria, pertussis, *Chlamydia*, erythrasma, *N. gonorrhoeae*, *E. histolytica*, syphilis and nongonococcal urethritis, and *Campylobacter* gastroenteritis; used in conjunction with neomycin for decontaminating the bowel

Unlabeled Use Treatment of gastroparesis, chancroid; preoperative gut sterilization

Mechanism of Action/Effect Inhibits RNA-dependent protein synthesis

Contraindications Hypersensitivity to erythromycin, any macrolide antibiotics, or any component of the formulation

Concomitant use with pimozide, cisapride, ergotamine or dihydroergotamine, terfenadine, astemizole

Warnings/Precautions Use caution with hepatic impairment with or without jaundice has occurred, it may be accompanied by malaise, nausea, vomiting, abdominal colic, and fever; discontinue use if these occur. Use caution with other medication relying on CYP3A4 metabolism; high potential for drug interactions exists. Prolonged use may result in fungal or bacterial superinfection, including *C. difficile*-associated diarrhea (CDAD) and pseudomembranous colitis; CDAD has been observed >2 months postantibiotic treatment. Use in infants has been associated with infantile hypertrophic pyloric stenosis (IHPS). Macrolides have been associated with rare QT_c prolongation and ventricular arrhythmias, including torsade de pointes. Use caution in elderly patients, as risk of adverse events may be increased. Use caution in myasthenia gravis patients; erythromycin may aggravate muscular weakness.

Drug Interactions

Avoid Concomitant Use

Avoid concomitant use of Erythromycin (Systemic) with any of the following: Artemether; BCG; Cisapride; Conivaptan; Disopyramide; Dronedarone; Lincosamide Antibiotics; Lumefantrine; Nilotinib; Pimozide; QUEtiapine; QuiNINE; Silodosin; Terfenadine; Tetrabenazine; Thioridazine; Topotecan; Toremifene; Vandetanib; Vemurafenib; Ziprasidone

Decreased Effect

Erythromycin (Systemic) may decrease the levels/effects of: BCG; Clopidogrel; Typhoid Vaccine; Zafirlukast

The levels/effects of Erythromycin (Systemic) may be decreased by: CYP3A4 Inducers (Strong); Deferasirox; Etravirine; Lincosamide Antibiotics; P-glycoprotein/ABCB1 Inducers; Tocilizumab

Increased Effect/Toxicity

Erythromycin (Systemic) may increase the levels/effects of: Alfentanil; Antifungal Agents (Azole Derivatives, Systemic); Antineoplastic Agents (Vinca Alkaloids); ARIPiprazole; Benzodiazepines (metabolized by oxidation); Budesonide (Systemic, Oral Inhalation); BusPIRone; Calcium Channel Blockers; CarBAMazepine; Cardiac Glycosides; Cilostazol; Cisapride; CloZAPine; Colchicine; Corticosteroids (Systemic); CycloSPORINE; CycloSPORINE (Systemic); CYP3A4 Substrates; Dabigatran Etexilate; Disopyramide; Dronedarone; Eletriptan; Eplerenone; Ergot Derivatives; Everolimus; FentaNYL; Fexofenadine; HMG-CoA Reductase Inhibitors; Lurasidone; P-glycoprotein/ABCB1 Substrates; Pimecrolimus; Pimozide; Prucalopride; QTc-Prolonging Agents; QuiNIDine; QuiNINE; Repaglinide; Rifamycin Derivatives; Rivaroxaban; Salmeterol; Selective Serotonin Reuptake Inhibitors; Silodosin; Sirolimus; Tacrolimus; Tacrolimus (Systemic); Tacrolimus (Topical); Temsirolimus; Terfenadine; Tetrabenazine; Theophylline Derivatives; Thioridazine; Topotecan; Toremifene; Vandetanib; Vemurafenib; Vitamin K Antagonists; Ziprasidone; Zopiclone

The levels/effects of Erythromycin (Systemic) may be increased by: Alfuzosin; Antifungal Agents (Azole Derivatives, Systemic); Artemether; Chloroquine; Ciprofloxacin; Ciprofloxacin (Systemic); Conivaptan; CYP3A4 Inhibitors (Moderate); CYP3A4 Inhibitors (Strong); Gadobutrol; Indacaterol; Lumefantrine; Nilotinib; P-glycoprotein/ABCB1 Inhibitors; QUEtiapine; QuiNINE

Nutritional/Ethanol Interactions

Ethanol: Ethanol may decrease absorption of erythromycin or enhance effects of ethanol. Management: Avoid ethanol.

Food: Erythromycin serum levels may be altered if taken with food (formulation-dependent). GI upset, including diarrhea, is common. Management: May be taken with food to decrease GI upset, otherwise take around-the-clock with a full glass of water. Do not give with milk or acidic beverages (eg, soda, juice).

Herb/Nutraceutical: St John's wort may decrease erythromycin levels. Management: Avoid St John's wort.

Adverse Reactions Frequency not defined. Incidence may vary with formulation.

Cardiovascular: QT_c prolongation, torsade de pointes, ventricular arrhythmia, ventricular tachycardia

Central nervous system: Seizure

Dermatologic: Erythema multiforme, pruritus, rash, Stevens-Johnson syndrome, toxic epidermal necrolysis

Gastrointestinal: Abdominal pain, anorexia, diarrhea, infantile hypertrophic pyloric stenosis, nausea, oral candidiasis, pancreatitis, pseudomembranous colitis, vomiting

Hepatic: Cholestatic jaundice (most common with estolate), hepatitis, liver function tests abnormal

Local: Phlebitis at the injection site, thrombophlebitis

Neuromuscular & skeletal: Weakness

Otic: Hearing loss

Miscellaneous: Allergic reactions, anaphylaxis, hypersensitivity reactions, interstitial nephritis, urticaria

Available Dosage Forms

Capsule, delayed release, enteric coated pellets, oral: 250 mg

Granules for suspension, oral:
E.E.S.®: 200 mg/5 mL (100 mL, 200 mL)
Injection, powder for reconstitution:
Erythrocin® Lactobionate-I.V.: 500 mg
Powder, for prescription compounding:
Erythro-RX: USP: 100% (50 g)
Powder for suspension, oral:
EryPed®: 200 mg/5 mL (100 mL); 400 mg/5 mL (100 mL)
Tablet, oral: 250 mg, 400 mg, 500 mg
E.E.S.®: 400 mg
Erythrocin®: 250 mg, 500 mg
Tablet, delayed release, enteric coated, oral:
Ery-Tab®: 250 mg, 333 mg, 500 mg
Tablet, polymer coated particles, oral:
PCE®: 333 mg, 500 mg

General Dosage Range

I.V.:
Children: 15-50 mg/kg/day divided every 6 hours (maximum: 4 g/day)
Adults: 15-20 mg/kg/day divided every 6 hours **or** 500 mg to 1 g every 6 hours or as a continuous infusion over 24 hours (maximum: 4 g/day)

Oral:
Children: 30-50 mg/kg/day in 2-4 divided doses (maximum base or stearate: 2 g/day; maximum ethylsuccinate: 3.2 g/day)
Adults: Base: 250-500 mg every 6-12 hours (maximum base or ethylsuccinate: 400-800 mg every 6-12 hours)

Administration

Oral Do not crush enteric coated drug product. GI upset, including diarrhea, is common. May be administered with food to decrease GI upset. Do not give with milk or acidic beverages.

I.V. Infuse 1 g over 20-60 minutes.

I.V. Detail I.V. infusion may be very irritating to the vein. If phlebitis/pain occurs with used dilution, consider diluting further (eg, 1:5) if fluid status of the patient will tolerate, or consider administering in larger available vein. The addition of lidocaine or bicarbonate does not decrease the irritation of erythromycin infusions.

pH: Erythromycin lactobionate: 6.5-7.5 (reconstituted with sterile water for injection or D_5W to a 50 mg/mL concentration)

Stability

Reconstitution Erythromycin lactobionate should be reconstituted with sterile water for injection without preservatives to avoid gel formation. I.V. form has the longest stability in NS and should be prepared in this base solution whenever possible. Do not use D_5W as a diluent unless sodium bicarbonate is added to solution. If I.V. must be prepared in D_5W, 0.5 mL of the 8.4% sodium bicarbonate solution should be added per each 100 mL of D_5W.

Standard diluent: 500 mg/250 mL D_5W/NS; 750 mg/250 mL D_5W/NS; 1 g/250 mL D_5W/NS.

Storage
Injection: Store unreconstituted vials at 15°C to 30°C (59°F to 86°F). Reconstituted solution is stable for 2 weeks when refrigerated or for 8 hours at room temperature. Erythromycin I.V. infusion solution is stable at pH 6-8; stability of lactobionate is pH dependent; I.V. form has longest stability in NS. Stability of parenteral admixture at room temperature (25°C) and at refrigeration temperature (4°C) is 24 hours.
Oral suspension:
Granules: After mixing, store under refrigeration and use within 10 days.
Powder: Erythromycin ethylsuccinate may be stored at room temperature if used within 14 days. Refrigerate to preserve taste.
Tablet and capsule formulations: Store at <30°C (<86°F).

Nursing Actions

Physical Assessment Results of culture and sensitivity tests and patient's previous allergy history should be assessed prior to therapy.

Patient Education Tablets/capsules: Take around-the-clock, with a full glass of water (not juice or milk); may take with food to reduce GI upset. Do not chew or crush extended release capsules or tablets. Avoid alcohol (may cause adverse response). May cause nausea, vomiting, or mouth sores. Report immediately any unusual malaise, nausea, vomiting, abdominal colic, or fever; skin rash or itching; easy bruising or bleeding; vaginal itching or discharge; watery or bloody diarrhea; yellowing of skin or eyes, pale stool or dark urine; persistent diarrhea; white plaques, sores, or fuzziness in mouth; or any change in hearing.

Dietary Considerations Drug may cause GI upset; may take with food. Some products may contain sodium.

Erythromycin (Topical) (er ith roe MYE sin)

Brand Names: U.S. Akne-mycin®; Ery

Pharmacologic Category Acne Products; Antibiotic, Macrolide; Antibiotic, Topical; Topical Skin Product; Topical Skin Product, Acne

Medication Safety Issues
Sound-alike/look-alike issues:
Erythromycin may be confused with azithromycin, clarithromycin

Pregnancy Risk Factor B

Lactation Use caution (AAP considers "compatible"; AAP 2001 update pending)

Use Treatment of acne vulgaris

Available Dosage Forms
Gel, topical: 2% (30 g, 60 g)
Ointment, topical:
Akne-mycin®: 2% (25 g)
Pledget, topical: 2% (60s)
Ery: 2% (60s)

Solution, topical: 2% (60 mL)

General Dosage Range Topical: *Children and Adults:* Apply over the affected area twice daily

Nursing Actions

Patient Education Apply as directed after skin has been cleansed and gently dried.

Escitalopram (es sye TAL oh pram)

Brand Names: U.S. Lexapro®

Index Terms Escitalopram Oxalate; Lu-26-054; S-Citalopram

Pharmacologic Category Antidepressant, Selective Serotonin Reuptake Inhibitor

Medication Safety Issues

Sound-alike/look-alike issues:

Lexapro® may be confused with Loxitane®

International issues:

Zavesca: Brand name for escitalopram [in multiple international markets; ISMP April 21, 2010], but also brand name for miglustat [Canada, U.S., and multiple international markets]

Medication Guide Available Yes

Pregnancy Risk Factor C

Lactation Enters breast milk/consider risk:benefit

Breast-Feeding Considerations Escitalopram and its metabolite are excreted into breast milk. Limited data is available concerning the effects escitalopram may have in the nursing infant and the long-term effects on development and behavior have not been studied. According to the manufacturer, the decision to continue or discontinue breast-feeding during therapy should take into account the risk of exposure to the infant and the benefits of treatment to the mother. Escitalopram is the S-enantiomer of the racemic derivative citalopram; also refer to the Citalopram monograph.

Use Treatment of major depressive disorder; generalized anxiety disorders (GAD)

Unlabeled Use Treatment of mild dementia-associated agitation in nonpsychotic patients

Mechanism of Action/Effect Escitalopram is the S-enantiomer of the racemic derivative citalopram, which selectively inhibits the reuptake of serotonin with little to no effect on norepinephrine or dopamine reuptake. It has no or very low affinity for 5-HT_{1-7}, alpha- and beta-adrenergic, D_{1-5}, H_{1-3}, M_{1-5}, and benzodiazepine receptors. Escitalopram does not bind to or has low affinity for Na^+, K^+, Cl^-, and Ca^{++} ion channels.

Contraindications Hypersensitivity to escitalopram, citalopram, or any component of the formulation; concomitant use with pimozide; concomitant use or within 2 weeks of MAO inhibitors

Warnings/Precautions [U.S. Boxed Warning]: Antidepressants increase the risk of suicidal thinking and behavior in children, adolescents, and young adults (18-24 years of age) with major depressive disorder (MDD) and other psychiatric disorders; consider risk prior to prescribing. Short-term studies did not show an increased risk in patients >24 years of age and showed a decreased risk in patients ≥65 years. Closely monitor patients for clinical worsening, suicidality, or unusual changes in behavior, particularly during the initial 1-2 months of therapy or during periods of dosage adjustments (increases or decreases); the patient's family or caregiver should be instructed to closely observe the patient and communicate condition with healthcare provider. A medication guide concerning the use of antidepressants should be dispensed with each prescription. **Escitalopram is not FDA approved for use in children <12 years of age.**

The possibility of a suicide attempt is inherent in major depression and may persist until remission occurs. Use caution in high-risk patients. Worsening depression and severe abrupt suicidality that are not part of the presenting symptoms may require discontinuation or modification of drug therapy. The patient's family or caregiver should be alerted to monitor patients for the emergence of suicidality and associated behaviors (such as agitation, irritability, hostility, impulsivity, and hypomania) and call healthcare provider.

May worsen psychosis in some patients or precipitate a shift to mania or hypomania in patients with bipolar disorder. Patients presenting with depressive symptoms should be screened for bipolar disorder. Monotherapy in patients with bipolar disorder should be avoided. Escitalopram is not FDA approved for the treatment of bipolar depression. Escitalopram is not FDA approved for the treatment of bipolar depression.

Serotonin syndrome and neuroleptic malignant syndrome (NMS)-like reactions have occurred with serotonin/norepinephrine reuptake inhibitors (SNRIs) and selective serotonin reuptake inhibitors (SSRIs) when used alone, and particularly when used in combination with serotonergic agents (eg, triptans) or antidopaminergic agents (eg, antipsychotics). Concurrent use or within 2 weeks of an MAO inhibitor is contraindicated. May increase the risks associated with electroconvulsive therapy. Has a low potential to impair cognitive or motor performance; caution operating hazardous machinery or driving.

Use caution with a previous seizure disorder or condition predisposing to seizures such as brain damage, alcoholism, or concurrent therapy with other drugs which lower the seizure threshold. May cause hyponatremia/SIADH (elderly at increased risk); volume depletion (diuretics may increase risk) may occur. May cause or exacerbate sexual dysfunction. Use caution with severe renal impairment or liver impairment; concomitant CNS depressants; pregnancy (high doses of citalopram have been associated with teratogenicity in animals). Use caution with concomitant use of aspirin,

NSAIDs, warfarin, or other drugs that affect coagulation; the risk of bleeding may be potentiated.

Upon discontinuation of escitalopram therapy, gradually taper dose. If intolerable symptoms occur following a decrease in dosage or upon discontinuation of therapy, then resuming the previous dose with a more gradual taper should be considered.

Safety and efficacy have not been established in children <12 years of age with major depressive disorder or in children <18 years with generalized anxiety disorder.

Drug Interactions

Avoid Concomitant Use

Avoid concomitant use of Escitalopram with any of the following: Conivaptan; Iobenguane I 123; MAO Inhibitors; Methylene Blue; Pimozide; Tryptophan

Decreased Effect

Escitalopram may decrease the levels/effects of: Iobenguane I 123; Ioflupane I 123

The levels/effects of Escitalopram may be decreased by: CarBAMazepine; CYP2C19 Inducers (Strong); CYP3A4 Inducers (Strong); Cyproheptadine; Deferasirox; NSAID (COX-2 Inhibitor); NSAID (Nonselective); Telaprevir; Tocilizumab

Increased Effect/Toxicity

Escitalopram may increase the levels/effects of: Alpha-/Beta-Blockers; Anticoagulants; Antidepressants (Serotonin Reuptake Inhibitor/Antagonist); Antiplatelet Agents; Aspirin; BusPIRone; CarBAMazepine; CloZAPine; Collagenase (Systemic); Desmopressin; Dextromethorphan; Drotrecogin Alfa (Activated); Ibritumomab; Lithium; Methadone; Methylene Blue; Metoclopramide; Mexiletine; NSAID (COX-2 Inhibitor); NSAID (Nonselective); Pimozide; RisperiDONE; Rivaroxaban; Salicylates; Serotonin Modulators; Thrombolytic Agents; Tositumomab and Iodine I 131 Tositumomab; TraMADol; Tricyclic Antidepressants; Vitamin K Antagonists

The levels/effects of Escitalopram may be increased by: Alcohol (Ethyl); Analgesics (Opioid); Antipsychotics; BusPIRone; Cimetidine; CNS Depressants; Conivaptan; CYP2C19 Inhibitors (Moderate); CYP2C19 Inhibitors (Strong); CYP3A4 Inhibitors (Moderate); CYP3A4 Inhibitors (Strong); Dasatinib; Glucosamine; Herbs (Anticoagulant/Antiplatelet Properties); Ivacaftor; Linezolid; Macrolide Antibiotics; MAO Inhibitors; Metoclopramide; Omega-3-Acid Ethyl Esters; Pentosan Polysulfate Sodium; Pentoxifylline; Prostacyclin Analogues; TraMADol; Tryptophan; Vitamin E

Nutritional/Ethanol Interactions

Ethanol: May increase CNS depression; monitor for increased effects with coadministration. Caution patients about effects.

Herb/Nutraceutical: Avoid valerian, St John's wort, SAMe, kava kava, and gotu kola (may increase CNS depression).

Adverse Reactions

>10%:

Central nervous system: Headache (24%), somnolence (6% to 13%), insomnia (9% to 12%)

Gastrointestinal: Nausea (15% to 18%)

Genitourinary: Ejaculation disorder (9% to 14%)

1% to 10%:

Central nervous system: Fatigue (5% to 8%), dizziness (5%), abnormal dreaming (3%), lethargy (3%), yawning (2%)

Endocrine & metabolic: Libido decreased (3% to 7%), anorgasmia (2% to 6%), menstrual disorder (2%)

Gastrointestinal: Xerostomia (6% to 9%), diarrhea (8%), constipation (3% to 5%), appetite decreased (3%), indigestion (3%), vomiting (3%), abdominal pain (2%), flatulence (2%), toothache (2%)

Genitourinary: Impotence (2% to 3%)

Neuromuscular & skeletal: Neck/shoulder pain (3%), paresthesia (2%)

Respiratory: Rhinitis (5%), sinusitis (3%)

Miscellaneous: Diaphoresis (4% to 5%), flu-like syndrome (5%)

Pharmacodynamics/Kinetics

Onset of Action Depression: The onset of action is within a week; however, individual response varies greatly and full response may not be seen until 8-12 weeks after initiation of treatment.

Available Dosage Forms

Solution, oral: 1 mg/mL (240 mL)

Lexapro®: 1 mg/mL (240 mL)

Tablet, oral: 5 mg, 10 mg, 20 mg

Lexapro®: 5 mg, 10 mg, 20 mg

General Dosage Range Dosage adjustment recommended in patients with hepatic impairment

Oral:

Children ≥12 years and Adults: Initial: 10 mg once daily; Maintenance: 10-20 mg once daily

Elderly: 10 mg once daily

Administration

Oral Administer once daily (morning or evening), with or without food.

Stability

Storage Store at 25°C (77°F); excursions permitted to 15°C to 30°C (59°F to 86°F).

Nursing Actions

Physical Assessment Assess therapeutic effectiveness (mental status for depression, suicide ideation, social functioning, mania, or panic attacks). Monitor for signs of clinical worsening or hypomania. Taper dosage slowly when discontinuing.

Patient Education Avoid alcohol. May cause fatigue, dizziness, lightheadedness, insomnia, impaired concentration, headache, nausea, vomiting, loss of appetite, diarrhea, sexual dysfunction (reversible when drug is discontinued), muscle pain, dry mouth, or tremor. Report immediately any CNS changes, such as increased depression, confusion, impaired concentration, severe headache, insomnia, nightmares, irritability, acute anxiety, panic attacks, suicide ideation, persistent GI changes, chest pain or palpitations, blurred vision or vision changes, or unusual bleeding (eg, blood in stool, urine, or vomitus; unusual bruising or nosebleeds).

Dietary Considerations May be taken with or without food.

Esmolol (ES moe lol)

Brand Names: U.S. Brevibloc

Index Terms Esmolol Hydrochloride

Pharmacologic Category Antiarrhythmic Agent, Class II; Beta Blocker, Beta-1 Selective

Medication Safety Issues

Sound-alike/look-alike issues:

Esmolol may be confused with Osmitrol®

Brevibloc® may be confused with Brevital®, Bumex®, Buprenex®

High alert medication:

The Institute for Safe Medication Practices (ISMP) includes this medication among its list of drugs which have a heightened risk of causing significant patient harm when used in error.

Pregnancy Risk Factor C

Lactation Excretion in breast milk unknown/use with caution

Breast-Feeding Considerations It is not known if esmolol is excreted into breast milk. The manufacturer recommends that caution be exercised when administering esmolol to nursing women. The short half-life and the fact that it is not intended for chronic use should limit any exposure to the nursing infant.

Use Treatment of supraventricular tachycardia (SVT) and atrial fibrillation/flutter (control ventricular rate); treatment of intraoperative and postoperative tachycardia and/or hypertension; treatment of noncompensatory sinus tachycardia

Unlabeled Use

Children: SVT and postoperative hypertension

Adults: Arrhythmia/rate control during acute coronary syndrome (eg, acute myocardial infarction, unstable angina), aortic dissection, intubation, thyroid storm, pheochromocytoma, electroconvulsive therapy

Mechanism of Action/Effect Class II antiarrhythmic: Beta$_1$-adrenergic receptor blocking agent that competes with beta$_1$-adrenergic agonists for available beta-receptor sites; it is a selective beta$_1$-antagonist with a very short duration of action; has little if any intrinsic sympathomimetic activity; and lacks membrane stabilizing action; it is administered intravenously and is used when beta-blockade of short duration is desired or in critically-ill patients in whom adverse effects of bradycardia, heart failure, or hypotension may necessitate rapid withdrawal of the drug

Contraindications Sinus bradycardia; heart block greater than first degree (except in patients with a functioning artificial pacemaker); cardiogenic shock; uncompensated cardiac failure

Warnings/Precautions Consider pre-existing conditions such as sick sinus syndrome before initiating. Hypotension is common; patients need close blood pressure monitoring. Administer cautiously in compensated heart failure and monitor for a worsening of the condition. Can precipitate or aggravate symptoms of arterial insufficiency in patients with PVD and Raynaud's disease. Use with caution and monitor for progression of arterial obstruction. Use caution with concurrent use of digoxin, verapamil or diltiazem; bradycardia or heart block can occur. Use with caution in patients receiving inhaled anesthetic agents known to depress myocardial contractility. Use beta-blockers cautiously in patients with bronchospastic disease; monitor pulmonary status closely. Use cautiously in patients with diabetes because it can mask prominent hypoglycemic symptoms. Bradycardia may be observed more frequently in elderly patients (>65 years of age); dosage reductions may be necessary. May mask signs of hyperthyroidism (eg, tachycardia); if hyperthyroidism is suspected, carefully manage and monitor; abrupt withdrawal may exacerbate symptoms of hyperthyroidism or precipitate thyroid storm. Use with caution in patients with myasthenia gravis. Use caution in patients with renal dysfunction (active metabolite retained). Adequate alpha-blockade is required prior to use of any beta-blocker for patients with untreated pheochromocytoma. Use caution with history of severe anaphylaxis to allergens; patients taking beta-blockers may become more sensitive to repeated challenges. Treatment of anaphylaxis (eg, epinephrine) in patients taking beta-blockers may be ineffective or promote undesirable effects. Beta-blocker therapy should not be withdrawn abruptly (particularly in patients with CAD), but gradually tapered to avoid acute tachycardia, hypertension, and/or ischemia. Do not use in the treatment of hypertension associated with vasoconstriction related to hypothermia. Extravasation can lead to skin necrosis and sloughing.

Drug Interactions

Avoid Concomitant Use

Avoid concomitant use of Esmolol with any of the following: Floctafenine; Methacholine

Decreased Effect

Esmolol may decrease the levels/effects of: Beta2-Agonists; Theophylline Derivatives

The levels/effects of Esmolol may be decreased by: Barbiturates; Herbs (Hypertensive Properties); Methylphenidate; Nonsteroidal Anti-Inflammatory Agents; Rifamycin Derivatives; Yohimbine

Increased Effect/Toxicity

Esmolol may increase the levels/effects of: Alpha-/Beta-Agonists (Direct-Acting); Alpha1-Blockers; Alpha2-Agonists; Amifostine; Antihypertensives; Antipsychotic Agents (Phenothiazines); Bupivacaine; Cardiac Glycosides; Cholinergic Agonists; Fingolimod; Hypotensive Agents; Insulin; Lidocaine; Lidocaine (Systemic); Lidocaine (Topical); Mepivacaine; Methacholine; Midodrine; RiTUXimab; Sulfonylureas

The levels/effects of Esmolol may be increased by: Acetylcholinesterase Inhibitors; Aminoquinolines (Antimalarial); Amiodarone; Anilidopiperidine Opioids; Antipsychotic Agents (Phenothiazines); Calcium Channel Blockers (Dihydropyridine); Calcium Channel Blockers (Nondihydropyridine); Diazoxide; Dipyridamole; Disopyramide; Dronedarone; Floctafenine; Herbs (Hypotensive Properties); MAO Inhibitors; Pentoxifylline; Phosphodiesterase 5 Inhibitors; Propafenone; Prostacyclin Analogues; QuiNIDine; Reserpine

Adverse Reactions

>10%:

Cardiovascular: Asymptomatic hypotension (dose related: 25% to 38%), symptomatic hypotension (dose related: 12%)

Miscellaneous: Diaphoresis (10%)

1% to 10%:

Cardiovascular: Peripheral ischemia (1%)

Central nervous system: Dizziness (3%), somnolence (3%), confusion (2%), headache (2%), agitation (2%), fatigue (1%)

Gastrointestinal: Nausea (7%), vomiting (1%)

Local: Pain on injection (8%), infusion site reaction

Pharmacodynamics/Kinetics

Onset of Action Beta-blockade: I.V.: 2-10 minutes (quickest when loading doses are administered)

Duration of Action Hemodynamic effects: 10-30 minutes; prolonged following higher cumulative doses, extended duration of use

Available Dosage Forms

Infusion, premixed in NS [preservative free]:

Brevibloc: 2000 mg (100 mL); 2500 mg (250 mL)

Injection, solution [preservative free]: 10 mg/mL (10 mL)

Brevibloc: 10 mg/mL (10 mL)

General Dosage Range I.V.: *Adults:* Bolus: 80 mg **or** 500 mcg/kg; Infusion: 50-200 mcg/kg/minute (maximum: 300 mcg/kg/minute)

Administration

I.V. Infusion into small veins or through a butterfly catheter should be avoided (can cause thrombophlebitis). Medication port of premixed bags should be used to withdraw only the initial bolus, if necessary (not to be used for withdrawal of additional bolus doses).

I.V. Detail Infusions must be administered with an infusion pump. Decrease or discontinue infusion if hypotension, congestive heart failure occur.

pH: 4.5-5.5

Stability

Storage Clear, colorless to light yellow solution which should be stored at 25°C (77°F); excursions permitted to 15°C to 30°C (59°F to 86°F); do not freeze. Protect from excessive heat.

Nursing Actions

Physical Assessment Requires continuous cardiac, hemodynamic, and infusion site monitoring (to prevent extravasation). Taper dosage slowly when discontinuing. Advise patients with diabetes to monitor glucose levels closely; beta-blockers may alter glucose tolerance.

Patient Education Esmolol is administered in emergencies; patient education should be appropriate to the situation.

Related Information

Management of Drug Extravasations *on page 1269*

Esomeprazole (es oh ME pray zol)

Brand Names: U.S. NexIUM®; NexIUM® I.V.

Index Terms Esomeprazole Magnesium; Esomeprazole Sodium

Pharmacologic Category Proton Pump Inhibitor; Substituted Benzimidazole

Medication Safety Issues

Sound-alike/look-alike issues:

Esomeprazole may be confused with ARIPiprazole

NexIUM® may be confused with NexAVAR®

Pregnancy Risk Factor B

Lactation Excretion in breast milk unknown/not recommended

Breast-Feeding Considerations Esomeprazole excretion into breast milk has not been studied. However, omeprazole is excreted in breast milk, and therefore considered likely that esomeprazole is similarly excreted; breast-feeding is not recommended.

Use

Oral: Short-term (4-8 weeks) treatment of erosive esophagitis; maintaining symptom resolution and healing of erosive esophagitis; treatment of symptomatic gastroesophageal reflux disease (GERD); as part of a multidrug regimen for *Helicobacter pylori* eradication in patients with duodenal ulcer disease (active or history of within the past 5 years); prevention of gastric ulcers in patients at risk (age ≥60 years and/or history of gastric ulcer) associated with continuous NSAID therapy; long-term treatment of pathological hypersecretory conditions including Zollinger-Ellison syndrome

Canadian labeling: Additional use (not in U.S. labeling): Oral: Treatment of nonerosive reflux disease (NERD)

I.V.: Short-term (≤10 days) treatment of gastroesophageal reflux disease (GERD) when oral therapy is not possible or appropriate

Unlabeled Use I.V.: Prevention of recurrent peptic ulcer bleeding postendoscopy

Mechanism of Action/Effect Prevents gastric acid secretion

Contraindications Hypersensitivity to esomeprazole, substituted benzimidazoles (eg, omeprazole, lansoprazole), or any component of the formulation

Warnings/Precautions Use of proton pump inhibitors (PPIs) may increase the risk of gastrointestinal infections (eg, *Salmonella, Campylobacter*). Relief of symptoms does not preclude the presence of a gastric malignancy. Atrophic gastritis (by biopsy) has been noted with long-term omeprazole therapy; this may also occur with esomeprazole. No reports of enterochromaffin-like (ECL) cell carcinoids, dysplasia, or neoplasia have occurred. Severe liver dysfunction may require dosage reductions. Safety and efficacy of I.V. therapy >10 days have not been established; transition from I.V. to oral therapy as soon possible. Bioavailability may be increased in Asian populations, the elderly, and patients with hepatic dysfunction. Decreased *H. pylori* eradication rates have been observed with short-term (≤7 days) combination therapy. The American College of Gastroenterology recommends 10-14 days of therapy (triple or quadruple) for eradication of *H. pylori* (Chey, 2007).

PPIs may diminish the therapeutic effect of clopidogrel, thought to be due to reduced formation of the active metabolite of clopidogrel. The manufacturer of clopidogrel recommends either avoidance of omeprazole or use of a PPI with less potent CYP2C19 inhibition (eg, pantoprazole); avoidance of esomeprazole would appear prudent. Others have recommended the continued use of PPIs, regardless of the degree of inhibition, in patients with a history of GI bleeding or multiple risk factors for GI bleeding who are also receiving clopidogrel since no evidence has established clinically meaningful differences in outcome; however, a clinically-significant interaction cannot be excluded in those who are poor metabolizers of clopidogrel (Abraham, 2010; Levine, 2011). Avoid concurrent use of CYP3A4 and 2C19 inducers (eg, St John's wort, rifampin) as esomeprazole's efficacy may be reduced.

Increased incidence of osteoporosis-related bone fractures of the hip, spine, or wrist may occur with PPI therapy. Patients on high-dose or long-term therapy should be monitored. Use the lowest effective dose for the shortest duration of time, use vitamin D and calcium supplementation, and follow appropriate guidelines to reduce risk of fractures in patients at risk.

Hypomagnesemia, reported rarely, usually with prolonged PPI use of >3 months (most cases >1 year of therapy); may be symptomatic or asymptomatic; severe cases may cause tetany, seizures, and cardiac arrhythmias. Consider obtaining serum magnesium concentrations prior to beginning long-term therapy, especially if taking concomitant digoxin, diuretics, or other drugs known to cause hypomagnesemia; and periodically thereafter. Hypomagnesemia may be corrected by magnesium supplementation, although discontinuation of esomeprazole may be necessary; magnesium levels typically return to normal within 1 week of stopping. Serum chromogranin A levels may be increased if assessed while patient on esomeprazole; may lead to diagnostic errors related to neuroendocrine tumors.

Drug Interactions

Avoid Concomitant Use

Avoid concomitant use of Esomeprazole with any of the following: Delavirdine; Erlotinib; Nelfinavir; Posaconazole; Rifampin; Rilpivirine; St Johns Wort

Decreased Effect

Esomeprazole may decrease the levels/effects of: Atazanavir; Bisphosphonate Derivatives; Cefditoren; Clopidogrel; Dabigatran Etexilate; Dasatinib; Delavirdine; Erlotinib; Gefitinib; Indinavir; Iron Salts; Itraconazole; Ketoconazole; Ketoconazole (Systemic); Mesalamine; Mycophenolate; Nelfinavir; Posaconazole; Rilpivirine; Vismodegib

The levels/effects of Esomeprazole may be decreased by: CYP2C19 Inducers (Strong); Rifampin; St Johns Wort; Tipranavir; Tocilizumab

Increased Effect/Toxicity

Esomeprazole may increase the levels/effects of: Amphetamines; Benzodiazepines (metabolized by oxidation); Cilostazol; Citalopram; CYP2C19 Substrates; Dexmethylphenidate; Methotrexate; Methylphenidate; Raltegravir; Saquinavir; Tacrolimus; Tacrolimus (Systemic); Vitamin K Antagonists; Voriconazole

The levels/effects of Esomeprazole may be increased by: Conivaptan; Fluconazole; Ketoconazole; Ketoconazole (Systemic)

Nutritional/Ethanol Interactions

Food: Absorption is decreased by 43% to 53% when taken with food. Management: Take at least 1 hour before meals at the same time each day, best if before breakfast.

Herb/Nutraceutical: St John's wort may decrease the efficacy of esomeprazole. Management: Avoid St John's wort.

Adverse Reactions Unless otherwise specified, percentages represent adverse reactions identified in clinical trials evaluating the oral formulation.

>10%: Central nervous system: Headache (I.V. 11%; oral ≤8%)

1% to 10%:

Cardiovascular: Hypertension (≤3%), chest pain (>1%)

Central nervous system: Pain (4%), dizziness (oral >1%; I.V. 3%), anxiety (2%), insomnia (2%), pyrexia (2%), fatigue (>1%)

Dermatologic: Rash (>1%), pruritus (I.V. ≤1%)

Endocrine & metabolic: Hypercholesterolemia (2%)

Gastrointestinal: Flatulence (oral ≤5%; I.V. 10%), diarrhea (oral ≤7%; I.V. 4%), abdominal pain (oral ≤6%; I.V. 6%), nausea (oral 5%; I.V. 6%), dyspepsia (oral >1%; I.V. 6%), gastritis (≤6%), constipation (oral 2%; I.V. 3%), vomiting (≤3%), benign GI neoplasm (>1%), dyspepsia (>1%), duodenitis (>1%), epigastric pain (>1%), esophageal disorder (>1%), gastroenteritis (>1%), GI mucosal discoloration (>1%), serum gastrin increased (>1%), xerostomia (1%)

Genitourinary: Urinary tract infection (4%)

Hematologic: Anemia (>1%)

Hepatic: Transaminases increased (>1%)

Local: Injection site reaction (I.V. 2%)

Neuromuscular & skeletal: Arthralgia (3%), back pain (>1%), fracture (>1%), arthropathy (1%), myalgia (1%)

Respiratory: Respiratory infection (oral ≤9%; I.V. 1%), bronchitis (4%), sinusitis (oral ≤4%; I.V. 2%), coughing (>1%), rhinitis (>1%), dyspnea (1%)

Miscellaneous: Accident/injury (≤8%), viral infection (4%), allergy (2%), ear infection (2%), hernia (>1%), flu-like syndrome (1%)

Available Dosage Forms

Capsule, delayed release, oral:

NexIUM®: 20 mg, 40 mg

Granules for suspension, delayed release, oral:

NexIUM®: 10 mg/packet (30s); 20 mg/packet (30s); 40 mg/packet (30s)

Injection, powder for reconstitution:

NexIUM® I.V.: 20 mg, 40 mg

General Dosage Range Dosage adjustment recommended in patients with hepatic impairment.

I.V.:

Children 1-11 months: 0.5 mg/kg once daily

Children 1-17 years: <55 kg: 10 mg once daily; ≥55 kg: 20 mg once daily

Adults: 20-40 mg once daily

Oral:

Children 1-11 years: <20 kg: 10 mg once daily; ≥20 kg: 10-20 mg once daily

Children 12-17 years: 20-40 mg once daily

Adults: 20-40 mg once daily **or** 80-240 mg/day in divided doses (hypersecretory conditions)

Administration

Oral

Capsule: Should be swallowed whole and taken at least 1 hour before eating (best if taken before breakfast). Capsule can be opened and contents mixed with 1 tablespoon of applesauce. Swallow immediately; mixture should not be chewed or warmed. For patients with difficulty swallowing, use of granules may be more appropriate.

Granules: Empty into container with 15 mL of water and stir; leave 2-3 minutes to thicken. Stir and drink within 30 minutes. If any medicine remains after drinking, add more water, stir and drink immediately.

Tablet (Canadian formulation, not available in U.S.): Swallow whole or may be dispersed in a half a glass of noncarbonated water. Stir until tablets disintegrate, leaving a liquid containing pellets. Drink contents within 30 minutes. Do not chew or crush pellets. After drinking, rinse glass with water and drink.

I.V. Flush line prior to and after administration with NS, LR, or D_5W.

Children: Administer by intermittent infusion (10-30 minutes); the manufacturer recommends that children receive intravenous esomeprazole by intermittent infusion only.

Adults: May be administered by injection (≥3 minutes), intermittent infusion (10-30 minutes), or continuous infusion for up to 72 hours (Sung, 2009).

I.V. Detail pH: 9-11

Other Nasogastric tube:

Capsule: Open capsule and place intact granules into a 60 mL catheter-tip syringe; mix with 50 mL of water. Replace plunger and shake vigorously for 15 seconds. Ensure that no granules remain in syringe tip. Do not administer if pellets dissolve or disintegrate. Use immediately after preparation. After administration, flush nasogastric tube with additional water.

Granules: Delayed release oral suspension granules can also be given by nasogastric or gastric tube. Add 15 mL of water to a catheter-tip syringe, add granules from packet. Shake the syringe, leave 2-3 minutes to thicken. Shake the syringe and administer through nasogastric or gastric tube (size 6 French or greater) within 30 minutes. Refill the syringe with 15 mL of water, shake and flush nasogastric/gastric tube.

Tablet (Canadian formulation, not available in U.S.): Disperse tablets in 50 mL of noncarbonated water. Stir until tablets disintegrate leaving a liquid containing pellets. After administration, flush with additional 25-50 mL of water to clear the syringe and tube.

Stability

Reconstitution Powder for injection:

For I.V. injection: Adults: Reconstitute powder with 5 mL NS.

For I.V. infusion:

Children: Initially reconstitute powder (20 mg or 40 mg) with 5 mL of NS, then further dilute to a final volume of 50 mL; withdraw the appropriate amount of the final solution to administer the intended dose.

Adults: Initially reconstitute powder with 5 mL of NS, LR, or D_5W, then further dilute to a final volume of 50 mL.

Storage

Capsule, granules: Store at 15°C to 30°C (59°F to 86°F). Keep container tightly closed.

Powder for injection: Store at 25°C (77°F); excursions permitted to 15°C to 30°C (59°F to 86°F). Protect from light. Per the manufacturer, following reconstitution, solution for injection prepared in NS, and solution for infusion prepared in NS or LR should be used within 12 hours. Following reconstitution, solution for infusion prepared in D_5W should be used within 6 hours. Refrigeration is not required following reconstitution.

Additional stability data: Following reconstitution, solutions for infusion prepared in D_5W, NS, or LR in PVC bags are chemically and physically stable for 48 hours at room temperature (25°C) and for at least 120 hours under refrigeration (4°C) (Kupiec, 2008).

Nursing Actions

Physical Assessment Monitor for rebleeding.

Patient Education Take as directed, 1 hour before eating at same time each day. Swallow capsule whole; do not crush or chew. If you cannot swallow capsule whole, open capsule, mix contents with 1 tablespoon of applesauce, and swallow immediately; do not chew mixture. Do not store for future use. You may experience headache, constipation, diarrhea, or abdominal pain. Report persistent headache, diarrhea, abdominal pain, gas, changes in urination or pain on urination, or persistent muscular aches or pain.

Dietary Considerations Take at least 1 hour before meals; best if taken before breakfast. The contents of the capsule may be mixed in applesauce or water; pellets also remain intact when exposed to orange juice, apple juice, and yogurt.

Estradiol (Systemic) (es tra DYE ole)

Brand Names: U.S. Alora®; Climara®; Delestrogen®; Depo®-Estradiol; Divigel®; Elestrin®; Estrace®; Estraderm®; Estrasorb®; EstroGel®; Evamist™; Femring®; Femtrace®; Menostar®; Vivelle-Dot®

Index Terms Estradiol; Estradiol Acetate; Estradiol Transdermal; Estradiol Valerate

Pharmacologic Category Estrogen Derivative

Medication Safety Issues

Sound-alike/look-alike issues:

Alora® may be confused with Aldara®

Elestrin® may be confused with alosetron

BEERS Criteria medication:

This drug may be inappropriate for use in geriatric patients (low severity risk).

Other safety issues:

Transdermal patch may contain conducting metal (eg, aluminum); remove patch prior to MRI.

International issues:

Vivelle: Brand name for estradiol [U.S. and multiple international markets, but also the brand name for ethinyl estradiol and norgestimate [Austria]

Pregnancy Risk Factor X

Lactation Enters breast milk/use caution

Use Treatment of moderate-to-severe vasomotor symptoms associated with menopause; treatment of moderate-to-severe vulvar and vaginal atrophy associated with menopause; hypoestrogenism (due to hypogonadism, castration, or primary ovarian failure); advanced prostatic cancer (palliation); metastatic breast cancer (palliation) in men and postmenopausal women; postmenopausal osteoporosis (prophylaxis)

Available Dosage Forms

Emulsion, topical:

Estrasorb®: 2.5 mg/g (56s)

Gel, topical:

Divigel®: 0.1% (30s)

Elestrin®: 0.06% (35 g, 70 g)

EstroGel®: 0.06% (50 g)

Injection, oil: 20 mg/mL (5 mL); 40 mg/mL (5 mL)

Delestrogen®: 10 mg/mL (5 mL); 20 mg/mL (5 mL); 40 mg/mL (5 mL)

Depo®-Estradiol: 5 mg/mL (5 mL)

Patch, transdermal: 0.025 mg/24 hours (4s); 0.0375 mg/24 hours (4s); 0.05 mg/24 hours (4s); 0.06 mg/24 hours (4s); 0.075 mg/24 hours (4s); 0.1 mg/24 hours (4s)

Alora®: 0.025 mg/24 hours (8s); 0.05 mg/24 hours (8s); 0.075 mg/24 hours (8s); 0.1 mg/24 hours (8s)

Climara®: 0.025 mg/24 hours (4s); 0.0375 mg/24 hours (4s); 0.05 mg/24 hours (4s); 0.06 mg/24 hours (4s); 0.075 mg/24 hours (4s); 0.1 mg/24 hours (4s)

Estraderm®: 0.05 mg/24 hours (8s); 0.1 mg/24 hours (8s)

Menostar®: 0.014 mg/24 hours (4s)

Vivelle-Dot®: 0.025 mg/24 hours (24s); 0.0375 mg/24 hours (24s); 0.05 mg/24 hours (24s); 0.075 mg/24 hours (24s); 0.1 mg/24 hours (24s)

Ring, vaginal:

Femring®: 0.05 mg/24 hours (1s); 0.1 mg/24 hours (1s)

Solution, topical:

Evamist™: 1.53 mg/spray (8.1 mL)

Tablet, oral: 0.5 mg, 1 mg, 2 mg

Estrace®: 0.5 mg, 1 mg, 2 mg

Femtrace®: 0.45 mg, 0.9 mg, 1.8 mg

General Dosage Range

I.M.:

Cypionate:

Adults (females): Hypoestrogenism: 1.5-2 mg monthly

Adults (females): Menopause: 1-5 mg every 3-4 weeks

Valerate:

Adults (females): Menopause: 10-20 mg every 4 weeks

Adults (males): Prostate cancer: 30 mg or more every 1-2 weeks

Oral:

Adults (females):

Estrace®: Breast cancer: 10 mg 3 times/day; Hypoestrogenism: 1-2 mg/day; Menopause: 0.5-2 mg/day

Femtrace®: Menopause: 0.45-1.8 mg/day

Adults (males): Estrace®: Prostate cancer: 1-2 mg 3 times/day; Breast cancer: 10 mg 3 times/day

Intravaginal: *Adults (females):* (Femring®): 0.05-0.1 mg, leave in place for 3 months

Topical: *Adults (females):*

Emulsion (Estrasorb®): 3.48 g applied once daily in the morning

Gel: 1.25 g/day (EstroGel®) or 0.87-1.7 g/day (Elestrin®) or 0.25-1 g/day (Divigel®) applied at the same time each day

Spray (Evamist™): 1 spray (1.53 mg) per day; dosing range: 1-3 sprays/day

Transdermal: *Adults (females):*

Alora®, Estraderm®, Vivelle-Dot®: Apply twice weekly continuously or cyclically (3 weeks on, 1 week off)

Climara®: Apply once weekly continuously or cyclically (3 weeks on, 1 week off)

Menostar®: Apply once weekly continuously

Administration

I.M. The use of a progestin should be considered when administering estrogens to postmenopausal women with an intact uterus.

Injection for intramuscular administration only. Estradiol valerate should be injected into the upper outer quadrant of the gluteal muscle; administer with a dry needle (solution may become cloudy with wet needle).

Topical The use of a progestin should be considered when administering estrogens to postmenopausal women with an intact uterus.

Emulsion (Estrasorb®): Apply to clean, dry skin while in a sitting position. Contents of two pouches (total 3.48 g) are to be applied individually, once daily in the morning. Apply contents of first pouch to left thigh; massage into skin of left thigh and calf until thoroughly absorbed (~3 minutes). Apply excess from both hands to the buttocks. Apply contents of second pouch to the right thigh; massage into skin of right thigh and calf until thoroughly absorbed (~3 minutes). Apply excess from both hands to buttocks. Wash hands with soap and water. Allow skin to dry before covering legs with clothing. Do not apply to other areas of body. Do not apply to red or irritated skin.

Gel: Apply to clean, dry, unbroken skin at the same time each day. Allow to dry for 5 minutes prior to dressing. Gel is flammable; avoid fire or flame until dry. After application, wash hands with soap and water. Prior to the first use, pump must be primed. Do not apply gel to breast.

Divigel®: Apply entire contents of packet to right or left upper thigh each day (alternate sites). Do not apply to face, breasts, vaginal area or irritated skin. Apply over an area ~5x7 inches. Do not wash application site for 1 hour. Allow gel to dry before dressing

Elestrin®: Apply to upper arm and shoulder area using two fingers to spread gel. Apply after bath or shower; allow at least 2 hours between applying gel and going swimming. Wait at least 25 minutes before applying sunscreen to application area. Do not apply sunscreen to application area for ≥7 days (may increase absorption of gel).

EstroGel®: Apply gel to the arm, from the wrist to the shoulder. Spread gel as thinly as possible over one arm.

Spray: Evamist™: Prior to first use, prime pump by spraying 3 sprays with the cover on. To administer dose, hold container upright and vertical and rest the plastic cone flat against the skin while spraying. Spray to the inner surface of the forearm, starting near the elbow. If more than one spray is needed, apply to adjacent but not overlapping areas. Apply at the same time each day. Allow spray to dry for ~2 minutes; do not rub into skin; do not cover with clothing until dry. Do not wash application site for at least 60 minutes. Apply to clean, dry, unbroken skin. Do not apply to skin other than that of the forearm. Make sure that children do not come in contact with any skin area where the drug was applied. If contact with children is unavoidable, wear a garment with long sleeves that covers the site of application. If direct exposure should occur, wash the child in the area of exposure with soap and water as soon as possible. Solution contained in the spray is flammable; avoid fire, flame, or smoking until spray has dried. If needed, sunscreen should be applied ~1 hour prior to application of Evamist™ .

Transdermal patch: Do not apply transdermal system to breasts, but place on trunk of body (preferably abdomen). Rotate application sites allowing a 1-week interval between applications at a particular site. Do not apply to oily, damaged or irritated skin; avoid waistline or other areas where tight clothing may rub the patch off. Apply patch immediately after removing from protective pouch. In general, if patch falls off, the same patch may be reapplied or a new system may be used for the remainder of the dosing interval (not recommended with all products) When replacing patch, reapply to a new site. Swimming, bathing or showering are not expected to affect use of the patch. Note the following exceptions:

Estraderm®: Do not apply to an area exposed to direct sunlight.

Climara®, Menostar®: Swimming, bathing, or wearing patch while in a sauna have not been studied; adhesion of patch may be decreased or delivery of estradiol may be affected. Remove patch slowly after use to avoid skin irritation. If any adhesive remains on the skin after removal, first allow skin to dry for 15 minutes, then gently rub area with an oil-based cream or lotion. If patch falls off, a new patch should be applied for the remainder of the dosing interval.

Other Vaginal ring: Exact positioning is not critical for efficacy; however, patient should not feel anything once inserted. In case of discomfort, ring should be pushed further into vagina. If ring is expelled prior to 90 days, it may be rinsed off and reinserted. Ensure proper vaginal placement of the ring to avoid inadvertent urinary bladder insertion. If vaginal infection develops, Femring® may remain in place during local treatment of a vaginal infection.

Nursing Actions

Physical Assessment Monitor for CNS changes, hypertension, thromboembolism, fluid retention, edema, CHF, and respiratory changes on a regular basis during therapy. Caution patients with diabetes to monitor glucose levels closely (may impair glucose tolerance). Remind patient about the importance of frequent self-breast exams and the need for annual gynecological exam.

Patient Education Follow directions for timing and application of your prescription. Women (menopausal symptoms): Annual gynecologic and regular self-breast exams are important. Men (prostate or breast cancer), women (breast cancer): Follow up with oncologist as directed. If you have diabetes, monitor glucose levels closely (may impair glucose tolerance). You may experience nausea, vomiting, abdominal pain, dizziness or mental depression, rash, headache, breast pain, or enlargement/tenderness of breasts. Report unusual swelling of extremities; sudden acute pain in legs or calves, chest, or abdomen; shortness of breath; severe headache; sudden blindness or change in visual acuity; weakness or numbness of arm or leg; unusual vaginal bleeding; yellowing of skin or eyes; unusual bruising or bleeding; or skin rash. You may become intolerant to wearing contact lenses; notify prescriber if this occurs.

Estradiol and Dienogest

(es tra DYE ole & dye EN oh jest)

Brand Names: U.S. Natazia®

Index Terms Dienogest and Estradiol; Estradiol Valerate and Dienogest

Pharmacologic Category Contraceptive; Estrogen and Progestin Combination

Lactation Enters breast milk/not recommended

Use Prevention of pregnancy

Unlabeled Use Treatment of hypermenorrhea (menorrhagia); pain associated with endometriosis; dysmenorrhea; dysfunctional uterine bleeding

Available Dosage Forms

Tablet, oral [four-phasic formulation]:

Natazia®:

Days 1-2: Estradiol valerate 3 mg [2 dark yellow tablets]

Days 3-7: Estradiol valerate 2 mg and dienogest 2 mg [5 medium red tablets]

Days 8-24: Estradiol valerate 2 mg and dienogest 3 mg [17 light yellow tablets]

Days 25-26: Estradiol valerate 1 mg [2 dark red tablets]

Days 27-28: 2 white inactive tablets (28s)

General Dosage Range Oral: *Children and Adults (females, postmenarche):* 1 tablet daily

Administration

Oral Tablets should be taken at the same time each day in the order presented in the blister pack. Do not delay administration by >12 hours. In case of vomiting or diarrhea within 3-4 hours of taking a colored tablet, treat as if the dose was missed (or can take another tablet of the same color from an extra blister pack). Patients should be instructed not to take more than 2 tablets in any one day. A nonhormonal contraceptive (eg, condom or spermicide) should be used for the first 9 days of therapy. If patient is unsure of number of tablets missed, they should continue taking one tablet each day and use a back-up form of contraception.

Nursing Actions

Physical Assessment See individual agents.

Patient Education See individual agents.

Estradiol and Norethindrone

(es tra DYE ole & nor eth IN drone)

Brand Names: U.S. Activella®; CombiPatch®; Mimvey™

Index Terms Norethindrone and Estradiol

Pharmacologic Category Estrogen and Progestin Combination

Lactation Enters breast milk/use caution

Use Women with an intact uterus:

Tablet: Treatment of moderate-to-severe vasomotor symptoms associated with menopause; treatment of vulvar and vaginal atrophy; prophylaxis for postmenopausal osteoporosis

Transdermal patch: Treatment of moderate-to-severe vasomotor symptoms associated with menopause; treatment of vulvar and vaginal atrophy; treatment of hypoestrogenism due to hypogonadism, castration, or primary ovarian failure

Available Dosage Forms

Patch, transdermal:

CombiPatch®:

0.05/0.14: Estradiol 0.05 mg and norethindrone 0.14 mg per day (8s) [9 sq cm]

0.05/0.25: Estradiol 0.05 mg and norethindrone 0.25 mg per day (8s) [16 sq cm]

Tablet, oral: Estradiol 1 mg and norethindrone acetate 0.5 mg (28s)

Activella® 0.5/0.1: Estradiol 0.5 mg and norethindrone acetate 0.1 mg (28s)

Activella® 1/0.5, Mimvey™: Estradiol 1 mg and norethindrone acetate 0.5 mg (28s)

General Dosage Range

Oral: *Adults (females):* 1 tablet daily

Transdermal: *Adults (females):* Apply 1 patch twice weekly

Administration

Other Transdermal patch: Apply to clean dry skin. Do not apply transdermal patch to breasts; apply to lower abdomen, avoiding waistline. Rotate application sites.

Nursing Actions

Physical Assessment See individual agents.

Patient Education See individual agents.

Related Information

Estradiol (Systemic) *on page 424*

Norethindrone *on page 840*

Estramustine (es tra MUS teen)

Brand Names: U.S. Emcyt®

Index Terms Estramustine Phosphate; Estramustine Phosphate Sodium; NSC-89199

Pharmacologic Category Antineoplastic Agent, Alkylating Agent; Antineoplastic Agent, Hormone; Antineoplastic Agent, Hormone (Estrogen/Nitrogen Mustard)

Medication Safety Issues

Sound-alike/look-alike issues:

Emcyt® may be confused with Eryc®

Estramustine may be confused with exemestane.

High alert medication:

The Institute for Safe Medication Practices (ISMP) includes this medication among its list of drug classes which have a heightened risk of causing significant patient harm when used in error.

Breast-Feeding Considerations Estramustine is not indicated for use in women.

Use Palliative treatment of progressive or metastatic prostate cancer

Mechanism of Action/Effect Combines the effects of estradiol and nitrogen mustard. It appears to bind to microtubule proteins, preventing normal tubulin function. The antitumor effect may be due solely to an estrogenic effect. Estramustine causes a marked decrease in plasma testosterone and an increase in estrogen levels.

Contraindications Hypersensitivity to estramustine, estradiol, nitrogen mustard, or any component of the formulation; active thrombophlebitis or thromboembolic disorders (except where tumor mass is the cause of thromboembolic disorder and the benefit may outweigh the risk)

Canadian labeling: Additional contraindications (not in the U.S. labeling): Severe hepatic or cardiac disease

Warnings/Precautions Hazardous agent - use appropriate precautions for handling and disposal. Glucose tolerance may be decreased; use with caution in patients with diabetes. Elevated blood pressure, peripheral edema (new-onset or exacerbation), or congestive heart disease may occur; use with caution in patients where fluid accumulation may be poorly tolerated, including cardiovascular disease (HF or hypertension), migraine, seizure disorder or renal dysfunction. Estrogen treatment for prostate cancer is associated with an increased risk of thrombosis and MI; use caution with history of cardiovascular disease (eg, thrombophlebitis, thrombosis, or thromboembolic disease) and cerebrovascular or coronary artery disease. Use with caution in patients with hepatic impairment (may be metabolized poorly) or with metabolic bone diseases. Allergic reactions and angioedema, including airway involvement, have been reported with use. Patients with prostate cancer and osteoblastic metastases should have their calcium monitored regularly. Estrogen use may cause gynecomastia and/or impotence. Avoid vaccination with live vaccines during treatment (risk of infection may be increased due to immunosuppression). Although the response to vaccines may be diminished, inactivated vaccines may be administered during treatment.

Drug Interactions

Avoid Concomitant Use

Avoid concomitant use of Estramustine with any of the following: BCG; Natalizumab; Pimecrolimus; Tacrolimus (Topical); Vaccines (Live)

Decreased Effect

Estramustine may decrease the levels/effects of: BCG; Coccidioidin Skin Test; Sipuleucel-T; Vaccines (Inactivated); Vaccines (Live)

The levels/effects of Estramustine may be decreased by: Calcium Salts; Echinacea

Increased Effect/Toxicity

Estramustine may increase the levels/effects of: Leflunomide; Natalizumab; Vaccines (Live)

The levels/effects of Estramustine may be increased by: Clodronate; Denosumab; Pimecrolimus; Roflumilast; Tacrolimus (Topical); Trastuzumab

Nutritional/Ethanol Interactions Food: Estramustine serum levels may be decreased if taken with milk or other dairy products, calcium supplements, and vitamins containing calcium. Management: Take on an empty stomach at least 1 hour before or 2 hours after eating.

Adverse Reactions

>10%:

Cardiovascular: Edema (20%)

Endocrine & metabolic: Gynecomastia (75%), breast tenderness (71%), libido decreased

Gastrointestinal: Nausea (16%), diarrhea (13%), gastrointestinal upset (12%)
Hepatic: LDH increased (2% to 33%), AST increased (2% to 33%)
Respiratory: Dyspnea (12%)

1% to 10%:
Cardiovascular: CHF (3%), MI (3%), cerebrovascular accident (2%), chest pain (1%), flushing (1%)
Central nervous system: Lethargy (4%), insomnia (3%), emotional lability (2%), anxiety (1%), headache (1%)
Dermatologic: Bruising (3%), dry skin (2%), pruritus (2%), hair thinning (1%), rash (1%), skin peeling (1%)
Gastrointestinal: Anorexia (4%), flatulence (2%), burning throat (1%), gastrointestinal bleeding (1%), thirst (1%), vomiting (1%)
Hematologic: Leukopenia (4%), thrombocytopenia (1%)
Hepatic: Bilirubin increased (1% to 2%)
Local: Thrombophlebitis (3%)
Neuromuscular & skeletal: Leg cramps (9%)
Ocular: Tearing (1%)
Respiratory: Pulmonary embolism (2%), upper respiratory discharge (1%), hoarseness (1%)

Available Dosage Forms

Capsule, oral:
Emcyt®: 140 mg

General Dosage Range Oral: *Adults (males):* 14 mg/kg/day (range: 10-16 mg/kg/day) in 3 or 4 divided doses

Administration

Oral Administer on an empty stomach, at least 1 hour before or 2 hours after eating.

Stability

Storage Refrigerate at 2°C to 8°C (36°F to 46°F).

Nursing Actions

Physical Assessment Monitor for CNS changes, hypertension, and thromboembolism on a regular basis. Caution patients with diabetes to monitor glucose carefully; glucose tolerance may be decreased.

Patient Education It may take several weeks to manifest effects of this medication. Take on empty stomach, 1 hour before or 2 hours after meals or any supplements containing calcium; do not take with milk or milk products. Patients with diabetes should use caution and monitor glucose carefully; glucose tolerance may be decreased. May cause nausea, vomiting, flatulence, diarrhea, decreased libido (reversible), or breast tenderness or enlargement. Report sudden acute pain or cramping in legs or calves, unusual swelling in legs or feet, chest pain, shortness of breath, weakness or numbness of arms or legs, or respiratory difficulty.

Dietary Considerations Should be taken at least 1 hour before or 2 hours after eating. Milk products and calcium-rich foods or supplements may impair the oral absorption of estramustine phosphate sodium.

Estrogens (Conjugated A/Synthetic)

(ES troe jenz KON joo gate ed aye sin THET ik)

Brand Names: U.S. Cenestin®

Pharmacologic Category Estrogen Derivative

Medication Safety Issues

Sound-alike/look-alike issues:
Cenestin® may be confused with Senexon®

BEERS Criteria medication:
This drug may be inappropriate for use in geriatric patients (low severity risk).

International issues:
Cenestin [U.S., Canada] may be confused with Canesten which is a brand name for clotrimazole [multiple international markets]

Lactation Enters breast milk/use caution

Use Treatment of moderate-to-severe vasomotor symptoms of menopause; treatment of vulvar and vaginal atrophy

Available Dosage Forms

Tablet, oral:
Cenestin®: 0.3 mg, 0.45 mg, 0.625 mg, 0.9 mg, 1.25 mg

General Dosage Range Oral: *Adults (females):* 0.3-1.25 mg once daily

Nursing Actions

Physical Assessment Monitor annual gynecological exam. Monitor for thromboembolism, hypertension, edema, and CNS changes on a regular basis during therapy. Caution patients with diabetes to monitor glucose levels closely (may impair glucose tolerance). Remind patient about the importance of frequent self-breast exams and the need for annual gynecological exam.

Patient Education Annual gynecologic and regular self-breast exams are important. If you have diabetes, monitor glucose levels closely (may impair glucose tolerance). You may experience nausea, vomiting, abdominal pain, dizziness, mental depression, rash, headache, breast pain, or enlargement/tenderness of breasts. Report significant swelling of extremities; sudden acute pain in legs or calves, chest, or abdomen; shortness of breath; severe headache; sudden blindness; weakness or numbness of arm or leg; unusual vaginal bleeding; yellowing of skin or eyes; or unusual bruising or bleeding. You may become intolerant to wearing contact lenses; notify prescriber if this occurs.

Estrogens (Conjugated B/Synthetic)

(ES troe jenz KON joo gate ed bee sin THET ik)

Brand Names: U.S. Enjuvia™

Pharmacologic Category Estrogen Derivative

Medication Safety Issues

Sound-alike/look-alike issues:

Enjuvia™ may be confused with Januvia®

BEERS Criteria medication:

This drug may be inappropriate for use in geriatric patients (low severity risk).

Lactation Enters breast milk/use caution

Use Treatment of moderate-to-severe vasomotor symptoms of menopause; treatment of vulvar and vaginal atrophy associated with menopause; treatment of moderate-to-severe vaginal dryness and pain with intercourse associated with menopause

Available Dosage Forms

Tablet, oral:

Enjuvia™: 0.3 mg, 0.45 mg, 0.625 mg, 0.9 mg, 1.25 mg

General Dosage Range Oral: *Adults (females):* 0.3-1.25 mg once daily

Nursing Actions

Physical Assessment Monitor annual gynecological exam. Monitor for thromboembolism, hypertension, edema, and CNS changes on a regular basis during therapy. Caution patients with diabetes to monitor glucose levels closely (may impair glucose tolerance). Remind patient about the importance of frequent self-breast exams and the need for annual gynecological exam.

Patient Education Annual gynecologic and regular self-breast exams are important. If you have diabetes, monitor glucose levels closely (may impair glucose tolerance). You may experience nausea, vomiting, abdominal pain, dizziness, depression, rash, headache, breast pain, or enlargement/tenderness of breasts. Report significant swelling of extremities; sudden acute pain in legs or calves, chest, or abdomen; shortness of breath; severe headache; sudden blindness; weakness or numbness of arm or leg; unusual vaginal bleeding; yellowing of skin or eyes; or unusual bruising or bleeding. You may become intolerant to wearing contact lenses; notify prescriber if this occurs.

Estrogens (Conjugated/Equine, Systemic) (ES troe jenz KON joo gate ed, EE kwine)

Brand Names: U.S. Premarin®

Index Terms C.E.S.; CE; CEE; Conjugated Estrogen; Estrogenic Substances, Conjugated

Pharmacologic Category Estrogen Derivative

Medication Safety Issues

Sound-alike/look-alike issues:

Premarin® may be confused with Primaxin®, Provera®, Remeron®

BEERS Criteria medication:

This drug may be inappropriate for use in geriatric patients (low severity risk).

Lactation Enters breast milk/use caution

Breast-Feeding Considerations Estrogen has been shown to decrease the quantity and quality of human milk. Use only if clearly needed. Monitor the growth of the infant closely.

Use Treatment of moderate-to-severe vasomotor symptoms associated with menopause; treatment of vulvar and vaginal atrophy due to menopause; hypoestrogenism (due to hypogonadism, castration, or primary ovarian failure); prostatic cancer (palliation); breast cancer (palliation); postmenopausal osteoporosis (prophylaxis); abnormal uterine bleeding

Unlabeled Use Uremic bleeding

Mechanism of Action/Effect Estrogens modulate the pituitary secretion of gonadotropins, luteinizing hormone, and follicle-stimulating hormone through a negative feedback system; estrogen replacement reduces elevated levels of these hormones in postmenopausal women

Contraindications Angioedema or anaphylactic reaction to estrogens or any component of the formulation; undiagnosed abnormal vaginal bleeding; history of or current thrombophlebitis or venous thromboembolic disorders (including DVT, PE); active or history of arterial thromboembolic disease (eg, stroke, MI); carcinoma of the breast (except in appropriately selected patients being treated for metastatic disease); estrogen-dependent tumor; hepatic dysfunction or disease; known protein C, protein S, antithrombin deficiency or other known thrombophilic disorders; pregnancy

Canadian labeling: Additional contraindications (not in U.S. labeling): Endometrial hyperplasia; partial or complete vision loss due to ophthalmic vascular disease; migraine with aura

Warnings/Precautions

Anaphylaxis requiring emergency medical management has been reported within minutes to hours of taking conjugated estrogen (CE) tablets. Angioedema involving the face, feet, hands, larynx, and tongue has also been reported. Exogenous estrogens may exacerbate symptoms in women with hereditary angioedema.

[U.S. Boxed Warning]: Estrogens may increase the risk of breast cancer. An increased risk of invasive breast cancer was observed in postmenopausal women using conjugated estrogens (CE) in combination with medroxyprogesterone acetate (MPA); a smaller increase in risk was seen with estrogen therapy alone in observational studies. An increase in abnormal mammogram findings has also been reported with estrogen alone or in combination with progestin therapy. Estrogen use may lead to severe hypercalcemia in patients with breast cancer and bone metastases; discontinue estrogen if hypercalcemia occurs. **[U.S. Boxed Warning]: The use of unopposed estrogen in women with an intact uterus is associated with an increased risk of endometrial cancer. The addition of a**

progestin to estrogen therapy may decrease the risk of endometrial hyperplasia, a precursor to endometrial cancer. Adequate diagnostic measures, including endometrial sampling if indicated, should be performed to rule out malignancy in postmenopausal women with undiagnosed abnormal vaginal bleeding. Estrogens may exacerbate endometriosis. Malignant transformation of residual endometrial implants has been reported posthysterectomy with unopposed estrogen therapy. Consider adding a progestin in women with residual endometriosis posthysterectomy. Postmenopausal estrogen therapy and combined estrogen/progesterone therapy may increase the risk of ovarian cancer; however, the absolute risk to an individual woman is small. Although results from various studies are not consistent, risk does not appear to be significantly associated with the duration, route, or dose of therapy. In one study, the risk decreased after 2 years following discontinuation of therapy (Mørch, 2009). Although the risk of ovarian cancer is rare, women who are at an increased risk (eg, family history) should be counseled about the association (NAMS, 2012).

[U.S. Boxed Warning]: Estrogens with or without progestin should not be used to prevent cardiovascular disease. Using data from the Women's Health Initiative (WHI) studies, an increased risk of deep vein thrombosis (DVT) and stroke has been reported with CE and an increased risk of DVT, stroke, pulmonary emboli (PE) and myocardial infarction (MI) has been reported with CE with MPA in postmenopausal women. Additional risk factors include diabetes mellitus, hypercholesterolemia, hypertension, SLE, obesity, tobacco use, and/or history of venous thromboembolism (VTE). Adverse cardiovascular events have also been reported in males taking estrogens for prostate cancer. Risk factors should be managed appropriately; discontinue use if adverse cardiovascular events occur or are suspected. Women with inherited thrombophilias (eg, protein C or S deficiency) may have increased risk of venous thromboembolism (DeSancho, 2010; van Vlijmen, 2011). Use is contraindicated in women with protein C, protein S, antithrombin deficiency, or other known thrombophilic disorders.

[U.S. Boxed Warning]: Estrogens with or without progestin should not be used to prevent dementia. In the Women's Health Initiative Memory Study (WHIMS), an increased incidence of dementia was observed in women ≥65 years of age taking CE alone or in combination with MPA.

Estrogen compounds are generally associated with lipid effects such as increased HDL-cholesterol and decreased LDL-cholesterol. Triglycerides may also be increased; discontinue if pancreatitis occurs. Use with caution in patients with familial defects of lipoprotein metabolism. Estrogens may increase thyroid-binding globulin (TBG) levels leading to increased circulating total thyroid hormone levels. Women on thyroid replacement therapy may require higher doses of thyroid hormone while receiving estrogens. Use caution in patients with hypoparathyroidism; estrogen-induced hypocalcemia may occur. May have adverse effects on glucose tolerance; use caution in women with diabetes. Use caution in patients with asthma, epilepsy, hepatic hemangiomas, porphyria, or SLE; may exacerbate disease. Use with caution in patients with diseases which may be exacerbated by fluid retention, including cardiac or renal dysfunction. Use of postmenopausal estrogen may be associated with an increased risk of gallbladder disease requiring surgery. Use caution with migraine; may exacerbate disease. Canadian labeling contraindicates use in migraine with aura. Estrogens may cause retinal vascular thrombosis; discontinue if migraine, loss of vision, proptosis, diplopia, or other visual disturbances occur; discontinue permanently if papilledema or retinal vascular lesions are observed on examination.

Estrogens are poorly metabolized in patients with hepatic dysfunction. Use caution with a history of cholestatic jaundice associated with prior estrogen use or pregnancy. Discontinue if jaundice develops or if acute or chronic hepatic disturbances occur. Use is contraindicated with hepatic disease.

Whenever possible, estrogens should be discontinued at least 4-6 weeks prior to elective surgery associated with an increased risk of thromboembolism or during periods of prolonged immobilization. May be inappropriate for use in the elderly due to potential of increased risk of breast and endometrial cancers and lack of proven cardioprotection (Beers Criteria). Prior to puberty, estrogens may cause premature closure of the epiphyses, premature breast development in girls or gynecomastia in boys. Vaginal bleeding and vaginal cornification may also be induced in girls.

[U.S. Boxed Warning]: Estrogens with or without progestin should be used for the shortest duration possible at the lowest effective dose consistent with treatment goals. Before prescribing estrogen therapy to postmenopausal women, the risks and benefits must be weighed for each patient. Women should be informed of these risks and benefits, as well as possible effects of progestin when added to estrogen therapy. Patients should be reevaluated as clinically appropriate to determine if treatment is still necessary. Available data related to treatment risks are from Women's Health Initiative (WHI) studies, which evaluated oral CE 0.625 mg with or without MPA 2.5 mg relative to placebo in postmenopausal women. Other combinations and dosage forms of estrogens and progestins were not studied. **Outcomes reported from clinical trials using CE with or**

without MPA should be assumed to be similar for other doses and other dosage forms of estrogens and progestins until comparable data becomes available.

Vulvar and vaginal atrophy use: Moderate-to-severe symptoms of vulvar and vaginal atrophy include vaginal dryness, dyspareunia, and atrophic vaginitis. When used solely for the treatment of vulvar and vaginal atrophy, topical vaginal products should be considered (NAMS, 2007).

Osteoporosis use: For use only in women at significant risk of osteoporosis and for who other nonestrogen medications are not considered appropriate.

Drug Interactions

Avoid Concomitant Use

Avoid concomitant use of Estrogens (Conjugated/Equine, Systemic) with any of the following: Anastrozole; Axitinib

Decreased Effect

Estrogens (Conjugated/Equine, Systemic) may decrease the levels/effects of: Anastrozole; ARIPiprazole; Axitinib; Chenodiol; Saxagliptin; Somatropin; Thyroid Products; Ursodiol

The levels/effects of Estrogens (Conjugated/Equine, Systemic) may be decreased by: CYP1A2 Inducers (Strong); CYP3A4 Inducers (Strong); Cyproterone; Deferasirox; Herbs (CYP3A4 Inducers); Peginterferon Alfa-2b; Tipranavir; Tocilizumab

Increased Effect/Toxicity

Estrogens (Conjugated/Equine, Systemic) may increase the levels/effects of: Corticosteroids (Systemic); ROPINIRole; Tipranavir

The levels/effects of Estrogens (Conjugated/Equine, Systemic) may be increased by: Ascorbic Acid; Conivaptan; Herbs (Estrogenic Properties)

Nutritional/Ethanol Interactions

Ethanol: Avoid ethanol (routine use increases estrogen plasma concentrations and risk of breast cancer). Ethanol may also increase the risk of osteoporosis.

Food: Folic acid absorption may be decreased.

Herb/Nutraceutical: St John's wort may decrease levels. Herbs with estrogenic properties may enhance the adverse/toxic effect of estrogen derivatives; examples include alfalfa, black cohosh, bloodroot, hops, kudzu, licorice, red clover, saw palmetto, soybean, thyme, wild yam, yucca.

Adverse Reactions

Note: Percentages reported in postmenopausal women following oral use.

>10%:

Central nervous system: Headache (26% to 32%; placebo 28%), pain (17% to 20%; placebo 18%)

Endocrine & metabolic: Breast pain (7% to 12%; placebo 9%)

Gastrointestinal: Abdominal pain (15% to 17%), diarrhea (6% to 7%; placebo 6%)

Genitourinary: Vaginal hemorrhage (2% to 14%)

Neuromuscular & skeletal: Back pain (13% to 14%), arthralgia (7% to 14%; placebo 12%)

Respiratory: Pharyngitis (10% to 12%; placebo 11%), sinusitis: (6% to 11%; placebo 7%)

1% to 10%:

Central nervous system: Depression (5% to 8%), dizziness (4% to 6%), nervousness (2% to 5%)

Dermatologic: Pruritus (4% to 5%)

Gastrointestinal: Flatulence (6% to 7%)

Genitourinary: Vaginitis (5% to 7%), leukorrhea (4% to 7%), vaginal moniliasis (5% to 6%)

Neuromuscular & skeletal: Weakness (7% to 8%), leg cramps (3% to 7%)

Respiratory: Cough increased (4% to 7%)

Additional adverse reactions reported with injection; frequency not defined: Local: injection site: Edema, pain, phlebitis

Available Dosage Forms

Injection, powder for reconstitution:

Premarin®: 25 mg

Tablet, oral:

Premarin®: 0.3 mg, 0.45 mg, 0.625 mg, 0.9 mg, 1.25 mg

General Dosage Range

I.M., I.V.: *Children (postmenarche) and Adults (females):* Abnormal uterine bleeding: 25 mg, may repeat in 6-12 hours if needed

Oral:

Adolescents and Adult (females): 0.3-1.25 mg daily or cyclically **or** 10 mg 3 times/day [breast cancer]

Adults (males): Breast cancer: 10 mg 3 times/day; Prostate cancer: 1.25-2.5 mg 3 times/day

Administration

Oral Administer at bedtime to minimize adverse effects. May be administered without regard to meals.

Abnormal uterine bleeding: High-dose therapy (eg. 10-20 mg/day) may cause nausea; consider concomitant use of an antiemetic

I.M. May be administered intramuscularly.

I.V. Administer I.V. doses slowly to avoid a flushing reaction.

Stability

Reconstitution Injection: Reconstitute with sterile water for injection; slowly inject diluent against side wall of the vial. Agitate gently; do not shake violently.

Storage

Injection: Refrigerate at 2°C to 8°C (36°F to 46°F) prior to reconstitution. Use immediately following reconstitution.

Tablets: Store at room temperature 20°C to 25°C (68°F to 77°F).

Nursing Actions

Physical Assessment Monitor results of annual gynecological exam. Monitor for thromboembolism, hypertension, edema, and CNS changes on a regular basis during therapy. Caution patients with diabetes to monitor glucose levels closely (may impair glucose tolerance). Remind patient about the importance of frequent self-breast exams and the need for annual gynecological exam. Determine that patient is not pregnant before starting therapy. Do not give to females of childbearing age unless patient is capable of complying with contraceptive use. Advise patient about appropriate contraceptive measures as appropriate.

Patient Education Annual gynecologic exams and regular self-breast exams are important. If you have diabetes, monitor glucose levels closely (may impair glucose tolerance). You may experience nausea, vomiting, bloating, abdominal pain, dizziness, depression, rash, headache, breast pain, or enlargement/tenderness of breasts. Report significant swelling of extremities; sudden acute pain in legs, chest, or abdomen; shortness of breath; severe headache; CNS changes (dementia, mood disturbances, irritability, nervousness); sudden blindness; weakness or numbness of arm or leg; unusual vaginal bleeding; yellowing of skin or eyes; or unusual bruising or bleeding. You may become intolerant to wearing contact lenses; notify prescriber if this occurs.

Dietary Considerations Ensure adequate calcium and vitamin D intake when used for the prevention of osteoporosis. Powder for reconstitution for injection (25 mg) contains lactose 200 mg.

Estrogens (Conjugated/Equine, Topical) (ES troe jenz KON joo gate ed, EE kwine)

Brand Names: U.S. Premarin®

Index Terms C.E.S.; CE; CEE; Conjugated Estrogen; Estrogenic Substances, Conjugated

Pharmacologic Category Estrogen Derivative

Medication Safety Issues

Sound-alike/look-alike issues:

Premarin® may be confused with Primaxin®, Provera®, Remeron®

Lactation Enters breast milk/use caution

Use Treatment of atrophic vaginitis and kraurosis vulvae; moderate-to-severe dyspareunia (pain during intercourse) due to vaginal/vulvar atrophy of menopause

Available Dosage Forms

Cream, vaginal:

Premarin®: 0.625 mg/g (42.5 g)

General Dosage Range Intravaginal: *Adults (females):*

Atrophic vaginitis, kraurosis vulvae: 0.5-2 g/day given cyclically

Moderate-to-severe dyspareunia due to menopause: 0.5 g twice weekly (eg, Monday and Thursday) **or** once daily cyclically

Administration

Other Administer at bedtime to minimize adverse effects. Applicator calibrated in 0.5 g increments up to 2 g. To clean applicator, remove plunger from barrel. Wash with mild soap and warm water; do not boil or use hot water.

Nursing Actions

Physical Assessment Monitor results of annual gynecological exam. Monitor for thromboembolism, hypertension, edema, and CNS changes on a regular basis during therapy. Caution patients with diabetes to monitor glucose levels closely (may impair glucose tolerance). Remind patient about the importance of frequent self-breast exams and the need for annual gynecological exam. Determine that patient is not pregnant before starting therapy.

Patient Education Annual gynecologic exams and regular self-breast exams are important. If you have diabetes, monitor glucose levels closely (may impair glucose tolerance). You may experience nausea, vomiting, bloating, abdominal pain, dizziness, depression, rash, headache, breast pain, or enlargement/tenderness of breasts. Report significant swelling of extremities; sudden acute pain in legs, chest, or abdomen; shortness of breath; severe headache; CNS changes (dementia, mood disturbances, irritability, nervousness); sudden blindness; weakness or numbness of arm or leg; unusual vaginal bleeding; yellowing of skin or eyes; or unusual bruising or bleeding. You may become intolerant to wearing contact lenses; notify prescriber if this occurs.

Estrogens (Conjugated/Equine) and Medroxyprogesterone

(ES troe jenz KON joo gate ed/EE kwine & me DROKS ee proe JES te rone)

Brand Names: U.S. Premphase®; Prempro®

Index Terms Medroxyprogesterone and Estrogens (Conjugated); MPA and Estrogens (Conjugated)

Pharmacologic Category Estrogen and Progestin Combination

Lactation Enters breast milk/use caution

Use Women with an intact uterus: Treatment of moderate-to-severe vasomotor symptoms associated with menopause; treatment of moderate-to-severe vulvar and vaginal atrophy due to menopause; postmenopausal osteoporosis (prophylaxis)

Available Dosage Forms

Tablet:

Premphase® [therapy pack contains two separate tablet formulations]: Conjugated estrogens 0.625 mg [14 maroon tablets] and conjugated estrogen 0.625 mg/medroxyprogesterone 5 mg [14 light blue tablets] (28s)

Prempro®:

0.3/1.5: Conjugated estrogens 0.3 mg and medroxyprogesterone 1.5 mg (28s)

0.45/1.5: Conjugated estrogens 0.45 mg and medroxyprogesterone 1.5 mg (28s)
0.625/2.5: Conjugated estrogens 0.625 mg and medroxyprogesterone 2.5 mg (28s)
0.625/5: Conjugated estrogens 0.625 mg and medroxyprogesterone 5 mg (28s)

General Dosage Range Oral: *Adults (females):* Prempro®: Conjugated estrogen 0.3-0.625 mg/mPA 1.5-5 mg once daily **or** Premphase®: One 0.625 mg tablet daily on days 1 through 14 and 1 conjugated estrogen 0.625 mg/mPA 5 mg tablet daily on days 15 through 28

Nursing Actions

Physical Assessment See individual agents.

Patient Education See individual agents.

Related Information

Estrogens (Conjugated/Equine, Systemic) *on page 429*

MedroxyPROGESTERone *on page 725*

Estrogens (Esterified)

(ES troe jenz es TER i fied)

Brand Names: U.S. Menest®

Index Terms Esterified Estrogens

Pharmacologic Category Estrogen Derivative

Medication Safety Issues

Beers Criteria medication:

This drug may be inappropriate for use in geriatric patients (low severity risk).

Lactation Enters breast milk/use caution

Use Treatment of moderate-to-severe vasomotor symptoms associated with menopause; treatment of moderate-to-severe vulvar and vaginal atrophy associated with menopause; hypoestrogenism (due to hypogonadism, castration, or primary ovarian failure); advanced prostatic cancer (palliation), metastatic breast cancer (palliation) in men and postmenopausal women

Available Dosage Forms

Tablet, oral:

Menest®: 0.3 mg, 0.625 mg, 1.25 mg, 2.5 mg

General Dosage Range

Oral:

Adults (females): Hypogonadism: 2.5-7.5 mg/day for 20 days followed by a 10-day rest, repeat until response; Castration or ovarian failure: 1.25 mg/day, cyclically; Menopause 0.3-1.25 mg/day given cyclically; Breast cancer: 10 mg 3 times/day

Adults (males): Breast cancer: 10 mg 3 times/day; Prostate cancer: 1.25-2.5 mg 3 times/day

Administration

Oral Administer with food at same time each day.

Nursing Actions

Physical Assessment Assess results of annual gynecological exam. Monitor for thromboembolism, hypertension, edema, and CNS changes on a regular basis during therapy. Caution patients with diabetes to monitor glucose levels closely (may impair glucose tolerance). Remind patient about the importance of frequent self-breast exams and the need for annual gynecological exam.

Patient Education Annual gynecologic and regular self-breast exams are important. If you have diabetes, monitor glucose levels closely (may impair glucose tolerance). You may experience nausea, vomiting, abdominal pain, dizziness, mental depression, rash, hair loss, headache, breast pain, increased/decreased libido, enlargement/tenderness of breasts, or difficult/painful menstrual cycles. Report significant swelling of extremities; sudden acute pain in legs or calves, chest, or abdomen; shortness of breath; severe headache; sudden blindness; weakness or numbness of arm or leg; unusual vaginal bleeding; yellowing of skin or eyes; or unusual bruising or bleeding. You may become intolerant to wearing contact lenses; notify prescriber if this occurs.

Eszopiclone (es zoe PIK lone)

Brand Names: U.S. Lunesta®

Pharmacologic Category Hypnotic, Nonbenzodiazepine

Medication Safety Issues

Sound-alike/look-alike issues:

Lunesta® may be confused with Neulasta®

Medication Guide Available Yes

Pregnancy Risk Factor C

Lactation Excretion in breast milk unknown/use caution

Use Treatment of insomnia

Mechanism of Action/Effect Interact with the GABA-receptor complex to promote sleep.

Contraindications There are no contraindications listed within the manufacturer's labeling.

Warnings/Precautions Symptomatic treatment of insomnia should be initiated only after careful evaluation of potential causes of sleep disturbance. Tolerance did not develop over 6 months of use. Use with caution in patients with depression or a history of drug dependence. Abrupt discontinuance may lead to withdrawal symptoms. Use with caution in patients receiving other CNS depressants or psychoactive medications. Hypnotics/sedatives have been associated with abnormal thinking and behavior changes including decreased inhibition, aggression, bizarre behavior, agitation, hallucinations, and depersonalization. These changes may occur unpredictably and may indicate previously unrecognized psychiatric disorders; evaluate appropriately. Amnesia may occur. May impair physical and mental capabilities. Postmarketing studies have indicated that the use of hypnotic/sedative agents for sleep has been associated with hypersensitivity reactions including anaphylaxis as well as angioedema. An increased risk for hazardous sleep-related activities such as sleep-driving (as well as cooking and eating food and making phone calls while asleep) has also been noted. Use caution in patients with respiratory compromise, hepatic dysfunction, elderly or those taking strong CYP3A4 inhibitors. Because of the rapid onset of action, administer immediately prior to bedtime or after the patient has gone to bed and is having difficulty falling asleep.

Drug Interactions

Avoid Concomitant Use

Avoid concomitant use of Eszopiclone with any of the following: Conivaptan

Decreased Effect

The levels/effects of Eszopiclone may be decreased by: CYP3A4 Inducers (Strong); Cyproterone; Deferasirox; Flumazenil; Herbs (CYP3A4 Inducers); Tocilizumab

Increased Effect/Toxicity

Eszopiclone may increase the levels/effects of: Alcohol (Ethyl); CNS Depressants; Methotrimeprazine; Selective Serotonin Reuptake Inhibitors

The levels/effects of Eszopiclone may be increased by: Antifungal Agents (Azole Derivatives, Systemic); Conivaptan; CYP3A4 Inhibitors (Moderate); CYP3A4 Inhibitors (Strong); Dasatinib; Droperidol; HydrOXYzine; Ivacaftor; Methotrimeprazine

Nutritional/Ethanol Interactions

Ethanol: Ethanol may increase CNS depression. Management: Avoid ethanol.

Food: Onset of action may be reduced if taken with or immediately after a heavy meal. Management: Take immediately prior to bedtime, not with or immediately after a heavy or high-fat meal.

Herb/Nutraceutical: Some herbal medications may increase CNS depression. Management: Avoid valerian, St John's wort, kava kava, and gotu kola.

Adverse Reactions

>10%:

Central nervous system: Headache (15% to 21%)

Gastrointestinal: Unpleasant taste (8% to 34%)

1% to 10%:

Cardiovascular: Chest pain, peripheral edema

Central nervous system: Somnolence (8% to 10%), dizziness (5% to 7%), pain (4% to 5%), nervousness (up to 5%), depression (1% to 4%), confusion (up to 3%), hallucinations (1% to 3%), anxiety (1% to 3%), abnormal dreams (1% to 3%), migraine

Dermatologic: Rash (3% to 4%), pruritus (1% to 4%)

Endocrine & metabolic: Libido decreased (up to 3%), dysmenorrhea (up to 3%), gynecomastia (males up to 3%)

Gastrointestinal: Xerostomia (3% to 7%), dyspepsia (2% to 6%), nausea (4% to 5%), diarrhea (2% to 4%), vomiting (up to 3%)

Genitourinary: Urinary tract infection (up to 3%)

Neuromuscular & skeletal: Neuralgia (up to 3%)

Miscellaneous: Infection (5% to 10%), viral infection (3%), accidental injury (up to 3%)

Controlled Substance C-IV

Available Dosage Forms

Tablet, oral:

Lunesta®: 1 mg, 2 mg, 3 mg

General Dosage Range Dosage adjustment recommended in patients with hepatic impairment or on concomitant therapy

Oral:

Adults: Initial: 1-2 mg immediately before bedtime (maximum: 3 mg/day)

Elderly: Maximum: 2 mg/day

Administration

Oral Because of the rapid onset of action, eszopiclone should be administered immediately prior to bedtime or after the patient has gone to bed and is having difficulty falling asleep. Do not take with, or immediately following, a high-fat meal. Do not crush or break tablet.

Stability

Storage Store at controlled room temperature of 25°C (77°F).

Nursing Actions

Physical Assessment Evaluate potential causes of insomnia prior to initiating medication. Monitor for excessive CNS depression, abnormal thinking, and behavior changes. For inpatient use, institute safety measures (side rails, night light, call bell, assistance with ambulation).

Patient Education Drug may cause physical and/ or psychological dependence. While using this medication, do not use alcohol. Take immediately prior to bedtime (quick onset) or when having difficulty falling asleep. Do not use unless you are able to get 8 or more hours of sleep before you must be active again. Swallow whole; do not crush or break tablet. You may experience drowsiness, dizziness, lightheadedness, difficulty with coordination, headache, or unpleasant taste. Report CNS changes (confusion, depression, increased sedation, excitation, severe headache, abnormal thinking, insomnia, or nightmares); respiratory difficulty; or unusual swelling, especially on face or neck.

Dietary Considerations Avoid taking after a heavy meal; may delay onset.

Etanercept (et a NER sept)

Brand Names: U.S. Enbrel®; Enbrel® SureClick®

Pharmacologic Category Antirheumatic, Disease Modifying; Tumor Necrosis Factor (TNF) Blocking Agent

Medication Safety Issues

Sound-alike/look-alike issues:

Enbrel® may be confused with Levbid®

Medication Guide Available Yes

Pregnancy Risk Factor B

Lactation Excretion in breast milk unknown/not recommended

Breast-Feeding Considerations It is not known whether etanercept is excreted in human milk. Because many drugs and immunoglobulins are excreted in human milk and the potential for serious adverse reactions exists, a decision should be made whether to discontinue nursing or to discontinue the drug, taking into account the importance of the drug to the mother.

Use Treatment of moderately- to severely-active rheumatoid arthritis (RA); moderately- to severely-active polyarticular juvenile idiopathic arthritis (JIA); psoriatic arthritis; active ankylosing spondylitis (AS); moderate-to-severe chronic plaque psoriasis

Mechanism of Action/Effect Etanercept is a recombinant DNA-derived protein composed of tumor necrosis factor receptor (TNFR) linked to the Fc portion of human IgG1. Etanercept binds tumor necrosis factor (TNF) and blocks its interaction with cell surface receptors. TNF plays an important role in the inflammatory processes and the resulting joint pathology of rheumatoid arthritis (RA), polyarticular-course juvenile idiopathic arthritis (JIA), ankylosing spondylitis (AS), and plaque psoriasis.

Contraindications Hypersensitivity to etanercept or any component of the formulation; patients with sepsis (mortality may be increased)

Warnings/Precautions **[U.S. Boxed Warning]: Patients receiving etanercept are at increased risk for serious infections which may result in hospitalization and/or fatality; infections usually developed in patients receiving concomitant immunosuppressive agents (eg, methotrexate or corticosteroids) and may present as disseminated (rather than local) disease. Active tuberculosis (or reactivation of latent tuberculosis), invasive fungal (including aspergillosis, blastomycosis, candidiasis, coccidioidomycosis, histoplasmosis, and pneumocystosis) and bacterial, viral or other opportunistic infections (including legionellosis and listeriosis) have been reported in patients receiving TNF-blocking agents, including etanercept. Monitor closely for signs/symptoms of infection. Discontinue for serious infection or sepsis. Consider risks versus benefits prior to use in patients with a history of chronic or recurrent infection. Consider empiric antifungal therapy in patients who are at risk for invasive fungal infection and develop severe systemic illness.** Caution should be exercised when considering use in the elderly or in patients with conditions that predispose them to infections (eg, diabetes) or residence/travel from areas of endemic mycoses (blastomycosis, coccidioidomycosis, histoplasmosis), or with latent or localized infections. Do not initiate etanercept therapy with clinically important active infection. Patients who develop a new infection while undergoing treatment should be monitored closely. **[U.S. Boxed Warning]: Tuberculosis (disseminated or extrapulmonary) has been reported in patients receiving etanercept; both reactivation of latent infection and new infections have been reported.** Patients should be evaluated for tuberculosis risk factors and for latent tuberculosis infection with a tuberculin skin test prior to starting therapy. Treatment of latent tuberculosis should be initiated before etanercept therapy; consider antituberculosis treatment if adequate course of treatment cannot be confirmed in patients with a history of latent or active tuberculosis or with risk factors despite negative skin test. Some patients who tested negative prior to therapy have developed active infection; monitor for signs and symptoms of tuberculosis in all patients. Rare reactivation of hepatitis B virus (HBV) has occurred in chronic virus carriers; use with caution; evaluate prior to initiation and during treatment. Patients should be brought up to date with all immunizations before initiating therapy. Live vaccines should not be given concurrently with etanercept. Patients with a significant exposure to varicella virus should temporarily discontinue etanercept. Treatment with varicella zoster immune globulin should be considered.

[U.S. Boxed Warning]: Lymphoma and other malignancies have been reported in children and adolescent patients receiving TNF-blocking agents, including etanercept. Half of the malignancies reported in children were lymphomas (Hodgkin's and non-Hodgkin's) while other cases varied and included malignancies not typically observed in this population. The impact of etanercept on the development and course of malignancy is not fully defined. Compared to the general population, an increased risk of lymphoma has been noted in clinical trials; however, rheumatoid arthritis alone has been previously associated with an increased rate of lymphoma. Lymphomas and other malignancies were also observed (at rates higher than expected for the general population) in adult patients receiving etanercept. Etanercept is not recommended for use in patients with Wegener's granulomatosis who are receiving immunosuppressive therapy. Treatment may result in the formation of autoimmune antibodies; cases of autoimmune disease have not been described. Non-neutralizing antibodies to etanercept may also be formed. Rarely, a reversible lupus-like syndrome has occurred.

Allergic reactions may occur; if an anaphylactic reaction or other serious allergic reaction occurs, administration should be discontinued immediately and appropriate therapy initiated. Use with caution in patients with pre-existing or recent onset CNS demyelinating disorders; rare cases of new onset or exacerbation of CNS demyelinating disorders have occurred; may present with mental status ▶

changes and some may be associated with permanent disability. Optic neuritis, transverse myelitis, multiple sclerosis, and new onset or exacerbation of seizures have been reported. Use with caution in patients with heart failure or decreased left ventricular function; worsening and new-onset heart failure has been reported. Use caution in patients with a history of significant hematologic abnormalities; has been associated with pancytopenia and aplastic anemia (rare). Discontinue if significant hematologic abnormalities are confirmed. Use with caution in patients with moderate to severe alcoholic hepatitis. Compared to placebo, the mortality rate in patients treated with etanercept was similar at one month but significantly higher after 6 months Due to a higher incidence of serious infections, concomitant use with anakinra is not recommended. Some dosage forms may contain dry natural rubber (latex). Some dosage forms may contain benzyl alcohol which has been associated with "gasping syndrome" in neonates.

Drug Interactions

Avoid Concomitant Use

Avoid concomitant use of Etanercept with any of the following: Abatacept; Anakinra; BCG; Belimumab; Canakinumab; Certolizumab Pegol; Cyclophosphamide; Natalizumab; Pimecrolimus; Rilonacept; Tacrolimus (Topical); Vaccines (Live)

Decreased Effect

Etanercept may decrease the levels/effects of: BCG; Coccidioidin Skin Test; Sipuleucel-T; Vaccines (Inactivated); Vaccines (Live)

The levels/effects of Etanercept may be decreased by: Echinacea

Increased Effect/Toxicity

Etanercept may increase the levels/effects of: Abatacept; Anakinra; Belimumab; Canakinumab; Certolizumab Pegol; Cyclophosphamide; Leflunomide; Natalizumab; Rilonacept; Vaccines (Live)

The levels/effects of Etanercept may be increased by: Denosumab; Pimecrolimus; Roflumilast; Tacrolimus (Topical); Trastuzumab

Nutritional/Ethanol Interactions Herb/Nutraceutical: Echinacea may decrease the therapeutic effects of etanercept (avoid concurrent use).

Adverse Reactions Percentages reported for adults except where specified.

>10%:

Central nervous system: Headache (17%; children 19%)

Dermatologic: Rash (3% to 13%)

Gastrointestinal: Abdominal pain (5%; children 19%), vomiting (3%; children 13%)

Local: Injection site reaction (14% to 43%; bleeding, bruising, erythema, itching, pain or swelling)

Respiratory: Respiratory tract infection (upper; 38% to 65%), rhinitis (12%)

Miscellaneous: Infection (50% to 81%; children 62%), positive ANA (11%), positive antidouble-stranded DNA antibodies (15% by RIA, 3% by *Crithidia luciliae* assay)

≥3% to 10%:

Central nervous system: Dizziness (7%)

Dermatologic: Pruritus (2% to 5%)

Gastrointestinal: Nausea (children 9%), dyspepsia (4%), diarrhea (3%)

Neuromuscular & skeletal: Weakness (5%)

Respiratory: Pharyngitis (7%), cough (6%), respiratory disorder (5%), sinusitis (3%)

Pharmacodynamics/Kinetics

Onset of Action ~2-3 weeks; RA: 1-2 weeks

Available Dosage Forms

Injection, powder for reconstitution:

Enbrel®: 25 mg

Injection, solution [preservative free]:

Enbrel®: 50 mg/mL (0.51 mL, 0.98 mL)

Enbrel® SureClick®: 50 mg/mL (0.98 mL)

General Dosage Range SubQ:

Children 2-17 years: 0.8 mg/kg (maximum: 50 mg) once weekly **or** 0.4 mg/kg (maximum: 25 mg) twice weekly

Adults: 50 mg once weekly **or** 25-50 mg twice weekly

Administration

Other Administer subcutaneously. Rotate injection sites. New injections should be given at least one inch from an old site and never into areas where the skin is tender, bruised, red, or hard. **Note:** If the physician determines that it is appropriate, patients may self-inject after proper training in injection technique.

Powder for reconstitution: Follow package instructions carefully for reconstitution. The maximum amount injected at any single site should not exceed 25 mg.

Solution for injection: May be allowed to reach room temperature prior to injection.

Stability

Reconstitution Reconstitute lyophilized powder aseptically with 1 mL sterile bacteriostatic water for injection, USP (supplied); swirl gently, do not shake. Do not filter reconstituted solution during preparation or administration.

Storage

Prefilled syringes, autoinjectors: Store prefilled syringes and autoinjectors 2°C to 8°C (36°F to 46°F); do not freeze. Protect from light; do not shake. The following stability information has also been reported: May be stored at room temperature for up to 4 days (Cohen, 2007).

Powder for reconstitution: Must be refrigerated at 2°C to 8°C (36°F to 46°F); do not freeze. The following stability information has also been reported: May be stored at room temperature for up to 7 days (Cohen, 2007).

Nursing Actions

Physical Assessment Monitor for signs and symptoms of infection, especially respiratory infections. Perform tuberculin skin test prior to initiating therapy; monitor for signs of tuberculosis throughout therapy. Assess for liver dysfunction (unusual fatigue, easy bruising or bleeding, jaundice). Monitor effectiveness of therapy (eg, pain, range of motion, mobility, ADL function, inflammation). If self-administered, teach patient appropriate injection technique and needle disposal.

Patient Education If self-injecting, follow instructions for injection and disposal of needles exactly. If redness, swelling, or irritation appears at the injection site, contact prescriber. You may experience headache or dizziness. If stomach pain or cramping; unusual bleeding or bruising; difficulty breathing; persistent fever; paleness; or blood in vomitus, stool, or urine occurs, stop medication and contact prescriber immediately. Also immediately report skin rash, unusual muscle or bone weakness, or signs of respiratory flu or other infection (eg, chills, fever, sore throat, easy bruising or bleeding, mouth sores, unhealed sores).

Ethacrynic Acid (eth a KRIN ik AS id)

Brand Names: U.S. Edecrin®; Sodium Edecrin®

Index Terms Ethacrynate Sodium

Pharmacologic Category Diuretic, Loop

Medication Safety Issues

Sound-alike/look-alike issues:

Edecrin® may be confused with Eulexin, Ecotrin®

BEERS Criteria medication:

This drug may be inappropriate for use in geriatric patients (low severity risk).

Pregnancy Risk Factor B

Lactation Contraindicated

Use Management of edema associated with congestive heart failure; hepatic cirrhosis or renal disease; short-term management of ascites due to malignancy, idiopathic edema, and lymphedema

Available Dosage Forms

Injection, powder for reconstitution:

Sodium Edecrin®: 50 mg

Tablet, oral:

Edecrin®: 25 mg

General Dosage Range

I.V.: *Adults:* 0.5-1 mg/kg/dose (maximum: 100 mg/dose)

Oral:

Children: 1-3 mg/kg/day

Adults: 50-400 mg/day in 1-2 divided doses

Elderly: Initial: 25-50 mg/day

Administration

I.V. Injection should **not** be given SubQ or I.M. due to local pain and irritation. Single I.V. doses should not exceed 100 mg. Administer each 10 mg over a minute.

I.V. Detail If a second dose is needed, it is recommended to use a new injection site to avoid possible thrombophlebitis.

pH: 6.3-7.7

Nursing Actions

Physical Assessment Monitor for dehydration and electrolyte imbalance on a regular basis.

Patient Education Take prescribed dose with food early in day. Include potassium-rich foods in your diet, but do not take potassium supplements without consulting prescriber. May cause dizziness, drowsiness, or diarrhea. Report hearing changes (ringing in ears); persistent headache; unusual confusion or nervousness; abdominal pain; palpitations or chest pain; flu-like symptoms; skin rash; blurred vision; swelling of ankles or feet; weight changes; increased fatigue; or joint/muscle swelling, pain, cramping, or trembling.

Ethambutol (e THAM byoo tole)

Brand Names: U.S. Myambutol®

Index Terms Ethambutol Hydrochloride

Pharmacologic Category Antitubercular Agent

Medication Safety Issues

Sound-alike/look-alike issues:

Myambutol® may be confused with Nembutal®

Pregnancy Risk Factor C

Lactation Enters breast milk/use caution (AAP considers "compatible"; AAP 2001 update pending)

Breast-Feeding Considerations The manufacturer suggests use during breast-feeding only if benefits to the mother outweigh the possible risk to the infant. Some references suggest that exposure to the infant is low and does not produce toxicity, and breast-feeding should not be discouraged. Other references recommend if breast-feeding, monitor the infant for rash, malaise, nausea, or vomiting.

Use Treatment of pulmonary tuberculosis in conjunction with other antituberculosis agents

Unlabeled Use Other mycobacterial diseases in conjunction with other antimycobacterial agents

Mechanism of Action/Effect Inhibits arabinosyl transferase resulting in impaired mycobacterial cell wall synthesis

Contraindications Hypersensitivity to ethambutol or any component of the formulation; optic neuritis (risk vs benefit decision); use in young children, unconscious patients, or any other patient who may be unable to discern and report visual changes

Warnings/Precautions May cause optic neuritis (unilateral or bilateral), resulting in decreased visual acuity or other vision changes. Discontinue promptly in patients with changes in vision, color blindness, or visual defects (effects normally reversible, but reversal may require up to a year). Irreversible blindness has been reported. Monitor visual acuity prior to and during therapy. Evaluation of visual acuity changes may be more difficult in patients with cataracts, optic neuritis, diabetic retinopathy, and inflammatory conditions of the eye; consideration should be given to whether or not visual changes are related to disease progression or effects of therapy. Use only in children whose visual acuity can accurately be determined and monitored (not recommended for use in children <13 years of age unless the benefit outweighs the risk). Dosage modification is required in patients with renal insufficiency; monitor renal function prior to and during treatment. Hepatic toxicity has been reported, possibly due to concurrent therapy; monitor liver function prior to and during treatment.

Drug Interactions

Avoid Concomitant Use There are no known interactions where it is recommended to avoid concomitant use.

Decreased Effect

The levels/effects of Ethambutol may be decreased by: Aluminum Hydroxide

Increased Effect/Toxicity There are no known significant interactions involving an increase in effect.

Adverse Reactions Frequency not defined.

Cardiovascular: Myocarditis, pericarditis

Central nervous system: Confusion, disorientation, dizziness, fever, hallucinations, headache, malaise

Dermatologic: Dermatitis, erythema multiforme, exfoliative dermatitis, pruritus, rash

Endocrine & metabolic: Acute gout or hyperuricemia

Gastrointestinal: Abdominal pain, anorexia, GI upset, nausea, vomiting

Hematologic: Eosinophilia, leukopenia, lymphadenopathy, neutropenia, thrombocytopenia

Hepatic: Hepatitis, hepatotoxicity (possibly related to concurrent therapy), LFTs abnormal

Neuromuscular & skeletal: Arthralgia, peripheral neuritis

Ocular: Optic neuritis; symptoms may include decreased acuity, scotoma, color blindness, or visual defects (usually reversible with discontinuation, irreversible blindness has been described)

Renal: Nephritis

Respiratory: Infiltrates (with or without eosinophilia), pneumonitis

Miscellaneous: Anaphylaxis, anaphylactoid reaction; hypersensitivity syndrome (cutaneous reactions, eosinophilia, and organ-specific inflammation)

Available Dosage Forms

Tablet, oral: 100 mg, 400 mg

Myambutol®: 100 mg, 400 mg

General Dosage Range Dosage adjustment recommended in patients with renal impairment

Oral:

Children: 15-20 mg/kg/day (maximum: 1 g/day) **or** 50 mg/kg twice weekly (maximum: 2.5 g/dose)

Adults: Daily therapy: 1.5-2.5 g/kg/day (maximum dose: 1.5-2.5 g); 3 times/week DOT: 25-30 mg/kg/dose (maximum dose: 2.4 g/dose); Twice weekly DOT: 50 mg/kg/dose (maximum dose: 4 g/dose)

Stability

Storage Store at controlled room temperature of 20°C to 25°C (68°F to 77°F).

Nursing Actions

Physical Assessment Monitor for CNS changes, neuritis, and ocular changes on a regular basis during therapy. Teach patient need to adhere to dosing program and importance of regular laboratory tests and ophthalmic evaluations.

Patient Education Take with meals. May cause GI distress, dizziness, disorientation, and drowsiness. You will need to have frequent ophthalmic exams and periodic medical check-ups to evaluate drug effects. Report vision changes, numbness or tingling of extremities, or persistent loss of appetite.

Dietary Considerations May be taken with food as absorption is not affected, may cause gastric irritation.

Ethinyl Estradiol and Desogestrel

(ETH in il es tra DYE ole & des oh JES trel)

Brand Names: U.S. Apri®; Azurette™; Caziant®; Cyclessa®; Desogen®; Emoquette™; Kariva®; Mircette®; Ortho-Cept®; Reclipsen®; Velivet™

Index Terms Desogestrel and Ethinyl Estradiol; Ortho Cept

Pharmacologic Category Contraceptive; Estrogen and Progestin Combination

Medication Safety Issues

Sound-alike/look-alike issues:

Apri® may be confused with Apriso™

Ortho-Cept® may be confused with Ortho-Cyclen®

Pregnancy Risk Factor X

Lactation Enters breast milk/not recommended

Use Prevention of pregnancy

Unlabeled Use Treatment of hypermenorrhea (menorrhagia); pain associated with endometriosis; dysmenorrhea; dysfunctional uterine bleeding

Available Dosage Forms

Tablet, low-dose formulations:

Azurette™:

Day 1-21: Ethinyl estradiol 0.02 mg and desogestrel 0.15 mg [21 white tablets]

Day 22-23: 2 inactive green tablets

Day 24-28: Ethinyl estradiol 0.01 mg [5 blue tablets] (28s)

Kariva®:

Day 1-21: Ethinyl estradiol 0.02 mg and desogestrel 0.15 mg [21 white tablets]

Day 22-23: 2 inactive light green tablets

Day 24-28: Ethinyl estradiol 0.01 mg [5 light blue tablets] (28s)

Mircette®:

Day 1-21: Ethinyl estradiol 0.02 mg and desogestrel 0.15 mg [21 white tablets]

Day 22-23: 2 inactive green tablets

Day 24-28: Ethinyl estradiol 0.01 mg [5 yellow tablets] (28s)

Tablet, monophasic formulations:

Apri® 28: Ethinyl estradiol 0.03 mg and desogestrel 0.15 mg (28s) [21 rose tablets and 7 white inactive tablets]

Desogen®, Reclipsen®: Ethinyl estradiol 0.03 mg and desogestrel 0.15 mg (28s) [21 white tablets and 7 green inactive tablets]

Emoquette™: Ethinyl estradiol 0.03 mg and desogestrel 0.15 mg (28s) [21 white tablets and 7 light green inactive tablets]

Ortho-Cept® 28: Ethinyl estradiol 0.03 mg and desogestrel 0.15 mg (28s) [21 light orange tablets and 7 green inactive tablets]

Tablet, triphasic formulations:

Caziant®:

Day 1-7: Ethinyl estradiol 0.025 mg and desogestrel 0.1 mg [7 white tablets]

Day 8-14: Ethinyl estradiol 0.025 mg and desogestrel 0.125 mg [7 light blue tablets]

Day 15-21: Ethinyl estradiol 0.025 mg and desogestrel 0.15 mg [7 blue tablets]

Day 22-28: 7 green inactive tablets (28s)

Cyclessa®:

Day 1-7: Ethinyl estradiol 0.025 mg and desogestrel 0.1 mg [7 light yellow tablets]

Day 8-14: Ethinyl estradiol 0.025 mg and desogestrel 0.125 mg [7 orange tablets]

Day 15-21: Ethinyl estradiol 0.025 mg and desogestrel 0.15 mg [7 red tablets]

Day 22-28: 7 green inactive tablets (28s)

Velivet™:

Day 1-7: Ethinyl estradiol 0.025 mg and desogestrel 0.1 mg [7 beige tablets]

Day 8-14: Ethinyl estradiol 0.025 mg and desogestrel 0.125 mg [7 orange tablets]

Day 15-21: Ethinyl estradiol 0.025 mg and desogestrel 0.15 mg [7 pink tablets]

Day 22-28: 7 white inactive tablets (28s)

General Dosage Range Oral: *Children and Adults (females, postmenarche):* 1 tablet daily

Administration

Oral Administer at the same time each day.

Nursing Actions

Physical Assessment Monitor blood pressure on a regular basis. Teach importance of regular (monthly) blood pressure checks and annual physical assessment, Pap smear, and vision assessment. Teach importance of maintaining prescribed schedule of dosing.

Patient Education Oral contraceptives do not protect against HIV infection or other sexually-transmitted diseases. You are at risk of becoming pregnant if doses are missed. Detailed and complete information on dosing and missed doses can be found in the package insert. Be aware that some medications may reduce the effectiveness of oral contraceptives; an alternate form of contraception may be needed. It is important that you check your blood pressure monthly and that you have an annual physical assessment, Pap smear, and vision exam while taking this medication. Avoid smoking while taking this medication; smoking increases risk of adverse effects, including thromboembolic events and heart attacks. You may experience loss of appetite or constipation. Report immediately pain or muscle soreness; warmth, swelling, pain, or redness in calves; shortness of breath; sudden loss of vision; unresolved leg/foot swelling; change in menstrual pattern (unusual bleeding, amenorrhea, breakthrough spotting); breast tenderness that does not go away; acute abdominal cramping; signs of vaginal infection (drainage, pain, itching); CNS changes (blurred vision, confusion, acute anxiety, or unresolved depression); chest pain; severe headache or vomiting; weakness in arm or leg; severe abdominal pain or tenderness; jaundice; or weight gain. Notify prescriber of changes in contact lens tolerance.

Ethinyl Estradiol and Drospirenone

(ETH in il es tra DYE ole & droh SPYE re none)

Brand Names: U.S. Gianvi™; Loryna™; Ocella™; Syeda™; Vestura™; Yasmin®; Yaz®; Zarah®

Index Terms Drospirenone and Ethinyl Estradiol

Pharmacologic Category Contraceptive; Estrogen and Progestin Combination

Medication Safety Issues

Sound-alike/look-alike issues:

Yaz® may be confused with Beyaz™, Yasmin®

Pregnancy Risk Factor X

Lactation Enters breast milk/not recommended

Use Prevention of pregnancy; treatment of premenstrual dysphoric disorder (PMDD); treatment of acne

Unlabeled Use Treatment of hypermenorrhea (menorrhagia); pain associated with endometriosis; dysmenorrhea; dysfunctional uterine bleeding

Available Dosage Forms

Tablet, oral:

Gianvi™: Ethinyl estradiol 0.03 mg and drospirenone 3 mg (28s) [24 light pink active tablets and 4 white inactive tablets]

Loryna™: Ethinyl estradiol 0.02 mg and drospirenone 3 mg (28s) [24 peach active tablets and 4 white inactive tablets]

Ocella™, Syeda™, Yasmin®: Ethinyl estradiol 0.03 mg and drospirenone 3 mg (28s) [21 yellow active tablets and 7 white inactive tablets]

Vestura™: Ethinyl estradiol 0.02 mg and drospirenone 3 mg (28s) [24 pink active tablets and 4 peach inactive tablets]

Yaz®: Ethinyl estradiol 0.02 mg and drospirenone 3 mg (28s) [24 light pink active tablets and 4 white inactive tablets]

Zarah®: Ethinyl estradiol 0.03 mg and drospirenone 3 mg (28s) [21 blue active tablets and 7 peach inactive tablets]

General Dosage Range Oral: *Children and Adults (females, postmenarche):* 1 tablet daily

Administration

Oral Dose should be taken at the same time each day, either after the evening meal or at bedtime. If severe vomiting or diarrhea occurs, additional contraception (nonhormonal) should be used. If vomiting occurs within 3-4 hours of dosing, consider the dose to be missed.

Nursing Actions

Physical Assessment Monitor blood pressure on a regular (monthly) basis. Teach patient the importance of annual physical examinations (including Pap smear and vision exam) and the importance of maintaining prescribed schedule of dosing.

Patient Education Oral contraceptives do not protect against HIV infection or other sexually-transmitted diseases. You are at risk of becoming pregnant if doses are missed. Detailed and complete information on dosing and missed doses can be found in the package insert. Be aware that some medications may reduce the effectiveness of oral contraceptives; an alternate form of contraception may be needed. It is important that you check your blood pressure monthly and that you have an annual physical assessment, Pap smear, and vision exam while taking this medication. Avoid smoking while taking this medication; smoking increases risk of adverse effects, including thromboembolic events and heart attacks. You may experience loss of appetite or constipation. Report immediately pain or muscle soreness; warmth, swelling, pain, or redness in calves; shortness of breath; sudden loss of vision; unresolved leg/foot swelling; change in menstrual pattern (unusual bleeding, amenorrhea, breakthrough spotting); breast tenderness that does not go away; acute abdominal cramping; signs of vaginal infection (drainage, pain, itching); CNS changes (blurred vision, confusion, acute anxiety, or unresolved depression); chest pain; severe headache or vomiting; weakness in arm or leg; severe abdominal pain or tenderness; jaundice; or weight gain. Notify prescriber of changes in contact lens tolerance.

Ethinyl Estradiol and Ethynodiol Diacetate

(ETH in il es tra DYE ole & e thye noe DYE ole dye AS e tate)

Brand Names: U.S. Kelnor™; Zovia®

Index Terms Ethynodiol Diacetate and Ethinyl Estradiol

Pharmacologic Category Contraceptive; Estrogen and Progestin Combination

Medication Safety Issues

Sound-alike/look-alike issues:

Demulen® may be confused with Dalmane®, Demerol®

Pregnancy Risk Factor X

Lactation Enters breast milk/not recommended

Use Prevention of pregnancy

Unlabeled Use Treatment of hypermenorrhea (menorrhagia); pain associated with endometriosis; dysmenorrhea; dysfunctional uterine bleeding

Available Dosage Forms

Tablet, monophasic formulations:

Kelnor™ 1/35: Ethinyl estradiol 0.035 mg and ethynodiol diacetate 1 mg [21 light yellow tablets and 7 white inactive tablets] (28s)

Zovia® 1/35-28: Ethinyl estradiol 0.035 mg and ethynodiol diacetate 1 mg [21 light pink tablets and 7 white inactive tablets] (28s)

Zovia® 1/50-28: Ethinyl estradiol 0.05 mg and ethynodiol diacetate 1 mg [21 pink tablets and 7 white inactive tablets] (28s)

General Dosage Range Oral: *Children and Adults (females, postmenarche):* 1 tablet daily

Administration

Oral Administer at the same time each day.

Nursing Actions

Physical Assessment Assess blood pressure on a regular basis. Monitor for thromboembolic disease, visual changes, and neuromuscular weakness. Teach importance of regular (monthly) blood pressure checks and annual physical assessment, Pap smear, and vision assessment. Teach importance of maintaining prescribed schedule of dosing.

Patient Education Oral contraceptives do not protect against HIV or other sexually-transmitted diseases. You are at risk of becoming pregnant if doses are missed. Be aware that some medications may reduce the effectiveness of oral contraceptives; an alternate form of contraception may be needed. It is important that you check your blood pressure monthly (on same day each month) and that you have an annual physical assessment, Pap smear, and vision assessment while taking this medication. Avoid smoking while taking this medication; smoking increases risk of adverse effects, including thromboembolic events and heart attacks. You may experience loss of appetite or constipation. If you have diabetes, use accurate serum glucose testing to identify any changes in glucose tolerance; notify prescriber of significant changes so antidiabetic medication can be adjusted if necessary. Report immediately pain or muscle soreness; warmth, swelling, pain, or redness in calves; shortness of breath; sudden loss of vision; unresolved leg/foot swelling; change in menstrual pattern (unusual bleeding, amenorrhea, breakthrough spotting); breast tenderness that does not go away; acute abdominal cramping; signs of vaginal infection (drainage, pain, itching); CNS changes (blurred vision, confusion, acute anxiety, or unresolved depression); chest pain; severe headache or vomiting; weakness in arm or leg; severe abdominal pain or tenderness; jaundice; or weight gain. Notify prescriber of changes in contact lens tolerance.

Ethinyl Estradiol and Levonorgestrel

(ETH in il es tra DYE ole & LEE voe nor jes trel)

Brand Names: U.S. Altavera™; Amethia™; Amethia™ Lo; Amethyst™; Aviane™; camrese™; Enpresse®; Introvale™; Jolessa™; Lessina®; Levora®; LoSeasonique®; Lutera®; Lybrel®; Nordette® 28; Orsythia™; Portia®; Quasense®; Seasonale®; Seasonique®; Sronyx®; Trivora®

Index Terms Levonorgestrel and Ethinyl Estradiol

Pharmacologic Category Contraceptive; Estrogen and Progestin Combination

Medication Safety Issues

Sound-alike/look-alike issues:

Nordette® may be confused with Nicorette®
Portia® may be confused with Potiga™
Seasonale® may be confused with Seasonique®
Tri-Levlen® may be confused with Trilafon®

Pregnancy Risk Factor X

Lactation Enters breast milk/not recommended

Use Prevention of pregnancy; postcoital contraception

Unlabeled Use Treatment of hypermenorrhea (menorrhagia); pain associated with endometriosis; dysmenorrhea; dysfunctional uterine bleeding

Available Dosage Forms

Tablet, oral [low-dose formulation]:

Aviane™: Ethinyl estradiol 0.02 mg and levonorgestrel 0.1 mg (28s) [21 orange tablets and 7 light green inactive tablets]

Lutera®, Sronyx®: Ethinyl estradiol 0.02 mg and levonorgestrel 0.1 mg (28s) [21 white tablets and 7 peach inactive tablets]

Orsythia™: Ethinyl estradiol 0.02 mg and levonorgestrel 0.1 mg (28s) [21 pink tablets and 7 light green inactive tablets]

Tablet, oral [monophasic formulation]:

Altavera™: Ethinyl estradiol 0.03 mg and levonorgestrel 0.15 mg (28s) [21 peach tablets and 7 white inactive tablets]

Levora®: Ethinyl estradiol 0.03 mg and levonorgestrel 0.15 mg (28s) [21 white tablets and 7 peach inactive tablets]

Nordette® 28: Ethinyl estradiol 0.03 mg and levonorgestrel 0.15 mg (28s) [21 light orange tablets and 7 pink inactive tablets]

Portia® 28: Ethinyl estradiol 0.03 mg and levonorgestrel 0.15 mg (28s) [21 pink tablets and 7 white inactive tablets]

Tablet, oral [extended cycle regimen]: Ethinyl estradiol 0.02 mg and levonorgestrel 0.1 mg [84 tablets] and ethinyl estradiol 0.01 mg [7 tablets] (91s)

Amethia™:Ethinyl estradiol 0.03 mg and levonorgestrel 0.15 mg (91s) [84 white tablets] and ethinyl estradiol 0.01 mg [7 light blue tablets]

Amethia™ Lo: Ethinyl estradiol 0.02 mg and levonorgestrel 0.1 mg (91s) [84 white tablets] and ethinyl estradiol 0.01 mg [7 blue tablets]

camrese™: Ethinyl estradiol 0.03 mg and levonorgestrel 0.15 mg (91s) [84 light blue-green tablets] and ethinyl estradiol 0.01 mg [7 yellow tablets]

Introvale™: Ethinyl estradiol 0.03 mg and levonorgestrel 0.15 mg (91s) [84 peach tablets and 7 white inactive tablets]

Jolessa™, Seasonale®: Ethinyl estradiol 0.03 mg and levonorgestrel 0.15 mg (91s) [84 pink tablets and 7 white inactive tablets]

LoSeasonique®: Ethinyl estradiol 0.02 mg and levonorgestrel 0.1 mg (91s) [84 orange tablets] and ethinyl estradiol 0.01 mg [7 yellow tablets]

Quasense®: Ethinyl estradiol 0.03 mg and levonorgestrel 0.15 mg] (91s) [84 white tablets and 7 peach inactive tablets]

Seasonique®: Ethinyl estradiol 0.03 mg and levonorgestrel 0.15 mg (91s) [84 light blue-green tablets] and ethinyl estradiol 0.01 mg [7 yellow tablets]

Tablet, oral [noncyclic regimen]:

Amethyst™: Ethinyl estradiol 0.02 mg and levonorgestrel 0.09 mg (28s) [28 white tablets]

Lybrel®: Ethinyl estradiol 0.02 mg and levonorgestrel 0.09 mg (28s) [28 yellow tablets]

Tablet, oral [triphasic formulation]:

Enpresse®:

Day 1-6: Ethinyl estradiol 0.03 mg and levonorgestrel 0.05 mg [6 pink tablets]

Day 7-11: Ethinyl estradiol 0.04 mg and levonorgestrel 0.075 mg [5 white tablets]

Day 12-21: Ethinyl estradiol 0.03 mg and levonorgestrel 0.125 mg [10 orange tablets]

Day 22-28: 7 light green inactive tablets (28s)

Trivora®:

Day 1-6: Ethinyl estradiol 0.03 mg and levonorgestrel 0.05 mg [6 blue tablets]

Day 7-11: Ethinyl estradiol 0.04 mg and levonorgestrel 0.075 mg [5 white tablets]

Day 12-21: Ethinyl estradiol 0.03 mg and levonorgestrel 0.125 mg [10 pink tablets]

Day 22-28: 7 peach inactive tablets (28s)

General Dosage Range Oral: *Children and Adults (females, postmenarche):* 1 tablet daily **or** 2 tablets as soon as possible (but within 72 hours of unprotected intercourse), followed by 2 tablets 12 hours later

Administration

Oral Administer at the same time each day.

Nursing Actions

Physical Assessment See individual agents.

Patient Education See individual agents.

Related Information

Levonorgestrel *on page 691*

Ethinyl Estradiol and Norethindrone

(ETH in il es tra DYE ole & nor eth IN drone)

Brand Names: U.S. Aranelle®; Balziva™; Brevicon®; Cyclafem™ 1/35; Cyclafem™ 7/7/7; Estrostep® Fe; Femcon® Fe; femhrt®; femhrt® Lo; Generess™ Fe; Gildess® FE 1.5/30; Gildess® FE 1/20; Jevantique™; Jinteli™; Junel® 1.5/30; Junel® 1/20; Junel® Fe 1.5/30; Junel® Fe 1/20; Leena®; Lo Loestrin™ Fe; Loestrin® 21 1.5/30; Loestrin® 21 1/20; Loestrin® 24 Fe; Loestrin® Fe 1.5/30; Loestrin® Fe 1/20; Microgestin® 1.5/30; Microgestin® 1/20; Microgestin® Fe 1.5/30; Microgestin® Fe 1/20; Modicon®; Necon® 0.5/35; Necon® 1/35; Necon® 10/11; Necon® 7/7/7; Norinyl® 1+35; Nortrel® 0.5/35; Nortrel® 1/35; Nortrel® 7/7/7; Ortho-Novum® 1/35; Ortho-Novum® 7/7/7; Ovcon® 35; Ovcon® 50; Tilia™ Fe; Tri-Legest™ Fe; Tri-Norinyl®; Zenchent Fe™; Zenchent™; Zeosa™

Index Terms Norethindrone Acetate and Ethinyl Estradiol; Ortho Novum

Pharmacologic Category Contraceptive; Estrogen and Progestin Combination

Medication Safety Issues

Sound-alike/look-alike issues:

femhrt® may be confused with Femara®

Lo Loestrin™ Fe may be confused with Loestrin® Fe

Modicon® may be confused with Mylicon®

Norinyl® may be confused with Nardil®

Pregnancy Risk Factor X

Lactation Enters breast milk/not recommended

Use Prevention of pregnancy; treatment of acne; moderate-to-severe vasomotor symptoms associated with menopause; prevention of osteoporosis (in women at significant risk only)

Unlabeled Use Treatment of hypermenorrhea (menorrhagia); pain associated with endometriosis, dysmenorrhea; dysfunctional uterine bleeding

Available Dosage Forms

Tablet, oral:

femhrt® 1/5: Ethinyl estradiol 0.005 mg and norethindrone acetate 1 mg (28s, 90s) [white tablets]

femhrt® Lo 0.5/2.5: Ethinyl estradiol 0.0025 mg and norethindrone acetate 0.5 mg (28s, 90s) [white tablets]

Tablet, oral, monophasic formulations:

Balziva™: Ethinyl estradiol 0.035 mg and norethindrone 0.4 mg (28s) [21 light peach tablets and 7 white inactive tablets]

Brevicon®: Ethinyl estradiol 0.035 mg and norethindrone 0.5 mg (28s) [21 blue tablets and 7 orange inactive tablets]

Cyclafem™ 1/35: Ethinyl estradiol 0.035 mg and norethindrone 1 mg [21 pink tablets and 7 light green inactive tablets] (28s)

Gildess® FE 1/20: Ethinyl estradiol 0.02 mg and norethindrone acetate 1 mg [21 white tablets] and ferrous fumarate 75 mg [7 white-speckled brown tablets] (28s)

Gildess® FE 1.5/30: Ethinyl estradiol 0.03 mg and norethindrone acetate 1.5 mg [21 light green tablets] and ferrous fumarate 75 mg [7 white-speckled brown tablets] (28s)

Junel® 1/20: Ethinyl estradiol 0.02 mg and norethindrone acetate 1 mg (21s) [yellow tablets]

Junel® 1.5/30, Loestrin® 21 1.5/30: Ethinyl estradiol 0.03 mg and norethindrone acetate 1.5 mg (21s) [pink tablets]

Junel® Fe 1/20: Ethinyl estradiol 0.02 mg and norethindrone acetate 1 mg [21 yellow tablets] and ferrous fumarate 75 mg [7 brown tablets] (28s)

Junel® Fe 1.5/30, Loestrin® Fe 21 1.5/30: Ethinyl estradiol 0.03 mg and norethindrone acetate 1.5 mg [21 pink tablets] and ferrous fumarate 75 mg [7 brown tablets] (28s)

Loestrin® 21 1/20: Ethinyl estradiol 0.02 mg and norethindrone acetate 1 mg (21s) [light yellow tablets]

Lo Loestrin™ Fe: Ethinyl estradiol 0.01 mg and norethindrone acetate 1mg [24 blue tablets] and ethinyl estradiol 0.01 mg [2 white tablets] and ferrous fumarate 75 mg [2 brown tablets] (28s)

Loestrin® 24 Fe: Ethinyl estradiol 0.02 mg and norethindrone acetate 1 mg [24 white tablets] and ferrous fumarate 75 mg [4 brown tablets] (28s)

Loestrin® Fe 1/20: Ethinyl estradiol 0.02 mg and norethindrone acetate 1 mg [21 light yellow tablets] and ferrous fumarate 75 mg [7 brown tablets] (28s)

Loestrin® Fe 1.5/30: Ethinyl estradiol 0.03 mg and norethindrone acetate 1.5 mg [21 pink tablets] and ferrous fumarate 75 mg [7 brown tablets] (28s)

Microgestin® 1/20: Ethinyl estradiol 0.02 mg and norethindrone acetate 1 mg (21s) [white tablets]

Microgestin® 1.5/30: Ethinyl estradiol 0.03 mg and norethindrone acetate 1.5 mg (21s) [green tablets]

Microgestin® Fe 1/20: Ethinyl estradiol 0.02 mg and norethindrone acetate 1 mg [21 white tablets] and ferrous fumarate 75 mg [7 brown tablets] (28s)

Microgestin® Fe 1.5/30: Ethinyl estradiol 0.03 mg and norethindrone acetate 1.5 mg [21 green tablets] and ferrous fumarate 75 mg [7 brown tablets] (28s)

Modicon®: Ethinyl estradiol 0.035 mg and norethindrone 0.5 mg (28s) [21 white tablets and 7 green inactive tablets]

Necon® 0.5/35, Nortrel® 0.5/35: Ethinyl estradiol 0.035 mg and norethindrone 0.5 mg (28s) [21 light yellow tablets and 7 white inactive tablets]

Necon® 1/35: Ethinyl estradiol 0.035 mg and norethindrone 1 mg (28s) [21 dark yellow tablets and 7 white inactive tablets]

Norinyl® 1+35: Ethinyl estradiol 0.035 mg and norethindrone 1 mg (28s) [21 yellow-green tablets and 7 orange inactive tablets]

Nortrel® 1/35:

Ethinyl estradiol 0.035 mg and norethindrone 1 mg (21s) [yellow tablets]

Ethinyl estradiol 0.035 mg and norethindrone 1 mg (28s) [21 yellow tablets and 7 white inactive tablets]

Ortho-Novum® 1/35: Ethinyl estradiol 0.035 mg and norethindrone 1 mg (28s) [21 peach tablets and 7 green inactive tablets]

Ovcon® 35: Ethinyl estradiol 0.035 mg and norethindrone 0.4 mg (28s) [21 light peach tablets and 7 green inactive tablets]

Ovcon® 50: Ethinyl estradiol 0.05 mg and norethindrone 1 mg (28s) [21 yellow tablets and 7 green inactive tablets]

Zenchent™: Ethinyl estradiol 0.035 mg and norethindrone 0.4 mg (28s) [21 orange tablets and 7 white inactive tablets]

Tablet, chewable, oral, monophasic formulations: Ethinyl estradiol 0.035 mg and norethindrone 0.4 mg [21 tablets] and ferrous fumarate 75 mg [7 tablets] (28s)

Femcon® Fe: Ethinyl estradiol 0.035 mg and norethindrone 0.4 mg [21 white tablets] and ferrous fumarate 75 mg [7 brown tablets] (28s)

Generess™ Fe: Ethinyl estradiol 0.025 mg and norethindrone 0.8 mg [24 light green tablets] and ferrous fumarate 75 mg [4 brown tablets] (28s)

Zenchent Fe™, Zeosa™: Ethinyl estradiol 0.035 mg and norethindrone 0.4 mg [21 light yellow tablets] and ferrous fumarate 75 mg [7 brown tablets] (28s)

Tablet, oral, biphasic formulations:

Necon® 10/11:

Day 1-10: Ethinyl estradiol 0.035 mg and norethindrone 0.5 mg [10 light yellow tablets]

Day 11-21: Ethinyl estradiol 0.035 mg and norethindrone 1 mg [11 dark yellow tablets]

Day 22-28: 7 white inactive tablets (28s)

Tablet, oral, triphasic formulations:

Aranelle®:

Day 1-7: Ethinyl estradiol 0.035 mg and norethindrone 0.5 mg [7 light yellow tablets]

Day 8-16: Ethinyl estradiol 0.035 mg and norethindrone 1 mg [9 white tablets]

Day 17-21: Ethinyl estradiol 0.035 mg and norethindrone 0.5 mg [5 light yellow tablets]

Day 22-28: 7 peach inactive tablets (28s)

Cyclafem™ 7/7/7:

Day 1-7: Ethinyl estradiol 0.035 mg and norethindrone 0.5 mg [7 white tablets]

Day 8-14: Ethinyl estradiol 0.035 mg and norethindrone 0.75 mg [7 light pink tablets]

Day 15-21: Ethinyl estradiol 0.035 mg and norethindrone 1 mg [7 pink tablets]

Day 22-28: 7 light green inactive tablets (28s)

Estrostep® Fe, Tilia™ Fe:

Day 1-5: Ethinyl estradiol 0.02 mg and norethindrone acetate 1 mg [5 white triangular tablets]

Day 6-12: Ethinyl estradiol 0.03 mg and norethindrone acetate 1 mg [7 white square tablets]

Day 13-21: Ethinyl estradiol 0.035 mg and norethindrone acetate 1 mg [9 white round tablets]

Day 22-28: Ferrous fumarate 75 mg [7 brown tablets] (28s)

Leena®:

Day 1-7: Ethinyl estradiol 0.035 mg and norethindrone 0.5 mg [7 light blue tablets]

Day 8-16: Ethinyl estradiol 0.035 mg and norethindrone 1 mg [9 light yellow-green tablets]

Day 17-21: Ethinyl estradiol 0.035 mg and norethindrone 0.5 mg [5 light blue tablets]

Day 22-28: 7 orange inactive tablets (28s)

Necon® 7/7/7, Ortho-Novum® 7/7/7:

Day 1-7: Ethinyl estradiol 0.035 mg and norethindrone 0.5 mg [7 white tablets]

Day 8-14: Ethinyl estradiol 0.035 mg and norethindrone 0.75 mg [7 light peach tablets]

Day 15-21: Ethinyl estradiol 0.035 mg and norethindrone 1 mg [7 peach tablets]

Day 22-28: 7 green inactive tablets (28s)

Nortrel® 7/7/7:

Day 1-7: Ethinyl estradiol 0.035 mg and norethindrone 0.5 mg [7 light yellow tablets]

Day 8-14: Ethinyl estradiol 0.035 mg and norethindrone 0.75 mg [7 blue tablets]

Day 15-21: Ethinyl estradiol 0.035 mg and norethindrone 1 mg [7 peach tablets]

Day 22-28: 7 white inactive tablets (28s)

Tri-Legest™ Fe:

Day 1-5: Ethinyl estradiol 0.02 mg and norethindrone acetate 1 mg [5 light pink tablets]

Day 6-12: Ethinyl estradiol 0.03 mg and norethindrone acetate 1 mg [7 light yellow tablets]

Day 13-21: Ethinyl estradiol 0.035 mg and norethindrone acetate 1 mg [9 light blue tablets]

Day 22-28: Ferrous fumarate 75 mg [7 brown tablets] (28s)

Tri-Norinyl®:

Day 1-7: Ethinyl estradiol 0.035 mg and norethindrone 0.5 mg [7 blue tablets]

Day 8-16: Ethinyl estradiol 0.035 mg and norethindrone 1 mg [9 yellow-green tablets]

Day 17-21: Ethinyl estradiol 0.035 mg and norethindrone 0.5 mg [5 blue tablets]

Day 22-28: 7 orange inactive tablets (28s)

General Dosage Range Oral: *Children and Adults (females, postmenarche):* 1 tablet daily

Administration

Oral Administer at the same time each day; without regard to meals.

Lo Loestrin™ Fe: If vomiting or diarrhea occurs within 3-4 hours of a dose, consider the dose to be missed.

Nursing Actions

Physical Assessment See individual agents.

Patient Education See individual agents.

Related Information

Norethindrone *on page 840*

Ethinyl Estradiol and Norgestimate

(ETH in il es tra DYE ole & nor JES ti mate)

Brand Names: U.S. MonoNessa®; Ortho Tri-Cyclen®; Ortho Tri-Cyclen® Lo; Ortho-Cyclen®; Sprintec®; Tri-Sprintec®; TriNessa®

Index Terms Ethinyl Estradiol and NGM; Norgestimate and Ethinyl Estradiol; Ortho Cyclen; Ortho Tri Cyclen

Pharmacologic Category Contraceptive; Estrogen and Progestin Combination

Medication Safety Issues

Sound-alike/look-alike issues:

Ortho-Cyclen® may be confused with Ortho-Cept®

Ortho Tri-Cyclen® may be confused with Ortho Tri-Cyclen® Lo

International issues:

Vivelle: Brand name for ethinyl estradiol/norgestimate [Austria], but also a brand name for estradiol [U.S. (discontinued), Belgium]

Pregnancy Risk Factor X

Lactation Enters breast milk/not recommended

Use Prevention of pregnancy; treatment of acne

Unlabeled Use Treatment of hypermenorrhea (menorrhagia); pain associated with endometriosis; dysmenorrhea; dysfunctional uterine bleeding

Available Dosage Forms

Tablet, monophasic formulations:

MonoNessa®, Ortho-Cyclen®: Ethinyl estradiol 0.035 mg and norgestimate 0.25 mg (28s) [21 blue tablets and 7 green inactive tablets]

Sprintec®: Ethinyl estradiol 0.035 mg and norgestimate 0.25 mg (28s) [21 blue tablets and 7 white inactive tablets]

Tablet, triphasic formulations:

Ortho Tri-Cyclen®, TriNessa®:

Day 1-7: Ethinyl estradiol 0.035 mg and norgestimate 0.18 mg [7 white tablets]

Day 8-14: Ethinyl estradiol 0.035 mg and norgestimate 0.215 mg [7 light blue tablets]

Day 15-21: Ethinyl estradiol 0.035 mg and norgestimate 0.25 mg [7 blue tablets]

Day 22-28: 7 green inactive tablets (28s)

Tri-Sprintec®:

Day 1-7: Ethinyl estradiol 0.035 mg and norgestimate 0.18 mg [7 gray tablets]

Day 8-14: Ethinyl estradiol 0.035 mg and norgestimate 0.215 mg [7 light blue tablets]

Day 15-21: Ethinyl estradiol 0.035 mg and norgestimate 0.25 mg [7 blue tablets]

Day 22-28: 7 white inactive tablets (28s)

Ortho Tri-Cyclen® Lo:

Day 1-7: Ethinyl estradiol 0.025 mg and norgestimate 0.18 mg [7 white tablets]

Day 8-14: Ethinyl estradiol 0.025 mg and norgestimate 0.215 mg [7 light blue tablets]

Day 15-21: Ethinyl estradiol 0.025 mg and norgestimate 0.25 mg [7 dark blue tablets]

Day 22-28: 7 green inactive tablets (28s)

General Dosage Range Oral: *Children and Adults (females, postmenarche):* 1 tablet daily

Administration

Oral Administer at the same time each day.

Nursing Actions

Physical Assessment Emphasize importance of regular (monthly) blood pressure checks and annual physical assessment, Pap smear, and vision assessment. Teach importance of maintaining prescribed schedule of dosing.

Patient Education Oral contraceptives do not protect against HIV or other sexually-transmitted diseases. You are at risk of becoming pregnant if doses are missed. Be aware that some medications may reduce the effectiveness of oral contraceptives; an alternate form of contraception may be needed. It is important that you check your blood pressure monthly and that you have an annual physical assessment, Pap smear, and vision assessment while taking this medication. Avoid smoking while taking this medication; smoking increases risk of adverse effects, including thromboembolic events and heart attacks. You may experience loss of appetite or constipation. Report immediately pain or muscle soreness; warmth, swelling, pain, or redness in calves; shortness of breath; sudden loss of vision; unresolved leg/foot swelling; change in menstrual pattern (unusual bleeding, amenorrhea, breakthrough spotting); breast tenderness that does not go away; acute abdominal cramping; signs of vaginal infection (drainage, pain, itching); CNS changes (blurred vision, confusion, acute anxiety, or unresolved depression); chest pain; severe headache or vomiting; weakness in arm or leg; severe abdominal pain or tenderness; jaundice; or weight gain. Notify prescriber of changes in contact lens tolerance.

Ethinyl Estradiol, Drospirenone, and Levomefolate

(ETH in il es tra DYE ole, droh SPYE re none, & lee voe me FOE late)

Brand Names: U.S. Beyaz™; Safyral™

Index Terms Drospirenone, Ethinyl Estradiol, and Levomefolate Calcium; Ethinyl Estradiol, Drospirenone, and Levomefolate Calcium; Levomefolate

Calcium, Drospirenone, and Ethinyl Estradiol; Levomefolate, Drospirenone, and Ethinyl Estradiol

Pharmacologic Category Contraceptive; Estrogen and Progestin Combination

Medication Safety Issues

Sound-alike/look-alike issues:

Beyaz™ may be confused with Yaz®

Lactation Enters breast milk/not recommended

Use Prevention of pregnancy; treatment of premenstrual dysphoric disorder (PMDD); treatment of acne; folate supplementation

Unlabeled Use Treatment of hypermenorrhea (menorrhagia); pain associated with endometriosis; dysmenorrhea; dysfunctional uterine bleeding

Available Dosage Forms

Tablet, oral:

Beyaz™: Ethinyl estradiol 0.02 mg, drospirenone 3 mg, and levomefolate calcium 0.451 mg [24 pink tablets] and levomefolate calcium 0.451 mg [4 light orange tablets] (28s)

Safyral™: Ethinyl estradiol 0.03 mg, drospirenone 3 mg, and levomefolate calcium 0.451 mg [21 orange tablets] and levomefolate calcium 0.451 mg [7 light orange tablets] (28s)

General Dosage Range Oral: *Children ≥14 years and Adults:* 1 tablet daily

Administration

Oral May be administered with or without food, but must be taken at the same time each day, preferably after the evening meal or at bedtime. If severe vomiting or diarrhea occurs, additional contraception (nonhormonal) should be used. If vomiting occurs within 3-4 hours of dosing, consider the dose to be missed.

Etodolac (ee toe DOE lak)

Index Terms Etodolic Acid; Lodine

Pharmacologic Category Nonsteroidal Anti-inflammatory Drug (NSAID), Oral

Medication Safety Issues

Sound-alike/look-alike issues:

Lodine may be confused with codeine, iodine, Lopid®

Medication Guide Available Yes

Pregnancy Risk Factor C

Lactation Excretion in breast milk unknown/not recommended

Use Acute and long-term use in the management of signs and symptoms of osteoarthritis; rheumatoid arthritis and juvenile idiopathic arthritis (JIA); management of acute pain

Available Dosage Forms

Capsule, oral: 200 mg, 300 mg

Tablet, oral: 400 mg, 500 mg

Tablet, extended release, oral: 400 mg, 500 mg, 600 mg

General Dosage Range Oral:

Extended release:

Children 6-16 years and 20-30 kg: 400 mg once daily

Children 6-16 years and 31-45 kg: 600 mg once daily

Children 6-16 years and 46-60 kg: 800 mg once daily

Children 6-16 years and >60 kg: 1000 mg once daily

Adults: 400-1000 mg once daily

Regular release: *Adults:* 200-400 mg every 6-12 hours as needed **or** 500 mg 2 times/day (maximum: 1 g/day)

Administration

Oral May be administered with food to decrease GI upset.

Nursing Actions

Physical Assessment Monitor blood pressure at the beginning of therapy and periodically during use. Monitor for adverse gastrointestinal effects, cardiovascular complaints, and ototoxicity at beginning of therapy and periodically throughout.

Patient Education Do not crush tablets or break capsules. Take with food or milk to reduce GI distress. Do not use alcohol. You may experience anorexia, nausea, vomiting, heartburn, drowsiness, dizziness, nervousness, headache, or fluid retention; GI bleeding, ulceration, or perforation can occur with or without pain; discontinue medication and contact prescriber if persistent abdominal pain or cramping or blood in stool occurs. Report respiratory difficulty or unusual cough; chest pain, rapid heartbeat, or palpitations; bruising/bleeding; blood in urine, stool, mouth, or vomitus; swollen extremities; skin rash; fever; jaundice; abdominal tenderness; flu-like symptoms; or ringing in ears.

Etonogestrel (e toe noe JES trel)

Brand Names: U.S. Implanon®; Nexplanon®

Index Terms 3-Keto-desogestrel; ENG

Pharmacologic Category Contraceptive; Progestin

Lactation Enters breast milk/use caution

Breast-Feeding Considerations Etonogestrel was not found to affect the quality or quantity of breast milk. Do not insert <21 days postpartum. Levels of etonogestrel are highest during the first month following insertion (~2.2% of the weight-adjusted maternal daily dose). Breast-fed infants of mothers with an etonogestrel implant were not found to have adverse physical or psychomotor development in comparison to those infants of mothers using nonhormonal contraception.

Use Prevention of pregnancy; for use in women who request long-acting (up to 3 years) contraception

Mechanism of Action/Effect Etonogestrel is the active metabolite of desogestrel. It prevents pregnancy by suppressing ovulation, increasing the viscosity of cervical mucous, and inhibiting endometrial proliferation.

Contraindications Hypersensitivity to etonogestrel or any component of the formulation; undiagnosed abnormal genital bleeding; active hepatic disease or tumors; thrombosis or thromboembolic disorders (current or history of); known/suspected or history of carcinoma of the breast; pregnancy

Warnings/Precautions Use does not protect against HIV infection or other sexually-transmitted diseases. Insert intradermally; should be palpable after implanted. Improper insertion may lead to unintended pregnancy or may cause difficult or impossible removal. Failure to properly remove may lead to infertility, ectopic pregnancy, or continued adverse reactions. Following removal of the implant, alternative contraception should be initiated immediately. Pregnancies have been observed as early as 7-14 days following implant removal. A nonhormonal contraceptive should be used until the presence of the implant has been confirmed. Menstrual bleeding patterns are likely to be altered; patients should be counseled prior to implant insertion. Abnormal bleeding should be evaluated as required to exclude pathologic conditions or pregnancy. Ectopic pregnancy (rare) may occur more commonly than in women using no contraception. Follicular development may occur and may continue to increase in size beyond what may occur in a normal cycle; generally ovarian cysts resolve spontaneously without intervention; however, surgery may rarely be required. Contraceptive therapy with etonogestrel commonly results in an average weight gain of ~2.8 pounds after 1 year and ~3.7 pounds after 2 years of treatment. Use caution in overweight women; women >130% of ideal body weight were not included in clinical studies.

May increase the risk of thromboembolism; prior to implantation, carefully consider use in women with known risk factors for arterial/venous thromboembolism. Consider removal during periods of prolonged immobilization due to surgery or illness. Due to risk of thromboembolism associated with pregnancy and the postpartum period, do not use etonogestrel prior to 21 days postpartum. Women with a history of hypertension-related diseases should be encouraged to use a nonhormonal form of contraception. In women with hypertension that is well-controlled, use may be considered; monitor blood pressure closely. Estrogens may cause retinal vascular thrombosis; discontinue if migraine, loss of vision, proptosis, diplopia, or other visual disturbances occur; discontinue permanently if papilledema or retinal vascular lesions are observed on examination. Not for use prior to menarche.

Hormonal contraception should be avoided in women with active or a history of breast cancer. Combination hormonal contraception use has been associated with a slight increase in frequency of breast cancer; however, studies are not consistent. Use with caution in patients with diabetes, patients treated for hyperlipidemia, a history of depression, or in patients with diseases which may be exacerbated by fluid retention, including asthma, epilepsy, migraine, diabetes, or renal dysfunction. Use with caution in patients with renal impairment; women with renal disease should be encouraged to use a nonhormonal form of contraception. Use is contraindicated active hepatic disease; remove implant if jaundice develops or if liver function becomes abnormal. Extremely rare hepatic adenomas have been reported in association with long-term combination oral contraceptive use; risk with progestin only contraceptives is not known. The manufacturer does not recommend use in women chronically taking hepatic enzyme inducers. Etonogestrel serum levels and contraceptive efficacy may be significantly decreased by potent hepatic enzyme inducers. Any changes with lens tolerance or vision in contact lens wearers should be evaluated by an ophthalmologist.

Additional warnings based on combination hormonal (estrogen and progestin) contraceptives: The risk of cardiovascular side effects increases in women who smoke cigarettes, especially those who are >35 years of age; women who use combination hormonal contraceptives should be strongly advised not to smoke. Combination hormonal contraceptives may lead to increased risk of myocardial infarction; use with caution in patients with risk factors for coronary artery disease. Combination hormonal contraceptives may have a dose-related risk of gallbladder disease.

Drug Interactions

Avoid Concomitant Use

Avoid concomitant use of Etonogestrel with any of the following: Griseofulvin

Decreased Effect

Etonogestrel may decrease the levels/effects of: Vitamin K Antagonists

The levels/effects of Etonogestrel may be decreased by: Acitretin; Aminoglutethimide; Aprepitant; Artemether; Barbiturates; Bexarotene; Bexarotene (Systemic); Bile Acid Sequestrants; Bosentan; CarBAMazepine; Clobazam; Efavirenz; Felbamate; Fosaprepitant; Fosphenytoin; Griseofulvin; LamoTRIgine; Mycophenolate; Nevirapine; OXcarbazepine; Phenytoin; Prucalopride; Retinoic Acid Derivatives; Rifamycin Derivatives; St Johns Wort; Telaprevir; Tocilizumab; Topiramate

Increased Effect/Toxicity

Etonogestrel may increase the levels/effects of: Benzodiazepines (metabolized by oxidation); Selegiline; Tranexamic Acid; Voriconazole

The levels/effects of Etonogestrel may be increased by: Boceprevir; Conivaptan; Herbs (Progestogenic Properties); Voriconazole

Nutritional/Ethanol Interactions

Herb/Nutraceutical: St John's wort (an enzyme inducer) may decrease serum levels of etonogestrel. Concomitant use is not recommended. Bloodroot, chasteberry, damiana, oregano, and yucca may enhance the adverse/toxic effect of progestins.

Adverse Reactions

>10%:

Central nervous system: Headache (25%)

Dermatologic: Acne (14%)

Endocrine & metabolic: Infrequent menstrual bleeding (<3 episodes/90 days: 34%), amenorrhea (no bleeding in 90 days: 22%), prolonged menstrual bleeding (lasting >14 days: 18%), breast pain (13%), menstrual bleeding irregularities requiring discontinuation (11%)

Gastrointestinal: Weight gain (14%), abdominal pain (11%)

Genitourinary: Vaginitis (15%)

Respiratory: Upper respiratory tract infection (13%), pharyngitis (11%)

5% to 10%:

Central nervous system: Dizziness (7%), emotional lability (7%), depression (6%), nervousness (6%), pain (6%)

Endocrine & metabolic: Dysmenorrhea (7%), frequent menstrual bleeding (>5 episodes/90 days: 7%)

Gastrointestinal: Nausea (6%)

Genitourinary: Leukorrhea (10%)

Local: Implant site reactions (9%), insertion site pain (5%)

Neuromuscular & skeletal: Back pain (7%)

Respiratory: Sinusitis (6%)

Miscellaneous: Flu-like syndrome (8%), hypersensitivity (5%)

Pharmacodynamics/Kinetics

Onset of Action Serum levels sufficient to inhibit ovulation: ≤8 hours of implant

Duration of Action Implant: Each rod maintains etonogestrel levels sufficient to inhibit ovulation for 3 years

Available Dosage Forms

Rod, subdermal:

Implanon®: 68 mg

Nexplanon®: 68 mg

General Dosage Range Subdermal: *Adults (females, postmenarche):* Implant 1 rod for up to 3 years

Administration

Other Subdermal: For insertion under local anesthesia by healthcare providers trained in the insertion and removal procedure. Rod should be inserted ~8-10 cm (3-4 inches) above the medial epicondyle of the humerus just under the skin. Rod must be palpable after insertion. Deep insertion may require surgery to remove. A pressure bandage should be applied and left in place for 24 hours after insertion to decrease bruising; a small bandage placed over the insertion site should remain in place for 3-5 days.

If rod is impalpable:

Implanon®: Ultrasound should be used to locate the rod; MRI may also be useful if ultrasound is not successful. Implanon® is not radiopaque and cannot be visualized by x-ray or CT scan. If ultrasound and MRI are unsuccessful, call 1-877-467-5266 for more information.

Nexplanon®: Two-dimensional x-ray should be used to locate the rod; other methods for localization include x-ray computer tomography (CT), ultrasound scanning (USS) with a high-frequency linear array transducer (≥10 MHz), or MRI. If these methods are unsuccessful, call 1-877-467-5266.

Stability

Storage Store at controlled room temperature of 25°C (77°F); excursions permitted to 15°C to 30°C (59°F to 86°F). Implanon®: Protect from light.

Nursing Actions

Physical Assessment Assess insertion site.

Patient Education Does not protect against HIV or other sexually transmitted diseases. Regular gynecological and self-breast exams are important. Changes in menstrual periods may occur (change in frequency, length, or spotting between periods). Use of a backup method of birth control is recommended for 7 days after insertion. Periodically check for the presence of the device. If the device cannot be felt, use an alternative form of birth control until your prescriber confirms its presence. You will be given a user card to document the insertion of the device. Keep track of the removal date. You may experience acne, breast pain, weight gain, vaginal discharge, back pain, dizziness, or nausea. Report excessive vaginal bleeding, depression or severe mood swings, persistent or severe headaches, chest pain, coughing up blood, shortness of breath, pain in legs, or abdominal pain.

Etoposide (e toe POE side)

Brand Names: U.S. Toposar®

Index Terms EPEG; Epipodophyllotoxin; VePesid; VP-16; VP-16-213

Pharmacologic Category Antineoplastic Agent, Podophyllotoxin Derivative; Antineoplastic Agent, Topoisomerase II Inhibitor

Medication Safety Issues

Sound-alike/look-alike issues:

Etoposide may be confused with teniposide

Etoposide may be confused with etoposide phosphate (a prodrug of etoposide which is rapidly converted in the plasma to etoposide)

VePesid may be confused with Versed

High alert medication:

This medication is in a class the Institute for Safe Medication Practices (ISMP) includes among its list of drug classes which have a heightened risk of causing significant patient harm when used in error.

Pregnancy Risk Factor D

Lactation Excretion in breast milk unknown/not recommended

Use Treatment of refractory testicular tumors (injectable formulation); treatment of small cell lung cancer

Unlabeled Use Treatment of acute lymphocytic leukemia (ALL), refractory acute myeloid leukemia (AML), recurrent or metastatic breast cancer, central nervous system tumors, Ewing's sarcoma, gestational trophoblastic disease, Hodgkin's lymphoma, merkel cell cancer, refractory multiple myeloma, neuroblastoma, neuroendocrine tumors (adrenal gland and carcinoid tumors), non-Hodgkin's lymphomas, nonsmall-cell lung cancer (NSCLC), osteosarcoma, ovarian cancer, prostate cancer, retinoblastoma, metastatic soft tissue sarcoma, thymic malignancies, unknown-primary adenocarcinoma, Wilms' tumor; conditioning regimen for hematopoietic cell transplantation

Mechanism of Action/Effect Inhibits DNA synthesis leading to cell death.

Contraindications Hypersensitivity to etoposide or any component of the formulation

Warnings/Precautions Hazardous agent - use appropriate precautions for handling and disposal. **[U.S. Boxed Warning]: Severe dose-limiting and dose-related myelosuppression with resulting infection or bleeding may occur.** Treatment should be withheld for platelets <50,000/mm^3 or absolute neutrophil count (ANC) <500/mm^3. May cause anaphylactic-like reactions manifested by chills, fever, tachycardia, bronchospasm, dyspnea, and hypotension. In addition, facial/tongue swelling, coughing, chest tightness, cyanosis, laryngospasm, diaphoresis, hypertension, and flushing have also been reported less commonly. Incidence is primarily associated with intravenous administration (up to 2%) compared to oral administration (<1%). Infusion should be interrupted and medications for the treatment of anaphylaxis should be available for immediate use. High drug concentration and rate of infusion, as well as presence of polysorbate 80 and benzyl alcohol in the etoposide intravenous formulation have been suggested as contributing factors to the development of hypersensitivity reactions. Etoposide intravenous formulations may contain polysorbate 80 and/or benzyl alcohol, while etoposide phosphate (the water soluble prodrug of etoposide) intravenous formulation does not contain either vehicle. Case reports have suggested that etoposide phosphate has been used successfully in patients with previous hypersensitivity reactions to etoposide (Collier, 2008; Siderov, 2002). The use of concentrations higher than recommended were associated with higher rates of anaphylactic-like reactions in children.

Secondary acute leukemias have been reported with etoposide, either as monotherapy or in combination with other chemotherapy agents. Must be diluted; do not give I.V. push, infuse over at least 30-60 minutes; hypotension is associated with rapid infusion. If hypotension occurs, interrupt infusion and administer I.V. hydration and supportive care; decrease infusion upon reinitiation. Dosage should be adjusted in patients with hepatic or renal impairment. Use with caution in patients with low serum albumin; may increase risk for toxicities. Use with caution in elderly patients; may be more likely to develop severe myelosuppression and/or GI effects (eg, nausea/vomiting). **[U.S. Boxed Warning]: Should be administered under the supervision of an experienced cancer chemotherapy physician.** Injectable formulation contains polysorbate 80; do not use in premature infants. May contain benzyl alcohol; do not use in newborn infants.

Drug Interactions

Avoid Concomitant Use

Avoid concomitant use of Etoposide with any of the following: BCG; CloZAPine; Conivaptan; Natalizumab; Pimecrolimus; Pimozide; Tacrolimus (Topical); Vaccines (Live)

Decreased Effect

Etoposide may decrease the levels/effects of: BCG; Coccidioidin Skin Test; Sipuleucel-T; Vaccines (Inactivated); Vaccines (Live); Vitamin K Antagonists

The levels/effects of Etoposide may be decreased by: Barbiturates; CYP3A4 Inducers (Strong); Cyproterone; Deferasirox; Echinacea; Fosphenytoin; P-glycoprotein/ABCB1 Inducers; Phenytoin; Tocilizumab

Increased Effect/Toxicity

Etoposide may increase the levels/effects of: ARIPiprazole; CloZAPine; Leflunomide; Natalizumab; Pimozide; Vaccines (Live); Vitamin K Antagonists

The levels/effects of Etoposide may be increased by: Atovaquone; Conivaptan; CycloSPORINE; CycloSPORINE (Systemic); CYP3A4 Inhibitors (Moderate); CYP3A4 Inhibitors (Strong); Dasatinib; Denosumab; P-glycoprotein/ABCB1 Inhibitors; Pimecrolimus; Roflumilast; Tacrolimus (Topical); Trastuzumab

Nutritional/Ethanol Interactions

Ethanol: Avoid ethanol (may increase GI irritation).
Herb/Nutraceutical: Avoid concurrent St John's wort; may decrease etoposide levels.

Adverse Reactions Note: The following may occur with higher doses used in stem cell transplantation: Alopecia, ethanol intoxication, hepatitis, hypotension (infusion-related), metabolic acidosis, mucositis, nausea and vomiting (severe), secondary malignancy, skin lesions (resembling Stevens-Johnson syndrome).

>10%:

- Dermatologic: Alopecia (8% to 66%)
- Gastrointestinal: Nausea/vomiting (31% to 43%), anorexia (10% to 13%), diarrhea (1% to 13%)
- Hematologic: Leukopenia (60% to 91%; grade 4: 3% to 17%; nadir: 7-14 days; recovery: by day 20), thrombocytopenia (22% to 41%; grades 3/4: 1% to 20%; nadir 9-16 days; recovery: by day 20), anemia (≤33%)

1% to 10%:

- Cardiovascular: Hypotension (1% to 2%; due to rapid infusion)
- Gastrointestinal: Stomatitis (1% to 6%), abdominal pain (up to 2%)
- Hepatic: Hepatic toxicity (up to 3%)
- Neuromuscular & skeletal: Peripheral neuropathy (1% to 2%)
- Miscellaneous: Anaphylactic-like reaction (I.V. infusion 1% to 2%; oral capsules <1%; including chills, fever, tachycardia, bronchospasm, dyspnea)

Available Dosage Forms

Capsule, softgel, oral: 50 mg

Injection, solution: 20 mg/mL (5 mL, 25 mL, 50 mL, 100 mL)

Toposar®: 20 mg/mL (5 mL, 25 mL, 50 mL)

General Dosage Range Dosage adjustment recommended in patients with hepatic or renal impairment

I.V., oral: *Adults:* Dosage varies greatly depending on indication

Administration

Oral Doses ≤400 mg/day as a single once daily dose; doses >400 mg should be given in 2-4 divided doses. If necessary, the injection may be used for oral administration.

I.M. Do not administer I.M. or SubQ (severe tissue necrosis).

I.V. Irritant.

Administer standard doses over at least 30-60 minutes to minimize the risk of hypotension. Higher (unlabeled) doses used in transplantation may be infused over longer time periods depending on the protocol. Etoposide injection contains polysorbate 80 which may cause leaching of diethylhexyl phthalate (DEHP), a plasticizer contained in polyvinyl chloride (PVC) tubing. Administration through non-PVC (low sorbing) tubing will minimize patient exposure to DEHP.

Concentrations >0.4 mg/mL are very unstable and may precipitate within a few minutes. For large doses, where dilution to ≤0.4 mg/mL is not feasible, consideration should be given to slow infusion of the undiluted drug through a running normal saline, dextrose or saline/dextrose infusion; or use of etoposide phosphate. Etoposide solutions of 0.1-0.4 mg/mL may be filtered through a 0.22 micron filter without damage to the filter; etoposide solutions of 0.2 mg/mL may be filtered through a 0.22 micron filter without significant loss of drug.

I.V. Detail

pH: 3-4

Stability

Reconstitution Etoposide should be diluted to a concentration of 0.2-0.4 mg/mL in D_5W or NS for administration. Diluted solutions have concentration-dependent stability: More concentrated solutions have shorter stability times. Precipitation may occur with concentrations >0.4 mg/mL. Use appropriate precautions for handling and disposal.

Storage

Capsules: Store oral capsules under refrigeration at 2°C to 8°C (36°F to 46°F); do not freeze.

Injection: Store intact vials of injection at room temperature of 25°C (77°F); do not freeze. Protect from light. Diluted solutions for infusion, at room temperature, in D_5W or NS in polyvinyl chloride, are stable as follows, depending on the concentration:

0.2 mg/mL: 96 hours

0.4 mg/mL: 24 hours

Etoposide injection contains polysorbate 80 which may cause leaching of diethylhexyl phthalate (DEHP), a plasticizer contained in polyvinyl chloride (PVC) bags and tubing. Higher concentrations and longer storage time after preparation in PVC bags may increase DEHP leaching. Preparation in glass or polyolefin containers will minimize patient exposure to DEHP. When undiluted etoposide injection is stored in acrylic or ABS (acrylonitrile, butadiene and styrene) plastic containers, may crack and leak.

Nursing Actions

Physical Assessment Patient should be monitored closely for anaphylactic reaction (chills, fever, tachycardia, bronchospasm, dyspnea, hypotension). Emergency equipment should be available. Assess renal function prior to each treatment and on a regular basis.

Patient Education This medication may be administered by infusion. Report immediately any swelling, pain, burning, or redness at infusion site; swelling of extremities; palpitations, rapid heartbeat, sudden difficulty breathing or swallowing; chest pain; or chills. It is important to maintain adequate nutrition and hydration, unless instructed to restrict fluid intake. You will be more susceptible to infection. May cause nausea, vomiting, diarrhea, loss of hair (reversible), or mouth sores. Report extreme fatigue, pain or numbness in extremities, severe GI upset or diarrhea, bleeding or bruising, fever, sore throat, vaginal discharge, yellowing of eyes or skin, or any changes in color of urine or stool.

Related Information

Management of Drug Extravasations *on page 1269*

Etoposide Phosphate (e toe POE side FOS fate)

Brand Names: U.S. Etopophos®

Index Terms Epipodophyllotoxin; ETOP

Pharmacologic Category Antineoplastic Agent, Podophyllotoxin Derivative; Antineoplastic Agent, Topoisomerase II Inhibitor

Medication Safety Issues

Sound-alike/look-alike issues:

Etoposide phosphate may be confused with etoposide, teniposide

Etoposide phosphate is a prodrug of etoposide and is rapidly converted in the plasma to etoposide. To avoid confusion or dosing errors, **dosage should be expressed as the desired etoposide dose,** not as the etoposide phosphate dose (eg, etoposide phosphate equivalent to ___ mg etoposide).

High alert medication:

This medication is in a class the Institute for Safe Medication Practices (ISMP) includes among its list of drug classes which have a heightened risk of causing significant patient harm when used in error.

Pregnancy Risk Factor D

Lactation Excretion in breast milk unknown/not recommended

Breast-Feeding Considerations Due to the potential for serious adverse reactions in the nursing infant, breast feeding is not recommended.

Use Treatment of refractory testicular tumors; treatment of small cell lung cancer

Mechanism of Action/Effect Etoposide phosphate is converted *in vivo* to the active moiety, etoposide, by dephosphorylation. Etoposide inhibits mitotic activity; inhibits cells from entering prophase; inhibits DNA synthesis. Initially thought to be mitotic inhibitors similar to podophyllotoxin, but actually have no effect on microtubule assembly. However, later shown to induce DNA strand breakage and inhibition of topoisomerase II (an enzyme which breaks and repairs DNA); etoposide acts in late S or early G2 phases.

Contraindications Hypersensitivity to etoposide, etoposide phosphate, or any component of the formulation

Warnings/Precautions Hazardous agent - use appropriate precautions for handling and disposal. **[U.S. Boxed Warning]: Severe dose-limiting and dose-related myelosuppression with resulting infection or bleeding may occur.** Treatment should be withheld for platelets <50,000/mm^3 or absolute neutrophil count (ANC) <500/mm^3. May cause anaphylactic-like reactions manifested by chills, fever, tachycardia, bronchospasm, dyspnea, and hypotension. In addition, facial/tongue swelling, coughing, throat tightness, cyanosis, laryngospasm, diaphoresis, back pain, hypertension, flushing, apnea and loss of consciousness have also been reported less commonly. Anaphylactic-type reactions have occurred with the first infusion. Infusion should be interrupted and medications for the treatment of anaphylaxis should be available for immediate use. Underlying mechanisms behind the development of hypersensitivity reactions is unknown, but have been attributed to high drug concentration and rate of infusion. Another possible mechanism may be due to the differences between available etoposide intravenous formulations. Etoposide intravenous formulation contains polysorbate 80 and benzyl alcohol, while etoposide phosphate (the water soluble prodrug of etoposide) intravenous formulation does not contain either vehicle. Case reports have suggested that etoposide phosphate has been used successfully in patients with previous hypersensitivity reactions to etoposide (Collier, 2008; Siderov, 2002).

Secondary acute leukemias have been reported with etoposide, either as monotherapy or in combination with other chemotherapy agents. Dosage should be adjusted in patients with hepatic or renal impairment. Use with caution in patients with low serum albumin; may increase risk for toxicities. Doses of etoposide phosphate >175 mg/m^2 have not been evaluated. Use caution in elderly patients (may be more likely to develop severe myelosuppression and/or GI effects. Administer by slow I.V. infusion; hypotension has been reported with etoposide phosphate administration, generally associated with rapid I.V. infusion. Injection site reactions may occur; monitor infusion site closely. **[U.S. Boxed Warning]: Should be administered under the supervision of an experienced cancer chemotherapy physician.**

Drug Interactions

Avoid Concomitant Use

Avoid concomitant use of Etoposide Phosphate with any of the following: BCG; CloZAPine; Conivaptan; Natalizumab; Pimecrolimus; Pimozide; Tacrolimus (Topical); Vaccines (Live)

Decreased Effect

Etoposide Phosphate may decrease the levels/effects of: BCG; Coccidioidin Skin Test; Sipuleucel-T; Vaccines (Inactivated); Vaccines (Live)

The levels/effects of Etoposide Phosphate may be decreased by: Barbiturates; CYP3A4 Inducers (Strong); Cyproterone; Deferasirox; Echinacea; Fosphenytoin; P-glycoprotein/ABCB1 Inducers; Phenytoin; Tocilizumab

Increased Effect/Toxicity

Etoposide Phosphate may increase the levels/effects of: ARIPiprazole; CloZAPine; Leflunomide; Natalizumab; Pimozide; Vaccines (Live)

The levels/effects of Etoposide Phosphate may be increased by: Conivaptan; CycloSPORINE; CycloSPORINE (Systemic); CYP3A4 Inhibitors (Moderate); CYP3A4 Inhibitors (Strong); Dasatinib; Denosumab; P-glycoprotein/ABCB1 Inhibitors; Pimecrolimus; Roflumilast; Tacrolimus (Topical); Trastuzumab

Nutritional/Ethanol Interactions
Ethanol: Avoid ethanol (may increase GI irritation).
Herb/Nutraceutical: Avoid St John's wort (may decrease etoposide levels).

Adverse Reactions Note: Also see Adverse Reactions for **etoposide;** etoposide phosphate is converted to etoposide, adverse reactions experienced with etoposide would also be expected with etoposide phosphate.

>10%:
- Central nervous system: Chills/fever (24%)
- Dermatologic: Alopecia (33% to 44%)
- Gastrointestinal: Nausea/vomiting (37%), anorexia (16%), mucositis (11%)
- Hematologic: Leukopenia (91%; grade 4: 17%; nadir: day 15-22; recovery: usually by day 21), neutropenia (88%; grade 4: 37%; nadir: day 12-19; recovery: usually by day 21), anemia (72%; grades 3/4: 19%), thrombocytopenia (23%; grade 4: 9%; nadir: day 10-15; recovery: usually by day 21)
- Neuromuscular & skeletal: Weakness/malaise (39%)

1% to 10%:
- Cardiovascular: Hypotension (1% to 5%), hypertension (3%), facial flushing (2%)
- Central nervous system: Dizziness (5%)
- Dermatologic: Skin rash (3%)
- Gastrointestinal: Constipation (8%), abdominal pain (7%), diarrhea (6%), taste perversion (6%)
- Local: Extravasation/phlebitis (5%; including swelling, pain, cellulitis, necrosis, and/or skin necrosis at site of infiltration)
- Miscellaneous: Anaphylactic-type reactions (3%; including chills, diaphoresis, fever, rigor, tachycardia, bronchospasm, dyspnea, pruritus)

Available Dosage Forms
Injection, powder for reconstitution:
Etopophos®: 100 mg

General Dosage Range Dosage adjustment recommended in patients with hepatic or renal impairment

I.V.: *Adults:* Dosage varies greatly depending on indication

Administration

I.V. Infuse by slow I.V. infusion over 5-210 minutes; risk of hypotension may increase with rate of infusion. Do not administer as a bolus injection.

I.V. Detail
pH: 2.9 (reconstituted with sterile water for injection)

Stability

Reconstitution Reconstitute vials with 5 mL or 10 mL SWFI, D_5W, NS, bacteriostatic SWFI, or bacteriostatic NS to a concentration of 20 mg/mL or 10 mg/mL etoposide equivalent. These solutions may be administered without further dilution or may be diluted in 50-500 mL of D_5W or NS to a concentration as low as 0.1 mg/mL. Use appropriate precautions for handling and disposal.

Storage Store intact vials under refrigeration at 2°C to 8°C (36°F to 46°F). Protect from light. Reconstituted solution is stable refrigerated at 2°C to 8°C (36°F to 46°F) for 7 days. At room temperature of 20°C to 25°C (68°F to 77°F), reconstituted solutions are stable for 24 hours when reconstituted with SWFI, D_5W, or NS, or for 48 hours when reconstituted with bacteriostatic SWFI or bacteriostatic NS. Further diluted solutions for infusion are stable at room temperature 20°C to 25°C (68°F to 77°F) or under refrigeration 2°C to 8°C (36°F to 46°F) for up to 24 hours.

Nursing Actions

Physical Assessment Use caution in presence of hepatic or renal impairment. Assess renal function prior to each treatment and on a regular basis.

Patient Education This medication is administered by infusion. Report immediately any swelling, pain, burning, or redness at infusion site. Avoid alcohol. It is important to maintain adequate nutrition and hydration, unless instructed to restrict fluid intake. You will be more susceptible to infection. May cause nausea, vomiting, diarrhea, loss of hair (reversible), or mouth sores. Report immediately chest pain, swelling of extremities, respiratory difficulty, palpitations, or rapid heartbeat. Report extreme fatigue, pain or numbness in extremities, severe GI upset or diarrhea, bleeding or bruising, fever, chills, sore throat, vaginal discharge, respiratory difficulty, yellowing of eyes or skin, or changes in color of urine or stool.

Etravirine (et ra VIR een)

Brand Names: U.S. Intelence®

Index Terms TMC125

Pharmacologic Category Antiretroviral Agent, Reverse Transcriptase Inhibitor (Non-nucleoside)

Medication Safety Issues

International issues:
Etravirine [U.S. and multiple international markets] may be confused with ethaverine [multiple international markets]

Pregnancy Risk Factor B

Lactation Excretion in breast milk unknown/contraindicated

Breast-Feeding Considerations Maternal or infant antiretroviral therapy does not completely eliminate the risk of postnatal HIV transmission. In addition, multiclass-resistant virus has been detected in breast-feeding infants despite maternal therapy. Therefore, in the United States, where formula is accessible, affordable, safe, and sustainable, and the risk of infant mortality due to diarrhea and respiratory infections is low, complete avoidance of breast-feeding by HIV-infected women is recommended to decrease potential transmission of HIV (DHHS [perinatal], 2011).

Use Treatment of HIV-1 infection in combination with at least two additional antiretroviral agents in treatment-experienced patients exhibiting viral replication with documented non-nucleoside reverse transcriptase inhibitor (NNRTI) resistance

Mechanism of Action/Effect As a non-nucleoside reverse transcriptase inhibitor, etravirine has activity against HIV-1 by binding to reverse transcriptase. It consequently blocks the RNA-dependent and DNA-dependent DNA polymerase activities, including HIV-1 replication. It does not require intracellular phosphorylation for antiviral activity.

Contraindications There are no contraindications listed in the manufacturer's labeling.

Warnings/Precautions Severe and possibly life-threatening skin reactions (including Stevens-Johnson syndrome, toxic epidermal necrolysis, erythema multiforme, and hypersensitivity reactions [ranging from rash and/or constitutional symptoms to occasional organ dysfunction, including hepatic failure]) have been reported; discontinue immediately with signs or symptoms of severe skin reaction or hypersensitivity. Self-limiting (with continued therapy) mild-to-moderate rashes (higher incidence in women) were also observed in clinical trials, usually during second week of therapy initiation. Not for use in treatment-naive patients, or experienced patients without evidence of viral mutations conferring resistance to NNRTIs and PIs. May cause redistribution of fat (eg, buffalo hump, peripheral wasting with increased abdominal girth, cushingoid appearance). Patients may develop immune reconstitution syndrome resulting in the occurrence of an inflammatory response to an indolent or residual opportunistic infection; further evaluation and treatment may be required.

Use with caution in patients taking major CYP3A4, 2C9 or 2C19 substrates (see Drug Interactions); consider alternative agents that avoid or lessen the potential for CYP-mediated interactions. Not recommended for use with other NNRTIs, unboosted protease inhibitors, high-dose ritonavir, tipranavir/ritonavir, fosamprenavir/ritonavir, atazanavir/ritonavir, enzyme-inducing anticonvulsants, macrolides (except azithromycin), St John's wort, rifampin, or rifapentine.

Drug Interactions

Avoid Concomitant Use

Avoid concomitant use of Etravirine with any of the following: Atazanavir; Axitinib; Bortezomib; CarBAMazepine; Clopidogrel; Crizotinib; Dienogest; Dronedarone; Everolimus; Fosamprenavir; Fosphenytoin; Lapatinib; Lurasidone; Nilotinib; Nisoldipine; Pazopanib; PHENobarbital; Phenytoin; Praziquantel; Ranolazine; Reverse Transcriptase Inhibitors (Non-Nucleoside); Rifamycin Derivatives; Rilpivirine; Ritonavir; Rivaroxaban; Roflumilast; RomiDEPsin; SORAfenib; St Johns Wort; Ticagrelor; Tipranavir; Tolvaptan; Toremifene; Vandetanib

Decreased Effect

Etravirine may decrease the levels/effects of: Amiodarone; Antifungal Agents (Azole Derivatives, Systemic); ARIPiprazole; Atazanavir; Axitinib; Bepridil [Off Market]; Boceprevir; Bortezomib; Brentuximab Vedotin; Buprenorphine; Clopidogrel; Crizotinib; CYP3A4 Substrates; Dasatinib; Dienogest; Disopyramide; Dronedarone; Everolimus; Exemestane; Flecainide; Gefitinib; GuanFACINE; HMG-CoA Reductase Inhibitors; Imatinib; Ixabepilone; Lapatinib; Lidocaine; Lidocaine (Systemic); Linagliptin; Lurasidone; Macrolide Antibiotics; Maraviroc; Methadone; Mexiletine; NIFEdipine; Nilotinib; Nisoldipine; Pazopanib; Phosphodiesterase 5 Inhibitors; Praziquantel; Propafenone; QuiNIDine; Ranolazine; Rilpivirine; Rivaroxaban; Roflumilast; RomiDEPsin; Saxagliptin; SORAfenib; SUNItinib; Ticagrelor; Tolvaptan; Toremifene; Ulipristal; Vandetanib; Vemurafenib; Zuclopenthixol

The levels/effects of Etravirine may be decreased by: CarBAMazepine; CYP2C19 Inducers (Strong); CYP2C9 Inducers (Strong); CYP3A4 Inducers (Strong); Deferasirox; Fosphenytoin; Peginterferon Alfa-2b; PHENobarbital; Phenytoin; Protease Inhibitors; Reverse Transcriptase Inhibitors (Non-Nucleoside); Rifabutin; Rifamycin Derivatives; Ritonavir; St Johns Wort; Tipranavir; Tocilizumab

Increased Effect/Toxicity

Etravirine may increase the levels/effects of: Antifungal Agents (Azole Derivatives, Systemic); Carvedilol; Citalopram; CYP2C19 Substrates; CYP2C9 Substrates; Digoxin; Fosamprenavir; PACLitaxel; Protease Inhibitors; Rilpivirine

The levels/effects of Etravirine may be increased by: Antifungal Agents (Azole Derivatives, Systemic); Atazanavir; Reverse Transcriptase Inhibitors (Non-Nucleoside)

Nutritional/Ethanol Interactions

Food: Food increases absorption of etravirine by ~50%. Management: Take after meals and maintain adequate hydration, unless instructed to restrict fluid intake.

Herb/Nutraceutical: St John's wort may decrease the levels/effects of etravirine. Management: Avoid St John's wort.

Adverse Reactions

>10%:

Dermatologic: Rash (≥ grade 2: 10%)

Endocrine & metabolic: Cholesterol (total) increased (≤300 mg/dL: 20%; >300 mg/dL: 8%), hyperglycemia (≤250 mg/dL: 15%;

251-500 mg/dL: 4%), LDL increased (≤190 mg/dL: 13%)
Gastrointestinal: Nausea
2% to 10%:
Endocrine & metabolic: Triglycerides increased (≤750 mg/dL: 9%; >750 mg/dL: 4% to 6%)
Hepatic: ALT increased (≤5 x ULN: 6%; >5 x ULN: 3%), AST increased (≤5 x ULN: 6%; >5 x ULN: 3%)
Neuromuscular & skeletal: Peripheral neuropathy (≥ grade 2: 4%)
Renal: Creatinine increased (≤1.8 x ULN: 6%; >1.8 x ULN: 2%)

Available Dosage Forms
Tablet, oral:
Intelence®: 100 mg, 200 mg

General Dosage Range Oral: *Adults:* 200 mg twice daily

Administration
Oral Administer after meals. Dose is given as two 100 mg or one 200 mg tablet. If unable to swallow tablets, may disperse tablets in glass of water; stir well prior to drinking (swallow completely) and rinse glass several times to ensure administration of complete dose.

Stability
Storage Store at USP controlled room temperature of 25°C (77°F); excursions permitted to 15°C to 30°C (59°F to 86°F). Protect from moisture.

Nursing Actions
Physical Assessment Assess adherence to therapy. Monitor for rash and gastrointestinal upset. Teach patient proper timing of multiple medications.

Patient Education This drug will not cure HIV, nor has it been found to reduce transmission of HIV; use appropriate precautions to prevent spread to other persons. This drug is prescribed as one part of a multi-drug combination; take exactly as directed for full course of therapy. Take after meals. Maintain adequate hydration, unless instructed to restrict fluid intake. Frequent blood tests may be required. You may experience nausea, vomiting, or changes in body fat (increased in upper back and neck and around trunk; decreased from extremities and face). Report immediately any sign of skin rash.

Dietary Considerations Take after meals. May disperse tablets in glass of water; stir well prior to drinking and rinse glass several times to ensure administration of complete dose.

Everolimus (e ver OH li mus)

Brand Names: U.S. Afinitor®; Zortress®
Index Terms RAD001
Pharmacologic Category Antineoplastic Agent, mTOR Kinase Inhibitor; Immunosuppressant Agent; mTOR Kinase Inhibitor

Medication Safety Issues
Sound-alike/look-alike issues:
Everolimus may be confused with sirolimus, tacrolimus, temsirolimus
High alert medication:
This medication is in a class the Institute for Safe Medication Practices (ISMP) includes among its list of drug classes which have a heightened risk of causing significant patient harm when used in error.

Medication Guide Available Yes

Pregnancy Risk Factor D (Afinitor®) / C (Zortress®)

Lactation Excretion in breast milk unknown/not recommended

Breast-Feeding Considerations Due to the potential for serious adverse reactions in the nursing infant, breast-feeding is not recommended.

Use Treatment of advanced renal cell cancer (RCC), after sunitinib or sorafenib failure (Afinitor®); treatment of subependymal giant cell astrocytoma (SEGA) associated with tuberous sclerosis, in patients who are not candidates for curative surgical resection (Afinitor®); treatment of advanced, metastatic or unresectable pancreatic neuroendocrine tumors (PNET) (Afinitor®); prophylaxis of organ rejection in patients at low-moderate immunologic risk receiving renal transplants (Zortress®)

Unlabeled Use Prophylaxis of organ rejection in heart transplant recipients; treatment of relapsed or refractory Waldenström's macroglobulinemia (WM)

Mechanism of Action/Effect Everolimus is a macrolide immunosuppressant and an m-TOR inhibitor which has antiproliferative and antiangiogenic properties; reduces protein synthesis and cell proliferation by binding to the intracellular protein, FK binding protein-12 (FKBP-12) to form a complex that inhibits activation of mTOR (mammalian target of rapamycin) protein kinase activity. Also reduces angiogenesis by inhibiting vascular endothelial growth factor (VEGF) and hypoxia-inducible factor (HIF-1) expression.

Contraindications Hypersensitivity to everolimus, sirolimus, other rapamycin derivatives, or any component of the formulation.

Warnings/Precautions Hazardous agent - use appropriate precautions for handling and disposal. Noninfectious pneumonitis (sometimes fatal) has been observed with mTOR inhibitors including everolimus; symptoms include dyspnea, cough, hypoxia and/or pleural effusion; promptly evaluate worsening respiratory symptoms; may require dosage modification (pneumonitis has developed even with reduced doses) or corticosteroid therapy; severe symptoms may require discontinuation. Imaging may overestimate the incidence of clinical pneumonitis. **[U.S. Boxed Warning]: Everolimus has immunosuppressant properties which may result in infection;** the risk of developing bacterial (including mycobacterial), viral, fungal and protozoal infections and for local, opportunistic (including polyomavirus infection), systemic infections, and/or sepsis is increased. BK virus-associated nephropathy, which may result in serious cases of deteriorating renal function and renal graft loss, has been observed with use. Reactivation of hepatitis B has been observed in patients with RCC. Resolve pre-existing invasive fungal infections prior to treatment initiation. Monitor for signs and symptoms of infection during treatment. Discontinue if invasive systemic fungal infection is diagnosed (and manage with appropriate antifungal therapy).

[U.S. Boxed Warning]: Immunosuppressant use may result in the development of malignancy, including lymphoma and skin cancer. The risk is associated with treatment intensity and the duration of therapy. To minimize the risk for skin cancer, limit exposure to sunlight and ultraviolet light; wear protective clothing and use effective sunscreen.

[U.S. Boxed Warning]: Due to the increased risk for nephrotoxicity in renal transplantation, avoid standard doses of cyclosporine in combination with everolimus; reduced cyclosporine doses are recommended when everolimus is used in combination with cyclosporine. Therapeutic monitoring of cyclosporine and everolimus concentrations is recommended. Monitor for proteinuria; the risk of proteinuria is increased when everolimus is used in combination with cyclosporine, and with higher serum everolimus concentrations. Everolimus and cyclosporine combination therapy may increase the risk for thrombotic microangiopathy/thrombotic thrombocytopenic purpura/hemolytic uremic syndrome (TMA/TTP/HUS); monitor blood counts. Elevations in serum creatinine (generally mild), renal failure, and proteinuria have been also observed with everolimus use; monitor renal function (BUN, creatinine, and/or urinary protein). Avoid concomitant use with strong CYP3A4 inducers (eg, dexamethasone, phenytoin, carbamazepine, rifampin, rifabutin, rifapentine, phenobarbital) and strong CYP3A4 inhibitors (eg, ketoconazole, itraconazole, voriconazole, clarithromycin, telithromycin, atazanavir, saquinavir, ritonavir, indinavir, delavirdine, fosamprenavir, nelfinavir, nefazodone, grapefruit juice). Dosage modification may be needed if concomitant use with strong CYP3A4 inducers cannot be avoided. Use with caution with concomitant moderate CYP3A4 inhibitors and/or P-gp inhibitors; decreased everolimus doses are recommended. Use is associated with mouth ulcers, mucositis and stomatitis; avoid the use of alcohol or peroxide based mouthwashes (due to the high potential for drug interactions, avoid the use of systemic antifungals unless fungal infection has been diagnosed). In renal transplantation, avoid the use of HMG-CoA reductase inhibitors; may increase the risk for rhabdomyolysis due to the potential interaction with cyclosporine (which is given in combination with everolimus for renal transplantation). **[U.S. Boxed Warning]: An increased risk of renal arterial and venous thrombosis has been reported with use in renal transplantation, generally within the first 30 days after transplant; may result in graft loss.**

Everolimus is associated with the development of angioedema; concomitant use with other agents known to cause angioedema (eg, ACE inhibitors) may increase the risk. Everolimus use may delay wound healing and increase the occurrence of wound-related complications (eg, wound dehiscence, infection, incisional hernia, lymphocele, seroma); may require surgical intervention. Generalized edema, including peripheral edema and lymphedema, and local fluid accumulation (eg, pericardial effusion, pleural effusion, ascites) may also occur.

Everolimus exposure is increased in patients with moderate hepatic impairment; dosage reductions are recommended. Use is not recommended in patients with severe impairment (has not been studied). Use with caution in patients with hyperlipidemia; may increase serum lipids (cholesterol and triglycerides); higher serum concentrations are associated with an increased risk for hyperlipidemia; use has not been studied in patients with baseline cholesterol >350 mg/dL. Decreases in hemoglobin, neutrophils, platelets, and lymphocytes have been reported with use. Increases in serum glucose are common; may alter insulin and/or oral hypoglycemic therapy requirements in patients with diabetes; the risk for new onset diabetes is increased with everolimus use after transplantation. Patients should not be immunized with live viral vaccines during or shortly after treatment and should avoid close contact with recently vaccinated (live vaccine) individuals; consider the timing of routine immunizations prior to the start of therapy in pediatric patients treated for SEGA. Continue treatment with everolimus for renal cell cancer as long as clinical benefit is demonstrated or until occurrence of unacceptable toxicity. Safety and efficacy have not been established for the use of everolimus in the treatment of carcinoid tumors.

Azoospermia and oligospermia have been observed in males. Avoid use in patients with hereditary galactose intolerance, Lapp lactase deficiency, or glucose-galactose malabsorption; may result in diarrhea and malabsorption. The safety and efficacy of everolimus in patients with high-immunologic risk in renal transplantation or in solid organ transplant other than renal have not been established. **[U.S. Boxed Warning]: In renal transplantation, everolimus should only be used by physicians experienced in immunosuppressive therapy and management of transplant patients. Adequate laboratory and supportive medical resources must be readily available.**

Drug Interactions

Avoid Concomitant Use

Avoid concomitant use of Everolimus with any of the following: BCG; CloZAPine; CYP3A4 Inducers (Strong); CYP3A4 Inhibitors (Strong); Grapefruit Juice; Natalizumab; Pimecrolimus; St Johns Wort; Tacrolimus (Topical); Vaccines (Live)

Decreased Effect

Everolimus may decrease the levels/effects of: BCG; Coccidioidin Skin Test; Sipuleucel-T; Vaccines (Inactivated); Vaccines (Live)

The levels/effects of Everolimus may be decreased by: CYP3A4 Inducers (Strong); Deferasirox; Echinacea; Efavirenz; P-glycoprotein/ABCB1 Inducers; St Johns Wort; Tocilizumab

Increased Effect/Toxicity

Everolimus may increase the levels/effects of: ACE Inhibitors; CloZAPine; Leflunomide; Natalizumab; Vaccines (Live)

The levels/effects of Everolimus may be increased by: CycloSPORINE; CycloSPORINE (Systemic); CYP3A4 Inhibitors (Moderate); CYP3A4 Inhibitors (Strong); Dasatinib; Denosumab; Grapefruit Juice; P-glycoprotein/ABCB1 Inhibitors; Pimecrolimus; Roflumilast; Tacrolimus (Topical); Trastuzumab

Nutritional/Ethanol Interactions

Food: Grapefruit juice may increase levels of everolimus. Absorption with food may be variable. Management: Avoid grapefruit juice. Take with or without food, but be consistent with regard to food. Swallow whole with a glass of water.

Herb/Nutraceutical: St John's wort may decrease the levels of everolimus. Management: Avoid St John's wort.

Adverse Reactions

>10%:

Cardiovascular: Peripheral edema (4% to 45%), hypertension (4% to 30%)

Central nervous system: Fatigue (7% to 45%), fever (19% to 32%), headache (18% to 30%), seizure (SEGA: 29%), personality change (SEGA:18%), insomnia (9% to 17%), dizziness (7% to 14%)

Dermatologic: Rash (18% to 59%), acneiform dermatitis (SEGA: 25%; RCC: 3%), cellulitis (SEGA: 21%), nail disorders (5% to 22%), pruritus (14% to 21%), dry skin (13% to 18%), contact dermatitis (14%), excoriation (14%), acne (11%)

Endocrine & metabolic: Hypercholesterolemia (17% to 77%), hyperglycemia (12% to 75%; grades 3/4: <1% to 17%), hypertriglyceridemia (≤73%), bicarbonate decreased (≤56%), hypophosphatemia (13% to 40%), hypocalcemia (17% to 37%), hypoglycemia (≤32%), hypokalemia (12% to 23%), hyperlipidemia (renal transplant: 21%), hyperkalemia (renal transplant: 18%), dyslipidemia (renal transplant: 15%), hypomagnesemia (renal transplant: 14%), hyponatremia (≤16%), albumin decreased (≤13%)

Gastrointestinal: Stomatitis (oncology uses: 44% to 86%; grade 3: 4% to 7%; grade 4: <1%; renal transplant: 8%), diarrhea (19% to 50%; grade 3: ≤5%; grade 4: <1%), constipation (11% to 38%), abdominal pain (3% to 36%), nausea (26% to 32%: grade 3: 1% to 2%), anorexia (1% to 30%), vomiting (15% to 29%; grade 3: 1% to 2%), weight loss (9% to 28%), taste alteration (10% to 19%), gastroenteritis (1% to 18%), xerostomia (8% to 11%)

Genitourinary: Urinary tract infection (renal transplant: 16% to 22%; RCC 5%), dysuria (renal transplant: 11%)

Hematologic: Anemia (26% to 92%; grades 3/4; 13% to 15%), leukopenia (oncology uses: 26% to 54%; renal transplant 3%), lymphocytopenia (45% to 51%; grades 3/4: 16% to 18%), thrombocytopenia (21% to 45%; grade 3: 1% to 3%; renal transplant <10%), neutropenia (14% to 30%; grades 3/4: ≤4%)

Hepatic: AST increased (25% to 89%; grade 3: <4%; grade 4: <1%), alkaline phosphatase increased (PNET: 74%), ALT increased (21% to 48%; grade 3: 1%)

Neuromuscular & skeletal: Weakness (19% to 33%), arthralgia (≤15%), back pain (11% to 15%), limb pain (10% to 14%)

Otic: Otitis (SEGA: 14% to 36%)

Renal: Creatinine increased (11% to 50%), hematuria (renal transplant: 12%)

Respiratory: Upper respiratory infection (16% to 82%), sinusitis (3% to 39%), cough (7% to 30%), dyspnea (20% to 24%; grade 3: 2% to 6%; grade 4: ≤1%), epistaxis (≤22%), pneumonitis (includes alveolitis, interstitial lung disease, lung infiltrate, pulmonary alveolar hemorrhage, pulmonary toxicity; 14% to 17%; grade 3: 3% to 4%), nasal congestion (14%), rhinitis (14%), pharyngitis (4% to 11%)

Miscellaneous: Infection (RCC: All infections: 37%; grade 3: 7%; grade 4: 3%; renal transplant: 62%)

1% to 10%:

Cardiovascular: Chest pain (5%), tachycardia (3%), heart failure (1%), angina, atrial fibrillation, chest discomfort, deep vein thrombosis, edema (generalized), hypotension, palpitation, syncope

Central nervous system: Chills (4%), agitation, anxiety, depression, hallucination, hemiparesis, hypesthesia, malaise, somnolence

Dermatologic: Palmar-plantar erythrodysesthesia syndrome ([hand-foot syndrome] 5%), erythema 4%, onychoclasis (4%), pityriasis rosea (4%), skin lesions (4%), alopecia, hirsutism, incision complications, hyperhydrosis, hypertrichosis

Endocrine & metabolic: Diabetes mellitus (exacerbation: 2%; new-onset: <10%), cushingoid syndrome, dehydration, gout, hypercalcemia, hyperparathyroidism, hyperphosphatemia, hyperuricemia, iron deficiency, vitamin B_{12} deficiency

Gastrointestinal: Gastritis (7%), hemorrhoids (5%), dyspepsia (4%), dysphagia (4%), abdominal distention, epigastric discomfort, flatulence, gastroesophageal reflux, gingival hypertrophy, hematemesis, ileus, peritonitis

Genitourinary: Bladder spasm, erectile dysfunction, ovarian cysts, pollakiuria, polyuria, pyuria, scrotal edema, urinary retention, urinary urgency

Hematologic: Hemorrhage (3%), leukocytosis, lymphadenopathy, thrombocythemia

Hepatic: Bilirubin increased (3% to 10%; grades 3/4: ≤1%)

Neuromuscular & skeletal: Muscle spasm (≤10%), tremor (8%), paresthesia (5%), jaw pain (3%), joint swelling, musculoskeletal pain, myalgia, osteonecrosis, osteopenia, osteoporosis, spondylitis

Ocular: Eyelid edema (4%), ocular hyperemia (4%), conjunctivitis (2%), blurred vision, cataract

Renal: Renal failure (3%), BUN increased, hydronephrosis, interstitial nephritis, proteinuria, renal artery thrombosis, renal impairment

Respiratory: Pleural effusion (7%), nasopharyngitis (6%), pneumonia (6%), bronchitis (4%), pharyngolaryngeal pain (4%), rhinorrhea (3%), atelectasis, nasal congestion, pulmonary edema, sinus congestion, wheezing

Miscellaneous: BK virus infection, candidiasis, night sweats

Available Dosage Forms

Tablet, oral:

Afinitor®: 2.5 mg, 5 mg, 10 mg

Zortress®: 0.25 mg, 0.5 mg, 0.75 mg

General Dosage Range Dosage adjustment recommended in patients with hepatic impairment, on concomitant therapy, or who develop toxicities

Oral: *Children ≥3 years and Adults:* Dosage varies greatly depending on indication

Administration

Oral May be taken with or without food; to reduce variability, take consistently with regard to food. Swallow whole with a glass of water. Do not chew or crush. If unable to swallow tablet whole, immediately prior to administration, disperse completely in 30 mL water with gentle stirring; rinse container with additional 30 mL water and swallow. Avoid contact with or exposure to crushed or broken tablets.

Pancreatic neuroendocrine tumors, renal cell cancer, subependymal giant cell astrocytoma: Administer at the same time each day.

Renal transplantation: Administer consistently ~12 hours apart; administer at the same time as cyclosporine.

Stability

Storage Store at room temperature of 25°C (77°F); excursions permitted to 15°C to 30°C (59°F to 86°F). Protect from light; protect from moisture.

Nursing Actions

Physical Assessment This drug is an mTor kinase inhibitor, which works intracellularly for the treatment of pancreatic neuroendocrine tumors. Instruct patients on avoiding grapefruit juice due to interference in absorption and potentiating toxicities. Dose reduction or temporary discontinuation of everolimus is in correlation with toxicities. Instruct patient of importance of using sunscreen and avoiding direct sunlight due to photosensitivity.

Patient Education Patients should avoid grapefruit and grapefruit juice; grapefruit alters the level of drug in the system, which can increase the side effects of the medication. Do not crush or break tablets. Dissolve medication in a glass of water, then rinse glass to ensure medication is received. Patients will be more prone to infections and need to avoid others with infections and those who have had live vaccines. Common side effects include decreased appetite, taste changes, dry skin, nosebleeds, or mouth sores. Side effects that are more serious and need to be reported include chest pain; dizziness; difficulty breathing; eye, lip, or tongue swelling; unusual bleeding or bruising; and fevers or chills. Instruct patients to protect their skin by using sunblock and protective clothing. Patients should notify their prescriber prior to dental work.

Dietary Considerations Avoid grapefruit juice. May be taken with or without food, although should be administered consistently with regard to food.

Exemestane (ex e MES tane)

Brand Names: U.S. Aromasin®

Pharmacologic Category Antineoplastic Agent, Aromatase Inactivator

Medication Safety Issues

Sound-alike/look-alike issues:

Aromasin® may be confused with Arimidex®

Exemestane may be confused with estramustine.

Pregnancy Risk Factor X

Lactation Excretion in breast milk unknown/not recommended

Use Treatment of advanced breast cancer in postmenopausal women whose disease has progressed following tamoxifen therapy; adjuvant treatment of postmenopausal estrogen receptor-positive early breast cancer following 2-3 years of tamoxifen (for a total of 5 years of adjuvant therapy)

Unlabeled Use Risk reduction for invasive breast cancer in postmenopausal women; treatment of endometrial cancer; treatment of uterine sarcoma

Mechanism of Action/Effect Exemestane prevents conversion of androgens to estrogens (aromatase inhibitor) and lowers circulating estrogen levels in postmenopausal breast cancers.

Contraindications Hypersensitivity to exemestane or any component of the formulation; use in women who are or may become pregnant; use in premenopausal women

Warnings/Precautions Hazardous agent - use appropriate precautions for handling and disposal. Due to decreased circulating estrogen levels, exemestane is associated with a reduction in bone mineral density; decreases (from baseline) in lumbar spine and femoral neck density have been observed. Grade 3 or 4 lymphopenia has been observed with exemestane use, although most patients had preexisting lower grade lymphopenia. Increases in bilirubin, alkaline phosphatase and serum creatinine have been observed. Not to be given with estrogen-containing agents. Dose adjustment recommended with concomitant CYP3A4 inducers.

Drug Interactions

Avoid Concomitant Use

Avoid concomitant use of Exemestane with any of the following: Axitinib

Decreased Effect

Exemestane may decrease the levels/effects of: ARIPiprazole; Axitinib; Saxagliptin

The levels/effects of Exemestane may be decreased by: CYP3A4 Inducers (Strong); Deferasirox; Herbs (CYP3A4 Inducers); Rifampin; Tocilizumab

Increased Effect/Toxicity

The levels/effects of Exemestane may be increased by: Conivaptan

Nutritional/Ethanol Interactions

Food: Plasma levels increased by 40% when exemestane was taken with a fatty meal.

Herb/Nutraceutical: St John's wort may decrease exemestane levels. Avoid black cohosh, dong quai in estrogen-dependent tumors.

Adverse Reactions

>10%:

Cardiovascular: Hypertension (5% to 15%)

Central nervous system: Fatigue (8% to 22%), insomnia (11% to 14%), pain (13%), headache (7% to 13%), depression (6% to 13%)

Dermatological: Hyperhidrosis (4% to 18%), alopecia (15%)

Endocrine & metabolic: Hot flashes (13% to 33%)

Gastrointestinal: Nausea (9% to 18%), abdominal pain (6% to 11%)

Hepatic: Alkaline phosphatase increased (14% to 15%)

Neuromuscular & skeletal: Arthralgia (15% to 29%)

1% to 10%:

Cardiovascular: Edema (6% to 7%); cardiac ischemic events (2%: MI, angina, myocardial ischemia); chest pain

Central nervous system: Dizziness (8% to 10%), anxiety (4% to 10%), fever (5%), confusion, hypoesthesia

Dermatologic: Dermatitis (8%), itching, rash

Endocrine & metabolic: Weight gain (8%)

Gastrointestinal: Diarrhea (4% to 10%), vomiting (7%), anorexia (6%), constipation (5%), appetite increased (3%), dyspepsia

Genitourinary: Urinary tract infection (2% to 5%)

Hepatic: Bilirubin increased (5% to 7%)

Neuromuscular & skeletal: Back pain (9%), limb pain (9%), myalgia (6%), osteoarthritis (6%), weakness (6%), osteoporosis (5%), pathological fracture (4%), paresthesia (3%), carpal tunnel syndrome (2%), cramps (2%)

Ocular: Visual disturbances (5%)

Renal: Creatinine increased (6%)

Respiratory: Dyspnea (10%), cough (6%), bronchitis, pharyngitis, rhinitis, sinusitis, upper respiratory infection

Miscellaneous: Flu-like syndrome (6%), lymphedema, infection

A dose-dependent decrease in sex hormone-binding globulin has been observed with daily doses of ≥2.5 mg. Serum luteinizing hormone and follicle-stimulating hormone levels have increased with this medicine.

Available Dosage Forms

Tablet, oral: 25 mg

Aromasin®: 25 mg

General Dosage Range Dosage adjustment recommended in patients on concomitant therapy

Oral: *Adults (postmenopausal females):* 25 mg once daily

Administration

Oral Administer after a meal.

Stability

Storage Store at 25°C (77°F); excursions permitted to 15°C to 30°C (59°F to 86°F).

Nursing Actions

Physical Assessment Monitor for new or unusual bone pain and swelling of face, lips, or throat. Monitor blood pressure; may cause hypertension.

Patient Education Take after meals at approximately the same time each day; may cause indigestion. You may be more susceptible to infection. May cause headache, dizziness, confusion, fatigue, anxiety, insomnia, nausea, vomiting, loss of appetite, or hot flashes. Report chest pain; palpitations; acute headache, visual disturbances; unresolved GI problems; itching or burning on urination, vaginal discharge; acute joint, back, bone, or muscle pain; respiratory difficulty; unusual cough; or respiratory infection.

Dietary Considerations Take after a meal; patients on aromatase inhibitor therapy should receive vitamin D and calcium supplements.

Exenatide (ex EN a tide)

Brand Names: U.S. Bydureon™; Byetta®

Index Terms AC 2993; AC002993; Exendin-4; LY2148568

Pharmacologic Category Antidiabetic Agent, Glucagon-Like Peptide-1 (GLP-1) Receptor Agonist

Medication Guide Available Yes

Pregnancy Risk Factor C

Lactation Excretion in breast milk unknown/use caution

Breast-Feeding Considerations It is not known if exenatide is present in breast milk. The manufacturer recommends that caution be exercised when administering exenatide to nursing women.

Use Treatment of type 2 diabetes mellitus (noninsulin dependent, NIDDM) to improve glycemic control

Mechanism of Action/Effect Exenatide is an analog of the hormone incretin (glucagon-like peptide 1 or GLP-1) which increases glucose-dependent insulin secretion, decreases inappropriate glucagon secretion, increases B-cell growth/replication, slows gastric emptying, and decreases food intake. Exenatide administration results in decreases in hemoglobin A_{1c} by approximately 0.5% to 1% (immediate release) or 1.5% to 1.9% (extended release).

Contraindications Hypersensitivity to exenatide or any component of the formulation

Bydureon™: Additional contraindications: History of or family history of medullary thyroid carcinoma (MTC); patients with multiple endocrine neoplasia syndrome type 2 (MEN2)

Warnings/Precautions Bydureon™: **[U.S. Boxed Warning] Dose- and duration- dependent thyroid C-cell tumors have developed in animal studies with exenatide extended release therapy; relevance in humans unknown.** Patients should be counseled on the risk and symptoms (eg, neck mass, dysphagia, dyspnea, persistent hoarseness) of thyroid tumors. Consultation with an endocrinologist is recommended in patients who develop elevated calcitonin concentrations or have thyroid nodules detected during imaging studies or physical exam. Use is contraindicated in patients with a personal or a family history of medullary thyroid cancer and in patients with multiple endocrine neoplasia syndrome type 2 (MEN2). All cases of MTC should be reported to the applicable state cancer registry.

Mechanism requires the presence of insulin, therefore use in type 1 diabetes (insulin dependent, IDDM) or diabetic ketoacidosis is not recommended; it is not a substitute for insulin in insulin-requiring patients. Concurrent use with insulin therapy has not been evaluated and is not recommended. (Exception: Safety and efficacy of concurrent insulin glargine and immediate release exenatide has been demonstrated in a clinical trial.) May increase the risk of hypoglycemia in patients receiving concomitant insulin secretagogues (eg, sulfonylureas, meglitinides); dosage reduction of sulfonylureas may be required. Clinicians should note that the risk of hypoglycemia is not increased when exenatide is added to metformin monotherapy. Avoid concurrent use of extended release (weekly) and immediate release (daily) exenatide formulations. Bydureon™ is not recommended for first-line therapy in patients inadequately controlled on diet and exercise alone.

Exenatide is frequently associated with gastrointestinal adverse effects and is not recommended for use in patients with gastroparesis or severe gastrointestinal disease. Gastrointestinal effects may be dose-related and may decrease in frequency/severity with gradual titration and continued use. Due to its effects on gastric emptying, exenatide may reduce the rate and extent of absorption of orally-administered drugs; use with caution in patients receiving medications with a narrow therapeutic window or require rapid absorption from the GI tract. Administer medications 1 hour prior to the use of immediate release (daily) exenatide when optimal drug absorption and peak levels are important to the overall therapeutic effect (eg, antibiotics, oral contraceptives); effects of extended release (weekly) exenatide on drug absorption have not been evaluated; use caution. Cases of acute pancreatitis (including hemorrhagic and necrotizing with some fatalities) have been reported; monitor for unexplained severe abdominal pain and if pancreatitis suspected, discontinue use. Do not resume unless an alternative etiology of pancreatitis is confirmed. Consider alternative antidiabetic therapy in patients with a history of pancreatitis. Use may be associated with the development of anti-exenatide antibodies. Low titers are not associated with a loss of efficacy; however, high titers (observed in 6% of patients in clinical studies) may result in an attenuation of response. May be associated with weight loss (due to reduced intake) independent of the change in hemoglobin A_{1c}.

Not recommended in severe renal impairment (Cl_{cr} <30 mL/minute) or end-stage renal disease (ESRD). Patients with ESRD receiving dialysis may be more susceptible to GI effects (eg, nausea, vomiting) which may result in hypovolemia and further reductions in renal function. Use with caution in patients with renal transplantation or in patients with moderate renal impairment (Cl_{cr} 30-50 mL/minute). Cases of acute renal failure and chronic renal failure exacerbation, including severe cases requiring hemodialysis, have been reported, predominately in patients with nausea/vomiting/diarrhea or dehydration; renal dysfunction was usually reversible with appropriate corrective measures, including discontinuation of exenatide. Risk may be increased in patients receiving concomitant medications affecting renal function and/or hydration status.

Drug Interactions

Avoid Concomitant Use There are no known interactions where it is recommended to avoid concomitant use.

Decreased Effect

The levels/effects of Exenatide may be decreased by: Corticosteroids (Orally Inhaled); Corticosteroids (Systemic); Luteinizing Hormone-Releasing Hormone Analogs; Somatropin; Thiazide Diuretics

Increased Effect/Toxicity

Exenatide may increase the levels/effects of: Sulfonylureas; Vitamin K Antagonists

The levels/effects of Exenatide may be increased by: Pegvisomant

Nutritional/Ethanol Interactions

Ethanol: Ethanol may cause hypoglycemia. Management: Consume ethanol with caution.

Food: Administer Byetta® within 60 minutes of meals, not after meals. May administer Bydureon™ without regard to meals or time of day.

Adverse Reactions Percentages as reported for combination therapy (sulfonylurea and/or metformin; thiazolidinedione and/or metformin) unless otherwise noted:

>10%:

Endocrine & metabolic: Hypoglycemia (monotherapy 4% to 5%; combination therapy: sulfonylurea - 14% to 36%; metformin - similar to placebo; thiazolidinedione - 11%)

Gastrointestinal: Nausea (monotherapy 8%; combination therapy 40% to 44%; dose-dependent), vomiting (monotherapy 4%; combination therapy 13%), diarrhea (monotherapy <2%; combination therapy 6% to 13%)

Miscellaneous: Anti-exenatide antibodies (low titers 38%, high titers 6%)

1% to 10%:

Central nervous system: Dizziness (monotherapy <2%; combination therapy 9%), headache (9%)

Dermatologic: Hyperhidrosis (3%)

Endocrine & metabolic: Appetite decreased (<2%)

Gastrointestinal: Dyspepsia (monotherapy 3%; combination therapy 6% to 7%), GERD (3%)

Neuromuscular & skeletal: Weakness (4%)

Miscellaneous: Feeling jittery (9%)

Available Dosage Forms

Injection, microspheres for suspension, extended release:

Bydureon™: 2 mg (1s)

Injection, solution:

Byetta®: 250 mcg/mL (1.2 mL, 2.4 mL)

General Dosage Range SubQ: *Adults:*

Immediate release: Initial: 5 mcg twice daily; Maintenance: 5-10 mcg twice daily

Extended release: 2 mg once weekly

Administration

Other SubQ:

Immediate release: Use only if clear, colorless, and free of particulate matter. Administer via injection in the upper arm, thigh, or abdomen. Administer within 60 minutes prior to morning and evening meal (or prior to the 2 main meals of the day, approximately ≥6 hours apart). Set up each new pen before the first use by priming it. See pen user manual for further details. Dial the dose into the dose window before each administration.

Extended release: Administer via injection in the upper arm, thigh, or abdomen; rotate injection sites weekly. Administer immediately after reconstitution. May administer without regard to meals or time of day.

Stability

Reconstitution Bydureon™: Reconstitute vial using provided diluent; use immediately.

Storage

Bydureon™: Store under refrigeration at 2°C to 8°C (36°F to 46°F); vials may be stored at ≤25°C (≤77°F) for up to 4 weeks. Do not freeze (discard if freezing occurs). Protect from light.

Byetta®: Prior to initial use, store under refrigeration at 2°C to 8°C (36°F to 46°F); after initial use, may store at ≤25°C (≤77°F). Do not freeze (discard if freezing occurs). Protect from light. Pen should be discarded 30 days after initial use.

Nursing Actions

Physical Assessment Monitor for signs and symptoms of hyperglycemia. Teach appropriate subcutaneous injection technique and disposal of needles. Assess gastrointestinal side effects of medication; can improve with use or with lower dose.

Patient Education Administer Byetta® within 60 minutes of meals; do not administer after meals. Note a difference between the products: Bydureon™ is given once a week without regard to meals; Byetta® is given twice a day. Ensure patient is aware of product directions. It is important to follow dietary and lifestyle recommendations of prescriber. Patient may experience nausea, vomiting, diarrhea, or decreased appetite. Have patient report increased urination, severe abdominal pain, neck mass, swallowing difficulty, breathing problems, hoarseness, very low blood sugars, or persistent nausea, diarrhea, or dizziness.

Ezetimibe (ez ET i mibe)

Brand Names: U.S. Zetia®

Pharmacologic Category Antilipemic Agent, 2-Azetidinone

Medication Safety Issues

Sound-alike/look-alike issues:

Ezetimibe may be confused with ezogabine

Zetia® may be confused with Zebeta®, Zestril®

Pregnancy Risk Factor C

Lactation Excretion in breast milk unknown/not recommended

Use Use in combination with dietary therapy for the treatment of primary hypercholesterolemia (as monotherapy or in combination with HMG-CoA reductase inhibitors); homozygous sitosterolemia; homozygous familial hypercholesterolemia (in combination with atorvastatin or simvastatin); mixed hyperlipidemia (in combination with fenofibrate)

Mechanism of Action/Effect Inhibits absorption of cholesterol at the brush border of the small intestine, leading to a decreased delivery of cholesterol to the liver, reduction of hepatic cholesterol stores and an increased clearance of cholesterol from the blood; decreases total C, LDL-C, ApoB, and triglycerides while increasing HDL-C

Contraindications Hypersensitivity to ezetimibe or any component of the formulation; concomitant use with an HMG-CoA reductase inhibitor in patients with active hepatic disease, unexplained persistent elevations in serum transaminases; pregnancy; breast-feeding

Warnings/Precautions Secondary causes of hyperlipidemia should be ruled out prior to therapy. Use caution with severe renal (Cl_{cr} <30 mL/minute) or mild hepatic impairment (Child-Pugh class A); not recommended for use with moderate or severe hepatic impairment (Child-Pugh classes B and C). Concurrent use of ezetimibe and fibric acid derivatives may increase the risk of cholelithiasis.

Drug Interactions

Avoid Concomitant Use There are no known interactions where it is recommended to avoid concomitant use.

Decreased Effect

The levels/effects of Ezetimibe may be decreased by: Bile Acid Sequestrants

Increased Effect/Toxicity

Ezetimibe may increase the levels/effects of: CycloSPORINE; CycloSPORINE (Systemic)

The levels/effects of Ezetimibe may be increased by: CycloSPORINE; CycloSPORINE (Systemic); Eltrombopag; Fibric Acid Derivatives

Nutritional/Ethanol Interactions Food: Ezetimibe did not cause meaningful reductions in fat-soluble vitamin concentrations during a 2-week clinical trial. Effects of long-term therapy have not been evaluated.

Adverse Reactions 1% to 10%:

Central nervous system: Fatigue (2%)

Gastrointestinal: Diarrhea (4%)

Hepatic: Transaminases increased (with HMG-CoA reductase inhibitors) (≥3 x ULN, 1%)

Neuromuscular & skeletal: Arthralgia (3%), pain in extremity (3%)

Respiratory: Upper respiratory tract infection (4%), sinusitis (3%)

Miscellaneous: Influenza (2%)

Available Dosage Forms

Tablet, oral:

Zetia®: 10 mg

General Dosage Range Oral: *Children ≥10 years and Adults:* 10 mg once daily

Administration

Oral May be administered without regard to meals. May be taken at the same time as HMG-CoA reductase inhibitors. Administer ≥2 hours before or ≥4 hours after bile acid sequestrants.

Stability

Storage Store at controlled room temperature of 25°C (77°F). Protect from moisture.

Nursing Actions

Physical Assessment Assess lipid profile at beginning of and at regular intervals during therapy. Teach patient to report signs of hepatic or muscle reactions.

Patient Education Take at the same time of day, without regard for meals. Take 2 hours before or 4 hours after bile acid binding agents (eg, Questran®). This medication does not replace the need for dietary and exercise recommendations of prescriber. May cause headache, dizziness, fatigue, diarrhea, or abdominal pain. Report yellowing of skin or sclera; dark urine or pale stools; excessive tiredness; chest pain or palpitations; muscle, skeletal, or joint pain; twitching or numbness; increased perspiration; or changes in urinary pattern.

Dietary Considerations May be taken without regard to meals. Before initiation of therapy, patients should be placed on a standard cholesterol-lowering diet for 6 weeks and the diet should be continued during drug therapy.

Ezetimibe and Simvastatin

(ez ET i mibe & SIM va stat in)

Brand Names: U.S. Vytorin®

Index Terms Simvastatin and Ezetimibe

Pharmacologic Category Antilipemic Agent, 2-Azetidinone; Antilipemic Agent, HMG-CoA Reductase Inhibitor

Medication Safety Issues

Sound-alike/look-alike issues:

Vytorin® may be confused with Vyvanse®

Pregnancy Risk Factor X

Lactation Excretion in breast milk unknown/contraindicated

Use Used in combination with dietary modification for the treatment of primary hypercholesterolemia and homozygous familial hypercholesterolemia

Available Dosage Forms

Tablet:

Vytorin®:

10/10: Ezetimibe 10 mg and simvastatin 10 mg
10/20: Ezetimibe 10 mg and simvastatin 20 mg
10/40: Ezetimibe 10 mg and simvastatin 40 mg
10/80: Ezetimibe 10 mg and simvastatin 80 mg

General Dosage Range Dosage adjustment recommended in patients with renal impairment or on concomitant therapy

Oral: *Adults:* Ezetimibe 10 mg and simvastatin 10-40 mg once daily

Administration

Oral May be administered without regard to meals. Administer in the evening for maximal efficacy.

Nursing Actions

Physical Assessment See individual agents.

Patient Education See individual agents.

Ezogabine (e ZOG a been)

Brand Names: U.S. Potiga™

Index Terms D-23129; EZG; Potiga™; Retigabine; RTG

Pharmacologic Category Anticonvulsant, Neuronal Potassium Channel Opener

Medication Safety Issues

Sound-alike/look-alike issues:

Ezogabine may be confused with ezetimibe.

Potiga™ may be confused with Portia®

Medication Guide Available Yes

Pregnancy Risk Factor C

Lactation Excretion in breast milk unknown/not recommended

Breast-Feeding Considerations According to the manufacturer, the decision to continue or discontinue breast-feeding during therapy should take into account the risk of exposure to the infant and the benefits to the mother.

Use Adjuvant treatment of partial-onset seizures

Mechanism of Action/Effect Ezogabine binds the KCNQ (Kv7.2-7.5) voltage-gated potassium channels. As a result, neuronal excitability is regulated and epileptiform activity is suppressed.

Contraindications There are no contraindications listed in the manufacturer's labeling.

Warnings/Precautions Urinary retention, including retention requiring catheterization, has been reported, generally within the first 6 months of treatment. All patients should be monitored for urologic symptoms; close monitoring is recommended in patients with other risk factors for urinary retention (eg, benign prostatic hyperplasia), patients unable to communicate clinical symptoms, or patients who use concomitant medications that may affect voiding (eg, anticholinergics). Dose-related neuropsychiatric disorders, including confusion, psychotic symptoms, and hallucinations, have been reported, generally within the first 8 weeks of treatment; some patients required hospitalization. Symptoms resolved in most patients within 7 days of discontinuation of ezogabine. The risk appears to be greatest with rapid titration at greater than the recommended doses. Dose-related dizziness and somnolence (generally mild-to-moderate) have been reported; effects generally occur during dose titration and appear to diminish with continued use. Patients must be cautioned about performing tasks which require mental alertness (eg, operating machinery or driving). QT prolongation has been observed; monitor EKG in patients with electrolyte abnormalities (eg, hypokalemia, hypomagnesemia), hypothyroidism, familial long QT syndrome, concomitant medications which may augment QT prolongation, or any underlying cardiac abnormality which may also potentiate risk (eg, congestive heart failure, ventricular hypertrophy). Pooled analysis of trials involving various antiepileptics (regardless of indication) showed an increased risk of suicidal thoughts/behavior (incidence rate: 0.43% treated patients compared to 0.24% of patients receiving placebo); risk observed as early as 1 week after initiation and continued through duration of trials (most trials ≤24 weeks). Monitor all patients for notable changes in behavior that might indicate suicidal thoughts or depression; notify healthcare provider immediately if symptoms occur.

Dosage adjustment recommended in hepatic impairment; ezogabine exposure increases in moderate-to-severe impairment. Dosage adjustment recommended in renal impairment; ezogabine undergoes significant renal elimination. Use caution in elderly due to potential for urinary retention, particularly in older men with symptomatic BPH. Systemic exposure is increased in the elderly; dosage adjustment is recommended in patients ≥65 years of age.

Anticonvulsants should not be discontinued abruptly because of the possibility of increasing seizure frequency; therapy should be withdrawn gradually over a period of ≥3 weeks to minimize the potential of increased seizure frequency, unless safety concerns require a more rapid withdrawal.

Adverse Reactions

>10%: Central nervous system: Dizziness (dose related; 23%), somnolence (dose related; 22%), fatigue (15%)

2% to 10%:

Central nervous system: Confusion (dose related; 9%), vertigo (8%), coordination impaired (dose related; 7%), attention disturbance (6%), memory impairment (dose related; 6%), aphasia (dose related; 4%), balance disorder (dose related; 4%), anxiety (3%), amnesia (2%), disorientation (2%)

Gastrointestinal: Nausea (7%), constipation (dose related; 3%), weight gain (dose related; 3%), dysphagia (2%)

Ocular: Diplopia (7%), blurred vision (dose related; 5%)

Neuromuscular & skeletal: Tremor (dose related; 8%), weakness (5%), abnormal gait (dose related; 4%), dysarthria (4%), paresthesia (3%)

Renal: Chromaturia (dose related; 2%), dysuria (dose related; 2%), hematuria (2%), urinary hesitation (2%)

Miscellaneous: Influenza infection (3%)

Product Availability Potiga™: FDA approved June 2011; availability expected by the end of 2011

General Dosage Range Dosage adjustment recommended in patients with renal impairment or hepatic impairment.

Oral:

Adults: Initial: 100 mg 3 times/day; Maintenance: 200-400 mg 3 times/day (maximum: 1200 mg/day)

Elderly: Initial: 50 mg 3 times/day; Maintenance: 250 mg 3 times/day (maximum: 750 mg/day)

Administration

Oral May be administered with or without food; swallow tablets whole. If therapy is discontinued, gradually reduce dose over ≥3 weeks unless safety concerns require abrupt withdrawal.

Stability

Storage Store at 25°C (77°F); excursions permitted to 15°C to 30°C (59°F to 86°F).

Dietary Considerations May be taken with or without food.

Factor VIIa (Recombinant)

(FAK ter SEV en aye ree KOM be nant)

Brand Names: U.S. NovoSeven® RT

Index Terms Coagulation Factor VIIa; Eptacog Alfa (Activated); rFVIIa

Pharmacologic Category Antihemophilic Agent

Pregnancy Risk Factor C

Lactation Excretion in breast milk unknown/not recommended

Use Treatment of bleeding episodes and prevention of bleeding in surgical interventions in patients with either hemophilia A or B with inhibitors to factor VIII or factor IX, acquired hemophilia, or congenital factor VII deficiency

Unlabeled Use Reduction of hematoma growth in patients with acute intracerebral hemorrhage, warfarin-related intracerebral hemorrhage; treatment of refractory bleeding after cardiac surgery in nonhemophiliac patients

Available Dosage Forms

Injection, powder for reconstitution [preservative free]:

NovoSeven® RT: 1 mg, 2 mg, 5 mg, 8 mg

General Dosage Range I.V.: *Children and Adults:* Dosage varies greatly depending on indication

Administration

I.V. I.V. administration only; bolus over 2-5 minutes. Administer within 3 hours after reconstitution.

I.V. Detail pH: 5.5

Nursing Actions

Physical Assessment Monitor patient closely (eg, vital signs, cardiac and CNS status, hemolytic status, hypersensitivity) during and after infusion.

Patient Education This medication can only be administered by infusion. Report immediately any swelling, pain, burning, or itching at infusion site. Report acute headache, visual changes, pain in joints or muscles, respiratory difficulty, chills, back pain, dizziness, or nausea.

Famciclovir (fam SYE kloe veer)

Brand Names: U.S. Famvir®

Pharmacologic Category Antiviral Agent

Medication Safety Issues

Sound-alike/look-alike issues:

Famvir® may be confused with Femara®

Pregnancy Risk Factor B

Lactation Excretion in breast milk unknown/not recommended

Breast-Feeding Considerations There is no specific data describing the excretion of famciclovir in breast milk. Breast-feeding is not recommended by the manufacturer unless the potential benefits outweigh any possible risk. If herpes lesions are on breast, breast-feeding should be avoided in order to avoid transmission to infant.

Use Treatment of acute herpes zoster (shingles); treatment and suppression of recurrent episodes of genital herpes in immunocompetent patients; treatment of herpes labialis (cold sores) in immunocompetent patients; treatment of recurrent mucocutaneous/genital herpes simplex in HIV-infected patients

Mechanism of Action/Effect The prodrug famciclovir undergoes rapid biotransformation to the active compound, penciclovir, then intracellular conversion to triphosphate which is active against HSV-1, HSV-2, VZV, and EBV infected cells.

Contraindications Hypersensitivity to famciclovir, penciclovir, or any component of the formulation

Warnings/Precautions Has not been studied in immunocompromised patients or patients with ophthalmic, disseminated zoster, or with initial episode of genital herpes. Dosage adjustment is required in patients with renal insufficiency. Tablets contain lactose; do not use with galactose intolerance, severe lactase deficiency, or glucose-galactose malabsorption syndromes.

Drug Interactions

Avoid Concomitant Use

Avoid concomitant use of Famciclovir with any of the following: Zoster Vaccine

Decreased Effect

Famciclovir may decrease the levels/effects of: Zoster Vaccine

Increased Effect/Toxicity There are no known significant interactions involving an increase in effect.

Nutritional/Ethanol Interactions Food: Rate of absorption and/or conversion to penciclovir and peak concentration are reduced with food, but bioavailability is not affected.

Adverse Reactions Note: Frequencies vary with dose and duration. Single-dose treatment (herpes labialis) was associated only with headache (10%), diarrhea (2%), fatigue (1%), and dysmenorrhea (1%).

>10%:

Central nervous system: Headache (14% to 39%)

Gastrointestinal: Nausea (3% to 13%)

1% to 10%:

Central nervous system: Fatigue (1% to 5%), migraine (1% to 3%)

Dermatologic: Pruritus (≤4%), rash (≤3%)

Endocrine & metabolic: Dysmenorrhea (≤8%)

Gastrointestinal: Diarrhea (5% to 9%), abdominal pain (≤8%), flatulence (1% to 5%), vomiting (1% to 5%)

Hematologic: Neutropenia (3%)

Hepatic: Transaminases increased (2% to 3%), bilirubin increased (2%)

Neuromuscular & skeletal: Paresthesia (≤3%)

Available Dosage Forms

Tablet, oral: 125 mg, 250 mg, 500 mg

Famvir®: 125 mg, 250 mg, 500 mg

General Dosage Range

Dosage adjustment recommended in patients with renal impairment

Oral: *Adults:* 250-1000 mg twice daily **or** 500 mg every 8 hours **or** 1500 mg once

Administration

Oral May be administered without regard to meals.

Stability

Storage Store at 25°C (77°F); excursions permitted to 15°C to 30°C (59°F to 86°F).

Nursing Actions

Physical Assessment Monitor for persistent fatigue and gastrointestinal upset.

Patient Education This is not a cure for genital herpes. May cause mild GI disturbances (eg, nausea, vomiting, constipation, diarrhea), fatigue, headache, or muscle aches and pains. If these are severe, contact prescriber.

Dietary Considerations May be taken without regard to meals.

Famotidine (fa MOE ti deen)

Brand Names: U.S. Heartburn Relief Maximum Strength [OTC]; Heartburn Relief [OTC]; Pepcid®; Pepcid® AC Maximum Strength [OTC]; Pepcid® AC [OTC]

Pharmacologic Category Histamine H_2 Antagonist

Medication Safety Issues

Sound-alike/look-alike issues:

Famotidine may be confused with FLUoxetine, furosemide

Pregnancy Risk Factor B

Lactation Enters breast milk/not recommended

Breast-Feeding Considerations Famotidine is excreted into breast milk with peak concentrations occurring ~6 hours after the maternal dose. According to the manufacturer, the decision to continue or discontinue breast-feeding during therapy should take into account the risk of exposure to the infant and the benefits of treatment to the mother.

Use Maintenance therapy and treatment of duodenal ulcer; treatment of gastroesophageal reflux disease (GERD), active benign gastric ulcer; pathological hypersecretory conditions

OTC labeling: Relief of heartburn, acid indigestion, and sour stomach

Unlabeled Use Part of a multidrug regimen for *H. pylori* eradication to reduce the risk of duodenal ulcer recurrence; stress ulcer prophylaxis in critically-ill patients; symptomatic relief in gastritis

Mechanism of Action/Effect Competitive inhibition of histamine at H_2 receptors of the gastric parietal cells, which inhibits gastric acid secretion

Contraindications Hypersensitivity to famotidine, other H_2 antagonists, or any component of the formulation

Warnings/Precautions Modify dose in patients with moderate-to-severe renal impairment. Prolonged QT interval has been reported in patients with renal dysfunction. The FDA has received reports of torsade de pointes occurring with famotidine (Poluzzi, 2009). Relief of symptoms does not preclude the presence of a gastric malignancy. Reversible confusional states, usually clearing within 3-4 days after discontinuation, have been linked to use. Increased age (>50 years) and renal or hepatic impairment are thought to be associated. Multidose vials for injection contain benzyl alcohol.

OTC labeling: When used for self-medication, patients should be instructed not to use if they have difficulty swallowing, are vomiting blood, or have bloody or black stools. Not for use with other acid reducers.

Drug Interactions

Avoid Concomitant Use

Avoid concomitant use of Famotidine with any of the following: Delavirdine

Decreased Effect

Famotidine may decrease the levels/effects of: Atazanavir; Cefditoren; Cefpodoxime; Cefuroxime; Dasatinib; Delavirdine; Erlotinib; Fosamprenavir; Gefitinib; Indinavir; Iron Salts; Itraconazole; Ketoconazole; Ketoconazole (Systemic);

Mesalamine; Nelfinavir; Posaconazole; Rilpivirine; Vismodegib

Increased Effect/Toxicity

Famotidine may increase the levels/effects of: Dexmethylphenidate; Methylphenidate; Saquinavir; Varenicline

Nutritional/Ethanol Interactions

Ethanol: Avoid ethanol (may cause gastric mucosal irritation).

Food: Famotidine bioavailability may be increased if taken with food.

Adverse Reactions

Note: Agitation and vomiting have been reported in up to 14% of pediatric patients <1 year of age.

1% to 10%:

Central nervous system: Headache (5%), dizziness (1%)

Gastrointestinal: Diarrhea (2%), constipation (1%)

Pharmacodynamics/Kinetics

Onset of Action Antisecretory effect: Oral: Within 1 hour; I.V.: Within 30 minutes

Peak effect: Antisecretory effect: Oral: Within 1-3 hours (dose-dependent)

Duration of Action Antisecretory effect: I.V., Oral: 10-12 hours

Available Dosage Forms

Infusion, premixed in NS [preservative free]: 20 mg (50 mL)

Injection, solution: 10 mg/mL (4 mL, 20 mL, 50 mL)

Injection, solution [preservative free]: 10 mg/mL (2 mL)

Powder for suspension, oral: 40 mg/5 mL (50 mL)

Pepcid®: 40 mg/5 mL (50 mL)

Tablet, oral: 10 mg, 20 mg, 40 mg

Heartburn Relief [OTC]: 10 mg

Heartburn Relief Maximum Strength [OTC]: 20 mg

Pepcid®: 20 mg, 40 mg

Pepcid® AC [OTC]: 10 mg

Pepcid® AC Maximum Strength [OTC]: 20 mg

Tablet, chewable, oral:

Pepcid® AC Maximum Strength [OTC]: 20 mg

General Dosage Range Dosage adjustment recommended in patients with renal impairment

I.V.:

Children 1-16 years: 0.25 mg/kg every 12 hours (maximum: 40 mg/day)

Adults: 20 mg every 12 hours

Oral:

Children <3 months: 0.5 mg/kg once daily

Children 3-12 months: 0.5 mg/kg twice daily

Children 1-11 years: 0.5-1 mg/kg/day in 1-2 divided doses (maximum: 80 mg/day)

Children 12-16 years: 0.5-1 mg/kg/day in 1-2 divided doses (maximum: 80 mg/day) **or** 10-20 mg every 12 hours (OTC dosing)

Adults: 20-40 mg/day in 1-2 divided doses **or** 20-160 mg every 6 hours [hypersecretory conditions]

Administration

Oral May administer with antacids.

Suspension: Shake vigorously before use. May be taken without regard to meals.

Tablet: May be taken without regard to meals.

I.V.

I.V. push: Inject over at least 2 minutes.

Solution for infusion: Administer over 15-30 minutes.

I.V. Detail pH: 5.7-6.4 (premixed solution); 5.0-5.6 (injection)

Stability

Reconstitution Solution for injection:

I.V. push: Dilute famotidine with NS (or another compatible solution) to a total of 5-10 mL (some centers also administer undiluted).

Infusion: Dilute with D_5W 100 mL or another compatible solution.

Storage

Oral:

Powder for oral suspension: Prior to mixing, dry powder should be stored at controlled room temperature of 25°C (77°F). Reconstituted oral suspension is stable for 30 days at room temperature; do not freeze.

Tablet: Store controlled room temperature. Protect from moisture.

I.V.:

Solution for injection: Prior to use, store at 2°C to 8°C (36°F to 46°F). If solution freezes, allow to solubilize at controlled room temperature. May be stored at room temperature for up to 3 months (data on file [Bedford Laboratories, 2011]).

I.V. push: Following preparation, solutions for I.V. push should be used immediately, or may be stored in refrigerator and used within 48 hours.

Infusion: Following preparation, the manufacturer states may be stored for up to 48 hours under refrigeration; however, solutions for infusion have been found to be physically and chemically stable for 7 days at room temperature.

Solution for injection, premixed bags: Store at controlled room temperature of 25°C (77°F); avoid excessive heat.

Nursing Actions

Physical Assessment Teach patient proper timing of administration.

Patient Education OTC: Do not use for more than 14 days unless recommended by prescriber. May cause drowsiness, dizziness, constipation, or diarrhea. Report acute headache, unresolved constipation or diarrhea, palpitations, black tarry stools, abdominal pain, rash, worsening of condition being treated, or recurrence of symptoms after therapy is completed.

Dietary Considerations May be taken without regard to meals.

Fat Emulsion (fat e MUL shun)

Brand Names: U.S. Intralipid®; Liposyn® III
Index Terms Intravenous Fat Emulsion
Pharmacologic Category Caloric Agent
Pregnancy Risk Factor C
Lactation Use with caution
Use Source of calories and essential fatty acids for patients requiring parenteral nutrition of extended duration; prevention and treatment of essential fatty acid deficiency (EFAD)
Unlabeled Use Treatment of local anesthetic-induced cardiac arrest unresponsive to conventional resuscitation
Available Dosage Forms
Injection, emulsion:
Intralipid®: 20% (100 mL, 250 mL, 500 mL, 1000 mL); 30% (500 mL)
Liposyn® III: 10% (250 mL, 500 mL); 20% (250 mL, 500 mL); 30% (500 mL)
General Dosage Range I.V.:
Infants: Initial: 1-2 g/kg/day; Maintenance: Up to 3 g/kg/day
Children: 1-2 g/kg/day; Maintenance: Up to 2-3 g/kg/day **or** 8% to 10% of caloric intake given 2-3 times weekly
Adolescents and Adults: Initial: 1 g/kg/day; Maintenance: Up to 2.5 g/kg/day **or** 8% to 10% of caloric intake given 2-3 times weekly

Administration

I.V. Can be administered in a peripheral line or by central venous infusion. At the onset of therapy, the patient should be observed for any immediate allergic reactions such as dyspnea, cyanosis, and fever. Change tubing after each infusion. May be simultaneously infused with amino acid dextrose mixtures by means of Y-connector located near infusion site or administered in total nutrient mixtures (3-in-1) with amino acids, dextrose, and other nutrients. Hang fat emulsion higher than other fluids (has low specific gravity and could run up into other lines). Infuse via a pump using either a peripheral or central venous line.
Intralipid®: Do not use <1.2 micron filter
Liposyn® III: Do not use a filter.
Caloric source/EFAD:
Children: Initiate infusions of 10% emulsions at ≤0.1 mL/minute for 10-15 minutes; if no untoward effects occur, the infusion rate may be increased to 1 mL/kg/hour. Initiate infusions of 20% emulsions at ≤0.05 mL/minute for 10-15 minutes; if no untoward effects occur, the infusion rate may be increased to 0.5 mL/kg/hour. **Note:** Premature and/or septic infants may require reduced infusion rates. Do not exceed 1 g fat/kg in 4 hours in this population.
Adults: Initiate infusions of 10% emulsions at 1 mL/minute for 15-30 minutes; if no untoward effects occur, the infusion rate may be increased to 2 mL/minute. Initiate infusions of 20% emulsions at 0.5 mL/minute for 15-30 minutes; if no untoward effects occur, the infusion rate may be increased to 1 mL/minute.
Local anesthetic toxicity: Administer initial bolus over 2-3 minutes followed by a continuous infusion. Chest compressions should continue during administration. Continue the infusion until hemodynamic stability is restored. The infusion rate may be increased if hemodynamic instability recurs (ACMT, 2010).
I.V. Detail
pH: ~6-9
Osmolality: ~300-350 mOsmol/kg water

Nursing Actions

Physical Assessment Assess for allergy to eggs prior to initiating therapy. Inspect emulsion before administering. Do not administer if oil separation or oiliness is noted. Monitor closely for allergic reactions or fluid overload.
Patient Education Report pain at infusion site or respiratory difficulty.

Febuxostat (feb UX oh stat)

Brand Names: U.S. Uloric®
Index Terms TEI-6720; TMX-67
Pharmacologic Category Antigout Agent; Xanthine Oxidase Inhibitor
Pregnancy Risk Factor C
Lactation Excretion in breast milk unknown/use caution
Use Chronic management of hyperuricemia in patients with gout
Mechanism of Action/Effect Selectively inhibits xanthine oxidase, the enzyme responsible for the conversion of hypoxanthine to xanthine to uric acid thereby decreasing uric acid.
Contraindications Concurrent use with azathioprine or mercaptopurine

Canadian labeling: Additional contraindications (not in U.S. labeling): Hypersensitivity to febuxostat or any component of the formulation; concomitant administration with theophylline
Warnings/Precautions Administer concurrently with an NSAID or colchicine (up to 6 months) to prevent gout flare upon initiation of therapy. Do not use to treat asymptomatic or secondary hyperuricemia. Significant hepatic transaminase elevations (>3 x ULN), MI, stroke and cardiovascular deaths have been reported in controlled trials (causal relationship not established). Monitor patients for signs/symptoms of MI and stroke. Liver function tests should be monitored 2 and 4 months after initiation of therapy and then periodically. Use with caution in patients with severe hepatic impairment (Child-Pugh class C); not studied. Use with caution in patients with severe renal impairment (Cl_{cr} <30 mL/minute); insufficient data.

Drug Interactions

Avoid Concomitant Use

Avoid concomitant use of Febuxostat with any of the following: AzaTHIOprine; Didanosine; Mercaptopurine

Decreased Effect There are no known significant interactions involving a decrease in effect.

Increased Effect/Toxicity

Febuxostat may increase the levels/effects of: AzaTHIOprine; Didanosine; Mercaptopurine; Theophylline Derivatives

Adverse Reactions 1% to 10%:

Dermatologic: Rash (1% to 2%)

Hepatic: Liver function abnormalities (5% to 7%)

Neuromuscular & skeletal: Arthralgia (1%)

Available Dosage Forms

Tablet, oral:

Uloric®: 40 mg, 80 mg

General Dosage Range Oral: *Adults:* 40-80 mg once daily

Administration

Oral Administer with or without meals or antacids.

Stability

Storage Store at 25°C (77°F); excursions permitted to 15°C to 30°C (59°F to 86°F). Protect from light.

Nursing Actions

Patient Education Report unusual fatigue, easy bruising or bleeding, jaundice, chest pain, shortness of breath, numbness or loss of function in extremities, or change in neurological status.

Dietary Considerations Take with or without meals or antacids.

Felodipine (fe LOE di peen)

Index Terms Plendil

Pharmacologic Category Calcium Channel Blocker; Calcium Channel Blocker, Dihydropyridine

Medication Safety Issues

Sound-alike/look-alike issues:

Plendil® may be confused with Isordil®, pindolol, Pletal®, PriLOSEC®, Prinivil®

Pregnancy Risk Factor C

Lactation Excretion in breast milk unknown/not recommended

Use Treatment of hypertension

Unlabeled Use Pediatric hypertension

Mechanism of Action/Effect Inhibits calcium ions from entering the "slow channels" or select voltage-sensitive areas of vascular smooth muscle and myocardium during depolarization

Contraindications Hypersensitivity to felodipine, any component of the formulation, or other calcium channel blocker

Warnings/Precautions Increased angina and/or MI has occurred with initiation or dosage titration of dihydropyridine calcium channel blockers, reflex tachycardia may occur resulting in angina and/or MI in patients with obstructive coronary disease especially in the absence of concurrent beta-blockade. Use with extreme caution in patients with severe aortic stenosis. Use caution in patients with heart failure and/or hypertrophic cardiomyopathy with outflow tract obstruction. Elderly patients and patients with hepatic impairment should start off with a lower dose. Peripheral edema (dose dependent) is the most common side effect (occurs within 2-3 weeks of starting therapy). Symptomatic hypotension with or without syncope can rarely occur; blood pressure must be lowered at a rate appropriate for the patient's clinical condition. Dosage titration should occur after 14 days on a given dose.

Drug Interactions

Avoid Concomitant Use

Avoid concomitant use of Felodipine with any of the following: Conivaptan; Pimozide

Decreased Effect

Felodipine may decrease the levels/effects of: Clopidogrel

The levels/effects of Felodipine may be decreased by: Barbiturates; Calcium Salts; CarBAMazepine; CYP3A4 Inducers (Strong); Deferasirox; Herbs (CYP3A4 Inducers); Herbs (Hypertensive Properties); Methylphenidate; Nafcillin; Rifamycin Derivatives; Tocilizumab; Yohimbine

Increased Effect/Toxicity

Felodipine may increase the levels/effects of: Amifostine; Antihypertensives; ARIPiprazole; Beta-Blockers; Calcium Channel Blockers (Nondihydropyridine); CYP2C8 Substrates; Fosphenytoin; Hypotensive Agents; Magnesium Salts; Neuromuscular-Blocking Agents (Nondepolarizing); Nitroprusside; Phenytoin; Pimozide; RiTUXimab; Tacrolimus; Tacrolimus (Systemic)

The levels/effects of Felodipine may be increased by: Alpha1-Blockers; Antifungal Agents (Azole Derivatives, Systemic); Calcium Channel Blockers (Nondihydropyridine); Cimetidine; Conivaptan; CycloSPORINE; CycloSPORINE (Systemic); CYP3A4 Inhibitors (Moderate); CYP3A4 Inhibitors (Strong); Dasatinib; Diazoxide; Fluconazole; Grapefruit Juice; Herbs (Hypotensive Properties); Ivacaftor; Macrolide Antibiotics; Magnesium Salts; MAO Inhibitors; Pentoxifylline; Phosphodiesterase 5 Inhibitors; Prostacyclin Analogues; Protease Inhibitors

Nutritional/Ethanol Interactions

Ethanol: Ethanol increases felodipine absorption. Management: Monitor for a greater hypotensive effect if ethanol is consumed.

Food: Compared to a fasted state, felodipine peak plasma concentrations are increased up to two-fold when taken after a meal high in fat or carbohydrates. Grapefruit juice similarly increases felodipine C_{max} by twofold. Increased therapeutic and vasodilator side effects, including severe hypotension and myocardial ischemia, may occur. Management: May be taken with a small meal that is low in fat and carbohydrates; avoid grapefruit juice during therapy.

Herb/Nutraceutical: St John's wort may decrease felodipine levels. Dong quai has estrogenic activity. Some herbal medications may worsen hypertension (eg, ephedra); garlic may have additional antihypertensive effects. Management: Avoid dong quai if using for hypertension. Avoid ephedra, yohimbe, ginseng, and garlic.

Adverse Reactions

>10%: Central nervous system: Headache (11% to 15%)

2% to 10%: Cardiovascular: Peripheral edema (2% to 17%), tachycardia (0.4% to 2.5%), flushing (4% to 7%)

Pharmacodynamics/Kinetics

Onset of Action Antihypertensive: 2-5 hours

Duration of Action Antihypertensive effect: 24 hours

Available Dosage Forms

Tablet, extended release, oral: 2.5 mg, 5 mg, 10 mg

General Dosage Range Dosage adjustment recommended in patients with hepatic impairment

Oral:

Adults: Initial: 2.5-10 mg once daily; Maintenance: 2.5-20 mg once daily (maximum: 20 mg/day)

Elderly: Initial: 2.5 mg/day

Administration

Oral Swallow tablet whole; tablet should not be divided, crushed, or chewed. May be administered without food or with a small meal that is low in fat and carbohydrates.

Nursing Actions

Physical Assessment When discontinuing, taper dose gradually.

Patient Education Take without food. Avoid concurrent alcohol (may cause dangerous hypotension). Swallow whole; do not crush or chew. May cause headache, constipation, or swelling of ankles. Report irregular heartbeat, chest pain or palpitations, persistent headache, severe constipation, peripheral swelling, weight gain, dyspnea, or respiratory changes.

Dietary Considerations May be taken with a small meal that is low in fat and carbohydrates.

Fenofibrate (fen oh FYE brate)

Brand Names: U.S. Antara®; Fenoglide®; Lipofen®; Lofibra®; TriCor®; Triglide®

Index Terms Procetofene; Proctofene

Pharmacologic Category Antilipemic Agent, Fibric Acid

Medication Safety Issues

Sound-alike/look-alike issues:

TriCor® may be confused with Fibricor®, Tracleer®

Pregnancy Risk Factor C

Lactation Excretion in breast milk unknown/not recommended

Breast-Feeding Considerations Tumor formation was observed in animal studies; nursing is not recommended if the medication cannot be discontinued.

Use Adjunct to dietary therapy for the treatment of adults with elevations of serum triglyceride levels (types IV and V hyperlipidemia); adjunct to dietary therapy for the reduction of low density lipoprotein cholesterol (LDL-C), total cholesterol (total-C), triglycerides, and apolipoprotein B (apo B), and to increase high density lipoprotein cholesterol (HDL-C) in adult patients with primary hypercholesterolemia or mixed dyslipidemia (Fredrickson types IIa and IIb)

Mechanism of Action/Effect Fenofibric acid increases VLDL catabolism by enhancing the synthesis of lipoprotein lipase; as a result of a decrease in VLDL levels, total plasma triglycerides are reduced by 30% to 60%. Modest increase in HDL occurs in some hypertriglyceridemic patients.

Contraindications Hypersensitivity to fenofibrate or any component of the formulation; hepatic dysfunction including primary biliary cirrhosis and unexplained persistent liver function abnormalities; severe renal dysfunction; pre-existing gallbladder disease; breast-feeding (only Fenoglide®)

Canadian labeling: Additional contraindications (not in U.S. labeling): Pregnancy; breast-feeding; known photoallergy or phototoxic reaction during treatment with fibrates or ketoprofen; allergy to soya lecithin or peanut or arachis oil

Warnings/Precautions Secondary causes of hyperlipidemia should be ruled out prior to therapy. Hepatic transaminases can become significantly elevated (dose-related); hepatocellular, chronic active, and cholestatic hepatitis have been reported. Regular monitoring of liver function tests is required. Increases in serum creatinine (>2 mg/dL) have been observed with use; monitor renal function in patients with renal impairment and consider monitoring patients with increased risk for developing renal impairment. May cause cholelithiasis. Use with caution in patient taking oral anticoagulants (eg, warfarin); adjustments in anticoagulation therapy may be required. Use caution with HMG-CoA reductase inhibitors (may lead to myopathy, rhabdomyolysis). In combination with HMG-CoA reductase inhibitors, fenofibrate is generally regarded as safer than gemfibrozil due to limited pharmacokinetic interaction with statins. Therapy should be withdrawn if an adequate response is not obtained after 2-3 months of therapy at the maximal daily dose. The occurrence of pancreatitis may represent a failure of efficacy in patients with severely elevated triglycerides. May cause mild-to-moderate decreases in hemoglobin, hematocrit, and WBC upon initiation of therapy which usually stabilizes with long-term therapy. Agranulocytosis and thrombocytopenia have rarely been reported. Periodic monitoring of blood counts is recommended during the first year of therapy.

Rare hypersensitivity reactions may occur. Use has been associated with pulmonary embolism (PE) and deep vein thrombosis (DVT). Use with caution in patients with risk factors for VTE. Dose adjustment is required for renal impairment and may be required for elderly patients.

Drug Interactions

Avoid Concomitant Use There are no known interactions where it is recommended to avoid concomitant use.

Decreased Effect

Fenofibrate may decrease the levels/effects of: Chenodiol; CycloSPORINE; CycloSPORINE (Systemic); Ursodiol

The levels/effects of Fenofibrate may be decreased by: Bile Acid Sequestrants; Tocilizumab

Increased Effect/Toxicity

Fenofibrate may increase the levels/effects of: Colchicine; Ezetimibe; HMG-CoA Reductase Inhibitors; Sulfonylureas; Vitamin K Antagonists; Warfarin

The levels/effects of Fenofibrate may be increased by: Conivaptan; CycloSPORINE; CycloSPORINE (Systemic)

Adverse Reactions

>10%: Hepatic: Liver function tests increased (dose related; 3% to 13%)

1% to 10%:

Central nervous system: Headache (3%)

Gastrointestinal: Abdominal pain (5%), constipation (2%), nausea (2%)

Neuromuscular & skeletal: Back pain (3%), CPK increased (3%)

Respiratory: Respiratory disorder (6%), rhinitis (2%)

Available Dosage Forms

Capsule, oral: 67 mg, 134 mg, 200 mg

Antara®: 43 mg, 130 mg

Lipofen®: 50 mg, 150 mg

Lofibra®: 67 mg, 134 mg, 200 mg

Tablet, oral: 54 mg, 160 mg

Fenoglide®: 40 mg, 120 mg

Lofibra®: 54 mg, 160 mg

TriCor®: 48 mg, 145 mg

Triglide®: 50 mg, 160 mg

General Dosage Range Dosage adjustment recommended in patients with renal impairment

Oral: *Adults and Elderly:* Dosage varies greatly depending on product

Administration

Oral 6-8 weeks of therapy is required to determine efficacy.

Fenoglide®, Lofibra® (capsules [micronized] and tablets), Lipofen®: Administer with meals.

Antara®, TriCor®: May be administered with or without food.

Triglide®: Do not consume chipped or broken tablets. May be administered with or without food.

Canadian products [not available in U.S.]:

Lipidil Micro®, Lipidil Supra®: Administer with meals.

Lipidil EZ®: May be administered with or without food.

Stability

Storage Store at 15°C to 30°C (59°F to 86°F). Protect from light and moisture. Store tablets in moisture-protective container.

Nursing Actions

Physical Assessment Monitor LFTs and blood counts on a regular basis throughout therapy. Monitor for myopathy, rhabdomyolysis, gastrointestinal upset, and myalgia.

Patient Education Maintain diet and exercise program as prescribed. If you are a diabetic taking a sulfonylurea, monitor blood sugars closely; this medication may alter the effects of your antidiabetic medication. You may experience mild GI disturbances (eg, abdominal pain, constipation, nausea); inform prescriber if these are severe. Report immediately unusual muscle pain or weakness; skin rash or irritation; insomnia; persistent dizziness; chest pain or palpitations; difficult respirations; or pain, swelling, redness, or heat in extremities.

Dietary Considerations

Fenoglide®, Lofibra® (capsules [micronized] and tablets), Lipofen®: Take with meals.

Antara®, TriCor®, Triglide®: May be taken with or without food.

Canadian products [not available in U.S.]:

Lipidil Micro®, Lipidil Supra®: Take with meals.

Lipidil EZ®: May be taken with or without food.

Fenofibric Acid (fen oh FYE brik AS id)

Brand Names: U.S. Fibricor®; TriLipix®

Index Terms ABT-335; Choline Fenofibrate

Pharmacologic Category Antilipemic Agent, Fibric Acid

Medication Safety Issues

Sound-alike/look-alike issues:

Fibricor® may be confused with Tricor®

TriLipix® may be confused with Trileptal®, TriLyte®

Medication Guide Available Yes

Pregnancy Risk Factor C

Lactation Excretion in breast milk unknown/contraindicated

Use Adjunct to dietary therapy for the treatment of severely elevated serum triglyceride levels; adjunct to dietary therapy for the reduction of low density lipoprotein cholesterol (LDL-C), total cholesterol (total-C), triglycerides, and apolipoprotein B (apo B) and to increase high density lipoprotein cholesterol (HDL-C) in patients with primary hypercholesterolemia or mixed dyslipidemia

TriLipix™ is also indicated as adjunct to dietary therapy concomitantly with a statin to reduce triglyceride levels and increase HDL-C levels in patients with mixed dyslipidemia and coronary heart disease (CHD) or at risk for CHD

Mechanism of Action/Effect Fenofibric acid increases VLDL catabolism by enhancing the synthesis of lipoprotein lipase; as a result of a decrease in VLDL levels, total plasma triglycerides are reduced by 30% to 60%; modest increased in HDL occurs in some hypertriglyceridemia patients.

Contraindications Hypersensitivity to fenofibric acid, choline fenofibrate, fenofibrate, or any component of the formulation; hepatic dysfunction including primary biliary cirrhosis and unexplained persistent liver function abnormalities; severe renal dysfunction (including patients on dialysis); preexisting gallbladder disease; breast-feeding

Warnings/Precautions Secondary causes of hyperlipidemia should be ruled out prior to therapy. Has been associated with rare myositis or rhabdomyolysis; patients should be monitored closely. Risk increased in the elderly, patients with diabetes mellitus, renal failure, or hypothyroidism. Patients should be instructed to report unexplained muscle pain, tenderness, weakness, or brown urine. Hepatic transaminases can become significantly elevated (dose-related); hepatocellular, chronic active, and cholestatic hepatitis have been reported. Regular monitoring of liver function tests is required. Increases in serum creatinine (>2 mg/dL) have been observed with use; monitor renal function in patients with renal impairment and consider monitoring patients with increased risk for developing renal impairment. May cause cholelithiasis discontinue if gallstones found upon gallbladder studies. Use caution with oral anticoagulants; adjustments in therapy may be required.

Use caution with HMG-CoA reductase inhibitors (may lead to myopathy, rhabdomyolysis). In combination with HMG-CoA reductase inhibitors, fenofibric acid derivatives are generally regarded as safer than gemfibrozil due to limited pharmacokinetic interaction. Therapy should be withdrawn if an adequate response is not obtained after 2-3 months of therapy at the maximal daily dose. The occurrence of pancreatitis may represent a failure of efficacy in patients with severely elevated triglycerides. May cause mild-to-moderate decreases in hemoglobin, hematocrit, and WBC upon initiation of therapy, which usually stabilizes with long-term therapy. Rare hypersensitivity reactions may occur. Use has been associated with pulmonary embolism (PE) and deep vein thrombosis (DVT). Use with caution in patients with risk factors for VTE. Dose adjustment is required for renal impairment and elderly patients.

Drug Interactions

Avoid Concomitant Use There are no known interactions where it is recommended to avoid concomitant use.

Decreased Effect

Fenofibric Acid may decrease the levels/effects of: Chenodiol; CycloSPORINE; CycloSPORINE (Systemic); Ursodiol

The levels/effects of Fenofibric Acid may be decreased by: Bile Acid Sequestrants

Increased Effect/Toxicity

Fenofibric Acid may increase the levels/effects of: Carvedilol; Colchicine; CYP2C9 Substrates; Ezetimibe; HMG-CoA Reductase Inhibitors; Sulfonylureas; Vitamin K Antagonists; Warfarin

The levels/effects of Fenofibric Acid may be increased by: CycloSPORINE; CycloSPORINE (Systemic)

Adverse Reactions Adverse reactions and frequency reported as observed during monotherapy and concurrent administration with a statin (HMG-CoA reductase inhibitor).

>10%: Central nervous system: Headache (12% to 13%)

1% to 10%:

Central nervous system: Dizziness (3% to 4%), pain (1% to 4%), fatigue (2% to 3%)

Gastrointestinal: Nausea (4% to 6%), dyspepsia (3% to 5%), diarrhea (3% to 4%), constipation (3%)

Hepatic: ALT increased (monotherapy: 1%; coadministered with statin: 3%)

Neuromuscular & skeletal: Back pain (4% to 6%), pain in extremities (3% to 5%), arthralgia (4%), myalgia (3% to 4%), muscle spasm (2% to 3%)

Respiratory: Nasopharyngitis (4% to 5%), upper respiratory infection (4% to 5%), sinusitis (3% to 4%)

Additional adverse reactions when fenofibric acid coadministered with a statin (frequency not defined): AST increased, bronchitis, cough, CPK increased, hepatic enzymes increased, hypertension, influenza, insomnia, musculoskeletal pain, pharyngolaryngeal pain, urinary tract infection

Available Dosage Forms

Capsule, delayed release, oral:

TriLipix®: 45 mg, 135 mg

Tablet, oral: 35 mg, 105 mg

Fibricor®: 35 mg, 105 mg

General Dosage Range Dosage adjustment recommended in patients with renal impairment

Oral: *Adults:* Fibricor®: 35-105 mg once daily (maximum: 105 mg/day); TriLipix™: 45-135 mg once daily (maximum: 135 mg/day)

Administration

Oral May be administered with or without food.

Stability

Storage Store at 25°C (77°F); excursions permitted to 15°C to 30°C (59°F to 86°F). Protect from light and moisture.

Nursing Actions

Physical Assessment Teach patient to report signs of myopathy, rhabdomyolysis, and liver dysfunction.

Patient Education May take with or without food. Maintain diet and exercise program as prescribed. If you have diabetes and are taking a sulfonylurea, monitor blood sugars closely; this medication may improve the effects of your antidiabetic medication. You will require scheduled blood tests to determine appropriate dosage and to reduce potential for adverse effects; maintaining laboratory testing schedule is vital. May cause mild GI disturbances (eg, gas, diarrhea, constipation, nausea); inform prescriber if these are severe. Report immediately unusual muscle, back, or joint pain, spasms, or weakness; yellowing of skin or eyes; unusual or increased bruising or bleeding; or persistent fatigue.

Dietary Considerations May be taken with or without food. Patients should follow appropriate lipid-lowering diet.

Fenoprofen (fen oh PROE fen)

Brand Names: U.S. Nalfon®

Index Terms Fenoprofen Calcium

Pharmacologic Category Nonsteroidal Anti-inflammatory Drug (NSAID), Oral

Medication Safety Issues

Sound-alike/look-alike issues:

Fenoprofen may be confused with flurbiprofen

Medication Guide Available Yes

Pregnancy Risk Factor C

Lactation Enters breast milk/not recommended

Use Symptomatic treatment of acute and chronic rheumatoid arthritis and osteoarthritis; relief of mild-to-moderate pain

Available Dosage Forms

Capsule, oral:

Nalfon®: 200 mg, 400 mg

Tablet, oral: 600 mg

General Dosage Range Oral: *Adults:* 200 mg every 4-6 hours as needed **or** 300-600 mg 3-4 times/day (maximum: 3.2 g/day)

Administration

Oral Do not crush tablets. Swallow whole with a full glass of water. Take with food to minimize stomach upset.

Nursing Actions

Physical Assessment Monitor blood pressure at the beginning of therapy and periodically during use. Monitor for adverse gastrointestinal effects or ototoxicity at beginning of therapy and periodically throughout.

Patient Education Do not crush tablets or break capsules. Take with food or milk to reduce GI distress. Do not use alcohol. You may experience drowsiness, dizziness, nervousness, headache, anorexia, nausea, vomiting, heartburn, or fluid retention; GI bleeding, ulceration, or perforation can occur with or without pain; discontinue medication and contact prescriber if persistent abdominal pain or cramping or blood in stool occurs. Report respiratory difficulty or unusual cough; chest pain, rapid heartbeat, or palpitations; bruising/bleeding; blood in urine, stool, mouth, or vomitus; swollen extremities; skin rash; weakness in one side or part of body; slurred speech; persistent nausea; yellowing of skin or eyes; abdominal pain; or ringing in ears.

FentaNYL (FEN ta nil)

Brand Names: U.S. Abstral®; Actiq®; Duragesic®; Fentora®; Lazanda®; Onsolis™

Index Terms Fentanyl Citrate; Fentanyl Hydrochloride; Fentanyl Patch; OTFC (Oral Transmucosal Fentanyl Citrate); Subsys®

Pharmacologic Category Analgesic, Opioid; Anilidopiperidine Opioid; General Anesthetic

Medication Safety Issues

Sound-alike/look-alike issues:

FentaNYL may be confused with alfentanil, SUFentanil

High alert medication:

The Institute for Safe Medication Practices (ISMP) includes this medication among its list of drug classes which have a heightened risk of causing significant patient harm when used in error.

Administration issues:

Fentanyl transdermal system patches: Leakage of fentanyl gel from the patch has been reported; patch may be less effective; do not use. Thoroughly wash any skin surfaces coming into direct contact with gel with water (do not use soap). May contain conducting metal (eg, aluminum); remove patch prior to MRI.

Other safety concerns:

Dosing of transdermal fentanyl patches may be confusing. Transdermal fentanyl patches should always be prescribed in mcg/hour, not size. Patch dosage form of Duragesic®-12 actually delivers 12.5 mcg/hour of fentanyl. Use caution, as orders may be written as "Duragesic 12.5" which can be erroneously interpreted as a 125 mcg dose.

Fentora®, Onsolis™, Abstral®, and Actiq® are not interchangeable; do not substitute doses on a mcg-per-mcg basis.

Medication Guide Available Yes

Pregnancy Risk Factor C

Lactation Enters breast milk/not recommended (AAP rates "compatible"; AAP 2001 update pending)

Breast-Feeding Considerations Fentanyl is excreted in low concentrations into breast milk. Breast-feeding is considered acceptable following single doses to the mother; however, limited information is available when used long-term. **Note:** Transdermal patch, transmucosal lozenge, sublingual tablet, buccal tablet (Fentora®), and buccal film (Onsolis™) are not recommended in nursing women due to potential for sedation and/or respiratory depression. Symptoms of opioid withdrawal may occur in infants following the cessation of breast-feeding.

Use

Injection: Relief of pain, preoperative medication, adjunct to general or regional anesthesia

Iontophoretic transdermal system (Ionsys™): Short-term, in-hospital management of acute postoperative pain

Transdermal patch (eg, Duragesic®): Management of persistent moderate-to-severe chronic pain

Transmucosal lozenge (eg, Actiq®), buccal tablet (Fentora®), buccal film (Onsolis™), nasal spray (Lazanda®), sublingual tablet (Abstral®): Management of breakthrough cancer pain in opioid-tolerant patients

Mechanism of Action/Effect Binds with stereospecific receptors at many sites within the CNS, increases pain threshold, alters pain reception, inhibits ascending pain pathways

Contraindications Hypersensitivity to fentanyl or any component of the formulation

Transdermal system: Severe respiratory disease or depression including acute asthma (unless patient is mechanically ventilated); paralytic ileus; patients requiring short-term therapy, management of intermittent pain

Transmucosal buccal tablets (Fentora®), buccal films (Onsolis™), lozenges (eg, Actiq®), sublingual tablets (Abstral®), nasal spray (Lazanda®), and/or transdermal patches (eg, Duragesic®): Contraindicated in the management of acute or postoperative pain (including headache, migraine, dental pain, or use in emergency room), and in patients who are not opioid tolerant

Canadian labeling: Additional contraindication (not in U.S. labeling): Sublingual tablets (Abstral™): Severe respiratory depression or severe obstructive lung disease

Warnings/Precautions An opioid-containing analgesic regimen should be tailored to each patient's needs and based upon the type of pain being treated (acute versus chronic), the route of administration, degree of tolerance for opioids (naive versus chronic user), age, weight, and medical condition. The optimal analgesic dose varies widely among patients. Doses should be titrated to pain relief/prevention. May cause CNS depression, which may impair physical or mental abilities; patients must be cautioned about performing tasks which require mental alertness (eg, operating machinery or driving). When using with other CNS depressants, reduce dose of one or both agents. Fentanyl shares the toxic potentials of opiate agonists, and precautions of opiate agonist therapy should be observed; use with caution in patients with bradycardia or bradyarrhythmias; rapid I.V. infusion may result in skeletal muscle and chest wall rigidity leading to respiratory distress and/or apnea, bronchoconstriction, laryngospasm; inject slowly over 3-5 minutes. **[U.S. Boxed Warning]: Healthcare provider should be alert to problems of abuse, misuse, and diversion.** Tolerance or drug dependence may result from extended use. The elderly may be particularly susceptible to the CNS depressant and constipating effects of narcotics. Use extreme caution in patients with COPD or other chronic respiratory conditions. Use caution with head injuries, morbid obesity, renal impairment, or hepatic dysfunction. **[U.S. Boxed Warning]: Use with strong or moderate CYP3A4 inhibitors may result in increased effects and potentially fatal respiratory depression.** Use is not recommended with MAO inhibitors or within 14 days of MAO inhibitor use; severe and unpredictable adverse effects may result. Concurrent use of agonist/antagonist analgesics may precipitate withdrawal symptoms and/or reduced analgesic efficacy in patients following prolonged therapy with mu opioid agonists. Abrupt discontinuation following prolonged use may also lead to withdrawal symptoms.

[U.S. Boxed Warning]: Safety and efficacy of the transdermal patch have been limited to children ≥2 years of age who are opioid-tolerant. [U.S. Boxed Warning]: Buccal film (Onsolis™), nasal spray (Lazanda®), sublingual tablet (Abstral®): Not indicated for use in cancer patients <18 years of age. Indicated only for cancer patients who are opioid tolerant and are ≥18 years of age. [U.S. Boxed Warning]: Buccal film, buccal tablet, nasal spray, sublingual tablet, and lozenge preparations contain an amount of medication that can be fatal to children. Keep all used and unused products out of the reach of children at all times and discard products properly. Patients and caregivers should be counseled on the dangers to children including the risk of exposure to partially-consumed products.

[U.S. Boxed Warning] Abstral®, Actiq®, Duragesic®, Fentora®, Lazanda®, Onsolis™: May cause potentially life-threatening hypoventilation, respiratory depression, and/or death; Abstral®, Actiq®, Duragesic®, Fentora®, Lazanda®, or Onsolis™ should only be prescribed for opioid-tolerant patients. Risk of respiratory depression increased in elderly patients, debilitated patients, and patients with conditions associated with hypoxia or hypercapnia; usually occurs after administration of initial dose in nontolerant patients or when given with other drugs that depress respiratory function.

Nasal spray (Lazanda®): **[U.S. Boxed Warning]: Should be used only for the care of opioid-tolerant cancer patients with breakthrough pain who are already receiving opioid therapy for their underlying persistent cancer pain. Intended to be prescribed only by health care professionals who are knowledgeable in treating cancer pain. Use is contraindicated in opioid nontolerant patients or in the management of acute or postoperative pain, including headache/migraine, dental pain, or use in the ER. [U.S. Boxed Warning]: Available only through the Lazanda REMS program. Prescribers who prescribe to outpatients, pharmacies (inpatient and outpatient), outpatients, and distributors are required to enroll in the program. [U.S. Boxed Warning]: Due to differing pharmacokinetics of fentanyl in the nasal spray formulation, do not substitute Lazanda® on a mcg-per-mcg basis for any other fentanyl product. Serious adverse events, including death, may occur when used inappropriately (improper dose or patient selection). All patients must begin therapy with a 100 mcg dose and titrate, if needed. During therapy, patients must wait at least 2 hours before taking another dose of nasal spray.** Allergic rhinitis is not expected to alter fentanyl absorption following nasal administration; however, use of nasal decongestants (eg, oxymetazoline) during episodes of rhinitis may result in lower peak concentrations and delayed T_{max}, therefore, titration of the nasal spray is not recommended during use of nasal decongestants.

Transmucosal: Lozenge (eg, Actiq®), buccal tablet (Fentora®), buccal film (Onsolis™), sublingual tablet (Abstral®): **[U.S. Boxed Warning]: Should be used only for the care of opioid-tolerant cancer patients with breakthrough pain and is intended for use by specialists who are knowledgeable in treating cancer pain.** Not approved for use in management of acute or postoperative pain.

Transmucosal: Buccal film (eg, Onsolis™): **[U.S. Boxed Warning]: Available only through the FOCUS Program, a restricted distribution program with prescriber, pharmacy, and patient required enrollment. [U.S. Boxed Warning]: Onsolis™ is contraindicated in the management of acute or postoperative pain, including headache/migraine. [U.S. Boxed Warning]: Due to higher bioavailability of fentanyl in the buccal film formulation, do not substitute Onsolis™ on a mcg-per-mcg basis for any other fentanyl product. Serious adverse events, including death, may occur when used inappropriately (improper dose or patient selection). All patients must begin therapy with a 200 mcg dose and titrate, if needed. During therapy, patients must wait at least 2 hours before taking another dose.**

Transmucosal: Buccal tablet (Fentora®): **[U.S. Boxed Warning]: Available only through the FENTORA REMS program. Prescribers who prescribe to outpatients, outpatients, pharmacies, and distributors are required to enroll in the program. [U.S. Boxed Warning]: Due to the higher bioavailability of fentanyl in Fentora®, when converting patients from oral transmucosal fentanyl citrate (OTFC, Actiq®) to Fentora®, do not substitute Fentora®): on a mcg-per-mcg basis for any other fentanyl product. [U.S. Boxed Warning]: Fentora® is contraindicated in the management of acute or postoperative pain, including headache/migraine. Serious adverse events, including death, have been reported when used inappropriately (improper dose or patient selection). [U.S. Boxed Warning]: Patients using Fentora® who experience breakthrough pain may only take one additional dose using the same strength and must wait four hours before taking another dose.**

Transmucosal: Lozenge (Actiq®): **[U.S. Boxed Warning]: Available only through the ACTIQ REMS program. Prescribers who prescribe to outpatients, outpatients, pharmacies, and distributors are required to enroll in the program. [U.S. Boxed Warning]: The substitution of Actiq® for any other fentanyl product may result in a fatal overdose. Do not convert patients on a mcg-per-mcg basis to Actiq® from other fentanyl products. Do not substitute Actiq® for any other fentanyl product. [U.S. Boxed Warning]: Patients using fentanyl lozenges who experience breakthrough pain may only take 1 additional dose using the same strength and must wait 4 hours before taking another dose.**

Transmucosal: Sublingual tablet (Abstral®): **[U.S. Boxed Warning]: Available only through the ABSTRAL REMS program. Prescribers who prescribe to outpatients, outpatients, pharmacies, and distributors are required to enroll in the program. [U.S. Boxed Warning]: Abstral® is contraindicated in opioid nontolerant patients. [U.S. Boxed Warning]: Due to differing pharmacokinetics of fentanyl in the sublingual tablet formulation, do not substitute Abstral® on a mcg-per-mcg basis for any other fentanyl product. Serious adverse events, including death, may occur when used inappropriately (improper dose or patient selection). All patients must begin therapy with a 100 mcg dose. During therapy, patients must wait at least 2 hours before treating another episode of breakthrough pain.**

Transdermal patches (eg, Duragesic®): **[U.S. Boxed Warning]: Indicated for the management of persistent moderate-to-severe pain when around the clock pain control is needed for an extended time period. Should only be used in patients who are already receiving opioid therapy, are opioid tolerant, and who require a total daily dose equivalent to 25 mcg/hour transdermal patch. Contraindicated in patients who are not opioid tolerant, in the management of short-term analgesia, or in the management of postoperative pain. Should be applied only to intact skin. Use of a patch that has been cut, damaged, or altered in any way may result in overdosage.** Serum fentanyl concentrations may increase approximately one-third for patients with a body temperature of 40°C secondary to a temperature-dependent increase in fentanyl release from the patch and increased skin permeability. **[U.S. Boxed Warning]: Avoid exposure of application site and surrounding area to direct external heat sources.** Patients who experience fever or increase in core temperature should be monitored closely. Patients who experience adverse reactions should be monitored for at least 24 hours after removal of the patch. Transdermal patch may contain conducting metal (eg, aluminum); remove patch prior to MRI.

Drug Interactions

Avoid Concomitant Use

Avoid concomitant use of FentaNYL with any of the following: Crizotinib; MAO Inhibitors; Pimozide

Decreased Effect

FentaNYL may decrease the levels/effects of: Ioflupane I 123; Pegvisomant

The levels/effects of FentaNYL may be decreased by: Alpha-/Beta-Agonists (Indirect-Acting); Alpha1-Agonists; Ammonium Chloride; Mixed Agonist / Antagonist Opioids; Rifamycin Derivatives; Tocilizumab

Increased Effect/Toxicity

FentaNYL may increase the levels/effects of: Alcohol (Ethyl); Alvimopan; ARIPiprazole; Beta-Blockers; Calcium Channel Blockers (Nondihydropyridine); CNS Depressants; Desmopressin; MAO Inhibitors; Pimozide; Selective Serotonin Reuptake Inhibitors; Thiazide Diuretics

The levels/effects of FentaNYL may be increased by: Amphetamines; Antipsychotic Agents (Phenothiazines); Crizotinib; CYP3A4 Inhibitors (Moderate); CYP3A4 Inhibitors (Strong); Dasatinib; Droperidol; HydrOXYzine; Ivacaftor; MAO Inhibitors; Succinylcholine

Nutritional/Ethanol Interactions

Ethanol: Ethanol may increase CNS depression. Management: Monitor for increased effects with coadministration. Caution patients about effects.

Food: Fentanyl concentrations may be increased by grapefruit juice. Management: Avoid concurrent intake of large quantities (>1 quart/day) of grapefruit juice.

Herb/Nutraceutical: St John's wort may decrease fentanyl levels; gotu kola, valerian, and kava kava may increase CNS depression. Management: Avoid St John's wort, gotu kola, valerian, and kava kava.

Adverse Reactions

>10%:

Cardiovascular: Bradycardia, edema

Central nervous system: CNS depression, confusion, dizziness, drowsiness, fatigue, headache, sedation

Endocrine & metabolic: Dehydration

Gastrointestinal: Constipation, nausea, vomiting, xerostomia

Local: Application-site reaction erythema

Neuromuscular & skeletal: Chest wall rigidity (high dose I.V.), muscle rigidity, weakness

Ocular: Miosis

Respiratory: Dyspnea, respiratory depression

Miscellaneous: Diaphoresis

1% to 10%:

Cardiovascular: Cardiac arrhythmia, cardiorespiratory arrest, chest pain, DVT, flushing, hyper-/hypotension, orthostatic hypotension, pallor, palpitation, peripheral edema, syncope, tachycardia, vasodilation

Central nervous system: Abnormal dreams, abnormal thinking, agitation, amnesia, anxiety, attention disturbance, depression, disorientation, dysphoria, euphoria, fever, hallucinations, hypoesthesia, insomnia, lethargy, malaise, mental status change, migraine, nervousness, paranoid reaction, somnolence, stupor, vertigo

Dermatologic: Alopecia, bruising, cellulitis, decubitus ulcer, erythema, hyperhidrosis, papules, pruritus, rash

Endocrine & metabolic: Breast pain, dehydration, hot flashes, hyper-/hypocalcemia, hyper-/hypoglycemia, hypoalbuminemia, hypokalemia, hypomagnesemia

Gastrointestinal: Abdominal pain, abnormal taste, anorexia, appetite decreased, biliary tract spasm, diarrhea, dyspepsia, dysphagia (buccal tablet/film), flatulence, gastritis, GI hemorrhage, gingival pain (buccal tablet), gingivitis (lozenge), glossitis (lozenge), ileus, intestinal obstruction (buccal film), periodontal abscess (lozenge/buccal tablet), proctalgia, stomatitis (lozenge/buccal tablet/sublingual tablet), tongue disorder (sublingual tablet), ulceration (gingival, lip, mouth; transmucosal use/nasal spray), weight loss

Genitourinary: Dysuria, erectile dysfunction, urinary incontinence, urinary retention, urinary tract infection, vaginitis, vaginal hemorrhage

Hematologic: Anemia, leukopenia, neutropenia, thrombocytopenia

Hepatic: Alkaline phosphatase increased, ascites, jaundice

Local: Application site pain, application site irritation

Neuromuscular & skeletal: Abnormal coordination, abnormal gait, arthralgia, back pain, limb pain, myalgia, neuropathy, paresthesia, rigors, tremor

Ocular: Blurred vision, diplopia, dry eye, swelling, ptosis, strabismus

Renal: Renal failure

Respiratory: Apnea, asthma, bronchitis, cough, epistaxis, hemoptysis, hypoventilation, hypoxia, nasal congestion (nasal spray), nasal discomfort (nasal spray), nasopharyngitis, pharyngolaryngeal pain, pharyngitis, pneumonia, postnasal drip (nasal spray), pulmonary embolism (nasal spray), rhinitis, rhinorrhea (nasal spray), sinusitis, upper respiratory infection, wheezing

Miscellaneous: Flu-like syndrome, hiccups, hypersensitivity, lymphadenopathy, night sweats, parosmia, speech disorder, withdrawal syndrome

Pharmacodynamics/Kinetics

Onset of Action Analgesic: I.M.: 7-8 minutes; I.V.: Almost immediate; Transdermal (initial placement): 6 hours; Transmucosal: 5-15 minutes

Peak effect: Analgesic: Transdermal (initial placement): 12 hours; Transmucosal: 15-30 minutes

Duration of Action I.M.: 1-2 hours; I.V.: 0.5-1 hour; Transdermal (removal of patch/no replacement): 12 hours; Transmucosal: Related to blood level; respiratory depressant effect may last longer than analgesic effect

Product Availability

Subsys® sublingual spray: FDA approved January 2012; availability is currently undetermined. Consult prescribing information for additional information.

Subsys® is a fentanyl sublingual spray formulation indicated for the management of breakthrough cancer pain in opioid-tolerant patients.

Controlled Substance C-II

Available Dosage Forms

Film, for buccal application:

Onsolis™: 200 mcg (30s); 400 mcg (30s); 600 mcg (30s); 800 mcg (30s); 1200 mcg (30s)

Injection, solution [preservative free]: 0.05 mg/mL (2 mL, 5 mL, 10 mL, 20 mL, 30 mL, 50 mL)

Lozenge, oral: 200 mcg (30s); 400 mcg (30s); 600 mcg (30s); 800 mcg (30s); 1200 mcg (30s); 1600 mcg (30s)

Actiq®: 200 mcg (30s); 400 mcg (30s); 600 mcg (30s); 800 mcg (30s); 1200 mcg (30s); 1600 mcg (30s)

Patch, transdermal: 12 [delivers 12.5 mcg/hr] (5s); 25 [delivers 25 mcg/hr] (5s); 50 [delivers 50 mcg/hr] (5s); 75 [delivers 75 mcg/hr] (5s); 100 [delivers 100 mcg/hr] (5s)

Duragesic®: 12 [delivers 12.5 mcg/hr] (5s); 25 [delivers 25 mcg/hr] (5s); 50 [delivers 50 mcg/hr] (5s); 75 [delivers 75 mcg/hr] (5s); 100 [delivers 100 mcg/hr] (5s)

Powder, for prescription compounding: USP: 100% (1 g)

Solution, intranasal, as citrate [spray]:

Lazanda®: 100 mcg/spray (5 mL); 400 mcg/spray (5 mL) [delivers 8 metered sprays]

Tablet, for buccal application:

Fentora®: 100 mcg (28s); 200 mcg (28s); 400 mcg (28s); 600 mcg (28s); 800 mcg (28s)

Tablet, sublingual:

Abstral®: 100 mcg (12s, 32s); 200 mcg (12s, 32s); 300 mcg (12s, 32s); 400 mcg (12s, 32s); 600 mcg (32s); 800 mcg (32s)

General Dosage Range

I.M.: *Adults:* 50-100 mcg/dose as a single dose

I.V.:

Children 2-12 years: 2-3 mcg/kg/dose every 1-2 hours

Children >12 years and Adults: 25-100 mcg as a single dose

Adults: Mechanically-ventilated patients (based on 70 kg patient) (unlabeled): 0.35-1.5 mcg/kg every 30-60 minutes as needed; Infusion: 0.7-10 mcg/kg/**hour**

Nasal: *Adults:* Initial 100 mcg; Maintenance dose range: 100-800 mcg; maximum single dose: 800 mcg; maximum frequency: 4 administrations/day

Transmucosal:

Buccal film (Onsolis™): *Adults:* Initial: 200 mcg; Maintenance dose range: 200-1200 mcg; maximum dose: 1200 mcg film; maximum frequency: 4 applications/day

Buccal tablet (Fentora®): *Adults:* Initial: 100 mcg; may repeat (maximum: 2 doses per breakthrough pain episode every 4 hours)

Lozenge (Actiq®): *Children ≥16 years and Adults:* Initial: 200 mcg; may repeat (maximum: 2 doses per breakthrough pain episode every 4 hours; maximum daily dose: 4 units/day)

Sublingual tablet (Abstral®): *Adults:* Initial: 100 mcg; may repeat (maximum: 2 doses per breakthrough pain episode every 2 hours); usual maximum: 800 mcg/dose

Transdermal: *Children ≥2 years and Adults:* 12.5-300 mcg/hour applied every 72 hours

Administration

Oral

Lozenge: Foil overwrap should be removed just prior to administration. Place the unit in mouth between the cheek and gum and allow it to dissolve. Do not chew. Lozenge may be moved from one side of the mouth to the other. The unit should be consumed over a period of 15 minutes. Handle should be removed after the lozenge is consumed; early removal should be considered if the patient has achieved an adequate response and/or shows signs of respiratory depression.

Buccal film: Foil overwrap should be removed just prior to administration. Prior to placing film, wet inside of cheek using tongue or by rinsing with water. Place film inside mouth with the pink side of the unit against the inside of the moistened cheek. With finger, press the film against cheek and hold for 5 seconds. The film should stick to the inside of cheek after 5 seconds. The film should be left in place until it dissolves (usually within 15-30 minutes after application). Liquids may be consumed after 5 minutes of application. Food can be eaten after film dissolves. If using more than 1 film simultaneously (during titration period), apply films on either side of mouth (do not apply on top of each other). Do not chew or swallow film. Do not cut or tear the film. All patients must initiate therapy using the 200 mcg film.

Buccal tablet: Patient should not open blister until ready to administer. The blister backing should be peeled back to expose the tablet; tablet should not be pushed out through the blister. Immediately use tablet once removed from blister. Place entire tablet in the buccal cavity (above a rear molar, between the upper cheek and gum). Tablet should not be broken, sucked, chewed, or swallowed. Should dissolve in about 14-25 minutes when left between the cheek and the gum. If remnants remain they may be swallowed with water.

Sublingual tablet: Remove from the blister unit immediately prior to administration. Place tablet directly under the tongue on the floor of the mouth and allow to completely dissolve; do not chew, suck, or swallow. Do not eat or drink anything until tablet is completely dissolved. In patients with a dry mouth, water may be used to moisten the buccal mucosa just before administration. All patients must initiate therapy using the 100 mcg tablet.

I.V. Administer as slow I.V. infusion over 1-2 minutes. May also be administered as continuous infusion or PCA (unlabeled use) routes. Muscular rigidity may occur with rapid I.V. administration.

I.V. Detail pH: 4.0-7.5

Topical

Nasal spray: Prior to initial use, prime device by spraying 4 sprays into the provided pouch (the counting window will show a green bar when the bottle is ready for use). Insert nozzle a short distance into the nose (~1/2 inch or 1 cm) and point towards the bridge of the nose (while closing off the other nostril using 1 finger). Press on finger grips until a "click" sound is heard and the number in the counting window advances by one. The "click" sound and dose counter are the only reliable methods for ensuring a dose has been administered (spray is not always felt on the nasal mucosa). Patient should remain seated for at least 1 minute following administration. Do not blow nose for ≥30 minutes after administration. Wash hands before and after use. There are 8 full therapeutic sprays in each bottle; do not continue to use bottle after "8" sprays have been used. Dispose of bottle and contents if ≥5 days have passed since last use or if it has been ≥4 days since bottle was primed. Spray the remaining contents into the provided pouch, seal in the child-resistant container, and dispose of in the trash.

Transdermal patch (eg, Duragesic®): Apply to nonirritated and nonirradiated skin, such as chest, back, flank, or upper arm. Do not shave skin; hair at application site should be clipped. Prior to application, clean site with clear water and allow to dry completely. Do not use damaged, cut or leaking patches; patch may be less effective. Skin exposure from fentanyl gel leaking from patch may lead to serious adverse effects; thoroughly wash affected skin surfaces with water (do not use soap). Firmly press in place and hold for 30 seconds. Change patch every 72 hours. Do **not** use soap, alcohol, or other solvents to remove transdermal gel if it accidentally touches skin; use copious amounts of water. Avoid exposing application site to external heat sources (eg, heating pad, electric blanket, heat lamp, hot tub). If there is difficulty with patch adhesion, the edges of the system may be taped in place with first-aid tape. If there is continued difficulty with adhesion, an adhesive film dressing (eg, Bioclusive®, Tegaderm®) may be applied over the system.

Stability

Storage

Injection formulation: Store at controlled room temperature of 20°C to 25°C (68°F to 77°F). Protect from light.

Nasal spray: Do not store above 25°C (77°F); do not freeze. Protect from light. Bottle should be stored in the provided child-resistant container when not in use and kept out of the reach of children at all times.

Transdermal patch: Do not store above 25°C (77°F). Keep out of the reach of children.

Transmucosal (buccal film, buccal tablet, lozenge, sublingual tablet): Store at controlled room temperature of 20°C to 25°C (68°F to 77°F). Protect from freezing and moisture. Keep out of the reach of children.

Nursing Actions

Physical Assessment Monitor effectiveness of pain relief. Monitor blood pressure, CNS and respiratory status, and degree of sedation prior to treatment and periodically throughout. Monitor closely for signs of withdrawal for 24 hours after transdermal product is removed. For inpatients, implement safety measures (eg, side rails up, call light within reach, instructions to call for assistance). Assess patient's physical and/or psychological dependence. Discontinue slowly after prolonged use.

Patient Education Do not use alcohol, sedatives, tranquilizers, antihistamines, or pain medications without consulting prescriber. Avoid drinking large quantities of grapefruit juice (eg, >1 quart/day). Keep out of the reach of children. Maintain adequate hydration, unless instructed to restrict fluid intake. May cause hypotension, dizziness, drowsiness, impaired coordination, or blurred vision; nausea or vomiting; or constipation (if unresolved, consult prescriber about use of stool softeners). Notify prescriber of dizziness, chest pain, slow or rapid heartbeat, or headache; confusion or changes in mentation; changes in voiding frequency or amount; swelling of extremities or unusual weight gain; temperature >102°F (38.8°C); shortness of breath or respiratory difficulty; or vision changes. Notify prescriber of poor pain control.

Transdermal patch: Apply to clean, dry skin immediately after removing from package. Firmly press in place and hold for 30 seconds. Do not use damaged, cut, or leaking patches. If fentanyl gel should leak, wash affected skin surfaces with water; do not use soap. Remove patch while having MRI scan; can cause burns. Avoid exposing application site to external heat sources (eg, heating pad, electric blanket, hot tub, heat lamp).

Transmucosal lozenge (eg, Actiq®): Contains an amount of medication that can be fatal to children. Keep all units, both used and unused, out of the reach of children and discard any open units properly. Actiq® Child Safety Kits are available which contain educational materials, safe storage, and disposal instructions. Using this product may make you more at risk for dental caries due to the sugar content. Maintain good oral hygiene.

Nasal spray (eg, Lazanda®): Not to be substituted for another fentanyl product. Have patient avoid blowing nose for 30 minutes after administration.

Dietary Considerations Transmucosal lozenge contains 2 g sugar per unit.

Related Information

Compatibility of Drugs *on page 1264*

Ferrous Gluconate (FER us GLOO koe nate)

Brand Names: U.S. Ferate [OTC]; Fergon® [OTC]

Index Terms Iron Gluconate

Pharmacologic Category Iron Salt

Lactation Enters breast milk

Use Prevention and treatment of iron-deficiency anemias

Available Dosage Forms For available OTC formulations, consult specific product labeling.

General Dosage Range Oral:

Children: 1-6 mg Fe/kg/day in 1-3 divided doses

Adults: 60 mg 1-4 times/day

Administration

Oral Administer 2 hours before or 4 hours after antacids. Administration of iron preparations to premature infants with vitamin E deficiency may cause increased red cell hemolysis and hemolytic anemia, therefore, vitamin E deficiency should be corrected if possible.

Nursing Actions

Patient Education May color stool black. Take between meals for maximum absorption; take with food if GI upset occurs. Do not take with milk or antacids.

Ferrous Sulfate (FER us SUL fate)

Brand Names: U.S. Feosol® [OTC]; Fer-In-Sol® [OTC]; Fer-iron [OTC]; MyKidz Iron 10™ [OTC]; Slow FE® [OTC]; Slow Release [OTC]

Index Terms $FeSO_4$; Iron Sulfate

Pharmacologic Category Iron Salt

Medication Safety Issues

Sound-alike/look-alike issues:

Feosol® may be confused with Fer-In-Sol®

Fer-In-Sol® may be confused with Feosol®

Slow FE® may be confused with Slow-K®

BEERS Criteria medication:

This drug may be inappropriate for use in geriatric patients (dosage dependent, low severity risk).

Administration issues:

Fer-In-Sol® (manufactured by Mead Johnson) and a limited number of generic products are available at a concentration of 15 mg/mL. However, many other generics and brand name products of ferrous sulfate oral liquid drops are available at a concentration of 15 mg/0.6 mL. Check concentration closely prior to dispensing. Prescriptions written in milliliters (mL) should be clarified.

Lactation Enters breast milk

Use Prevention and treatment of iron-deficiency anemias

Available Dosage Forms For available OTC formulations, consult specific product labeling.

General Dosage Range Oral:

Extended release: *Adults:* 250 mg 1-2 times/day

Immediate release:

Children: 1-6 mg Fe/kg/day in 1-3 divided doses (maximum: 15 mg/day [prophylaxis dosing])

Adults: 300 mg 1-4 times/day

Administration

Oral Should be taken with water or juice on an empty stomach; administer ferrous sulfate 2 hours prior to, or 4 hours after antacids

Nursing Actions

Physical Assessment May cause GI irritation. Monitor GI function (observe for epigastric pain, nausea, dark stools, vomiting, stomach cramping, constipation).

Patient Education May color stool black. Take between meals for maximum absorption; take with food if GI upset occurs. Do not take with milk or antacids. You may experience constipation, nausea, vomiting, abdominal pain, and other GI complaints.

Ferumoxytol (fer ue MOX i tol)

Brand Names: U.S. Feraheme®

Pharmacologic Category Iron Salt

Medication Safety Issues

Sound-alike/look-alike issues:

Ferumoxytol may be confused with ferric gluconate, iron dextran complex, iron sucrose

Pregnancy Risk Factor C

Lactation Excretion in breast milk unknown/not recommended

Use Treatment of iron-deficiency anemia in chronic kidney disease

Available Dosage Forms

Injection, solution:

Feraheme®: Elemental iron 30 mg/mL (17 mL)

General Dosage Range I.V.: *Adults:* 510 mg (17 mL) as a single dose; repeat once 3-8 days later

Administration

I.V. Administer intravenously as an undiluted injection at a rate ≤1 mL/second (30 mg of elemental iron/second). Do not administer if solution has particulate matter or is discolored (solution is black to reddish-brown).

Hemodialysis patients should receive injection after at least 1 hour of hemodialysis has been completed and once blood pressure has stabilized.

Nursing Actions

Physical Assessment Monitor closely during administration and for at least 60 minutes following for hypersensitive reactions. Resuscitation equipment should be available. Monitor blood pressure closely; can cause hypotension.

Patient Education You may experience dizziness or lightheadedness. Hypersensitivity reactions can occur. Healthcare personnel will need to monitor you for 60 minutes following the administration of this drug. Report itching, rash, wheezing, or respiratory difficulty immediately.

Fesoterodine (fes oh TER oh deen)

Brand Names: U.S. Toviaz™

Index Terms FESO; Fesoterodine Fumarate

Pharmacologic Category Anticholinergic Agent

Medication Safety Issues

Sound-alike/look-alike issues:

Fesoterodine may be confused with fexofenadine, tolterodine

Pregnancy Risk Factor C

Lactation Excretion in breast milk unknown/not recommended

Use Treatment of patients with an overactive bladder with symptoms of urinary frequency, urgency, or urge incontinence.

Available Dosage Forms

Tablet, extended release, oral:

Toviaz™: 4 mg, 8 mg

General Dosage Range Dosage adjustment recommended in patients with renal impairment or on concomitant therapy

Oral: *Adults:* 4-8 mg once daily

Administration

Oral May be administered with or without food. Swallow whole; do not chew, crush, or divide.

Nursing Actions

Patient Education You may experience drowsiness. Avoid alcohol; may increase drowsiness. May cause dry mouth or constipation. Report to prescriber problems urinating.

Fexofenadine (feks oh FEN a deen)

Brand Names: U.S. Allegra®; Allegra® Allergy 12 Hour [OTC]; Allegra® Allergy 24 Hour [OTC]; Allegra® Children's Allergy ODT [OTC]; Allegra® Children's Allergy [OTC]; Allegra® ODT [DSC]

Index Terms Fexofenadine Hydrochloride

Pharmacologic Category Histamine H_1 Antagonist; Histamine H_1 Antagonist, Second Generation; Piperidine Derivative

Medication Safety Issues

Sound-alike/look-alike issues:

Fexofenadine may be confused with fesoterodine

Allegra® may be confused with Viagra®

International issues:

Allegra [U.S, Canada, and multiple international markets] may be confused with Allegro brand name for fluticasone [Israel] and frovatriptan [Germany]

Pregnancy Risk Factor C

Lactation Excretion in breast milk unknown/use caution (AAP rates "compatible"; AAP 2001 update pending)

Breast-Feeding Considerations It is not known if fexofenadine is excreted in breast milk. The manufacturer recommends that caution be exercised when administering fexofenadine to nursing women.

Use Relief of symptoms associated with seasonal allergic rhinitis; treatment of chronic idiopathic urticaria

OTC labeling: Relief of symptoms associated with allergic rhinitis

Mechanism of Action/Effect Fexofenadine is an active metabolite of terfenadine and like terfenadine it competes with histamine for H_1-receptor sites on effector cells in the GI tract, blood vessels, and respiratory tract; binds to lung receptors significantly greater than it binds to cerebellar receptors, resulting in a greatly reduced sedative potential

Contraindications Hypersensitivity to fexofenadine or any component of the formulation

Warnings/Precautions Use with caution in patients with renal impairment; dosage adjustment recommended. Safety and efficacy in children <6 months of age have not been established; orally disintegrating tablet not recommended for use in children <6 years of age. Orally disintegrating tablet contains phenylalanine.

Drug Interactions

Avoid Concomitant Use There are no known interactions where it is recommended to avoid concomitant use.

Decreased Effect

Fexofenadine may decrease the levels/effects of: Acetylcholinesterase Inhibitors (Central); Benzylpenicilloyl Polylysine; Betahistine

The levels/effects of Fexofenadine may be decreased by: Acetylcholinesterase Inhibitors (Central); Amphetamines; Antacids; Grapefruit Juice; P-glycoprotein/ABCB1 Inducers; Rifampin; Tocilizumab

Increased Effect/Toxicity

Fexofenadine may increase the levels/effects of: Alcohol (Ethyl); Anticholinergics; ARIPiprazole; CNS Depressants; Methotrimeprazine; Selective Serotonin Reuptake Inhibitors

The levels/effects of Fexofenadine may be increased by: Conivaptan; Droperidol; Eltrombopag; Erythromycin; Erythromycin (Systemic); HydrOXYzine; Itraconazole; Ketoconazole; Ketoconazole (Systemic); Methotrimeprazine; P-glycoprotein/ABCB1 Inhibitors; Pramlintide; Verapamil

Nutritional/Ethanol Interactions

Ethanol: Ethanol may increase CNS depression. Management: Avoid ethanol.

Food: Fruit juice (apple, grapefruit, orange) may decrease bioavailability of fexofenadine by ~36%. Management: Administer with water only, avoid fruit juice.

Herb/Nutraceutical: St John's wort may decrease fexofenadine levels.

Adverse Reactions

>10%:

Central nervous system: Headache (5% to 11%)

Gastrointestinal: Vomiting (children 6 months to 5 years: 4% to 12%)

1% to 10%:

Central nervous system: Fatigue (1% to 3%), somnolence (1% to 3%), dizziness (2%), fever (2%), pain (2%), drowsiness (1%)

Endocrine & metabolic: Dysmenorrhea (2%)

Gastrointestinal: Diarrhea (3% to 4%), nausea (2%), dyspepsia (1% to 2%)

Neuromuscular & skeletal: Myalgia (3%), back pain (2% to 3%), pain in extremities (2%)

Otic: Otitis media (2% to 4%)

Respiratory: Upper respiratory tract infection (3% to 4%), cough (2% to 4%), rhinorrhea (1% to 2%)

Miscellaneous: Viral infection (3%)

Pharmacodynamics/Kinetics

Onset of Action 60 minutes

Duration of Action Antihistaminic effect: ≥12 hours

Available Dosage Forms

Suspension, oral:

Allegra®: 6 mg/mL (300 mL)

Allegra® Children's Allergy [OTC]: 6 mg/mL (120 mL)

Tablet, oral: 30 mg, 60 mg, 180 mg

Allegra® Allergy 12 Hour [OTC]: 60 mg

Allegra® Allergy 24 Hour [OTC]: 180 mg

Allegra® Children's Allergy [OTC]: 30 mg

Tablet, orally disintegrating, oral:

Allegra® Children's Allergy ODT [OTC]: 30 mg

General Dosage Range Dosage adjustment recommended in patients with renal impairment

Oral:

Children 6 months to <2 years: 15 mg twice daily

Children 2-11 years: 30 mg twice daily

Children ≥12 years and Adults: 60 mg twice daily **or** 180 mg once daily

Administration

Oral

Suspension, tablet: Administer with water only; do not administer with fruit juices. Shake suspension well before use.

Orally disintegrating tablet: Take on an empty stomach. Do not remove from blister pack until administered. Using dry hands, place immediately on tongue. Tablet will dissolve within seconds, and may be swallowed with or without liquid (do not administer with fruit juices). Do not split or chew.

Stability

Storage Store at controlled room temperature of 20°C to 25°C (68°F to 77°F). Protect from excessive moisture.

Nursing Actions

Patient Education Avoid use of alcohol. You may experience mild drowsiness, dizziness, or nausea. Report persistent sedation or drowsiness, lack of improvement, or worsening of condition.

Dietary Considerations Some products may contain phenylalanine and/or sodium. Take suspension and tablets with water only; do not administer with fruit juices.

Fexofenadine and Pseudoephedrine

(feks oh FEN a deen & soo doe e FED rin)

Brand Names: U.S. Allegra-D® 12 Hour; Allegra-D® 24 Hour

Index Terms Pseudoephedrine and Fexofenadine

Pharmacologic Category Alpha/Beta Agonist; Decongestant; Histamine H_1 Antagonist; Histamine H_1 Antagonist, Second Generation; Piperidine Derivative

Medication Safety Issues

Sound-alike/look-alike issues:

Allegra-D® may be confused with Viagra®

International issues:

Allegra-D [U.S, Canada, and multiple international markets] may be confused with Allegro brand name for fluticasone [Israel] and frovatriptan [Germany]

Pregnancy Risk Factor C

Lactation Enters breast milk/use caution (AAP rates "compatible"; AAP 2001 update pending)

Use Relief of symptoms associated with seasonal allergic rhinitis in adults and children ≥12 years of age

Available Dosage Forms

Tablet, extended release: Fexofenadine 60 mg [immediate release] and pseudoephedrine 120 mg [extended release]; fexofenadine 180 mg [immediate release] and pseudoephedrine 240 mg [extended release]

Allegra-D® 12 Hour: Fexofenadine 60 mg [immediate release] and pseudoephedrine 120 mg [extended release]

Allegra-D® 24 Hour: Fexofenadine 180 mg [immediate release] and pseudoephedrine 240 mg [extended release]

General Dosage Range Dosage adjustment recommended in patients with renal impairment

Oral: *Children ≥12 years and Adults:* 1 tablet (fexofenadine 60 mg/pseudoephedrine 120 mg) twice daily **or** 1 tablet (fexofenadine 180 mg/ pseudoephedrine 240 mg) once daily

Administration

Oral Tablets should be swallowed whole; do not crush or chew. Administer on an empty stomach with water; avoid administration with food. The inactive ingredients may be eliminated in the feces in a form resembling the original tablet.

Nursing Actions

Physical Assessment See individual agents.

Patient Education See individual agents.

Related Information

Fexofenadine *on page 477*

Pseudoephedrine *on page 961*

Fidaxomicin (fye DAX oh mye sin)

Brand Names: U.S. Dificid™

Index Terms Difimicin; Lipiarrmycin; OPT-80; PAR-101; Tiacumicin B

Pharmacologic Category Antibiotic, Macrolide

Pregnancy Risk Factor B

Lactation Excretion in breast milk unknown/use caution

Use Treatment of *Clostridium difficile*-associated diarrhea (CDAD)

Mechanism of Action/Effect Inhibits protein synthesis in susceptible organisms including *C. difficile*; bactericidal

Contraindications There are no contraindications listed in the manufacturer's labeling.

Warnings/Precautions Do not use for systemic infections; fidaxomicin systemic absorption is negligible. Use only in patients with proven or strongly suspected *Clostridium difficile (C. difficile)* infections.

Drug Interactions

Avoid Concomitant Use There are no known interactions where it is recommended to avoid concomitant use.

Decreased Effect There are no known significant interactions involving a decrease in effect.

Increased Effect/Toxicity There are no known significant interactions involving an increase in effect.

Adverse Reactions

>10%: Gastrointestinal: Nausea (11%)

2% to 10%:

Gastrointestinal: Gastrointestinal hemorrhage (4%), abdominal pain, vomiting

Hematologic: Anemia (2%), neutropenia (2%)

Available Dosage Forms

Tablet, oral:

Dificid™: 200 mg

General Dosage Range No dosage adjustment recommended in patients with hepatic or renal impairment.

Oral: *Adults:* 200 mg twice daily

Administration

Oral May be administered with or without food.

Stability

Storage Store at 20°C to 25°C (68°F to 77°F); excursions permitted to 15°C to 30°C (59°F to 86°F).

Dietary Considerations May be taken without regard to food.

Filgrastim (fil GRA stim)

Brand Names: U.S. Neupogen®

Index Terms G-CSF; Granulocyte Colony Stimulating Factor

Pharmacologic Category Colony Stimulating Factor

Medication Safety Issues

Sound-alike/look-alike issues:

Neupogen® may be confused with Epogen®, Neulasta®, Neumega®, Nutramigen®

International issues:

Neupogen [U.S., Canada, and multiple international markets] may be confused with Neupro brand name for rotigotine {multiple international markets]

Pregnancy Risk Factor C

Lactation Excretion in breast milk unknown/use caution

Use

Cancer patients (nonmyeloid malignancies) receiving myelosuppressive chemotherapy to decrease the incidence of infection (febrile neutropenia) in regimens associated with a high incidence of neutropenia with fever

Acute myelogenous leukemia (AML) following induction or consolidation chemotherapy to shorten time to neutrophil recovery and reduce the duration of fever

Cancer patients (nonmyeloid malignancies) receiving bone marrow transplant to shorten the duration of neutropenia and neutropenia-related events (eg, neutropenic fever)

Peripheral stem cell transplantation to mobilize hematopoietic progenitor cells for leukapheresis collection

Severe chronic neutropenia (SCN; chronic administration) to reduce the incidence and duration of neutropenic complications (fever, infections, oropharyngeal ulcers) in symptomatic patients with congenital, cyclic, or idiopathic neutropenia

Unlabeled Use Treatment of anemia in myelodysplastic syndrome (in combination with epoetin); mobilization of hematopoietic stem cells (HSC) for collection and subsequent autologous transplantation (in combination with plerixafor) in patients with non-Hodgkin's lymphoma (NHL) and multiple myeloma (MM); treatment of neutropenia in HIV-infected patients receiving zidovudine; hepatitis C treatment-associated neutropenia

Mechanism of Action/Effect Stimulates the production, maturation, and activation of neutrophils, filgrastim activates neutrophils to increase both their migration and cytotoxicity. Natural proteins which stimulate hematopoietic stem cells to proliferate, prolong cell survival, stimulate cell differentiation, and stimulate functional activity of mature cells. CSFs are produced by a wide variety of cell types. Specific mechanisms of action are not yet fully understood, but possibly work by a second-messenger pathway with resultant protein production.

Contraindications Hypersensitivity to filgrastim, *E. coli*-derived proteins, or any component of the formulation

Warnings/Precautions Do not use filgrastim in the period 24 hours before to 24 hours after administration of cytotoxic chemotherapy because of the potential sensitivity of rapidly dividing myeloid cells to cytotoxic chemotherapy. May potentially act as a growth factor for any tumor type, particularly myeloid malignancies; caution should be exercised in the usage of filgrastim in any malignancy with myeloid characteristics. Increases circulating leukocytes when used in conjunction with plerixafor for stem cell mobilization; monitor WBC; use with caution in patients with neutrophil count >50,000/mm^3; tumor cells released from marrow could be collected in leukapheresis product; potential effect of tumor cell reinfusion is unknown. Reports of alveolar hemorrhage, manifested as pulmonary infiltrates and hemoptysis, have occurred in healthy donors undergoing PBPC collection (not FDA approved for use in healthy donors); hemoptysis resolved upon discontinuation. Safety and efficacy have not been established with patients receiving radiation therapy (avoid concurrent radiation therapy with filgrastim), or chemotherapy associated with delayed myelosuppression (eg, nitrosoureas, mitomycin C).

Allergic-type reactions (rash, urticaria, facial edema, wheezing, dyspnea, tachycardia, and/or hypotension) have occurred with first or subsequent doses. Reactions tended to involve ≥2 body systems and occur more frequently with intravenous administration and generally within 30 minutes of administration; may recur with rechallenge. Rare cases of acute respiratory distress syndrome (ARDS) have been reported (possibly due to influx of neutrophils to sites of lung inflammation); withhold or discontinue filgrastim if ARDS occurs; patients must be instructed to report respiratory distress; monitor for fever, infiltrates, or respiratory distress. Rare cases of splenic rupture have been reported (may be fatal); patients must be instructed to report left upper quadrant pain or shoulder tip pain. Cutaneous vasculitis has been reported, generally occurring in severe chronic neutropenia (SCN) patients on long-term therapy; symptoms generally developed with increasing absolute neutrophil count (ANC) and subsided when the ANC decreased; dose reductions may improve symptoms to allow for continued therapy. Use caution in patients with sickle cell disorders; severe sickle cell crises (sometimes resulting in fatalities) have been reported following filgrastim therapy. Filgrastim use prior to appropriate diagnosis of SCN may impair proper evaluation and treatment for neutropenia not due to SCN. Cytogenetic abnormalities, transformation to myelodysplastic syndrome (MDS) and acute myeloid leukemia (AML) have been observed in patients treated with filgrastim for congenital neutropenia; a longer duration of treatment and poorer ANC response appear to increase the risk. Carefully consider the risk of continuing filgrastim in patients who develop abnormal cytogenetics or MDS. The packaging of some forms may contain latex.

Drug Interactions

Avoid Concomitant Use There are no known interactions where it is recommended to avoid concomitant use.

Decreased Effect There are no known significant interactions involving a decrease in effect.

Increased Effect/Toxicity

Filgrastim may increase the levels/effects of: Bleomycin; Topotecan

Adverse Reactions

>10%:

Central nervous system: Fever (12%)

Dermatologic: Petechiae (≤17%), rash (≤12%)

Endocrine & metabolic: LDH increased, uric acid increased

Gastrointestinal: Splenomegaly (severe chronic neutropenia: 30%; rare in other patients)

Hepatic: Alkaline phosphatase increased (21%)

Neuromuscular & skeletal: Bone/skeletal pain (22% to 33%; dose related), commonly in the lower back, posterior iliac crest, and sternum

Respiratory: Epistaxis (9% to 15%)

1% to 10%:

Cardiovascular: Hyper-/hypotension (4%), myocardial infarction/arrhythmias (3%)

Central nervous system: Headache (7%)

Gastrointestinal: Nausea (10%), vomiting (7%), peritonitis (≤2%)

Hematologic: Leukocytosis (2%)

Miscellaneous: Transfusion reaction (≤10%)

Pharmacodynamics/Kinetics

Onset of Action ~24 hours; plateaus in 3-5 days

Duration of Action Neutrophil counts generally return to baseline within 4 days

Available Dosage Forms

Injection, solution [preservative free]:

Neupogen®: 300 mcg/mL (1 mL, 1.6 mL); 600 mcg/mL (0.5 mL, 0.8 mL)

General Dosage Range

I.V.: *Children and Adults:* 5-10 mcg/kg/day

SubQ: *Children and Adults:* 5-10 mcg/kg/day **or** 6 mcg/kg twice daily

Administration

I.V. May be administered I.V. as a short infusion over 15-30 minutes (chemotherapy-induced neutropenia) or by continuous infusion (chemotherapy-induced neutropenia) or as a 4- or 24-hour infusion (bone marrow transplantation). Do not administer earlier than 24 hours after or in the 24 hours prior to cytotoxic chemotherapy.

I.V. Detail pH: 4

Other May be administered by SubQ injection, either as a bolus injection (chemotherapy-induced neutropenia) or as a continuous infusion (chemotherapy-induced neutropenia, bone marrow transplantation, and peripheral blood progenitor cell collection). Do not administer earlier than 24 hours after or in the 24 hours prior to cytotoxic chemotherapy.

Stability

Reconstitution Do not dilute with saline at any time; product may precipitate. Filgrastim may be diluted with D_5W to a concentration of 5-15 mcg/mL for I.V. infusion administration (minimum concentration: 5 mcg/mL). Concentrations 5-15 mcg/mL require addition of albumin (final albumin concentration of 2 mg/mL) to prevent adsorption to plastics. Dilution to <5 mcg/mL is not recommended. Do not shake.

Storage Intact vials and prefilled syringes should be stored under refrigeration at 2°C to 8°C (36°F to 46°F) and protected from direct sunlight. Filgrastim should be protected from freezing and temperatures >30°C to avoid aggregation.

Filgrastim vials and prefilled syringes are stable for 24 hours at 9°C to 30°C (47°F to 86°F).

Undiluted filgrastim is stable for 24 hours at 15°C to 30°C (59°F to 86°F) and for up to 14 days at 2°C to 8°C (36°F to 46°F) (data on file, Amgen Medical Information) in BD tuberculin syringes; however, sterility has only been assessed and maintained for up to 7 days when prepared under strict aseptic conditions (Jacobson, 1996; Singh, 1994). The manufacturer recommends using syringes within 24 hours due to the potential for bacterial contamination.

Filgrastim diluted with D_5W for I.V. infusion (5-15 mcg/mL) is stable for 7 days at 2°C to 8°C (36°F to 46°F), however, should be used within 24 hours due to the possibility for bacterial contamination.

Nursing Actions

Physical Assessment Hypersensitivity to *E. coli* products should be assessed prior to beginning therapy. Allergic-type reactions have occurred in patients receiving G-CSF. If self-administered, teach patient proper storage, administration, and syringe/needle disposal. Instruct patient to report upper quadrant pain, shoulder tip pain, or respiratory distress.

Patient Education If self-administered, follow directions for proper storage and administration of SubQ medication. Never reuse syringes or needles. May cause bone pain, nausea, vomiting, hair loss (reversible), or sore mouth. Report immediately any respiratory difficulty or pain in left shoulder, chest, or back. Report unusual fever or chills; unhealed sores; severe bone pain; pain, redness, or swelling at injection site; unusual swelling of extremities; or chest pain and palpitations.

Dietary Considerations Some products may contain sodium.

Finasteride (fi NAS teer ide)

Brand Names: U.S. Propecia®; Proscar®

Pharmacologic Category 5 Alpha-Reductase Inhibitor

Medication Safety Issues

Sound-alike/look-alike issues:

Finasteride may be confused with furosemide

Proscar® may be confused with ProSom, Provera®, PROzac®

Pregnancy Risk Factor X

Lactation Excretion in breast milk unknown/contraindicated in women of childbearing potential

Breast-Feeding Considerations Not indicated for use in women.

Use

Propecia®: Treatment of male pattern hair loss in **men only**. Safety and efficacy were demonstrated in men between 18-41 years of age.

Proscar®: Treatment of symptomatic benign prostatic hyperplasia (BPH); can be used in combination with an alpha-blocker, doxazosin

Unlabeled Use Treatment of female hirsutism

Mechanism of Action/Effect Finasteride inhibits conversion of testosterone to dihydrotestosterone and markedly suppresses serum dihydrotestosterone levels

Contraindications Hypersensitivity to finasteride or any component of the formulation; pregnancy; not for use in children

Warnings/Precautions Hazardous agent - use appropriate precautions for handling and disposal. Other urological diseases (including prostate cancer) should be ruled out before initiating. For BPH, a minimum of 6 months of treatment may be necessary to determine whether an individual will respond to finasteride; for male pattern hair loss, daily use for 3 months or longer may be required before benefit is observed. Reduces prostate specific antigen (PSA) by ~50%; in patients treated for ≥6 months the PSA value should be doubled when comparing to normal ranges in untreated patients (for interpretation of serial PSAs, a new PSA baseline should be established ≥6 months after treatment initiation and PSA monitored periodically thereafter). Failure to demonstrate a meaningful PSA decrease (<50%) or a PSA increase while on this medication may be associated with an increased risk for prostate cancer (NCCN prostate cancer early detection guidelines, v.1.2011). Patients on a 5-alpha-reductase inhibitor (5-ARI) with any increase in PSA levels, even if within normal limits, should be evaluated; may indicate presence of prostate cancer. Use with caution in patients with hepatic dysfunction; finasteride is extensively metabolized in the liver. When compared to placebo, 5-ARIs have been shown to reduce the overall incidence of prostate cancer, although an increase in the incidence of high-grade prostate cancers has been observed; 5-ARIs are not FDA-approved for the prevention of prostate cancer. Carefully monitor patients with a large residual urinary volume or severely diminished urinary flow for obstructive uropathy; these patients may not be candidates for finasteride therapy. Rare reports of male breast cancer have been observed with finasteride use. Patients should promptly report any breast changes, including breast enlargement, lumps, tenderness, pain, or nipple discharge to their healthcare provider. Active ingredient can be absorbed through the skin; women should always use caution whenever handling. Pregnant women or women trying to conceive should not handle the product; finasteride may negatively impact fetal development. Not indicated for use in children.

Drug Interactions

Avoid Concomitant Use There are no known interactions where it is recommended to avoid concomitant use.

Decreased Effect

The levels/effects of Finasteride may be decreased by: Tocilizumab

Increased Effect/Toxicity

The levels/effects of Finasteride may be increased by: Conivaptan

Nutritional/Ethanol Interactions Herb/Nutraceutical: St John's wort may decrease finasteride levels. Avoid saw palmetto (concurrent use has not been adequately studied).

Adverse Reactions Note: "Combination therapy" refers to finasteride and doxazosin.

>10%:

- Endocrine & metabolic: Impotence (5% to 19%; combination therapy 23%), libido decreased (2% to 10%; combination therapy 12%)
- Neuromuscular & skeletal: Weakness (5%; combination therapy 17%)

1% to 10%:

- Cardiovascular: Postural hypotension (9%; combination therapy 18%), edema (1%; combination therapy 3%)
- Central nervous system: Dizziness (7%; combination therapy 23%), somnolence (2%; combination therapy 3%)
- Dermatologic: Rash (1%)
- Genitourinary: Ejaculation disturbances (<1% to 7%; combination therapy 14%), decreased volume of ejaculate (2% to 4%)
- Endocrine & metabolic: Gynecomastia (1% to 2%), breast tenderness (≤1%)
- Respiratory: Dyspnea (1%; combination therapy 2%), rhinitis (1%; combination therapy 2%)

Pharmacodynamics/Kinetics

Onset of Action BPH: 6 months; Male pattern hair loss: ≥3 months of daily use.

Duration of Action

After a single oral dose as small as 0.5 mg: 65% depression of plasma dihydrotestosterone levels persists 5-7 days

After 6 months of treatment with 5 mg/day: Circulating dihydrotestosterone levels are reduced to castrate levels without significant effects on circulating testosterone; levels return to normal within 14 days of discontinuation of treatment

Available Dosage Forms

Tablet, oral: 5 mg

Propecia®: 1 mg

Proscar®: 5 mg

General Dosage Range Oral: *Adults:* 1 mg or 5 mg once daily

Administration

Oral May be administered without regard to meals. Women of childbearing age should not touch or handle broken tablets.

Stability

Storage

Propecia®: Store at 15°C to 30°C (59°F to 86°F). Protect from moisture.

Proscar®: Store below 30°C (86°F). Protect from light.

Nursing Actions

Physical Assessment Assess urinary pattern prior to therapy and periodically during therapy. A minimum of 6 months of treatment may be necessary to evaluate response.

Patient Education Take with or without meals. May cause decreased libido or impotence during therapy. Report any changes in urinary pattern (significant increase or decrease in volume or voiding patterns). Report changes in breast condition (pain, lumps, or nipple discharge) in male and female patients.

Dietary Considerations May be taken without regard to meals.

Fingolimod (fin GOL i mod)

Brand Names: U.S. Gilenya®

Index Terms FTY720

Pharmacologic Category Sphingosine 1-Phosphate (S1P) Receptor Modulator

Medication Guide Available Yes

Pregnancy Risk Factor C

Lactation Excretion in breast milk unknown/not recommended

Use Treatment of relapsing forms of multiple sclerosis (MS) to reduce the frequency of clinical exacerbations and delay disability progression

Available Dosage Forms

Capsule, oral:

Gilenya®: 0.5 mg

General Dosage Range Oral: *Adults:* 0.5 mg once daily

Administration

Oral May be administered with or without food.

Flecainide (fle KAY nide)

Brand Names: U.S. Tambocor™

Index Terms Flecainide Acetate

Pharmacologic Category Antiarrhythmic Agent, Class Ic

Medication Safety Issues

Sound-alike/look-alike issues:

Flecainide may be confused with fluconazole

Tambocor™ may be confused with Pamelor™, Temodar®, tamoxifen, Tamiflu®

Pregnancy Risk Factor C

Lactation Enters breast milk/compatible

Use Prevention and suppression of documented life-threatening ventricular arrhythmias (eg, sustained ventricular tachycardia); controlling symptomatic, disabling supraventricular tachycardias in patients without structural heart disease in whom other agents fail

Available Dosage Forms

Tablet, oral: 50 mg, 100 mg, 150 mg

Tambocor™: 50 mg, 100 mg, 150 mg

General Dosage Range Dosage adjustment recommended in patients with renal impairment

Oral:

Children: Initial: 3 mg/kg/day **or** 50-100 mg/m²/day in 3 divided doses; Maintenance: 3-6 mg/kg/day **or** 100-150 mg/m²/day in 3 divided doses (maximum: 11 mg/kg/day; 200 mg/m²/day)

Adults: Initial: 50-100 mg every 12 hours; Maintenance: 100-400 mg/day in 2 divided doses (maximum: 400 mg/day)

Administration

Oral Administer around-the-clock to promote less variation in peak and trough serum levels.

Nursing Actions

Physical Assessment Monitor cardiac status. Flecainide has a low toxic:therapeutic ratio and overdose may easily produce severe and life-threatening reactions.

Patient Education Take around-the-clock. You will require frequent monitoring while taking this medication. You may experience dizziness, visual disturbances, or nausea. Report palpitations, chest pain, or excessively slow or rapid heartbeat; acute nervousness, headache, or fatigue; unusual weight gain; unusual cough; respiratory difficulty; swelling of hands or ankles; or muscle tremor, numbness, or weakness.

Floctafenine (flok ta FEN een)

Index Terms Floctafenina; Floctafeninum

Pharmacologic Category Nonsteroidal Anti-inflammatory Drug (NSAID), Oral

Lactation Enters breast milk/not recommended

Use Short-term management of acute, mild-to-moderate pain

Product Availability Not available in U.S.

General Dosage Range Dosage adjustment recommended in patients with renal impairment

Oral: *Adults:* 200-400 mg every 6-8 hours as needed (maximum: 1200 mg/day)

Administration

Oral Administer after food or meal with glass of water.

Nursing Actions

Physical Assessment Assess for allergic reactions to salicylates or other NSAIDs. Monitor blood pressure at the beginning of therapy and periodically throughout. With long-term therapy, periodic ophthalmic exams are recommended.

Patient Education Take with food or milk to avoid GI irritation. Maintain adequate hydration, unless instructed to restrict fluid intake. Do not use alcohol. You may experience drowsiness, ▶

dizziness, nausea, vomiting, or gastric discomfort; GI bleeding, ulceration, and perforation can occur with or without pain. Stop taking medication and report occurrence immediately. Report ringing in ears, changes in hearing or vision, unresolved nausea or vomiting, difficulty breathing or shortness of breath, cramping or stomach pain, unusual bruising or bleeding (blood in urine, stool, mouth, or vomitus), unusual swelling of extremities or weight gain, chest pain, rapid heartbeat, or skin rash.

Floxuridine (floks YOOR i deen)

Index Terms Fluorodeoxyuridine; FUDR

Pharmacologic Category Antineoplastic Agent, Antimetabolite (Pyrimidine Analog)

Medication Safety Issues

Sound-alike/look-alike issues:

Floxuridine may be confused with Fludara®, fludarabine

FUDR® may be confused with Fludara®

High alert medication:

This medication is in a class the Institute for Safe Medication Practices (ISMP) includes among its list of drug classes which have a heightened risk of causing significant patient harm when used in error.

Pregnancy Risk Factor D

Lactation Excretion in breast milk unknown/not recommended

Use Management of hepatic metastases of colorectal and gastric cancers

Available Dosage Forms

Injection, powder for reconstitution: 500 mg

General Dosage Range Dosage adjustment recommended in patients with hepatic impairment

Intra-arterial: *Adults:* 0.1-0.6 mg/kg/day

Administration

I.V. Continuous intra-arterial or I.V. infusion (unlabeled use)

I.V. Detail pH: 4.0-5.5

Nursing Actions

Physical Assessment Use caution with impaired liver or kidney function. Monitor for CNS changes and acute gastrointestinal reactions (intractable vomiting or diarrhea may be dose limiting) on a regular basis. Teach patient or caregiver use and care of implantable pump.

Patient Education This drug can only be administered by infusion. Follow instructions of prescriber for care of implantable pump. Avoid alcohol. It is important to maintain adequate nutrition and hydration, unless instructed to restrict fluid intake. You will be more susceptible to infection. May cause nausea or vomiting, loss of hair (reversible), diarrhea, mouth sores, or sterility. Increased emotional or physical stress will adversely affect the response to this medication. Notify prescriber if you are experiencing unusual or elevated levels of stress. Report extreme fatigue; pain or numbness in extremities; severe GI upset or diarrhea; bleeding or bruising; fever, chills, or sore throat; vaginal discharge; or signs of fluid retention (eg, swelling of extremities, respiratory difficulty, unusual weight gain).

Related Information

Management of Drug Extravasations *on page 1269*

Fluconazole (floo KOE na zole)

Brand Names: U.S. Diflucan®

Pharmacologic Category Antifungal Agent, Oral; Antifungal Agent, Parenteral

Medication Safety Issues

Sound-alike/look-alike issues:

Fluconazole may be confused with flecainide, FLUoxetine, furosemide, itraconazole

Diflucan® may be confused with diclofenac, Diprivan®, disulfiram

International issues:

Canesten Oral [Great Britain] may be confused with Canesten brand name for clotrimazole [multiple international markets]; Cenestin brand name estrogens (conjugated A/synthetic) [U.S., Canada]

Pregnancy Risk Factor C (single dose for vaginal candidiasis)/D (all other indications)

Lactation Enters breast milk/not recommended (AAP rates "compatible"; AAP 2001 update pending)

Breast-Feeding Considerations Fluconazole is found in breast milk at concentration similar to plasma.

Use Treatment of candidiasis (vaginal, oropharyngeal, esophageal, urinary tract infections, peritonitis, pneumonia, and systemic infections); cryptococcal meningitis; antifungal prophylaxis in allogeneic bone marrow transplant recipients

Unlabeled Use Cryptococcal pneumonia; candidal intertrigo

Mechanism of Action/Effect Interferes with cytochrome P450 activity, decreasing ergosterol synthesis (principal sterol in fungal cell membrane) and inhibiting cell membrane formation

Contraindications Hypersensitivity to fluconazole or any component of the formulation (cross-reaction with other azole antifungal agents may occur, but has not been established; use caution); concomitant administration with cisapride or terfenadine

Warnings/Precautions Should be used with caution in patients with renal and hepatic dysfunction or previous hepatotoxicity from other azole derivatives. Patients who develop abnormal liver function tests during fluconazole therapy should be monitored closely and discontinued if symptoms consistent with liver disease develop. Rare exfoliative skin disorders have been observed; monitor closely if rash develops and discontinue if lesions progress. The manufacturer reports rare cases of QT_C prolongation and torsade de pointes associated with fluconazole use and advises caution in patients with concomitant medications or conditions which are arrhythmogenic. However, given the limited number of cases and the presence of multiple confounding variables, the likelihood that fluconazole causes conduction abnormalities appears remote. Oral suspension contains sucrose; avoid use in patients with fructose intolerance, glucose-galactose malabsorption, or sucrase-isomaltase insufficiency.

Drug Interactions

Avoid Concomitant Use

Avoid concomitant use of Fluconazole with any of the following: Artemether; Cisapride; Clopidogrel; Conivaptan; Dofetilide; Dronedarone; Lumefantrine; Nilotinib; Pimozide; QUEtiapine; QuiNIDine; QuiNINE; Ranolazine; Tetrabenazine; Thioridazine; Tolvaptan; Toremifene; Vandetanib; Vemurafenib; Voriconazole; Ziprasidone

Decreased Effect

Fluconazole may decrease the levels/effects of: Amphotericin B; Clopidogrel; Saccharomyces boulardii

The levels/effects of Fluconazole may be decreased by: Didanosine; Etravirine; Fosphenytoin; Phenytoin; Rifamycin Derivatives; Sucralfate

Increased Effect/Toxicity

Fluconazole may increase the levels/effects of: Alfentanil; Aprepitant; ARIPiprazole; Benzodiazepines (metabolized by oxidation); Bosentan; Budesonide (Systemic, Oral Inhalation); BusPIRone; Busulfan; Calcium Channel Blockers; CarBAMazepine; Carvedilol; Cilostazol; Cinacalcet; Cisapride; Citalopram; Colchicine; Conivaptan; Corticosteroids (Systemic); CycloSPORINE; CycloSPORINE (Systemic); CYP2C19 Substrates; CYP2C9 Substrates; CYP3A4 Substrates; Diclofenac; DOCEtaxel; Dofetilide; Dronedarone; Eletriptan; Eplerenone; Erlotinib; Eszopiclone; Etravirine; Everolimus; FentaNYL; Fosaprepitant; Fosphenytoin; Gefitinib; HMG-CoA Reductase Inhibitors; Imatinib; Irbesartan; Irinotecan; Ivacaftor; Losartan; Lurasidone; Macrolide Antibiotics; Methadone; Nevirapine; Phenytoin; Phosphodiesterase 5 Inhibitors; Pimecrolimus; Pimozide; Protease Inhibitors; Proton Pump Inhibitors; QTc-Prolonging Agents; QuiNIDine; QuiNINE; Ramelteon; Ranolazine; Repaglinide; Rifamycin Derivatives; Salmeterol; Saxagliptin; Sirolimus; Solifenacin; Sulfonylureas; SUNItinib; Tacrolimus; Tacrolimus (Systemic); Tacrolimus (Topical); Temsirolimus; Tetrabenazine; Thioridazine; Tolterodine; Tolvaptan; Toremifene; Vandetanib; Vemurafenib; Vilazodone; Vitamin K Antagonists; Voriconazole; Zidovudine; Ziprasidone; Zolpidem

The levels/effects of Fluconazole may be increased by: Alfuzosin; Artemether; Chloroquine; Ciprofloxacin; Ciprofloxacin (Systemic); Etravirine; Gadobutrol; Grapefruit Juice; Indacaterol; Lumefantrine; Macrolide Antibiotics; Nilotinib; Protease Inhibitors; QUEtiapine; QuiNINE

Adverse Reactions Frequency not always defined.

Cardiovascular: Angioedema, pallor, QT prolongation (rare, case reports), torsade de pointes (rare, case reports)

Central nervous system: Headache (2% to 13%), dizziness (1%), seizure

Dermatologic: Rash (2%), alopecia, toxic epidermal necrolysis, Stevens-Johnson syndrome

Endocrine & metabolic: Hypercholesterolemia, hypertriglyceridemia, hypokalemia

Gastrointestinal: Nausea (2% to 7%), abdominal pain (2% to 6%), vomiting (2% to 5%), diarrhea (2% to 3%), dyspepsia (1%), taste perversion (1%)

Hematologic: Agranulocytosis, leukopenia, neutropenia, thrombocytopenia

Hepatic: Alkaline phosphatase increased, ALT increased, AST increased, cholestasis, hepatic failure (rare), hepatitis, jaundice

Respiratory: Dyspnea

Miscellaneous: Anaphylactic reactions (rare)

Available Dosage Forms

Infusion, premixed iso-osmotic dextrose solution: 200 mg (100 mL); 400 mg (200 mL)

Infusion, premixed iso-osmotic sodium chloride solution: 100 mg (50 mL); 200 mg (100 mL); 400 mg (200 mL)

Infusion, premixed iso-osmotic sodium chloride solution [preservative free]: 200 mg (100 mL); 400 mg (200 mL)

Powder for suspension, oral: 10 mg/mL (35 mL); 40 mg/mL (35 mL)

Diflucan®: 10 mg/mL (35 mL); 40 mg/mL (35 mL)

Tablet, oral: 50 mg, 100 mg, 150 mg, 200 mg

Diflucan®: 50 mg, 100 mg, 150 mg, 200 mg

General Dosage Range Dosage adjustment recommended in patients with renal impairment

I.V., oral:

Children: Loading dose: 6-12 mg/kg; Maintenance: 3-12 mg/kg/day

Adults: 100-800 mg once daily **or** 150 mg as a single dose

Administration

Oral May be administered without regard to meals.

I.V. Do not use if cloudy or precipitated. Infuse over approximately 1-2 hours; do not exceed 200 mg/hour.

I.V. Detail pH: 4-8 (sodium chloride diluent); 3.5-6.5 (dextrose)

Stability

Storage

Tablet: Store at <30°C (86°F).

Powder for oral suspension: Store dry powder at <30°C (86°F). Following reconstitution, store at 5°C to 30°C (41°F to 86°F). Discard unused portion after 2 weeks. Do not freeze.

Injection: Store injection in glass at 5°C to 30°C (41°F to 86°F). Store injection in Viaflex® at 5°C to 25°C (41°F to 77°F). Do not freeze. Do not unwrap unit until ready for use.

Nursing Actions

Physical Assessment Cultures should be obtained and allergy history assessed prior to beginning therapy. Assess renal and hepatic function. Monitor for hepatotoxicity (jaundice), skin disorders, and abdominal pain on a regular basis.

Patient Education Frequent blood tests may be required. Maintain adequate hydration, unless instructed to restrict fluid intake. May cause headache, dizziness, drowsiness, nausea, vomiting, or diarrhea. Report skin rash, persistent GI upset, urinary pattern changes, excessively dry eyes or mouth, or changes in color of stool or urine.

Dietary Considerations Take without regard to meals.

Related Information

Compatibility of Drugs *on page 1264*

Flucytosine (floo SYE toe seen)

Brand Names: U.S. Ancobon®

Index Terms 5-FC; 5-Fluorocytosine; 5-Flurocytosine

Pharmacologic Category Antifungal Agent, Oral

Medication Safety Issues

Sound-alike/look-alike issues:

Flucytosine may be confused with fluorouracil

Ancobon® may be confused with Oncovin

High alert medication:

The Institute for Safe Medication Practices (ISMP) includes this medication among its list of drugs which have a heightened risk of causing significant patient harm when used in error.

Pregnancy Risk Factor C

Lactation Excretion in breast milk unknown/not recommended

Use Adjunctive treatment of systemic fungal infections (eg, septicemia, endocarditis, UTI, meningitis, or pulmonary) caused by susceptible strains of *Candida* or *Cryptococcus*

Mechanism of Action/Effect Penetrates fungal cells and interferes with fungal RNA and protein synthesis

Contraindications Hypersensitivity to flucytosine or any component of the formulation

Warnings/Precautions [U.S. Boxed Warning]: Use with extreme caution in patients with renal dysfunction; dosage adjustment required. Avoid use as monotherapy; resistance rapidly develops. Use with caution in patients with bone marrow depression; patients with hematologic disease or who have been treated with radiation or drugs that suppress the bone marrow may be at greatest risk. Bone marrow toxicity can be irreversible. **[U.S. Boxed Warning]: Closely monitor hematologic, renal, and hepatic status.** Hepatotoxicity and bone marrow toxicity appear to be dose related; monitor levels closely and adjust dose accordingly.

Drug Interactions

Avoid Concomitant Use

Avoid concomitant use of Flucytosine with any of the following: CloZAPine

Decreased Effect

Flucytosine may decrease the levels/effects of: Saccharomyces boulardii

The levels/effects of Flucytosine may be decreased by: Cytarabine (Conventional)

Increased Effect/Toxicity

Flucytosine may increase the levels/effects of: CloZAPine

The levels/effects of Flucytosine may be increased by: Amphotericin B

Nutritional/Ethanol Interactions Food: Food decreases the rate, but not the extent of absorption.

Adverse Reactions Frequency not defined.

Cardiovascular: Cardiac arrest, myocardial toxicity, ventricular dysfunction, chest pain

Central nervous system: Ataxia, confusion, dizziness, drowsiness, fatigue, hallucinations, headache, parkinsonism, psychosis, pyrexia, sedation, seizure, vertigo

Dermatologic: Rash, photosensitivity, pruritus, toxic epidermal necrolysis, urticaria

Endocrine & metabolic: Hypoglycemia, hypokalemia

Gastrointestinal: Abdominal pain, diarrhea, dry mouth, duodenal ulcer, hemorrhage, loss of appetite, nausea, ulcerative colitis, vomiting

Hematologic: Agranulocytosis, anemia, aplastic anemia, eosinophilia, leukopenia, pancytopenia, thrombocytopenia

Hepatic: Acute hepatic injury, bilirubin increased, hepatic dysfunction, jaundice, liver enzymes increased

Neuromuscular & skeletal: Paresthesia, peripheral neuropathy, weakness

Otic: Hearing loss

Renal: Azotemia, BUN increased, crystalluria, renal failure, serum creatinine increased

Respiratory: Dyspnea, respiratory arrest

Miscellaneous: Allergic reaction

Available Dosage Forms

Capsule, oral: 250 mg, 500 mg

Ancobon®: 250 mg, 500 mg

General Dosage Range Dosage adjustment recommended in patients with renal impairment

Oral: *Adults:* 50-150 mg/kg/day in divided doses every 6 hours

Administration

Oral Administer around-the-clock to promote less variation in peak and trough serum levels. To avoid nausea and vomiting, administer a few capsules at a time over 15 minutes until full dose is taken.

Stability

Storage Store at room temperature of 15°C to 30°C (59°F to 86°F). Protect from light.

Nursing Actions

Physical Assessment Hematologic, renal, and hepatic status must be closely monitored; dose adjustments may be necessary. Monitor for cardiac incidents, CNS changes, bone marrow suppression, jaundice, skin reactions, and hearing loss on a regular basis.

Patient Education Take capsules one at a time over a few minutes with food to reduce GI upset. Frequent blood tests may be required. May cause nausea and vomiting. Report rash; respiratory difficulty; CNS changes (eg, confusion, hallucinations, ataxia, acute headache); yellowing of skin or eyes; changes in frequency of stool or urine; unresolved diarrhea or anorexia; or unusual bleeding, fatigue, or weakness.

Fludarabine (floo DARE a been)

Brand Names: U.S. Fludara®; Oforta™ [DSC]

Index Terms 2F-ara-AMP; Fludarabine Phosphate

Pharmacologic Category Antineoplastic Agent, Antimetabolite (Purine Analog)

Medication Safety Issues

Sound-alike/look-alike issues:

Fludarabine may be confused with cladribine, floxuridine, Flumadine®

Fludara® may be confused with FUDR®

High alert medication:

This medication is in a class the Institute for Safe Medication Practices (ISMP) includes among its list of drug classes which have a heightened risk of causing significant patient harm when used in error.

Pregnancy Risk Factor D

Lactation Excretion in breast milk unknown/not recommended

Breast-Feeding Considerations Due to the potential for serious adverse reactions in the nursing infant, breast-feeding is not recommended.

Use Treatment of progressive or refractory B-cell chronic lymphocytic leukemia (CLL)

Canadian labeling: Second-line treatment of chronic lymphocytic leukemia (CLL); second-line treatment of low-grade, refractory non-Hodgkin's lymphoma (NHL)

Unlabeled Use Treatment of non-Hodgkin's lymphomas (NHL); acute myeloid leukemia (AML), either refractory or in poor risk patients; relapsed acute lymphocytic leukemia (ALL) or AML in pediatric patients; Waldenström's macroglobulinemia (WM); reduced-intensity conditioning regimens prior to allogeneic hematopoietic stem cell transplantation (generally administered in combination with busulfan or cyclophosphamide and antithymocyte globulin or lymphocyte immune globulin, or in combination with melphalan and alemtuzumab)

Mechanism of Action/Effect Inhibits DNA synthesis by inhibition of DNA polymerase and ribonucleotide reductase; also inhibits DNA primase and DNA ligase I

Contraindications Hypersensitivity of fludarabine or any component of the formulation

Canadian labeling: Additional contraindications (not in U.S. labeling): Severe renal impairment (Cl_{cr} <30 mL/minute); decompensated hemolytic anemia; concurrent use with pentostatin

Warnings/Precautions Hazardous agent - use appropriate precautions for handling and disposal. Use with caution in patients with renal insufficiency (clearance of the primary metabolite 2-fluoro-ara-A is reduced); dosage reductions are recommended (monitor closely for excessive toxicity); use of the I.V. formulation is not recommended if Cl_{cr} <30 mL/minute. Use with caution in patients with pre-existing hematological disorders (particularly granulocytopenia) or pre-existing central nervous system disorder (epilepsy), spasticity, or peripheral neuropathy. **[U.S. Boxed Warning]: Higher than recommended doses are associated with severe neurologic toxicity (delayed blindness, coma, death); similar neurotoxicity (agitation, coma, confusion and seizure) has been reported with standard CLL doses.** Neurotoxicity symptoms due to high doses appear from 21-60 days following the last fludarabine dose, although neurotoxicity has been reported as early as 7 days and up to 225 days. Possible neurotoxic effects of chronic administration are unknown. Caution patients about performing tasks which require mental alertness (eg, operating machinery or driving).

[U.S. Boxed Warning]: Life-threatening (and sometimes fatal) autoimmune effects, including hemolytic anemia, autoimmune thrombocytopenia/thrombocytopenic purpura (ITP), Evans syndrome, and acquired hemophilia have occurred; monitor closely for hemolysis; discontinue fludarabine if hemolysis occurs; the hemolytic effects usually recur with fludarabine rechallenge. **[U.S. Boxed Warning]: Severe bone marrow suppression (anemia, thrombocytopenia, and neutropenia) may occur;** may be cumulative. Severe myelosuppression (trilineage bone marrow hypoplasia/aplasia) has been reported (rare) with a duration of significant cytopenias ranging from 2 months to 1 year. First-line combination therapy is associated with prolonged cytopenias, with anemia lasting up to 7 months, neutropenia up to 9 months, and thrombocytopenia up to 10 months; increased age is predictive for prolonged cytopenias (Gill, 2010).

Use with caution in patients with documented infection, fever, immunodeficiency, or with a history of opportunistic infection; prophylactic anti-infectives should be considered for patients with an increased risk for developing opportunistic infections. Progressive multifocal leukoencephalopathy

(PML) due to JC virus (usually fatal) has been reported with use; usually in patients who had received prior and/or other concurrent chemotherapy; onset ranges from a few weeks to 1 year; evaluate any neurological change promptly. Avoid vaccination with live vaccines during and after fludarabine treatment. May cause tumor lysis syndrome; risk is increased in patients with large tumor burden prior to treatment. Patients receiving blood products should only receive irradiated blood products due to the potential for transfusion related GVHD. **[U.S. Boxed Warnings]: Do not use in combination with pentostatin; may lead to severe, even fatal pulmonary toxicity. Should be administered under the supervision of an experienced cancer chemotherapy physician.**

Drug Interactions

Avoid Concomitant Use

Avoid concomitant use of Fludarabine with any of the following: BCG; CloZAPine; Natalizumab; Pentostatin; Pimecrolimus; Tacrolimus (Topical); Vaccines (Live)

Decreased Effect

Fludarabine may decrease the levels/effects of: BCG; Coccidioidin Skin Test; Sipuleucel-T; Vaccines (Inactivated); Vaccines (Live)

The levels/effects of Fludarabine may be decreased by: Echinacea; Imatinib

Increased Effect/Toxicity

Fludarabine may increase the levels/effects of: CloZAPine; Leflunomide; Natalizumab; Pentostatin; Vaccines (Live)

The levels/effects of Fludarabine may be increased by: Denosumab; Pentostatin; Pimecrolimus; Roflumilast; Tacrolimus (Topical); Trastuzumab

Nutritional/Ethanol Interactions Ethanol: Avoid ethanol (due to GI irritation).

Adverse Reactions

>10%:

Cardiovascular: Edema (8% to 19%)

Central nervous system: Fever (11% to 69%), fatigue (10% to 38%), pain (5% to 22%), chills (11% to 19%)

Dermatologic: Rash (4% to 15%)

Gastrointestinal: Nausea/vomiting (1% to 36%), anorexia (≤34%), diarrhea (5% to 15%), gastrointestinal bleeding (3% to 13%)

Genitourinary: Urinary tract infection (2% to 15%)

Hematologic: Myelosuppression (nadir: 10-14 days; recovery: 5-7 weeks; dose-limiting toxicity), anemia (14% to 60%), neutropenia (grade 4: 37% to 59%; nadir: ~13 days), thrombocytopenia (17% to 55%; nadir: ~16 days)

Neuromuscular & skeletal: Weakness (9% to 65%), myalgia (4% to 16%), paresthesia (4% to 12%)

Ocular: Visual disturbance (3% to 15%)

Respiratory: Cough (≤44%), pneumonia (3% to 22%), dyspnea (1% to 22%), upper respiratory infection (2% to 16%), rhinitis (≤11%)

Miscellaneous: Infection (12% to 44%), diaphoresis (≤14%)

1% to 10%:

Cardiovascular: Peripheral edema (≤7%), angina (≤6%), chest pain (≤5%), CHF (≤3%), arrhythmia (≤3%), cerebrovascular accident (≤3%), MI (≤3%), supraventricular tachycardia (≤3%), deep vein thrombosis (1% to 3%), phlebitis (1% to 3%), aneurysm (≤1%), transient ischemic attack (≤1%)

Central nervous system: Headache (≤9%), malaise (6% to 8%), sleep disorder (1% to 3%), cerebellar syndrome (≤1%), depression (≤1%), mentation impaired (≤1%)

Dermatologic: Alopecia (≤3%), pruritus (1% to 3%), seborrhea (≤1%)

Endocrine & metabolic: Hyperglycemia (1% to 6%), LDH increased (≤6%), dehydration (≤1%)

Gastrointestinal: Abdominal pain (≤10%), stomatitis (≤9%), weight loss (≤6%), esophagitis (≤3%), constipation (1% to 3%), mucositis (≤2%), dysphagia (≤1%)

Genitourinary: Dysuria (3% to 4%), hesitancy (≤3%)

Hematologic: Hemorrhage (≤1%), myelodysplastic syndrome/acute myeloid leukemia (usually associated with prior or concurrent treatment with other anticancer agents)

Hepatic: Cholelithiasis (≤3%), liver function tests abnormal (1% to 3%), liver failure (≤1%)

Neuromuscular & skeletal: Back pain (≤9%), osteoporosis (≤2%), arthralgia (≤1%)

Otic: Hearing loss (2% to 6%)

Renal: Hematuria (2% to 3%), renal failure (≤1%), renal function test abnormal (≤1%), proteinuria (≤1%)

Respiratory: Bronchitis (≤9%), pharyngitis (≤9%), allergic pneumonitis (≤6%), hemoptysis (1% to 6%), sinusitis (≤5%), epistaxis (≤1%), hypoxia (≤1%)

Miscellaneous: Flu-like syndrome (5% to 8%), herpes simplex infection (≤8%), anaphylaxis (≤1%), tumor lysis syndrome (1%)

Available Dosage Forms

Injection, powder for reconstitution: 50 mg

Fludara®: 50 mg

Injection, solution [preservative free]: 25 mg/mL (2 mL)

General Dosage Range Dosage adjustment recommended in patients with renal impairment or who develop toxicities.

Oral: *Adults:* 40 mg/m²/day for 5 days every 28 days

I.V.: *Adults:* 25 mg/m²/day for 5 days every 28 days

Administration

Oral Tablet may be administered with or without food; should be swallowed whole with water; do not chew, break, or crush.

I.V. Administer I.V. over 30 minutes; continuous infusions (unlabeled administration rate) are occasionally used

I.V. Detail pH: 7.2-8.2

Stability

Reconstitution Use appropriate precautions for handling and disposal. Reconstitute vials with SWI, NS, or D_5W to a concentration of 10-25 mg/mL. Standard I.V. dilution: 100-125 mL D_5W or NS.

Storage

I.V.: Store intact vials under refrigeration at 2°C to 8°C (36°F to 46°F). Reconstituted vials are stable for 16 days at room temperature of 15°C to 30°C (59°F to 86°F) or refrigerated, although the manufacturer recommends use within 8 hours. Solutions diluted in saline or dextrose are stable for 48 hours at room temperature or under refrigeration.

Tablet: Store at 25°C (77°F); excursions permitted to 15°C to 30°C (59°F to 86°F); should be kept within packaging until use.

Nursing Actions

Patient Education If this drug is administered by infusion, report any burning, pain, redness, or swelling at infusion site. It is important to maintain adequate nutrition and hydration, unless instructed to restrict fluid intake. You will be more susceptible to infection. May cause fatigue, weakness, visual disturbances, nausea, vomiting, loss of hair (reversible), or mouth sores. Report severe or persistent GI upset or diarrhea; extreme fatigue or weakness; pain or numbness in muscles; any unusual bleeding or bruising; fever, chills, or sore throat; vaginal discharge; difficulty or pain on urination; unusual cough or respiratory difficulty; or changes in vision.

Dietary Considerations Tablet may be taken with or without food.

Fludrocortisone (floo droe KOR ti sone)

Index Terms 9α-Fluorohydrocortisone Acetate; Florinef; Fludrocortisone Acetate; Fluohydrisone Acetate; Fluohydrocortisone Acetate

Pharmacologic Category Corticosteroid, Systemic

Medication Safety Issues

Sound-alike/look-alike issues:

Florinef® may be confused with Fioricet®, Fiorinal®

Pregnancy Risk Factor C

Lactation Excretion in breast milk unknown/use caution

Breast-Feeding Considerations Corticosteroids are excreted in human milk; information specific to fludrocortisone has not been located.

Use Partial replacement therapy for primary and secondary adrenocortical insufficiency in Addison's disease; treatment of salt-losing adrenogenital syndrome

Mechanism of Action/Effect Promotes increased reabsorption of sodium and loss of potassium from renal distal tubules

Contraindications Hypersensitivity to fludrocortisone or any component of the formulation; systemic fungal infections

Warnings/Precautions May cause hypercorticism or suppression of hypothalamic-pituitary-adrenal (HPA) axis, particularly in younger children or in patients receiving high doses for prolonged periods. HPA axis suppression may lead to adrenal crisis. Withdrawal and discontinuation of a corticosteroid should be done slowly and carefully. Fludrocortisone is primarily a mineralocorticoid agonist, but may also inhibit the HPA axis. May increase risk of infection and/or limit response to vaccinations; close observation is required in patients with latent tuberculosis and/or TB reactivity. Restrict use in active TB (only in conjunction with antituberculosis treatment). Use with caution in patients with sodium retention and potassium loss, hepatic impairment, myocardial infarction, osteoporosis, and/or renal impairment. Use with caution in the elderly. Withdraw therapy with gradual tapering of dose.

Drug Interactions

Avoid Concomitant Use

Avoid concomitant use of Fludrocortisone with any of the following: Aldesleukin; BCG; Natalizumab; Pimecrolimus; Tacrolimus (Topical)

Decreased Effect

Fludrocortisone may decrease the levels/effects of: Aldesleukin; Antidiabetic Agents; BCG; Calcitriol; Coccidioidin Skin Test; Corticorelin; Isoniazid; Salicylates; Sipuleucel-T; Telaprevir; Vaccines (Inactivated)

The levels/effects of Fludrocortisone may be decreased by: Aminoglutethimide; Antacids; Barbiturates; Bile Acid Sequestrants; Echinacea; Mitotane; Primidone; Rifamycin Derivatives

Increased Effect/Toxicity

Fludrocortisone may increase the levels/effects of: Acetylcholinesterase Inhibitors; Amphotericin B; Deferasirox; Leflunomide; Loop Diuretics; Natalizumab; NSAID (COX-2 Inhibitor); NSAID (Nonselective); Thiazide Diuretics; Vaccines (Live); Warfarin

The levels/effects of Fludrocortisone may be increased by: Antifungal Agents (Azole Derivatives, Systemic); Aprepitant; Calcium Channel Blockers (Nondihydropyridine); Denosumab; Estrogen Derivatives; Fluconazole; Fosaprepitant; Indacaterol; Macrolide Antibiotics;

Neuromuscular-Blocking Agents (Nondepolarizing); Pimecrolimus; Quinolone Antibiotics; Roflumilast; Salicylates; Tacrolimus (Topical); Telaprevir; Trastuzumab

Adverse Reactions Frequency not defined.

Cardiovascular: CHF, edema, hypertension

Central nervous system: Dizziness, headache, seizures

Dermatologic: Acne, bruising, rash

Endocrine & metabolic: HPA axis suppression, hyperglycemia, hypokalemic alkalosis, suppression of growth

Gastrointestinal: Peptic ulcer

Neuromuscular & skeletal: Muscle weakness

Ocular: Cataracts

Miscellaneous: Anaphylaxis (generalized), diaphoresis

Available Dosage Forms

Tablet, oral: 0.1 mg

General Dosage Range Oral:

Children: 0.05-0.1 mg/day

Adults: 0.05-0.2 mg/day (range: 0.1 mg 3 times/week to 0.2 mg/day)

Administration

Oral Administration in conjunction with a glucocorticoid is preferable.

Nursing Actions

Physical Assessment Teach patients to report opportunistic infection and adrenal suppression. Instruct patients with diabetes to monitor serum glucose levels closely; corticosteroids can alter glycemic response. Dose may need to be increased if patient is experiencing higher than normal levels of stress. When discontinuing, taper dose and frequency slowly.

Patient Education Take with or after meals. Take once-a-day dose with food in the morning. Limit intake of caffeine or stimulants. Maintain adequate nutrition; consult prescriber for possibility of special dietary recommendations. If you have diabetes, monitor serum glucose closely and notify prescriber of changes; this medication can alter glycemic response. Notify prescriber if you are experiencing higher than normal levels of stress; medication may need adjustment. Periodic ophthalmic examinations will be necessary. You will be susceptible to infection. You may experience insomnia or nervousness. Report weakness, change in menstrual pattern, vision changes, signs of hyperglycemia, signs of infection (eg, fever, chills, mouth sores, perianal itching, vaginal discharge), or worsening of condition.

Dietary Considerations Systemic use of mineralocorticoids/corticosteroids may require a diet with increased potassium, vitamins A, B_6, C, D, folate, calcium, zinc, and phosphorus, and decreased sodium. With fludrocortisone, a decrease in dietary sodium is often not required as the increased retention of sodium is usually the desired therapeutic effect.

Flumazenil (FLOO may ze nil)

Brand Names: U.S. Romazicon®

Pharmacologic Category Antidote

Medication Safety Issues

Sound-alike/look-alike issues:

Flumazenil may be confused with influenza virus vaccine

Pregnancy Risk Factor C

Lactation Excretion in breast milk unknown/use caution

Use Benzodiazepine antagonist; reverses sedative effects of benzodiazepines used in conscious sedation and general anesthesia; treatment of benzodiazepine overdose

Mechanism of Action/Effect Competitively inhibits the activity at the benzodiazepine receptor site on the GABA/benzodiazepine receptor complex. Flumazenil does not antagonize the CNS effect of drugs affecting GABA-ergic neurons by means other than the benzodiazepine receptor (ethanol, barbiturates, general anesthetics) and does not reverse the effects of opioids.

Contraindications Hypersensitivity to flumazenil, benzodiazepines, or any component of the formulation; patients given benzodiazepines for control of potentially life-threatening conditions (eg, control of intracranial pressure or status epilepticus); patients who are showing signs of serious cyclic-antidepressant overdosage

Warnings/Precautions [U.S. Boxed Warning]: Benzodiazepine reversal may result in seizures in some patients. Patients who may develop seizures include patients on benzodiazepines for long-term sedation, tricyclic antidepressant overdose patients, concurrent major sedative-hypnotic drug withdrawal, recent therapy with repeated doses of parenteral benzodiazepines, myoclonic jerking or seizure activity prior to flumazenil administration. Flumazenil may not reliably reverse respiratory depression/hypoventilation. Flumazenil is not a substitute for evaluation of oxygenation; establishing an airway and assisting ventilation, as necessary, is always the initial step in overdose management. Resedation occurs more frequently in patients where a large single dose or cumulative dose of a benzodiazepine is administered along with a neuromuscular-blocking agent and multiple anesthetic agents. Flumazenil should be used with caution in the intensive care unit because of increased risk of unrecognized benzodiazepine dependence in such settings. Should not be used to diagnose benzodiazepine-induced sedation. Reverse neuromuscular blockade before considering use. Flumazenil does not antagonize the CNS effects of other GABA agonists (such as ethanol, barbiturates, or general anesthetics); nor does it reverse narcotics. Flumazenil does not consistently reverse amnesia; patient may not recall verbal instructions after procedure.

Use with caution in patients with a history of panic disorder; may provoke panic attacks. Use caution in drug and ethanol-dependent patients; these patients may also be dependent on benzodiazepines. Not recommended for treatment of benzodiazepine dependence. Use with caution in head injury patients. Use caution in patients with mixed drug overdoses; toxic effects of other drugs taken may emerge once benzodiazepine effects are reversed. Use caution in hepatic dysfunction and in patients relying on a benzodiazepine for seizure control. Safety and efficacy have not been established in children <1 year of age.

Drug Interactions

Avoid Concomitant Use There are no known interactions where it is recommended to avoid concomitant use.

Decreased Effect

Flumazenil may decrease the levels/effects of: Hypnotics (Nonbenzodiazepine)

Increased Effect/Toxicity There are no known significant interactions involving an increase in effect.

Adverse Reactions

>10%: Gastrointestinal: Vomiting, nausea

1% to 10%:

Cardiovascular: Vasodilation (1% to 3%), palpitation

Central nervous system: Dizziness (10%), agitation (3% to 9%), emotional lability (1% to 3%), fatigue (1% to 3%), headache (1% to 3%)

Gastrointestinal: Xerostomia

Local: Pain at injection site (3% to 9%)

Neuromuscular & skeletal: Tremor, weakness, paresthesia (1% to 3%)

Ocular: Abnormal vision, blurred vision (3% to 9%)

Respiratory: Dyspnea, hyperventilation (3% to 9%)

Miscellaneous: Diaphoresis

Pharmacodynamics/Kinetics

Onset of Action 1-3 minutes; 80% response within 3 minutes; Peak effect: 6-10 minutes

Duration of Action Resedation: ~1 hour; duration related to dose given and benzodiazepine plasma concentrations; reversal effects of flumazenil may wear off before effects of benzodiazepine

Available Dosage Forms

Injection, solution: 0.1 mg/mL (5 mL, 10 mL)

Romazicon®: 0.1 mg/mL (5 mL, 10 mL)

General Dosage Range I.V.:

Children: Initial: 0.01 mg/kg (maximum dose: 0.2 mg), may repeat 0.01 mg/kg (maximum dose: 0.2 mg) as needed (maximum cumulative total: 1 mg or 0.05 mg/kg, whichever is lower)

Adults: Benzodiazepine overdose: Initial: 0.2 mg, may repeat with 0.3 mg, then 0.5 mg (maximum cumulative total dose: 5 mg); Reversal of conscious sedation/general anesthesia: Initial: 0.2 mg, may repeat (maximum total dose: 1 mg)

Administration

I.V. Administer in freely-running I.V. into large vein. Inject over 15 seconds for conscious sedation and general anesthesia and over 30 seconds for overdose.

I.V. Detail pH: 4 (injection)

Stability

Reconstitution For I.V. use only. Once drawn up in the syringe or mixed with solution use within 24 hours. Discard any unused solution after 24 hours.

Storage Store at 15°C to 30°C (59°F to 86°F).

Nursing Actions

Physical Assessment Assess level of consciousness frequently. Monitor vital signs and airway closely. Observe continually for resedation, respiratory depression, seizure activity, or other residual benzodiazepine effects.

Patient Education Flumazenil does not consistently reverse amnesia. Do not engage in activities requiring alertness for 18-24 hours after discharge. Avoid alcohol. Resedation may occur in patients on long-acting benzodiazepines.

Flunisolide (Nasal) (floo NISS oh lide)

Pharmacologic Category Corticosteroid, Nasal

Medication Safety Issues

Sound-alike/look-alike issues:

Flunisolide may be confused with Flumadine®, fluocinonide

Pregnancy Risk Factor C

Lactation Excretion in breast milk unknown/use caution

Use Seasonal or perennial rhinitis

Available Dosage Forms

Solution, intranasal: 25 mcg/actuation (25 mL); 29 mcg/actuation (25 mL)

General Dosage Range Intranasal:

Children 6-14 years: 1-2 sprays 2-3 times/day (maximum: 4 sprays/day in each nostril)

Children ≥15 years and Adults: 2 sprays twice daily (maximum: 8 sprays/day in each nostril)

Administration

Inhalation Before first use, prime by pressing pump 5-6 times or until a fine spray appears. Repeat priming if ≥5 days between use, or if dissembled for cleaning. Administer at regular intervals. Blow nose to clear nostrils. Insert applicator into nostril, keeping bottle upright, and close off the other nostril. Breathe in through nose. While inhaling, press pump to release spray.

Nursing Actions

Patient Education Full benefit of regular use may not be seen for 2-4 weeks. Review use of spray with prescriber.

Fluocinolone (Otic) (floo oh SIN oh lone)

Brand Names: U.S. DermOtic®

Index Terms Fluocinolone Acetonide

Pharmacologic Category Corticosteroid, Otic

Medication Safety Issues

Sound-alike/look-alike issues:

Fluocinolone may be confused with fluocinonide

Pregnancy Risk Factor C

Lactation Excretion in breast milk unknown/use caution

Use Relief of chronic eczematous external otitis

Available Dosage Forms

Oil, otic: 0.01% (20 mL)

DermOtic®: 0.01% (20 mL)

General Dosage Range Otic: *Children ≥2 years and Adults:* 5 drops into affected ear twice daily

Fluocinolone (Topical) (floo oh SIN oh lone)

Brand Names: U.S. Capex®; Derma-Smoothe/FS®

Index Terms Fluocinolone Acetonide

Pharmacologic Category Corticosteroid, Topical

Medication Safety Issues

Sound-alike/look-alike issues:

Fluocinolone may be confused with fluocinonide

Pregnancy Risk Factor C

Lactation Excretion in breast milk unknown/use caution

Use Relief of susceptible inflammatory dermatosis [low, medium corticosteroid]; dermatitis or psoriasis of the scalp; atopic dermatitis in adults and children ≥3 months of age

Available Dosage Forms

Cream, topical: 0.01% (15 g, 60 g); 0.025% (15 g, 60 g)

Oil, topical: 0.01% (118 mL)

Derma-Smoothe/FS®: 0.01% (120 mL)

Ointment, topical: 0.025% (15 g, 60 g)

Shampoo, topical:

Capex®: 0.01% (120 mL)

Solution, topical: 0.01% (60 mL)

General Dosage Range Topical:

Children ≥3 months: Apply a thin layer to affected area 2-4 times/day

Adults: Body: Apply thin layer to affected area 2-4 times/day; Scalp: 1 ounce daily (Capex®) **or** massage into wet hair and leave on for at least 4 hours (Derma-Smoothe/FS®)

Administration

Topical Apply thin film to affected area; avoid eyes.

Nursing Actions

Patient Education For external use only. Inform prescriber if you are allergic to peanuts. Do not use for eyes, mucous membranes, or open wounds. Before using, wash and dry area gently. Apply in a thin layer (may rub in lightly). Apply light dressing (if necessary) to area being treated. Do not use occlusive dressing unless so advised by prescriber. Avoid prolonged or excessive use around sensitive tissues or genital or rectal areas. Avoid exposing treated area to direct sunlight. Inform prescriber if condition worsens (redness, swelling, irritation, signs of infection, or open sores) or fails to improve after 2 weeks.

Fluocinonide (floo oh SIN oh nide)

Brand Names: U.S. Vanos®

Index Terms Lidex

Pharmacologic Category Corticosteroid, Topical

Medication Safety Issues

Sound-alike/look-alike issues:

Fluocinonide may be confused with flunisolide, fluocinolone

Lidex® may be confused with Lasix®, Videx®

Pregnancy Risk Factor C

Lactation Excretion unknown/not recommended

Use Anti-inflammatory, antipruritic; treatment of plaque-type psoriasis (up to 10% of body surface area) [high-potency topical corticosteroid]

Available Dosage Forms

Cream, topical:

Vanos®: 0.1% (30 g, 60 g, 120 g)

Cream, anhydrous, emollient, topical: 0.05% (15 g, 30 g, 60 g, 120 g)

Cream, aqueous, emollient, topical: 0.05% (15 g, 30 g, 60 g)

Gel, topical: 0.05% (15 g, 30 g, 60 g)

Ointment, topical: 0.05% (15 g, 30 g, 60 g)

Solution, topical: 0.05% (20 mL, 60 mL)

General Dosage Range Topical:

Children <12 years: Apply thin layer of 0.05% cream to affected area 2-4 times/day

Children ≥12 years and Adults: Apply thin layer of 0.05% cream to affected area 2-4 times/day **or** apply a thin layer of 0.1% cream once or twice daily to affected area

Nursing Actions

Patient Education For external use only. Do not use for eyes, mucous membranes, or open wounds. Before using, wash and dry area gently. Apply in a thin layer (may rub in lightly). Apply light dressing (if necessary) to area being treated. Do not use occlusive dressing unless so advised by prescriber. Avoid prolonged or excessive use around sensitive tissues or genital or rectal areas. Avoid exposing treated area to direct sunlight. Inform prescriber if condition worsens (redness, swelling, irritation, signs of infection, or open sores) or fails to improve.

Fluorometholone (flure oh METH oh lone)

Brand Names: U.S. Flarex®; FML Forte®; FML®

Pharmacologic Category Corticosteroid, Ophthalmic

Medication Safety Issues

International issues:

Flarex [U.S., Canada, and multiple international markets] may be confused with Fluarix brand name for influenza virus vaccine (inactivated) [U.S. and multiple international markets] and Fluorex brand name for fluoride [France]

Pregnancy Risk Factor C

Lactation Excretion in breast milk unknown/use caution

Use Treatment of steroid-responsive inflammatory conditions of the eye

Available Dosage Forms

Ointment, ophthalmic:

FML®: 0.1% (3.5 g)

Suspension, ophthalmic: 0.1% (5 mL, 10 mL, 15 mL)

Flarex®: 0.1% (5 mL)

FML Forte®: 0.25% (5 mL, 10 mL)

FML®: 0.1% (5 mL, 10 mL, 15 mL)

General Dosage Range Ophthalmic:

Ointment: *Children >2 years and Adults:* Apply small amount (~1/2" ribbon) every 4 hours (initial: 24-48 hours) **or** 1-3 times/day

Suspension:

Children >2 years: Instill 1 drop every 4 hours (initial: 24-48 hours) **or** 1 drop 2-4 times/day

Adults: Instill 2 drops (initial: 24-48 hours) **or** 1-2 drops 2-4 times/day

Administration

Other Contact lenses should be removed before instillation. Shake suspension well before use.

Nursing Actions

Physical Assessment Monitor intraocular pressure in patients with glaucoma or when used for ≥10 days; monitor for presence of secondary infections (including the development of fungal infections and exacerbation of viral infections).

Patient Education For ophthalmic use only. Wash hands before using. Wipe away excess from skin around eye. Do not use any other eye preparation for at least 10 minutes. Do not touch tip of applicator to eye or any other surface. May cause sensitivity to bright light; temporary stinging or blurred vision may occur. Do not wear contacts during administration and for 15 minutes after. Inform prescriber if you experience eye pain, redness, burning, watering, dryness, double vision, puffiness around eye, vision changes, worsening of condition, or lack of improvement.

Ointment: Gently squeeze the tube to apply to inside of lower lid. Close eye for 1-2 minutes and roll eyeball in all directions.

Suspension: Shake well before using. Tilt head back and look upward. Gently pull down lower lid and put drop(s) in inner corner of eye. Close eye and roll eyeball in all directions. Do not blink for 30 seconds. Apply gentle pressure to inner corner of eye for 30 seconds.

Fluorouracil (Systemic) (flure oh YOOR a sil)

Brand Names: U.S. Adrucil®

Index Terms 5-Fluorouracil; 5-FU; FU

Pharmacologic Category Antineoplastic Agent, Antimetabolite (Pyrimidine Analog)

Medication Safety Issues

Sound-alike/look-alike issues:

Fluorouracil may be confused with flucytosine

High alert medication:

This medication is in a class the Institute for Safe Medication Practices (ISMP) includes among its list of drugs which have a heightened risk of causing significant patient harm when used in error.

Pregnancy Risk Factor D

Lactation Excretion in breast milk unknown/not recommended

Use Treatment of carcinomas of the breast, colon, rectum, pancreas, or stomach

Unlabeled Use Treatment of head and neck cancer, esophageal cancer, anal cancer, cervical cancer, bladder cancer, renal cell cancer, and unknown primary cancer

Mechanism of Action/Effect Interferes with DNA synthesis by blocking the methylation of deoxyuricytic acid.

Contraindications Hypersensitivity to fluorouracil or any component of the formulation; poor nutritional states; depressed bone marrow function; potentially serious infections

Warnings/Precautions Hazardous agent - use appropriate precautions for handling and disposal. Use with caution in patients with impaired kidney or liver function. The drug should be discontinued if intractable vomiting or diarrhea, precipitous falls in leukocyte or platelet counts, gastrointestinal ulcer or bleeding, stomatitis, or esophagopharyngitis, hemorrhage, or myocardial ischemia occurs. Use with caution in patients who have had high-dose pelvic radiation or previous use of alkylating agents. Palmar-plantar erythrodysesthesia (hand-foot) syndrome has been associated with use.

Administration to patients with a genetic deficiency of dihydropyrimidine dehydrogenase (DPD) has been associated with prolonged clearance and increased toxicity following administration (diarrhea, neutropenia, and neurotoxicity); rechallenge has resulted in recurrent toxicity (despite dose reduction). **[U.S. Boxed Warning]: Should be administered under the supervision of an experienced cancer chemotherapy physician.**

Drug Interactions

Avoid Concomitant Use

Avoid concomitant use of Fluorouracil (Systemic) with any of the following: BCG; Natalizumab; Pimecrolimus; Tacrolimus (Topical); Vaccines (Live)

Decreased Effect

Fluorouracil (Systemic) may decrease the levels/effects of: BCG; Coccidioidin Skin Test; Sipuleucel-T; Vaccines (Inactivated); Vaccines (Live); Vitamin K Antagonists

The levels/effects of Fluorouracil (Systemic) may be decreased by: Echinacea; SORAfenib

Increased Effect/Toxicity

Fluorouracil (Systemic) may increase the levels/effects of: Carvedilol; CYP2C9 Substrates; Diclofenac; Fosphenytoin; Leflunomide; Natalizumab; Phenytoin; Vaccines (Live); Vitamin K Antagonists

The levels/effects of Fluorouracil (Systemic) may be increased by: Denosumab; Gemcitabine; Leucovorin Calcium-Levoleucovorin; MetroNIDAZOLE; MetroNIDAZOLE (Systemic); Pimecrolimus; Roflumilast; SORAfenib; Tacrolimus (Topical); Trastuzumab

Nutritional/Ethanol Interactions

Ethanol: Avoid ethanol (due to GI irritation).

Herb/Nutraceutical: Avoid black cohosh, dong quai in estrogen-dependent tumors.

Adverse Reactions Toxicity depends on duration of treatment

Cardiovascular: Angina, arrhythmia, heart failure, MI, myocardial ischemia, vasospasm, ventricular ectopy

Central nervous system: Acute cerebellar syndrome, confusion, disorientation, euphoria, headache, nystagmus, stroke

Dermatologic: Alopecia, dermatitis, dry skin, fissuring, palmar-plantar erythrodysesthesia syndrome, pruritic maculopapular rash, photosensitivity, Stevens-Johnson syndrome, toxic epidermal necrolysis, vein pigmentations

Gastrointestinal: Anorexia, bleeding, diarrhea, esophagopharyngitis, mesenteric ischemia (acute), nausea, sloughing, stomatitis, ulceration, vomiting

Hematologic: Myelosuppression (nadir: 9-14 days; recovery by day 30), agranulocytosis, anemia, leukopenia, pancytopenia, thrombocytopenia

Local: Thrombophlebitis

Ocular: Lacrimation, lacrimal duct stenosis, photophobia, visual changes

Respiratory: Epistaxis

Miscellaneous: Anaphylaxis, generalized allergic reactions, nail loss

Pharmacodynamics/Kinetics

Duration of Action ~3 weeks

Available Dosage Forms

Injection, solution: 50 mg/mL (10 mL, 20 mL, 50 mL, 100 mL)

Adrucil®: 50 mg/mL (10 mL, 50 mL, 100 mL)

General Dosage Range Dosage adjustment recommended in patients with hepatic or renal impairment

I.V.: *Adults:* Dosage varies greatly depending on indication

Administration

I.V. Irritant. Direct I.V. push injection (50 mg/mL solution needs no further dilution) or by I.V. infusion. Doses >1000 mg/m^2 are usually administered as a 24-hour infusion, although some protocols may be continuous infusion with lower doses. Toxicity may be reduced by giving the drug as a constant infusion. Bolus doses may be administered by slow IVP or IVPB.

I.V. Detail After vial has been entered, any unused portion should be discarded within 1 hour. Continuous infusions may be administered in D_5W or NS. Solution should be protected from direct sunlight. Fluorouracil may also be administered intra-arterially or intrahepatically (refer to specific protocols).

pH: 9.2 (adjusted)

Stability

Reconstitution Dilute in 50-1000 mL NS, D_5W, or bacteriostatic NS for infusion.

Storage Store intact vials at room temperature. Protect from light. Slight discoloration does not usually denote decomposition. If exposed to cold, a precipitate may form; **gentle** heating to 60°C will dissolve the precipitate without impairing the potency. Solutions in 50-1000 mL NS or D_5W, or undiluted solutions in syringes are stable for 72 hours at room temperature.

Nursing Actions

Physical Assessment Assess cardiovascular, respiratory, and renal function prior to each infusion and on a regular basis. Inform prescriber if intractable vomiting or diarrhea, precipitous fall in leukocyte or platelet counts, or myocardial ischemia occurs (drug may be discontinued). Teach patient proper use of oral solution (rinse mouth thoroughly) and importance of adequate hydration.

Patient Education Avoid excessive alcohol (may increase gastrointestinal irritation). Maintain adequate nutrition and hydration, unless instructed to restrict fluid intake. May cause sensitivity to sunlight, susceptibility to infection, nausea, vomiting, diarrhea, loss of appetite, weakness, lethargy, dizziness, decreased vision, or headache. Report signs and symptoms of infection (eg, fever, chills, sore throat, burning urination, vaginal itching or discharge, fatigue, mouth sores); bleeding (eg, black or tarry stools, easy bruising, unusual bleeding); vision changes; unremitting nausea, vomiting, or abdominal pain; CNS changes; respiratory difficulty; or chest pain or palpitations.

Oral solution: May be mixed in water, grape juice, or carbonated beverage. It is generally best to drink undiluted solution, then rinse mouth thoroughly. CocaCola® has been recommended as the best rinse following oral fluorouracil.

Dietary Considerations Increase dietary intake of thiamine.

Related Information

Management of Drug Extravasations *on page 1269*

FLUoxetine (floo OKS e teen)

Brand Names: U.S. PROzac®; PROzac® Weekly™; Sarafem®; Selfemra® [DSC]

Index Terms Fluoxetine Hydrochloride

Pharmacologic Category Antidepressant, Selective Serotonin Reuptake Inhibitor

Medication Safety Issues

Sound-alike/look-alike issues:

FLUoxetine may be confused with DULoxetine, famotidine, Feldene®, fluconazole, fluvastatin, fluvoxaMINE, fosinopril, furosemide, PARoxetine, thiothixene

PROzac® may be confused with Paxil®, Prelone®, PriLOSEC®, Prograf®, Proscar®, ProSom, Provera®

Sarafem® may be confused with Serophene®

BEERS Criteria medication:

This drug may be inappropriate for use in geriatric patients (high severity risk).

International issues:

Reneuron [Spain] may be confused with Remeron brand name for mirtazapine [U.S., Canada, and multiple international markets]

Medication Guide Available Yes

Pregnancy Risk Factor C

Lactation Enters breast milk/not recommended (AAP rates "of concern"; AAP 2001 update pending)

Breast-Feeding Considerations Fluoxetine and its metabolite are excreted into breast milk and can be detected in the serum of breast-feeding infants. Concentrations in breast milk are variable. Colic, irritability, slow weight gain, and feeding and sleep disorders have been reported in nursing infants. Breast-feeding is not recommended by the manufacturer.

Because the long-term effects on development and behavior have not been studied and adverse effects have been noted in some infants exposed, one should prescribe fluoxetine to a mother who is breast-feeding only when the benefits outweigh the potential risks.

Use Treatment of major depressive disorder (MDD); treatment of binge-eating and vomiting in patients with moderate-to-severe bulimia nervosa; obsessive-compulsive disorder (OCD); premenstrual dysphoric disorder (PMDD); panic disorder with or without agoraphobia; in combination with olanzapine for treatment-resistant or bipolar I depression

Unlabeled Use Selective mutism; treatment of mild dementia-associated agitation in nonpsychotic patients; post-traumatic stress disorder (PTSD); social anxiety disorder; fibromyalgia; Raynaud's phenomenon

Mechanism of Action/Effect Inhibits CNS neuron serotonin reuptake; minimal or no effect on reuptake of norepinephrine or dopamine; does not significantly bind to alpha-adrenergic, histamine or cholinergic receptors

Contraindications Hypersensitivity to fluoxetine or any component of the formulation; patients currently receiving MAO inhibitors, pimozide, or thioridazine

Note: MAO inhibitor therapy must be stopped for 14 days before fluoxetine is initiated. Treatment with MAO inhibitors or thioridazine should not be initiated until 5 weeks after the discontinuation of fluoxetine.

Warnings/Precautions [U.S. Boxed Warning]: Antidepressants increase the risk of suicidal thinking and behavior in children, adolescents, and young adults (18-24 years of age) with major depressive disorder (MDD) and other psychiatric disorders; consider risk prior to prescribing. Short-term studies did not show an increased risk in patients >24 years of age and showed a decreased risk in patients ≥65 years. Closely monitor patients for clinical worsening, suicidality, or unusual changes in behavior, particularly during the initial 1-2 months of therapy or during periods of dosage adjustments (increases or decreases); the patient's family or caregiver should be instructed to closely observe the patient and communicate condition with healthcare provider. A medication guide concerning the use of antidepressants should be dispensed with each prescription. **Fluoxetine is FDA approved for the treatment of OCD in children ≥7 years of age and MDD in children ≥8 years of age.**

The possibility of a suicide attempt is inherent in major depression and may persist until remission occurs. Use caution in high-risk patients. Worsening depression and severe abrupt suicidality that are not part of the presenting symptoms may require discontinuation or modification of drug therapy. The patient's family or caregiver should be alerted to monitor patients for the emergence of suicidality and associated behaviors (such as agitation, irritability, hostility, impulsivity, and hypomania) and call healthcare provider.

May worsen psychosis in some patients or precipitate a shift to mania or hypomania in patients with bipolar disorder. Patients presenting with depressive symptoms should be screened for bipolar disorder. Monotherapy in patients with bipolar disorder should be avoided. **Fluoxetine monotherapy is not FDA approved for the treatment of bipolar depression.** May cause insomnia, anxiety, nervousness, or anorexia. Use with caution in patients where weight loss is undesirable. May impair cognitive or motor performance; caution operating hazardous machinery or driving.

Serotonin syndrome and neuroleptic malignant syndrome (NMS)-like reactions have occurred with ▶

serotonin/norepinephrine reuptake inhibitors (SNRIs) and selective serotonin reuptake inhibitors (SSRIs) when used alone, and particularly when used in combination with serotonergic agents (eg, triptans) or antidopaminergic agents (eg, antipsychotics). Concurrent use with MAO inhibitors is contraindicated. Fluoxetine may elevate plasma levels of thioridazine or pimozide and increase the risk of QT_c interval prolongation. This may lead to serious ventricular arrhythmias, such as torsade de pointes-type arrhythmias, and sudden death. Fluoxetine use has been associated with occurrences of significant rash and allergic events, including vasculitis, lupus-like syndrome, laryngospasm, anaphylactoid reactions, and pulmonary inflammatory disease. Discontinue if underlying cause of rash cannot be identified.

Use caution in patients with a previous seizure disorder or condition predisposing to seizures such as brain damage, alcoholism, or concurrent therapy with other drugs which lower the seizure threshold. Use with caution in patients with hepatic or severe renal dysfunction and in elderly patients. Fluoxetine (daily) may be inappropriate for use in the elderly due to risk of agitation, sleep disturbances, and excessive CNS stimulation, attributed to this drug's long half-life (Beers Criteria). May cause hyponatremia/SIADH (elderly at increased risk); volume depletion (diuretics may increase risk). May increase the risks associated with electroconvulsive treatment. Use caution with concomitant use of NSAIDs, ASA, or other drugs that affect coagulation; the risk of bleeding may be potentiated. Use caution with history of MI or unstable heart disease; use in these patients is limited. May alter glycemic control in patients with diabetes. Due to the long half-life of fluoxetine and its metabolites, the effects and interactions noted may persist for prolonged periods following discontinuation. May cause or exacerbate sexual dysfunction. May cause mydriasis; use caution in patients at risk of acute narrow-angle glaucoma or with increased intraocular pressure. Discontinuation symptoms (eg, dysphoric mood, irritability, agitation, confusion, anxiety, insomnia, hypomania) may occur upon abrupt discontinuation. Taper dose when discontinuing therapy.

Drug Interactions

Avoid Concomitant Use

Avoid concomitant use of FLUoxetine with any of the following: Artemether; Clopidogrel; Dronedarone; Iobenguane I 123; Lumefantrine; MAO Inhibitors; Methylene Blue; Nilotinib; Pimozide; QUEtiapine; QuiNINE; Tamoxifen; Tetrabenazine; Thioridazine; Toremifene; Tryptophan; Vandetanib; Vemurafenib; Ziprasidone

Decreased Effect

FLUoxetine may decrease the levels/effects of: Clopidogrel; Iobenguane I 123; Ioflupane I 123

The levels/effects of FLUoxetine may be decreased by: CarBAMazepine; CYP2C9 Inducers (Strong); Cyproheptadine; Cyproterone; NSAID (COX-2 Inhibitor); NSAID (Nonselective); Peginterferon Alfa-2b; Tocilizumab

Increased Effect/Toxicity

FLUoxetine may increase the levels/effects of: Alpha-/Beta-Blockers; Anticoagulants; Antidepressants (Serotonin Reuptake Inhibitor/Antagonist); Antiplatelet Agents; Aspirin; Atomoxetine; Benzodiazepines (metabolized by oxidation); Beta-Blockers; BusPIRone; CarBAMazepine; CloZAPine; Collagenase (Systemic); CYP1A2 Substrates; CYP2C19 Substrates; CYP2D6 Substrates; Desmopressin; Dextromethorphan; Dronedarone; Drotrecogin Alfa (Activated); Fesoterodine; Fosphenytoin; Galantamine; Haloperidol; Ibritumomab; Lithium; Methadone; Methylene Blue; Metoclopramide; Mexiletine; NIFEdipine; NiMODipine; NSAID (COX-2 Inhibitor); NSAID (Nonselective); Phenytoin; Pimozide; Propafenone; QTc-Prolonging Agents; QuiNIDine; QuiNINE; RisperiDONE; Rivaroxaban; Salicylates; Serotonin Modulators; Tamoxifen; Tetrabenazine; Thioridazine; Thrombolytic Agents; Toremifene; Tositumomab and Iodine I 131 Tositumomab; TraMADol; Tricyclic Antidepressants; Vandetanib; Vemurafenib; Vitamin K Antagonists; Ziprasidone

The levels/effects of FLUoxetine may be increased by: Abiraterone Acetate; Alcohol (Ethyl); Alfuzosin; Analgesics (Opioid); Antipsychotics; Artemether; BusPIRone; Chloroquine; Cimetidine; Ciprofloxacin; Ciprofloxacin (Systemic); CNS Depressants; Conivaptan; CYP2C9 Inhibitors (Moderate); CYP2C9 Inhibitors (Strong); CYP2D6 Inhibitors (Moderate); CYP2D6 Inhibitors (Strong); Darunavir; Gadobutrol; Glucosamine; Herbs (Anticoagulant/Antiplatelet Properties); Indacaterol; Linezolid; Lumefantrine; Macrolide Antibiotics; MAO Inhibitors; Metoclopramide; Nilotinib; Omega-3-Acid Ethyl Esters; Pentosan Polysulfate Sodium; Pentoxifylline; Prostacyclin Analogues; QUEtiapine; QuiNINE; TraMADol; Tryptophan; Vitamin E

Nutritional/Ethanol Interactions

Ethanol: May increase CNS depression; monitor for increased effects with coadministration. Caution patients about effects.

Herb/Nutraceutical: Avoid valerian, St John's wort, kava kava, gotu kola (may increase CNS depression).

Adverse Reactions Percentages listed for adverse effects as reported in placebo-controlled trials and were generally similar in adults and children; actual frequency may be dependent upon diagnosis and in some cases the range presented may be lower than or equal to placebo for a particular disorder.

>10%:

Central nervous system: Insomnia (10% to 33%), headache (21%), somnolence (5% to 17%), anxiety (6% to 15%), nervousness (8% to 14%)

Endocrine & metabolic: Libido decreased (1% to 11%)

Gastrointestinal: Nausea (12% to 29%), diarrhea (8% to 18%), anorexia (4% to 17%), xerostomia (4% to 12%)

Neuromuscular & skeletal: Weakness (7% to 21%), tremor (3% to 13%)

Respiratory: Pharyngitis (3% to 11%), yawn (≤11%)

1% to 10%:

Cardiovascular: Vasodilation (1% to 5%), chest pain, hemorrhage, hypertension, palpitation

Central nervous system: Dizziness (9%), abnormal dreams (1% to 5%), abnormal thinking (2%), agitation, amnesia, chills, confusion, emotional lability, sleep disorder

Dermatologic: Rash (2% to 6%), pruritus (4%)

Endocrine & metabolic: Ejaculation abnormal (≤7%), impotence (≤7%), menorrhagia (≥2%)

Gastrointestinal: Dyspepsia (6% to 10%), constipation (5%), flatulence (3%), vomiting (3%), thirst (≥2%), weight loss (2%), appetite increased, taste perversion, weight gain

Genitourinary: Urinary frequency

Neuromuscular & skeletal: Hyperkinesia (≥2%)

Ocular: Vision abnormal (2%)

Otic: Ear pain, tinnitus

Respiratory: Sinusitis (1% to 6%)

Miscellaneous: Flu-like syndrome (3% to 10%), diaphoresis (2% to 8%), epistaxis (≥2%)

Pharmacodynamics/Kinetics

Onset of Action Depression: The onset of action is within a week; however, individual response varies greatly and full response may not be seen until 8-12 weeks after initiation of treatment.

Available Dosage Forms

Capsule, oral: 10 mg, 20 mg, 40 mg

PROzac®: 10 mg, 20 mg, 40 mg

Capsule, delayed release, enteric coated pellets, oral: 90 mg

PROzac® Weekly™: 90 mg

Solution, oral: 20 mg/5 mL (5 mL, 120 mL)

Tablet, oral: 10 mg, 20 mg, 60 mg

Sarafem®: 10 mg, 15 mg, 20 mg

General Dosage Range Dosage adjustment recommended in patients with hepatic impairment

Oral:

Children 7-18 years: Initial: 10-20 mg once daily; Maintenance: 10-60 mg once daily

Adults: 10-80 mg once daily **or** 90 mg once weekly

Elderly: 10 mg/day

Administration

Oral Administer without regard to meals.

Bipolar I disorder and treatment-resistant depression: Take once daily in the evening.

Major depressive disorder and obsessive compulsive disorder: Once daily doses should be taken in the morning, or twice daily (morning and noon).

Bulimia: Take once daily in the morning.

Stability

Storage All dosage forms should be stored at controlled room temperature. Protect from light.

Nursing Actions

Physical Assessment Assess therapeutic response (eg, mental status, mode, affect) at beginning of therapy and periodically throughout. Monitor for CNS and gastrointestinal disturbances. Taper dosage slowly when discontinuing. Assess mental status for depression, signs of clinical worsening, suicide ideation, anxiety, social functioning, mania, or panic attack.

Patient Education It may take 2-3 weeks to achieve desired results. Take once-a-day dose in the morning to reduce incidence of insomnia. Avoid alcohol. Maintain adequate hydration, unless instructed to restrict fluid intake. You may experience drowsiness, lightheadedness, weakness, impaired coordination, dizziness, blurred vision, constipation, anorexia, or postural hypotension. Report persistent CNS effects (nervousness, restlessness, insomnia, anxiety, excitation, headache, sedation); suicide ideation; rash or skin irritation; muscle cramping, tremors, or change in gait; respiratory depression or respiratory difficulty; or worsening of condition.

Dietary Considerations May be taken without regard to meals.

Fluphenazine (floo FEN a zeen)

Index Terms Fluphenazine Decanoate; Fluphenazine Hydrochloride

Pharmacologic Category Antipsychotic Agent, Typical, Phenothiazine

Medication Safety Issues

Sound-alike/look-alike issues:

FluPHENAZine may be confused with fluvoxaMINE

International issues:

Prolixin [Turkey] may be confused with Prolixan brand name for azapropazone [Greece]

Use Management of manifestations of psychotic disorders and schizophrenia; depot formulation may offer improved outcome in individuals with psychosis who are nonadherent with oral antipsychotics

Unlabeled Use Psychosis/agitation related to Alzheimer's dementia

Available Dosage Forms

Elixir, oral: 2.5 mg/5 mL (60 mL, 473 mL)

Injection, oil: 25 mg/mL (5 mL)

Injection, solution: 2.5 mg/mL (10 mL)

Solution, oral: 5 mg/mL (118 mL)

Tablet, oral: 1 mg, 2.5 mg, 5 mg, 10 mg

General Dosage Range

I.M. (hydrochloride): *Adults:* Initial: 1.25 mg as a single dose; Maintenance: 2.5-10 mg/day in divided doses every 6-8 hours

I.M., SubQ (Depot): *Adults:* Initial: 6.25-25 mg every 2-4 weeks (maximum: 100 mg)

Oral: *Adults:* 1-20 mg/day in divided doses every 6-8 hours (maximum: 40 mg/day)

Administration

Oral Avoid contact of oral solution or injection with skin (contact dermatitis). Oral liquid should be diluted into at least 60 mL (2 fl oz) of the following **only**: Water, saline, homogenized milk, carbonated orange beverages, pineapple, apricot, prune, orange, tomato, and grapefruit juices. Do **not** dilute in beverages containing caffeine, tannics (eg, tea), or pectinate (eg, apple juice).

I.M. The hydrochloride or decanoate formulation may be administered intramuscularly. Watch for hypotension when administering I.M. Use a dry syringe and needle of ≥21 gauge to administer the fluphenazine decanoate; a wet needle/syringe may cause the solution to become cloudy.

I.V. Detail pH: 4.8-5.2

Other SubQ: Only the decanoate formulation may be administered subcutaneously. Use a dry syringe and needle of ≥21 gauge to administer the fluphenazine decanoate; a wet needle/syringe may cause the solution to become cloudy.

Nursing Actions

Physical Assessment Monitor for anticholinergic and extrapyramidal symptoms. With I.M. or SubQ use, monitor closely for hypotension. Avoid skin contact with oral or injection medication; may cause contact dermatitis (wash immediately with warm, soapy water). Initiate at lower doses and taper dosage slowly when discontinuing.

Patient Education Dilute with water, milk, orange juice, or grapefruit juice; do not dilute with beverages containing caffeine, tannin, or pectinate (eg, coffee, colas, tea, or apple juice). Avoid alcohol. Avoid skin contact with liquid medication; may cause contact dermatitis (wash immediately with warm, soapy water). Maintain adequate hydration, unless instructed to restrict fluid intake. You may experience excess drowsiness, lightheadedness, dizziness, blurred vision, dry mouth, upset stomach, nausea, vomiting, constipation, urinary retention, ejaculatory dysfunction (reversible), decreased perspiration, or photosensitivity. Report persistent CNS effects (eg, trembling fingers, altered gait or balance, excessive sedation, seizures, unusual movements, anxiety, confusion); chest pain or palpitations; severe dizziness; unresolved urinary retention; altered menstrual pattern; change in libido; swelling or pain in breasts (male or female); vision changes; skin rash or yellowing of skin; or worsening of condition.

Flurazepam (flure AZ e pam)

Index Terms Flurazepam Hydrochloride

Pharmacologic Category Hypnotic, Benzodiazepine

Medication Safety Issues

Sound-alike/look-alike issues:

Flurazepam may be confused with temazepam

Dalmane® may be confused with Demulen®

BEERS Criteria medication:

This drug may be inappropriate for use in geriatric patients (high severity risk).

Medication Guide Available Yes

Lactation Excretion in breast milk unknown

Use Short-term treatment of insomnia

Controlled Substance C-IV

Available Dosage Forms

Capsule, oral: 15 mg, 30 mg

General Dosage Range Oral:

Children ≥15 years and Elderly: 15 mg at bedtime

Adults: 15-30 mg at bedtime

Nursing Actions

Physical Assessment For short-term use. Assess for history of addiction; long-term use can result in dependence, abuse, or tolerance. Be alert to possibility of anaphylaxis any time during therapy. Evaluate periodically need for continued use. Monitor for CNS changes. For inpatient use, institute safety measures to prevent falls.

Patient Education Drug may cause physical and/or psychological dependence. While using this medication, do not use alcohol. You may experience drowsiness, dizziness, lightheadedness, blurred vision, dry mouth, nausea, vomiting, difficulty urinating, or altered libido (resolves when medication is discontinued). Report CNS changes (confusion, depression, increased sedation, excitation, headache, abnormal thinking, insomnia, or nightmares, memory impairment, impaired coordination); muscle pain or weakness; respiratory difficulty; persistent dizziness, chest pain, or palpitations; unusual swelling, especially on face or neck; alterations in normal gait; vision changes; ringing in ears; or ineffectiveness of medication.

Flutamide (FLOO ta mide)

Index Terms 4′-Nitro-3′-Trifluoromethylisobutyrantide; Eulexin; Niftolid; NSC-147834; SCH 13521

Pharmacologic Category Antineoplastic Agent, Antiandrogen

Medication Safety Issues

Sound-alike/look-alike issues:

Flutamide may be confused with Flumadine®, thalidomide

Eulexin® may be confused with Edecrin®, Eurax®

Pregnancy Risk Factor D

Use Treatment of metastatic prostatic carcinoma in combination therapy with LHRH agonist analogues

Unlabeled Use Female hirsutism

Available Dosage Forms

Capsule, oral: 125 mg

General Dosage Range Oral: *Adults:* 250 mg 3 times/day

Administration

Oral Usually administered orally in 3 divided doses. Contents of capsule may be opened and mixed with applesauce, pudding, or other soft foods. Mixing with a beverage is not recommended.

Nursing Actions

Physical Assessment Assess serum transaminase levels prior to and periodically during therapy. Monitor for galactorrhea, CNS changes, ataxia, anorexia, vomiting, lacrimation, and anemia on a regular basis. Monitor liver function. Teach patient to report chest pain, respiratory difficulty, abdominal pain, and signs of liver dysfunction.

Patient Education This medication will be prescribed in conjunction with another medication; take both exactly as directed; do not discontinue without consulting prescriber. May cause decreased libido, impotence, swelling of breasts, hot flashes, decreased appetite, or diarrhea. Report chest pain or palpitation; acute abdominal pain; pain, tingling, or numbness of extremities; swelling of extremities or unusual weight gain; respiratory difficulty; yellowing of skin or sclera; dark urine; pale stool; or unusual fatigue.

Fluticasone (Oral Inhalation)

(floo TIK a sone)

Brand Names: U.S. Flovent® Diskus®; Flovent® HFA

Index Terms Flovent; Fluticasone Propionate

Pharmacologic Category Corticosteroid, Inhalant (Oral)

Medication Safety Issues

Sound-alike/look-alike issues:

Flovent® may be confused with Flonase®

International issues:

Allegro: Brand name for fluticasone [Israel], but also the brand name for frovatriptan [Germany]

Allegro [Israel] may be confused with Allegra and Allegra-D brand names for fexofenadine and fexofenadine/pseudoephedrine, respectively, [U.S., Canada, and multiple international markets]

Flovent [U.S., Canada] may be confused with Flogen brand name for naproxen [Mexico]; Flogene brand name for piroxicam [Brazil]

Pregnancy Risk Factor C

Lactation Excretion in breast milk unknown/use caution

Breast-Feeding Considerations Systemic corticosteroids are excreted in human milk. It is not known if sufficient quantities of fluticasone are absorbed following inhalation to produce detectable amounts in breast milk. The use of inhaled corticosteroids is not considered a contraindication to breast feeding.

Use Maintenance treatment of asthma as prophylactic therapy; also indicated for patients requiring oral corticosteroid therapy for asthma to assist in total discontinuation or reduction of total oral dose

Mechanism of Action/Effect Fluticasone belongs to a group of corticosteroids which utilizes a fluorocarbothioate ester linkage at the 17 carbon position; extremely potent vasoconstrictive and anti-inflammatory activity. The effectiveness of inhaled fluticasone is due to its direct local effect.

Contraindications Hypersensitivity to fluticasone or any component of the formulation; primary treatment of status asthmaticus or acute bronchospasm

Warnings/Precautions May cause hypercorticism or suppression of hypothalamic-pituitary-adrenal (HPA) axis, particularly in younger children or in patients receiving high doses for prolonged periods. HPA axis suppression may lead to adrenal crisis. Withdrawal and discontinuation of a corticosteroid should be done slowly and carefully. Particular care is required when patients are transferred from systemic corticosteroids to inhaled products due to possible adrenal insufficiency or withdrawal from steroids, including an increase in allergic symptoms. Patients receiving ≥20 mg per day of prednisone (or equivalent) may be most susceptible. Concurrent use of ritonavir (and potentially other strong inhibitors of CYP3A4) may increase fluticasone levels and effects on HPA suppression. Fatalities have occurred due to adrenal insufficiency in asthmatic patients during and after transfer from systemic corticosteroids to aerosol steroids; aerosol steroids do **not** provide the systemic steroid needed to treat patients having trauma, surgery, or infections.

Bronchospasm may occur with wheezing after inhalation; if this occurs, stop steroid and treat with a fast-acting bronchodilator. Supplemental steroids (oral or parenteral) may be needed during stress or severe asthma attacks. Corticosteroid use may cause psychiatric disturbances, including depression, euphoria, insomnia, mood swings, and personality changes. Pre-existing psychiatric conditions may be exacerbated by corticosteroid use. Prolonged use of corticosteroids may also increase the incidence of secondary infection, mask acute infection (including fungal infections), prolong or exacerbate viral infections, or limit response to vaccines. Exposure to chickenpox should be avoided; corticosteroids should not be used to treat ocular herpes simplex. Corticosteroids should not be used for cerebral malaria. Close observation is required in patients with latent tuberculosis and/or TB reactivity; restrict use in active TB (only in conjunction with antituberculosis treatment). Rare cases of vasculitis (Churg-Strauss syndrome) or other eosinophilic conditions can occur. Prolonged treatment with corticosteroids has been associated with the development of Kaposi's sarcoma (case reports); if noted, discontinuation of therapy should be considered.

Use with caution in patients with thyroid disease, hepatic impairment, renal impairment, cardiovascular disease, diabetes, glaucoma, cataracts, myasthenia gravis, patients at risk for osteoporosis, patients at risk for seizures, or GI diseases (diverticulitis, peptic ulcer, ulcerative colitis) due to perforation risk. Use caution following acute MI (corticosteroids have been associated with myocardial rupture). Because of the risk of adverse effects, systemic corticosteroids should be used cautiously in the elderly in the smallest possible effective dose for the shortest duration.

Orally-inhaled corticosteroids may cause a reduction in growth velocity in pediatric patients (~1 centimeter per year [range: 0.3-1.8 cm per year] and related to dose and duration of exposure). To minimize the systemic effects of orally-inhaled corticosteroids, each patient should be titrated to the lowest effective dose. Growth should be routinely monitored in pediatric patients.

Not to be used in status asthmaticus or for the relief of acute bronchospasm. Flovent® Diskus® contains lactose; very rare anaphylactic reactions have been reported in patients with severe milk protein allergy. There have been reports of systemic corticosteroid withdrawal symptoms (eg, joint/muscle pain, lassitude, depression) when withdrawing oral inhalation therapy. Local yeast infections (eg, oral pharyngeal candidiasis) may occur. Lower respiratory tract infections, including pneumonia, have been reported in patients with COPD with an even higher incidence in the elderly.

Drug Interactions

Avoid Concomitant Use

Avoid concomitant use of Fluticasone (Oral Inhalation) with any of the following: Aldesleukin; BCG; CYP3A4 Inhibitors (Strong); Natalizumab; Pimecrolimus; Tacrolimus (Topical)

Decreased Effect

Fluticasone (Oral Inhalation) may decrease the levels/effects of: Aldesleukin; Antidiabetic Agents; BCG; Coccidioidin Skin Test; Corticorelin; Sipuleucel-T; Telaprevir; Vaccines (Inactivated)

The levels/effects of Fluticasone (Oral Inhalation) may be decreased by: Echinacea; Tocilizumab

Increased Effect/Toxicity

Fluticasone (Oral Inhalation) may increase the levels/effects of: Amphotericin B; Deferasirox; Leflunomide; Loop Diuretics; Natalizumab; Thiazide Diuretics

The levels/effects of Fluticasone (Oral Inhalation) may be increased by: CYP3A4 Inhibitors (Moderate); CYP3A4 Inhibitors (Strong); Dasatinib; Denosumab; Ivacaftor; Pimecrolimus; Tacrolimus (Topical); Telaprevir; Trastuzumab

Nutritional/Ethanol Interactions Herb/Nutraceutical: In theory, St John's wort may decrease serum levels of fluticasone by inducing CYP3A4 isoenzymes.

Adverse Reactions

>10%:

- Central nervous system: Headache (2% to 14%)
- Respiratory: Upper respiratory tract infection (14% to 21%), throat irritation (3% to 22%)

3% to 10%:

- Central nervous system: Fever (1% to 7%)
- Gastrointestinal: Oral candidiasis (≤9%), nausea/vomiting (1% to 8%), gastrointestinal infection (including viral; 1% to 5%), gastrointestinal discomfort/pain (1% to 4%)
- Neuromuscular & skeletal: Musculoskeletal pain (2% to 5%), muscle injury (1% to 5%)
- Respiratory: Sinusitis/sinus infection (4% to 10%), lower respiratory tract infections/pneumonia (1% to 7%; COPD diagnosis and age >65 years increase risk), cough (1% to 6%), bronchitis (≤8%), hoarseness/dysphonia (2% to 6%), upper respiratory tract inflammation (≤5%), viral respiratory infection (1% to 5%), rhinitis (1% to 4%)
- Miscellaneous: Viral infection (≤5%)

1% to 3%:

- Cardiovascular: Chest symptoms, edema, palpitation
- Central nervous system: Cranial nerve paralysis, dizziness, fatigue, malaise, migraine, mood disorders, pain, sleep disorder
- Dermatologic: Acne, dermatitis/dermatosis, eczema, folliculitis, photodermatitis, infection (fungal, viral), pruritus, rash, urticaria
- Endocrine & metabolic: Fluid disturbance, goiter, uric acid metabolism disturbance
- Gastrointestinal: Abdominal discomfort/pain, appetite changes, dental discomfort/pain, diarrhea, dyspepsia, gastroenteritis, hyposalivation, oral discomfort/pain, oral erythema/rash, oral ulcerations, oropharyngeal plaques, tooth decay, weight gain
- Genitourinary: Reproductive organ infections (bacterial), urinary tract infection
- Hematologic: Hematoma
- Hepatic: Cholecystitis
- Neuromuscular & skeletal: Arthralgia, articular rheumatism, muscle cramps/spasms, muscle pain, muscle stiffness/tightness/rigidity, musculoskeletal inflammation
- Ocular: Blepharoconjunctivitis, conjunctivitis, keratitis
- Otic: Otitis
- Respiratory: Epistaxis, hoarseness/dysphonia, laryngitis, nasal sinus disorder, pharyngitis/throat infection, rhinorrhea/postnasal drip, throat constriction

Miscellaneous: Infection (bacterial, fungal); injuries (including muscle, soft tissue); polyps (ear, nose, throat); tonsillitis

Pharmacodynamics/Kinetics

Onset of Action Maximal benefit may take 1-2 weeks or longer

Available Dosage Forms

Aerosol, for oral inhalation:

Flovent® HFA: 44 mcg/inhalation (10.6 g); 110 mcg/inhalation (12 g); 220 mcg/inhalation (12 g)

Powder, for oral inhalation:

Flovent® Diskus®: 50 mcg (60s); 100 mcg (60s); 250 mcg (60s)

General Dosage Range Inhalation:

Flovent® HFA:

Children 4-11 years: 88 mcg twice daily (maximum: >352 mcg/day in 2 divided doses)

Children ≥12 years and Adults: 88-880 mcg twice daily

Flovent® Diskus®:

Children 4-11 years: 50-100 mcg twice daily

Children >11 years and Adults: 100-1000 mcg twice daily

Administration

Inhalation

Aerosol inhalation: Flovent® HFA: Shake container thoroughly before using. Take 3-5 deep breaths. Use inhaler on inspiration. Allow 1 full minute between inhalations. Rinse mouth with water after use to reduce aftertaste and incidence of candidiasis; do not swallow. Flovent® HFA inhaler must be primed before first use, when not used for 7 days, or if dropped. To prime the first time, release 4 sprays into air; shake well before each spray and spray away from face. If dropped or not used for 7 days, prime by releasing a single test spray. Patient should contact pharmacy for refill when the dose counter reads "020". Discard device when the dose counter reads "000". Do not use "float" test to determine contents.

Powder for oral inhalation: Flovent® Diskus®: Do not use with a spacer device. Do not exhale into Diskus®. Do not wash or take apart. Use in horizontal position. Mouth should be rinsed with water after use (do not swallow). Discard after 6 weeks once removed from protective pouch or when the dose counter reads "0", whichever comes first (device is not reusable).

Stability

Storage

Flovent® HFA: Store at 15°C to 30°C (59°F to 86°F). Discard device when the dose counter reads "000". Store with mouthpiece down.

Flovent® Diskus®: Store at 20°C to 25°C (68°F to 77°F) in a dry place away from direct heat or sunlight. Discard after 6 weeks from removal from protective foil pouch or when the dose counter reads "0" (whichever comes first); device is not reusable.

Nursing Actions

Physical Assessment May take as long as 2 weeks before full benefit of medication is known. Encourage regular eye exams with long-term use. Monitor for possible eosinophilic conditions (including Churg-Strauss syndrome) and signs/symptoms of HPA axis suppression/adrenal insufficiency. Assess growth in adolescents and children.

Patient Education Although you may see improvement within a few hours of use, the full benefit of the medication may not be achieved for several days. Avoid exposure to chickenpox or measles. If exposed, inform your prescriber as soon as possible. May cause headache. Report signs of infection or change in vision to prescriber.

Metered-dose inhalation: Sit when using. Take deep breaths for 3-5 minutes and clear nasal passages before administration (use decongestant as needed). Hold breath for 5-10 seconds after use and wait 1-3 minutes between inhalations. If also using inhaled bronchodilator, use before fluticasone. Rinse mouth and throat after use to reduce aftertaste and prevent candidiasis.

Powder for oral inhalation: Flovent® Diskus®: Do not attempt to take device apart. Do not use with a spacer device. Do not exhale into the Diskus®; use in a level horizontal position. Do not wash the mouthpiece.

Dietary Considerations Flovent® Diskus® contains lactose; very rare anaphylactic reactions have been reported in patients with severe milk protein allergy.

Fluticasone (Nasal) (floo TIK a sone)

Brand Names: U.S. Flonase®; Veramyst®

Index Terms Fluticasone Furoate; Fluticasone Propionate

Pharmacologic Category Corticosteroid, Nasal

Medication Safety Issues

Sound-alike/look-alike issues:

Flonase® may be confused with Flovent®

International issues:

Allegro: Brand name for fluticasone [Israel], but also the brand name for frovatriptan [Germany]

Allegro [Israel] may be confused with Allegra and Allegra-D brand names for fexofenadine and fexofenadine/pseudoephedrine, respectively, [U.S., Canada, and multiple international markets]

Pregnancy Risk Factor C

Lactation Excretion in breast milk unknown/use caution

Use

Flonase®: Management of seasonal and perennial allergic rhinitis and nonallergic rhinitis

Veramyst®, Avamys® [CAN]: Management of seasonal and perennial allergic rhinitis

Available Dosage Forms

Suspension, intranasal: 50 mcg/inhalation (16 g)

Flonase®: 50 mcg/inhalation (16 g)

Veramyst®: 27.5 mcg/inhalation (10 g)

General Dosage Range Intranasal:

Propionate (Flonase®):

Children ≥4 years: Initial: 1 spray (50 mcg/spray) per nostril once daily; Maintenance: 1-2 sprays (100 mcg) per nostril once daily (maximum: 2 sprays in each nostril [200 mcg]/day)

Adults: Initial: 2 sprays (50 mcg/spray) per nostril once daily; Maintenance: 1-2 sprays per nostril once daily

Furoate (Veramyst®):

Children 2-11 years: Initial: 1 spray (27.5 mcg/spray) per nostril once daily; Maintenance 1-2 sprays per nostril once daily (55-110 mcg/day) (maximum: 2 sprays in each nostril [110 mcg]/day)

Children ≥12 years and Adults: Initial: 2 sprays (27.5 mcg/spray) per nostril once daily; Maintenance 1-2 sprays per nostril once daily (55-110 mcg/day) (maximum: 2 sprays in each nostril [110 mcg]/day)

Administration

Inhalation Nasal spray: Administer at regular intervals. Shake bottle gently before using. Blow nose to clear nostrils. Insert applicator into nostril, keeping bottle upright, and close off the other nostril. Breathe in through nose. While inhaling, press pump to release spray. Discard after labeled number of doses has been used, even if bottle is not completely empty.

Flonase®: Prime pump (press 6 times until fine spray appears) prior to first use or if spray unused for ≥7 days. Once weekly, nasal applicator may be removed and rinsed with warm water to clean.

Veramyst®, Avamys® [CAN]: Prime pump (press 6 times until fine spray appears) prior to first use, if spray unused for ≥30 days, or if cap left off bottle for ≥5 days. After each use, nozzle should be wiped with a clean, dry tissue. Once weekly, inside of cap should be cleaned with a clean, dry tissue.

Nursing Actions

Physical Assessment May take as long as 2 weeks before full benefit of medication is known. Encourage regular eye exams with long-term use. Monitor growth in adolescents and children. Assess signs/symptoms of HPA axis suppression/adrenal insufficiency.

Patient Education Shake gently before use. Report unusual cough; persistent nasal bleeding, burning, or irritation; or worsening of condition.

Fluticasone (Topical) (floo TIK a sone)

Brand Names: U.S. Cutivate®

Index Terms Fluticasone Propionate

Pharmacologic Category Corticosteroid, Topical

Medication Safety Issues

Sound-alike/look-alike issues:

Cutivate® may be confused with Ultravate®

International issues:

Allegro: Brand name for fluticasone [Israel], but also the brand name for frovatriptan [Germany]

Allegro [Israel] may be confused with Allegra and Allegra-D brand names for fexofenadine and fexofenadine/pseudoephedrine, respectively, [U.S., Canada, and multiple international markets]

Pregnancy Risk Factor C

Lactation Excretion in breast milk unknown/use caution

Use Relief of inflammation and pruritus associated with corticosteroid-responsive dermatoses; atopic dermatitis

Available Dosage Forms

Cream, topical: 0.05% (15 g, 30 g, 60 g)

Cutivate®: 0.05% (30 g, 60 g)

Lotion, topical:

Cutivate®: 0.05% (120 mL)

Ointment, topical: 0.005% (15 g, 30 g, 60 g)

Cutivate®: 0.005% (30 g, 60 g)

General Dosage Range Topical:

Cream: *Children ≥3 months and Adults:* Apply sparingly to affected area once or twice daily

Lotion:

Children ≥1 year: Apply sparingly to affected area once daily

Adults: Apply sparingly to affected area once or twice daily

Administration

Topical Apply sparingly in a thin film. Rub in lightly. Unless otherwise directed by healthcare professional, do not use with occlusive dressing; do not use on children's skin covered by diapers or plastic pants.

Nursing Actions

Physical Assessment May take as long as 2 weeks before full benefit of medication is known. Monitor for possible eosinophilic conditions (including Churg-Strauss syndrome) and signs/symptoms of HPA axis suppression/adrenal insufficiency. Assess growth in adolescents and children.

Patient Education For external use only. Apply thin film to affected area only; rub in lightly. Do not apply occlusive covering unless advised by prescriber. Wash hand thoroughly after use; avoid contact with eyes. Notify prescriber if skin condition persists or worsens. Do not use for treatment of diaper dermatitis or under diapers or plastic pants.

Fluticasone and Salmeterol

(floo TIK a sone & sal ME te role)

Brand Names: U.S. Advair Diskus®; Advair® HFA

Index Terms Fluticasone Propionate and Salmeterol Xinafoate; Salmeterol and Fluticasone

Pharmacologic Category Beta$_2$ Agonist; Beta$_2$-Adrenergic Agonist, Long-Acting; Corticosteroid, Inhalant (Oral)

Medication Safety Issues

Sound-alike/look-alike issues:

Advair® may be confused with Adcirca®, Advicor®

Medication Guide Available Yes

Pregnancy Risk Factor C

Lactation

Fluticasone: Excretion in breast milk unknown/use caution

Salmeterol: Enters breast milk/use caution

Use Maintenance treatment of asthma; maintenance treatment of COPD

Available Dosage Forms

Aerosol, for oral inhalation:

Advair® HFA:

45/21: Fluticasone propionate 45 mcg and salmeterol 21 mcg (8 g, 12 g) [chlorofluorocarbon free]

115/21: Fluticasone propionate 115 mcg and salmeterol 21 mcg (8 g, 12 g) [chlorofluorocarbon free]

230/21: Fluticasone propionate 230 mcg and salmeterol 21 mcg (8 g, 12 g) [chlorofluorocarbon free]

Powder, for oral inhalation:

Advair Diskus®:

100/50: Fluticasone propionate 100 mcg and salmeterol 50 mcg (14s, 60s)

250/50: Fluticasone propionate 250 mcg and salmeterol 50 mcg (60s)

500/50: Fluticasone propionate 500 mcg and salmeterol 50 mcg (60s)

General Dosage Range Oral inhalation:

Children 4-11 years: Advair Diskus®: Fluticasone 100 mcg/salmeterol 50 mcg/inhalation: One inhalation twice daily (maximum dose)

Children ≥12 years:

Advair Diskus®: Fluticasone 100-500 mcg/salmeterol 50 mcg/inhalation: One inhalation twice daily. Maximum: Fluticasone 500 mcg/salmeterol 50 mcg/inhalation twice daily

Advair® HFA: Fluticasone 45-230 mcg/salmeterol 21 mcg/inhalation: Two inhalations twice daily

Adults:

Advair Diskus®: Initial, maximum: Fluticasone 250 mcg/salmeterol 50 mcg twice daily [COPD]; Maximum dose: Fluticasone 500 mcg/salmeterol 50 mcg/inhalation: One inhalation twice daily [Asthma]

Advair® HFA: Fluticasone 45-230 mcg/salmeterol 50 mcg/inhalation: Two inhalations twice daily

Administration

Inhalation

Advair Diskus®: After removing from box and foil pouch, write the "Pouch opened" and "Use by" dates on the label on top of the Diskus®. The "Use by" date is 1 month from date of opening the pouch. Every time the lever is pushed back, a dose is ready to be inhaled. Do not close or tilt the Diskus® after the lever is pushed back. Do not play with the lever or move the lever more than once. The dose indicator tells you how many doses are left. When the numbers 5 to 0 appear in red, only a few doses remain. Discard device 1 month after you remove it from the foil pouch or when the dose counter reads "0" (whichever comes first). Rinse mouth with water after use and spit to reduce risk of oral candidiasis.

Advair® HFA: Shake well for 5 seconds before each spray. Prime with 4 test sprays (into air and away from face) before using for the first time. If canister is dropped or not used for >4 weeks, prime with 2 sprays. Patient should contact pharmacy for refill when the dose counter reads "020". Discard device when the dose counter reads "000". Do not spray in eyes. Rinse mouth with water after use and spit to reduce risk of oral candidiasis.

Nursing Actions

Physical Assessment See individual agents.

Patient Education See individual agents.

Related Information

Fluticasone (Oral Inhalation) *on page 499*

Salmeterol *on page 1021*

Fluvastatin (FLOO va sta tin)

Brand Names: U.S. Lescol®; Lescol® XL

Pharmacologic Category Antilipemic Agent, HMG-CoA Reductase Inhibitor

Medication Safety Issues

Sound-alike/look-alike issues:

Fluvastatin may be confused with fluoxetine, nystatin, pitavastatin

Pregnancy Risk Factor X

Lactation Enters breast milk/contraindicated

Use To be used as a component of multiple risk factor intervention in patients at risk for atherosclerosis vascular disease due to hypercholesterolemia

Adjunct to dietary therapy to reduce elevated total cholesterol (total-C), LDL-C, triglyceride, and apolipoprotein B (apo-B) levels and to increase HDL-C in primary hypercholesterolemia and mixed dyslipidemia (Fredrickson types IIa and IIb); to slow the progression of coronary atherosclerosis in patients with coronary heart disease; reduce risk of coronary revascularization procedures in patients with coronary heart disease

Available Dosage Forms

Capsule, oral:

Lescol®: 20 mg, 40 mg

Tablet, extended release, oral:

Lescol® XL: 80 mg

General Dosage Range Oral:

Extended release: *Adolescents 10-16 years (females 1 year postmenarche) and Adults:* 80 mg once daily

Immediate release:

Adolescents 10-16 years (females 1 year postmenarche): Initial: 20 mg once daily; Maintenance: Up to 80 mg/day in 2 divided doses

Adults: Initial: 20-40 mg once daily; Maintenance: Up to 80 mg/day in 2 divided doses

Administration

Oral Patient should be placed on a standard cholesterol-lowering diet before and during treatment. Fluvastatin may be taken without regard to meals. Adjust dosage as needed in response to periodic lipid determinations during the first 4 weeks after a dosage change; lipid-lowering effects are additive when fluvastatin is combined with a bile-acid binding resin or niacin, however, it must be administered at least 2 hours following these drugs. Do not break, chew, or crush extended release tablets; do not open capsules.

Nursing Actions

Physical Assessment Rule out secondary causes of hyperlipidemia prior to initiation. Assess risk potential for interactions with other prescriptions or herbal products patient may be taking that may increase risk of rhabdomyolysis or acute renal failure. Assess LFTs and cholesterol panel prior to treatment and at regular intervals.

Patient Education Take as directed, with or without food. If taking other cholesterol-lowering medication, check with prescriber for appropriate timing. Do not chew, crush, or dissolve extended release tablets; swallow whole. Follow prescribed diet and exercise regimen. You will need periodic laboratory tests to evaluate response. Avoid excessive alcohol. Report unusual muscle cramping or weakness, yellowing of skin or eyes, easy bruising or bleeding, or unusual fatigue.

Fluvoxamine (floo VOKS a meen)

Brand Names: U.S. Luvox® CR

Index Terms Luvox

Pharmacologic Category Antidepressant, Selective Serotonin Reuptake Inhibitor

Medication Safety Issues

Sound-alike/look-alike issues:

FluvoxaMINE may be confused with flavoxATE, FLUoxetine, fluPHENAZine

Luvox may be confused with Lasix®, Levoxyl®, Lovenox®

Medication Guide Available Yes

Pregnancy Risk Factor C

Lactation Enters breast milk/consider risk:benefit (AAP rates "of concern"; AAP 2001 update pending)

Breast-Feeding Considerations Fluvoxamine is excreted in breast milk. Based on case reports, the dose the infant receives is relatively small and adverse events have not been observed. According to the manufacturer, the decision to continue or discontinue breast-feeding during therapy should take into account the risk of exposure to the infant and the benefits of treatment to the mother.

The long-term effects on development and behavior have not been studied; therefore, fluvoxamine should be prescribed to a mother who is breast-feeding only when the benefits outweigh the potential risks.

Use Treatment of obsessive-compulsive disorder (OCD)

Unlabeled Use Treatment of major depression; panic disorder; anxiety disorders in children; treatment of mild dementia-associated agitation in nonpsychotic patients; post-traumatic stress disorder (PTSD); social anxiety disorder (SAD)

Mechanism of Action/Effect Inhibits CNS neuron serotonin uptake; minimal or no effect on reuptake of norepinephrine or dopamine; does not significantly bind to alpha-adrenergic, histamine or cholinergic receptors

Contraindications Hypersensitivity to fluvoxamine or any component of the formulation; concurrent use with alosetron, pimozide, ramelteon, thioridazine, or tizanidine; use with or within 14 days of MAO inhibitors

Warnings/Precautions [U.S. Boxed Warning]: Antidepressants increase the risk of suicidal thinking and behavior in children, adolescents, and young adults (18-24 years of age) with major depressive disorder (MDD) and other psychiatric disorders; consider risk prior to prescribing. Short-term studies did not show an increased risk in patients >24 years of age and showed a decreased risk in patients ≥65 years. Closely monitor patients for clinical worsening, suicidality, or unusual changes in behavior, particularly during the initial 1-2 months of therapy or during periods of dosage adjustments (increases or decreases); the patient's family or caregiver should be instructed to closely observe the patient and communicate condition with healthcare provider. A medication guide concerning the use of antidepressants should be dispensed with each prescription. **Fluvoxamine is FDA approved for the treatment of OCD in children ≥8 years of age; extended release capsules are not FDA approved for use in children.**

The possibility of a suicide attempt is inherent in major depression and may persist until remission occurs. Use caution in high-risk patients. Worsening depression and severe abrupt suicidality that are not part of the presenting symptoms may require discontinuation or modification of drug therapy. The patient's family or caregiver should be alerted to monitor patients for the emergence of suicidality and associated behaviors (such as agitation, irritability, hostility, impulsivity, and hypomania) and call healthcare provider.

May worsen psychosis in some patients or precipitate a shift to mania or hypomania in patients with bipolar disorder. Patients presenting with depressive symptoms should be screened for bipolar disorder. Monotherapy in patients with bipolar disorder should be avoided. **Fluvoxamine is not FDA approved for the treatment of bipolar depression.**

Serotonin syndrome and neuroleptic malignant syndrome (NMS)-like reactions have occurred with serotonin/norepinephrine reuptake inhibitors (SNRIs) and selective serotonin reuptake inhibitors (SSRIs) when used alone, and particularly when used in combination with serotonergic agents (eg, triptans) or antidopaminergic agents (eg, antipsychotics). Concurrent use with MAO inhibitors is contraindicated. Fluvoxamine has a low potential to impair cognitive or motor performance; caution operating hazardous machinery or driving. Use caution in patients with a previous seizure disorder or condition predisposing to seizures such as brain damage, alcoholism, or concurrent therapy with other drugs which lower the seizure threshold. Fluvoxamine may significantly increase alosetron concentrations; concurrent use **contraindicated.** Potential for QT_c prolongation and arrhythmia with thioridazine and pimozide; concurrent use of fluvoxamine with either of these agents is **contraindicated.** Concomitant use with tizanidine may cause a significant decrease in blood pressure and increase in drowsiness; concurrent use is **contraindicated.** Fluvoxamine levels may be lower in patients who smoke.

May increase the risks associated with electroconvulsive therapy. Use with caution in patients with hepatic dysfunction and in elderly patients. May cause hyponatremia/SIADH (elderly at increased risk); volume depletion (diuretics may increase risk). Use with caution in patients at risk of bleeding or receiving concurrent anticoagulant therapy, although not consistently noted, fluvoxamine may cause impairment in platelet function. May cause or exacerbate sexual dysfunction.

Drug Interactions

Avoid Concomitant Use

Avoid concomitant use of FluvoxaMINE with any of the following: Alosetron; Clopidogrel; Iobenguane I 123; MAO Inhibitors; Methylene Blue; Pimozide; Ramelteon; Thioridazine; TiZANidine; Tryptophan

Decreased Effect

FluvoxaMINE may decrease the levels/effects of: Clopidogrel; Iobenguane I 123; Ioflupane I 123

The levels/effects of FluvoxaMINE may be decreased by: CarBAMazepine; CYP1A2 Inducers (Strong); Cyproheptadine; Cyproterone; NSAID (COX-2 Inhibitor); NSAID (Nonselective); Peginterferon Alfa-2b

Increased Effect/Toxicity

FluvoxaMINE may increase the levels/effects of: Alosetron; Anticoagulants; Antidepressants (Serotonin Reuptake Inhibitor/Antagonist); Antiplatelet Agents; Asenapine; Aspirin; Bendamustine; Benzodiazepines (metabolized by oxidation); Bromazepam; BusPIRone; CarBAMazepine; CloZAPine; Collagenase (Systemic); CYP1A2 Substrates; CYP2C19 Substrates; Desmopressin; Drotrecogin Alfa (Activated); DULoxetine; Erlotinib; Fosphenytoin; Haloperidol; Ibritumomab; Lithium; Methadone; Methylene Blue; Metoclopramide; Mexiletine; NSAID (COX-2 Inhibitor); NSAID (Nonselective); OLANZapine; Phenytoin; Pimozide; Propafenone; Propranolol; QuiNIDine; Ramelteon; Rivaroxaban; Roflumilast; Ropivacaine; Salicylates; Serotonin Modulators; Theophylline Derivatives; Thioridazine; Thrombolytic Agents; TiZANidine; Tositumomab and Iodine I 131 Tositumomab; TraMADol; Tricyclic Antidepressants; Vitamin K Antagonists

The levels/effects of FluvoxaMINE may be increased by: Abiraterone Acetate; Alcohol (Ethyl); Analgesics (Opioid); Antipsychotics; BusPIRone; Cimetidine; CNS Depressants; CYP1A2 Inhibitors (Moderate); CYP1A2 Inhibitors (Strong); CYP2D6 Inhibitors (Moderate); CYP2D6 Inhibitors (Strong); Darunavir; Dasatinib; Deferasirox; Glucosamine; Herbs (Anticoagulant/Antiplatelet Properties); Linezolid; MAO Inhibitors; Metoclopramide; Omega-3-Acid Ethyl Esters; Pentosan Polysulfate Sodium; Pentoxifylline; Prostacyclin Analogues; TraMADol; Tryptophan; Vitamin E

Nutritional/Ethanol Interactions

Ethanol: May increase CNS depression; monitor for increased effects with coadministration. Caution patients about effects.

Food: The bioavailability of melatonin has been reported to be increased by fluvoxamine.

Herb/Nutraceutical: Avoid valerian, St John's wort, SAMe, kava kava (may increase risk of serotonin syndrome and/or excessive sedation). Avoid alfalfa, anise, bilberry, bladderwrack, bromelain, cat's claw, celery, chamomile, coleus, cordyceps, dong quai, evening primrose, fenugreek, feverfew, garlic, ginger, ginkgo biloba, ginseng (American), ginseng (Panax), ginseng (Siberian), grape seed, green tea, guggul, horse chestnuts, horseradish, licorice, prickly ash, red clover, reishi, SAMe (S-adenosylmethionine), sweet clover, turmeric, white willow (all have additional antiplatelet activity).

Adverse Reactions Frequency varies by dosage form and indication. Adverse reactions reported as a composite of all indications.

>10%:
- Central nervous system: Headache (22% to 35%), insomnia (21% to 35%), somnolence (22% to 27%), dizziness (11% to 15%), nervousness (10% to 12%)
- Gastrointestinal: Nausea (34% to 40%), diarrhea (11% to 18%), xerostomia (10% to 14%), anorexia (6% to 14%)
- Genitourinary: Ejaculation abnormal (8% to 11%)
- Neuromuscular & skeletal: Weakness (14% to 26%)

1% to 10%:
- Cardiovascular: Chest pain (3%), palpitation (3%), vasodilation (2% to 3%), hypertension (1% to 2%), edema (≤1%), hypotension (≤1%), syncope (≤1%), tachycardia (≤1%)
- Central nervous system: Pain (10%), anxiety (5% to 8%), abnormal dreams (3%), abnormal thinking (3%), agitation (2% to 3%), apathy (≥1% to 3%), chills (2%), CNS stimulation (2%), depression (2%), neurosis (2%), amnesia, malaise, manic reaction, psychotic reaction
- Dermatologic: Bruising (4%), acne (2%)
- Endocrine & metabolic: Libido decreased (2% to 10%; incidence higher in males), anorgasmia (2% to 5%), sexual function abnormal (2% to 4%), menorrhagia (3%)
- Gastrointestinal: Dyspepsia (8% to 10%), constipation (4% to 10%), vomiting (4% to 6%), abdominal pain (5%), flatulence (4%), taste perversion (2% to 3%), toothache and dental caries (2% to 3%), dysphagia (2%), gingivitis (2%), weight loss (≤1% to 2%), weight gain
- Genitourinary: Polyuria (2% to 3%), impotence (2%), urinary tract infection (2%), urinary retention (1%)
- Hepatic: Liver function tests abnormal (≥1% to 2%)
- Neuromuscular & skeletal: Tremor (5% to 8%), myalgia (5%), paresthesia (3%), hypertonia (2%), twitching (2%), hyper-/hypokinesia, myoclonus
- Ocular: Amblyopia (2% to 3%)
- Respiratory: Upper respiratory infection (9%), pharyngitis (6%), yawn (2% to 5%), laryngitis (3%), bronchitis (2%), dyspnea (2%), epistaxis (2%), cough increased, sinusitis
- Miscellaneous: Diaphoresis (6% to 7%), flu-like syndrome (3%), viral infection (2%)

Pharmacodynamics/Kinetics

Onset of Action Depression: The onset of action is within a week; however, individual response varies greatly and full response may not be seen until 8-12 weeks after initiation of treatment.

Available Dosage Forms

Capsule, extended release, oral:
Luvox® CR: 100 mg, 150 mg

Tablet, oral: 25 mg, 50 mg, 100 mg

General Dosage Range Dosage adjustment recommended in patients with hepatic impairment

Oral:

Children 8-11 years: Initial: 25 mg at bedtime; Maintenance: 50-200 mg/day (maximum: 200 mg/day)

Children 12-17 years: Initial: 25 mg at bedtime; Maintenance: 50-200 mg/day (maximum: 300 mg/day)

Adults: Initial: 50-100 mg at bedtime; Maintenance: 100-300 mg/day in 1-2 divided doses

Administration

Oral May be administered with or without food. Do not crush, open, or chew extended release capsules.

Stability

Storage Protect from high humidity and store at controlled room temperature 25°C (77°F).

Nursing Actions

Physical Assessment Monitor for CNS and gastrointestinal disturbances. Taper dosage slowly when discontinuing. Assess mental status for depression, signs of clinical worsening, suicide ideation, anxiety, social functioning, mania, or panic attack.

Patient Education It may take 2-3 weeks to achieve desired results. Avoid alcohol. Maintain adequate hydration, unless instructed to restrict fluid intake. You may experience drowsiness, lightheadedness, impaired coordination, dizziness, weakness, blurred vision, nausea, vomiting, dry mouth, anorexia, diarrhea, postural hypotension, or decreased sexual function or libido (reversible). Report persistent CNS effects (insomnia, anxiety, suicide ideation, sedation, seizures, mania, abnormal thinking); rash; tremors; chest pain or palpitations; or worsening of condition.

Dietary Considerations May be taken with or without food.

Folic Acid (FOE lik AS id)

Brand Names: U.S. Folacin-800 [OTC]

Index Terms Folacin; Folate; Pteroylglutamic Acid

Pharmacologic Category Vitamin, Water Soluble

Medication Safety Issues

Sound-alike/look-alike issues:

Folic acid may be confused with folinic acid

Pregnancy Risk Factor A

Lactation Enters breast milk/compatible

Use Treatment of megaloblastic and macrocytic anemias due to folate deficiency; dietary supplement to prevent neural tube defects

Unlabeled Use Adjunctive cofactor therapy in methanol toxicity (alternative to leucovorin calcium)

Available Dosage Forms

Injection, solution: 5 mg/mL (10 mL)

Tablet, oral: 0.4 mg, 0.8 mg, 1 mg
Folacin-800 [OTC]: 0.8 mg

General Dosage Range

I.M., I.V., SubQ:

Infants: 0.1 mg/day

Children <4 years: Up to 0.3 mg/day

Children ≥4 years and Adults: 0.4 mg/day

Pregnant and lactating women: 0.8 mg/day

Oral:

Infants: 0.1 mg/day

Children <4 years: Up to 0.3 mg/day

Children ≥4 years and Adults: 0.4 mg/day

Pregnant and lactating women: 0.8 mg/day (anemia) **or** 4 mg/day (prevention of neural tube defects)

Females of childbearing potential: Prevention of neural tube defects: 0.4-0.8 mg/day

Administration

I.M. May also be administered by deep I.M. injection.

I.V. May administer ≤5 mg dose undiluted over ≥1 minute **or** may dilute ≤5 mg in 50 mL of NS or D_5W and infuse over 30 minutes. May also be added to I.V. maintenance solutions and given as an infusion.

I.V. Detail pH: 8-11

Nursing Actions

Patient Education Increased intake of foods high in folic acid may be recommended by prescriber. Excessive use of alcohol increases requirement for folic acid. Report skin rash.

Follitropin Alfa (foe li TRO pin AL fa)

Brand Names: U.S. Gonal-f®; Gonal-f® RFF; Gonal-f® RFF Pen

Index Terms Follicle Stimulating Hormone, Recombinant; FSH; rFSH-alpha; rhFSH-alpha

Pharmacologic Category Gonadotropin; Ovulation Stimulator

Pregnancy Risk Factor X

Lactation Excretion in breast milk unknown/not recommended

Use

Gonal-f®: Induction of ovulation in anovulatory infertile patients in whom the cause of infertility is functional and not caused by primary ovarian failure; development of multiple follicles with Assisted Reproductive Technology (ART); induction of spermatogenesis in men with primary and secondary hypogonadotropic hypogonadism in whom the cause of infertility is not due to primary testicular failure.

Gonal-f® RFF: Induction of ovulation in oligo-anovulatory infertile patients in whom the cause of infertility is functional and not caused by primary ovarian failure; development of multiple follicles with ART

Mechanism of Action/Effect Follitropin alfa is a human FSH preparation of recombinant DNA origin. Follitropins stimulate ovarian follicular growth in women who do not have primary ovarian failure, and stimulate spermatogenesis in men with hypogonadotrophic hypogonadism. FSH is required for normal follicular growth, maturation, gonadal steroid production, and spermatogenesis.

Contraindications Hypersensitivity to follitropins or any component of the formulation; high levels of FSH indicating primary gonadal failure (ovarian or testicular); uncontrolled thyroid or adrenal dysfunction; tumor of the ovary, breast, uterus, hypothalamus, testis, or pituitary gland; abnormal vaginal bleeding of undetermined origin; ovarian cysts or enlargement not due to polycystic ovary syndrome; pregnancy

Warnings/Precautions These medications should only be used by physicians who are thoroughly familiar with infertility problems and their management. To minimize risks, use only at the lowest effective dose. Monitor ovarian response with serum estradiol and vaginal ultrasound on a regular basis.

Ovarian enlargement, which may be accompanied by abdominal distention or abdominal pain, occurs in ~20% of those treated with urofollitropin and hCG, and generally regresses without treatment within 2-3 weeks. If ovaries are abnormally enlarged on the last day of treatment, withhold hCG to reduce the risk of ovarian hyperstimulation syndrome (OHSS). OHSS is reported in about 7% of patients; it is characterized by severe ovarian enlargement, abdominal pain/distention, nausea, vomiting, diarrhea, dyspnea, and oliguria, and may be accompanied by ascites, pleural effusion, hypovolemia, electrolyte imbalance, hemoperitoneum, and thromboembolic events. If hyperstimulation occurs, stop treatment and hospitalize patient. This syndrome develops rapidly within 24 hours to several days and generally occurs after treatment has ended and reaches its maximum on days 7-10 days following treatment. Hemoconcentration associated with fluid loss into the abdominal cavity has occurred and should be assessed by fluid intake and output, weight, hematocrit, serum and urinary electrolytes, urine specific gravity, BUN and creatinine, and abdominal girth. Determinations should be performed daily or more often if the need arises. Treatment is primarily symptomatic and consists of bedrest, fluid and electrolyte replacement, and analgesics. The ascitic, pleural, and pericardial fluids should not be removed unless needed to relieve symptoms of cardiopulmonary distress.

Serious pulmonary conditions (atelectasis, acute respiratory distress syndrome, and exacerbation of asthma) have been reported. Thromboembolic events, both in association with and separate from ovarian hyperstimulation syndrome, have been reported.

Multiple births may result from the use of these medications; advise patient of the potential risk of multiple births before starting the treatment.

Drug Interactions

Avoid Concomitant Use There are no known interactions where it is recommended to avoid concomitant use.

Decreased Effect There are no known significant interactions involving a decrease in effect.

Increased Effect/Toxicity There are no known significant interactions involving an increase in effect.

Adverse Reactions Percentage may vary by indication, product formulation

>10%:

Central nervous system: Headache
Dermatologic: Acne (males)
Endocrine & metabolic: Breast pain (males), ovarian cyst
Gastrointestinal: Abdomen enlarged, abdominal pain, nausea
Miscellaneous: Upper respiratory infection

1% to 10%:

Cardiovascular: Chest pain, hypotension, palpitation
Central nervous system: Anxiety, dizziness, emotional lability, fatigue, fever, malaise, migraine, nervousness, pain, somnolence
Dermatologic: Acne (females), pruritus
Endocrine & metabolic: Breast pain (females), cervix lesion, dysmenorrhea, gynecomastia, hot flashes, intermenstrual bleeding, menstrual disorder, ovarian disorder, ovarian hyperstimulation
Gastrointestinal: Anorexia, constipation, diarrhea, dyspepsia, flatulence, stomatitis (ulcerative), toothache, vomiting, weight gain
Genitourinary: Cystitis, leukorrhea, micturition frequency, pelvic pain, urinary tract infection, uterine hemorrhage, vaginal hemorrhage
Local: Injection site bruising, edema, inflammation, pain, reaction
Neuromuscular & skeletal: Back pain, myalgia, paresthesia
Respiratory: Asthma, cough, dyspnea, pharyngitis, rhinitis, sinusitis
Miscellaneous: Flu-like syndrome, infection, moniliasis, thirst increased

Pharmacodynamics/Kinetics

Onset of Action Peak effect:

Spermatogenesis, median: 6.8-12.4 months (range: 2.7-18.1 months)
Follicle development: Within cycle

Available Dosage Forms

Injection, powder for reconstitution:

Gonal-f®: 450 int. units, 1050 int. units
Gonal-f® RFF: 75 int. units

Injection, solution:

Gonal-f® RFF Pen: 300 int. units/0.5 mL (0.5 mL); 450 int. units/0.75 mL (0.75 mL); 900 int. units/1.5 mL (1.5 mL)

General Dosage Range SubQ:

Adults (females): Initial: 75-225 int. units/day; Maximum: Up to 300-450 int. units/day

Adults (males): Gonal-f®: Initial: 150 int. units 3 times/week; Maximum: Up to 300 int. units 3 times/week

Administration

Other Gonal-f®, Gonal-f® RFF: Administer SubQ. Contents of multidose vials should be administered using the calibrated syringes provided by the manufacturer. Do not shake solution; allow any bubbles to settle prior to administration.

Stability

Reconstitution

Gonal-f®: Dissolve the contents of vial by slowly injecting provided diluent; do not shake. If bubbles appear, allow to settle prior to use. Final concentration: 600 int. units/mL.

Gonal-f® RFF: Powder: Dissolve contents of one or more vials using diluent provided in prefilled syringe. (Total concentration should not exceed 450 int. units/mL.) Slowly inject diluent into vial, and gently rotate vial until powder is dissolved; do not shake vial. If bubbles appear, allow to settle prior to use. Use immediately after reconstitution.

Storage

Gonal-f®: Store powder refrigerated or at room temperature of 2°C to 25°C (36°F to 77°F). Protect from light; do not freeze. Following reconstitution, multidose vials may be stored under refrigeration or at room temperature for up to 28 days.

Gonal-f® RFF:

Powder: Store at room temperature or under refrigeration of 2°C to 25°C (36°F to 77°F). Protect from light. Discard unused drug.

Solution (pen): Prior to dispensing, store under refrigeration at 2°C to 8°C (36°F to 46°F). Upon dispensing, patient may store under refrigeration until product expiration date or at room temperature of 20°C to 25°C (68°F to 77°F) for up to 3 months. Do not freeze. Protect from light. After first use, discard unused portion after 28 days.

Nursing Actions

Physical Assessment This medication should only be prescribed by a fertility specialist. Teach patient appropriate injection technique and syringe disposal.

Patient Education This medication can only be administered by injection. If you are using this medication at home, follow exact instructions for administering injections and disposal of syringes. Frequent laboratory tests will be required while you are on this therapy; do not miss appointments for laboratory tests or ultrasound. You may experience headache, dizziness, fever, nausea, or vomiting. Report immediately abdominal pain/distension or bloating; persistent nausea, vomiting, or diarrhea; dyspnea; respiratory difficulty or exacerbation of asthma; swelling, pain, or redness of extremities; itching or burning on urination; menstrual irregularity, acute backache; or rash, pain, or inflammation at injection site.

Follitropin Beta (foe li TRO pin BAY ta)

Brand Names: U.S. Follistim® AQ; Follistim® AQ Cartridge

Index Terms Follicle Stimulating Hormone, Recombinant; FSH; rFSH-beta; rhFSH-beta

Pharmacologic Category Gonadotropin; Ovulation Stimulator

Pregnancy Risk Factor X

Lactation Excretion in breast milk unknown/not recommended

Use

Females: Induction of ovulation and pregnancy in anovulatory infertile patients in whom the cause of infertility is functional and not caused by primary ovarian failure; induction of pregnancy in normal ovulatory women undergoing Assisted Reproductive Technology (ART) (eg, *in vitro* fertilization [IVF], intracytoplasmic sperm injection [ICSI])

Males: Induction of spermatogenesis in men with primary and secondary hypogonadotropic hypogonadism in whom the cause of infertility is not due to primary testicular failure.

Mechanism of Action/Effect Follitropin beta is a human FSH preparation of recombinant DNA origin. Follitropins stimulate ovarian follicular growth in women who do not have primary ovarian failure and stimulate spermatogenesis in men with hypogonadotrophic hypogonadism. FSH is required for normal follicular growth, maturation, gonadal steroid production, and spermatogenesis.

Contraindications Hypersensitivity to follitropins or any component of the formulation; high levels of FSH indicating primary gonadal failure; uncontrolled nongonadal endocrinopathies (eg, adrenal, pituitary, or thyroid disorders); tumor of the ovary, breast, uterus, testis, hypothalamus, or pituitary gland

Females: Additional contraindications: Abnormal vaginal bleeding of undetermined origin; ovarian cysts or enlargement not due to polycystic ovary syndrome; pregnancy

Warnings/Precautions These medications should only be used by physicians who are thoroughly familiar with infertility problems and their management. To minimize risks, use only at the lowest effective dose. Monitor ovarian response with serum estradiol and vaginal ultrasound on a regular basis.

If ovaries are abnormally enlarged on the last day of treatment, withhold hCG to reduce the risk of ovarian hyperstimulation syndrome (OHSS). OHSS is characterized by severe ovarian enlargement, abdominal pain/distention, nausea, vomiting, diarrhea, dyspnea, and oliguria, and may be accompanied by ascites, pleural effusion, hypovolemia, electrolyte imbalance, hemoperitoneum, and thromboembolic events. If hyperstimulation occurs, stop treatment and hospitalize patient. This syndrome develops rapidly within 24 hours to several days and generally occurs after treatment has ended and reaches its maximum on days 7-10 following treatment. Hemoconcentration associated with fluid loss into the abdominal cavity has occurred and should be assessed by fluid intake and output, weight, hematocrit, serum and urinary electrolytes, urine specific gravity, BUN and creatinine, and abdominal girth. Determinations should be performed daily or more often if the need arises. Treatment is primarily symptomatic and consists of bedrest, fluid and electrolyte replacement, and analgesics. The ascitic, pleural, and pericardial fluids should not be removed unless needed to relieve symptoms of cardiopulmonary distress. Ovarian torsion may occur in relation to OHSS, pregnancy, previous or current ovarian cyst and polycystic ovaries, previous abdominal surgery, and previous history of ovarian torsion

Serious pulmonary conditions (atelectasis, acute respiratory distress syndrome, and exacerbation of asthma) have been reported. Thromboembolic events, both in association with and separate from ovarian hyperstimulation syndrome, have been reported.

Multiple births may result from the use of these medications; advise patient of the potential risk of multiple births before starting the treatment. May contain trace amounts of neomycin or streptomycin.

Drug Interactions

Avoid Concomitant Use There are no known interactions where it is recommended to avoid concomitant use.

Decreased Effect There are no known significant interactions involving a decrease in effect.

Increased Effect/Toxicity There are no known significant interactions involving an increase in effect.

Adverse Reactions Frequency may vary based on indication.

Central nervous system: Headache (7%), fatigue (2%)

Dermatologic: Acne (7%), rash (3%)

Endocrine & metabolic: Pelvic discomfort (8%), ovarian hyperstimulation (6% to 8%), pelvic pain (6%), gynecomastia (3%), ovarian cyst (3%)

Gastrointestinal: Nausea (4%), abdominal pain/discomfort (2% to 3%)

Local: Injection site pain (7%), injection site reaction (7%)

Postmarketing and/or case reports: Abdominal distension, breast tenderness, constipation, diarrhea, metrorrhagia, miscarriage, ovarian enlargement, ovarian neoplasm, ovarian torsion, thromboembolism, vaginal hemorrhage

Pharmacodynamics/Kinetics

Onset of Action Peak effect: Females: Follicle development: Within cycle

Available Dosage Forms

Injection, solution:

Follistim® AQ: 75 int. units/0.5 mL (0.5 mL); 150 int. units/0.5 mL (0.5 mL)

Follistim® AQ Cartridge: 350 int. units/0.42 mL (0.42 mL); 650 int. units/0.78 mL (0.78 mL); 975 int. units/1.17 mL (1.17 mL)

General Dosage Range

I.M., SubQ: *Adults (females):* Initial: 75-225 int. units/day; Maintenance: Up to 175-600 int. units/day

SubQ: *Adults (males):* 450 int. units/week

Administration

I.M. Follistim® AQ may be administered by I.M. or SubQ injection.

Other

Follistim® AQ may be administered by I.M. or SubQ injection. Follistim® AQ cartridge may be administered only by SubQ injection using the Follistim Pen® which can be set to deliver the appropriate dose.

Stability

Storage Prior to dispensing, store refrigerated at 2°C to 8°C (36°F to 46°F). After dispensed, may be stored under refrigeration or ≤25°C (77°F) for up to 3 months. Once cartridge is pierced, must be stored at 2°C to 25°C (36°F to 77°F) and used within 28 days. Do not freeze. Protect from light.

Nursing Actions

Physical Assessment This medication should only be prescribed by a fertility specialist. Teach patient appropriate injection technique and syringe disposal.

Patient Education This medication can only be administered by injection. If you are using this medication at home, follow exact instruction for administering injections and disposal of syringes. Frequent laboratory tests will be required while you are on this therapy; do not miss appointments for laboratory tests or ultrasound. You may experience headache, dizziness, fever, nausea, or vomiting. Report immediately abdominal pain/distension or bloating; persistent nausea, vomiting, or diarrhea; dyspnea; respiratory difficulty; swelling, pain, or redness of extremities; acute backache; or rash, pain, or inflammation at injection site.

Fondaparinux (fon da PARE i nuks)

Brand Names: U.S. Arixtra®

Index Terms Fondaparinux Sodium

Pharmacologic Category Factor Xa Inhibitor

Medication Safety Issues

High alert medication:

The Institute for Safe Medication Practices (ISMP) includes this medication among its list of drugs which have a heightened risk of causing significant patient harm when used in error.

Pregnancy Risk Factor B

Lactation Excretion in breast milk unknown/use caution

Use Prophylaxis of deep vein thrombosis (DVT) in patients undergoing surgery for hip replacement, knee replacement, hip fracture (including extended prophylaxis following hip fracture surgery), or abdominal surgery (in patients at risk for thromboembolic complications); treatment of acute pulmonary embolism (PE); treatment of acute DVT without PE

Canadian labeling: Additional uses (not approved in U.S.): Unstable angina or non-ST segment elevation myocardial infarction (UA/NSTEMI) for the prevention of death and subsequent MI; ST segment elevation MI (STEMI) for the prevention of death and myocardial reinfarction

Unlabeled Use Prophylaxis of DVT in patients with a history of heparin-induced thrombocytopenia (HIT)

Mechanism of Action/Effect Fondaparinux prevents factor Xa from binding with antithrombin III and inhibits thrombin formation and thrombus development.

Contraindications Hypersensitivity to fondaparinux or any component of the formulation; severe renal impairment (Cl_{cr} <30 mL/minute); body weight <50 kg (prophylaxis); active major bleeding; bacterial endocarditis; thrombocytopenia associated with a positive *in vitro* test for antiplatelet antibody in the presence of fondaparinux

Warnings/Precautions **[U.S. Boxed Warning]: Spinal or epidural hematomas, including subsequent paralysis, may occur with recent or anticipated neuraxial anesthesia (epidural or spinal anesthesia) or spinal puncture in patients anticoagulated with LMWH, heparinoids, or fondaparinux.** Consider risk versus benefit prior to spinal procedures; risk is increased by the use of concomitant agents which may alter hemostasis, the use of indwelling epidural catheters for analgesia, a history of spinal deformity or spinal surgery, as well as a history of traumatic or repeated epidural or spinal punctures. Patient should be observed closely for bleeding and signs and symptoms of neurological impairment if therapy is administered during or immediately following diagnostic lumbar puncture, epidural anesthesia, or spinal anesthesia.

Not to be used interchangeably (unit-for-unit) with heparin, low molecular weight heparins (LMWHs), or heparinoids. Use caution in patients with moderate renal dysfunction (Cl_{cr} 30-50 mL/minute); contraindicated in patients with Cl_{cr} <30 mL/minute. Discontinue if severe dysfunction or labile function develops.

Use caution in congenital or acquired bleeding disorders; bacterial endocarditis; renal impairment; hepatic impairment; active ulcerative or angiodysplastic gastrointestinal disease; hemorrhagic stroke; shortly after brain, spinal, or ophthalmologic surgery; or in patients taking platelet inhibitors. Risk of major bleeding may be increased if initial dose is administered earlier than recommended (initiation recommended at 6-8 hours following surgery). Discontinue agents that may enhance the risk of hemorrhage if possible. Although considered an insensitive measure of fondaparinux activity, there have been postmarketing reports of bleeding associated with elevated aPTT. Thrombocytopenia has occurred with administration, including reports of thrombocytopenia with thrombosis similar to heparin-induced thrombocytopenia. Monitor patients closely and discontinue therapy if platelets fall to <100,000/mm^3.

For subcutaneous administration; not for I.M. administration. Do not use interchangeably (unit for unit) with low molecular weight heparins, heparin, or heparinoids. Use caution in patients <50 kg who are being treated for DVT/PE; dosage reduction recommended. Contraindicated in patients <50 kg when used for prophylactic therapy. Use with caution in the elderly. The needle guard contains natural latex rubber.

The administration of fondaparinux is **not recommended** prior to and during primary PCI in patients with STEMI, due to an increased risk for guiding-catheter thrombosis. Patients with UA/NSTEMI or STEMI undergoing any PCI should not receive fondaparinux as the sole anticoagulant. Use of an anticoagulant with antithrombin activity (eg, unfractionated heparin) is recommended as adjunctive therapy to PCI even if prior treatment with fondaparinux (must take into account whether GP IIb/IIIa antagonists have been administered) (Levine, 2011). Do not administer with other agents that increase the risk of hemorrhage unless they are essential for the management of the underlying condition (eg, warfarin for treatment of VTE).

Drug Interactions

Avoid Concomitant Use

Avoid concomitant use of Fondaparinux with any of the following: Rivaroxaban

Decreased Effect There are no known significant interactions involving a decrease in effect.

Increased Effect/Toxicity

Fondaparinux may increase the levels/effects of: Anticoagulants; Collagenase (Systemic); Deferasirox; Ibritumomab; Rivaroxaban; Tositumomab and Iodine I 131 Tositumomab

The levels/effects of Fondaparinux may be increased by: Antiplatelet Agents; Dasatinib; Drotrecogin Alfa (Activated); Herbs (Anticoagulant/Antiplatelet Properties); Nonsteroidal Anti-Inflammatory Agents; Pentosan Polysulfate Sodium; Prostacyclin Analogues; Salicylates; Thrombolytic Agents

Nutritional/Ethanol Interactions Herb/Nutraceutical: Avoid alfalfa, anise, bilberry, bladderwrack, bromelain, cat's claw, celery, coleus, cordyceps, dong quai, evening primrose oil, fenugreek, feverfew, garlic, ginger, ginkgo biloba, ginseng (American/Panax/Siberian), grapeseed, green tea, guggul, horse chestnut seed, horseradish, licorice, prickly ash, red clover, reishi, sweet clover, turmeric, white willow (all possess anticoagulant or antiplatelet activity and as such, may enhance the anticoagulant effects of fondaparinux).

Adverse Reactions As with all anticoagulants, bleeding is the major adverse effect. Hemorrhage may occur at any site. Risk appears increased by a number of factors including renal dysfunction, age (>75 years), and weight (<50 kg).

>10%:
- Central nervous system: Fever (4% to 14%)
- Gastrointestinal: Nausea (11%)
- Hematologic: Anemia (20%)

1% to 10%:
- Cardiovascular: Edema (9%), hypotension (4%), thrombosis PCI catheter (without heparin 1%)
- Central nervous system: Insomnia (5%), dizziness (4%), headache (2% to 5%), confusion (3%), pain (2%)
- Dermatologic: Rash (8%), purpura (4%), bullous eruption (3%)
- Endocrine & metabolic: Hypokalemia (1% to 4%)
- Gastrointestinal: Constipation (5% to 9%), nausea (3%), vomiting (6%), diarrhea (3%), dyspepsia (2%)
- Genitourinary: Urinary tract infection (4%), urinary retention (3%)
- Hematologic: Moderate thrombocytopenia (50,000-100,000/mm^3: 3%), major bleeding (1% to 3%), minor bleeding (2% to 4%), hematoma (3%); risk of major bleeding increased as high as 5% in patients receiving initial dose <6 hours following surgery
- Hepatic: ALT increased (≤3%), AST increased (≤2%)
- Local: Injection site reaction (bleeding, rash, pruritus)
- Miscellaneous: Wound drainage increased (5%)

Available Dosage Forms

Injection, solution [preservative free]: 2.5 mg/0.5 mL (0.5 mL); 5 mg/0.4 mL (0.4 mL); 7.5 mg/0.6 mL (0.6 mL); 10 mg/0.8 mL (0.8 mL)

Arixtra®: 2.5 mg/0.5 mL (0.5 mL); 5 mg/0.4 mL (0.4 mL); 7.5 mg/0.6 mL (0.6 mL); 10 mg/0.8 mL (0.8 mL)

General Dosage Range SubQ:

Adults <50 kg: Treatment: 5 mg once daily

Adults 50-100 kg: Prophylaxis: 2.5 mg once daily; Treatment: 7.5 mg once daily

Adults >100 kg: Prophylaxis: 2.5 mg once daily; Treatment: 10 mg once daily

Administration

I.M. Do **not** administer I.M.

I.V. Canadian labeling only: STEMI patients: I.V. push or mixed in 25-50 mL of NS and infused over 2 minutes. Flush tubing with NS after infusion to ensure complete administration of fondaparinux. Infusion bag should not be mixed with other agents.

Other For SubQ administration only. Do not mix with other injections or infusions. Do not expel air bubble from syringe before injection. Administer according to recommended regimen; early initiation (before 6 hours after surgery) has been associated with increased bleeding.

To convert from I.V. unfractionated heparin (UFH) infusion to SubQ fondaparinux (Nutescu, 2007): Calculate specific dose for fondaparinux based on indication, discontinue UFH, and begin fondaparinux within 1 hour

To convert from SubQ fondaparinux to I.V. UFH infusion (Nutescu, 2007): Discontinue fondaparinux; calculate specific dose for I.V. UFH infusion based on indication; omit heparin bolus/loading dose

For subQ fondaparinux dosed every 24 hours: Start I.V. UFH infusion 22-23 hours after last dose of fondaparinux

Stability

Reconstitution Canadian labeling: For I.V. administration: May mix with 25 mL or 50 mL NS

Storage Store at 25°C (77°F); excursions permitted to 15°C to 30°C (59°F to 86°F).

Canadian labeling: For I.V. administration: Manufacturer recommends immediate use once diluted in NS, but is stable for up to 24 hours at 15°C to 30°C (59°F to 86°F).

Nursing Actions

Physical Assessment Assess closely for bleeding; bleeding precautions should be observed. Teach appropriate injection technique, syringe/needle disposal, and bleeding precautions.

Patient Education This drug can only be administered by injection. Report pain, burning, redness, or swelling at injection site. You may have a tendency to bleed easily while taking this drug. May cause bleeding problems, anemia, nausea, and fever. Report unusual bleeding or bruising (bleeding gums, nosebleed, blood in urine, dark stool), pain in joints or back, CNS changes (severe headache, confusion), any falls or accidents, or rash.

Formoterol (for MOH te rol)

Brand Names: U.S. Foradil® Aerolizer®; Perforomist®

Index Terms Formoterol Fumarate; Formoterol Fumarate Dihydrate

Pharmacologic Category $Beta_2$ Agonist; $Beta_2$-Adrenergic Agonist, Long-Acting

Medication Safety Issues

Sound-alike/look-alike issues:

Foradil® may be confused with Toradol®

Administration issues:

Foradil® capsules for inhalation are for administration via Aerolizer™ inhaler and are **not** for oral use.

International issues:

Foradil [U.S., Canada, and multiple international markets] may be confused with Theradol brand name for tramadol [Netherlands]

Medication Guide Available Yes

Pregnancy Risk Factor C

Lactation Excretion in breast milk unknown/use caution

Use Maintenance treatment of asthma and prevention of bronchospasm (as concomitant therapy) in patients ≥5 years of age with reversible obstructive airway disease, including patients with symptoms of nocturnal asthma; maintenance treatment of bronchoconstriction in patients with COPD; prevention of exercise-induced bronchospasm in patients ≥5 years of age (monotherapy may be indicated in patients without persistent asthma)

Canadian labeling: Oxeze®: Also approved for acute relief of symptoms ("on demand" treatment) in patients ≥6 years of age

Mechanism of Action/Effect Relaxes bronchial smooth muscle

Contraindications Hypersensitivity to formoterol or any component of the formulation (Foradil® only); monotherapy in the treatment of asthma (ie, use without a concomitant long-term asthma control medication, such as an inhaled corticosteroid)

Canadian labeling: Oxeze®: Hypersensitivity to formoterol, inhaled lactose, or any component of the formulation; presence of tachyarrhythmias

Warnings/Precautions [U.S. Boxed Warning]: Long-acting $beta_2$-agonists (LABAs) increase the risk of asthma-related deaths. Formoterol should only be used in asthma patients as adjuvant therapy in patients who are currently receiving but are not adequately controlled on a long-term asthma control medication (ie, an inhaled corticosteroid). Monotherapy with an LABA is contraindicated in the treatment of asthma. In a large, randomized, placebo-controlled U.S. clinical trial (SMART, 2006), salmeterol was associated with an increase in asthma-related deaths (when added to usual asthma therapy); risk is considered a class effect among all LABAs. Data are not available to determine if the addition of an inhaled corticosteroid lessens this increased risk of death associated with LABA use. Assess patients at regular intervals once asthma control is maintained on combination therapy to determine if step-down therapy is appropriate and the LABA can be discontinued (without loss of asthma control), and the patient can be maintained on an inhaled corticosteroid. LABAs are not appropriate in patients whose asthma is adequately controlled on low- or medium-dose inhaled corticosteroids. Do **not** use for acute bronchospasm. Short-acting beta$_2$-agonist (eg, albuterol) should be used for acute symptoms and symptoms occurring between treatments. Do **not** initiate in patients with significantly worsening or acutely deteriorating asthma; reports of severe (sometimes fatal) respiratory events have been reported when formoterol has been initiated in this situation. Corticosteroids should not be stopped or reduced when formoterol is initiated. Formoterol is not a substitute for inhaled or systemic corticosteroids and should not be used as monotherapy. During initiation, watch for signs of worsening asthma. **[U.S. Boxed Warning]: LABAs may increase the risk of asthma-related hospitalization in pediatric and adolescent patients**. In general, a combination product containing a LABA and an inhaled corticosteroid is preferred in patients <18 years of age to ensure compliance.

Because LABAs may disguise poorly controlled persistent asthma, frequent or chronic use of LABAs for exercise-induced bronchospasm is discouraged by the NIH Asthma Guidelines (NIH, 2007). The safety and efficacy of Perforomist™ in the treatment of asthma have not been established. Oxeze® is a formulation of formoterol (available outside the U.S. [eg, Canada]) approved for acute treatment of asthmatic symptoms. The labelings for U.S. approved formulations (Foradil®, Perforomist™) state that formoterol is not meant to relieve acute asthmatic symptoms.

Do **not** use for acute episodes of COPD. Do **not** initiate in patients with significantly worsening or acutely deteriorating COPD. Data are not available to determine if LABA use increases the risk of death in patients with COPD. Increased use and/or ineffectiveness of short-acting beta$_2$-agonists may indicate rapidly deteriorating disease and should prompt re-evaluation of the patient's condition.

Immediate hypersensitivity reactions (urticaria, angioedema, rash, bronchospasm) have been reported. Do not exceed recommended dose or frequency; serious adverse events (including serious asthma exacerbations and fatalities) have been associated with excessive use of inhaled sympathomimetics. Beta$_2$-agonists may increase risk of arrhythmias, decrease serum potassium, prolong QT_c interval, or increase serum glucose. These effects may be exacerbated in hypoxemia. Use caution in patients with cardiovascular disease (arrhythmia, coronary insufficiency, hypertension, or HF), seizures, diabetes, hyperthyroidism, or hypokalemia. Beta-agonists may cause elevation in blood pressure and heart rate, and result in CNS stimulation/excitation. Tolerance to the bronchodilator effect, measured by FEV_1, has been observed in studies.

Powder for oral inhalation contains lactose; very rare anaphylactic reactions have been reported in patients with severe milk protein allergy. The contents of the Foradil® capsules are for inhalation via the Aerolizer™ device. There have been reports of incorrect administration (swallowing of the capsules).

Drug Interactions

Avoid Concomitant Use

Avoid concomitant use of Formoterol with any of the following: Beta-Blockers (Nonselective); Iobenguane I 123

Decreased Effect

Formoterol may decrease the levels/effects of: Iobenguane I 123

The levels/effects of Formoterol may be decreased by: Alpha-/Beta-Blockers; Beta-Blockers (Beta1 Selective); Beta-Blockers (Nonselective); Betahistine

Increased Effect/Toxicity

Formoterol may increase the levels/effects of: Loop Diuretics; Sympathomimetics; Thiazide Diuretics

The levels/effects of Formoterol may be increased by: Atomoxetine; Caffeine; Cannabinoids; MAO Inhibitors; Theophylline Derivatives; Tricyclic Antidepressants

Adverse Reactions

1% to 10%:

- Cardiovascular: Chest pain (2% to 3%), palpitation
- Central nervous system: Anxiety (2%), dizziness (2%), fever (2%), insomnia (2%), dysphonia (1%), headache
- Dermatologic: Pruritus (2%), rash (1%)
- Gastrointestinal: Diarrhea (5%), nausea (5%), xerostomia (1% to 3%), vomiting (2%), abdominal pain, dyspepsia, gastroenteritis
- Neuromuscular & skeletal: Muscle cramps (2%), tremor
- Respiratory: Infection (3% to 7%), asthma exacerbation (age 5-12 years: 5% to 6%; age >12 years: <4%), bronchitis (5%), pharyngitis (3% to 4%), sinusitis (3%), dyspnea (2%), tonsillitis (1%)

Pharmacodynamics/Kinetics

Onset of Action Powder for inhalation: Within 3 minutes

Peak effect: Powder for inhalation: 80% of peak effect within 15 minutes; Solution for nebulization: 2 hours

Duration of Action Improvement in FEV_1 observed for 12 hours in most patients

Available Dosage Forms

Powder, for oral inhalation:

Foradil® Aerolizer®: 12 mcg/capsule (12s, 60s)

Solution, for nebulization:
Perforomist®: 20 mcg/2 mL (60s)

General Dosage Range Inhalation:

Foradil®: *Children ≥5 years and Adults:* 12 mcg capsule inhaled every 12 hours (maximum: 24 mcg/day) **or** 12 mcg capsule inhaled prior to exercise

Perforomist™: *Adults:* 20 mcg twice daily (maximum dose: 40 mcg/day)

Administration

Inhalation

Foradil®: Remove capsule from foil blister **immediately** before use. Place capsule in the capsule-chamber in the base of the Aerolizer™ Inhaler. Must only use the Aerolizer™ Inhaler. Press both buttons **once only** and then release. Keep inhaler in a level, horizontal position. Exhale fully. Do not exhale into inhaler. Tilt head slightly back and inhale (rapidly, steadily, and deeply). Hold breath as long as possible. If any powder remains in capsule, exhale and inhale again. Repeat until capsule is empty. Throw away empty capsule; do not leave in inhaler. Do not use a spacer with the Aerolizer™ Inhaler. Always keep capsules and inhaler dry.

Perforomist™: Remove unit-dose vial from foil pouch **immediately** before use. Solution does not require dilution prior to administration; do not mix other medications with formoterol solution. Place contents of unit-dose vial into the reservoir of a standard jet nebulizer connected to an air compressor; assemble nebulizer based on the manufacturer's instructions and turn nebulizer on; breathe deeply and evenly until all of the medication has been inhaled. Discard any unused medication immediately; do not ingest contents of vial. Clean nebulizer after use.

Oxeze® Turbuhaler® [CAN; not available in U.S.]: Hold inhaler upright. Turn colored grip as far as it will go in one direction and then turn back to original position; a clicking sound should be heard which means the inhaler is ready for use. Exhale fully. Do not exhale into mouthpiece of inhaler. Place mouthpiece to lips and inhale forcefully and deeply. Do not chew or bite on mouthpiece. Clean outside of mouthpiece once weekly with a dry tissue. Avoid getting inhaler wet.

Stability

Storage

Foradil®: Prior to dispensing, store in refrigerator at 2°C to 8°C (36°F to 46°F). After dispensing, store at room temperature at 20°C to 25°C (68°F to 77°F). Protect from heat and moisture. Capsules should always be stored in the blister and only removed immediately before use. Always check expiration date. Use within 4 months of purchase date or product expiration date, whichever comes first.

Perforomist™: Prior to dispensing, store in refrigerator at 2°C to 8°C (36°F to 46°F). After dispensing, store at 2°C to 25°C (36°F to 77°F) for up to 3 months. Protect from heat. Unit-dose vials should always be stored in the foil pouch and only removed immediately before use.

Nursing Actions

Physical Assessment Teach patient how to properly use.

Patient Education Do not swallow capsules; this medication can only be used in the Aerolizer™ Inhaler. It is recommended that you wear identification (Med-Alert bracelet) if you have asthma. You may experience nervousness, dizziness, insomnia, dry mouth, nausea, or GI discomfort. Report any unresolved GI upset, nervousness or dizziness, muscle cramping, chest pain or palpitations, skin rash, or worsening of condition.

Administration: Wash hands prior to treatment and sit in comfortable position for treatment. Place capsule in the capsule-chamber in the base of the Aerolizer™ Inhaler. Press both buttons once only and then release. Hold inhaler in a level, horizontal position, exhale fully. Tilt head slightly back and inhale from inhaler rapidly, steadily, and deeply. Hold breath as long as possible. If any powder remains in capsule, exhale and inhale again. Repeat until capsule is empty. Throw away empty capsule. Do not use a spacer with Aerolizer™. Do not wash inhaler; store in dry place.

Fosamprenavir (FOS am pren a veer)

Brand Names: U.S. Lexiva®

Index Terms Fosamprenavir Calcium; GW433908G

Pharmacologic Category Antiretroviral Agent, Protease Inhibitor

Medication Safety Issues

Sound-alike/look-alike issues:

Lexiva® may be confused with Levitra®

Pregnancy Risk Factor C

Lactation Excretion in breast milk unknown/contraindicated

Breast-Feeding Considerations Maternal or infant antiretroviral therapy does not completely eliminate the risk of postnatal HIV transmission. In addition, multiclass-resistant virus has been detected in breast-feeding infants despite maternal therapy. Therefore, in the United States, where formula is accessible, affordable, safe, and sustainable, and the risk of infant mortality due to diarrhea and respiratory infections is low, complete avoidance of breast-feeding by HIV-infected women is recommended to decrease potential transmission of HIV (DHHS [perinatal], 2011).

Use Treatment of HIV infections in combination with at least two other antiretroviral agents

Mechanism of Action/Effect Fosamprenavir is rapidly and almost completely converted to amprenavir *in vivo*. Amprenavir blocks the site of HIV-1

protease activity, resulting in the formation of immature, noninfectious viral particles.

Contraindications Clinically-significant hypersensitivity (eg, Stevens-Johnson syndrome) to fosamprenavir, amprenavir, or any component of the formulation; concurrent therapy with CYP3A4 substrates with a narrow therapeutic window; concomitant use with alfuzosin, cisapride, delavirdine, ergot derivatives, lovastatin, midazolam, pimozide, rifampin, simvastatin, St John's wort, and triazolam; use of flecainide and propafenone with concomitant ritonavir therapy; sildenafil (when used for pulmonary artery hypertension [eg, Revatio®])

Warnings/Precautions Use with caution in patients taking strong CYP3A4 inhibitors, moderate or strong CYP3A4 inducers, and major CYP3A4 substrates (see Drug Interactions); consider alternative agents that avoid or lessen the potential for CYP-mediated interactions. Do not use with hormonal contraceptives. Do not coadminister colchicine in patient with renal or hepatic impairment; avoid concurrent use with salmeterol.

Use with caution in patients with diabetes mellitus or sulfonamide allergy. Use caution with hepatic impairment (dosage adjustment required) or underlying hepatitis B or C. Redistribution of fat may occur (eg, buffalo hump, peripheral wasting, cushingoid appearance). Dosage adjustment is required for combination therapies (ritonavir and/or efavirenz); in addition, the risk of hyperlipidemia may be increased during concurrent therapy. Protease inhibitors have been associated with a variety of hypersensitivity events (some severe), including rash, anaphylaxis (rare), angioedema, bronchospasm, erythema multiforme, and/or Stevens-Johnson syndrome (rare). It is generally recommended to discontinue treatment if severe rash or moderate symptoms accompanied by other systemic symptoms occur. Acute hemolytic anemia has been reported in association with amprenavir use. Cases of nephrolithiasis have been reported in postmarketing surveillance; temporary or permanent discontinuation of therapy should be considered if symptoms develop. Spontaneous bleeding has been reported in patients with hemophilia A or B following treatment with protease inhibitors; use caution. Immune reconstitution syndrome may develop resulting in the occurrence of an inflammatory response to an indolent or residual opportunistic infection; further evaluation and treatment may be necessary. Safety and efficacy have not been established in children <2 years of age.

Drug Interactions

Avoid Concomitant Use

Avoid concomitant use of Fosamprenavir with any of the following: Alfuzosin; Amiodarone; Axitinib; Cisapride; Conivaptan; Crizotinib; Delavirdine; Dronedarone; Eplerenone; Ergot Derivatives; Etravirine; Everolimus; Fluticasone (Oral Inhalation); Halofantrine; Lapatinib; Lovastatin; Lurasidone; Midazolam; Nilotinib; Nisoldipine; Pimozide; QuiNIDine; Ranolazine; Rifampin; Rivaroxaban; RomiDEPsin; Salmeterol; Silodosin; Simvastatin; St Johns Wort; Tamsulosin; Telaprevir; Ticagrelor; Tolvaptan; Toremifene; Triazolam

Decreased Effect

Fosamprenavir may decrease the levels/effects of: Abacavir; Boceprevir; Clarithromycin; Contraceptives (Estrogens); Delavirdine; Divalproex; Fosphenytoin; Lopinavir; Meperidine; Methadone; PARoxetine; Phenytoin; Posaconazole; Prasugrel; Raltegravir; Telaprevir; Ticagrelor; Valproic Acid; Zidovudine

The levels/effects of Fosamprenavir may be decreased by: Antacids; Boceprevir; CarBAMazepine; CYP3A4 Inducers (Strong); Deferasirox; Efavirenz; Garlic; H2-Antagonists; Nevirapine; Peginterferon Alfa-2b; P-glycoprotein/ABCB1 Inducers; Raltegravir; Rifampin; St Johns Wort; Telaprevir; Tenofovir; Tocilizumab

Increased Effect/Toxicity

Fosamprenavir may increase the levels/effects of: Alfuzosin; Almotriptan; Alosetron; ALPRAZolam; Amiodarone; Antifungal Agents (Azole Derivatives, Systemic); ARIPiprazole; Axitinib; Bortezomib; Brentuximab Vedotin; Brinzolamide; Budesonide (Nasal); Budesonide (Systemic, Oral Inhalation); Calcium Channel Blockers (Dihydropyridine); Calcium Channel Blockers (Nondihydropyridine); CarBAMazepine; Ciclesonide; Cisapride; Clarithromycin; Clorazepate; Colchicine; Conivaptan; Corticosteroids (Orally Inhaled); Crizotinib; CycloSPORINE; CycloSPORINE (Systemic); CYP3A4 Substrates; Diazepam; Dienogest; Digoxin; Dronedarone; Dutasteride; Enfuvirtide; Eplerenone; Ergot Derivatives; Everolimus; FentaNYL; Fesoterodine; Flurazepam; Fluticasone (Nasal); Fluticasone (Oral Inhalation); Fusidic Acid; GuanFACINE; Halofantrine; HMG-CoA Reductase Inhibitors; Iloperidone; Ivacaftor; Ixabepilone; Lapatinib; Lovastatin; Lumefantrine; Lurasidone; Maraviroc; Meperidine; MethylPREDNISolone; Midazolam; Nefazodone; Nilotinib; Nisoldipine; Paricalcitol; Pazopanib; Pimecrolimus; Pimozide; Propafenone; Protease Inhibitors; QuiNIDine; Ranolazine; Rifabutin; Rivaroxaban; RomiDEPsin; Ruxolitinib; Salmeterol; Saxagliptin; Sildenafil; Silodosin; Simvastatin; Sirolimus; SORAfenib; Tacrolimus; Tacrolimus (Systemic); Tacrolimus (Topical); Tadalafil; Tamsulosin; Temsirolimus; Tenofovir; Ticagrelor; Tolterodine; Tolvaptan; Toremifene; TraZODone; Triazolam; Tricyclic Antidepressants; Vardenafil; Vemurafenib; Vilazodone; Warfarin; Zuclopenthixol

The levels/effects of Fosamprenavir may be increased by: Antifungal Agents (Azole Derivatives, Systemic); Clarithromycin; CycloSPORINE; CycloSPORINE (Systemic); Delavirdine; Efavirenz; Enfuvirtide; Etravirine; Fosphenytoin; Fusidic

Acid; P-glycoprotein/ABCB1 Inhibitors; Phenytoin; Posaconazole; Rifabutin

Nutritional/Ethanol Interactions

Food: Management:

Oral suspension: Administer without food to adults or with food to pediatric patients.

Tablet: Administer with food if taken with ritonavir. May be administered without regard to food if not taken with ritonavir.

Herb/Nutraceutical: Serum concentration may be decreased by St John's wort. Management: Avoid St John's wort; concurrent use is contraindicated.

Adverse Reactions

>10%:

Dermatologic: Rash (≤19%; onset: ~11 days; duration: ~13 days)

Endocrine & metabolic: Hypertriglyceridemia (>750 mg/dL: ≤11%)

Gastrointestinal: Diarrhea (moderate-to-severe; 5% to 13%)

1% to 10%:

Central nervous system: Headache (moderate-to-severe; 2% to 4%), fatigue (moderate-to-severe; 2% to 4%)

Dermatologic: Pruritus (7% to 8%)

Endocrine & metabolic: Hyperglycemia (>251 mg/dL: ≤2%)

Gastrointestinal: Serum lipase increased (>2 times ULN: 5% to 8%), nausea (moderate-to-severe; 3% to 7%), vomiting (moderate-to-severe; 2% to 6%), abdominal pain (moderate-to-severe; ≤2%)

Hematologic: Neutropenia (<750 cells/mm^3: 3%)

Hepatic: Transaminases increased (>5 times ULN: 4% to 8%)

Frequency not defined: Diabetes mellitus, fat redistribution, and immune reconstitution syndrome have been associated with protease inhibitor therapy. Spontaneous bleeding has been reported in patients with hemophilia A or B following treatment with protease inhibitors. Acute hemolytic anemia has been reported in association with amprenavir use.

Available Dosage Forms

Suspension, oral:

Lexiva®: 50 mg/mL (225 mL)

Tablet, oral:

Lexiva®: 700 mg

General Dosage Range Dosage adjustment recommended in patients with hepatic impairment or on concomitant therapy

Oral:

Children 2-5 years: 30 mg/kg/dose twice daily (maximum: 1400 mg twice daily)

Children ≥6 years:

Unboosted regimen: 30 mg/kg/dose twice daily (maximum: 1400 mg twice daily)

Ritonavir-boosted regimen: 18 mg/kg/dose twice daily (maximum: 700 mg twice daily)

Adults:

Unboosted regimen: 1400 mg twice daily

Ritonavir-boosted regimen: 700 mg twice daily **or** 1400 mg once daily

Administration

Oral

Oral suspension: Administer **without** food to adults; administer **with** food to pediatric patients. Readminister dose of suspension if emesis occurs within 30 minutes after dosing. Shake suspension vigorously prior to use.

Tablet: Administer with food if taken with ritonavir. May be administered without regard to food if not taken with ritonavir.

Stability

Storage

Lexiva®: Store tablets at 25°C (77°F); excursions permitted to 15°C to 30°C (59°F to 86°F). Store oral suspension at 5°C to 30°C (41°F to 86°F). Do not freeze.

Telzir®: Store tablets 2°C to 30°C; do not freeze and discard 25 days after opening.

Nursing Actions

Physical Assessment Monitor for adherence to regimen. Monitor for hypersensitivity, gastrointestinal disturbance (nausea, vomiting, diarrhea) that can lead to dehydration and weight loss, hyperglycemia, and cardiac status. Caution patients to monitor glucose levels closely; protease inhibitors may cause hyperglycemia or new-onset diabetes. Teach patient proper timing of multiple medications and drugs that should not be used concurrently. Instruct patient on glucose testing (protease inhibitors may cause hyperglycemia), exacerbation or new-onset diabetes.

Patient Education This is not a cure for HIV, nor has it been found to reduce transmission of HIV; use appropriate precautions to prevent spread to other persons. Maintain adequate hydration, unless instructed to restrict fluid intake. This medication will be prescribed with a combination of other medications; time these medications as directed by prescriber. You may be advised to check your glucose levels; this class of drugs can cause hyperglycemia. Frequent blood tests may be required. May cause body changes due to redistribution of body fat (buffalo hump, peripheral wasting, cushingoid appearance may occur), dizziness or fatigue, nausea or vomiting, diarrhea, back pain, or arthralgia. Inform prescriber if you experience muscle numbness or tingling; unresolved persistent vomiting, diarrhea, or abdominal pain; respiratory difficulty or chest pain; unusual skin rash, blistering, or peeling of skin; or change in color of stool or urine.

Dietary Considerations Tablets may be taken with or without food. Adults should take oral suspension **without** food; however, children should take oral suspension **with** food.

Fosaprepitant (fos a PRE pi tant)

Brand Names: U.S. Emend® for Injection

Index Terms Aprepitant Injection; Fosaprepitant Dimeglumine; L-758,298; MK 0517

Pharmacologic Category Antiemetic; Substance P/Neurokinin 1 Receptor Antagonist

Medication Safety Issues

Sound-alike/look-alike issues:

Fosaprepitant may be confused with aprepitant, fosamprenavir, fospropofol

Emend® for Injection (fosaprepitant) may be confused with Emend® (aprepitant) which is an oral capsule formulation.

Pregnancy Risk Factor B

Lactation Excretion in breast milk unknown/not recommended

Use Prevention of acute and delayed nausea and vomiting associated with moderately- and highly-emetogenic chemotherapy (in combination with other antiemetics)

Mechanism of Action/Effect Fosaprepitant is a prodrug of aprepitant, a substance P/neurokinin 1 (NK1) receptor antagonist. It is rapidly converted to aprepitant which prevents acute and delayed vomiting by inhibiting the substance P/neurokinin 1 (NK1) receptor; augments the antiemetic activity of the 5-HT_3 receptor antagonist and corticosteroid activity and inhibits chemotherapy-induced emesis.

Contraindications Hypersensitivity to fosaprepitant, aprepitant, polysorbate 80, or any component of the formulation; concurrent use with pimozide or cisapride

Canadian labeling: Additional contraindications (not in U.S. labeling): Concurrent use with astemizole or terfenadine

Warnings/Precautions Fosaprepitant is rapidly converted to aprepitant, which has a high potential for drug interactions. Use caution with agents primarily metabolized via CYP3A4; aprepitant is a 3A4 inhibitor. Effect on orally administered 3A4 substrates is greater than those administered intravenously. Immediate hypersensitivity has been reported (rarely) with fosaprepitant; stop infusion with hypersensitivity symptoms (dyspnea, erythema, flushing, or anaphylaxis); do not reinitiate. Use caution with hepatic impairment; has not been studied in patients with severe hepatic impairment (Child-Pugh class C). Not studied for treatment of existing nausea and vomiting. Chronic continuous administration of fosaprepitant is not recommended.

Drug Interactions

Avoid Concomitant Use

Avoid concomitant use of Fosaprepitant with any of the following: Astemizole; Axitinib; Cisapride; Conivaptan; Pimozide; Terfenadine; Tolvaptan

Decreased Effect

Fosaprepitant may decrease the levels/effects of: ARIPiprazole; Axitinib; Contraceptives (Estrogens); Contraceptives (Progestins); PARoxetine; Saxagliptin; TOLBUTamide; Warfarin

The levels/effects of Fosaprepitant may be decreased by: CYP3A4 Inducers (Strong); Cyproterone; Deferasirox; Herbs (CYP3A4 Inducers); PARoxetine; Rifampin; Tocilizumab

Increased Effect/Toxicity

Fosaprepitant may increase the levels/effects of: ARIPiprazole; Astemizole; Benzodiazepines (metabolized by oxidation); Budesonide (Systemic, Oral Inhalation); Cisapride; Colchicine; Corticosteroids (Systemic); CYP3A4 Substrates; Diltiazem; Eplerenone; Everolimus; FentaNYL; Halofantrine; Ivacaftor; Lurasidone; Pimecrolimus; Pimozide; Propafenone; Ranolazine; Salmeterol; Saxagliptin; Terfenadine; Tolvaptan; Vilazodone; Zuclopenthixol

The levels/effects of Fosaprepitant may be increased by: Antifungal Agents (Azole Derivatives, Systemic); Conivaptan; CYP3A4 Inhibitors (Moderate); CYP3A4 Inhibitors (Strong); Dasatinib; Diltiazem; Ivacaftor

Nutritional/Ethanol Interactions

Food: Aprepitant serum concentration may be increased when taken with grapefruit juice; avoid concurrent use.

Herb/Nutraceutical: Avoid St John's wort (may decrease aprepitant levels).

Adverse Reactions Adverse reactions reported with aprepitant and fosaprepitant (as part of a combination chemotherapy regimen) occurring at a higher frequency than standard antiemetic therapy:

1% to 10%:

Central nervous system: Fatigue (1% to 3%), headache (2%)

Gastrointestinal: Anorexia (2%), constipation 2%), dyspepsia (2%), diarrhea (1%), eructation (1%)

Hepatic: ALT increased (1% to 3%), AST increased (1%)

Local: Injection site reactions (3%; includes erythema, induration, pain, pruritus, or thrombophlebitis)

Neuromuscular & skeletal: Weakness (3%)

Miscellaneous: Hiccups (5%)

Available Dosage Forms

Injection, powder for reconstitution:

Emend® for Injection: 150 mg

General Dosage Range I.V.: *Adults:* 115 or 150 mg as a single dose

Administration

I.V.

115 mg: Infuse over 15 minutes 30 minutes prior to chemotherapy

150 mg: Infuse over 20-30 minutes ~30 minutes prior to chemotherapy

Stability

Reconstitution Reconstitute either vial size with 5 mL of sodium chloride 0.9%, directing diluent down side of vial to avoid foaming; swirl gently.

Add reconstituted contents of the 150 mg vial to 145 mL sodium chloride 0.9% (add 115 mg vial to 110 mL), resulting in a final concentration of 1 mg/mL; gently invert bag to mix.

Storage Store intact vials at 2°C to 8°C (36°F to 46°F). Solutions diluted for infusion are stable for 24 hours at room temperature of ≤25°C (≤77°F).

Nursing Actions

Physical Assessment Monitor patient closely for immediate hypersensitivity reaction (dyspnea, erythema, and/or flushing); if reaction occurs, stop infusion (do not restart) and notify prescriber.

Patient Education This medication is intended to prevent or treat nausea/vomiting. Report immediately any pain or burning at infusion site, swelling of mouth, difficulty swallowing, difficulty breathing, or flushing.

Foscarnet (fos KAR net)

Index Terms PFA; Phosphonoformate; Phosphonoformic Acid

Pharmacologic Category Antiviral Agent

Pregnancy Risk Factor C

Lactation Excretion in breast milk unknown/contraindicated

Use Treatment of acyclovir-resistant mucocutaneous herpes simplex virus (HSV) infections in immunocompromised persons (eg, with advanced AIDS); treatment of CMV retinitis in persons with HIV

Unlabeled Use Other CMV infections (eg, colitis, esophagitis, neurological disease); CMV prophylaxis for cancer patients receiving alemtuzumab therapy or allogeneic stem cell transplant

Available Dosage Forms

Injection, solution [preservative free]: 24 mg/mL (250 mL, 500 mL)

General Dosage Range Dosage adjustment recommended in patients with renal impairment

I.V.: *Children >12 years and Adults:* Induction: CMV: 180 mg/kg/day in 2-3 evenly divided doses; HSV: 40 mg/kg/dose every 8-12 hours; Maintenance: CMV: 90-120 mg/kg once daily

Administration

I.V. Use an infusion pump, at a rate not exceeding 1 mg/kg/minute. Adult induction doses of 60 mg/kg are administered over 1 hour. Adult maintenance doses of 90-120 mg/kg are infused over 2 hours. The manufacturer recommends 750-1000 mL of NS or D_5W be administered prior to first infusion to establish diuresis. With subsequent infusions of 90-120 mg/kg, this volume would be repeated. If the dose were 40-60 mg/kg, then the volume could be reduced to 500 mL. After the first dose, the hydration fluid should be administered concurrently with foscarnet.

I.V. Detail Undiluted (24 mg/mL) solution can be administered without further dilution when using a central venous catheter for infusion. For peripheral vein administration, the solution **must** be diluted to a final concentration **not to exceed** 12 mg/mL. The recommended dosage, frequency, and rate of infusion should not be exceeded.

pH: 7.4 (adjusted)

Nursing Actions

Physical Assessment Evaluate electrolytes, renal status, and dental status prior to beginning therapy. Monitor for nephrotoxicity, electrolyte imbalance, and seizures. Teach patient need for regular dental evaluations.

Patient Education While on therapy, it is important to maintain adequate nutrition and hydration, unless instructed to restrict fluid intake. Regular dental check-ups are recommended. May cause dizziness, confusion, nausea, vomiting, or diarrhea. Report any change in sensorium or seizures; unresolved diarrhea or vomiting; unusual fever, chills, or sore throat; unhealed sores; swollen lymph glands; or malaise.

Fosinopril (foe SIN oh pril)

Index Terms Fosinopril Sodium; Monopril

Pharmacologic Category Angiotensin-Converting Enzyme (ACE) Inhibitor

Medication Safety Issues

Sound-alike/look-alike issues:

Fosinopril may be confused with FLUoxetine, Fosamax®, furosemide, lisinopril

Monopril may be confused with Accupril®, minoxidil, moexipril, Monoket®, Monurol®, ramipril

Pregnancy Risk Factor C (1st trimester); D (2nd and 3rd trimesters)

Lactation Enters breast milk/not recommended

Breast-Feeding Considerations Fosinoprilat is excreted in breast milk. Breast-feeding is not recommended by the manufacturer.

Use Treatment of hypertension, either alone or in combination with other antihypertensive agents; treatment of heart failure (HF)

Mechanism of Action/Effect Competitive inhibitor of angiotensin-converting enzyme (ACE); prevents conversion of angiotensin I to angiotensin II, a potent vasoconstrictor; results in lower levels of angiotensin II which causes an increase in plasma renin activity and a reduction in aldosterone secretion; a CNS mechanism may also be involved in hypotensive effect as angiotensin II increases adrenergic outflow from CNS; vasoactive kallikreins may be decreased in conversion to active hormones by ACE inhibitors, thus reducing blood pressure

Contraindications Hypersensitivity to fosinopril, any other ACE inhibitor, or any component of the formulation; angioedema related to previous treatment with an ACE inhibitor

Warnings/Precautions Anaphylactic reactions may occur rarely with ACE inhibitors. At any time during treatment (especially following first dose), angioedema may occur rarely with ACE inhibitors; it may involve the head and neck (potentially compromising airway) or the intestine (presenting with abdominal pain). African-Americans may be at an increased risk and patients with idiopathic or hereditary angioedema may be at an increased risk. Prolonged frequent monitoring may be required especially if tongue, glottis, or larynx are involved as they are associated with airway obstruction. Patients with a history of airway surgery may have a higher risk of airway obstruction. Aggressive early and appropriate management is critical. Use in patients with previous angioedema associated with ACE inhibitor therapy is contraindicated. Severe anaphylactoid reactions may be seen during hemodialysis (eg, CVVHD) with high-flux dialysis membranes (eg, AN69), and rarely, during low density lipoprotein apheresis with dextran sulfate cellulose. Rare cases of anaphylactoid reactions have been reported in patients undergoing sensitization treatment with hymenoptera (bee, wasp) venom while receiving ACE inhibitors.

Symptomatic hypotension with or without syncope can occur with ACE inhibitors (usually with the first several doses); effects are most often observed in volume-depleted patients; correct volume depletion prior to initiation; close monitoring of patient is required especially with initial dosing and dosing increases; blood pressure must be lowered at a rate appropriate for the patient's clinical condition. Initiation of therapy in patients with ischemic heart disease or cerebrovascular disease warrants close observation due to the potential consequences posed by falling blood pressure (eg, MI, stroke). Use with caution in hypertrophic cardiomyopathy with outflow tract obstruction, severe aortic stenosis, or before, during, or immediately after major surgery. **[U.S. Boxed Warning]: Based on human data, ACEIs can cause injury and death to the developing fetus when used in the second and third trimesters. ACEIs should be discontinued as soon as possible once pregnancy is detected.**

Hyperkalemia may occur with ACE inhibitors; risk factors include renal dysfunction, diabetes mellitus, concomitant use of potassium-sparing diuretics, potassium supplements, and/or potassium-containing salts. Use cautiously, if at all, with these agents and monitor potassium closely. Cough may occur with ACE inhibitors. Other causes of cough should be considered (eg, pulmonary congestion in patients with heart failure) and excluded prior to discontinuation.

May be associated with deterioration of renal function and/or increases in serum creatinine, particularly in patients with low renal blood flow (eg, renal artery stenosis, heart failure) whose glomerular filtration rate (GFR) is dependent on efferent arteriolar vasoconstriction by angiotensin II; deterioration may result in oliguria, acute renal failure, and progressive azotemia. Small increases in serum creatinine may occur following initiation; consider discontinuation only in patients with progressive and/or significant deterioration in renal function. Use with caution in patients with unstented unilateral/bilateral renal artery stenosis. When unstented bilateral renal artery stenosis is present, use is generally avoided due to the elevated risk of deterioration in renal function unless possible benefits outweigh risks. Concurrent use of angiotensin receptor blockers may increase the risk of clinically-significant adverse events (eg, renal dysfunction, hyperkalemia).

Rare toxicities associated with ACE inhibitors include cholestatic jaundice (which may progress to fulminant hepatic necrosis), agranulocytosis, neutropenia or leukopenia with myeloid hypoplasia. Patients with collagen vascular diseases (especially with concomitant renal impairment) or renal impairment alone may be at increased risk for hematologic toxicity; periodically monitor CBC with differential in these patients.

Drug Interactions

Avoid Concomitant Use There are no known interactions where it is recommended to avoid concomitant use.

Decreased Effect

The levels/effects of Fosinopril may be decreased by: Antacids; Aprotinin; Herbs (Hypertensive Properties); Icatibant; Lanthanum; Methylphenidate; Nonsteroidal Anti-Inflammatory Agents; Salicylates; Yohimbine

Increased Effect/Toxicity

Fosinopril may increase the levels/effects of: Allopurinol; Amifostine; Antihypertensives; AzaTHIOprine; CycloSPORINE; CycloSPORINE (Systemic); Ferric Gluconate; Gold Sodium Thiomalate; Hypotensive Agents; Iron Dextran Complex; Lithium; Nonsteroidal Anti-Inflammatory Agents; RiTUXimab; Sodium Phosphates

The levels/effects of Fosinopril may be increased by: Alfuzosin; Angiotensin II Receptor Blockers; Diazoxide; DPP-IV Inhibitors; Eplerenone; Everolimus; Herbs (Hypotensive Properties); Loop Diuretics; MAO Inhibitors; Pentoxifylline; Phosphodiesterase 5 Inhibitors; Potassium Salts; Potassium-Sparing Diuretics; Prostacyclin Analogues; Sirolimus; Temsirolimus; Thiazide Diuretics; TiZANidine; Tolvaptan; Trimethoprim

Nutritional/Ethanol Interactions

Food: Potassium supplements and/or potassium-containing salts may cause or worsen hyperkalemia. Management: Consult prescriber before consuming a potassium-rich diet, potassium supplements, or salt substitutes.

Herb/Nutraceutical: Some herbal medications may worsen hypertension (eg, licorice); others may increase the antihypertensive effect of fosinopril (eg, shepherd's purse). Management: Avoid bayberry, blue cohosh, cayenne, ephedra, ginger, ginseng (American), kola, licorice, and yohimbe. Avoid black cohosh, california poppy, coleus, golden seal, hawthorn, mistletoe, periwinkle, quinine, and shepherd's purse.

Adverse Reactions Note: Frequency ranges include data from hypertension and heart failure trials. Higher rates of adverse reactions have generally been noted in patients with CHF. However, the frequency of adverse effects associated with placebo is also increased in this population.

>10%: Central nervous system: Dizziness (2% to 12%)

1% to 10%:

Cardiovascular: Orthostatic hypotension (1% to 2%), palpitation (1%)

Central nervous system: Dizziness (1% to 2%; up to 12% in CHF patients), headache (3%), fatigue (1% to 2%)

Endocrine & metabolic: Hyperkalemia (2.6%)

Gastrointestinal: Diarrhea (2%), nausea/vomiting (1.2% to 2.2%)

Hepatic: Transaminases increased

Neuromuscular & skeletal: Musculoskeletal pain (<1% to 3%), noncardiac chest pain (<1% to 2%), weakness (1%)

Renal: Serum creatinine increased, renal function worsening (in patients with bilateral renal artery stenosis or hypovolemia)

Respiratory: Cough (2% to 10%)

Miscellaneous: Upper respiratory infection (2%)

>1% but ≤ frequency in patients receiving placebo: Sexual dysfunction, fever, flu-like syndrome, dyspnea, rash, headache, insomnia

Other events reported with ACE inhibitors: Neutropenia, agranulocytosis, eosinophilic pneumonitis, cardiac arrest, pancytopenia, hemolytic anemia, anemia, aplastic anemia, thrombocytopenia, acute renal failure, hepatic failure, jaundice, symptomatic hyponatremia, bullous pemphigus, exfoliative dermatitis, Stevens-Johnson syndrome. In addition, a syndrome which may include fever, myalgia, arthralgia, interstitial nephritis, vasculitis, rash, eosinophilia and positive ANA, and elevated ESR has been reported for other ACE inhibitors.

Pharmacodynamics/Kinetics

Onset of Action 1 hour

Duration of Action 24 hours

Available Dosage Forms

Tablet, oral: 10 mg, 20 mg, 40 mg

General Dosage Range Oral:

Children ≥6 years and >50 kg: Initial: 5-10 mg once daily (maximum: 40 mg/day)

Adults: Initial: 10 mg once daily; Maintenance: 10-40 mg/day in 1-2 divided doses (maximum: 80 mg/day)

Stability

Storage Store at 25°C (77°F); excursions permitted to 15°C to 30°C (59°F to 86°F). Protect from moisture by keeping bottle tightly closed.

Nursing Actions

Physical Assessment Assess potential for interactions with other pharmacological agents or herbal products that may impact fluid balance or cardiac status. Monitor for anaphylactic reactions, hypovolemia, angioedema, and postural hypotension.

Patient Education Do not use potassium supplement or salt substitutes without consulting prescriber. This drug does not eliminate need for diet or exercise regimen as recommended by prescriber. May cause dizziness, fainting, lightheadedness, postural hypotension, nausea, vomiting, abdominal pain, dry mouth, or loss of appetite - report if these persist. Report chest pain or palpitations; mouth sores; fever or chills; swelling of extremities, face, mouth, or tongue; skin rash; numbness, tingling, or pain in muscles; respiratory difficulty; or unusual cough.

Dietary Considerations Should not take a potassium salt supplement without the advice of healthcare provider.

Fosphenytoin (FOS fen i toyn)

Brand Names: U.S. Cerebyx®

Index Terms Fosphenytoin Sodium

Pharmacologic Category Anticonvulsant, Hydantoin

Medication Safety Issues

Sound-alike/look-alike issues:

Cerebyx® may be confused with CeleBREX®, CeleXA®, Cerezyme®, Cervarix®

Fosphenytoin may be confused with fospropofol

Administration issues:

Overdoses have occurred due to confusion between the **mg per mL concentration** of fosphenytoin (50 mg PE/mL) and **total drug content per vial** (either 100 mg PE/2 mL vial or 500 mg PE/10 mL vial). ISMP recommends that the total drug content per container is identified instead of the concentration in mg per mL to avoid confusion and potential overdosages. Additionally, since most errors have occurred with overdoses in children, they recommend that pediatric hospitals should consider stocking only the 2 mL vial.

Pregnancy Risk Factor D

Lactation Excretion in breast milk unknown/not recommended

Breast-Feeding Considerations Fosphenytoin is the prodrug of phenytoin. It is not known if fosphenytoin is excreted in breast milk prior to conversion to phenytoin. Refer to Phenytoin monograph for additional information.

Use Used for the control of generalized convulsive status epilepticus and prevention and treatment of seizures occurring during neurosurgery; indicated for short-term parenteral administration when other means of phenytoin administration are unavailable, inappropriate, or deemed less advantageous (the safety and effectiveness of fosphenytoin use for more than 5 days has not been systematically evaluated)

Mechanism of Action/Effect Diphosphate ester salt of phenytoin which acts as a water soluble prodrug of phenytoin; after administration, plasma esterases convert fosphenytoin to phosphate, formaldehyde, and phenytoin as the active moiety; phenytoin works by stabilizing neuronal membranes and decreasing seizure activity by increasing efflux or decreasing influx of sodium ions across cell membranes in the motor cortex during generation of nerve impulses

Contraindications Hypersensitivity to phenytoin, other hydantoins, or any component of the formulation; patients with sinus bradycardia, sinoatrial block, second- and third-degree AV block, or Adams-Stokes syndrome; occurrence of rash during treatment (should not be resumed if rash is exfoliative, purpuric, or bullous); treatment of absence seizures

Warnings/Precautions Doses of fosphenytoin are expressed as their phenytoin sodium equivalent (PE). Antiepileptic drugs should not be abruptly discontinued. Hypotension may occur, especially after I.V. administration at high doses and high rates of administration. Administration of phenytoin has been associated with atrial and ventricular conduction depression and ventricular fibrillation. Careful cardiac monitoring is needed when administering I.V. loading doses of fosphenytoin. Acute hepatotoxicity associated with a hypersensitivity syndrome characterized by fever, skin eruptions, and lymphadenopathy has been reported to occur within the first 2 months of treatment. Discontinue if skin rash or lymphadenopathy occurs. A spectrum of hematologic effects have been reported with use (eg, neutropenia, leukopenia, thrombocytopenia, pancytopenia, and anemias). Use with caution in patients with hypotension, severe myocardial insufficiency, diabetes mellitus, porphyria, hypoalbuminemia, hypothyroidism, fever, or hepatic or renal dysfunction. Effects with other sedative drugs or ethanol may be potentiated. Severe reactions, including toxic epidermal necrolysis and Stevens-Johnson syndromes, although rarely reported, have resulted in fatalities; drug should be discontinued if there are any signs of rash. Patients of Asian descent with the variant *HLA-B*1502* may be at an increased risk of developing Stevens-Johnson syndrome and/or toxic epidermal necrolysis.

Drug Interactions

Avoid Concomitant Use

Avoid concomitant use of Fosphenytoin with any of the following: Axitinib; Boceprevir; Bortezomib; Crizotinib; Darunavir; Delavirdine; Dronedarone; Etravirine; Everolimus; Lapatinib; Lurasidone; Nilotinib; Pazopanib; Praziquantel; Ranolazine; Rilpivirine; Rivaroxaban; Roflumilast; RomiDEPsin; SORAfenib; Telaprevir; Ticagrelor; Tolvaptan; Toremifene; Vandetanib

Decreased Effect

Fosphenytoin may decrease the levels/effects of: Acetaminophen; Amiodarone; Antifungal Agents (Azole Derivatives, Systemic); ARIPiprazole; Axitinib; Boceprevir; Bortezomib; Brentuximab Vedotin; Busulfan; CarBAMazepine; Chloramphenicol; Clarithromycin; CloZAPine; Contraceptives (Estrogens); Contraceptives (Progestins); Crizotinib; CycloSPORINE; CycloSPORINE (Systemic); CYP2B6 Substrates; CYP2C19 Substrates; CYP2C8 Substrates; CYP2C9 Substrates; CYP3A4 Substrates; Darunavir; Dasatinib; Deferasirox; Delavirdine; Diclofenac; Disopyramide; Divalproex; Doxycycline; Dronedarone; Efavirenz; Ethosuximide; Etoposide; Etoposide Phosphate; Etravirine; Everolimus; Exemestane; Felbamate; Flunarizine; Gefitinib; GuanFACINE; HMG-CoA Reductase Inhibitors; Imatinib; Irinotecan; Ixabepilone; Lacosamide; LamoTRIgine; Lapatinib; Levodopa; Linagliptin; Loop Diuretics; Lopinavir; Lurasidone; Maraviroc; Mebendazole; Meperidine; Methadone; MethylPREDNISolone; MetroNIDAZOLE; MetroNIDAZOLE (Systemic); Metyrapone; Mexiletine; Nelfinavir; Nilotinib; OXcarbazepine; Pazopanib; Praziquantel; PrednisoLONE; PrednisoLONE (Systemic); PredniSONE; Primidone; QUEtiapine; QuiNIDine; QuiNINE; Ranolazine; Rilpivirine; Ritonavir; Rivaroxaban; Roflumilast; RomiDEPsin; Rufinamide; Saxagliptin; Sertraline; Sirolimus; SORAfenib; SUNItinib; Tacrolimus; Tacrolimus (Systemic); Tadalafil; Telaprevir; Temsirolimus; Teniposide; Theophylline Derivatives; Thyroid Products; Ticagrelor; Tipranavir; Tolvaptan; Topiramate; Toremifene; TraZODone; Treprostinil; Ulipristal; Valproic Acid; Vandetanib; Vecuronium; Vemurafenib; Zonisamide; Zuclopenthixol

The levels/effects of Fosphenytoin may be decreased by: Alcohol (Ethyl); Antacids; Barbiturates; CarBAMazepine; Ciprofloxacin; Ciprofloxacin (Systemic); CISplatin; CYP2C19 Inducers (Strong); CYP2C9 Inducers (Strong); Diazoxide; Divalproex; Folic Acid; Fosamprenavir; Ketorolac; Ketorolac (Nasal); Ketorolac (Systemic); Leucovorin Calcium-Levoleucovorin; Levomefolate; Lopinavir; Mefloquine; Methylfolate; Peginterferon Alfa-2b; Pyridoxine; Rifamycin Derivatives; Ritonavir; Telaprevir; Theophylline Derivatives; Tipranavir; Tocilizumab; Valproic Acid; Vigabatrin ▶

Increased Effect/Toxicity

Fosphenytoin may increase the levels/effects of: Barbiturates; Clarithromycin; CNS Depressants; Fosamprenavir; Lithium; Methotrimeprazine; Selective Serotonin Reuptake Inhibitors; Vecuronium; Vitamin K Antagonists

The levels/effects of Fosphenytoin may be increased by: Alcohol (Ethyl); Allopurinol; Amiodarone; Antifungal Agents (Azole Derivatives, Systemic); Barbiturates; Benzodiazepines; Calcium Channel Blockers; Capecitabine; CarBAMazepine; Carbonic Anhydrase Inhibitors; CeFAZolin; Chloramphenicol; Cimetidine; Clarithromycin; Conivaptan; CYP2C19 Inhibitors (Moderate); CYP2C19 Inhibitors (Strong); CYP2C9 Inhibitors (Moderate); CYP2C9 Inhibitors (Strong); Delavirdine; Dexmethylphenidate; Disulfiram; Droperidol; Efavirenz; Ethosuximide; Felbamate; Floxuridine; Fluconazole; Fluorouracil; Fluorouracil (Systemic); Fluorouracil (Topical); FLUoxetine; FluvoxaMINE; Halothane; HydrOXYzine; Isoniazid; Methotrimeprazine; Methylphenidate; MetroNIDAZOLE; MetroNIDAZOLE (Systemic); OXcarbazepine; Proton Pump Inhibitors; Rufinamide; Sertraline; Sulfonamide Derivatives; Tacrolimus; Tacrolimus (Systemic); Telaprevir; Ticlopidine; Topiramate; TraZODone; Trimethoprim; Vitamin K Antagonists

Nutritional/Ethanol Interactions Ethanol:

Acute use: Avoid or limit ethanol (inhibits metabolism of phenytoin). Ethanol may also increase CNS depression; monitor for increased effects with coadministration. Caution patients about effects.

Chronic use: Avoid or limit ethanol (stimulates metabolism of phenytoin).

Adverse Reactions The more important adverse clinical events caused by the I.V. use of fosphenytoin or phenytoin are cardiovascular collapse and/or central nervous system depression. Hypotension can occur when either drug is administered rapidly by the I.V. route.

The adverse clinical events most commonly observed with the use of fosphenytoin in clinical trials were nystagmus, dizziness, pruritus, paresthesia, headache, somnolence, and ataxia. Paresthesia and pruritus were seen more often following fosphenytoin (versus phenytoin) administration and occurred more often with I.V. fosphenytoin than with I.M. administration. These events were dose and rate related (adult doses ≥15 mg/kg at a rate of 150 mg/minute). These sensations, generally described as itching, burning, or tingling are usually not at the infusion site. The location of the discomfort varied with the groin mentioned most frequently. The paresthesia and pruritus were transient events that occurred within several minutes of the start of infusion and generally resolved within 10 minutes after completion of infusion.

Transient pruritus, tinnitus, nystagmus, somnolence, and ataxia occurred 2-3 times more often at adult doses ≥15 mg/kg and rates ≥150 mg/minute.

I.V. administration (maximum dose/rate):

>10%:

Central nervous system: Nystagmus, dizziness, somnolence, ataxia

Dermatologic: Pruritus

1% to 10%:

Cardiovascular: Hypotension, vasodilation, tachycardia

Central nervous system: Stupor, incoordination, paresthesia, extrapyramidal syndrome, tremor, agitation, hypoesthesia, dysarthria, vertigo, brain edema, headache

Gastrointestinal: Nausea, tongue disorder, dry mouth, vomiting

Neuromuscular & skeletal: Pelvic pain, muscle weakness, back pain

Ocular: Diplopia, amblyopia

Otic: Tinnitus, deafness

Miscellaneous: Taste perversion

I.M. administration (substitute for oral phenytoin):

1% to 10%:

Central nervous system: Nystagmus, tremor, ataxia, headache, incoordination, somnolence, dizziness, paresthesia, reflexes decreased

Dermatologic: Pruritus

Gastrointestinal: Nausea, vomiting

Hematologic/lymphatic: Ecchymosis

Neuromuscular & skeletal: Muscle weakness

Available Dosage Forms

Injection, solution: 75 mg/mL (2 mL, 10 mL)

Cerebyx®: 75 mg/mL (2 mL)

Injection, solution [preservative free]: 75 mg/mL (2 mL)

General Dosage Range

I.M.: *Adults:* Loading: 15-20 mg PE/kg; Maintenance: 4-6 mg PE/kg/day

I.V.: *Adults:* Loading: 10-20 mg PE/kg; Maintenance: 4-6 mg PE/kg/day

Administration

I.M. I.M. may be administered as a single daily dose using either 1 or 2 injection sites.

I.V. Rates of infusion:

Children: 1-3 mg PE/kg/minute (maximum rate: 150 mg PE/minute)

Adults: Should not exceed 150 mg PE/minute. For nonemergent situations, may administer loading dose over 30 minutes.

Stability

Reconstitution Must be diluted to concentrations of 1.5-25 mg PE/mL, in normal saline or D_5W, for I.V. infusion.

Storage Refrigerate at 2°C to 8°C (36°F to 46°F). Do not store at room temperature for more than 48 hours. Do not use vials that develop particulate matter.

Nursing Actions

Physical Assessment Continuous hemodynamic monitoring and respiratory status are essential during infusion and for 30 minutes following infusion. Monitor closely for adverse reactions during and following infusion.

Patient Education Patients may not be in a position to evaluate their response. If conscious or alert, advise patient to report signs or symptoms of palpitations, slow heartbeat, respiratory difficulty, faintness, CNS disturbances (eg, somnolence, ataxia), and visual disturbances.

Dietary Considerations Provides phosphate 0.0037 mmol/mg PE fosphenytoin

Frovatriptan (froe va TRIP tan)

Brand Names: U.S. Frova®

Index Terms Frovatriptan Succinate

Pharmacologic Category Antimigraine Agent; Serotonin 5-$HT_{1B,\ 1D}$ Receptor Agonist

Medication Safety Issues

International issues:

Allegro: Brand name for frovatriptan [Germany], but also the brand name for fluticasone [Israel]

Allegro [Germany] may be confused with Allegra and Allegra-D brand names for fexofenadine and fexofenadine/pseudoehedrine, respectively, in the [U.S., Canada, and multiple international markets]

Pregnancy Risk Factor C

Lactation Excretion in breast milk unknown/use caution

Use Acute treatment of migraine with or without aura

Mechanism of Action/Effect Selective agonist for serotonin receptor in cranial arteries; causes vasoconstriction and relief of migraine

Contraindications Hypersensitivity to frovatriptan or any component of the formulation; patients with ischemic heart disease or signs or symptoms of ischemic heart disease (including Prinzmetal's angina, angina pectoris, myocardial infarction, silent myocardial ischemia); cerebrovascular syndromes (including strokes, transient ischemic attacks); peripheral vascular syndromes (including ischemic bowel disease); uncontrolled hypertension; use within 24 hours of ergotamine derivatives; use within 24 hours of another 5-HT_1 agonist; management of hemiplegic or basilar migraine

Canadian labeling: Additional contraindications (not in U.S. labeling): Cardiac arrhythmias, valvular heart disease, congenital heart disease, atherosclerotic disease; management of ophthalmoplegic migraine; severe hepatic impairment

Warnings/Precautions Not intended for migraine prophylaxis, or treatment of cluster headaches, hemiplegic or basilar migraines. Rule out underlying neurologic disease in patients with atypical headache, migraine (with no prior history of migraine) or inadequate clinical response to initial dosing. Cardiac events (coronary artery vasospasm, transient ischemia, MI, ventricular tachycardia/fibrillation, cardiac arrest, and death), cerebral/subarachnoid hemorrhage, stroke, peripheral vascular ischemia, and colonic ischemia have been reported with 5-HT_1 agonist administration. Patients who experience sensations of chest pain/pressure/tightness or symptoms suggestive of angina following dosing should be evaluated for coronary artery disease or Prinzmetal's angina before receiving additional doses; if dosing is resumed and similar symptoms recur, monitor with ECG. May cause vasospastic reactions resulting in colonic, peripheral, or coronary ischemia. Do not give to patients with risk factors for CAD until a cardiovascular evaluation has been performed; if evaluation is satisfactory, the healthcare provider should administer the first dose (consider ECG monitoring) and cardiovascular status should be periodically evaluated. Significant elevation in blood pressure, including hypertensive crisis, has also been reported on rare occasions in patients using other 5-HT_{1D} agonists with and without a history of hypertension. May lower seizure threshold, use caution in epilepsy or structural brain lesions. Symptoms of agitation, confusion, hallucinations, hyper-reflexia, myoclonus, shivering, and tachycardia (serotonin syndrome) may occur with concomitant proserotonergic drugs (ie, SSRIs/SNRIs or triptans) or agents which reduce frovatriptan's metabolism. Concurrent use of serotonin precursors (eg, tryptophan) is not recommended. If concomitant administration with SSRIs is warranted, monitor closely, especially at initiation and with dose increases. Safety and efficacy in pediatric patients have not been established.

Drug Interactions

Avoid Concomitant Use

Avoid concomitant use of Frovatriptan with any of the following: Ergot Derivatives

Decreased Effect

The levels/effects of Frovatriptan may be decreased by: Cyproterone

Increased Effect/Toxicity

Frovatriptan may increase the levels/effects of: Ergot Derivatives; Metoclopramide; Serotonin Modulators

The levels/effects of Frovatriptan may be increased by: Antipsychotics; Ergot Derivatives

Nutritional/Ethanol Interactions Food: Food does not affect frovatriptan bioavailability.

Adverse Reactions 1% to 10%:

Cardiovascular: Flushing (4%), chest pain (2%), palpitation (1%)

Central nervous system: Dizziness (8%), fatigue (5%), headache (4%), hot or cold sensation (3%), somnolence (≥2%), anxiety (1%), dysesthesia (1%), hypoesthesia (1%), insomnia (1%), pain (1%)

Gastrointestinal: Xerostomia (3%), nausea (≥2%), dyspepsia (2%), abdominal pain (1%), diarrhea (1%), vomiting (1%)
Neuromuscular & skeletal: Paresthesia (4%), skeletal pain (3%)
Ocular: Vision abnormal (1%)
Otic: Tinnitus (1%)
Respiratory: Rhinitis (1%), sinusitis (1%)
Miscellaneous: Diaphoresis (1%)

Available Dosage Forms

Tablet, oral:
Frova®: 2.5 mg

General Dosage Range Oral: *Adults:* 2.5 mg as a single dose, may repeat after 2 hours (maximum: 7.5 mg/day)

Administration

Oral Administer with fluids.

Stability

Storage Store at controlled room temperature of 25°C (77°F); excursions permitted to 15°C to 30°C (59°F to 86°F). Protect from moisture.

Nursing Actions

Physical Assessment Monitor cardiovascular status periodically; monitor for hypertension and cardiac events. Teach patient proper use (treatment of acute migraine).

Patient Education This drug is to be used to reduce your migraine, not to prevent or reduce the number of attacks. If first dose brings relief, a second dose may be taken anytime after 2 hours if migraine returns. May cause dizziness, fatigue, insomnia, drowsiness, dry mouth, skin flushing or hot flashes, mild abdominal discomfort, or vomiting. Report immediately any chest pain, palpitations, or irregular heartbeat; severe dizziness; acute headache; stiff or painful neck; facial swelling; muscle weakness or pain; feeling of tingling in extremities; changes in mental acuity; blurred vision, eye pain, or ringing in ears; changes in urinary pattern; or respiratory difficulty.

Fulvestrant (fool VES trant)

Brand Names: U.S. Faslodex®

Index Terms ICI-182,780; ZD9238

Pharmacologic Category Antineoplastic Agent, Estrogen Receptor Antagonist

Pregnancy Risk Factor D

Lactation Excretion in breast milk unknown/not recommended

Breast-Feeding Considerations Approved for use only in postmenopausal women.

Use Treatment of hormone receptor positive metastatic breast cancer in postmenopausal women with disease progression following antiestrogen therapy

Mechanism of Action/Effect Estrogen receptor antagonist; competitively binds to estrogen receptors on tumors and other tissue targets, producing a nuclear complex that causes a dose-related down-regulation of estrogen receptors and inhibits tumor growth.

Contraindications Hypersensitivity to fulvestrant or any component of the formulation

Warnings/Precautions Hazardous agent - use appropriate precautions for handling and disposal. Use caution in hepatic impairment; dosage adjustment is recommended in patients with moderate hepatic impairment. Safety and efficacy have not been established in severe hepatic impairment. Use with caution in patients with a history of bleeding disorders (including thrombocytopenia) and/or patients on anticoagulant therapy; bleeding/hematoma may occur from I.M. administration.

Drug Interactions

Avoid Concomitant Use There are no known interactions where it is recommended to avoid concomitant use.

Decreased Effect

The levels/effects of Fulvestrant may be decreased by: Tocilizumab

Increased Effect/Toxicity

The levels/effects of Fulvestrant may be increased by: Conivaptan

Adverse Reactions Adverse reactions reported with 500 mg dose.

>10%:
Endocrine & metabolic: Hot flushes (7% to 13%)
Hepatic: Alkaline phosphatase increased (>15%; grades 3/4: 1% to 2%), transaminases increased (>15%; grades 3/4: 1% to 2%)
Local: Injection site pain (12% to 14%)
Neuromuscular & skeletal: Joint disorders (14% to 19%)

1% to 10%:
Cardiovascular: Ischemic disorder (1%)
Central nervous system: Fatigue (8%), headache (8%)
Gastrointestinal: Nausea (10%), anorexia (6%), vomiting (6%), constipation (5%), weight gain (≤1%)
Genitourinary: Urinary tract infection (2% to 4%)
Neuromuscular & skeletal: Bone pain (9%), arthralgia (8%), back pain (8%), extremity pain (7%), musculoskeletal pain (6%), weakness (6%)
Respiratory: Cough (5%), dyspnea (4%)

<1%, postmarketing, and/or case reports (reported with 250 mg or 500 mg dose): Angioedema, hypersensitivity reactions, leukopenia, myalgia, osteoporosis, thrombosis, urticaria, vaginal bleeding, vertigo

Pharmacodynamics/Kinetics

Duration of Action I.M.: Steady state concentrations reached within first month, when administered with additional dose given 2 weeks following the initial dose; plasma levels maintained for at least 1 month

Available Dosage Forms

Injection, solution:
Faslodex®: 50 mg/mL (5 mL)

General Dosage Range Dosage adjustment recommended in patients with hepatic impairment

I.M.: *Adults (postmenopausal women):* Initial: 500 mg on days 1, 15, and 29; Maintenance: 500 mg once monthly

Administration

I.M. For I.M. administration only; do not administer I.V., SubQ, or intra-arterially. Administer 500 mg dose as two 5 mL injections (one in each buttocks) slowly over 1-2 minutes per injection.

Stability

Storage Store in original carton under refrigeration at 2°C to 8°C (36°F to 46°F). Protect from light.

Nursing Actions

Physical Assessment Monitor for thromboembolism, vasodilation, edema, gastrointestinal disturbances, dyspnea, and pain on a regular basis throughout.

Patient Education This medication is administered by injection; report immediately any redness, swelling, burning, or pain at injection site. You may experience bone or muscle pain, back pain, or headache; nausea, vomiting, or loss of appetite; dizziness; or hot flashes. Report any chest pain or palpitations, swelling of extremities or weight gain, cough, or respiratory difficulty.

Furosemide (fyoor OH se mide)

Brand Names: U.S. Lasix®

Index Terms Frusemide

Pharmacologic Category Diuretic, Loop

Medication Safety Issues

Sound-alike/look-alike issues:

Furosemide may be confused with famotidine, finasteride, fluconazole, FLUoxetine, fosinopril, loperamide, torsemide

Lasix® may be confused with Lanoxin®, Lidex®, Lomotil®, Lovenox®, Luvox®, Luxiq®

International issues:

Lasix [U.S., Canada, and multiple international markets] may be confused with Esidrex brand name for hydrochlorothiazide [multiple international markets]; Esidrix brand name for hydrochlorothiazide [Germany]

Urex [Australia, Hong Kong, Turkey] may be confused with Eurax brand name for crotamiton [U.S., Canada, and multiple international markets]

Pregnancy Risk Factor C

Lactation Enters breast milk/use caution

Breast-Feeding Considerations Crosses into breast milk; may suppress lactation

Use Management of edema associated with heart failure and hepatic or renal disease; acute pulmonary edema; treatment of hypertension (alone or in combination with other antihypertensives)

Canadian labeling: Additional use: Furosemide Special Injection and Lasix® Special (products not available in the U.S.): Adjunctive treatment of oliguria in patients with severe renal impairment

Mechanism of Action/Effect Inhibits reabsorption of sodium and chloride in the ascending loop of Henle and distal renal tubule, interfering with the chloride-binding cotransport system, thus causing increased excretion of water, sodium, chloride, magnesium, and calcium

Contraindications Hypersensitivity to furosemide or any component of the formulation; anuria

Canadian labeling: Additional contraindications (not in U.S. labeling): Hypersensitivity to sulfonamide-derived drugs; complete renal shutdown; hepatic coma and precoma; uncorrected states of electrolyte depletion, hypovolemia, or hypotension; jaundiced newborn infants or infants with disease(s) capable of causing hyperbilirubinemia and possibly kernicterus; breast-feeding. **Note:** Manufacturer labeling for Lasix® Special and Furosemide Special Injection also includes: GFR <5 mL/minute or GFR >20 mL/minute; hepatic cirrhosis; renal failure accompanied by hepatic coma and precoma; renal failure due to poisoning with nephrotoxic or hepatotoxic substances.

Warnings/Precautions [U.S. Boxed Warning]: If given in excessive amounts, furosemide, similar to other loop diuretics, can lead to profound diuresis, resulting in fluid and electrolyte depletion; close medical supervision and dose evaluation are required. Watch for and correct electrolyte disturbances; adjust dose to avoid dehydration. When electrolyte depletion is present, therapy should not be initiated unless serum electrolytes, especially potassium, are normalized. In cirrhosis, avoid electrolyte and acid/base imbalances that might lead to hepatic encephalopathy; correct electrolyte and acid/base imbalances prior to initiation when hepatic coma is present. Coadministration of antihypertensives may increase the risk of hypotension.

Monitor fluid status and renal function in an attempt to prevent oliguria, azotemia, and reversible increases in BUN and creatinine; close medical supervision of aggressive diuresis is required. May increase risk of contrast-induced nephropathy. Rapid I.V. administration, renal impairment, excessive doses, hypoproteinemia, and concurrent use of other ototoxins is associated with ototoxicity. Asymptomatic hyperuricemia has been reported with use; rarely, gout may precipitate. Photosensitization may occur.

Use with caution in patients with prediabetes or diabetes mellitus; may see a change in glucose control. Use with caution in patients with systemic lupus erythematosus (SLE); may cause SLE exacerbation or activation. Use with caution in patients with prostatic hyperplasia/urinary stricture; may cause urinary retention. May lead to ▶

nephrocalcinosis or nephrolithiasis in premature infants or in children <4 years of age with chronic use. May prevent closure of patent ductus arteriosus in premature infants. Chemical similarities are present among sulfonamides, sulfonylureas, carbonic anhydrase inhibitors, thiazides, and loop diuretics (except ethacrynic acid). A risk of cross-reaction exists in patients with allergy to any of these compounds; avoid use when previous reaction has been severe. Discontinue if signs of hypersensitivity are noted.

Drug Interactions

Avoid Concomitant Use

Avoid concomitant use of Furosemide with any of the following: Chloral Hydrate; Ethacrynic Acid

Decreased Effect

Furosemide may decrease the levels/effects of: Lithium; Neuromuscular-Blocking Agents

The levels/effects of Furosemide may be decreased by: Aliskiren; Bile Acid Sequestrants; Fosphenytoin; Herbs (Hypertensive Properties); Methotrexate; Methylphenidate; Nonsteroidal Anti-Inflammatory Agents; Phenytoin; Probenecid; Salicylates; Sucralfate; Yohimbine

Increased Effect/Toxicity

Furosemide may increase the levels/effects of: ACE Inhibitors; Allopurinol; Amifostine; Aminoglycosides; Antihypertensives; Cardiac Glycosides; Chloral Hydrate; CISplatin; Dofetilide; Ethacrynic Acid; Hypotensive Agents; Lithium; Methotrexate; Neuromuscular-Blocking Agents; RisperiDONE; RiTUXimab; Salicylates; Sodium Phosphates

The levels/effects of Furosemide may be increased by: Alfuzosin; Beta2-Agonists; Corticosteroids (Orally Inhaled); Corticosteroids (Systemic); CycloSPORINE (Systemic); Diazoxide; Herbs (Hypotensive Properties); Licorice; MAO Inhibitors; Methotrexate; Pentoxifylline; Phosphodiesterase 5 Inhibitors; Probenecid; Prostacyclin Analogues

Nutritional/Ethanol Interactions

Food: Furosemide serum levels may be decreased if taken with food.

Herb/Nutraceutical: Avoid bayberry, blue cohosh, cayenne, ephedra, ginger, ginseng (American), kola, licorice (may worsen hypertension). Avoid black cohosh, California poppy, coleus, golden seal, hawthorn, mistletoe, periwinkle, quinine, shepherd's purse (may increase antihypertensive effect). Licorice may also cause or worsen hypokalemia.

Adverse Reactions Frequency not defined.

Cardiovascular: Acute hypotension, chronic aortitis, necrotizing angiitis, orthostatic hypotension, vasculitis

Central nervous system: Dizziness, fever, headache, hepatic encephalopathy, lightheadedness, restlessness, vertigo

Dermatologic: Bullous pemphigoid, cutaneous vasculitis, erythema multiforme, exfoliative dermatitis, photosensitivity, pruritus, purpura, rash, Stevens-Johnson syndrome, toxic epidermal necrolysis, urticaria

Endocrine & metabolic: Cholesterol and triglycerides increased, glucose tolerance test altered, gout, hyperglycemia, hyperuricemia, hypocalcemia, hypochloremia, hypokalemia, hypomagnesemia, hyponatremia, metabolic alkalosis

Gastrointestinal: Anorexia, constipation, cramping, diarrhea, nausea, oral and gastric irritation, pancreatitis, vomiting

Genitourinary: Urinary bladder spasm, urinary frequency

Hematological: Agranulocytosis (rare), anemia, aplastic anemia (rare), eosinophilia, hemolytic anemia, leukopenia, thrombocytopenia

Hepatic: Intrahepatic cholestatic jaundice, ischemic hepatitis, liver enzymes increased

Local: Injection site pain (following I.M. injection), thrombophlebitis

Neuromuscular & skeletal: Muscle spasm, paresthesia, weakness

Ocular: Blurred vision, xanthopsia

Otic: Hearing impairment (reversible or permanent with rapid I.V. or I.M. administration), tinnitus

Renal: Allergic interstitial nephritis, fall in glomerular filtration rate and renal blood flow (due to overdiuresis), glycosuria, transient rise in BUN

Miscellaneous: Anaphylaxis (rare), exacerbate or activate systemic lupus erythematosus

Pharmacodynamics/Kinetics

Onset of Action Diuresis: Oral, S.L.: 30-60 minutes; I.M.: 30 minutes; I.V.: ~5 minutes

Symptomatic improvement with acute pulmonary edema: Within 15-20 minutes; occurs prior to diuretic effect

Peak effect: Oral: 1-2 hours

Duration of Action Oral, S.L.: 6-8 hours; I.V.: 2 hours

Available Dosage Forms

Injection, solution [preservative free]: 10 mg/mL (2 mL, 4 mL, 10 mL)

Solution, oral: 40 mg/5 mL (5 mL, 500 mL); 10 mg/mL (4 mL, 60 mL, 120 mL)

Tablet, oral: 20 mg, 40 mg, 80 mg

Lasix®: 20 mg, 40 mg, 80 mg

General Dosage Range

I.M.:

Children: Initial: 1 mg/kg/dose; Maintenance: Up to 6 mg/kg/dose every 6-12 hours

Adults: Initial: 20-40 mg/dose; Usual maintenance dose interval: 6-12 hours (maximum: 200 mg/dose)

Elderly: Initial: 20 mg/day

I.V.:

Children: Initial: 1 mg/kg/dose; Maintenance: Up to 6 mg/kg/dose every 6-12 hours

Adults: Initial: 20-40 mg/dose; Usual maintenance dose interval: 6-12 hours (maximum: 200 mg/dose) **or** 40 mg, followed by 80 mg within 1 hour if inadequate response **or** 20-40 mg bolus, followed by continuous I.V. infusion doses of 10-40 mg/hour, doubled as needed up to a maximum 160 mg/hour

Elderly: Initial: 20 mg/day

Oral:

Children: Initial: 2 mg/kg/dose every 6-8 hours (maximum: 6 mg/kg/dose)

Adults: Initial: 20-80 mg/dose every 6-8 hours; Usual maintenance dose interval: Once or twice daily (maximum: 600 mg/day)

Elderly: Initial: 20 mg/day

Administration

Oral Administer on an empty stomach (Bard, 2004). May be administered with food or milk if GI distress occurs; however, this may reduce diuretic efficacy.

I.V. I.V. injections should be given slowly. In adults, undiluted direct I.V. injections may be administered at a rate of 20-40 mg per minute; maximum rate of administration for short-term intermittent infusion is 4 mg/minute; exceeding this rate increases the risk of ototoxicity. In children, a maximum rate of 0.5 mg/kg/minute has been recommended.

I.V. Detail pH: 8-9.3

Other When I.V. or oral administration is not possible, the sublingual route may be used. Place 1 tablet under tongue for at least 5 minutes to allow for maximal absorption. Patients should be advised not to swallow during disintegration time (Haegeli, 2007).

Stability

Reconstitution I.V. infusion solution mixed in NS or D_5W solution is stable for 24 hours at room temperature. May also be diluted for infusion to 1-2 mg/mL (maximum: 10 mg/mL).

Storage

Injection: Store at room temperature of 15°C to 30°C (59°F to 86°F). Protect from light. Exposure to light may cause discoloration; do not use furosemide solutions if they have a yellow color. Furosemide solutions are unstable in acidic media, but very stable in basic media. Refrigeration may result in precipitation or crystallization; however, resolubilization at room temperature or warming may be performed without affecting the drug's stability.

Tablet: Store at 25°C (77°F); excursions permitted to 15°C to 30°C (59°F to 89°F). Protect from light.

Nursing Actions

Physical Assessment Allergy history should be assessed before beginning therapy. Monitor for dehydration, electrolyte imbalance, and postural hypotension on a regular basis during therapy.

Patient Education For daily administration, may be taken with food or milk early in the day to reduce GI distress; if taken twice daily, take last dose in early afternoon in order to avoid sleep disturbance and to achieve maximum therapeutic effect. Follow dietary advice of prescriber; include potassium-rich foods in daily diet. Do not take potassium supplements without advice of prescriber. Weigh yourself each day at the same time when beginning therapy and weekly for long-term therapy. Report unusual or unanticipated weight gain or loss. May cause dizziness, blurred vision, drowsiness, or sensitivity to sunlight. Report signs of edema (eg, weight gain; swollen ankles, feet, or hands), trembling, numbness or fatigue, cramping or muscle weakness, chest pain or palpitations, unresolved nausea or vomiting, or any change in hearing.

Dietary Considerations May cause potassium loss; potassium supplement or dietary changes may be required.

Related Information

Compatibility of Drugs *on page 1264*

Gabapentin (GA ba pen tin)

Brand Names: U.S. Gralise™; Neurontin®

Pharmacologic Category Anticonvulsant, Miscellaneous; GABA Analog

Medication Safety Issues

Sound-alike/look-alike issues:

Neurontin® may be confused with Motrin®, Neoral®, nitrofurantoin, Noroxin®, Zarontin®

Medication Guide Available Yes

Pregnancy Risk Factor C

Lactation Enters breast milk/use caution

Breast-Feeding Considerations Gabapentin is excreted in human breast milk. A nursed infant could be exposed to ~1 mg/kg/day of gabapentin; the effect on the child is not known. Use in breast-feeding women only if the benefits to the mother outweigh the potential risk to the infant.

Use Adjunct for treatment of partial seizures with and without secondary generalized seizures in patients >12 years of age with epilepsy; adjunct for treatment of partial seizures in pediatric patients 3-12 years of age; management of postherpetic neuralgia (PHN) in adults

Unlabeled Use Neuropathic pain, diabetic peripheral neuropathy, fibromyalgia, postoperative pain, restless legs syndrome (RLS), vasomotor symptoms

Mechanism of Action/Effect Although structurally related to GABA, it does not interact with GABA receptors. Interacts with calcium channels to inhibit neurotransmission related to seizure activity and pain perception.

Contraindications Hypersensitivity to gabapentin or any component of the formulation

Warnings/Precautions Antiepileptics are associated with an increased risk of suicidal behavior/thoughts with use (regardless of indication); patients should be monitored for signs/symptoms of depression, suicidal tendencies, and other unusual behavior changes during therapy and instructed to inform their healthcare provider immediately if symptoms occur. Avoid abrupt withdrawal, may precipitate seizures; Gralise™ should be withdrawn over ≥1 week. Use cautiously in patients with severe renal dysfunction; male rat studies demonstrated an association with pancreatic adenocarcinoma (clinical implication unknown). May cause CNS depression, which may impair physical or mental abilities. Patients must be cautioned about performing tasks which require mental alertness (eg, operating machinery or driving). Effects with other sedative drugs or ethanol may be potentiated. Pediatric patients (3-12 years of age) have shown increased incidence of CNS-related adverse effects, including emotional lability, hostility, thought disorder, and hyperkinesia. Gabapentin immediate release and extended release (Gralise™) products are not interchangeable with each other **or** with gabapentin encarbil (Horizant™). The safety and efficacy of extended release gabapentin (Gralise™) has not been studied in patients with epilepsy. Potentially serious, sometimes fatal multiorgan hypersensitivity (also known as drug reaction with eosinophilia and systemic symptoms [DRESS]) has been reported with some antiepileptic drugs, including gabapentin; may affect lymphatic, hepatic, renal, cardiac, and/or hematologic systems; fever, rash, and eosinophilia may also be present. Discontinue immediately if suspected.

Drug Interactions

Avoid Concomitant Use There are no known interactions where it is recommended to avoid concomitant use.

Decreased Effect

The levels/effects of Gabapentin may be decreased by: Antacids; Ketorolac; Ketorolac (Nasal); Ketorolac (Systemic); Mefloquine

Increased Effect/Toxicity

Gabapentin may increase the levels/effects of: Alcohol (Ethyl); CNS Depressants; Methotrimeprazine; Selective Serotonin Reuptake Inhibitors

The levels/effects of Gabapentin may be increased by: Droperidol; HydrOXYzine; Methotrimeprazine

Nutritional/Ethanol Interactions

Ethanol: May increase CNS depression; monitor for increased effects with coadministration. Caution patients about effects.

Food: Tablet, solution (immediate release): No significant effect on rate or extent of absorption; tablet (extended release): Increases rate and extent of absorption.

Herb/Nutraceutical: Avoid evening primrose (seizure threshold decreased). Avoid valerian, St John's wort, kava kava, gotu kola (may increase CNS depression).

Adverse Reactions As reported for immediate release (IR) formulations in patients >12 years of age, unless otherwise noted in children (3-12 years) or with use of extended release (ER) formulation

>10%:

Central nervous system: Dizziness (IR: 17% to 28%; children 3%; ER: 11%), somnolence (IR: 19% to 21%; children 8%; ER: 5%), ataxia (3% to 13%), fatigue (11%; children 3%)

Miscellaneous: Viral infection (children 11%)

1% to 10%:

Cardiovascular: Peripheral edema (2% to 8%), vasodilatation (1%)

Central nervous system: Fever (children 10%), hostility (children 5% to 8%), emotional lability (children 4% to 6%), headache (IR: 3%; ER: 4%), abnormal thinking (2% to 3%; children 2%), amnesia (2%), depression (2%), nervousness (2%), abnormal coordination (1% to 2%), pain (ER: 1% to 2%), hyperesthesia (1%), lethargy (ER: 1%), twitching (1%), vertigo (ER: 1%)

Dermatologic: Pruritus (1%), rash (1%)

Endocrine & metabolic: Hyperglycemia (1%)

Gastrointestinal: Diarrhea (IR: 6%; ER: 3%), nausea/vomiting (3% to 4%; children 8%), abdominal pain (3%), xerostomia (2% to 5%), constipation (1% to 4%), weight gain (adults and children 2% to 3%), dyspepsia (IR: 2%; ER: 1%), flatulence (2%), dry throat (2%), dental abnormalities (2%), appetite stimulation (1%)

Genitourinary: Impotence (2%), urinary tract infection (ER: 2%)

Hematologic: Decreased WBC (1%), leukopenia (1%)

Neuromuscular & skeletal: Tremor (7%), weakness (6%), hyperkinesia (children 3% to 5%), abnormal gait (2%), back pain (2%), dysarthria (2%), myalgia (2%), fracture (1%)

Ocular: Nystagmus (8%), diplopia (1% to 6%), blurred vision (3% to 4%), conjunctivitis (1%)

Otic: Otitis media (1%)

Respiratory: Rhinitis (4%), bronchitis (children 3%), respiratory infection (children 3%), pharyngitis (1% to 3%), cough (2%)

Miscellaneous: Infection (5%)

Available Dosage Forms

Capsule, oral: 100 mg, 300 mg, 400 mg

Neurontin®: 100 mg, 300 mg, 400 mg

Solution, oral: 250 mg/5 mL (470 mL)

Neurontin®: 250 mg/5 mL (470 mL)

Tablet, oral: 600 mg, 800 mg

Gralise™: 300 mg, 600 mg, 300 mg (9s) [white tablets; contains soybean lecithin] and 600 mg (69s) [beige tablets]

Neurontin®: 600 mg, 800 mg

General Dosage Range Dosage adjustment recommended in patients with renal impairment

Oral:

Children 3-4 years: Initial: 10-15 mg/kg/day in 3 divided doses; Usual dose: 40 mg/kg/day in 3 divided doses (maximum: 50 mg/kg/day)

Children 5-12 years: Initial: 10-15 mg/kg/day in 3 divided doses; Usual dose: 25-35 mg/kg/day in 3 divided doses (maximum: 50 mg/kg/day)

Children >12 years: Initial: 300 mg 3 times/day; Usual dose: 900-1800 mg/day in 3 divided doses (maximum: 3600 mg/day [short-term])

Adults:

Immediate release: Initial: 300 mg 1-3 times/day; Maintenance: 900-3600 mg/day in 3 divided doses (maximum: 3600 mg/day [short-term])

Extended release: Initial: 300 mg; Maintenance: 1800 mg once daily

Administration

Oral

Tablet, solution (immediate release): Administer first dose on first day at bedtime to avoid somnolence and dizziness. Dosage must be adjusted for renal function; when given 3 times daily, the maximum time between doses should not exceed 12 hours.

Tablet (extended release): Take with evening meal. Swallow whole; do not chew, crush, or split.

Stability

Storage

Capsules and tablets: Store at 25°C (77°F); excursions permitted to 15°C to 30°C (59°F to 86°F).

Oral solution: Store refrigerated at 2°C to 8°C (36°F to 46°F).

Nursing Actions

Physical Assessment Monitor therapeutic response (seizure activity, force, type, duration) at beginning of therapy and periodically throughout. Assess for CNS depression. Taper dosage slowly when discontinuing. If treating seizures, observe and teach seizure/safety precautions.

Patient Education Avoid alcohol. You may experience drowsiness, lightheadedness, impaired coordination, dizziness, blurred vision, nausea, vomiting, anorexia, constipation, diarrhea, postural hypotension, or decreased sexual function or libido (reversible). Notify prescriber of persistent CNS effects (nervousness, restlessness, insomnia, anxiety, excitation, headache, sedation, worsening seizures or change in quality, mania, abnormal thinking), severe dizziness or passing out, suicide ideation or depression, rash or skin irritation, change in gait, bruising or bleeding, or worsening of condition.

Dietary Considerations Immediate release tablet and solution may be taken without regard to meals; extended release tablet should be taken with food.

Gabapentin Enacarbil

(gab a PEN tin en a KAR bil)

Brand Names: U.S. Horizant™

Index Terms GSK 1838262; Horizant™; Solzira; XP13512

Pharmacologic Category Anticonvulsant, Miscellaneous

Medication Guide Available Yes

Pregnancy Risk Factor C

Lactation Excretion in breast milk unknown/not recommended

Breast-Feeding Considerations It is not known if gabapentin enacarbil is excreted in human breast milk; however, other gabapentin products are excreted in human breast milk. A nursed infant could be exposed to ~1 mg/kg/day of gabapentin; the effect on the child is not known. Use in breast-feeding women only if the benefits to the mother outweigh the potential risk to the infant.

Use Treatment of moderate-to-severe restless leg syndrome (RLS)

Mechanism of Action/Effect Gabapentin enacarbil is a prodrug of gabapentin. Although gabapentin is structurally related to GABA, it does not interact with GABA receptors. Interacts with calcium channels to inhibit neurotransmission. These effects on RLS are unknown.

Contraindications There are no contraindication listed within the manufacturer's labeling.

Warnings/Precautions

Gabapentin and other antiepileptics are associated with an increased risk of suicidal behavior/thoughts with use (regardless of indication); gabapentin enacarbil is a prodrug of gabapentin and may also increase patient's risk. Patients should be monitored for signs/symptoms of depression, suicidal tendencies, and other unusual behavior changes during therapy and instructed to inform their health-care provider immediately if symptoms occur. Doses >600 mg/day (not included in approved labeling) should be reduced to 600 mg daily for 1 week prior to stopping. Rat studies demonstrated an association with pancreatic adenocarcinoma (clinical implication unknown). May cause CNS depression, which may impair physical or mental abilities. Patients must be cautioned about performing tasks which require mental alertness (eg, operating machinery or driving). Effects with other sedative drugs or ethanol may be potentiated. Use with caution in patients with renal impairment; use not recommended in patients with severe impairment (Cl_{cr} <30 mL/minute). Gabapentin enacarbil (Horizant™) and other gabapentin products are not interchangeable due to differences in formulation, indications and pharmacokinetics.

Drug Interactions

Avoid Concomitant Use There are no known interactions where it is recommended to avoid concomitant use.

Decreased Effect

The levels/effects of Gabapentin Enacarbil may be decreased by: Ketorolac; Ketorolac (Nasal); Ketorolac (Systemic); Mefloquine

Increased Effect/Toxicity

Gabapentin Enacarbil may increase the levels/effects of: Alcohol (Ethyl); CNS Depressants; Methotrimeprazine; Selective Serotonin Reuptake Inhibitors

The levels/effects of Gabapentin Enacarbil may be increased by: Droperidol; HydrOXYzine; Methotrimeprazine

Nutritional/Ethanol Interactions

Ethanol: Avoid ethanol (may increase CNS depression).

Herb/Nutraceutical: Avoid evening primrose (seizure threshold decreased). Avoid valerian, St John's wort, kava kava, gotu kola (may increase CNS depression).

Adverse Reactions Percentages reported are for 600 mg/day dosing.

>10%: Central nervous system: Sedation/somnolence (20%), dizziness (13%), headache (12%)

1% to 10%:

Central nervous system: Fatigue (6%), irritability (4%), balance disorder (<2%), disorientation (<2%), lethargy (<2%), drunk feeling (1%), vertigo (1%)

Gastrointestinal: Nausea (6%), flatulence (3%), xerostomia (3%), appetite increased (2%), weight gain (2%)

Ocular: Blurred vision (<2%)

Available Dosage Forms

Tablet, extended release, oral:

Horizant™: 600 mg

General Dosage Range Dosage adjustment recommended in patients with renal impairment.

Oral: *Adults:* 600 mg once daily

Administration

Oral Administer with food at ~5:00 pm daily; tablet should be swallowed whole; do not break, chew, cut, or crush.

Stability

Storage Store at 25°C (77°F); excursions permitted to 15°C to 30°C (59°F to 86°F). Protect from moisture. Do not remove from original container.

Dietary Considerations Take with food.

Galantamine (ga LAN ta meen)

Brand Names: U.S. Razadyne®; Razadyne® ER

Index Terms Galantamine Hydrobromide

Pharmacologic Category Acetylcholinesterase Inhibitor (Central)

Medication Safety Issues

Sound-alike/look-alike issues:

Razadyne® may be confused with Rozerem®

International issues:

Reminyl [Canada and multiple international markets] may be confused with Amarel brand name for glimepiride [France]; Amaryl brand name for glimepiride [U.S., Canada, and multiple international markets]; Robinul brand name for glycopyrrolate [U.S. and multiple international markets]

Pregnancy Risk Factor B

Lactation Excretion in breast milk unknown/not recommended

Use Treatment of mild-to-moderate dementia of Alzheimer's disease

Unlabeled Use Severe dementia associated with Alzheimer's disease; mild-to-moderate dementia associated with Parkinson's disease; Lewy body dementia

Mechanism of Action/Effect Increases the concentration of acetylcholine in the brain by slowing its metabolism.

Contraindications Hypersensitivity to galantamine or any component of the formulation

Warnings/Precautions Use caution in patients with supraventricular conduction delays (without a functional pacemaker in place); Alzheimer's treatment guidelines consider bradycardia to be a relative contraindication for use of centrally-active cholinesterase inhibitors. Use caution in patients taking medicines that slow conduction through SA or AV node. Use caution in peptic ulcer disease (or in patients at risk); seizure disorder; asthma; COPD; mild-to-moderate liver dysfunction; moderate renal dysfunction. May cause bladder outflow obstruction. May exaggerate neuromuscular blockade effects of succinylcholine and like agents.

Drug Interactions

Avoid Concomitant Use There are no known interactions where it is recommended to avoid concomitant use.

Decreased Effect

Galantamine may decrease the levels/effects of: Anticholinergics; Neuromuscular-Blocking Agents (Nondepolarizing)

The levels/effects of Galantamine may be decreased by: Anticholinergics; Dipyridamole; Peginterferon Alfa-2b; Tocilizumab

Increased Effect/Toxicity

Galantamine may increase the levels/effects of: Antipsychotics; Beta-Blockers; Cholinergic Agonists; Succinylcholine

The levels/effects of Galantamine may be increased by: Conivaptan; Corticosteroids (Systemic); Selective Serotonin Reuptake Inhibitors

Nutritional/Ethanol Interactions

Ethanol: Avoid ethanol (may increase CNS adverse events).

Herb/Nutraceutical: St John's wort may decrease galantamine serum levels; avoid concurrent use.

Adverse Reactions

>10%: Gastrointestinal: Nausea (13% to 24%), vomiting (6% to 13%), diarrhea (6% to 12%)

1% to 10%:

Cardiovascular: Bradycardia (2% to 3%), hypertension (≥2%), peripheral edema (≥2%), syncope (0.4% to 2.2%: dose related), chest pain (≥1% to 2%)

Central nervous system: Dizziness (9%), headache (8%), depression (7%), fatigue (5%), insomnia (5%), somnolence (4%), agitation (≥2%), anxiety (≥2%), confusion (≥2%), hallucination (≥2%), fever (≥1%), malaise (≥1%)

Dermatologic: Purpura (≥2%)

Gastrointestinal: Anorexia (7% to 9%), weight loss (5% to 7%), abdominal pain (5%), dyspepsia (5%), constipation (≥2%), flatulence (≥1%)

Genitourinary: Urinary tract infection (8%), hematuria (<1% to 3%), incontinence (≥1% to 2%)

Hematologic: Anemia (3%)

Neuromuscular & skeletal: Tremor (3%), back pain (≥2%), fall (≥2%), weakness (≥1% to 2%)

Respiratory: Rhinitis (4%), bronchitis (≥2%), cough (≥2%), upper respiratory tract infection (≥2%)

Pharmacodynamics/Kinetics

Duration of Action 3 hours; maximum inhibition of erythrocyte acetylcholinesterase ~40% at 1 hour post 8 mg oral dose; levels return to baseline at 30 hours

Available Dosage Forms

Capsule, extended release, oral: 8 mg, 16 mg, 24 mg

Razadyne® ER: 8 mg, 16 mg, 24 mg

Solution, oral: 4 mg/mL (100 mL)

Razadyne®: 4 mg/mL (100 mL)

Tablet, oral: 4 mg, 8 mg, 12 mg

Razadyne®: 4 mg, 8 mg, 12 mg

General Dosage Range Dosage adjustment recommended in patients with hepatic or renal impairment

Oral:

Extended-release: *Adults:* Initial: 8 mg once daily; Maintenance: 16-24 mg once daily

Immediate release: *Adults:* Initial: 4 mg twice daily; Maintenance: 16-24 mg/day in 2 divided doses

Administration

Oral Administer oral solution or tablet with breakfast and dinner; administer extended release capsule with breakfast. If therapy is interrupted for ≥3 days, restart at the lowest dose and increase to current dose. If using oral solution, mix dose with 3-4 ounces of any nonalcoholic beverage; mix well and drink immediately.

Stability

Storage Store at 25°C (77°F); excursions permitted to 15°C to 30°C (59°F to 86°F). Do not freeze oral solution.

Nursing Actions

Physical Assessment Assess bladder and sphincter adequacy prior to treatment. Monitor for cholinergic crisis.

Patient Education This medication will not cure Alzheimer's disease, but may help reduce symptoms. May cause dizziness, sedation, hypotension, or tremor; diarrhea; or nausea or vomiting. Report persistent GI disturbances; significantly increased salivation, sweating, or tearing; excessive fatigue, insomnia, dizziness, or depression; increased muscle, joint, or body pain or spasms; vision changes; respiratory changes, wheezing, or signs of dyspnea; chest pain or palpitations; or other adverse reactions.

Dietary Considerations Administration with food is preferred, but not required; should be taken with breakfast and dinner (tablet or solution) or with breakfast (capsule).

Ganciclovir (Systemic) (gan SYE kloe veer)

Brand Names: U.S. Cytovene®-IV

Index Terms DHPG Sodium; GCV Sodium; Nordeoxyguanosine

Pharmacologic Category Antiviral Agent

Medication Safety Issues

Sound-alike/look-alike issues:

Cytovene® may be confused with Cytosar®, Cytosar-U

Ganciclovir may be confused with acyclovir

Pregnancy Risk Factor C

Lactation Excretion in breast milk unknown/not recommended

Breast-Feeding Considerations Due to the carcinogenic and teratogenic effects observed in animal studies, the possibility of adverse events in a nursing infant is considered likely. Therefore, nursing should be discontinued during therapy. In addition, the CDC recommends **not** to breast-feed if diagnosed with HIV to avoid postnatal transmission of the virus.

Use Treatment of CMV retinitis in immunocompromised individuals, including patients with acquired immunodeficiency syndrome; prophylaxis of CMV infection in transplant patients

Unlabeled Use CMV retinitis: May be given in combination with foscarnet in patients who relapse after monotherapy with either drug

Mechanism of Action/Effect Ganciclovir is phosphorylated to a substrate which competitively inhibits the binding of deoxyguanosine triphosphate to DNA polymerase resulting in inhibition of viral DNA synthesis.

Contraindications Hypersensitivity to ganciclovir, acyclovir, or any component of the formulation

Warnings/Precautions Hazardous agent - use appropriate precautions for handling and disposal. **[U.S. Boxed Warning]: Granulocytopenia (neutropenia), anemia, and thrombocytopenia may occur.** Dosage adjustment or interruption of ganciclovir therapy may be necessary in patients with neutropenia and/or thrombocytopenia and patients with impaired renal function. **[U.S. Boxed**

Warning]: Animal studies have demonstrated carcinogenic and teratogenic effects, and inhibition of spermatogenesis; contraceptive precautions for female and male patients need to be followed during and for at least 90 days after therapy with the drug; take care to administer only into veins with good blood flow. **[U.S. Boxed Warning]: Indicated only for treatment of CMV retinitis in the immunocompromised patient and CMV prevention in transplant patients at risk.**

Drug Interactions

Avoid Concomitant Use

Avoid concomitant use of Ganciclovir (Systemic) with any of the following: Imipenem

Decreased Effect There are no known significant interactions involving a decrease in effect.

Increased Effect/Toxicity

Ganciclovir (Systemic) may increase the levels/effects of: Imipenem; Mycophenolate; Reverse Transcriptase Inhibitors (Nucleoside); Tenofovir

The levels/effects of Ganciclovir (Systemic) may be increased by: Mycophenolate; Probenecid; Tenofovir

Adverse Reactions

>10%:

Central nervous system: Fever (48%)

Gastrointestinal: Diarrhea (44%), anorexia (14%), vomiting (13%)

Hematologic: Thrombocytopenia (57%), leukopenia (41%), anemia (16% to 26%), neutropenia with ANC <500/mm^3 (12% to 14%)

Ocular: Retinal detachment (11%; relationship to ganciclovir not established)

Renal: Serum creatinine increased (2% to 14%)

Miscellaneous: Sepsis (15%), diaphoresis (12%)

1% to 10%:

Central nervous system: Chills (10%), neuropathy (9%)

Dermatologic: Pruritus (5%)

<1%, postmarketing, and/or case reports (limited to important or life-threatening): Allergic reaction (including anaphylaxis), alopecia, arrhythmia, bronchospasm, cardiac arrest, cataracts, cholestasis, coma, dyspnea, edema, encephalopathy, exfoliative dermatitis, extrapyramidal symptoms, hepatitis, hepatic failure, pancreatitis, pancytopenia, pulmonary fibrosis, psychosis, rhabdomyolysis, seizure, alopecia, urticaria, eosinophilia, hemorrhage, Stevens-Johnson syndrome, torsade de pointes, renal failure, SIADH, visual loss

Available Dosage Forms

Injection, powder for reconstitution: 500 mg

Cytovene®-IV: 500 mg

General Dosage Range Dosage adjustment recommended in patients with renal impairment

I.V.: *Children and Adults:* Induction: 5 mg/kg every 12 hours; Maintenance: 30-35 mg/kg/week, given as once-daily dose for 5-7 days per week

Administration

I.V. Should not be administered by I.M., SubQ, or rapid IVP. Administer by slow I.V. infusion over at least 1 hour. Too rapid infusion can cause increased toxicity and excessive plasma levels.

I.V. Detail Flush line well with NS before and after administration.

pH: 11

Stability

Reconstitution Reconstitute powder with unpreserved sterile water not bacteriostatic water because parabens may cause precipitation. Dilute in 250-1000 mL D_5W or NS to a concentration ≤10 mg/mL for infusion.

Storage Intact vials should be stored at room temperature and protected from temperatures >40°C. Reconstituted solution is stable for 12 hours at room temperature, however, conflicting data indicates that reconstituted solution is stable for 60 days under refrigeration (4°C). Stability of parenteral admixture at room temperature (25°C) and at refrigeration temperature (4°C) is 5 days.

Nursing Actions

Physical Assessment I.V.: Monitor for paresthesia, neutropenia, anemia, and nephrotoxicity throughout therapy. Teach patient importance of contraceptive precautions during and for 90 days following therapy.

Patient Education Ganciclovir is not a cure for CMV retinitis. You will need frequent blood tests and regular ophthalmic exams while taking this drug. You may experience increased susceptibility to infection. You may experience confusion, headache, nausea, vomiting, anorexia, diarrhea, or photosensitivity. Report rash, infection (fever, chills, unusual bleeding or bruising, or unhealed sores or white plaques in mouth); abdominal pain; tingling, weakness, or pain in extremities; or pain, redness, or swelling at injection site.

Dietary Considerations Some products may contain sodium.

Ganirelix (ga ni REL ix)

Index Terms Antagon; Ganirelix Acetate

Pharmacologic Category Gonadotropin Releasing Hormone Antagonist

Medication Safety Issues

International issues:

Antagon former U.S. brand name for ganirelix, but also the brand name for ranitidine in Brazil

Pregnancy Risk Factor X

Lactation Excretion in breast milk unknown/not recommended

Use Inhibits premature luteinizing hormone (LH) surges in women undergoing controlled ovarian hyperstimulation

Mechanism of Action/Effect Suppresses gonadotropin secretion and luteinizing hormone secretion to prevent ovulation until the follicles are of adequate size.

Contraindications Hypersensitivity to ganirelix or any component of the formulation; hypersensitivity to gonadotropin-releasing hormone (GnRH) or any other GnRH analog; known or suspected pregnancy

Warnings/Precautions Should only be prescribed by fertility specialists. Hypersensitivity reactions, including anaphylactoid reactions, have been reported; may occur with the first dose. The packaging contains natural rubber latex (may cause allergic reactions). Pregnancy must be excluded before starting medication.

Drug Interactions

Avoid Concomitant Use There are no known interactions where it is recommended to avoid concomitant use.

Decreased Effect There are no known significant interactions involving a decrease in effect.

Increased Effect/Toxicity There are no known significant interactions involving an increase in effect.

Adverse Reactions 1% to 10%:

Central nervous system: Headache (3%)

Endocrine & metabolic: Ovarian hyperstimulation syndrome (2%)

Gastrointestinal: Abdominal pain (1%), nausea (1%)

Genitourinary: Pelvic pain (5%), vaginal bleeding (2%)

Local: Injection site reaction (1%)

Pharmacodynamics/Kinetics

Duration of Action <48 hours

Available Dosage Forms

Injection, solution: 250 mcg/0.5 mL (0.5 mL)

General Dosage Range SubQ: *Adults:* 250 mcg/day

Administration

Other Administer SubQ in abdomen (around upper navel) or upper thigh; rotate injection site.

Stability

Storage Store at controlled room temperature of 25°C (77°F); excursions permitted to 15°C to 30°C (59°F to 86°F). Protect from light.

Nursing Actions

Physical Assessment This medication should only be prescribed by a fertility specialist. Teach patient proper injection procedures and syringe disposal.

Patient Education This drug can only be given by injection. You must keep all scheduled ultrasound appointments. You may experience headache or nausea. Report immediately any sudden or acute abdominal pain; vaginal bleeding; or pain, itching, or signs of infection at injection site.

Gatifloxacin (gat i FLOKS a sin)

Brand Names: U.S. Zymar® [DSC]; Zymaxid™

Pharmacologic Category Antibiotic, Ophthalmic; Antibiotic, Quinolone

Pregnancy Risk Factor C

Lactation Excretion in breast milk unknown/use caution

Breast-Feeding Considerations Other quinolones are known to be excreted in breast milk. The manufacturer recommends using caution if gatifloxacin is administered while nursing.

Use Treatment of bacterial conjunctivitis

Mechanism of Action/Effect Inhibits bacterial DNA

Contraindications

Zymar®: Hypersensitivity to gatifloxacin, other quinolone antibiotics, or any component of the formulation

Zymaxid™: There are no contraindications listed in the manufacturer's labeling.

Warnings/Precautions Severe hypersensitivity reactions, including anaphylaxis, have occurred with systemic quinolone therapy. Reactions may present as typical allergic symptoms after a single dose, or may manifest as severe idiosyncratic dermatologic, vascular, pulmonary, renal, hepatic, and/or hematologic events, usually after multiple doses. Prompt discontinuation of drug should occur if skin rash or other symptoms arise. Prolonged use may result in fungal or bacterial superinfection. For topical ophthalmic use only. Do not inject ophthalmic solution subconjunctivally or introduce directly into the anterior chamber of the eye. Contact lenses should not be worn during treatment of ophthalmic infections.

Drug Interactions

Avoid Concomitant Use There are no known interactions where it is recommended to avoid concomitant use.

Decreased Effect There are no known significant interactions involving a decrease in effect.

Increased Effect/Toxicity There are no known significant interactions involving an increase in effect.

Adverse Reactions 1% to 10%:

Central nervous system: Headache

Gastrointestinal: Taste disturbance

Ocular: Chemosis, conjunctival hemorrhage, conjunctival irritation, discharge, dry eye, edema, irritation, keratitis, lacrimation increased, pain, papillary conjunctivitis, visual acuity decreased

Available Dosage Forms

Solution, ophthalmic:

Zymaxid™: 0.5% (2.5 mL)

General Dosage Range Ophthalmic: *Children ≥1 year and Adults:* 1 drop into affected eye(s) every 2 hours while awake (maximum: 8 times/day) for 1-2 days; followed by 1 drop into affected eye(s) 2-4 times/day

Administration

Other For topical ophthalmic use only; avoid touching tip of applicator to eye, fingers, or other surfaces.

Stability

Storage Store between 15°C to 25°C (59°F to 77°F); do not freeze.

Nursing Actions

Patient Education Tilt head back and instill prescribed number of drops in affected eye as often as directed for length of time prescribed. Do not allow dropper to touch any surface, including the eyes or hands. Apply light pressure to the inside corner of the eye (near the nose) after each drop. Avoid wearing contact lenses during treatment. May cause headache or dizziness. May cause temporary eye discomfort (stinging, burning, itching, pain, tearing) or a bad taste in mouth after instillation. Report persistent adverse reactions, visual disturbances, or if condition worsens. If you experience signs of allergic reaction (eg, itching, rash, respiratory difficulty, facial edema, difficulty swallowing), discontinue use immediately and report to prescriber.

Gefitinib (ge FI tye nib)

Brand Names: U.S. Iressa®

Index Terms ZD1839

Pharmacologic Category Antineoplastic Agent, Tyrosine Kinase Inhibitor

Medication Safety Issues

Sound-alike/look-alike issues:

Gefitinib may be confused with axitinib, crizotinib, erlotinib, imatinib, SORAfenib, SUNItinib, vandetanib

High alert medication:

This medication is in a class the Institute for Safe Medication Practices (ISMP) includes among its list of drug classes which have a heightened risk of causing significant patient harm when used in error.

Pregnancy Risk Factor D

Lactation Excretion in breast milk unknown/not recommended

Use Treatment of locally advanced or metastatic nonsmall cell lung cancer (NSCLC) after failure of platinum-based and docetaxel therapies. Treatment is limited to patients who are benefiting or have benefited from treatment with gefitinib.

Note: Due to the lack of improved survival data from clinical trials of gefitinib, and in response to positive survival data with another EGFR inhibitor, according to the U.S. labeling, physicians are advised to use treatment options other than gefitinib in patients with advanced nonsmall cell lung cancer following one or two prior chemotherapy regimens when they are refractory/intolerant to their most recent regimen.

Canada labeling: First-line treatment of locally advanced or metastatic NSCLC with activating mutations of EGFR-TK

Unlabeled Use First-line treatment of NSCLC with known EGFR mutation

Available Dosage Forms

Tablet, oral:

Iressa®: 250 mg

General Dosage Range Dosage adjustment recommended in patients on concomitant therapy or who develop toxicities.

Oral: *Adults:* 250 mg once daily

Administration

Oral May administer with or without food.

For patients unable to swallow tablets or for administration via NG tube: Tablets may be dispersed in noncarbonated drinking water. Drop whole tablet (do not crush) into 1/2 glass of water; stir until tablet is dispersed (~10 minutes). Drink immediately. Rinse glass with 1/2 glass of water and drink.

Nursing Actions

Physical Assessment Assess results of liver function tests on a regular basis.

Patient Education Take with or without food. Do not take with grapefruit juice. You will need periodic laboratory tests while taking this medication. Maintain adequate hydration, unless instructed to restrict fluid intake. You may experience loss of appetite, nausea, vomiting, or diarrhea. Report immediately persistent diarrhea; skin rash; unusual or persistent respiratory difficulty or wheezing; chest pain or cough; any change in vision, eye pain, or signs of eye infection; unusual weakness; or joint pain.

Gemcitabine (jem SITE a been)

Brand Names: U.S. Gemzar®

Index Terms dFdC; dFdCyd; Difluorodeoxycytidine Hydrochlorothiazide; Gemcitabine Hydrochloride; LY-188011

Pharmacologic Category Antineoplastic Agent, Antimetabolite (Pyrimidine Analog)

Medication Safety Issues

Sound-alike/look-alike issues:

Gemcitabine may be confused with gemtuzumab

Gemzar® may be confused with Zinecard®

High alert medication:

This medication is in a class the Institute for Safe Medication Practices (ISMP) includes among its list of drug classes which have a heightened risk of causing significant patient harm when used in error.

Pregnancy Risk Factor D

Lactation Excretion in breast milk unknown/not recommended

Breast-Feeding Considerations According to the manufacturer, the decision to continue or discontinue breast-feeding during therapy should take into account the risk of exposure to the infant and the benefits of treatment to the mother.

Use Treatment of metastatic breast cancer; inoperable locally-advanced or metastatic nonsmall cell lung cancer (NSCLC); locally advanced or metastatic pancreatic cancer; advanced, relapsed ovarian cancer

Unlabeled Use Treatment of biliary tract cancers (advanced), bladder cancer, cervical cancer (recurrent or persistent), Ewing's sarcoma (refractory), head and neck cancer (nasopharyngeal), Hodgkin lymphoma (relapsed), non-Hodgkin lymphomas (refractory), malignant pleural mesothelioma, osteosarcoma (refractory), renal cell cancer (metastatic), small cell lung cancer (refractory or relapsed), soft tissue sarcoma (advanced), testicular cancer (refractory germ cell tumors), thymic malignancies, uterine sarcoma, and unknown-primary adenocarcinoma

Mechanism of Action/Effect A pyrimidine antimetabolite that inhibits DNA synthesis by inhibition of DNA polymerase and ribonucleotide reductase, cell cycle-specific for the S-phase of the cycle (also blocks cellular progression at G1/S phase).

Contraindications Hypersensitivity to gemcitabine or any component of the formulation

Warnings/Precautions Hazardous agent - use appropriate precautions for handling and disposal. Prolongation of the infusion time >60 minutes and more frequent than weekly dosing have been shown to increase toxicity. Gemcitabine may suppress bone marrow function (leukopenia, thrombocytopenia, and anemia); myelosuppression is usually the dose-limiting toxicity; monitor blood counts; dosage adjustments are frequently required. Gemcitabine may cause fever in the absence of clinical infection. Pulmonary toxicity has occurred; discontinue if severe and institute supportive measures.

Hemolytic uremic syndrome (and/or renal failure) has been reported; monitor for evidence of microangiopathic hemolysis (elevation of bilirubin or LDH, reticulocytosis, severe thrombocytopenia, and/or renal failure); use with caution in patients with pre-existing renal impairment. Serious hepatotoxicity (including liver failure and death) has been reported (when used alone or in combination with other hepatotoxic medications). Use with caution in patients with hepatic impairment (history of cirrhosis, hepatitis, or alcoholism) or in patients with hepatic metastases; may lead to exacerbation of hepatic impairment; dose adjustments may be considered with elevated bilirubin.

Pulmonary toxicity has been observed; discontinue if severe and institute supportive measures. Use caution with concurrent radiation therapy; radiation toxicity, including tissue injury, severe mucositis, esophagitis, or pneumonitis, has been reported with concurrent and nonconcurrent administration; may have radiosensitizing activity when gemcitabine and radiation therapy are given ≤7 days apart; lower doses with concurrent radiation therapy may produce less severe toxicity; however, an optimum regimen for combination therapy has not been determined for all tumor types; radiation recall may occur when gemcitabine and radiation therapy are given >7 days apart. Prolongation of the infusion time >60 minutes and more frequent than weekly dosing have been shown to increase toxicity; has been administered at a fixed-dose rate (FDR) infusion rate of 10 mg/m^2/minute in studies (unlabeled); prolonged infusion times increase the accumulation of the active metabolite, gemcitabine triphosphate, optimizing the pharmacokinetics (Ko, 2006; Tempero, 2003); patients who receive gemcitabine FDR experience more grade 3/4 hematologic toxicity (Ko, 2006; Poplin, 2009). Use caution in the elderly; clearance is affected by age.

Drug Interactions

Avoid Concomitant Use

Avoid concomitant use of Gemcitabine with any of the following: BCG; CloZAPine; Natalizumab; Pimecrolimus; Tacrolimus (Topical); Vaccines (Live)

Decreased Effect

Gemcitabine may decrease the levels/effects of: BCG; Coccidioidin Skin Test; Sipuleucel-T; Vaccines (Inactivated); Vaccines (Live); Vitamin K Antagonists

The levels/effects of Gemcitabine may be decreased by: Echinacea

Increased Effect/Toxicity

Gemcitabine may increase the levels/effects of: Bleomycin; CloZAPine; Fluorouracil; Fluorouracil (Systemic); Fluorouracil (Topical); Leflunomide; Natalizumab; Vaccines (Live); Vitamin K Antagonists

The levels/effects of Gemcitabine may be increased by: Denosumab; Pimecrolimus; Roflumilast; Tacrolimus (Topical); Trastuzumab

Nutritional/Ethanol Interactions Ethanol: Avoid ethanol (due to GI irritation).

Adverse Reactions Frequency of adverse reactions reported for single-agent use of gemcitabine only.

>10%:

Cardiovascular: Peripheral edema (20%), edema (13%)

Central nervous system: Fever (38% to 41%), somnolence (11%)

Dermatologic: Rash (28% to 30%), alopecia (15% to 16%), pruritus (13%)

Gastrointestinal: Nausea/vomiting (69% to 71%; grade 3: 10% to 13%; grade 4: 1% to 2%), diarrhea (19% to 30%), stomatitis (10% to 11%)

Hematologic: Anemia (68% to 73%; grade 4: 1% to 2%), leukopenia (62% to 64%; grade 4: ≤1%), neutropenia (61% to 63%; grade 4: 6% to 7%), thrombocytopenia (24% to 36%; grade 4: ≤1%), hemorrhage (4% to 17%; grades 3: ≤2%; grade 4: <1%); myelosuppression is the dose-limiting toxicity

Hepatic: AST increased (67% to 78%; grade 3: 6% to 12%; grade 4: 2% to 5%), alkaline phosphatase increased (55% to 77%; grade 3: 7% to 16%; grade 4: 2% to 4%), ALT increased (68% to 72%; grade 3: 8% to 10%; grade 4: 1% to 2%), bilirubin increased (13% to 26%; grade 3: 2% to 6%; grade 4: ≤2%)

Renal: Proteinuria (32% to 45%; grades 3/4: <1%), hematuria (23% to 35%; grades 3/4: <1%), BUN increased (15% to 16%)

Respiratory: Dyspnea (10% to 23%)

Miscellaneous: Flu-like syndrome (19%), infection (10% to 16%; grade 3: 1% to 2%; grade 4: <1%)

1% to 10%:

Local: Injection site reactions (4%)

Neuromuscular & skeletal: Paresthesia (10%)

Renal: Creatinine increased (6% to 8%)

Respiratory: Bronchospasm (<2%)

Available Dosage Forms

Injection, powder for reconstitution: 200 mg, 1 g, 2 g

Gemzar®: 200 mg, 1 g

Injection, solution: 38 mg/mL (5.26 mL, 26.3 mL, 52.6 mL)

General Dosage Range Dosage adjustment recommended in patients with hepatic impairment or who develop toxicities

I.V.: *Adults:* Dosage varies greatly depending on indication

Administration

I.V. Infuse over 30 minutes; for unlabeled uses, infusion times may vary (refer to specific references). **Note:** Prolongation of the infusion time >60 minutes has been shown to increase toxicity. Gemcitabine has been administered at a fixed-dose rate (FDR) infusion rate of 10 mg/m^2/minute (unlabeled); prolonged infusion times increase the accumulation of the active metabolite, gemcitabine triphosphate, optimizing the pharmacokinetics (Ko, 2006; Tempero, 2003). Patients who receive gemcitabine FDR experience more grade 3/4 hematologic toxicity (Ko, 2006; Poplin, 2009).

Other For intravesicular (bladder) instillation, gemcitabine was diluted in 50-100 mL normal saline; patients were instructed to retain in the bladder for 1 hour (Addeo, 2010; Dalbaghi, 2006)

Stability

Reconstitution Use appropriate precautions for handling and disposal. Reconstitute lyophilized powder with preservative free NS; add 5 mL to the 200 mg vial, add 25 mL to the 1000 mg vial, or add 50 mL to the 2000 mg vial, resulting in a reconstituted concentration of 38 mg/mL (solutions must be reconstituted to ≤40 mg/mL to completely dissolve).

Further dilute for infusion in NS 50-500 mL injection; to concentrations as low as 0.1 mg/mL.

Storage

Lyophilized powder: Store intact vials at room temperature of 20°C to 25°C (68°F to 77°F); excursions permitted to 15°C to 30°C (59°F to 86°F). Reconstituted vials are stable for 24 hours at room temperature. Do not refrigerate (may form crystals).

Solution for injection: Store intact vials refrigerated at 2°C to 8°C (36°F to 46°F); do not freeze. Solutions diluted for infusion in NS are stable for 24 hours at room temperature. Do not refrigerate.

Nursing Actions

Physical Assessment Monitor hepatic and renal function. Monitor for fever, CNS changes, rash, gastrointestinal upset, myelosuppression, anemia, dyspnea, and infection prior to each treatment and on a regular basis.

Patient Education You will be monitored during infusion. Report immediately any pain, burning, or swelling at infusion site; sudden chest pain or palpitations; difficulty breathing or swallowing; or chills. Between infusions, maintain adequate nutrition and hydration, unless instructed to restrict fluid intake. You may be more susceptible to infection. You may experience new fatigue, lethargy, somnolence, nausea, vomiting, loss of hair (reversible), or mouth sores. Report extreme fatigue; severe GI upset, constipation, or diarrhea; unusual bleeding or bruising; fever, chills, or sore throat; vaginal discharge; signs of fluid retention (swelling of extremities, respiratory difficulty, unusual weight gain); yellowing of skin or eyes; change in color of urine or stool; or muscle or skeletal pain or weakness.

Related Information

Management of Drug Extravasations *on page 1269*

Gemfibrozil (jem FI broe zil)

Brand Names: U.S. Lopid®

Index Terms CI-719

Pharmacologic Category Antilipemic Agent, Fibric Acid

Medication Safety Issues

Sound-alike/look-alike issues:

Lopid® may be confused with Levbid®, Lipitor®, Lodine

Pregnancy Risk Factor C

Lactation Excretion in breast milk unknown/not recommended

Use Treatment of hypertriglyceridemia in Fredrickson types IV and V hyperlipidemia for patients who are at greater risk for pancreatitis and who have not responded to dietary intervention; to reduce the risk of CHD development in Fredrickson type IIb patients without a history or symptoms of existing CHD who have not responded to dietary and other interventions (including pharmacologic treatment) and who have decreased HDL, increased LDL, and increased triglycerides

Mechanism of Action/Effect Inhibits lipolysis and decreases subsequent hepatic fatty acid uptake and hepatic secretion of VLDL; decreases serum levels of VLDL and increases HDL levels

Contraindications Hypersensitivity to gemfibrozil or any component of the formulation; hepatic or severe renal dysfunction; primary biliary cirrhosis; pre-existing gallbladder disease; concurrent use with repaglinide

Warnings/Precautions Secondary causes of hyperlipidemia should be ruled out prior to therapy. Possible increased risk of malignancy and cholelithiasis. Anemia, leukopenia, thrombocytopenia, and bone marrow hypoplasia have rarely been reported. Periodic monitoring recommended during the first year of therapy. Elevations in serum transaminases can be seen. Discontinue if lipid response not seen. Be careful in patient selection; this is not a first- or second-line choice. Other agents may be more suitable. Adjustments in warfarin therapy may be required with concurrent use. Has been associated with rare myositis or rhabdomyolysis; patients should be monitored closely. Patients should be instructed to report unexplained muscle pain, tenderness, weakness, or brown urine. Use caution when combining gemfibrozil with HMG-CoA reductase inhibitors (may lead to myopathy, rhabdomyolysis). Use with caution in patients with mild-to-moderate renal impairment; contraindicated in patients with severe impairment. Renal function deterioration has been seen when used in patients with a serum creatinine >2 mg/dL.

Drug Interactions

Avoid Concomitant Use

Avoid concomitant use of Gemfibrozil with any of the following: Bexarotene; Bexarotene (Systemic); Clopidogrel; Lovastatin; Repaglinide; Simvastatin

Decreased Effect

Gemfibrozil may decrease the levels/effects of: Chenodiol; Clopidogrel; CycloSPORINE; CycloSPORINE (Systemic); Ursodiol

The levels/effects of Gemfibrozil may be decreased by: Bile Acid Sequestrants; Tocilizumab

Increased Effect/Toxicity

Gemfibrozil may increase the levels/effects of: Antidiabetic Agents (Thiazolidinedione); Atorvastatin; Bexarotene; Bexarotene (Systemic); Carvedilol; Citalopram; Colchicine; CYP1A2 Substrates; CYP2C19 Substrates; CYP2C8 Substrates; CYP2C9 Substrates; Diclofenac; Ezetimibe; Fluvastatin; Lovastatin; Pitavastatin; Pravastatin; Repaglinide; Rosuvastatin; Simvastatin; Sulfonylureas; Treprostinil; Vitamin K Antagonists

The levels/effects of Gemfibrozil may be increased by: Conivaptan; CycloSPORINE; CycloSPORINE (Systemic)

Nutritional/Ethanol Interactions

Ethanol: Avoid ethanol to decrease triglycerides.

Food: When given after meals, the AUC of gemfibrozil is decreased.

Adverse Reactions

>10%: Gastrointestinal: Dyspepsia (20%)

1% to 10%:

Cardiovascular: Atrial fibrillation (1%)

Central nervous system: Fatigue (4%), vertigo (2%)

Dermatologic: Eczema (2%), rash (2%)

Gastrointestinal: Abdominal pain (10%), nausea/vomiting (3%)

Reports where causal relationship has not been established: Alopecia, anaphylaxis, cataracts, colitis, confusion, decreased fertility (male), drug-induced lupus-like syndrome, extrasystoles, hepatoma, intracranial hemorrhage, pancreatitis, peripheral vascular disease, photosensitivity, positive ANA, renal dysfunction, retinal edema, seizure, syncope, thrombocytopenia, vasculitis, weight loss

Pharmacodynamics/Kinetics

Onset of Action May require several days

Available Dosage Forms

Tablet, oral: 600 mg

Lopid®: 600 mg

General Dosage Range Oral: *Adults:* 600 mg twice daily

Administration

Oral Administer 30 minutes prior to breakfast and dinner.

Stability

Storage Store at controlled room temperature of 20°C to 25°C (68°F to 77°F). Protect from light and moisture.

Nursing Actions

Physical Assessment Assess serum cholesterol and LFTs.

Patient Education Should be taken 30 minutes before meals. Take with milk or meals if GI upset occurs. Avoid alcohol. Follow dietary recommendations of prescriber. You will need check-ups and blood work to assess effectiveness of therapy. You may experience loss of appetite, flatulence, or diarrhea. Report severe stomach pain, nausea, and vomiting.

Dietary Considerations Before initiation of therapy, patients should be placed on a standard cholesterol-lowering diet for 3-6 months and the diet should be continued during drug therapy. Should be taken 30 minutes prior to breakfast and dinner

Gemifloxacin (je mi FLOKS a sin)

Brand Names: U.S. Factive®

Index Terms DW286; Gemifloxacin Mesylate; LA 20304a; SB-265805

Pharmacologic Category Antibiotic, Quinolone; Respiratory Fluoroquinolone

Medication Guide Available Yes

Pregnancy Risk Factor C

Lactation Excretion in breast milk unknown/not recommended

Breast-Feeding Considerations It is not known if gemifloxacin is excreted in breast milk. Breast-feeding is not recommended by the manufacturer. Nondose-related effects could include modification of bowel flora.

Use Treatment of acute exacerbation of chronic bronchitis; treatment of community-acquired pneumonia (CAP), including pneumonia caused by multidrug-resistant strains of *S. pneumoniae* (MDRSP)

Unlabeled Use Acute sinusitis

Mechanism of Action/Effect Gemifloxacin is a DNA gyrase inhibitor and also inhibits topoisomerase IV. These enzymes are required for DNA replication and transcription, DNA repair, recombination, and transposition; quinolones are bactericidal

Contraindications Hypersensitivity to gemifloxacin, other fluoroquinolones, or any component of the formulation

Warnings/Precautions [U.S. Boxed Warning]: There have been reports of tendon inflammation and/or rupture with quinolone antibiotics; risk may be increased with concurrent corticosteroids, organ transplant recipients, and in patients >60 years of age. Rupture of the Achilles tendon sometimes requiring surgical repair has been reported most frequently; but other tendon sites (eg, rotator cuff, biceps) have also been reported. Strenuous physical activity, rheumatoid arthritis, and renal impairment may be an independent risk factor for tendonitis. Discontinue at first sign of tendon inflammation or pain. May occur even after discontinuation of therapy. Use with caution in patients with rheumatoid arthritis; may increase risk of tendon rupture. Fluoroquinolones may prolong QT_c interval; avoid use of gemifloxacin in patients with a history of QT_c prolongation, uncorrected hypokalemia, hypomagnesemia, or concurrent administration of other medications known to prolong the QT interval (including Class Ia and Class III antiarrhythmics, cisapride, erythromycin, antipsychotics, and tricyclic antidepressants). Use with caution in patients with significant bradycardia or acute myocardial ischemia. CNS effects may occur (tremor, restlessness, confusion, and very rarely hallucinations, increased intracranial pressure [including pseudotumor cerebri] or seizures). Use with caution in patients with known or suspected CNS disorder. Potential for seizures, although very rare, may be increased with concomitant NSAID therapy. Use with caution in individuals at risk of seizures. Use caution in renal dysfunction; dosage adjustment required for Cl_{cr} ≤40 mL/minute.

Fluoroquinolones have been associated with the development of serious, and sometimes fatal, hypoglycemia, most often in elderly diabetics, but also in patients without diabetes. This occurred most frequently with gatifloxacin (no longer available systemically) but may occur at a lower frequency with other quinolones.

Severe hypersensitivity reactions, including anaphylaxis, have occurred with quinolone therapy. Reactions may present as typical allergic symptoms after a single dose, or may manifest as severe idiosyncratic dermatologic, vascular, pulmonary, renal, hepatic, and/or hematologic events, usually after multiple doses. May cause maculopapular rash, usually 8-10 days after treatment initiation; risk factors may include age <40 years, female gender (including postmenopausal women on HRT), and treatment duration >7 days. Prompt discontinuation of drug should occur if skin rash or other symptoms arise. **[U.S. Boxed Warning]: Quinolones may exacerbate myasthenia gravis; avoid use (rare, potentially life-threatening weakness of respiratory muscles may occur).** Avoid excessive sunlight and take precautions to limit exposure (eg, loose fitting clothing, sunscreen); may cause moderate-to-severe phototoxicity reactions. Discontinue use if photosensitivity occurs. Prolonged use may result in fungal or bacterial superinfection, including *C. difficile*-associated diarrhea (CDAD) and pseudomembranous colitis; CDAD has been observed >2 months post-antibiotic treatment. Peripheral neuropathy has been linked to the use of quinolones; these cases were rare. Hemolytic reactions may (rarely) occur with quinolone use in patients with latent or actual G6PD deficiency.

Drug Interactions

Avoid Concomitant Use

Avoid concomitant use of Gemifloxacin with any of the following: BCG

Decreased Effect

Gemifloxacin may decrease the levels/effects of: BCG; Mycophenolate; Sulfonylureas; Typhoid Vaccine

The levels/effects of Gemifloxacin may be decreased by: Antacids; Calcium Salts; Didanosine; Iron Salts; Magnesium Salts; Quinapril; Sevelamer; Sucralfate; Zinc Salts

Increased Effect/Toxicity

Gemifloxacin may increase the levels/effects of: Corticosteroids (Systemic); Porfimer; Sulfonylureas; Varenicline; Vitamin K Antagonists

The levels/effects of Gemifloxacin may be increased by: Insulin; Nonsteroidal Anti-Inflammatory Agents; Probenecid

Nutritional/Ethanol Interactions Herb/Nutraceutical: Avoid dong quai, St John's wort (may also cause photosensitization).

Adverse Reactions 1% to 10%:

Central nervous system: Headache (4%), dizziness (2%)

Dermatologic: Rash (4%)

Gastrointestinal: Diarrhea (5%), nausea (4%), abdominal pain (2%), vomiting (2%)

Hepatic: Transaminases increased (1% to 4%)

Important adverse effects reported with other agents in this drug class include (not reported for gemifloxacin): Allergic reactions, CNS stimulation, hepatitis, jaundice, peripheral neuropathy, pneumonitis (eosinophilic), seizure; sensorimotor-axonal neuropathy (paresthesia, hypoesthesias, dysesthesias, weakness); severe dermatologic reactions (toxic epidermal necrolysis, Stevens-Johnson syndrome); torsade de pointes, vasculitis

Available Dosage Forms

Tablet, oral:

Factive®: 320 mg

General Dosage Range Dosage adjustment recommended in patients with renal impairment

Oral: *Adults:* 320 mg once daily

Administration

Oral May be administered with or without food, milk, or calcium supplements. Gemifloxacin should be taken 3 hours before or 2 hours after supplements (including multivitamins) containing iron, zinc, or magnesium.

Stability

Storage Store at 25°C (77°F). Protect from light.

Nursing Actions

Physical Assessment Allergy history should be ascertained prior to initiating therapy. Monitor for hypersensitivity, opportunistic infection, pseudomembraneous colitis, and tendon inflammation. Teach patient proper use (timing of meals, supplements, or other medications).

Patient Education Should be taken at least 3 hours before or 2 hours after antacids or other products containing aluminum, iron, magnesium, or zinc (including multivitamins). Maintain adequate hydration, unless instructed to restrict fluid intake. May cause headache, dizziness, nausea, vomiting, abdominal discomfort, or diarrhea. Discontinue use immediately and report to prescriber if signs of tendon inflammation or pain occur or if you experience signs of allergic reaction (eg, itching, rash, respiratory difficulty, facial edema, difficulty swallowing). Report CNS changes (eg, hallucinations, suicide ideation, seizures) or signs of opportunistic infection (unusual fever or chills, vaginal itching or foul-smelling vaginal discharge, easy bruising or bleeding).

Dietary Considerations May take tablets with or without food, milk, or calcium supplements. Gemifloxacin should be taken 3 hours before or 2 hours after supplements (including multivitamins) containing iron, zinc, or magnesium.

Gentamicin (Systemic) (jen ta MYE sin)

Index Terms Gentamicin Sulfate

Pharmacologic Category Antibiotic, Aminoglycoside

Medication Safety Issues

Sound-alike/look-alike issues:

Gentamicin may be confused with gentian violet, kanamycin, vancomycin

High alert medication:

The Institute for Safe Medication Practices (ISMP) includes this medication (intrathecal administration) among its list of drug classes which have a heightened risk of causing significant patient harm when used in error.

Pregnancy Risk Factor D

Lactation Enters breast milk/use caution (AAP rates "compatible"; AAP 2001 update pending)

Breast-Feeding Considerations Gentamicin is excreted into breast milk; however, it is not well absorbed when taken orally. This limited oral absorption may minimize exposure to the nursing infant. Nondose-related effects could include modification of bowel flora.

Use Treatment of susceptible bacterial infections, normally gram-negative organisms, including *Pseudomonas*, *Proteus*, *Serratia*, and gram-positive *Staphylococcus*; treatment of bone infections, respiratory tract infections, skin and soft tissue infections, as well as abdominal and urinary tract infections, and septicemia; treatment of infective endocarditis

Mechanism of Action/Effect Bactericidal; interferes with bacterial protein synthesis resulting in cell death

Contraindications Hypersensitivity to gentamicin or other aminoglycosides

Warnings/Precautions [U.S. Boxed Warning]: Aminoglycosides may cause neurotoxicity and/or nephrotoxicity; usual risk factors include pre-existing renal impairment, concomitant neuro-/nephrotoxic medications, advanced age and dehydration. Ototoxicity may be directly proportional to the amount of drug given and the duration of treatment; tinnitus or vertigo are indications of vestibular injury and impending hearing loss; renal damage is usually reversible. May cause neuromuscular blockade and respiratory paralysis; especially when given soon after anesthesia or muscle relaxants.

Not intended for long-term therapy due to toxic hazards associated with extended administration; use caution in pre-existing renal insufficiency, vestibular or cochlear impairment, myasthenia gravis, hypocalcemia, conditions which depress neuromuscular transmission. Dosage modification required in patients with impaired renal function. Prolonged use may result in fungal or bacterial superinfection, including *C. difficile*-associated diarrhea (CDAD) and pseudomembranous colitis; CDAD has been observed >2 months postantibiotic treatment.

Drug Interactions

Avoid Concomitant Use

Avoid concomitant use of Gentamicin (Systemic) with any of the following: Agalsidase Alfa; Agalsidase Beta; BCG; Gallium Nitrate

Decreased Effect

Gentamicin (Systemic) may decrease the levels/effects of: Agalsidase Alfa; Agalsidase Beta; BCG; Typhoid Vaccine

The levels/effects of Gentamicin (Systemic) may be decreased by: Penicillins

Increased Effect/Toxicity

Gentamicin (Systemic) may increase the levels/effects of: AbobotulinumtoxinA; Bisphosphonate Derivatives; CARBOplatin; Colistimethate; CycloSPORINE; CycloSPORINE (Systemic); Gallium Nitrate; Neuromuscular-Blocking Agents; OnabotulinumtoxinA; RimabotulinumtoxinB

The levels/effects of Gentamicin (Systemic) may be increased by: Amphotericin B; Capreomycin; Cephalosporins (2nd Generation); Cephalosporins (3rd Generation); Cephalosporins (4th Generation); CISplatin; Loop Diuretics; Nonsteroidal Anti-Inflammatory Agents; Vancomycin

Adverse Reactions

>10%:

Central nervous system: Neurotoxicity (vertigo, ataxia)

Neuromuscular & skeletal: Gait instability

Otic: Ototoxicity (auditory), ototoxicity (vestibular)

Renal: Nephrotoxicity, decreased creatinine clearance

1% to 10%: Cardiovascular: Edema

Available Dosage Forms

Infusion, premixed in NS: 60 mg (50 mL); 80 mg (50 mL, 100 mL); 100 mg (50 mL, 100 mL); 120 mg (50 mL, 100 mL)

Injection, solution: 40 mg/mL (2 mL, 20 mL, 50 mL)

Injection, solution [preservative free]: 10 mg/mL (2 mL)

General Dosage Range Dosage adjustment recommended for the I.M. and I.V. routes in patients with renal impairment

I.M., I.V.:

Children <5 years: 2.5 mg/kg/dose every 8 hours

Children ≥5 years: 2-2.5 mg/kg/dose every 8 hours

Adults: 1-2.5 mg/kg/dose every 8-12 hours **or** 4-7 mg/kg once daily

Intrathecal: *Adults:* 4-8 mg/day

Administration

I.M. Administer by deep I.M. route if possible. Slower absorption and lower peak concentrations, probably due to poor circulation in the atrophic muscle, may occur following I.M. injection; in paralyzed patients, suggest I.V. route.

I.V. Some penicillins (eg, carbenicillin, ticarcillin, and piperacillin) have been shown to inactivate aminoglycosides *in vitro*. This has been observed to a greater extent with tobramycin and gentamicin, while amikacin has shown greater stability against inactivation. Concurrent use of these agents may pose a risk of reduced antibacterial efficacy *in vivo*, particularly in the setting of profound renal impairment. However, definitive clinical evidence is lacking. If combination penicillin/aminoglycoside therapy is desired in a patient with renal dysfunction, separation of doses (if feasible), and routine monitoring of aminoglycoside levels, CBC, and clinical response should be considered.

I.V. Detail pH: 3.0-5.5 (I.V./I.M. injection); pH: 4 (premixed infusion in sodium chloride)

Stability

Storage Gentamicin is a colorless to slightly yellow solution which should be stored between 2°C to 30°C, but refrigeration is not recommended. I.V. infusion solutions mixed in NS or D_5W solution are stable for 24 hours at room temperature and refrigeration. Premixed bag: Manufacturer expiration date; remove from overwrap stability: 30 days.

Nursing Actions

Physical Assessment Assess patient's hearing level before, during, and following therapy; report changes to prescriber immediately. Monitor for neurotoxicity (vertigo, ataxia), ototoxicity, decreased renal function, and opportunistic infection (eg, fever, mouth, and vaginal sores or plaques).

Patient Education Drink adequate amounts of water unless instructed to restrict fluid intake. You may experience ringing in ears, dizziness, blurred vision, GI upset, loss of appetite, or photosensitivity. Report severe headache, changes in hearing acuity, ringing in ears, change in balance, changes in urine pattern, persistent diarrhea, respiratory difficulty, rash, fever, unhealed sores, sores in mouth, vaginal drainage, muscle or bone pain, change in gait, or worsening of condition.

Dietary Considerations Calcium, magnesium, potassium: Renal wasting may cause hypocalcemia, hypomagnesemia, and/or hypokalemia.

Related Information

Peak and Trough Guidelines *on page 1276*

Gentamicin (Ophthalmic) (jen ta MYE sin)

Brand Names: U.S. Garamycin®; Gentak®

Index Terms Gentamicin Sulfate

Pharmacologic Category Antibiotic, Aminoglycoside; Antibiotic, Ophthalmic

Medication Safety Issues

Sound-alike/look-alike issues:

Gentamicin may be confused with gentian violet, kanamycin, vancomycin

Pregnancy Risk Factor C

Use Treatment of ophthalmic infections caused by susceptible bacteria

Available Dosage Forms

Ointment, ophthalmic:

Gentak®: 0.3% (3.5 g)

Ointment, ophthalmic [preservative free]:

Garamycin®: 0.3% (3.5 g)

Solution, ophthalmic: 0.3% (5 mL, 15 mL)

Garamycin®: 0.3% (5 mL)

Gentak®: 0.3% (5 mL)

General Dosage Range Ophthalmic: *Children and Adults:* Ointment: Instill 1/2" (1.25 cm) 2-3 times/day to every 3-4 hours; Solution: Instill 1-2 drops every 4 hours, up to 2 drops every hour for severe infections

Administration

Other Avoid contaminating tip of the solution container or ointment tube.

Nursing Actions

Patient Education Wash hands before instilling. Sit or lie down to instill. Open eye, look at ceiling, and instill prescribed amount of solution; for ointment, pull lower lid down gently, instill thin ribbon of ointment inside lid. Close eye, roll eye in all directions, and apply gentle pressure to inner corner of eye. Do not let tip of applicator touch eye; do not contaminate tip of applicator (may cause eye infection, eye damage, or vision loss). Temporary stinging or blurred vision may occur. Report persistent pain, burning, vision changes, swelling, itching, or worsening of condition.

Glatiramer Acetate (gla TIR a mer AS e tate)

Brand Names: U.S. Copaxone®

Index Terms Copolymer-1

Pharmacologic Category Biological, Miscellaneous

Medication Safety Issues

Sound-alike/look-alike issues:

Copaxone® may be confused with Compazine

Pregnancy Risk Factor B

Lactation Excretion in breast milk unknown/use caution

Use Management of relapsing-remitting type multiple sclerosis, including patients with a first clinical episode with MRI features consistent with multiple sclerosis

Mechanism of Action/Effect Glatiramer is a mixture of random polymers of four amino acids; L-alanine, L-glutamic acid, L-lysine, and L-tyrosine, the resulting mixture is antigenically similar to myelin basic protein, which is an important component of the myelin sheath of nerves; glatiramer is thought to induce and activate T-lymphocyte suppressor cells specific for a myelin antigen, it is also proposed that glatiramer interferes with the antigen-presenting function of certain immune cells opposing pathogenic T-cell function

Contraindications Hypersensitivity to glatiramer acetate, mannitol, or any component of the formulation

Warnings/Precautions For SubQ use only, **not for I.V. administration**. Glatiramer acetate is antigenic, and may interfere with recognition of foreign antigens affecting tumor surveillance and infection defense systems. Immediate postinjection systemic reactions occur in a substantial percentage of patients (~16% in studies); symptoms may begin within minutes of injection and are usually self-limiting. Most patients only have one reaction despite repeated administration. Chest pain (transient pain resolving in minutes) may occur as part of the postinjection systemic reaction, but can also occur alone. Lipoatrophy may occur at injection site; proper injection site rotation may prevent. Safety and efficacy has not been established in patients with renal impairment, in the elderly, or in patients <18 years of age.

Drug Interactions

Avoid Concomitant Use

Avoid concomitant use of Glatiramer Acetate with any of the following: BCG; Natalizumab; Pimecrolimus; Tacrolimus (Topical); Vaccines (Live)

Decreased Effect

Glatiramer Acetate may decrease the levels/effects of: BCG; Coccidioidin Skin Test; Sipuleucel-T; Vaccines (Inactivated); Vaccines (Live)

The levels/effects of Glatiramer Acetate may be decreased by: Echinacea

Increased Effect/Toxicity

Glatiramer Acetate may increase the levels/effects of: Leflunomide; Natalizumab; Vaccines (Live)

The levels/effects of Glatiramer Acetate may be increased by: Denosumab; Pimecrolimus; Roflumilast; Tacrolimus (Topical); Trastuzumab

Adverse Reactions

>10%:

Cardiovascular: Vasodilation (20%), chest pain (13%)

Central nervous system: Pain (20%), anxiety (13%)

Dermatologic: Rash (19%)

Gastrointestinal: Nausea (15%)
Local: Injection site reactions: Inflammation (49%), erythema (43%), pain (40%), pruritus (27%), mass (27%)
Neuromuscular & skeletal: Weakness (22%), back pain (12%)
Respiratory: Dyspnea (14%)
Miscellaneous: Infection (30%), flu-like syndrome (14%), diaphoresis (15%)

1% to 10%:
Cardiovascular: Edema (8%; includes peripheral and facial), palpitation (7%), tachycardia (5%), syncope (3%), hypertension (1%)
Central nervous system: Fever (6%), migraine (4%), chills (3%), nervousness (2%), speech disorder (2%), abnormal dreams (1%), emotional lability (1%), stupor (1%)
Dermatologic: Bruising (8%), pruritus (5%), erythema (4%), urticaria (3%), skin nodule (2%), eczema (1%), pustular rash (1%)
Endocrine & metabolic: Amenorrhea (1%), impotence (1%), menorrhagia (1%)
Gastrointestinal: Vomiting (7%), gastroenteritis (6%), weight gain (3%), dysphagia (2%), dental caries (1%)
Genitourinary: Urinary urgency (5%), vaginal moniliasis (4%)
Local: Injection site reactions: Hemorrhage (5%), hypersensitivity (4%), fibrosis (2%), lipoatrophy (2%), abscess (1%), edema (1%)
Neuromuscular & skeletal: Neck pain (8%), tremor (4%)
Ocular: Diplopia (3%), visual field defect (1%)
Respiratory: Rhinitis (7%), bronchitis (6%), cough (6%), laryngismus (5%), hyperventilation (1%)
Miscellaneous: Lymphadenopathy (7%), hypersensitivity (3%)

Available Dosage Forms

Injection, solution [preservative free]:
Copaxone®: 20 mg/mL (1 mL)

General Dosage Range SubQ: *Adults:* 20 mg daily

Administration

Other For SubQ administration in the arms, abdomen, hips, or thighs; rotate injection sites to prevent lipoatrophy. Bring to room temperature prior to use. Visually inspect the solution; discard if solution is cloudy or contains any particulate matter.

Stability

Storage Store in refrigerator at 2°C to 8°C (36°F to 46°F); excursions to room temperature for up to 1 month do not have a negative impact on potency. Avoid heat; protect from intense light.

Nursing Actions

Physical Assessment Monitor for postinjection reactions (eg, self-resolving flushing, chest tightness, dyspnea, and palpitations). Teach patient proper use (reconstitution, injection technique, and syringe/needle disposal).

Patient Education This drug will not cure MS, but may help relieve the severity and frequency of attacks. This drug can only be given by subcutaneous injection. Your prescriber will instruct you in proper injection technique and syringe/needle disposal. May cause a transient reaction after injection, including flushing, chest tightness, dyspnea, or palpitations. May cause weakness, dizziness, confusion, nervousness, anxiety, nausea, or vomiting. Report chest pain or pounding heartbeat; persistent diarrhea or GI upset; infection (vaginal itching or drainage, sores in mouth, unusual fever or chills) or flu-like symptoms (swollen glands, chills, excessive sweating); bruising, rash, or skin irritation; joint pain or neck pain; swelling of puffiness of face; vision changes or ear pain; unusual cough or respiratory difficulty; alterations in menstrual pattern; or redness, pain, or swelling at injection site.

Glimepiride (GLYE me pye ride)

Brand Names: U.S. Amaryl®

Pharmacologic Category Antidiabetic Agent, Sulfonylurea

Medication Safety Issues

Sound-alike/look-alike issues:
Glimepiride may be confused with glipiZIDE
Amaryl® may be confused with Altace®, Amerge®

High alert medication:
The Institute for Safe Medication Practices (ISMP) includes this medication among its list of drugs which have a heightened risk of causing significant patient harm when used in error.

International issues:
Amarel [France], Amaryl [U.S., Canada, and multiple international markets] may be confused with Reminyl brand name for galantamine [multiple international markets]
Amaryl [U.S., Canada, and multiple international markets] may be confused with Almarl brand name for arotinolol [Japan]

Pregnancy Risk Factor C

Lactation Excretion in breast milk unknown/not recommended

Breast-Feeding Considerations It is not known if glimepiride is excreted in breast milk. Breast-feeding is not recommended by the manufacturer. Potentially, hypoglycemia may occur in a nursing infant exposed to a sulfonylurea via breast milk.

Use Management of type 2 diabetes mellitus (noninsulin dependent, NIDDM) as an adjunct to diet and exercise to lower blood glucose; may be used in combination with metformin or insulin in patients whose hyperglycemia cannot be controlled by diet and exercise in conjunction with a single oral hypoglycemic agent

Mechanism of Action/Effect Stimulates insulin release from the pancreatic beta cells; reduces glucose output from the liver; insulin sensitivity is increased at peripheral target sites

Contraindications Hypersensitivity to glimepiride, any component of the formulation, or sulfonamides; diabetic ketoacidosis (with or without coma)

Warnings/Precautions All sulfonylurea drugs are capable of producing severe hypoglycemia. Hypoglycemia is more likely to occur when caloric intake is deficient, after severe or prolonged exercise, when ethanol is ingested, or when more than one glucose-lowering drug is used. It is also more likely in elderly patients, malnourished patients and in patients with impaired renal or hepatic function; use with caution. Autonomic neuropathy, advanced age, and concomitant use of beta-blockers or other sympatholytic agents may impair the patient's ability to recognize the signs and symptoms of hypoglycemia; use with caution.

Loss of efficacy may be observed following prolonged use as a result of the progression of type 2 diabetes mellitus which results in continued beta cell destruction. In patients who were previously responding to sulfonylurea therapy, consider additional factors which may be contributing to decreased efficacy (eg, inappropriate dose, nonadherence to diet and exercise regimen). If no contributing factors can be identified, consider discontinuing use of the sulfonylurea due to secondary failure of treatment. Additional antidiabetic therapy (eg, insulin) will be required. It may be necessary to discontinue therapy and administer insulin if the patient is exposed to stress (fever, trauma, infection, surgery).

Chemical similarities are present among sulfonamides, sulfonylureas, carbonic anhydrase inhibitors, thiazides, and loop diuretics (except ethacrynic acid). Use in patients with sulfonamide allergy is not specifically contraindicated in product labeling, however, a risk of cross-reaction exists in patients with allergy to any of these compounds; avoid use when previous reaction has been severe. Patients with G6PD deficiency may be at an increased risk of sulfonylurea-induced hemolytic anemia; however, cases have also been described in patients without G6PD deficiency during postmarketing surveillance. Use with caution and consider a nonsulfonylurea alternative in patients with G6PD deficiency.

Product labeling states oral hypoglycemic drugs may be associated with an increased cardiovascular mortality as compared to treatment with diet alone or diet plus insulin. Data to support this association are limited, and several studies, including a large prospective trial (UKPDS) have not supported an association.

Drug Interactions

Avoid Concomitant Use There are no known interactions where it is recommended to avoid concomitant use.

Decreased Effect

The levels/effects of Glimepiride may be decreased by: Corticosteroids (Orally Inhaled); Corticosteroids (Systemic); CYP2C9 Inducers (Strong); Luteinizing Hormone-Releasing Hormone Analogs; Peginterferon Alfa-2b; Quinolone Antibiotics; Rifampin; Somatropin; Thiazide Diuretics

Increased Effect/Toxicity

Glimepiride may increase the levels/effects of: Alcohol (Ethyl); Hypoglycemic Agents; Porfimer

The levels/effects of Glimepiride may be increased by: Beta-Blockers; Chloramphenicol; Cimetidine; Cyclic Antidepressants; CYP2C9 Inhibitors (Moderate); CYP2C9 Inhibitors (Strong); Fibric Acid Derivatives; Fluconazole; GLP-1 Agonists; Herbs (Hypoglycemic Properties); Pegvisomant; Quinolone Antibiotics; Ranitidine; Salicylates; Sulfonamide Derivatives; Voriconazole

Nutritional/Ethanol Interactions

Ethanol: Caution with ethanol (may cause hypoglycemia).

Herb/Nutraceutical: Caution with chromium, garlic, gymnema (may cause hypoglycemia).

Adverse Reactions 1% to 10%:

Central nervous system: Dizziness (2%), headache (2%)

Endocrine & metabolic: Hypoglycemia (1% to 2%)

Gastrointestinal: Nausea (1%)

Neuromuscular & skeletal: Weakness (2%)

Pharmacodynamics/Kinetics

Onset of Action Peak effect: Blood glucose reductions: 2-3 hours

Duration of Action 24 hours

Available Dosage Forms

Tablet, oral: 1 mg, 2 mg, 4 mg

Amaryl®: 1 mg, 2 mg, 4 mg

General Dosage Range Dosage adjustment recommended in patients with renal impairment

Oral:

Adults: Initial: 1-2 mg once daily; Maintenance: 1-4 mg once daily (maximum: 8 mg/day)

Elderly: Initial: 1 mg/day

Administration

Oral Administer once daily with breakfast or first main meal of the day. Patients that are NPO or require decreased caloric intake may need doses held to avoid hypoglycemia.

Nursing Actions

Physical Assessment Allergy history should be assessed prior to beginning therapy.

Patient Education This medication is used to control diabetes; it is not a cure. Monitor glucose as recommended by prescriber. Other important components of treatment plan may include prescribed diet and exercise regimen (consult prescriber or diabetic educator). Always carry quick source of sugar with you. Take with breakfast or the first main meal of the day. Avoid alcohol while taking this medication; could cause severe reaction. If you experience hypoglycemic reaction, contact prescriber immediately. You may experience side effects during first weeks of therapy (eg, headache, nausea); consult prescriber if these persist. Report severe or persistent side effects (eg, hypoglycemia: palpitations, sweaty palms, lightheadedness; extended vomiting or flu-like symptoms; skin rash; easy bruising or bleeding; or change in color of urine or stool).

Dietary Considerations Administer with breakfast or the first main meal of the day. Individualized medical nutrition therapy (MNT) based on ADA recommendations is an integral part of therapy.

GlipiZIDE (GLIP i zide)

Brand Names: U.S. Glucotrol XL®; Glucotrol®

Index Terms Glydiazinamide

Pharmacologic Category Antidiabetic Agent, Sulfonylurea

Medication Safety Issues

Sound-alike/look-alike issues:

GlipiZIDE may be confused with glimepiride, glyBURIDE

Glucotrol® may be confused with Glucophage®, Glucotrol® XL, glyBURIDE

High alert medication:

The Institute for Safe Medication Practices (ISMP) includes this medication among its list of drugs which have a heightened risk of causing significant patient harm when used in error.

Pregnancy Risk Factor C

Lactation Excretion in breast milk unknown/not recommended

Breast-Feeding Considerations Data from initial studies note that glipizide was not detected in breast milk. Breast-feeding is not recommended by the manufacturer. Potentially, hypoglycemia may occur in a nursing infant exposed to a sulfonylurea via breast milk.

Use Management of type 2 diabetes mellitus (noninsulin dependent, NIDDM)

Mechanism of Action/Effect Stimulates insulin release from the pancreatic beta cells; reduces glucose output from the liver; insulin sensitivity is increased at peripheral target sites

Contraindications Hypersensitivity to glipizide or any component of the formulation, other sulfonamides; type 1 diabetes mellitus (insulin dependent, IDDM); diabetic ketoacidosis

Warnings/Precautions All sulfonylurea drugs are capable of producing severe hypoglycemia. Hypoglycemia is more likely to occur when caloric intake is deficient, after severe or prolonged exercise, when ethanol is ingested, or when more than one glucose-lowering drug is used. It is also more likely in elderly patients, malnourished patients and in patients with impaired renal or hepatic function; use with caution.

Use with caution in patients with severe hepatic disease. It may be necessary to discontinue therapy and administer insulin if the patient is exposed to stress (fever, trauma, infection, surgery). Loss of efficacy may be observed following prolonged use as a result of the progression of type 2 diabetes mellitus which results in continued beta cell destruction. In patients who were previously responding to sulfonylurea therapy, consider additional factors which may be contributing to decreased efficacy (eg, inappropriate dose, nonadherence to diet and exercise regimen). If no contributing factors can be identified, consider discontinuing use of the sulfonylurea due to secondary failure of treatment. Additional antidiabetic therapy (eg, insulin) will be required. Chemical similarities are present among sulfonamides, sulfonylureas, carbonic anhydrase inhibitors, thiazides, and loop diuretics (except ethacrynic acid). Use in patients with sulfonamide allergy is specifically contraindicated in product labeling, however, a risk of cross-reaction exists in patients with allergy to any of these compounds; avoid use when previous reaction has been severe. Patients with G6PD deficiency may be at an increased risk of sulfonylurea-induced hemolytic anemia; however, cases have also been described in patients without G6PD deficiency during postmarketing surveillance. Use with caution and consider a nonsulfonylurea alternative in patients with G6PD deficiency.

Product labeling states oral hypoglycemic drugs may be associated with an increased cardiovascular mortality as compared to treatment with diet alone or diet plus insulin. Data to support this association are limited, and several studies, including a large prospective trial (UKPDS) have not supported an association. Avoid use of extended release tablets (Glucotrol XL®) in patients with known stricture/narrowing of the GI tract.

Drug Interactions

Avoid Concomitant Use There are no known interactions where it is recommended to avoid concomitant use.

Decreased Effect

The levels/effects of GlipiZIDE may be decreased by: Corticosteroids (Orally Inhaled); Corticosteroids (Systemic); CYP2C9 Inducers (Strong); Luteinizing Hormone-Releasing Hormone Analogs; Peginterferon Alfa-2b; Quinolone Antibiotics; Rifampin; Somatropin; Thiazide Diuretics

Increased Effect/Toxicity

GlipiZIDE may increase the levels/effects of: Alcohol (Ethyl); Hypoglycemic Agents; Porfimer

The levels/effects of GlipiZIDE may be increased by: Beta-Blockers; Chloramphenicol; Cimetidine; Clarithromycin; Cyclic Antidepressants; CYP2C9 Inhibitors (Moderate); CYP2C9 Inhibitors (Strong); Fibric Acid Derivatives; Fluconazole; GLP-1 Agonists; Herbs (Hypoglycemic Properties); Pegvisomant; Posaconazole; Quinolone

Antibiotics; Ranitidine; Salicylates; Sulfonamide Derivatives; Voriconazole

Nutritional/Ethanol Interactions

Ethanol: Caution with ethanol (may cause hypoglycemia or rare disulfiram reaction).

Food: A delayed release of insulin may occur if glipizide is taken with food. Immediate release tablets should be administered 30 minutes before meals to avoid erratic absorption.

Herb/Nutraceutical: Herbs with hypoglycemic properties may enhance the hypoglycemic effect of glipizide. This includes alfalfa, aloe, bilberry, bitter melon, burdock, celery, damiana, fenugreek, garcinia, garlic, ginger, ginseng (American), gymnema, marshmallow, stinging nettle

Adverse Reactions Frequency not defined.

Cardiovascular: Edema, syncope

Central nervous system: Anxiety, depression, dizziness, drowsiness, headache, hypoesthesia, insomnia, nervousness, pain

Dermatologic: Eczema, erythema, maculopapular eruptions, morbilliform eruptions, photosensitivity, pruritus, rash, urticaria

Endocrine & metabolic: Disulfiram-like reaction, hypoglycemia, hyponatremia, SIADH (rare)

Gastrointestinal: Anorexia, constipation, diarrhea, epigastric fullness, flatulence, gastralgia, heartburn, nausea, vomiting

Hematologic: Agranulocytopenia, aplastic anemia, blood dyscrasias, hemolytic anemia, leukopenia, pancytopenia, porphyria cutanea tarda, thrombocytopenia

Hepatic: Hepatic porphyria

Neuromuscular & skeletal: Arthralgia, leg cramps, myalgia, paresthesia, tremor

Ocular: Blurred vision

Renal: Diuretic effect (minor)

Respiratory: Rhinitis

Miscellaneous: Diaphoresis

Pharmacodynamics/Kinetics

Duration of Action 12-24 hours

Available Dosage Forms

Tablet, oral: 5 mg, 10 mg

Glucotrol®: 5 mg, 10 mg

Tablet, extended release, oral: 2.5 mg, 5 mg, 10 mg

Glucotrol XL®: 2.5 mg, 5 mg, 10 mg

General Dosage Range Dosage adjustment recommended in patients with hepatic impairment

Oral:

Immediate release:

Adults: Initial: 5 mg/day; Maintenance: Up to 40 mg/day

Elderly: Initial: 2.5 mg/day

Extended release: *Adults:* Initial: 5 mg/day; Maintenance: Up to 20 mg/day

Administration

Oral Administer immediate release tablets 30 minutes before a meal to achieve greatest reduction in postprandial hyperglycemia. Extended release tablets should be given with breakfast. Patients that are NPO or require decreased caloric intake may need doses held to avoid hypoglycemia.

Nursing Actions

Physical Assessment Monitor for hypoglycemia during therapy.

Patient Education This medication is used to control diabetes; it is not a cure. Monitor glucose as recommended by prescriber. Other important components of treatment plan may include prescribed diet and exercise regimen (consult prescriber or diabetic educator). Always carry quick source of sugar with you. Immediate release tablets should be taken 30 minutes before meals, at the same time each day. Extended release tablets should be taken with breakfast. Do not chew or crush extended release tablets. Avoid alcohol while taking this medication; could cause severe reaction. If you experience hypoglycemic reaction, contact prescriber immediately. You may experience more sensitivity to sunlight, headache, or nausea. Report severe or persistent side effects (eg, hypoglycemia: palpitations, sweaty palms, lightheadedness; extended vomiting; diarrhea or constipation; flu-like symptoms; skin rash; easy bruising or bleeding; or change in color of urine or stool).

Dietary Considerations Take immediate release tablets 30 minutes before meals; extended release tablets should be taken with breakfast. Individualized medical nutrition therapy (MNT) based on ADA recommendations is an integral part of therapy.

Glipizide and Metformin

(GLIP i zide & met FOR min)

Brand Names: U.S. Metaglip™

Index Terms Glipizide and Metformin Hydrochloride; Metformin and Glipizide

Pharmacologic Category Antidiabetic Agent, Biguanide; Antidiabetic Agent, Sulfonylurea

Medication Safety Issues

High alert medication:

The Institute for Safe Medication Practices (ISMP) includes this medication among its list of drugs which have a heightened risk of causing significant patient harm when used in error.

Pregnancy Risk Factor C

Lactation

Glipizide: Excretion in breast milk unknown/not recommended

Metformin: Enters breast milk/not recommended

Use Indicated as an adjunct to diet and exercise to improve glycemic control in adults with type 2 diabetes mellitus (noninsulin dependent, NIDDM)

Available Dosage Forms

Tablet, oral: 2.5/250: Glipizide 2.5 mg and metformin 250 mg; 2.5/500: Glipizide 2.5 mg and metformin 500 mg; 5/500: Glipizide 5 mg and metformin 500 mg

Metaglip™: 2.5/500: Glipizide 2.5 mg and metformin 500 mg; 5/500: Glipizide 5 mg and metformin 500 mg

General Dosage Range Oral: *Adults:* Initial: Glipizide 2.5 mg and metformin 250 mg once daily; Maintenance: Up to glipizide 20 mg/day and metformin 2000 mg/day in divided doses

Administration

Oral All doses should be administered with a meal. Twice-daily dosing should be administered with the morning and evening meals. Patients that are NPO or require decreased caloric intake may need doses held to avoid hypoglycemia.

Nursing Actions

Physical Assessment See individual agents.

Patient Education See individual agents.

Related Information

GlipiZIDE *on page 544*
MetFORMIN *on page 746*

Glucagon (GLOO ka gon)

Brand Names: U.S. GlucaGen®; GlucaGen® Diagnostic Kit; GlucaGen® HypoKit®; Glucagon Emergency Kit

Index Terms Glucagon Hydrochloride

Pharmacologic Category Antidote; Antidote, Hypoglycemia; Diagnostic Agent

Pregnancy Risk Factor B

Lactation Excretion in breast milk unknown/use caution

Breast-Feeding Considerations Glucagon is not absorbed from the GI tract and therefore, it is unlikely adverse effects would occur in a breast-feeding infant.

Use Management of hypoglycemia; diagnostic aid in radiologic examinations to temporarily inhibit GI tract movement

Unlabeled Use Beta-blocker- or calcium channel blocker-induced myocardial depression (with or without hypotension) unresponsive to standard measures; suspected or documented hypoglycemia secondary to insulin or sulfonylurea overdose (as adjunct to dextrose)

Mechanism of Action/Effect Stimulates adenylate cyclase to produce increased cyclic AMP, which promotes hepatic glycogenolysis and gluconeogenesis, causing a raise in blood glucose levels

Contraindications Hypersensitivity to glucagon or any component of the formulation; insulinoma; pheochromocytoma

Warnings/Precautions Use of glucagon is contraindicated in insulinoma; exogenous glucagon may cause an initial rise in blood glucose followed by rebound hypoglycemia. Use of glucagon is contraindicated in pheochromocytoma; exogenous glucagon may cause the release of catecholamines, resulting in an increase in blood pressure. Use caution with prolonged fasting, starvation, adrenal insufficiency or chronic hypoglycemia; levels of glucose stores in liver may be decreased. Supplemental carbohydrates should be given to patients who respond to glucagon for severe hypoglycemia to prevent secondary hypoglycemia. Monitor blood glucose levels closely.

In patients with hypoglycemia secondary to insulin or sulfonylurea overdose, dextrose should be immediately administered; if I.V. access cannot be established or if dextrose is not available, glucagon may be considered as alternative acute treatment until dextrose can be administered.

May contain lactose; avoid administration in hereditary galactose intolerance, Lapp lactase deficiency, or glucose-galactose malabsorption.

Drug Interactions

Avoid Concomitant Use There are no known interactions where it is recommended to avoid concomitant use.

Decreased Effect There are no known significant interactions involving a decrease in effect.

Increased Effect/Toxicity

Glucagon may increase the levels/effects of: Vitamin K Antagonists

Nutritional/Ethanol Interactions Glucagon depletes glycogen stores.

Adverse Reactions Frequency not defined.

Cardiovascular: Hypotension (up to 2 hours after GI procedures), hypertension, tachycardia

Gastrointestinal: Nausea, vomiting (high incidence with rapid administration of high doses)

Miscellaneous: Hypersensitivity reactions, anaphylaxis

Pharmacodynamics/Kinetics

Onset of Action Peak effect: Blood glucose levels: Parenteral: I.V.: 5-20 minutes; I.M.: 30 minutes; SubQ: 30-45 minutes

Duration of Action Glucose elevation: SubQ: 60-90 minutes; I.V.: 30 minutes

Available Dosage Forms

Injection, powder for reconstitution:

GlucaGen®: 1 mg
GlucaGen® Diagnostic Kit: 1 mg
GlucaGen® HypoKit®: 1 mg
Glucagon Emergency Kit: 1 mg

General Dosage Range

I.M.:

Children <20 kg: 0.5 mg **or** 20-30 mcg/kg/dose, may repeat

Children ≥20 kg: 1 mg, may repeat

Adults: 1 mg, may repeat **or** 1-2 mg prior to gastrointestinal procedure

I.V.:

Children <20 kg: 0.5 mg or 20-30 mcg/kg/dose, may repeat

Children ≥20 kg: 1 mg, may repeat

Adults: 1 mg, may repeat in 20 minutes **or** 0.25-2 mg 10 minutes prior to gastrointestinal procedure

SubQ:

Children <20 kg: 0.5 mg **or** 20-30 mcg/kg/dose, may repeat

Children ≥20 kg and Adults: 1 mg, may repeat

Administration

I.V. Bolus may be associated with nausea and vomiting.

Beta-blocker/calcium channel blocker toxicity: Administer bolus over 3-5 minutes; continuous infusions may be used. Ensure adequate supply available to continue therapy.

Stability

Reconstitution Reconstitute powder for injection by adding 1 mL of sterile diluent to a vial containing 1 unit of the drug, to provide solutions containing 1 mg of glucagon/mL. Gently roll vial to dissolve. Solution for infusion may be prepared by reconstitution with and further dilution in NS or D_5W (Love, 1998).

Storage Prior to reconstitution, store at controlled room temperature of 20°C to 25° (69°F to 77°F); do not freeze. Use reconstituted solution immediately. May be kept at 5°C for up to 48 hours if necessary.

Nursing Actions

Physical Assessment Arouse patient from hypoglycemic or insulin shock as soon as possible and administer carbohydrates. Instruct patient (or significant other) in appropriate administration procedures for emergency use of glucagon.

Patient Education Identify appropriate support person to administer glucagon if necessary.

Dietary Considerations Administer carbohydrates to patient as soon as possible after response to treatment.

Glucarpidase (gloo KAR pid ase)

Index Terms Carboxypeptidase-G2; CPDG2; CPG2; Voraxaze

Pharmacologic Category Antidote; Enzyme

Pregnancy Risk Factor C

Lactation Excretion in breast milk unknown/use caution

Use Treatment of toxic plasma methotrexate concentrations (>1 micromole/L) in patients with delayed clearance due to renal impairment

Note: Due to the risk of subtherapeutic methotrexate exposure, glucarpidase is **NOT** indicated when methotrexate clearance is within expected range (plasma methotrexate concentration ≤2 standard deviations of mean methotrexate excretion curve specific for dose administered) **or** with normal renal function or mild renal impairment.

Unlabeled Use Rescue agent to reduce methotrexate toxicity in patients with accidental intrathecal methotrexate overdose

Product Availability

Voraxaze®: FDA approved January 2012; availability is currently undetermined; consult prescribing information for additional information

Prior to FDA approval, glucarpidase was available for I.V. use under an Open-Label Treatment protocol. Information and participation requirements are available from the Voraxaze® 24-hour access call center (Clinical Trials and Consulting Services, Inc) at 1-877-398-9829. Further information may be found at http://www.btgplc.com/products/voraxazeae-us-treatment-ind.

Glucarpidase is available for intrathecal (I.T.) use through an Emergency Use IND. Information is available from BTG International at 1-888-327-1027. For FDA Emergency Use IND information and procedures, refer to http://www.fda.gov/RegulatoryInformation/Guidances/ucm126491.htm. For further information on intrathecal use, please also refer to http://www.btgplc.com/products/voraxazeae-us-treatment-ind.

Available Dosage Forms

Injection, powder for reconstitution:

Voraxaze®: 1000 units

General Dosage Range I.V.: *Children and Adults:* 50 units/kg

Administration

I.V. Infuse over 5 minutes. Flush I.V. line before and after glucarpidase administration.

Other Intrathecal (for intrathecal methotrexate overdose; unlabeled use): Glucarpidase was administered within 3-9 hours of accidental intrathecal methotrexate overdose in conjunction with lumbar drainage or ventriculolumbar perfusion (Widemann, 2004). Administered over 5 minutes via lumbar route, ventriculostomy, Ommaya reservoir, or lumbar and ventriculostomy (O'Marcaigh, 1996; Widemann, 2004). In one case report, 1000 units was administered through the ventricular catheter over 5 minutes and another 1000 units was administered through the lumbar catheter (O'Marcaigh, 1996).

Nursing Actions

Physical Assessment Assess patient tolerance during infusion.

Patient Education Patients tolerate this medication very well. Side effects include flushing, low blood pressure, headache, nausea, vomiting, and paresthesias. Call prescriber for any immediate signs of a bad reaction (wheezing, chest tightness, fever, itching, cough, difficulty breathing; swelling of face, lips, tongue, or throat).

GlyBURIDE (GLYE byoor ide)

Brand Names: U.S. DiaBeta®; Glynase® PresTab®

Index Terms Diabeta; Glibenclamide; Glybenclamide; Glybenzcyclamide; Micronase

Pharmacologic Category Antidiabetic Agent, Sulfonylurea

Medication Safety Issues

Sound-alike/look-alike issues:

GlyBURIDE may be confused with glipiZIDE, Glucotrol®

Diaβeta® may be confused with Zebeta®

Micronase may be confused with microK®, miconazole, Micronor®, Microzide®

High alert medication:

The Institute for Safe Medication Practices (ISMP) includes this medication among its list of drugs which have a heightened risk of causing significant patient harm when used in error.

Pregnancy Risk Factor B/C (manufacturer dependent)

Lactation Does not enter breast milk/use caution

Breast-Feeding Considerations Data from initial studies note that glyburide was not detected in breast milk. Breast-feeding is not recommended by the manufacturer. Potentially, hypoglycemia may occur in a nursing infant exposed to a sulfonylurea via breast milk.

Use Adjunct to diet and exercise for the management of type 2 diabetes mellitus (noninsulin dependent, NIDDM)

Unlabeled Use Alternative to insulin in women for the treatment of gestational diabetes mellitus (GDM) (11-33 weeks gestation)

Mechanism of Action/Effect Stimulates insulin release from the pancreatic beta cells; reduces glucose output from the liver; insulin sensitivity is increased at peripheral target sites

Contraindications Hypersensitivity to glyburide or any component of the formulation; type 1 diabetes mellitus (insulin dependent, IDDM), diabetic ketoacidosis; concomitant use with bosentan

Warnings/Precautions All sulfonylurea drugs are capable of producing severe hypoglycemia. Hypoglycemia is more likely to occur when caloric intake is deficient, after severe or prolonged exercise, when ethanol is ingested, or when more than one glucose-lowering drug is used. It is also more likely in elderly patients, malnourished patients and in patients with impaired renal or hepatic function; use with caution.

It may be necessary to discontinue therapy and administer insulin if the patient is exposed to stress (fever, trauma, infection, surgery). Loss of efficacy may be observed following prolonged use as a result of the progression of type 2 diabetes mellitus which results in continued beta cell destruction. In patients who were previously responding to sulfonylurea therapy, consider additional factors which may be contributing to decreased efficacy (eg, inappropriate dose, nonadherence to diet and exercise regimen). If no contributing factors can be identified, consider discontinuing use of the sulfonylurea due to secondary failure of treatment. Additional antidiabetic therapy (eg, insulin) will be required.

Elderly: Rapid and prolonged hypoglycemia (>12 hours) despite hypertonic glucose injections have been reported; age and hepatic and renal impairment are independent risk factors for hypoglycemia; dosage titration should be made at weekly intervals.

Chemical similarities are present among sulfonamides, sulfonylureas, carbonic anhydrase inhibitors, thiazides, and loop diuretics (except ethacrynic acid). Use in patients with sulfonamide allergy is not specifically contraindicated in product labeling, however, a risk of cross-reaction exists in patients with allergy to any of these compounds; avoid use when previous reaction has been severe.

Product labeling states oral hypoglycemic drugs may be associated with an increased cardiovascular mortality as compared to treatment with diet alone or diet plus insulin. Data to support this association are limited, and several studies, including a large prospective trial (UKPDS) have not supported an association.

Patients with G6PD deficiency may be at an increased risk of sulfonylurea-induced hemolytic anemia; however, cases have also been described in patients without G6PD deficiency during postmarketing surveillance. Use with caution and consider a nonsulfonylurea alternative in patients with G6PD deficiency.

Micronized glyburide tablets are **not** bioequivalent to *conventional* glyburide tablets; retitration should occur if patients are being transferred to a different glyburide formulation (eg, micronized-to-conventional or vice versa) or from other hypoglycemic agents.

Drug Interactions

Avoid Concomitant Use

Avoid concomitant use of GlyBURIDE with any of the following: Bosentan; Pimozide

Decreased Effect

GlyBURIDE may decrease the levels/effects of: Bosentan

The levels/effects of GlyBURIDE may be decreased by: Bosentan; Colesevelam; Corticosteroids (Orally Inhaled); Corticosteroids (Systemic); CycloSPORINE; CycloSPORINE (Systemic); CYP2C9 Inducers (Strong); Luteinizing Hormone-Releasing Hormone Analogs; Peginterferon Alfa-2b; Quinolone Antibiotics; Rifampin; Somatropin; Thiazide Diuretics

Increased Effect/Toxicity

GlyBURIDE may increase the levels/effects of: Alcohol (Ethyl); ARIPiprazole; Bosentan; CycloSPORINE; CycloSPORINE (Systemic); Hypoglycemic Agents; Pimozide; Porfimer

The levels/effects of GlyBURIDE may be increased by: Beta-Blockers; Chloramphenicol; Cimetidine; Clarithromycin; Cyclic

Antidepressants; CYP2C9 Inhibitors (Moderate); CYP2C9 Inhibitors (Strong); Fibric Acid Derivatives; Fluconazole; GLP-1 Agonists; Herbs (Hypoglycemic Properties); Pegvisomant; Quinolone Antibiotics; Ranitidine; Salicylates; Sulfonamide Derivatives; Voriconazole

Nutritional/Ethanol Interactions

Ethanol: Caution with ethanol (may cause hypoglycemia).

Herb/Nutraceutical: Herbs with hypoglycemic properties may enhance the hypoglycemic effect of glyburide. This includes alfalfa, aloe, bilberry, bitter melon, burdock, celery, damiana, fenugreek, garcinia, garlic, ginger, ginseng (American), gymnema, marshmallow, stinging nettle

Adverse Reactions Frequency not defined.

Cardiovascular: Vasculitis

Central nervous system: Dizziness, headache

Dermatologic: Angioedema, erythema, maculopapular eruptions, morbilliform eruptions, photosensitivity reaction, pruritus, purpura, rash, urticaria

Endocrine & metabolic: Disulfiram-like reaction, hypoglycemia, hyponatremia (SIADH reported with other sulfonylureas)

Gastrointestinal: Anorexia, constipation, diarrhea, epigastric fullness, heartburn, nausea

Genitourinary: Nocturia

Hematologic: Agranulocytosis, aplastic anemia, hemolytic anemia, leukopenia, pancytopenia, porphyria cutanea tarda, thrombocytopenia

Hepatic: Cholestatic jaundice, hepatitis, liver failure, transaminase increased

Neuromuscular & skeletal: Arthralgia, myalgia, paresthesia

Ocular: Blurred vision

Renal: Diuretic effect (minor)

Miscellaneous: Allergic reaction

Pharmacodynamics/Kinetics

Onset of Action Serum insulin levels begin to increase 15-60 minutes after a single dose

Duration of Action ≤24 hours

Available Dosage Forms

Tablet, oral: 1.25 mg, 1.5 mg, 2.5 mg, 3 mg, 5 mg, 6 mg

DiaBeta®: 1.25 mg, 2.5 mg, 5 mg

Glynase® PresTab®: 1.5 mg, 3 mg, 6 mg

General Dosage Range Oral:

Regular tablets: *Adults:* Initial: 1.25-5 mg once daily; Maintenance: 1.25-20 mg/day as single or divided doses (maximum: 20 mg/day)

Micronized tablets: *Adults:* Initial: 0.75-3 mg once daily; Maintenance: 0.75-12 mg/day as single or divided doses (maximum: 12 mg/day)

Administration

Oral Administer with meals at the same time each day (twice-daily dosing may be beneficial if conventional glyburide doses are >10 mg or micronized glyburide doses are >6 mg). Patients that are NPO or require decreased caloric intake may need doses held to avoid hypoglycemia.

Nursing Actions

Physical Assessment Allergy history should be evaluated prior to beginning therapy. Monitor for hypoglycemia during therapy.

Patient Education This medication is used to control diabetes; it is not a cure. Monitor glucose as recommended by prescriber. Other important components of treatment plan may include prescribed diet and exercise regimen (consult prescriber or diabetic educator). If you experience hypoglycemic reaction, contact prescriber immediately. Always carry quick source of sugar with you. Take 30 minutes before meals at the same time each day. Avoid alcohol while taking this medication; could cause severe reaction. You may experience more sensitivity to sunlight, headache, or nausea. Report hypoglycemia (palpitations, sweaty palms, lightheadedness); extended vomiting, diarrhea, or constipation; flu-like symptoms; skin rash; easy bruising or bleeding; or change in color of urine or stool.

Dietary Considerations Should be taken with meals at the same time each day (twice-daily dosing may be beneficial if conventional glyburide doses are >10 mg or micronized glyburide doses are >6 mg). Individualized medical nutrition therapy (MNT) based on ADA recommendations is an integral part of therapy.

Glyburide and Metformin

(GLYE byoor ide & met FOR min)

Brand Names: U.S. Glucovance®

Index Terms Glyburide and Metformin Hydrochloride; Metformin and Glyburide

Pharmacologic Category Antidiabetic Agent, Biguanide; Antidiabetic Agent, Sulfonylurea

Medication Safety Issues

Sound-alike/look-alike issues:

Glucovance® may be confused with Vyvanse®

High alert medication:

The Institute for Safe Medication Practices (ISMP) includes this medication among its list of drugs which have a heightened risk of causing significant patient harm when used in error.

Pregnancy Risk Factor B

Lactation Excretion in breast milk unknown/not recommended

Use Adjunct to diet and exercise for the management of type 2 diabetes mellitus (noninsulin dependent, NIDDM)

Available Dosage Forms

Tablet: Glyburide 1.25 mg and metformin 250 mg; glyburide 2.5 mg and metformin 500 mg; glyburide 5 mg and metformin 500 mg

Glucovance®: 2.5 mg/500 mg: Glyburide 2.5 mg and metformin 500 mg; 5 mg/500 mg: Glyburide 5 mg and metformin 500 mg

General Dosage Range Oral: *Adults:* Initial: Glyburide 1.25-5 mg and metformin 250-500 mg once or twice daily; Maintenance: Up to glyburide 20 mg/day and metformin 2000 mg/day

Administration

Oral All doses should be administered with a meal. Twice-daily dosing should be administered with the morning and evening meals. Patients that are NPO or require decreased caloric intake may need doses held to avoid hypoglycemia.

Nursing Actions

Physical Assessment See individual agents.

Patient Education See individual agents.

Related Information

GlyBURIDE *on page 547*
MetFORMIN *on page 746*

Glycopyrrolate (glye koe PYE roe late)

Brand Names: U.S. Cuvposa™; Robinul®; Robinul® Forte

Index Terms Glycopyrronium Bromide

Pharmacologic Category Anticholinergic Agent

Medication Safety Issues

International issues:

Robinul [U.S. and multiple international markets] may be confused with Reminyl brand name for galantamine [Canada and multiple international markets]

Pregnancy Risk Factor B (injection) / C (oral solution)

Lactation Excretion in breast milk unknown/use caution

Use Inhibit salivation and excessive secretions of the respiratory tract preoperatively; control of upper airway secretions; intraoperatively to counteract drug-induced or vagal mediated bradyarrhythmias; adjunct in treatment of peptic ulcer (indication listed in product labeling but currently has no place in management of peptic ulcer disease)

Cuvposa™: Reduce chronic, severe drooling in those with neurologic conditions (eg, cerebral palsy) associated with drooling

Unlabeled Use Adjunct with acetylcholinesterase inhibitors (eg, neostigmine, edrophonium, pyridostigmine) to antagonize cholinergic effects

Available Dosage Forms

Injection, solution: 0.2 mg/mL (1 mL, 2 mL, 5 mL, 20 mL)

Robinul®: 0.2 mg/mL (1 mL, 2 mL, 5 mL, 20 mL)

Solution, oral:

Cuvposa™: 1 mg/5 mL (473 mL)

Tablet, oral: 1 mg, 2 mg

Robinul®: 1 mg

Robinul® Forte: 2 mg

General Dosage Range

I.M.:

Children <2 years: 4-9 mcg/kg once **or** 4-10 mcg/kg every 3-4 hours (maximum: 0.2 mg/dose; 0.8 mg/day)

Children ≥2 years: 4 mcg/kg once **or** 4-10 mcg/kg every 3-4 hours (maximum: 0.2 mg/dose; 0.8 mg/day)

Adults: 4 mcg/kg once **or** 0.1-0.2 mg 3-4 times/day

I.V.:

Children: 4-10 mcg/kg every 3-4 hours (maximum: 0.2 mg/dose; 0.8 mg/day) **or** 4 mcg/kg (maximum: 0.1 mg); repeat as needed

Adults: 0.1-0.2 mg 3-4 times/day **or** 0.1 mg repeated as needed

Oral: *Children 3-16 years:* 0.02-0.1 mg/kg/dose 3 times/day (maximum 3 mg/dose)

Administration

Oral Administer oral solution on an empty stomach, 1 hour before or 2 hours after meals

I.M. Administer undiluted.

I.V. Administer at a rate of 0.2 mg over 1-2 minutes.

I.V. Detail May administer undiluted. May also be administered via the tubing of a running I.V. infusion of a compatible solution. May be administered in the same syringe with neostigmine or pyridostigmine.

pH: 2-3

Nursing Actions

Physical Assessment Assess potential for interactions with any drugs that may add to anticholinergic effects.

Patient Education Take before meals. Void before taking medication. You may experience dizziness, blurred vision, dry mouth, photosensitivity, decreased ability to sweat, or impotence (temporary). Report excessive and persistent anticholinergic effects (blurred vision, headache, flushing, tachycardia, nervousness, constipation, dizziness, insomnia, mental confusion or excitement, dry mouth, altered taste perception, dysphagia, palpitations, bradycardia, urinary hesitancy or retention, impotence, decreased sweating).

Golimumab (goe LIM ue mab)

Brand Names: U.S. Simponi®

Index Terms CNTO-148

Pharmacologic Category Antipsoriatic Agent; Antirheumatic, Disease Modifying; Monoclonal Antibody; Tumor Necrosis Factor (TNF) Blocking Agent

Medication Guide Available Yes

Pregnancy Risk Factor B

Lactation Excretion in breast milk unknown/not recommended

Breast-Feeding Considerations It is not known whether golimumab is secreted in human milk. Because many immunoglobulins are secreted in milk and the potential for serious adverse reactions exists, a decision should be made whether to discontinue nursing or discontinue the drug, taking into account the importance of the drug to the mother.

Use Treatment of active rheumatoid arthritis (moderate-to-severe), active psoriatic arthritis, and active ankylosing spondylitis

Mechanism of Action/Effect Monoclonal antibody that binds to human tumor necrosis factor alpha (TNFα), thereby decreasing inflammatory and other responses

Contraindications There are no contraindications listed in the FDA-approved manufacturer's labeling.

Canadian labeling: Hypersensitivity to golimumab, latex, or any other component of formulation or packaging; patients with severe infections (eg, sepsis, tuberculosis, opportunistic infections)

Warnings/Precautions [U.S. Boxed Warning]: Patients receiving golimumab are at increased risk for serious infections which may result in hospitalization and/or fatality; infections usually developed in patients receiving concomitant immunosuppressive agents (eg, methotrexate or corticosteroids) and may present as disseminated (rather than local) disease. Active tuberculosis (or reactivation of latent tuberculosis), invasive fungal (including aspergillosis, blastomycosis, candidiasis, coccidioidomycosis, histoplasmosis, and pneumocystosis) and bacterial, viral or other opportunistic infections (including legionellosis and listeriosis) have been reported in patients receiving TNF-blocking agents, including golimumab. Monitor closely for signs/ symptoms of infection. Discontinue for serious infection or sepsis. Consider risks versus benefits prior to use in patients with a history of chronic or recurrent infection. Consider empiric antifungal therapy in patients who are at risk for invasive fungal infection and develop severe systemic illness. Caution should be exercised when considering use in the elderly or in patients with conditions that predispose them to infections (eg, diabetes) or residence/travel from areas of endemic mycoses (blastomycosis, coccidioidomycosis, histoplasmosis), or with latent or localized infections. Do not initiate golimumab therapy with clinically important active infection. Patients who develop a new infection while undergoing treatment should be monitored closely.

[U.S. Boxed Warning]: Tuberculosis (disseminated or extrapulmonary) has been reported in patients receiving golimumab; both reactivation of latent infection and new infections have been reported. Patients should be evaluated for tuberculosis risk factors and latent tuberculosis infection (with a tuberculin skin test) prior to therapy. Treatment of latent tuberculosis should be initiated before use. Patients with initial negative tuberculin skin tests should receive continued monitoring for tuberculosis throughout treatment; active tuberculosis has developed in this population during treatment with TNF-blocking agents. Use with caution in patients who have resided in regions where tuberculosis is endemic. Consider antituberculosis therapy if an adequate course of treatment cannot be confirmed in patients with a history of latent or active tuberculosis or for patients with risk factors despite negative skin test.

Rare reactivation of hepatitis B virus (HBV) has occurred in chronic virus carriers; use with caution; evaluate prior to initiation and during treatment. Patients should be brought up to date with all immunizations before initiating therapy. Live vaccines should not be given concurrently. In clinical trials, humoral response to pneumococcal vaccine was not suppressed in psoriatic arthritis patients.

[U.S. Boxed Warning]: Lymphoma and other malignancies have been reported in children and adolescent patients receiving TNF-blocking agents. Half of the malignancies reported in children were lymphomas (Hodgkin's and non-Hodgkin's) while other cases varied and included malignancies not typically observed in this population. The impact of golimumab on the development and course of malignancy is not fully defined. Compared to the general population, an increased risk of lymphoma has been noted in clinical trials; however, rheumatoid arthritis alone has been previously associated with an increased rate of lymphoma. Lymphomas and other malignancies were also observed (at rates higher than expected for the general population) in adult patients receiving TNF-blocking agents. Treatment may result in the formation of autoimmune antibodies; cases of autoimmune disease have not been described. Neutralizing antibodies to golimumab may also be formed. Rarely, a reversible lupus-like syndrome has occurred with use of TNF blockers.

Use with caution in patients with peripheral or central nervous system demyelinating disorders; rare cases of new onset or exacerbation of demyelinating disorders (eg, multiple sclerosis, Guillain-Barré syndrome) have occurred with use of TNF-blockers, including golimumab. Consider discontinuing use in patients who develop peripheral or central nervous system demyelinating disorders during treatment. Optic neuritis, transverse myelitis, multiple sclerosis, and new onset or exacerbation of seizures has been reported. Use with caution in patients with heart failure or decreased left ventricular function and discontinue use with new onset or worsening of symptoms. Use caution in patients with a history of significant hematologic abnormalities (cytopenias).

Avoid concomitant use with abatacept (increased incidence of serious infections) or anakinra (increased incidence of neutropenia and serious infection). Use caution when switching between biological disease-modifying antirheumatic drugs (DMARDs); overlapping of biological activity may increase the risk for infection. Use with caution in the elderly (general incidence of infection is higher). Packaging (prefilled syringe and needle cover) contains dry natural rubber (latex). Some dosage forms may contain dry natural rubber (latex) and/or polysorbate 80.

Drug Interactions

Avoid Concomitant Use

Avoid concomitant use of Golimumab with any of the following: Abatacept; Anakinra; BCG; Belimumab; Canakinumab; Certolizumab Pegol; Natalizumab; Pimecrolimus; Rilonacept; Tacrolimus (Topical); Vaccines (Live)

Decreased Effect

Golimumab may decrease the levels/effects of: BCG; Coccidioidin Skin Test; Sipuleucel-T; Vaccines (Inactivated); Vaccines (Live)

The levels/effects of Golimumab may be decreased by: Echinacea

Increased Effect/Toxicity

Golimumab may increase the levels/effects of: Abatacept; Anakinra; Belimumab; Canakinumab; Certolizumab Pegol; Leflunomide; Natalizumab; Rilonacept; Vaccines (Live)

The levels/effects of Golimumab may be increased by: Abciximab; Denosumab; Pimecrolimus; Roflumilast; Tacrolimus (Topical); Trastuzumab

Adverse Reactions

>10%:

Respiratory: Upper respiratory tract infection (16%; includes laryngitis, nasopharyngitis, pharyngitis, and rhinitis)

Miscellaneous: Infection (28%)

1% to 10%:

Cardiovascular: Hypertension (3%)

Central nervous system: Dizziness (2%), fever (1%)

Gastrointestinal: Constipation (1%)

Hepatic: ALT increased (4%), AST increased (3%)

Local: Injection site reactions (6%)

Neuromuscular & skeletal: Paresthesia (2%)

Respiratory: Bronchitis (2%), sinusitis (2%)

Miscellaneous: Viral infection (5%; includes herpes and influenza), antibody formation (4%), fungal infection (superficial; 2%)

Available Dosage Forms

Injection, solution [preservative free]:

Simponi®: 50 mg/0.5 mL (0.5 mL)

General Dosage Range SubQ: *Adults:* 50 mg once per month

Administration

Other Subcutaneous injection: Prior to administration, allow syringe to sit at room temperature for 30 minutes. Solution should be clear to slightly opalescent and colorless to light yellow. Discard if solution is cloudy, discolored, or has foreign particles. Hold autoinjector firmly against skin and inject subcutaneously into thigh, lower abdomen (below navel), or upper arm. A loud click is heard when injection has begun. Continue to hold autoinjector against skin until second click is heard (may take 3-15 seconds). Following second click, lift autoinjector from injection site. Discard any unused portion. Rotate injection sites and avoid injecting into tender, red, hard, or bruised skin.

Stability

Storage Store under refrigeration at 2°C to 8°C (36°F to 46°F); do not freeze. Do not shake. Protect from light.

Nursing Actions

Physical Assessment Perform tuberculin skin test prior to initiating therapy. Monitor for signs of tuberculosis throughout therapy. Do not initiate therapy if active infection is present. Monitor closely for signs and symptoms of infection. Identify history of latex or polysorbate 80 allergy; some dosage containers may contain latex and/or polysorbate 80. Assess for liver dysfunction. Assess results of laboratory tests (PDD) at regular intervals during treatment. If self-injected, teach patient appropriate injection technique and syringe/needle disposal.

Patient Education Inform prescriber of any allergies, history of tuberculosis, or any kind of infection you have. If self-administered, follow directions for injection and needle/syringe disposal exactly. You may be more susceptible to infection. May cause dizziness. Report persistent fever; increased bruising or bleeding; respiratory tract infection; unhealed or infected wounds; urinary tract infection; flu-like symptoms; unexplained weight loss; persistent cough; respiratory difficulty; unusual bump or sore that does not heal; weight gain; swelling of extremities; or redness, swelling, or pain at injection site.

Goserelin (GOE se rel in)

Brand Names: U.S. Zoladex®

Index Terms Goserelin Acetate; ICI-118630; ZDX

Pharmacologic Category Antineoplastic Agent, Gonadotropin-Releasing Hormone Agonist; Gonadotropin Releasing Hormone Agonist

Pregnancy Risk Factor X (endometriosis, endometrial thinning); D (advanced breast cancer)

Lactation Excretion in breast milk unknown/not recommended

Breast-Feeding Considerations Goserelin is inactivated when used orally. Breast-feeding is not recommended by the manufacturer.

Use Treatment of locally confined prostate cancer; palliative treatment of advanced prostate cancer; palliative treatment of advanced breast cancer in pre- and perimenopausal women; treatment of endometriosis, including pain relief and reduction of endometriotic lesions; endometrial thinning agent as part of treatment for dysfunctional uterine bleeding

Mechanism of Action/Effect LHRH synthetic analog of luteinizing hormone-releasing hormone also known as gonadotropin-releasing hormone (GnRH)

Contraindications Hypersensitivity to goserelin, GnRH, GnRH agonist analogues, or any component of the formulation; pregnancy (except if using for palliative treatment of advanced breast cancer)

Warnings/Precautions Hazardous agent - use appropriate precautions for handling and disposal. Allergic hypersensitivity reactions (including anaphylaxis) and antibody formation may occur; monitor. Androgen-deprivation therapy may increase the risk for cardiovascular disease (Levine, 2010). Transient increases in serum testosterone (in men with prostate cancer) and estrogen (in women with breast cancer) may result in a worsening of disease signs and symptoms (tumor flare) during the first few weeks of treatment. Urinary tract obstruction or spinal cord compression have been reported when used for prostate cancer; closely observe patients for weakness, paresthesias, and urinary tract obstruction in first few weeks of therapy. Decreased bone density has been reported in women and may be irreversible; use caution if other risk factors are present; evaluate and institute preventative treatment if necessary.

Women of childbearing potential should not receive therapy until pregnancy has been excluded. Nonhormonal contraception is recommended for premenopausal women during therapy and for 12 weeks after therapy is discontinued. Cervical resistance may be increased; use caution when dilating the cervix. The 3-month implant currently has no approved indications for use in women. Rare cases of pituitary apoplexy (frequently secondary to pituitary adenoma) have been observed with GnRH administration (onset from 1 hour to usually <2 weeks); may present as sudden headache, vomiting, visual or mental status changes, and infrequently cardiovascular collapse; immediate medical attention required. Hyperglycemia has been reported in males and may manifest as diabetes or worsening of pre-existing diabetes. Decreased AUC may be observed when using the 3-month implant in obese patients. Monitor testosterone levels if desired clinical response is not observed. Safety and efficacy have not been established in pediatric patients.

Drug Interactions

Avoid Concomitant Use There are no known interactions where it is recommended to avoid concomitant use.

Decreased Effect

Goserelin may decrease the levels/effects of: Antidiabetic Agents

Increased Effect/Toxicity There are no known significant interactions involving an increase in effect.

Adverse Reactions Percentages reported with the 1-month implant:

>10%:

Cardiovascular: Peripheral edema (female 21%)

Central nervous system: Headache (female 32% to 75%; male 1% to 5%), emotional lability (female 60%), depression (female 54%; male 1% to 5%), pain (female 17%; male 8%), insomnia (female 11%; male 5%)

Dermatologic: Acne (female 42%), seborrhea (female 26%)

Endocrine & metabolic: Hot flashes (female 57% to 96%; male 62%), libido decreased (female 48% to 61%), sexual dysfunction (male 21%), breast atrophy (female 33%), breast enlargement (female 18%), erections decreased (18%), libido increased (female 12%)

Gastrointestinal: Nausea (female 8% to 11%; male 5%), abdominal pain (female 7% to 11%)

Genitourinary: Vaginitis (75%), pelvic symptoms (female 9% to 18%), dyspareunia (female 14%), lower urinary symptoms (male 13%)

Neuromuscular & skeletal: Bone mineral density decreased (female 23%; ~4% decrease from baseline in 6 months; postmarketing reports in males), weakness (female 11%)

Miscellaneous: Diaphoresis (female 16% to 45%; male 6%), tumor flare (female: 23%), infection (female 13%)

1% to 10%:

Cardiovascular: Arrhythmia, cerebrovascular accident, chest pain, edema, heart failure, hypertension, MI, palpitation, peripheral vascular disorder, tachycardia

Central nervous system: Abnormal thinking, anxiety, chills, dizziness, fever, lethargy, malaise, migraine, nervousness, somnolence

Dermatologic: Alopecia, bruising, dry skin, hair disorder, hirsutism, pruritus, rash, skin discoloration

Endocrine & metabolic: Breast pain, breast swelling/tenderness, dysmenorrhea, gout, hyperglycemia

Gastrointestinal: Anorexia, appetite increased, constipation, diarrhea, dyspepsia, flatulence, ulcer, vomiting, weight gain/loss, xerostomia

Genitourinary: Urinary frequency, urinary obstruction, urinary tract infection, vaginal hemorrhage, vulvovaginitis

Hematologic: Anemia, hemorrhage

Local: Application site reaction

Neuromuscular & skeletal: Arthralgia, back pain, hypertonia, joint disorder, leg cramps, myalgia, paresthesia
Ocular: Amblyopia, dry eyes
Renal: Renal insufficiency
Respiratory: Bronchitis, COPD, cough, epistaxis, pharyngitis, rhinitis, sinusitis, upper respiratory tract infection
Miscellaneous: Allergic reaction, flu-like syndrome, voice alteration

Pharmacodynamics/Kinetics

Onset of Action

Females: Estradiol suppression reaches postmenopausal levels within 3 weeks and FSH and LH are suppressed to follicular phase levels within 4 weeks of initiation.
Males: Testosterone suppression reaches castrate levels within 2-4 weeks after initiation.

Duration of Action

Females: Estradiol, LH and FSH generally return to baseline levels within 12 weeks following the last monthly implant.
Males: Testosterone levels maintained at castrate levels throughout the duration of therapy.

Available Dosage Forms

Implant, subcutaneous:
Zoladex®: 3.6 mg (1s); 10.8 mg (1s)

General Dosage Range SubQ: *Adults:* 3.6 mg every 28 days **or** 10.8 mg every 12 weeks

Administration

Other SubQ: Administer implant by inserting needle at a 30-45 degree angle into the anterior abdominal wall below the navel line. Goserelin is an implant; therefore, do not attempt to eliminate air bubbles prior to injection (may displace implant). Do not attempt to aspirate prior to injection; if a large vessel is penetrated, blood will be visualized in the syringe chamber (if vessel is penetrated, withdraw needle and inject elsewhere with a new syringe). Do not penetrate into muscle or peritoneum. Implant may be detected by ultrasound if removal is required.

Stability

Storage Zoladex® should be stored at room temperature not to exceed 25°C (77°F). Protect from light.

Nursing Actions

Physical Assessment Observe patients for weakness and paresthesias in the first few weeks of therapy. Monitor for symptoms of hypoglycemia.

Patient Education This drug must be implanted under the skin of your abdomen every 28 days or every 3 months; it is important to maintain appointment schedule. If you have diabetes, monitor blood sugar frequently; can cause loss of glycemic control/hyperglycemia. Males or females, you may experience systemic hot flashes; headache; depression; mood swings; insomnia; acne; increased sweating, especially in women; constipation; sexual dysfunction (decreased libido, decreased erection for males, vaginal dryness for females); or bone pain. Symptoms may worsen temporarily during first weeks of therapy. Report chest pain, palpitations, or respiratory difficulty; swelling of extremities; unusual persistent nausea, vomiting, or constipation; infections; unresolved dizziness; skin rash; or paresthesias or muscle weakness.

Granisetron (gra NI se tron)

Brand Names: U.S. Granisol™; Kytril®; Sancuso®

Index Terms BRL 43694

Pharmacologic Category Antiemetic; Selective 5-HT_3 Receptor Antagonist

Medication Safety Issues

Sound-alike/look-alike issues:

Granisetron may be confused with dolasetron, ondansetron, palonosetron

Pregnancy Risk Factor B

Lactation Excretion in breast milk unknown/use caution

Use Prophylaxis of nausea and vomiting associated with emetogenic chemotherapy and radiation therapy; prophylaxis and treatment of postoperative nausea and vomiting (PONV)

Unlabeled Use Breakthrough treatment of nausea and vomiting associated with chemotherapy

Mechanism of Action/Effect Selective 5-HT_3 receptor antagonist, blocking serotonin, both peripherally on vagal nerve terminals and centrally in the chemoreceptor trigger zone.

Contraindications Hypersensitivity to granisetron or any component of the formulation

Warnings/Precautions Use with caution in patients with congenital long QT syndrome or other risk factors for QT prolongation (eg, medications known to prolong QT interval, electrolyte abnormalities, and cumulative high-dose anthracycline therapy). 5-HT_3 antagonists have been associated with a number of dose-dependent increases in ECG intervals (eg, PR, QRS duration, QT/QT_c, JT), usually occurring 1-2 hours after I.V. administration. In general, these changes are not clinically relevant, however, when used in conjunction with other agents that prolong these intervals, arrhythmia may occur. When used with agents that prolong the QT interval (eg, Class I and III antiarrhythmics), clinically relevant QT interval prolongation may occur resulting in torsade de pointes. I.V. formulations of 5-HT_3 antagonists have more association with ECG interval changes, compared to oral formulations.

For chemotherapy-related emesis, **granisetron should be used on a scheduled basis, not on an "as needed" (PRN) basis**, since data support the use of this drug in the prevention of nausea and vomiting and not in the rescue of nausea and vomiting. Granisetron should be used only in the first 24-48 hours of receiving chemotherapy or radiation. Data do not support any increased efficacy of granisetron in delayed nausea and vomiting.

Use with caution in patients allergic to other 5-HT_3 receptor antagonists; cross-reactivity has been reported. Routine prophylaxis for PONV is not recommended in patients where there is little expectation of nausea and vomiting postoperatively. In patients where nausea and vomiting must be avoided postoperatively, administer to all patients even when expected incidence of nausea and vomiting is low. Use caution following abdominal surgery or in chemotherapy-induced nausea and vomiting; may mask progressive ileus or gastric distention. Application site reactions, generally mild, have occurred with transdermal patch use; if skin reaction is severe or generalized, remove patch. Cover patch application site with clothing to protect from natural or artificial sunlight exposure while patch is applied and for 10 days following removal; granisetron may potentially be affected by natural or artificial sunlight. Do not apply patch to red, irritated, or damaged skin. Injection contains benzyl alcohol (1 mg/mL) and should not be used in neonates.

Drug Interactions

Avoid Concomitant Use

Avoid concomitant use of Granisetron with any of the following: Apomorphine; Artemether; Dronedarone; Lumefantrine; Nilotinib; Pimozide; QUEtiapine; QuiNINE; Tetrabenazine; Thioridazine; Toremifene; Vandetanib; Vemurafenib; Ziprasidone

Decreased Effect

The levels/effects of Granisetron may be decreased by: Tocilizumab

Increased Effect/Toxicity

Granisetron may increase the levels/effects of: Apomorphine; Dronedarone; Pimozide; QTc-Prolonging Agents; QuiNINE; Tetrabenazine; Thioridazine; Toremifene; Vandetanib; Vemurafenib; Ziprasidone

The levels/effects of Granisetron may be increased by: Alfuzosin; Artemether; Chloroquine; Ciprofloxacin; Ciprofloxacin (Systemic); Conivaptan; Gadobutrol; Indacaterol; Lumefantrine; Nilotinib; QUEtiapine; QuiNINE

Adverse Reactions

>10%:

Central nervous system: Headache (3% to 21%; transdermal patch: 1%)

Gastrointestinal: Constipation (3% to 18%)

Neuromuscular & skeletal: Weakness (5% to 18%)

1% to 10%:

Cardiovascular: QT_c prolongation (1% to 3%), hypertension (1% to 2%)

Central nervous system: Pain (10%), fever (3% to 9%), dizziness (4% to 5%), insomnia (<2% to 5%), somnolence (1% to 4%), anxiety (2%), agitation (<2%), CNS stimulation (<2%)

Dermatologic: Rash (1%)

Gastrointestinal: Diarrhea (3% to 9%), abdominal pain (4% to 6%), dyspepsia (3% to 6%), taste perversion (2%)

Hepatic: Liver enzymes increased (5% to 6%)

Renal: Oliguria (2%)

Respiratory: Cough (2%)

Miscellaneous: Infection (3%)

Pharmacodynamics/Kinetics

Duration of Action Oral, I.V.: Generally up to 24 hours

Available Dosage Forms

Injection, solution: 1 mg/mL (1 mL, 4 mL)

Injection, solution [preservative free]: 0.1 mg/mL (1 mL); 1 mg/mL (1 mL)

Patch, transdermal:

Sancuso®: 3.1 mg/24 hours (1s)

Solution, oral:

Granisol™: 2 mg/10 mL (30 mL)

Tablet, oral: 1 mg

Kytril®: 1 mg

General Dosage Range

I.V.:

Children ≥2 years: 10 mcg/kg/dose (maximum: 1 mg/dose) as a single dose or every 12 hours

Adults: 10 mcg/kg/dose (maximum: 1 mg/dose) as a single dose or every 12 hours **or** 1 mg as a single dose

Oral: *Adults:* 2 mg/day in 1-2 divided dose

Transdermal: *Adults:* 1 patch prior to chemotherapy; Maximum duration: Patch may be worn up to 7 days

Administration

Oral Doses should be given up to 1 hour prior to initiation of chemotherapy/radiation

I.V. Administer I.V. push over 30 seconds or as a 5- to 10-minute infusion

Prevention of PONV: Administer before induction of anesthesia or immediately before reversal of anesthesia.

Treatment of PONV: Administer undiluted over 30 seconds.

I.V. Detail pH: 4.7-7.3

Topical Transdermal (Sancuso®): Apply patch to clean, dry, intact skin on upper outer arm. Do not use on red, irritated or damaged skin. Remove patch from pouch immediately before application. Do not cut patch.

Stability

Storage

I.V.: Store at 15°C to 30°C (59°F to 86°F). Protect from light. Do not freeze vials. Stable when mixed in NS or D_5W for 7 days under refrigeration and for 3 days at room temperature.

Oral: Store tablet or oral solution at 15°C to 30°C (59°F to 86°F). Protect from light.

Transdermal patch: Store at 20°C to 25°C (68°F to 77°F). Keep patch in original packaging until immediately prior to use.

Nursing Actions

Physical Assessment Allergy history to selective 5-HT_3 receptor antagonists should be assessed prior to administering. Assess other drugs patient may be taking that may prolong QT interval. I.V.: Follow infusion specifics. Oral, I.V., and transdermal formulations have different doses and schedules and should not be administered on a PRN basis.

Patient Education This drug is given to prevent nausea and vomiting. If this medication is given by intravenous infusion you will be monitored during infusion. Report immediately any chest pain, respiratory difficulty, or pain or itching at infusion site. Remove patch from packaging pouch immediately before application; do not cut patch. Apply to clean, dry, intact skin on upper outer arm. You may experience headache, drowsiness, or dizziness. Report chest pain or palpitations, persistent headache, excessive drowsiness, fever, or changes in elimination patterns (constipation or diarrhea).

Griseofulvin (gri see oh FUL vin)

Brand Names: U.S. Grifulvin V®; Gris-PEG®

Index Terms Griseofulvin Microsize; Griseofulvin Ultramicrosize

Pharmacologic Category Antifungal Agent, Oral

Pregnancy Risk Factor C

Lactation Excretion in breast milk unknown/use caution

Use Treatment of susceptible tinea infections of the skin, hair, and nails

Available Dosage Forms

Suspension, oral: 125 mg/5 mL (118 mL, 120 mL)

Tablet, oral:

Grifulvin V®: 500 mg

Gris-PEG®: 125 mg, 250 mg

General Dosage Range Oral:

Microsize:

Children >2 years: 10-20 mg/kg/day in single or divided doses

Adults: 500-1000 mg/day in single or divided doses

Ultramicrosize:

Children >2 years: 5-15 mg/kg/day in single dose or 2 divided doses (maximum: 750 mg/day)

Adults: 375-750 mg/day in single or divided doses

Administration

Oral Administer with a fatty meal (peanuts or ice cream) to increase absorption, or with food or milk to avoid GI upset

Gris-PEG® tablets: May be swallowed whole or crushed and sprinkled onto 1 tablespoonful of applesauce and swallowed immediately without chewing.

Nursing Actions

Physical Assessment Assess renal and hepatic function with long-term use. Monitor for CNS changes, gastrointestinal upset, rash, and opportunistic infection periodically during therapy.

Patient Education Avoid alcohol while taking this drug (disulfiram reactions). You may experience confusion, dizziness, drowsiness, nausea, vomiting, diarrhea, or increased sensitivity to sun. Report skin rash, respiratory difficulty, CNS changes (confusion, dizziness, acute headache), changes in color of stool or urine, or worsening of condition.

GuaiFENesin (gwye FEN e sin)

Brand Names: U.S. Allfen [OTC]; Bidex®-400 [OTC]; Diabetic Siltussin DAS-Na [OTC]; Diabetic Tussin® EX [OTC]; Fenesin IR [OTC]; Ganidin® NR [OTC] [DSC]; Geri-Tussin [OTC]; Humibid® Maximum Strength [OTC]; Mucinex® Kid's Mini-Melts™ [OTC]; Mucinex® Kid's [OTC]; Mucinex® Maximum Strength [OTC]; Mucinex® [OTC]; Mucus Relief [OTC]; Organidin® NR [OTC] [DSC]; Refenesen™ 400 [OTC]; Refenesen™ [OTC]; Robafen [OTC]; Scot-Tussin® Expectorant [OTC]; Siltussin SA [OTC]; Vicks® Casero™ Chest Congestion Relief [OTC]; Vicks® DayQuil® Mucus Control [OTC]; Xpect™ [OTC]

Index Terms Cheratussin; GG; Glycerol Guaiacolate

Pharmacologic Category Expectorant

Medication Safety Issues

Sound-alike/look-alike issues:

GuaiFENesin may be confused with guanFACINE

Mucinex® may be confused with Mucomyst®

Lactation Excretion in breast milk unknown

Use Help loosen phlegm and thin bronchial secretions to make coughs more productive

Available Dosage Forms

Caplet, oral:

Fenesin IR [OTC]: 400 mg

Refenesen™ 400 [OTC]: 400 mg

Granules, oral:

Mucinex® Kid's Mini-Melts™ [OTC]: 50 mg/packet (12s); 100 mg/packet (12s)

Liquid, oral:

Diabetic Tussin® EX [OTC]: 100 mg/5 mL (118 mL)

Mucinex® Kid's [OTC]: 100 mg/5 mL (118 mL)

Scot-Tussin® Expectorant [OTC]: 100 mg/5 mL (120 mL)

Vicks® Casero™ Chest Congestion Relief [OTC]: 100 mg/6.25 mL (120 mL, 240 mL)

Vicks® DayQuil® Mucus Control [OTC]: 200 mg/15 mL (295 mL)

Syrup, oral: 100 mg/5 mL (5 mL, 10 mL, 15 mL, 118 mL, 120 mL, 240 mL, 473 mL, 480 mL)
Diabetic Siltussin DAS-Na [OTC]: 100 mg/5 mL (118 mL)
Geri-Tussin [OTC]: 100 mg/5 mL (480 mL)
Robafen [OTC]: 100 mg/5 mL (120 mL, 240 mL, 480 mL)
Siltussin SA [OTC]: 100 mg/5 mL (120 mL, 240 mL, 480 mL)

Tablet, oral: 400 mg
Allfen [OTC]: 400 mg
Bidex®-400 [OTC]: 400 mg
Mucus Relief [OTC]: 400 mg
Refenesen™ [OTC]: 200 mg
Xpect™ [OTC]: 400 mg

Tablet, extended release, oral:
Humibid® Maximum Strength [OTC]: 1200 mg
Mucinex® [OTC]: 600 mg
Mucinex® Maximum Strength [OTC]: 1200 mg

General Dosage Range Oral:
Extended release: *Children ≥12 years and Adults:* 600-1200 mg every 12 hours (maximum: 2.4 g/day)
Immediate release:
Children 6 months to 2 years: 25-50 mg every 4 hours (maximum: 300 mg/day)
Children 2-5 years: 50-100 mg every 4 hours (maximum: 600 mg/day)
Children 6-11 years: 100-200 mg every 4 hours (maximum: 1.2 g/day)
Children ≥12 years and Adults: 200-400 mg every 4 hours (maximum: 2.4 g/day)

Administration
Oral Do not crush, chew, or break extended release tablets. Administer with a full glass of water.

Nursing Actions
Patient Education Do not chew or crush extended release tablet; take with a full glass of water. Maintain adequate hydration, unless instructed to restrict fluid intake. Report excessive drowsiness, respiratory difficulty, lack of improvement, or worsening of condition.

Guaifenesin and Codeine
(gwye FEN e sin & KOE deen)

Brand Names: U.S. Allfen CD; Allfen CDX; Codar® GF; Dex-Tuss; ExeClear-C; Gani-Tuss® NR [DSC]; Guaiatussin AC; Iophen C-NR; M-Clear; M-Clear WC; Mar-Cof® CG; Robafen AC
Index Terms Codeine and Guaifenesin; Robitussin AC
Pharmacologic Category Antitussive; Cough Preparation; Expectorant
Use Temporary control of cough due to minor throat and bronchial irritation
Controlled Substance Capsule: C-V; Liquid products: C-V; Tablet: C-III

Available Dosage Forms
Capsule, oral:
M-Clear: Guaifenesin 200 mg and codeine 9 mg
Liquid, oral:
Codar® GF: Guaifenesin 200 mg and codeine 8 mg per 5 mL
Dex-Tuss: Guaifenesin 300 mg and codeine 10 mg per 5 mL
Iophen C-NR: Guaifenesin 100 mg and codeine 10 mg per 5 mL
M-Clear WC: Guaifenesin 100 mg and codeine 6.33 mg per 5 mL
Solution, oral: Guaifenesin 100 mg and codeine 10 mg per 5 mL
Mar-Cof® CG: Guaifenesin 225 mg and codeine 7.5 mg per 5 mL
Syrup, oral: Guaifenesin 100 mg and codeine 10 mg per 5 mL (473 mL)
ExeClear-C: Guaifenesin 200 mg and codeine 10 mg per 5 mL
Guaiatussin AC, Robafen AC: Guaifenesin 100 mg and codeine 10 mg per 5 mL
Tablet, oral:
Allfen CD: Guaifenesin 400 mg and codeine 10 mg
Allfen CDX: Guaifenesin 400 mg and codeine 20 mg

General Dosage Range Oral: *Children ≥6 years and Adults:* Dosage varies greatly depending on product

Nursing Actions
Physical Assessment See individual agents.
Patient Education See individual agents.

Related Information
Codeine *on page 268*
GuaiFENesin *on page 556*

Haemophilus b Conjugate and Hepatitis B Vaccine
(he MOF i lus bee KON joo gate & hep a TYE tis bee vak SEEN)

Brand Names: U.S. Comvax®
Index Terms *Haemophilus* b (meningococcal protein conjugate) Conjugate Vaccine; Hepatitis B Vaccine (Recombinant); Hib Conjugate Vaccine; Hib-HepB
Pharmacologic Category Vaccine, Inactivated (Bacterial); Vaccine, Inactivated (Viral)

Medication Safety Issues
Sound-alike/look-alike issues:
Comvax® may be confused with Recombivax [Recombivax HB®]

Pregnancy Risk Factor C
Use
Immunization against invasive disease caused by *H. influenzae* type b and against infection caused by all known subtypes of hepatitis B virus in infants 6 weeks to 15 months of age born of hepatitis B surface antigen (HB_sAg)-negative mothers

Infants born of HB_sAg-positive mothers or mothers of unknown HB_sAg status should receive hepatitis B vaccine (recombinant) at birth and should complete the hepatitis B vaccination series given according to a particular schedule (refer to current ACIP recommendations).

Available Dosage Forms

Injection, suspension [preservative free]:

Comvax®: *Haemophilus* b capsular polysaccharide 7.5 mcg and hepatitis B surface antigen 5 mcg per 0.5 mL (0.5 mL)

General Dosage Range I.M.: *Infants ≥6 weeks:* 0.5 mL (series includes 3 doses)

Administration

I.M. Shake well prior to use. Administer 0.5 mL I.M. into anterolateral thigh [data suggests that injections given in the buttocks frequently are given into fatty tissue instead of into muscle and result in lower seroconversion rates]; **do not administer intravenously, intradermally, or subcutaneously.**

For patients at risk of hemorrhage following intramuscular injection, the ACIP recommends "it should be administered intramuscularly if, in the opinion of the physician familiar with the patients bleeding risk, the vaccine can be administered with by this route with reasonable safety. If the patient receives antihemophilia or other similar therapy, intramuscular vaccination can be scheduled shortly after such therapy is administered. A fine needle (23 gauge or smaller) can be used for the vaccination and firm pressure applied to the site (without rubbing) for at least 2 minutes. The patient should be instructed concerning the risk of hematoma from the injection." Patients on anticoagulant therapy should be considered to have the same bleeding risks and treated as those with clotting factor disorders (CDC, 2011).

Simultaneous administration of vaccines helps ensure the patients will be fully vaccinated by the appropriate age. Simultaneous administration of vaccines is defined as administering >1 vaccine on the same day at different anatomic sites. The use of licensed combination vaccines is generally preferred over separate injections of the equivalent components. Separate vaccines should not be combined in the same syringe unless indicated by product specific labeling. Separate needles and syringes should be used for each injection. The ACIP prefers each dose of a specific vaccine in a series come from the same manufacturer when possible. Adolescents and adults should be vaccinated while seated or lying down. In general, preterm infants should be vaccinated at the same chronological age as full-term infants (CDC, 2011).

Antipyretics have not been shown to prevent febrile seizures. Antipyretics may be used to treat fever or discomfort following vaccination (CDC, 2011). One study reported that routine prophylactic administration of acetaminophen to prevent fever prior to vaccination decreased the immune response of some vaccines; the clinical significance of this reduction in immune response has not been established (Prymula, 2009).

Nursing Actions

Physical Assessment U.S. federal law requires entry into the patient's medical record.

Patient Education See individual agents.

Related Information

Immunization Administration Recommendations *on page 1243*

Immunization Recommendations *on page 1248*

Haemophilus b Conjugate Vaccine

(he MOF fi lus bee KON joo gate vak SEEN)

Brand Names: U.S. ActHIB®; Hiberix®; PedvaxHIB®

Index Terms *Haemophilus* b Oligosaccharide Conjugate Vaccine; *Haemophilus* b Polysaccharide Vaccine; Diphtheria Toxoid Conjugate; HbCV; Hib; Hib Conjugate Vaccine; Hib Polysaccharide Conjugate; PRP-OMP; PRP-T

Pharmacologic Category Vaccine, Inactivated (Bacterial)

Pregnancy Risk Factor C

Use Routine immunization of children against invasive disease caused by *H. influenzae* type b

The Advisory Committee on Immunization Practices (ACIP) recommends routine vaccination of all children through age 59 months. Efficacy data are not available for use in older children and adults with chronic conditions associated with an increased risk of Hib disease. However, a single dose may also be considered for older children, adolescents, and adults who did not receive the childhood series and who have a chronic condition associated with an increased risk of Hib disease (eg, splenectomy, sickle cell disease, leukemia, HIV infection).

Available Dosage Forms

Injection, powder for reconstitution [preservative free]:

ActHIB® *Haemophilus* b capsular polysaccharide 10 mcg per 0.5 mL

Hiberix®: *Haemophilus* b capsular polysaccharide 10 mcg per 0.5 mL

Injection, suspension:

PedvaxHIB®: *Haemophilus* b capsular polysaccharide 7.5 mcg

General Dosage Range I.M.: *Children:* 0.5 mL (number of doses determined by age at first dose)

Administration

I.M. For I.M. administration; do not inject I.V.

Hiberix®: Shake well prior to use. Administer into the anterolateral thigh or deltoid. If Hiberix® is inadvertently administered during the primary vaccination series, the dose can be counted as a valid PRP-T dose that does not need to be repeated if administered according to schedule. In this case, a total of 3 doses completes the primary series.

ActHIB®, PedvaxHIB®: Shake well prior to use. Administer into the anterolateral thigh or deltoid. Do not administer into buttocks due to potential risk of injury to sciatic nerve.

For patients at risk of hemorrhage following intramuscular injection, the ACIP recommends "it should be administered intramuscularly if, in the opinion of the physician familiar with the patients bleeding risk, the vaccine can be administered by this route with reasonable safety. If the patient receives antihemophilia or other similar therapy, intramuscular vaccination can be scheduled shortly after such therapy is administered. A fine needle (23 gauge or smaller) can be used for the vaccination and firm pressure applied to the site (without rubbing) for at least 2 minutes. The patient should be instructed concerning the risk of hematoma from the injection." Patients on anticoagulant therapy should be considered to have the same bleeding risks and treated as those with clotting factor disorders (CDC, 2011).

Simultaneous administration of vaccines helps ensure the patients will be fully vaccinated by the appropriate age. Simultaneous administration of vaccines is defined as administering >1 vaccine on the same day at different anatomic sites. The use of licensed combination vaccines is generally preferred over separate injections of the equivalent components. Separate vaccines should not be combined in the same syringe unless indicated by product specific labeling. Separate needles and syringes should be used for each injection. The ACIP prefers each dose of a specific vaccine in a series come from the same manufacturer when possible. Adolescents and adults should be vaccinated while seated or lying down. In general, preterm infants should be vaccinated at the same chronological age as full-term infants (CDC, 2011).

Antipyretics have not been shown to prevent febrile seizures. Antipyretics may be used to treat fever or discomfort following vaccination (CDC, 2011). One study reported that routine prophylactic administration of acetaminophen to prevent fever prior to vaccination decreased the immune response of some vaccines; the clinical significance of this reduction in immune response has not been established (Prymula, 2009).

Nursing Actions

Physical Assessment U.S. federal law requires entry into the patient's medical record.

Related Information

Immunization Administration Recommendations *on page 1243*

Immunization Recommendations *on page 1248*

Halcinonide (hal SIN oh nide)

Brand Names: U.S. Halog®

Pharmacologic Category Corticosteroid, Topical

Medication Safety Issues

Sound-alike/look-alike issues:

Halcinonide may be confused with Halcion®

Halog® may be confused with Haldol®

Pregnancy Risk Factor C

Lactation Excretion in breast milk unknown/use caution

Use Inflammation of corticosteroid-responsive dermatoses [high potency topical corticosteroid]

Available Dosage Forms

Cream, topical:

Halog®: 0.1% (30 g, 60 g, 216 g)

Ointment, topical:

Halog®: 0.1% (30 g, 60 g)

General Dosage Range Topical: *Children and Adults:* Apply sparingly 1-3 times/day

Nursing Actions

Patient Education For external use only. Do not use for eyes, mucous membranes, or open wounds. Before using, wash and dry area gently. Apply in a thin layer (may rub in lightly). Apply light dressing (if necessary) to area being treated. Do not use occlusive dressing unless so advised by prescriber. Avoid prolonged or excessive use around sensitive tissues or genital or rectal areas. Avoid exposing treated area to direct sunlight. Inform prescriber if condition worsens (redness, swelling, irritation, signs of infection, or open sores) or fails to improve.

Haloperidol (ha loe PER i dole)

Brand Names: U.S. Haldol®; Haldol® Decanoate

Index Terms Haloperidol Decanoate; Haloperidol Lactate

Pharmacologic Category Antipsychotic Agent, Typical

Medication Safety Issues

Sound-alike/look-alike issues:

Haldol® may be confused with Halcion®, Halog®, Stadol

International issues:

Haldol [U.S. and multiple international markets] may be confused with Halotestin brand name for fluoxymesterone [Great Britain]

Pregnancy Risk Factor C

Lactation Enters breast milk/not recommended (AAP rates "of concern"; AAP 2001 update pending)

Breast-Feeding Considerations Haloperidol is found in breast milk and has been detected in the plasma and urine of nursing infants. Developmental decline was observed in 3 nursing infants following maternal use of haloperidol in combination with chlorpromazine. Breast engorgement, gynecomastia, and lactation are known side effects with the use of haloperidol.

Use Management of schizophrenia; control of tics and vocal utterances of Tourette's disorder in children and adults; severe behavioral problems in children

Unlabeled Use Treatment of nonschizophrenia psychosis; may be used for the emergency sedation of severely-agitated or delirious patients; adjunctive treatment of ethanol dependence; postoperative nausea and vomiting (alternative therapy); psychosis/agitation related to Alzheimer's dementia

Mechanism of Action/Effect Haloperidol is a butyrophenone antipsychotic which blocks postsynaptic mesolimbic dopaminergic D_1 and D_2 receptors in the brain; depresses the release of hypothalamic and hypophyseal hormones; believed to depress the reticular activating system thus affecting basal metabolism, body temperature, wakefulness, vasomotor tone, and emesis

Contraindications Hypersensitivity to haloperidol or any component of the formulation; Parkinson's disease; severe CNS depression; coma

Warnings/Precautions [U.S. Boxed Warning]: Elderly patients with dementia-related psychosis treated with antipsychotics are at an increased risk of death compared to placebo. Most deaths appeared to be either cardiovascular (eg, heart failure, sudden death) or infectious (eg, pneumonia) in nature. Haloperidol is not approved for the treatment of dementia-related psychosis. Hypotension may occur, particularly with parenteral administration. Although the short-acting form (lactate) is used clinically, the I.V. use of the injection is not an FDA-approved route of administration; the decanoate form should never be administered intravenously.

May alter cardiac conduction and prolong QT interval; life-threatening arrhythmias have occurred with therapeutic doses of antipsychotics but risk may be increased with doses exceeding recommendations and/or intravenous administration (unlabeled route). Use caution or avoid use in patients with electrolyte abnormalities (eg, hypokalemia, hypomagnesemia), hypothyroidism, familial long QT syndrome, concomitant medications which may augment QT prolongation, or any underlying cardiac abnormality which may also potentiate risk. Monitor ECG closely for dose-related QT effects. Adverse effects of decanoate may be prolonged. Avoid in thyrotoxicosis.

Leukopenia, neutropenia, and agranulocytosis (sometimes fatal) have been reported in clinical trials and postmarketing reports with antipsychotic use; presence of risk factors (eg, pre-existing low WBC or history of drug-induced leuko-/neutropenia) should prompt periodic blood count assessment. Discontinue therapy at first signs of blood dyscrasias or if absolute neutrophil count <1000/mm^3.

May be sedating, use with caution in disorders where CNS depression is a feature. Effects may be potentiated when used with other sedative drugs or ethanol. Caution in patients with severe cardiovascular disease, predisposition to seizures, subcortical brain damage, or renal disease. Esophageal dysmotility and aspiration have been associated with antipsychotic use - use with caution in patients at risk of pneumonia (eg, Alzheimer's disease). Use associated with increased prolactin levels; clinical significance of hyperprolactinemia in patients with breast cancer or other prolactin-dependent tumors is unknown. May alter temperature regulation or mask toxicity of other drugs due to antiemetic effects. May cause orthostatic hypotension; use with caution in patients at risk of this effect or those who would tolerate transient hypotensive episodes (cerebrovascular disease, cardiovascular disease, or other medications which may predispose). Some tablets contain tartrazine. Antipsychotics have been associated with pigmentary retinopathy.

May cause anticholinergic effects (confusion, agitation, constipation, xerostomia, blurred vision, urinary retention). Therefore, they should be used with caution in patients with decreased gastrointestinal motility, urinary retention, BPH, xerostomia, or visual problems. Conditions which also may be exacerbated by cholinergic blockade include narrow-angle glaucoma and worsening of myasthenia gravis. Relative to other neuroleptics, haloperidol has a low potency of cholinergic blockade.

May cause extrapyramidal symptoms (EPS), including pseudoparkinsonism, acute dystonic reactions, akathisia, and tardive dyskinesia. Risk of dystonia (and possibly other EPS) may be greater with increased doses, use of conventional antipsychotics, males, and younger patients. May be associated with neuroleptic malignant syndrome (NMS). Use with caution in the elderly.

Drug Interactions

Avoid Concomitant Use

Avoid concomitant use of Haloperidol with any of the following: Artemether; Conivaptan; Dronedarone; Lumefantrine; Metoclopramide; Nilotinib; Pimozide; QUEtiapine; QuiNINE; Tetrabenazine; Thioridazine; Tolvaptan; Toremifene; Vandetanib; Vemurafenib; Ziprasidone

Decreased Effect

Haloperidol may decrease the levels/effects of: Amphetamines; Codeine; Quinagolide

The levels/effects of Haloperidol may be decreased by: Anti-Parkinson's Agents (Dopamine Agonist); CarBAMazepine; CYP3A4

Inducers (Strong); Cyproterone; Deferasirox; Glycopyrrolate; Lithium formulations; Peginterferon Alfa-2b; Tocilizumab

Increased Effect/Toxicity

Haloperidol may increase the levels/effects of: Alcohol (Ethyl); Anticholinergics; Anti-Parkinson's Agents (Dopamine Agonist); ARIPiprazole; Budesonide (Systemic, Oral Inhalation); ChlorproMAZINE; CNS Depressants; Colchicine; CYP2D6 Substrates; CYP3A4 Substrates; Dronedarone; Eplerenone; Everolimus; FentaNYL; Fesoterodine; Ivacaftor; Lurasidone; Methylphenidate; Nebivolol; Pimecrolimus; Pimozide; QTc-Prolonging Agents; QuiNIDine; QuiNINE; Salmeterol; Saxagliptin; Serotonin Modulators; Tamoxifen; Tetrabenazine; Thioridazine; Tolvaptan; Toremifene; Vandetanib; Vemurafenib; Ziprasidone

The levels/effects of Haloperidol may be increased by: Abiraterone Acetate; Acetylcholinesterase Inhibitors (Central); Alfuzosin; Artemether; Chloroquine; ChlorproMAZINE; Ciprofloxacin; Ciprofloxacin (Systemic); Conivaptan; CYP2D6 Inhibitors (Moderate); CYP2D6 Inhibitors (Strong); CYP3A4 Inhibitors (Moderate); CYP3A4 Inhibitors (Strong); Darunavir; FLUoxetine; FluvoxaMINE; Gadobutrol; HydrOXYzine; Indacaterol; Ivacaftor; Lithium formulations; Lumefantrine; Methylphenidate; Metoclopramide; Nilotinib; Nonsteroidal Anti-Inflammatory Agents; Pramlintide; QUEtiapine; QuiNIDine; QuiNINE; Tetrabenazine

Nutritional/Ethanol Interactions

Ethanol: May increase CNS depression; monitor for increased effects with coadministration. Caution patients about effects.

Herb/Nutraceutical: Avoid valerian, St John's wort, kava kava, gotu kola (may increase CNS depression).

Adverse Reactions Frequency not defined.

Cardiovascular: Abnormal T waves with prolonged ventricular repolarization, arrhythmia, hyper-/hypotension, QT prolongation, sudden death, tachycardia, torsade de pointes

Central nervous system: Agitation, akathisia, altered central temperature regulation, anxiety, confusion, depression, drowsiness, dystonic reactions, euphoria, extrapyramidal reactions, headache, insomnia, lethargy, neuroleptic malignant syndrome (NMS), pseudoparkinsonian signs and symptoms, restlessness, seizure, tardive dyskinesia, tardive dystonia, vertigo

Dermatologic: Alopecia, contact dermatitis, hyperpigmentation, photosensitivity (rare), pruritus, rash

Endocrine & metabolic: Amenorrhea, breast engorgement, galactorrhea, gynecomastia, hyper-/hypoglycemia, hyponatremia, lactation, mastalgia, menstrual irregularities, sexual dysfunction

Gastrointestinal: Anorexia, constipation, diarrhea, dyspepsia, hypersalivation, nausea, vomiting, xerostomia

Genitourinary: Priapism, urinary retention

Hematologic: Cholestatic jaundice, obstructive jaundice

Ocular: Blurred vision

Respiratory: Bronchospasm, laryngospasm

Miscellaneous: Diaphoresis, heat stroke

Pharmacodynamics/Kinetics

Onset of Action Sedation: I.M., I.V.: 30-60 minutes

Duration of Action Decanoate: ~3 weeks

Available Dosage Forms

Injection, oil: 50 mg/mL (1 mL, 5 mL); 100 mg/mL (1 mL, 5 mL)

Haldol® Decanoate: 50 mg/mL (1 mL); 100 mg/mL (1 mL)

Injection, solution: 5 mg/mL (1 mL, 10 mL)

Haldol®: 5 mg/mL (1 mL)

Solution, oral: 2 mg/mL (5 mL, 15 mL, 120 mL)

Tablet, oral: 0.5 mg, 1 mg, 2 mg, 5 mg, 10 mg, 20 mg

General Dosage Range

I.M.:

Decanoate: *Adults:* Initial: 10-20 times daily oral dose at 4-week intervals; Maintenance: 10-15 times initial oral dose

Lactate:

Children 6-12 years: 1-3 mg/dose every 4-8 hours (maximum: 0.15 mg/kg/day)

Adults: 2-5 mg every 4-8 hours as needed

Oral:

Children 3-12 years (15-40 kg): Initial: 0.5 mg/day in 2-3 divided doses; Maintenance: 0.05-0.15 mg/kg/day in 2-3 divided doses

Adults: Initial: 0.5-5 mg 2-3 times/day; Maintenance: Up to 30 mg/day in 2-3 divided doses

Administration

Oral Dilute the oral concentrate with water or juice before administration. **Note:** Avoid skin contact with oral medication; may cause contact dermatitis.

I.M. The decanoate injectable formulation should be administered I.M. only; **do not give decanoate I.V.**

I.V.

Decanoate: Do **not** administer I.V.

Lactate: May be administered I.V. (unlabeled route) or I.M.

I.V. Detail

pH: 3.0-3.6

Stability

Reconstitution Haloperidol lactate may be administered IVPB or I.V. infusion in D_5W solutions. NS solutions should not be used due to reports of decreased stability and incompatibility.

Standardized dose: 0.5-100 mg/50-100 mL D_5W.

Storage Protect oral dosage forms from light. Haloperidol lactate injection should be stored at controlled room temperature; do not freeze or expose to temperatures >40°C. Protect from light; exposure to light may cause discoloration and the development of a grayish-red precipitate over several weeks. Stability of standardized solutions is 38 days at room temperature (24°C).

Nursing Actions

Physical Assessment Monitor for sedation and anticholinergic and extrapyramidal symptoms. With I.M. or I.V. use, monitor closely for hypotension and cardiac irregularities. Initiate at lower doses and taper dosage slowly when discontinuing. Avoid skin contact with oral medication; may cause contact dermatitis (wash immediately with warm, soapy water).

Patient Education It may take 2-3 weeks to achieve desired results. Dilute oral concentration with water or juice. Avoid alcohol. Maintain adequate hydration, unless instructed to restrict fluid intake. Avoid skin contact with medication; may cause contact dermatitis (wash immediately with warm, soapy water). You may experience excess drowsiness, restlessness, dizziness, blurred vision, nausea, vomiting, constipation, postural hypotension, urinary retention, or decreased perspiration. Report persistent CNS effects (eg, trembling fingers, altered gait or balance, excessive sedation, seizures, unusual movements, anxiety, abnormal thoughts, confusion, personality changes), chest pain, palpitations, rapid heartbeat, severe dizziness, unresolved urinary retention or changes in urinary pattern, vision changes, skin rash or yellowing of skin, respiratory difficulty, or worsening of condition.

Heparin (HEP a rin)

Brand Names: U.S. Hep-Lock; Hep-Lock U/P; HepFlush®-10

Index Terms Heparin Calcium; Heparin Lock Flush; Heparin Sodium

Pharmacologic Category Anticoagulant

Medication Safety Issues

Sound-alike/look-alike issues:

Heparin may be confused with Hespan®

High alert medication:

The Institute for Safe Medication Practices (ISMP) includes this medication among its list of drugs which have a heightened risk of causing significant patient harm when used in error.

National Patient Safety Goals:

The Joint Commission (TJC) requires healthcare organizations that provide anticoagulant therapy to have a process in place to reduce the risk of anticoagulant-associated patient harm. Patients receiving anticoagulants should receive individualized care through a defined process that includes standardized ordering, dispensing, administration, monitoring and education. This does not apply to routine short-term use of anticoagulants for prevention of venous thromboembolism when the expectation is that the patient's laboratory values will remain within or close to normal values (NPSG.03.05.01).

Administration issues:

The 100 unit/mL concentration should not be used to flush heparin locks, I.V. lines, or intra-arterial lines in neonates or infants <10 kg (systemic anticoagulation may occur). The 10 unit/mL flush concentration may inadvertently cause systemic anticoagulation in infants <1 kg who receive frequent flushes.

Other safety concerns:

Heparin sodium injection 10,000 units/mL and Hep-Lock U/P 10 units/mL have been confused with each other. Fatal medication errors have occurred between the two whose labels are both blue. **Never rely on color as a sole indicator to differentiate product identity.**

Heparin lock flush solution is intended only to maintain patency of I.V. devices and is **not** to be used for anticoagulant therapy.

Pregnancy Risk Factor C

Lactation Does not enter breast milk

Breast-Feeding Considerations Some products contain benzyl alcohol as a preservative; their use in breast-feeding women is contraindicated by some manufacturers due to the association of gasping syndrome in premature infants.

Use Prophylaxis and treatment of thromboembolic disorders; as an anticoagulant for extracorporeal and dialysis procedures

Note: Heparin lock flush solution is intended only to maintain patency of I.V. devices and is **not** to be used for systemic anticoagulant therapy.

Unlabeled Use ST-elevation myocardial infarction (STEMI) as an adjunct to thrombolysis; unstable angina/non-STEMI (UA/NSTEMI); anticoagulant used during percutaneous coronary intervention (PCI)

Mechanism of Action/Effect Potentiates the action of antithrombin III and thereby inactivates thrombin (as well as activated coagulation factors IX, X, XI, XII, and plasmin) and prevents the conversion of fibrinogen to fibrin; heparin also stimulates release of lipoprotein lipase (lipoprotein lipase hydrolyzes triglycerides to glycerol and free fatty acids)

Contraindications Hypersensitivity to heparin or any component of the formulation (unless a life-threatening situation necessitates use and use of an alternative anticoagulant is not possible); severe thrombocytopenia; uncontrolled active bleeding except when due to disseminated intravascular coagulation (DIC); not for use when appropriate blood coagulation tests cannot be obtained at appropriate intervals (applies to full-dose heparin only)

Note: Some products contain benzyl alcohol as a preservative; their use in neonates, infants, or pregnant or nursing mothers is contraindicated by some manufacturers.

Warnings/Precautions Hypersensitivity reactions can occur. Only in life-threatening situations when use of an alternative anticoagulant is not possible should heparin be cautiously used in patients with a documented hypersensitivity reaction. Hemorrhage is the most common complication. Monitor for signs and symptoms of bleeding. Certain patients are at increased risk of bleeding. Risk factors for bleeding include bacterial endocarditis; congenital or acquired bleeding disorders; active ulcerative or angiodysplastic GI diseases; continuous GI tube drainage; severe uncontrolled hypertension; history of hemorrhagic stroke; or use shortly after brain, spinal, or ophthalmology surgery; patient treated concomitantly with platelet inhibitors; conditions associated with increased bleeding tendencies (hemophilia, vascular purpura); recent GI bleeding; thrombocytopenia or platelet defects; severe liver disease; hypertensive or diabetic retinopathy; renal failure; or in patients undergoing invasive procedures including spinal tap or spinal anesthesia. Many concentrations of heparin are available ranging from 1 unit/mL to 20,000 units/mL. Clinicians **must** carefully examine each prefilled syringe or vial prior to use ensuring that the correct concentration is chosen; fatal hemorrhages have occurred related to heparin overdose especially in pediatric patients. A higher incidence of bleeding has been reported in patients >60 years of age, particularly women. They are also more sensitive to the dose. Discontinue heparin if hemorrhage occurs; severe hemorrhage or overdosage may require protamine.

May cause thrombocytopenia; monitor platelet count closely. Patients who develop HIT may be at risk of developing a new thrombus (heparin-induced thrombocytopenia and thrombosis [HITT]). Discontinue therapy and consider alternatives if platelets are <100,000/mm^3 and/or thrombosis develops. HIT or HITT may be delayed and can occur up to several weeks after discontinuation of heparin. Osteoporosis may occur with prolonged use (>6 months) due to a reduction in bone mineral density. Monitor for hyperkalemia; can cause hyperkalemia by suppressing aldosterone production. Patients >60 years of age may require lower doses of heparin.

[U.S. Boxed Warning]: Some products contain benzyl alcohol as a preservative; use of these products is contraindicated in neonates. In neonates, large amounts of benzyl alcohol (>100 mg/kg/day) have been associated with fatal toxicity (gasping syndrome). Use in neonates, infants, or pregnant or nursing mothers is contraindicated by some manufacturers; the use of preservative-free heparin is, therefore, recommended in these populations. Some preparations contain sulfite which may cause allergic reactions.

Heparin resistance may occur in patients with antithrombin deficiency, increased heparin clearance, elevations in heparin-binding proteins, elevations in factor VIII and/or fibrinogen; frequently encountered in patients with fever, thrombosis, thrombophlebitis, infections with thrombosing tendencies, MI, cancer, and in postsurgical patients; measurement of anticoagulant effects using anti-factor Xa levels may be of benefit.

Drug Interactions

Avoid Concomitant Use

Avoid concomitant use of Heparin with any of the following: Corticorelin; Rivaroxaban

Decreased Effect

The levels/effects of Heparin may be decreased by: Nitroglycerin

Increased Effect/Toxicity

Heparin may increase the levels/effects of: Anticoagulants; Collagenase (Systemic); Corticorelin; Deferasirox; Drotrecogin Alfa (Activated); Ibritumomab; Rivaroxaban; Tositumomab and Iodine I 131 Tositumomab

The levels/effects of Heparin may be increased by: 5-ASA Derivatives; Antiplatelet Agents; Aspirin; Dasatinib; Herbs (Anticoagulant/Antiplatelet Properties); Nonsteroidal Anti-Inflammatory Agents; Pentosan Polysulfate Sodium; Pentoxifylline; Prostacyclin Analogues; Salicylates; Thrombolytic Agents

Nutritional/Ethanol Interactions Herb/Nutraceutical: Avoid cat's claw, dong quai, evening primrose, feverfew, red clover, horse chestnut, garlic, green tea, ginseng, ginkgo (all have additional antiplatelet activity).

Adverse Reactions Frequency not defined.

Cardiovascular: Allergic vasospastic reaction (possibly related to thrombosis), chest pain, hemorrhagic shock, shock, thrombosis

Central nervous system: Chills, fever, headache

Dermatologic: Alopecia (delayed, transient), bruising (unexplained), cutaneous necrosis, dysesthesia pedis, erythematous plaques (case reports), eczema, urticaria, purpura

Endocrine & metabolic: Adrenal hemorrhage, hyperkalemia (suppression of aldosterone synthesis), ovarian hemorrhage, rebound hyperlipidemia on discontinuation

Gastrointestinal: Constipation, hematemesis, nausea, tarry stools, vomiting

Genitourinary: Frequent or persistent erection

Hematologic: Bleeding from gums, epistaxis, hemorrhage, ovarian hemorrhage, retroperitoneal hemorrhage, thrombocytopenia (see note)

Hepatic: Liver enzymes increased

Local: Irritation, erythema, pain, hematoma, and ulceration have been rarely reported with deep SubQ injections; I.M. injection (not recommended) is associated with a high incidence of these effects

Neuromuscular & skeletal: Peripheral neuropathy, osteoporosis (chronic therapy effect)

Ocular: Conjunctivitis (allergic reaction), lacrimation

Renal: Hematuria

Respiratory: Asthma, bronchospasm (case reports), hemoptysis, pulmonary hemorrhage, rhinitis

Miscellaneous: Allergic reactions, anaphylactoid reactions, heparin resistance, hypersensitivity (including chills, fever, and urticaria)

Note: Thrombocytopenia has been reported to occur at an incidence between 0% and 30%. It is often of no clinical significance. However, immunologically mediated heparin-induced thrombocytopenia (HIT) has been estimated to occur in 1% to 2% of patients, and is marked by a progressive fall in platelet counts and, in some cases, thromboembolic complications (skin necrosis, pulmonary embolism, gangrene of the extremities, stroke, or MI).

Pharmacodynamics/Kinetics

Onset of Action Anticoagulation: I.V.: Immediate; SubQ: ~20-30 minutes

Available Dosage Forms

Infusion, premixed in 1/2 NS: 25,000 units (250 mL, 500 mL)

Infusion, premixed in D_5W: 10,000 units (100 mL, 250 mL); 12,500 units (250 mL); 20,000 units (500 mL); 25,000 units (250 mL, 500 mL)

Infusion, premixed in NS: 1000 units (500 mL); 2000 units (1000 mL)

Infusion, premixed in NS [preservative free]: 1000 units (500 mL); 2000 units (1000 mL)

Injection, solution: 10 units/mL (1 mL, 2 mL, 3 mL, 5 mL, 10 mL, 30 mL); 100 units/mL (1 mL, 2 mL, 3 mL, 5 mL, 10 mL, 30 mL); 1000 units/mL (1 mL, 10 mL, 30 mL); 5000 units/mL (1 mL, 10 mL); 10,000 units/mL (1 mL, 4 mL, 5 mL); 20,000 units/mL (1 mL)

Hep-Lock: 10 units/mL (1 mL, 2 mL, 10 mL, 30 mL); 100 units/mL (1 mL, 2 mL, 10 mL, 30 mL)

Injection, solution [preservative free]: 1 units/mL (2 mL, 3 mL, 5 mL); 2 units/mL (3 mL); 10 units/mL (1 mL, 2 mL, 2.5 mL, 3 mL, 5 mL, 6 mL, 10 mL); 100 units/mL (1 mL, 2 mL, 2.5 mL, 3 mL, 5 mL, 10 mL); 1000 units/mL (2 mL); 5000 units/mL (0.5 mL); 10,000 units/mL (0.5 mL)

Hep-Lock U/P: 10 units/mL (1 mL); 100 units/mL (1 mL)

HepFlush®-10: 10 units/mL (10 mL)

General Dosage Range

I.V.:

Children: Bolus: 50-100 units/kg; Initial infusion: 15-25 units/kg/hour; Maintenance: Increase dose by 2-4 units/kg/hour every 6-8 hours as needed **or** 50-100 units/kg every 4 hours intermittently

Adults: Bolus: 60-80 units/kg; Infusion: 10-30 units/kg/hour **or** 10,000 units (initially), then 50-70 units/kg (5000-10,000 units) every 4-6 hours intermittently

SubQ: *Adults:* Thromboprophylaxis: 5000 units every 8-12 hours; Treatment: 17,500 units every 12 hours

Administration

I.M. Do not administer I.M. due to pain, irritation, and hematoma formation.

I.V.

Continuous infusion: Infuse via infusion pump.

Heparin lock: Inject via injection cap using positive pressure flushing technique. Heparin lock flush solution is intended only to maintain patency of I.V. devices and is **not** to be used for anticoagulant therapy.

Other SubQ: Inject in subcutaneous tissue only (not muscle tissue). Injection sites should be rotated (usually left and right portions of the abdomen, above iliac crest).

Stability

Reconstitution

Standard concentration/diluent: 25,000 units/500 mL D_5W (premixed). If preparing solution, mix thoroughly prior to administration.

Minimum volume: 250 mL D_5W.

Storage Heparin solutions are colorless to slightly yellow. Minor color variations do not affect therapeutic efficacy. Heparin should be stored at controlled room temperature. Protect from freezing and temperatures >40°C.

Stability at room temperature and refrigeration:

Prepared bag: 24-72 hours (specific to solution, concentration, and/or study conditions)

Premixed bag: After seal is broken. 4 days.

Out of overwrap stability: 30 days.

Nursing Actions

Physical Assessment Assess potential for interactions with any drugs that will affect coagulation or platelet function. Note specific infusion directions in Administration. Bleeding precautions must be observed at all times during heparin therapy. Monitor laboratory tests regularly (dosing adjustments may be necessary). Monitor patient closely for hypersensitivity reaction, bleeding, chest pain, hyperkalemia, and peripheral neuropathy. For I.V. bolus, emergency treatment for hypersensitivity reactions should be immediately available. Teach patient bleeding precautions.

Patient Education This drug can only be administered by infusion or injection. You may have a tendency to bleed easily while taking this drug (brush teeth with soft brush, floss with waxed floss, use electric razor, avoid scissors or sharp knives and potentially harmful activities). Report immediately any chest pain; difficulty breathing or unusual cough; bleeding or bruising (bleeding gums, nosebleed, blood in urine, dark stool); pain in joints or back; CNS changes (fever, confusion); unusual fever; persistent nausea or GI upset; change in vision, or swelling, pain, or redness at injection site.

Related Information

Compatibility of Drugs *on page 1264*

Hepatitis A and Hepatitis B Recombinant Vaccine

(hep a TYE tis aye & hep a TYE tis bee ree KOM be nant vak SEEN)

Brand Names: U.S. Twinrix®

Index Terms Engerix-B® and Havrix®; Havrix® and Engerix-B®; HepA-HepB; Hepatitis B and Hepatitis A Vaccine

Pharmacologic Category Vaccine, Inactivated (Viral)

Pregnancy Risk Factor C

Lactation Excretion in breast milk unknown/use caution

Use Active immunization against disease caused by hepatitis A virus and hepatitis B virus (all known subtypes) in populations desiring protection against or at high risk of exposure to these viruses.

Populations include travelers or people living in or relocating to areas of intermediate/high endemicity for **both** HAV and HBV and are at increased risk of HBV infection due to behavioral or occupational factors; patients with chronic liver disease; laboratory workers who handle live HAV and HBV; health-care workers, police, and other personnel who render first-aid or medical assistance; workers who come in contact with sewage; employees of day care centers and correctional facilities; patients/staff of hemodialysis units; men who have sex with men; patients frequently receiving blood products; military personnel; users of injectable illicit drugs; close household contacts of patients with hepatitis A and hepatitis B infection; residents of drug and alcohol treatment centers

Available Dosage Forms

Injection, suspension [preservative free]:

Twinrix®: Hepatitis A virus antigen 720 ELISA units and hepatitis B surface antigen 20 mcg per mL (1 mL)

General Dosage Range I.M.: *Adults:* 3 doses (1 mL each) given on a 0-, 1-, and 6-month schedule

Administration

I.M. Shake well prior to use. Do not dilute prior to administration. Discard if the suspension is discolored or does not appear homogenous after shaking or if there are cracks in the vial or syringe. Administer in the deltoid region; do not administer in the gluteal region (may give suboptimal response). Administer in the anterolateral thigh in infants (Canadian labeling). Do not administer at the same site, or using the same syringe, as additional vaccines or immunoglobulins.

For patients at risk of hemorrhage following intramuscular injection, the ACIP recommends "it should be administered intramuscularly if, in the opinion of the physician familiar with the patients bleeding risk, the vaccine can be administered by this route with reasonable safety. If the patient receives antihemophilia or other similar therapy, intramuscular vaccination can be scheduled shortly after such therapy is administered. A fine needle (23 gauge or smaller) can be used for the vaccination and firm pressure applied to the site (without rubbing) for at least 2 minutes. The patient should be instructed concerning the risk of hematoma from the injection." Patients on anticoagulant therapy should be considered to have the same bleeding risks and treated as those with clotting factor disorders (CDC, 2011).

Simultaneous administration of vaccines helps ensure the patients will be fully vaccinated by the appropriate age. Simultaneous administration of vaccines is defined as administering >1 vaccine on the same day at different anatomic sites. The use of licensed combination vaccines is generally preferred over separate injections of the equivalent components. Separate vaccines should not be combined in the same syringe unless indicated by product specific labeling. Separate needles and syringes should be used for each injection. The ACIP prefers each dose of a specific vaccine in a series come from the same manufacturer when possible. Adolescents and adults should be vaccinated while seated or lying down. In general, preterm infants should be vaccinated at the same chronological age as full-term infants (CDC, 2011).

Antipyretics have not been shown to prevent febrile seizures. Antipyretics may be used to treat fever or discomfort following vaccination (CDC, 2011). One study reported that routine prophylactic administration of acetaminophen to prevent fever prior to vaccination decreased the immune response of some vaccines; the clinical significance of this reduction in immune response has not been established (Prymula, 2009).

Nursing Actions

Physical Assessment Have emergency treatment for anaphylactoid or hypersensitivity reaction available. Observe patient for 15 minutes following administration. All serious adverse reactions must be reported to the U.S. DHHS. U.S. federal law also requires entry into the patient's medical record.

Patient Education You may experience fever, fatigue, nausea, vomiting, diarrhea, and redness and tenderness at injection site. Notify prescriber if symptoms persist.

Related Information

Immunization Administration Recommendations *on page 1243*

Immunization Recommendations *on page 1248*

Hepatitis A Vaccine (hep a TYE tis aye vak SEEN)

Brand Names: U.S. Havrix®; VAQTA®

Index Terms HepA

Pharmacologic Category Vaccine, Inactivated (Viral)

Medication Safety Issues

International issues:

Avaxim [Canada and multiple international markets] may be confused with Avastin brand name for bevacizumab [U.S., Canada, and multiple international markets]

Pregnancy Risk Factor C

Lactation Excretion in breast milk unknown/use caution

Use

Active immunization against disease caused by hepatitis A virus (HAV)

The Advisory Committee on Immunization Practices (ACIP) recommends routine vaccination for:

- All children ≥12 months of age
- All unvaccinated adults requesting protection from HAV infection
- All unvaccinated adults at risk for HAV infection, such as:

  Behavioral risks: Men who have sex with men; injection drug users

  Occupational risks: Persons who work with HAV-infected primates or with HAV in a research laboratory setting

  Medical risks: Persons with chronic liver disease; patients who receive clotting-factor concentrates
- Other risks: International travelers to regions with high or intermediate levels of endemic HAV infection (a list of countries is available at http://wwwn.cdc.gov/travel/contentdiseases.-aspx)
- Unvaccinated persons who anticipate close personal contact with international adoptee from a country of intermediate to high endemicity of HAV, during their first 60 days of arrival into the United States (eg, household contacts, babysitters)

Available Dosage Forms

Injection, suspension [preservative free]:

Havrix®: Hepatitis A virus antigen 720 ELISA units/0.5 mL (0.5 mL); Hepatitis A virus antigen 1440 ELISA units/mL (1 mL)

VAQTA®: Hepatitis A virus antigen 25 units/0.5 mL (0.5 mL); Hepatitis A virus antigen 50 units/mL (1 mL)

General Dosage Range I.M.:

Children 12 months to 18 years: 0.5 mL

Adults: 1 mL

Administration

I.M. The deltoid muscle is the preferred site for injection for older children and adults; administer to the anterolateral aspect of the thigh in infants and young children. Do not administer to the gluteal region; may decrease efficacy. Do not administer intravenously, intradermally, or subcutaneously. Shake well prior to use; discard if the suspension is discolored or does not appear homogenous after shaking, or if there are cracks in the vial or syringe. When used for primary immunization, the vaccine should be given at least 2 weeks prior to expected HAV exposure. When used for postexposure prophylaxis, the vaccine should be given as soon as possible. For patients at risk of hemorrhage following intramuscular injection, the ACIP recommends "it should be administered intramuscularly if, in the opinion of the physician familiar with the patients bleeding risk, the vaccine can be administered by this route with reasonable safety. If the patient receives antihemophilia or other similar therapy, intramuscular vaccination can be scheduled shortly after such therapy is administered. A fine needle (23 gauge or smaller) can be used for the vaccination and firm pressure applied to the site (without rubbing) for at least 2 minutes. The patient should be instructed concerning the risk of hematoma from the injection." Patients on anticoagulant therapy should be considered to have the same bleeding risks and treated as those with clotting factor disorders (CDC, 2011).

Simultaneous administration of vaccines helps ensure the patients will be fully vaccinated by the appropriate age. Simultaneous administration of vaccines is defined as administering >1 vaccine on the same day at different anatomic sites. The use of licensed combination vaccines is generally preferred over separate injections of the equivalent components. Separate vaccines should not be combined in the same syringe unless indicated by product specific labeling. Separate needles and syringes should be used for each injection. The ACIP prefers each dose of a specific vaccine in a series come from the same manufacturer when possible. Adolescents and adults should be vaccinated while seated or lying down. In general, preterm infants should be vaccinated at the same chronological age as full-term infants (CDC, 2011).

Antipyretics have not been shown to prevent febrile seizures. Antipyretics may be used to treat fever or discomfort following vaccination (CDC, 2011). One study reported that routine prophylactic administration of acetaminophen to prevent fever prior to vaccination decreased the immune response of some vaccines; the clinical significance of this reduction in immune response has not been established (Prymula, 2009).

Nursing Actions

Physical Assessment All serious adverse reactions must be reported to the U.S. DHHS. U.S. federal law also requires entry into the patient's medical record.

Patient Education Inform healthcare provider if you have a high fever, change in behavior, or a rash.

Related Information

Immunization Administration Recommendations *on page 1243*

Immunization Recommendations *on page 1248*

Hepatitis B Vaccine (Recombinant)

(hep a TYE tis bee vak SEEN ree KOM be nant)

Brand Names: U.S. Engerix-B®; Recombivax HB®

Index Terms Hepatitis B Inactivated Virus Vaccine (recombinant DNA); HepB

Pharmacologic Category Vaccine, Inactivated (Viral)

Medication Safety Issues

Sound-alike/look-alike issues:

Engerix-B® adult may be confused with Engerix-B® pediatric/adolescent

Recombivax HB® may be confused with Comvax®

Pregnancy Risk Factor C

Lactation Excretion in breast milk unknown/use caution

Use Immunization against infection caused by all known subtypes of hepatitis B virus (HBV)

The Advisory Committee on Immunization Practices (ACIP) recommends routine vaccination for the following (CDC, 2005; CDC, 2006; CDC, 2011):

- All infants at birth
- All infants and children (post-birth dose; refer to recommended vaccination schedule)
- All unvaccinated adults requesting protection from HBV infection
- All unvaccinated adults at risk for HBV infection such as those with:

Behavioral risks: Sexually-active persons with >1 partner in a 6-month period; persons seeking evaluation or treatment for a sexually-transmitted disease; men who have sex with men; injection drug users

Occupational risks: Healthcare and public safety workers with reasonably anticipated risk for exposure to blood or blood contaminated body fluids

Medical risks: Persons with end-stage renal disease (including predialysis, hemodialysis, peritoneal dialysis, and home dialysis); persons with HIV infection; persons with chronic liver disease. Adults (19 through 59 years of age) with diabetes mellitus type 1 or type 2 should be vaccinated as soon as possible following diagnosis. Adults ≥60 years with diabetes mellitus may also be vaccinated at the discretion of their treating clinician.

Other risks: Household contacts and sex partners of persons with chronic HBV infection; residents and staff of facilities for developmentally disabled persons; international travelers to regions with high or intermediate levels of endemic HBV infection

In addition, the ACIP recommends vaccination for any persons who are wounded in bombings or similar mass casualty events who have penetrating injuries or nonintact skin exposure, or who have contact with mucous membranes (exception - superficial contact with intact skin), and who cannot confirm receipt of a hepatitis B vaccination (CDC, 2008).

Available Dosage Forms

Injection, suspension [preservative free]:

Engerix-B®: Hepatitis B surface antigen 10 mcg/0.5 mL (0.5 mL); Hepatitis B surface antigen 20 mcg/mL (1 mL)

Recombivax HB®: Hepatitis B surface antigen 5 mcg/0.5 mL (0.5 mL); Hepatitis B surface antigen 10 mcg/mL (1 mL); Hepatitis B surface antigen 40 mcg/mL (1 mL)

General Dosage Range Dosage adjustment recommended in patients with renal impairment.

I.M.:

Birth to 19 years: 0.5 mL

Adults ≥20 years: 1 mL

Administration

I.M. Pediatric/adolescent formulations of hepatitis B vaccine products differ by concentration (mcg/mL). However, when dosed in terms of volume (mL), the dose of Engerix-B® and Recombivax HB® are the same (both 0.5 mL). Adult formulations of hepatitis B vaccine products also differ by concentration (mcg/mL), but when dosed in terms of volume (mL), the dose of Engerix-B® and Recombivax HB® are the same (both 1 mL). It is possible to interchange the vaccines for completion of a series or for booster doses; the antibody produced in response to each type of vaccine is comparable, however, the quantity of the vaccine will vary.

I.M. injection only; in adults, the deltoid muscle is the preferred site; the anterolateral thigh is the recommended site in infants and young children. Not for gluteal administration. Shake well prior to withdrawal and use.

For patients at risk of hemorrhage following intramuscular injection, hepatitis B vaccine may be administered subcutaneously although lower titers and/or increased incidence of local reactions may result. The ACIP recommends "it should be administered intramuscularly if, in the opinion of the physician familiar with the patients bleeding risk, the vaccine can be administered by this route with reasonable safety. If the patient receives antihemophilia or other similar therapy, intramuscular vaccination can be scheduled shortly after such therapy is administered. A fine needle (23 gauge or smaller) can be used for the vaccination and firm pressure applied to the site (without rubbing) for at least 2 minutes. The patient should be instructed concerning the risk of hematoma from the injection." Patients on anticoagulant therapy should be considered to have the same bleeding risks and treated as those with clotting factor disorders (CDC, 2011).

Simultaneous administration of vaccines helps ensure the patients will be fully vaccinated by the appropriate age. Simultaneous administration of vaccines is defined as administering >1 vaccine on the same day at different anatomic sites. The use of licensed combination vaccines is generally preferred over separate injections of the equivalent components. Separate vaccines should not be combined in the same syringe unless indicated by product specific labeling. Separate needles and syringes should be used for each injection. The ACIP prefers each dose of a specific vaccine in a series come from the same manufacturer when possible. Adolescents and adults should be vaccinated while seated or lying down. In general, preterm infants should be vaccinated at the same chronological age as full-term infants (CDC, 2011).

Antipyretics have not been shown to prevent febrile seizures. Antipyretics may be used to treat fever or discomfort following vaccination (CDC, 2011). One study reported that routine prophylactic administration of acetaminophen to prevent fever prior to vaccination decreased the immune response of some vaccines; the clinical significance of this reduction in immune response has not been established (Prymula, 2009).

Vaccination at the time of HB_sAg testing: For persons in whom vaccination is recommended, the first dose of hepatitis B vaccine can be given after blood is drawn to test for HB_sAg.

Nursing Actions

Physical Assessment All serious adverse reactions must be reported to the U.S. DHHS. U.S. federal law also requires entry into the patient's medical record.

Patient Education Common side effects include soreness where the shot is given and mild fever. Have patient call prescriber for a high fever or unusual behavior, difficulty breathing, hoarseness, wheezing, hives, paleness, weakness, a fast heartbeat, or dizziness.

Related Information

Immunization Administration Recommendations *on page 1243*

Immunization Recommendations *on page 1248*

Hetastarch (HET a starch)

Brand Names: U.S. Hespan®; Hextend®

Index Terms HES; Hydroxyethyl Starch

Pharmacologic Category Plasma Volume Expander, Colloid

Medication Safety Issues

Sound-alike/look-alike issues:

Hespan® may be confused with heparin

Pregnancy Risk Factor C

Lactation Excretion in breast milk unknown/use caution

Use Blood volume expander used in treatment of hypovolemia; adjunct in leukapheresis to improve harvesting and increase the yield of granulocytes by centrifugation (Hespan®)

Unlabeled Use Priming fluid in pump oxygenators during cardiopulmonary bypass; plasma volume expansion during cardiopulmonary bypass

Available Dosage Forms

Infusion:

Hextend®: 6% (500 mL)

Infusion, premixed in NS: 6% (500 mL)

Hespan®: 6% (500 mL)

General Dosage Range Dosage adjustment recommended in patients with renal impairment

I.V.: *Adults:* 500-1500 mL/day **or** 20 mL/kg/day (up to 1500 mL/day)

Leukapheresis: *Adults:* 250-700 mL

Administration

I.V. Volume expansion: Administer I.V. only; may be administered via infusion pump or pressure infusion. Administration rates vary depending upon the extent of blood loss, age, and clinical condition of patient, but, *in general*, should not exceed 1.2 g/kg/hour (20 mL/kg/hour); *however,* **rates up to 1000 mL over 7-8 minutes via pressure infusion have been studied in otherwise healthy subjects (McIlroy, 2003)**. Anaphylactoid reactions can occur, have epinephrine and resuscitative equipment available. If administered by pressure infusion, air should be withdrawn or expelled from bag prior to infusion to prevent air embolus. Do not administer Hextend® with blood through the same administration set. Change I.V. tubing or flush copiously with normal saline before administering blood through the same line. Change I.V. tubing at least every 24 hours.

I.V. Detail Do not use if crystalline precipitate forms or is turbid deep brown.

pH: 3.5-7

Other Leukapheresis: Mix Hespan® and citrate well. Administer to the input line of the centrifuge apparatus at a ration of 1:8 to 1:13 to venous whole blood.

Nursing Actions

Physical Assessment Patient's allergy history must be assessed prior to therapy (patients allergic to corn may have a cross allergy to hetastarch). Monitor patient closely for hypersensitivity reaction and circulatory overload. Vital signs, CVP, and urine output should be monitored frequently (every 5-15 minutes) during first hour and at regular intervals thereafter.

Patient Education Report immediately any chest pain or palpitations, respiratory difficulty, acute headache, chills, or itching.

HydrALAZINE (hye DRAL a zeen)

Index Terms Apresoline [DSC]; Hydralazine Hydrochloride

Pharmacologic Category Vasodilator

Medication Safety Issues

Sound-alike/look-alike issues:

HydrALAZINE may be confused with hydrOXYzine

Pregnancy Risk Factor C

Lactation Enters breast milk/use caution (AAP rates "compatible"; AAP 2001 update pending)

Breast-Feeding Considerations In a case report, following a maternal dose of hydralazine 50 mg three times daily, exposure to the infant was calculated to be 0.013 mg per 75mL breast milk.

Use Management of moderate-to-severe hypertension

Unlabeled Use Heart failure; hypertension secondary to pre-eclampsia/eclampsia

Mechanism of Action/Effect Direct vasodilation of arterioles (with little effect on veins) with decreased systemic resistance

Contraindications Hypersensitivity to hydralazine or any component of the formulation; mitral valve rheumatic heart disease

Warnings/Precautions May cause peripheral neuritis or a drug-induced lupus-like syndrome (more likely on larger doses, longer duration). Discontinue hydralazine in patients who develop SLE-like syndrome or positive ANA. Use with caution in patients with severe renal disease or cerebral vascular accidents or with known or suspected coronary artery disease; monitor blood pressure closely with I.V. use. Slow acetylators, patients with decreased renal function, and patients receiving >200 mg/day (chronically) are at higher risk for SLE. Titrate dosage cautiously to patient's response. Hypotensive effect after I.V. administration may be delayed and unpredictable in some patients. Usually administered with diuretic and a beta-blocker to counteract side effects of sodium and water retention and reflex tachycardia. Adjust dose in severe renal dysfunction. Use with caution in CAD (increase in tachycardia may increase myocardial oxygen demand). Use with caution in pulmonary hypertension (may cause hypotension). Patients may be poorly compliant because of frequent dosing. Hydralazine-induced fluid and sodium retention may require addition or increased dosage of a diuretic.

Drug Interactions

Avoid Concomitant Use

Avoid concomitant use of HydrALAZINE with any of the following: Pimozide

Decreased Effect

The levels/effects of HydrALAZINE may be decreased by: Herbs (Hypertensive Properties); Methylphenidate; Nonsteroidal Anti-Inflammatory Agents; Yohimbine

Increased Effect/Toxicity

HydrALAZINE may increase the levels/effects of: Amifostine; Antihypertensives; ARIPiprazole; Hypotensive Agents; Pimozide; RiTUXimab

The levels/effects of HydrALAZINE may be increased by: Alfuzosin; Diazoxide; Herbs (Hypotensive Properties); MAO Inhibitors; Pentoxifylline; Phosphodiesterase 5 Inhibitors; Prostacyclin Analogues

Nutritional/Ethanol Interactions

Ethanol: Avoid ethanol (may increase CNS depression).

Food: Food enhances bioavailability of hydralazine.

Herb/Nutraceutical: Avoid dong quai if using for hypertension (has estrogenic activity). Avoid ephedra, yohimbe, ginseng (may worsen hypertension). Avoid garlic (may have increased antihypertensive effect).

Adverse Reactions Frequency not defined.

Cardiovascular: Angina pectoris, flushing, orthostatic hypotension, palpitations, paradoxical hypertension, peripheral edema, tachycardia, vascular collapse

Central nervous system: Anxiety, chills, depression, disorientation, dizziness, fever, headache, increased intracranial pressure (I.V.; in patient with pre-existing increased intracranial pressure), psychotic reaction

Dermatologic: Pruritus, rash, urticaria

Gastrointestinal: Anorexia, constipation, diarrhea, nausea, paralytic ileus, vomiting

Genitourinary: Dysuria, impotence

Hematologic: Agranulocytosis, eosinophilia, erythrocyte count reduced, hemoglobin decreased, hemolytic anemia, leukopenia, thrombocytopenia (rare)

Neuromuscular & skeletal: Muscle cramps, peripheral neuritis, rheumatoid arthritis, tremor, weakness

Ocular: Conjunctivitis, lacrimation

Respiratory: Dyspnea, nasal congestion

Miscellaneous: Diaphoresis, drug-induced lupus-like syndrome (dose related; fever, arthralgia, splenomegaly, lymphadenopathy, asthenia, myalgia, malaise, pleuritic chest pain, edema, positive

ANA, positive LE cells, maculopapular facial rash, positive direct Coombs' test, pericarditis, pericardial tamponade)

Pharmacodynamics/Kinetics

Onset of Action Oral: 20-30 minutes; I.V.: 5-20 minutes

Duration of Action Oral: Up to 8 hours; I.V.: 1-4 hours; **Note:** May vary depending on acetylator status of patient

Available Dosage Forms

Injection, solution: 20 mg/mL (1 mL)

Tablet, oral: 10 mg, 25 mg, 50 mg, 100 mg

General Dosage Range Dosage adjustment recommended in patients with renal impairment

I.M., I.V.:

Children: 0.1-0.2 mg/kg/dose (not to exceed 20 mg) every 4-6 hours as needed (maximum: 3.5 mg/kg/day in 4-6 divided doses)

Adults: Initial: 10-20 mg/dose every 4-6 hours as needed; Maintenance: Up to 40 mg/dose every 4-6 hours **or** Eclampsia/pre-eclampsia: 5 mg/dose then 5-10 mg every 20-30 minutes as needed

Oral:

Children: Initial: 0.75-1 mg/kg/day in 2-4 divided doses; Maintenance: Up to 7.5 mg/kg/day in 2-4 divided doses (maximum: 200 mg/day)

Adults: Initial: 10-25 mg 3-4 times/day; Maintenance: 25-300 mg/day (target dose: 225-300 mg/day for CHF) in 2-4 divided doses (maximum: 300 mg/day)

Elderly: Initial: 10 mg 2-3 times/day, increase by 10-25 mg/day every 2-5 days; Target dose: 225-300 mg/day for CHF

Administration

I.V. Solution for injection: Administer as a slow I.V. push; maximum rate: 5 mg/minute

I.V. Detail pH: 3.4-4.0

Stability

Reconstitution Hydralazine should be diluted in NS for IVPB administration due to decreased stability in D_5W. Stability of IVPB solution in NS is 4 days at room temperature.

Storage Intact ampuls/vials of hydralazine should not be stored under refrigeration because of possible precipitation or crystallization.

Nursing Actions

Physical Assessment Orthostatic precautions should be observed and patient monitored closely during and following infusion. Monitor for hypotension and fluid retention periodically during therapy.

Patient Education Take with meals. Avoid alcohol. This medication does not replace other antihypertensive interventions; follow prescriber's instructions for diet and lifestyle changes. Weigh daily for the first 2 weeks and weekly thereafter. Report weight gain or swelling of feet or ankles. May cause dizziness, weakness, nausea, vomiting, or headache. Report skin rash, severe dizziness or loss of consciousness, significant weight gain, joint pain or swelling, or persistent GI problems.

Dietary Considerations Administer tablet with meals.

Hydrochlorothiazide

(hye droe klor oh THYE a zide)

Brand Names: U.S. Microzide®

Index Terms HCTZ (error-prone abbreviation); Hydrodiuril

Pharmacologic Category Diuretic, Thiazide

Medication Safety Issues

Sound-alike/look-alike issues:

HCTZ is an error-prone abbreviation (mistaken as hydrocortisone)

Hydrochlorothiazide may be confused with hydrocortisone, Viskazide®

Microzide™ may be confused with Maxzide®, Micronase®

International issues:

Esidrex [multiple international markets] may be confused with Lasix brand name for furosemide [U.S., Canada, and multiple international markets]

Esidrix [Germany] may be confused with Lasix brand name for furosemide [U.S., Canada, and multiple international markets]

Pregnancy Risk Factor B

Lactation Enters breast milk/not recommended (AAP rates "compatible"; AAP 2001 update pending)

Breast-Feeding Considerations Thiazide diuretics are found in breast milk. Following a single oral maternal dose of hydrochlorothiazide 50 mg, the mean breast milk concentration was 80 ng/mL (samples collected over 24 hours) and hydrochlorothiazide was not detected in the blood of the breast feeding infant (limit of detection 20 ng/mL). Peak plasma concentrations reported in adults following hydrochlorothiazide 12.5-100 mg are 70-490 ng/mL.

Use Management of mild-to-moderate hypertension; treatment of edema in heart failure and nephrotic syndrome

Unlabeled Use Treatment of lithium-induced diabetes insipidus

Mechanism of Action/Effect Inhibits sodium reabsorption in the distal tubules causing increased excretion of sodium and water as well as potassium and hydrogen ions

Contraindications Hypersensitivity to hydrochlorothiazide or any component of the formulation, thiazides, or sulfonamide-derived drugs; anuria; renal decompensation; pregnancy

Warnings/Precautions Avoid in severe renal disease (ineffective as a diuretic). Electrolyte disturbances (hypokalemia, hypochloremic alkalosis, hyponatremia) can occur. Use with caution in severe hepatic dysfunction; hepatic encephalopathy can be caused by electrolyte disturbances. Gout may be precipitated in certain patients with a history of gout, a familial predisposition to gout, or chronic renal failure. Thiazide diuretics reduce calcium excretion; pathologic changes in the parathyroid glands with hypercalcemia and hypophosphatemia have been observed with prolonged use. Use with caution in patients with prediabetes and diabetes; may alter glucose control. May cause SLE exacerbation or activation. Use with caution in patients with moderate or high cholesterol concentrations. Photosensitization may occur. Correct hypokalemia before initiating therapy. Thiazide diuretics may decrease renal calcium excretion; consider avoiding use in patients with hypercalcemia. May cause acute transient myopia and acute angle-closure glaucoma, typically occurring within hours to weeks following initiation; discontinue therapy immediately in patients with acute decreases in visual acuity or ocular pain. Risk factors may include a history of sulfonamide or penicillin allergy.

Chemical similarities are present among sulfonamides, sulfonylureas, carbonic anhydrase inhibitors, thiazides, and loop diuretics (except ethacrynic acid). Use in patients with sulfonamide allergy is specifically contraindicated in product labeling, however, a risk of cross-reaction exists in patients with allergy to any of these compounds; avoid use when previous reaction has been severe. Discontinue if signs of hypersensitivity are noted.

Drug Interactions

Avoid Concomitant Use

Avoid concomitant use of Hydrochlorothiazide with any of the following: Dofetilide

Decreased Effect

Hydrochlorothiazide may decrease the levels/effects of: Antidiabetic Agents

The levels/effects of Hydrochlorothiazide may be decreased by: Benazepril; Bile Acid Sequestrants; Herbs (Hypertensive Properties); Methylphenidate; Nonsteroidal Anti-Inflammatory Agents; Yohimbine

Increased Effect/Toxicity

Hydrochlorothiazide may increase the levels/effects of: ACE Inhibitors; Allopurinol; Amifostine; Antihypertensives; Benazepril; Calcium Salts; CarBAMazepine; Dofetilide; Hypotensive Agents; Lithium; OXcarbazepine; Porfimer; RiTUXimab; Sodium Phosphates; Topiramate; Toremifene; Valsartan; Vitamin D Analogs

The levels/effects of Hydrochlorothiazide may be increased by: Alcohol (Ethyl); Alfuzosin; Analgesics (Opioid); Barbiturates; Beta2-Agonists; Corticosteroids (Orally Inhaled); Corticosteroids (Systemic); Herbs (Hypotensive Properties); Licorice; MAO Inhibitors; Pentoxifylline; Phosphodiesterase 5 Inhibitors; Prostacyclin Analogues; Valsartan

Nutritional/Ethanol Interactions

Food: Hydrochlorothiazide peak serum levels may be decreased if taken with food. This product may deplete potassium, sodium, and magnesium.

Herb/Nutraceutical: Avoid herbs with *hypertensive* properties (bayberry, blue cohosh, cayenne, ephedra, ginger, ginseng [American], kola, licorice); may diminish the antihypertensive effect of hydrochlorothiazide. Avoid herbs with *hypotensive* properties (black cohosh, California poppy, coleus, golden seal, hawthorn, mistletoe, periwinkle, quinine, shepherd's purse); may enhance the hypotensive effect of hydrochlorothiazide.

Adverse Reactions Frequency not defined; adverse events reported were observed at doses ≥25 mg:

Cardiovascular: Hypotension, orthostatic hypotension

Central nervous system: Dizziness, fever, headache, vertigo

Dermatologic: Alopecia, erythema multiforme, exfoliative dermatitis, photosensitivity, purpura, rash, Stevens-Johnson syndrome, toxic epidermal necrolysis, urticaria

Endocrine & metabolic: Hyperglycemia, hypokalemia, hyperuricemia

Gastrointestinal: Anorexia, constipation, cramping, diarrhea, epigastric distress, gastric irritation, nausea, pancreatitis, sialadenitis, vomiting

Genitourinary: Glycosuria, impotence

Hematologic: Agranulocytosis, aplastic anemia, hemolytic anemia, leukopenia, thrombocytopenia

Hepatic: Jaundice

Neuromuscular & skeletal: Muscle spasm, paresthesia, restlessness, weakness

Ocular: Blurred vision (transient), xanthopsia

Renal: Interstitial nephritis, renal dysfunction, renal failure

Respiratory: Respiratory distress, pneumonitis, pulmonary edema

Miscellaneous: Anaphylactic reactions, necrotizing angiitis

Pharmacodynamics/Kinetics

Onset of Action Diuresis: ~2 hours; Peak effect: 4-6 hours

Duration of Action 6-12 hours

Available Dosage Forms

Capsule, oral: 12.5 mg

Microzide®: 12.5 mg

Tablet, oral: 12.5 mg, 25 mg, 50 mg

General Dosage Range Oral:

Children <6 months: 1-3 mg/kg/day in 2 divided doses

Children >6 months to 2 years: 1-3 mg/kg/day in 2 divided doses (maximum: 37.5 mg/day)

Children >2-17 years: Initial: 1 mg/kg/day (maximum: 3 mg/kg/day [50 mg/day])

Adults: 12.5-100 mg/day in 1-2 divided doses (maximum: 200 mg/day)

Elderly: 12.5-25 once daily

Administration

Oral May be administered with food or milk. Take early in day to avoid nocturia. Take the last dose of multiple doses no later than 6 PM unless instructed otherwise.

Nursing Actions

Physical Assessment Allergy history should be identified prior to beginning therapy (sulfonamides). Monitor for hypotension and hypokalemia.

Patient Education Follow prescriber's instructions for diet and lifestyle changes. Take with meals early in the day to avoid nocturia. Your physician may prescribe a potassium supplement or recommend that you eat foods high in potassium. Do not change your diet on your own while taking this medication, especially if you are taking potassium supplements or medications to reduce potassium loss. May cause dizziness, postural hypotension, or photosensitivity. Report palpitations, muscle cramping, or skin rash.

Dietary Considerations May be taken with food or milk.

Hydrochlorothiazide and Spironolactone

(hye droe klor oh THYE a zide & speer on oh LAK tone)

Brand Names: U.S. Aldactazide®

Index Terms Spironolactone and Hydrochlorothiazide

Pharmacologic Category Diuretic, Thiazide; Selective Aldosterone Blocker

Medication Safety Issues

Sound-alike/look-alike issues:

Aldactazide® may be confused with Aldactone®

Pregnancy Risk Factor C

Lactation Enters breast milk/not recommended

Use Management of mild-to-moderate hypertension; treatment of edema in congestive heart failure and nephrotic syndrome, and cirrhosis of the liver accompanied by edema and/or ascites

Available Dosage Forms

Tablet: Hydrochlorothiazide 25 mg and spironolactone 25 mg

Aldactazide®: 25/25: Hydrochlorothiazide 25 mg and spironolactone 25 mg; 50/50: Hydrochlorothiazide 50 mg and spironolactone 50 mg

General Dosage Range Oral: *Adults:* 12.5-50 mg hydrochlorothiazide and 12.5-50 mg spironolactone/day in 1-2 divided doses

Administration

Oral Administer in the morning; administer the last dose of multiple doses before 6 PM unless instructed otherwise.

Nursing Actions

Physical Assessment See individual agents.

Patient Education See individual agents.

Related Information

Hydrochlorothiazide *on page 570*

Spironolactone *on page 1059*

Hydrochlorothiazide and Triamterene

(hye droe klor oh THYE a zide & trye AM ter een)

Brand Names: U.S. Dyazide®; Maxzide®; Maxzide®-25

Index Terms Triamterene and Hydrochlorothiazide

Pharmacologic Category Diuretic, Potassium-Sparing; Diuretic, Thiazide

Medication Safety Issues

Sound-alike/look-alike issues:

Dyazide® may be confused with diazoxide, Dynacin®

Maxzide® may be confused with Maxidex®, Microzide®

Pregnancy Risk Factor C

Lactation Enters breast milk/not recommended

Use Treatment of hypertension or edema (not recommended for initial treatment) when hypokalemia has developed on hydrochlorothiazide alone or when the development of hypokalemia must be avoided

Available Dosage Forms

Capsule: Hydrochlorothiazide 25 mg and triamterene 37.5 mg; hydrochlorothiazide 25 mg and triamterene 50 mg

Dyazide®: Hydrochlorothiazide 25 mg and triamterene 37.5 mg

Tablet: Hydrochlorothiazide 25 mg and triamterene 37.5 mg; hydrochlorothiazide 50 mg and triamterene 75 mg

Maxzide®: Hydrochlorothiazide 50 mg and triamterene 75 mg [scored]

Maxzide®-25: Hydrochlorothiazide 25 mg and triamterene 37.5 mg [scored]

General Dosage Range Oral: *Adults:* 25-50 mg hydrochlorothiazide and 37.5-75 mg triamterene once daily

Nursing Actions

Physical Assessment See individual agents.

Patient Education See individual agents.

Related Information

Hydrochlorothiazide *on page 570*

Hydrocodone and Acetaminophen

(hye droe KOE done & a seet a MIN oh fen)

Brand Names: U.S. hycet®; Lorcet® 10/650; Lorcet® Plus; Lortab®; Margesic® H; Maxidone®; Norco®; Stagesic™; Vicodin®; Vicodin® ES; Vicodin® HP; Xodol® 10/300; Xodol® 5/300; Xodol® 7.5/300; Zamicet™; Zolvit®; Zydone®

Index Terms Acetaminophen and Hydrocodone

Pharmacologic Category Analgesic Combination (Opioid)

Medication Safety Issues

Sound-alike/look-alike issues:

Lorcet® may be confused with Fioricet®

Lortab® may be confused with Cortef®

Vicodin® may be confused with Hycodan, Indocin®

Zydone® may be confused with Vytone

High alert medication:

The Institute for Safe Medication Practices (ISMP) includes this medication among its list of drug classes which have a heightened risk of causing significant patient harm when used in error.

Other safety concerns:

Duplicate therapy issues: This product contains acetaminophen, which may be a component of other combination products. Do not exceed the maximum recommended daily dose of acetaminophen.

Pregnancy Risk Factor C

Lactation Enters breast milk/not recommended

Use Relief of moderate-to-severe pain

Controlled Substance C-III

Available Dosage Forms

Capsule, oral: Hydrocodone 5 mg and acetaminophen 500 mg

Margesic® H, Stagesic™: Hydrocodone 5 mg and acetaminophen 500 mg

Elixir, oral:

Lortab®: Hydrocodone 7.5 mg and acetaminophen 500 mg per 15 mL

Solution, oral: Hydrocodone 7.5 mg and acetaminophen 325 mg per 15 mL; hydrocodone 7.5 mg and acetaminophen 500 mg per 15 mL; hydrocodone 10 mg and acetaminophen 325 mg per 15 mL

hycet®: Hydrocodone 7.5 mg and acetaminophen 325 mg per 15 mL

Zamicet™: Hydrocodone 10 mg and acetaminophen 325 mg per 15 mL

Zolvit®: Hydrocodone 10 mg and acetaminophen 300 mg per 15 mL (480 mL)

Tablet, oral:

Generics:

Hydrocodone 2.5 mg and acetaminophen 500 mg

Hydrocodone 5 mg and acetaminophen 300 mg

Hydrocodone 5 mg and acetaminophen 325 mg

Hydrocodone 5 mg and acetaminophen 500 mg

Hydrocodone 7.5 mg and acetaminophen 300 mg

Hydrocodone 7.5 mg and acetaminophen 325 mg

Hydrocodone 7.5 mg and acetaminophen 500 mg

Hydrocodone 7.5 mg and acetaminophen 650 mg

Hydrocodone 7.5 mg and acetaminophen 750 mg

Hydrocodone 10 mg and acetaminophen 300 mg

Hydrocodone 10 mg and acetaminophen 325 mg

Hydrocodone 10 mg and acetaminophen 500 mg

Hydrocodone 10 mg and acetaminophen 650 mg

Hydrocodone 10 mg and acetaminophen 660 mg

Hydrocodone 10 mg and acetaminophen 750 mg

Brands:

Lorcet® 10/650: Hydrocodone 10 mg and acetaminophen 650 mg

Lorcet® Plus: Hydrocodone 7.5 mg and acetaminophen 650 mg

Lortab®: 5/500: Hydrocodone 5 mg and acetaminophen 500 mg; 7.5/500: Hydrocodone 7.5 mg and acetaminophen 500 mg; 10/500: Hydrocodone 10 mg and acetaminophen 500 mg

Maxidone®: Hydrocodone 10 mg and acetaminophen 750 mg

Norco®: Hydrocodone 5 mg and acetaminophen 325 mg; hydrocodone 7.5 mg and acetaminophen 325 mg; hydrocodone 10 mg and acetaminophen 325 mg

Vicodin®: Hydrocodone 5 mg and acetaminophen 500 mg

Vicodin® ES: Hydrocodone 7.5 mg and acetaminophen 750 mg

Vicodin® HP: Hydrocodone 10 mg and acetaminophen 660 mg

Xodol®: 5/300: Hydrocodone 5 mg and acetaminophen 300 mg; 7.5/300: Hydrocodone 7.5 mg and acetaminophen 300 mg; 10/300: Hydrocodone 10 mg and acetaminophen 300 mg

Zydone®: Hydrocodone 5 mg and acetaminophen 400 mg; hydrocodone 7.5 mg and acetaminophen 400 mg; hydrocodone 10 mg and acetaminophen 400 mg

General Dosage Range Oral:

Children 2-13 years or <50 kg: Hydrocodone 0.1-0.2 mg/kg/dose every 4-6 hours (maximum: 6 doses/day or maximum recommended dose of acetaminophen for age/weight)

Children ≥50 kg and Adults: Hydrocodone 2.5-10 mg every 4-6 hours (maximum: 4 g/day [acetaminophen])

Elderly: Hydrocodone 2.5-5 mg every 4-6 hours

Nursing Actions

Physical Assessment Assess patient for history of liver disease or ethanol abuse (acetaminophen and any ethanol may have adverse liver effects). Ensure adult patients keep daily dose to ≤4 g/day. Monitor for effectiveness of pain relief. Monitor blood pressure, CNS and respiratory status, and degree of sedation prior to treatment and periodically throughout. For inpatients, implement safety measures (eg, side rails up, call light within reach, instructions to call for assistance). Assess patient's physical and/or psychological dependence. Discontinue slowly after prolonged use.

Patient Education Oral: Take with food or milk. While using this medication, avoid alcohol and other prescription or OTC medications that contain acetaminophen. Keep dose to below accepted maximum level for specific age group or weight. Encourage patient to report if he/she took more than maximum dose. This medication will not reduce inflammation; consult prescriber for anti-inflammatory, if needed. Report unusual bleeding (stool, mouth, urine) or bruising, unusual fatigue and weakness, belly pain, yellow eyes or skin, or lack of appetite.

May cause physical and/or psychological dependence. Do not use sedatives, tranquilizers, antihistamines, or pain medications without consulting prescriber. Maintain adequate hydration, unless instructed to restrict fluid intake. May cause dizziness, drowsiness, confusion, agitation, impaired coordination, or blurred vision; nausea or vomiting; loss of appetite; or constipation (if unresolved, consult prescriber about use of stool softeners). Report confusion, excessive sedation or drowsiness, acute GI upset, respiratory difficulty or shortness of breath, rapid heartbeat, or palpitations.

Related Information

Acetaminophen *on page 23*

Hydrocodone and Ibuprofen

(hye droe KOE done & eye byoo PROE fen)

Brand Names: U.S. Ibudone™; Reprexain™; Vicoprofen®

Index Terms Hydrocodone Bitartrate and Ibuprofen; Ibuprofen and Hydrocodone

Pharmacologic Category Analgesic, Opioid; Nonsteroidal Anti-inflammatory Drug (NSAID), Oral

Medication Safety Issues

Sound-alike/look-alike issues:

Reprexain™ may be confused with ZyPREXA®

High alert medication:

The Institute for Safe Medication Practices (ISMP) includes this medication among its list of drug classes which have a heightened risk of causing significant patient harm when used in error.

Medication Guide Available Yes

Pregnancy Risk Factor C/D (3rd trimester)

Lactation Enters breast milk/not recommended

Use Short-term (generally <10 days) management of moderate-to-severe acute pain; is not indicated for treatment of such conditions as osteoarthritis or rheumatoid arthritis

Controlled Substance C-III

Available Dosage Forms

Tablet: Hydrocodone 5 mg and ibuprofen 200 mg; hydrocodone 7.5 mg and ibuprofen 200 mg

Ibudone™: 5/200: Hydrocodone 5 mg and ibuprofen 200 mg; 10/200: Hydrocodone 10 mg and ibuprofen 200 mg

Reprexain™: 2.5/200: Hydrocodone 2.5 mg and ibuprofen 200 mg; 5/200: Hydrocodone 5 mg and ibuprofen 200 mg; 10/200: Hydrocodone 10 mg and ibuprofen 200 mg

Vicoprofen®: 7.5/200: Hydrocodone 7.5 mg and ibuprofen 200 mg

General Dosage Range Oral: *Adults:* 1 tablet every 4-6 hours (maximum: 5 tablets/day; <10 days total therapy)

Nursing Actions

Physical Assessment Assess patient for allergic reaction to salicylates or other NSAIDs. Monitor blood pressure and for adverse gastrointestinal response prior to treatment and periodically throughout. Monitor for effectiveness of pain relief. Monitor CNS and respiratory status and degree of sedation prior to treatment and periodically throughout. For inpatients, implement safety measures (eg, side rails up, call light within reach, instructions to call for assistance). Assess patient's physical and/or psychological dependence. Discontinue slowly after prolonged use.

Patient Education Consult your prescriber before use if you have hypertension or heart failure. Do not take longer than 3 days for fever or 10 days for pain without consulting prescriber. Take with food or milk. Do not use alcohol. Maintain adequate hydration, unless instructed to restrict fluid intake. You may experience nausea, vomiting, or gastric discomfort. GI bleeding, ulceration, or perforation can occur with or without pain. Stop taking medication and report ringing in ears, persistent cramping or stomach pain, unresolved nausea or vomiting, respiratory difficulty or shortness of breath, unusual bruising or bleeding (mouth, urine, stool), skin rash, unusual swelling of extremities, chest pain, or palpitations. May cause physical and/or psychological dependence. Do not use sedatives, tranquilizers, antihistamines, or pain medications without consulting prescriber. May cause dizziness, drowsiness, confusion, agitation, impaired coordination, or blurred vision; loss of appetite; or constipation (if unresolved, consult prescriber about use of stool softeners). Report confusion, excessive sedation or drowsiness, acute GI upset, respiratory difficulty or shortness of breath, rapid heartbeat, or palpitations.

Related Information

Ibuprofen *on page* 588

Hydrocortisone (Systemic)

(hye droe KOR ti sone)

Brand Names: U.S. A-Hydrocort®; Cortef®; Solu-CORTEF®

Index Terms A-hydroCort; Compound F; Cortisol; Hydrocortisone Sodium Succinate

Pharmacologic Category Corticosteroid, Systemic

Medication Safety Issues

Sound-alike/look-alike issues:

Hydrocortisone may be confused with hydrocodone, hydroxychloroquine, hydrochlorothiazide

Cortef® may be confused with Coreg®, Lortab®

HCT (occasional abbreviation for hydrocortisone) is an error-prone abbreviation (mistaken as hydrochlorothiazide)

Solu-CORTEF® may be confused with Solu-MEDROL®

Pregnancy Risk Factor C

Lactation Enters breast milk/use caution

Breast-Feeding Considerations Corticosteroids are excreted in breast milk and endogenous hydrocortisone is also found in human milk; the effect of maternal hydrocortisone intake is not known.

Use Management of adrenocortical insufficiency; anti-inflammatory or immunosuppressive

Unlabeled Use Management of septic shock when blood pressure is poorly responsive to fluid resuscitation and vasopressor therapy; treatment of thyroid storm

Mechanism of Action/Effect Decreases inflammation by suppression of migration of polymorphonuclear leukocytes and reversal of increased capillary permeability

Contraindications Hypersensitivity to hydrocortisone or any component of the formulation; serious infections, except septic shock or tuberculous meningitis; viral, fungal, or tubercular skin lesions; I.M. administration contraindicated in idiopathic thrombocytopenia purpura; intrathecal administration of injection

Warnings/Precautions Use with caution in patients with thyroid disease, hepatic impairment, renal impairment, heart failure, hypertension, diabetes, glaucoma, cataracts, myasthenia gravis, patients at risk for osteoporosis, patients at risk for seizures, or GI diseases (diverticulitis, peptic ulcer, ulcerative colitis) due to perforation risk. Use caution following acute MI (corticosteroids have been associated with myocardial rupture). Because of the risk of adverse effects, systemic corticosteroids should be used cautiously in the elderly in the smallest possible effective dose for the shortest duration. May affect growth velocity; growth should be routinely monitored in pediatric patients. Withdraw therapy with gradual tapering of dose.

May cause hypercorticism or suppression of hypothalamic-pituitary-adrenal (HPA) axis, particularly in younger children or in patients receiving high doses for prolonged periods. HPA axis suppression may lead to adrenal crisis. Withdrawal and discontinuation of a corticosteroid should be done slowly and carefully. Particular care is required when patients are transferred from systemic corticosteroids to inhaled products due to possible adrenal insufficiency or withdrawal from steroids, including an increase in allergic symptoms. Patients receiving >20 mg per day of prednisone (or equivalent) may be most susceptible. Fatalities have occurred due to adrenal insufficiency in asthmatic patients during and after transfer from systemic corticosteroids to aerosol steroids; aerosol steroids do not provide the systemic steroid needed to treat patients having trauma, surgery, or infections.

Acute myopathy has been reported with high dose corticosteroids, usually in patients with neuromuscular transmission disorders; may involve ocular and/or respiratory muscles; monitor creatine kinase; recovery may be delayed. Corticosteroid use may cause psychiatric disturbances, including depression, euphoria, insomnia, mood swings, and personality changes. Pre-existing psychiatric conditions may be exacerbated by corticosteroid use. Prolonged use of corticosteroids may also increase the incidence of secondary infection, mask acute infection (including fungal infections), prolong or exacerbate viral infections, or limit response to vaccines. Exposure to chickenpox should be avoided; corticosteroids should not be used to treat ocular herpes simplex. Corticosteroids should not be used for cerebral malaria or viral hepatitis. Oral steroid treatment is not recommended for the treatment of acute optic neuritis. Close observation is required in patients with latent tuberculosis and/or TB reactivity; restrict use in active TB (only in conjunction with antituberculosis treatment). Prolonged treatment with corticosteroids has been associated with the development of Kaposi's sarcoma (case reports); if noted, discontinuation of therapy should be considered. High-dose corticosteroids should not be used to manage acute head injury. Some dosage forms contain benzyl alcohol which has been associated with "gasping syndrome" in neonates.

Drug Interactions

Avoid Concomitant Use

Avoid concomitant use of Hydrocortisone (Systemic) with any of the following: Aldesleukin; Axitinib; BCG; Natalizumab; Pimecrolimus; Tacrolimus (Topical)

Decreased Effect

Hydrocortisone (Systemic) may decrease the levels/effects of: Aldesleukin; Antidiabetic Agents; ARIPiprazole; Axitinib; BCG; Calcitriol; Coccidioidin Skin Test; Corticorelin; Isoniazid; Salicylates; Sipuleucel-T; Telaprevir; Vaccines (Inactivated)

The levels/effects of Hydrocortisone (Systemic) may be decreased by: Aminoglutethimide; Antacids; Barbiturates; Bile Acid Sequestrants; Echinacea; Mitotane; P-glycoprotein/ABCB1 Inducers; Primidone; Rifamycin Derivatives; Tocilizumab

Increased Effect/Toxicity

Hydrocortisone (Systemic) may increase the levels/effects of: Acetylcholinesterase Inhibitors; Amphotericin B; Deferasirox; Leflunomide; Loop Diuretics; Natalizumab; NSAID (COX-2 Inhibitor); NSAID (Nonselective); Thiazide Diuretics; Vaccines (Live); Warfarin

The levels/effects of Hydrocortisone (Systemic) may be increased by: Antifungal Agents (Azole Derivatives, Systemic); Aprepitant; Calcium Channel Blockers (Nondihydropyridine); Conivaptan; Denosumab; Estrogen Derivatives; Fluconazole; Fosaprepitant; Indacaterol; Macrolide Antibiotics; Neuromuscular-Blocking Agents (Nondepolarizing); P-glycoprotein/ABCB1 Inhibitors; Pimecrolimus; Quinolone Antibiotics; Roflumilast; Salicylates; Tacrolimus (Topical); Telaprevir; Trastuzumab

Nutritional/Ethanol Interactions

Ethanol: Avoid ethanol (may enhance gastric mucosal irritation).

Food: Hydrocortisone interferes with calcium absorption.

Herb/Nutraceutical: St John's wort may decrease hydrocortisone levels. Avoid cat's claw, echinacea (have immunostimulant properties).

Adverse Reactions Frequency not defined.

Cardiovascular: Arrhythmias, bradycardia, cardiac arrest, cardiomegaly, circulatory collapse, congestive heart failure, edema, fat embolism, hypertension, hypertrophic cardiomyopathy (premature infants), myocardial rupture (post MI), syncope, tachycardia, thromboembolism, vasculitis

Central nervous system: Delirium, depression, emotional instability, euphoria, hallucinations, headache, insomnia, intracranial pressure increased, malaise, mood swings, nervousness, neuritis, neuropathy, personality changes, pseudotumor cerebri, psychic disorders, psychoses, seizure, vertigo

Dermatologic: Acne, allergic dermatitis, alopecia, bruising, burning/tingling, dry scaly skin, edema, erythema, hirsutism, hyper-/hypopigmentation, impaired wound healing, petechiae, rash, skin atrophy, skin test reaction impaired, sterile abscess, striae, urticaria

Endocrine & metabolic: Adrenal suppression, alkalosis, amenorrhea, carbohydrate intolerance increased, Cushing's syndrome, diabetes mellitus, glucose intolerance, growth suppression, hyperglycemia, hyperlipidemia, hypokalemia, hypokalemic alkalosis, menstrual irregularities, negative nitrogen balance, pituitary-adrenal axis suppression, potassium loss, protein catabolism, sodium and water retention, sperm motility increased/decreased, spermatogenesis increased/decreased

Gastrointestinal: Abdominal distention, appetite increased, bowel dysfunction (intrathecal administration), indigestion, nausea, pancreatitis, peptic ulcer, gastrointestinal perforation, ulcerative esophagitis, vomiting, weight gain

Genitourinary: Bladder dysfunction (intrathecal administration)

Hematologic: Leukocytosis (transient)

Hepatic: Hepatomegaly, transaminases increased

Local: Atrophy (at injection site), postinjection flare (intra-articular use), thrombophlebitis

Neuromuscular & skeletal: Arthralgia, necrosis (femoral and humoral heads), Charcot-like arthropathy, fractures, muscle mass loss, muscle weakness, myopathy, osteoporosis, tendon rupture, vertebral compression fractures

Ocular: Cataracts, exophthalmoses, glaucoma, intraocular pressure increased

Miscellaneous: Abnormal fat deposits, anaphylaxis, avascular necrosis, diaphoresis, hiccups, hypersensitivity reactions, infection, secondary malignancy

Pharmacodynamics/Kinetics

Onset of Action Hydrocortisone sodium succinate (water soluble): Rapid

Available Dosage Forms

Injection, powder for reconstitution:

A-Hydrocort®: 100 mg

Solu-CORTEF®: 100 mg

Injection, powder for reconstitution [preservative free]:

Solu-CORTEF®: 100 mg, 250 mg, 500 mg, 1000 mg

Tablet, oral: 5 mg, 10 mg, 20 mg

Cortef®: 5 mg, 10 mg, 20 mg

General Dosage Range

I.M., I.V.: *Children and Adults:* Dosage varies greatly depending on indication

Oral:

Children: 0.5-10 mg/kg/day **or** 10-300 mg/m^2/day divided every 6-8 hours

Adolescents: 0.5-10 mg/kg/day **or** 10-300 mg/m^2/day divided every 6-8 hours **or** 15-240 mg every 12 hours

Adults: 20-480 mg/day in divided doses every 8-12 hours **or** 10-20 mg/m^2/day in 3 divided doses

Administration

Oral Administer with food or milk to decrease GI upset.

I.V.

Parenteral: Hydrocortisone sodium succinate may be administered by I.M. or I.V. routes.

Dermal and/or subdermal skin depression may occur at the site of injection. Avoid injection into deltoid muscle (high incidence of subcutaneous atrophy).

I.V. bolus: Dilute to 50 mg/mL and administer over 30 seconds or over 10 minutes for doses ≥500 mg

I.V. intermittent infusion: Dilute to 1 mg/mL and give over 20-30 minutes.

Note: Should be administered in a 0.1-1 mg/mL concentration due to stability problems.

I.V. Detail pH: Hydrocortisone sodium succinate: 7-8

Stability

Reconstitution

Sodium succinate: Reconstitute 100 mg vials with bacteriostatic water (not >2 mL). Act-O-Vial (self-contained powder for injection plus diluent) may be reconstituted by pressing the activator to force diluent into the powder compartment. Following gentle agitation, solution may be withdrawn via syringe through a needle inserted into the center of the stopper. May be administered (I.V. or I.M.) without further dilution.

Solutions for I.V. infusion: Reconstituted solutions may be added to an appropriate volume of compatible solution for infusion. Concentration should generally not exceed 1 mg/mL. However, in cases where administration of a small volume of fluid is desirable, 100-3000 mg may be added to 50 mL of D_5W or NS (stability limited to 4 hours).

Storage Store at controlled room temperature 20°C to 25°C (68°F to 77°F). Protect from light. Hydrocortisone sodium phosphate and hydrocortisone sodium succinate are clear, light yellow solutions which are heat labile.

Sodium succinate: After initial reconstitution, hydrocortisone sodium succinate solutions are stable for 3 days at room temperature or under refrigeration when protected from light. Stability of parenteral admixture (Solu-Cortef®) at room temperature (25°C) and at refrigeration temperature (4°C) is concentration-dependent:

Stability of concentration 1 mg/mL: 24 hours.

Stability of concentration 2 mg/mL to 60 mg/mL: At least 4 hours.

Nursing Actions

Physical Assessment Assess for signs of fluid retention, signs of hyperglycemia, or infection. Taper dosage slowly when discontinuing if patient has been on for a period of time; assess tolerance of taper (BP, pulse, mentation, energy level). Do not use with existing fungal infections.

Patient Education Dosage is usually tapered off gradually. Take oral dose with food to reduce GI upset. Avoid alcohol. Hydrocortisone may cause immunosuppression and mask symptoms of infection; avoid exposure to contagion and notify prescriber of any signs of infection (eg, fever, chills, sore throat, injury) and notify dentist or surgeon (if necessary) that you are taking this medication. Notify prescriber if exposed to chicken pox or measles. Avoid live vaccines during this time. Call for help immediately with shortness of breath; swelling of face, lips, tongue, or throat; abdominal pain; vomiting; or bloody or tarry stools. You may experience increased appetite, indigestion, or increased nervousness. Notify prescriber with weight gain, blurred vision, swelling of extremities, fatigue, anorexia, weakness, increased urination, or unusual mood swings.

Dietary Considerations Systemic use of corticosteroids may require a diet with increased potassium, vitamins A, B_6, C, D, folate, calcium, zinc, phosphorus, and decreased sodium. Some products may contain sodium.

Hydrocortisone (Topical)

(hye droe KOR ti sone)

Brand Names: U.S. Ala-Cort; Ala-Scalp; Anu-med HC; Anucort-HC™; Anusol-HC®; Aquanil HC® [OTC]; Beta-HC® [OTC]; Caldecort® [OTC]; Colocort®; Cortaid® Advanced [OTC]; Cortaid® Intensive Therapy [OTC]; Cortaid® Maximum Strength [OTC]; Cortenema®; CortiCool® [OTC]; Cortifoam®; Cortizone-10® Hydratensive Healing [OTC]; Cortizone-10® Hydratensive Soothing [OTC]; Cortizone-10® Intensive Healing Eczema [OTC]; Cortizone-10® Maximum Strength Cooling Relief [OTC]; Cortizone-10® Maximum Strength Easy Relief [OTC]; Cortizone-10® Maximum Strength Intensive Healing Formula [OTC]; Cortizone-10® Maximum Strength [OTC]; Cortizone-10® Plus Maximum Strength [OTC]; Dermarest® Eczema Medicated [OTC]; Hemril® -30; Hydrocortisone Plus [OTC]; Hydroskin® [OTC]; Locoid Lipocream®; Locoid®; Pandel®; Pediaderm™ HC; Preparation H® Hydrocortisone [OTC]; Procto-Pak™; Proctocort®; ProctoCream®-HC; Proctosol-HC®; Proctozone-HC 2.5%™; Recort [OTC]; Scalpana [OTC]; Texacort™; U-Cort®; Westcort®

Index Terms A-hydroCort; Compound F; Cortisol; Hemorrhoidal HC; Hydrocortisone Acetate; Hydrocortisone Butyrate; Hydrocortisone Probutate; Hydrocortisone Valerate; Nutracort

Pharmacologic Category Corticosteroid, Rectal; Corticosteroid, Topical

Medication Safety Issues

Sound-alike/look-alike issues:

Hydrocortisone may be confused with hydrocodone, hydroxychloroquine, hydrochlorothiazide

Anusol® may be confused with Anusol-HC®, Aplisol®, Aquasol®

Cortizone® may be confused with cortisone

HCT (occasional abbreviation for hydrocortisone) is an error-prone abbreviation (mistaken as hydrochlorothiazide)

Hytone® may be confused with Vytone®

Proctocort® may be confused with ProctoCream®

International issues:

Nutracort [multiple international markets] may be confused with Nitrocor brand name of nitroglycerin [Italy, Russia, and Venezuela]

Pregnancy Risk Factor C

Lactation Enters breast milk/use caution

Use Relief of inflammation of corticosteroid-responsive dermatoses (low and medium potency topical corticosteroid); adjunctive treatment of ulcerative colitis; mild-to-moderate atopic dermatitis; inflamed hemorrhoids, postirradiation (factitial) proctitis, and other inflammatory conditions of anorectum and pruritus ani

Available Dosage Forms

Aerosol, foam, rectal:

Cortifoam®: 10% (15 g)

Cream, topical: 0.1% (15 g, 45 g); 0.2% (15 g, 45 g, 60 g); 0.5% (0.9 g, 15 g, 28.4 g, 30 g, 60 g); 1% (0.9 g, 1 g, 1.5 g, 15 g, 20 g, 28.35 g, 28.4 g, 30 g, 114 g, 120 g, 454 g); 2% (43 g); 2.5% (20 g, 28 g, 28.35 g, 30 g, 454 g)

Ala-Cort: 1% (28.4 g, 85.2 g)

Anusol-HC®: 2.5% (30 g)

Caldecort® [OTC]: 1% (28.4 g)

Cortaid® Advanced [OTC]: 1% (42 g)

Cortaid® Intensive Therapy [OTC]: 1% (37 g, 56 g)

Cortaid® Maximum Strength [OTC]: 1% (14 g, 28 g, 37 g, 56 g)

Cortizone-10® Maximum Strength [OTC]: 1% (15 g, 28 g, 56 g)

Cortizone-10® Maximum Strength Intensive Healing Formula [OTC]: 1% (28 g, 56 g)

Cortizone-10® Plus Maximum Strength [OTC]: 1% (28 g, 56 g)

Hydrocortisone Plus [OTC]: 1% (28.4 g)

Hydroskin® [OTC]: 1% (28 g)

Locoid Lipocream®: 0.1% (15 g, 45 g, 60 g)

Locoid®: 0.1% (15 g, 45 g)

Pandel®: 0.1% (15 g, 45 g, 80 g)

Preparation H® Hydrocortisone [OTC]: 1% (26 g)

Procto-Pak™: 1% (28.4 g)

Proctocort®: 1% (28.35 g)

ProctoCream®-HC: 2.5% (30 g)

Proctosol-HC®: 2.5% (28.35 g)

Proctozone-HC 2.5%™: 2.5% (30 g)

Recort [OTC]: 1% (30 g)

U-Cort®: 1% (28 g)

Gel, topical:

CortiCool® [OTC]: 1% (0.9 g, 42.5 g)

Cortizone-10® Maximum Strength Cooling Relief [OTC]: 1% (28 g)

Liquid, topical:

Cortizone-10® Maximum Strength Easy Relief [OTC]: 1% (36 mL)

Scalpana [OTC]: 1% (85.5 mL)

Lotion, topical: 1% (114 g, 118 mL, 120 mL); 2.5% (59 mL, 60 mL, 118 mL)

Ala-Scalp: 2% (29.6 mL)

Aquanil HC® [OTC]: 1% (120 mL)

Beta-HC® [OTC]: 1% (60 mL)

Cortaid® Intensive Therapy [OTC]: 1% (98 g)

Cortizone-10® Hydratensive Healing [OTC]: 1% (113 g)

Cortizone-10® Hydratensive Soothing [OTC]: 1% (113 g)

Cortizone-10® Intensive Healing Eczema [OTC]: 1% (99 g)

Dermarest® Eczema Medicated [OTC]: 1% (118 mL)

Hydroskin® [OTC]: 1% (118 mL)

Locoid®: 0.1% (60 mL)

Pediaderm™ HC: 2% (29.6 mL)

Ointment, topical: 0.1% (15 g, 45 g); 0.2% (15 g, 45 g, 60 g); 0.5% (30 g); 1% (25 g, 28.4 g, 30 g, 110 g, 430 g, 454 g); 2.5% (20 g, 28.35 g, 30 g, 454 g)

Cortaid® Maximum Strength [OTC]: 1% (28 g, 37 g)

Cortizone-10® Maximum Strength [OTC]: 1% (28 g, 56 g)

Locoid®: 0.1% (15 g, 45 g)

Westcort®: 0.2% (45 g, 60 g)

Powder, for prescription compounding: USP: 100% (10 g, 25 g, 50 g, 100 g, 1000 g)

Solution, topical: 0.1% (20 mL, 60 mL)

Cortaid® Intensive Therapy [OTC]: 1% (59 mL)

Locoid®: 0.1% (20 mL, 60 mL)

Texacort™: 2.5% (30 mL)

Suppository, rectal: 25 mg (12s, 24s, 1000s); 30 mg (12s)

Anu-med HC: 25 mg (12s)

Anucort-HC™: 25 mg (12s, 24s, 100s)

Anusol-HC®: 25 mg (12s, 24s)

Hemril® -30: 30 mg (12s, 24s)

Proctocort®: 30 mg (12s, 24s)

Suspension, rectal: 100 mg/60 mL (60 mL)

Colocort®: 100 mg/60 mL (60 mL)

Cortenema®: 100 mg/60 mL (60 mL)

General Dosage Range

Rectal: *Adults:* Foam: One applicatorful 1-2 times/day; Suppository: 1-2 suppositories 2-3 times/day; Suspension: One enema at bedtime

Topical: *Children and Adults:* Apply thin film to affected area 2-4 times/day

Administration

Topical

Topical cream, lotion, ointment: Apply a thin film to clean, dry skin and rub in gently.

Rectal foam: Shake vigorously for 5-10 seconds prior to use. Do not remove cap during use. Hold container upright to fill applicator. Gently insert applicator tip into anus. Only use applicator provided by manufacturer; do not insert any part of the aerosol container in the anus. Clean applicator after each use.

Rectal suppository: Remove foil from rectal suppository and insert pointed end first. Avoid handling unwrapped suppository for too long.

Rectal suspension: Shake bottle well. Remove protective sheath from applicator tip. Lie on left side with left leg extended and right leg flexed forward. Gently insert lubricated applicator tip into rectum, pointed slightly toward navel. Grasp bottle firmly and squeeze slowly to instill the medication. After administering, withdraw and discard the used unit. Remain in position for at least 30 minutes. Retain the enema all night if possible.

Nursing Actions

Physical Assessment Topical absorption may be minimal.

Patient Education

Topical: Before applying, wash area gently and thoroughly. Apply a thin film to cleansed area and rub in gently until medication vanishes. Avoid use of occlusive dressings over topical application unless directed by a prescriber. Avoid use on weeping or exudative lesions. Avoid exposing affected area to sunlight; you will be more sensitive and severe sunburn may occur.

Rectal: Gently insert suppository as high as possible with gloved finger while lying down. Remain in resting position for 10 minutes after insertion.

Enema: When patient is in the proper position, insert applicator tip rectally. Slowly squeeze to instill medication. Maintain patient in position for at least 30 minutes.

HYDROmorphone (hye droe MOR fone)

Brand Names: U.S. Dilaudid-HP®; Dilaudid®; Exalgo™

Index Terms Dihydromorphinone; Hydromorphone Hydrochloride

Pharmacologic Category Analgesic, Opioid

Medication Safety Issues

Sound-alike/look-alike issues:

Dilaudid® may be confused with Demerol®, Dilantin®

HYDROmorphone may be confused with morphine; significant overdoses have occurred when hydromorphone products have been inadvertently administered instead of morphine sulfate. Commercially available prefilled syringes of both products looks similar and are often stored in close proximity to each other. **Note:** Hydromorphone 1 mg oral is approximately equal to morphine 4 mg oral; hydromorphone 1 mg I.V. is approximately equal to morphine 5 mg I.V.

High alert medication:

The Institute for Safe Medication Practices (ISMP) includes this medication among its list of drug classes which have a heightened risk of causing significant patient harm when used in error.

Administration issues:

Dilaudid®, Dilaudid-HP®: Extreme caution should be taken to avoid confusing the highly-concentrated (Dilaudid-HP®) injection with the less-concentrated (Dilaudid®) injectable product.

Exalgo™: Extreme caution should be taken to avoid confusing the extended release Exalgo™ 8 mg tablets with immediate release hydromorphone 8 mg tablets.

Significant differences exist between oral and I.V. dosing. Use caution when converting from one route of administration to another.

Medication Guide Available Yes

Pregnancy Risk Factor C

Lactation Enters breast milk/not recommended

Breast-Feeding Considerations Low concentrations of hydromorphone can be found in breast milk. Withdrawal symptoms may be observed in breast-feeding infants when opioid analgesics are discontinued. Breast-feeding is not recommended.

Use Management of moderate-to-severe pain

Exalgo™: Management of moderate-to-severe pain in opioid-tolerant patients (requiring around-the-clock analgesia for an extended period of time)

Mechanism of Action/Effect Binds to opiate receptors in the CNS, causing inhibition of ascending pain pathways, altering the perception of and response to pain; causes cough supression by direct central action in the medulla; produces generalized CNS depression

Contraindications Hypersensitivity to hydromorphone, any component of the formulation; acute or severe asthma, severe respiratory depression (in absence of resuscitative equipment or ventilatory support); severe CNS depression

Additional product-specific contraindications:

Dilaudid®, Dilaudid-HP®: Obstetrical analgesia

Exalgo™: Opioid nontolerant patients, paralytic ileus, preexisting GI surgery or diseases resulting in narrowing of GI tract, loops in the GI tract or GI obstruction

Warnings/Precautions Use with caution in patients with hypersensitivity reactions to other phenanthrene derivative opioid agonists (codeine, hydrocodone, levorphanol, oxycodone, oxymorphone). Hydromorphone shares toxic potential of opiate agonists, including CNS depression and respiratory depression. Precautions associated with opiate agonist therapy should be observed. May cause CNS depression, which may impair physical or mental abilities; patients must be cautioned about performing tasks which require mental alertness (eg, operating machinery or driving). Myoclonus and seizures have been reported with high doses. Critical respiratory depression may occur, even at therapeutic dosages, particularly in elderly or debilitated patients or in patients with pre-existing respiratory compromise (hypoxia and/or hypercapnia). Use caution in COPD or other obstructive pulmonary disease. Use with caution in patients with hypersensitivity to other phenanthrene opiates, kyphoscoliosis, cardiovascular disease, morbid obesity, adrenocortical insufficiency, hypothyroidism, acute alcoholism, delirium tremens, toxic psychoses, prostatic hyperplasia and/or urinary stricture, or severe liver or renal failure. Use with caution in patients with biliary tract dysfunction. Hydromorphone may increase biliary tract pressure following spasm in sphincter of Oddi. Use caution in patients with inflammatory or obstructive bowel disorder, acute pancreatitis secondary to biliary tract disease, and patients undergoing biliary surgery. Use extreme caution in patients with head injury, intracranial lesions, or elevated intracranial pressure; exaggerated elevation of ICP may occur (in addition, hydromorphone may complicate neurologic evaluation due to pupillary dilation and CNS depressant effects). Use with caution in patients with depleted blood volume or drugs which may exaggerate hypotensive effects (including phenothiazines or general anesthetics). May obscure diagnosis or clinical course of patients with acute abdominal conditions.

[U.S. Boxed Warning]: Hydromorphone has a high potential for abuse. Those at risk for opioid abuse include patients with a history of substance abuse or mental illness. Tolerance or drug dependence may result from extended use; however, concerns for abuse should not prevent effective management of pain. In general, abrupt discontinuation of therapy in dependent patients should be avoided.

An opioid-containing analgesic regimen should be tailored to each patient's needs and based upon the type of pain being treated (acute versus chronic), the route of administration, degree of tolerance for opioids (naive versus chronic user), age, weight, and medical condition. The optimal analgesic dose varies widely among patients. Doses should be titrated to pain relief/prevention. I.M. use may result in variable absorption and a lag time to peak effect.

Dosage form specific warnings:

[U.S. Boxed Warning]: Dilaudid-HP®: Extreme caution should be taken to avoid confusing the highly-concentrated (Dilaudid-HP®) injection with the less-concentrated (Dilaudid®) injectable product. Dilaudid-HP® should only be used in patients who are opioid-tolerant.

Controlled release: Capsules should only be used when continuous analgesia is required over an extended period of time. Controlled release products are not to be used on an "as needed" (PRN) basis.

Extended release tablets (Exalgo™): **[U.S. Boxed Warning]: For use in opioid tolerant patients only; fatal respiratory depression may occur in patient who are not opioid tolerant. Indicated for the management of moderate-to-severe pain when around the clock pain control is needed for an extended time period. Not for use as an as-needed analgesic or for the management of acute or postoperative pain. Tablets should be swallowed whole; do not crush, break, chew, dissolve or inject; doing so may lead to rapid release and absorption of a potentially fatal dose of hydromorphone. Accidental consumption may lead to fatal overdose, especially in children.** Exalgo™ tablets are nondeformable; do not administer to patients with preexisting severe gastrointestinal narrowing (eg, esophageal motility, small bowel inflammatory disease, short gut syndrome, history of peritonitis, cystic fibrosis, chronic intestinal pseudo-obstruction, Meckel's diverticulum); obstruction may occur. Exalgo™ is not recommended for use within 14 days of MAO inhibitors; severe and unpredictable potentiation by MAO inhibitors has been reported with opioid analgesics

Some dosage forms contain trace amounts of sodium metabisulfite which may cause allergic reactions in susceptible individuals.

Drug Interactions

Avoid Concomitant Use

Avoid concomitant use of HYDROmorphone with any of the following: MAO Inhibitors

Decreased Effect

HYDROmorphone may decrease the levels/effects of: Pegvisomant

The levels/effects of HYDROmorphone may be decreased by: Ammonium Chloride; Mixed Agonist / Antagonist Opioids

Increased Effect/Toxicity

HYDROmorphone may increase the levels/effects of: Alcohol (Ethyl); Alvimopan; CNS Depressants; Desmopressin; Selective Serotonin Reuptake Inhibitors; Thiazide Diuretics

The levels/effects of HYDROmorphone may be increased by: Amphetamines; Antipsychotic Agents (Phenothiazines); Droperidol; HydrOXYzine; MAO Inhibitors; Succinylcholine

Nutritional/Ethanol Interactions

Ethanol: Ethanol may increase CNS depression. Management: Monitor for increased effects with coadministration. Caution patients about effects.

Herb/Nutraceutical: Gotu kola, valerian, and kava kava may increase CNS depression. Management: Avoid gotu kola, valerian, and kava kava.

Adverse Reactions Frequency not defined.

Cardiovascular: Bradycardia, extrasystoles, flushing of face, hyper-/hypotension, palpitation, peripheral edema, peripheral vasodilation, syncope, tachycardia

Central nervous system: Abnormal dreams, abnormal feelings, agitation, aggression, apprehension, attention disturbances, chills, coordination impaired, CNS depression, confusion, cognitive disorder, crying, dizziness, drowsiness, dysphoria, encephalopathy, euphoria, fatigue, hallucinations, headache, hyper-reflexia, hypo/hyperesthesia, hypothermia, increased intracranial pressure, insomnia, lightheadedness, listlessness, malaise, memory impairment, mental depression, mood alterations, nervousness, panic attacks, paranoia, psychomotor hyperactivity, restlessness, sedation, seizure, somnolence, suicide ideation, vertigo

Dermatologic: Hyperhidrosis, pruritus, rash, urticaria

Endocrine & metabolic: Amylase decreased, dehydration, erectile dysfunction, fluid retention, hyperuricemia, hypogonadism, hypokalemia, libido decreased, sexual dysfunction, testosterone decreased

Gastrointestinal: Abdominal distention, anal fissure, anorexia, appetite increased, bezoar (Exalgo™), biliary tract spasm, constipation, diarrhea, diverticulum, diverticulitis, duodenitis, dysgeusia, dysphagia, eructation, flatulence, gastric emptying impaired, gastrointestinal motility disorder (Exalgo™), gastroenteritis, hematochezia, ileus, intestinal obstruction (Exalgo™), large intestine perforation (Exalgo™), nausea, painful defecation, paralytic ileus, stomach cramps, taste perversion, vomiting, weight loss, xerostomia

Genitourinary: Dysuria, micturition disorder, ureteral spasm, urinary frequency, urinary hesitation, urinary retention, urinary tract spasm, urination decreased

Hepatic: LFTs increased

Local: Pain at injection site (I.M.), wheal/flare over vein (I.V.)

Neuromuscular & skeletal: Arthralgia, dysarthria, dyskinesia, muscle rigidity, muscle spasms, myalgia, myoclonus, paresthesia, trembling, tremor, uncoordinated muscle movements, weakness

Ocular: Blurred vision, diplopia, dry eyes, miosis, nystagmus

Otic: Tinnitus

Respiratory: Apnea, bronchospasm, dyspnea, hyperventilation, hypoxia, laryngospasm, oxygen saturation decreased, respiratory depression/distress, rhinorrhea

Miscellaneous: Antidiuretic effects, balance disorder, diaphoresis, difficulty walking, histamine release, physical and psychological dependence

Pharmacodynamics/Kinetics

Onset of Action Analgesic: Immediate release formulations:

Oral: 15-30 minutes; Peak effect: 30-60 minutes

I.V.: 5 minutes; Peak effect: 10-20 minutes

Duration of Action Immediate release formulations: Oral, I.V.: 4-5 hours

Controlled Substance C-II

Available Dosage Forms

Injection, powder for reconstitution:

Dilaudid-HP®: 250 mg

Injection, solution: 1 mg/mL (1 mL); 2 mg/mL (1 mL, 20 mL); 4 mg/mL (1 mL); 10 mg/mL (1 mL, 5 mL, 50 mL)

Dilaudid-HP®: 10 mg/mL (1 mL, 5 mL, 50 mL)

Dilaudid®: 1 mg/mL (1 mL); 2 mg/mL (1 mL); 4 mg/mL (1 mL)

Injection, solution [preservative free]: 10 mg/mL (1 mL, 5 mL, 50 mL)

Liquid, oral:

Dilaudid®: 1 mg/mL (473 mL)

Powder, for prescription compounding: USP: 100% (972 mg)

Suppository, rectal: 3 mg (6s)

Tablet, oral: 2 mg, 4 mg, 8 mg

Dilaudid®: 2 mg, 4 mg, 8 mg

Tablet, extended release, oral:

Exalgo™: 8 mg, 12 mg, 16 mg

General Dosage Range Dosage adjustment recommended in patients with hepatic or renal impairment

I.M., SubQ: *Children >50 kg and Adults:* 0.8-2 mg every 4-6 hours

I.V.:

Children ≥6 months and <50 kg: 0.015 mg/kg/dose every 3-6 hours as needed

Children >50 kg and Adults: 0.2-0.6 mg every 2-3 hours as needed

Adults (mechanically ventilated): Infusion: 0.5-1 mg/**hour** (based on 70 kg patient) **or** 7-15 mcg/kg/**hour**

Epidural PCA: *Children >50 kg and Adults:* Bolus: 0.4-1 mg; Infusion: 0.03-0.3 mg/**hour**; Demand dose: 0.02-0.5 mg; Lockout interval: 10-15 minutes

Oral:

Children ≥6 months and <50 kg: 0.03-0.08 mg/kg/dose every 3-4 hours as needed

Children >50 kg: 2-8 mg every 3-4 hours as needed

Adults: 2-8 mg every 3-4 hours as needed; Extended release: 8-64 mg every 24 hours

Elderly: 1-2 mg every 3-6 hours

PCA:

Children <50 kg: Usual concentration: 0.2 mg/mL; Demand dose: 0.003-0.005 mg/kg/dose; Lockout interval: 6-10 minutes; Usual basal rate: 0-0.004 mg/kg/hour

Children >50 kg and Adults: Usual concentration: 0.2 mg/mL; Demand dose: 0.05-0.4 mg; Lockout interval: 5-10 minutes

Rectal: *Children >50 kg and Adults:* 3 mg every 6-8 hours as needed

Administration

Oral Hydromorphone is available in an 8 mg immediate release tablet and an 8 mg extended release tablet. Extreme caution should be taken to avoid confusing dosage forms.

Exalgo™: Tablets should be swallowed whole; do not crush, break, chew, dissolve or inject. May be taken with or without food.

Hydromorph Contin®: Capsule should be swallowed whole; do not crush or chew; contents may be sprinkled on soft food and swallowed

I.M. May be given SubQ or I.M.; vial stopper contains latex

I.V. For IVP, must be given slowly over 2-3 minutes (rapid IVP has been associated with an increase in side effects, especially respiratory depression and hypotension)

I.V. Detail pH: 4.0-5.5

Other May be given SubQ or I.M.

Stability

Storage Store injection and oral dosage forms at 15°C to 30°C (59°F to 86°F). Protect tablets from light. A slightly yellowish discoloration has not been associated with a loss of potency.

Nursing Actions

Physical Assessment Monitor for effectiveness of pain relief. Monitor blood pressure, CNS and respiratory status, and degree of sedation prior to treatment and periodically throughout. Assess patient's physical and/or psychological dependence. For inpatients, implement safety measures (eg, side rails up, call light within reach, instructions to call for assistance). Discontinue slowly after prolonged use.

Patient Education Exalgo™ tablets should be swallowed whole; do not crush, break, chew, dissolve, or inject. May cause physical and/or psychological dependence. Do not use alcohol, sedatives, tranquilizers, antihistamines, or pain medications without consulting prescriber. Maintain adequate hydration, unless instructed to restrict fluid intake. May cause dizziness, drowsiness, impaired coordination, or blurred vision; loss of appetite, nausea, or vomiting; or constipation (if unresolved, consult prescriber about use of stool softeners). Report chest pain, slow or rapid heartbeat, dizziness, or persistent headache; confusion or respiratory difficulties; or severe constipation.

Hydroquinone (HYE droe kwin one)

Brand Names: U.S. Aclaro PD®; Aclaro®; Alphaquin HP®; Eldopaque Forte®; Eldopaque® [OTC]; Eldoquin Forte®; Eldoquin® [OTC]; EpiQuin® Micro; Esoterica® Daytime [OTC]; Esoterica® Nighttime [OTC]; Lustra-AF®; Lustra-Ultra™; Lustra®; Melanex® [DSC]; Melpaque HP®; Melquin HP®; Melquin-3®; NeoStrata® HQ Skin Lightening [OTC]; Nuquin HP®; Palmer's® Skin Success® Eventone® Fade Cream [OTC]; Palmer's® Skin Success® Eventone® Fade Milk [OTC]; Palmer's® Skin Success® Eventone® Ultra Fade Serum [OTC]

Index Terms Hydroquinol; Quinol

Pharmacologic Category Depigmenting Agent

Medication Safety Issues

Sound-alike/look-alike issues:

Eldopaque® may be confused with Eldoquin®

Eldopaque Forte® may be confused with Eldoquin Forte®

Pregnancy Risk Factor C

Lactation Excretion in breast milk unknown/use caution

Use Gradual bleaching of hyperpigmented skin conditions

Available Dosage Forms

Cream, topical: 4% (28.35 g, 28.4 g, 30 g)

Alphaquin HP®: 4% (28.4 g, 56.7 g)

Eldopaque Forte®: 4% (28.35 g)

Eldopaque® [OTC]: 2% (28.35 g)

Eldoquin Forte®: 4% (28.4 g)

Eldoquin® [OTC]: 2% (28.35 g)

EpiQuin® Micro: 4% (40 g)

Esoterica® Daytime [OTC]: 2% (70 g, 85 g)

Esoterica® Nighttime [OTC]: 2% (85 g)

Lustra-AF®: 4% (56.8 g)

Lustra-Ultra™: 4% (56.8 g)

Lustra®: 4% (56.8 g)

Melpaque HP®: 4% (14.2 g, 28.4 g)

Melquin HP®: 4% (14.2 g, 28.4 g)

Nuquin HP®: 4% (14.2 g, 28.4 g, 56.7 g)

Palmer's® Skin Success® Eventone® Fade Cream [OTC]: 2% (75 g, 125 g)

Emulsion, topical:

Aclaro PD®: 4% (42.5 g)

Aclaro®: 4% (48.2 g)

Gel, topical: 4% (28.35 g, 30 g)

NeoStrata® HQ Skin Lightening [OTC]: 2% (30 g)

Nuquin HP®: 4% (14.2 g, 28.4 g)

Lotion, topical:

Palmer's® Skin Success® Eventone® Fade Milk [OTC]: 2% (250 mL)

Solution, topical:

Melquin-3®: 3% (29.57 mL)

Palmer's® Skin Success® Eventone® Ultra Fade Serum [OTC]: 2% (30 mL)

General Dosage Range Topical: *Children >12 years and Adults:* Apply thin layer and rub in twice daily

Administration

Topical For external use only; avoid contact with eyes

Nursing Actions

Physical Assessment When applied to large areas or for extensive periods of time, monitor for skin irritation.

Patient Education Therapeutic effect may take several weeks. Test response by applying to small area of unbroken skin and check in 24 hours; if irritation or blistering occurs do not use. Avoid contact with eyes. Do not apply to open wounds or weeping areas. Before using, wash and dry area gently. Apply a thin film to affected area and rub in gently. Avoid direct sunlight or use sunblock or protective clothing to prevent repigmentation. Report rash, itching, or worsening of condition.

Hydroxocobalamin (hye droks oh koe BAL a min)

Brand Names: U.S. Cyanokit®

Index Terms Vitamin B_{12a}

Pharmacologic Category Antidote; Vitamin, Water Soluble

Pregnancy Risk Factor C

Lactation Excretion in breast milk unknown/use caution

Use Treatment of pernicious anemia, vitamin B_{12} deficiency due to dietary deficiencies or malabsorption diseases, inadequate secretion of intrinsic factor, and inadequate utilization of B_{12} (eg, during neoplastic treatment); diagnostic agent for Schilling test

Cyanokit®: Treatment of cyanide poisoning (known or suspected)

Unlabeled Use Neuropathies

Available Dosage Forms

Injection, powder for reconstitution:

Cyanokit®: 5 g

Injection, solution: 1000 mcg/mL (30 mL)

General Dosage Range

I.M.:

Children: 1-5 mg given in single daily doses of 100 mcg over 2 or more weeks, followed by 30-50 mcg/month

Adults: 30 mcg/day for 5-10 days, followed by 100-200 mcg/month

I.V.: *Adults:* 5 g as single infusion; may repeat if needed (maximum: 10 g cumulative dose)

Administration

I.M. Solution for I.M. injection: Administer 1000 mcg/mL solution I.M. only

I.V. Cyanokit®: Administer by I.V. infusion over 15 minutes; if repeat dose needed, administer second dose over 15 minutes to 2 hours

Nursing Actions

Physical Assessment Teach patient appropriate injection technique and needle disposal and appropriate nutrition. Cyanide toxicity: Monitor blood pressure and heart rate during infusion.

Patient Education Pernicious anemia may require monthly injections for life. Report skin rash; swelling, pain, or redness in extremities; or acute persistent diarrhea. Cyanokit®: May cause headache, redness of skin (can last up to 2 weeks; avoid exposure to sun while skin is red), skin lesions (can appear 7-28 days after infusion), and red urine (can last for 5 weeks).

Hydroxychloroquine (hye droks ee KLOR oh kwin)

Brand Names: U.S. Plaquenil®

Index Terms Hydroxychloroquine Sulfate

Pharmacologic Category Aminoquinoline (Antimalarial)

Medication Safety Issues

Sound-alike/look-alike issues:

Hydroxychloroquine may be confused with hydrocortisone

Plaquenil® may be confused with Platinol

Lactation Enters breast milk (AAP considers "compatible"; AAP 2001 update pending)

Use Suppression and treatment of acute attacks of malaria; treatment of systemic lupus erythematosus (SLE) and rheumatoid arthritis

Unlabeled Use Porphyria cutanea tarda, polymorphous light eruptions

Available Dosage Forms

Tablet, oral: 200 mg

Plaquenil®: 200 mg

General Dosage Range Oral:

Children: 13 mg/kg for 1-2 doses, followed by 6.5 mg/kg for 3 doses or once weekly

Adults: Initial: 400-800 mg/day divided 1-2 times/day; Maintenance: 200-400 mg/day **or** 800 mg for 1-2 doses, followed by 400 mg for 3 doses or once weekly

Administration

Oral Administer with food or milk.

Nursing Actions

Physical Assessment Evaluate results of CBC, liver function tests, and ophthalmic exam prior to treatment and periodically throughout. Monitor for dermatologic, neuromuscular [deep tendon reflexes, muscle weakness], and ocular changes throughout.

Patient Education It is important to complete full course of therapy. May be taken with meals to decrease GI upset and bitter aftertaste. Avoid excessive alcohol. You should have regular ophthalmic exams (every 3 months) if using this medication over extended periods. You may experience skin discoloration (blue/black), hair bleaching, or skin rash. If you have psoriasis, you may experience exacerbation. You may experience dizziness, headache, nervousness, abnormal color vision, lightheadedness, nausea, vomiting, loss of appetite, or increased sensitivity to sunlight. Report any changes in hearing acuity or ringing in ears, any changes in vision (visual disturbances, blurred vision), weakness, numbness, tingling, tremors in muscles, skin rash or itching, persistent GI disturbances, chest pain or palpitation, CNS changes, unusual fatigue, or easy bruising or bleeding.

Hydroxyprogesterone Caproate (hye droks ee proe JES te rone CAP ro ate)

Brand Names: U.S. Makena™

Index Terms 17OHPC

Pharmacologic Category Progestin

Medication Safety Issues

Sound-alike/look-alike issues:

Hydroxyprogesterone caproate may be confused with medroxyPROGESTERone

Pregnancy Risk Factor B

Use To reduce the risk of preterm birth in women with singleton pregnancies who have a history of spontaneous preterm birth (delivery <37 weeks gestation) with previous singleton pregnancies

Available Dosage Forms

Injection, solution:

Makena™: 250 mg/mL (5 mL)

General Dosage Range I.M.: *Pregnant females:* 250 mg every 7 days

Administration

I.M. For I.M. administration into the upper outer quadrant of the gluteus maximus. Withdraw dose using an 18 gauge needle; inject dose using a 21 gauge 1 1/2 inch needle. Administer by slow injection (≥1 minute). Solution is viscous and oily; do not use if solution is cloudy or contains solid particles. Apply pressure to injection site to decrease bruising and swelling.

Nursing Actions

Patient Education Maintain a regular schedule of injections as prescribed. This drug can only be given deep I.M. injection. If diabetic, monitor serum glucose closely. Report rash, alopecia, radically increased weight gain or swelling, anorexia, muscular weakness, fever, or unresolved nausea or vomiting. Report immediately any swelling or warmth in calves, chest pain or respiratory difficulty, severe headache or acute dizziness, numbness and/or tingling in extremities.

Hydroxyurea (hye droks ee yoor EE a)

Brand Names: U.S. Droxia®; Hydrea®

Index Terms Hydroxycarbamide; Hydurea

Pharmacologic Category Antineoplastic Agent, Antimetabolite

Medication Safety Issues

Sound-alike/look-alike issues:

Hydroxyurea may be confused with hydrOXYzine

High alert medication:

This medication is in a class the Institute for Safe Medication Practices (ISMP) includes among its list of drugs which have a heightened risk of causing significant patient harm when used in error.

International issues:

Hydrea [U.S., Canada, and multiple international markets] may be confused with Hydra brand name for isoniazid [Japan]

Pregnancy Risk Factor D

Lactation Enters breast milk/not recommended

Breast-Feeding Considerations Due to the potential for serious adverse reactions in the nursing infant, breast-feeding is not recommended.

Use Treatment of melanoma, refractory chronic myelocytic leukemia (CML); recurrent, metastatic, or inoperable ovarian cancer; radiosensitizing agent in the treatment of squamous cell head and neck cancer (excluding lip cancer); adjunct in the management of sickle cell patients who have had at least three painful crises in the previous 12 months (to reduce frequency of these crises and the need for blood transfusions)

Unlabeled Use Treatment of essential thrombocythemia, polycythemia vera, hypereosinophilic syndrome; management of hyperleukocytosis due to acute myeloid leukemia; treatment of cervical cancer, treatment of meningiomas

Mechanism of Action/Effect Antimetabolite which selectively inhibits ribonucleoside diphosphate reductase, preventing the conversion of ribonucleotides to deoxyribonucleotides, halting the cell cycle at the G1/S phase and therefore has radiation sensitizing activity by maintaining cells in the G_1 phase and interfering with DNA repair. In sickle cell anemia, hydroxyurea increases red blood cell (RBC) hemoglobin F levels, RBC water content, deformability of sickled cells, and alters adhesion of RBCs to endothelium.

Contraindications Hypersensitivity to hydroxyurea or any component of the formulation; severe bone marrow suppression (WBC <2500/mm^3 or platelet count <100,000/mm^3) or severe anemia (in patients with sickle cell anemia; use is not recommended if neutrophils <2000/mm^3, platelets <80,000/mm^3, hemoglobin <4.5 g/dL, or reticulocytes <80,000/mm^3 when hemoglobin <9 g/dL)

Warnings/Precautions Hazardous agent - use appropriate precautions for handling and disposal; to decrease risk of exposure, wear gloves when handling and wash hands before and after contact. Leukopenia may commonly occur (thrombocytopenia and anemia are less common; reversible with treatment interruption. Use with caution in patients with a history of prior chemotherapy or radiation therapy; myelosuppression is more common. Correct severe anemia prior to initiating treatment. Patients with a history of radiation therapy are also at risk for exacerbation of post irradiation erythema. Self-limiting megaloblastic erythropoiesis may be seen early in treatment (may resemble pernicious anemia, but is unrelated to vitamin B_{12} or folic acid deficiency). Plasma iron clearance may be delayed and iron utilization rate (by erythrocytes) may be reduced. When treated concurrently with hydroxyurea and antiretroviral agents (including didanosine), HIV-infected patients are at higher risk for potentially fatal pancreatitis, hepatotoxicity, hepatic failure, and severe peripheral neuropathy. Hyperuricemia may occur with treatment; adequate hydration and initiation or dosage adjustment of uricosuric agents (eg, allopurinol) may be necessary.

In patients with sickle cell anemia, use is not recommended if neutrophils <2000/mm^3, platelets <80,000/mm^3, hemoglobin <4.5 g/dL, or reticulocytes <80,000/mm^3 when hemoglobin <9 g/dL. May cause macrocytosis, which can mask folic acid deficiency; prophylactic fold acid supplementation is recommended. **[U.S. Boxed Warning]: Hydroxyurea is mutagenic and clastogenic. Treatment of myeloproliferative disorders (eg, polycythemia vera, thrombocythemia) with long-term hydroxyurea is associated with secondary leukemia;** it is unknown if this is drug-related or disease-related. Cutaneous vasculitic toxicities (vasculitic ulceration and gangrene) have been reported with hydroxyurea treatment, most often in patients with a history of or receiving concurrent interferon therapy; discontinue hydroxyurea and consider alternate cytoreductive therapy if cutaneous vasculitic toxicity develops. Use caution with renal dysfunction; may require dose reductions. Elderly patients may be more sensitive to the effects of hydroxyurea; may require lower doses. **[U.S. Boxed Warning]: Should be administered under the supervision of a physician experienced in the treatment of sickle cell anemia** or in cancer chemotherapy.

Drug Interactions

Avoid Concomitant Use

Avoid concomitant use of Hydroxyurea with any of the following: BCG; CloZAPine; Didanosine; Natalizumab; Pimecrolimus; Stavudine; Tacrolimus (Topical); Vaccines (Live)

Decreased Effect

Hydroxyurea may decrease the levels/effects of: BCG; Coccidioidin Skin Test; Sipuleucel-T; Vaccines (Inactivated); Vaccines (Live)

The levels/effects of Hydroxyurea may be decreased by: Echinacea

Increased Effect/Toxicity

Hydroxyurea may increase the levels/effects of: CloZAPine; Didanosine; Leflunomide; Natalizumab; Stavudine; Vaccines (Live)

The levels/effects of Hydroxyurea may be increased by: Denosumab; Didanosine; Pimecrolimus; Roflumilast; Stavudine; Tacrolimus (Topical); Trastuzumab

Adverse Reactions Frequency not defined.

Cardiovascular: Edema

Central nervous system: Chills, disorientation, dizziness, drowsiness (dose-related), fever, hallucinations, headache, malaise, seizure

Dermatologic: Alopecia, cutaneous vasculitic toxicities, dermatomyositis-like skin changes, facial erythema, gangrene, hyperpigmentation, maculopapular rash, nail atrophy, nail discoloration, peripheral erythema, scaling, skin atrophy, skin cancer, skin ulcer, vasculitis ulcerations, violet papules

Endocrine & metabolic: Hyperuricemia

Gastrointestinal: Anorexia, constipation, diarrhea, gastrointestinal irritation and mucositis, (potentiated with radiation therapy), nausea, pancreatitis, stomatitis, vomiting

Genitourinary: Dysuria

Hematologic: Myelosuppression (anemia, leukopenia [common; reversal of WBC count occurs rapidly], thrombocytopenia); macrocytosis, megaloblastic erythropoiesis, secondary leukemias (long-term use)

Hepatic: Hepatic enzymes increased, hepatotoxicity

Neuromuscular & skeletal: Peripheral neuropathy, weakness

Renal: BUN increased, creatinine increased

Respiratory: Acute diffuse pulmonary infiltrates (rare), dyspnea, pulmonary fibrosis (rare)

Pharmacodynamics/Kinetics

Onset of Action Sickle cell anemia: Fetal hemoglobin increase: 4-12 weeks

Available Dosage Forms

Capsule, oral: 500 mg

Droxia®: 200 mg, 300 mg, 400 mg

Hydrea®: 500 mg

General Dosage Range Dosage adjustment recommended in patients with renal impairment

Oral: *Adults:* 15-35 mg/kg/day **or** 500-3000 mg/day as single or divided dose **or** 80 mg/kg as a single dose every third day

Administration

Oral The manufacturer does not recommend opening the capsules; observe proper handling procedures (eg, wear gloves)

Stability

Storage Store at room temperature of 25°C (77°F); excursions permitted between 15°C and 30°C (59°F and 86°F).

Nursing Actions

Physical Assessment Monitor closely for CNS changes, gastrointestinal upset. hepatotoxicity, and peripheral neuropathy. Teach proper use and need for frequent monitoring.

Patient Education Take capsules exactly as directed by prescriber (dosage and timing will be specific to purpose of therapy). Contents of capsule may be emptied into a glass of water and taken immediately. You will require frequent monitoring and blood tests while taking this medication to assess effectiveness and monitor adverse reactions. You will be susceptible to infection. May cause nausea, vomiting, loss of appetite, constipation, diarrhea, or mouth sores. Report persistent vomiting, diarrhea, constipation, stomach pain, or mouth sores; skin rash, redness, irritation, or sores; painful or difficult urination; anemia (unusual fatigue, lethargy), CNS changes (increased confusion, depression, hallucinations, or seizures); opportunistic infection (persistent fever or chills, white plaques in mouth, vaginal discharge, or unhealed sores); unusual lassitude, muscle tremors or weakness; easy bruising/ bleeding; or blood in vomitus, stool, or urine. People not taking hydroxyurea should not be exposed to it. If powder from capsule is spilled, wipe up with damp, disposable towel immediately, and discard the towel in a closed container, such as a plastic bag. Wash hands thoroughly.

Dietary Considerations In sickle cell patients, supplemental administration of folic acid is recommended; hydroxyurea may mask development of folic acid deficiency.

HydrOXYzine (hye DROKS i zeen)

Brand Names: U.S. Vistaril®

Index Terms Hydroxyzine Hydrochloride; Hydroxyzine Pamoate

Pharmacologic Category Antiemetic; Histamine H_1 Antagonist; Histamine H_1 Antagonist, First Generation; Piperazine Derivative

Medication Safety Issues

Sound-alike/look-alike issues:

HydrOXYzine may be confused with hydrALAZINE, hydroxyurea

Atarax® may be confused with Ativan®

Vistaril® may be confused with Restoril™, Versed, Zestril®

BEERS Criteria medication:

This drug may be inappropriate for use in geriatric patients (high severity risk).

International issues:

Vistaril [U.S. and Turkey] may be confused with Vastarel brand name for trimetazidine [multiple international markets]

Lactation Excretion in breast milk unknown/not recommended

Use Treatment of anxiety/agitation (including adjunctive therapy in alcoholism); adjunct to pre- and postoperative analgesia and anesthesia; antipruritic; antiemetic

Available Dosage Forms

Capsule, oral: 25 mg, 50 mg, 100 mg

Vistaril®: 25 mg, 50 mg

Injection, solution: 25 mg/mL (1 mL); 50 mg/mL (1 mL, 2 mL, 10 mL)

Solution, oral: 10 mg/5 mL (473 mL)

Syrup, oral: 10 mg/5 mL (118 mL, 473 mL, 480 mL)

Tablet, oral: 10 mg, 25 mg, 50 mg

General Dosage Range Dosage adjustment recommended in patients with hepatic impairment

I.M.:

Children: 1.1 mg/kg/dose

Adults: 25-100 mg/dose

Oral:

Children: 0.6 mg/kg/dose (sedation)

Children <6 years: 50 mg/day in divided doses

Children ≥6 years: 50-100 mg/day in divided doses

Adults: 25-100 mg/dose

Administration

Oral Shake suspension vigorously prior to use.

I.M. For I. M. use only. Do not administer I.V., SubQ, or intra-arterially. Administer I.M. deep in large muscle. In adults, the preferred site is the upper outer quadrant of the buttock or midlateral thigh. In children, the preferred site is the midlateral thigh. The upper outer quadrant of the gluteal region should be used only when necessary to minimize potential damage to the sciatic nerve. With I.V. administration, extravasation can result in sterile abscess and marked tissue induration.

I.V. Extravasation can result in sterile abscess and marked tissue induration.

I.V. Detail pH: 3.5-6.0

Nursing Actions

Physical Assessment Ensure patient safety to prevent falls (side rails up, call light within reach).

Patient Education Will cause drowsiness. Do not use alcohol. Report hallucinations, seizure activity, tremors or involuntary movements, or loss of sensation.

Ibandronate (eye BAN droh nate)

Brand Names: U.S. Boniva®

Index Terms Ibandronate Sodium; Ibandronic Acid

Pharmacologic Category Bisphosphonate Derivative

Medication Guide Available Yes

Pregnancy Risk Factor C

Lactation Excretion in breast milk unknown/use caution

Use Treatment and prevention of osteoporosis in postmenopausal females

Unlabeled Use Hypercalcemia of malignancy; corticosteroid-induced osteoporosis; Paget's disease; reduce bone pain and skeletal complications from metastatic bone disease

Mechanism of Action/Effect A bisphosphonate which inhibits bone resorption via actions on osteoclasts or on osteoclast precursors; decreases the rate of bone resorption, leading to an indirect increase in bone mineral density.

Contraindications Hypersensitivity to ibandronate or any component of the formulation; hypocalcemia; oral tablets are also contraindicated in patients unable to stand or sit upright for at least 60 minutes and in patients with abnormalities of the esophagus which delay esophageal emptying, such as stricture or achalasia

Warnings/Precautions Hypocalcemia must be corrected before therapy initiation. Ensure adequate calcium and vitamin D intake. Osteonecrosis of the jaw (ONJ) has been reported in patients receiving bisphosphonates. Risk factors include invasive dental procedures (eg, tooth extraction, dental implants, boney surgery); a diagnosis of cancer, with concomitant chemotherapy or corticosteroids; poor oral hygiene, ill-fitting dentures; and comorbid disorders (anemia, coagulopathy, infection, pre-existing dental disease). Most reported cases occurred after I.V. bisphosphonate therapy; however, cases have been reported following oral therapy. A dental exam and preventative dentistry should be performed prior to placing patients with risk factors on chronic bisphosphonate therapy.

The manufacturer's labeling states that discontinuing bisphosphonates in patients requiring invasive dental procedures may reduce the risk of ONJ. However, other experts suggest that there is no evidence that discontinuing therapy reduces the risk of developing ONJ (Assael, 2009). The benefit/risk must be assessed by the treating physician and/or dentist/surgeon prior to any invasive dental procedure. Patients developing ONJ while on bisphosphonates should receive care by an oral surgeon.

Atypical femur fractures have been reported in patients receiving bisphosphonates for treatment/prevention of osteoporosis. The fractures include subtrochanteric femur (bone just below the hip joint) and diaphyseal femur (long segment of the thigh bone). Some patients experience prodromal pain weeks or months before the fracture occurs. It is unclear if bisphosphonate therapy is the cause for these fractures, although the majority have been reported in patients taking bisphosphonates. Patients receiving long-term (>3-5 years) therapy may be at an increased risk. Discontinue bisphosphonate therapy in patients who develop a femoral shaft fracture.

Infrequently, severe (and occasionally debilitating) bone, joint, and/or muscle pain have been reported during bisphosphonate treatment. The onset of pain ranged from a single day to several months. Consider discontinuing therapy in patients who experience severe symptoms; symptoms usually resolve upon discontinuation. Some patients experienced recurrence when rechallenged with same drug or another bisphosphonate; avoid use in patients with a history of these symptoms in association with bisphosphonate therapy.

Oral bisphosphonates may cause dysphagia, esophagitis, esophageal or gastric ulcer; risk may increase in patients unable to comply with dosing instructions; discontinue use if new or worsening symptoms develop. Intravenous bisphosphonates may cause transient decreases in serum calcium and have also been associated with renal toxicity.

Use not recommended with severe renal impairment (Cl_{cr} <30 mL/minute).

Drug Interactions

Avoid Concomitant Use There are no known interactions where it is recommended to avoid concomitant use.

Decreased Effect

The levels/effects of Ibandronate may be decreased by: Antacids; Calcium Salts; Iron Salts; Magnesium Salts; Proton Pump Inhibitors

Increased Effect/Toxicity

Ibandronate may increase the levels/effects of: Deferasirox; Phosphate Supplements

The levels/effects of Ibandronate may be increased by: Aminoglycosides; Nonsteroidal Anti-Inflammatory Agents

Nutritional/Ethanol Interactions

Ethanol: Ethanol may increase risk of osteoporosis. Management: Avoid ethanol.

Food: May reduce absorption; mean oral bioavailability is decreased up to 90% when given with food. Management: Take with a full glass (6-8 oz) of plain water, at least 60 minutes prior to any food, beverages, or medications. Mineral water with a high calcium content should be avoided. Wait at least 60 minutes after taking ibandronate before taking anything else.

Adverse Reactions Percentages vary based on frequency of administration (daily vs monthly). Unless specified, percentages are reported with oral use.

>10%:

Gastrointestinal: Dyspepsia (6% to 12%)

Neuromuscular & skeletal: Back pain (4% to 14%)

1% to 10%:

Cardiovascular: Hypertension (6% to 7%)

Central nervous system: Headache (3% to 7%), dizziness (1% to 4%), insomnia (1% to 2%)

Dermatologic: Rash (1% to 2%)

Endocrine & metabolic: Hypercholesterolemia (5%)

Gastrointestinal: Abdominal pain (5% to 8%), diarrhea (4% to 7%), nausea (5%), constipation (3% to 4%), vomiting (3%)

Genitourinary: Urinary tract infection (2% to 6%)

Hepatic: Alkaline phosphatase decreased (frequency not defined)

Local: Injection site reaction (<2%)

Neuromuscular & skeletal: Pain in extremity (1% to 8%), arthralgia (4% to 6%), myalgia (1% to 6%), joint disorder (4%), osteonecrosis of the jaw (4%), weakness (4%), osteoarthritis (localized; 1% to 3%), muscle cramp (2%)

Respiratory: Bronchitis (3% to 10%), pneumonia (6%), pharyngitis/nasopharyngitis (3% to 4%), upper respiratory infection (2%)

Miscellaneous: Acute phase reaction (I.V. 10%; oral 3% to 9%), infection (4%), flu-like syndrome (1% to 4%), allergic reaction (3%)

Available Dosage Forms

Injection, solution:

Boniva®: 1 mg/mL (3 mL)

Tablet, oral:

Boniva®: 150 mg

General Dosage Range

I.V.: *Adults:* 3 mg every 3 months

Oral: *Adults:* 2.5 mg once daily **or** 150 mg once a month

Administration

Oral Should be administered 60 minutes before the first food or drink of the day (other than water) and prior to taking any oral medications or supplements (eg, calcium, antacids, vitamins). Ibandronate should be taken in an upright position with a full glass (6-8 oz) of plain water and the patient should avoid lying down for 60 minutes to minimize the possibility of GI side effects. Mineral water with a high calcium content should be avoided. The tablet should be swallowed whole; do not chew or suck. Do not eat or drink anything (except water) for 60 minutes following administration of ibandronate.

Once-monthly dosing: The 150 mg tablet should be taken on the same date each month. In case of a missed dose, do not take two 150 mg tablets within the same week. If the next scheduled dose is 1-7 days away, wait until the next scheduled dose to take the tablet. If the next scheduled dose is >7 days away, take the dose the morning it is remembered, and then resume taking the once-monthly dose on the originally scheduled day.

I.V. Administer as a 15-30 second bolus. Do not mix with calcium-containing solutions or other drugs. For osteoporosis, do not administer more frequently than every 3 months. Infuse over 1 hour for metastatic bone disease and over 2 hours for hypercalcemia of malignancy.

Stability

Storage Store at controlled room temperature of 25°C (77°F); excursions permitted to 15°C to 30°C (59°F to 86°F).

Nursing Actions

Physical Assessment Monitor for unusual or acute musculoskeletal pain. Monitor blood pressure at the beginning of therapy and periodically during use. Patients at risk for osteonecrosis of the jaw (eg, chemotherapy, corticosteroids, poor oral hygiene) should have dental exams; necessary preventive dentistry should be done before beginning bisphosphonate therapy. Assess ability of patient to comply with administration directions. Teach patient appropriate administration of medication. Instruct patient in lifestyle and dietary changes.

Patient Education Oral: Take with a full glass of water first thing in the morning and at least 60 minutes before the first food or beverage of the day. Wait at least 60 minutes after taking Ibandronate before taking anything else. Stay in sitting or standing position for 60 minutes following administration and until after the first food of the day to reduce potential for esophageal irritation. Consult prescriber to determine necessity of lifestyle changes (eg, decreased smoking, decreased alcohol intake). Certain dental procedures should be avoided if possible while you are taking this medication. You may experience temporary flatulence, bloating, nausea, acid regurgitation, or temporary bone pain. Report persistent muscle or bone pain, leg cramps, acute headache, persistent gastric pain or unresolved GI upset, unusual fever, chills, rash, or pain in mouth.

Dietary Considerations Ensure adequate calcium and vitamin D intake; women and men >50 years of age should consume 1200-1500 mg/day of elemental calcium and 800-1000 int. units/day of vitamin D. Ibandronate tablet should be taken with a full glass (6-8 oz) of plain water, at least 60 minutes prior to any food, beverages, or medications. Mineral water with a high calcium content should be avoided.

Ibuprofen (eye byoo PROE fen)

Brand Names: U.S. Addaprin [OTC]; Advil® Children's [OTC]; Advil® Infants' [OTC]; Advil® Migraine [OTC]; Advil® [OTC]; Caldolor™; I-Prin [OTC]; Ibu-200 [OTC]; Ibu®; Midol® Cramps & Body Aches [OTC]; Motrin® Children's [OTC]; Motrin® IB [OTC]; Motrin® Infants' [OTC]; Motrin® Junior [OTC]; NeoProfen®; Proprinal® [OTC]; TopCare® Junior Strength [OTC]; Ultraprin [OTC]

Index Terms *p*-Isobutylhydratropic Acid; Ibuprofen Lysine

Pharmacologic Category Nonsteroidal Anti-inflammatory Drug (NSAID), Oral; Nonsteroidal Anti-inflammatory Drug (NSAID), Parenteral

Medication Safety Issues

Sound-alike/look-alike issues:

Haltran® may be confused with Halfprin®

Motrin® may be confused with Neurontin®

Administration issues:

Injectable formulations: Both ibuprofen and ibuprofen lysine are available for parenteral use. Ibuprofen lysine is **only** indicated for closure of a clinically-significant patent ductus arteriosus.

Medication Guide Available Yes

Pregnancy Risk Factor C/D ≥30 weeks gestation

Lactation Enters breast milk/not recommended (AAP rates "compatible"; AAP 2001 update pending)

Use

Oral: Inflammatory diseases and rheumatoid disorders including juvenile idiopathic arthritis (JIA), mild-to-moderate pain, fever, dysmenorrhea, osteoarthritis

Ibuprofen injection (Caldolor™): Management of mild-to-moderate pain; management moderate-to-severe pain when used concurrently with an opioid analgesic; reduction of fever

Ibuprofen lysine injection (NeoProfen®): To induce closure of a clinically-significant patent ductus arteriosus (PDA) in premature infants weighing between 500-1500 g and who are ≤32 weeks gestational age (GA) when usual treatments are ineffective

Unlabeled Use Cystic fibrosis, gout, ankylosing spondylitis, acute migraine headache

Available Dosage Forms

Caplet, oral: 200 mg

Advil® [OTC]: 200 mg

Motrin® IB [OTC]: 200 mg

Motrin® Junior [OTC]: 100 mg

Capsule, liquid filled, oral: 200 mg

Advil® [OTC]: 200 mg

Advil® Migraine [OTC]: 200 mg

Capsule, softgel, oral: 200 mg

Gelcap, oral:
Advil® [OTC]: 200 mg
Injection, solution:
Caldolor™: 100 mg/mL (4 mL, 8 mL)
Injection, solution [preservative free]:
NeoProfen®: 17.1 mg/mL (2 mL)
Suspension, oral: 100 mg/5 mL (5 mL, 10 mL, 120 mL, 480 mL); 40 mg/mL (15 mL)
Advil® Children's [OTC]: 100 mg/5 mL (120 mL)
Advil® Infants' [OTC]: 40 mg/mL (15 mL)
Motrin® Children's [OTC]: 100 mg/5 mL (60 mL, 120 mL)
Motrin® Infants' [OTC]: 40 mg/mL (15 mL)
Tablet, oral: 200 mg, 400 mg, 600 mg, 800 mg
Addaprin [OTC]: 200 mg
Advil® [OTC]: 200 mg
I-Prin [OTC]: 200 mg
Ibu-200 [OTC]: 200 mg
Ibu®: 400 mg, 600 mg, 800 mg
Midol® Cramps & Body Aches [OTC]: 200 mg
Motrin® IB [OTC]: 200 mg
Proprinal® [OTC]: 200 mg
Ultraprin [OTC]: 200 mg
Tablet, chewable, oral:
Motrin® Junior [OTC]: 100 mg
TopCare® Junior Strength [OTC]: 100 mg

General Dosage Range

I.V. (ibuprofen [Caldolor™]): *Adults:* 100-400 mg every 4-6 hours or 400-800 mg every 6 hours (maximum: 3.2 g/day)

I.V. (ibuprofen lysine [NeoProfen®]): *Infants between 500-1500 g and ≤32 weeks GA:* Initial: 10 mg/kg, followed by two doses of 5 mg/kg at 24 and 48 hours; **Note:** Dose should be based on birth weight.

Oral:
Analgesic/antipyretic:
Children 6-11 months and 12-17 lbs: 50 mg every 6-8 hours (maximum: 4 doses/day) **or** 4-10 mg/kg every 6-8 hours (maximum: 40 mg/kg/day)
Children 12-23 months and 18-23 lbs: 75 mg every 6-8 hours (maximum: 4 doses/day) **or** 4-10 mg/kg every 6-8 hours (maximum: 40 mg/kg/day)
Children 2-3 years and 24-35 lbs: 100 mg every 6-8 hours (maximum: 4 doses/day) **or** 4-10 mg/kg every 6-8 hours (maximum: 40 mg/kg/day)
Children 4-5 years and 36-47 lbs: 150 mg every 6-8 hours (maximum: 4 doses/day) **or** 4-10 mg/kg every 6-8 hours (maximum: 40 mg/kg/day)
Children 6-8 years and 48-59 lbs: 200 mg every 6-8 hours (maximum: 4 doses/day) **or** 4-10 mg/kg every 6-8 hours (maximum: 40 mg/kg/day)
Children 9-10 years and 60-71 lbs: 250 mg every 6-8 hours (maximum: 4 doses/day) **or** 4-10 mg/kg every 6-8 hours (maximum: 40 mg/kg/day)
Children 11-12 years and 72-95 lbs: 300 mg every 6-8 hours (maximum: 4 doses/day) **or** 4-10 mg/kg every 6-8 hours (maximum: 40 mg/kg/day)
Children >12 years: 200 mg every 4-6 hours as needed (maximum: 1200 mg/day) **or** 4-10 mg/kg every 6-8 hours (maximum: 40 mg/kg/day)
Adults: 200-400 mg every 4-6 hours
Inflammatory disease: *Adults:* 400-800 mg 3-4 times/day (maximum: 3200 mg/day)
JIA: *Children >6 months:* 30-50 mg/kg/day divided every 8 hours (maximum: 2.4 g/day)

Administration

Oral Administer with food.

I.V.
Caldolor™: For I.V. administration only; must be diluted to a final concentration of ≤4 mg/mL prior to administration; infuse over at least 30 minutes
NeoProfen® (ibuprofen lysine): For I.V. administration only; administration via umbilical arterial line has not been evaluated. Infuse over 15 minutes through port closest to insertion site. Avoid extravasation. Do not administer simultaneously via same line with TPN. If needed, interrupt TPN for 15 minutes prior to and after ibuprofen administration, keeping line open with dextrose or saline.

I.V. Detail
Caldolor™: pH: 7.4
NeoProfen®: pH: 7.0

Nursing Actions

Physical Assessment Assess patient for allergic reaction to salicylates or other NSAIDs. Monitor blood pressure prior to treatment and periodically throughout. Monitor for adverse gastrointestinal response prior to treatment and periodically throughout. Periodic ophthalmic exams are recommended.

Patient Education Consult your prescriber before use if you have hypertension or heart failure. Do not take longer than 3 days for fever or 10 days for pain without consulting prescriber. Take with food or milk. Do not use alcohol. Maintain adequate hydration, unless instructed to restrict fluid intake. You may experience nausea, vomiting, or gastric discomfort. GI bleeding, ulceration, or perforation can occur with or without pain. Stop taking medication and report ringing in ears, persistent cramping or stomach pain, unresolved nausea or vomiting, respiratory difficulty or shortness of breath, unusual bruising or bleeding (mouth, urine, stool), skin rash, unusual swelling of extremities, chest pain, or palpitations.

Ibuprofen and Famotidine

(eye byoo PROE fen & fa MOE ti deen)

Brand Names: U.S. Duexis®

Index Terms Famotidine and Ibuprofen; HZT-501

Pharmacologic Category Histamine H_2 Antagonist; Nonsteroidal Anti-inflammatory Drug (NSAID), Oral

Medication Guide Available Yes

Pregnancy Risk Factor C

Lactation Enters breast milk/not recommended

Use Reduction of the risk of NSAID-associated gastric ulcers in patients who require an NSAID for the treatment of rheumatoid arthritis or osteoarthritis

Available Dosage Forms

Tablet, oral:

Duexis®: Ibuprofen 800 mg and famotidine 26.6 mg

General Dosage Range Oral: *Adults:* One tablet (800 mg ibuprofen/26.6 mg famotidine) 3 times daily

Administration

Oral Administer with or without food. Tablets should be swallowed whole; do not chew, crush, or split.

Nursing Actions

Physical Assessment See individual agents.

Patient Education Do not take if you had an asthma attack, hives, or other allergic reaction after taking aspirin or other NSAID medicine; for pain right before or after heart bypass surgery; if you are in the late stages of pregnancy (after 30 weeks of pregnancy); or if you are allergic to any other histamine H_2 receptor antagonist. Take the pill whole, do not crush.

Ibutilide (i BYOO ti lide)

Brand Names: U.S. Corvert®

Index Terms Ibutilide Fumarate

Pharmacologic Category Antiarrhythmic Agent, Class III

Medication Safety Issues

High alert medication:

The Institute for Safe Medication Practices (ISMP) includes this medication among its list of drugs which have a heightened risk of causing significant patient harm when used in error.

Pregnancy Risk Factor C

Lactation Enters breast milk/contraindicated

Use Acute termination of atrial fibrillation or flutter of recent onset; the effectiveness of ibutilide has not been determined in patients with arrhythmias >90 days in duration

Mechanism of Action/Effect Exact mechanism of action is unknown; prolongs the action potential in cardiac tissue

Contraindications Hypersensitivity to ibutilide or any component of the formulation; QT_c >440 msec

Warnings/Precautions **[U.S. Boxed Warning]: Potentially fatal arrhythmias (eg, polymorphic ventricular tachycardia) can occur with ibutilide, usually in association with torsade de pointes (QT prolongation).** Studies indicate a 1.7% incidence of arrhythmias in treated patients. The drug should be given in a setting of continuous ECG monitoring and by personnel trained in treating arrhythmias particularly polymorphic ventricular tachycardia. **[U.S. Boxed Warning]: Patients with chronic atrial fibrillation may not be the best candidates for ibutilide since they often revert after conversion and the risks of treatment may not be justified when compared to alternative management.** Dosing adjustments are not required in patients with renal or hepatic dysfunction. Safety and efficacy in children have not been established. Use caution in elderly patients. Avoid concurrent use of any drug that can prolong QT interval. Correct hyperkalemia and hypomagnesemia before using. Monitor for heart block.

Drug Interactions

Avoid Concomitant Use

Avoid concomitant use of Ibutilide with any of the following: Artemether; Dronedarone; Lumefantrine; Nilotinib; Pimozide; QUEtiapine; QuiNINE; Tetrabenazine; Thioridazine; Toremifene; Vandetanib; Vemurafenib; Ziprasidone

Decreased Effect There are no known significant interactions involving a decrease in effect.

Increased Effect/Toxicity

Ibutilide may increase the levels/effects of: Dronedarone; Lidocaine (Topical); Pimozide; QTc-Prolonging Agents; QuiNINE; Tetrabenazine; Thioridazine; Toremifene; Vandetanib; Vemurafenib; Ziprasidone

The levels/effects of Ibutilide may be increased by: Alfuzosin; Artemether; Chloroquine; Ciprofloxacin; Ciprofloxacin (Systemic); Eribulin; Fingolimod; Gadobutrol; Indacaterol; Lidocaine (Topical); Lumefantrine; Nilotinib; QUEtiapine; QuiNINE

Adverse Reactions 1% to 10%:

Cardiovascular: Ventricular extrasystoles (5.1%), nonsustained monomorphic ventricular tachycardia (4.9%), nonsustained polymorphic ventricular tachycardia (2.7%), tachycardia/supraventricular tachycardia (2.7%), hypotension (2%), bundle branch block (1.9%), sustained polymorphic ventricular tachycardia (eg, torsade de pointes) (1.7%, often requiring cardioversion), AV block (1.5%), bradycardia (1.2%), QT segment prolongation, hypertension (1.2%), palpitation (1%)

Central nervous system: Headache (3.6%)

Gastrointestinal: Nausea (>1%)

Pharmacodynamics/Kinetics

Onset of Action ~90 minutes after start of infusion (1/2 of conversions to sinus rhythm occur during infusion)

Available Dosage Forms

Injection, solution: 0.1 mg/mL (10 mL)

Corvert®: 0.1 mg/mL (10 mL)

General Dosage Range I.V.:

Adults <60 kg: 0.01 mg/kg; may repeat once

Adults ≥60 kg: 1 mg; may repeat once

Administration

I.V. May be administered undiluted or diluted in 50 mL diluent (0.9% NS or D_5W). Infuse over 10 minutes.

I.V. Detail Observe patient with continuous ECG monitoring for at least 4 hours following infusion or until QT_c has returned to baseline. Skilled personnel and proper equipment should be available during administration of ibutilide and subsequent monitoring of the patient.

Stability

Reconstitution May be administered undiluted or diluted in 50 mL diluent (0.9% NS or D_5W).

Storage Admixtures are chemically and physically stable for 24 hours at room temperature and for 48 hours at refrigerated temperatures.

Nursing Actions

Physical Assessment Requires infusion pump and continuous cardiac and hemodynamic monitoring during and for 4 hours following infusion.

Patient Education This drug is only given I.V. and you will be on continuous cardiac monitoring during and for several hours following administration. You may experience headache or irregular heartbeat during infusion. Report chest pain or respiratory difficulty immediately.

Icatibant (eye KAT i bant)

Brand Names: U.S. Firazyr®

Index Terms HOE 140; Icatibant Acetate

Pharmacologic Category Selective Bradykinin B2 Receptor Antagonist

Pregnancy Risk Factor C

Lactation Excretion unknown/use caution

Use Treatment of acute attacks of hereditary angioedema (HAE)

Mechanism of Action/Effect Icatibant is a selective competitive antagonist for the bradykinin B_2 receptor. Icatibant inhibits bradykinin from binding at the B_2 receptor, thereby treating the symptoms associated with acute attack.

Contraindications There are no contraindications listed in the manufacturer's labeling.

Warnings/Precautions Airway obstruction may occur during acute laryngeal attacks of HAE. Patients with laryngeal attacks should be instructed to seek medical attention immediately in addition to treatment with icatibant. Icatibant may potentially attenuate the antihypertensive effect of ACE inhibitors; patients taking ACE inhibitors were excluded from initial clinical trials.

Drug Interactions

Avoid Concomitant Use There are no known interactions where it is recommended to avoid concomitant use.

Decreased Effect

Icatibant may decrease the levels/effects of: ACE Inhibitors

Increased Effect/Toxicity There are no known significant interactions involving an increase in effect.

Adverse Reactions

>10%: Local: Injection site reaction (97%)

1% to 10%:

Central nervous system: Pyrexia (4%), dizziness (3%)

Hepatic: Transaminase increased (4%)

Pharmacodynamics/Kinetics

Onset of Action Median time to 50% decrease of symptoms: ~2 hours

Duration of Action Inhibits symptoms caused by bradykinin for ~6 hours

Available Dosage Forms

Injection, solution [preservative free]:

Firazyr®: 10 mg/mL (3 mL)

General Dosage Range SubQ: *Adults:* 30 mg/dose; maximum: 3 doses/24 hours

Administration

Other For SubQ injection only. Inject into the abdomen over ≥30 seconds, using the 25 gauge needle provided. Inject 2-4 inches below belly button and away from any scars; do not inject into an area that is bruised, swollen, or painful.

Stability

Storage Store between 2°C to 25°C (36°F to 77°F); do not freeze. Store in original container until time of administration.

Nursing Actions

Physical Assessment Monitor for laryngeal symptoms or airway obstruction. Report adverse reactions to the FDA at 1-866-880-0660.

Patient Education This medication is given as an injection under the skin. Give no more than 3 injections in a 24-hour period. Do not use if medication is cloudy in appearance. Less serious side effects include dizziness, drowsiness, nausea, vomiting, headaches, or redness at injection site. Serious side effects that require immediate attention include chest pain, feeling as if you will pass out, trouble breathing, and swelling of the throat or tongue.

IDArubicin (eye da ROO bi sin)

Brand Names: U.S. Idamycin PFS®

Index Terms 4-Demethoxydaunorubicin; 4-DMDR; Idarubicin Hydrochloride; IDR; IMI 30; SC 33428

Pharmacologic Category Antineoplastic Agent, Anthracycline; Antineoplastic Agent, Antibiotic

Medication Safety Issues

Sound-alike/look-alike issues:

IDArubicin may be confused with DOXOrubicin, DAUNOrubicin, epirubicin

Idamycin PFS® may be confused with Adriamycin

High alert medication:
The Institute for Safe Medication Practices (ISMP) includes this medication among its list of drugs which have a heightened risk of causing significant patient harm when used in error.

Pregnancy Risk Factor D

Lactation Excretion in breast milk unknown/not recommended

Use Treatment of acute myeloid leukemia (AML)

Unlabeled Use Acute lymphocytic leukemia (ALL)

Mechanism of Action/Effect Similar to daunorubicin, idarubicin exhibits inhibitory effects on DNA and RNA polymerase.

Contraindications Hypersensitivity to idarubicin, other anthracyclines, or any component of the formulation; bilirubin >5 mg/dL

Warnings/Precautions Hazardous agent - use appropriate precautions for handling and disposal. **[U.S. Boxed Warning]: May cause myocardial toxicity (HF, arrhythmias or cardiomyopathies) and is more common in patients who have previously received anthracyclines or have pre-existing cardiac disease.** The risk of myocardial toxicity is also increased in patients with concomitant or prior mediastinal/pericardial irradiation, patients with anemia, bone marrow depression, infections, leukemic pericarditis or myocarditis. Monitor cardiac function during treatment.

[U.S. Boxed Warnings]: May cause severe myelosuppression; use caution in patients with pre-existing myelosuppression from prior treatment or radiation. Use caution with renal or hepatic impairment; may required dosage reductions. For I.V. administration only; may cause severe local tissue damage and necrosis if extravasation occurs. Rapid lysis of leukemic cells may lead to hyperuricemia. Systemic infections should be managed prior to initiation of treatment. **[U.S. Boxed Warning]: Should be administered under the supervision of an experienced cancer chemotherapy physician. Safety and efficacy in children have not been established.**

Drug Interactions

Avoid Concomitant Use

Avoid concomitant use of IDArubicin with any of the following: BCG; CloZAPine; Natalizumab; Pimecrolimus; Tacrolimus (Topical); Vaccines (Live)

Decreased Effect

IDArubicin may decrease the levels/effects of: BCG; Cardiac Glycosides; Coccidioidin Skin Test; Sipuleucel-T; Vaccines (Inactivated); Vaccines (Live)

The levels/effects of IDArubicin may be decreased by: Cardiac Glycosides; Echinacea; P-glycoprotein/ABCB1 Inducers

Increased Effect/Toxicity

IDArubicin may increase the levels/effects of: CloZAPine; Leflunomide; Natalizumab; Vaccines (Live)

The levels/effects of IDArubicin may be increased by: Bevacizumab; Denosumab; P-glycoprotein/ABCB1 Inhibitors; Pimecrolimus; Roflumilast; Tacrolimus (Topical); Taxane Derivatives; Trastuzumab

Adverse Reactions

>10%:

Cardiovascular: Transient ECG abnormalities (supraventricular tachycardia, S-T wave changes, atrial or ventricular extrasystoles); generally asymptomatic and self-limiting. CHF, dose related. The relative cardiotoxicity of idarubicin compared to doxorubicin is unclear. Some investigators report no increase in cardiac toxicity at cumulative oral idarubicin doses up to 540 mg/m^2; other reports suggest a maximum cumulative intravenous dose of 150 mg/m^2.

Central nervous system: Headache

Dermatologic: Alopecia (25% to 30%), radiation recall, skin rash (11%), urticaria

Gastrointestinal: Nausea, vomiting (30% to 60%); diarrhea (9% to 22%); stomatitis (11%); GI hemorrhage (30%)

Genitourinary: Discoloration of urine (darker yellow)

Hematologic: Myelosuppression (nadir: 10-15 days; recovery: 21-28 days), primarily leukopenia; thrombocytopenia and anemia. Effects are generally less severe with oral dosing.

Hepatic: Bilirubin and transaminases increased (44%)

1% to 10%:

Central nervous system: Seizure

Neuromuscular & skeletal: Peripheral neuropathy

Available Dosage Forms

Injection, solution [preservative free]: 1 mg/mL (5 mL, 10 mL, 20 mL)

Idamycin PFS®: 1 mg/mL (5 mL, 10 mL, 20 mL)

General Dosage Range Dosage adjustment recommended in patients with hepatic or renal impairment

I.V.: *Adults:* Induction: 12 mg/m^2/day for 3 days, Consolidation: 10-12 mg/m^2/day for 2 days

Administration

I.V. Do not administer I.M. or SubQ; administer as slow push over 3-5 minutes, preferably into the side of a freely-running saline or dextrose infusion **or** as intermittent infusion over 10-15 minutes into a free-flowing I.V. solution of NS or D_5W; also occasionally administered as a bladder lavage.

I.V. Detail Administer into a free-flowing I.V. solution of NS or D_5W. Avoid extravasation - potent vesicant. Local erythematous streaking along the vein may indicate rapid administration. Unless specific data is available, do not mix with other drugs.

Extravasation management: Topical cooling may be achieved using ice packs or cooling pad with circulating ice water. Cooling of site for 24 hours as tolerated by the patient. Elevate and rest extremity 24-48 hours, then resume normal activity as tolerated. Application of cold inhibits vesicant's cytotoxicity. **Application of heat can be harmful and is contraindicated.** If pain, erythema, and/or swelling persist beyond 48 hours, refer patient immediately to plastic surgeon for consultation and possible debridement.

pH: 5-7

Stability

Storage Store intact vials of solution under refrigeration at 2°C to 8°C (36°F to 46°F). Protect from light. Solutions diluted in D_5W or NS for infusion are stable for 4 weeks at room temperature, protected from light. Syringe and IVPB solutions are stable for 72 hours at room temperature and 7 days under refrigeration.

Nursing Actions

Physical Assessment Infusion site must be closely monitored; extravasation can cause severe cellulitis or tissue necrosis (eg, do not apply heat). Monitor for cardiac toxicity, myelosuppression, and peripheral neuropathy frequently during therapy.

Patient Education This medication is only administered by intravenous infusion; report immediately any swelling, pain, burning, or redness at infusion site or sudden onset of chest pain, breathing or swallowing difficulty, or chills. It is important to maintain adequate nutrition and hydration, unless instructed to restrict fluid intake. You will be more susceptible to infection. You may experience nausea or vomiting, diarrhea, or loss of hair (reversible). Urine may turn darker color (normal). Report immediately chest pain, swelling of extremities, respiratory difficulty, palpitations, or rapid heartbeat. Report unresolved nausea, vomiting, or diarrhea; alterations in urinary pattern (increased or decreased); opportunistic infection (eg, fever, chills, unusual bruising or bleeding, signs of infection fatigue, purulent vaginal discharge, unhealed mouth sores); abdominal pain or blood in stools; excessive fatigue; yellowing of eyes or skin; swelling of extremities; respiratory difficulty; or unresolved diarrhea.

Related Information

Management of Drug Extravasations *on page* 1269

Ifosfamide (eye FOSS fa mide)

Brand Names: U.S. Ifex

Index Terms Isophosphamide; Z4942

Pharmacologic Category Antineoplastic Agent, Alkylating Agent; Antineoplastic Agent, Alkylating Agent (Nitrogen Mustard)

Medication Safety Issues

Sound-alike/look-alike issues:

Ifosfamide may be confused with cyclophosphamide

High alert medication:

The Institute for Safe Medication Practices (ISMP) includes this medication among its list of drugs which have a heightened risk of causing significant patient harm when used in error.

Pregnancy Risk Factor D

Lactation Enters breast milk/not recommended

Use Treatment of testicular cancer

Unlabeled Use Treatment of bladder cancer, cervical cancer, ovarian cancer, nonsmall cell lung cancer, small cell lung cancer, Hodgkin's and non-Hodgkin's lymphoma; acute lymphocytic leukemia; Ewing's sarcoma, osteosarcoma, and soft tissue sarcomas

Mechanism of Action/Effect Inhibits protein synthesis and DNA synthesis

Contraindications Hypersensitivity to ifosfamide or any component of the formulation; patients with severely depressed bone marrow function

Warnings/Precautions Hazardous agent - use appropriate precautions for handling and disposal. **[U.S. Boxed Warning]: Urotoxic side effects, primarily hemorrhagic cystitis, may occur (dose-limiting toxicity).** Hydration (at least 2 L/day) and/or mesna administration will protect against hemorrhagic cystitis. **[U.S. Boxed Warning]: Severe bone marrow suppression may occur (dose-limiting toxicity);** use is contraindicated in patients with severely depressed bone marrow function. **[U.S. Boxed Warning]: May cause CNS toxicity, including confusion and coma;** usually reversible upon discontinuation of treatment. Encephalopathy, ranging from mild somnolence to hallucinations and/or coma may occur; risk factors may include hypoalbuminemia, renal dysfunction and prior history of ifosfamide-induced encephalopathy. Use with caution in patients with impaired renal function or those with compromised bone marrow reserve. May interfere with wound healing. **[U.S. Boxed Warning]: Should be administered under the supervision of an experienced cancer chemotherapy physician.** Safety and efficacy in children have not been established.

Drug Interactions

Avoid Concomitant Use

Avoid concomitant use of Ifosfamide with any of the following: BCG; CloZAPine; Conivaptan; Natalizumab; Pimecrolimus; Pimozide; Tacrolimus (Topical); Vaccines (Live)

Decreased Effect

Ifosfamide may decrease the levels/effects of: BCG; Coccidioidin Skin Test; Sipuleucel-T; Vaccines (Inactivated); Vaccines (Live); Vitamin K Antagonists

The levels/effects of Ifosfamide may be decreased by: CYP2A6 Inducers (Strong); CYP2C19 Inducers (Strong); CYP3A4 Inducers (Strong); Deferasirox; Echinacea; Herbs (CYP3A4 Inducers); Tocilizumab

Increased Effect/Toxicity

Ifosfamide may increase the levels/effects of: ARIPiprazole; CloZAPine; Leflunomide; Natalizumab; Pimozide; Vaccines (Live); Vitamin K Antagonists

The levels/effects of Ifosfamide may be increased by: Conivaptan; CYP2A6 Inhibitors (Moderate); CYP2A6 Inhibitors (Strong); CYP2C19 Inhibitors (Moderate); CYP2C19 Inhibitors (Strong); CYP3A4 Inhibitors (Moderate); CYP3A4 Inhibitors (Strong); Dasatinib; Denosumab; Ivacaftor; Pimecrolimus; Roflumilast; Tacrolimus (Topical); Trastuzumab

Nutritional/Ethanol Interactions Herb/Nutraceutical: St John's wort may decrease ifosfamide levels.

Adverse Reactions

>10%:

- Central nervous system: CNS toxicity or encephalopathy (10% to 30%; includes somnolence, agitation, confusion, delirium, hallucinations, depressive psychosis, incontinence, palsy, diplopia, aphasia, or coma)
- Dermatologic: Alopecia (83%)
- Endocrine & metabolic: Metabolic acidosis (31%)
- Gastrointestinal: Nausea/vomiting (58%), may be more common with higher doses or bolus infusion
- Hematologic: Myelosuppression (onset: 7-14 days; nadir: 21-28 days; recovery: 21-28 days), leukopenia (50% to ≤100%; grade 4: ≤50%), thrombocytopenia (20%; grades 3/4: 8%)
- Renal: Hematuria (6% to 92%; grade 2 [gross hematuria]: 8% to 12%)

1% to 10%:

- Central nervous system: Fever
- Hepatic: Bilirubin increased (3%), liver dysfunction (3%), transaminases increased (3%)
- Local: Phlebitis (2%)
- Renal: Renal impairment (6%)
- Miscellaneous: Infection (8%)

Available Dosage Forms

Injection, powder for reconstitution: 1 g, 3 g

Ifex: 1 g, 3 g

Injection, solution: 50 mg/mL (20 mL, 60 mL)

General Dosage Range Dosage adjustment recommended in patients with hepatic or renal impairment

I.V.: *Adults:* 4000-5000 mg/m²/day for 1 day every 14-28 days **or** 1000-3000 mg/m²/day for 2-5 days every 21-28 days

Administration

I.V. Administer I.V. over 30 minutes to several hours or continuous intravenous infusion over 5 days.

I.V. Detail Adequate hydration (at least 2 L/day) of the patient before and for 72 hours after therapy is recommended to minimize the risk of hemorrhagic cystitis.

pH: 6

Stability

Reconstitution Dilute powder with SWFI or bacteriostatic SWFI to a concentration of 50 mg/mL. Further dilution in 50-1000 mL D_5W or NS (to a final concentration of 0.6-20 mg/mL) is recommended for I.V. infusion.

Storage Store intact vials of powder for injection at room temperature of 20°C to 25°C (68°F to 77°F). Store intact vials of solution under refrigeration at 2°C to 8°C (36°F to 46°F). Reconstituted solutions may be stored under refrigeration for up to 21 days. Solutions diluted for administration are stable for 7 days at room temperature and for 6 weeks under refrigeration.

Nursing Actions

Physical Assessment To prevent bladder toxicity, maintain adequate hydration for 72 hours prior to infusion to minimize risk of hemorrhagic cystitis. Premedication with antiemetic may be ordered. Monitor vital signs prior to each infusion and regularly during therapy. Monitor for CNS depression or psychoses, hematuria (hemorrhagic cystitis), and myelosuppression (anemia) throughout therapy. Teach patient importance of adequate hydration.

Patient Education This drug can only be administered by infusion. Report immediately any swelling, redness, or pain at infusion site. Maintain adequate hydration, unless instructed to restrict fluid intake, for at least 3 days prior to infusion and each day of therapy. You will be more susceptible to infection. May cause loss of hair (reversible, although regrowth hair may be different color or texture), fertility or amenorrhea, nausea or vomiting, headache, or mouth sores. Report any difficulty or pain with urination, chest pain, rapid heartbeat, palpitations, CNS changes (eg, hallucinations, confusion, somnolence), unusual rash, persistent nausea or vomiting, swelling of extremities, respiratory difficulty, unusual fatigue, or opportunistic infection (eg, fever, chills, easy bruising, or unusual bleeding).

Related Information

Management of Drug Extravasations *on page 1269*

Iloperidone (eye loe PER i done)

Brand Names: U.S. Fanapt®

Pharmacologic Category Antipsychotic Agent, Atypical

Medication Safety Issues

Sound-alike/look-alike issues:

Fanapt® may be confused with Xanax®

Iloperidone may be confused with domperidone

Pregnancy Risk Factor C

Lactation Excretion in breast milk unknown/not recommended

Use Acute treatment of schizophrenia

Mechanism of Action/Effect Iloperidone is an atypical antipsychotic which blocks serotonin and dopamine receptors. Results in improvement of psychoses with lower incidence of extrapyramidal side effects.

Contraindications Hypersensitivity to iloperidone or any component of the formulation

Warnings/Precautions [U.S. Boxed Warning]: Elderly patients with dementia-related psychosis treated with antipsychotics are at an increased risk of death compared to placebo. Most deaths appeared to be either cardiovascular (eg, heart failure, sudden death) or infectious (eg, pneumonia) in nature. In addition, an increased incidence of cerebrovascular effects (eg, transient ischemic attack, cerebrovascular accidents) has been reported in studies of placebo-controlled trials of antipsychotics in elderly patients with dementia-related psychosis. Iloperidone is not approved for the treatment of dementia-related psychosis.

May be sedating; use with caution in disorders where CNS depression is a feature. Caution in patients with predisposition to seizures. Use is not recommended in patients with hepatic impairment. Esophageal dysmotility and aspiration have been associated with antipsychotic use; use with caution in patients at risk of aspiration pneumonia (ie, Alzheimer's disease). Use is associated with increased prolactin levels; clinical significance of hyperprolactinemia in patients with breast cancer or other prolactin-dependent tumors is unknown. May alter temperature regulation. Leukopenia, neutropenia, and agranulocytosis (sometimes fatal) have been reported in clinical trials and postmarketing reports; presence of risk factors (eg, pre-existing low WBC or history of drug-induced leuko-/neutropenia) should prompt periodic blood count assessment and discontinuation at first signs of blood dyscrasias.

May alter cardiac conduction and prolong the QT_c interval; life-threatening arrhythmias have occurred with therapeutic doses of antipsychotics. Risks may be increased by conditions or concomitant medications which cause bradycardia, hypokalemia, and/or hypomagnesemia. Avoid use in combination with QT_c-prolonging drugs and in patients with congenital long QT syndrome, history of cardiac arrhythmia, recent MI, or uncompensated heart failure. Discontinue treatment in patients found to have persistent QT_c intervals >500 msec. Further cardiac evaluation is warranted in patients with symptoms of dizziness, palpitations, or syncope. May cause orthostatic hypotension; use with caution in patients at risk of this effect (eg, concurrent medication use which may predispose to hypotension/bradycardia or presence of hypovolemia) or in those who would not tolerate transient hypotensive episodes. Use with caution in patients with cardiovascular diseases (eg, heart failure, history of myocardial infarction or ischemia, cerebrovascular disease, conduction abnormalities).

May cause anticholinergic effects (confusion, agitation, constipation, xerostomia, blurred vision, urinary retention); therefore, use with caution in patients with decreased gastrointestinal motility, urinary retention, BPH, xerostomia, or visual problems (including narrow-angle glaucoma). May cause extrapyramidal symptoms (EPS), including pseudoparkinsonism, acute dystonic reactions, akathisia, and tardive dyskinesia. Risk of dystonia (and probably other EPS) may be greater with increased doses, use of conventional antipsychotics, males, and younger patients. Risk of neuroleptic malignant syndrome (NMS) may be increased in patients with Parkinson's disease or Lewy body dementia. May cause hyperglycemia; in some cases may be extreme and associated with ketoacidosis, hyperosmolar coma, or death. Use with caution in patients with diabetes or other disorders of glucose regulation; monitor for worsening of glucose control. Significant weight gain has been observed with antipsychotic therapy; incidence varies with product. Monitor waist circumference and BMI. Rare cases of priapism have been reported.

Dosage adjustments are recommended for iloperidone when given concomitantly with strong CYP2D6 or CYP3A4 inhibitors or in poor metabolizers of CYP2D6. The possibility of a suicide attempt is inherent in psychotic illness; use caution in high-risk patients during initiation of therapy. Prescriptions should be written for the smallest quantity consistent with good patient care. Continued use for >6 weeks has not been evaluated.

Drug Interactions

Avoid Concomitant Use

Avoid concomitant use of Iloperidone with any of the following: Artemether; Dronedarone; Lumefantrine; Metoclopramide; Nilotinib; Pimozide; QUEtiapine; QuiNINE; Tetrabenazine; Thioridazine; Toremifene; Vandetanib; Vemurafenib; Ziprasidone

Decreased Effect

Iloperidone may decrease the levels/effects of: Amphetamines; Anti-Parkinson's Agents (Dopamine Agonist); Quinagolide

The levels/effects of Iloperidone may be decreased by: CYP2D6 Inhibitors (Strong); Lithium formulations; Peginterferon Alfa-2b; Tocilizumab

Increased Effect/Toxicity

Iloperidone may increase the levels/effects of: Alcohol (Ethyl); CNS Depressants; Dronedarone; Methylphenidate; Pimozide; QTc-Prolonging ▶

Agents; QuiNINE; Serotonin Modulators; Tetrabenazine; Thioridazine; Toremifene; Vandetanib; Vemurafenib; Ziprasidone

The levels/effects of Iloperidone may be increased by: Abiraterone Acetate; Acetylcholinesterase Inhibitors (Central); Alfuzosin; Artemether; Chloroquine; Ciprofloxacin; Ciprofloxacin (Systemic); CYP2D6 Inhibitors (Moderate); CYP2D6 Inhibitors (Strong); CYP3A4 Inhibitors (Strong); Gadobutrol; HydrOXYzine; Indacaterol; Lithium formulations; Lumefantrine; MAO Inhibitors; Methylphenidate; Metoclopramide; Nilotinib; QUEtiapine; QuiNINE; Tetrabenazine

Nutritional/Ethanol Interactions

Ethanol: May increase CNS depression; monitor for increased effects with coadministration. Caution patients about effects.

Herb/Nutraceutical: Avoid St John's wort (may decrease serum levels of iloperidone). Avoid kava kava, gotu kola, valerian, St John's wort (may increase CNS depression).

Adverse Reactions

>10%:

Cardiovascular: Tachycardia (3% to 12%; dose related)

Central nervous system: Dizziness (10% to 20%; dose related), somnolence (9% to 15%)

1% to 10%:

Cardiovascular: Orthostatic hypotension (3% to 5%), hypotension (<1% to 3%; dose related), palpitations (≥1%)

Central nervous system: Fatigue (4% to 6%), extrapyramidal symptoms (4% to 5%), tremor (3%), lethargy (1% to 3%), akathisia (2%), aggression (≥1%), delusion (≥1%), restlessness (≥1%)

Dermatologic: Rash (2% to 3%)

Gastrointestinal: Nausea (≤10%), xerostomia (8% to 10%), weight gain (1% to 9%; dose related), diarrhea (5% to 7%), abdominal discomfort (≤3%; dose related), weight loss (≥1%)

Genitourinary: Ejaculation failure (2%), erectile dysfunction (≥1%), urinary incontinence (≥1%)

Neuromuscular & skeletal: Arthralgia (3%), stiffness (1% to 3%; dose related), dyskinesia (<2%), muscle spasm (≥1%), myalgia (≥1%)

Ocular: Blurred vision (≤3%), conjunctivitis (≥1%)

Respiratory: Nasal congestion (5% to 8%), nasopharyngitis (≤4%), upper respiratory tract infection (2% to 3%), dyspnea (2%)

Available Dosage Forms

Tablet, oral:

Fanapt®: 1 mg, 2 mg, 4 mg, 6 mg, 8 mg, 10 mg, 12 mg, 1 mg (2s), 2 mg (2s), 4 mg (2s), and 6 mg (2s)

General Dosage Range Oral: *Adults:* Initial: 1 mg twice daily; Dosage range: 6-12 mg twice daily (maximum: 24 mg/day)

Administration

Oral May be administered with or without food.

Stability

Storage Store at 25°C (77°F); excursions permitted to 15°C to 30°C (59°F to 86°F). Protect from light and moisture.

Nursing Actions

Physical Assessment Monitor weight prior to initiating therapy and at least monthly; can cause weight gain. Be alert to the potential for suicide ideation and orthostatic hypotension, especially during the titration phase. Initiate at lower doses and titrate to target dose. Taper dosage slowly when discontinuing.

Patient Education It may take several weeks to achieve desired results. Avoid alcohol. Maintain adequate hydration. Avoid overheating. If you have diabetes, you may experience increased blood sugars; monitor blood sugars closely. You may experience excess sedation, drowsiness, restlessness, dizziness, or blurred vision; dry mouth, nausea, or GI upset; postural hypotension; or urinary retention. Report persistent CNS effects (eg, trembling fingers, altered gait or balance, excessive sedation, seizures, unusual muscle or skeletal movements, anxiety, abnormal thoughts [especially suicide ideation], confusion, personality changes); chest pain, palpitations, irregular or rapid heartbeat, feeling faint, or severe dizziness; signs of infection or fever; vision changes; respiratory difficulty; or worsening of condition.

Dietary Considerations May be given with or without food.

Imatinib (eye MAT eh nib)

Brand Names: U.S. Gleevec®

Index Terms CGP-57148B; Glivec; Imatinib Mesylate; STI-571

Pharmacologic Category Antineoplastic Agent, Tyrosine Kinase Inhibitor

Medication Safety Issues

Sound-alike/look-alike issues:

Imatinib may be confused with axitinib, dasatinib, erlotinib, gefitinib, nilotinib, SORAfenib, SUNItinib, vandetanib

High alert medication:

This medication is in a class the Institute for Safe Medication Practices (ISMP) includes among its list of drug classes which have a heightened risk of causing significant patient harm when used in error.

Pregnancy Risk Factor D

Lactation Enters breast milk/not recommended

Breast-Feeding Considerations Imatinib and its active metabolite are found in human breast milk; the milk/plasma ratio is 0.5 for imatinib and 0.9 for the active metabolite. Based on body weight, up to 10% of a therapeutic maternal dose could potentially be received by a breastfed infant, the decision to discontinue breast-feeding during therapy or to discontinue imatinib should take into account the benefits of treatment to the mother.

Use Treatment of:

Gastrointestinal stromal tumors (GIST) kit-positive (CD117), including unresectable and/or metastatic malignant and adjuvant treatment following complete resection

Philadelphia chromosome-positive (Ph+) chronic myeloid leukemia (CML) in chronic phase (newly-diagnosed)

Ph+ CML in blast crisis, accelerated phase, or chronic phase after failure of interferon therapy

Ph+ acute lymphoblastic leukemia (ALL) (relapsed or refractory)

Aggressive systemic mastocytosis (ASM) without D816V c-Kit mutation (or c-Kit mutation status unknown)

Dermatofibrosarcoma protuberans (DFSP) (unresectable, recurrent and/or metastatic)

Hypereosinophilic syndrome (HES) and/or chronic eosinophilic leukemia (CEL)

Myelodysplastic/myeloproliferative disease (MDS/MPD) associated with platelet-derived growth factor receptor (PDGFR) gene rearrangements

Canadian labeling (not an approved indication in the U.S.): Ph+ ALL induction therapy (newly diagnosed)

Unlabeled Use Treatment of desmoid tumors or chordoma (soft tissue sarcomas); post-stem cell transplant (allogeneic) follow-up treatment for recurrence in CML; treatment of Ph+ acute lymphoblastic lymphoma

Mechanism of Action/Effect Inhibits a specific enzyme (Bcr-Abl tyrosine kinase) produced by the Philadelphia chromosome found in many patients with chronic myeloid leukemia (CML). Inhibition of this enzyme blocks proliferation and induces cell death in leukemic cells. Also inhibits tyrosine kinase for platelet-derived growth factor (SCF), c-Kit, and cellular events mediated by PDGF and SCF.

Contraindications There are no contraindications listed within the FDA-approved manufacturer's labeling.

Canadian labeling: Hypersensitivity to imatinib or any component of the formulation

Warnings/Precautions Hazardous agent - use appropriate precautions for handling and disposal. Often associated with fluid retention, weight gain, and edema (probability increases with higher doses and age >65 years); occasionally serious and may lead to significant complications, including pleural effusion, pericardial effusion, pulmonary edema, and ascites. Monitor for rapid weight gain or other signs/symptoms of fluid retention. Use with caution in patients where fluid accumulation may be poorly tolerated, such as in cardiovascular disease (heart failure [HF] or hypertension) and pulmonary disease. Severe HF and left ventricular dysfunction (LVD) have been reported occasionally, usually in patients with comorbidities and/or risk factors; carefully monitor patients with pre-existing cardiac disease or risk factors for HF or history of renal failure. With initiation of imatinib treatment, cardiogenic shock and/or LVD have been reported in patients with hypereosinophilic syndrome and cardiac involvement (reversible with systemic steroids, circulatory support and temporary cessation of imatinib). Patients with high eosinophil levels and an abnormal echocardiogram or abnormal serum troponin level may benefit from prophylactic systemic steroids (for 1-2 weeks) with the initiation of imatinib.

Severe bullous dermatologic reactions (including erythema multiforme and Stevens-Johnson syndrome) have been reported; recurrence has been described with rechallenge. Case reports of successful resumption at a lower dose (with corticosteroids and/or antihistamine) have been described; however, some patients may experience recurrent reactions.

Hepatotoxicity may occur (may be severe); fatal hepatic failure and severe hepatic injury have been reported with both short- and long-term use; monitor; therapy interruption or dose reduction may be necessary. Transaminase and bilirubin elevations, and acute liver failure have been observed with imatinib in combination with chemotherapy. Use with caution in patients with pre-existing hepatic impairment; dosage adjustment recommended in patients with severe impairment. Use with caution in renal impairment; dosage adjustment recommended for moderate and severe impairment. Tumor lysis syndrome (TLS), including fatalities, has been reported in patients with ALL, CML eosinophilic leukemias, and GIST; risk for TLS is higher in patients with a high tumor burden or high proliferation rate; monitor closely; correct clinically significant dehydration and treat high uric acid levels prior to initiation of imatinib.

May cause GI irritation, severe hemorrhage (grades 3 and 4; including gastrointestinal hemorrhage and/or tumor hemorrhage; hemorrhage incidence is higher in patients with GIST [gastrointestinal tumors may have been hemorrhage source]), or hematologic toxicity (anemia, neutropenia, and thrombocytopenia); monitor blood counts; median duration of neutropenia is 2-3 weeks; median duration of thrombocytopenia is 3-4 weeks; in CML, cytopenias are more common in accelerated or blast phase than in chronic phase. Hypothyroidism has been reported in patients who were receiving thyroid hormone replacement therapy prior to the initiation of imatinib; monitor thyroid function; the average onset for imatinib-induced hypothyroidism is 2 weeks; consider doubling levothyroxine doses upon initiation of imatinib (Hamnvik, 2011). Use with caution in patients receiving concurrent therapy with drugs which alter cytochrome P450 activity or require metabolism by these isoenzymes; avoid concomitant use of strong CYP3A4 inducers. Imatinib exposure may be reduced in patients who have had gastric surgery (eg, bypass, major gastrectomy, or resection); monitor imatinib trough concentrations (Liu, 2011; Pavlovsky, 2009; Yoo, 2010). Growth retardation has been reported in children receiving imatinib for the treatment of CML; generally where treatment was initiated in prepubertal children; growth velocity was usually restored as pubertal age was reached (Shima, 2010); monitor growth closely. Reports of accidents have been received but it is unclear if imatinib has been the direct cause in any case; use caution when driving/operating motor vehicles and heavy machinery.

Drug Interactions

Avoid Concomitant Use

Avoid concomitant use of Imatinib with any of the following: Alfuzosin; Axitinib; BCG; CloZAPine; Conivaptan; Crizotinib; Dronedarone; Eplerenone; Everolimus; Fluticasone (Oral Inhalation); Halofantrine; Lapatinib; Lovastatin; Lurasidone; Natalizumab; Nilotinib; Nisoldipine; Pimecrolimus; Pimozide; Ranolazine; Rivaroxaban; RomiDEPsin; Salmeterol; Silodosin; Simvastatin; Tacrolimus (Topical); Tamsulosin; Thioridazine; Ticagrelor; Tolvaptan; Toremifene; Vaccines (Live)

Decreased Effect

Imatinib may decrease the levels/effects of: BCG; Cardiac Glycosides; Coccidioidin Skin Test; Codeine; Fludarabine; Prasugrel; Sipuleucel-T; Ticagrelor; TraMADol; Vaccines (Inactivated); Vaccines (Live); Vitamin K Antagonists

The levels/effects of Imatinib may be decreased by: CYP3A4 Inducers (Strong); Cyproterone; Deferasirox; Echinacea; Peginterferon Alfa-2b; P-glycoprotein/ABCB1 Inducers; Rifamycin Derivatives; St Johns Wort; Tocilizumab

Increased Effect/Toxicity

Imatinib may increase the levels/effects of: Acetaminophen; Alfuzosin; Almotriptan; Alosetron; ARIPiprazole; Axitinib; Bortezomib; Brentuximab Vedotin; Brinzolamide; Budesonide (Nasal); Budesonide (Systemic, Oral Inhalation); Ciclesonide; CloZAPine; Colchicine; Conivaptan; Corticosteroids (Orally Inhaled); Crizotinib; CycloSPORINE; CycloSPORINE (Systemic); CYP2D6 Substrates; CYP3A4 Substrates; Dienogest; Dronedarone; Dutasteride; Eplerenone; Everolimus; FentaNYL; Fesoterodine; Fluticasone (Nasal); Fluticasone (Oral Inhalation); GuanFACINE; Halofantrine; Iloperidone; Ivacaftor; Ixabepilone; Lapatinib; Leflunomide; Lovastatin; Lumefantrine; Lurasidone; Maraviroc; MethylPREDNISolone; Natalizumab; Nebivolol; Nilotinib; Nisoldipine; Paricalcitol; Pazopanib; Pimecrolimus; Pimozide; Propafenone; Ranolazine; Rivaroxaban; RomiDEPsin; Ruxolitinib; Salmeterol; Saxagliptin; Sildenafil; Silodosin; Simvastatin; SORAfenib; Tadalafil; Tamsulosin; Thioridazine; Ticagrelor; Tolterodine; Tolvaptan; Topotecan; Toremifene; Vaccines (Live); Vardenafil; Vemurafenib; Vilazodone; Vitamin K Antagonists; Warfarin; Zuclopenthixol

The levels/effects of Imatinib may be increased by: Acetaminophen; Antifungal Agents (Azole Derivatives, Systemic); CYP3A4 Inhibitors (Moderate); CYP3A4 Inhibitors (Strong); Dasatinib; Denosumab; Lansoprazole; P-glycoprotein/ABCB1 Inhibitors; Pimecrolimus; Roflumilast; Tacrolimus (Topical); Trastuzumab

Nutritional/Ethanol Interactions

Ethanol: Management: Avoid ethanol.

Food: Food may reduce GI irritation. Grapefruit juice may increase imatinib plasma concentration. Management: Take with a meal and a large glass of water. Avoid grapefruit juice. Maintain adequate hydration, unless instructed to restrict fluid intake.

Herb/Nutraceutical: St John's wort may increase metabolism and decrease imatinib plasma concentration. Management: Avoid St John's wort.

Adverse Reactions Note: Adverse reactions listed as a composite of data across many trials, except where noted for a specific indication.

>10%:

Cardiovascular: Edema/fluid retention (11% to 86%; grades 3/4: 3% to 13%; includes aggravated edema, anasarca, ascites, pericardial effusion, peripheral edema, pleural effusion, pulmonary edema and superficial edema); facial edema (≤17%), chest pain (7% to 11%)

Central nervous system: Fatigue (29% to 75%), pain (≤47%), fever (6% to 41%), headache (8% to 37%), dizziness (5% to 19%), insomnia (10% to 15%), depression (≤15%), anxiety (8% to 12%), chills (≤11%)

Dermatologic: Rash (9% to 50%; grades 3/4: 1% to 9%), dermatitis (GIST ≤39%), pruritus (8% to 26%), alopecia (GIST 10% to 15%)

Endocrine & metabolic: LDH increased (GIST ≤60%), hypoproteinemia (≤32%), albumin decreased (≤21%; grade 3: ≤4%), hypokalemia (6% to 13%)

Gastrointestinal: Nausea (42% to 73%), diarrhea (25% to 59%), vomiting (11% to 58%), abdominal pain (3% to 57%), anorexia (≤36%), weight gain (5% to 32%), dyspepsia (11% to 27%), flatulence (≤25%), abdominal distension (≤19%), constipation (9% to 16%), taste disturbance (≤13%)

Hematologic: Anemia (25% to 80%; grade 3: 1% to 42%; grade 4: ≤11%), leukopenia (GIST 5% to 47%), hemorrhage (3% to 53%; grades 3/4 ≤19%), neutropenia (grade 3: 7% to 27%; grade 4: 3% to 48%), thrombocytopenia (grade 3: 1% to 31%; grade 4: <1% to 33%)

Hepatic: AST increased (≤38%; grade 3: 2% to 5%; grade 4: ≤3%), ALT increased (≤34%; grade 3: 2% to 7%; grade 4: <3%), alkaline phosphatase increased (≤17%; grade 3: ≤6%; grade 4: <1%), bilirubin increased (≤13%; grade 3: 1% to 4%; grade 4: ≤3%)

Neuromuscular & skeletal: Muscle cramps (16% to 62%), arthralgia (≤40%), joint pain (11% to 31%), myalgia (9% to 32%), weakness (≤21%), musculoskeletal pain (children 21%; adults 38% to 47%), rigors (10% to 12%), paresthesia (≤12%), bone pain (≤11%)

Ocular: Periorbital edema (DFSP 33%; MPD 29%; GIST ≤74%), lacrimation increased (DFSP 25%; GIST ≤18%), blurred vision (≤11%)

Renal: Serum creatinine increased (≤44%; grade 3: ≤3%; DFSP: grade 4: 8%)

Respiratory: Nasopharyngitis (1% to 31%), cough (11% to 27%), dyspnea (≤21%), upper respiratory tract infection (3% to 21%), pharyngolaryngeal pain (≤18%), rhinitis (DFSP 17%), pharyngitis (CML 10% to 15%), pneumonia (CML 4% to 13%), sinusitis (4% to 11%)

Miscellaneous: Infection (GIST ≤28%), night sweats (CML 13% to 17%), influenza (1% to 14%), diaphoresis (GIST ≤13%)

1% to 10%:

Cardiovascular: Flushing, palpitation (≤5%)

Central nervous system: CNS/cerebral hemorrhage (≤9%), depression (≤8%), hypoesthesia

Dermatologic: Dry skin, erythema, photosensitivity reaction

Endocrine & metabolic: Hyperglycemia (≤10%), hypocalcemia (GIST ≤6%)

Gastrointestinal: Stomatitis/mucositis (≤10%), weight loss (≤10%), gastrointestinal hemorrhage (2% to 8%), gastritis, gastroesophageal reflux, xerostomia

Hematologic: Lymphopenia (GIST ≤10%), neutropenic fever, pancytopenia

Neuromuscular & skeletal: Back pain (GIST ≤7%), limb pain (GIST ≤7%), peripheral neuropathy, joint swelling

Ocular: Conjunctival hemorrhage, conjunctivitis, dry eyes, eyelid edema

Respiratory: Epistaxis

Available Dosage Forms

Tablet, oral:

Gleevec®: 100 mg, 400 mg

General Dosage Range Dosage adjustment recommended in patients with hepatic or renal impairment, on concomitant therapy, and/or who develop toxicities

Oral:

Children ≥2 years: 340 mg/m²/day in 1-2 divided doses (maximum: 600 mg/day)

Adults: 100-800 mg/day in 1-2 divided doses

Administration

Oral Should be administered with a meal and a large glass of water. Tablets may be dispersed in water or apple juice (using ~50 mL for 100 mg tablet, ~200 mL for 400 mg tablet); stir until dissolved and use immediately. For daily dosing ≥800 mg, the 400 mg tablets should be used in order to reduce iron exposure.

Stability

Storage Store at 25°C (77°F); excursions permitted between 15°C to 30°C (59°F to 86°F). Protect from moisture.

Nursing Actions

Physical Assessment Monitor weight and fluid status. Monitor for hemorrhage, paresthesia, and respiratory or CNS changes.

Patient Education Avoid chronic use of acetaminophen or aspirin unless approved by prescriber. Take with food or a large glass of water. If you have difficulty swallowing tablets, tablet may be dispersed in water or apple juice (using ~50 mL for 100 mg tablet or ~200 mL for 400 mg tablet); stir until dissolved and use immediately. Maintain adequate hydration, unless instructed to restrict fluid intake. You will be required to have regularly scheduled laboratory tests while on this medication. You will be more susceptible to infection. You may experience headache, dizziness, fatigue, loss of appetite, nausea, vomiting, mouth sores, or constipation. Report chest pain, palpitations, or swelling of extremities; cough, difficulty breathing, or wheezing; weight gain; skin rash; muscle or bone pain, tremors, or cramping; persistent fatigue or weakness; easy bruising or unusual bleeding (eg, tarry stools, blood in vomitus, stool, urine, or mouth); or persistent GI problems or pain. Take caution when driving a car or operating heavy machinery.

Dietary Considerations Should be taken with food and a large glass of water to decrease gastrointestinal irritation. Avoid grapefruit juice.

Imipenem and Cilastatin

(i mi PEN em & sye la STAT in)

Brand Names: U.S. Primaxin® I.V.

Index Terms Imipemide; Primaxin® I.M. [DSC]

Pharmacologic Category Antibiotic, Carbapenem

Medication Safety Issues

Sound-alike/look-alike issues:

Imipenem may be confused with ertapenem, meropenem

Primaxin® may be confused with Premarin®, Primacor®

Pregnancy Risk Factor C

Lactation Enters breast milk/use caution

Use Treatment of lower respiratory tract, urinary tract, intra-abdominal, gynecologic, bone and joint, skin and skin structure, endocarditis (caused by *Staphylococcus aureus*) and polymicrobic infections as well as bacterial septicemia. Antibacterial activity includes gram-positive bacteria (methicillin-sensitive *S. aureus* and *Streptococcus* spp), resistant gram-negative bacilli (including extended spectrum beta-lactamase-producing *Escherichia coli* and *Klebsiella* spp, *Enterobacter* spp, and *Pseudomonas aeruginosa*), and anaerobes.

Unlabeled Use Hepatic abscess; neutropenic fever; melioidosis

Available Dosage Forms

Injection, powder for reconstitution: Imipenem 250 mg and cilastatin 250 mg; imipenem 500 mg and cilastatin 500 mg

Primaxin® I.V.: Imipenem 250 mg and cilastatin 250 mg; imipenem 500 mg and cilastatin 500 mg

General Dosage Range Dosage adjustment recommended in patients with renal impairment

I.V.:

Children >3 months: 15-25 mg/kg every 6 hours (maximum: 4 g/day)

Adults 30 to <70 kg: 125 mg every 12 hours up to 1000 mg every 8 hours

Adults ≥70 kg: 250-1000 mg every 6-8 hours (maximum: 50 mg/kg/day; 4 g/day)

Administration

I.V. Do not administer I.V. push. Infuse doses ≤500 mg over 20-30 minutes; infuse doses ≥750 mg over 40-60 minutes.

I.V. Detail Vial contents must be transferred to 100 mL of infusion solution. If nausea and/or vomiting occur during administration, decrease the rate of I.V. infusion. Do not mix with or physically add to other antibiotics; however, may administer concomitantly.

pH: 6.5-8.5 (buffered)

Nursing Actions

Physical Assessment Results of culture and sensitivity tests and patient's allergy history should be assessed prior to beginning therapy. Advise patients with diabetes about use of Clinitest®.

Patient Education This medication can only be administered by injection or infusion. Report immediately any warmth, swelling, pain, or redness at infusion or injection site. Maintain adequate hydration, unless instructed to restrict fluid intake, and nutrition. May cause false test results with Clinitest®; use of another type of glucose testing is preferable. Report immediately any CNS changes (dizziness, hallucinations, anxiety, visual disturbances); swelling of throat, tongue, lips, or face; chills or fever; persistent diarrhea; or unusual discharge or foul-smelling urine.

Imipramine (im IP ra meen)

Brand Names: U.S. Tofranil-PM®; Tofranil®

Index Terms Imipramine Hydrochloride; Imipramine Pamoate

Pharmacologic Category Antidepressant, Tricyclic (Tertiary Amine)

Medication Safety Issues

Sound-alike/look-alike issues:

Imipramine may be confused with amitriptyline, desipramine, Norpramin®

Medication Guide Available Yes

Lactation Enters breast milk/not recommended (AAP rates "of concern"; AAP 2001 update pending)

Use Treatment of depression; treatment of nocturnal enuresis in children

Unlabeled Use Analgesic for certain chronic and neuropathic pain (including diabetic neuropathy); panic disorder; attention-deficit/hyperactivity disorder (ADHD); post-traumatic stress disorder (PTSD)

Available Dosage Forms

Capsule, oral: 75 mg, 100 mg, 125 mg, 150 mg

Tofranil-PM®: 75 mg, 100 mg, 125 mg, 150 mg

Tablet, oral: 10 mg, 25 mg, 50 mg

Tofranil®: 10 mg, 25 mg, 50 mg

General Dosage Range Oral:

Children ≥6-12 years: Initial: 25 mg at bedtime, may increase to 50 mg at bedtime if no response (maximum: 2.5 mg/kg/day; 50 mg/day)

Children >12 years: Initial: 25 mg at bedtime, may increase to 75 mg at bedtime if not response (maximum: 75 mg/day) **or** 30-40 mg/day, increase gradually, to a maximum of 100 mg/day in single or divided doses

Adults: Initial: 75-150 mg/day, increase gradually to a maximum of 200 mg/day (outpatients) or 300 mg/day (inpatients) in divided doses or a single dose at bedtime

Elderly: Initial: 25-50 mg at bedtime (maximum: 100 mg/day)

Nursing Actions

Physical Assessment Perform careful cardiovascular assessment prior to initiating therapy. Monitor therapeutic response (eg, mental status, mood, affect, suicide ideation) at the beginning of therapy and periodically throughout. Taper dosage slowly when discontinuing.

Patient Education It may take 2-3 weeks to achieve desired results. Take in the evening. Avoid alcohol. Maintain adequate hydration, unless instructed to restrict fluid intake. You may experience drowsiness, lightheadedness, impaired coordination, dizziness, blurred vision, nausea, vomiting, altered taste, dry mouth, constipation, diarrhea, postural hypotension, or urinary retention. Report persistent insomnia; muscle cramping or tremors; chest pain, palpitations, rapid heartbeat, swelling of extremities, or severe dizziness; unresolved urinary retention; rash or skin irritation; yellowing of eyes or skin; pale stools/dark urine; worsening of condition; and suicide ideation.

Related Information

Peak and Trough Guidelines *on page 1276*

Imiquimod (i mi KWI mod)

Brand Names: U.S. Aldara®; Zyclara®

Pharmacologic Category Skin and Mucous Membrane Agent; Topical Skin Product

Medication Safety Issues

Sound-alike/look-alike issues:

Aldara® may be confused with Alora®, Lialda®

Pregnancy Risk Factor C

Lactation Excretion in breast milk unknown/use caution

Use Treatment of external genital and perianal warts/condyloma acuminata; nonhyperkeratotic actinic keratosis on face or scalp; superficial basal cell carcinoma (sBCC) with a maximum tumor diameter of 2 cm located on the trunk, neck, or extremities (excluding hands or feet)

Unlabeled Use Treatment of common warts

Available Dosage Forms

Cream, topical: 5% (24s)

Aldara®: 5% (24s)

Zyclara®: 3.75% (28s)

General Dosage Range Topical:

Children ≥12 years: Apply a thin layer 3 times/week on alternate days, leave on for 6-10 hours

Adults:

Actinic keratosis: Apply twice weekly or once daily at bedtime for 2 treatment cycles (14 days each) separated by a 14-day rest period with no treatment; leave on for 8 hours

External genital and/or perianal warts/condyloma acuminata: Apply a thin layer 3 times/week on alternate days; leave on for 6-10 hours

Superficial basal cell carcinoma: Apply once daily at bedtime 5 days/week; leave on for 8 hours before washing

Administration

Topical Topical: Wash hands prior to and following application. Do not occlude the application site. Partially used packets should be discarded and not reused.

Actinic keratosis: Apply Aldara® over a single contiguous area (approximately 25 cm^2) on the face or scalp or Zyclara® 3.75% over an area <200 cm^2 on the face or scalp; the treatment area should be washed and thoroughly dried prior to application. Both areas should not be treated concurrently. Apply a thin layer to the affected area and rub in until the cream is no longer visible. Avoid contact with the eyes, lips, and nostrils.

External genital warts: Aldara®: Instruct patients to apply to external or perianal warts; not for vaginal use. Apply a thin layer to the wart area and rub in until the cream is no longer visible. Single-use packets contain sufficient cream to cover a wart area of up to 20 cm^2; avoid use of excessive amounts of cream. Nonocclusive dressings (such as cotton gauze or cotton underwear) may be used in the management of skin reactions.

Superficial basal cell carcinoma: Aldara®: Treatment area should have a maximum diameter no more than 2 cm on the trunk, neck, or extremities (excluding the hands, feet, and anogenital skin). Treatment area should include a 1 cm margin around the tumor. Wash and thoroughly dry treatment area prior to application; apply a thin layer to the affected area (and margin) and rub in until the cream is no longer visible. Avoid contact with the eyes, lips, and nostrils.

Nursing Actions

Patient Education This medication will not eliminate nor prevent the transmission of the virus. For external use only; avoid contact with eyes, mouth, nostrils, or vagina. Exposure to sun should be avoided or minimized. Use sunscreen or wear protective clothing if sun exposure is unavoidable. Sexual contact (vaginal, anal, or oral) should be avoided while cream is on skin. May cause pain, itching, redness, burning, flaking, swelling, or scabbing in treated area. If these effects persist or become severe or open sores develop, stop treatment and notify prescriber. Report fever, malaise, myalgia, or flu-like symptoms. Prescriber may recommend a rest period of several days before resuming treatment. Apply treatment just prior to sleeping and leave on 6-10 hours. Wash hands thoroughly before and after application. Wash and dry area to be treated before applying cream. After treatment period, remove cream with mild soap and water. Apply a thin layer to external warts and rub in until cream is no longer visible. Avoid use of excessive cream. May cover area with light gauze dressing or cotton underwear; do not apply occlusive dressing.

Immune Globulin (i MYUN GLOB yoo lin)

Brand Names: U.S. Carimune® NF; Flebogamma® DIF; GamaSTAN™ S/D; Gammagard S/D®; Gammagard® Liquid; Gammaked™; Gammaplex®; Gamunex® [DSC]; Gamunex®-C; Hizentra®; Octagam®; Privigen®; Vivaglobin® [DSC]

Index Terms Gamma Globulin; IG; IGIM; IGIV; Immune Globulin Subcutaneous (Human); Immune Serum Globulin; ISG; IV Immune Globulin; IVIG; Panglobulin; SCIG

Pharmacologic Category Blood Product Derivative; Immune Globulin

Medication Safety Issues

Sound-alike/look-alike issues:

Gamimune® N may be confused with CytoGam®

Immune globulin (intravenous) may be confused with hepatitis B immune globulin

Pregnancy Risk Factor C

Lactation Excretion in breast milk unknown/use caution

Use

Treatment of primary humoral immunodeficiency syndromes (congenital agammaglobulinemia, severe combined immunodeficiency syndromes [SCIDS], common variable immunodeficiency, X-linked immunodeficiency, Wiskott-Aldrich syndrome) (Carimune® NF, Flebogamma® DIF, Gammagard® Liquid, Gammagard S/D®, Gammaked™, Gammaplex®, Gamunex®, Gamunex®-C, Hizentra®, Octagam®, Privigen®, Vivaglobin®)

Treatment of acute and chronic immune (idiopathic) thrombocytopenic purpura (ITP) (Carimune® NF, Gammagard S/D®, Gammaked™, Gamunex®, Gamunex®-C, Privigen® [chronic only])

Treatment of chronic inflammatory demyelinating polyneuropathy (CIDP) (Gammaked™, Gamunex®, Gamunex®-C)

Prevention of coronary artery aneurysms associated with Kawasaki syndrome (in combination with aspirin) (Gammagard S/D®)

Prevention of bacterial infection in patients with hypogammaglobulinemia and/or recurrent bacterial infections with B-cell chronic lymphocytic leukemia (CLL) (Gammagard S/D®)

Prevention of serious infection in immunoglobulin deficiency (select agammaglobulinemias) (GamaSTAN™ S/D)

Provision of passive immunity in the following susceptible individuals (GamaSTAN™ S/D):

Hepatitis A: Pre-exposure prophylaxis; postexposure: within 14 days and/or prior to manifestation of disease

Measles: For use within 6 days of exposure in an unvaccinated person, who has not previously had measles

Rubella: Postexposure prophylaxis (within 72 hours) to reduce the risk of infection and fetal damage in exposed pregnant women who will not consider therapeutic abortion

Varicella: For immunosuppressed patients when varicella zoster immune globulin is not available

Unlabeled Use Acquired hypogammaglobulinemia secondary to malignancy; Guillain-Barré syndrome; hematopoietic stem cell transplantation (HSCT), to prevent bacterial infections among allogeneic recipients with severe hypogammaglobulinemia (IgG <400 mg/dL) at <100 days post transplant (CDC guidelines); HIV-associated thrombocytopenia; multiple sclerosis (relapsing, remitting when other therapies cannot be used); myasthenia gravis; refractory dermatomyositis/polymyositis

Mechanism of Action/Effect Replacement therapy for primary and secondary immunodeficiencies, and IgG antibodies against bacteria, viral, parasitic and mycoplasma antigens; interference with F_c receptors on the cells of the reticuloendothelial system for autoimmune cytopenias and ITP; provides passive immunity by increasing the antibody titer and antigen-antibody reaction potential

Contraindications Hypersensitivity to immune globulin or any component of the formulation; selective IgA deficiency; hyperprolinemia (Hizentra®, Privigen®); severe thrombocytopenia or coagulation disorders; severe thrombocytopenia or coagulation disorders where IM injections are contraindicated

Warnings/Precautions [U.S. Boxed Warning]: I.V. formulation only: Acute renal dysfunction (increased serum creatinine, oliguria, acute renal failure, osmotic nephrosis) can rarely occur; usually within 7 days of use (more likely with products stabilized with sucrose). Use with caution in the elderly, patients with renal disease, diabetes mellitus, volume depletion, sepsis, paraproteinemia, and nephrotoxic medications due to risk of renal dysfunction. In patients at risk of renal dysfunction, the rate of infusion and concentration of solution should be minimized. Discontinue if renal function deteriorates. High-dose regimens (1 g/kg for 1-2 days) are not recommended for individuals with fluid overload or where fluid volume may be of concern. Hypersensitivity and anaphylactic reactions can occur; a severe fall in blood pressure may rarely occur with anaphylactic reaction; immediate treatment (including epinephrine 1:1000) should be available. Product of human plasma; may potentially contain infectious agents which could transmit disease. Screening of donors, as well as testing and/or inactivation or removal of certain viruses, reduces the risk. Infections thought to be transmitted by this product should be reported to the manufacturer. Aseptic meningitis may occur with high doses (≥1-2 g/kg [product-dependent]) and/or rapid infusion; syndrome usually appears within several hours to 2 days following treatment; usually resolves within several days after product is discontinued; patients with a migraine history may be at higher risk for AMS. Increased risk of hypersensitivity, especially in patients with anti-IgA antibodies. Increased risk of hematoma formation when administered subcutaneously for the treatment of ITP.

Intravenous immune globulin has been associated with antiglobulin hemolysis; monitor for signs of hemolytic anemia. Patients should be adequately hydrated prior to initiation of therapy. Hyperproteinemia, increased serum viscosity and hyponatremia may occur; distinguish hyponatremia from pseudohyponatremia to prevent volume depletion, a further increase in serum viscosity, and a higher risk of thrombotic events. Use caution in patients with a history of thrombotic events or a history of atherosclerosis or cardiovascular disease or patients with known/suspected hyperviscosity; there is clinical evidence of a possible association between thrombotic events and administration of intravenous immune globulin and subcutaneous immune globulin. Consider a baseline assessment of blood viscosity in patients at risk for hyperviscosity. Patients should be monitored for adverse events during and after the infusion. Stop administration with signs of infusion reaction (fever, chills, nausea, vomiting, and rarely shock). Risk may be increased with initial treatment, when switching brands of immune globulin, and with treatment interruptions of >8 weeks. Monitor for transfusion-related acute lung injury (TRALI); noncardiogenic pulmonary edema has been reported with intravenous immune globulin use. TRALI is characterized by severe respiratory distress, pulmonary edema, hypoxemia, and fever (in the presence of normal left ventricular function) and usually occurs within 1-6 hours after infusion. Response to live vaccinations may be impaired. Some clinicians may administer intravenous immune globulin products as a subcutaneous infusion based on patient tolerability and clinical judgment. SubQ infusion should begin 1 week after the last I.V. dose; dose should be individualized based on clinical response and serum IgG trough concentrations; consider premedicating with acetaminophen and diphenhydramine.

Some products may contain maltose, which may result in falsely-elevated blood glucose readings; maltose-containing products are contraindicated in patients with an allergy to corn. Some products may contain polysorbate 80, sodium, and/or sucrose. Some products may contain sorbitol; do not use in patients with fructose intolerance. Hizentra® and Privigen® contain the stabilizer L-proline and are contraindicated in patients with hyperprolinemia. Packaging of some products may contain natural latex/natural rubber; skin testing should not be performed with GamaSTAN™ S/D as local irritation can occur and be misinterpreted as a positive reaction.

Drug Interactions

Avoid Concomitant Use There are no known interactions where it is recommended to avoid concomitant use.

Decreased Effect

Immune Globulin may decrease the levels/effects of: Vaccines (Live)

Increased Effect/Toxicity There are no known significant interactions involving an increase in effect.

Adverse Reactions Frequency not defined.

Cardiovascular: Angioedema, chest tightness, edema, flushing of the face, hyper-/hypotension, palpitation, tachycardia

Central nervous system: Anxiety, aseptic meningitis syndrome, chills, dizziness, drowsiness, fatigue, fever, headache, irritability, lethargy, lightheadedness, malaise, migraine, pain

Dermatologic: Bruising, contact dermatitis, eczema, erythema, hyperhidrosis, petechiae, pruritus, purpura, rash, urticaria

Gastrointestinal: Abdominal cramps, abdominal pain, diarrhea, discomfort, dyspepsia, gastroenteritis, nausea, sore throat, toothache, vomiting

Hematologic: Anemia, autoimmune hemolytic anemia, hematocrit decreased, hematoma, hemolysis (mild), hemorrhage, thrombocytopenia

Hepatic: Bilirubin increased, LDH increased, liver function test increased

Local: Muscle stiffness at I.M. site; pain, swelling, redness or irritation at the infusion site

Neuromuscular & skeletal: Arthralgia, back or hip pain, leg cramps, muscle cramps, myalgia, neck pain, rigors, weakness

Ocular: Conjunctivitis

Otic: Ear pain

Renal: Acute renal failure, acute tubular necrosis, anuria, BUN increased, creatinine increased, oliguria, proximal tubular nephropathy, osmotic nephrosis

Respiratory: Asthma aggravated, bronchitis, cough, dyspnea, epistaxis, nasal congestion, oropharyngeal pain, pharyngeal pain, pharyngitis, rhinitis, rhinorrhea, sinus headache, sinusitis, upper respiratory infection, wheezing

Miscellaneous: Anaphylaxis, diaphoresis, flu-like syndrome, hypersensitivity reactions, infusion reaction, thermal burn

Pharmacodynamics/Kinetics

Onset of Action I.V.: Provides immediate antibody levels

Duration of Action I.M., I.V.: Immune effects: 3-4 weeks (variable)

Available Dosage Forms

Injection, powder for reconstitution [preservative free]:

Carimune® NF: 3 g, 6 g, 12 g

Gammagard S/D®: 2.5 g, 5 g, 10 g

Injection, solution [preservative free]:

Flebogamma® DIF: 5% [50 mg/mL] (10 mL, 50 mL, 100 mL, 200 mL, 400 mL); 10% [100 mg/mL] (100 mL, 200 mL)

GamaSTAN™ S/D: 15% to 18% [150 to 180 mg/mL] (2 mL, 10 mL)

Gammagard® Liquid: 10% [100 mg/mL] (10 mL, 25 mL, 50 mL, 100 mL, 200 mL)

Gammaked™: 10% [100 mg/mL] (10 mL, 25 mL, 50 mL, 100 mL, 200 mL)

Gammaplex®: 5% [50 mg/mL] (50 mL, 100 mL, 200 mL)

Gamunex®-C: 10% [100 mg/mL] (10 mL, 25 mL, 50 mL, 100 mL, 200 mL)

Hizentra®: 200 mg/mL (5 mL, 10 mL, 20 mL)

Octagam®: 5% [50 mg/mL] (20 mL, 50 mL, 100 mL, 200 mL)

Privigen®: 10% [100 mg/mL] (50 mL, 100 mL, 200 mL)

General Dosage Range

I.M.: *Children and Adults:*

Hepatitis A:

Pre-exposure prophylaxis upon travel into endemic areas:

0.02 mL/kg for anticipated risk of exposure <3 months

0.06 mL/kg for anticipated risk of exposure ≥3 months

Postexposure prophylaxis: 0.02 mL/kg

Measles:

Postexposure, immunocompetent: 0.25 mL/kg

Postexposure, immunocompromised: 0.5 mL/kg (maximum dose: 15 mL)

Rubella: Prophylaxis during pregnancy: 0.55 mL/kg

Varicella: Prophylaxis: 0.6-1.2 mL/kg

Immune globulin deficiency: 0.66 mL/kg; administer a double dose at onset of therapy

I.V.: *Children and Adults:*

B-cell chronic lymphocytic leukemia (CLL): 400 mg/kg

Chronic inflammatory demyelinating polyneuropathy (CIDP): Loading dose: 2000 mg/kg; Maintenance: 500-1000 mg/kg

Immune (idiopathic) thrombocytopenic purpura (ITP): Dosage varies greatly depending on product

Kawasaki syndrome: 400-2000 mg/kg

Measles: >400 mg/kg

Primary humoral immunodeficiency disorders: 200-800 mg/kg

SubQ: *Children and Adults:*

Measles: ≥200 mg/kg

Primary humoral immunodeficiency disorders: Dosage varies greatly depending on product

Administration

I.M. Note: If plasmapheresis employed for treatment of condition, administer immune globulin **after** completion of plasmapheresis session.

Administer I.M. in the anterolateral aspects of the upper thigh or deltoid muscle of the upper arm. Avoid gluteal region due to risk of injury to sciatic nerve. Divide doses >10 mL and inject in multiple sites.

GamaSTAN™ S/D is for I.M. administration only.

I.V. Note: If plasmapheresis employed for treatment of condition, administer immune globulin **after** completion of plasmapheresis session.

Infuse over 2-24 hours; administer in separate infusion line from other medications; if using primary line, flush with saline prior to administration. Decrease dose, rate and/or concentration of infusion in patients who may be at risk of renal failure. Decreasing the rate or stopping the infusion may help relieve some adverse effects (flushing, changes in pulse rate, changes in blood pressure). Epinephrine should be available during administration.

For initial treatment or in the elderly, a lower concentration and/or a slower rate of infusion should be used. Initial rate of administration and titration is specific to each IVIG product. Consult specific product prescribing information for detailed recommendations. Refrigerated product should be warmed to room temperature prior to infusion. Some products require filtration; refer to individual product labeling. Antecubital veins should be used, especially with concentrations ≥10% to prevent injection site discomfort.

I.V. Detail

Carimune® NF: pH 6.4-6.8

Flebogamma® DIF: pH 5.0-6.0

GamaSTAN™ S/D: pH 6.4-7.2

Gammagard® Liquid: pH 4.6-5.1

Gammagard S/D® 5%: pH 6.4-7.2

Gammaked™: pH 4.0-4.5

Gammaplex®: pH 4.8-5.0

Gamunex®, Gamunex-C®: pH 4.0-4.5

Hizentra®: pH: 4.6-5.2

Octagam®: pH 5.1-6.0

Privigen®: pH 4.6-5.0

Vivaglobin®: pH: 6.4-7.2

Other SubQ infusion: Initial dose should be administered in a healthcare setting capable of providing monitoring and treatment in the event of hypersensitivity. Using aseptic technique, follow the infusion device manufacturer's instructions for filling the reservoir and preparing the pump. Remove air from administration set and needle by priming. Appropriate injection sites include the abdomen, thigh, upper arm, lower back, and/or lateral hip; dose may be infused into multiple sites (spaced ≥2 inches apart) simultaneously. After the sites are clean and dry, insert subcutaneous needle and prime administration set. Attach sterile needle to administration set, gently pull back on the syringe to assure a blood vessel has not been inadvertently accessed (do not use needle and tubing if blood present). Repeat for each injection site; deliver the dose following instructions for the infusion device. Rotate the site(s) weekly. Treatment may be transitioned to the home/home care setting in the absence of adverse reactions.

Gammagard® Liquid:

Injection sites: ≤8 simultaneous injection sites

Initial infusion rate:

<40 kg: 15 mL/hour per injection site (maximum volume: 20 mL per injection site)

≥40 kg: 20 mL/hour per injection site (maximum volume: 30 mL per injection site)

Maintenance infusion rate:

<40 kg: 15-20 mL/hour per injection site (maximum volume: 20 mL per injection site)

≥40 kg: 20-30 mL/hour per injection site (maximum volume: 30 mL per injection site)

Gammaked™, Gamunex-C®:

Injection sites: ≤8 simultaneous injection sites

Recommended infusion rate: 20 mL/hour per injection site

Hizentra®:

Injection sites: ≤4 simultaneous injection sites

Maximum infusion rate: First infusion: 15 mL/hour per injection site; subsequent infusions: 25 mL/hour per injection site (maximum: 50 mL/hour for all simultaneous sites combined)

Maximum infusion volume: First 4 infusions: 15 mL per injection site; subsequent infusions: 20 mL per injection site (maximum: 25 mL per site as tolerated)

Vivaglobin®:

Injection sites: Children <45 kg: ≤3 simultaneous injection sites; Adults ≤65 years: ≤6 simultaneous injection sites; Adults >65 years: ≤4 simultaneous injection sites

Maximum infusion rate: 20 mL/hour per injection site (maximum: 3 mg/kg/minute [1.13 mL/kg/hour] for all simultaneous sites combined)

Maximum infusion volume: 15 mL per injection site

Stability

Reconstitution Dilution is dependent upon the manufacturer and brand. Gently swirl; do not shake; avoid foaming. Do not mix products from different manufacturers together. Discard unused portion of vials.

Carimune® NF: In a sterile laminar air flow environment, reconstitute with NS, D_5W, or SWFI. Complete dissolution may take up to 20 minutes. Begin infusion within 24 hours.

Flebogamma® DIF: Dilution is not recommended.

Gammagard® Liquid: May dilute in D_5W only.

Gammagard S/D®: Reconstitute with SWFI.

Gammaked™: May dilute in D_5W only.

Gamunex®, Gamunex®-C: May dilute in D_5W only.

Privigen®: If necessary to further dilute, D_5W may be used.

Storage Stability is dependent upon the manufacturer and brand. Do not freeze.

Carimune® NF: Prior to reconstitution, store at or below 30°C (86°F). Reconstitute with NS, D_5W, or SWFI. Following reconstitution in a sterile laminar air flow environment, store under refrigeration. Begin infusion within 24 hours.

Flebogamma® DIF: Store at 2°C to 25°C (36°F to 77°F); do not freeze.

GamaSTAN™ S/D: Store under refrigeration at 2°C to 8°C (36°F to 46°F). The following stability information has also been reported for GamaSTAN™ S/D: May be exposed to room temperature for a cumulative 7 days (Cohen, 2007).

Gammagard® Liquid: Prior to use, store at 2°C to 8°C (36°F to 46°F); do not freeze. May store at room temperature of 25°C (77°F) within the first 24 months of manufacturing. Storage time at room temperature varies with length of time previously refrigerated; refer to product labeling for details.

Gammagard S/D®: Store at ≤25°C (≤77°F). May store diluted solution under refrigeration at 2°C to 8°C (36°F to 46°F) for up to 24 hours if originally prepared in a sterile laminar air flow environment.

Gammaked™: Store at 2°C to 8°C (36°F to 46°F); may be stored at ≤25°C (≤77°F) for up to 6 months.

Gammaplex®: Store at 2°C to 25°C (36°F to 77°F); do not freeze. Protect from light.

Gamunex®, Gamunex®-C: Store at 2°C to 8°C (36°F to 46°F); may be stored at ≤25°C (≤77°F) for up to 6 months.

Hizentra®: Store at ≤25°C (≤77°F); do not freeze or use product if previously frozen. Do not shake.

Octagam®: Store at 2°C to 25°C (36°F to 77°F).

Privigen®: Store at ≤25°C (≤77°F); do not freeze (do not use if previously frozen). Protect from light.

Vivaglobin®: Store at 2°C to 8°C (36°F to 46°F); do not freeze or use product if previously frozen. Do not shake.

Nursing Actions

Physical Assessment Assess for history of previous allergic reactions. Monitor vital signs during infusion or injection and observe for adverse or allergic reactions. Hypersensitivity and anaphylaxis can occur. Medications for the treatment of hypersensitivity reactions should be available for immediate use. Teach patient adverse symptoms to report.

Patient Education This medication can be administered I.M., I.V. or SubQ. You will be monitored closely during the I.V. or SubQ infusion. If you experience nausea ask for assistance, do not get up alone. Immediately report chills; chest pain, tightness, or rapid heartbeat; acute back pain; or respiratory difficulty during infusion. Also report decrease in urine output, swelling of extremities, or weight gain; fever and other signs of infection; trouble breathing; increased heart rate, yellowing of skin or eyes, dark urine; stiff neck, severe headache, unexplained drowsiness, or sensitivity to light.

Dietary Considerations Some products may contain sodium.

Related Information

Immunization Administration Recommendations *on page 1243*

Immunization Recommendations *on page 1248*

Indacaterol (in da KA ter ol)

Index Terms Indacaterol Maleate; OnBrez Breezehaler; QAB149

Pharmacologic Category $Beta_2$ Agonist; $Beta_2$-Adrenergic Agonist, Long-Acting

Medication Guide Available Yes

Pregnancy Risk Factor C

Lactation Excretion unknown/use caution

Use Long-term maintenance treatment of airflow obstruction in chronic obstructive pulmonary disease (COPD) including chronic bronchitis and/or emphysema

Mechanism of Action/Effect Relaxes bronchial smooth muscle by selective action on beta$_2$-receptors with little effect on heart rate; acts locally in the lung.

Contraindications Monotherapy in the treatment of asthma (ie, use without a concomitant long-term asthma control medication, such as an inhaled corticosteroid). **Note:** Indacaterol is not FDA approved for treatment of asthma.

Warnings/Precautions Asthma-related deaths: **[U.S. Boxed Warning]: Long-acting beta$_2$-agonists (LABAs) increase the risk of asthma-related deaths. Indacaterol is not indicated for treatment of asthma and should not be used.** In a large, randomized, placebo-controlled U.S. clinical trial (SMART, 2006), salmeterol was associated with an increase in asthma-related deaths (when added to usual asthma therapy); risk is considered a class effect among all LABAs. It is unknown if indacaterol increases asthma-related deaths. Do not use for acutely deteriorating COPD or as rescue therapy in acute episodes. Short-acting beta$_2$-agonists (eg, albuterol) should be used for acute symptoms and symptoms occurring between treatments. If deterioration develops, prompt evaluation of the COPD regimen is warranted. Do not increase the dose or frequency of indacaterol. Data are not available to determine if LABA use increases the risk of death in patients with COPD. Do not use more than once daily or at a higher dose than indicated; do not combine use with other long-acting beta$_2$-agonists. Deaths and significant cardiovascular effects have been reported with excessive sympathomimetic use. Rarely, paradoxical bronchospasm may occur with use of inhaled bronchodilators; this should be distinguished from inadequate response.

Use caution in patients with cardiovascular disease (eg, arrhythmias, coronary insufficiency, hypertension), diabetes mellitus, hyperthyroidism, seizure disorders, or hypokalemia. Beta-agonists may cause elevation in blood pressure, heart rate, CNS stimulation/excitation, increased risk of arrhythmia, increase serum glucose, or decrease serum potassium.

Drug Interactions

Avoid Concomitant Use

Avoid concomitant use of Indacaterol with any of the following: Beta-Blockers (Nonselective); Iobenguane I 123

Decreased Effect

Indacaterol may decrease the levels/effects of: Iobenguane I 123

The levels/effects of Indacaterol may be decreased by: Alpha-/Beta-Blockers; Beta-Blockers (Beta1 Selective); Beta-Blockers (Nonselective); Betahistine; Peginterferon Alfa-2b; Tocilizumab

Increased Effect/Toxicity

Indacaterol may increase the levels/effects of: Corticosteroids (Systemic); Loop Diuretics; QTc-Prolonging Agents; Sympathomimetics; Thiazide Diuretics

The levels/effects of Indacaterol may be increased by: Atomoxetine; Caffeine; Cannabinoids; Conivaptan; MAO Inhibitors; Theophylline Derivatives; Tricyclic Antidepressants

Adverse Reactions

>10%: Respiratory: Cough (post inhalation 7% to 24%)

1% to 10%:

Central nervous system: Headache (5%)

Gastrointestinal: Nausea (2%)

Respiratory: Nasopharyngitis (5%), oropharyngeal pain (2%)

Pharmacodynamics/Kinetics

Onset of Action 5 minutes; Peak effect: 1-4 hours

Duration of Action 24 hours

Available Dosage Forms

Powder, for oral inhalation [capsule]:

Arcapta™ Neohaler™: 75 mcg/capsule (30s)

General Dosage Range Inhalation: *Adults:* One inhalation once daily

Administration

Inhalation For inhalation using Neohaler™ inhaler only. Do **not** swallow indacaterol capsules. Use the new inhaler included with each prescription. Do not remove capsules from blister until immediately before use. Use at the same time each day. Not to be used for the relief of acute attacks. Not for use with a spacer device. Do not wash mouthpiece; Neohaler™ should be kept dry. Discard any capsules that are exposed to air and not used immediately.

Stability

Storage Store capsules at controlled room temperature of 25°C (77°F); excursions permitted to 15°C to 30°C (59°F to 86°F). Protect from direct sunlight and moisture. Remove from blister pack immediately before use; discard capsule if not used immediately.

Nursing Actions

Physical Assessment Monitor pulmonary function tests regularly. Instruct patient to expect a mild cough up to 15 seconds after use. Report immediately hives; difficulty breathing; wheezing; swelling of the face, lips, tongue, or throat; or development of chest pain. Other symptoms to report include tremors or lower extremity swelling. Monitor blood sugars and electrolytes. Instruct patient to monitor for symptoms of hyperglycemia.

Patient Education Patient to inform prescriber of history of heart disease, hypertension, DM, seizures, or lactose intolerance. For best results, take at the same daily. Instruct patient to notify prescriber if medication is ineffective. Inform patient that for best effect medication should be taken at the same time daily and is not to be used during ongoing bronchospasm. This is not a rescue drug. Report immediately hives; difficulty breathing; wheezing; swelling of the face, lips, tongue, or throat; or development of chest pain. Other symptoms to notify include tremors or lower extremity swelling. Instruct patients to monitor for symptoms of hyperglycemia.

Indapamide (in DAP a mide)

Pharmacologic Category Diuretic, Thiazide-Related

Medication Safety Issues

Sound-alike/look-alike issues:

Indapamide may be confused with Iopidine®

International issues:

Pretanix [Hungary] may be confused with Protonix brand name for pantoprazole [U.S., Canada]

Pregnancy Risk Factor B

Lactation Excretion in breast milk unknown/not recommended

Use Management of mild-to-moderate hypertension; treatment of edema in heart failure

Unlabeled Use Nephrotic syndrome (Tanaka, 2005)

Available Dosage Forms

Tablet, oral: 1.25 mg, 2.5 mg

General Dosage Range Oral: *Adults:* 1.25-5 mg once daily

Administration

Oral May be administered without regard to meals (Caruso, 1983); however, administration with food or milk may to decrease GI adverse effects. Administer early in day to avoid nocturia.

Nursing Actions

Physical Assessment Allergy history should be assessed prior to beginning therapy (sulfonamides, thiazides). Monitor for hypotension, hypokalemia, and photosensitivity at regular intervals during therapy.

Patient Education Take early in the day. Follow prescriber's instructions for diet and lifestyle changes. Monitor weight on a regular basis. Report weight gain, swelling of ankles or hands, or respiratory difficulty. You may experience dizziness, weakness, sensitivity to sunlight, or dry mouth.

Indinavir (in DIN a veer)

Brand Names: U.S. Crixivan®

Index Terms Indinavir Sulfate

Pharmacologic Category Antiretroviral Agent, Protease Inhibitor

Medication Safety Issues

Sound-alike/look-alike issues:

Indinavir may be confused with Denavir®

Pregnancy Risk Factor C

Lactation Excretion in breast milk unknown/contraindicated

Breast-Feeding Considerations Maternal or infant antiretroviral therapy does not completely eliminate the risk of postnatal HIV transmission. In addition, multiclass-resistant virus has been detected in breast-feeding infants despite maternal therapy. Therefore, in the United States, where formula is accessible, affordable, safe, and sustainable, and the risk of infant mortality due to diarrhea and respiratory infections is low, complete avoidance of breast-feeding by HIV-infected women is recommended to decrease potential transmission of HIV (DHHS [perinatal], 2011).

Use Treatment of HIV infection; should always be used as part of a multidrug regimen (at least three antiretroviral agents)

Mechanism of Action/Effect Blocks the site of HIV-1 protease activity, resulting in the formation of immature, noninfectious viral particles.

Contraindications Hypersensitivity to indinavir or any component of the formulation; concurrent use of alfuzosin, alprazolam, amiodarone, cisapride, triazolam, midazolam (oral), pimozide, or ergot alkaloids; sildenafil (when used for pulmonary artery hypertension [eg, Revatio®]), simvastatin, St John's wort, or triazolam

Warnings/Precautions Because indinavir may cause nephrolithiasis/urolithiasis the drug should be discontinued if signs and symptoms occur. Adequate hydration is recommended. May cause tubulointerstitial nephritis (rare); severe asymptomatic leukocyturia may warrant evaluation. Use with caution in patients taking strong CYP3A4 inhibitors, moderate or strong CYP3A4 inducers and major CYP3A4 substrates (see Drug Interactions); consider alternative agents that avoid or lessen the potential for CYP-mediated interactions. Do not coadminister colchicine in patient with renal or hepatic impairment; avoid concurrent use with salmeterol.

Patients with hepatic insufficiency due to cirrhosis should have dose reduction. Warn patients about fat redistribution that can occur. Indinavir has been associated with hemolytic anemia (discontinue if diagnosed), hepatitis, hyperbilirubinemia, and hyperglycemia (exacerbation or new-onset diabetes). Treatment may result in immune reconstitution syndrome (acute inflammatory response to indolent or residual opportunistic infections). Use caution in patients with hemophilia; spontaneous bleeding has been reported.

Drug Interactions

Avoid Concomitant Use

Avoid concomitant use of Indinavir with any of the following: Alfuzosin; ALPRAZolam; Amiodarone; Atazanavir; Axitinib; Cisapride; Conivaptan; Crizotinib; Dronedarone; Eplerenone; Ergot Derivatives; Everolimus; Fluticasone (Oral Inhalation); Halofantrine; Lapatinib; Lovastatin; Lurasidone; Midazolam; Nilotinib; Nisoldipine; Pimozide; QuiNIDine; Ranolazine; Rifampin; Rivaroxaban; RomiDEPsin; Salmeterol; Silodosin; Simvastatin; St Johns Wort; Tamsulosin; Ticagrelor; Tolvaptan; Toremifene; Triazolam

Decreased Effect

Indinavir may decrease the levels/effects of: Abacavir; Boceprevir; Clarithromycin; Delavirdine; Divalproex; Etravirine; Meperidine; Prasugrel; Theophylline Derivatives; Ticagrelor; Valproic Acid; Zidovudine

The levels/effects of Indinavir may be decreased by: Antacids; Atovaquone; Boceprevir; Bosentan; CarBAMazepine; CYP3A4 Inducers (Strong); Deferasirox; Didanosine; Efavirenz; Garlic; H2-Antagonists; Nevirapine; Peginterferon Alfa-2b; P-glycoprotein/ABCB1 Inducers; Proton Pump Inhibitors; Rifabutin; Rifampin; St Johns Wort; Tenofovir; Tocilizumab; Venlafaxine

Increased Effect/Toxicity

Indinavir may increase the levels/effects of: Alfuzosin; Almotriptan; Alosetron; ALPRAZolam; Amiodarone; Antifungal Agents (Azole Derivatives, Systemic); ARIPiprazole; Atazanavir; Axitinib; Bortezomib; Bosentan; Brentuximab Vedotin; Brinzolamide; Budesonide (Nasal); Budesonide (Systemic, Oral Inhalation); Calcium Channel Blockers (Dihydropyridine); Calcium Channel Blockers (Nondihydropyridine); CarBAMazepine; Ciclesonide; Cisapride; Clarithromycin; Colchicine; Conivaptan; Corticosteroids (Orally Inhaled); Crizotinib; CycloSPORINE; CycloSPORINE (Systemic); CYP3A4 Substrates; Dienogest; Digoxin; Dronedarone; Dutasteride; Enfuvirtide; Eplerenone; Ergot Derivatives; Everolimus; FentaNYL; Fesoterodine; Fluticasone (Nasal); Fluticasone (Oral Inhalation); Fusidic Acid; GuanFACINE; Halofantrine; HMG-CoA Reductase Inhibitors; Iloperidone; Ivacaftor; Ixabepilone; Lapatinib; Lovastatin; Lumefantrine; Lurasidone; Maraviroc; Meperidine; MethylPREDNISolone; Midazolam; Nefazodone; Nilotinib; Nisoldipine; Paricalcitol; Pazopanib; Pimecrolimus; Pimozide; Propafenone; Protease Inhibitors; QuiNIDine; Ranolazine; Rifabutin; Rivaroxaban; RomiDEPsin; Ruxolitinib; Salmeterol; Saxagliptin; Sildenafil; Silodosin; Simvastatin; Sirolimus; SORAfenib; Tacrolimus; Tacrolimus (Systemic); Tacrolimus (Topical); Tadalafil; Tamsulosin; Temsirolimus; Tenofovir; Ticagrelor; Tolterodine; Tolvaptan; Toremifene; TraZODone; Triazolam; Tricyclic Antidepressants; Vardenafil; Vemurafenib; Vilazodone; Zuclopenthixol

The levels/effects of Indinavir may be increased by: Antifungal Agents (Azole Derivatives, Systemic); Atazanavir; Clarithromycin; CycloSPORINE; CycloSPORINE (Systemic); Delavirdine; Efavirenz; Enfuvirtide; Etravirine; Fusidic Acid; P-glycoprotein/ABCB1 Inhibitors

Nutritional/Ethanol Interactions

Food: Indinavir bioavailability may be decreased if taken with food. Meals high in calories, fat, and protein result in a significant decrease in drug levels. Indinavir serum concentrations may be decreased by grapefruit juice. Management: Administer with water 1 hour before or 2 hours after a meal. May also be administered with other liquids (eg, skim milk, juice, coffee, tea) or a light meal (eg, toast, corn flakes). Administer around-the-clock to avoid significant fluctuation in serum levels. Drink at least 48 oz of water daily. May be taken with food when administered in combination with ritonavir.

Herb/Nutraceutical: Garlic may decrease the levels/effects of protease inhibitors. St John's wort appears to induce CYP3A enzymes and has lead to 57% reductions in indinavir AUCs and 81% reductions in trough serum concentrations, which may lead to treatment failures. Management: Avoid garlic and St John's wort while taking indinavir.

Adverse Reactions

>10%:

Gastrointestinal: Abdominal pain (17%), nausea (12%)

Hepatic: Hyperbilirubinemia (14%; dose dependent)

Renal: Nephrolithiasis/urolithiasis, including flank pain with/without hematuria (29%, pediatric patients; 12% adult patients; dose dependent)

1% to 10%:

Central nervous system: Headache (5%), dizziness (3%), somnolence (2%), fever (2%), malaise (2%), fatigue (2%)

Dermatologic: Pruritus (4%), rash (1%)

Endocrine & metabolic: Hyperglycemia (1%)

Gastrointestinal: Vomiting (8%), diarrhea (3%), taste perversion (3%), acid reflux (3%), anorexia (3%), appetite increased (2%), dyspepsia (2%), serum amylase increased (2%)

Hematologic: Neutropenia (2%), anemia (1%), thrombocytopenia (1%)

Hepatic: Transaminases increased (4% to 5%), jaundice (2%)

Neuromuscular & skeletal: Back pain (8%), weakness (2%)

Renal: Dysuria (2%)

Respiratory: Cough (2%)

Available Dosage Forms

Capsule, oral:

Crixivan®: 100 mg, 200 mg, 400 mg

General Dosage Range Dosage adjustment recommended in patients with hepatic impairment or on concomitant therapy

Oral: *Adults:* 800 mg every 8 hours; Boosted regimen: 800 mg every 12 hours

Administration

Oral Drink at least 48 oz of water daily. Administer with water, 1 hour before or 2 hours after a meal. May also be administered with other liquids (eg, skim milk, juice, coffee, tea) or a light meal (eg, toast, corn flakes). Administer around-the-clock to avoid significant fluctuation in serum levels. May be taken with food when administered in combination with ritonavir.

Stability

Storage Medication should be stored at 15°C to 30°C (59°F to 86°F), and used in the original container and the desiccant should remain in the bottle. Capsules are sensitive to moisture.

Nursing Actions

Physical Assessment Monitor for adherence to regimen. Monitor for gastrointestinal disturbance (nausea, vomiting, diarrhea) that can lead to dehydration and weight loss, hyperlipidemia and redistribution of body fat, rash, CNS effects (malaise, insomnia, abnormal thinking), and electrolyte imbalance at regular intervals during therapy. Teach patient proper timing of multiple medications. Instruct patient on glucose testing (protease inhibitors may cause hyperglycemia, exacerbation or new-onset diabetes).

Patient Education This is not a cure for HIV, nor has it been found to reduce transmission of HIV; use appropriate precautions to prevent spread to other persons. Take with meals. Maintain adequate hydration, unless instructed to restrict fluid intake. This medication will be prescribed with a combination of other medications; time these medications as directed by prescriber. You may be advised to check your glucose levels; this class of drug can cause hyperglycemia. Frequent blood tests may be required. May cause body changes due to redistribution of body fat, facial atrophy, or breast enlargement (normal effects of drug); headache, dizziness, or fatigue; nausea or vomiting; diarrhea; back pain, or arthralgia. Inform prescriber if you experience muscle numbness or tingling; unresolved persistent vomiting, diarrhea, or abdominal pain; respiratory difficulty or chest pain; unusual skin rash; or change in color of stool or urine.

Dietary Considerations Should be taken without food but with water 1 hour before or 2 hours after a meal. Administration with lighter meals (eg, dry toast, skim milk, corn flakes) resulted in little/no change in indinavir concentration. If taking with ritonavir, may take with food. Patient should drink at least 48 oz of water daily.

Indomethacin (in doe METH a sin)

Brand Names: U.S. Indocin®; Indocin® I.V.

Index Terms Indometacin; Indomethacin Sodium Trihydrate

Pharmacologic Category Nonsteroidal Anti-inflammatory Drug (NSAID), Oral; Nonsteroidal Anti-inflammatory Drug (NSAID), Parenteral

Medication Safety Issues

Sound-alike/look-alike issues:

Indocin® may be confused with Imodium®, Lincocin®, Minocin®, Vicodin®

BEERS Criteria medication:

This drug may be inappropriate for use in geriatric patients (high severity risk).

Medication Guide Available Yes

Pregnancy Risk Factor C

Lactation Enters breast milk/not recommended (AAP rates "compatible"; AAP 2001 update pending)

Breast-Feeding Considerations Indomethacin is excreted into breast milk and low amounts have been measured in the plasma of nursing infants. Seizures in a nursing infant were observed in one case report, although adverse events have not been noted in other cases. Breast-feeding is not recommended by the manufacturer. (The therapeutic use of indomethacin is contraindicated in neonates with significant renal failure.) Hypertensive crisis and psychiatric side effects have been noted in case reports following use of indomethacin for analgesia in postpartum women. Use with caution in nursing women with hypertensive disorders of pregnancy or pre-existing renal disease.

Use Acute gouty arthritis, acute bursitis/tendonitis, moderate-to-severe osteoarthritis, rheumatoid arthritis, ankylosing spondylitis; I.V. form used as alternative to surgery for closure of patent ductus arteriosus in neonates

Unlabeled Use Management of preterm labor

Mechanism of Action/Effect Reversibly inhibits cyclooxygenase-1 and 2 (COX-1 and 2) enzymes, which results in decreased formation of prostaglandin precursors; has antipyretic, analgesic, and anti-inflammatory properties

Contraindications Hypersensitivity to indomethacin, aspirin, other NSAIDs, or any component of the formulation; perioperative pain in the setting of coronary artery bypass graft (CABG) surgery; patients with a history of proctitis or recent rectal bleeding (suppositories)

Neonates: Necrotizing enterocolitis; impaired renal function; active bleeding (including intracranial hemorrhage and gastrointestinal bleeding), thrombocytopenia, coagulation defects; untreated infection; congenital heart disease where patent ductus arteriosus is necessary

Warnings/Precautions [U.S. Boxed Warning]: NSAIDs are associated with an increased risk of adverse cardiovascular thrombotic events, including MI and stroke. Risk may be increased with duration of use or pre-existing cardiovascular risk factors or disease. May cause new-onset hypertension or worsening of existing hypertension. Use caution with fluid retention. Avoid use in heart failure. Concurrent administration of ibuprofen, and potentially other nonselective NSAIDs, may interfere with aspirin's cardioprotective effect. **[U.S. Boxed Warning]: Use is contraindicated for treatment of perioperative pain in the setting of coronary artery bypass graft (CABG) surgery.** Risk of MI and stroke may be increased with use following CABG surgery.

Platelet adhesion and aggregation may be decreased; may prolong bleeding time; patients with coagulation disorders or who are receiving anticoagulants should be monitored closely. Anemia may occur; patients on long-term NSAID therapy should be monitored for anemia. Rarely, NSAID use may cause severe blood dyscrasias (eg, agranulocytosis, aplastic anemia, thrombocytopenia).

NSAID use may compromise existing renal function; dose-dependent decreases in prostaglandin synthesis may result from NSAID use, reducing renal blood flow which may cause renal decompensation. NSAID use may increase the risk for hyperkalemia. Patients with impaired renal function, dehydration, heart failure, liver dysfunction, those taking diuretics, and ACE inhibitors are at greater risk of renal toxicity and hyperkalemia. Rehydrate patient before starting therapy; monitor renal function closely. Not recommended for use in patients with advanced renal disease. Long-term NSAID use may result in renal papillary necrosis.

The elderly are at increased risk for adverse effects (especially peptic ulceration, CNS effects, renal toxicity) from NSAIDs even at low doses. Risk of CNS adverse events may be higher with indomethacin compared to other NSAIDs; avoid use in this age group (Beers Criteria).

[U.S. Boxed Warning]: NSAIDs may increase risk of gastrointestinal irritation, inflammation, ulceration, bleeding, and perforation. Use caution with a history of GI disease (bleeding or ulcers), concurrent therapy with aspirin, anticoagulants and/or corticosteroids, smoking, use of alcohol, the elderly or debilitated patients. When used concomitantly with ≤325 mg of aspirin, a substantial increase in the risk of gastrointestinal complications (eg, ulcer) occurs; concomitant gastroprotective therapy (eg, proton pump inhibitors) is recommended (Bhatt, 2008).

Use the lowest effective dose for the shortest duration of time, consistent with individual patient goals, to reduce risk of cardiovascular or GI adverse events. Alternate therapies should be considered for patients at high risk.

NSAIDS may cause drowsiness, dizziness, blurred vision and other neurologic effects which may impair physical or mental abilities; patients must be cautioned about performing tasks which require mental alertness (eg, operating machinery or driving). Discontinue use with blurred or diminished vision and perform ophthalmologic exam. Monitor vision with long-term therapy.

NSAIDs may cause serious skin adverse events including exfoliative dermatitis, Stevens-Johnson syndrome (SJS) and toxic epidermal necrolysis (TEN); discontinue use at first sign of skin rash or hypersensitivity. Anaphylactoid reactions may occur, even without prior exposure; patients with "aspirin triad" (bronchial asthma, aspirin intolerance, rhinitis) may be at increased risk. Do not use in patients who experience bronchospasm, asthma, rhinitis, or urticaria with NSAID or aspirin therapy. Use caution in other forms of asthma.

Use with caution in patients with decreased hepatic function. Closely monitor patients with any abnormal LFT. Severe hepatic reactions (eg, fulminant hepatitis, liver failure) have occurred with NSAID use, rarely; discontinue if signs or symptoms of liver disease develop, or if systemic manifestations occur. The elderly are at increased risk for adverse effects (especially peptic ulceration, CNS effects, renal toxicity) from NSAIDs even at low doses. Prolonged use may cause corneal deposits and retinal disturbances; discontinue if visual changes are observed. Use caution with depression, epilepsy, or Parkinson's disease.

Withhold for at least 4-6 half-lives prior to surgical or dental procedures.

Oral: Safety and efficacy have not been established in children <14 years of age. Hepatotoxicity has been reported in younger children treated for juvenile idiopathic arthritis (JIA). Closely monitor if use is needed in children ≥2 years of age.

Drug Interactions

Avoid Concomitant Use

Avoid concomitant use of Indomethacin with any of the following: Floctafenine; Ketorolac; Ketorolac (Nasal); Ketorolac (Systemic)

Decreased Effect

Indomethacin may decrease the levels/effects of: ACE Inhibitors; Aliskiren; Angiotensin II Receptor Blockers; Antiplatelet Agents; Beta-Blockers; Eplerenone; HydrALAZINE; Loop Diuretics; Potassium-Sparing Diuretics; Salicylates; Selective Serotonin Reuptake Inhibitors; Thiazide Diuretics

The levels/effects of Indomethacin may be decreased by: Bile Acid Sequestrants; Nonsteroidal Anti-Inflammatory Agents; Salicylates

Increased Effect/Toxicity

Indomethacin may increase the levels/effects of: Aliskiren; Aminoglycosides; Anticoagulants; Antiplatelet Agents; Bisphosphonate Derivatives; Collagenase (Systemic); CycloSPORINE; CycloSPORINE (Systemic); Deferasirox; Desmopressin; Digoxin; Drotrecogin Alfa (Activated); Eplerenone; Haloperidol; Ibritumomab; Lithium; Methotrexate; Nonsteroidal Anti-Inflammatory Agents; PEMEtrexed; Porfimer; Potassium-Sparing Diuretics; PRALAtrexate; Quinolone Antibiotics; Rivaroxaban; Salicylates; Thrombolytic Agents; Tiludronate; Tositumomab and Iodine I 131 Tositumomab; Triamterene; Vancomycin; Vitamin K Antagonists

The levels/effects of Indomethacin may be increased by: ACE Inhibitors; Angiotensin II Receptor Blockers; Antidepressants (Tricyclic, Tertiary Amine); Corticosteroids (Systemic); CycloSPORINE; CycloSPORINE (Systemic); Dasatinib; Floctafenine; Glucosamine; Herbs (Anticoagulant/Antiplatelet Properties); Ketorolac; Ketorolac (Nasal); Ketorolac (Systemic); Nonsteroidal Anti-Inflammatory Agents; Omega-3-Acid Ethyl Esters; Pentosan Polysulfate Sodium; Pentoxifylline; Probenecid; Prostacyclin Analogues; Selective Serotonin Reuptake Inhibitors; Serotonin/Norepinephrine Reuptake Inhibitors; Sodium Phosphates; Treprostinil; Vitamin E

Nutritional/Ethanol Interactions

Ethanol: Avoid ethanol (may enhance gastric mucosal irritation).

Food: Food may decrease the rate but not the extent of absorption. Indomethacin peak serum levels may be delayed if taken with food.

Herb/Nutraceutical: Avoid alfalfa, anise, bilberry, bladderwrack, bromelain, cat's claw, celery, chamomile, coleus, cordyceps, dong quai, evening primrose, fenugreek, feverfew, garlic, ginger, ginkgo biloba, ginseng (American, Panax, Siberian), grapeseed, green tea, guggul, horse chestnut seed, horseradish, licorice, prickly ash, red clover, reishi, SAMe (S-adenosylmethionine), sweet clover, turmeric, white willow (all have additional antiplatelet activity).

Adverse Reactions

>10%: Central nervous system: Headache (12%)

1% to 10%:

Central nervous system: Dizziness (3% to 9%), depression (<3%), fatigue (<3%), malaise (<3%), somnolence (<3%), vertigo (<3%)

Gastrointestinal: Dyspepsia (3% to 9%), epigastric pain (3% to 9%), heartburn (3% to 9%), indigestion (3% to 9%), nausea (3% to 9%), abdominal pain/cramps/distress (<3%), constipation (<3%), diarrhea (<3%), rectal irritation (suppository), tenesmus (suppository), vomiting

Otic: Tinnitus (<3%)

Pharmacodynamics/Kinetics

Onset of Action ~30 minutes

Duration of Action 4-6 hours

Available Dosage Forms

Capsule, oral: 25 mg, 50 mg

Capsule, extended release, oral: 75 mg

Injection, powder for reconstitution: 1 mg

Indocin® I.V.: 1 mg

Suppository, rectal:

Indocin®: 50 mg (30s)

Suspension, oral:

Indocin®: 25 mg/5 mL (237 mL)

General Dosage Range

I.V.:

Neonates <48 hours old at time of first dose: Initial: 0.2 mg/kg, followed by 2 doses of 0.1 mg/kg at 12- to 24-hour intervals

Neonates 2-7 days old at time of first dose: Initial: 0.2 mg/kg, followed by 2 doses of 0.2 mg/kg at 12- to 24-hour intervals

Neonates >7 days old at time of first dose: Initial: 0.2 mg/kg, followed by 2 doses of 0.25 mg/kg at 12- to 24-hour intervals

Oral:

Extended release: *Children >14 years and Adults:* 75-150 mg/day in 1-2 divided doses (maximum: 150 mg/day)

Immediate release:

Children ≥2 years: 1-2 mg/kg/day in 2-4 divided doses (maximum: 4 mg/kg/day; 200 mg/day)

Adults: 50-150 mg/day in 2-4 divided doses (maximum: 200 mg/day)

Administration

Oral Administer with food, milk, or antacids to decrease GI adverse effects. Extended release capsules must be swallowed whole; do not crush.

I.V. Administer over 20-30 minutes. Reconstitute I.V. formulation just prior to administration; discard any unused portion; avoid I.V. bolus administration or infusion via an umbilical catheter into vessels near the superior mesenteric artery as these may cause vasoconstriction and can compromise blood flow to the intestines. Do not administer intra-arterially.

I.V. Detail pH: 6.0-7.5

Stability

Reconstitution Reconstitute with 1-2 mL preservative free NS or SWFI just prior to administration. Discard any unused portion. Do not use preservative-containing diluents for reconstitution.

Storage I.V.: Store below 30°C (86°F). Protect from light.

Nursing Actions

Physical Assessment Monitor blood pressure prior to treatment and periodically throughout. Regular ophthalmic evaluations are recommended.

Patient Education Do not crush, break, or chew extended-release capsules. Take with food or milk to reduce GI distress. Maintain adequate hydration, unless instructed to restrict fluid intake. May cause drowsiness, dizziness, nervousness, headache, anorexia, nausea, vomiting, heartburn, or fluid retention (weigh yourself weekly and report unusual weight gain). GI bleeding, ulceration, or perforation can occur with or without pain; discontinue medication and contact prescriber if persistent abdominal pain or cramping or blood in stool occurs. Report difficult breathing or unusual cough; chest pain, rapid heartbeat, or palpitations; unusual bruising or bleeding; blood in urine, gums, or vomitus; swollen extremities; skin rash, irritation, or itching; acute persistent fatigue; vision changes; or ringing in ears.

Dietary Considerations May cause GI upset; take with food or milk to minimize

InFLIXimab (in FLIKS e mab)

Brand Names: U.S. Remicade®

Index Terms Avakine; Infliximab, Recombinant

Pharmacologic Category Antirheumatic, Disease Modifying; Gastrointestinal Agent, Miscellaneous; Immunosuppressant Agent; Monoclonal Antibody; Tumor Necrosis Factor (TNF) Blocking Agent

Medication Safety Issues

Sound-alike/look-alike issues:

InFLIXimab may be confused with riTUXimab

Remicade® may be confused with Renacidin®, Rituxan®

Medication Guide Available Yes

Pregnancy Risk Factor B

Lactation Excretion in breast milk unknown/not recommended

Breast-Feeding Considerations It is not known whether infliximab is secreted in human milk. Because many immunoglobulins are secreted in milk and the potential for serious adverse reactions exists, a decision should be made whether to discontinue nursing or discontinue the drug, taking into account the importance of the drug to the mother.

Use

Treatment of moderately- to severely-active rheumatoid arthritis (with methotrexate)

Treatment of moderately- to severely-active Crohn's disease with inadequate response to conventional therapy (to reduce signs/symptoms and induce and maintain clinical remission) or to reduce the number of draining enterocutaneous and rectovaginal fistulas and maintain fistula closure

Treatment of psoriatic arthritis (to reduce signs/symptoms of active arthritis and inhibit progression of structural damage and improve physical function)

Treatment of chronic severe plaque psoriasis

Treatment of active ankylosing spondylitis (reduce signs/symptoms)

Treatment of moderately- to severely-active ulcerative colitis with inadequate response to conventional therapy (reduce signs/symptoms and induce and maintain clinical remission, mucosal healing and eliminate corticosteroid use)

Mechanism of Action/Effect Infliximab is a monoclonal antibody that binds to human tumor necrosis factor alpha (TNFα), thereby decreasing inflammatory and other responses.

Contraindications Hypersensitivity to infliximab, murine proteins or any component of the formulation; doses >5 mg/kg in patients with moderate or severe heart failure (NYHA Class III/IV)

Canadian labeling: Additional contraindications (not in U.S. labeling): Severe infections (eg, sepsis, abscesses, tuberculosis, and opportunistic infections)

Warnings/Precautions [U.S. Boxed Warning]: Patients receiving infliximab are at increased risk for serious infections which may result in hospitalization and/or fatality; infections usually developed in patients receiving concomitant immunosuppressive agents (eg, methotrexate or corticosteroids) and may present as disseminated (rather than local) disease. Active tuberculosis (or reactivation of latent tuberculosis), invasive fungal (including aspergillosis, blastomycosis, candidiasis, coccidioidomycosis, histoplasmosis, and pneumocystosis) and bacterial, viral or other opportunistic infections (including legionellosis and listeriosis) have been reported in patients receiving TNF-blocking agents, including infliximab. Monitor closely for signs/symptoms of infection. Discontinue for serious infection or sepsis. Consider risks versus benefits prior to use in patients with a history of chronic or recurrent infection. Consider empiric antifungal therapy in patients who are at risk for invasive fungal infection and develop severe systemic illness. Caution should be exercised when considering use the elderly or in patients with conditions that predispose them to infections (eg, diabetes) or residence/travel from areas of endemic mycoses (blastomycosis, coccidioidomycosis, histoplasmosis), or with latent or localized infections. Do not initiate infliximab therapy with clinically important active infection. Patients who develop a new infection while undergoing treatment should be monitored closely. Serious infections have been reported when anakinra or abatacept have been used concurrently with other TNF-blocking agents; concurrent use of infliximab with anakinra or abatacept is not recommended. Use caution when switching from one biologic disease-modifying antirheumatic drug (DMARD) to another; overlapping biological activities may further increase the risk of infection.

[U.S. Boxed Warning]: Infliximab treatment has been associated with active tuberculosis (may be disseminated or extrapulmonary) or reactivation of latent infections; evaluate patients for tuberculosis risk factors and latent

tuberculosis infection (with a tuberculin skin test) prior to and during therapy; treatment of latent tuberculosis should be initiated before use. Patients with initial negative tuberculin skin tests should receive continued monitoring for tuberculosis throughout treatment. Most cases of reactivation have been reported within the first 3-6 months of treatment. Caution should be exercised when considering the use of infliximab in patients who have been exposed to tuberculosis.

Patients should be brought up to date with all immunizations before initiating therapy. Live vaccines should not be given concurrently; there is no data available concerning secondary transmission of live vaccines in patients receiving therapy. Rare reactivation of hepatitis B virus (HBV) has occurred in chronic virus carriers; use with caution; evaluate prior to initiation and during treatment.

[U.S. Boxed Warning]: Lymphoma and other malignancies have been reported in children and adolescent patients receiving TNF-blocking agents including infliximab. Half the cases are lymphomas (Hodgkin's and non-Hodgkin's). **[U.S. Boxed Warning]: Hepatosplenic T-cell lymphoma has been reported in patients with Crohn's disease or ulcerative colitis treated with infliximab and concurrent or prior azathioprine or mercaptopurine use, usually reported in adolescent and young adult males.** The impact of infliximab on the development and course of malignancies is not fully defined, but may be dose dependent. As compared to the general population, an increased risk of lymphoma has been noted in clinical trials; however, rheumatoid arthritis alone has been previously associated with an increased rate of lymphoma. Use caution in patients with a history of COPD, higher rates of malignancy were reported in COPD patients treated with infliximab. Psoriasis patients with a history of phototherapy had a higher incidence of nonmelanoma skin cancers.

Severe hepatic reactions (including hepatitis, jaundice, acute hepatic failure, and cholestasis) have been reported during treatment; discontinue with jaundice or marked increase in liver enzymes (≥5 times ULN). Use caution with heart failure; if a decision is made to use with heart failure, monitor closely and discontinue if exacerbated or new symptoms occur. Doses >5 mg/kg should not be administered in patients with moderate-to-severe heart failure (NYHA Class III/IV). Use caution with history of hematologic abnormalities; hematologic toxicities (eg, leukopenia, neutropenia, thrombocytopenia, pancytopenia) have been reported; discontinue if significant abnormalities occur. Autoimmune antibodies and a lupus-like syndrome have been reported. If antibodies to double-stranded DNA are confirmed in a patient with lupus-like symptoms, infliximab should be discontinued. Rare cases of optic neuritis and demyelinating disease (including multiple sclerosis, systemic vasculitis, and Guillain-Barré syndrome) have been reported; use with caution in patients with pre-existing or recent onset CNS demyelinating disorders, or seizures; discontinue if significant CNS adverse reactions develop.

Acute infusion reactions may occur. Hypersensitivity reaction may occur within 2 hours of infusion. Medication and equipment for management of hypersensitivity reaction should be available for immediate use. Interruptions and/or reinstitution at a slower rate may be required (consult protocols). Pretreatment may be considered, and may be warranted in all patients with prior infusion reactions. Serum sickness-like reactions have occurred; may be associated with a decreased response to treatment. The development of antibodies to infliximab may increase the risk of hypersensitivity and/or infusion reactions; concomitant use of immunosuppressants may lessen the development of anti-infliximab antibodies. The risk of infusion reactions may be increased with retreatment after an interruption or discontinuation of prior maintenance therapy. Retreatment in psoriasis patients should be resumed as a scheduled maintenance regimen without any induction doses; use of an induction regimen should be used cautiously for retreatment of all other patients.

Efficacy was not established in a study to evaluate infliximab use in juvenile idiopathic arthritis (JIA). Safety and efficacy for use in pediatric plaque psoriasis or pediatric ulcerative colitis have not been established. **Note:** For use in Crohn's disease: Safety and efficacy have not been established in children <6 years of age (U.S. labeling) and in children <9 years of age (Canadian labeling).

Drug Interactions

Avoid Concomitant Use

Avoid concomitant use of InFLIXimab with any of the following: Abatacept; Anakinra; BCG; Belimumab; Canakinumab; Certolizumab Pegol; Natalizumab; Pimecrolimus; Rilonacept; Tacrolimus (Topical); Vaccines (Live)

Decreased Effect

InFLIXimab may decrease the levels/effects of: BCG; Coccidioidin Skin Test; Sipuleucel-T; Vaccines (Inactivated); Vaccines (Live)

The levels/effects of InFLIXimab may be decreased by: Echinacea

Increased Effect/Toxicity

InFLIXimab may increase the levels/effects of: Abatacept; Anakinra; Belimumab; Canakinumab; Certolizumab Pegol; Leflunomide; Natalizumab; Rilonacept; Vaccines (Live)

The levels/effects of InFLIXimab may be increased by: Abciximab; Denosumab; Pimecrolimus; Roflumilast; Tacrolimus (Topical); Trastuzumab

Nutritional/Ethanol Interactions Herb/Nutraceutical: Avoid echinacea (may diminish the therapeutic effect of infliximab).

Adverse Reactions Although profile is similar, frequency of adverse effects may vary with disease state. Except where noted, percentages reported in adults with rheumatoid arthritis:

>10%:

Central nervous system: Headache (18%)

Gastrointestinal: Nausea (21%), diarrhea (12%), abdominal pain (12%, Crohn's 26%)

Hepatic: ALT increased (risk increased with concomitant methotrexate)

Respiratory: Upper respiratory tract infection (32%), sinusitis (14%), cough (12%), pharyngitis (12%)

Miscellaneous: Development of antinuclear antibodies (~50%), infection (36%), infusion reactions (20%; severe <1%), development of antibodies to double-stranded DNA (20%), development of new abscess (Crohn's patients with fistulizing disease: 15%), anti-infliximab antibodies (variable; ~10% to 15% [range: 6% to 61%]; Mayer, 2006)

5% to 10%:

Cardiovascular: Hypertension (7%)

Central nervous system: Fatigue (9%), pain (8%), fever (7%)

Dermatologic: Rash (1% to 10%), pruritus (7%)

Gastrointestinal: Dyspepsia (10%)

Genitourinary: Urinary tract infection (8%)

Neuromuscular & skeletal: Arthralgia (1% to 8%), back pain (8%)

Respiratory: Bronchitis (10%), rhinitis (8%), dyspnea (6%)

Miscellaneous: Moniliasis (5%)

The following adverse events were reported in children with Crohn's disease and were found more frequently in children than adults:

>10%:

Hepatic: Liver enzymes increased (18%; ≥5 times ULN: 1%)

Hematologic: Anemia (11%)

Miscellaneous: Infections (56%; more common with every 8-week versus every 12-week infusions)

1% to 10%:

Central nervous system: Flushing (9%)

Gastrointestinal: Blood in stool (10%)

Hematologic: Leukopenia (9%), neutropenia (7%)

Neuromuscular & skeletal: Bone fracture (7%)

Respiratory: Respiratory tract allergic reaction (6%)

Miscellaneous: Viral infection (8%), bacterial infection (6%), antibodies to infliximab (3%)

Pharmacodynamics/Kinetics

Onset of Action Crohn's disease: ~2 weeks

Available Dosage Forms

Injection, powder for reconstitution:

Remicade®: 100 mg

General Dosage Range Dosage adjustment is required in heart failure patients.

I.V.:

Children ≥6 years: Initial: 5 mg/kg at 0, 2, and 6 weeks; Maintenance: 5 mg/kg every 8 weeks

Adults: Initial: 3-10 mg/kg at 0, 2, and 6 weeks; Maintenance: 3-10 mg/kg every 8 weeks **or** 5 mg/kg every 6 weeks

Administration

I.V. Infuse over at least 2 hours; do not infuse with other agents; use in-line low protein binding filter (≤1.2 micron). Temporarily discontinue or decrease infusion rate with infusion-related reactions. Antihistamines (H_1-antagonist +/- H_2-antagonist), acetaminophen and/or corticosteroids may be used to manage reactions. Infusion may be reinitiated at a lower rate upon resolution of mild-to-moderate symptoms.

Canadian labeling (not approved in U.S. labeling): Infusion of doses ≤6 mg/kg over not less than 1 hour may be considered in patients treated for rheumatoid arthritis who have initially tolerated 3 infusions each over 2 hours. Safety of shortened infusion has not been studied with doses >6 mg/kg.

Guidelines for the treatment and prophylaxis of infusion reactions: (Note: Limited to adult patients and dosages used in Crohn's; prospective data for other populations [pediatrics, other indications/dosing] are not available).

A protocol for the treatment of infusion reactions, as well as prophylactic therapy for repeat infusions, has been published (Mayer, 2006).

Treatment of infusion reactions: Medications for the treatment of hypersensitivity reactions should be available for immediate use. For mild reactions, the rate of infusion should be decreased to 10 mL/hour. Initiate a normal saline infusion (500-1000 mL/hour) and appropriate symptomatic treatment (eg, acetaminophen and diphenhydramine); monitor vital signs every 10 minutes until normal. After 20 minutes, the infusion may be increased at 15-minute intervals, as tolerated, to completion (initial increase to 20 mL/hour, then 40 mL/hour, then 80 mL/hour, etc [maximum of 125 mL/hour]). For moderate reactions, the infusion should be stopped or slowed. Initiate a normal saline infusion (500-1000 mL/hour) and appropriate symptomatic treatment. Monitor vital signs every 5 minutes until normal. After 20 minutes, the infusion may be reinstituted at 10 mL/hour; then increased at 15-minute intervals, as tolerated, to completion (initial increase 20 mL/hour, then

40 mL/hour, then 80 mL/hour, etc [maximum of 125 mL/hour]). For severe reactions, the infusion should be stopped with administration of appropriate symptomatic treatment (eg, hydrocortisone/methylprednisolone, diphenhydramine and epinephrine) and frequent monitoring of vitals (consult institutional policies, if available). Retreatment after a severe reaction should only be done if the benefits outweigh the risks and with appropriate prophylaxis. Delayed infusion reactions typically occur 1-7 days after an infusion. Treatment should consist of appropriate symptomatic treatment (eg. acetaminophen, antihistamine, methylprednisolone).

Prophylaxis of infusion reactions: Premedication with acetaminophen and diphenhydramine 90 minutes prior to infusion may be considered in all patients with prior infusion reactions, and in patients with severe reactions corticosteroid administration is recommended. Steroid dosing may be oral (prednisone 50 mg orally every 12 hours for 3 doses prior to infusion) or intravenous (a single dose of hydrocortisone 100 mg or methylprednisolone 20-40 mg administered 20 minutes prior to the infusion). On initiation of the infusion, begin with a test dose at 10 mL/hour for 15 minutes. Thereafter, the infusion may be increased at 15-minute intervals, as tolerated, to completion (initial increase 20 mL/hour, then 40 mL/hour, then 80 mL/hour, etc). A maximum rate of 125 mL/hour is recommended in patients who experienced prior mild-moderate reactions and 100 mL/hour is recommended in patients who experienced prior severe reactions. In patients with cutaneous flushing, aspirin may be considered (Becker, 2004). For delayed infusion reactions, premedicate with acetaminophen and diphenhydramine 90 minutes prior to infusion. On initiation of the infusion, begin with a test dose at 10 mL/hour for 15 minutes. Thereafter, the infusion may be increased to infuse over 3 hours. Postinfusion therapy with acetaminophen for 3 days and an antihistamine for 7 days is recommended.

I.V. Detail Do not infuse with other agents. Use in-line low protein binding filter (≤1.2 micron).

pH ~7.2

Stability

Reconstitution Reconstitute vials with 10 mL sterile water for injection. Swirl vial gently to dissolve powder; do not shake. Allow solution to stand for 5 minutes. Total dose of reconstituted product should be further diluted to 250 mL of 0.9% sodium chloride injection to a final concentration of 0.4-4 mg/mL. Infusion of dose should begin within 3 hours of preparation.

Storage Store vials at 2°C to 8°C (36°F to 46°F).

Nursing Actions

Physical Assessment Monitor for hypersensitivity and respiratory effects. Infusion reactions may occur. Premedication may be helpful. Treatment for hypersensitivity reactions should be available. Monitor for signs or symptoms of infection. Assess for signs of liver dysfunction (eg, unusual fatigue, dark urine, decreased urine output, abdominal pain, easy bruising or bleeding, jaundice). Report immediately chest pain; bloody or mucus-producing cough; or neck stiffness. Monitor labs throughout treatment. Do not use with live vaccines, such as BCG or influenza, or past allergies to mouse proteins.

Patient Education This drug can only be administered by infusion. You will be more prone to infection. Report immediately any headache or unusual fatigue; increased nausea or abdominal pain; bruising or bleeding easily; cough, runny nose, or respiratory difficulty; chest pain or persistent dizziness; mouth sores; vaginal itching or discharge; and frequent infections or unhealed sores. Common reactions include fatigue, muscle pain or weakness, back pain, fever, or chills. Do not receive live vaccines such as BCG or influenza during treatment.

Influenza Virus Vaccine (H5N1)

(in floo EN za VYE rus vak SEEN H5N1)

Index Terms Avian Influenza Virus Vaccine; Bird Flu Vaccine; H5N1 Influenza Vaccine; Influenza Virus Vaccine (Monovalent)

Pharmacologic Category Vaccine, Inactivated (Viral)

Medication Safety Issues

Sound-alike/look-alike issues:

Influenza virus vaccine (H5N1) may be confused with the nonavian strain of influenza virus vaccine

Pregnancy Risk Factor C

Lactation Excretion in breast milk unknown/use caution

Use Active immunization of adults at increased risk of exposure to the H5N1 viral subtype of influenza

Available Dosage Forms

Injection, suspension: Hemagglutinin (H5N1strain) 90 mcg/mL (5 mL)

General Dosage Range I.M.: *Adults 18-64 years:* 1 mL, followed by second 1 mL dose given 28 days later

Administration

I.M. For I.M. administration only. Inspect for particulate matter and discoloration prior to administration. Vaccinate in the deltoid muscle using a ≥1 inch needle length. Suspension should be shaken well prior to use. **Note:** For patients at risk of hemorrhage following intramuscular injection, the ACIP recommends "it should be administered intramuscularly if, in the opinion of the physician familiar with the patients bleeding risk, the vaccine can be administered by this route with reasonable safety. If the patient receives antihemophilia or other similar therapy, intramuscular vaccination can be scheduled shortly after such therapy is administered. A fine needle (23 gauge or smaller) can be used for the vaccination and firm pressure applied to the site (without rubbing) for at least 2 minutes. The patient should be instructed concerning the risk of hematoma from the injection." Patients on anticoagulant therapy should be considered to have the same bleeding risks and treated as those with clotting factor disorders (CDC, 2011).

Simultaneous administration of vaccines helps ensure the patients will be fully vaccinated by the appropriate age. Simultaneous administration of vaccines is defined as administering >1 vaccine on the same day at different anatomic sites. Separate vaccines should not be combined in the same syringe unless indicated by product specific labeling. Separate needles and syringes should be used for each injection. The ACIP prefers each dose of a specific vaccine in a series come from the same manufacturer when possible. Adolescents and adults should be vaccinated while seated or lying down. In general, preterm infants should be vaccinated at the same chronological age as full-term infants (CDC, 2011).

Antipyretics have not been shown to prevent febrile seizures. Antipyretics may be used to treat fever or discomfort following vaccination (CDC, 2011). One study reported that routine prophylactic administration of acetaminophen to prevent fever prior to vaccination decreased the immune response of some vaccines; the clinical significance of this reduction in immune response has not been established (Prymula, 2009).

Nursing Actions

Physical Assessment Patient should be evaluated for contraindications prior to treatment. Treatment for anaphylactic/anaphylactoid reaction should be immediately available during vaccine use. All serious adverse reactions must be reported to the U.S. DHHS. U.S. federal law also requires entry into the patient's medical record.

Patient Education Notify prescriber immediately of any acute reaction to vaccination (eg, difficulty breathing, chest pain, acute headache, rash, difficulty swallowing). May cause mild headache, fever, muscle pain, or some redness, pain, or swelling at injection site; consult prescriber if excessive or persisting. All serious adverse reactions must be reported to the U.S. DHHS. U.S. federal law also requires entry into the patient's medical record.

Related Information

Immunization Administration Recommendations *on page 1243*

Immunization Recommendations *on page 1248*

Influenza Virus Vaccine (Inactivated)

(in floo EN za VYE rus vak SEEN, in ak ti VAY ted)

Brand Names: U.S. Afluria®; Fluarix®; FluLaval®; Fluvirin®; Fluzone®; Fluzone® High-Dose; Fluzone® Intradermal

Index Terms H1N1 Influenza Vaccine; Influenza Vaccine; Influenza Virus Vaccine (Purified Surface Antigen); Influenza Virus Vaccine (Split-Virus); TIV; Trivalent Inactivated Influenza Vaccine

Pharmacologic Category Vaccine, Inactivated (Viral)

Medication Safety Issues

Sound-alike/look-alike issues:

Fluarix® may be confused with Flarex®

Influenza virus vaccine may be confused with flumazenil

Influenza virus vaccine may be confused with tetanus toxoid and tuberculin products. Medication errors have occurred when tuberculin skin tests (PPD) have been inadvertently administered instead of tetanus toxoid products and influenza virus vaccine. These products are refrigerated and often stored in close proximity to each other.

International issues:

Fluarix [U.S., Canada, and multiple international markets] may be confused with Flarex brand name for fluorometholone [U.S. and multiple international markets] and Fluorex brand name for fluoride [France]

Pregnancy Risk Factor B/C (manufacturer specific)

Lactation Excretion in breast milk unknown/use caution

Use Provide active immunity to influenza virus strains contained in the vaccine

The Advisory Committee on Immunization Practices (ACIP) recommends annual vaccination with the seasonal trivalent inactivated influenza vaccine (TIV) (injection) for all persons ≥6 months of age.

When vaccine supply is limited, target groups for vaccination (those at higher risk of complications from influenza infection and their close contacts) include the following:

- Persons ≥50 years of age
- Residents of nursing homes and other chronic-care facilities that house persons of any age with chronic medical conditions
- Adults and children with chronic disorders of the pulmonary or cardiovascular systems (except hypertension), including asthma
- Adults and children who have chronic metabolic diseases (including diabetes mellitus), hepatic disease, renal dysfunction, hematologic

disorders, or immunosuppression (including immunosuppression caused by medications or HIV)

- Adults and children with cognitive or neurologic/neuromuscular conditions (including conditions such as spinal cord injuries or seizure disorders) which may compromise respiratory function, the handling of respiratory secretions, or that can increase the risk of aspiration
- Children and adolescents (6 months to 18 years of age) who are receiving long-term aspirin therapy, and therefore, may be at risk for developing Reye's syndrome after influenza
- Women who are or will be pregnant during the influenza season
- Children 6-59 months of age
- Healthcare personnel
- Household contacts and caregivers of children <5 years (particularly children <6 months) and adults ≥50 years
- Household contacts and caregivers of persons with medical conditions which put them at high risk of complications from influenza infection
- American Indians/Alaska Natives
- Morbidly obese (BMI ≥40)

The Advisory Committee on Immunization Practices (ACIP) states that healthy, nonpregnant persons aged 2-49 years may receive vaccination with either the seasonal live, attenuated influenza vaccine (LAIV) (nasal spray) or the seasonal trivalent inactivated influenza vaccine (TIV) (injection).

Available Dosage Forms

Injection, suspension:
Afluria®: Hemagglutinin 45 mcg/0.5 mL (5 mL)
FluLaval®: Hemagglutinin 45 mcg/0.5 mL (5 mL)
Fluvirin®: Hemagglutinin 45 mcg/0.5 mL (5 mL)
Fluzone®: Hemagglutinin 45 mcg/0.5 mL (5 mL)

Injection, suspension [preservative free]:
Afluria®: Hemagglutinin 45 mcg/0.5 mL (0.5 mL)
Fluarix®: Hemagglutinin 45 mcg/0.5 mL (0.5 mL)
Fluvirin®: Hemagglutinin 45 mcg/0.5 mL (0.5 mL)
Fluzone®: Hemagglutinin 22.5 mcg/0.25 mL (0.25 mL); Hemagglutinin 45 mcg/0.5 mL (0.5 mL)
Fluzone® High-Dose: Hemagglutinin 180 mcg/0.5 mL (0.5 mL)
Fluzone® Intradermal: Hemagglutinin 27 mcg/0.1 mL (0.1 mL)

General Dosage Range

I.M.:
Children 6-35 months: 0.25 mL/dose (1 or 2 doses per season)
Children 3-9 years: 0.5 mL/dose (1 or 2 doses per season)
Children ≥9 years and Adults: 0.5 mL/dose (1 dose per season)

Intradermal: *Adults:* 18-64 years: 0.1 mL/dose (1 dose per season)

Administration

I.M. *Afluria®, Agriflu™ [CAN], Fluad™ [CAN], Fluarix®, FluLaval®, Fluviral® [CAN], Fluvirin®, Fluzone®, Fluzone® High-Dose, Vaxigrip® [CAN]:* For I.M. administration only. Inspect for particulate matter and discoloration prior to administration. Adults and older children should be vaccinated in the deltoid muscle using a ≥1 inch needle length. Infants and young children <12 months of age should be vaccinated in the anterolateral aspect of the thigh using a 7/8 inch to 1 inch needle length. Young children with adequate deltoid muscle mass should be vaccinated using a 7/8 inch to 1.25 inch needle. Do not inject into the gluteal region or areas where there may be a major nerve trunk. Suspensions should be shaken well prior to use.

Influvac® [CAN]: May be administered by I.M. injection. Shake well prior to use.

If a pediatric vaccine (0.25 mL) is inadvertently administered to an adult, an additional 0.25 mL should be administered to provide the full adult dose (0.5 mL). If the error is discovered after the patient has left, an adult dose should be given as soon as the patient can return. If an adult vaccine (0.5 mL) is inadvertently given to a child, no action needs to be taken. *Agriflu™ [CAN]:* If 0.25 mL dose is to be given, discard half the contained syringe volume prior to administration.

Note: For patients at risk of hemorrhage following intramuscular injection, the ACIP recommends "it should be administered intramuscularly if, in the opinion of the physician familiar with the patients bleeding risk, the vaccine can be administered by this route with reasonable safety. If the patient receives antihemophilia or other similar therapy, intramuscular vaccination can be scheduled shortly after such therapy is administered. A fine needle (23 gauge or smaller) can be used for the vaccination and firm pressure applied to the site (without rubbing) for at least 2 minutes. The patient should be instructed concerning the risk of hematoma from the injection." Patients on anticoagulant therapy should be considered to have the same bleeding risks and treated as those with clotting factor disorders (CDC, 2011).

Simultaneous administration of vaccines helps ensure the patients will be fully vaccinated by the appropriate age. Simultaneous administration of vaccines is defined as administering >1 vaccine on the same day at different anatomic sites. Separate vaccines should not be combined in the same syringe unless indicated by product specific labeling. Separate needles and syringes should be used for each injection. However, in general, vaccination should not be deferred if the brand name or route of the previous dose is not available or not known (CDC, 2011). Adolescents and adults should be vaccinated while seated or lying down. In general, preterm infants should be vaccinated at the same chronological age as full-term infants (CDC, 2011).

Antipyretics have not been shown to prevent febrile seizures. Antipyretics may be used to treat fever or discomfort following vaccination (CDC, 2011). One study reported that routine prophylactic administration of acetaminophen to prevent fever prior to vaccination decreased the immune response of some vaccines; the clinical significance of this reduction in immune response has not been established (Prymula, 2009).

Other

Fluzone® Intradermal, Intanza® [CAN] For intradermal administration over the deltoid muscle only. Fluzone® Intradermal should be shaken gently prior to use. Intanza® should not be shaken prior to use. Hold system using the thumb and middle finger (do not place fingers on windows). Insert needle perpendicular to the skin; inject using index finger to push on plunger. Do not aspirate.

Influvac® [CAN]: May be administered by deep subcutaneous injection. Shake well prior to use.

Simultaneous administration of vaccines helps ensure the patients will be fully vaccinated by the appropriate age. Simultaneous administration of vaccines is defined as administering >1 vaccine on the same day at different anatomic sites. Separate vaccines should not be combined in the same syringe unless indicated by product specific labeling. Separate needles and syringes should be used for each injection. However, in general, vaccination should not be deferred if the brand name or route of the previous dose is not available or not known (CDC, 2011). Adolescents and adults should be vaccinated while seated or lying down. In general, preterm infants should be vaccinated at the same chronological age as full-term infants (CDC, 2011).

Antipyretics have not been shown to prevent febrile seizures. Antipyretics may be used to treat fever or discomfort following vaccination (CDC, 2011). One study reported that routine prophylactic administration of acetaminophen to prevent fever prior to vaccination decreased the immune response of some vaccines; the clinical significance of this reduction in immune response has not been established (Prymula, 2009).

Nursing Actions

Physical Assessment Have emergency treatment for anaphylactoid or hypersensitivity reaction available. Evaluate for allergies (some products are manufactured with chicken egg protein, gentamicin, neomycin, polymyxin, and/or thimerosal), previous adverse reactions (especially Guillain-Barré syndrome), bleeding disorders, presence of acute illness, and immunosuppressed status. All serious adverse reactions must be reported to the U.S. DHHS. U.S. federal law also requires entry into the patient's medical record.

Patient Education The vaccination is not effective immediately. The full effect of the vaccine is generally reached approximately 3 weeks after vaccination. You may experience nausea, vomiting, diarrhea, flu-like symptoms (eg, cough, rhinitis, fever, muscle or joint pain, fatigue, headache), and redness and tenderness at injection site. Notify prescriber if symptoms persist.

Related Information

Immunization Administration Recommendations *on page 1243*

Immunization Recommendations *on page 1248*

Influenza Virus Vaccine (Live/Attenuated) (in floo EN za VYE rus vak SEEN)

Brand Names: U.S. FluMist®

Index Terms H1N1 Influenza Vaccine; Influenza Vaccine; Influenza Virus Vaccine (Trivalent, Live); LAIV; Live Attenuated Influenza Vaccine

Pharmacologic Category Vaccine, Live (Viral)

Medication Safety Issues

Sound-alike/look-alike issues:

Influenza virus vaccine may be confused with flumazenil

Pregnancy Risk Factor C

Lactation Excretion in breast milk unknown/use caution

Use Provide active immunity to influenza virus strains contained in the vaccine

The Advisory Committee on Immunization Practices (ACIP) states that healthy, nonpregnant persons aged 2-49 years may receive vaccination with either the seasonal live, attenuated influenza vaccine (LAIV) (nasal spray) or the seasonal trivalent inactivated influenza vaccine (TIV) (injection).

Product Availability FluMist® Quadrivalent Vaccine: FDA approved February 2012; availability anticipated for the 2013-2014 flu season. Consult prescribing information for additional information.

Available Dosage Forms

Solution, intranasal [preservative free]:

FluMist®: (0.2 mL)

General Dosage Range Intranasal:

Children 2-8 years: 0.2 mL/dose (1 or 2 doses per season)

Children ≥9 years and Adults ≤49 years: 0.2 mL/dose (1 dose per season)

Administration

Other LAIV: Intranasal: Half the dose (0.1 mL) is administered to each nostril; patient should be in upright position. A dose divider clip is provided. Severely-immunocompromised persons should not administer the live vaccine. If recipient sneezes following administration, the dose should not be repeated.

Simultaneous administration of vaccines helps ensure the patients will be fully vaccinated by the appropriate age. Simultaneous administration of vaccines is defined as administering >1 vaccine on the same day at different anatomic sites. The ACIP prefers each dose of a specific vaccine in a series come from the same manufacturer when possible. However, in general, vaccination should not be deferred if the brand name or route of the previous dose is not available or not known (CDC, 2011).

Antipyretics have not been shown to prevent febrile seizures. Antipyretics may be used to treat fever or discomfort following vaccination (CDC, 2011). One study reported that routine prophylactic administration of acetaminophen to prevent fever prior to vaccination decreased the immune response of some vaccines; the clinical significance of this reduction in immune response has not been established (Prymula, 2009).

Vaccine administration with oral influenza antiviral medications: Live influenza virus vaccine (LAIV) should not be given until 48 hours after the completion of influenza antiviral therapy (influenza A and B). Influenza antiviral therapy (influenza A and B) should not be administered for 2 weeks after receiving LAIV. If influenza antiviral therapy (influenza A and B) and LAIV are administered concomitantly, revaccination should be considered.

Nursing Actions

Physical Assessment U.S. federal law requires entry into the patient's medical record.

Related Information

Immunization Administration Recommendations *on page 1243*

Immunization Recommendations *on page 1248*

Ingenol Mebutate (IN je nol MEB u tate)

Index Terms *Euphorbia peplus* Derivative; PEP005; Picato®

Pharmacologic Category Topical Skin Product

Pregnancy Risk Factor C

Use Topical treatment of actinic keratosis

Product Availability Picato® gel: FDA approved January 2012; availability expected in March 2012. Consult prescribing information for additional information.

Available Dosage Forms

Gel, topical:

Picato®: 0.015% (3s); 0.05% (2s)

General Dosage Range Topical: *Adults:* Apply once daily for 2 days (0.05%) or 3 days (0.015%)

Administration

Topical Apply to one contiguous affected area of skin using one unit-dose tube; one unit-dose tube will cover ~5 cm x 5 cm (~25 cm^2 or ~2 inch x 2 inch). Spread evenly then allow gel to dry for 15 minutes. Do not cover with bandages or occlusive dressings. Wash hands immediately after applying and avoid transferring gel to any other areas. Avoid washing or touching the treatment area for at least 6 hours, and following this period of time, patients may wash the area with a mild soap. Not for oral, ophthalmic, or intravaginal use.

Nursing Actions

Physical Assessment Educate patient about sun avoidance and ways to protect skin against further sun damage.

Patient Education The treatment length is 2-3 days only; the gel will be applied to the skin once daily for 2-3 days in a row. Wash hands immediately after applying. Do not use on broken skin until healed. Do not touch or wash the skin for 6 hours after applying. Side effects include skin irritation, change in skin to hard and thick, and headache. Instruct the patient to call the prescriber if severe skin irritation (or any rash) occurs.

Insulin Aspart (IN soo lin AS part)

Brand Names: U.S. NovoLOG®; NovoLOG® FlexPen®; NovoLOG® Penfill®

Index Terms Aspart Insulin

Pharmacologic Category Insulin, Rapid-Acting

Medication Safety Issues

Sound-alike/look-alike issues:

NovoLOG® may be confused with HumaLOG®, HumuLIN® R, NovoLIN® N, NovoLIN® R, NovoLOG® Mix 70/30

High alert medication:

The Institute for Safe Medication Practices (ISMP) includes this medication among its list of drugs which have a heightened risk of causing significant patient harm when used in error. ***Due to the number of insulin preparations, it is essential to identify/clarify the type of insulin to be used.***

Other safety concerns:

Cross-contamination may occur if insulin pens are shared among multiple patients. Steps should be taken to prohibit sharing of insulin pens.

Pregnancy Risk Factor B

Lactation Excretion in breast milk unknown/compatible

Breast-Feeding Considerations It is not known if insulin aspart is found in breast milk. Endogenous insulin can be found in breast milk. Plasma glucose concentrations in the mother affect glucose concentrations in breast milk. The gastrointestinal tract destroys insulin when administered orally; therefore, insulin is not expected to be absorbed intact by the breast-feeding infant. All types of insulin are safe for use while breast-feeding. Due to increased calorie expenditure, women with diabetes may require less insulin while nursing.

Use Treatment of type 1 diabetes mellitus (insulin dependent, IDDM) and type 2 diabetes mellitus (noninsulin dependent, NIDDM) to improve glycemic control

Unlabeled Use Gestational diabetes mellitus (GDM); mild-to-moderate diabetic ketoacidosis (DKA); mild-to-moderate hyperosmolar hyperglycemic state (HHS)

Mechanism of Action/Effect Insulin aspart is a rapid-acting insulin analog.

Refer to Insulin Regular on page 629.

Contraindications Hypersensitivity to insulin aspart or any component of the formulation; during episodes of hypoglycemia

Warnings/Precautions Refer to Insulin Regular on page 629.

Due to short duration of action, a longer acting insulin is needed to maintain adequate glucose control. Administration should be immediately followed by a meal. Insulin aspart may be administered I.V. in selected clinical situations to control hyperglycemia.

Drug Interactions

Avoid Concomitant Use There are no known interactions where it is recommended to avoid concomitant use.

Decreased Effect

The levels/effects of Insulin Aspart may be decreased by: Corticosteroids (Orally Inhaled); Corticosteroids (Systemic); Luteinizing Hormone-Releasing Hormone Analogs; Somatropin; Thiazide Diuretics

Increased Effect/Toxicity Refer to Insulin Regular on page 629.

Nutritional/Ethanol Interactions Refer to Insulin Regular on page 629.

Pharmacodynamics/Kinetics

Onset of Action 0.2-0.3 hours; Peak effect: 1-3 hours

Duration of Action 3-5 hours

Available Dosage Forms

Injection, solution:

NovoLOG®: 100 units/mL (10 mL)
NovoLOG® FlexPen®: 100 units/mL (3 mL)
NovoLOG® Penfill®: 100 units/mL (3 mL)

General Dosage Range Note: Insulin aspart is a rapid-acting insulin analog which is normally administered as a premeal component of the insulin regimen. It is normally used along with a long-acting (basal) form of insulin

SubQ:

Children: Refer to Insulin Regular on page 629. When used in a meal-related treatment regimen, 50% to 70% of total daily insulin requirement may be provided by insulin aspart and the remainder provided by an intermediate or long-acting insulin.

Adults: Refer to Insulin Regular on page 629. When used in a meal-related treatment regimen, 50% to 70% of total daily insulin requirement may be provided by insulin aspart and the remainder provided by an intermediate or long-acting insulin.

SubQ infusion pump:

Children: Refer to Insulin Regular on page 629. Approximately 50% of total dose given as meal related bolus and ~50% of total dose given as basal infusion; adjust dose as necessary.

Adults: Refer to Insulin Regular on page 629. Approximately 50% of total dose given as meal related bolus and ~50% of total dose given as basal infusion; adjust dose as necessary.

Administration

I.V. Do not use if solution is viscous or cloudy; use only if clear and colorless. May be administered I.V. with close monitoring of blood glucose and serum potassium; appropriate medical supervision is required. **Do not administer insulin mixtures intravenously.**

I.V. Detail I.V. infusions: To minimize adsorption to I.V. solution bag: **Note:** Refer to institution-specific protocols where appropriate.

*If new tubing is **not** needed:* Wait a minimum of 30 minutes between the preparation of the solution and the initiation of the infusion

If new tubing is needed: After receiving the insulin drip solution, the administration set should be attached to the I.V. container and the entire line should be flushed with a priming infusion of 20-50 mL of the insulin solution (Goldberg, 2006; Hirsch, 2006). Wait 30 minutes, and then flush the line again with the insulin solution prior to initiating the infusion.

Because of adsorption, the actual amount of insulin being administered via I.V. infusion could be substantially less than the apparent amount. Therefore, adjustment of the I.V. infusion rate should be based on effect and not solely on the apparent insulin dose. The apparent dose may be used as a starting point for determining the subsequent SubQ dosing regimen (Moghissi, 2009); however, the transition to SubQ administration requires continuous medical supervision, frequent monitoring of blood glucose, and careful adjustment of therapy. In addition, SubQ insulin should be given 1-4 hours prior to the discontinuation of I.V. insulin to prevent hyperglycemia (Moghissi, 2009).

pH: 7.2-7.6

Other

SubQ administration: Do not use if solution is viscous or cloudy; use only if clear and colorless. Insulin aspart should be administered immediately (within 5-10 minutes) before a meal. Cold injections should be avoided. SubQ administration is usually made into the thighs, arms, buttocks, or abdomen; rotate injection sites. When mixing insulin aspart with other preparations of insulin (eg, insulin NPH), insulin aspart should be drawn into syringe first. Do not dilute or mix other insulin formulations with insulin aspart contained in a cartridge or prefilled pen.

CSII administration: Do not use if solution is viscous or cloudy; use only if clear and colorless. Patients should be trained in the proper use of their external insulin pump and in intensive insulin therapy. Infusion sets and infusion set insertion sites should be changed at least every 3 days; rotate infusion sites. Do not dilute or mix other insulin formulations with insulin aspart that is to be used in an external insulin pump.

Stability

Reconstitution

For SubQ administration: *NovoLog® vials:* May be diluted with Insulin Diluting Medium for NovoLog® to a concentration of 10 units/mL (U-10) or 50 units/mL (U-50). Do not dilute insulin contained in a cartridge, prefilled pen, or external insulin pump.

For I.V. infusion: May be diluted in NS, D_5W, or $D_{10}W$ to concentrations of 0.05-1 unit/mL.

Storage Unopened vials, cartridges, and prefilled pens may be stored under refrigeration between 2°C and 8°C (36°F to 46°F) until the expiration date or at room temperature <30°C (<86°F) for 28 days; do not freeze; keep away from heat and sunlight. Once punctured (in use), vials may be stored under refrigeration or at room temperature <30°C (<86°F); use within 28 days. Cartridges and prefilled pens that have been punctured (in use) should be stored at temperatures <30°C (<86°F) and used within 28 days; do not freeze or refrigerate. When used for CSII, insulin aspart contained within an external insulin pump reservoir should be replaced at least every 6 days; discard if exposed to temperatures >37°C (>98.6°F).

For SubQ administration: *NovoLog® vials:* According to the manufacturer, diluted insulin should be stored at temperatures <30°C (<86°F) and used within 28 days.

For I.V. infusion: Stable for 24 hours at room temperature.

Nursing Actions

Physical Assessment Monitor for hypoglycemia at regular intervals during therapy. Teach patient proper use, including appropriate injection technique and syringe/needle disposal, and monitoring requirements.

Patient Education Do not share pens, cartridges, or needles with others. This medication is used to control diabetes; it is not a cure. It is imperative to follow other components of prescribed treatment (eg, diet and exercise regimen). With insulin aspart (NovoLog®), you must start eating within 5-10 minutes after injection. If you experience hypoglycemic reaction, contact prescriber immediately. Always carry quick source of sugar with you. Monitor glucose levels as directed by prescriber. Report adverse side effects, including chest pain or palpitations; persistent fatigue, confusion, headache; skin rash or redness; numbness of mouth, lips, or tongue; muscle weakness or tremors; vision changes; respiratory difficulty; or nausea, vomiting, or flu-like symptoms.

Dietary Considerations Individualized medical nutrition therapy (MNT) based on ADA recommendations is an integral part of therapy.

Related Information

Insulin Regular *on page 629*

Insulin Aspart Protamine and Insulin Aspart (IN soo lin AS part PROE ta meen & IN soo lin AS part)

Brand Names: U.S. NovoLOG® Mix 70/30; NovoLOG® Mix 70/30 FlexPen®

Index Terms Insulin Aspart and Insulin Aspart Protamine; NovoLog 70/30

Pharmacologic Category Insulin, Combination

Medication Safety Issues

Sound-alike/look-alike issues:

NovoLOG® Mix 70/30 may be confused with HumaLOG® Mix 75/25™, HumuLIN® 70/30, NovoLIN® 70/30, NovoLOG®

High alert medication:

The Institute for Safe Medication Practices (ISMP) includes this medication among its list of drugs which have a heightened risk of causing significant patient harm when used in error. ***Due to the number of insulin preparations, it is essential to identify/clarify the type of insulin to be used.***

Other safety concerns:

Cross-contamination may occur if insulin pens are shared among multiple patients. Steps should be taken to prohibit sharing of insulin pens.

Pregnancy Risk Factor B

Lactation Excretion in breast milk unknown/compatible

Use Treatment of type 1 diabetes mellitus (insulin dependent, IDDM) and type 2 diabetes mellitus (noninsulin dependent, NIDDM) to improve glycemic control

Available Dosage Forms

Injection, suspension:

NovoLOG® Mix 70/30: Insulin aspart protamine suspension 70% [intermediate acting] and insulin aspart solution 30% [rapid acting]: 100 units/mL (10 mL)

NovoLOG® Mix 70/30 FlexPen®: Insulin aspart protamine suspension 70% [intermediate acting] and insulin aspart solution 30% [rapid acting]: 100 units/mL (3 mL)

General Dosage Range Note: Fixed ratio insulins (such as insulin aspart protamine and insulin aspart combination) are normally administered in 2 daily doses.

SubQ:

Children: Dosage not established

Adults: Refer to Insulin Regular on page 629

Administration

Other SubQ administration: In order to properly resuspend the insulin, vials and prefilled pens should be gently rolled between the palms ten times; in addition, prefilled pens should be inverted 180° ten times. Properly resuspended insulin should look uniformly cloudy or milky; do not use if any white insulin substance remains at the bottom of the container, if any clumps are present, if the insulin remains clear after adequate mixing, or if white particles are stuck to the bottom or wall of the container. Cold injections should be avoided. Insulin aspart protamine and insulin aspart combination products should be administered within 15 minutes before a meal (type 1 diabetes) or 15 minutes before or after a meal (type 2 diabetes); typically given twice daily. SubQ administration is usually made into the thighs, arms, buttocks, or abdomen; rotate injection sites. Do not dilute or mix with any other insulin formulation or solution; not recommended for use in external SubQ insulin infusion pump.

Nursing Actions

Physical Assessment See individual agents.

Patient Education See individual agents.

Related Information

Insulin Regular *on page 629*

Insulin Detemir (IN soo lin DE te mir)

Brand Names: U.S. Levemir®; Levemir® FlexPen®

Index Terms Detemir Insulin

Pharmacologic Category Insulin, Intermediate- to Long-Acting

Medication Safety Issues

High alert medication:

The Institute for Safe Medication Practices (ISMP) includes this medication among its list of drugs which have a heightened risk of causing significant patient harm when used in error. ***Due to the number of insulin preparations, it is essential to identify/clarify the type of insulin to be used.***

Administration issues:

Insulin detemir is a clear solution, but it is NOT intended for I.V. or I.M. administration.

Other safety concerns:

Cross-contamination may occur if insulin pens are shared among multiple patients. Steps should be taken to prohibit sharing of insulin pens.

Pregnancy Risk Factor C

Lactation Excretion in breast milk unknown/compatible

Breast-Feeding Considerations It is not known if insulin detemir is found in breast milk. Endogenous insulin can be found in breast milk. Plasma glucose concentrations in the mother affect glucose concentrations in breast milk. The gastrointestinal tract destroys insulin when administered orally; therefore, insulin is not expected to be absorbed intact by the breast-feeding infant. All types of insulin are safe for use while breast-feeding. Due to increased calorie expenditure, women with diabetes may require less insulin while nursing.

Use Treatment of type 1 diabetes mellitus (insulin dependent, IDDM) and type 2 diabetes mellitus (noninsulin dependent, NIDDM) to improve glycemic control

Mechanism of Action/Effect Insulin detemir is an intermediate- to long-acting insulin analog.

Refer to Insulin Regular on page 629.

Contraindications Hypersensitivity to insulin detemir or any component of the formulation

Warnings/Precautions Refer to Insulin Regular on page 629. Safety and efficacy not established in children <6 years of age.

Careful adjustment of dosage and timing is required to achieve glycemic targets. Adjustment of other antidiabetic therapy (short-acting or oral antidiabetic agents) may be required. The duration of of action of insulin detemir is dose-dependent and this factor must be considered during dosage adjustment and titration. Insulin detemir is a clear solution, but it is not for intravenous administration.

Drug Interactions

Avoid Concomitant Use There are no known interactions where it is recommended to avoid concomitant use.

Decreased Effect

The levels/effects of Insulin Detemir may be decreased by: Corticosteroids (Orally Inhaled); Corticosteroids (Systemic); Luteinizing Hormone-Releasing Hormone Analogs; Somatropin; Thiazide Diuretics

Increased Effect/Toxicity Refer to Insulin Regular on page 629.

Nutritional/Ethanol Interactions Refer to Insulin Regular on page 629.

Adverse Reactions Refer to Insulin Regular on page 629.

Pharmacodynamics/Kinetics

Onset of Action 3-4 hours; Peak effect: 3-9 hours (Plank, 2005)

Duration of Action Dose dependent: 6-23 hours; **Note:** Duration is dose-dependent. At lower dosages (0.1-0.2 units/kg), mean duration is variable (5.7-12.1 hours). At 0.4 units/kg, the mean duration was 19.9 hours. At high dosages (≥0.8 units/kg) the duration is longer and less variable (mean of 22-23 hours) (Plank, 2005).

Available Dosage Forms

Injection, solution:

Levemir®: 100 units/mL (10 mL)

Levemir® FlexPen®: 100 units/mL (3 mL)

General Dosage Range Dosage adjustment recommended in patients with renal impairment

SubQ:

Children ≥6 years: Refer to Insulin Regular on page 629

Adults: Refer to Insulin Regular on page 629; 0.1-0.2 units/kg once daily **or** 10 units once- or twice daily (manufacturer recommendations)

Administration

Other SubQ administration: Do not use if solution is viscous or cloudy; use only if clear and colorless with no visible particles. Insulin detemir should be administered once or twice daily. When given once daily, administer with the evening meal or at bedtime. When given twice daily, administer the evening dose with the evening meal, at bedtime, or 12 hours following the morning dose. Cold injections should be avoided. SubQ administration is usually made into the thighs, arms, buttocks, or abdomen; rotate injection sites. Do not dilute or mix insulin detemir with any other insulin formulation or solution; **not** recommended for use in external SubQ insulin infusion pump.

Stability

Storage Unopened vials, cartridges, and prefilled pens may be stored under refrigeration between 2°C and 8°C (36°F to 46°F) until the expiration date or at room temperature <30°C (<86°F) for 42 days; do not freeze; keep away from heat and sunlight. Once punctured (in use), vials may be stored under refrigeration or at room temperature <30°C (<86°F); use within 42 days. Cartridges and prefilled pens that have been punctured (in use) should be stored at temperatures <30°C (<86°F) and used within 42 days; do not freeze or refrigerate.

Nursing Actions

Physical Assessment Monitor for hypoglycemia at regular intervals during therapy. Teach patient proper use, including appropriate injection technique and syringe/needle disposal, and monitoring requirements.

Patient Education Do not share pens, cartridges, or needles with others. This medication is used to control diabetes; it is not a cure. It is imperative to follow other components of prescribed treatment (eg, diet and exercise regimen). If you experience hypoglycemic reaction, contact prescriber immediately. Always carry quick source of sugar with you. Monitor glucose levels as directed by prescriber. Report adverse side effects, including chest pain or palpitations; persistent fatigue, confusion, headache; skin rash or redness; numbness of mouth, lips, or tongue; muscle weakness or tremors; vision changes; respiratory difficulty; or nausea, vomiting, or flu-like symptoms.

Dietary Considerations Individualized medical nutrition therapy (MNT) based on ADA recommendations is an integral part of therapy.

Related Information

Insulin Regular *on page* 629

Insulin Glargine (IN soo lin GLAR jeen)

Brand Names: U.S. Lantus®; Lantus® Solostar®

Index Terms Glargine Insulin

Pharmacologic Category Insulin, Long-Acting

Medication Safety Issues

Sound-alike/look-alike issues:

Insulin glargine may be confused with insulin glulisine

Lantus® may be confused with latanoprost, Latuda®, Xalatan®

High alert medication:

The Institute for Safe Medication Practices (ISMP) includes this medication among its list of drugs which have a heightened risk of causing significant patient harm when used in error. ***Due to the number of insulin preparations, it is essential to identify/clarify the type of insulin to be used.***

Administration issues:

Insulin glargine is a clear solution, but it is NOT intended for I.V. or I.M. administration.

Other safety concerns:

Cross-contamination may occur if insulin pens are shared among multiple patients. Steps should be taken to prohibit sharing of insulin pens.

International issues:

Lantus [U.S., Canada, and multiple international markets] may be confused with Lanvis brand name for thioguanine [Canada and multiple international markets]

Pregnancy Risk Factor C

Lactation Excretion in breast milk unknown/compatible

Breast-Feeding Considerations It is not known if significant amounts of insulin glargine are found in breast milk. Endogenous insulin can be found in breast milk. Plasma glucose concentrations in the mother affect glucose concentrations in breast milk. The gastrointestinal tract destroys insulin when administered orally; therefore, insulin is not expected to be absorbed intact by the breast-feeding infant. All types of insulin are safe for use while breast-feeding. Due to increased calorie expenditure, women with diabetes may require less insulin while nursing.

Use Treatment of type 1 diabetes mellitus (insulin dependent, IDDM) and type 2 diabetes mellitus (noninsulin dependent, NIDDM) to improve glycemic control

Mechanism of Action/Effect Insulin glargine is a long-acting insulin analog.

Refer to Insulin Regular on page 629.

Contraindications Hypersensitivity to insulin glargine or any component of the formulation

Warnings/Precautions Refer to Insulin Regular on page 629. Safety and efficacy not established in children <6 years of age.

In type 1 diabetes mellitus (insulin dependent, IDDM), insulin lispro (Humalog®) and insulin glulisine (Apidra™) should be used in combination with a long-acting insulin. However, in type 2 diabetes mellitus (noninsulin dependent, NIDDM), insulin lispro (Humalog®) may be used without a long-acting insulin when used in combination with a sulfonylurea.

Drug Interactions

Avoid Concomitant Use There are no known interactions where it is recommended to avoid concomitant use.

Decreased Effect

The levels/effects of Insulin Glargine may be decreased by: Corticosteroids (Orally Inhaled); Corticosteroids (Systemic); Luteinizing Hormone-Releasing Hormone Analogs; Somatropin; Thiazide Diuretics

Increased Effect/Toxicity Refer to Insulin Regular on page 629.

Nutritional/Ethanol Interactions Refer to Insulin Regular on page 629.

Adverse Reactions Refer to Insulin Regular on page 629.

Pharmacodynamics/Kinetics

Onset of Action 3-4 hours; Peak effect: No pronounced peak

Duration of Action Generally 24 hours or longer; reported range: 10.8 to >24 hours (up to 32 hours documented in some studies)

Available Dosage Forms

Injection, solution:

Lantus®: 100 units/mL (3 mL, 10 mL)

Lantus® Solostar®: 100 units/mL (3 mL)

General Dosage Range

SubQ:

Children:

Type 1 diabetes: Refer to Insulin Regular on page 629

Type 2 diabetes: Initial: 10 units once daily; Range: 2-100 units/day; **Note:** When changing from once-daily NPH or Ultralente®, initial dose should be the same but when changing from twice daily NPH the total dose should be reduced by 20% and adjusted according to patient response.

Adults:

Type 1 diabetes: Refer to Insulin Regular on page 629

Type 2 diabetes: Initial: 10 units once daily; Range: 2-100 units/day; **Note:** When changing from once-daily NPH or Ultralente®, initial dose should be the same but when changing from twice daily NPH the total dose should be reduced by 20% and adjusted according to patient response.

Administration

Other SubQ administration: Do not use if solution is viscous or cloudy; use only if clear and colorless with no visible particles. Insulin glargine should be administered once daily, at any time of day; however, administer at the same time each day. Cold injections should be avoided. SubQ administration is usually made into the thighs, arms, buttocks, or abdomen; rotate injection sites. Do not dilute or mix insulin glargine with any other insulin formulation or solution.

Stability

Storage Unopened vials, cartridges, and prefilled pens may be stored under refrigeration between 2°C and 8°C (36°F to 46°F) until the expiration date or at room temperature <30°C (<86°F) for 28 days; do not freeze; keep away from heat and sunlight. Once punctured (in use), vials may be stored under refrigeration or at room temperature <30°C (<86°F); use within 28 days. Cartridges within the OptiClik® system and prefilled pens (SoloStar®) that have been punctured (in use) should be stored at temperatures <30°C (<86°F) and used within 28 days; do not freeze or refrigerate.

Nursing Actions

Physical Assessment Monitor for hypoglycemia at regular intervals during therapy. Teach patient proper use, including appropriate injection technique and syringe/needle disposal, and monitoring requirements.

Patient Education Do not share pens, cartridges, or needles with others. This medication is used to control diabetes; it is not a cure. It is imperative to follow other components of prescribed treatment (eg, diet and exercise regimen). If you experience hypoglycemic reaction, contact prescriber immediately. Always carry quick source of sugar with you. Monitor glucose levels as directed by prescriber. Report adverse side effects, including chest pain or palpitations; persistent fatigue, confusion, headache; skin rash or redness; numbness of mouth, lips, or tongue; muscle weakness or tremors; vision changes; respiratory difficulty; or nausea, vomiting, or flu-like symptoms.

Dietary Considerations Individualized medical nutrition therapy (MNT) based on ADA recommendations is an integral part of therapy.

Related Information

Insulin Regular *on page 629*

Insulin Glulisine (IN soo lin gloo LIS een)

Brand Names: U.S. Apidra®; Apidra® SoloStar®

Index Terms Glulisine Insulin

Pharmacologic Category Insulin, Rapid-Acting

Medication Safety Issues

Sound-alike/look-alike issues:

Insulin glulisine may be confused with insulin glargine

High alert medication:

The Institute for Safe Medication Practices (ISMP) includes this medication among its list of drugs which have a heightened risk of causing significant patient harm when used in error. ***Due to the number of insulin preparations, it is essential to identify/clarify the type of insulin to be used.***

Other safety concerns:

Cross-contamination may occur if insulin pens are shared among multiple patients. Steps should be taken to prohibit sharing of insulin pens.

Pregnancy Risk Factor C

Lactation Excretion in breast milk unknown/compatible

Use Treatment of type 1 diabetes mellitus (insulin dependent, IDDM) and type 2 diabetes mellitus (noninsulin dependent, NIDDM) to improve glycemic control

Available Dosage Forms

Injection, solution:

Apidra®: 100 units/mL (3 mL, 10 mL)

Apidra® SoloStar®: 100 units/mL (3 mL)

General Dosage Range

SubQ:

Children: Refer to Insulin Regular on page 629

Adults: Refer to Insulin Regular on page 629

Administration

I.V.

Do not use if solution is viscous or cloudy; use only if clear and colorless. May be administered I.V. with close monitoring of blood glucose and serum potassium; appropriate medical supervision is required. **Do not administer insulin mixtures intravenously.**

I.V. Detail

I.V. infusions: To minimize adsorption to I.V. solution bag: **Note:** Refer to institution-specific protocols where appropriate.

*If new tubing is **not** needed:* Wait a minimum of 30 minutes between the preparation of the solution and the initiation of the infusion.

If new tubing is needed: After receiving the insulin drip solution, the administration set should be attached to the I.V. container and the entire line should be flushed with a priming infusion of 20-50 mL of the insulin solution (Goldberg, 2006; Hirsch, 2006). Wait 30 minutes, and then flush the line again with the insulin solution prior to initiating the infusion.

Because of adsorption, the actual amount of insulin being administered via I.V. infusion could be substantially less than the apparent amount. Therefore, adjustment of the I.V. infusion rate should be based on effect and not solely on the apparent insulin dose. The apparent dose may be used as a starting point for determining the subsequent SubQ dosing regimen (Moghissi, 2009); however, the transition to SubQ administration requires continuous medical supervision, frequent monitoring of blood glucose, and careful adjustment of therapy. In addition, SubQ insulin should be given 1-4 hours prior to the discontinuation of I.V. insulin to prevent hyperglycemia (Moghissi, 2009).

pH: ~7.3

Other

SubQ administration: Do not use if solution is viscous or cloudy; use only if clear and colorless. Insulin glulisine should be administered within 15 minutes before or within 20 minutes after starting a meal. Cold injections should be avoided. SubQ administration is usually made into the thighs, arms, buttocks, or abdomen; rotate injection sites. When mixing insulin glulisine with other preparations of insulin (eg, insulin NPH), insulin glulisine should be drawn into syringe first. Do not mix other insulin formulations with insulin glulisine contained in a cartridge or prefilled pen.

CSII administration: Do not use if solution is viscous or cloudy; use only if clear and colorless. Patients should be trained in the proper use of their external insulin pump and in intensive insulin therapy. Infusion sets, reservoirs, and infusion set insertion sites should be changed every 48 hours; rotate infusion sites. Do not dilute or mix other insulin formulations with insulin glulisine that is to be used in an external insulin pump.

Nursing Actions

Physical Assessment Monitor for hypoglycemia at regular intervals during therapy. Teach patient proper use, including appropriate injection technique and syringe/needle disposal, and monitoring requirements.

Patient Education Do not share pens, cartridges, or needles with others. This medication is used to control diabetes; it is not a cure. It is imperative to follow other components of prescribed treatment (eg, diet and exercise regimen). Insulin glulisine (Apidra®) should be administered within 15 minutes before or within 20 minutes after start of a meal. If you experience hypoglycemic reaction, contact prescriber immediately. Always carry quick source of sugar with you. Monitor glucose levels as directed by prescriber. Report adverse side effects, including chest pain or palpitations; persistent fatigue, confusion, headache; skin rash or redness; numbness of mouth, lips, or tongue; muscle weakness or tremors; vision changes; respiratory difficulty; or nausea, vomiting, or flu-like symptoms.

Related Information

Insulin Regular *on page* 629

Insulin Lispro (IN soo lin LYE sproe)

Brand Names: U.S. HumaLOG®; HumaLOG® KwikPen™

Index Terms Lispro Insulin

Pharmacologic Category Insulin, Rapid-Acting

Medication Safety Issues

Sound-alike/look-alike issues:

HumaLOG® may be confused with HumaLOG® Mix 50/50, Humira®, HumuLIN® N, HumuLIN® R, NovoLOG®

High alert medication:

The Institute for Safe Medication Practices (ISMP) includes this medication among its list of drugs which have a heightened risk of causing significant patient harm when used in error. ***Due to the number of insulin preparations, it is essential to identify/clarify the type of insulin to be used.***

Other safety concerns:

Cross-contamination may occur if insulin pens are shared among multiple patients. Steps should be taken to prohibit sharing of insulin pens.

Pregnancy Risk Factor B

Lactation Excretion in breast milk unknown/compatible

Breast-Feeding Considerations It is not known if significant amounts of insulin lispro are found in breast milk. Endogenous insulin can be found in breast milk. Plasma glucose concentrations in the mother affect glucose concentrations in breast milk. The gastrointestinal tract destroys insulin when administered orally; therefore, insulin is not expected to be absorbed intact by the breast-feeding infant. All types of insulin are safe for use while breast-feeding. Due to increased calorie expenditure, women with diabetes may require less insulin while nursing.

Use Treatment of type 1 diabetes mellitus (insulin dependent, IDDM) and type 2 diabetes mellitus (noninsulin dependent, NIDDM) to improve glycemic control

Unlabeled Use Gestational diabetes mellitus (GDM); mild-to-moderate diabetic ketoacidosis (DKA); mild-to-moderate hyperosmolar hyperglycemic state (HHS)

Mechanism of Action/Effect Refer to Insulin Regular on page 629. Insulin lispro is a rapid-acting form of insulin.

Contraindications Hypersensitivity to insulin lispro or any component of the formulation; during episodes of hypoglycemia

Warnings/Precautions Refer to Insulin Regular on page 629.

In type 1 diabetes mellitus (insulin dependent, IDDM), insulin lispro (Humalog®) and insulin glulisine (Apidra™) should be used in combination with a long-acting insulin. However, in type 2 diabetes mellitus (noninsulin dependent, NIDDM), insulin lispro (Humalog®) may be used without a long-acting insulin when used in combination with a sulfonylurea.

Drug Interactions

Avoid Concomitant Use There are no known interactions where it is recommended to avoid concomitant use.

Decreased Effect

The levels/effects of Insulin Lispro may be decreased by: Corticosteroids (Orally Inhaled); Corticosteroids (Systemic); Luteinizing Hormone-Releasing Hormone Analogs; Somatropin; Thiazide Diuretics

Increased Effect/Toxicity Refer to Insulin Regular on page 629.

Nutritional/Ethanol Interactions Refer to Insulin Regular on page 629.

Adverse Reactions Refer to Insulin Regular on page 629.

Pharmacodynamics/Kinetics

Onset of Action 0.25-0.5 hours; Peak effect: 0.5-2.5 hours

Duration of Action ≤5 hours

Available Dosage Forms

Injection, solution:

HumaLOG®: 100 units/mL (3 mL, 10 mL)

HumaLOG® KwikPen™: 100 units/mL (3 mL)

General Dosage Range Note: Insulin lispro is equipotent to insulin regular, but has a more rapid onset

SubQ:

Children: Refer to Insulin Regular on page 629

Adults: Refer to Insulin Regular on page 629

Administration

I.V. I.V. administration (unlabeled use): Do not use if solution is viscous or cloudy; use only if clear and colorless. May be administered I.V. with close monitoring of blood glucose and serum potassium; appropriate medical supervision is required. Do not administer insulin mixtures intravenously.

I.V. Detail I.V. infusions: To minimize adsorption to I.V. solution bag: **Note:** Refer to institution-specific protocols where appropriate.

*If new tubing is **not** needed:* Wait a minimum of 30 minutes between the preparation of the solution and the initiation of the infusion.

If new tubing is needed: After receiving the insulin drip solution, the administration set should be attached to the I.V. container and the entire line should be flushed with a priming infusion of 20-50 mL of the insulin solution (Goldberg, 2006; Hirsch, 2006). Wait 30 minutes, and then flush the line again with the insulin solution prior to initiating the infusion.

Because of adsorption, the actual amount of insulin being administered via I.V. infusion could be substantially less than the apparent amount. Therefore, adjustment of the I.V. infusion rate should be based on effect and not solely on the apparent insulin dose. The apparent dose may be used as a starting point for determining the subsequent SubQ dosing regimen (Moghissi, 2009); however, the transition to SubQ administration requires continuous medical supervision, frequent monitoring of blood glucose, and careful adjustment of therapy. In addition, SubQ insulin should be given 1-4 hours prior to the discontinuation of I.V. insulin to prevent hyperglycemia (Moghissi, 2009).

pH: 7.0-7.8

Other

SubQ administration: Do not use if solution is viscous or cloudy; use only if clear and colorless. Insulin lispro should be administered within 15 minutes before or immediately after a meal. Cold injections should be avoided. SubQ administration is usually made into the thighs, arms, buttocks, or abdomen; rotate injection sites. When mixing insulin lispro with other preparations of insulin (eg, insulin NPH), insulin lispro should be drawn into syringe first. Do not dilute or mix other insulin formulations with insulin lispro contained in a cartridge or prefilled pen.

CSII administration: Do not use if solution is viscous or cloudy; use only if clear and colorless. Patients should be trained in the proper use of their external insulin pump and in intensive insulin therapy. Infusion sets and infusion set insertion sites should be changed every 3 days; rotate infusion sites. Insulin in reservoir should be changed every 7 days. Do not dilute or mix other insulin formulations with insulin lispro contained in an external insulin pump.

Stability

Reconstitution

For SubQ administration: *Humalog® vials:* May be diluted with the universal diluent, Sterile Diluent for Humalog®, Humulin® N, Humulin® R, Humulin® 70/30, and Humulin® R U-500, to a concentration of 10 units/mL (U-10) or 50 units/mL (U-50). Do not dilute insulin contained in a cartridge, prefilled pen, or external insulin pump.

For I.V. infusion (unlabeled use): May be diluted in NS or D_5W to concentrations of 0.025-2 units/mL.

Storage Unopened vials, cartridges, and prefilled pens may be stored under refrigeration between 2°C and 8°C (36°F to 46°F) until the expiration date or at room temperature <30°C (<86°F) for 28 days; do not freeze; keep away from heat and sunlight. Once punctured (in use), vials may be stored under refrigeration or at room temperature <30°C (<86°F); use within 28 days. Cartridges and prefilled pens that have been punctured (in use) should be stored at temperatures <30°C (<86°F) and used within 28 days; do not freeze or refrigerate. When used for CSII, insulin lispro contained within an external insulin pump reservoir should be changed every 7 days and insulin lispro contained within a 3 mL cartridge should be discarded after 7 days; discard if exposed to temperatures >37°C (>98.6°F).

For SubQ administration: *Humalog® vials:* According to the manufacturer, diluted insulin should be stored at 30°C (86°F) and used within 14 days or 5°C (41°F) and used within 28 days.

For I.V. infusion (unlabeled use): Stable for 48 hours at room temperature.

Nursing Actions

Physical Assessment Monitor for hypoglycemia at regular intervals during therapy. Teach patient proper use, including appropriate injection technique and syringe/needle disposal, and monitoring requirements.

Patient Education Do not share pens, cartridges, or needles with others. This medication is used to control diabetes; it is not a cure. It is imperative to follow other components of prescribed treatment (eg, diet and exercise regimen). If you experience hypoglycemic reaction, contact prescriber immediately. Always carry quick source of sugar with you. Monitor glucose levels as directed by prescriber. Report adverse side effects, including chest pain or palpitations; persistent fatigue, confusion, headache; skin rash or redness; numbness of mouth, lips, or tongue; muscle weakness or tremors; vision changes; respiratory difficulty; or nausea, vomiting, or flu-like symptoms.

Dietary Considerations Individualized medical nutrition therapy (MNT) based on ADA recommendations is an integral part of therapy.

Related Information

Insulin Regular *on page* 629

Insulin Lispro Protamine and Insulin Lispro

(IN soo lin LYE sproe PROE ta meen & IN soo lin LYE sproe)

Brand Names: U.S. HumaLOG® Mix 50/50™; HumaLOG® Mix 50/50™ KwikPen™; HumaLOG® Mix 75/25™; HumaLOG® Mix 75/25™ KwikPen™

Index Terms Insulin Lispro and Insulin Lispro Protamine

Pharmacologic Category Insulin, Combination

Medication Safety Issues

Sound-alike/look-alike issues:

HumaLOG® Mix 50/50™ may be confused with HumaLOG®

HumaLOG® Mix 75/25™ may be confused with HumuLIN® 70/30, NovoLIN® 70/30, and NovoLOG® Mix 70/30

High alert medication:

The Institute for Safe Medication Practices (ISMP) includes this medication among its list of drugs which have a heightened risk of causing significant patient harm when used in error. ***Due to the number of insulin preparations, it is essential to identify/clarify the type of insulin to be used.***

Other safety concerns:

Cross-contamination may occur if insulin pens are shared among multiple patients. Steps should be taken to prohibit sharing of insulin pens.

Pregnancy Risk Factor B

Lactation Excretion in breast milk unknown/compatible

Use Treatment of type 1 diabetes mellitus (insulin dependent, IDDM) and type 2 diabetes mellitus (noninsulin dependent, NIDDM) to improve glycemic control

Available Dosage Forms

Injection, suspension:

HumaLOG® Mix 50/50™: Insulin lispro protamine suspension 50% [intermediate acting] and insulin lispro solution 50% [rapid acting]: 100 units/mL (10 mL)

HumaLOG® Mix 50/50™ KwikPen™: Insulin lispro protamine suspension 50% [intermediate acting] and insulin lispro solution 50% [rapid acting]: 100 units/mL (3 mL)

HumaLOG® Mix 75/25™: Insulin lispro protamine suspension 75% [intermediate acting] and insulin lispro solution 25% [rapid acting]: 100 units/mL (10 mL)

HumaLOG® Mix 75/25™ KwikPen™: Insulin lispro protamine suspension 75% [intermediate acting] and insulin lispro solution 25% [rapid acting]: 100 units/mL (3 mL)

General Dosage Range Note: Fixed ratio insulins (such as insulin lispro protamine and insulin lispro) are normally administered in 2 daily doses.

SubQ:

Children: Dosage not established

Adults: Refer to Insulin Regular on page 629

Administration

Other SubQ administration: In order to properly resuspend the insulin, vials should be carefully shaken or rolled several times and prefilled pens should be rolled between the palms ten times and inverted 180° ten times. Properly resuspended insulin should look uniformly cloudy or milky; do not use if any white insulin substance remains at the bottom of the container, if any clumps are present, if the insulin remains clear after adequate mixing, or if white particles are stuck to the bottom or wall of the container. Cold injections should be avoided. Insulin lispro protamine and insulin lispro combination products should be administered within 15 minutes before a meal; typically given once- or twice daily. SubQ administration is usually made into the thighs, arms, buttocks, or abdomen; rotate injection sites. Do not dilute or mix with any other insulin formulation or solution; **not** recommended for use in external SubQ insulin infusion pump.

Nursing Actions

Physical Assessment See individual agents.

Patient Education See individual agents.

Related Information

Insulin Regular *on page 629*

Insulin NPH (IN soo lin N P H)

Brand Names: U.S. HumuLIN® N; NovoLIN® N

Index Terms Isophane Insulin; NPH Insulin

Pharmacologic Category Insulin, Intermediate-Acting

Medication Safety Issues

Sound-alike/look-alike issues:

HumuLIN® N may be confused with HumuLIN® R, HumaLOG®, Humira®

NovoLIN® N may be confused with NovoLIN® R, NovoLOG®

High alert medication:

The Institute for Safe Medication Practices (ISMP) includes this medication among its list of drugs which have a heightened risk of causing significant patient harm when used in error. ***Due to the number of insulin preparations, it is essential to identify/clarify the type of insulin to be used.***

Other safety concerns:

Cross-contamination may occur if insulin pens are shared among multiple patients. Steps should be taken to prohibit sharing of insulin pens.

Lactation Excretion in breast milk unknown/compatible

Use Treatment of type 1 diabetes mellitus (insulin dependent, IDDM) and type 2 diabetes mellitus (noninsulin dependent, NIDDM) to improve glycemic control

Unlabeled Use Gestational diabetes mellitus (GDM)

Available Dosage Forms

Injection, suspension:

HumuLIN® N: 100 units/mL (3 mL, 10 mL)

NovoLIN® N: 100 units/mL (10 mL)

General Dosage Range Note: Usually administered 1-2 times daily

SubQ:

Children: Refer to Insulin Regular on page 629

Adults: Refer to Insulin Regular on page 629

Administration

Other SubQ administration: In order to properly resuspend the insulin, vials should be carefully shaken or rolled several times, prefilled pens should be rolled between the palms ten times and inverted 180° ten times, and cartridges should be inverted 180° at least ten times. Properly resuspended insulin NPH should look uniformly cloudy or milky; do not use if any white insulin substance remains at the bottom of the container, if any clumps are present, or if white particles are stuck to the bottom or wall of the container. Cold injections should be avoided. SubQ administration is usually made into the thighs, arms, buttocks, or abdomen; rotate injection sites. When mixing insulin NPH with other preparations of insulin (eg, insulin aspart, insulin glulisine, insulin lispro, insulin regular), insulin NPH should be drawn into the syringe **after** the other insulin preparations. Do not dilute or mix other insulin formulations with insulin NPH contained in a cartridge or prefilled pen. Insulin NPH is **not** recommended for use in external SubQ insulin infusion pump.

Nursing Actions

Physical Assessment Monitor for hypoglycemia at regular intervals during therapy. Teach patient proper use, including appropriate injection technique and syringe/needle disposal, and monitoring requirements.

Patient Education Do not share pens, cartridges, or needles with others. This medication is used to control diabetes; it is not a cure. It is imperative to follow other components of prescribed treatment (eg, diet and exercise regimen). If you experience hypoglycemic reaction, contact prescriber immediately. Always carry quick source of sugar with you. Monitor glucose levels as directed by prescriber. Report adverse side effects, including chest pain or palpitations; persistent fatigue, confusion, headache; skin rash or redness; numbness of mouth, lips, or tongue; muscle weakness or tremors; vision changes; respiratory difficulty; or nausea, vomiting, or flu-like symptoms.

Related Information

Insulin Regular *on page* 629

Insulin NPH and Insulin Regular

(IN soo lin N P H & IN soo lin REG yoo ler)

Brand Names: U.S. HumuLIN® 70/30; NovoLIN® 70/30

Index Terms Insulin Regular and Insulin NPH; Isophane Insulin and Regular Insulin; NPH Insulin and Regular Insulin

Pharmacologic Category Insulin, Combination

Medication Safety Issues

Sound-alike/look-alike issues:

HumuLIN® 70/30 may be confused with HumaLOG® Mix 75/25, HumuLIN® R, NovoLIN® 70/30, NovoLOG® Mix 70/30

NovoLIN® 70/30 may be confused with HumaLOG® Mix 75/25, HumuLIN® 70/30, HumuLIN® R, NovoLIN® R, and NovoLOG® Mix 70/30

High alert medication:

The Institute for Safe Medication Practices (ISMP) includes this medication among its list of drugs which have a heightened risk of causing significant patient harm when used in error. ***Due to the number of insulin preparations, it is essential to identify/clarify the type of insulin to be used.***

Other safety concerns:

Cross-contamination may occur if insulin pens are shared among multiple patients. Steps should be taken to prohibit sharing of insulin pens.

Use Treatment of type 1 diabetes mellitus (insulin dependent, IDDM) and type 2 diabetes mellitus (noninsulin dependent, NIDDM) to improve glycemic control

Unlabeled Use Gestational diabetes mellitus (GDM)

Available Dosage Forms

Injection, suspension:

HumuLIN® 70/30: Insulin NPH suspension 70% [intermediate acting] and insulin regular solution 30% [short acting]: 100 units/mL (3 mL, 10 mL)

NovoLIN® 70/30: Insulin NPH suspension 70% [intermediate acting] and insulin regular solution 30% [short acting]: 100 units/mL (10 mL)

General Dosage Range

Note: Fixed ratio insulins are normally administered in 1-2 daily doses

SubQ:

Children: Refer to Insulin Regular on page 629

Adults: Refer to Insulin Regular on page 629

Administration

Other SubQ administration: In order to properly resuspend the insulin, vials should be carefully shaken or rolled several times, prefilled pens should be rolled between the palms ten times and inverted 180° ten times, and cartridges should be inverted 180° at least ten times. Properly resuspended insulin should look uniformly cloudy or milky; do not use if any white insulin substance remains at the bottom of the container, if any clumps are present, if the insulin remains clear after adequate mixing, or if white particles are stuck to the bottom or wall of the container. Cold injections should be avoided. Insulin NPH and insulin regular combination products should be administered within 30 minutes before a meal; typically given once- or twice daily. SubQ administration is usually made into the thighs, arms, buttocks, or abdomen; rotate injection sites. Do not mix with any other insulin formulation. Do not dilute combination product (insulin NPH and insulin regular) contained in a cartridge or prefilled pen. Combination insulin products are not recommended for use in an external SubQ insulin infusion pump.

Nursing Actions

Physical Assessment See individual agents.

Patient Education See individual agents.

Related Information

Insulin Regular *on page* 629

Insulin Regular

(IN soo lin REG yoo ler)

Brand Names: U.S. HumuLIN® R; HumuLIN® R U-500; NovoLIN® R

Index Terms Regular Insulin

Pharmacologic Category Insulin, Short-Acting

Medication Safety Issues

Sound-alike/look-alike issues:

HumuLIN® R may be confused with HumaLOG®, Humira®, HumuLIN® 70/30, HumuLIN® N, NovoLIN® 70/30, NovoLIN® R, NovoLOG®

NovoLIN® R may be confused with HumuLIN® R, NovoLIN® 70/30, NovoLIN® N, NovoLOG®

High alert medication:

The Institute for Safe Medication Practices (ISMP) includes this medication among its list of drugs which have a heightened risk of causing significant patient harm when used in error. ***Due to the number of insulin preparations, it is essential to identify/clarify the type of insulin to be used.***

Administration issues:

Concentrated solutions (eg, U-500) should not be available in patient care areas. U-500 regular insulin should be stored, dispensed, and administered separately from U-100 regular insulin. For patients who receive U-500 insulin in the hospital setting, highlighting the strength prominently on the patient's medical chart and medication record may help to reduce dispensing errors.

Other safety concerns:

Cross-contamination may occur if insulin pens are shared among multiple patients. Steps should be taken to prohibit sharing of insulin pens.

Lactation Excretion in breast milk unknown/compatible

Breast-Feeding Considerations Endogenous insulin can be found in breast milk. Plasma glucose concentrations in the mother affect glucose concentrations in breast milk. The gastrointestinal tract destroys insulin when administered orally; therefore, insulin is not expected to be absorbed intact by the breast-feeding infant. All types of insulin are safe for use while breast-feeding. Due to increased calorie expenditure, women with diabetes may require less insulin while nursing.

Use Treatment of type 1 diabetes mellitus (insulin dependent, IDDM) and type 2 diabetes mellitus (noninsulin dependent, NIDDM) to improve glycemic control

Unlabeled Use Hyperkalemia; gestational diabetes mellitus (GDM), diabetic ketoacidosis (DKA); hyperosmolar hyperglycemic state (HHS); adjunct of parenteral nutrition

Mechanism of Action/Effect Insulin acts via specific membrane-bound receptors on target tissues to regulate metabolism of carbohydrate, protein, and fats. Target organs for insulin include the liver, skeletal muscle, and adipose tissue.

Within the liver, insulin stimulates hepatic glycogen synthesis. Insulin promotes hepatic synthesis of fatty acids, which are released into the circulation as lipoproteins. Skeletal muscle effects of insulin include increased protein synthesis and increased glycogen synthesis. Within adipose tissue, insulin stimulates the processing of circulating lipoproteins to provide free fatty acids, facilitating triglyceride synthesis and storage by adipocytes; also directly inhibits the hydrolysis of triglycerides. In addition, insulin stimulates the cellular uptake of amino acids and increases cellular permeability to several ions, including potassium, magnesium, and phosphate. By activating sodium-potassium ATPases, insulin promotes the intracellular movement of potassium.

Insulins are categorized based on the onset, peak, and duration of effect (eg, rapid-, short-, intermediate-, and long-acting insulin).

Contraindications Hypersensitivity to regular insulin or any component of the formulation; during episodes of hypoglycemia

Warnings/Precautions Hypoglycemia is the most common adverse effect of insulin. The timing of hypoglycemia differs among various insulin formulations. Hypoglycemia may result from increased work or exercise without eating; use of long-acting insulin preparations (eg, insulin detemir, insulin glargine) may delay recovery from hypoglycemia. Profound and prolonged episodes of hypoglycemia may result in convulsions, unconsciousness, temporary or permanent brain damage or even death. Insulin requirements may be altered during illness, emotional disturbances or other stressors. Insulin may produce hypokalemia which, if left untreated, may result in respiratory paralysis, ventricular arrhythmia and even death. Use with caution in patients at risk for hypokalemia (eg, I.V. insulin use). Use with caution in renal or hepatic impairment.

Human insulin differs from animal-source insulin. Any change of insulin should be made cautiously; changing manufacturers, type, and/or method of manufacture may result in the need for a change of dosage. U-500 regular insulin is a concentrated insulin formulation which contains 500 units of insulin per mL; for SubQ administration only using a U-100 insulin syringe or tuberculin syringe; **not for I.V. administration**. To avoid dosing errors when using a U-100 insulin syringe, the prescribed dose should be written in actual insulin units and as unit markings on the U-100 insulin syringe (eg, 50 units [10 units on a U-100 insulin syringe]). To avoid dosing errors when using a tuberculin syringe, the prescribed dose should be written in actual insulin units and as a volume (eg, 50 units [0.1 mL]). Mixing U-500 regular insulin with other insulin formulations is not recommended.

Regular insulin may be administered I.V. or I.M. in selected clinical situations; close monitoring of blood glucose and serum potassium, as well as medical supervision, is required.

The general objective of exogenous insulin therapy is to approximate the physiologic pattern of insulin secretion which is characterized by two distinct phases. Phase 1 insulin secretion suppresses hepatic glucose production and phase 2 insulin secretion occurs in response to carbohydrate ingestion; therefore, exogenous insulin therapy may consist of basal insulin (eg, intermediate- or long-acting insulin or via continuous subcutaneous insulin infusion [CSII]) and/or preprandial insulin (eg, short- or rapid-acting insulin). Patients with type 1 diabetes do not produce endogenous insulin; therefore, these patients require both basal and preprandial insulin administration. Patients with type 2 diabetes retain some beta-cell function in the early stages of their disease; however, as the disease progresses, phase 1 insulin secretion may become completely impaired and phase 2 insulin secretion becomes delayed and/or inadequate in response to meals. Therefore, patients with type 2 diabetes may be treated with oral antidiabetic agents, basal insulin, and/or preprandial insulin depending on the stage of disease and current glycemic control. Since treatment regimens often consist of multiple agents, dosage adjustments must address the specific phase of insulin release that is primarily contributing to the patient's impaired glycemic control. Diabetes self-management education (DSME) is essential to maximize the effectiveness of therapy. Treatment and monitoring regimens must be individualized.

Drug Interactions

Avoid Concomitant Use There are no known interactions where it is recommended to avoid concomitant use.

Decreased Effect

The levels/effects of Insulin Regular may be decreased by: Corticosteroids (Orally Inhaled); Corticosteroids (Systemic); Luteinizing Hormone-Releasing Hormone Analogs; Somatropin; Thiazide Diuretics

Increased Effect/Toxicity

Insulin Regular may increase the levels/effects of: Antidiabetic Agents (Thiazolidinedione); Hypoglycemic Agents; Quinolone Antibiotics

The levels/effects of Insulin Regular may be increased by: Beta-Blockers; Edetate CALCIUM Disodium; Edetate Disodium; Herbs (Hypoglycemic Properties); Pegvisomant

Nutritional/Ethanol Interactions

Ethanol: Use caution with ethanol; may increase risk of hypoglycemia.

Herb/Nutraceutical: Use caution with alfalfa, aloe, bilberry, bitter melon, burdock, celery, damiana, fenugreek, garcinia, garlic, ginger, ginseng (American), gymnema, marshmallow, stinging nettle; may increase risk of hypoglycemia.

Adverse Reactions Primarily symptoms of hypoglycemia

Cardiovascular: Pallor, palpitation, tachycardia

Central nervous system: Fatigue, headache, hypothermia, loss of consciousness, mental confusion

Dermatologic: Redness, urticaria

Endocrine & metabolic: Hypoglycemia, hypokalemia

Gastrointestinal: Hunger, nausea, numbness of mouth

Local: Atrophy or hypertrophy of SubQ fat tissue; edema, itching, pain or warmth at injection site; stinging

Neuromuscular & skeletal: Muscle weakness, paresthesia, tremor

Ocular: Transient presbyopia or blurred vision

Miscellaneous: Anaphylaxis, diaphoresis, local and/or systemic hypersensitivity reactions

Pharmacodynamics/Kinetics

Onset of Action SubQ: 0.5 hours; Peak effect: SubQ: 2.5-5 hours

Duration of Action SubQ:

U-100: 4-12 hours (may increase with dose)

U-500: Up to 24 hours

Available Dosage Forms

Injection, solution:

HumuLIN® R: 100 units/mL (3 mL, 10 mL)

HumuLIN® R U-500: 500 units/mL (20 mL)

NovoLIN® R: 100 units/mL (10 mL)

General Dosage Range Dosage adjustment recommended in patients with renal impairment

I.V., SubQ: *Children and Adults:*

Diabetes mellitus, type 1: Initial: 0.5-1 unit/kg/day in divided doses; Usual maintenance: 0.5-1.2 units/kg/day in divided doses. **Note:** Generally, 50% to 75% of the total daily dose (TDD) is given as an intermediate- or long-acting form of insulin (1-2 daily injections) and the remaining portion is then divided and administered before or at mealtime (depending on the formulation) as a rapid-acting or short-acting form of insulin.

Diabetes mellitus, type 2: Initial basal insulin dose: 0.2 units/kg or 10 units/day given as an intermediate- or long-acting insulin at bedtime or long-acting insulin given in the morning

Administration

I.M. Do not use if solution is viscous or cloudy; use only if clear and colorless. May be administered I.M. in selected clinical situations; close monitoring of blood glucose and serum potassium as well as medical supervision is required.

I.V. Do not use if solution is viscous or cloudy; use only if clear and colorless. May be administered I.V. with close monitoring of blood glucose and serum potassium; appropriate medical supervision is required. If possible, avoid I.V. bolus administration in pediatric patients with DKA; may increase risk of cerebral edema. **Do not administer mixtures of insulin formulations intravenously.** I.V. administration of U-500 regular insulin is not recommended.

I.V. Detail I.V. infusions: To minimize adsorption to I.V. solution bag (**Note:** Refer to institution-specific protocols where appropriate):

*If new tubing is **not** needed:* Wait a minimum of 30 minutes between the preparation of the solution and the initiation of the infusion.

If new tubing is needed: After receiving the insulin drip solution, the administration set should be attached to the I.V. container and the entire line should be flushed with a priming infusion of 20-50 mL of the insulin solution (Goldberg, 2006; Hirsch, 2006). Wait 30 minutes, then flush the line again with the insulin solution prior to initiating the infusion.

If insulin is required prior to the availability of the insulin drip, regular insulin should be administered by I.V. push injection.

Because of adsorption, the actual amount of insulin being administered via I.V. infusion could be substantially less than the apparent amount. Therefore, adjustment of the I.V. infusion rate should be based on effect and not solely on the apparent insulin dose. The apparent dose may be used as a starting point for determining the subsequent SubQ dosing regimen (Moghissi, 2009); however, the transition to SubQ administration requires continuous medical supervision, frequent monitoring of blood glucose, and careful adjustment of therapy. In addition, SubQ insulin should be given 1-4 hours prior to the discontinuation of I.V. insulin to prevent hyperglycemia (Moghissi, 2009).

pH: 7.0-7.8

Other SubQ administration: Do not use if solution is viscous or cloudy; use only if clear and colorless. Regular insulin should be administered within 30-60 minutes before a meal. Cold injections should be avoided. SubQ administration is usually made into the thighs, arms, buttocks, or abdomen; rotate injection sites. When mixing regular insulin with other preparations of insulin, regular insulin should be drawn into syringe first. Regular insulin is not recommended for use in external SubQ insulin infusion pump.

Stability

Reconstitution

For SubQ administration:

Humulin® R: May be diluted with the universal diluent, Sterile Diluent for Humalog®, Humulin® N, Humulin® R, Humulin® 70/30, and Humulin® R U-500, to a concentration of 10 units/mL (U-10) or 50 units/mL (U-50).

Novolin® R: Insulin Diluting Medium for NovoLog® is **not** intended for use with Novolin® R or any insulin product other than insulin aspart.

For I.V. infusion:

Humulin® R: May be diluted in NS or D_5W to concentrations of 0.1-1 unit/mL.

Novolin® R: May be diluted in NS, D_5W, or $D_{10}W$ with 40 mEq/L potassium chloride at concentrations of 0.05-1 unit/mL.

Storage

Humulin® R, Humulin® R U-500: Store unopened vials in refrigerator between 2°C and 8°C (36°F to 46°F); do not freeze; keep away from heat and sunlight. Once punctured (in use), vials may be stored for up to 31 days in the refrigerator between 2°C and 8°C (36°F to 46°F) or at room temperature of ≤30°C (≤86°F).

Novolin® R: Store unopened vials in refrigerator between 2°C and 8°C (36°F to 46°F) until product expiration date or at room temperature ≤25°C (≤77°F) for up to 42 days; do not freeze; keep away from heat and sunlight. Once punctured (in use), store vials at room temperature ≤25°C (≤77°F) for up to 42 days (this includes any days stored at room temperature prior to opening vial); refrigeration of in-use vials is not recommended.

Canadian labeling (not in U.S. labeling): All products: Unopened vials, cartridges, and pens should be stored under refrigeration between 2°C and 8°C (36°F to 46°F) until the expiration date; do not freeze; keep away from heat and sunlight. Once punctured (in use), Humulin® vials, cartridges, and pens should be stored at room temperature <25°C (<77°F) for up to 4 weeks. Once punctured (in use), Novolin® ge vials, cartridges, and pens may be stored for up to 1 month at room temperature <25°C (<77°F) for vials or <30°C (<86°F) for pens/cartridges; do not refrigerate.

For SubQ administration:

Humulin® R: According to the manufacturer, diluted insulin should be stored at 30°C (86°F) and used within 14 days **or** at 5°C (41°F) and used within 28 days.

For I.V. infusion:

Humulin® R: Stable for 48 hours at room temperature or for 48 hours under refrigeration followed by 48 hours at room temperature.

Novolin® R: Stable for 24 hours at room temperature

Nursing Actions

Physical Assessment Monitor for hypoglycemia at regular intervals during therapy. Teach patient proper use, including appropriate injection technique and syringe/needle disposal, and monitoring requirements.

Patient Education Do not share pens, cartridges, or needles with others. This medication is used to control diabetes; it is not a cure. It is imperative to follow other components of prescribed treatment (eg, diet and exercise regimen). If you experience hypoglycemic reaction, contact prescriber immediately. Always carry quick source of sugar with you. Monitor glucose levels as directed by prescriber. Report adverse side effects, including chest pain or palpitations; persistent fatigue, confusion, headache; skin rash or redness; numbness of mouth, lips, or tongue; muscle weakness or tremors; vision changes; respiratory difficulty; or nausea, vomiting, or flu-like symptoms.

Dietary Considerations Individualized medical nutrition therapy (MNT) based on ADA recommendations is an integral part of therapy.

Related Information

Insulin Aspart *on page 619*
Insulin Aspart Protamine and Insulin Aspart *on page 621*
Insulin Detemir *on page 622*
Insulin Glargine *on page 623*
Insulin Glulisine *on page 624*
Insulin Lispro *on page 625*
Insulin Lispro Protamine and Insulin Lispro *on page 627*
Insulin NPH *on page 628*
Insulin NPH and Insulin Regular *on page 629*

Interferon Alfa-2b (in ter FEER on AL fa too bee)

Brand Names: U.S. Intron® A

Index Terms INF-alpha 2; Interferon Alpha-2b; rLFN-α2; α-2-interferon

Pharmacologic Category Interferon

Medication Safety Issues

Sound-alike/look-alike issues:

Interferon alfa-2b may be confused with interferon alfa-2a, interferon alfa-n3, pegylated interferon alfa-2b

Intron® A may be confused with PEG-Intron

International issues:

Interferon alfa-2b may be confused with interferon alpha multi-subtype which is available in international markets

Medication Guide Available Yes

Pregnancy Risk Factor C / X in combination with ribavirin

Lactation Enters breast milk/not recommended (AAP rates "compatible"; AAP 2001 update pending)

Use

Patients ≥1 year of age: Chronic hepatitis B

Patients ≥3 years of age: Chronic hepatitis C (in combination with ribavirin)

Patients ≥18 years of age: Condyloma acuminata, chronic hepatitis B, chronic hepatitis C, hairy cell leukemia, malignant melanoma, AIDS-related Kaposi's sarcoma, follicular non-Hodgkin's lymphoma

Unlabeled Use AIDS-related thrombocytopenia, cutaneous ulcerations of Behçet's disease, neuroendocrine tumors (including carcinoid syndrome and islet cell tumor), cutaneous T-cell lymphoma, desmoid tumor, lymphomatoid granulomatosis, hepatitis D, chronic myelogenous leukemia (CML), non-Hodgkin's lymphomas (other than follicular lymphoma, see approved use), multiple myeloma, renal cell carcinoma, West Nile virus

Available Dosage Forms

Injection, powder for reconstitution [preservative free]:

Intron® A: 10 million int. units, 18 million int. units, 50 million int. units

Injection, solution:

Intron® A: 6 million int. units/mL (3 mL); 10 million int. units/mL (2.5 mL); 3 million int. units/0.2 mL (1.2 mL); 5 million int. units/0.2 mL (1.2 mL); 10 million int. units/0.2 mL (1.2 mL)

General Dosage Range Dosage adjustment is recommended in patients who develop toxicities

I.M.:

Children 1-17 years: 3-5 million units/m² 3 times/week (maximum: 3 million units/dose)

Adults: Dosage varies greatly depending on indication

I.V.: *Adults:* 20 million units/m² for 5 consecutive days per week

Intralesional: *Adults:* 1 million units/lesion 3 times/week, on alternate days (maximum: 5 lesions/treatment)

SubQ:

Children 1-17 years: Initial: 3 million units/m² 3 times/week for 1 week; Maintenance: 6 million units/m² 3 times/week (maximum: 10 million units 3 times/week)

Adults: Dosage varies greatly depending on indication

Administration

I.M. Administer in evening (if possible)

I.V. Infuse over ~20 minutes

I.V. Detail pH: 6.9-7.5

Other

SubQ: SubQ administration is suggested for those who are at risk for bleeding or are thrombocytopenic. Rotate SubQ injection site. Administer in evening (if possible). Patient should be well hydrated. Reconstitute with recommended amount of SWFI and agitate gently; do not shake. **Note:** Different vial strengths require different amounts of diluent. Not every dosage form is appropriate for every indication; refer to manufacturer's labeling.

Intralesional: Inject at an angle nearly parallel to the plane of the skin, directing the needle to center of the base of the wart to infiltrate the lesion core and cause a small wheal. Only infiltrate the keratinized layer; avoid administration which is too deep or shallow.

Nursing Actions

Physical Assessment Monitor for neuropsychiatric changes, especially depression, suicidal or homicidal ideation, psychosis, or mania; decreased pulmonary function; or ophthalmic changes. Evaluate immediately any reported changes in vision. Teach appropriate reconstitution, injection, and needle disposal.

Patient Education Maintain adequate hydration, unless instructed to restrict fluid intake. You may experience flu-like syndrome, nausea, vomiting, dizziness, or abnormal thinking. Inform prescriber immediately if you feel depressed or have any thoughts of suicide or homicide. Report unusual bruising or bleeding; persistent abdominal disturbances; unusual fatigue; muscle pain or tremors;

fever; chest pain or palpitation; swelling of extremities or unusual weight gain; respiratory difficulty; pain, swelling, or redness at injection site; or sudden change in vision.

Interferon Alfacon-1
(in ter FEER on AL fa con one)

Brand Names: U.S. Infergen®

Pharmacologic Category Interferon

Medication Safety Issues

Sound-alike/look-alike issues:

Interferon alfacon-1 may be confused with interferon alfa-2a, interferon alfa-2b, interferon alfa-n3, peginterferon alfa-2b

International issues:

Interferon alfacon-1 may be confused with interferon alpha multi-subtype which is available in international markets

Medication Guide Available Yes

Pregnancy Risk Factor C

Lactation Excretion in breast milk unknown/use caution (AAP rates "compatible"; AAP 2001 update pending)

Use Treatment of chronic hepatitis C virus (HCV) infection in patients ≥18 years of age with compensated liver disease and anti-HCV serum antibodies or HCV RNA; concurrent use with ribavirin in HCV-infected patients who have failed treatment with pegylated interferon/ribavirin (Bacon, 2009)

Available Dosage Forms

Injection, solution [preservative free]:

Infergen®: 30 mcg/mL (0.3 mL, 0.5 mL)

General Dosage Range Dosage adjustment recommended in patients who develop toxicities

SubQ: *Adults:* 9-15 mcg 3 times/week; may increase to 15 mcg 3 times/week

Administration

Other Interferon alfacon-1 is given by SubQ injection, 3 times/week, with at least 48 hours between doses. Allow to reach room temperature just prior to administration.

Nursing Actions

Physical Assessment Monitor for signs of depression and suicide ideation. Patient with pre-existing diabetes mellitus or hypertension should have an ophthalmic exam prior to beginning treatment. If self-administered, instruct patient in appropriate storage, injection technique, and syringe disposal.

Patient Education If self-administered, follow exact instructions for injection and syringe disposal. You will need frequent laboratory tests during course of therapy. If you have diabetes or hypertension, you should have ophthalmic exam prior to beginning therapy. You may experience dizziness; nausea, vomiting, or diarrhea; flu-like symptoms, such as headache, fatigue, or muscle or joint pain; or hair loss. Promptly report any persistent GI upset, depression or suicide ideation, chest pain or palpitations, respiratory difficulties, unusual bruising or bleeding, yellowing of skin, or vision changes.

Interferon Beta-1a (in ter FEER on BAY ta won aye)

Brand Names: U.S. Avonex®; Rebif®

Index Terms rIFN beta-1a

Pharmacologic Category Interferon

Medication Safety Issues

Sound-alike/look-alike issues:

Avonex® may be confused with Avelox®

Medication Guide Available Yes

Pregnancy Risk Factor C

Lactation Excretion in breast milk unknown/not recommended

Breast-Feeding Considerations Potential for serious adverse reactions. Because its use has not been evaluated during lactation, a decision should be made to either discontinue breast-feeding or discontinue the drug.

Use Treatment of relapsing forms of multiple sclerosis (MS)

Mechanism of Action/Effect Mechanism in the treatment of MS is unknown; slows the accumulation of physical disability and decreases frequency of clinical MS exacerbations

Contraindications Hypersensitivity to natural or recombinant interferons, human albumin, or any other component of the formulation

Warnings/Precautions Interferons have been associated with severe psychiatric adverse events (psychosis, mania, depression, suicidal behavior/ideation) in patients with and without previous psychiatric symptoms, avoid use in severe psychiatric disorders and use caution in patients with a history of depression; patients exhibiting depressive symptoms should be closely monitored and discontinuation of therapy should be considered.

Autoimmune disorders including idiopathic thrombocytopenia, hyper- and hypothyroidism and rarely autoimmune hepatitis have been reported. Allergic reactions, including anaphylaxis, have been reported. Caution should be used in patients with hepatic impairment or in those who abuse alcohol. Rare cases of severe hepatic injury, including hepatic failure, have been reported in patients receiving interferon beta-1a; risk may be increased by ethanol use or concurrent therapy with hepatotoxic drugs. Treatment should be suspended if jaundice or symptoms of hepatic dysfunction occur. Transaminase elevations may be asymptomatic, so monitoring is important. Dose adjustment may be necessary with hepatic impairment. Hematologic effects, including pancytopenia (rare) and thrombocytopenia, have been reported. Associated with a high incidence of flu-like adverse effects; use of analgesics and/or antipyretics on treatment days may be helpful. Use caution in patients with pre-existing cardiovascular disease, including angina, HF, and/or arrythmia. Rare cases of new-onset cardiomyopathy and/or HF have been reported. Use caution in patients with seizure disorders, or myelosuppression. Safety and efficacy in patients with chronic progressive MS or in patients <18 years of age have not been established. Albumin is a component of some formulations (contraindicated in albumin-sensitive patients); rare risk of CJD or viral transmission.

Drug Interactions

Avoid Concomitant Use There are no known interactions where it is recommended to avoid concomitant use.

Decreased Effect There are no known significant interactions involving a decrease in effect.

Increased Effect/Toxicity

Interferon Beta-1a may increase the levels/effects of: Theophylline Derivatives; Zidovudine

Adverse Reactions Note: Adverse reactions reported as a composite of both commercially-available products. Spectrum and incidence of reactions is generally similar between products, but consult individual product labels for specific incidence.

>10%:

Central nervous system: Headache (58% to 70%), fatigue (33% to 41%), fever (20% to 28%), pain (23%), chills (19%), depression (18% to 25%), dizziness (14%)

Gastrointestinal: Nausea (23%), abdominal pain (8% to 22%)

Genitourinary: Urinary tract infection (17%)

Hematologic: Leukopenia (28% to 36%)

Hepatic: ALT increased (20% to 27%), AST increased (10% to 17%)

Local: Injection site reaction (3% to 92%)

Neuromuscular & skeletal: Myalgia (25% to 29%), back pain (23% to 25%), weakness (24%), skeletal pain (10% to 15%), rigors (6% to 13%)

Ocular: Vision abnormal (7% to 13%)

Respiratory: Sinusitis (14%), upper respiratory tract infection (14%)

Miscellaneous: Flu-like syndrome (49% to 59%), neutralizing antibodies (significance not known; Avonex® 5%; Rebif® 24%), lymphadenopathy (11% to 12%)

1% to 10%:

Cardiovascular: Chest pain (5% to 6%), vasodilation (2%)

Central nervous system: Migraine (5%), somnolence (4% to 5%), malaise (4% to 5%), seizure (1% to 5%)

Dermatologic: Erythematous rash (5% to 7%), maculopapular rash (4% to 5%), alopecia (4%), urticaria

Endocrine & metabolic: Thyroid disorder (4% to 6%)

Gastrointestinal: Xerostomia (1% to 5%), toothache (3%)

Genitourinary: Micturition frequency (2% to 7%), urinary incontinence (2% to 4%)

Hematologic: Thrombocytopenia (2% to 8%), anemia (3% to 5%)

Hepatic: Bilirubinemia (2% to 3%)

Local: Injection site pain (8%), injection site bruising (6%), injection site necrosis (1% to 3%), injection site inflammation

Neuromuscular & skeletal: Arthralgia (9%), hypertonia (6% to 7%), coordination abnormal (4% to 5%)

Ocular: Eye disorder (4%), xerophthalmia (1% to 3%)

Respiratory: Bronchitis (8%)

Miscellaneous: Infection (7%)

Pharmacodynamics/Kinetics

Onset of Action Avonex®: 12 hours (based on biological response markers)

Duration of Action Avonex®: 4 days (based on biological response markers)

Product Availability Avonex® Pen Autoinjector: FDA approved February 2012; availability anticipated in May 2012. Consult prescribing information for additional information.

Available Dosage Forms

Injection, powder for reconstitution [preservative free]:

Avonex®: 33 mcg [contains albumin (human); 6.6 million units; provides 30 mcg/mL following reconstitution; supplied with diluent]

Injection, solution:

Avonex®: 30 mcg/0.5 mL (0.5 mL)

Injection, solution [preservative free]:

Rebif®: 22 mcg/0.5 mL (0.5 mL), 44 mcg/0.5 mL (0.5 mL)

Injection, solution [preservative free, combination package]:

Rebif®: Titration Pack: 22 mcg/0.5 mL (6s) and 8.8 mcg/0.2 mL (6s)

General Dosage Range Dosage adjustment recommended in patients who develop toxicities

I.M.: *Adults:* 30 mcg once weekly

SubQ: *Adults:* Initial: 4.4 or 8.8 mcg 3 times/week for 2 weeks; Titration: 11 or 22 mcg 3 times/week for 2 weeks; Maintenance: 22 or 44 mcg 3 times/week

Administration

I.M. Avonex®: Must be given by I.M. injection.

Other Rebif®: Administer SubQ at the same time of day on the same 3 days each week (ie, late afternoon/evening Mon, Wed, Fri). Rotate injection sites.

Stability

Reconstitution Avonex®: Reconstitute with 1.1 mL of diluent and swirl gently to dissolve. Do not shake. The reconstituted product contains no preservative and is for single-use only; discard unused portion.

Storage

Avonex®:

Prefilled syringe: Store at 2°C to 8°C (36°F to 46°F); do not freeze. Protect from light. Allow to warm to room temperature prior to use (do not use external heat source). If refrigeration is not available, product may be stored at ≤25°C (77°F) for up to 7 days.

Vial: Store unreconstituted vial at 2°C to 8°C (36°F to 46°F). If refrigeration is not available, may be stored at 25°C (77°F) for up to 30 days; do not freeze. Protect from light. Following reconstitution, use immediately, but may be stored up to 6 hours at 2°C to 8°C (36°F to 46°F); do not freeze.

Rebif®: Store at 2°C to 8°C (36°F to 46°F); do not freeze. Protect from light. May also be stored ≤25°C (77°F) for up to 30 days if protected from heat and light.

Nursing Actions

Physical Assessment Monitor for signs of depression and suicide ideation. Instruct patient/caregiver on appropriate reconstitution, injection, and needle disposal.

Patient Education This is not a cure for MS; you will continue to receive regular treatment and follow-up for MS. Maintain adequate hydration, unless instructed to restrict fluid intake. You may experience flu-like syndrome, nausea, vomiting, dizziness, or abnormal thinking. Inform prescriber immediately if you feel depressed or have suicide ideation. Report unusual bruising or bleeding; persistent abdominal disturbances; chest pain or palpitations; shortness of breath; swelling of extremities; visual disturbances; or pain, swelling, or redness at injection site.

Interferon Beta-1b (in ter FEER on BAY ta won bee)

Brand Names: U.S. Betaseron®; Extavia®

Index Terms rIFN beta-1b

Pharmacologic Category Interferon

Medication Guide Available Yes

Pregnancy Risk Factor C

Lactation Excretion in breast milk unknown/not recommended

Breast-Feeding Considerations Because its use has not been evaluated during lactation, breast-feeding is not recommended.

Use Treatment of relapsing forms of multiple sclerosis (MS); treatment of first clinical episode with MRI features consistent with MS

Canadian labeling: Additional use (not in U.S. labeling): Treatment of secondary-progressive MS

Mechanism of Action/Effect Alters the expression and response to cell surface antigens and can enhance immune cell activities; mechanism in MS in unknown

Contraindications Hypersensitivity to *E. coli*-derived products, natural or recombinant interferon beta, albumin human or any other component of the formulation

Canadian labeling: Additional contraindication (not in U.S. labeling): Pregnancy

Warnings/Precautions Anaphylaxis has been reported rarely with use. Associated with a high incidence of flu-like adverse effects; improvement in symptoms occurs over time. Hepatotoxicity has been reported with beta interferons, including rare reports of hepatitis (autoimmune) and hepatic failure requiring transplant. Interferons have been associated with severe psychiatric adverse events (psychosis, mania, depression, suicidal behavior/ideation) in patients with and without previous psychiatric symptoms, avoid use in severe psychiatric disorders and use caution in patients with a history of depression; patients exhibiting symptoms of depression should be closely monitored and discontinuation of therapy should be considered. Use caution in patients with pre-existing cardiovascular disease, pulmonary disease, seizure disorders, renal impairment or hepatic impairment. Use caution in myelosuppression; routine monitoring for leukopenia is recommended; dose reduction may be required. Thyroid dysfunction has rarely been reported with use. Severe injection site reactions (necrosis) may occur, which may or may not heal with continued therapy; patient and/or caregiver competency in injection technique should be confirmed and periodically re-evaluated. Contains albumin, which may carry a remote risk of transmitting viral diseases.

Drug Interactions

Avoid Concomitant Use There are no known interactions where it is recommended to avoid concomitant use.

Decreased Effect There are no known significant interactions involving a decrease in effect.

Increased Effect/Toxicity

Interferon Beta-1b may increase the levels/effects of: Theophylline Derivatives; Zidovudine

Adverse Reactions Note: Flu-like syndrome (including at least two of the following - headache, fever, chills, malaise, diaphoresis, and myalgia) are reported in the majority of patients (60%) and decrease over time (average duration ~1 week).

>10%:

Cardiovascular: Peripheral edema (15%), chest pain (11%)

Central nervous system: Headache (57%), fever (36%), pain (51%), chills (25%), dizziness (24%), insomnia (24%)

Dermatologic: Rash (24%), skin disorder (12%)

Endocrine & metabolic: Metrorrhagia (11%)

Gastrointestinal: Nausea (27%), diarrhea (19%), abdominal pain (19%), constipation (20%), dyspepsia (14%)

Genitourinary: Urinary urgency (13%)

Hematologic: Lymphopenia (88%), neutropenia (14%), leukopenia (14%)

Local: Injection site reaction (85%), inflammation (53%), pain (18%)

Neuromuscular & skeletal: Weakness (61%), myalgia (27%), hypertonia (50%), myasthenia (46%), arthralgia (31%), incoordination (21%)
Miscellaneous: Flu-like syndrome (decreases over treatment course; 60%), neutralizing antibodies (≤45%; significance not known)

1% to 10%:

Cardiovascular: Palpitation (4%), vasodilation (8%), hypertension (7%), tachycardia (4%), peripheral vascular disorder (6%)
Central nervous system: Anxiety (10%), malaise (8%), nervousness (7%)
Dermatologic: Alopecia (4%)
Endocrine & metabolic: Menorrhagia (8%), dysmenorrhea (7%)
Gastrointestinal: Weight gain (7%)
Genitourinary: Impotence (9%), pelvic pain (6%), cystitis (8%), urinary frequency (7%), prostatic disorder (3%)
Hematologic: Lymphadenopathy (8%)
Hepatic: ALT increased >5x baseline (10%), AST increased >5x baseline (3%)
Local: Injection site necrosis (4% to 5%), edema (3%), mass (2%)
Neuromuscular & skeletal: Leg cramps (4%)
Respiratory: Dyspnea (7%)
Miscellaneous: Diaphoresis (8%), hypersensitivity (3%)

Available Dosage Forms

Injection, powder for reconstitution:
Betaseron®: 0.3 mg [~9.6 million int. units]

Injection, powder for reconstitution [preservative free]:
Extavia®: 0.3 mg [~9.6 million int. units]

General Dosage Range SubQ: *Adults:* 0.0625-0.25 mg (2-8 million units) every other day

Administration

Other SubQ: Withdraw 1 mL of reconstituted solution from the vial into a sterile syringe fitted with a 27-gauge needle and inject the solution subcutaneously. Sites for self-injection include outer surface of the arms, abdomen, hips, and thighs. Rotate SubQ injection site. Patient should be well hydrated.

Stability

Reconstitution To reconstitute solution, inject 1.2 mL of diluent (provided); gently swirl to dissolve, do not shake. Reconstituted solution provides 0.25 mg/mL (8 million units). Use product within 3 hours of reconstitution. Discard unused portion of vial.

Storage Store at room temperature of 25°C (77°F); excursions permitted to 15°C to 30°C (59°F to 86°F). If not used immediately following reconstitution, refrigerate solution at 2°C to 8°C (36°F to 46°F) and use within 3 hours; do not freeze or shake solution. Discard unused portion of vial.

Nursing Actions

Physical Assessment Assess for psychiatric or suicide histories (eg, psychosis, mania, depression, suicide behavior/ideation). Monitor injection sites for signs of necrosis. Teach proper administration for SubQ injections and disposal of needles if appropriate. Emphasize the need for adequate hydration. Monitor for opportunistic infection.

Patient Education This is not a cure for MS; you will continue to receive regular treatment and follow-up for MS. Rotate injection site with each injection. Maintain adequate hydration, unless instructed to restrict fluid intake. You may experience flu-like syndrome, nausea, vomiting, diarrhea, dizziness, or abnormal thinking. Inform prescriber immediately if you feel depressed or have suicide ideation. Report unusual bruising or bleeding; persistent abdominal disturbances; chest pain or palpitations; swelling of extremities; visual disturbances; or pain, swelling, or redness at injection site.

Interferon Gamma-1b

(in ter FEER on GAM ah won bee)

Brand Names: U.S. Actimmune®

Pharmacologic Category Interferon

Pregnancy Risk Factor C

Lactation Excretion in breast milk unknown/not recommended

Breast-Feeding Considerations Potential for serious adverse reactions. Because its use has not been evaluated during lactation, breast-feeding is not recommended

Use Reduce frequency and severity of serious infections associated with chronic granulomatous disease; delay time to disease progression in patients with severe, malignant osteopetrosis

Mechanism of Action/Effect Interferon gamma participates in immunoregulation. The exact mechanism of action for the treatment of chronic granulomatous disease or osteopetrosis has not been defined.

Contraindications Hypersensitivity to interferon gamma, *E. coli* derived proteins, or any component of the formulation

Warnings/Precautions Hypersensitivity reactions have been reported (rarely). Transient cutaneous rashes may occur. Dose-related bone marrow toxicity has been reported; use caution in patients with myelosuppression. May cause hepatotoxicity and the incidence may be increased in children <1 year of age. Doses >10 times the weekly recommended dose (used in studies for unlabeled indications) have been associated with a different pattern/frequency of adverse effects. Flu-like symptoms which may exacerbate pre-existing cardiovascular disorders (including ischemia, HF, or arrhythmias) and the development of neurologic disorders have been noted at the higher doses. Caution should also be used in patients with seizure disorders or compromised CNS function.

Drug Interactions

Avoid Concomitant Use There are no known interactions where it is recommended to avoid concomitant use.

Decreased Effect There are no known significant interactions involving a decrease in effect.

Increased Effect/Toxicity

Interferon Gamma-1b may increase the levels/effects of: Theophylline Derivatives; Zidovudine

Adverse Reactions Based on 50 mcg/m^2 dose administered 3 times weekly for chronic granulomatous disease

>10%:

Central nervous system: Fever (52%), headache (33%), chills (14%), fatigue (14%)

Dermatologic: Rash (17%)

Gastrointestinal: Diarrhea (14%), vomiting (13%)

Local: Injection site erythema or tenderness (14%)

1% to 10%:

Central nervous system: Depression (3%)

Gastrointestinal: Nausea (10%), abdominal pain (8%)

Neuromuscular & skeletal: Myalgia (6%), arthralgia (2%), back pain (2%)

Additional adverse reactions noted at doses >100 mcg/m^2 administered 3 times weekly: ALT increased, AST increased, autoantibodies increased, bronchospasm, chest discomfort, confusion, dermatomyositis exacerbation, disorientation, DVT, gait disturbance, GI bleeding, hallucinations, heart block, heart failure, hepatic insufficiency, hyperglycemia, hypertriglyceridemia, hyponatremia, hypotension, interstitial pneumonitis, lupus-like syndrome, MI, neutropenia, pancreatitis (may be fatal), Parkinsonian symptoms, PE, proteinuria, renal insufficiency (reversible), seizure, syncope, tachyarrhythmia, tachypnea, thrombocytopenia, TIA

Available Dosage Forms

Injection, solution [preservative free]:

Actimmune®: 100 mcg (0.5 mL)

General Dosage Range Dosage adjustment recommended in patients who develop toxicities

SubQ: *Children and Adults:*

BSA ≤0.5 m^2: 1.5 mcg/kg/dose 3 times/week

BSA >0.5 m^2: 50 mcg/m^2 (1 million int. units/m^2) 3 times/week

Administration

Other Administer by SubQ injection into the right and left deltoid or anterior thigh.

Stability

Storage Store in refrigerator at 2°C to 8°C (36°F to 46°F); do not freeze. Do not shake. Discard if left unrefrigerated for >12 hours.

Nursing Actions

Physical Assessment Teach patient/caregiver appropriate reconstitution, injection, and needle disposal.

Patient Education Maintain adequate hydration, unless instructed to restrict fluid intake. You may experience flu-like syndrome, nausea, vomiting, or abnormal thinking. Report unusual bruising or bleeding; persistent abdominal disturbances; unusual fatigue; muscle pain or tremors; chest pain or palpitations; swelling of extremities; visual disturbances; or pain, swelling, or redness at injection site.

Ipilimumab (ip i LIM u mab)

Brand Names: U.S. Yervoy™

Index Terms MDX-010; MDX-CTLA-4; MOAB-CTLA-4

Pharmacologic Category Antineoplastic Agent, Monoclonal Antibody; Monoclonal Antibody

Medication Safety Issues

High alert medication:

This medication is in a class the Institute for Safe Medication Practices (ISMP) includes among its list of drug classes which have a heightened risk of causing significant patient harm when used in error.

Medication Guide Available Yes

Pregnancy Risk Factor C

Lactation Excretion in breast milk unknown/not recommended

Use Treatment of unresectable or metastatic melanoma

Available Dosage Forms

Injection, solution [preservative free]:

Yervoy™: 5 mg/mL (10 mL, 40 mL)

General Dosage Range Dosage adjustment recommended in patients who develop toxicities.

I.V.: *Adults:* 3 mg/kg every 3 weeks

Administration

I.V. I.V.: Infuse over 90 minutes through a low protein-binding in-line filter. Flush with NS or D_5W at the end of infusion

I.V. Detail pH: 7; may contain translucent or white amorphous ipilimumab particles

Ipratropium (Oral Inhalation)
(i pra TROE pee um)

Brand Names: U.S. Atrovent® HFA

Index Terms Ipratropium Bromide

Pharmacologic Category Anticholinergic Agent

Medication Safety Issues

Sound-alike/look-alike issues:

Atrovent® may be confused with Alupent, Serevent®

Ipratropium may be confused with tiotropium

Pregnancy Risk Factor B

Lactation Excretion in breast milk unknown/use caution

Use Anticholinergic bronchodilator used in bronchospasm associated with COPD, bronchitis, and emphysema

Mechanism of Action/Effect Blocks the action of acetylcholine at parasympathetic sites in bronchial smooth muscle causing bronchodilation; local application to nasal mucosa inhibits serous and seromucous gland secretions.

Contraindications Hypersensitivity to ipratropium, atropine (and its derivatives), or any component of the formulation

Warnings/Precautions Immediate hypersensitivity reactions (urticaria, angioedema, rash, bronchospasm) have been reported. Rarely, paradoxical bronchospasm may occur with use of inhaled bronchodilating agents; this should be distinguished from inadequate response. Not indicated for the initial treatment of acute episodes of bronchospasm where rescue therapy is required for rapid response. Should only be used in acute exacerbations of asthma in conjunction with short-acting beta-adrenergic agonists for acute episodes. Use with caution in patients with myasthenia gravis, narrow-angle glaucoma, benign prostatic hyperplasia (BPH), or bladder neck obstruction

Drug Interactions

Avoid Concomitant Use There are no known interactions where it is recommended to avoid concomitant use.

Decreased Effect

Ipratropium (Oral Inhalation) may decrease the levels/effects of: Acetylcholinesterase Inhibitors (Central); Secretin

The levels/effects of Ipratropium (Oral Inhalation) may be decreased by: Acetylcholinesterase Inhibitors (Central)

Increased Effect/Toxicity

Ipratropium (Oral Inhalation) may increase the levels/effects of: AbobotulinumtoxinA; Anticholinergics; Cannabinoids; OnabotulinumtoxinA; Potassium Chloride; RimabotulinumtoxinB

The levels/effects of Ipratropium (Oral Inhalation) may be increased by: Pramlintide

Adverse Reactions

>10%: Respiratory: Upper respiratory tract infection (9% to 34%), bronchitis (10% to 23%), sinusitis (1% to 11%)

1% to 10%:

Cardiovascular: Chest pain (3%), palpitation

Central nervous system: Headache (6% to 7%), dizziness (2% to 3%)

Gastrointestinal: Dyspepsia (1% to 5%), nausea (4%), xerostomia (2% to 4%)

Genitourinary: Urinary tract infection (2% to 10%)

Neuromuscular & skeletal: Back pain (2% to 7%)

Respiratory: Dyspnea (7% to 10%), rhinitis (2% to 6%), cough (3% to 5%), pharyngitis (4%), bronchospasm (2%), sputum increased (1%)

Miscellaneous: Flu-like syndrome (4% to 8%)

Pharmacodynamics/Kinetics

Onset of Action Bronchodilation: Within 15 minutes; Peak effect: 1-2 hours

Duration of Action 2-5 hours

Available Dosage Forms

Aerosol, for oral inhalation:

Atrovent® HFA: 17 mcg/actuation (12.9 g)

Solution, for nebulization: 0.02% [500 mcg/2.5 mL] (25s, 30s, 60s)

Solution, for nebulization [preservative free]: 0.02% [500 mcg/2.5 mL] (25s, 30s, 60s)

General Dosage Range

Inhalation: *Children >12 years and Adults:* 2 inhalations 4 times/day (maximum: 12 inhalations/day)

Nebulization: *Children >12 years and Adults:* 500 mcg every 6-8 hours

Administration

Inhalation Atrovent® HFA: Prior to initial use, prime inhaler by releasing 2 test sprays into the air. If the inhaler has not been used for >3 days, reprime.

Stability

Storage

Aerosol: Store at controlled room temperature of 25°C (77°F). Do not store near heat or open flame.

Solution: Store at 15°C to 30°C (59°F to 86°F). Protect from light.

Nursing Actions

Physical Assessment Teach patient importance of proper administration.

Patient Education Use care to avoid direct contact with eyes. Do not use more often than recommended. Maintain adequate hydration, unless instructed to restrict fluid intake. May cause sensitivity to heat, nervousness, dizziness, fatigue, dry mouth, unpleasant taste, stomach upset, or difficulty urinating (always void before treatment). Report unresolved GI upset, dizziness or fatigue, vision changes, palpitations, persistent inability to void, nervousness, or insomnia.

Inhaler: Close eyes when administering ipratropium; blurred vision may result if sprayed into eyes. Effects are enhanced by holding breath 10 seconds after inhalation; wait at least 1 full minute between inhalations.

Nebulizer: Wash hands before and after treatment. Wash and dry nebulizer after each treatment. Twist open the top of one unit dose vial and squeeze the contents into the nebulizer reservoir. Connect the nebulizer reservoir to the mouthpiece or face mask. Connect nebulizer to compressor. Sit in a comfortable, upright position. Place mouthpiece in your mouth or put on the face mask and turn on the compressor. If a face mask is used, avoid leakage around the mask (temporary blurring of vision, worsening of narrow-angle glaucoma, or eye pain may occur if mist gets into eyes). Breathe calmly and deeply until no more mist is formed in the nebulizer (about 5 minutes). At this point, treatment is finished.

Ipratropium (Nasal) (i pra TROE pee um)

Brand Names: U.S. Atrovent®

Index Terms Ipratropium Bromide

Pharmacologic Category Anticholinergic Agent

Medication Safety Issues

Sound-alike/look-alike issues:

Atrovent® may be confused with Alupent, Serevent®

Ipratropium may be confused with tiotropium

Pregnancy Risk Factor B

Lactation Excretion in breast milk unknown/use caution

Use Symptomatic relief of rhinorrhea associated with the common cold and allergic and nonallergic rhinitis

Available Dosage Forms

Solution, intranasal: 0.03% (30 mL); 0.06% (15 mL)

Atrovent®: 0.03% (30 mL); 0.06% (15 mL)

General Dosage Range Intranasal:

0.03% solution: *Children ≥6 years and Adults:* 2 sprays in each nostril 2-3 times/day

0.06% solution: *Children ≥5 years and Adults:* 2 sprays in each nostril 3-4 times/day

Administration

Inhalation Prior to initial use, prime inhaler by releasing 7 test sprays into the air. If the inhaler has not been used for >24 hours, reprime by releasing 2 test sprays into the air.

Nursing Actions

Physical Assessment Teach patient importance of proper administration.

Patient Education Use care to avoid direct contact with eyes. Do not use more often than recommended. Store solution away from light. May cause dry mouth, unpleasant taste, or stomach upset. Report unresolved GI upset or persistent inability to void.

Ipratropium and Albuterol
(i pra TROE pee um & al BYOO ter ole)

Brand Names: U.S. Combivent®; DuoNeb®

Index Terms Albuterol and Ipratropium; Salbutamol and Ipratropium

Pharmacologic Category Anticholinergic Agent; Beta$_2$-Adrenergic Agonist

Medication Safety Issues

Sound-alike/look-alike issues:

Combivent® may be confused with Combivir®, Serevent®

DuoNeb® may be confused with DuoTrav™, Duovent® UDV

Pregnancy Risk Factor C

Use Treatment of COPD in those patients who are currently on a regular bronchodilator who continue to have bronchospasms and require a second bronchodilator

Product Availability

Combivent® Respimat®: FDA approved October 2011; availability expected mid-2012

Combivent® Respimat® spray is a non-CFC ipratropium and albuterol inhalation formulation approved for the treatment of COPD and will replace Combivent® inhalation aerosol, which is being phased out in accordance with the Montreal Protocol on Substances that Deplete the Ozone Layer.

Available Dosage Forms

Aerosol for oral inhalation:

Combivent®: Ipratropium bromide 18 mcg and albuterol (base) 90 mcg per inhalation (14.7 g) [200 metered actuations]

Solution for nebulization: Ipratropium 0.5 mg and albuterol (base) 2.5 mg per 3 mL (30s, 60s)

DuoNeb®: Ipratropium 0.5 mg and albuterol (base) 2.5 mg per 3 mL (30s, 60s)

General Dosage Range

Inhalation: *Adults:* 2 inhalations 4 times/day (maximum: 12 inhalations/day)

Nebulization: *Adults:* 3 mL every 4-6 hours

Administration

Inhalation Nebulization: Administer via jet nebulizer to an air compressor with an adequate air flow, equipped with a mouthpiece or face mask. MDI: Shake canister vigorously for ≥10 seconds. Prior to first use (or if not used for >24 hours) a test spray of 3 sprays is recommended. Avoid spraying into eyes.

Nursing Actions

Physical Assessment See individual agents.

Patient Education See individual agents.

Related Information

Albuterol *on page 36*

Ipratropium (Oral Inhalation) *on page 638*

Irbesartan (ir be SAR tan)

Brand Names: U.S. Avapro®

Pharmacologic Category Angiotensin II Receptor Blocker

Medication Safety Issues

Sound-alike/look-alike issues:

Avapro® may be confused with Anaprox®

Pregnancy Risk Factor D

Lactation Excretion in breast milk unknown/contraindicated

Use Treatment of hypertension alone or in combination with other antihypertensives; treatment of diabetic nephropathy in patients with type 2 diabetes mellitus (noninsulin dependent, NIDDM) and hypertension

Unlabeled Use To slow the rate of progression of aortic-root dilation in pediatric patients with Marfan's syndrome

Mechanism of Action/Effect Irbesartan is an angiotensin receptor antagonist. Angiotensin II acts as a vasoconstrictor and stimulates the release of aldosterone, which results in reabsorption of sodium and water. These effects result in an elevation in blood pressure. Irbesartan blocks the AT1 angiotensin II receptor, thereby blocking the vasoconstriction and the aldosterone secreting effects of angiotensin II.

Contraindications Hypersensitivity to irbesartan or any component of the formulation

Warnings/Precautions [U.S. Boxed Warning]: Drugs that act on the renin-angiotensin system can cause injury and death to the developing fetus. Discontinue as soon as possible once pregnancy is detected. May cause hyperkalemia; avoid potassium supplementation unless specifically required by healthcare provider. May be associated with deterioration of renal function and/or increases in serum creatinine, particularly in patients with low renal blood flow (eg, renal artery stenosis, heart failure) whose glomerular filtration rate (GFR) is dependent on efferent arteriolar vasoconstriction by angiotensin II. Avoid use or use a much smaller dose in patients who are intravascularly volume-depleted; use caution in patients with unstented unilateral or bilateral renal artery stenosis. When unstented bilateral renal artery stenosis is present, use is generally avoided due to the elevated risk of deterioration in renal function unless possible benefits outweigh risks. AUCs of irbesartan (not the active metabolite) are about 50% greater in patients with Cl_{cr} <30 mL/minute and are doubled in hemodialysis patients. Concurrent use of ACE inhibitors may increase the risk of clinically-significant adverse events (eg, renal dysfunction, hyperkalemia).

Drug Interactions

Avoid Concomitant Use

Avoid concomitant use of Irbesartan with any of the following: Pimozide

Decreased Effect

The levels/effects of Irbesartan may be decreased by: Herbs (Hypertensive Properties); Methylphenidate; Nonsteroidal Anti-Inflammatory Agents; Rifamycin Derivatives; Yohimbine

Increased Effect/Toxicity

Irbesartan may increase the levels/effects of: ACE Inhibitors; Amifostine; Antihypertensives; ARIPiprazole; Carvedilol; CYP2C8 Substrates; CYP2C9 Substrates; Hypotensive Agents; Lithium; Nonsteroidal Anti-Inflammatory Agents; Pimozide; Potassium-Sparing Diuretics; RiTUXimab; Sodium Phosphates

The levels/effects of Irbesartan may be increased by: Alfuzosin; Diazoxide; Eplerenone; Fluconazole; Herbs (Hypotensive Properties); MAO Inhibitors; Pentoxifylline; Phosphodiesterase 5 Inhibitors; Potassium Salts; Prostacyclin Analogues; Tolvaptan; Trimethoprim

Nutritional/Ethanol Interactions Herb/Nutraceutical: Dong quai has estrogenic activity. Some herbal medications may worsen hypertension (eg, ephedra); garlic may have additional antihypertensive effects. Management: Avoid dong quai if using for hypertension. Avoid ephedra, yohimbe, ginseng, and garlic.

Adverse Reactions Unless otherwise indicated, percentage of incidence is reported for patients with hypertension.

>10%: Endocrine & metabolic: Hyperkalemia (19%, diabetic nephropathy; rarely seen in HTN)

1% to 10%:

Cardiovascular: Orthostatic hypotension (5%, diabetic nephropathy)

Central nervous system: Fatigue (4%), dizziness (10%, diabetic nephropathy)

Gastrointestinal: Diarrhea (3%), dyspepsia (2%)

Respiratory: Upper respiratory infection (9%), cough (2.8% versus 2.7% in placebo)

Pharmacodynamics/Kinetics

Onset of Action Peak levels in 1-2 hours

Duration of Action >24 hours

Available Dosage Forms

Tablet, oral:

Avapro®: 75 mg, 150 mg, 300 mg

General Dosage Range Oral:

Children 6-12 years: Initial: 75 mg once daily; Maintenance: 75-150 mg once daily

Children ≥13 years and Adults: Initial: 75-150 mg once daily; Maintenance: 75 to 300 mg once daily

Stability

Storage Store at room temperature of 15°C to 30°C (59°F to 86°F).

Nursing Actions

Physical Assessment Assess potential for interactions with other pharmacological agents or herbal products (risk of hyperkalemia or toxicity). Monitor for hypotension at regular intervals during therapy.

Patient Education May be taken with or without food. Take first dose at bedtime. This medication does not replace other antihypertensive interventions; follow prescriber's instructions for diet and lifestyle changes. May cause dizziness, fainting, lightheadedness, nausea, vomiting, abdominal pain, or diarrhea. Report chest pain or palpitations, skin rash, fluid retention (swelling of extremities), or respiratory difficulty or unusual cough.

Dietary Considerations May be taken with or without food.

Irbesartan and Hydrochlorothiazide

(ir be SAR tan & hye droe klor oh THYE a zide)

Brand Names: U.S. Avalide®

Index Terms Avapro® HCT; Hydrochlorothiazide and Irbesartan

Pharmacologic Category Angiotensin II Receptor Blocker; Diuretic, Thiazide

Medication Safety Issues

Sound-alike/look-alike issues:

Avalide® may be confused with Avandia®

Pregnancy Risk Factor D

Lactation Enters breast milk/not recommended

Use Combination therapy for the management of hypertension; may be used as initial therapy in patients likely to need multiple drugs to achieve blood pressure goals

Available Dosage Forms

Tablet:

Avalide®: Irbesartan 150 mg and hydrochlorothiazide 12.5 mg; irbesartan 300 mg and hydrochlorothiazide 12.5 mg

General Dosage Range Oral: *Adults:* Irbesartan 150-300 mg and hydrochlorothiazide 12.5-25 mg once daily

Nursing Actions

Physical Assessment See individual agents.

Patient Education See individual agents.

Related Information

Hydrochlorothiazide *on page 570*

Irbesartan *on page 640*

Irinotecan (eye rye no TEE kan)

Brand Names: U.S. Camptosar®

Index Terms Camptothecin-11; CPT-11; Irinotecan HCl; Irinotecan Hydrochloride

Pharmacologic Category Antineoplastic Agent, Camptothecin; Antineoplastic Agent, Natural Source (Plant) Derivative; Antineoplastic Agent, Topoisomerase I Inhibitor

Medication Safety Issues

Sound-alike/look-alike issues:

Irinotecan may be confused with topotecan

High alert medication:

This medication is in a class the Institute for Safe Medication Practices (ISMP) includes among its list of drug classes which have a heightened risk of causing significant patient harm when used in error.

Pregnancy Risk Factor D

Lactation Excretion in breast milk unknown/not recommended

Breast-Feeding Considerations Due to the potential for serious adverse reactions in the nursing infant, breast-feeding is not recommended.

Use Treatment of metastatic carcinoma of the colon or rectum

Unlabeled Use Treatment of cervical cancer (recurrent or metastatic), central nervous system tumors (recurrent glioblastoma), esophageal cancer, Ewing's sarcoma (recurrent or progressive), gastric cancer (metastatic or locally advanced), nonsmall cell lung cancer (advanced), ovarian cancer (recurrent), pancreatic cancer (advanced), small cell lung cancer (extensive stage)

Mechanism of Action/Effect Irinotecan and its active metabolite (SN-38) bind reversibly to topoisomerase I-DNA complex preventing religation of the cleaved DNA strand. This results in the accumulation of cleavable complexes and double-strand DNA breaks. As mammalian cells cannot efficiently repair these breaks, cell death consistent with S-phase cell cycle specificity occurs, leading to termination of cellular replication.

Contraindications Hypersensitivity to irinotecan or any component of the formulation

Warnings/Precautions Hazardous agent - use appropriate precautions for handling and disposal. Severe hypersensitivity reactions (including anaphylaxis) have occurred. For I.V. use only; monitor infusion site; may cause local tissue necrosis or thrombophlebitis if extravasation occurs.

[U.S. Boxed Warning]: Severe diarrhea may be dose-limiting and potentially fatal; early-onset and late-onset diarrhea may occur. Early diarrhea occurs during or within 24 hours of receiving irinotecan and is characterized by cholinergic symptoms (eg, increased salivation, diaphoresis, flushing, abdominal cramping, lacrimation); may be prevented or treated with atropine. Late diarrhea occurs more than 24 hours after treatment which may lead to dehydration, electrolyte imbalance, or sepsis; may be life-threatening and should be promptly treated with loperamide; dose reductions may be recommended for future doses within the current cycle. Antibiotics may be necessary if patient develops ileus, fever, or severe neutropenia. Patients with diarrhea should be carefully monitored and treated promptly; may require fluid and electrolyte therapy. Colitis, complicated by ulceration, bleeding, ileus, and infection has been reported; initiate antibiotics promptly in patients with ileus.

[U.S. Boxed Warning]: May cause severe myelosuppression. Deaths due to sepsis following severe neutropenia have been reported. Complications due to neutropenia should be promptly managed with antibiotics. Therapy should be temporarily discontinued if neutropenic fever occurs or if the absolute neutrophil count is <1000/mm^3. The dose of irinotecan should be reduced if there is a clinically significant decrease in the total WBC (<200/mm^3), neutrophil count (<1500/mm^3), hemoglobin (<8 g/dL), or platelet count (<100,000/mm^3). Routine administration of a colony-stimulating factor is generally not necessary, but may be considered for patients experiencing significant neutropenia. Fatal cases of Interstitial Pulmonary Disease (IPD)-like events have been reported with single-agent and combination therapy. Promptly evaluate changes in baseline pulmonary symptoms or any new-onset pulmonary symptoms. Discontinue therapy if IPD is diagnosed.

Patients with even modest elevations in total serum bilirubin levels (1-2 mg/dL) have a significantly greater likelihood of experiencing first-course grade 3 or 4 neutropenia than those with bilirubin levels that were <1 mg/dL. Patients with abnormal glucuronidation of bilirubin, such as those with Gilbert's syndrome, may also be at greater risk of myelosuppression when receiving therapy with irinotecan. Use caution when treating patients with known hepatic dysfunction or hyperbilirubinemia exposure to the active metabolite (SN-38) is increased; toxicities may be increased. Dosage adjustments should be considered.

Patients homozygous for the UGT1A1*28 allele are at increased risk of neutropenia; initial one-level dose reduction should be considered for both single-agent and combination regimens. Heterozygous carriers of the UGT1A1*28 allele may also be at increased risk; however, most patients have tolerated normal starting doses. Avoid vaccination with live vaccines during treatment (risk of infection may be increased due to immunosuppression). Although the response to vaccines may be diminished, inactivated vaccines may be administered during treatment.

Renal impairment and acute renal failure have been reported, possibly due to dehydration secondary to diarrhea. Use with caution in patients with renal impairment; not recommended in patients on dialysis. Patients with bowel obstruction should not be treated with irinotecan until resolution of obstruction. Use caution in patients who previously received pelvic/abdominal radiation, elderly patients with comorbid conditions, or baseline performance status of 2; close monitoring and dosage adjustments are recommended. Contains sorbitol; do not use in patients with hereditary fructose intolerance. **[U.S. Boxed Warning]: Should be administered under the supervision of an experienced cancer chemotherapy physician.** Except as part of a clinical trial, use in combination with fluorouracil and leucovorin "Mayo Clinic" regimen is not recommended. Increased toxicity has also been noted in patients with a baseline performance status of 2 in other combination regimens containing irinotecan, leucovorin, and fluorouracil. High potential for CYP-mediated drug interactions; enzyme inducers may decrease exposure to irinotecan and SN-38 (active metabolite); enzyme inhibitors may increase exposure; for use in patients with CNS tumors (unlabeled use), selection of antiseizure medications which are not enzyme inducers is preferred.

Drug Interactions

Avoid Concomitant Use

Avoid concomitant use of Irinotecan with any of the following: Atazanavir; BCG; CloZAPine; Conivaptan; Natalizumab; Pimecrolimus; St Johns Wort; Tacrolimus (Topical); Vaccines (Live)

Decreased Effect

Irinotecan may decrease the levels/effects of: BCG; Coccidioidin Skin Test; Sipuleucel-T; Vaccines (Inactivated); Vaccines (Live)

The levels/effects of Irinotecan may be decreased by: CarBAMazepine; CYP2B6 Inducers (Strong); CYP3A4 Inducers (Strong); Deferasirox; Echinacea; Fosphenytoin; P-glycoprotein/ABCB1 Inducers; PHENobarbital; Phenytoin; St Johns Wort; Tocilizumab

Increased Effect/Toxicity

Irinotecan may increase the levels/effects of: CloZAPine; Leflunomide; Natalizumab; Vaccines (Live)

The levels/effects of Irinotecan may be increased by: Antifungal Agents (Azole Derivatives, Systemic); Atazanavir; Bevacizumab; Conivaptan; CYP2B6 Inhibitors (Moderate); CYP2B6 Inhibitors (Strong); CYP3A4 Inhibitors (Moderate); CYP3A4 Inhibitors (Strong); Dasatinib; Denosumab; Eltrombopag; P-glycoprotein/ABCB1 Inhibitors; Pimecrolimus; Quazepam; Roflumilast; SORAfenib; Tacrolimus (Topical); Trastuzumab

Nutritional/Ethanol Interactions Herb/Nutraceutical: Avoid St John's wort (decreases the efficacy of irinotecan).

Adverse Reactions Frequency of adverse reactions reported for single-agent use of irinotecan only.

>10%:

Cardiovascular: Vasodilation (9% to 11%)

Central nervous system: Cholinergic toxicity (47% - includes rhinitis, increased salivation, miosis, lacrimation, diaphoresis, flushing and intestinal hyperperistalsis); fever (44% to 45%), pain (23% to 24%), dizziness (15% to 21%), insomnia (19%), headache (17%), chills (14%)

Dermatologic: Alopecia (46% to 72%), rash (13% to 14%)

Endocrine & metabolic: Dehydration (15%)

Gastrointestinal: Diarrhea, late (83% to 88%; grade 3/4: 14% to 31%), diarrhea, early (43% to 51%; grade 3/4: 7% to 22%), nausea (70% to 86%), abdominal pain (57% to 68%), vomiting (62% to 67%), cramps (57%), anorexia (44% to 55%), constipation (30% to 32%), mucositis (30%), weight loss (30%), flatulence (12%), stomatitis (12%)

Hematologic: Anemia (60% to 97%; grades 3/4: 5% to 7%), leukopenia (63% to 96%, grades 3/4: 14% to 28%), thrombocytopenia (96%, grades 3/4: 1% to 4%), neutropenia (30% to 96%; grades 3/4: 14% to 31%)

Hepatic: Bilirubin increased (84%), alkaline phosphatase increased (13%)

Neuromuscular & skeletal: Weakness (69% to 76%), back pain (14%)

Respiratory: Dyspnea (22%), cough (17% to 20%), rhinitis (16%)

Miscellaneous: Diaphoresis (16%), infection (14%)

1% to 10%:

Cardiovascular: Edema (10%), hypotension (6%), thromboembolic events (5%)

Central nervous system: Somnolence (9%), confusion (3%)
Gastrointestinal: Abdominal fullness (10%), dyspepsia (10%)
Hematologic: Neutropenic fever (grades 3/4: 2% to 6%), hemorrhage (grades 3/4: 1% to 5%), neutropenic infection (grades 3/4: 1% to 2%)
Hepatic: AST increased (10%), ascites and/or jaundice (grades 3/4: 9%)
Respiratory: Pneumonia (4%)

Note: In limited pediatric experience, dehydration (often associated with severe hypokalemia and hyponatremia) was among the most significant grade 3/4 adverse events, with a frequency up to 29%. In addition, grade 3/4 infection was reported in 24%.

Available Dosage Forms

Injection, solution: 20 mg/mL (2 mL, 5 mL, 25 mL)
Camptosar®: 20 mg/mL (2 mL, 5 mL, 15 mL)

General Dosage Range Dosage adjustment recommended in patients with hepatic impairment or who develop toxicities

I.V.: *Adults:* Dosage varies greatly depending on indication

Administration

I.V. Administer by I.V. infusion, usually over 90 minutes. Premedication with dexamethasone and a 5-HT_3 blocker is recommended 30 minutes prior to administration; prochlorperazine may be considered for subsequent use. Consider premedication of atropine 0.25-1 mg I.V. or SubQ in patients with cholinergic symptoms (eg, increased salivation, diaphoresis, abdominal cramping) or diarrhea.

The recommended regimen to manage late diarrhea is loperamide 4 mg orally at onset of late diarrhea, followed by 2 mg every 2 hours (or 4 mg every 4 hours at night) until 12 hours have passed without a bowel movement. If diarrhea recurs, then repeat administration. Loperamide should not be used for more than 48 consecutive hours.

I.V. Detail pH: 3-3.8

Stability

Reconstitution Use appropriate precautions for handling and disposal. Dilute in 250-500 mL D_5W or NS to a final concentration of 0.12-2.8 mg/mL. Due to the relatively acidic pH, irinotecan appears to be more stable in D_5W than NS.

Storage Store intact vials of injection at room temperature. Protect from light. Solutions diluted in NS may precipitate if refrigerated. Solutions diluted in D_5W are stable for 24 hours at room temperature or 48 hours under refrigeration at 2°C to 8°C, although the manufacturer recommends use within 6 hours at room temperature and 24 hours if refrigerated. Do not freeze.

Nursing Actions

Physical Assessment Premedication with antiemetic may be ordered (emetic potential moderate). Monitor infusion site closely to prevent extravasation. Monitor for immediate or delayed diarrhea (can be fatal), neutropenia, sepsis. mucositis, and/or stomatitis.

Patient Education This drug can only be administered by infusion. Report immediately any burning, pain, redness, or swelling at infusion site. Maintain adequate hydration, unless instructed to restrict fluid intake. May cause severe diarrhea; follow instructions for taking antidiarrheal medication (do not use antidiarrheal medication for longer than 48 consecutive hours). Report immediately if diarrhea persists or you experience signs of dehydration (eg, fainting, dizziness, lightheadedness). You may be more susceptible to infection. You may experience nausea, vomiting, or hair loss (will regrow after treatment is completed). Report immediately persistent diarrhea, unresolved nausea or vomiting, alterations in urinary pattern (increased or decreased), opportunistic infection (fever, chills, unusual bruising or bleeding, fatigue, purulent vaginal discharge, unhealed mouth sores), chest pain, or respiratory difficulty.

Dietary Considerations Contains sorbitol; do not use in patients with hereditary fructose intolerance.

Related Information

Management of Drug Extravasations *on page 1269*

Iron Dextran Complex

(EYE ern DEKS tran KOM pleks)

Brand Names: U.S. Dexferrum®; INFeD®

Index Terms High-Molecular-Weight Iron Dextran (DexFerrum®); Imferon; Iron Dextran; Low-Molecular-Weight Iron Dextran (INFeD®)

Pharmacologic Category Iron Salt

Medication Safety Issues

Sound-alike/look-alike issues:

Dexferrum® may be confused with Desferal®
Iron dextran complex may be confused with ferumoxytol

Pregnancy Risk Factor C

Lactation Enters breast milk/use caution

Use Treatment of iron deficiency in patients in whom oral administration is infeasible or ineffective

Unlabeled Use Cancer-/chemotherapy-associated anemia

Available Dosage Forms

Injection, solution:
Dexferrum®: Elemental iron 50 mg/mL (1 mL, 2 mL)
INFeD®: Elemental iron 50 mg/mL (2 mL)

General Dosage Range Note: A 0.5 mL test dose (0.25 mL in infants) should be given prior to starting iron dextran therapy.

I.M., I.V.:

Children <5 kg and >4 months: Replacement iron (mg) = blood loss (mL) x Hct; **Note:** Total dose should be divided daily at not more than 25 mg/day

Children 5-15 kg and >4 months: Total Dose (mL) = 0.0442 (desired Hgb [usually 12 g/dL] - observed Hgb) x W (in kg) + (0.26 x W [in kg]) **or** replacement iron (mg) = blood loss (mL) x hematocrit; **Note:** Total dose should be divided daily at not more than 50 mg/day (5-10 kg) or 100 mg/day (10-15 kg)

Children >15 kg: Total Dose (mL) = 0.0442 (desired Hgb [usually 14.8 g/dL] - observed Hgb) x LBW + (0.26 x LBW) **or** replacement iron (mg) = blood loss (mL) x Hct; **Note:** Total dose should be divided daily at not more than 100 mg/day

Adults: Total Dose (mL) = 0.0442 (desired Hgb [usually 14.8 g/dL] - observed Hgb) x LBW + (0.26 x LBW) **or** replacement iron (mg) = blood loss (mL) x Hct; **Note:** Total dose should be divided daily at not more than 100 mg/day

Administration

I.M. Note: Test dose: A test dose should be given on the first day of therapy; patient should be observed for 1 hour for hypersensitivity reaction, then the remaining dose (dose minus test dose) should be given. Resuscitation equipment and trained personnel should be available. An uneventful test dose does not ensure an anaphylactic-type reaction will not occur during administration of the therapeutic dose.

I.M. (INFeD®): Use Z-track technique (displacement of the skin laterally prior to injection); injection should be deep into the upper outer quadrant of buttock; alternate buttocks with subsequent injections. Administer test dose at same recommended site using the same technique.

I.V. Test dose should be given gradually over at least 30 seconds (INFeD®) or 5 minutes (Dexferrum®). Subsequent dose(s) may be administered by I.V. bolus undiluted at a rate not to exceed 50 mg/minute or diluted in 250-1000 mL NS and infused over 1-6 hours (initial 25 mL should be given slowly and patient should be observed for allergic reactions); avoid dilutions with dextrose (increased incidence of local pain and phlebitis). Resuscitation equipment and trained personnel should be available. An uneventful test dose does not ensure an anaphylactic-type reaction will not occur during administration of the therapeutic dose.

I.V. Detail pH: 4.2-7

Nursing Actions

Physical Assessment Be alert to the potential for anaphylaxis. Resuscitation equipment should be available. Note that adverse response may occur some time (1-4 days) after administration. Assess patients with rheumatoid arthritis for exacerbated swelling and joint pain; adjust medications as needed.

Patient Education You will need frequent blood tests while on this therapy. If you have rheumatoid arthritis, you may experience increased swelling or joint pain; consult prescriber for medication adjustment. You may experience dizziness, severe headache, nausea, metallic taste, or increased sweating. Large doses can sometimes be associated with a delayed reaction (muscle pain, backache, headache, chills, fever, nausea, or vomiting) occurring 24-48 hours after administration and usually lasting 3-4 days. Report acute GI problems, fever, respiratory difficulty, rapid heartbeat, yellowing of skin or eyes, or swelling of hands and feet.

Iron Sucrose (EYE ern SOO krose)

Brand Names: U.S. Venofer®

Pharmacologic Category Iron Salt

Medication Safety Issues

Sound-alike/look-alike issues:

Iron sucrose may be confused with ferumoxytol

Pregnancy Risk Factor B

Lactation Excretion in breast milk unknown/use caution

Use Treatment of iron-deficiency anemia in chronic renal failure, including nondialysis-dependent patients (with or without erythropoietin therapy) and dialysis-dependent patients receiving erythropoietin therapy

Unlabeled Use Cancer-/chemotherapy-associated anemia

Available Dosage Forms

Injection, solution [preservative free]:

Venofer®: Elemental iron 20 mg/mL (2.5 mL, 5 mL, 10 mL)

General Dosage Range I.V.: *Adults:* 100 mg (5 mL) 1-3 times/week during dialysis **or** 200 mg on 5 different occasions within a 14-day period **or** two 300 mg infusion 14 days apart, followed by a single 400 mg infusion 14 days later (maximum: 1000 mg cumulative total)

Administration

I.V. Not for rapid I.V. injection; inject slowly over 2-5 minutes. Can be administered through dialysis line. Do not mix with other medications or parenteral nutrient solutions.

Slow I.V. injection: May administer undiluted by slow I.V. injection (100 mg over 2-5 minutes in hemodialysis-dependent patients **or** 200 mg over 2-5 minutes in nondialysis-dependent patients)

Infusion: Dilute 100 mg in maximum of 100 mL normal saline; infuse over at least 15 minutes; 300 mg/250 mL should be infused over at least 1.5 hours; 400 mg/250 mL should be infused over at least 2.5 hours; 500 mg/250 mL should be infused over at least 3.5 hours

Nursing Actions

Physical Assessment Facilities for cardiopulmonary resuscitation must be available during administration. Monitor blood pressure closely during infusion.

Patient Education You will be watched closely during infusion. You will need frequent blood tests while on this therapy. You may experience hypotension, black stools, nausea, vomiting, or constipation. Report immediately severe unresolved nausea, headache, dizziness, leg cramps, chest pain or palpations, or swelling of extremities.

Isoniazid (eye soe NYE a zid)

Index Terms INH; Isonicotinic Acid Hydrazide

Pharmacologic Category Antitubercular Agent

Medication Safety Issues

International issues:

Hydra [Japan] may be confused with Hydrea brand name for hydroxyurea [U.S., Canada, and multiple international markets]

Pregnancy Risk Factor C

Lactation Enters breast milk/compatible

Breast-Feeding Considerations Small amounts of isoniazid are excreted in breast milk. However, women with tuberculosis should not be discouraged from breast-feeding. Pyridoxine supplementation is recommended for the mother and infant.

Use Treatment of susceptible tuberculosis infections; treatment of latent tuberculosis infection (LTBI)

Mechanism of Action/Effect Unknown, but may include the inhibition of mycolic acid synthesis resulting in disruption of the bacterial cell wall

Contraindications Hypersensitivity to isoniazid or any component of the formulation; acute liver disease; previous history of hepatic damage during isoniazid therapy; previous severe adverse reaction (drug fever, chills, arthritis) to isoniazid

Warnings/Precautions Use with caution in patients with severe renal impairment and liver disease. **[U.S. Boxed Warning]: Severe and sometimes fatal hepatitis may occur; usually occurs within the first 3 months of treatment, although may develop even after many months of treatment.** The risk of developing hepatitis is age-related, although isoniazid-induced hepatotoxicity has been reported in children; daily ethanol consumption may also increase the risk. Patients must report any prodromal symptoms of hepatitis, such as fatigue, weakness, malaise, anorexia, nausea, abdominal pain, jaundice, or vomiting. Patients should be instructed to immediately discontinue therapy if any of these symptoms occur, even if a clinical evaluation has yet to be conducted. Treatment with isoniazid for latent tuberculosis infection should be deferred in patients with acute hepatic diseases. Periodic ophthalmic examinations are recommended even when usual symptoms do not occur. Pyridoxine (10-50 mg/day) is recommended in individuals at risk for development of peripheral neuropathies (eg, HIV infection, nutritional deficiency, diabetes, pregnancy). Children with low milk and low meat intake should receive concomitant pyridoxine therapy. Multidrug regimens should be utilized for the treatment of active tuberculosis to prevent the emergence of drug resistance.

Drug Interactions

Avoid Concomitant Use

Avoid concomitant use of Isoniazid with any of the following: Clopidogrel; Pimozide; Thioridazine

Decreased Effect

Isoniazid may decrease the levels/effects of: Clopidogrel; Codeine; TraMADol

The levels/effects of Isoniazid may be decreased by: Antacids; Corticosteroids (Systemic); Cyproterone

Increased Effect/Toxicity

Isoniazid may increase the levels/effects of: Acetaminophen; ARIPiprazole; Benzodiazepines (metabolized by oxidation); CarBAMazepine; Chlorzoxazone; Citalopram; CycloSERINE; CYP2A6 Substrates; CYP2C19 Substrates; CYP2D6 Substrates; CYP2E1 Substrates; Fesoterodine; Fosphenytoin; Nebivolol; Phenytoin; Pimozide; Tamoxifen; Theophylline Derivatives; Thioridazine

The levels/effects of Isoniazid may be increased by: Ethionamide; Propafenone; Rifamycin Derivatives

Nutritional/Ethanol Interactions

Ethanol: Ethanol increases the risk of hepatitis. Management: Avoid ethanol.

Food: Serum levels may be decreased if taken with food. Has some ability to inhibit tyramine metabolism; several case reports of mild reactions (flushing, palpitations) after ingestion of cheese (with or without wine). Reactions resembling allergic symptoms following ingestion of fish high in histamine content have been reported. Isoniazid decreases folic acid absorption. Isoniazid alters pyridoxine metabolism. Management: Take on an empty stomach 1 hour before or 2 hours after a meal, increase dietary intake of folate, niacin, and magnesium. Avoid tyramine-containing foods (eg, aged or matured cheese, air-dried or cured meats including sausages and salamis; fava or broad bean pods, tap/draft beers, Marmite concentrate, sauerkraut, soy sauce, and other soybean condiments). Food's freshness is also an important concern; improperly stored or spoiled food can create an environment in which tyramine concentrations may increase. Avoid histamine-containing foods.

Adverse Reactions Frequency not defined.

Cardiovascular: Hypertension, palpitation, tachycardia, vasculitis

Central nervous system: Depression, dizziness, encephalopathy, fever, lethargy, memory impairment, psychosis, seizure, slurred speech, toxic encephalopathy
Dermatologic: Flushing, rash (morbilliform, maculopapular, pruritic, or exfoliative)
Endocrine & metabolic: Gynecomastia, hyperglycemia, metabolic acidosis, pellagra, pyridoxine deficiency
Gastrointestinal: Anorexia, epigastric distress, nausea, stomach pain, vomiting
Hematologic: Agranulocytosis, anemia (sideroblastic, hemolytic, or aplastic), eosinophilia, thrombocytopenia
Hepatic: LFTs mildly increased (10% to 20%), hyperbilirubinemia, bilirubinuria, jaundice, hepatic dysfunction, hepatitis (may involve progressive liver damage; risk increases with age; 2.3% in patients >50 years)
Neuromuscular & skeletal: Arthralgia, hyperreflexia, paresthesia, peripheral neuropathy (dose-related incidence, 10% to 20% incidence with 10 mg/kg/day), weakness
Ocular: Blurred vision, loss of vision, optic neuritis and atrophy
Miscellaneous: Lupus-like syndrome, lymphadenopathy, rheumatic syndrome

Available Dosage Forms

Injection, solution: 100 mg/mL (10 mL)
Solution, oral: 50 mg/5 mL (473 mL)
Tablet, oral: 100 mg, 300 mg

General Dosage Range Oral, I.M.:

Children: 10-20 mg/kg/day once daily (maximum: 300 mg/day) **or** 20-40 mg/kg 2-3 times/week (maximum: 900 mg/dose)
Adults: 300 mg (5 mg/kg) once daily **or** 900 mg (15 mg/kg) 2-3 times/week

Administration

Oral Should be administered 1 hour before or 2 hours after meals on an empty stomach.

Stability

Storage

Tablet: Store at 20°C to 25°C (68°F to 77°F). Protect from light.
Oral solution: Store at 15°C to 30°C (59°F to 86°F). Protect from light.

Nursing Actions

Physical Assessment Monitor for liver damage, nausea, vomiting, peripheral neuropathy, and CNS changes at regular intervals during therapy. Teach patient importance of proper diet and ophthalmic examinations.

Patient Education Best if taken on an empty stomach, 1 hour before or 2 hours after meals. Avoid excessive alcohol and tyramine-containing foods. Increase dietary intake of folate, niacin, and magnesium. You will need to have frequent ophthalmic exams and periodic medical checkups to evaluate drug effects. If you experience nausea, vomiting, loss of appetite, weakness, fatigue, abdominal pain, dark-colored urine or change in color of stool, or yellowing of eyes/skin, discontinue and contact prescriber as soon as possible. Report chest pain, rapid heart beat, or palpitations; tingling, numbness, or loss of sensation in hands or feet; CNS changes (depression, dizziness, memory impairment, slurred speech, seizure); unusual weakness or fatigue; persistent gastrointestinal upset; change in vision; or skin rash.

Dietary Considerations Should be taken 1 hour before or 2 hours after meals on an empty stomach; increase dietary intake of folate, niacin, magnesium. Avoid tyramine-containing foods; some examples include aged or matured cheese, air-dried or cured meats (including sausages and salamis), fava or broad bean pods, tap/draft beers, Marmite concentrate, sauerkraut, soy sauce and other soybean condiments. Avoid histamine-containing foods.

Isoproterenol (eye soe proe TER e nole)

Brand Names: U.S. Isuprel®

Index Terms Isoproterenol Hydrochloride

Pharmacologic Category $Beta_1$- & $Beta_2$-Adrenergic Agonist Agent

Medication Safety Issues

Sound-alike/look-alike issues:

Isuprel® may be confused with Disophrol®, Isordil®

Pregnancy Risk Factor C

Lactation Excretion in breast milk unknown

Use Manufacturer's labeled indications (see **"Note"**): Mild or transient episodes of heart block that do not require electric shock or pacemaker therapy; serious episodes of heart block and Adams-Stokes attacks (except when caused by ventricular tachycardia or fibrillation); cardiac arrest until electric shock or pacemaker therapy is available; bronchospasm during anesthesia; adjunct to fluid and electrolyte replacement therapy and other drugs and procedures in the treatment of hypovolemic or septic shock and low cardiac output states (eg, decompensated heart failure, cardiogenic shock)

Note: The use of isoproterenol in advanced cardiac life support (ACLS) has largely been supplanted by the use of other adrenergic agents (eg, epinephrine and dopamine). The use of isoproterenol for bronchospasm during anesthesia and cardiogenic, hypovolemic, or septic shock is no longer recommended. See *Unlabeled Use* for more appropriate, yet unlabeled, uses.

Unlabeled Use Pharmacologic overdrive pacing for refractory torsade de pointes; pharmacologic provocation during tilt table testing for syncope; temporary control of bradycardia in denervated heart transplant patients unresponsive to atropine; ventricular arrhythmias due to AV nodal block; beta-blocker overdose; electrical storm associated with Brugada syndrome

Available Dosage Forms

Injection, solution:

Isuprel®: 0.2 mg/mL (1 mL, 5 mL)

General Dosage Range Continuous I.V. infusion:

Children: 0.05-2 mcg/**kg**/minute; titrate to patient response

Adults: 2-10 mcg/minute; titrate to patient response

Administration

I.V. I.V. infusion administration requires the use of an infusion pump.

I.V. Detail pH: 2.5-4.5

Nursing Actions

Physical Assessment Monitor cardiac, respiratory, and hemodynamic status when used in acute or emergency situations.

Patient Education You may experience nervousness, dizziness, fatigue, dry mouth, nausea, or vomiting. Report chest pain, rapid heartbeat or palpitations, unresolved/persistent GI upset, dizziness, fatigue, trembling, increased anxiety, sleeplessness, or respiratory difficulty.

Isosorbide Dinitrate

(eye soe SOR bide dye NYE trate)

Brand Names: U.S. Dilatrate®-SR; Isordil® Titradose™

Index Terms ISD; ISDN

Pharmacologic Category Antianginal Agent; Vasodilator

Medication Safety Issues

Sound-alike/look-alike issues:

Isordil® may be confused with Inderal®, Isuprel®, Plendil®

Pregnancy Risk Factor C

Lactation Excretion in breast milk unknown

Use Prevention and treatment of angina pectoris

Note: Due to slower onset of action, not the drug of choice to abort an acute anginal episode.

Unlabeled Use Patients with heart failure (HF) who do not tolerate an ACE inhibitor or an angiotensin receptor blocker (ARB); African-American (self-identified) patients with HF remaining symptomatic despite optimal standard therapy; esophageal spastic disorders

Mechanism of Action/Effect Relaxes vascular smooth muscles, decreases arterial resistance and venous return which reduces cardiac oxygen demand. Additionally, coronary artery dilation improves collateral flow to ischemic regions.

Contraindications Hypersensitivity to isosorbide dinitrate or any component of the formulation; hypersensitivity to organic nitrates; concurrent use with phosphodiesterase-5 (PDE-5) inhibitors (sildenafil, tadalafil, or vardenafil)

Warnings/Precautions Severe hypotension can occur; paradoxical bradycardia and increased angina pectoris can accompany hypotension. Postural hypotension can also occur; ethanol may potentiate this effect. Use with caution in volume depletion and moderate hypotension, and use with extreme caution with inferior wall MI and suspected right ventricular infarctions. Nitrates may reduce preload, exacerbating obstruction and cause hypotension or syncope and/or worsening of heart failure (Gibbons, 2003). Avoid use in patients with hypertrophic cardiomyopathy (HCM).

Use of isosorbide dinitrate sublingual tablets to treat acute angina attacks is recommended only in patients unresponsive to sublingual nitroglycerin; however, current clinical practice guidelines do not recommend use during an acute anginal episode. Avoid use of extended release formulations in acute MI or acute HF; cannot easily reverse effects if adverse events develop. Nitrates may precipitate or aggravate increased intracranial pressure and subsequently may worsen clinical outcomes in patients with neurologic injury (eg, intracranial hemorrhage, traumatic brain injury). Appropriate dosing intervals are needed to minimize tolerance development. Tolerance can only be overcome by short periods of nitrate absence from the body. Dose escalation does not overcome this effect. When used for HF in combination with hydralazine, tolerance is less of a concern (Gogia, 1995).

Avoid concurrent use with PDE-5 inhibitors (eg, sildenafil, tadalafil, vardenafil). When nitrate administration becomes medically necessary, may administer nitrates only if 24 hours have elapsed after use of sildenafil or vardenafil (48 hours after tadalafil use) (Trujillo, 2007).

Drug Interactions

Avoid Concomitant Use

Avoid concomitant use of Isosorbide Dinitrate with any of the following: Conivaptan; Phosphodiesterase 5 Inhibitors

Decreased Effect

The levels/effects of Isosorbide Dinitrate may be decreased by: CYP3A4 Inducers (Strong); Deferasirox; Herbs (CYP3A4 Inducers); Tocilizumab

Increased Effect/Toxicity

Isosorbide Dinitrate may increase the levels/effects of: Hypotensive Agents; Prilocaine; Rosiglitazone

The levels/effects of Isosorbide Dinitrate may be increased by: Conivaptan; CYP3A4 Inhibitors (Moderate); CYP3A4 Inhibitors (Strong); Dasatinib; Ivacaftor; Phosphodiesterase 5 Inhibitors

Nutritional/Ethanol Interactions

Ethanol: Caution with ethanol (may increase risk of hypotension).

Herb/Nutraceutical: Avoid black cohosh, California poppy, coleus, golden seal, hawthorn, mistletoe, periwinkle, quinine, shepherd's purse (may cause hypotension).

Adverse Reactions Frequency not defined.

Cardiovascular: Crescendo angina (uncommon), hypotension, postural hypotension, rebound hypertension (uncommon), syncope (uncommon)

Central nervous system: Headache (most common), lightheadedness (related to blood pressure changes)

Hematologic: Methemoglobinemia (rare, overdose)

Pharmacodynamics/Kinetics

Onset of Action Sublingual tablet: ~3 minutes; Oral tablet and capsule (includes extended-release formulations): ~1 hour

Duration of Action Sublingual tablet: 1-2 hours; Oral tablet and capsule (includes extended-release formulations): Up to 8 hours

Available Dosage Forms

Capsule, sustained release, oral:
Dilatrate®-SR: 40 mg

Tablet, oral: 5 mg, 10 mg, 20 mg, 30 mg
Isordil® Titradose™: 5 mg, 40 mg

Tablet, sublingual: 2.5 mg, 5 mg

Tablet, extended release, oral: 40 mg

General Dosage Range

Oral:

Immediate release: *Adults:* 5-40 mg 2-3 times/day

Sustained release: *Adults:* 40-160 mg/day in divided doses

Sublingual: *Adults:* 2.5-5 mg every 5-10 minutes for maximum of 3 doses in 15-30 minutes **or** 2.5-5 mg 15 minutes prior to activities which may provoke an anginal episode.

Administration

Oral May consider administration of first dose in physician office; observe for maximal cardiovascular dynamic effects and adverse effects (orthostatic hypotension, headache). Do not administer around the clock; allow nitrate-free interval ≥14 hours (immediate release products) and >18 hours (sustained release products). Do not crush sublingual tablets or extended release formulations.

Immediate release products: When prescribed twice daily, consider administering at 8 AM and 1 PM. For 3 times/day dosing, consider 8 AM, 1 PM, and 6 PM.

Sustained release products: Consider once daily in morning or twice-daily dosing at 8 AM and between 1-2 PM.

Nursing Actions

Physical Assessment Assess blood pressure and monitor for hypotension and tolerance at regular intervals during therapy. Teach patient importance of maintaining dosing schedule to provide drug-free period.

Patient Education Take at the same time each day, with last dose in early evening. Do not chew or swallow sublingual tablets; allow them to dissolve under your tongue. Do not crush or chew sustained release or extended release products; swallow whole with water. Avoid excessive alcohol; combination may cause severe hypotension. May cause headache, dizziness, and flushed feeling. If chest pain occurs, seek emergency medical help at once. Report severe headache, dizziness, loss of consciousness, or any rash.

Isosorbide Mononitrate

(eye soe SOR bide mon oh NYE trate)

Brand Names: U.S. Imdur®; Ismo®; Monoket®

Index Terms ISMN

Pharmacologic Category Antianginal Agent; Vasodilator

Medication Safety Issues

Sound-alike/look-alike issues:

Imdur® may be confused with Imuran®, Inderal® LA, K-Dur®

Monoket® may be confused with Monopril®

Pregnancy Risk Factor B/C (manufacturer dependent)

Lactation Excretion in breast milk unknown/use caution

Use Prevention of angina pectoris

Available Dosage Forms

Tablet, oral: 10 mg, 20 mg
Ismo®: 20 mg
Monoket®: 10 mg, 20 mg

Tablet, extended release, oral: 30 mg, 60 mg, 120 mg
Imdur®: 30 mg, 60 mg, 120 mg

General Dosage Range Oral:

Extended release: *Adults:* Initial: 30-60 mg once daily; Maintenance: 30-240 mg once daily (maximum: 240 mg/day)

Regular release: *Adults:* 5-20 mg twice daily

Administration

Oral Do not administer around-the-clock. Immediate release tablet should be scheduled twice daily with doses 7 hours apart (8 AM and 3 PM); extended release tablet may be administered once daily in the morning upon rising with a half-glassful of fluid and should not be chewed or crushed.

Nursing Actions

Physical Assessment Tolerance to nitrates will develop and proper timing of doses is needed to minimize tolerance. Monitor for hypotension and GI disturbance when beginning therapy, when dose is adjusted, and at regular intervals during therapy. Teach patient importance of maintaining dosing schedule.

Patient Education Take at same time(s) each day. Do not crush or chew extended release tablets; swallow whole with water. Avoid excess alcohol intake; combination may cause severe hypotension. May cause dizziness, headache, and flushed feeling. Report severe headache, persistent dizziness, loss of consciousness, or any rash. If chest pain occurs, seek emergency medical help at once.

Isotretinoin (eye soe TRET i noyn)

Brand Names: U.S. Amnesteem®; Claravis™; Sotret®

Index Terms 13-*cis*-Retinoic Acid; 13-*cis*-Vitamin A Acid; 13-CRA; *Cis*-Retinoic Acid; Accutane; Isotretinoinum

Pharmacologic Category Acne Products; Antineoplastic Agent, Miscellaneous; Retinoic Acid Derivative

Medication Safety Issues

Sound-alike/look-alike issues:

Accutane® may be confused with Accolate®, Accupril®

Claravis™ may be confused with Cleviprex®

ISOtretinoin may be confused with tretinoin

Medication Guide Available Yes

Pregnancy Risk Factor X

Lactation Excretion in breast milk unknown/contraindicated

Breast-Feeding Considerations Due to the potential for adverse reactions, breast-feeding is not recommended.

Use Treatment of severe recalcitrant nodular acne unresponsive to conventional therapy

Unlabeled Use Management of moderate degrees of treatment-resistant acne, management of acne that produces physical or psychological scarring; treatment of cutaneous T-cell lymphomas (mycosis fungoides and Sézary syndrome); prevention of squamous cell skin cancers (in high-risk patients); treatment of high-risk neuroblastoma in children

Mechanism of Action/Effect Reduces sebaceous gland size and reduces sebum production in acne treatment; in neuroblastoma, decreases cell proliferation and induces differentiation

Contraindications Hypersensitivity to isotretinoin or any component of the formulation; sensitivity to parabens, vitamin A, or other retinoids; pregnancy

Warnings/Precautions This medication should only be prescribed by prescribers competent in treating severe recalcitrant nodular acne and experienced with the use of systemic retinoids. **[U.S. Boxed Warnings]: Birth defects (facial, eye, ear, skull, central nervous system, cardiovascular, thymus and parathyroid gland abnormalities) have been noted following isotretinoin exposure during pregnancy; low IQ scores have also been reported. The risk for spontaneous abortion and premature births is increased. Because of the high likelihood of teratogenic effects, all patients (male and female), prescribers, wholesalers, and dispensing pharmacists must register and be active in the iPLEDGE™ risk management program; do not prescribe isotretinoin for women who are or who are likely to become pregnant while using the drug.** Women of childbearing potential must be capable of complying with effective contraceptive measures. Patients must select and commit to two forms of contraception. Therapy is begun after two negative pregnancy tests; effective contraception must be used for at least 1 month before beginning therapy, during therapy, and for 1 month after discontinuation of therapy. Prescriptions should be written for no more than a 30-day supply, and pregnancy testing and counseling should be repeated monthly.

May cause depression, psychosis, aggressive or violent behavior, and changes in mood; use with extreme caution in patients with psychiatric disorders. Rarely, suicidal thoughts and actions have been reported during isotretinoin usage. All patients should be observed closely for symptoms of depression or suicidal thoughts. Discontinuation of treatment alone may not be sufficient, further evaluation may be necessary. Cases of pseudotumor cerebri (benign intracranial hypertension) have been reported, some with concomitant use of tetracycline (avoid using together). Patients with papilledema, headache, nausea, vomiting, and visual disturbances should be referred to a neurologist and treatment with isotretinoin discontinued. Hearing impairment, which can continue after therapy is discontinued, may occur. Clinical hepatitis, elevated liver enzymes, inflammatory bowel disease, skeletal hyperostosis, premature epiphyseal closure, vision impairment, corneal opacities, and decreased night vision have also been reported with the use of isotretinoin. Rare postmarketing cases of severe skin reactions (eg, Stevens-Johnson syndrome, erythema multiforme) have been reported with use.

Use with caution in patients with diabetes mellitus; impaired glucose control has been reported. Use caution in patients with hypertriglyceridemia; acute pancreatitis and fatal hemorrhagic pancreatitis (rare) have been reported. Bone mineral density may decrease; use caution in patients with a genetic predisposition to bone disorders (ie osteoporosis, osteomalacia) and with disease states or concomitant medications that can induce bone disorders. Patients may be at risk when participating in activities with repetitive impact (such as sports). Patients should be instructed not to donate blood during therapy and for 1 month following discontinuation of therapy due to risk of donated blood being given to a pregnant female. Safety of long-term use is not established and is not recommended.

Drug Interactions

Avoid Concomitant Use

Avoid concomitant use of ISOtretinoin with any of the following: Tetracycline Derivatives; Vitamin A

Decreased Effect

ISOtretinoin may decrease the levels/effects of: Contraceptives (Estrogens); Contraceptives (Progestins)

Increased Effect/Toxicity

ISOtretinoin may increase the levels/effects of: Porfimer; Vitamin A

The levels/effects of ISOtretinoin may be increased by: Alcohol (Ethyl); Tetracycline Derivatives

Nutritional/Ethanol Interactions

Ethanol: Avoid or limit ethanol (may increase triglyceride levels if taken in excess).

Food: Isotretinoin bioavailability increased if taken with food or milk.

Herb/Nutraceutical: Avoid dong quai, St John's wort (may also cause photosensitization and may decrease the effectiveness of oral contraceptives). Additional vitamin A supplements may lead to vitamin A toxicity (dry skin, irritation, arthralgias, myalgias, abdominal pain, hepatic changes); avoid use.

Adverse Reactions Frequency not always defined.

Cardiovascular: Chest pain, edema, flushing, palpitation, stroke, syncope, tachycardia, vascular thrombotic disease

Central nervous system: Aggressive behavior, depression, dizziness, drowsiness, emotional instability, fatigue, headache, insomnia, lethargy, malaise, nervousness, paresthesia, pseudotumor cerebri, psychosis, seizure, stroke, suicidal ideation, suicide attempts, suicide, violent behavior

Dermatologic: Abnormal wound healing acne fulminans, alopecia, bruising, cheilitis, cutaneous allergic reactions, dry nose, dry skin, eczema, eruptive xanthomas, facial erythema, fragility of skin, hair abnormalities, hirsutism, hyperpigmentation, hypopigmentation, increased sunburn susceptibility, nail dystrophy, paronychia, peeling of palms, peeling of soles, photoallergic reactions, photosensitizing reactions, pruritus, purpura, rash

Endocrine & metabolic: Triglycerides increased (25%), abnormal menses, blood glucose increased, cholesterol increased, HDL decreased, hyperuricemia

Gastrointestinal: Bleeding and inflammation of the gums, colitis, esophagitis, esophageal ulceration, inflammatory bowel disease, nausea, nonspecific gastrointestinal symptoms, pancreatitis, weight loss, xerostomia

Genitourinary: Nonspecific urogenital findings

Hematologic: Agranulocytosis (rare), anemia, neutropenia, pyogenic granuloma, thrombocytopenia

Hepatic: Alkaline phosphatase increased, ALT increased, AST increased, GGTP increased, hepatitis, LDH increased

Neuromuscular & skeletal: Back pain (29% in pediatric patients), arthralgia, arthritis, bone abnormalities, bone mineral density decreased, calcification of tendons and ligaments, CPK increased, myalgia, premature epiphyseal closure, skeletal hyperostosis, tendonitis, weakness

Ocular: Cataracts, color vision disorder, conjunctivitis, corneal opacities, dry eyes, eyelid inflammation, keratitis, night vision decreased, optic neuritis, photophobia, visual disturbances

Otic: Hearing impairment, tinnitus

Renal: Glomerulonephritis, hematuria, proteinuria, pyuria, vasculitis

Respiratory: Bronchospasms, epistaxis, respiratory infection, voice alteration, Wegener's granulomatosis

Miscellaneous: Allergic reactions, anaphylactic reactions, disseminated herpes simplex, diaphoresis, infection, lymphadenopathy

Available Dosage Forms

Capsule, oral:

Claravis™: 10 mg, 20 mg, 30 mg, 40 mg

Capsule, softgel, oral:

Amnesteem®: 10 mg, 20 mg, 40 mg

Sotret®: 10 mg, 20 mg, 30 mg, 40 mg

General Dosage Range Dosage adjustments recommended in patients with hepatic impairment

Oral:

Children 12-17 years: 0.5-1 mg/kg/day in 2 divided doses

Adults: 0.5-2 mg/kg/day in 2 divided doses

Administration

Oral Administer orally with a meal. According to the manufacturers' labeling, capsules should be swallowed whole with a full glass of liquid. For patients unable to swallow capsule whole, an oral liquid may be prepared; may irritate esophagus if contents are removed from the capsule.

Stability

Storage Store at room temperature of 59°F to 86°F (15°C to 30°C). Protect from light.

Nursing Actions

Physical Assessment Monitor patients with diabetes closely; monitor skin for unusual reactions. Observe for depression or suicide ideation.

Patient Education A patient information/consent form must be signed before this medication is prescribed. Do not sign (and do not take this medication) if you do not understand all of the information on the form. Prescriptions will be written for a 1-month supply and must be filled within 7 days; they will not be honored if filled after that time or if they do not have the appropriate yellow qualification sticker attached. Capsule should be swallowed whole, however, may be opened with a large needle and contents sprinkled on applesauce or ice cream (may irritate esophagus when contents are removed from the capsule). Whole capsules should be swallowed with a full glass of liquid. Do not take any other vitamin A products, limit vitamin A intake, and increase exercise during therapy. Limit or avoid alcohol intake. Exacerbations of acne may occur during first weeks of therapy. You may experience headache; loss of night vision; muscle aches; lethargy; visual disturbances; photosensitivity; dry mouth; nausea; dryness, redness, or itching of skin; eye irritation; or increased sensitivity to contact lenses. Report depression, suicide ideation, or severe skin reactions. Discontinue therapy and report acute vision changes, ringing in the ears or changes in hearing, rectal bleeding, abdominal cramping, or unresolved diarrhea.

Dietary Considerations Should be taken with food. Limit intake of vitamin A; avoid use of other vitamin A products. Some formulations may contain soybean oil.

Isradipine (iz RA di peen)

Brand Names: U.S. DynaCirc CR®

Pharmacologic Category Calcium Channel Blocker; Calcium Channel Blocker, Dihydropyridine

Medication Safety Issues

Sound-alike/look-alike issues:

DynaCirc® may be confused with Dynacin®

Pregnancy Risk Factor C

Lactation Excretion in breast milk unknown/not recommended

Use Treatment of hypertension

Unlabeled Use Pediatric hypertension

Available Dosage Forms

Capsule, oral: 2.5 mg, 5 mg

Tablet, controlled release, oral:

DynaCirc CR®: 5 mg, 10 mg

General Dosage Range Dosage adjustment recommended in patients with hepatic or renal impairment

Oral: *Adults:*

Capsule: Initial: 2.5 mg twice daily; Usual range: 2.5-10 mg/day

Controlled release tablet: Initial: 5 mg once daily; Maintenance: 5-20 mg once daily (maximum: 20 mg/day)

Administration

Oral May be administered without regard to meals. Controlled release tablets should be swallowed whole; do not divide or chew

Nursing Actions

Physical Assessment Monitor for tachycardia, hypotension, edema, and dyspnea at regular intervals during therapy. When discontinuing, dose should be tapered slowly.

Patient Education Take with or without food. Do not crush extended release tablets. Follow prescriber's instructions for diet and lifestyle changes. You may experience headache, constipation, dizziness, or ankle swelling. Report unrelieved headache, severe constipation, chest pain, palpitations, swelling of feet or weight gain, or chest pain or pressure.

Itraconazole (i tra KOE na zole)

Brand Names: U.S. Sporanox®

Pharmacologic Category Antifungal Agent, Oral

Medication Safety Issues

Sound-alike/look-alike issues:

Itraconazole may be confused with fluconazole

Sporanox® may be confused with Suprax®, Topamax®

Pregnancy Risk Factor C

Lactation Enters breast milk/not recommended

Use

Oral capsules: Treatment of susceptible fungal infections in immunocompromised and immunocompetent patients including blastomycosis and histoplasmosis; indicated for aspergillosis (in patients intolerant/refractory to amphotericin B), and onychomycosis of the toenail and fingernail (in nonimmunocompromised patients)

Oral solution: Treatment of oral and esophageal candidiasis

Mechanism of Action/Effect Interferes with cytochrome P450 activity, decreasing ergosterol synthesis (principal sterol in fungal cell membrane) and inhibiting cell membrane formation

Contraindications Hypersensitivity to itraconazole (use caution in patients with a history of hypersensitivity to other azoles), any component of the formulation; concurrent administration with cisapride, dofetilide, ergot derivatives, levomethadyl, lovastatin, midazolam (oral), nisoldipine, pimozide, quinidine, simvastatin, or triazolam; treatment of onychomycosis (or other non-life-threatening indications) in patients with evidence of ventricular dysfunction, heart failure (HF) or a history of HF; treatment of onychomycosis in patients who are pregnant or intend on becoming pregnant

Warnings/Precautions [U.S. Boxed Warning]: Negative inotropic effects have been observed following intravenous administration. Discontinue or reassess use if signs or symptoms of HF (heart failure) occur during treatment. [U.S. Boxed Warning]: Not recommended for treatment of onychomycosis in patients with ventricular dysfunction or a history of HF. HF has been reported, particularly in patients receiving a total daily oral dose of 400 mg. Use with caution in patients with risk factors for HF (COPD, renal failure, edematous disorders, ischemic or valvular disease). Discontinue if signs or symptoms of HF or neuropathy occur during treatment. **[U.S. Boxed Warning]: Serious cardiovascular adverse events including, QT prolongation, ventricular tachycardia, torsade de pointes, cardiac arrest and/or sudden death have been observed due**

to increased cisapride, pimozide, quinidine or levomethadyl concentrations induced by itraconazole; concurrent use contraindicated. Additionally, the following drugs metabolized by the CYP 3A4 isoenzyme system are also contraindicated: Ergot derivatives, lovastatin, midazolam (oral), simvastatin, and triazolam.

Calcium channel blockers (CCBs) may cause additive negative inotropic effects when used concurrently with itraconazole. Itraconazole may also inhibit the metabolism of CCBs. Use caution with concurrent use of itraconazole and CCBs due to an increased risk of HF. Concurrent use of itraconazole and nisoldipine is contraindicated.

Use with caution in patients with renal impairment. Rare cases of serious hepatotoxicity (including liver failure and death) have been reported (including some cases occurring within the first week of therapy); hepatotoxicity was reported in some patients without pre-existing liver disease or risk factors. Use with caution in patients with pre-existing hepatic impairment; monitor liver function closely and dosage adjustment may be warranted. Not recommended for use in patients with active liver disease, elevated liver enzymes, or prior hepatotoxic reactions to other drugs unless the expected benefit exceeds the risk of hepatotoxicity. Transient or permanent hearing loss has been reported. Quinidine (a contraindicated drug) was used concurrently in several of these cases. Hearing loss usually resolves after discontinuation, but may persist in some patients.

Large differences in itraconazole pharmacokinetic parameters have been observed in cystic fibrosis patients receiving the solution; if a patient with cystic fibrosis does not respond to therapy, alternate therapies should be considered. Due to differences in bioavailability, oral capsules and oral solution cannot be used interchangeably. Only the oral solution has proven efficacy for oral and esophageal candidiasis. Initiation of treatment with oral solution is not recommended in patients at immediate risk for systemic candidiasis (eg, patients with severe neutropenia).

Drug Interactions

Avoid Concomitant Use

Avoid concomitant use of Itraconazole with any of the following: Alfuzosin; Aliskiren; Axitinib; Cisapride; Conivaptan; Crizotinib; Dofetilide; Dronedarone; Eplerenone; Ergot Derivatives; Everolimus; Fluticasone (Oral Inhalation); Halofantrine; Lapatinib; Lovastatin; Lurasidone; Nevirapine; Nilotinib; Nisoldipine; Pimozide; QuiNIDine; Ranolazine; Rivaroxaban; RomiDEPsin; Salmeterol; Silodosin; Simvastatin; Tamsulosin; Ticagrelor; Tolvaptan; Topotecan; Toremifene

Decreased Effect

Itraconazole may decrease the levels/effects of: Amphotericin B; Prasugrel; Saccharomyces boulardii; Ticagrelor

The levels/effects of Itraconazole may be decreased by: Antacids; CYP3A4 Inducers (Strong); Deferasirox; Didanosine; Efavirenz; Etravirine; Fosphenytoin; H2-Antagonists; Herbs (CYP3A4 Inducers); Nevirapine; Phenytoin; Proton Pump Inhibitors; Rifamycin Derivatives; Sucralfate; Tocilizumab

Increased Effect/Toxicity

Itraconazole may increase the levels/effects of: Alfentanil; Alfuzosin; Aliskiren; Almotriptan; Alosetron; Aprepitant; ARIPiprazole; Axitinib; Benzodiazepines (metabolized by oxidation); Boceprevir; Bortezomib; Bosentan; Brentuximab Vedotin; Brinzolamide; Budesonide (Nasal); Budesonide (Systemic, Oral Inhalation); BusPIRone; Busulfan; Calcium Channel Blockers; CarBAMazepine; Cardiac Glycosides; Ciclesonide; Cilostazol; Cisapride; Colchicine; Conivaptan; Corticosteroids (Orally Inhaled); Corticosteroids (Systemic); Crizotinib; CycloSPORINE; CycloSPORINE (Systemic); CYP3A4 Substrates; Dabigatran Etexilate; Dienogest; DOCEtaxel; Dofetilide; Dronedarone; Dutasteride; Eletriptan; Eplerenone; Ergot Derivatives; Erlotinib; Eszopiclone; Etravirine; Everolimus; FentaNYL; Fesoterodine; Fexofenadine; Fluticasone (Nasal); Fluticasone (Oral Inhalation); Fosaprepitant; Fosphenytoin; Gefitinib; GuanFACINE; Halofantrine; HMG-CoA Reductase Inhibitors; Iloperidone; Imatinib; Irinotecan; Ivacaftor; Ixabepilone; Lapatinib; Losartan; Lovastatin; Lumefantrine; Lurasidone; Macrolide Antibiotics; Maraviroc; Methadone; MethylPREDNISolone; Nilotinib; Nisoldipine; Paliperidone; Paricalcitol; Pazopanib; P-glycoprotein/ABCB1 Substrates; Phenytoin; Phosphodiesterase 5 Inhibitors; Pimecrolimus; Pimozide; Propafenone; Protease Inhibitors; Prucalopride; QuiNIDine; Ramelteon; Ranolazine; Repaglinide; Rifamycin Derivatives; Rivaroxaban; RomiDEPsin; Ruxolitinib; Salmeterol; Saxagliptin; Sildenafil; Silodosin; Simvastatin; Sirolimus; Solifenacin; SORAfenib; SUNItinib; Tacrolimus; Tacrolimus (Systemic); Tacrolimus (Topical); Tadalafil; Tamsulosin; Telaprevir; Temsirolimus; Ticagrelor; Tolterodine; Tolvaptan; Topotecan; Toremifene; Vardenafil; Vemurafenib; Vilazodone; VinBLAStine; VinCRIStine; Vinorelbine; Vitamin K Antagonists; Ziprasidone; Zolpidem; Zuclopenthixol

The levels/effects of Itraconazole may be increased by: Boceprevir; Etravirine; Grapefruit Juice; Macrolide Antibiotics; Protease Inhibitors; Telaprevir

Nutritional/Ethanol Interactions

Food:

Capsules: Absorption enhanced by food and possibly by gastric acidity. Cola drinks have been shown to increase the absorption of the capsules in patients with achlorhydria or those taking H_2-receptor antagonists or other gastric acid suppressors. Grapefruit/grapefruit juice may increase serum levels. Management: Take capsules immediately after meals. Avoid grapefruit juice.

Solution: Food decreases the bioavailability and increases the time to peak concentration. Management: Take solution on an empty stomach 1 hour before or 2 hours after meals.

Herb/Nutraceutical: St John's wort may decrease itraconazole levels.

Adverse Reactions

>10%: Gastrointestinal: Nausea (11%), diarrhea (3% to 11%)

1% to 10%:

Cardiovascular: Edema (4%), hypertension (3%), chest pain (3%)

Central nervous system: Fever (3% to 7%), headache (4%), fatigue (2% to 3%), dizziness (2%), depression (2%)

Dermatologic: Rash (4% to 9%), pruritus (3%)

Endocrine & metabolic: Hypokalemia (2%)

Gastrointestinal: Vomiting (5% to 7%), abdominal pain (2% to 6%), constipation (2%)

Hepatic: LFTs abnormal (3%)

Respiratory: Rhinitis (5% to 9%), cough (4%), dyspnea (2%), pneumonia (2%), sinusitis (2%), sputum increased (2%)

Miscellaneous: Diaphoresis increased (3%)

Available Dosage Forms

Capsule, oral: 100 mg

Sporanox®: 100 mg

Solution, oral:

Sporanox®: 10 mg/mL (150 mL)

General Dosage Range Dosage adjustment recommended in patients with renal impairment

Oral: *Adults:* 100-800 mg/day; doses >200 mg/day are given in 2-3 divided doses

Administration

Oral Doses >200 mg/day are given in 2 divided doses; do not administer with antacids. Capsule and oral solution formulations are not bioequivalent and thus are not interchangeable. Capsule absorption is best if taken with food, therefore, it is best to administer itraconazole after meals; solution should be taken on an empty stomach. When treating oropharyngeal and esophageal candidiasis, solution should be swished vigorously in mouth, then swallowed.

Stability

Storage

Capsule: Store at room temperature, 15°C to 25°C (59°F to 77°F). Protect from light and moisture.

Oral solution: Store at ≤25°C (77°F); do not freeze.

Nursing Actions

Patient Education Treatment for some fungal infections may take several weeks or months. Take capsule immediately after meals; take solution on empty stomach (1 hour before or 2 hours after meals). Frequent blood tests may be required with prolonged therapy. May cause dizziness, drowsiness, nausea, vomiting, or anorexia. Report any rash, any change in hearing acuity, difficulty breathing, or chest pain. Report any signs and symptoms of liver dysfunction (eg, unusual fatigue, anorexia, nausea and/or vomiting, jaundice [yellowing of skin or sclera], dark urine, pale stool) so that the appropriate laboratory testing can be done.

Dietary Considerations

Capsule: Take with food.

Solution: Take without food, if possible.

Ivacaftor (eye va KAF tor)

Brand Names: U.S. Kalydeco™

Index Terms VX-770

Pharmacologic Category Cystic Fibrosis Transmembrane Conductance Regulator Potentiator

Pregnancy Risk Factor B

Lactation Excretion unknown/use caution

Use Treatment of cystic fibrosis (CF) in patients who have a G551D mutation in the cystic fibrosis transmembrane conductance regulator (CFTR) gene

Note: Not effective in patients with CF who are homozygous for the F508del mutation in the CTFR gene

Available Dosage Forms

Tablet, oral:

Kalydeco™: 150 mg

General Dosage Range Dosage adjustment recommended in patients with hepatic impairment or on concomitant therapy.

Oral: *Children ≥6 years and Adults:* 150 mg every 12 hours

Administration

Oral Administer with high-fat-containing foods (eg, butter, cheese pizza, eggs, peanut butter).

Nursing Actions

Physical Assessment Monitor for liver function tests on a routine basis; educate patient about need to take with fatty foods. Assess pulmonary exam with use.

Patient Education Educate patient about need to take with fatty foods; avoid grapefruit juice and Seville oranges. Side effects include headache, abdominal pain, nausea, vomiting, diarrhea, sore throat, and runny nose. Instruct patient to call prescriber if there is a bad reaction to the drug, abdominal pain, nausea or vomiting, dark urine, yellow skin or eyes, not able to eat, or development of a rash.

Ketoconazole (Systemic)
(kee toe KOE na zole)

Pharmacologic Category Antifungal Agent, Oral

Medication Safety Issues

Sound-alike/look-alike issues:

Nizoral® may be confused with Nasarel, Neoral®, Nitrol®

Pregnancy Risk Factor C

Lactation Enters breast milk/not recommended

Use Treatment of susceptible fungal infections, including candidiasis, oral thrush, blastomycosis, histoplasmosis, paracoccidioidomycosis, coccidioidomycosis, chromomycosis, candiduria, chronic mucocutaneous candidiasis, as well as certain recalcitrant cutaneous dermatophytoses

Unlabeled Use Treatment of prostate cancer (androgen synthesis inhibitor)

Available Dosage Forms

Tablet, oral: 200 mg

General Dosage Range Oral:

Children ≥2 years: 3.3-6.6 mg/kg once daily

Adults: 200-400 mg once daily

Administration

Oral Administer oral tablets 2 hours prior to antacids to prevent decreased absorption due to the high pH of gastric contents.

Nursing Actions

Physical Assessment Monitor liver function on a regular basis. Teach patient necessity of completing full therapy and importance of adequate hydration.

Patient Education Maintain adequate hydration unless instructed to restrict fluid intake. Cream, foam, gel, and shampoo are for external use only. Use full course of medication; some infections may require long periods of therapy. May cause nausea and vomiting. Report unresolved headache, rash or itching, yellowing of eyes or skin, changes in color of urine or stool, chest pain or palpitations, sense of fullness or ringing in ears, or if condition worsens.

Ketoconazole (Topical) (kee toe KOE na zole)

Brand Names: U.S. Extina®; Nizoral®; Nizoral® A-D [OTC]; Xolegel®

Pharmacologic Category Antifungal Agent, Topical

Medication Safety Issues

Sound-alike/look-alike issues:

Nizoral® may be confused with Nasarel, Neoral®, Nitrol®

Pregnancy Risk Factor C

Lactation Excretion in breast milk unknown/use caution

Use

Cream: Treatment of tinea corporis, tinea cruris, tinea versicolor, cutaneous candidiasis, seborrheic dermatitis

Foam, gel: Treatment of seborrheic dermatitis

Shampoo: Treatment of dandruff, seborrheic dermatitis, tinea versicolor

Unlabeled Use Cream: Treatment of susceptible fungal infections in the oral cavity including candidiasis, oral thrush, and chronic mucocutaneous candidiasis

Available Dosage Forms

Aerosol, foam, topical: 2% (50 g, 100 g)

Extina®: 2% (50 g, 100 g)

Cream, topical: 2% (15 g, 30 g, 60 g)

Gel, topical:

Xolegel®: 2% (45 g)

Shampoo, topical: 2% (120 mL)

Nizoral®: 2% (120 mL)

Nizoral® A-D [OTC]: 1% (120 mL, 210 mL)

General Dosage Range Topical:

Cream: *Children ≥12 years and Adults:* Rub gently into the affected area 1-2 times daily

Foam: *Children ≥12 years and Adults:* Apply to affected area twice daily

Gel: *Children ≥12 years and Adults:* Apply gently to affected area once daily

Shampoo: *Children ≥12 years and Adults:* Apply up to twice weekly

Administration

Topical Cream, foam, gel, and shampoo are for external use only. Avoid exposure to flame or smoking immediately following application of gel or foam; do not apply directly to hands.

Nursing Actions

Physical Assessment Teach patient proper administration or application and necessity of completing full therapy.

Patient Education Cream, foam, gel, and shampoo are for external use only.

Cream, foam, and gel: Wash hands thoroughly before and after applying; keep away from eyes or mouth. Keep Extina foam can away from open fire, flame, or direct heat (Extina foam is flammable). You may experience some burning, dryness, irritation, or rash at site of application. Report severe or persistent adverse effects or if condition worsens.

Shampoo: May cause some temporary hair loss, scalp irritation, itching, or change in hair texture. Report severe or persistent adverse effects or if condition worsens.

Ketoprofen (kee toe PROE fen)

Pharmacologic Category Nonsteroidal Anti-inflammatory Drug (NSAID), Oral

Medication Safety Issues

Sound-alike/look-alike issues:

Ketoprofen may be confused with ketotifen

Medication Guide Available Yes

Pregnancy Risk Factor C

Lactation Enters breast milk

Use Acute and long-term treatment of rheumatoid arthritis and osteoarthritis; primary dysmenorrhea; mild-to-moderate pain

Available Dosage Forms

Capsule, oral: 50 mg, 75 mg

Capsule, extended release, oral: 200 mg

General Dosage Range Dosage adjustment recommended in patients with hepatic and renal impairment

Oral:

Extended release: *Adults:* 200 mg once daily

Regular release: *Adults:* 25-50 mg 4 times/day or 75 mg 3 times/day (maximum: 300 mg/day)

Administration

Oral May take with food to reduce GI upset. Do not crush or break extended release capsules.

Nursing Actions

Physical Assessment Monitor blood pressure at the beginning of therapy and periodically during use. Monitor for GI effects, hepatotoxicity, and ototoxicity at beginning of therapy and periodically throughout therapy. Schedule ophthalmic evaluations for patients who develop eye complaints during long-term NSAID therapy.

Patient Education Do not break capsules. Take with food or milk to reduce GI distress. Do not use alcohol. You may experience drowsiness, dizziness, nervousness, headache, anorexia, nausea, vomiting, heartburn, or fluid retention; GI bleeding, ulceration, or perforation can occur with or without pain; discontinue medication and contact prescriber if persistent abdominal pain or cramping or blood in stool occurs. Report respiratory difficulty or unusual cough; chest pain or rapid heartbeat; bruising/bleeding; blood in urine, stool, mouth, or vomitus; swollen extremities; skin rash or itching; hearing changes (ringing in ears); jaundice; right upper quadrant tenderness; or flu-like symptoms.

Ketorolac (Systemic) (KEE toe role ak)

Index Terms Ketorolac Tromethamine; Toradol

Pharmacologic Category Nonsteroidal Anti-inflammatory Drug (NSAID), Oral; Nonsteroidal Anti-inflammatory Drug (NSAID), Parenteral

Medication Safety Issues

Sound-alike/look-alike issues:

Ketorolac may be confused with Ketalar®

Toradol® may be confused with Foradil®, Inderal®, TEGretol®, traMADol, tromethamine

Beers Criteria medication:

This drug may be inappropriate for use in geriatric patients (high severity risk).

International issues:

Toradol [Canada and multiple international markets] may be confused with Theradol brand name for tramadol [Netherlands]

Medication Guide Available Yes

Pregnancy Risk Factor C

Lactation Enters breast milk/contraindicated (per manufacturer's labeling)

Breast-Feeding Considerations Low concentrations of ketorolac are found in breast milk (milk concentrations were <1% of the weight-adjusted maternal dose in one study). **[U.S. Boxed Warning]: Inhibition of prostaglandin synthesis may adversely affect neonates; use of systemic ketorolac is contraindicated in breast-feeding women.** The manufacturer of the ophthalmic product recommends that caution be used if administered to a breast-feeding woman. The maternal pharmacokinetics of ketorolac were not found to change immediately postpartum.

Use Short-term (≤5 days) management of moderate-to-severe acute pain requiring analgesia at the opioid level

Mechanism of Action/Effect Reversibly inhibits cyclooxygenase-1 and 2 (COX-1 and 2) enzymes, which results in decreased formation of prostaglandin precursors; has antipyretic, analgesic, and anti-inflammatory properties

Contraindications Hypersensitivity to ketorolac, aspirin, other NSAIDs, or any component of the formulation; active or history of peptic ulcer disease; recent or history of GI bleeding or perforation; patients with advanced renal disease or risk of renal failure (due to volume depletion); prophylaxis before major surgery; suspected or confirmed cerebrovascular bleeding; hemorrhagic diathesis, incomplete hemostasis, or high risk of bleeding; concurrent ASA or other NSAIDs; concomitant probenecid or pentoxifylline; epidural or intrathecal administration; perioperative pain in the setting of coronary artery bypass graft (CABG) surgery; labor and delivery; breast-feeding

Warnings/Precautions [U.S. Boxed Warning]: May inhibit platelet function; contraindicated in patients with cerebrovascular bleeding (suspected or confirmed), hemorrhagic diathesis, incomplete hemostasis and patients at high risk for bleeding. Effects on platelet adhesion and aggregation may prolong bleeding time. Anemia may occur; patients on long-term NSAID therapy should be monitored for anemia. Rarely, NSAID use has been associated with potentially severe blood dyscrasias (eg, agranulocytosis, thrombocytopenia, aplastic anemia).

[U.S. Boxed Warning]: NSAIDs are associated with an increased risk of adverse cardiovascular thrombotic events, including MI and stroke. Risk may be increased with duration of use or pre-existing cardiovascular risk factors or disease. Carefully evaluate individual cardiovascular risk profiles prior to prescribing. May cause new-onset hypertension or worsening of existing hypertension. Use caution with fluid retention. Avoid use in heart failure. Concurrent administration of ibuprofen, and potentially other nonselective NSAIDs, may interfere with aspirin's cardioprotective effect. **[U.S. Boxed Warning]: Use is contraindicated as prophylactic analgesic before any major**

surgery and is contraindicated for treatment of perioperative pain in the setting of coronary artery bypass graft (CABG) surgery. Risk of MI and stroke may be increased with use following CABG surgery. Wound bleeding and postoperative hematomas have been associated with ketorolac use in the perioperative setting. Withhold for at least 4-6 half-lives prior to surgical or dental procedures.

[U.S. Boxed Warning]: Ketorolac is contraindicated in patients with advanced renal impairment and in patients at risk for renal failure due to volume depletion. NSAID use may compromise existing renal function; dose-dependent decreases in prostaglandin synthesis may result from NSAID use, reducing renal blood flow which may cause renal decompensation. NSAID use may increase the risk for hyperkalemia. Patients with impaired renal function, dehydration, heart failure, liver dysfunction, those taking diuretics and ACE inhibitors, and the elderly are at greater risk of renal toxicity. Use with caution in patients with impaired renal function or history of kidney disease; dosage adjustment is required in patients with moderate elevation in serum creatinine. Monitor renal function closely. Acute renal failure, interstitial nephritis, and nephrotic syndrome have been reported with ketorolac use; papillary necrosis and renal injury have been reported with the use of NSAIDs. Use of NSAIDs can compromise existing renal function. Rehydrate patient before starting therapy.

[U.S. Boxed Warning]: NSAIDs may increase risk of gastrointestinal irritation, inflammation, ulceration, bleeding, and perforation. These events may occur at any time during therapy and without warning. Use caution with a history of GI disease (bleeding, ulcers, inflammatory bowel disease), concurrent therapy with aspirin, anticoagulants and/or corticosteroids, smoking, use of alcohol, the elderly, or debilitated patients. When used concomitantly with ≤325 mg of aspirin, a substantial increase in the risk of gastrointestinal complications (eg, ulcer) occurs; concomitant gastroprotective therapy (eg, proton pump inhibitors) is recommended (Bhatt, 2008).

NSAIDs may cause serious skin adverse events including exfoliative dermatitis, Stevens-Johnson syndrome (SJS), and toxic epidermal necrolysis (TEN); discontinue use at first sign of skin rash or hypersensitivity. Hypersensitivity or anaphylactoid reactions may occur, even without prior exposure; patients with "aspirin triad" (bronchial asthma, aspirin intolerance, rhinitis) may be at increased risk. Do not use in patients who experience bronchospasm, asthma, rhinitis, or urticaria with NSAID or aspirin therapy. **[U.S. Boxed Warning]: Ketorolac injection is contraindicated in patients with prior hypersensitivity reaction to aspirin or NSAIDs.** Use caution in other forms of asthma.

Use with caution in patients with hepatic impairment or a history of liver disease. Closely monitor patients with any abnormal LFT. Rarely, severe hepatic reactions (eg, fulminant hepatitis, hepatic necrosis, liver failure) have occurred with NSAID use; discontinue if signs or symptoms of liver disease develop, or if systemic manifestations occur.

[U.S. Boxed Warning]: Dosage adjustment is required for patients ≥65 years of age. The elderly are at increased risk for adverse effects (especially peptic ulceration, CNS effects, renal toxicity) from NSAIDs, even at low doses. Avoid immediate and long-term use (Beers Criteria). **[U.S. Boxed Warning]: Dosage adjustment is required for patients weighing <50 kg (<110 pounds). [U.S. Boxed Warning]: May inhibit uterine contractions and affect fetal circulation; inhibits prostaglandin synthesis in neonates; use is contraindicated in labor and delivery and breast-feeding women.** Avoid use in late pregnancy. **[U.S. Boxed Warning]: Concurrent use of ketorolac with aspirin or other NSAIDs is contraindicated due to the increased risk of adverse reactions.**

[U.S. Boxed Warning]: Contraindicated for epidural or intrathecal administration. [U.S. Boxed Warning]: Systemic ketorolac is indicated for short term (≤5 days) use in adults for treatment of moderately severe acute pain requiring opioid-level analgesia. Low doses of narcotics may be needed for breakthrough pain. **[U.S. Boxed Warning]: Oral therapy is only indicated for use as continuation treatment, following parenteral ketorolac and is not indicated for minor or chronic painful conditions. The maximum daily oral dose is 40 mg (adults); doses above 40 mg/day do not improve efficacy but may increase the risk of serious adverse effects.** The combined therapy duration (oral and parenteral) should not exceed 5 days. Use the lowest effective dose for the shortest duration of time, consistent with individual patient goals, to reduce risk of cardiovascular or GI adverse events. Alternate therapies should be considered for patients at high risk. **[U.S. Boxed Warning]: Oral ketorolac is not indicated for use in children.**

NSAIDS may cause drowsiness, dizziness, blurred vision and other neurologic effects which may impair physical or mental abilities; patients must be cautioned about performing tasks which require mental alertness (eg, operating machinery or driving). Discontinue use with blurred or diminished vision and perform ophthalmologic exam. Monitor vision with long-term therapy.

Drug Interactions

Avoid Concomitant Use

Avoid concomitant use of Ketorolac (Systemic) with any of the following: Aspirin; Floctafenine; Ketorolac; Ketorolac (Nasal); Nonsteroidal Anti-Inflammatory Agents; Pentoxifylline; Probenecid

Decreased Effect

Ketorolac (Systemic) may decrease the levels/effects of: ACE Inhibitors; Aliskiren; Angiotensin II Receptor Blockers; Anticonvulsants; Antiplatelet Agents; Beta-Blockers; Eplerenone; HydrALAZINE; Loop Diuretics; Potassium-Sparing Diuretics; Salicylates; Selective Serotonin Reuptake Inhibitors; Thiazide Diuretics

The levels/effects of Ketorolac (Systemic) may be decreased by: Bile Acid Sequestrants; Salicylates

Increased Effect/Toxicity

Ketorolac (Systemic) may increase the levels/effects of: Aliskiren; Aminoglycosides; Anticoagulants; Antiplatelet Agents; Aspirin; Bisphosphonate Derivatives; Collagenase (Systemic); CycloSPORINE; CycloSPORINE (Systemic); Deferasirox; Desmopressin; Digoxin; Drotrecogin Alfa (Activated); Eplerenone; Haloperidol; Ibritumomab; Lithium; Methotrexate; Neuromuscular-Blocking Agents (Nondepolarizing); Nonsteroidal Anti-Inflammatory Agents; PEMEtrexed; Pentoxifylline; Porfimer; Potassium-Sparing Diuretics; PRALAtrexate; Quinolone Antibiotics; Rivaroxaban; Salicylates; Thrombolytic Agents; Tositumomab and Iodine I 131 Tositumomab; Vancomycin; Vitamin K Antagonists

The levels/effects of Ketorolac (Systemic) may be increased by: ACE Inhibitors; Angiotensin II Receptor Blockers; Antidepressants (Tricyclic, Tertiary Amine); Corticosteroids (Systemic); CycloSPORINE; CycloSPORINE (Systemic); Dasatinib; Floctafenine; Glucosamine; Herbs (Anticoagulant/Antiplatelet Properties); Ketorolac; Ketorolac (Nasal); Omega-3-Acid Ethyl Esters; Pentosan Polysulfate Sodium; Probenecid; Prostacyclin Analogues; Selective Serotonin Reuptake Inhibitors; Serotonin/Norepinephrine Reuptake Inhibitors; Sodium Phosphates; Treprostinil; Vitamin E

Nutritional/Ethanol Interactions

Ethanol: Avoid ethanol (may enhance gastric mucosal irritation).

Food: Oral: High-fat meals may delay time to peak (by ~1 hour) and decrease peak concentrations.

Herb/Nutraceutical: Avoid alfalfa, anise, bilberry, bladderwrack, bromelain, cat's claw, celery, chamomile, coleus, cordyceps, dong quai, evening primrose, fenugreek, feverfew, garlic, ginger, ginkgo biloba, ginseng (American, Panax, Siberian), grapeseed, green tea, guggul, horse chestnut seed, horseradish, licorice, prickly ash, red clover, reishi, SAMe (S-adenosylmethionine), sweet clover, turmeric, and white willow (all have additional antiplatelet activity).

Adverse Reactions

Frequencies noted for parenteral administration:

>10%:

Central nervous system: Headache (17%)

Gastrointestinal: Gastrointestinal pain (13%), dyspepsia (12%), nausea (12%)

>1% to 10%:

Cardiovascular: Edema (4%), hypertension

Central nervous system: Dizziness (7%), drowsiness (6%)

Dermatologic: Pruritus, purpura, rash

Gastrointestinal: Diarrhea (7%), constipation, flatulence, GI bleeding, GI fullness, GI perforation, GI ulcer, heartburn, stomatitis, vomiting

Hematologic: Anemia, bleeding time increased

Hepatic: Liver enzymes increased

Local: Injection site pain (2%)

Otic: Tinnitus

Renal: Renal function abnormal

Miscellaneous: Diaphoresis

Pharmacodynamics/Kinetics

Onset of Action Analgesic: I.M.: ~10 minutes; Peak effect: Analgesic: 2-3 hours

Duration of Action Analgesic: 6-8 hours

Available Dosage Forms

Injection, solution: 15 mg/mL (1 mL, 2 mL); 30 mg/mL (1 mL, 2 mL, 10 mL)

Tablet, oral: 10 mg

General Dosage Range

Dosage adjustment recommended in patients with renal impairment

I.M.:

Children ≥16 years and Adults <50 kg and Elderly ≥65 years: 30 mg as a single dose **or** 15 mg every 6 hours (maximum: 60 mg/day)

Children ≥16 years and Adults ≥50 kg: 60 mg as a single dose **or** 30 mg every 6 hours (maximum: 120 mg/day)

I.V.:

Children ≥16 years and Adults <50 kg and Elderly ≥65 years: 15 mg as a single dose **or** 15 mg every 6 hours (maximum: 60 mg/day)

Children ≥16 years and Adults ≥50 kg: 30 mg as a single dose **or** 30 mg every 6 hours (maximum: 120 mg/day)

Oral:

Children ≥17 years and Adults <50 kg and Elderly ≥65 years: 10 mg every 4-6 hours (maximum: 40 mg/day)

Children ≥17 years and Adults ≥50 kg: 20 mg, followed by 10 mg every 4-6 hours (maximum: 40 mg/day)

Administration

Oral May take with food to reduce GI upset.

I.M. Administer slowly and deeply into the muscle. Analgesia begins in 30 minutes and maximum effect within 2 hours.

I.V. Administer I.V. bolus over a minimum of 15 seconds; onset within 30 minutes; peak analgesia within 2 hours.

I.V. Detail pH: 6.9-7.9

Stability

Storage

Injection: Store at room temperature of 15°C to 30°C (59°F to 86°F). Protect from light. Injection is clear and has a slight yellow color. Precipitation may occur at relatively low pH values.

Tablet: Store at room temperature of 15°C to 30°C (59°F to 86°F).

Nursing Actions

Physical Assessment Assess allergy history prior to treatment. I.V./I.M.: Monitor vital signs on a regular basis during infusion or following injection. Oral: Monitor blood pressure prior to treatment and periodically throughout.

Patient Education Do not take aspirin-containing products or any other NSAIDs during therapy unless approved by prescriber. Oral doses may be taken with food or milk. Avoid alcohol. Maintain adequate hydration unless instructed to restrict fluid intake. May cause nausea or vomiting. Report blood in vomitus or stool or other signs of unusual bleeding, abdominal pain, weakness, slurring of speech, ringing in ears, unresolved nausea or vomiting, respiratory difficulty or shortness of breath, skin rash, unusual swelling of extremities, unexplained weight gain, chest pain, or palpitations.

Dietary Considerations Administer tablet with food or milk to decrease gastrointestinal distress.

Ketorolac (Nasal) (KEE toe role ak)

Brand Names: U.S. Sprix®

Index Terms Ketorolac Tromethamine

Pharmacologic Category Nonsteroidal Anti-inflammatory Drug (NSAID), Nasal

Medication Safety Issues

Sound-alike/look-alike issues:

Ketorolac may be confused with Ketalar®

BEERS Criteria medication:

This drug may be inappropriate for use in geriatric patients (high severity risk).

Medication Guide Available Yes

Pregnancy Risk Factor C/D ≥30 weeks gestation

Lactation Enters breast milk/contraindicated (per manufacturer's labeling)

Use Short-term (≤5 days) management of moderate-to-moderately-severe acute pain requiring analgesia at the opioid level

Available Dosage Forms

Solution, intranasal [preservative free]:

Sprix®: 15.75 mg/spray (1.7 g)

General Dosage Range Dosage adjustment recommended in patients with renal impairment.

Intranasal:

Adults <65 years and ≥50 kg: one spray (15.75 mg) in each nostril (total dose: 31.5 mg) every 6-8 hours; maximum dose: 4 doses (126 mg)/day

Adults <50 kg and/or Elderly ≥65 years: One spray (15.75 mg) in 1 nostril (total dose: 15.75 mg) every 6-8 hours; maximum dose: 4 doses (63 mg)/day

Administration

Inhalation Each nasal spray contains medication for 1 day of therapy. Before first use of a nasal spray container, prime by pressing pump 5 times. There is no need to prime the pump again if more doses are administered during the next 24 hours using the same nasal container. Repeat priming each day prior to first use of each new nasal spray. Blow nose to clear nostrils. Sit up straight or stand; tilt head slightly forward. Insert tip of container into nostril, keeping bottle upright, and point container away from the center of nose. Spray once, pressing down evenly on both sides of container.

Discard container within 24 hours of priming even if there is unused medication.

Ketorolac (Ophthalmic) (KEE toe role ak)

Brand Names: U.S. Acular LS®; Acular®; Acuvail®

Index Terms Ketorolac Tromethamine

Pharmacologic Category Nonsteroidal Anti-inflammatory Drug (NSAID), Ophthalmic

Medication Safety Issues

Sound-alike/look-alike issues:

Acular® may be confused with Acthar®, Ocular

Ketorolac may be confused with Ketalar®

Pregnancy Risk Factor C

Lactation Use caution

Use Temporary relief of ocular itching due to seasonal allergic conjunctivitis; postoperative inflammation following cataract extraction; reduction of ocular pain and photophobia following incisional refractive surgery; reduction of ocular pain, burning, and stinging following corneal refractive surgery

Available Dosage Forms

Solution, ophthalmic: 0.4% (5 mL); 0.5% (3 mL, 5 mL, 10 mL)

Acular LS®: 0.4% (5 mL)

Acular®: 0.5% (5 mL)

Solution, ophthalmic [preservative free]:

Acuvail®: 0.45% (0.4 mL)

General Dosage Range Ophthalmic: *Children ≥3 years and Adults:* Instill 1 drop (0.25 mg) 4 times/day to eye(s)

Administration

Other Contact lenses should be removed before instillation. Acular® and Acular LS® have been safely administered with other ophthalmic medications including antibiotics, beta-blockers, carbonic anhydrase inhibitors, cycloplegics, and mydriatics.

Nursing Actions

Patient Education Wash hands before instilling. Sit or lie down to instill. Open eye, look at ceiling, and instill prescribed amount of solution. Close eye and roll eye in all directions. Apply gentle pressure to inner corner of eye for 1-2 minutes after instillation. Do not let tip of applicator touch eye; do not contaminate tip of applicator (may cause eye infection, eye damage, or vision loss). Temporary stinging or blurred vision may occur. Do not wear soft contact lenses. Report persistent pain, burning, double vision, swelling, itching, or worsening of condition.

Ketotifen (Systemic) (kee toe TYE fen)

Index Terms Ketotifen Fumarate

Pharmacologic Category Histamine H_1 Antagonist; Histamine H_1 Antagonist, Second Generation; Mast Cell Stabilizer; Piperidine Derivative

Medication Safety Issues

Sound-alike/look-alike issues:

Ketotifen may be confused with ketoprofen

Zaditen® may be confused with Zaditor®

Lactation Enters breast milk/not recommended

Use Adjunctive therapy in the chronic treatment of pediatric patients ≥6 months of age with mild, atopic asthma

Mechanism of Action/Effect Relatively selective, noncompetitive H_1-receptor antagonist and mast cell stabilizer, inhibiting the release of mediators from cells involved in hypersensitivity reactions

Contraindications Hypersensitivity to ketotifen or any component of the formulation; use of ketotifen syrup in patients sensitive to benzoate compounds

Warnings/Precautions Indicated for prophylactic treatment; not effective for the prevention or treatment of acute asthma attacks. Therapy for acute symptoms of asthma (eg, corticosteroids, beta2-agonists, xanthine derivatives) should be maintained and gradually reduced. Several weeks of oral ketotifen therapy may be needed to observe clinical response while maximum therapeutic response usually requires duration of therapy ≥10 weeks. Therapy should be maintained for at least 2-3 months to determine effectiveness. If therapy requires discontinuation, gradually reduce over 2-4 weeks. Oral dosage forms may cause sedation early in therapy. Sedative effects may be reduced by initiating therapy at one-half the recommended daily dose with gradual increase over 5 days to maintenance dose.

Caution patients about performing tasks which require mental alertness (eg, driving or operating machinery). Thrombocytopenia has occurred rarely when used concomitantly with oral antidiabetic agents. Use with caution in epileptic patients; may lower seizure threshold. Use caution in diabetics and individuals with benzoate allergies as the syrup preparation contains carbohydrates and benzoate compounds.

Adverse Reactions 1% to 10%:

Central nervous system: Sedation (8%; less than placebo), headache (1%), sleep disturbance (1%)

Dermatologic: Rash (4%), urticaria (1%)

Gastrointestinal: Weight gain (5%), abdominal pain (1%), appetite increased (1%)

Respiratory: Respiratory infection (4%), epistaxis (1%)

Miscellaneous: Flu (3%), puffy eyelid (1%)

Product Availability Not available in the U.S.

General Dosage Range Oral:

Children 6 months to 3 years: Initial: 0.05 mg/kg once daily or in 2 divided doses for 5 days; Maintenance: 0.05 mg/kg twice daily (maximum dose: 1 mg twice daily)

Children >3 years: Initial: 1 mg once daily or in 2 divided doses for 5 days; Maintenance: 1 mg twice daily

Administration

Oral Administer without regards to meals.

Stability

Storage

Syrup: Store at up to 25°C (up to 77°F).

Tablet: Store at up to 25°C (up to 77°F). Protect from moisture.

Dietary Considerations May be taken without regard to meals. Syrup contains carbohydrate 4 g/5 mL.

Labetalol (la BET a lole)

Brand Names: U.S. Trandate®

Index Terms Ibidomide Hydrochloride; Labetalol Hydrochloride

Pharmacologic Category Beta Blocker With Alpha-Blocking Activity

Medication Safety Issues

Sound-alike/look-alike issues:

Labetalol may be confused with betaxolol, lamoTRIgine, Lipitor®

Normodyne® may be confused with Norpramin®

Trandate® may be confused with traMADol, TRENtal®

High alert medication:

The Institute for Safe Medication Practices (ISMP) includes this medication among its list of drugs which have a heightened risk of causing significant patient harm when used in error.

Administration issues:

Significant differences exist between oral and I.V. dosing. Use caution when converting from one route of administration to another.

Pregnancy Risk Factor C

Lactation Enters breast milk/use caution (AAP rates "compatible"; AAP 2001 update pending)

Breast-Feeding Considerations Low amounts of labetalol are found in breast milk and can be detected in the serum of nursing infants. The manufacturer recommends that caution be exercised when administering labetalol to nursing women.

Use Treatment of mild-to-severe hypertension; I.V. for severe hypertension (eg, hypertensive emergencies)

Unlabeled Use Pediatric hypertension; management of pre-eclampsia; severe hypertension in pregnancy; hypertension during acute ischemic stroke

Mechanism of Action/Effect Blocks alpha-, $beta_1$-, and $beta_2$-adrenergic receptor sites; elevated renins are reduced. The ratios of alpha- to beta-blockade differ depending on the route of administration: 1:3 (oral) and 1:7 (I.V.).

Contraindications Hypersensitivity to labetalol or any component of the formulation; severe bradycardia; heart block greater than first degree (except in patients with a functioning artificial pacemaker); cardiogenic shock; bronchial asthma; uncompensated cardiac failure; conditions associated with severe and prolonged hypotension

Warnings/Precautions Consider pre-existing conditions such as sick sinus syndrome before initiating. Symptomatic hypotension with or without syncope may occur with labetalol; close monitoring of patient is required especially with initial dosing and dosing increases; blood pressure must be lowered at a rate appropriate for the patient's clinical condition. Initiation with a low dose and gradual up-titration may help to decrease the occurrence of hypotension or syncope. Patients should be advised to avoid driving or other hazardous tasks during initiation of therapy due to the risk of syncope. Orthostatic hypotension may occur with I.V. administration; patient should remain supine during and for up to 3 hours after I.V. administration. Use with caution in impaired hepatic function; bioavailability is increased due to decreased first-pass metabolism. Severe hepatic injury including some fatalities have also been rarely reported with use: periodically monitor LFTs with prolonged use. Use with caution in patients with diabetes mellitus; may potentiate hypoglycemia and/or mask signs and symptoms. Bradycardia may be observed more frequently in elderly patients (>65 years of age); dosage reductions may be necessary. May also reduce release of insulin in response to hyperglycemia; dosage of antidiabetic agents may need to be adjusted. May mask signs of hyperthyroidism (eg, tachycardia); if hyperthyroidism is suspected, carefully manage and monitor; abrupt withdrawal may exacerbate symptoms of hyperthyroidism or precipitate thyroid storm. Elimination of labetalol is reduced in elderly patients; lower maintenance doses may be required.

Use only with extreme caution in compensated heart failure and monitor for a worsening of the condition. Beta-blocker therapy should not be withdrawn abruptly (particularly in patients with CAD), but gradually tapered to avoid acute tachycardia, hypertension, and/or ischemia. Chronic beta-blocker therapy should not be routinely withdrawn prior to major surgery. Use caution with concurrent use of digoxin, verapamil, or diltiazem; bradycardia or heart block can occur. Use with caution in patients receiving inhaled anesthetic agents known to depress myocardial contractility. Patients with bronchospastic disease should not receive beta-blockers; if used at all, should be used cautiously with close monitoring. Use with caution in patients with myasthenia gravis or psychiatric disease (may cause or exacerbate CNS depression). Can precipitate or aggravate symptoms of arterial insufficiency in patients with PVD and Raynaud's disease; use with caution and monitor for progression of arterial obstruction. If possible, obtain diagnostic tests for pheochromocytoma prior to use. May induce or exacerbate psoriasis. Labetalol has been shown to be effective in lowering blood pressure and relieving symptoms in patients with pheochromocytoma. However, some patients have experienced paradoxical hypertensive responses; use with caution in patients with pheochromocytoma. Additional alpha-blockade may be required during use of labetalol. Use caution with history of severe anaphylaxis to allergens; patients taking beta-blockers may become more sensitive to repeated challenges. Treatment of anaphylaxis (eg, epinephrine) in patients taking beta-blockers may be ineffective or promote undesirable effects.

Drug Interactions

Avoid Concomitant Use

Avoid concomitant use of Labetalol with any of the following: Beta2-Agonists; Floctafenine; Methacholine

Decreased Effect

Labetalol may decrease the levels/effects of: Beta2-Agonists; Theophylline Derivatives

The levels/effects of Labetalol may be decreased by: Barbiturates; Herbs (Hypertensive Properties); Methylphenidate; Nonsteroidal Anti-Inflammatory Agents; Rifamycin Derivatives; Yohimbine

Increased Effect/Toxicity

Labetalol may increase the levels/effects of: Alpha-/Beta-Agonists (Direct-Acting); Alpha1-Blockers; Alpha2-Agonists; Amifostine; Antihypertensives; Antipsychotic Agents (Phenothiazines); Bupivacaine; Cardiac Glycosides; Cholinergic Agonists; Fingolimod; Hypotensive Agents; Insulin; Lidocaine; Lidocaine (Systemic); Lidocaine (Topical); Mepivacaine; Methacholine; Midodrine; RiTUXimab; Sulfonylureas

The levels/effects of Labetalol may be increased by: Acetylcholinesterase Inhibitors; Aminoquinolines (Antimalarial); Amiodarone; Anilidopiperidine Opioids; Antipsychotic Agents (Phenothiazines); Calcium Channel Blockers

(Dihydropyridine); Calcium Channel Blockers (Nondihydropyridine); Diazoxide; Dipyridamole; Disopyramide; Dronedarone; Floctafenine; Herbs (Hypotensive Properties); MAO Inhibitors; Pentoxifylline; Phosphodiesterase 5 Inhibitors; Propafenone; Prostacyclin Analogues; QuiNIDine; Reserpine; Selective Serotonin Reuptake Inhibitors

Nutritional/Ethanol Interactions

Food: Labetalol serum concentrations may be increased if taken with food.

Herb/Nutraceutical: Avoid dong quai if using for hypertension (has estrogenic activity). Avoid ephedra, yohimbe, ginseng (may worsen hypertension). Avoid natural licorice (causes sodium and water retention and increases potassium loss). Avoid garlic (may have increased antihypertensive effect).

Adverse Reactions

>10%:

Cardiovascular: Postural hypotension (I.V. use; ≤58%)

Central nervous system: Dizziness (1% to 20%), fatigue (1% to 11%)

Gastrointestinal: Nausea (≤19%)

1% to 10%:

Cardiovascular: Hypotension (1% to 5%), edema (≤2%), flushing (1%), ventricular arrhythmia (I.V. use; 1%)

Central nervous system: Somnolence (3%), headache (2%), vertigo (1% to 2%)

Dermatologic: Scalp tingling (≤7%), pruritus (1%), rash (1%)

Gastrointestinal: Dyspepsia (≤4%), vomiting (≤3%), taste disturbance (1%)

Genitourinary: Ejaculatory failure (≤5%), impotence (1% to 4%)

Hepatic: Transaminases increased (4%)

Neuromuscular & skeletal: Paresthesia (≤5%), weakness (1%)

Ocular: Vision abnormal (1%)

Renal: BUN increased (≤8%)

Respiratory: Nasal congestion (1% to 6%), dyspnea (2%)

Miscellaneous: Diaphoresis (≤4%)

Other adverse reactions noted with beta-adrenergic blocking agents include mental depression, catatonia, disorientation, short-term memory loss, emotional lability, clouded sensorium, intensification of pre-existing AV block, laryngospasm, respiratory distress, agranulocytosis, thrombocytopenic purpura, nonthrombocytopenic purpura, mesenteric artery thrombosis, and ischemic colitis.

Pharmacodynamics/Kinetics

Onset of Action Oral: 20 minutes to 2 hours; I.V.: 2-5 minutes; Peak effect: Oral: 1-4 hours; I.V.: 5-15 minutes

Duration of Action Blood pressure response:

Oral: 8-12 hours (dose dependent)

I.V.: 2-18 hours (dose dependent; based on single and multiple sequential doses of 0.25-0.5 mg/kg with cumulative dosing up to 3.25 mg/kg)

Available Dosage Forms

Injection, solution: 5 mg/mL (4 mL, 8 mL, 20 mL, 40 mL)

Trandate®: 5 mg/mL (20 mL, 40 mL)

Tablet, oral: 100 mg, 200 mg, 300 mg

Trandate®: 100 mg, 200 mg, 300 mg

General Dosage Range

I.V.:

Children: 0.3-1 mg/kg/dose intermittently **or** 0.4-1 mg/kg/hour infusion (maximum: 3 mg/kg/hour)

Adults: Bolus: 20 mg, may give 40-80 mg at 10-minute intervals; Infusion: 2 mg/minute (maximum: 300 mg total cumulative dose)

Oral: *Adults:* Initial: 100 mg twice daily; Maintenance: 200-800 mg/day in 2 divided doses (maximum: 2.4 g/day)

Administration

I.V. Bolus dose may be administered I.V. push at a rate of 10 mg/minute; may follow with continuous I.V. infusion

I.V. Detail pH: 3-4

Stability

Reconstitution

Standard concentration: 500 mg/250 mL D_5W.

Minimum volume: 250 mL D_5W.

Storage

Tablets: Store at room temperature (refer to manufacturer's labeling for detailed storage requirements). Protect from light and excessive moisture.

Injectable: Store at room temperature (refer to manufacturer's labeling for detailed storage requirements); do not freeze. Protect from light. The solution is clear to slightly yellow.

Parenteral admixture: Stability of parenteral admixture at room temperature (25°C) and refrigeration temperature (4°C): 3 days.

Nursing Actions

Physical Assessment Monitor blood pressure and heart rate prior to and following first dose and with any change in dosage. Caution patients with diabetes to monitor glucose levels closely; beta-blockers may alter glucose tolerance. Monitor for CHF.

Patient Education Take with meals. This medication does not replace other antihypertensive interventions; follow prescriber's instructions for diet and lifestyle changes. If you have diabetes, monitor serum glucose closely and notify prescriber of changes (this medication can alter glycemic response). You may experience drowsiness, dizziness, postural hypotension, or dry mouth. Report altered CNS status (eg, fatigue, depression, numbness or tingling of fingers, toes, or skin), palpitations or slowed heartbeat, respiratory difficulty, edema, or cold extremities.

Lacosamide (la KOE sa mide)

Brand Names: U.S. Vimpat®

Index Terms ADD 234037; Harkoseride; LCM; SPM 927

Pharmacologic Category Anticonvulsant, Miscellaneous

Medication Safety Issues

Sound-alike/look-alike issues:

Lacosamide may be confused with zonisamide

Vimpat® may be confused with Vimovo™

Medication Guide Available Yes

Pregnancy Risk Factor C

Lactation Excretion in breast milk unknown/not recommended

Breast-Feeding Considerations It is unknown if lacosamide is excreted in human milk. Use during lactation only if the potential benefits to the mother outweigh the potential risks to the infant.

Use Adjunctive therapy in the treatment of partial-onset seizures

Mechanism of Action/Effect Lacosamide stabilizes hyperexcitable neuronal membranes and inhibits repetitive neuronal firing to decrease epileptiform activity.

Contraindications There are no contraindications listed in manufacturer's labeling.

Warnings/Precautions Antiepileptics are associated with an increased risk of suicidal behavior/ thoughts with use (regardless of indication); patients should be monitored for signs/symptoms of depression, suicidal tendencies, and other unusual behavior changes during therapy and instructed to inform their healthcare provider immediately if symptoms occur. CNS effects may occur; patients should be cautioned about performing tasks which require alertness (eg, operating machinery or driving). Lacosamide may prolong PR interval; use caution in patients with conduction problems (eg, first/second degree atrioventricular block and sick sinus syndrome without pacemaker), myocardial ischemia, heart failure, or if concurrent use with other drugs that prolong the PR interval; ECG is recommended prior to initiating therapy and when at steady state. During investigational trials, atrial fibrillation/flutter, or syncope occurred slightly more often in patients with diabetic neuropathy and/or cardiovascular disease. Use caution with renal or hepatic impairment; dosage adjustment may be necessary. Multiorgan hypersensitivity reactions can occur (rare); monitor patient and discontinue therapy if necessary. Withdraw therapy gradually (≥1 week) to minimize the potential of increased seizure frequency. Effects with ethanol may be potentiated. Some products may contain phenylalanine.

Drug Interactions

Avoid Concomitant Use There are no known interactions where it is recommended to avoid concomitant use.

Decreased Effect

The levels/effects of Lacosamide may be decreased by: CarBAMazepine; Fosphenytoin; PHENobarbital; Phenytoin

Increased Effect/Toxicity There are no known significant interactions involving an increase in effect.

Nutritional/Ethanol Interactions Ethanol: Avoid ethanol (may increase CNS depression).

Adverse Reactions

>10%:

Central nervous system: Dizziness (31%), headache (13%)

Gastrointestinal: Nausea (11%)

Ocular: Diplopia (11%)

1% to 10%:

Cardiovascular: Syncope (1%; dose-related: >400 mg/day)

Central nervous system: Fatigue (9%), ataxia (8%), somnolence (7%), coordination impaired (4%), vertigo (4%), depression (2%), memory impairment (2%)

Dermatologic: Pruritus (2%)

Gastrointestinal: Vomiting (9%), diarrhea (4%)

Hepatic: ALT increased (1%)

Local: Contusion (3%), skin laceration (3%), injection site pain/discomfort (2.5%), irritation (1%)

Neuromuscular & skeletal: Tremor (7%), gait instability (2%), weakness (2%)

Ocular: Blurred vision (8%), nystagmus (5%)

Controlled Substance C-V

Available Dosage Forms

Injection, solution:

Vimpat®: 10 mg/mL (20 mL)

Solution, oral:

Vimpat®: 10 mg/mL (465 mL)

Tablet, oral:

Vimpat®: 50 mg, 100 mg, 150 mg, 200 mg

General Dosage Range Dosage adjustment recommended in patients with hepatic or renal impairment

Oral: *Adolescents ≥17 years and Adults:* Initial: 50 mg twice daily; Maintenance dose: 200-400 mg/day

Administration

Oral Oral solution, tablets: May be administered with or without food. Oral solution should be administered with a calibrated measuring device (not a household teaspoon or tablespoon).

I.V. Administer over 30-60 minutes. Twice daily I.V. infusions have been used for up to 5 days.

I.V. Detail Can be administered without further dilution or may be mixed with compatible diluents (NS, LR, D_5W). Should not be admixed with other solutions. If diluted, stable for ≤24 hours when stored in glass or PVC bags at room temperature. Discard any unused portion.

pH: 3.5-5

Stability

Reconstitution Injection solution: Can be administered without further dilution or may be mixed with compatible diluents (NS, LR, D_5W).

Storage

Injection: Store at 20°C to 25°C (68°F to 77°F); excursions permitted between 15°C to 30°C (59°F to 86°F). Do not freeze. Stable when mixed with compatible diluents for ≤24 hours in glass or PVC at room temperature of 15°C to 30°C (59°F to 86°F). Any unused portion should be discarded.

Oral solution, tablets: Store at 20°C to 25°C (68°F to 77°F); excursions permitted between 15°C to 30°C (59°F to 86°F). Do not freeze oral solution. Discard any unused portion of oral solution after 7 weeks.

Nursing Actions

Physical Assessment Taper dosage slowly when discontinuing. Do not discontinue abruptly. Monitor for depression. Be alert to suicide ideation. Teach patient safety and seizure precautions.

Patient Education Avoid alcohol. You may experience dizziness, lightheadedness, excessive drowsiness, headaches, nausea, vomiting, tremors, or change in vision. Contact prescriber if symptoms persist. Report signs of suicide ideation or depression.

Dietary Considerations Oral solution and tablets may be taken with or without food. Some products may contain phenylalanine.

Lactulose (LAK tyoo lose)

Brand Names: U.S. Constulose; Enulose; Generlac; Kristalose®

Pharmacologic Category Ammonium Detoxicant; Laxative, Osmotic

Medication Safety Issues

Sound-alike/look-alike issues:

Lactulose may be confused with lactose

Pregnancy Risk Factor B

Lactation Excretion in breast milk unknown/use caution

Use Prevention and treatment of portal-systemic encephalopathy (including hepatic precoma and coma); treatment of constipation

Available Dosage Forms

Crystals for solution, oral:

Kristalose®: 10 g/packet (30s); 20 g/packet (30s)

Solution, oral: 10 g/15 mL (15 mL, 30 mL, 237 mL, 240 mL, 473 mL, 480 mL, 500 mL, 946 mL, 960 mL, 1000 mL, 1890 mL, 1892 mL, 1920 mL)

Constulose: 10 g/15 mL (946 mL)

Enulose: 10 g/15 mL (473 mL)

Solution, oral/rectal: 10 g/15 mL (237 mL, 473 mL, 946 mL, 1920 mL)

Generlac: 10 g/15 mL (473 mL, 1892 mL)

General Dosage Range

Oral:

Infants: 1.7-6.7 g/day (2.5-10 mL/day) in divided doses

Older Children and Adolescents: 26.7-60 g/day (40-90 mL/day) in divided doses

Adults: PSE: 20-30 g (30-45 mL) every hour initially, then 3-4 times/day; Constipation: 10-40 g (15-60 mL) daily

Rectal: *Adults:* Constipation: 200 g (300 mL); may repeat every 4-6 hours

Administration

Oral

Oral solution: May mix with fruit juice, water, or milk.

Crystals for oral solution: Dissolve contents of packet in 120 mL water.

Other Rectal: Mix with water or normal saline; administer as retention enema using a rectal balloon catheter; retain for 30-60 minutes. Transition to oral lactulose when appropriate (able to take oral medication and no longer a risk for aspiration) prior to discontinuing rectal administration.

Nursing Actions

Physical Assessment Monitor therapeutic effectiveness (soft formed stools or resolution of CNS status in PSE). Monitor for CHF. Monitor frequency/consistency of stools. May need to adjust dose for severe diarrhea.

Patient Education Not for long-term use. Take alone or diluted with water, juice or milk, or take with food. Laxative results may not occur for 24-48 hours; do not take more often than recommended or for a longer time than recommended. Do not use any other laxatives while taking lactulose. Do not use if experiencing abdominal pain, nausea, or vomiting. Diarrhea may indicate need to decrease dose. May cause flatulence, belching, or abdominal cramping. Report persistent or severe diarrhea or abdominal cramping.

LamiVUDine (la MI vyoo deen)

Brand Names: U.S. Epivir-HBV®; Epivir®

Index Terms 3TC

Pharmacologic Category Antiretroviral Agent, Reverse Transcriptase Inhibitor (Nucleoside)

Medication Safety Issues

Sound-alike/look-alike issues:

LamiVUDine may be confused with lamoTRIgine

Epivir® may be confused with Combivir®

Pregnancy Risk Factor C

Lactation Enters breast milk/contraindicated

Breast-Feeding Considerations Lamivudine is excreted into breast milk and can be detected in the serum of nursing infants.

Maternal or infant antiretroviral therapy does not completely eliminate the risk of postnatal HIV transmission. In addition, multiclass-resistant virus has been detected in breast-feeding infants despite maternal therapy. Therefore, in the United States, where formula is accessible, affordable, safe, and sustainable, and the risk of infant mortality due to diarrhea and respiratory infections is low, complete avoidance of breast-feeding by HIV-infected women is recommended to decrease potential transmission of HIV (DHHS [perinatal], 2011).

Use

Epivir®: Treatment of HIV infection when antiretroviral therapy is warranted; should always be used as part of a multidrug regimen (at least three antiretroviral agents)

Epivir-HBV®: Treatment of chronic hepatitis B associated with evidence of hepatitis B viral replication and active liver inflammation. Resistance develops rapidly in hepatitis B; consider use only if other anti-HBV antiviral agents with more favorable resistance patterns cannot be used.

Unlabeled Use Postexposure prophylaxis for HIV exposure as part of a multidrug regimen

Mechanism of Action/Effect Lamivudine is a cytosine analog. *In vitro*, lamivudine is phosphorylated to its active 5′-triphosphate metabolite (L-TP), which inhibits HIV reverse transcription via viral DNA chain termination; L-TP also inhibits the RNA- and DNA-dependent DNA polymerase activities of reverse transcriptase. The monophosphate form is incorporated into viral DNA by hepatitis B polymerase, resulting in DNA chain termination.

Contraindications Hypersensitivity to lamivudine or any component of the formulation

Warnings/Precautions Use caution with renal impairment; dosage reduction recommended. Use with extreme caution in children with history of pancreatitis or risk factors for development of pancreatitis. Pancreatitis has been reported, particularly in HIV-infected children with a history of nucleoside use. Do not use as monotherapy in treatment of HIV. Lamivudine combined with emtricitabine is not recommended as a dual-NRTI combination due to similar resistance patterns and negligible additive antiviral activity; lamivudine and tenofovir combination is preferred as the NRTIs in a fully suppressive antiretroviral regimen (DHHS, 2011). Treatment of HBV in patients with unrecognized/untreated HIV may lead to rapid HIV resistance. In addition, treatment of HIV in patients with unrecognized/untreated HBV may lead to rapid HBV resistance. Use with caution in combination with interferon alfa with or without ribavirin in HIV/HBV coinfected patients; monitor closely for hepatic decompensation, anemia, or neutropenia; dose reduction or discontinuation of interferon and/or ribavirin may be required if toxicity evident. In HIV/HBV coinfection, lamivudine and tenofovir are a preferred NRTI backbone in a fully suppressive antiretroviral regimen to provide activity against both HIV and HBV (DHHS, 2011). **[U.S. Boxed Warning]: Do not use Epivir-HBV® tablets or Epivir-HBV® oral solution for the treatment of HIV.**

[U.S. Boxed Warning]: Lactic acidosis and severe hepatomegaly with steatosis have been reported, including fatal cases. Use caution in hepatic impairment. Pregnancy, obesity, and/or prolonged therapy may increase the risk of lactic acidosis and liver damage.

Immune reconstitution syndrome may develop resulting in the occurrence of an inflammatory response to an indolent or residual opportunistic infection. May be associated with fat redistribution.

[U.S. Boxed Warning]: Monitor patients closely for several months following discontinuation of therapy for chronic hepatitis B; clinical exacerbations may occur.

Not recommended as first-line therapy of chronic HBV due to high rate of resistance. Consider use only if other anti-HBV antiviral regimens with more favorable resistance patterns cannot be used. May be appropriate for short-term treatment of acute HBV (Lok, 2009). Potential compliance problems, frequency of administration, and adverse effects should be discussed with patients before initiating therapy to help prevent the emergence of resistance.

Drug Interactions

Avoid Concomitant Use

Avoid concomitant use of LamiVUDine with any of the following: Emtricitabine

Decreased Effect There are no known significant interactions involving a decrease in effect.

Increased Effect/Toxicity

LamiVUDine may increase the levels/effects of: Emtricitabine

The levels/effects of LamiVUDine may be increased by: Ganciclovir-Valganciclovir; Ribavirin; Trimethoprim

Nutritional/Ethanol Interactions Food: Food decreases the rate of absorption and C_{max}; however, there is no change in the systemic AUC. Therefore, may be taken with or without food.

Adverse Reactions Reported for treatment of HIV or HBV in adults. Incidence data include patients on combination therapy with other antiretroviral agents.

>10%:

Central nervous system: Headache (21% to 35%), fatigue (24% to 27%), insomnia (11%)

Gastrointestinal: Nausea (15% to 33%), diarrhea (14% to 18%), pancreatitis (range: 0.3% to 18%; higher percentage in pediatric patients), abdominal pain (9% to 16%), vomiting (13% to 15%)

Hematologic: Neutropenia (7% to 15%)

Hepatic: Transaminases increased (2% to 11%)

Neuromuscular & skeletal: Myalgia (8% to 14%), neuropathy (12%), musculoskeletal pain (12%)
Respiratory: Nasal signs and symptoms (20%), cough (18%), sore throat (13%)
Miscellaneous: Infections (25%; includes ear, nose, and throat)

1% to 10%:

Central nervous system: Dizziness (10%), depression (9%), fever (7% to 10%), chills (7% to 10%)
Dermatologic: Rash (5% to 9%)
Gastrointestinal: Anorexia (10%), lipase increased (10%), abdominal cramps (6%), dyspepsia (5%), amylase increased (<1% to 4%), heartburn
Hematologic: Thrombocytopenia (1% to 4%), hemoglobinemia (2% to 3%)
Neuromuscular & skeletal: Creatine phosphokinase increased (9%), arthralgia (5% to 7%)

Available Dosage Forms

Solution, oral:
Epivir-HBV®: 5 mg/mL
Epivir®: 10 mg/mL

Tablet, oral: 150 mg, 300 mg
Epivir-HBV®: 100 mg
Epivir®: 150 mg, 300 mg

General Dosage Range Dosage adjustment recommended in patients with renal impairment

Oral:

Infants 1-3 months: HIV (DHHS [pediatric], 2010): 4 mg/kg/dose twice daily

Children 3 months to 2 years: HIV: 4 mg/kg/dose twice daily (maximum: 150 mg/dose twice daily)

Children 2-16 years and >16 years and <50 kg: Hepatitis B: 3 mg/kg/dose once daily (maximum: 100 mg/day); HIV: 4 mg/kg/dose twice daily (maximum: 150 mg/dose twice daily)

Children >16 years and ≥50 kg: Hepatitis B: 3 mg/kg/dose once daily (maximum: 100 mg/day); HIV: 150 mg twice daily **or** 300 mg once daily

Adults <50 kg: Hepatitis B: 100 mg/day; HIV (DHHS [pediatric], 2010): 4 mg/kg/dose twice daily (maximum: 150 mg/dose twice daily)

Adults ≥50 kg: Hepatitis B: 100 mg/day; HIV: 150 mg twice daily **or** 300 mg once daily

Administration

Oral May be administered without regard to meals. Adjust dosage in renal failure.

Stability

Storage

Oral solution:
Epivir®: Store at 25°C (77°F) tightly closed.
Epivir-HBV®: Store at 20°C to 25°C (68°F to 77°F) tightly closed.

Tablet: Store at 25°C (77°F); excursions permitted to 15°C to 30°C (59°F to 86°F).

Nursing Actions

Physical Assessment Monitor for headache, fatigue, and insomnia. Monitor patients closely for several months following discontinuation of therapy for chronic hepatitis B. Teach patient timing of multiple medications.

Patient Education Maintain adequate hydration unless instructed to restrict fluid intake. This medication may be prescribed with a combination of other medications; time these medications as directed by prescriber. Take with or without food. Frequent blood tests may be required. May cause nausea, vomiting, abdominal pain, diarrhea, dizziness, insomnia, headache, fever, or muscle pain. Report persistent lethargy or unusual fatigue, yellowing of eyes, pale stool and dark urine, acute headache, severe nausea or vomiting, respiratory difficulty, loss of sensation, or rash.

Dietary Considerations May be taken without regard to meals. Some products may contain sucrose.

Lamivudine and Zidovudine

(la MI vyoo deen & zye DOE vyoo deen)

Brand Names: U.S. Combivir®

Index Terms AZT + 3TC (error-prone abbreviation); Zidovudine and Lamivudine

Pharmacologic Category Antiretroviral Agent, Reverse Transcriptase Inhibitor (Nucleoside)

Medication Safety Issues

Sound-alike/look-alike issues:
Combivir® may be confused with Combivent® Epivir®

Other safety concerns:
AZT is an error-prone abbreviation (mistaken as azaTHIOprine, aztreonam)

Pregnancy Risk Factor C

Lactation See individual agents.

Use Treatment of HIV infection when therapy is warranted based on clinical and/or immunological evidence of disease progression

Available Dosage Forms

Tablet, oral: Lamivudine 150 mg and zidovudine 300 mg
Combivir®: Lamivudine 150 mg and zidovudine 300 mg [scored]

General Dosage Range Oral: *Adolescents ≥30 kg and Adults:* 1 tablet (lamivudine 150 mg/zidovudine 300 mg) twice daily

Nursing Actions

Physical Assessment See individual agents.

Patient Education See individual agents.

Related Information

LamiVUDine *on page 664*
Zidovudine *on page 1197*

LamoTRIgine

(la MOE tri jeen)

Brand Names: U.S. LaMICtal®; LaMICtal® ODT™; LaMICtal® XR™

Index Terms BW-430C; LTG

Pharmacologic Category Anticonvulsant, Miscellaneous

Medication Safety Issues

Sound-alike/look-alike issues:

LamoTRIgine may be confused with labetalol, LamISIL®, lamiVUDine, levothyroxine, Lomotil®

LaMICtal® may be confused with LamISIL®, Lomotil®

Administration issues:

Potential exists for medication errors to occur among different formulations of LaMICtal® (tablets, extended release tablets, orally disintegrating tablets, and chewable/dispersible tablets). Patients should be instructed to visually inspect tablets dispensed to verify receiving the correct medication and formulation. The medication guide includes illustrations to aid in tablet verification.

International issues:

Lamictal [U.S., Canada, and multiple international markets] may be confused with Ludiomil brand name for maprotiline [multiple international markets]

Lamotrigine [U.S., Canada, and multiple international markets] may be confused with Ludiomil brand name for maprotiline [multiple international markets]

Medication Guide Available Yes

Pregnancy Risk Factor C

Lactation Enters breast milk/not recommended (AAP rates "of concern"; AAP 2001 update pending)

Breast-Feeding Considerations Lamotrigine is found in breast milk. In one study, the relative dose to the infant was 9% (range: 2% to 20%) of the weight-adjusted maternal dose. Lamotrigine was measurable in the plasma of nursing infants; adverse events were not observed.

Use Adjunctive therapy in the treatment of generalized seizures of Lennox-Gastaut syndrome, primary generalized tonic-clonic seizures, and partial seizures; conversion to monotherapy in patients with partial seizures who are receiving treatment with valproic acid or a single enzyme-inducing antiepileptic drug (specifically carbamazepine, phenytoin, phenobarbital or primidone); maintenance treatment of bipolar I disorder

Mechanism of Action/Effect A triazine derivative which inhibits release of glutamate (an excitatory amino acid) and inhibits voltage-sensitive sodium channels, which stabilizes neuronal membranes. Lamotrigine has weak inhibitory effect on the $5HT_3$ receptor; *in vitro* inhibits dihydrofolate reductase.

Contraindications Hypersensitivity to lamotrigine or any component of the formulation

Warnings/Precautions [U.S. Boxed Warning]: Severe and potentially life-threatening skin rashes requiring hospitalization have been reported; incidence of serious rash is higher in pediatric patients than adults; risk may be increased by coadministration with valproic acid, higher than recommended starting doses, and exceeding recommended dose titration. The majority of cases occur in the first 8 weeks; however, isolated cases may occur after prolonged treatment or in patients without these risk factors. Discontinue at first sign of rash and do not reinitiate therapy unless rash is clearly not drug related. Rare cases of Stevens-Johnson syndrome, toxic epidermal necrolysis, and angioedema have been reported.

Antiepileptics are associated with an increased risk of suicidal behavior/thoughts with use (regardless of indication); patients should be monitored for signs/symptoms of depression, suicidal tendencies, and other unusual behavior changes during therapy and instructed to inform their healthcare provider immediately if symptoms occur.

A spectrum of hematologic effects have been reported with use (eg, neutropenia, leukopenia, thrombocytopenia, pancytopenia, anemias, and rarely, aplastic anemia and pure red cell aplasia); patients with a previous history of adverse hematologic reaction to any drug may be at increased risk. Early detection of hematologic change is important; advise patients of early signs and symptoms including fever, sore throat, mouth ulcers, infections, easy bruising, petechial or purpuric hemorrhage. May be associated with hypersensitivity syndrome (eg, anticonvulsant hypersensitivity syndrome). Multiorgan hypersensitivity reactions (drug reaction with eosinophilia and systemic symptoms [DRESS]) have been reported. Symptoms may include fever, rash, and/or lymphadenopathy; monitor for signs and symptoms of possible disparate manifestations associated with lymphatic, hepatic, renal, and/or hematologic organ systems. Evaluate patient with fever and lymphadenopathy, even if rash is not present; discontinuation and conversion to alternate therapy may be required. Increased risk of developing aseptic meningitis has been reported; symptoms (eg, headache, nuchal rigidity, fever, nausea/vomiting, rash, photophobia) have generally occurred within 1-45 days following therapy initiation. Use caution in patients with renal or hepatic impairment. Avoid abrupt cessation, taper over at least 2 weeks if possible.

May cause CNS depression, which may impair physical or mental abilities. Patients must be cautioned about performing tasks which require mental alertness (eg, operating machinery or driving). Effects with other sedative drugs or ethanol may be potentiated. Binds to melanin and may accumulate in the eye and other melanin-rich tissues; the clinical significance of this is not known. Safety and efficacy have not been established for use as initial monotherapy, conversion to monotherapy from antiepileptic drugs (AED) other than carbamazepine, phenytoin, phenobarbital, primidone or valproic acid or conversion to monotherapy from two or more AEDs. Patients treated for bipolar disorder should be monitored closely for clinical worsening or suicidality; prescriptions should be written for the smallest quantity consistent with good patient care. Hormonal contraceptives may cause a decrease in lamotrigine levels; dose adjustment of the lamotrigine maintenance dose may be required when initiating or discontinuing estrogen-containing oral contraceptives. Valproic acid may cause an increase in lamotrigine levels requiring dose adjustment. There is a potential for medication errors with similar-sounding medications and among different lamotrigine formulations; medication errors have occurred.

Drug Interactions

Avoid Concomitant Use There are no known interactions where it is recommended to avoid concomitant use.

Decreased Effect

LamoTRIgine may decrease the levels/effects of: Contraceptives (Progestins)

The levels/effects of LamoTRIgine may be decreased by: Barbiturates; CarBAMazepine; Contraceptives (Estrogens); Fosphenytoin; Ketorolac; Ketorolac (Nasal); Ketorolac (Systemic); Mefloquine; Phenytoin; Primidone; Rifampin; Ritonavir

Increased Effect/Toxicity

LamoTRIgine may increase the levels/effects of: Alcohol (Ethyl); CarBAMazepine; CNS Depressants; Desmopressin; Methotrimeprazine; OLANZapine; Selective Serotonin Reuptake Inhibitors

The levels/effects of LamoTRIgine may be increased by: Divalproex; Droperidol; HydrOXYzine; Methotrimeprazine; Valproic Acid

Nutritional/Ethanol Interactions

Ethanol: May increase CNS depression; monitor for increased effects with coadministration. Caution patients about effects.

Food: Has no effect on absorption.

Herb/Nutraceutical: Avoid evening primrose (seizure threshold decreased).

Adverse Reactions Percentages reported in adults on monotherapy for epilepsy or bipolar disorder.

>10%: Gastrointestinal: Nausea (7% to 14%)

1% to 10%:

Cardiovascular: Chest pain (5%), peripheral edema (2% to 5%), edema (1% to 5%)

Central nervous system: Insomnia (5% to 10%), somnolence (9%), fatigue (8%), coordination impaired (7%), dizziness (7%), anxiety (5%), pain (5%), ataxia (2% to 5%), irritability (2% to 5%), suicidal ideation (2% to 5%), agitation (1% to 5%), amnesia (1% to 5%), depression (1% to 5%), dream abnormality (1% to 5%), emotional lability (1% to 5%), fever (1% to 5%), hypoesthesia (1% to 5%), migraine (1% to 5%), thought abnormality (1% to 5%), confusion (1%)

Dermatologic: Rash (nonserious: 7%), dermatitis (2% to 5%), dry skin (2% to 5%)

Endocrine & metabolic: Dysmenorrhea (5%), libido increased (2% to 5%)

Gastrointestinal: Vomiting (5% to 9%), dyspepsia (7%), abdominal pain (6%), xerostomia (2% to 6%), constipation (5%), weight loss (5%), anorexia (2% to 5%), peptic ulcer (2% to 5%), rectal hemorrhage (2% to 5%), flatulence (1% to 5%), weight gain (1% to 5%)

Genitourinary: Urinary frequency (1% to 5%)

Neuromuscular & skeletal: Back pain (8%), weakness (2% to 5%), arthralgia (1% to 5%), myalgia (1% to 5%), neck pain (1% to 5%), paresthesia (1%)

Ocular: Nystagmus (2% to 5%), vision abnormal (2% to 5%), amblyopia (1%)

Respiratory: Rhinitis (7%), cough (5%), pharyngitis (5%), bronchitis (2% to 5%), dyspnea (2% to 5%), epistaxis (2% to 5%), sinusitis (1% to 5%)

Miscellaneous: Infection (5%), diaphoresis (2% to 5%), reflexes increased/decreased (2% to 5%), dyspraxia (1% to 5%)

Available Dosage Forms

Tablet, oral: 25 mg, 100 mg, 150 mg, 200 mg

LaMICtal®: 25 mg, 100 mg, 150 mg, 200 mg, 25 mg (42s) [white tablets] and 100 mg (7s) [peach tablets], 25 mg (84s) [white tablets] and 100 mg (14s) [peach tablets]

Tablet, chewable/dispersible, oral: 5 mg, 25 mg

LaMICtal®: 2 mg, 5 mg, 25 mg

Tablet, extended release, oral:

LaMICtal® XR™: 25 mg, 50 mg, 100 mg, 200 mg, 250 mg, 300 mg, 25 mg (21s) [yellow/white tablets] and 50 mg (7s) [green/white tablets], 50 mg (14s) [green/white tablets], 100 mg (14s) [orange/white tablets], and 200 mg (7s) [blue/white tablets], 25 mg (14s) [yellow/white tablets], 50 mg (14s) [green/white tablets], and 100 mg (7s) [orange/white tablets]

Tablet, orally disintegrating, oral:

LaMICtal® ODT™: 25 mg, 50 mg, 100 mg, 200 mg, 25 mg (21s) and 50 mg (7s), 50 mg (42s) and 100 mg (14s), 25 mg (14s), 50 mg (14s), and 100 mg (7s)

General Dosage Range Dosage adjustment recommended in patients with hepatic or renal impairment or on concomitant therapy

Oral:

Immediate release formulation:

Children 2-12 years: Dosage varies greatly depending on indication

Children ≥13 years and Adults: Dosage varies greatly depending on indication

Extended release formulation: *Children ≥13 years and Adults:* Dosage varies greatly depending on indication

Administration

Oral Doses should be rounded down to the nearest whole tablet.

Lamictal® chewable/dispersible tablets: May be chewed, dispersed in water or diluted fruit juice, or swallowed whole. To disperse tablets, add to a small amount of liquid (just enough to cover tablet); let sit ~1 minute until dispersed; swirl solution and consume immediately. Do not administer partial amounts of liquid. If tablets are chewed, a small amount of water or diluted fruit juice should be used to aid in swallowing.

Lamictal® ODT™: Place tablets on tongue and move around in the mouth. Tablets will dissolve rapidly and can be swallowed with or without food or water.

Lamictal® XR™: Administer without regard to meals. Swallow whole; do not chew, crush, or cut.

Stability

Storage Store at 25°C (77°F); excursions permitted to 15°C to 30°C (59°F to 86°F). Protect from light.

Nursing Actions

Physical Assessment Monitor therapeutic response (seizure activity, type, duration) at beginning of therapy and periodically throughout. Report presence of skin rash immediately. Monitor for suicide ideation, depression, or unusual behavior changes. Taper dosage slowly when discontinuing. Observe and teach seizure/safety precautions.

Patient Education Only whole tablets should be used for dosing, rounded down to the nearest whole tablet. While using this medication, do not use alcohol. Maintain adequate hydration unless instructed to restrict fluid intake. You may experience drowsiness, dizziness, blurred vision, nausea, vomiting, loss of appetite, heartburn, or dry mouth. Wear identification of epileptic status and medications. Report CNS changes, mentation changes, suicide ideation, depression, or changes in cognition; persistent GI symptoms (cramping, constipation, vomiting, anorexia); swelling of face, lips, or tongue; easy bruising or bleeding (mouth, urine, stool); vision changes; worsening of seizure activity, or loss of seizure control. A skin rash may indicate a serious medical problem; contact prescriber immediately if rash noted.

Lansoprazole (lan SOE pra zole)

Brand Names: U.S. First®-Lansoprazole; Prevacid®; Prevacid® 24 HR [OTC]; Prevacid® SoluTab™

Pharmacologic Category Proton Pump Inhibitor; Substituted Benzimidazole

Medication Safety Issues

Sound-alike/look-alike issues:

Lansoprazole may be confused with aripiprazole, dexlansoprazole

Prevacid® may be confused with Pravachol®, Prevpac®, PriLOSEC®, Prinivil®

Pregnancy Risk Factor B

Lactation Excretion in breast milk unknown/not recommended

Use Short-term treatment of active duodenal ulcers; maintenance treatment of healed duodenal ulcers; as part of a multidrug regimen for *H. pylori* eradication to reduce the risk of duodenal ulcer recurrence; short-term treatment of active benign gastric ulcer; treatment of NSAID-associated gastric ulcer; to reduce the risk of NSAID-associated gastric ulcer in patients with a history of gastric ulcer who require an NSAID; short-term treatment of symptomatic GERD; short-term treatment for all grades of erosive esophagitis; to maintain healing of erosive esophagitis; long-term treatment of pathological hypersecretory conditions, including Zollinger-Ellison syndrome

OTC labeling: Relief of frequent heartburn (≥2 days/week)

Mechanism of Action/Effect A proton pump inhibitor which decreases acid secretion in gastric parietal cells

Contraindications Hypersensitivity to lansoprazole or any component of the formulation

Warnings/Precautions Use of proton pump inhibitors (PPIs) may increase the risk of gastrointestinal infections (eg, *Salmonella, Campylobacter*). Relief of symptoms does not preclude the presence of a gastric malignancy. Atrophic gastritis (by biopsy) has been noted with long-term omeprazole therapy; this may also occur with lansoprazole. No reports of enterochromaffin-like (ECL) cell carcinoids, dysplasia, or neoplasia have occurred. Severe liver dysfunction may require dosage reductions. Decreased *H. pylori* eradication rates have been observed with short-term (≤7 days) combination therapy. The American College of Gastroenterology recommends 10-14 days of therapy (triple or quadruple) for eradication of *H. pylori* (Chey, 2007).

PPIs may diminish the therapeutic effect of clopidogrel thought to be due to reduced formation of the active metabolite of clopidogrel. The manufacturer of clopidogrel recommends either avoidance of omeprazole or use of a PPI with less potent CYP2C19 inhibition (eg, pantoprazole). Lansoprazole exhibits the most potent CYP2C19 inhibition; given the potency of lansoprazole's CYP2C19 inhibitory activity, avoidance of lansoprazole would appear prudent. Others have recommended the continued use of PPIs, regardless of the degree of inhibition, in patients with a history of GI bleeding or multiple risk factors for GI bleeding who are also receiving clopidogrel since no evidence has established clinically meaningful differences in outcome; however, a clinically-significant interaction cannot be excluded in those who are poor metabolizers of clopidogrel (Abraham, 2010; Levine, 2011).

Increased incidence of osteoporosis-related bone fractures of the hip, spine, or wrist may occur with PPI therapy. Patients on high-dose or long-term therapy should be monitored. Use the lowest effective dose for the shortest duration of time, use vitamin D and calcium supplementation, and follow appropriate guidelines to reduce risk of fractures in patients at risk. Lansoprazole has been shown to be ineffective for the treatment of symptomatic GERD in children 1 month to <1 year.

Hypomagnesemia, reported rarely, usually with prolonged PPI use of >3 months (most cases >1 year of therapy); may be symptomatic or asymptomatic; severe cases may cause tetany, seizures, and cardiac arrhythmias. Consider obtaining serum magnesium concentrations prior to beginning long-term therapy, especially if taking concomitant digoxin, diuretics, or other drugs known to cause hypomagnesemia; and periodically thereafter. Hypomagnesemia may be corrected by magnesium supplementation, although discontinuation of lansoprazole may be necessary; magnesium levels typically return to normal within 1 week of stopping.

When used for self-medication, patients should be instructed not to use if they have difficulty swallowing, are vomiting blood, or have bloody or black stools. Prior to use, patients should contact healthcare provider if they have liver disease, heartburn for >3 months, heartburn with dizziness, lightheadedness, or sweating, MI symptoms, frequent chest pain, frequent wheezing (especially with heartburn), unexplained weight loss, nausea/vomiting, stomach pain, or are taking antifungals, atazanavir, digoxin, tacrolimus, theophylline, or warfarin. Patients should stop use and consult a healthcare provider if heartburn continues or worsens, or if they need to take for >14 days or more often than every 4 months. Patients should be informed that it may take 1-4 days for full effect to be seen; should not be used for immediate relief.

Drug Interactions

Avoid Concomitant Use

Avoid concomitant use of Lansoprazole with any of the following: Delavirdine; Erlotinib; Nelfinavir; Pimozide; Posaconazole; Rilpivirine

Decreased Effect

Lansoprazole may decrease the levels/effects of: Atazanavir; Bisphosphonate Derivatives; Cefditoren; Clopidogrel; Dabigatran Etexilate; Dasatinib; Delavirdine; Erlotinib; Gefitinib; Indinavir; Iron Salts; Itraconazole; Ketoconazole; Ketoconazole (Systemic); Mesalamine; Mycophenolate; Nelfinavir; Posaconazole; Rilpivirine; Vismodegib

The levels/effects of Lansoprazole may be decreased by: CYP2C19 Inducers (Strong); CYP3A4 Inducers (Strong); Deferasirox; Herbs (CYP3A4 Inducers); Tipranavir; Tocilizumab

Increased Effect/Toxicity

Lansoprazole may increase the levels/effects of: Amphetamines; ARIPiprazole; Citalopram; CYP2C19 Substrates; Dexmethylphenidate; Imatinib; Methotrexate; Methylphenidate; Pimozide; Raltegravir; Saquinavir; Tacrolimus; Tacrolimus (Systemic); Vitamin K Antagonists; Voriconazole

The levels/effects of Lansoprazole may be increased by: Conivaptan; Fluconazole; Ketoconazole; Ketoconazole (Systemic)

Nutritional/Ethanol Interactions

Ethanol: Avoid ethanol (may cause gastric mucosal irritation).

Food: Lansoprazole serum concentrations may be decreased if taken with food.

Herb/Nutraceutical: Avoid St John's wort (may decrease the levels/effect of lansoprazole).

Adverse Reactions 1% to 10%:

Central nervous system: Headache (children 1-11 years 3%, 12-17 years 7%), dizziness (children 12-17 years 3%; adults <1%)

Gastrointestinal: Diarrhea (1% to 5%; 60 mg/day: 7%), abdominal pain (children 12-17 years 5%; adults 2%), constipation (children 1-11 years 5%; adults 1%), nausea (children 12-17 years 3%; adults 1%)

Pharmacodynamics/Kinetics

Onset of Action Gastric acid suppression: Oral: 1-3 hours

Duration of Action Gastric acid suppression: Oral: >1 day

Available Dosage Forms

Capsule, delayed release, oral: 15 mg, 30 mg
Prevacid®: 15 mg, 30 mg
Prevacid® 24 HR [OTC]: 15 mg

Powder for suspension, oral:
First®-Lansoprazole: 3 mg/mL (90 mL, 150 mL, 300 mL)

Tablet, delayed release, orally disintegrating, oral: 15 mg, 30 mg
Prevacid® SoluTab™: 15 mg, 30 mg

General Dosage Range Oral:

Children 1-11 years and ≤30 kg: 15 mg once daily (maximum: 30 mg twice daily)

Children 1-11 years and >30 kg: 30 mg once daily (maximum: 30 mg twice daily)

Children 12-17 years: 15-30 mg once daily

Adults: 15-180 mg/day in 1-2 divided doses

Administration

Oral

Administer before food; best if taken before breakfast. The intact granules should not be chewed or crushed; however, several options are available for those patients unable to swallow capsules:

Capsules may be opened and the intact granules sprinkled on 1 tablespoon of applesauce, Ensure® pudding, cottage cheese, yogurt, or strained pears. The granules should then be swallowed immediately.

Capsules may be opened and emptied into ~60 mL orange juice, apple juice, or tomato juice; mix and swallow immediately. Rinse the glass with additional juice and swallow to assure complete delivery of the dose.

Orally-disintegrating tablets: Should not be swallowed whole, broken, cut, or chewed. Place tablet on tongue; allow to dissolve (with or without water) until particles can be swallowed. Orally-disintegrating tablets may also be administered via an oral syringe: Place the 15 mg tablet in an oral syringe and draw up ~4 mL water, or place the 30 mg tablet in an oral syringe and draw up ~10 mL water. After tablet has dispersed, administer within 15 minutes. Refill the syringe with water (2 mL for the 15 mg tablet; 5 mL for the 30 mg tablet), shake gently, then administer any remaining contents.

Other Nasogastric tube administration:

Capsule: Capsule can be opened, the granules mixed (not crushed) with 40 mL of apple juice and then injected through the NG tube into the stomach, then flush tube with additional apple juice. Do not mix with other liquids.

Orally-disintegrating tablet: Nasogastric tube ≥8 French: Place a 15 mg tablet in a syringe and draw up ~4 mL water, or place the 30 mg tablet in a syringe and draw up ~10 mL water. After tablet has dispersed, administer within 15 minutes. Refill the syringe with ~5 mL water, shake gently, and then flush the nasogastric tube.

Stability

Storage Store at 25°C (77°F); excursions permitted to 15°C to 30°C (59°F to 86°F).

Nursing Actions

Physical Assessment Monitor effectiveness of ulcer symptom relief.

Patient Education Take before eating. Do not crush or chew granules. Patients who may have difficulty swallowing capsules may open the delayed-release capsules and sprinkle the contents on applesauce, pudding, cottage cheese, or yogurt. Avoid alcohol. Report unresolved diarrhea, persistent heartburn, or abdominal pain.

Dietary Considerations Should be taken before eating; best if taken before breakfast. Some products may contain phenylalanine.

Related Information

Compatibility of Drugs *on page 1264*

Lansoprazole, Amoxicillin, and Clarithromycin

(lan SOE pra zole, a moks i SIL in, & kla RITH roe mye sin)

Brand Names: U.S. Prevpac®

Index Terms Amoxicillin, Clarithromycin, and Lansoprazole; Clarithromycin, Lansoprazole, and Amoxicillin; Lansoprazole, Amoxicillin, and Clarithromycin

Pharmacologic Category Antibiotic, Macrolide Combination; Antibiotic, Penicillin; Gastrointestinal Agent, Miscellaneous; Proton Pump Inhibitor; Substituted Benzimidazole

Medication Safety Issues

Sound-alike/look-alike issues:

Prevpac® may be confused with Prevacid®

Pregnancy Risk Factor C (clarithromycin)

Lactation Excretion in breast milk unknown/not recommended

Use Eradication of *H. pylori* to reduce the risk of recurrent duodenal ulcer

Available Dosage Forms

Combination package [each administration card contains]:

Prevpac®:

Capsule: Amoxicillin 500 mg (4 capsules/day)

Capsule, delayed release (Prevacid®): Lansoprazole 30 mg (2 capsules/day)

Tablet (Biaxin®): Clarithromycin 500 mg (2 tablets/day)

General Dosage Range Oral: *Adults:* Lansoprazole 30 mg, amoxicillin 1 g, and clarithromycin 500 mg taken together twice daily

Nursing Actions

Physical Assessment See individual agents.

Patient Education See individual agents.

Related Information

Amoxicillin *on page 68*

Clarithromycin *on page 246*

Lansoprazole *on page 669*

Lapatinib (la PA ti nib)

Brand Names: U.S. Tykerb®

Index Terms GW572016; Lapatinib Ditosylate

Pharmacologic Category Antineoplastic Agent, Tyrosine Kinase Inhibitor; Epidermal Growth Factor Receptor (EGFR) Inhibitor

Medication Safety Issues

Sound-alike/look-alike issues:

Lapatinib may be confused with dasatinib, erlotinib, imatinib, SUNItinib, vandetanib

High alert medication:

This medication is in a class of medications the Institute for Safe Medication Practices (ISMP) includes among its list of drug classes which have a heightened risk of causing significant patient harm when used in error.

Pregnancy Risk Factor D

Lactation Excretion in breast milk unknown/not recommended

Breast-Feeding Considerations Due to the potential for serious adverse reactions in the nursing infant, breast-feeding is not recommended.

Use Treatment of HER2 overexpressing advanced or metastatic breast cancer (in combination with capecitabine) in patients who have received prior therapy (with an anthracycline, a taxane, and trastuzumab) and HER2 overexpressing hormone receptor positive metastatic breast cancer in postmenopausal women (in combination with letrozole)

Unlabeled Use Treatment (in combination with trastuzumab) of HER2 overexpressing metastatic breast cancer which had progressed on prior trastuzumab containing therapy

Mechanism of Action/Effect Tyrosine kinase (dual kinase) inhibitor that blocks HER2 and EGFR pathways.

Contraindications Hypersensitivity to lapatinib or any component of the formulation

Warnings/Precautions Decreases in left ventricular ejection fraction (LVEF) have been reported (usually within the first 3 months of treatment); baseline and periodic LVEF evaluations are recommended; interrupt therapy or decrease dose with decreased LVEF ≥grade 2 or LVEF < LLN. QT_c prolongation has been observed; use caution in patients with a history of QT_c prolongation or with medications known to prolong the QT interval; a baseline and periodic 12-lead ECG should be considered; correct electrolyte (potassium, calcium and magnesium) abnormalities prior to and during treatment. Use with caution in conditions which may impair left ventricular function and in patients with a history of or predisposed (prior treatment with anthracyclines, chest wall irradiation) to left ventricular dysfunction. Interstitial lung disease (ILD) and pneumonitis have been reported (with lapatinib monotherapy and with combination chemotherapy); monitor for pulmonary symptoms which may indicate ILD or pneumonitis; discontinue therapy for grade 3 (or higher) pulmonary symptoms indicative of ILD or pneumonitis (eg, dyspnea, dry cough).

[U.S. Boxed Warning]: Hepatotoxicity (ALT or AST >3 times ULN and total bilirubin >2 times ULN) has been reported with lapatinib; may be severe and/or fatal. Onset of hepatotoxicity may occur within days to several months after treatment initiation; monitor (at baseline and during treatment); discontinue with severe changes in liver function; do not retreat. Use caution in patients with hepatic dysfunction; Dose reductions should be considered in patients with severe (Child-Pugh class C) preexisting hepatic impairment. Avoid concurrent use with strong CYP3A4 inhibitors or inducers; if concomitant therapy cannot be avoided, lapatinib dosage adjustments should be considered. May cause diarrhea (may be severe); manage with antidiarrheal agents; severe diarrhea may require hydration, electrolytes, and or interruption of therapy.

Drug Interactions

Avoid Concomitant Use

Avoid concomitant use of Lapatinib with any of the following: Artemether; CYP3A4 Inducers (Strong); CYP3A4 Inhibitors (Strong); Dronedarone; Grapefruit Juice; Lumefantrine; Nilotinib; Pimozide; QUEtiapine; QuiNINE; Silodosin; St Johns Wort; Tetrabenazine; Thioridazine; Topotecan; Toremifene; Vandetanib; Vemurafenib; Ziprasidone

Decreased Effect

Lapatinib may decrease the levels/effects of: Cardiac Glycosides; Vitamin K Antagonists

The levels/effects of Lapatinib may be decreased by: CYP3A4 Inducers (Strong); Deferasirox; P-glycoprotein/ABCB1 Inducers; St Johns Wort; Tocilizumab

Increased Effect/Toxicity

Lapatinib may increase the levels/effects of: ARIPiprazole; Colchicine; CYP2C8 Substrates; Dabigatran Etexilate; Dronedarone; Everolimus; Pazopanib; P-glycoprotein/ABCB1 Substrates; Pimozide; Prucalopride; QTc-Prolonging Agents; QuiNINE; Rivaroxaban; Silodosin; Tetrabenazine; Thioridazine; Topotecan; Toremifene; Vandetanib; Vemurafenib; Vitamin K Antagonists; Ziprasidone

The levels/effects of Lapatinib may be increased by: Alfuzosin; Artemether; Chloroquine; Ciprofloxacin; Ciprofloxacin (Systemic); CYP3A4 Inhibitors (Moderate); CYP3A4 Inhibitors (Strong); Gadobutrol; Grapefruit Juice; Indacaterol; Lumefantrine; Nilotinib; P-glycoprotein/ABCB1 Inhibitors; QUEtiapine; QuiNINE

Nutritional/Ethanol Interactions

Food: Systemic exposure of lapatinib is increased when administered with food (AUC three- to fourfold higher). Grapefruit juice may increase the levels/effects of lapatinib. Management: Administer once daily on an empty stomach, 1 hour before or 1 hour after a meal at the same time each day. Avoid grapefruit juice. Maintain adequate hydration, unless instructed to restrict fluid intake.

Herb/Nutraceutical: St John's wort may increase metabolism and decrease lapatinib concentrations. Management: Avoid St John's wort.

Adverse Reactions Percentages reported for combination therapy.

>10%:

Central nervous system: Fatigue (10% to 20%), headache (≤14%)

Dermatologic: Palmar-plantar erythrodysesthesia (hand-and-foot syndrome) (with capecitabine: 53%; grade 3: 12%), rash (28% to 44%), dry skin (10% to 13%), alopecia (≤13%), pruritus (≤12%), nail disorder (≤11%)

Gastrointestinal: Diarrhea (64% to 65%; grade 3: 9% to 13%; grade 4: ≤1%), nausea (31% to 44%), vomiting (17% to 26%), abdominal pain (≤15%), mucosal inflammation (≤15%), stomatitis (≤14%), anorexia (≤11%), dyspepsia (≤11%)

Hematologic: Anemia (with capecitabine: 56%; grade 3: <1%), neutropenia (with capecitabine: 22%; grade 3: 3%; grade 4: <1%), thrombocytopenia (with capecitabine: 18%; grade 3: <1%)

Hepatic: AST increased (49% to 53%; grade 3: 2% to 6%; grade 4: <1%), ALT increased (37% to 46%; grade 3: 2% to 5%; grade 4: <1%) total bilirubin increased (22% to 45%; grade 3: ≤4%; grade 4: <1%)

Neuromuscular & skeletal: Limb pain (≤12%), weakness (≤12%), back pain (≤11%)

Respiratory:Dyspnea (≤12%), epistaxis (≤11%)

1% to 10%:

Cardiovascular: LVEF decreased (grades 1/2: 2% to 4%; grades 3/4: <1%)

Central nervous system: Insomnia (≤10%)

Available Dosage Forms

Tablet, oral:

Tykerb®: 250 mg

General Dosage Range Dosage adjustment recommended in patients with hepatic impairment, on concomitant therapy, or who develop toxicities

Oral: *Adults:* 1250-1500 mg once daily

Administration

Oral Administer once daily, on an empty stomach, 1 hour before or 1 hour after a meal. Take at the same time each day; dividing doses is not recommended.

Stability

Storage Store at room temperature of 25°C (77°F); excursions permitted between 15°C and 30°C (59°F and 86°F).

Nursing Actions

Physical Assessment Monitor CBC, LFTs, electrolytes, and left ventricular ejection fraction at baseline and on a regular basis. Monitor for cardiac changes, gastrointestinal disturbance (diarrhea may become severe), interstitial lung disease, and pneumonitis.

Patient Education Take on an empty stomach 1 hour before or 1 hour after a meal. Avoid grapefruit or grapefruit juice while taking this medication. Maintain adequate hydration unless instructed to restrict fluid intake. You may be required to have regularly scheduled laboratory tests while on this medication. You will be more susceptible to infection. You may experience diarrhea (contact prescriber if persistent or severe); insomnia or fatigue; nausea, vomiting, stomach pain, or dyspepsia; red, painful hands, feet, or limbs; or back pain. Report chest pain or palpitations, any unusual cough, respiratory difficulty or wheezing, easy bruising, or unusual bleeding.

Dietary Considerations Take on an empty stomach, 1 hour before or 1 hour after a meal. (**Note:** For combination with capecitabine treatment, capecitabine should be taken with food, or within 30 minutes after a meal.) Avoid grapefruit juice.

Latanoprost (la TA noe prost)

Brand Names: U.S. Xalatan®

Pharmacologic Category Ophthalmic Agent, Antiglaucoma; Prostaglandin, Ophthalmic

Medication Safety Issues

Sound-alike/look-alike issues:

Latanoprost may be confused with Lantus®

Xalatan® may be confused with Lantus®, Travatan®, Xalacom™, Zarontin®

Pregnancy Risk Factor C

Lactation Excretion in breast milk unknown/use caution

Use Reduction of elevated intraocular pressure in patients with open-angle glaucoma or ocular hypertension

Available Dosage Forms

Solution, ophthalmic: 0.005% (2.5 mL)

Xalatan®: 0.005% (2.5 mL)

General Dosage Range Ophthalmic: *Adults:* 1 drop (1.5 mcg) in the affected eye(s) once daily

Administration

Other If more than one topical ophthalmic drug is being used, administer the drugs at least 5 minutes apart. A delivery aid, Xal-Ease™, is available for administering Xalatan®.

Nursing Actions

Physical Assessment Monitor for blurred vision, burning and stinging, conjunctival hyperemia, foreign body sensation, itching, increased pigmentation of the iris, and punctate epithelial keratopathy.

Patient Education For use in eyes only. Iris color may change because of an increase of the brown pigment. Iris pigmentation changes may be more noticeable in patients with green-brown, blue/gray-brown, or yellow-brown irides. If any ocular reaction develops, particularly conjunctivitis and lid reactions, immediately notify prescriber. If more than one topical ophthalmic drug is being used, administer the drugs at least 5 minutes apart. Latanoprost contains benzalkonium chloride, which may be absorbed by contact lenses. Remove contact lenses prior to administration; lenses may be reinserted after 15 minutes. Do not let tip of applicator touch eye; do not contaminate tip of applicator (may cause eye infection, eye damage, or vision loss).

Leflunomide (le FLOO noh mide)

Brand Names: U.S. Arava®

Pharmacologic Category Antirheumatic, Disease Modifying

Pregnancy Risk Factor X

Lactation Excretion in breast milk unknown/not recommended

Breast-Feeding Considerations It is not known whether leflunomide is secreted in human milk. Because the potential for serious adverse reactions exists in the nursing infant, a decision should be made whether to discontinue nursing or discontinue the drug, taking into account the importance of the drug to the mother.

Use Treatment of active rheumatoid arthritis; indicated to reduce signs and symptoms, and to inhibit structural damage and improve physical function

Unlabeled Use Treatment of cytomegalovirus (CMV) disease in transplant recipients resistant to standard antivirals; prevention of acute and chronic rejection in recipients of solid organ transplants

Mechanism of Action/Effect Leflunomide is an immunodulatory agent that inhibits pyrimidine synthesis, resulting in antiproliferative and anti-inflammatory effects. Leflunomide is a prodrug; the active metabolite is responsible for activity. For CMV, may interfere with virion assembly.

Contraindications Hypersensitivity to leflunomide or any component of the formulation; pregnancy

Warnings/Precautions Hazardous agent - use appropriate precautions for handling and disposal. **[U.S. Boxed Warning]: Use has been associated with rare reports of hepatotoxicity, hepatic failure, and death. Treatment should not be initiated in patients with pre-existing acute or chronic liver disease or ALT >2 x ULN. Use caution in patients with concurrent exposure to potentially hepatotoxic drugs. Monitor ALT levels during therapy; discontinue if ALT >3 x ULN occurs and, if hepatotoxicity is likely leflunomide-induced, start drug elimination procedures** (eg, cholestyramine, activated charcoal).

Use has been associated (rarely) with interstitial lung disease; discontinue in patients who develop new onset or worsening of pulmonary symptoms. Drug elimination procedures should be considered (eg, cholestyramine, activated charcoal) if interstitial lung disease occurs; fatal outcomes have been reported. May increase susceptibility to infection, including opportunistic pathogens. Severe infections, sepsis, and fatalities have been reported. Not recommended in patients with severe immunodeficiency, bone marrow dysplasia, or severe, uncontrolled infections. Caution should be exercised when considering the use in patients with a history of new/recurrent infections, with conditions that predispose them to infections, or with chronic, latent, or localized infections. Patients who develop a new infection while undergoing treatment should be monitored closely; consider discontinuation of therapy and drug elimination procedures if infection is serious.

Use may affect defenses against malignancies; impact on the development and course of malignancies is not fully defined. As compared to the general population, an increased risk of lymphoma has been noted in clinical trials; however, rheumatoid arthritis has been previously associated with an increased rate of lymphoma. Use with caution in patients with a prior history of significant hematologic abnormalities; avoid use with bone marrow dysplasia. Use has been associated with rare pancytopenia, agranulocytosis, and thrombocytopenia, generally when given concurrently or recently with methotrexate or other immunosuppressive agents. Monitoring of hematologic function is required; discontinue if evidence of bone marrow suppression and begin drug elimination procedures (eg, cholestyramine or activated charcoal). Rare cases of dermatologic reactions (including Stevens-Johnson syndrome and toxic epidermal necrolysis) have been reported; discontinue if evidence of severe dermatologic reaction occurs, and begin drug elimination procedures (eg, cholestyramine or activated charcoal). Cases of peripheral neuropathy have been reported; use with caution in patients >60 years of age, receiving concomitant neurotoxic medications, or patients with diabetes; discontinue if evidence of peripheral neuropathy occurs and begin drug elimination procedures (eg, cholestyramine, activated charcoal).

Safety has not been established in patients with latent tuberculosis infection. Patients should be screened for tuberculosis and if necessary, treated prior to initiating therapy. Use with caution in patients with renal impairment. **[U.S. Boxed Warning]: Women of childbearing potential should not receive therapy until pregnancy has been excluded,** they have been counseled concerning fetal risk and reliable contraceptive measures have been confirmed. Women of childbearing potential should also undergo drug elimination procedures (eg, cholestyramine, activated charcoal) following discontinuation of therapy. Patients should be brought up to date with all immunizations before initiating therapy. Live vaccines should not be given concurrently; there is no data available concerning secondary transmission of live vaccines in patients receiving therapy. Due to variations in clearance, it may take up to 2 years to reach low levels of leflunomide metabolite serum concentrations. A drug elimination procedure using cholestyramine or activated charcoal is recommended when a more rapid elimination is needed.

Drug Interactions

Avoid Concomitant Use

Avoid concomitant use of Leflunomide with any of the following: BCG; Natalizumab; Pimecrolimus; Tacrolimus (Topical)

Decreased Effect

Leflunomide may decrease the levels/effects of: BCG; Coccidioidin Skin Test; Sipuleucel-T; Vaccines (Inactivated)

The levels/effects of Leflunomide may be decreased by: Bile Acid Sequestrants; Charcoal, Activated; Echinacea

Increased Effect/Toxicity

Leflunomide may increase the levels/effects of: Carvedilol; CYP2C9 Substrates; Natalizumab; TOLBUTamide; Vaccines (Live); Vitamin K Antagonists

The levels/effects of Leflunomide may be increased by: Denosumab; Immunosuppressants; Methotrexate; Pimecrolimus; Rifampin; Roflumilast; Tacrolimus (Topical); TOLBUTamide; Trastuzumab

Nutritional/Ethanol Interactions

Food: No interactions with food have been noted. Management: Maintain adequate hydration, unless instructed to restrict fluid intake.

Herb/Nutraceutical: Echinacea may diminish the therapeutic effect of leflunomide.

Adverse Reactions

>10%:

Gastrointestinal: Diarrhea (17%)

Respiratory: Respiratory tract infection (4% to 15%)

1% to 10%:

Cardiovascular: Hypertension (10%), chest pain (2%), edema (peripheral), palpitation, tachycardia, vasodilation, varicose vein, vasculitis

Central nervous system: Headache (7%), dizziness (4%), pain (2%), anxiety, depression, fever, insomnia, malaise, migraine, sleep disorder, vertigo

Dermatologic: Alopecia (10%), rash (10%), pruritus (4%), dry skin (2%), eczema (2%), acne, bruising, dermatitis, hair discoloration, hematoma, nail disorder, skin disorder/discoloration, skin ulcer, subcutaneous nodule

Endocrine & metabolic: Hypokalemia (1%), diabetes mellitus, hyperglycemia, hyperlipidemia, hyperthyroidism, menstrual disorder

Gastrointestinal: Nausea (9%), abdominal pain (5% to 6%), dyspepsia (5%), weight loss (4%), anorexia (3%), gastroenteritis (3%), mouth ulceration (3%), vomiting (3%), candidiasis (oral), colitis, constipation, esophagitis, flatulence, gastritis, gingivitis, melena, salivary gland enlarged, stomatitis, taste disturbance, xerostomia

Genitourinary: Urinary tract infection (5%), albuminuria, cystitis, dysuria, prostate disorder, urinary frequency, vaginal candidiasis

Hematologic: Anemia

Hepatic: Abnormal LFTs (5%), cholelithiasis

Local: Abscess

Neuromuscular & skeletal: Back pain (5%), joint disorder (4%), weakness (3%), tenosynovitis (3%), synovitis (2%), paresthesia (2%), arthralgia (1%), leg cramps (1%), arthrosis, bone necrosis, bone pain, bursitis, CPK increased, myalgia, neck pain, neuralgia, neuritis, pelvic pain, tendon rupture

Ocular: Blurred vision, cataract, conjunctivitis, eye disorder

Renal: Hematuria

Respiratory: Bronchitis (7%), cough (3%), pharyngitis (3%), pneumonia (2%), rhinitis (2%), sinusitis (2%), asthma, dyspnea, epistaxis

Miscellaneous: Accidental injury (5%), allergic reactions (2%), flu-like syndrome (2%), cyst, diaphoresis, hernia, herpes infection

Available Dosage Forms

Tablet, oral: 10 mg, 20 mg

Arava®: 10 mg, 20 mg

General Dosage Range Dosage adjustment recommended in patients who develop toxicities

Oral: *Adults:* Initial: 100 mg/day for 3 days; Maintenance range: 10-20 mg/day

Administration

Oral Administer without regard to meals.

Stability

Storage Store at 25°C (77°F); excursions permitted to 15°C to 30°C (59°F to 86°F). Protect from light.

Nursing Actions

Physical Assessment Monitor for reduction of rheumatoid arthritis signs and symptoms and structural damage. Place and read PPD prior to initiating. Monitor for signs and symptoms of severe infection, hypertension, or hepatic dysfunction. Monitor for new onset or worsening of pulmonary symptoms.

Patient Education Maintain adequate hydration unless instructed to restrict fluid intake. You will be more prone to infections. You may experience diarrhea, nausea, vomiting, loss of appetite, flatulence, or dizziness. If you have diabetes, monitor blood sugars closely; this medication may alter glucose levels. If you experience symptoms such as nausea, vomiting, stomach pain or swelling, jaundice, dark urine, or unusual tiredness, report these to your prescriber immediately. Report chest pain, palpitations, rapid heartbeat, or swelling of extremities; persistent GI problems; skin rash; mucous membrane lesions; frequent, painful, or difficult urination; genital itching; depression; acute headache; muscle tremors, cramping, or weakness; back pain; altered gait; cough, cold symptoms, wheezing, or respiratory difficulty; easy bruising/bleeding; or blood in vomitus, stool, or urine.

Dietary Considerations May be taken without regard to meals.

Lenalidomide (le na LID oh mide)

Brand Names: U.S. Revlimid®

Index Terms CC-5013; IMid-1

Pharmacologic Category Angiogenesis Inhibitor; Antineoplastic Agent; Immunomodulator, Systemic

Medication Safety Issues

Sound-alike/look-alike issues:

Lenalidomide may be confused with thalidomide

High alert medication:

This medication is in a class the Institute for Safe Medication Practices (ISMP) includes among its list of drug classes which have a heightened risk of causing significant patient harm when used in error.

Medication Guide Available Yes

Pregnancy Risk Factor X

Lactation Excretion in breast milk unknown/not recommended

Use Treatment of low- or intermediate-risk myelodysplastic syndrome (MDS) in patients with deletion 5q (del 5q) cytogenetic abnormality with transfusion-dependent anemia (with or without other cytogenetic abnormalities); treatment of multiple myeloma (in combination with dexamethasone) in patients who have received at least one prior therapy

Unlabeled Use Treatment of non-Hodgkin's lymphomas; systemic amyloidosis (light chain); lower-risk myelodysplastic syndrome (MDS) in transfusion-dependent patients without deletion 5q (del 5q); maintenance treatment for multiple myeloma (following autologous stem cell transplant)

Available Dosage Forms

Capsule, oral:

Revlimid®: 5 mg, 10 mg, 15 mg, 25 mg

General Dosage Range Dosage adjustment recommended in patients with renal impairment or who develop toxicities

Oral: *Adults:* 10 once daily **or** 25 mg once daily for 21 of 28 days

Administration

Oral Administer with water. Swallow capsule whole; do not break, open, or chew.

Nursing Actions

Physical Assessment Verify that patient is not pregnant prior to initiating therapy. Instruct patient on the need to use two reliable forms of contraception beginning 4 weeks prior to, during, and for 4 weeks after therapy and during therapy interruptions. Monitor for signs of thromboembolism (shortness of breath, chest pain, or arm or leg swelling), deep vein thrombosis (swelling and tenderness of extremities), rash, angioedema, infection, or bleeding.

Patient Education You will need frequent blood tests while taking this medication. Maintain adequate hydration unless instructed to restrict intake by prescriber. If you have diabetes, monitor blood glucose closely. Can cause hyperglycemia. You may be susceptible to infections. Avoid vaccinations unless approved by prescriber. Do not donate blood during treatment or for 4 weeks following completion of therapy. You may experience headache, fever, insomnia, fatigue, dizziness, swelling of extremities, rash, itching, nausea, diarrhea, constipation, abdominal pain, loss of appetite, change in taste, upper respiratory infections, urinary tract infection, or sore throat. Report rash, shortness of breath, chest pain, arm or leg swelling and tenderness, weight gain, extreme weakness or fatigue, muscle cramping, unusual bleeding or bruising, or nosebleeds.

Lepirudin (leh puh ROO din)

Brand Names: U.S. Refludan®

Index Terms Lepirudin (rDNA); Recombinant Hirudin

Pharmacologic Category Anticoagulant, Thrombin Inhibitor

Medication Safety Issues

High alert medication:

The Institute for Safe Medication Practices (ISMP) includes this medication among its list of drugs which have a heightened risk of causing significant patient harm when used in error.

Pregnancy Risk Factor B

Lactation Enters breast milk/consult prescriber

Use Indicated for anticoagulation in patients with heparin-induced thrombocytopenia (HIT) and associated thromboembolic disease in order to prevent further thromboembolic complications

Mechanism of Action/Effect Lepirudin is a highly specific direct thrombin inhibitor. Each molecule is capable of binding one molecule of thrombin and inhibiting its thrombogenic activity.

Contraindications Hypersensitivity to hirudins or any component of the formulation

Warnings/Precautions Hemorrhagic events: Intracranial bleeding following concomitant thrombolytic therapy with rt-PA or streptokinase may be life threatening. For patients with an increased risk of bleeding, a careful assessment weighing the risk of lepirudin administration versus its anticipated benefit has to be made by the treating physician. In particular, this includes the following conditions: Recent puncture of large vessels or organ biopsy; anomaly of vessels or organs; recent cerebrovascular accident, stroke, intracerebral surgery, or other neuroaxial procedures; severe uncontrolled hypertension; bacterial endocarditis; advanced renal impairment; hemorrhagic diathesis; recent major surgery; and recent major bleeding (eg, intracranial, gastrointestinal, intraocular, or pulmonary bleeding). With renal impairment, relative overdose might occur even with standard dosage regimen. The bolus dose and rate of infusion must be reduced in patients with known or suspected renal insufficiency.

Formation of antihirudin antibodies may increase the anticoagulant effect of lepirudin possibly due to delayed renal elimination of active lepirudin-antihirudin complexes. Therefore, strict monitoring of aPTT is necessary also during prolonged therapy. No evidence of neutralization of lepirudin or of allergic reactions associated with positive antibody test results was found. Allergic and hypersensitivity reactions, including anaphylaxis have been reported and may occur frequently in patients treated concomitantly with streptokinase; caution is warranted during re-exposure (anaphylaxis has been reported).

Serious liver injury (eg, liver cirrhosis) may enhance the anticoagulant effect of lepirudin due to coagulation defects secondary to reduced generation of vitamin K-dependent clotting factors.

Clinical trials have provided limited information to support any recommendations for re-exposure to lepirudin (anaphylaxis has been reported). Safety and efficacy have not been established in children.

Drug Interactions

Avoid Concomitant Use

Avoid concomitant use of Lepirudin with any of the following: Rivaroxaban

Decreased Effect There are no known significant interactions involving a decrease in effect.

Increased Effect/Toxicity

Lepirudin may increase the levels/effects of: Anticoagulants; Collagenase (Systemic); Deferasirox; Ibritumomab; Rivaroxaban; Tositumomab and Iodine I 131 Tositumomab

The levels/effects of Lepirudin may be increased by: Antiplatelet Agents; Dasatinib; Herbs (Anticoagulant/Antiplatelet Properties); Nonsteroidal Anti-Inflammatory Agents; Pentosan Polysulfate Sodium; Prostacyclin Analogues; Salicylates; Thrombolytic Agents

Nutritional/Ethanol Interactions Herb/Nutraceutical: Avoid cat's claw, dong quai, evening primrose, feverfew, garlic, ginger, ginkgo, red clover, horse chestnut, green tea, ginseng (all have additional antiplatelet activity)

Adverse Reactions As with all anticoagulants, bleeding is the most common adverse event associated with lepirudin. Hemorrhage may occur at virtually any site. Risk is dependent on multiple variables.

HIT patients:

>10%: Hematologic: Anemia (12%), bleeding from puncture sites (11%), hematoma (11%)

1% to 10%:

Cardiovascular: Heart failure (3%), pericardial effusion (1%), ventricular fibrillation (1%)

Central nervous system: Fever (7%)

Dermatologic: Maculopapular rash (4%), eczema (3%)

Gastrointestinal: GI bleeding/rectal bleeding (5%)

Genitourinary: Vaginal bleeding (2%)

Hepatic: Transaminases increased (6%)

Renal: Hematuria (4%)

Respiratory: Epistaxis (4%)

Non-HIT populations (including those receiving thrombolytics and/or contrast media):

1% to 10%: Respiratory: Bronchospasm/stridor/dyspnea/cough

Available Dosage Forms

Injection, powder for reconstitution:

Refludan®: 50 mg

General Dosage Range Dosage adjustment recommended in patients with renal impairment

I.V.: *Adults:* Bolus: 0.2-0.4 mg/kg; Infusion: 0.1-0.15 mg/kg/hour (maximum: 0.21 mg/kg/hour)

Administration

Oral Administer **only** intravenously

I.V. I.V. bolus: Inject slowly for continuous infusion; solutions with 0.2 or 0.4 mg/mL may be used.

Stability

Reconstitution

Intravenous bolus: Use a solution with a concentration of 5 mg/mL: Reconstitute one vial (50 mg) of lepirudin with 1 mL of sterile water for injection or 0.9% sodium chloride injection. The final concentration of 5 mg/mL is obtained by transferring the contents of the vial into a sterile, single-use syringe (of at least 10 mL capacity) and diluting the solution to a total volume of 10 mL using sterile water for injection, 0.9% sodium chloride, or 5% dextrose in water.

Intravenous infusion: For continuous intravenous infusion, solutions with concentrations of 0.2 or 0.4 mg/mL may be used. Reconstitute 2 vials (50 mg each) of lepirudin with 1 mL each using either sterile water for injection or 0.9% sodium chloride injection. The final concentration of 0.2 mg/mL or 0.4 mg/mL is obtained by transferring the contents of both vials into an infusion bag containing 500 mL or 250 mL of 0.9% sodium chloride injection or 5% dextrose injection.

Storage

Intact vials should be stored at 2°C to 25°C (36°F to 77°F). Manufacturer recommends using reconstituted solution immediately after preparation. Reconstituted solutions of lepirudin are stable for 24 hours at room temperature.

Nursing Actions

Physical Assessment Note Administration for infusion specifics. Bleeding precautions should be observed. Monitor for hypersensitivity reaction, bleeding, chest pain, and rash. Teach patient bleeding precautions.

Patient Education This drug can only be administered by infusion. Report immediately any pain, swelling, burning, or bleeding at infusion site. You may have a tendency to bleed easily while taking this drug (brush teeth with soft brush, floss with waxed floss, use electric razor, avoid scissors or sharp knives, and avoid potentially harmful activities). Report unusual bleeding or bruising (bleeding gums, nosebleed, blood in urine, dark stool), pain in joints or back, CNS changes (fever, confusion), unusual fever, persistent nausea or GI upset, or swelling or pain at injection site.

Letrozole (LET roe zole)

Brand Names: U.S. Femara®

Index Terms CGS-20267

Pharmacologic Category Antineoplastic Agent, Aromatase Inhibitor

Medication Safety Issues

Sound-alike/look-alike issues:

Femara® may be confused with Famvir®, femhrt®, Provera®

Letrozole may be confused with anastrozole

Pregnancy Risk Factor X

Lactation Excretion in breast milk unknown/not recommended

Use For use in postmenopausal women in the adjuvant treatment of hormone receptor positive early breast cancer, extended adjuvant treatment of early breast cancer after 5 years of tamoxifen, advanced breast cancer with disease progression following antiestrogen therapy, hormone receptor positive or hormone receptor unknown, locally-advanced, or first-line (or second-line) treatment of advanced or metastatic breast cancer

Unlabeled Use Treatment of ovarian (epithelial) cancer, endometrial cancer

Mechanism of Action/Effect Nonsteroidal competitive inhibitor of the aromatase enzyme system, which catalyzes conversion of androgens to estrogens. Inhibition leads to a significant reduction in plasma estrogen levels. Does not affect synthesis of adrenal or thyroid hormones, aldosterone, or androgens.

Contraindications Use in women who are or may become pregnant

Canadian labeling: Additional contraindications (not in U.S. labeling): Hypersensitivity to letrozole, other aromatase inhibitors, or any component of the formulation; use in patients <18 years of age; breast-feeding

Warnings/Precautions Hazardous agent - use appropriate precautions for handling and disposal. Use caution with hepatic impairment; dose adjustment recommended in patients with cirrhosis or severe hepatic dysfunction. May cause dizziness, fatigue, and somnolence; patients should be cautioned before performing tasks which require mental alertness (eg, operating machinery or driving). May increase total serum cholesterol; in patients treated with adjuvant therapy and cholesterol levels within normal limits, an increase of >1.5 x ULN in total cholesterol has been demonstrated in 8.2% of letrozole-treated patients (25% requiring lipid-lowering medications) vs 3.2% of tamoxifen-treated patients (16% requiring medications); monitor cholesterol panel; may require antihyperlipidemics. May cause decreases in bone mineral density (BMD); a decrease in hip BMD by 3.8% from baseline in letrozole-treated patients vs 2% in placebo at 2 years has been demonstrated; however, there was no statistical difference in changes to the lumbar spine BMD scores; monitor BMD.

Drug Interactions

Avoid Concomitant Use There are no known interactions where it is recommended to avoid concomitant use.

Decreased Effect

The levels/effects of Letrozole may be decreased by: Tamoxifen; Tocilizumab

Increased Effect/Toxicity

Letrozole may increase the levels/effects of: CYP2A6 Substrates

The levels/effects of Letrozole may be increased by: Conivaptan

Adverse Reactions

>10%:

Cardiovascular: Edema (7% to 18%)

Central nervous system: Headache (4% to 20%), dizziness (3% to 14%), fatigue (8% to 13%)

Endocrine & metabolic: Hypercholesterolemia (3% to 52%), hot flashes (6% to 50%)

Gastrointestinal: Nausea (9% to 17%), weight gain (2% to 13%), constipation (2% to 11%)

Neuromuscular & skeletal: Weakness (4% to 34%), arthralgia (8% to 25%), arthritis (7% to 25%), bone pain (5% to 22%), back pain (5% to 18%), bone mineral density decreased/osteoporosis (5% to 15%), bone fracture (10% to 14%)

Respiratory: Dyspnea (6% to 18%), cough (6% to 13%)

Miscellaneous: Diaphoresis (≤24%), night sweats (15%)

1% to 10%:

Cardiovascular: Chest pain (6% to 8%), hypertension (5% to 8%), chest wall pain (6%), peripheral edema (5%); cerebrovascular accident including hemorrhagic stroke, thrombotic stroke (2% to 3%); thromboembolic event including venous thrombosis, thrombophlebitis, portal vein thrombosis, pulmonary embolism (2% to 3%); MI (1% to 2%), angina (1% to 2%), transient ischemic attack

Central nervous system: Insomnia (6% to 7%), pain (5%), anxiety (<5%), depression (<5%), vertigo (<5%),somnolence (3%)

Dermatologic: Rash (5%), alopecia (3% to 5%), pruritus (1%)

Endocrine & metabolic: Breast pain (2% to 7%), hypercalcemia (<5%)

Gastrointestinal: Diarrhea (5% to 8%), vomiting (3% to 7%), weight loss (6% to 7%), abdominal pain (6%), anorexia (1% to 5%), dyspepsia (3%)

Genitourinary: Urinary tract infection (6%), vaginal bleeding (5%), vaginal dryness (5%), vaginal hemorrhage (5%), vaginal irritation (5%)

Neuromuscular & skeletal: Limb pain (4% to 10%), myalgia (7% to 9%)

Ocular: Cataract (2%)

Renal: Renal disorder (5%)

Respiratory: Pleural effusion (<5%)

Miscellaneous: Infection (7%), influenza (6%), viral infection (6%), secondary malignancy (2% to 4%)

Available Dosage Forms

Tablet, oral: 2.5 mg

Femara®: 2.5 mg

General Dosage Range Dosage adjustment recommended in patients with hepatic impairment

Oral: *Adults (postmenopausal females):* 2.5 mg once daily

Administration

Oral Administer with or without food.

Stability

Storage Store at room temperature of 25°C (77°F); excursions permitted to 15°C to 30°C (59°F to 86°F).

Nursing Actions

Physical Assessment For use in postmenopausal women only. Monitor for hypertension, pain, gastrointestinal upset, hot flashes, and dyspnea on a regular basis.

Patient Education You may experience nausea, vomiting, hot flashes, loss of appetite, musculoskeletal pain, headache, sleepiness, fatigue, dizziness, constipation, diarrhea, or loss of hair (will grow back). Report chest pain, pressure, palpitations, or swollen extremities; weakness, severe headache, numbness, or loss of strength in any part of the body; difficulty speaking; vaginal bleeding; unusual signs of bleeding or bruising; respiratory difficulty; severe nausea; muscle pain; or skin rash.

Dietary Considerations May be taken without regard to meals. Calcium and vitamin D supplementation are recommended.

Leucovorin Calcium (loo koe VOR in KAL see um)

Index Terms 5-Formyl Tetrahydrofolate; Calcium Folinate; Calcium Leucovorin; Citrovorum Factor; Folinate Calcium; Folinic Acid (error prone synonym); Leucovorin

Pharmacologic Category Antidote; Chemotherapy Modulating Agent; Rescue Agent (Chemotherapy); Vitamin, Water Soluble

Medication Safety Issues

Sound-alike/look-alike issues:

Leucovorin may be confused with Leukeran®, Leukine®, LEVOleucovorin

Folinic acid may be confused with folic acid

Folinic acid is an error prone synonym and should not be used

Pregnancy Risk Factor C

Lactation Excretion in breast milk unknown/use caution

Breast-Feeding Considerations Leucovorin is a biologically active form of folic acid. Adequate amounts of folic acid are recommended in breast-feeding women. Refer to Folic Acid monograph.

Use Antidote for folic acid antagonists (methotrexate, trimethoprim, pyrimethamine) and rescue therapy following high-dose methotrexate; in combination with fluorouracil in the treatment of colon cancer; treatment of megaloblastic anemias when folate is deficient as in infancy, sprue, pregnancy, and nutritional deficiency when oral folate therapy is not possible

Unlabeled Use Adjunctive cofactor therapy in methanol toxicity; prevention of pyrimethamine hematologic toxicity in HIV-positive patients

Mechanism of Action/Effect A reduced form of folic acid, leucovorin supplies the necessary cofactor blocked by methotrexate. Leucovorin actively competes with methotrexate for transport sites, displaces methotrexate from intracellular binding sites, and restores active folate stores required for DNA/RNA synthesis. Stabilizes the binding of 5-dUMP and thymidylate synthetase, enhancing the activity of fluorouracil. When administered with pyrimethamine for the treatment of opportunistic infections, leucovorin reduces the risk for hematologic toxicity.

Methanol toxicity treatment: Formic acid (methanol's toxic metabolite) is normally metabolized to carbon dioxide and water by 10-formyltetrahydrofolate dehydrogenase after being bound to tetrahydrofolate. Administering a source of tetrahydrofolate may aid the body in eliminating formic acid.

Contraindications Pernicious anemia or vitamin B_{12}-deficient megaloblastic anemias

Warnings/Precautions When used for the treatment of accidental weak folic acid antagonist overdose, administer as soon as possible. When used for the treatment of a methotrexate overdose, administer as soon as possible. Do not wait for the results of a methotrexate level before initiating therapy. It is important to adjust the leucovorin dose once a methotrexate level is known. When used for methotrexate rescue therapy, methotrexate serum concentrations should be monitored to determine dose and duration of leucovorin therapy. The dose may need to be increased or administration prolonged in situations where methotrexate excretion may be delayed (eg, ascites, pleural effusion, renal insufficiency, inadequate hydration); **never administer leucovorin intrathecally.** Combination of leucovorin and sulfamethoxazole-trimethoprim for the acute treatment of PCP in patients with HIV infection has been reported to cause increased rates of treatment failure. Leucovorin may increase the toxicity of 5-fluorouracil; dose of 5-fluorouracil may need decreased.

Powder for injection: When doses >10 mg/m² are required, reconstitute using sterile water for injection, not a solution containing benzyl alcohol.

Injection: Due to calcium content, do not administer I.V. solutions at a rate >160 mg/minute. Not intended for intrathecal use.

Drug Interactions

Avoid Concomitant Use

Avoid concomitant use of Leucovorin Calcium with any of the following: Raltitrexed

Decreased Effect

Leucovorin Calcium may decrease the levels/effects of: Fosphenytoin; PHENobarbital; Phenytoin; Primidone; Raltitrexed; Trimethoprim

Increased Effect/Toxicity

Leucovorin Calcium may increase the levels/effects of: Capecitabine; Fluorouracil; Fluorouracil (Systemic); Fluorouracil (Topical)

Adverse Reactions Frequency not defined. Toxicities (especially gastrointestinal toxicity) of fluorouracil is higher when used in combination with leucovorin.

Dermatologic: Rash, pruritus, erythema, urticaria

Hematologic: Thrombocytosis

Respiratory: Wheezing

Miscellaneous: Allergic reactions, anaphylactoid reactions

Available Dosage Forms

Injection, powder for reconstitution: 50 mg, 100 mg, 200 mg, 350 mg

Injection, solution [preservative free]: 10 mg/mL (50 mL)

Tablet, oral: 5 mg, 10 mg, 15 mg, 25 mg

General Dosage Range

I.M.: *Children and Adults:* ≤1 mg/day [folate deficient megaloblastic anemia] **or** 15 mg (~10 mg/m^2) every 6 hours for 10 doses [methotrexate rescue dose]

I.V.:

Children: 15 mg (~10 mg/m^2) every 6 hours for 10 doses

Adults: Initial: 15 mg (~10 mg/m^2) every 6 hours for 10 doses [methotrexate rescue dose] **or** 200 mg/m^2 **or** 20 mg/m^2 as a single dose [colorectal cancer]

Oral: *Children and Adults:* 5-15 mg/day [weak folic acid antagonist overdose] **or** 15 mg (~10 mg/m^2) every 6 hours for 10 doses [methotrexate rescue dose]

Administration

Oral Do not administer orally in the presence of nausea or vomiting. Doses >25 mg should be administered parenterally.

I.V. Due to calcium content, do not administer I.V. solutions at a rate >160 mg/minute; not intended for intrathecal use.

Refer to individual protocols. Should be administered I.M., I.V. push, or I.V. infusion (15 minutes to 2 hours). Leucovorin should not be administered concurrently with methotrexate. It is commonly initiated 24 hours after the start of methotrexate. Toxicity to normal tissues may be irreversible if leucovorin is not initiated by ~40 hours after the start of methotrexate.

As a rescue after folate antagonists: Administer by I.V. bolus, I.M., or orally.

In combination with fluorouracil: Fluorouracil activity, the fluorouracil is usually given after, or at the midpoint, of the leucovorin infusion. Leucovorin is usually administered by I.V. bolus injection or short (10-120 minutes) I.V. infusion. Other administration schedules have been used; refer to individual protocols.

I.V. Detail pH: 8.1 (vials)

Stability

Reconstitution Powder for injection: Reconstitute with SWFI or BWFI; dilute in 100-1000 mL NS, D_5W for infusion. When doses >10 mg/m^2 are required, reconstitute using sterile water for injection, not a solution containing benzyl alcohol.

Storage

Powder for injection: Store at room temperature of 25°C (77°F). Protect from light. Solutions reconstituted with bacteriostatic water for injection U.S.P., must be used within 7 days. Solutions reconstituted with SWFI must be used immediately. Parenteral admixture is stable for 24 hours stored at room temperature (25°C) and for 4 days when stored under refrigeration (4°C).

Solution for injection: Prior to dilution, store vials under refrigeration at 2°C to 8°C (36°F to 46°F). Protect from light.

Tablet: Store at room temperature of 15°C to 30°C (59°F to 86°F).

Nursing Actions

Patient Education Maintain hydration. Report respiratory difficulty, lethargy, rash, or itching.

Dietary Considerations Solutions for injection contain calcium 0.004 mEq per leucovorin 1 mg

Leuprolide (loo PROE lide)

Brand Names: U.S. Eligard®; Lupron Depot-Ped®; Lupron Depot®

Index Terms Abbott-43818; Leuprolide Acetate; Leuprorelin Acetate; TAP-144

Pharmacologic Category Antineoplastic Agent, Gonadotropin-Releasing Hormone Agonist; Gonadotropin Releasing Hormone Agonist

Medication Safety Issues

Sound-alike/look-alike issues:

Lupron Depot® (1-month or 3-month formulation) may be confused with Lupron Depot-Ped® (1-month or 3-month formulation)

Lupron Depot-Ped® is available in two formulations, a 1-month formulation and a 3-month formulation. Both formulations offer an 11.25 mg strength which may further add confusion.

Pregnancy Risk Factor X

Lactation Excretion in breast milk unknown/contraindicated

Use Palliative treatment of advanced prostate cancer; management of endometriosis; treatment of anemia caused by uterine leiomyomata (fibroids); central precocious puberty

Unlabeled Use Treatment of breast cancer; infertility

Mechanism of Action/Effect Leuprolide, is an agonist of luteinizing hormone-releasing hormone (LHRH). Acting as a potent inhibitor of gonadotropin secretion; continuous administration results in suppression of ovarian and testicular steroidogenesis due to decreased levels of LH and FSH with subsequent decrease in testosterone (male) and estrogen (female) levels. In males, testosterone levels are reduced to below castrate levels. Leuprolide may also have a direct inhibitory effect on the testes, and act by a different mechanism not directly related to reduction in serum testosterone.

Contraindications Hypersensitivity to leuprolide, GnRH, GnRH-agonist analogs, or any component of the formulation; undiagnosed abnormal vaginal bleeding; pregnancy; breast-feeding

Lupron Depot® 22.5 mg, 30 mg, and 45 mg are also not indicated for use in women

Warnings/Precautions Hazardous agent - use appropriate precautions for handling and disposal. Transient increases in testosterone serum levels (~50% above baseline) occur at the start of treatment. Androgen-deprivation therapy (ADT) may increase the risk for cardiovascular disease (Levine, 2010); sudden cardiac death and stroke have been reported in men receiving GnRH agonists; long-term ADT may prolong the QT interval; consider the benefits of ADT versus the risk for QT prolongation in patients with a history of QT_c prolongation, with medications known to prolong the QT interval, or with pre-existing cardiac disease. Tumor flare, bone pain, neuropathy, urinary tract obstruction, and spinal cord compression have been reported when used for prostate cancer; closely observe patients for weakness, paresthesias, hematuria, and urinary tract obstruction in first few weeks of therapy. Observe patients with metastatic vertebral lesions or urinary obstruction closely. Exacerbation of endometriosis or uterine leiomyomata may occur initially. Decreased bone density has been reported when used for ≥6 months; use caution in patients with additional risk factors for bone loss (eg, chronic alcohol use, corticosteroid therapy). In patients with prostate cancer, androgen deprivation therapy may increase the risk for cardiovascular disease, diabetes, insulin resistance, obesity, alterations in lipids, and fractures. Use caution in patients with a history of psychiatric illness; alteration in mood, memory impairment, and depression have been associated with use. Rare cases of pituitary apoplexy (frequently secondary to pituitary adenoma) have been observed with leuprolide administration (onset from 1 hour to usually <2 weeks); may present as sudden headache, vomiting, visual or mental status changes, and infrequently cardiovascular collapse; immediate medical attention required. Females treated for precocious puberty may experience menses or spotting during the first 2 months of treatment; notify healthcare provider if bleeding continues after the second month.

Some dosage forms may contain benzyl alcohol which has been associated with "gasping syndrome" in neonates; patients with benzyl alcohol allergy may demonstrate a hypersensitivity reaction (usually local) in the form of erythema and induration at the injection site. Vehicle used in depot injectable formulations (polylactide-co-glycolide microspheres) has rarely been associated with retinal artery occlusion in patients with abnormal arteriovenous anastomosis. Due to different release properties, combinations of dosage forms or fractions of dosage forms should not be interchanged.

Drug Interactions

Avoid Concomitant Use There are no known interactions where it is recommended to avoid concomitant use.

Decreased Effect

Leuprolide may decrease the levels/effects of: Antidiabetic Agents

Increased Effect/Toxicity There are no known significant interactions involving an increase in effect.

Adverse Reactions

Children (percentages based on 1-month and 3-month pediatric formulations combined):

>10%: Local: Injection site pain (≤20%)

2% to 10%:

Cardiovascular: Vasodilation (2%)

Central nervous system: Emotional lability (5%), mood altered (5%), headache (3% to 5%), pain (3%)

Dermatologic: Acne (3%), rash (3% including erythema multiforme), seborrhea (3%)

Gastrointestinal: Weight gain (≤7%)

Genitourinary: Vaginal bleeding (3%), vaginal discharge (3%), vaginitis (3%)

Local: Injection site reaction (≤9%)

Adults: Note: For prostate cancer treatment, an initial rise in serum testosterone concentrations may cause "tumor flare" or worsening of symptoms, including bone pain, neuropathy, hematuria, or ureteral or bladder outlet obstruction during the first 2 weeks. Similarly, an initial increase in estradiol levels, with a temporary worsening of symptoms, may occur in women treated with leuprolide.

Delayed release formulations:

>10%:

Cardiovascular: Edema (≤14%)

Central nervous system: Headache (≤65%), pain (<2% to 33%), depression (≤31%), insomnia (≤31%), fatigue (≤17%), dizziness/vertigo (≤16%)

Dermatologic: Skin reaction (≤12%)

Endocrine & metabolic: Hot flashes (25% to 98%), testicular atrophy (≤20%), hyperlipidemia (≤12%), libido decreased (≤11%)

Gastrointestinal: Nausea/vomiting (≤25%), bowel function altered (≤14%), weight gain/loss (≤13%)

Genitourinary: Vaginitis (11% to 28%), urinary disorder (13% to 15%)
Local: Injection site burning/stinging (transient: ≤35%)
Neuromuscular & skeletal: Weakness (≤18%), joint disorder (≤12%)
Miscellaneous: Flu-like syndrome (≤12%)
1% to 10% (limited to important or life-threatening):
Cardiovascular: Angina (<5%), arrhythmia (<5%), atrial fibrillation (<5%), bradycardia (<5%), CHF (<5%), deep thrombophlebitis (<5%), hyper-/hypotension (<5%), palpitation (<5%), syncope (<5%), tachycardia (<5%)
Central nervous system: Nervousness (≤8%), anxiety (≤6%), confusion (<5%), delusions (<5%), dementia (<5%), fever (<5%), seizure (<5%)
Dermatologic: Acne (≤10%), alopecia (≤5%), bruising (≤5%), cellulitis (<5%), pruritus (≤3%), rash (≤2%), hirsutism (<2%)
Endocrine & metabolic: Dehydration (≤8%), gynecomastia (≤7%), breast tenderness/pain (≤6%), bicarbonate decreased (≥5%), hyper-/hypocholesterolemia (≥5%), hyperglycemia (≥5%), hyperphosphatemia (≥5%), hyperuricemia (≥5%), hypoalbuminemia (≥5%), hypoproteinemia (≥5%), lactation (<5%), testicular pain (≤4%), menstrual disorder (≤2%)
Gastrointestinal: Dysphagia (<5%), gastrointestinal hemorrhage (<5%), intestinal obstruction (<5%), ulcer (<5%), constipation (≤3%), gastroenteritis/colitis (≤3%), diarrhea (≤2%)
Genitourinary: Prostatic acid phosphatase increased/decreased (≥5%), urine specific gravity increased/decreased (≥5%), impotence (≤5%), balanitis (<5%), incontinence (<5%), penile/testis disorder (<5%), urinary tract infection (<5%), nocturia (≤4%), polyuria (2% to 4%), dysuria (≤2%), bladder spasm (<2%), erectile dysfunction (<2%), hematuria (<2%), urinary retention (<2%), urinary urgency (<2%)
Hematologic: Eosinophilia (≥5%), leukopenia (≥5%), platelets increased (≥5%), anemia
Hepatic: Liver function tests abnormal (≥5%), partial thromboplastin time increased (≥5%), prothrombin time increased (≥5%), hepatomegaly (<5%)
Local: Injection site pain (2% to 5%), injection site erythema (1% to 3%)
Neuromuscular & skeletal: Myalgia (≤8%), paresthesia (≤8%), neuropathy (<5%), paralysis (<5%), pathologic fracture (<5%), bone pain (<2%), arthralgia (≤1%)
Renal: BUN increased (≥5%), creatinine increased (≥5%)
Respiratory: Emphysema (<5%), epistaxis (<5%), hemoptysis (<5%), pleural effusion (<5%), pulmonary edema (<5%), dyspnea (≤2%), cough (≤1%)
Miscellaneous: Diaphoresis (≤5%), allergic reaction (<5%), infection (5%), lymphadenopathy (<5%)

Immediate release formulation:

>10%:
Cardiovascular: ECG changes/ischemia (19%), peripheral edema (12%)
Central nervous system: Pain (13%)
Endocrine & metabolic: Hot flashes (55%)
1% to 10% (limited to important or life-threatening):
Cardiovascular: Hypertension (8%), murmur (3%), thrombosis/phlebitis (2%), CHF (1%), angina, arrhythmia, MI, syncope
Central nervous system: Headache (7%), insomnia (7%), dizziness/lightheadedness (5%), anxiety, depression, fatigue, fever, nervousness
Dermatologic: Dermatitis (5%), alopecia, bruising, itching, lesions, pigmentation
Endocrine & metabolic: Gynecomastia/breast tenderness/pain (7%), testicular size decreased (7%), diabetes, hypercalcemia, hypoglycemia, libido decreased, thyroid enlarged
Gastrointestinal: Constipation (7%), anorexia (6%), nausea/vomiting (5%), diarrhea, dysphagia, gastrointestinal bleeding, peptic ulcer, rectal polyps
Genitourinary: Urinary frequency/urgency (6%), impotence (4%), urinary tract infection (3%), bladder spasm, dysuria, incontinence, testicular pain, urinary obstruction
Hematologic: Anemia (5%)
Local: Injection site reaction
Neuromuscular & skeletal: Weakness (10%), bone pain (5%), peripheral neuropathy
Ocular: Blurred vision
Renal: Hematuria (6%), BUN increased, creatinine increased
Respiratory: Dyspnea (2%), cough, pneumonia, pulmonary embolus, pulmonary fibrosis
Miscellaneous: Infection, inflammation

Pharmacodynamics/Kinetics

Onset of Action Following transient increase, testosterone suppression occurs in ~2-4 weeks of continued therapy

Product Availability

Lupron Depot-Ped® 3-month formulation: FDA approved August 2011; availability expected August 2011

Lupron Depot-Ped® 3-month formulation will be available in two strengths, 11.25 mg and 30 mg.

Available Dosage Forms

Injection, powder for reconstitution [preservative free]:
Eligard®: 7.5 mg (monthly), 22.5 mg (3 month), 30 mg (4 month), 45 mg (6 month)
Lupron Depot-Ped®: 7.5 mg (monthly), 11.25 mg (3 month), 11.25 mg (monthly), 15 mg (monthly), 30 mg (3 month)

Lupron Depot®: 3.75 mg (monthly), 7.5 mg (monthly), 11.25 mg (3 month), 22.5 mg (3 month), 30 mg (4 month), 45 mg (6 month)

Injection, solution: 5 mg/mL (2.8 mL)

General Dosage Range I.M., SubQ: *Children and Adults:* Dosage varies greatly depending on indication

Administration

I.M. Lupron Depot®, Lupron Depot-Ped®: Administer as a single injection. Vary injection site periodically

Other SubQ:

Eligard®: Vary injection site; choose site with adequate subcutaneous tissue (eg, upper or mid-abdomen, upper buttocks); avoid areas that may be compressed or rubbed (eg, belt or waistband)

Leuprolide acetate 5 mg/mL solution: Vary injection site; if an alternate syringe from the syringe provided is required, insulin syringes should be used

Stability

Reconstitution

Eligard®: Packaged in two syringes; one contains the Atrigel® polymer system and the second contains leuprolide acetate powder; follow package instructions for mixing

Lupron Depot®, Lupron Depot-Ped®: Reconstitute only with diluent provided

Storage

Eligard®: Store at 2°C to 8°C (36°F to 46°C). Allow to reach room temperature prior to using; once mixed, must be administered within 30 minutes.

Lupron Depot®, Lupron Depot-Ped®: Store at room temperature of 25°C (77°F); excursions permitted to 15°C to 30°C (59°F to 86°F). Upon reconstitution, the suspension does not contain a preservative and should be used immediately; discard if not used within 2 hours.

Leuprolide acetate 5 mg/mL solution: Store at 20°C to 25°C (68°F to 77°F); excursions permitted to 15°C to 30°C (59°F to 86°F). Protect from light and store vial in carton until use. Do not freeze.

Nursing Actions

Physical Assessment Instruct patients with diabetes to monitor glucose levels closely; may impact effectiveness of antidiabetic agents. If self-administered, teach patient or caregiver proper storage, injection technique, and syringe/ needle disposal. Wash hands before and after injection. Observe patients for weakness and paresthesias in the first few weeks of therapy. Monitor for symptoms of hypoglycemia.

Patient Education This medication may be administered on a regular schedule; keep all appointments. If you have diabetes, monitor blood sugar frequently; can cause alteration in glycemic control. You may experience disease flare (increased bone pain) and urinary retention during early treatment (usually resolves); dizziness, headache, lethargy, or faintness; nausea or vomiting; constipation; hot flashes or flushing; breast swelling or tenderness; or decreased libido or impotence. Instruct patient to notify prescriber of chest pain; swelling of extremities; difficulty urinating; CNS changes (change in strength on one side is greater than the other, trouble speaking or thinking, change in balance, or blurred eyesight); behavioral changes, such as depression, mood swings, or insomnia; severe headache; menstruation over 2 months; severe nausea or vomiting; increase in bone pain after 2-4 weeks of care; severe back pain; feeling very tired or weak; or increased thirst, weight loss, or urination.

Levalbuterol (leve al BYOO ter ole)

Brand Names: U.S. Xopenex HFA™; Xopenex®

Index Terms Levalbuterol Hydrochloride; Levalbuterol Tartrate; R-albuterol

Pharmacologic Category Beta$_2$ Agonist

Medication Safety Issues

Sound-alike/look-alike issues:

Xopenex® may be confused with Xanax®

Pregnancy Risk Factor C

Lactation Excretion in breast milk unknown/use caution

Breast-Feeding Considerations It is not known whether levalbuterol is excreted in human milk. Plasma levels following oral inhalation are low. Racemic albuterol was shown to be tumorigenic in animal studies.

Use Treatment or prevention of bronchospasm in children and adults with reversible obstructive airway disease

Mechanism of Action/Effect Relaxes bronchial smooth muscle by action on beta$_2$-receptors with little effect on heart rate

Contraindications Hypersensitivity to levalbuterol, albuterol, or any component of the formulation

Warnings/Precautions Optimize anti-inflammatory treatment before initiating maintenance treatment with levalbuterol. Do not use as a component of chronic therapy without an anti-inflammatory agent. Only the mildest form of asthma (Step 1 and/or exercise-induced) would not require concurrent use based upon asthma guidelines. Patient must be instructed to seek medical attention in cases where acute symptoms are not relieved or a previous level of response is diminished. The need to increase frequency of use may indicate deterioration of asthma, and treatment must not be delayed. A spacer device or valved holding chamber is recommended when using a metered-dose inhaler.

Use caution in patients with cardiovascular disease (arrhythmia or hypertension or HF), convulsive disorders, diabetes, glaucoma, hyperthyroidism, or hypokalemia. Beta-agonists may cause elevation in blood pressure, heart rate, and result in CNS stimulation/excitation. $Beta_2$-agonists may increase risk of arrhythmia, increase serum glucose, or decrease serum potassium.

Immediate hypersensitivity reactions (urticaria, angioedema, rash, bronchospasm) have been reported. Do not exceed recommended dose; serious adverse events including fatalities, have been associated with excessive use of inhaled sympathomimetics. Rarely, paradoxical bronchospasm may occur with use of inhaled bronchodilating agents; this should be distinguished from inadequate response. Use with caution during labor and delivery. Safety and efficacy have not been established in patients <4 years of age.

Drug Interactions

Avoid Concomitant Use

Avoid concomitant use of Levalbuterol with any of the following: Beta-Blockers (Nonselective); Iobenguane I 123

Decreased Effect

Levalbuterol may decrease the levels/effects of: Iobenguane I 123

The levels/effects of Levalbuterol may be decreased by: Alpha-/Beta-Blockers; Beta-Blockers (Beta1 Selective); Beta-Blockers (Nonselective); Betahistine

Increased Effect/Toxicity

Levalbuterol may increase the levels/effects of: Loop Diuretics; Sympathomimetics; Thiazide Diuretics

The levels/effects of Levalbuterol may be increased by: Atomoxetine; Cannabinoids; MAO Inhibitors; Tricyclic Antidepressants

Adverse Reactions

>10%:

Endocrine & metabolic: Serum glucose increased, serum potassium decreased

Neuromuscular & skeletal: Tremor (≤7%)

Respiratory: Rhinitis (3% to 11%)

Miscellaneous: Viral infection (7% to 12%)

>2% to 10%:

Central nervous system: Headache (8% to 12%), nervousness (3% to 10%), dizziness (1% to 3%), anxiety (≤3%), migraine (≤3%), weakness (3%)

Cardiovascular: Tachycardia (~3%)

Dermatologic: Rash (≤8%)

Gastrointestinal: Diarrhea (2% to 6%), dyspepsia (1% to 3%)

Neuromuscular & skeletal: Leg cramps (≤3%)

Respiratory: Asthma (9%), pharyngitis (3% to 10%), cough (1% to 4%), sinusitis (1% to 4%), nasal edema (1% to 3%)

Miscellaneous: Flu-like syndrome (1% to 4%), accidental injury (≤3%)

Note: Immediate hypersensitivity reactions have occurred (including angioedema, oropharyngeal edema, urticaria, and anaphylaxis).

Pharmacodynamics/Kinetics

Onset of Action Measured as a 15% increase in FEV_1:

Aerosol: 5.5-10.2 minutes; Peak effect: ~77 minutes

Nebulization: 10-17 minutes; Peak effect: 1.5 hours

Duration of Action Measured as a 15% increase in FEV_1:

Aerosol: 3-4 hours (up to 6 hours in some patients)

Nebulization: 5-6 hours (up to 8 hours in some patients)

Available Dosage Forms

Aerosol, for oral inhalation:

Xopenex HFA™: 45 mcg/actuation (15 g)

Solution, for nebulization [preservative free]: 1.25 mg/0.5 mL (30s)

Xopenex®: 0.31 mg/3 mL (24s); 0.63 mg/3 mL (24s); 1.25 mg/3 mL (24s)

General Dosage Range

Inhalation (metered-dose inhaler): *Children ≥4 years and Adults:* 1-2 puffs every 4-6 hours

Nebulization (solution):

Children ≤4 years: 0.31-1.25 mg every 4-6 hours as needed

Children 5-11 years: 0.31-0.63 mg 3 times/day

Children ≥12 years and Adults: 0.63-1.25 mg every 8 hours as needed

Elderly: Initial: 0.63 mg

Administration

Inhalation

Metered-dose inhaler: Shake well before use; prime with 4 test sprays prior to first use or if inhaler has not been use of more than 3 days. Clean actuator (mouthpiece) weekly. A spacer device or valved holding chamber is recommended when using a metered-dose inhaler.

Solution for nebulization: Safety and efficacy were established when administered with the following nebulizers: PARI LC Jet™, PARI LC Plus™, as well as the following compressors: PARI Master®, Dura-Neb® 2000, and Dura-Neb® 3000. Concentrated solution should be diluted prior to use. Blow-by administration is not recommended, use a mask device if patient unable to hold mouthpiece in mouth for administration.

Stability

Reconstitution Concentrated solution should be diluted with 2.5 mL NS prior to use.

Storage

Aerosol: Store at room temperature of 20°C to 25°C (68°F to 77°F); protect from freezing and direct sunlight. Store with mouthpiece down. Discard after 200 actuations.

Solution for nebulization: Store in protective foil pouch at room temperature of 20°C to 25°C (68°F to 77°F). Protect from light and excessive heat. Vials should be used within 2 weeks after opening protective pouch. Use within 1 week and protect from light if removed from pouch. Vials of concentrated solution should be used immediately after removing from protective pouch.

Nursing Actions

Physical Assessment Teach patient safe use of nebulizer.

Patient Education Stress or excessive exercising may exacerbate wheezing or bronchospasm. You may experience tremor, anxiety, dizziness, headache, upset stomach, nausea, or vomiting. Paradoxical bronchospasm can occur. Notify prescriber if any of the following occur: Chest pain, tightness, palpitations, severe headache, increased nervousness, restlessness, trembling, or muscle cramps. Report unusual signs of flu or infection, leg or muscle cramps, unusual cough, persistent GI problems, or vision changes.

Levetiracetam (lee va tye RA se tam)

Brand Names: U.S. Keppra XR™; Keppra®

Pharmacologic Category Anticonvulsant, Miscellaneous

Medication Safety Issues

Sound-alike/look-alike issues:

Keppra® may be confused with Keflex®, Keppra XR™

LevETIRAcetam may be confused with levOCARNitine, levofloxacin

Potential for dispensing errors between Keppra® and Kaletra® (lopinavir/ritonavir)

Medication Guide Available Yes

Pregnancy Risk Factor C

Lactation Enters breast milk/not recommended

Use Adjunctive therapy in the treatment of partial onset, myoclonic, and/or primary generalized tonic-clonic seizures

Mechanism of Action/Effect The precise mechanism by which levetiracetam exerts its antiepileptic effect is unknown. However, several studies have suggested the mechanism may involve one or more central pharmacologic effects.

Contraindications There are no contraindications listed in the U.S. manufacturer's labeling.

Canadian labeling: Hypersensitivity to levetiracetam or any component of the formulation

Warnings/Precautions Antiepileptics are associated with an increased risk of suicidal behavior/thoughts with use (regardless of indication); patients should be monitored for signs/symptoms of depression, suicidal tendencies, and other unusual behavior changes during therapy and instructed to inform their healthcare provider immediately if symptoms occur.

Severe dermatologic reactions (toxic epidermal necrolysis and Stevens-Johnson syndrome) have been reported; onset usually within ~2 weeks of treatment initiation but may be delayed (>4 months); discontinue for any signs of a hypersensitivity reaction or unspecified rash.

Psychotic symptoms (psychosis, hallucinations) and behavioral symptoms (including aggression, anger, anxiety, depersonalization, depression, personality disorder) may occur; incidence may be increased in children. Dose reduction or discontinuation may be required. Levetiracetam should be withdrawn gradually, when possible, to minimize the potential of increased seizure frequency. Use caution with renal impairment; dosage adjustment may be necessary. Impaired coordination, weakness, dizziness, and somnolence may occur, most commonly during the first month of therapy; use caution when driving or operating heavy machinery. Although rare, decreases in red blood cell counts, hemoglobin, hematocrit, white blood cell counts and neutrophils have been observed. Safety and efficacy of I.V. and extended release tablet formulations have not been established in children <16 years of age. Isolated elevations in diastolic blood pressure measurements have been reported in children <4 years of age; however, no observable differences were noted in mean diastolic measurements of children receiving levetiracetam vs placebo. Similar effects have not been observed in older children and adults.

Drug Interactions

Avoid Concomitant Use There are no known interactions where it is recommended to avoid concomitant use.

Decreased Effect

The levels/effects of LevETIRAcetam may be decreased by: Ketorolac; Ketorolac (Nasal); Ketorolac (Systemic); Mefloquine

Increased Effect/Toxicity

LevETIRAcetam may increase the levels/effects of: Alcohol (Ethyl); CNS Depressants; Methotrimeprazine; Selective Serotonin Reuptake Inhibitors

The levels/effects of LevETIRAcetam may be increased by: Droperidol; HydrOXYzine; Methotrimeprazine

Nutritional/Ethanol Interactions

Ethanol: May increase CNS depression; monitor for increased effects with coadministration. Caution patients about effects.

Food: Food may delay, but does not affect the extent of absorption.

Adverse Reactions

>10%:

Central nervous system: Behavioral symptoms (agitation, aggression, anger, anxiety, apathy, depersonalization, depression, emotional lability, hostility, hyperkinesias, irritability, nervousness, neurosis and personality disorder: adults 5% to 13%; children 5% to 38%), somnolence (8% to 23%), headache (14%), hostility (2% to 12%)

Gastrointestinal: Vomiting (15%), anorexia (3% to 13%)

Neuromuscular & skeletal: Weakness (9% to 15%)

Respiratory: Pharyngitis (6% to 14%), rhinitis (4% to 13%), cough (2% to 11%)

Miscellaneous: Accidental injury (17%), infection (2% to 13%)

1% to 10%:

Cardiovascular: Facial edema (2%)

Central nervous system: Fatigue (10%), nervousness (4% to 10%), dizziness (5% to 9%), personality disorder (8%), pain (6% to 7%), agitation (6%), irritability (6% to 7%), emotional lability (2% to 6%), mood swings (5%), depression (3% to 5%), vertigo (3% to 5%), ataxia (3%), amnesia (2%), anxiety (2%), confusion (2%)

Dermatologic: Bruising (4%), pruritus (2%), rash (2%), skin discoloration (2%)

Endocrine & metabolic: Dehydration (2%)

Gastrointestinal: Diarrhea (8%), nausea (5%), gastroenteritis (4%), constipation (3%)

Genitourinary: Urine abnormality (2%)

Hematologic: Leukocytes decreased (2% to 3%)

Neuromuscular & skeletal: Neck pain (2% to 8%), paresthesia (2%), reflexes increased (2%)

Ocular: Conjunctivitis (3%), diplopia (2%), amblyopia (2%)

Otic: Ear pain (2%)

Renal: Albuminuria (4%)

Respiratory: Influenza (5%), asthma (2%), sinusitis (2%)

Miscellaneous: Flu-like syndrome (3% to 8%), viral infection (2%)

Pharmacodynamics/Kinetics

Onset of Action Peak effect: Oral: 1 hour

Available Dosage Forms

Infusion, premixed in sodium chloride 0.54%: 1500 mg (100 mL)

Infusion, premixed in sodium chloride 0.75%: 1000 mg (100 mL)

Infusion, premixed in sodium chloride 0.82%: 500 mg (100 mL)

Injection, solution: 100 mg/mL (5 mL)

Keppra®: 100 mg/mL (5 mL)

Solution, oral: 100 mg/mL (5 mL, 118 mL, 472 mL, 473 mL, 480 mL, 500 mL)

Keppra®: 100 mg/mL (480 mL)

Tablet, oral: 250 mg, 500 mg, 750 mg, 1000 mg

Keppra®: 250 mg, 500 mg, 750 mg

Tablet, extended release, oral: 500 mg, 750 mg

Keppra XR™: 500 mg, 750 mg

General Dosage Range Dosage adjustment recommended in patients with renal impairment

Oral:

Immediate release:

Children 1 to <6 months: Initial: 7 mg/kg twice daily; Maintenance: 7-21 mg/kg/dose twice daily (maximum: 42 mg/kg/day)

Children 6 months to <4 years: Initial: 10 mg/kg twice daily; Maintenance: 10-25 mg/kg twice daily (maximum: 50 mg/kg/day)

Children 4 to <16 years: Initial: 10 mg/kg twice daily; Maintenance: 10-30 mg/kg twice daily (maximum: 60 mg/kg/day or 3000 mg/day)

Children ≥12 years: Initial: 500 mg twice daily; Maintenance: 500-1500 mg twice daily (maximum: 3000 mg/day)

Adults: Initial: 500 mg twice daily; Maintenance: 500-1500 mg twice daily (maximum: 3000 mg/day)

Extended release: *Children ≥16 years and Adults:* Initial: 1000 mg once daily; Maintenance: 1000-3000 mg once daily (maximum: 3000 mg/day)

I.V.: *Children ≥16 years and Adults:* Initial: 500 mg twice daily; Maintenance: 500-1500 mg twice daily (maximum: 3000 mg/day)

Administration

Oral

May be administered without regard to meals.

Oral solution: Should be administered with a calibrated measuring device (not a household teaspoon or tablespoon)

Tablet (immediate release and extended release): Only administer as whole tablet; do not crush, break or chew.

I.V. Infuse over 15 minutes

I.V. Detail pH: 5.5

Stability

Reconstitution Vials for injection: Must dilute dose in 100 mL of NS, LR, or D_5W.

Storage

Oral solution, tablets: Store at 25°C (77°F); excursions permitted to 15°C to 30°C (59°F to 86°F).

Premixed solution for infusion: Store at 20°C to 25°C (68°F to 77°F).

Vials for injection: Store at 25°C (77°F); excursions permitted to 15°C to 30°C (59°F to 86°F). Admixed solution is stable for 24 hours in PVC bags kept at room temperature.

Nursing Actions

Physical Assessment Monitor therapeutic response (seizure activity, force, type, duration) at beginning of therapy and periodically throughout. Monitor for CNS depression (somnolence and fatigue), behavioral abnormalities (psychosis, hallucinations, psychotic depression), and other behavioral symptoms (agitation, anger, aggression, irritability, hostility, anxiety, apathy, emotional lability, depersonalization, and depression). Taper dosage slowly when discontinuing. Observe and teach seizure/safety precautions.

Patient Education While using this medication, do not use alcohol. Maintain adequate hydration unless instructed to restrict fluid intake. You may experience drowsiness, dizziness, blurred vision, nausea, vomiting, loss of appetite, or dry mouth. Wear identification of epileptic status and medications. Report CNS changes, mentation changes, suicide ideation, depression, or changes in cognition; muscle cramping, weakness, tremors, changes in gait; persistent GI symptoms (cramping, constipation, vomiting, anorexia); rash or skin irritations; unusual bruising or bleeding (mouth, urine, stool); or worsening of seizure activity or loss of seizure control.

Dietary Considerations May be taken without regard to meals.

Levocabastine (Nasal) (LEE voe kab as teen)

Index Terms Levocabastine Hydrochloride

Pharmacologic Category Histamine H_1 Antagonist; Histamine H_1 Antagonist, Second Generation; Piperidine Derivative

Medication Safety Issues

Sound-alike/look-alike issues:

Levocabastine may be confused with levobunolol, levOCARNitine

Livostin® may be confused with lovastatin

International issues:

Livostin [Canada and multiple international markets] may be confused with Limoxin brand name for ambroxol [Indonesia] and amoxicillin [Mexico]; Lovastin brand name for lovastatin [Malaysia, Poland, Singapore]

Use Symptomatic treatment of allergic rhinitis

Product Availability Not available in U.S.

General Dosage Range Intranasal: *Children ≥12 years and Adults ≤65 years:* 2 sprays in each nostril 2-4 times/day

Administration

Other Intranasal: Shake bottle well before each use. Prior to initial use, bottle should be primed until a fine spray is delivered. Instruct patients to blow nose and clear nasal passages before administering spray and to inhale nasally while spraying.

Levocabastine (Ophthalmic)
(LEE voe kab as teen)

Index Terms Levocabastine Hydrochloride

Pharmacologic Category Histamine H_1 Antagonist; Histamine H_1 Antagonist, Second Generation; Piperidine Derivative

Medication Safety Issues

Sound-alike/look-alike issues:

Levocabastine may be confused with levobunolol, levOCARNitine

Livostin® may be confused with lovastatin

International issues:

Livostin [Canada and multiple international markets] may be confused with Limoxin brand name for ambroxol [Indonesia] and amoxicillin [Mexico]; Lovastin brand name for lovastatin [Malaysia, Poland, Singapore]

Use Treatment of seasonal allergic conjunctivitis

Product Availability Not available in U.S.

General Dosage Range Ophthalmic: *Children ≥12 years and Adults ≤65 years:* Instill 1 drop in affected eye(s) 2-4 times/day

Administration

Other For topical ophthalmic use only. Shake bottle well. Wash hands prior to use. Avoid touching the dropper tip to surfaces to avoid contamination.

Nursing Actions

Patient Education For use in eyes only. Shake well before using. Do not let tip of applicator touch eye; do not contaminate tip of applicator (may cause eye infection, eye damage, or vision loss). Do not wear contact lenses during treatment. This medication may cause drowsiness in some patients.

Levocetirizine (LEE vo se TI ra zeen)

Brand Names: U.S. Xyzal®

Index Terms Levocetirizine Dihydrochloride

Pharmacologic Category Histamine H_1 Antagonist; Histamine H_1 Antagonist, Second Generation; Piperazine Derivative

Medication Safety Issues

Sound-alike/look-alike issues:

Levocetirizine may be confused with cetirizine

Pregnancy Risk Factor B

Lactation Excretion in breast milk unknown/not recommended

Use Relief of symptoms of perennial and seasonal allergic rhinitis; treatment of skin manifestations (uncomplicated) of chronic idiopathic urticaria

Available Dosage Forms

Solution, oral: 0.5 mg/mL (150 mL)

Xyzal®: 0.5 mg/mL (150 mL)

Tablet, oral: 5 mg

Xyzal®: 5 mg

General Dosage Range Dosage adjustment recommended in patients with renal impairment

Oral:

Children 6 months to 5 years: 1.25 mg once daily

Children 6-11 years: 2.5 mg once daily

Children ≥12 years and Adults: 2.5-5 mg once daily

Administration

Oral Administer in the evening. May be administered without regard to meals.

Nursing Actions

Patient Education You may experience drowsiness. Avoid alcohol; may increase drowsiness. Children may experience diarrhea or constipation. Report excessive sedation.

Levodopa, Carbidopa, and Entacapone

(lee voe DOE pa, kar bi DOE pa, & en TA ka pone)

Brand Names: U.S. Stalevo®

Index Terms Carbidopa, Entacapone, and Levodopa; Carbidopa, Levodopa, and Entacapone; Entacapone, Carbidopa, and Levodopa

Pharmacologic Category Anti-Parkinson's Agent, COMT Inhibitor; Anti-Parkinson's Agent, Decarboxylase Inhibitor; Anti-Parkinson's Agent, Dopamine Precursor

Medication Safety Issues

Administration issues:

Strengths listed in Stalevo® brand names correspond to the **levodopa** component of the formulation only. All strengths of Stalevo® contain a levodopa/carbidopa ratio of 4:1 plus entacapone 200 mg.

Pregnancy Risk Factor C

Lactation Excretion in breast milk unknown/use caution

Use Treatment of idiopathic Parkinson's disease

Available Dosage Forms

Tablet:

Stalevo®: 50: Levodopa 50 mg, carbidopa 12.5 mg, and entacapone 200 mg; 75: Levodopa 75 mg, carbidopa 18.75 mg, and entacapone 200 mg; 100: Levodopa 100 mg, carbidopa 25 mg, and entacapone 200 mg; 125: Levodopa 125 mg, carbidopa 31.25 mg, and entacapone 200 mg; 150: Levodopa 150 mg, carbidopa 37.5 mg, and entacapone 200 mg; 200: Levodopa 200 mg, carbidopa 50 mg, and entacapone 200 mg

General Dosage Range Oral: *Adults:* 1 tablet (50-200 mg levodopa/12.5-50 mg carbidopa/200 mg entacapone) at each dosing interval (maximum: 1600 mg/day entacapone or 300 mg/day carbidopa)

Administration

Oral Swallow tablet whole; do not crush, break, or chew. Only 1 tablet should be administered at each dosing interval. May be administered without regard to meals.

Nursing Actions

Physical Assessment See individual agents.

Patient Education See individual agents.

Related Information

Entacapone *on page 396*

Levofloxacin (Systemic)

(lee voe FLOKS a sin)

Brand Names: U.S. Levaquin®

Pharmacologic Category Antibiotic, Quinolone; Respiratory Fluoroquinolone

Medication Safety Issues

Sound-alike/look-alike issues:

Levaquin® may be confused with Levoxyl®, Levsin/SL®, Lovenox®

Levofloxacin may be confused with levETIRAcetam, levodopa, Levophed®, levothyroxine

Medication Guide Available Yes

Pregnancy Risk Factor C

Lactation Enters breast milk/not recommended

Breast-Feeding Considerations Based on data from a case report, small amounts of levofloxacin are excreted in breast milk. Breast-feeding is not recommended by the manufacturer. Levofloxacin is the L-isomer of ofloxacin. Ofloxacin has also been shown to have minimal concentrations in human milk. Nondose-related effects could include modification of bowel flora.

Use Treatment of community-acquired pneumonia, including multidrug resistant strains of *S. pneumoniae* (MDRSP); nosocomial pneumonia; chronic bronchitis (acute bacterial exacerbation); acute bacterial sinusitis; prostatitis, urinary tract infection (uncomplicated or complicated); acute pyelonephritis; skin or skin structure infections (uncomplicated or complicated); reduce incidence or disease progression of inhalational anthrax (post-exposure)

Unlabeled Use Diverticulitis, enterocolitis (*Shigella* spp), epididymitis (nongonococcal), gonococcal infections, complicated intra-abdominal infections (in combination with metronidazole), Legionnaires' disease, peritonitis, PID

Note: As of April 2007, the CDC no longer recommends the use of fluoroquinolones for the treatment of gonococcal disease.

Mechanism of Action/Effect Levofloxacin, a fluorinated quinolone, exerts a broad spectrum bactericidal effect. It inhibits DNA gyrase which is required for DNA replication and transcription, DNA repair, recombination, and transposition within the bacteria.

Contraindications Hypersensitivity to levofloxacin, any component of the formulation, or other quinolones

Warnings/Precautions **[U.S. Boxed Warning]: There have been reports of tendon inflammation and/or rupture with quinolone antibiotics; risk may be increased with concurrent corticosteroids, organ transplant recipients, and in patients >60 years of age.** Rupture of the Achilles tendon sometimes requiring surgical repair has been reported most frequently; but other tendon sites (eg, rotator cuff, biceps) have also been reported. Strenuous physical activity, rheumatoid arthritis, and renal impairment may be an independent risk factor for tendonitis. Discontinue at first sign of tendon inflammation or pain. May occur even after discontinuation of therapy. Use with caution in patients with rheumatoid arthritis; may increase risk of tendon rupture. Systemic use is only recommended in children <18 years of age for the prevention of inhalational anthrax (postexposure); increased incidence of musculoskeletal disorders (eg, arthralgia, tendon rupture) has been observed in children. CNS effects may occur (tremor, restlessness, confusion, and very rarely hallucinations, increased intracranial pressure [including pseudotumor cerebri] or seizures). Potential for seizures, although very rare, may be increased with concomitant NSAID therapy. Use with caution in individuals at risk of seizures, with known or suspected CNS disorders or renal dysfunction. Avoid excessive sunlight and take precautions to limit exposure (eg, loose fitting clothing, sunscreen); may cause moderate-to-severe phototoxicity reactions. Discontinue use if photosensitivity occurs.

Rare cases of torsade de pointes have been reported in patients receiving levofloxacin. Use caution in patients with known prolongation of QT interval, bradycardia, hypokalemia, hypomagnesemia, or in those receiving concurrent therapy with Class Ia or Class III antiarrhythmics.

Severe hypersensitivity reactions, including anaphylaxis, have occurred with quinolone therapy. Reactions may present as typical allergic symptoms after a single dose, or may manifest as severe idiosyncratic dermatologic, vascular, pulmonary, renal, hepatic, and/or hematologic events, usually after multiple doses. Prompt discontinuation of drug should occur if skin rash or other symptoms arise. Prolonged use may result in fungal or bacterial superinfection, including *C. difficile*-associated diarrhea (CDAD) and pseudomembranous colitis; CDAD has been observed >2 months postantibiotic treatment. Peripheral neuropathies have been linked to levofloxacin use; discontinue if numbness, tingling, or weakness develops. **[U.S. Boxed Warning]: Quinolones may exacerbate myasthenia gravis; avoid use (rare, potentially life-threatening weakness of respiratory muscles may occur).** Unrelated to hypersensitivity, severe hepatotoxicity (including acute hepatitis and fatalities) has been reported. Elderly patients may be at greater risk. Discontinue therapy immediately if signs and symptoms of hepatitis occur. Hemolytic reactions may (rarely) occur with quinolone use in patients with latent or actual G6PD deficiency.

Fluoroquinolones have been associated with the development of serious, and sometimes fatal, hypoglycemia, most often in elderly diabetics, but also in patients without diabetes. This occurred most frequently with gatifloxacin (no longer available systemically) but may occur at a lower frequency with other quinolones.

Drug Interactions

Avoid Concomitant Use

Avoid concomitant use of Levofloxacin (Systemic) with any of the following: Artemether; BCG; Dronedarone; Lumefantrine; Nilotinib; Pimozide; QUEtiapine; QuiNINE; Tetrabenazine; Thioridazine; Toremifene; Vandetanib; Vemurafenib; Ziprasidone

Decreased Effect

Levofloxacin (Systemic) may decrease the levels/effects of: BCG; Mycophenolate; Sulfonylureas; Typhoid Vaccine

The levels/effects of Levofloxacin (Systemic) may be decreased by: Antacids; Calcium Salts; Didanosine; Iron Salts; Lanthanum; Magnesium Salts; Quinapril; Sevelamer; Sucralfate; Zinc Salts

Increased Effect/Toxicity

Levofloxacin (Systemic) may increase the levels/effects of: Corticosteroids (Systemic); Dronedarone; Pimozide; Porfimer; QTc-Prolonging Agents; QuiNINE; Sulfonylureas; Tetrabenazine; Thioridazine; Toremifene; Vandetanib; Varenicline; Vemurafenib; Vitamin K Antagonists; Ziprasidone

The levels/effects of Levofloxacin (Systemic) may be increased by: Alfuzosin; Artemether; Chloroquine; Ciprofloxacin; Ciprofloxacin (Systemic); Gadobutrol; Indacaterol; Insulin; Lumefantrine; Nilotinib; Nonsteroidal Anti-Inflammatory Agents; Probenecid; QUEtiapine; QuiNINE

Adverse Reactions 1% to 10%:

Cardiovascular: Chest pain (1%), edema (1%)

Central nervous system: Headache (6%), insomnia (4%), dizziness (3%), fatigue (1%), pain (1%)

Dermatologic: Rash (2%), pruritus (1%)

Gastrointestinal: Nausea (7%), diarrhea (5%), constipation (3%), abdominal pain (2%), dyspepsia (2%), vomiting (2%)

Genitourinary: Vaginitis (1%)

Local: Injection site reaction (1%)

Respiratory: Pharyngitis (4%), dyspnea (1%)

Miscellaneous: Moniliasis (1%)

Available Dosage Forms

Infusion, premixed in D_5W [preservative free]: 250 mg (50 mL); 500 mg (100 mL); 750 mg (150 mL)

Levaquin®: 250 mg (50 mL); 500 mg (100 mL); 750 mg (150 mL)

Injection, solution [preservative free]: 25 mg/mL (20 mL, 30 mL)

Solution, oral: 25 mg/mL (100 mL, 200 mL, 480 mL)

Levaquin®: 25 mg/mL (480 mL)

Tablet, oral: 250 mg, 500 mg, 750 mg

Levaquin®: 250 mg, 500 mg, 750 mg

General Dosage Range Dosage adjustment recommended in patients with renal impairment

Oral, I.V.:

Infants ≥6 months and Children ≤50 kg: 8 mg/kg every 12 hours (maximum: 250 mg/dose)

Children >50 kg: 500 mg once daily

Adults: 250-750 mg once daily

Administration

Oral Tablets may be administered without regard to meals. Oral solution should be administered 1 hour before or 2 hours after meals. Maintain adequate hydration of patient to prevent crystalluria.

I.V. Infuse 250-500 mg I.V. solution over 60 minutes; infuse 750 mg I.V. solution over 90 minutes. Too rapid of infusion can lead to hypotension. Avoid administration through an intravenous line with a solution containing multivalent cations (eg, magnesium, calcium). Maintain adequate hydration of patient to prevent crystalluria.

I.V. Detail pH: 3.8-5.8

Stability

Reconstitution Solution for injection: Single-use vials must be further diluted in compatible solution to a final concentration of 5 mg/mL prior to infusion.

Storage

Solution for injection:

Vial: Store at room temperature. Protect from light. Diluted solution is stable for 72 hours when stored at room temperature; stable for 14 days when stored under refrigeration. When frozen, stable for 6 months; do not refreeze. Do not thaw in microwave or by bath immersion.

Premixed: Store at ≤25°C (77°F); do not freeze. Brief exposure to 40°C (104°F) does not affect product. Protect from light.

Tablet, oral solution: Store at 25°C (77°F); excursions permitted to 15°C to 30°C (59°F to 86°F).

Nursing Actions

Physical Assessment Results of culture and sensitivity tests and patient's allergy history should be assessed before initiating therapy. Monitor patient closely; if an allergic reaction occurs (itching, urticaria, dyspnea or facial edema, loss of consciousness, tingling, cardiovascular collapse), drug should be discontinued immediately and prescriber notified. Monitor for hypersensitivity reactions, opportunistic infection, tendon rupture, and persistent diarrhea (*C. difficile*-associated colitis can occur post-treatment).

Patient Education If administered by infusion, report immediately any chest or back pain; tightness in chest; difficulty swallowing; swelling of face or mouth; or redness, swelling, or pain at infusion site.

Oral: Take exactly as directed (timing with meals, dairy products, antacids, or products containing calcium, iron, or zinc differs with each formulation). If you have diabetes, monitor glucose levels closely; may cause hypoglycemia. May cause dizziness, lightheadedness, confusion, nausea, vomiting, or photosensitivity. Report chest pain or palpitations; persistent diarrhea, abdominal pain, or constipation; signs of infection (unusual fever or chills, vaginal itching, or foul-smelling vaginal discharge); or unusual bruising or bleeding. If tendon inflammation or pain occurs or you experience signs of an allergic reaction (eg, itching, skin rash, respiratory difficulty, facial edema, difficulty swallowing, chest pain, palpitations), discontinue use and contact prescriber immediately.

Dietary Considerations Tablets may be taken without regard to meals. Oral solution should be administered on an empty stomach (1 hour before or 2 hours after a meal). Take 2 hours before or 2 hours after multiple vitamins, antacids, or other products containing magnesium, aluminum, iron, or zinc.

Related Information

Compatibility of Drugs *on page 1264*

LEVOleucovorin (lee voe loo koe VOR in)

Brand Names: U.S. Fusilev™

Index Terms 6S-leucovorin; Calcium Levoleucovorin; L-leucovorin; Levo-folinic Acid; Levo-leucovorin; Levoleucovorin Calcium Pentahydrate; S-leucovorin

Pharmacologic Category Antidote; Chemotherapy Modulating Agent; Rescue Agent (Chemotherapy)

Medication Safety Issues

Sound-alike/look-alike issues:

LEVOleucovorin may be confused with leucovorin calcium, Leukeran®, Leukine®

Pregnancy Risk Factor C

Lactation Excretion in breast milk unknown/not recommended

Use Treatment of advanced, metastatic colorectal cancer (palliative) in combination with fluorouracil; rescue agent after high-dose methotrexate therapy in osteosarcoma; antidote for impaired methotrexate elimination and for inadvertent overdosage of folic acid antagonists

Product Availability

Fusilev™ solution for injection: FDA approved April 2011; availability expected in the third quarter of 2011

Fusilev™ solution for injection is a ready-to-use formulation and will be available in 175 mg/17.5 mL and 250 mg/25 mL presentations.

Available Dosage Forms

Injection, powder for reconstitution:

Fusilev™: 50 mg

General Dosage Range I.V.: *Children and Adults:* Dosing varies greatly depending on indication

Administration

I.V. For I.V. administration only; do not administer intrathecally. Administer by slow I.V. push or infusion over at least 3 minutes, not to exceed 160 mg/minute (due to calcium content).

For colorectal cancer: Levoleucovorin has also been administered (unlabeled administration rate) as I.V. infusion over 2 hours (Comella, 2000; Tournigand, 2006).

Other Do not administer intrathecally.

Nursing Actions

Physical Assessment Levoleucovorin is used in combination with the drug 5FU for the treatment of colorectal cancer. When it is given with 5FU, it is usually administered over 5 days. It is important to review the patient's medications and monitor if he or she takes sulfa medications, seizure medications (eg, phenytoin), or a multivitamin with folic acid.

Patient Education Instruct patients that they should not take this medication if they have allergies to levoleucovorin, folic acid, or folinic acid. Patients should inform their doctors if they have kidney or liver problems. Patients should monitor their mouth daily for white patches or sores. Notify doctor of decreased urine output, more than four to five watery, loose stools which lasts more than 24 hours, or increased thirst, dry skin, or fever and/or shaking chills.

Levonorgestrel (LEE voe nor jes trel)

Brand Names: U.S. Mirena®; Next Choice™; Plan B® One Step

Index Terms LNg 20; Plan B

Pharmacologic Category Contraceptive; Progestin

Lactation Enters breast milk/use caution

Use

Intrauterine device (IUD): Prevention of pregnancy; treatment of heavy menstrual bleeding in women who also choose to use an IUD for contraception

Oral: Emergency contraception following unprotected intercourse or possible contraceptive failure

Plan B® One-Step is approved for OTC use by women ≥17 years of age and available by prescription only for women <17 years of age. Next Choice™ (generic of the original Plan-B® 2-dose regimen) is also approved for OTC use by women ≥17 years of age and by prescription only for women <17 years of age.

Available Dosage Forms

Intrauterine device, intrauterine:

Mirena®: 52 mg/device

Tablet, oral: 0.75 mg

Next Choice™: 0.75 mg

Plan B® One Step: 1.5 mg

General Dosage Range

Intrauterine: *Adults:* Insert into uterine cavity, releases 20 mcg/day over 5 years

Oral: *Adults:* 0.75 mg every 12 hours for 2 doses **or** 1.5 mg as a single dose

Administration

Oral Oral (Plan B® One Step): Consider repeating the dose if vomiting occurs within 2 hours. If severe vomiting occurs, may consider administering the oral tablets vaginally (ACOG, 2010).

Other

Intrauterine device: Inserted in the uterine cavity, to a depth of 6-10 cm, with the provided insertion device; should not be forced into the uterus

Oral tablets: If severe vomiting occurs, may consider administering the oral tablets vaginally (ACOG, 2010).

Nursing Actions

Physical Assessment Pregnancy should be ruled out prior to insertion of IUD. Monitor for prolonged menstrual bleeding, amenorrhea, and irregularity of menses. Caution patient about need for annual medical exams.

Patient Education This drug does not protect against HIV infection or other sexually-transmitted diseases. Cigarette smoking is not recommended. You may experience cramping, headache, abdominal discomfort, hair loss, weight changes, or unusual menses (breakthrough bleeding, irregularity, excessive bleeding). Report sudden acute headache or visual disturbance, unusual nausea or vomiting, any loss of feeling in arms or legs, or lower abdominal pain.

Intrauterine device: This method provides up to 5 years of birth control. It will be inserted and removed by your prescriber. Notify your prescriber if the system comes out by itself or if you have heavy bleeding, unusual vaginal discharge, low abdominal pain, painful sexual intercourse, chills, or fever. There is an increased risk of ectopic pregnancy with this product. Thread placement should be checked following each menstrual cycle; do not pull thread.

Tablet: This method provides emergency contraception. It is used after your normal form of birth control has failed or following unprotected sexual intercourse. It should be used within 72 hours. Contact prescriber if you vomit within 2 hours of taking either dose.

Levorphanol (lee VOR fa nole)

Index Terms Levo-Dromoran; Levorphan Tartrate; Levorphanol Tartrate

Pharmacologic Category Analgesic, Opioid

Medication Safety Issues

High alert medication:

The Institute for Safe Medication Practices (ISMP) includes this medication among its list of drug classes which have a heightened risk of causing significant patient harm when used in error.

Pregnancy Risk Factor B/D (prolonged use or high doses at term)

Lactation Excretion in breast milk unknown/not recommended

Use Relief of moderate-to-severe pain; preoperative sedation/analgesia; management of chronic pain (eg, cancer) requiring opioid therapy

Controlled Substance C-II

Available Dosage Forms

Tablet, oral: 2 mg,

General Dosage Range Dosage adjustment recommended in patients with hepatic impairment

Oral: *Adults:* 2-4 mg every 6-8 hours as needed

Nursing Actions

Physical Assessment Monitor blood pressure, CNS and respiratory status, and degree of sedation at beginning of therapy and periodically thereafter. Assess patient's physical and/or psychological dependence. For inpatients, implement safety measures (eg, side rails up, call light within reach, instructions to call for assistance). Discontinue slowly after prolonged use.

Patient Education Drug may cause physical and/or psychological dependence. While using this medication, do not use alcohol and other prescription or OTC medications (especially sedatives, tranquilizers, antihistamines, or pain medications) without consulting prescriber. Maintain adequate hydration, unless instructed to restrict fluid intake. May cause hypotension, dizziness, drowsiness, impaired coordination, or blurred vision; loss of appetite, nausea, or vomiting; or constipation. Report chest pain, slow or rapid heartbeat, dizziness, or persistent headache; confusion or respiratory difficulties; or severe constipation.

Levothyroxine (lee voe thye ROKS een)

Brand Names: U.S. Levothroid®; Levoxyl®; Synthroid®; Tirosint®; Unithroid®

Index Terms *L*-Thyroxine Sodium; Levothyroxine Sodium; T_4

Pharmacologic Category Thyroid Product

Medication Safety Issues

Sound-alike/look-alike issues:

Levothyroxine may be confused with lamoTRIgine, Lanoxin®, levofloxacin, liothyronine

Levoxyl® may be confused with Lanoxin®, Levaquin®, Luvox®

Synthroid® may be confused with Symmetrel®

Administration issues:

Significant differences exist between oral and I.V. dosing. Use caution when converting from one route of administration to another.

Other safety concerns:

To avoid errors due to misinterpretation of a decimal point, always express dosage in mcg (**not** mg).

Pregnancy Risk Factor A

Lactation Enters breast milk/use caution

Breast-Feeding Considerations Thyroid hormones are minimally found in breast milk. The amount of endogenous thyroxine found in breast milk does not influence infant plasma thyroid values. Levothyroxine was not found to cause adverse events to the infant or mother during breast-feeding. Adequate thyroid hormone concentrations are required to maintain normal lactation. Appropriate levothyroxine doses should be continued during breast-feeding.

Use Replacement or supplemental therapy in hypothyroidism; pituitary TSH suppression

Unlabeled Use Management of hemodynamically unstable potential organ donors increasing the quantity of organs available for transplantation

Mechanism of Action/Effect It is believed the thyroid hormone exerts its many metabolic effects through control of DNA transcription and protein synthesis

Contraindications Hypersensitivity to levothyroxine sodium or any component of the formulation; acute MI; thyrotoxicosis of any etiology; uncorrected adrenal insufficiency

Capsule: Additional contraindication: Inability to swallow capsules

Warnings/Precautions [U.S. Boxed Warning]: Thyroid supplements are ineffective and potentially toxic when used for the treatment of obesity or for weight reduction, especially in euthyroid patients. High doses may produce serious or even life-threatening toxic effects particularly when used with some anorectic drugs (eg, sympathomimetic amines). Routine use of T_4 for TSH suppression is not recommended in patients with benign thyroid nodules. In patients deemed appropriate candidates, treatment should never be fully suppressive (TSH <0.1 mIU/L). Use with caution and reduce dosage in patients with angina pectoris or other cardiovascular disease; decrease initial dose. Use cautiously in the elderly since they may be more likely to have compromised cardiovascular functions. Patients with adrenal insufficiency, myxedema, diabetes mellitus and insipidus may have symptoms exaggerated or aggravated. Chronic hypothyroidism predisposes patients to coronary artery disease. Long-term therapy can decrease bone mineral density. Levoxyl® may rapidly swell and disintegrate causing choking or gagging (should be administered with a full glass of water); use caution in patients with dysphagia or other swallowing disorders.

Drug Interactions

Avoid Concomitant Use

Avoid concomitant use of Levothyroxine with any of the following: Sodium Iodide I131

Decreased Effect

Levothyroxine may decrease the levels/effects of: Sodium Iodide I131; Theophylline Derivatives

The levels/effects of Levothyroxine may be decreased by: Aluminum Hydroxide; Bile Acid Sequestrants; Calcium Polystyrene Sulfonate; Calcium Salts; CarBAMazepine; Estrogen Derivatives; Fosphenytoin; Iron Salts; Lanthanum; Orlistat; Phenytoin; Raloxifene; Rifampin; Sevelamer; Sodium Polystyrene Sulfonate; Sucralfate

Increased Effect/Toxicity

Levothyroxine may increase the levels/effects of: Vitamin K Antagonists

Nutritional/Ethanol Interactions Food: Taking levothyroxine with enteral nutrition may cause reduced bioavailability and may lower serum thyroxine levels leading to signs or symptoms of hypothyroidism. Soybean flour (infant formula), cottonseed meal, walnuts, and dietary fiber may decrease absorption of levothyroxine from the GI tract. Management: Take in the morning on an empty stomach at least 30 minutes before food. Consider an increase in dose if taken with enteral tube feed.

Adverse Reactions Frequency not defined.

Cardiovascular: Angina, arrhythmia, cardiac arrest, flushing, heart failure, hypertension, MI, palpitation, pulse increased, tachycardia

Central nervous system: Anxiety, emotional lability, fatigue, fever, headache, hyperactivity, insomnia, irritability, nervousness, pseudotumor cerebri (children), seizure (rare)

Dermatologic: Alopecia

Endocrine & metabolic: Fertility impaired, menstrual irregularities

Gastrointestinal: Abdominal cramps, appetite increased, diarrhea, vomiting, weight loss

Hepatic: Liver function tests increased

Neuromuscular & skeletal: Bone mineral density decreased, muscle weakness, tremor, slipped capital femoral epiphysis (children)

Respiratory: Dyspnea

Miscellaneous: Diaphoresis, heat intolerance, hypersensitivity (to inactive ingredients, symptoms include urticaria, pruritus, rash, flushing, angioedema, GI symptoms, fever, arthralgia, serum sickness, wheezing)

Levoxyl®: Choking, dysphagia, gagging

Pharmacodynamics/Kinetics

Onset of Action Therapeutic: Oral: 3-5 days; I.V. 6-8 hours; Peak effect: I.V.: 24 hours

Available Dosage Forms

Capsule, soft gelatin, oral:

Tirosint®: 13 mcg, 25 mcg, 50 mcg, 75 mcg, 88 mcg, 100 mcg, 112 mcg, 125 mcg, 137 mcg, 150 mcg

Injection, powder for reconstitution: 100 mcg, 500 mcg

Tablet, oral: 25 mcg, 50 mcg, 75 mcg, 88 mcg, 100 mcg, 112 mcg, 125 mcg, 137 mcg, 150 mcg, 175 mcg, 200 mcg, 300 mcg

Levothroid®: 25 mcg, 50 mcg, 75 mcg, 88 mcg, 100 mcg, 112 mcg, 125 mcg, 137 mcg, 150 mcg, 175 mcg, 200 mcg, 300 mcg

Levoxyl®: 25 mcg, 50 mcg, 75 mcg, 88 mcg, 100 mcg, 112 mcg, 125 mcg, 137 mcg, 150 mcg, 175 mcg, 200 mcg

Synthroid®: 25 mcg, 50 mcg, 75 mcg, 88 mcg, 100 mcg, 112 mcg, 125 mcg, 137 mcg, 150 mcg, 175 mcg, 200 mcg, 300 mcg

Unithroid®: 25 mcg, 50 mcg, 75 mcg, 88 mcg, 100 mcg, 112 mcg, 125 mcg, 150 mcg, 175 mcg, 200 mcg, 300 mcg

General Dosage Range

I.M.: *Children and Adults:* 50% of oral dose

I.V.:

Children: 50% of oral dose

Adults: 50% of oral dose or 200-500 mcg, then 100-300 mcg the next day if needed

Oral:

Children 1-3 months: 10-15 mcg/kg/day

Children 3-6 months: 8-10 mcg/kg/day

Children 6-12 months: 6-8 mcg/kg/day

Children 1-5 years: 5-6 mcg/kg/day

Children 6-12 years: 4-5 mcg/kg/day

Children >12 years: 2-3 mcg/kg/day

Adults: Initial: 12.5-25 mcg/day **or** 1.7 mcg/kg/day (usual doses are ≤200 mcg/day)

*Elderly >50 years without cardiac disease **or** <50 years with cardiac disease:* Initial: 25-50 mcg/day

Elderly >50 years with cardiac disease: Initial: 12.5-25 mcg/day

Administration

Oral Administer in the morning on an empty stomach, at least 30 minutes before food.

Capsule: Must be swallowed whole; do not cut, crush, or attempt to dissolve capsules in water to prepare a suspension

Tablet: May be crushed and suspended in 5-10 mL of water; suspension should be used immediately. Levoxyl® should be administered with a full glass of water to prevent gagging (due to tablet swelling).

I.V. Dilute vial with 5 mL normal saline; use immediately after reconstitution; should not be admixed with other solutions

Other Nasogastric tube: Bioavailability of levothyroxine is reduced if administered with enteral tube feeds. Since holding feedings for at least 1 hour before and after levothyroxine administration may not completely resolve the interaction, an increase in dose (eg, additional 25 mcg) may be necessary (Dickerson, 2010).

Stability

Reconstitution Dilute vial for injection with 5 mL normal saline. Reconstituted concentrations for the 100 mcg, 200 mcg and 500 mcg vials are 20 mcg/mL, 40 mcg/mL, and 100 mcg/mL, respectively. Shake well and use immediately after reconstitution (manufacturer recommendation); discard any unused portions.

Storage Store capsules, tablets, and injection at room temperature; excursions permitted to 15°C to 30°C (59°F to 86°F). Protect from light and moisture.

Additional stability data:

Stability in polypropylene syringes (100 mcg/mL in NS) at 5°C ± 1°C is 7 days (Gupta, 2000).

Stability in latex-free, PVC minibags protected from light and stored at 15°C to 30°C (59°F to 86°F) was 12 hours for a 2 mcg/mL concentration or 18 hours for a 0.4 mcg/mL concentration in NS. May be exposed to light; however, stability time is significantly reduced, especially for the 2 mcg/mL concentration (Strong, 2010).

Nursing Actions

Physical Assessment Monitor for hyper-/hypothyroidism on a regular basis during therapy.

Patient Education Thyroid replacement therapy is generally for life. Take in the morning, 30 minutes before breakfast. Do not take antacids or iron preparations within 4 hours of thyroid medication. Report chest pain, rapid heart rate, palpitations, heat intolerance, excessive sweating, increased nervousness, agitation, or lethargy.

Dietary Considerations Should be taken on an empty stomach, at least 30 minutes before food.

Lidocaine (Systemic) (LYE doe kane)

Brand Names: U.S. Xylocaine®; Xylocaine® Dental; Xylocaine® MPF

Index Terms Lidocaine Hydrochloride; Lignocaine Hydrochloride

Pharmacologic Category Antiarrhythmic Agent, Class Ib; Local Anesthetic

Medication Safety Issues

High alert medication:

The Institute for Safe Medication Practices (ISMP) includes this medication (epidural administration; I.V. formulation) among its list of drugs which have a heightened risk of causing significant patient harm when used in error.

International issues:

Lidosen [Italy] may be confused with Lincocin brand name for lincomycin [U.S., Canada, and multiple international markets]; Lodosyn brand name for carbidopa [U.S.]

Pregnancy Risk Factor B

Lactation Enters breast milk/use caution (AAP rates "compatible"; AAP 2001 update pending)

Breast-Feeding Considerations Small amounts of lidocaine and the MEGX metabolite are found in breast milk. The actual amount may depend on route and duration of administration. When administered topically at recommended doses, the amount of lidocaine available to the nursing infant would not be expected to cause adverse events. Cumulative exposure from all routes of administration should be considered.

Use Local and regional anesthesia by infiltration, nerve block, epidural, or spinal techniques; acute treatment of ventricular arrhythmias from myocardial infarction or cardiac manipulation

Unlabeled Use

ACLS guidelines: Hemodynamically stable monomorphic ventricular tachycardia (VT) (preserved ventricular function); polymorphic VT (preserved ventricular function); drug-induced monomorphic VT; when amiodarone is not available, pulseless VT or ventricular fibrillation (VF) (unresponsive to defibrillation, CPR, and vasopressor administration)

PALS guidelines: When amiodarone is not available, pulseless VT or VF (unresponsive to defibrillation, CPR, and epinephrine administration); consider in patients with cocaine overdose to prevent arrhythmias secondary to MI

I.V. infusion for chronic pain syndrome

Mechanism of Action/Effect Class Ib antiarrhythmic; suppresses automaticity of conduction tissue by increasing electrical stimulation threshold of ventricles, His-Purkinje system, and spontaneous depolarization of ventricles during diastole by direct action on tissues; blocks both initiation and conduction of nerve impulses by decreasing the neuronal membrane's permeability to sodium ions, which results in inhibition of depolarization with resultant blockade of conduction

Contraindications Hypersensitivity to lidocaine or any component of the formulation; hypersensitivity to another local anesthetic of the amide type; Adam-Stokes syndrome; severe degrees of SA, AV, or intraventricular heart block (except in patients with a functioning artificial pacemaker); premixed injection may contain corn-derived dextrose and its use is contraindicated in patients with allergy to corn-related products

Warnings/Precautions Use caution in patients with severe hepatic dysfunction or pseudocholinesterase deficiency; may have increased risk of lidocaine toxicity.

Intravenous: Constant ECG monitoring is necessary during I.V. administration. Use cautiously in hepatic impairment, any degree of heart block, Wolff-Parkinson-White syndrome, HF, marked hypoxia, severe respiratory depression, hypovolemia, history of malignant hyperthermia, or shock. Increased ventricular rate may be seen when administered to a patient with atrial fibrillation. Correct electrolyte disturbances, especially hypokalemia or hypomagnesemia, prior to use and throughout therapy. Correct any underlying causes of ventricular arrhythmias. Monitor closely for signs and symptoms of CNS toxicity. The elderly may be prone to increased CNS and cardiovascular side effects. Reduce dose in hepatic dysfunction and CHF.

Injectable anesthetic: Follow appropriate administration techniques so as not to administer any intravascularly. Continuous intra-articular infusion of local anesthetics after arthroscopic or other surgical procedures is **not** an approved use; chondrolysis (primarily in the shoulder joint) has occurred following infusion, with some cases requiring arthroplasty or shoulder replacement. Solutions containing antimicrobial preservatives should not be used for epidural or spinal anesthesia. Some solutions contain a bisulfite; avoid in patients who are allergic to bisulfite. Resuscitative equipment, medicine and oxygen should be available in case of emergency. Use products containing epinephrine cautiously in patients with significant vascular disease, compromised blood flow, or during or following general anesthesia (increased risk of arrhythmias). Adjust the dose for the elderly, pediatric, acutely ill, and debilitated patients.

Drug Interactions

Avoid Concomitant Use

Avoid concomitant use of Lidocaine (Systemic) with any of the following: Conivaptan; Saquinavir

Decreased Effect

The levels/effects of Lidocaine (Systemic) may be decreased by: CYP1A2 Inducers (Strong); CYP3A4 Inducers (Strong); Cyproterone; Deferasirox; Etravirine; Herbs (CYP3A4 Inducers); Tocilizumab

Increased Effect/Toxicity

Lidocaine (Systemic) may increase the levels/effects of: Prilocaine

The levels/effects of Lidocaine (Systemic) may be increased by: Abiraterone Acetate; Amiodarone; Beta-Blockers; Conivaptan; CYP1A2 Inhibitors (Moderate); CYP1A2 Inhibitors (Strong); CYP3A4 Inhibitors (Moderate); CYP3A4 Inhibitors (Strong); Darunavir; Dasatinib; Deferasirox; Disopyramide; Ivacaftor; Saquinavir; Telaprevir

Nutritional/Ethanol Interactions Herb/Nutraceutical: St John's wort may decrease lidocaine levels; avoid concurrent use.

Adverse Reactions Effects vary with route of administration. Many effects are dose related.

Frequency not defined.

Cardiovascular: Arrhythmia, bradycardia, arterial spasms, cardiovascular collapse, defibrillator threshold increased, edema, flushing, heart block, hypotension, sinus node supression, vascular insufficiency (periarticular injections)

Central nervous system: Agitation, anxiety, apprehension, coma, confusion, disorientation, dizziness, drowsiness, euphoria, hallucinations, headache, hyperesthesia, hypoesthesia, lethargy, lightheadedness, nervousness, psychosis, seizure, slurred speech, somnolence, unconsciousness

Gastrointestinal: Metallic taste, nausea, vomiting

Local: Thrombophlebitis

Neuromuscular & skeletal: Paresthesia, transient radicular pain (subarachnoid administration; up to 1.9%), tremor, twitching, weakness

Otic: Tinnitus

Respiratory: Bronchospasm, dyspnea, respiratory depression or arrest

Miscellaneous: Allergic reactions, anaphylactoid reaction, sensitivity to temperature extremes

Following spinal anesthesia: Positional headache (3%), shivering (2%) nausea, peripheral nerve symptoms, respiratory inadequacy and double vision (<1%), hypotension, cauda equina syndrome

Pharmacodynamics/Kinetics

Onset of Action Single bolus dose: 45-90 seconds

Duration of Action 10-20 minutes

Available Dosage Forms

Infusion, premixed in D_5W: 0.4% [4 mg/mL] (250 mL, 500 mL); 0.8% [8 mg/mL] (250 mL, 500 mL)

Injection, solution: 1% [10 mg/mL] (2 mL, 10 mL, 20 mL, 30 mL, 50 mL); 2% [20 mg/mL] (2 mL, 5 mL, 20 mL, 50 mL)

Xylocaine®: 0.5% [5 mg/mL] (50 mL); 1% [10 mg/mL] (10 mL, 20 mL, 50 mL); 2% [20 mg/mL] (10 mL, 20 mL, 50 mL)

Xylocaine® Dental: 2% [20 mg/mL] (1.8 mL)

Injection, solution [preservative free]: 0.5% [5 mg/mL] (50 mL); 1% [10 mg/mL] (2 mL, 5 mL, 30 mL); 1.5% [15 mg/mL] (20 mL); 2% [20 mg/mL] (2 mL, 5 mL, 10 mL); 4% [40 mg/mL] (5 mL)

Xylocaine®: 2% [20 mg/mL] (5 mL)

Xylocaine® MPF: 0.5% [5 mg/mL] (50 mL); 1% [10 mg/mL] (2 mL, 5 mL, 10 mL, 30 mL); 1.5% [15 mg/mL] (10 mL, 20 mL); 2% [20 mg/mL] (2 mL, 5 mL, 10 mL); 4% [40 mg/mL] (5 mL)

Injection, solution, premixed in $D_{7.5}W$ [preservative free]: 5% [50 mg/mL] (2 mL)

General Dosage Range Dosage adjustment recommended in patients with hepatic impairment.

I.V.:

Children: Loading dose: 1 mg/kg, may repeat 0.5-1 mg/kg; Infusion: 20-50 mcg/kg/minute

Adults: Bolus: 1-1.5 mg/kg, may repeat 0.5-0.75 mg/kg up to a total of 3 mg/kg; Infusion: 1-4 mg/minute

Local injection: *Children and Adults:* Maximum: 4.5 mg/kg/dose; do not repeat within 2 hours

Administration

I.V. Continuous I.V. infusion rates: 2 g/250 mL D_5W:

1 mg/minute: 7.5 mL/hour
2 mg/minute: 15 mL/hour
3 mg/minute: 22.5 mL/hour
4 mg/minute: 30 mL/hour

I.V. Detail Local thrombophlebitis may occur in patients receiving prolonged I.V. infusions.

pH: 5-7 (injection); 3.5-6.0 (premixed infusion solution in D_5W)

Other

Intraosseous (I.O.; unlabeled administration route): Intraosseous administration is a safe and effective alternative to venous access in children with cardiac arrest; the onset for most medications is similar to that of I.V. administration (PALS, 2010). In adults, I.O. administration is a reasonable alternative when quick I.V. access is not feasible (ACLS, 2010).

Intratracheal (unlabeled administration route): Dilute in NS or sterile water. Absorption is greater with sterile water and results in less impairment of PaO_2 (Hahnel, 1990). Stop compressions, spray drug quickly down tube. Flush with 5 mL of NS and follow immediately with several quick insufflations and continue chest compressions.

Local infiltration: Buffered lidocaine for injectable local anesthetic may be prepared: Add 2 mL of sodium bicarbonate 8.4% to 18 mL of lidocaine 1% (Christoph, 1988)

Stability

Reconstitution Standard diluent: 2 g/250 mL D_5W.

Storage Injection: Stable at room temperature. Stability of parenteral admixture at room temperature (25°C) is the expiration date on premixed bag; out of overwrap stability is 30 days.

Nursing Actions

Physical Assessment Dental/local anesthetic: Use caution to prevent gagging or choking. Avoid food or drink for 1 hour. **Antiarrhythmic: I.V.:** Monitor ECG, blood pressure, and respirations closely and continually. Keep patient supine to reduce hypotensive effects. Assess frequently for adverse reactions or signs of CNS toxicity (eg, drowsiness, lightheadedness, dizziness, tinnitus, blurred vision, vomiting, twitching, tremor, lethargy, coma, agitation, slurred speech, seizure, anxiety, euphoria, hallucinations, paresthesia, psychosis).

Patient Education I.V.: You will be monitored during infusion. Do not get up without assistance. Report dizziness, numbness, double vision, nausea, pain or burning at infusion site, nightmares, hearing strange noises, seeing unusual visions, or respiratory difficulty.

Dietary Considerations Premixed injection may contain corn-derived dextrose and its use is contraindicated in patients with allergy to corn-related products.

Related Information

Peak and Trough Guidelines *on page 1276*

Lidocaine (Topical) (LYE doe kane)

Brand Names: U.S. AneCream™ [OTC]; Anestafoam™ [OTC]; Band-Aid® Hurt Free™ Antiseptic Wash [OTC]; Burn Jel Plus [OTC]; Burn Jel® [OTC]; L-M-X® 4 [OTC]; L-M-X® 5 [OTC]; LidaMantle®; Lidoderm®; LTA® 360; Premjact®; Regenecare®; Regenecare® HA [OTC]; Solarcaine® cool aloe Burn Relief [OTC]; Topicaine® [OTC]; Unburn® [OTC]; Xylocaine®

Index Terms Lidocaine Hydrochloride; Lidocaine Patch; Lignocaine Hydrochloride; Viscous Lidocaine; Xylocaine Viscous

Pharmacologic Category Analgesic, Topical; Local Anesthetic

Pregnancy Risk Factor B

Lactation Enters breast milk/use caution (AAP rates "compatible"; AAP 2001 update pending)

Use

Rectal: Temporary relief of pain and itching due to anorectal disorders

Topical: Local anesthetic for oral mucous membrane; use in laser/cosmetic surgeries; minor burns, cuts, and abrasions of the skin

Oral topical solution (viscous): Topical anesthesia of irritated oral mucous membranes and pharyngeal tissue

Patch (Lidoderm®): Relief of allodynia (painful hypersensitivity) and chronic pain in postherpetic neuralgia

Available Dosage Forms

Aerosol, foam, topical:
Anestafoam™ [OTC]: 4% (30 g)

Aerosol, spray, topical:
Solarcaine® cool aloe Burn Relief [OTC]: 0.5% (127 g)

Cream, rectal:
L-M-X® 5 [OTC]: 5% (15 g, 30 g)

Cream, topical: 0.5% (0.9 g)
AneCream™ [OTC]: 4% (5 g, 15 g, 30 g)
L-M-X® 4 [OTC]: 4% (5 g, 15 g, 30 g)
LidaMantle®: 3% (85 g)

Gel, topical:
Burn Jel Plus [OTC]: 2.5% (118 mL)
Burn Jel® [OTC]: 2% (59 mL, 118 mL); 2% (3.5 g)
Regenecare®: 2% (14 g, 85 g)
Regenecare® HA [OTC]: 2% (85 g)
Solarcaine® cool aloe Burn Relief [OTC]: 0.5% (113 g, 226 g)
Topicaine® [OTC]: 4% (10 g, 30 g, 113 g); 5% (10 g, 30 g, 113 g)
Unburn® [OTC]: 2.5% (59 mL)

Jelly, topical: 2% (5 mL, 30 mL)
Xylocaine®: 2% (5 mL, 30 mL)

Jelly, topical [preservative free]: 2% (5 mL, 10 mL, 20 mL)
Lotion, topical:
LidaMantle®: 3% (177 mL)
Ointment, topical: 5% (30 g, 35.4 g, 50 g)
Patch, topical:
Lidoderm®: 5% (30s)
Solution, topical: 4% [40 mg/mL] (50 mL)
Band-Aid® Hurt Free™ Antiseptic Wash [OTC]: 2% [20 mg/mL] (177 mL)
LTA® 360: 4% [40 mg/mL] (4 mL)
Premjact®: 9.6% (13 mL)
Xylocaine®: 4% (50 mL)
Solution, topical [preservative free]: 4% [40 mg/mL] (4 mL)
Solution, viscous, oral topical: 2% [20 mg/mL] (20 mL, 100 mL, 500 mL)

General Dosage Range Topical:
Cream: *Children and Adults:* Dosage varies greatly depending on product
Gel, ointment, solution: *Adults:* Apply to affected area ≤4 times/day as needed (maximum: 4.5 mg/kg/dose; 300 mg/dose)
Jelly:
Children: Maximum: 4.5 mg/kg/dose
Adults: 3-30 mL (maximum: 30 mL [600 mg]/12-hour period)
Oral topical solution (viscous):
Infants and Children <3 years: 1.25 mL applied no more frequently than every 3 hours (maximum: 4 doses per 12-hour period)
Children ≥3 years: Should not exceed 4.5 mg/kg/dose (or 300 mg/dose); swished in the mouth and spit out no more frequently than every 3 hours
Adults: 15 mL swished in the mouth and spit out or gargled no more frequently than every 3 hours (maximum: 8 doses per 24-hour period)
Patch: *Adults:* Apply up to 3 patches in a single application for up to 12 hours in any 24-hour period

Administration

Topical

Gel (Topicaine®): Apply a moderately thick layer to affected area (~1/8 inch thick). Allow time for numbness to develop (~20-60 minutes after application). When used prior to laser surgery, avoid mucous membranes and remove prior to laser treatment.

Oral topical solution (viscous): Have patient swish medication around mouth and then spit it out; for pharyngeal anesthesia, patient should gargle and may swallow medication.

Patch: Apply to most painful area of skin immediately after removal from protective envelope. May be cut (with scissors, prior to removal of release liner) to appropriate size. Clothing may be worn over application area. After removal from skin, fold used patches so the adhesive side sticks to itself. Remove immediately if burning sensation occurs. Wash hands after application. Avoid exposing application site to external heat sources (eg, heating pad, electric blanket, heat lamp, hot tub).

Nursing Actions

Patient Education

Dermatologic: You will experience decreased sensation to pain, heat, or cold in the area and/or decreased muscle strength (depending on area of application) until effects wear off; use necessary caution to reduce incidence of possible injury until full sensation returns. Report irritation, pain, persistent numbness, tingling, swelling, restlessness, dizziness, acute weakness, blurred vision, ringing in ears, or respiratory difficulty.

Topical patch: Patch may be cut to appropriate size. Apply patch to most painful area. Up to 3 patches may be applied in a single application. Patch may remain in place for up to 12 hours in any 24-hour period. Remove immediately if burning sensation occurs. Wash hands after application. Remove patch while having MRI scan; can cause burns.

Oral topical solution (viscous): Instruct patient to swish medication around mouth and then spit it out; if unable to spit, can apply with cotton tip to painful area.

Lidocaine and Epinephrine

(LYE doe kane & ep i NEF rin)

Brand Names: U.S. Lignospan® Forte; Lignospan® Standard; Xylocaine® MPF With Epinephrine; Xylocaine® With Epinephrine

Index Terms Epinephrine and Lidocaine

Pharmacologic Category Local Anesthetic

Pregnancy Risk Factor B

Lactation Lidocaine enters breast milk/use caution

Use Local infiltration anesthesia; AVS for nerve block

Available Dosage Forms
Injection, solution:
Generics:
0.5% / 1:200,000: Lidocaine hydrochloride 0.5% [5 mg/mL] and epinephrine 1:200,000 (50 mL)
1% / 1:100,000: Lidocaine hydrochloride 1% [10 mg/mL] and epinephrine 1:100,000 (20 mL, 30 mL, 50 mL)
2% / 1:100,000: Lidocaine hydrochloride 2% [20 mg/mL] and epinephrine 1:100,000 (30 mL, 50 mL)
Brands:
Xylocaine® with Epinephrine:
0.5% / 1:200,000: Lidocaine hydrochloride 0.5% [5 mg/mL] and epinephrine 1:200,000 (50 mL)

1% / 1:100,000: Lidocaine hydrochloride 1% [10 mg/mL] and epinephrine 1:100,000 (10 mL, 20 mL, 50 mL)

2% / 1:100,000: Lidocaine hydrochloride 2% [20 mg/mL] and epinephrine 1:100,000 (10 mL, 20 mL, 50 mL)

Injection, solution [preservative free]:

Generics:

1.5% / 1:200,000: Lidocaine hydrochloride 1.5% [15 mg/mL] and epinephrine 1:200,000 (5 mL, 30 mL)

2% / 1:200,000: Lidocaine hydrochloride 2% [20 mg/mL] and epinephrine 1:200,000 (20 mL)

Brands:

Xylocaine®-MPF with Epinephrine:

1% / 1:200,000: Lidocaine hydrochloride 1% [10 mg/mL] and epinephrine 1:200,000 (5 mL, 10 mL, 30 mL)

1.5% / 1:200,000: Lidocaine hydrochloride 1.5% [15 mg/mL] and epinephrine 1:200,000 (5 mL, 10 mL, 30 mL)

2% / 1:200,000: Lidocaine hydrochloride 2% [20 mg/mL] and epinephrine 1:200,000 (5 mL, 10 mL, 20 mL)

Injection, solution [for dental use]:

Generics:

2% / 1:50,000: Lidocaine hydrochloride 2% [20 mg/mL] and epinephrine 1:50,000 (1.7 mL, 1.8 mL)

2% / 1:100,000: Lidocaine hydrochloride 2% [20 mg/mL] and epinephrine 1:100,000 (1.7 mL, 1.8 mL)

Brands:

Lignospan® Forte: 2% / 1:50,000: Lidocaine hydrochloride 2% [20 mg/mL] and epinephrine 1:50,000 (1.7 mL)

Lignospan® Standard: 2% / 1:100,000: Lidocaine hydrochloride 2% [20 mg/mL] and epinephrine 1:100,000 (1.7 mL)

General Dosage Range Conduction block or infiltration (dental):

Children <12 years: 20-30 mg (1-1.5 mL) of 2% lidocaine with epinephrine 1:100,000 (maximum: 4.5 mg/kg of lidocaine or 100-150 mg as a single dose)

Children ≥12 years and Adults: Do not exceed 7 mg/kg body weight up to a maximum range of 300 mg (usual dental practice) to 500 mg (approved product labeling) of lidocaine hydrochloride and 3 mcg (0.003 mg) of epinephrine/kg of body weight **or** 0.2 mg epinephrine per dental appointment.

Administration

Other Injection solution for infiltration: Before injecting, withdraw syringe plunger to ensure injection is not into vein or artery. Aspirate the syringe after tissue penetration and before injection to minimize chance of direct vascular injection.

Nursing Actions

Physical Assessment See individual agents.

Patient Education See individual agents.

Related Information

EPINEPHrine (Systemic, Oral Inhalation) *on page 397*

Lidocaine (Topical) *on page 696*

Linagliptin (lin a GLIP tin)

Brand Names: U.S. Tradjenta™

Index Terms BI-1356; Trajenta

Pharmacologic Category Antidiabetic Agent, Dipeptidyl Peptidase IV (DPP-IV) Inhibitor

Pregnancy Risk Factor B

Lactation Excretion in breast milk unknown/use caution

Breast-Feeding Considerations It is not known if linagliptin is excreted in breast milk. The manufacturer recommends that caution be used if administered to breast-feeding women.

Use Management of type 2 diabetes mellitus (noninsulin dependent, NIDDM) as an adjunct to diet and exercise as monotherapy or in combination with other antidiabetic agents

Mechanism of Action/Effect Linagliptin inhibits dipeptidyl peptidase IV (DPP-IV) enzyme resulting in increased insulin synthesis and release and decreased hepatic glucose production.

Contraindications Hypersensitivity to linagliptin or any component of the formulation

Canadian labeling: Additional contraindications: Use in type 1 diabetes mellitus or diabetic ketoacidosis

Warnings/Precautions Avoid use in type 1 diabetes mellitus (insulin dependent, IDDM) and diabetic ketoacidosis (DKA) due to lack of efficacy in these populations. Use caution if used in conjunction with insulin or insulin secretagogues; risk of hypoglycemia is increased. Monitor blood glucose closely; dosage adjustments of insulin or insulin secretagogues may be necessary. Diabetes self-management education (DSME) is essential to maximize the effectiveness of therapy.

Drug Interactions

Avoid Concomitant Use There are no known interactions where it is recommended to avoid concomitant use.

Decreased Effect

The levels/effects of Linagliptin may be decreased by: Corticosteroids (Orally Inhaled); Corticosteroids (Systemic); CYP3A4 Inducers (Strong); Deferasirox; Luteinizing Hormone-Releasing Hormone Analogs; P-glycoprotein/ABCB1 Inducers; Somatropin; Thiazide Diuretics; Tocilizumab

Increased Effect/Toxicity

Linagliptin may increase the levels/effects of: ACE Inhibitors; Hypoglycemic Agents

The levels/effects of Linagliptin may be increased by: Conivaptan; Herbs (Hypoglycemic Properties); Pegvisomant; P-glycoprotein/ABCB1 Inhibitors; Ritonavir

Nutritional/Ethanol Interactions

Ethanol: Caution with ethanol (may cause hypoglycemia).

Herb/Nutraceutical: Herbs with hypoglycemic properties may enhance the hypoglycemic effect of linagliptin. This includes alfalfa, aloe, bilberry, bitter melon, burdock, celery, damiana, fenugreek, garcinia, garlic, ginger, ginseng (American), gymnema, marshmallow, stinging nettle.

Adverse Reactions

>10%: Endocrine & metabolic: Hypoglycemia (combined with metformin/sulfonylurea [15%], metformin [<1%], pioglitazone [<1%]; monotherapy [<1%]) (Scott, 2011)

1% to 10%:

Central nervous system: Headache (6%)

Endocrine & metabolic: Hyperuricemia (3%), lipids increased (3%), triglycerides increased (2%), weight gain (2%)

Neuromuscular & skeletal: Arthralgia (6%), back pain (6%)

Respiratory: Nasopharyngitis (6%), cough (2%)

Available Dosage Forms

Tablet, oral:

Tradjenta™: 5 mg

General Dosage Range

Oral: *Adults:* 5 mg once daily

Administration

Oral May be administered with or without food.

Stability

Storage Store at 25°C (77°F); excursions permitted between 15°C to 30°C (59°F to 86°F).

Nursing Actions

Patient Education This medication will not cure diabetes and may be prescribed in conjunction with another antidiabetic medication. May be taken with or without food. It is important to follow dietary and lifestyle recommendations and glucose monitoring instructions of prescriber or diabetic educator. You will be instructed in signs of hyper-/hypoglycemia; always carry a source of glucose with you in event of hypoglycemia. You may experience mild headache, nasal irritation, muscular aches and pains, and cough. Notify prescriber of any signs of hypersensitivity reaction (swelling of face, lips, or mouth; severe skin rash or eruption; difficulty breathing).

Dietary Considerations May be taken without regard to food. Individualized medical nutrition therapy (MNT) based on ADA recommendations is an integral part of therapy.

Linagliptin and Metformin

(lin a GLIP tin & met FOR min)

Brand Names: U.S. Jentadueto™

Index Terms Linagliptin and Metformin Hydrochloride; Metformin and Linagliptin; Metformin Hydrochloride and Linagliptin

Pharmacologic Category Antidiabetic Agent, Biguanide; Antidiabetic Agent, Dipeptidyl Peptidase IV (DPP-IV) Inhibitor

Medication Safety Issues

Sound-alike/look-alike issues:

Linagliptin and Metformin may be confused with Sitagliptin and Metformin

Pregnancy Risk Factor B

Lactation

Linagliptin: Excretion in breast milk unknown/use caution

Metformin: Enters breast milk/not recommended

Use Management of type 2 diabetes mellitus (noninsulin dependent, NIDDM) as an adjunct to diet and exercise in patients not adequately controlled on metformin or linagliptin monotherapy

Available Dosage Forms

Tablet, oral:

Jentadueto™ 2.5/500: Linagliptin 2.5 mg and metformin 500 mg

Jentadueto™ 2.5/850: Linagliptin 2.5 mg and metformin 850 mg

Jentadueto™ 2.5/1000: Linagliptin 2.5 mg and metformin 1000 mg

General Dosage Range Oral: *Adults:* Linagliptin 2.5 mg and metformin 500-1000 mg twice daily (maximum: 5 mg/day [linagliptin], 2000 mg/day [metformin])

Administration

Oral Administer with meals, at the same time each day.

Nursing Actions

Physical Assessment See individual agents.

Patient Education See individual agents.

Lindane (LIN dane)

Index Terms Benzene Hexachloride; Gamma Benzene Hexachloride; Hexachlorocyclohexane

Pharmacologic Category Antiparasitic Agent, Topical; Pediculocide; Scabicidal Agent

Medication Guide Available Yes

Pregnancy Risk Factor C

Lactation Enters breast milk/contraindicated

Use Treatment of *Sarcoptes scabiei* (scabies), *Pediculus capitis* (head lice), and *Phthirus pubis* (crab lice); FDA recommends reserving lindane as a second-line agent or with inadequate response to other therapies

Available Dosage Forms

Lotion, topical: 1% (60 mL)

Shampoo, topical: 1% (60 mL)

General Dosage Range Topical:

Lotion: *Children and Adults:* Apply a thin layer; bathe and remove drug after 8-12 hours

Shampoo: *Children and Adults:* Apply to dry hair (maximum: 60 mL)

Administration

Oral Never administer orally.

Topical For topical use only. Caregivers should apply with gloves (avoid natural latex, may be permeable to lindane). Rinse off with warm (not hot) water.

Lotion: Apply to dry, cool skin; do not apply to face or eyes. Wait at least 1 hour after bathing or showering (wet or warm skin increases absorption). Skin should be clean and free of any other lotions, creams, or oil prior to lindane application.

Shampoo: Apply to clean, dry hair. Wait at least 1 hour after washing hair before applying lindane shampoo. Hair should be washed with a shampoo not containing a conditioner; hair and skin of head and neck should be free of any lotions, oils, or creams prior to lindane application.

Nursing Actions

Physical Assessment Assess head, hair, and skin surfaces for presence of lice and nits. Teach patient appropriate application.

Patient Education For external use only. Caregivers should apply with gloves on. Do not apply to face and avoid getting in eyes. Do not apply immediately after hot, soapy bath. For scabies, apply from neck to toes. For head lice or crab lice, massage into dry hair for 4 minutes; add water to hair to form lather, then rinse thoroughly. Clothing and bedding must be washed in hot water or dry cleaned to kill nits. Wash combs and brushes with lindane shampoo and thoroughly rinse. May need to treat all members of household and all sexual contacts concurrently. Report if condition persists or infection occurs.

Linezolid (li NE zoh lid)

Brand Names: U.S. Zyvox®

Pharmacologic Category Antibiotic, Oxazolidinone

Medication Safety Issues

Sound-alike/look-alike issues:

Zyvox® may be confused with Zosyn®, Zovirax®

Pregnancy Risk Factor C

Lactation Excretion in breast milk unknown/use caution

Breast-Feeding Considerations It is not known if linezolid is excreted in human milk. Linezolid has low protein binding and is 100% bioavailable orally which may increase the exposure to a nursing infant. The manufacturer advises caution if administering linezolid to a breast-feeding woman. Linezolid is used therapeutically in infants. Nondose-related effects could include modification of bowel flora.

Use Treatment of vancomycin-resistant *Enterococcus faecium* (VRE) infections, nosocomial pneumonia caused by *Staphylococcus aureus* (including MRSA) or *Streptococcus pneumoniae* (including multidrug-resistant strains [MDRSP]), complicated and uncomplicated skin and skin structure infections (including diabetic foot infections without concomitant osteomyelitis), and community-acquired pneumonia caused by susceptible gram-positive organisms

Mechanism of Action/Effect Inhibits bacterial protein synthesis by binding to bacterial 23S ribosomal RNA of the 50S subunit. This prevents the formation of a functional 70S initiation complex that is essential for the bacterial translation process. Linezolid is bacteriostatic against enterococci and staphylococci and bactericidal against most strains of streptococci.

Contraindications Hypersensitivity to linezolid or any other component of the formulation; concurrent use or within 2 weeks of MAO inhibitors; patients with uncontrolled hypertension, pheochromocytoma, thyrotoxicosis, and/or taking sympathomimetics (eg, pseudoephedrine), vasopressive agents (eg, epinephrine, norepinephrine), or dopaminergic agents (eg, dopamine, dobutamine) unless closely monitored for increased blood pressure; patients with carcinoid syndrome and/or taking SSRIs, tricyclic antidepressants, serotonin 5-$HT_{1B,1D}$ receptor agonists, meperidine, or buspirone unless closely monitored for sign/symptoms of serotonin syndrome

Warnings/Precautions Myelosuppression has been reported and may be dependent on duration of therapy (generally >2 weeks of treatment); use with caution in patients with pre-existing myelosuppression, in patients receiving other drugs which may cause bone marrow suppression, or in chronic infection (previous or concurrent antibiotic therapy). Weekly CBC monitoring is recommended. Consider discontinuation in patients developing myelosuppression (or in whom myelosuppression worsens during treatment).

Lactic acidosis has been reported with use. Linezolid exhibits mild MAO inhibitor properties and has the potential to have the same interactions as other MAO inhibitors; use with caution and monitor closely in patients with uncontrolled hypertension, pheochromocytoma, carcinoid syndrome, or untreated hyperthyroidism; use is contraindicated in the absence of close monitoring. Symptoms of agitation, confusion, hallucinations, hyper-reflexia, myoclonus, shivering, and tachycardia may occur with concomitant proserotonergic drugs (eg, SSRIs/SNRIs or triptans) or agents which reduce linezolid's metabolism; concurrent use with these medications is contraindicated unless patient is closely monitored for signs/symptoms of serotonin syndrome. Unnecessary use may lead to the development of resistance to linezolid; consider alternatives before initiating outpatient treatment.

Peripheral and optic neuropathy (with vision loss) has been reported and may occur primarily with extended courses of therapy >28 days; any symptoms of visual change or impairment warrant immediate ophthalmic evaluation and possible discontinuation of therapy. Seizures have been reported; use with caution in patients with a history of seizures. Prolonged use may result in fungal or bacterial superinfection, including *C. difficile*-associated diarrhea (CDAD) and pseudomembranous colitis; CDAD has been observed >2 months postantibiotic treatment.

Due to inconsistent concentrations in the CSF, empiric use in pediatric patients with CNS infections is not recommended by the manufacturer; however, there are multiple case reports describing successful treatment of documented VRE and *Staphylococcus aureus* CNS and shunt infections in the literature. Linezolid should not be used in the empiric treatment of catheter-related bloodstream infection (CRBSI), but may be appropriate for targeted therapy (Mermel, 2009). Oral suspension contains phenylalanine.

Drug Interactions

Avoid Concomitant Use

Avoid concomitant use of Linezolid with any of the following: Alpha-/Beta-Agonists (Indirect-Acting); Alpha1-Agonists; Alpha2-Agonists (Ophthalmic); Amphetamines; Anilidopiperidine Opioids; Antidepressants (Serotonin Reuptake Inhibitor/Antagonist); Atomoxetine; Bezafibrate; Buprenorphine; BuPROPion; BusPIRone; CarBAMazepine; CloZAPine; Cyclobenzaprine; Dexmethylphenidate; Dextromethorphan; Diethylpropion; HYDROmorphone; MAO Inhibitors; Maprotiline; Meperidine; Methyldopa; Methylene Blue; Methylphenidate; Mirtazapine; Oxymorphone; Pizotifen; Selective Serotonin Reuptake Inhibitors; Serotonin 5-HT1D Receptor Agonists; Serotonin/Norepinephrine Reuptake Inhibitors; Tapentadol; Tetrabenazine; Tetrahydrozoline; Tetrahydrozoline (Nasal); Tricyclic Antidepressants; Tryptophan

Decreased Effect There are no known significant interactions involving a decrease in effect.

Increased Effect/Toxicity

Linezolid may increase the levels/effects of: Alpha-/Beta-Agonists (Direct-Acting); Alpha-/Beta-Agonists (Indirect-Acting); Alpha1-Agonists; Alpha2-Agonists (Ophthalmic); Amphetamines; Antidepressants (Serotonin Reuptake Inhibitor/Antagonist); Antihypertensives; Atomoxetine; Beta2-Agonists; Bezafibrate; BuPROPion; CloZAPine; Dexmethylphenidate; Dextromethorphan; Diethylpropion; Doxapram; HYDROmorphone; Lithium; Meperidine; Methadone; Methyldopa; Methylene Blue; Methylphenidate; Metoclopramide; Mirtazapine; Nefazodone; Orthostatic Hypotension Producing Agents; Pizotifen; Reserpine; Selective Serotonin Reuptake Inhibitors; Serotonin 5-HT1D Receptor Agonists; Serotonin Modulators; Serotonin/Norepinephrine Reuptake Inhibitors; Sympathomimetics; Tetrahydrozoline; Tetrahydrozoline (Nasal); TraZODone; Tricyclic Antidepressants

The levels/effects of Linezolid may be increased by: Altretamine; Anilidopiperidine Opioids; Antipsychotics; Buprenorphine; BusPIRone; CarBAMazepine; COMT Inhibitors; Cyclobenzaprine; Levodopa; MAO Inhibitors; Maprotiline; Oxymorphone; Tapentadol; Tetrabenazine; TraMADol; Tryptophan

Nutritional/Ethanol Interactions

Ethanol: May cause additional CNS depressant effects and provide potential source of additional tyramine content. Management: Avoid ethanol.

Food: Concurrent ingestion of foods rich in tyramine may cause sudden and severe high blood pressure (hypertensive crisis). Food's freshness is also an important concern; improperly stored or spoiled food can create an environment where tyramine concentrations may increase. Management: Avoid tyramine-containing foods with MAOIs.

Herb/Nutraceutical: Ingestion of large quantities of supplements containing caffeine, tyrosine, tryptophan or phenylalanine.may increase the risk of severe side effects (eg, hypertensive reactions, serotonin syndrome). Management: Avoid supplements containing caffeine, tyrosine, tryptophan or phenylalanine.

Adverse Reactions Percentages as reported in adults; frequency similar in pediatric patients

>10%:

Central nervous system: Headache (<1% to 11%)

Gastrointestinal: Diarrhea (3% to 11%)

1% to 10%:

Central nervous system: Insomnia (3%), dizziness (≤2%), fever (2%)

Dermatologic: Rash (2%)

Gastrointestinal: Nausea (3% to 10%), lipase increased (3% to 4%), vomiting (1% to 4%), constipation (2%), taste alteration (1% to 2%), amylase increased (<1% to 2%), tongue discoloration (≤1%), oral moniliasis (≤1%), pancreatitis

Genitourinary: Vaginal moniliasis (1% to 2%)

Hematologic: Thrombocytopenia (<1% to 10%), hemoglobin decreased (1% to 7%), leukopenia (<1% to 2%), neutropenia (≤1%)

Hepatic: ALT increased (2% to 10%), AST increased (2% to 5%), alkaline phosphatase increased (<1% to 4%), bilirubin increased (≤1%)

Renal: BUN increased (≤2%)

Miscellaneous: Fungal infection (≤1% to 2%), lactate dehydrogenase increased (<1% to 2%)

Available Dosage Forms

Infusion, premixed:

Zyvox®: 200 mg (100 mL); 600 mg (300 mL)

Powder for suspension, oral:

Zyvox®: 100 mg/5 mL (150 mL)

Tablet, oral:

Zyvox®: 600 mg

General Dosage Range

I.V.:

Children ≤11 years: 10 mg/kg (maximum dose: 600 mg) every 8 hours

Children ≥12 years and Adults: 600 mg every 12 hours

Oral:

Children <5 years: 10 mg/kg every 8 hours (maximum: 600 mg/dose)

Children 5-11 years: 10 mg/kg every 8-12 hours (maximum: 600 mg/dose)

Children ≥12 years and Adults: 400-600 mg every 12 hours

Administration

Oral Oral suspension: Invert gently to mix prior to administration, do not shake. Administer without regard to meals.

I.V. Administer intravenous infusion over 30-120 minutes. Do not mix or infuse with other medications. When the same intravenous line is used for sequential infusion of other medications, flush line with D_5W, NS, or LR before and after infusing linezolid. The yellow color of the injection may intensify over time without affecting potency.

Stability

Reconstitution Oral suspension: Reconstitute with 123 mL of distilled water (in 2 portions); shake vigorously. Concentration is 100 mg/5 mL. Prior to administration mix gently by inverting bottle; do not shake.

Storage

Infusion: Store at 25°C (77°F); excursions permitted to 15°C to 30°C (59°F to 86°F). Protect from light. Keep infusion bags in overwrap until ready for use. Protect infusion bags from freezing.

Oral suspension: Following reconstitution, store at 25°C (77°F); excursions permitted to 15°C to 30°C (59°F to 86°F). Use reconstituted suspension within 21 days. Protect from light.

Tablet: Store at 25°C (77°F); excursions permitted to 15°C to 30°C (59°F to 86°F). Protect from light; protect from moisture.

Nursing Actions

Physical Assessment Previous drug allergies should be assessed before administering first dose. Serotonergic agents may increase resistance to linezolid and increase risk of serotonin syndrome, hypertension with adrenergic agents, or myelosuppression with other drugs that may cause bone marrow suppression. Monitor for myelosuppression (anemia), lactic acidosis, or peripheral or optic neuropathy. Instruct patient to follow a tyramine-free diet.

Patient Education

Oral suspension: Store at room temperature and use within 21 days. Maintain adequate hydration unless instructed to restrict fluid intake. Avoid alcohol. Avoid tyramine-containing foods (eg, pickles, aged cheese, wine).

Oral/I.V.: You may experience mild headache, GI discomfort, nausea, vomiting, taste alteration, or constipation. Report immediately unresolved, white plaques in mouth; skin rash or irritation; acute headache, dizziness, blurred vision, or changes in visual acuity; tingling or numbness in extremities; or persistent diarrhea.

Dietary Considerations Take without regard to meals. Some products may contain sodium and/or phenylalanine. Avoid consuming large amounts of tyramine-containing foods/beverages. Some examples include aged or matured cheese, air-dried or cured meats (including sausages and salamis), fava or broad bean pods, tap/draft beers, Marmite concentrate, sauerkraut, soy sauce, and other soybean condiments.

Liraglutide (lir a GLOO tide)

Brand Names: U.S. Victoza®

Index Terms NN2211

Pharmacologic Category Antidiabetic Agent, Glucagon-Like Peptide-1 (GLP-1) Receptor Agonist

Medication Safety Issues

Other safety concerns:

Cross-contamination may occur if pens are shared among multiple patients. Steps should be taken to prohibit sharing of pens.

Medication Guide Available Yes

Pregnancy Risk Factor C

Lactation Excretion in breast milk unknown/not recommended

Use Treatment of type 2 diabetes mellitus (noninsulin dependent, NIDDM) to improve glycemic control

Mechanism of Action/Effect Liraglutide is a long acting analog of human glucagon-like peptide-1 (GLP-1) (an incretin hormone) which increases glucose-dependent insulin secretion, decreases inappropriate glucagon secretion, increases B-cell growth/replication, slows gastric emptying, and decreases food intake. Liraglutide administration results in decreases in hemoglobin A_{1c} by approximately 1%.

Contraindications History of or family history of medullary thyroid carcinoma (MTC); patients with multiple endocrine neoplasia syndrome type 2 (MEN2)

Warnings/Precautions [U.S. Boxed Warning] Dose and duration dependent thyroid C-cell tumors have developed in animal studies with liraglutide therapy; relevance in humans unknown. During clinical studies a few cases of thyroid C-cell hyperplasia were reported. Due to the finding in animal studies, patients were monitored with serum calcitonin or thyroid ultrasound during clinical trials; however it us unknown if this is beneficial in decreasing the risk of thyroid tumors. Consultation with an endocrinologist is recommended in patients who develop elevated calcitonin concentrations. Patients should be counseled on the risk and symptoms of thyroid tumors. Use is contraindicated in patients with or a family history of medullary thyroid cancer and in patients with multiple endocrine neoplasia syndrome type 2 (MEN2). Cases of acute and chronic pancreatitis (including one case of fatal necrotizing pancreatitis) have been reported although conclusive evidence to liraglutide therapy has not been established; monitor for unexplained severe abdominal pain, and if pancreatitis is suspected, discontinue use. Do not resume unless an alternative etiology of pancreatitis is confirmed. Use with caution in patients with a history of pancreatitis, cholelithiasis, and/or alcohol abuse. Most common reactions are gastrointestinal related; these symptoms may be dose-related and may decrease in frequency/severity with gradual titration and continued use. Use may be associated with weight loss (likely due to reduced intake) independent of the change in hemoglobin A_{1c}. Use with caution in patients with hepatic or renal impairment; cases of acute renal failure and chronic renal failure exacerbation have been reported.

Concurrent use with insulin therapy has not been evaluated. Concomitant use of an insulin secretagogue (eg, sulfonylurea, meglitinide) may increase the risk of hypoglycemia; dosage reduction of secretagogues may be required during initiation of liraglutide. Due to its effects on gastric emptying, liraglutide may reduce the rate and extent of absorption of orally-administered drugs; use with caution in patients receiving medications with a narrow therapeutic window or require rapid absorption from the GI tract. Not recommended for first-line therapy; use as adjunct to diet and exercise. Do not use in patients with type 1 diabetes mellitus or for the treatment of diabetic ketoacidosis; not a substitute for insulin. Diabetes self-management education (DSME) is essential to maximize the effectiveness of therapy.

Drug Interactions

Avoid Concomitant Use There are no known interactions where it is recommended to avoid concomitant use.

Decreased Effect

The levels/effects of Liraglutide may be decreased by: Corticosteroids (Orally Inhaled); Corticosteroids (Systemic); Luteinizing Hormone-Releasing Hormone Analogs; Somatropin; Thiazide Diuretics

Increased Effect/Toxicity

Liraglutide may increase the levels/effects of: Sulfonylureas

The levels/effects of Liraglutide may be increased by: Pegvisomant

Nutritional/Ethanol Interactions Ethanol: Ethanol may cause hypoglycemia. Management: Avoid ethanol.

Adverse Reactions Percentages are as reported for monotherapy.

>10%: Gastrointestinal: Nausea (28%), diarrhea (17%), vomiting (11%)

1% to 10%:

Cardiovascular: Hypertension (3%)

Central nervous system: Headache (9%), dizziness (6%)

Gastrointestinal: Constipation (10%)

Genitourinary: Urinary tract infection (6%)

Hepatic: Hyperbilirubinemia (4%)

Local: Injection site reactions (2%; includes rash, erythema)

Neuromuscular & skeletal: Back pain (5%)

Respiratory: Upper respiratory infection (10%), sinusitis (6%), nasopharyngitis (5%)

Miscellaneous: Anti-liraglutide antibodies (low titers 9%, cross-reacting 7%), influenza (7%)

Available Dosage Forms

Injection, solution:

Victoza®: 6 mg/mL (3 mL)

General Dosage Range SubQ: *Adults:* Initial: 0.6 mg once daily; maintenance: 1.2-1.8 mg/day

Administration

Other SubQ: Use only if clear, colorless, and free of particulate matter. Administer via injection in the upper arm, thigh, or abdomen. Administer without regard to meals or time of day. Change needle with each administration. Do not share pens between patients even if needle is changed.

Stability

Storage Prior to initial use, store under refrigeration at 2°C to 8°C (36°F to 46°F); after initial use, may be stored in refrigerator or at room temperature of 15°C to 30°C (59°F to 86°F). Do not freeze (discard if freezing occurs). Protect from heat and light. Pen should be discarded 30 days after initial use.

Nursing Actions

Physical Assessment Assess for use-related cautions (eg, renal or hepatic impairment, history of patient or familial medullary thyroid cancer, multiple endocrine neoplasia syndrome type 2 [MEN 2]). Teach patient diabetes self-management and proper injection techniques and syringe/needle disposal.

Patient Education This medication is used to help control diabetes; it is not a cure. It is imperative that you follow other components of prescribed treatment regimen (eg, diet, regular exercise, glucose monitoring, laboratory testing). Follow directions for disposal of needles. May cause dizziness, headache, constipation, nausea, vomiting, or loss of appetite. Report persistent vomiting or diarrhea, severe or persistent abdominal pain, unusual lump or swelling of neck, difficulty swallowing, or unusual hoarseness.

Dietary Considerations Individualized medical nutrition therapy (MNT) based on ADA recommendations is an integral part of therapy.

Lisdexamfetamine (lis dex am FET a meen)

Brand Names: U.S. Vyvanse®

Index Terms Lisdexamfetamine Dimesylate; Lisdexamphetamine; NRP104

Pharmacologic Category Stimulant

Medication Safety Issues

Sound-alike/look-alike issues:

Vyvanse® may be confused with Visanne®, ViVAXIM®, Vytorin®, Glucovance®, Vivactil®

BEERS Criteria medication:

This drug may be inappropriate for use in geriatric patients (high severity risk).

Medication Guide Available Yes

Pregnancy Risk Factor C

Lactation Enters breast milk/not recommended

Breast-Feeding Considerations Manufacturer advises nursing mothers taking amphetamines to refrain from breast-feeding.

Use Treatment of attention-deficit/hyperactivity disorder (ADHD)

Mechanism of Action/Effect Lisdexamfetamine dimesylate is a prodrug that is converted to the active component dextroamphetamine. Amphetamines release catecholamines from storage sites in the nerve terminals.

Contraindications Known hypersensitivity or idiosyncratic reaction sympathomimetic amines; advanced arteriosclerosis, symptomatic cardiovascular disease, moderate-to-severe hypertension; hyperthyroidism; glaucoma; agitated states; history of drug abuse; concurrent use or within 2 weeks of use of MAO inhibitors

Warnings/Precautions [U.S. Boxed Warning]: Use has been associated with serious cardiovascular events including sudden death in patients with pre-existing structural cardiac abnormalities or other serious heart problems (sudden death in children and adolescents; sudden death, stroke and MI in adults. Use of this product should be avoided in the patients with known serious structural cardiac abnormalities, cardiomyopathy, serious heart rhythm abnormalities, coronary artery disease (adults), or other serious cardiac problems that could increase the risk of sudden death that these conditions alone carry. Patients should be carefully evaluated for these cardiac disorders prior to initiation of therapy.

Use with caution in patients with psychiatric or seizure disorders. May exacerbate symptoms of behavior and thought disorder in psychotic patients. Stimulants may unmask tics in individuals with coexisting Tourette's syndrome. **[U.S. Boxed Warning]: Potential for drug dependency exists; prolonged use may lead to drug dependency.** Use is contraindicated is patients with history of ethanol or drug abuse. Prescriptions should be written for the smallest quantity consistent with good patient care to minimize the possibility of overdose. Abrupt discontinuation following high doses or for prolonged periods may result in symptoms for withdrawal. Recommended to be used as part of a comprehensive treatment program for attention deficit disorders.

May be inappropriate for use in the elderly due to CNS stimulant adverse effects (Beers Criteria). Safety and efficacy of long-term use have not yet been established. Safety and efficacy in children <6 years of age have not been established. Appetite suppression may occur; monitor weight during therapy, particularly in children. Use of stimulants has been associated with slowing of growth rate; monitor growth rate during treatment. Treatment interruption may be necessary in patients who are not growing or gaining weight as expected.

Drug Interactions

Avoid Concomitant Use

Avoid concomitant use of Lisdexamfetamine with any of the following: Iobenguane I 123; MAO Inhibitors

Decreased Effect

Lisdexamfetamine may decrease the levels/effects of: Antihistamines; Ethosuximide; Iobenguane I 123; Ioflupane I 123; PHENobarbital; Phenytoin

The levels/effects of Lisdexamfetamine may be decreased by: Ammonium Chloride; Antipsychotics; Gastrointestinal Acidifying Agents; Lithium; Methenamine

Increased Effect/Toxicity

Lisdexamfetamine may increase the levels/effects of: Analgesics (Opioid); Sympathomimetics

The levels/effects of Lisdexamfetamine may be increased by: Alkalinizing Agents; Antacids; Atomoxetine; Cannabinoids; Carbonic Anhydrase Inhibitors; MAO Inhibitors; Proton Pump Inhibitors; Tricyclic Antidepressants

Nutritional/Ethanol Interactions

Ethanol: Ethanol may increase CNS depression. Caffeine use may worsen problems with sleeping, headache, irritability, dizziness, nausea, vomiting, abdominal pain, and decreased appetite. Management: Avoid ethanol and caffeine.

Food: High-fat meal prolongs T_{max} by ~1 hour.

Adverse Reactions

>10%:

Central nervous system: Headache (children 12%), insomnia (19% to 27%; 4% [initially])

Gastrointestinal: Appetite decreased (27% to 39%), xerostomia (children 5%; adults 26%), abdominal pain (children 12%)

1% to 10%:

Cardiovascular: Blood pressure increased (adults 3%), heart rate increased (adults 2%)

Central nervous system: Irritability (children 10%), anxiety (adults 6%), dizziness (children 5%), jitteriness (adults 4%), affect lability (children 3%), agitation (adults 3%), restlessness (adults 3%), fever (children 2%), somnolence (children 2%), tic (children 2%)

Dermatologic: Hyperhidrosis (adults 3%), rash (children 3%)

Gastrointestinal: Vomiting (children 9%), weight loss (children 9%), diarrhea (adults 7%), nausea (6% to 7%), anorexia (adults 5%)

Genitourinary: Erectile dysfunction (adults <2%), libido decreased (adults <2%)

Neuromuscular & skeletal: Tremor (adults 2%)

Respiratory: Dyspnea (adults 2%)

Additional adverse reaction associated with amphetamines; frequency not defined:

Cardiovascular: Cardiomyopathy, hypertension, MI, sudden death, tachycardia

Central nervous system: Exacerbation of motor and phonic tics, overstimulation, stroke, Tourette's syndrome

Dermatologic: Stevens-Johnson syndrome, toxic epidermal necrolysis

Gastrointestinal: Abnormal taste, constipation

Controlled Substance C-II

Available Dosage Forms

Capsule, oral:

Vyvanse®: 20 mg, 30 mg, 40 mg, 50 mg, 60 mg, 70 mg

General Dosage Range Oral: *Children ≥6 years and Adults:* Initial: 30 mg once daily; Maintenance: Up to 70 mg once daily

Administration

Oral Administer in the morning without regard to meals; swallow capsule whole, do not chew; capsule may be opened and the contents dissolved in glass of water; consume the resulting solution immediately; do not store solution.

Stability

Storage Store at controlled room temperature of 25°C (77°F) excursions permitted to 15°C to 30°C (59°F to 86°F). Protect from light.

Nursing Actions

Physical Assessment Perform careful cardiovascular assessment prior to initiating therapy. Monitor weight, blood pressure, and vital signs at beginning of therapy and periodically throughout. Children should also have height measured often while taking this medication.

Patient Education Avoid alcohol and caffeine use. May cause problems with sleeping, headache, irritability, dizziness, nausea, vomiting, abdominal pain, and decreased appetite. Report chest pain, difficulty breathing, fainting, abnormal thinking or behavior, increased aggression, hallucinations, or weight loss.

Dietary Considerations May be taken without regard to meals.

Lisinopril (lyse IN oh pril)

Brand Names: U.S. Prinivil®; Zestril®

Pharmacologic Category Angiotensin-Converting Enzyme (ACE) Inhibitor

Medication Safety Issues

Sound-alike/look-alike issues:

Lisinopril may be confused with fosinopril, Lioresal®, Lipitor®, RisperDAL®

Prinivil® may be confused with Plendil®, Pravachol®, Prevacid®, PriLOSEC®, Proventil®

Zestril® may be confused with Desyrel, Restoril™, Vistaril®, Zegerid®, Zerit®, Zetia®, Zostrix®, ZyPREXA®

International issues:

Acepril [Malaysia] may be confused with Accupril which is a brand name for quinapril [U.S.]

Acepril: Brand name for lisinopril [Malaysia], but also the brand name for captopril [Great Britain]; enalapril [Hungary, Switzerland]

Pregnancy Risk Factor C (1st trimester); D (2nd and 3rd trimesters)

Lactation Excretion in breast milk unknown/not recommended

Breast-Feeding Considerations It is not known if lisinopril is excreted in breast milk. Breast-feeding is not recommended by the manufacturer.

Use Treatment of hypertension, either alone or in combination with other antihypertensive agents; adjunctive therapy in treatment of heart failure (afterload reduction); treatment of acute myocardial infarction within 24 hours in hemodynamically-stable patients to improve survival; treatment of left ventricular dysfunction after myocardial infarction

Mechanism of Action/Effect Competitive inhibitor of angiotensin-converting enzyme (ACE); prevents conversion of angiotensin I to angiotensin II, a potent vasoconstrictor; results in lower levels of angiotensin II which causes an increase in plasma renin activity and a reduction in aldosterone secretion

Contraindications Hypersensitivity to lisinopril or any component of the formulation; angioedema related to previous treatment with an ACE inhibitor; patients with idiopathic or hereditary angioedema

Warnings/Precautions Anaphylactic reactions may occur rarely with ACE inhibitors. At any time during treatment (especially following first dose), angioedema may occur rarely with ACE inhibitors; it may involve the head and neck (potentially compromising airway) or the intestine (presenting with abdominal pain). African-Americans may be at an increased risk. Prolonged frequent monitoring may be required especially if tongue, glottis, or larynx are involved as they are associated with airway obstruction. Patients with a history of airway surgery may have a higher risk of airway obstruction. Aggressive early and appropriate management is critical. Use in patients with idiopathic or hereditary angioedema or previous angioedema associated with ACE inhibitor therapy is contraindicated. Severe anaphylactoid reactions may be seen during hemodialysis (eg, CVVHD) with high-flux dialysis membranes (eg, AN69), and rarely, during low density lipoprotein apheresis with dextran sulfate cellulose. Rare cases of anaphylactoid reactions have been reported in patients undergoing sensitization treatment with hymenoptera (bee, wasp) venom while receiving ACE inhibitors.

Symptomatic hypotension with or without syncope can occur with ACE inhibitors (usually with the first several doses); effects are most often observed in volume depleted patients; correct volume depletion prior to initiation; close monitoring of patient is required especially with initial dosing and dosing increases; blood pressure must be lowered at a rate appropriate for the patient's clinical condition. Initiation of therapy in patients with ischemic heart disease or cerebrovascular disease warrants close observation due to the potential consequences posed by falling blood pressure (eg, MI, stroke). Use with caution in hypertrophic cardiomyopathy with outflow tract obstruction, severe aortic stenosis, or before, during, or immediately after major surgery. **[U.S. Boxed Warning]: Based on human data, ACEIs can cause injury and death to the developing fetus when used in the second and third trimesters. ACEIs should be discontinued as soon as possible once pregnancy is detected.**

Hyperkalemia may occur with ACE inhibitors; risk factors include renal dysfunction, diabetes mellitus, concomitant use of potassium-sparing diuretics, potassium supplements, and/or potassium-containing salts. Use cautiously, if at all, with these agents and monitor potassium closely. Cough may occur with ACE inhibitors. Other causes of cough should be considered (eg, pulmonary congestion in patients with heart failure) and excluded prior to discontinuation.

May be associated with deterioration of renal function and/or increases in serum creatinine, particularly in patients with low renal blood flow (eg, renal artery stenosis, heart failure) whose glomerular filtration rate (GFR) is dependent on efferent arteriolar vasoconstriction by angiotensin II; deterioration may result in oliguria, acute renal failure, and progressive azotemia. Small increases in serum creatinine may occur following initiation; consider discontinuation only in patients with progressive and/or significant deterioration in renal function. Use with caution in patients with unstented unilateral/bilateral renal artery stenosis. When unstented bilateral renal artery stenosis is present, use is generally avoided due to the elevated risk of deterioration in renal function unless possible benefits outweigh risks. Concurrent use of angiotensin receptor blockers may increase the risk of clinically-significant adverse events (eg, renal dysfunction, hyperkalemia).

Rare toxicities associated with ACE inhibitors include cholestatic jaundice (which may progress to fulminant hepatic necrosis), agranulocytosis, neutropenia, or leukopenia with myeloid hypoplasia. Patients with collagen vascular diseases (especially with concomitant renal impairment) or renal impairment alone may be at increased risk for hematologic toxicity; periodically monitor CBC with differential in these patients. Safety and efficacy have not been established in children <6 years of age or children with a Cl_{cr} ≤30 mL/minute.

Drug Interactions

Avoid Concomitant Use There are no known interactions where it is recommended to avoid concomitant use.

Decreased Effect

The levels/effects of Lisinopril may be decreased by: Antacids; Aprotinin; Herbs (Hypertensive Properties); Icatibant; Lanthanum; Methylphenidate; Nonsteroidal Anti-Inflammatory Agents; Salicylates; Yohimbine

Increased Effect/Toxicity

Lisinopril may increase the levels/effects of: Allopurinol; Amifostine; Antihypertensives; AzaTHIOprine; CycloSPORINE; CycloSPORINE (Systemic); Ferric Gluconate; Gold Sodium Thiomalate; Hypotensive Agents; Iron Dextran Complex; Lithium; Nonsteroidal Anti-Inflammatory Agents; RiTUXimab; Sodium Phosphates

The levels/effects of Lisinopril may be increased by: Alfuzosin; Angiotensin II Receptor Blockers; Diazoxide; DPP-IV Inhibitors; Eplerenone; Everolimus; Herbs (Hypotensive Properties); Loop Diuretics; MAO Inhibitors; Pentoxifylline; Phosphodiesterase 5 Inhibitors; Potassium Salts; Potassium-Sparing Diuretics; Prostacyclin Analogues; Sirolimus; Temsirolimus; Thiazide Diuretics; TiZANidine; Tolvaptan; Trimethoprim

Nutritional/Ethanol Interactions

Food: Potassium supplements and/or potassium-containing salts may cause or worsen hyperkalemia. Management: Consult prescriber before consuming a potassium-rich diet, potassium supplements, or salt substitutes.

Herb/Nutraceutical: Some herbal medications may worsen hypertension (eg, licorice); others may increase the antihypertensive effect of lisinopril (eg, shepherd's purse). Management: Avoid bayberry, blue cohosh, cayenne, ephedra, ginger, ginseng (American), kola, licorice, and yohimbe. Avoid black cohosh, California poppy, coleus, golden seal, hawthorn, mistletoe, periwinkle, quinine, and shepherd's purse.

Adverse Reactions Note: Frequency ranges include data from hypertension and heart failure trials. Higher rates of adverse reactions have generally been noted in patients with CHF. However, the frequency of adverse effects associated with placebo is also increased in this population.

1% to 10%:
- Cardiovascular: Orthostatic effects (1%), hypotension (1% to 4%)
- Central nervous system: Headache (4% to 6%), dizziness (5% to 12%), fatigue (3%)
- Dermatologic: Rash (1% to 2%)
- Endocrine & metabolic: Hyperkalemia (2% to 5%)
- Gastrointestinal: Diarrhea (3% to 4%), nausea (2%), vomiting (1%), abdominal pain (2%)
- Genitourinary: Impotence (1%)
- Hematologic: Decreased hemoglobin (small)
- Neuromuscular & skeletal: Chest pain (3%), weakness (1%)
- Renal: BUN increased (2%); deterioration in renal function (in patients with bilateral renal artery stenosis or hypovolemia); serum creatinine increased (often transient)
- Respiratory: Cough (4% to 9%), upper respiratory infection (1% to 2%)

Pharmacodynamics/Kinetics

Onset of Action 1 hour; Peak effect: Hypotensive: Oral: ~6 hours

Duration of Action 24 hours

Available Dosage Forms

Tablet, oral: 2.5 mg, 5 mg, 10 mg, 20 mg, 30 mg, 40 mg

Prinivil®: 5 mg, 10 mg, 20 mg

Zestril®: 2.5 mg, 5 mg, 10 mg, 20 mg, 30 mg, 40 mg

General Dosage Range Dosage adjustment recommended in patients with renal impairment

Oral:

Children ≥6 years: Initial: 0.07 mg/kg once daily (up to 5 mg); Maintenance: Maximum: Doses >0.61 mg/kg or >40 mg have not been evaluated

Adults: Initial: 2.5-10 mg/day; Maintenance: 10-80 mg/day

Elderly: Initial: 2.5-5 mg/day (maximum: 40 mg/day)

Administration

Oral Watch for hypotensive effects within 1-3 hours of first dose or new higher dose.

Nursing Actions

Physical Assessment Assess potential for interactions with other pharmacological agents or herbal products that may impact fluid balance or cardiac status. Monitor for angioedema that may potentially affect airway or intestine, hypovolemia, postural hypotension, and anaphylactic reaction very closely following first dose, any increase in dose, and regularly during therapy.

Patient Education Take first dose at bedtime. Do not use potassium supplement or salt substitutes without consulting prescriber. This drug does not eliminate need for diet or exercise regimen as recommended by prescriber. May cause dizziness, fainting, lightheadedness, postural hypotension, nausea, vomiting, abdominal pain, dry mouth, or transient loss of appetite; report if these persist. Report chest pain or palpitations; mouth sores; fever or chills; swelling of extremities, face, mouth, or tongue; skin rash; numbness, tingling, or pain in muscles; or respiratory difficulty or unusual cough.

Dietary Considerations Use potassium-containing salt substitutes cautiously in patients with diabetes, patients with renal dysfunction, or those maintained on potassium supplements or potassium-sparing diuretics.

Lisinopril and Hydrochlorothiazide

(lyse IN oh pril & hye droe klor oh THYE a zide)

Brand Names: U.S. Prinzide®; Zestoretic®

Index Terms Hydrochlorothiazide and Lisinopril

Pharmacologic Category Angiotensin-Converting Enzyme (ACE) Inhibitor; Diuretic, Thiazide

Pregnancy Risk Factor C/D (2nd and 3rd trimesters)

Lactation Enters breast milk/not recommended

Use Treatment of hypertension

Available Dosage Forms

Tablet, oral: 10/12.5: Lisinopril 10 mg and hydrochlorothiazide 12.5 mg; 20/12.5: Lisinopril 20 mg and hydrochlorothiazide 12.5 mg; 20/25: Lisinopril 20 mg and hydrochlorothiazide 25 mg

Prinzide®:

- 10/12.5: Lisinopril 10 mg and hydrochlorothiazide 12.5 mg
- 20/12.5: Lisinopril 20 mg and hydrochlorothiazide 12.5 mg

Zestoretic®:

- 10/12.5: Lisinopril 10 mg and hydrochlorothiazide 12.5 mg
- 20/12.5: Lisinopril 20 mg and hydrochlorothiazide 12.5 mg
- 20/25: Lisinopril 20 mg and hydrochlorothiazide 25 mg

General Dosage Range Oral: *Adults:* Lisinopril 10-80 mg and hydrochlorothiazide 12.5-50 mg once daily

Nursing Actions

Physical Assessment See individual agents.

Patient Education See individual agents.

Related Information

Hydrochlorothiazide *on page 570*

Lisinopril *on page 705*

Lithium (LITH ee um)

Brand Names: U.S. Lithobid®

Index Terms Eskalith; Lithium Carbonate; Lithium Citrate

Pharmacologic Category Antimanic Agent

Medication Safety Issues

Sound-alike/look-alike issues:

Eskalith may be confused with Estratest

Lithium may be confused with lanthanum

Lithobid® may be confused with Levbid®, Lithostat®

Other safety concerns:

Do not confuse **mEq** (milliequivalent) with **mg** (milligram). **Note:** 300 mg lithium carbonate or citrate contain 8 mEq lithium. Dosage should be written in **mg** (milligrams) to avoid confusion.

Check prescriptions for unusually high volumes of the syrup for dosing errors.

Pregnancy Risk Factor D

Lactation Enters breast milk/contraindicated

Use Management of bipolar disorders; treatment of mania in individuals with bipolar disorder (maintenance treatment prevents or diminishes intensity of subsequent episodes)

Unlabeled Use Potential augmenting agent for antidepressants; aggression, post-traumatic stress disorder, conduct disorder in children

Mechanism of Action/Effect Stabilizes mood by actions on nerve cells of the central nervous system; involves serotonin, phosphatidylinositol cycle, and dopamine receptor sensitivity

Contraindications Hypersensitivity to lithium or any component of the formulation; avoid use in patients with severe cardiovascular or renal disease, or with severe debilitation, dehydration, or sodium depletion; pregnancy

Warnings/Precautions [U.S. Boxed Warning]: Lithium toxicity is closely related to serum levels and can occur at therapeutic doses; serum lithium determinations are required to monitor therapy. Use with caution in patients with thyroid disease, mild-moderate renal impairment, or mild-moderate cardiovascular disease. Use caution in patients receiving medications which alter sodium excretion (eg, diuretics, ACE inhibitors, NSAIDs), or in patients with significant fluid loss (protracted sweating, diarrhea, or prolonged fever); temporary reduction or cessation of therapy may be warranted. Some elderly patients may be extremely sensitive to the effects of lithium, see General Dosage Range. Chronic therapy results in diminished renal concentrating ability (nephrogenic DI); this is usually reversible when lithium is discontinued. Changes in renal function should be monitored, and re-evaluation of treatment may be necessary. Use caution in patients at risk of suicide (suicidal thoughts or behavior).

Use with caution in patients receiving neuroleptic medications - a syndrome resembling NMS has been associated with concurrent therapy. Lithium may impair the patient's alertness, affecting the ability to operate machinery or driving a vehicle. Neuromuscular-blocking agents should be administered with caution; the response may be prolonged.

Higher serum concentrations may be required and tolerated during an acute manic phase; however, the tolerance decreases when symptoms subside. Normal fluid and salt intake must be maintained during therapy.

Drug Interactions

Avoid Concomitant Use There are no known interactions where it is recommended to avoid concomitant use.

Decreased Effect

Lithium may decrease the levels/effects of: Amphetamines; Antipsychotics; Desmopressin

The levels/effects of Lithium may be decreased by: Calcitonin; Calcium Polystyrene Sulfonate; Carbonic Anhydrase Inhibitors; Loop Diuretics; Sodium Bicarbonate; Sodium Chloride; Sodium Polystyrene Sulfonate; Theophylline Derivatives

Increased Effect/Toxicity

Lithium may increase the levels/effects of: Antipsychotics; Metoclopramide; Neuromuscular-Blocking Agents; Serotonin Modulators; Tricyclic Antidepressants

The levels/effects of Lithium may be increased by: ACE Inhibitors; Angiotensin II Receptor Blockers; Antipsychotics; Calcium Channel Blockers (Nondihydropyridine); CarBAMazepine; Desmopressin; Fosphenytoin; Loop Diuretics; MAO Inhibitors; Methyldopa; Nonsteroidal Anti-Inflammatory Agents; Phenytoin; Potassium Iodide; Selective Serotonin Reuptake Inhibitors; Thiazide Diuretics; Topiramate

Nutritional/Ethanol Interactions Food: Limit caffeine.

Adverse Reactions Frequency not defined.

Cardiovascular: Cardiac arrhythmia, hypotension, sinus node dysfunction, flattened or inverted T waves (reversible), edema, bradycardia, syncope

Central nervous system: Blackout spells, coma, confusion, dizziness, dystonia, fatigue, headache, lethargy, pseudotumor cerebri, psychomotor retardation, restlessness, sedation, seizure, slowed intellectual functioning, slurred speech, stupor, tics, vertigo

Dermatologic: Dry or thinning of hair, folliculitis, alopecia, exacerbation of psoriasis, rash

Endocrine & metabolic: Euthyroid goiter and/or hypothyroidism, hyperthyroidism, hyperglycemia, diabetes insipidus

Gastrointestinal: Polydipsia, anorexia, nausea, vomiting, diarrhea, xerostomia, metallic taste, weight gain, salivary gland swelling, excessive salivation

Genitourinary: Incontinence, polyuria, glycosuria, oliguria, albuminuria

Hematologic: Leukocytosis

Neuromuscular & skeletal: Tremor, muscle hyperirritability, ataxia, choreoathetoid movements, hyperactive deep tendon reflexes, myasthenia gravis (rare)

Ocular: Nystagmus, blurred vision, transient scotoma

Miscellaneous: Coldness and painful discoloration of fingers and toes

Postmarketing and/or case reports: Drug-induced Brugada syndrome

Available Dosage Forms

Capsule, oral: 150 mg, 300 mg, 600 mg

Solution, oral: 300 mg/5 mL (5 mL, 473 mL, 500 mL)

Tablet, oral: 300 mg, 600 mg

Tablet, extended release, oral: 300 mg, 450 mg

Lithobid®: 300 mg

General Dosage Range Dosage adjustment recommended in patients with renal impairment

Oral:

Immediate release:

Adults: 900-2400 mg/day in 3-4 divided doses

Elderly: Initial: 300 mg twice daily (maximum: >900-1200 mg/day)

Extended release: *Adults:* 900-1800 mg/day in 2 divided doses

Administration

Oral Administer with meals to decrease GI upset. Extended release tablets must be swallowed whole; do not crush or chew.

Nursing Actions

Physical Assessment Monitor cardiovascular status; assess for fluid retention. Educate patient about signs and symptoms of toxicity.

Patient Education Do not crush or chew extended release tablets or capsules. Maintain adequate hydration unless instructed to restrict fluid intake. Avoid changes in sodium content (eg, low sodium diets); reduction of sodium can increase lithium toxicity. Frequent blood tests and monitoring will be necessary. You may experience decreased appetite, altered taste sensation, drowsiness, or dizziness, especially during early therapy. Immediately report unresolved diarrhea, abrupt changes in weight, muscular tremors or lack of coordination, fever, or changes in urinary volume.

Dietary Considerations May be taken with meals to avoid GI upset; maintain adequate fluid intake.

Related Information

Peak and Trough Guidelines *on page 1276*

Lodoxamide (loe DOKS a mide)

Brand Names: U.S. Alomide®

Index Terms Lodoxamide Tromethamine

Pharmacologic Category Mast Cell Stabilizer

Medication Safety Issues

International issues:

Thilomide [Greece, Turkey] may be confused with Thalomid brand name for thalidomide [U.S., Canada]

Pregnancy Risk Factor B

Lactation Excretion in breast milk unknown/use caution

Use Treatment of vernal keratoconjunctivitis, vernal conjunctivitis, and vernal keratitis

Available Dosage Forms

Solution, ophthalmic:

Alomide®: 0.1% (10 mL)

General Dosage Range Ophthalmic: *Children >2 years and Adults:* Instill 1-2 drops in eye(s) 4 times/day

Nursing Actions

Patient Education For use in eyes only. Avoid wearing soft contact lenses while using this medication. Wash hands before using. Lie down or tilt your head back and look upward. Hold dropper tip as near as possible to your eyelid without touching it. Pull the lower lid of eye down to form a pocket. Drop the prescribed number of drops into the pocket made by the lower lid and the eye (placing drops on the surface of the eyeball can cause stinging). Do not blink or rub eye. Close your eye and press lightly against the inside corner of your eye for about 1 minute. Repeat in other eye if directed by prescriber. You may experience temporary stinging or burning in the eyes, headache, increased eye tearing or dry eye, sneezing, or blurred vision. Inform prescriber if you experience eye pain, disturbance of vision, skin rash, swelling in or around the eyes, or if condition worsens or fails to improve. Do not use if solution has changed color, is cloudy, or contains particles.

Loperamide (loe PER a mide)

Brand Names: U.S. Anti-Diarrheal [OTC]; Diamode [OTC]; Imodium® A-D for children [OTC]; Imodium® A-D [OTC]

Index Terms Loperamide Hydrochloride

Pharmacologic Category Antidiarrheal

Medication Safety Issues

Sound-alike/look-alike issues:

Imodium® A-D may be confused with Indocin®

Loperamide may be confused with furosemide

International issues:

Indiaral [France] may be confused with Inderal and Inderal LA brand names for propranolol [U.S., Canada, and multiple international markets]

Lomotil: Brand name for loperamide [Mexico, Philippines], but also the brand name for diphenoxylate [U.S., Canada, and multiple international markets]

Lomotil [Mexico, Phillipines] may be confused with Ludiomil brand name for maprotiline [multiple international markets]

Pregnancy Risk Factor C

Lactation Enters breast milk/not recommended.

Use Treatment of chronic diarrhea associated with inflammatory bowel disease; acute nonspecific diarrhea; increased volume of ileostomy discharge

OTC labeling: Control of symptoms of diarrhea, including Traveler's diarrhea

Unlabeled Use Cancer treatment-induced diarrhea (eg, irinotecan induced); chronic diarrhea caused by bowel resection

Available Dosage Forms For available OTC formulations, consult specific product labeling.

General Dosage Range Oral:

Children 2-5 years (13-20 kg): Initial: 1 mg 3 times/day for first 24 hours; Maintenance: 0.1 mg/kg after each loose stool

Children 6-8 years (20-30 kg): Initial: 2 mg twice daily for first 24 hours; Maintenance: 0.1 mg/kg after each loose stool **or** 2 mg after first loose stool, followed by 1 mg after each subsequent stool (maximum: 4 mg/day)

Children 8-12 years (>30 kg): Initial: 2 mg 3 times/day for first 24 hours; Maintenance: 0.1 mg/kg after each loose stool

Children 9-11 years: 2 mg after first loose stool, followed by 1 mg after each subsequent stool (maximum: 6 mg/day)

Children ≥12 years: Initial: 4 mg after first loose stool, followed by 2 mg after each subsequent stool (maximum: 8 mg/day)

Adults: Initial: 4 mg followed by 2 mg after each loose stool (maximum: 8-16 mg/day) **or** 4-8 mg/day in divided doses

Nursing Actions

Physical Assessment Assess for cause of diarrhea before administering first dose.

Patient Education May cause drowsiness. If acute diarrhea lasts longer than 48 hours, consult prescriber. Do not take if diarrhea is bloody.

Lopinavir and Ritonavir

(loe PIN a veer & rit ON uh veer)

Brand Names: U.S. Kaletra®

Index Terms Ritonavir and Lopinavir

Pharmacologic Category Antiretroviral Agent, Protease Inhibitor

Medication Safety Issues

Sound-alike/look-alike issues:

Potential for dispensing errors between Kaletra® and Keppra® (levETIRAcetam)

Administration issues:

Children's doses are based on weight and calculated by milligrams of lopinavir. Care should be taken to accurately calculate the dose. The oral solution contains lopinavir 80 mg and ritonavir 20 mg per one mL. Children <12 years of age (and ≤40 kg) who are not taking certain concomitant antiretroviral medications will receive <5 mL of solution per dose.

Medication Guide Available Yes

Pregnancy Risk Factor C

Lactation Excretion in breast milk unknown/contraindicated

Use Treatment of HIV infection in combination with other antiretroviral agents

Available Dosage Forms

Solution, oral:

Kaletra®: Lopinavir 80 mg and ritonavir 20 mg per mL

Tablet:

Kaletra®:

Lopinavir 100 mg and ritonavir 25 mg

Lopinavir 200 mg and ritonavir 50 mg

General Dosage Range Dosage adjustment recommended in patients on concomitant therapy

Oral:

Children 14 days to 6 months: Lopinavir 16 mg/kg or 300 mg/m^2 twice daily

Children 6 months to 18 years and <15 kg: 12 mg lopinavir/kg twice daily (maximum dose: Lopinavir 400 mg/ritonavir 100 mg)

Children 6 months to 18 years and 15-40 kg: 10 mg lopinavir/kg twice daily (maximum dose: Lopinavir 400 mg/ritonavir 100 mg)

Children 6 months to 18 years and >40 kg: Lopinavir 400 mg/ritonavir 100 mg twice daily

Adults: Lopinavir 400 mg/ritonavir 100 mg twice daily **or** lopinavir 800 mg/ritonavir 200 mg once daily

Administration

Oral

Solution: Administer with food; if using didanosine, take didanosine 1 hour before or 2 hours after lopinavir/ritonavir. Administer using calibrated dosing syringe.

Tablet: May be taken with or without food. Swallow whole, do not break, crush, or chew. May be taken with didanosine when taken without food. Tablets are not recommended in patients <15 kg.

Nursing Actions

Physical Assessment See individual agents.

Patient Education See individual agents.

Related Information

Ritonavir *on page 1003*

Loratadine

(lor AT a deen)

Brand Names: U.S. Alavert® Allergy 24 Hour [OTC]; Alavert® Children's Allergy [OTC]; Claritin® 24 Hour Allergy [OTC]; Claritin® Children's Allergy [OTC]; Claritin® Liqui-Gels® 24 Hour Allergy [OTC]; Claritin® RediTabs® 24 Hour Allergy [OTC]; Loradamed [OTC]; Tavist® ND Allergy [OTC]

Pharmacologic Category Histamine H_1 Antagonist; Histamine H_1 Antagonist, Second Generation; Piperidine Derivative

Medication Safety Issues

Sound-alike/look-alike issues:

Claritin® may be confused with clarithromycin

Claritin® (loratadine) may be confused with Claritin™ Eye (ketotifen)

Use Relief of nasal and non-nasal symptoms of seasonal allergic rhinitis; treatment of chronic idiopathic urticaria

Available Dosage Forms For available OTC formulations, consult specific product labeling.

General Dosage Range Dosage adjustment recommended in patients with hepatic or renal impairment

Oral:

Children 2-5 years: 5 mg once daily

Children ≥6 years and Adults: 10 mg once daily

Administration

Oral May be administered without regard to meals.

Nursing Actions

Patient Education Avoid use of alcohol. You may experience drowsiness, dizziness, dry mouth, or nausea. Report persistent dizziness or sedation; swelling of face, mouth, lips, or tongue; respiratory difficulty; lack of improvement; or worsening of condition.

Rapidly-disintegrating tablets: Place tablet on tongue; it dissolves rapidly. May be used with or without water. Use within 6 months of opening foil pouch and immediately after opening individual tablet blister.

Loratadine and Pseudoephedrine

(lor AT a deen & soo doe e FED rin)

Brand Names: U.S. Alavert™ Allergy and Sinus [OTC]; Claritin-D® 12 Hour Allergy & Congestion [OTC]; Claritin-D® 24 Hour Allergy & Congestion [OTC]; Loratadine-D 12 Hour [OTC]

Index Terms Pseudoephedrine and Loratadine

Pharmacologic Category Alpha/Beta Agonist; Decongestant; Histamine H_1 Antagonist; Histamine H_1 Antagonist, Second Generation; Piperidine Derivative

Medication Safety Issues

Sound-alike/look-alike issues:

Claritin-D® may be confused with Claritin-D® 24

Claritin-D® 24 may be confused with Claritin-D®

Use Temporary relief of symptoms of seasonal allergic rhinitis, other upper respiratory allergies, or the common cold

Available Dosage Forms For available OTC formulations, consult specific product labeling.

General Dosage Range Dosage adjustment recommended in patients with renal impairment

Oral: *Children ≥12 years and Adults:* Alavert™ Allergy and Sinus, Claritin-D® 24-Hour: 1 tablet every 24 hours; Claritin-D® 12-Hour: 1 tablet every 12 hours

Nursing Actions

Physical Assessment See individual agents.

Patient Education See individual agents.

Related Information

Loratadine *on page 710*

Pseudoephedrine *on page 961*

LORazepam

(lor A ze pam)

Brand Names: U.S. Ativan®; Lorazepam Intensol™

Pharmacologic Category Benzodiazepine

Medication Safety Issues

Sound-alike/look-alike issues:

LORazepam may be confused with ALPRAZolam, clonazePAM, diazepam, KlonoPIN®, Lovaza®, temazepam, zolpidem

Ativan® may be confused with Ambien®, Atarax®, Atgam®, Avitene®

BEERS Criteria medication:

This drug may be inappropriate for use in geriatric patients (high severity risk).

Administration issues:

Injection dosage form contains propylene glycol. Monitor for toxicity when administering continuous lorazepam infusions.

Pregnancy Risk Factor D

Lactation Enters breast milk/not recommended (AAP rates "of concern"; AAP 2001 update pending)

Breast-Feeding Considerations Drowsiness, lethargy, or weight loss in nursing infants have been observed in case reports following maternal use of some benzodiazepines.

Use

Oral: Management of anxiety disorders or short-term (≤4 months) relief of the symptoms of anxiety, anxiety associated with depressive symptoms, or insomnia due to anxiety or transient stress

I.V.: Status epilepticus, amnesia, sedation

Unlabeled Use Ethanol detoxification; psychogenic catatonia; partial complex seizures; agitation (I.V.); antiemetic for chemotherapy; rapid tranquilization of the agitated patient

Mechanism of Action/Effect Binds to stereospecific benzodiazepine receptors on the postsynaptic GABA neuron at several sites within the central nervous system, including the limbic system, reticular formation. Enhancement of the inhibitory effect of GABA on neuronal excitability results by increased neuronal membrane permeability to chloride ions. This shift in chloride ions results in hyperpolarization (a less excitable state) and stabilization.

Contraindications Hypersensitivity to lorazepam or any component of the formulation (cross-sensitivity with other benzodiazepines may exist); acute narrow-angle glaucoma; sleep apnea (parenteral); intra-arterial injection of parenteral formulation; severe respiratory insufficiency (except during mechanical ventilation)

Warnings/Precautions Use with caution in elderly or debilitated patients, patients with hepatic disease (including alcoholics) or renal impairment. Due to increased sensitivity in the elderly, smaller doses of benzodiazepines may be safer and as effective; in this age group, avoid using doses >3 mg daily of lorazepam (Beers Criteria). Use with caution in patients with respiratory disease (COPD or sleep apnea) or limited pulmonary reserve, or impaired gag reflex. Initial doses in elderly or debilitated patients should be at the lower end of the dosing range. May worsen hepatic encephalopathy.

Causes CNS depression (dose-related) resulting in sedation, dizziness, confusion, or ataxia which may impair physical and mental capabilities. Patients must be cautioned about performing tasks which require mental alertness (eg, operating machinery or driving). Use with caution in patients receiving other CNS depressants or psychoactive agents. Effects with other sedative drugs or ethanol may be potentiated. Benzodiazepines have been associated with falls and traumatic injury and should be used with extreme caution in patients who are at risk of these events (especially the elderly).

Lorazepam may cause anterograde amnesia. Paradoxical reactions, including hyperactive or aggressive behavior have been reported with benzodiazepines, particularly in adolescent/pediatric or psychiatric patients. Does not have analgesic, antidepressant, or antipsychotic properties.

Use caution in patients with depression, particularly if suicidal risk may be present. Pre-existing depression may worsen or emerge during therapy. Not recommended for use in primary depressive or psychotic disorders. Use with caution in patients with a history of drug dependence, alcoholism, or significant personality disorders. Benzodiazepines have been associated with dependence and acute withdrawal symptoms on discontinuation or reduction in dose. Acute withdrawal, including seizures, may be precipitated after administration of flumazenil to patients receiving long-term benzodiazepine therapy.

As a hypnotic agent, should be used only after evaluation of potential causes of sleep disturbance. Failure of sleep disturbance to resolve after 7-10 days may indicate psychiatric or medical illness. A worsening of insomnia or the emergence of new abnormalities of thought or behavior may represent unrecognized psychiatric or medical illness and requires immediate and careful evaluation.

Parenteral formulation of lorazepam contains polyethylene glycol which has resulted in toxicity during high-dose and/or longer-term infusions. Parenteral formulation also contains propylene glycol (PG); may be associated with dose-related toxicity and can occur ≥48 hours after initiation of lorazepam. Limited data suggest increased risk of PG accumulation at doses of ≥6 mg/hour for 48 hours or more (Nelson, 2008). Consider monitoring for signs of toxicity which may include acute renal failure, lactic acidosis, and/or osmol gap. In high-risk patients requiring higher doses/extended treatment durations, use of enteral delivery of lorazepam tablets may be beneficial (Jacobi, 2002). Also contains benzyl alcohol; avoid in neonates.

Drug Interactions

Avoid Concomitant Use

Avoid concomitant use of LORazepam with any of the following: OLANZapine

Decreased Effect

The levels/effects of LORazepam may be decreased by: Theophylline Derivatives; Yohimbine

Increased Effect/Toxicity

LORazepam may increase the levels/effects of: Alcohol (Ethyl); CloZAPine; CNS Depressants; Fosphenytoin; Methotrimeprazine; Phenytoin; Selective Serotonin Reuptake Inhibitors

The levels/effects of LORazepam may be increased by: Divalproex; Droperidol; HydrOXYzine; Loxapine; Methotrimeprazine; OLANZapine; Probenecid; Valproic Acid

Nutritional/Ethanol Interactions

Ethanol: May increase CNS depression; monitor for increased effects with coadministration. Caution patients about effects.

Herb/Nutraceutical: Avoid valerian, St John's wort, kava kava, gotu kola (may increase CNS depression).

Adverse Reactions

>10%:

Central nervous system: Sedation

Respiratory: Respiratory depression

1% to 10%:

Cardiovascular: Hypotension

Central nervous system: Akathisia, amnesia, ataxia, confusion, depression, disorientation, dizziness, headache

Dermatologic: Dermatitis, rash

Gastrointestinal: Changes in appetite, nausea, weight gain/loss

Neuromuscular & skeletal: Weakness

Ocular: Visual disturbances

Respiratory: Apnea, hyperventilation, nasal congestion

Pharmacodynamics/Kinetics

Onset of Action Hypnosis: I.M.: 20-30 minutes; Sedation: I.V.: 5-20 minutes; Anticonvulsant: I.V.: 5 minutes, oral: 30-60 minutes

Duration of Action 6-8 hours

Controlled Substance C-IV

Available Dosage Forms

Injection, solution: 2 mg/mL (1 mL, 10 mL); 4 mg/mL (1 mL, 10 mL)

Ativan®: 2 mg/mL (1 mL, 10 mL); 4 mg/mL (1 mL, 10 mL)

Solution, oral: 2 mg/mL (30 mL)
Lorazepam Intensol™: 2 mg/mL (30 mL)
Tablet, oral: 0.5 mg, 1 mg, 2 mg
Ativan®: 0.5 mg, 1 mg, 2 mg

General Dosage Range

I.M.:
Children: 0.02-0.09 mg/kg as a single dose
Adults: 0.5-1 mg every 30-60 minutes as needed **or** 0.05 mg/kg as a single dose (maximum: 4 mg/dose)

I.V.: *Children and Adults:* Dosage varies greatly depending on indication

Oral:
Children: 0.02-0.09 mg/kg every 4-8 hours or as a single dose
Adults: Dosage varies greatly depending on indication

Administration

I.M. Should be administered deep into the muscle mass.

I.V. Continuous infusion solutions should have an in-line filter and the solution should be checked frequently for possible precipitation. Avoid intra-arterial administration. Monitor I.V. site for extravasation.

I.V. Detail Dilute I.V. dose with equal volume of compatible diluent (D_5W, NS, SWFI).

Stability

Reconstitution
Injection: Dilute with equal volume of compatible diluent (D_5W, NS, SWFI).
Infusion: Use 2 mg/mL injectable vial to prepare; there may be decreased stability when using 4 mg/mL vial. Dilute ≤1 mg/mL and mix in glass bottle. Precipitation may develop. Can also be administered undiluted via infusion.

Storage
I.V.: Intact vials should be refrigerated. Protect from light. Do not use discolored or precipitate-containing solutions. May be stored at room temperature for up to 3 months [data on file (Hospira Inc, 2010)]. Parenteral admixture is stable at room temperature (25°C) for 24 hours.
Tablet: Store at room temperature.

Nursing Actions

Physical Assessment Oral: Assess for history of addiction; long-term use can result in dependence, abuse, or tolerance; periodically evaluate need for continued use. For inpatient use, institute safety measures. Taper dosage slowly when discontinuing. **I.V./I.M.:** Monitor cardiac, respiratory, and CNS status and ability to void.

Patient Education Oral: Drug may cause physical and/or psychological dependence. Do not use alcohol. You may experience drowsiness, lightheadedness, impaired coordination, dizziness, blurred vision, nausea, vomiting, dry mouth, constipation, altered sexual drive or ability (reversible), or photosensitivity. Report persistent CNS effects (eg, confusion, depression, increased sedation, excitation, headache, agitation, insomnia or nightmares, dizziness, fatigue, impaired coordination, changes in personality, or changes in cognition); changes in urinary pattern; chest pain, palpitations, or rapid heartbeat; muscle cramping, weakness, tremors, or rigidity; ringing in ears or visual disturbances; excessive perspiration; excessive GI symptoms (cramping, constipation, vomiting, anorexia); or worsening of condition.

Related Information
Compatibility of Drugs *on page 1264*

Losartan (loe SAR tan)

Brand Names: U.S. Cozaar®

Index Terms DuP 753; Losartan Potassium; MK594

Pharmacologic Category Angiotensin II Receptor Blocker

Medication Safety Issues

Sound-alike/look-alike issues:
Cozaar® may be confused with Colace®, Coreg®, Hyzaar®, Zocor®
Losartan may be confused with valsartan

Pregnancy Risk Factor C (1st trimester); D (2nd and 3rd trimesters)

Lactation Excretion in breast milk unknown/not recommended

Breast-Feeding Considerations It is not known if losartan is found in breast milk; the manufacturer recommends discontinuing the drug or discontinuing nursing based on the importance of the drug to the mother.

Use Treatment of hypertension (HTN); treatment of diabetic nephropathy in patients with type 2 diabetes mellitus (noninsulin dependent, NIDDM) and a history of hypertension; stroke risk reduction in patients with HTN and left ventricular hypertrophy (LVH)

Unlabeled Use To slow the rate of progression of aortic-root dilation in pediatric patients with Marfan's syndrome

Mechanism of Action/Effect As a selective and competitive, nonpeptide angiotensin II receptor antagonist, losartan blocks the vasoconstrictor and aldosterone-secreting effects of angiotensin II. Losartan increases urinary flow rate and in addition to being natriuretic and kaliuretic, increases excretion of chloride, magnesium, uric acid, calcium, and phosphate.

Contraindications Hypersensitivity to losartan or any component of the formulation

Warnings/Precautions [U.S. Boxed Warning]: Drugs that act on the renin-angiotensin system can cause injury and death to the developing fetus. Discontinue as soon as possible once pregnancy is detected. Avoid use or use a much smaller dose in patients who are volume-depleted; correct depletion first. Use with caution in patients with significant aortic/mitral stenosis. May cause hyperkalemia; avoid potassium supplementation unless specifically required by healthcare provider. May be associated with deterioration of renal function and/or increases in serum creatinine, particularly in patients with low renal blood flow (eg, renal artery stenosis, heart failure) whose glomerular filtration rate (GFR) is dependent on efferent arteriolar vasoconstriction by angiotensin II. Use caution in patients with unstented unilateral/bilateral renal artery stenosis. When unstented bilateral renal artery stenosis is present, use is generally avoided due to the elevated risk of deterioration in renal function unless possible benefits outweigh risks. Use with caution with pre-existing renal insufficiency. AUCs of losartan (not the active metabolite) are about 50% greater in patients with Cl_{cr} <30 mL/minute and are doubled in hemodialysis patients. Concurrent use of ACE inhibitors may increase the risk of clinically-significant adverse events (eg, renal dysfunction, hyperkalemia).

At any time during treatment (especially following first dose), angioedema may occur rarely; may involve the head and neck (potentially compromising airway) or the intestine (presenting with abdominal pain). Patients with idiopathic or hereditary angioedema or previous angioedema associated with ACE-inhibitor therapy may be at an increased risk. Prolonged frequent monitoring may be required, especially if tongue, glottis, or larynx are involved, as they are associated with airway obstruction. Patients with a history of airway surgery may have a higher risk of airway obstruction. Aggressive early management is critical; intramuscular (I.M.) administration of epinephrine may be necessary.

When used to reduce the risk of stroke in patients with HTN and LVH, may not be effective in African-American population. Use caution with hepatic dysfunction, dose adjustment may be needed.

Drug Interactions

Avoid Concomitant Use

Avoid concomitant use of Losartan with any of the following: Pimozide

Decreased Effect

The levels/effects of Losartan may be decreased by: CYP2C9 Inducers (Strong); CYP3A4 Inducers (Strong); Deferasirox; Herbs (CYP3A4 Inducers); Herbs (Hypertensive Properties); Methylphenidate; Nonsteroidal Anti-Inflammatory Agents; Peginterferon Alfa-2b; Rifamycin Derivatives; Tocilizumab; Yohimbine

Increased Effect/Toxicity

Losartan may increase the levels/effects of: ACE Inhibitors; Amifostine; Antihypertensives; ARIPiprazole; Carvedilol; CYP2C8 Substrates; CYP2C9 Substrates; Hypoglycemic Agents; Hypotensive Agents; Lithium; Nonsteroidal Anti-Inflammatory Agents; Pimozide; Potassium-Sparing Diuretics; RiTUXimab; Sodium Phosphates

The levels/effects of Losartan may be increased by: Alfuzosin; Antifungal Agents (Azole Derivatives, Systemic); Conivaptan; CYP2C9 Inhibitors (Moderate); CYP2C9 Inhibitors (Strong); Diazoxide; Eplerenone; Fluconazole; Herbs (Hypoglycemic Properties); Herbs (Hypotensive Properties); MAO Inhibitors; Milk Thistle; Pentoxifylline; Phosphodiesterase 5 Inhibitors; Potassium Salts; Prostacyclin Analogues; Tolvaptan; Trimethoprim

Nutritional/Ethanol Interactions Herb/Nutraceutical: St John's wort may decrease levels of losartan. Some herbal medications may worsen hypertension (eg, licorice); others may increase the antihypertensive effect of losartan (eg, shepherd's purse). Some herbal medications may increase the hypoglycemic effects of losartan (eg, alfalfa). Management: Avoid St John's wort. Avoid bayberry, blue cohosh, ginseng (American), kola, licorice, and yohimbe. Avoid black cohosh, California poppy, coleus, golden seal, hawthorn, mistletoe, periwinkle, quinine, and shepherd's purse. Avoid alfalfa, aloe, bilberry, bitter melon, burdock, celery, damiana, fenugreek, garcinia, garlic, ginger, ginseng (American), gymnema, marshmallow, and stinging nettle.

Adverse Reactions Note: The incidence of some adverse reactions varied based on the underlying disease state. Notations are made, where applicable, for data derived from trials conducted in diabetic nephropathy and hypertensive patients, respectively.

>10%:

- Cardiovascular: Chest pain (12% diabetic nephropathy)
- Central nervous system: Fatigue (14% diabetic nephropathy)
- Endocrine: Hypoglycemia (14% diabetic nephropathy)
- Gastrointestinal: Diarrhea (2% hypertension to 15% diabetic nephropathy)
- Genitourinary: Urinary tract infection (13% diabetic nephropathy)
- Hematologic: Anemia (14% diabetic nephropathy)
- Neuromuscular & skeletal: Weakness (14% diabetic nephropathy), back pain (2% hypertension to 12% diabetic nephropathy)
- Respiratory: Cough (≤3% to 11%; similar to placebo; incidence higher in patients with previous cough related to ACE inhibitor therapy)

1% to 10%:

- Cardiovascular: Hypotension (7% diabetic nephropathy), orthostatic hypotension (4% hypertension to 4% diabetic nephropathy), first-dose hypotension (dose related: <1% with 50 mg, 2% with 100 mg)
- Central nervous system: Dizziness (4%), hypoesthesia (5% diabetic nephropathy), fever (4% diabetic nephropathy), insomnia (1%)
- Dermatology: Cellulitis (7% diabetic nephropathy)

Endocrine: Hyperkalemia (<1% hypertension to 7% diabetic nephropathy)

Gastrointestinal: Gastritis (5% diabetic nephropathy), weight gain (4% diabetic nephropathy), dyspepsia (1% to 4%), abdominal pain (2%), nausea (2%)

Neuromuscular & skeletal: Muscular weakness (7% diabetic nephropathy), knee pain (5% diabetic nephropathy), leg pain (1% to 5%), muscle cramps (1%), myalgia (1%)

Respiratory: Bronchitis (10% diabetic nephropathy), upper respiratory infection (8%), nasal congestion (2%), sinusitis (1% hypertension to 6% diabetic nephropathy)

Miscellaneous: Infection (5% diabetic nephropathy), flu-like syndrome (10% diabetic nephropathy)

Pharmacodynamics/Kinetics

Onset of Action 6 hours

Available Dosage Forms

Tablet, oral: 25 mg, 50 mg, 100 mg

Cozaar®: 25 mg, 50 mg, 100 mg

General Dosage Range Dosage adjustment recommended in patients with hepatic impairment

Oral:

Children 6-16 years: Initial: 0.7 mg/kg once daily (maximum: 50 mg/day); Maintenance: Maximum: ≤1.4 mg/kg; 100 mg

Adults: Initial: 25-50 mg once daily; Maintenance: 25-100 mg/day in 1-2 divided doses (maximum: 100 mg/day)

Administration

Oral May be administered without regard to meals.

Stability

Storage Store at 15°C to 30°C (59°F to 86°F). Protect from light.

Nursing Actions

Physical Assessment Monitor for hypotension on a regular basis during therapy. Caution patients with diabetes to monitor glucose levels closely; may alter glucose control.

Patient Education Preferable to take at same time each day without regard to meals. This drug does not eliminate need for diet or exercise regimen as recommended by prescriber. Do not use potassium supplement or salt substitutes without consulting prescriber. If you have diabetes, you may be cautioned to monitor glucose levels closely; may alter glucose control. May cause dizziness, fainting, lightheadedness, postural hypotension, or diarrhea. Report immediately swelling of face, lips, or mouth; difficulty swallowing; chest pain or palpitations; unrelenting headache; or CNS changes (delusions or depression).

Dietary Considerations May be taken without regard to meals. Some products may contain potassium.

Losartan and Hydrochlorothiazide

(loe SAR tan & hye droe klor oh THYE a zide)

Brand Names: U.S. Hyzaar®

Index Terms Hydrochlorothiazide and Losartan

Pharmacologic Category Angiotensin II Receptor Blocker; Diuretic, Thiazide

Medication Safety Issues

Sound-alike/look-alike issues:

Hyzaar® may be confused with Cozaar®

Pregnancy Risk Factor C/D (2nd and 3rd trimesters)

Lactation Enters breast milk/contraindicated

Use Treatment of hypertension; stroke risk reduction in patients with HTN and left ventricular hypertrophy (LVH)

Available Dosage Forms

Tablet: 50/12.5: Losartan 50 mg and hydrochlorothiazide 12.5 mg; 100/12.5: Losartan 100 mg and hydrochlorothiazide 12.5 mg; 100/25: Losartan 100 mg and hydrochlorothiazide 25 mg

Hyzaar®: 50/12.5: Losartan 50 mg and hydrochlorothiazide 12.5 mg; 100/12.5: Losartan 100 mg and hydrochlorothiazide 12.5 mg; 100/25: Losartan 100 mg and hydrochlorothiazide 25 mg

General Dosage Range Oral: *Adults:* Losartan 50-100 mg and hydrochlorothiazide 12.5-50 mg once daily

Nursing Actions

Physical Assessment See individual agents.

Patient Education See individual agents.

Related Information

Hydrochlorothiazide *on page 570*

Losartan *on page 713*

Loteprednol (loe te PRED nol)

Brand Names: U.S. Alrex®; Lotemax®

Index Terms Loteprednol Etabonate

Pharmacologic Category Corticosteroid, Ophthalmic

Pregnancy Risk Factor C

Lactation Excretion in breast milk unknown/use caution

Use

Ointment, 0.5% (Lotemax®): Treatment of postoperative inflammation and pain following ocular surgery

Suspension, 0.2% (Alrex®): Temporary relief of signs and symptoms of seasonal allergic conjunctivitis

Suspension, 0.5% (Lotemax®): Inflammatory conditions (treatment of steroid-responsive inflammatory conditions of the palpebral and bulbar conjunctiva, cornea, and anterior segment of the globe such as allergic conjunctivitis, acne rosacea, superficial punctate keratitis, herpes zoster keratitis, iritis, cyclitis, selected infective conjunctivitis, when the inherent hazard of steroid use is accepted to obtain an advisable diminution in edema and inflammation) and treatment of postoperative inflammation following ocular surgery

Product Availability

Lotemax® 0.5% ointment: FDA approved April 2011; expected availability undetermined

Lotemax® 0.5% ointment is a topical corticosteroid approved for the treatment of postoperative inflammation and pain following ocular surgery.

Available Dosage Forms

Ointment, ophthalmic:

Lotemax®: 0.5% (3.5 g)

Suspension, ophthalmic:

Alrex®: 0.2% (5 mL, 10 mL)

Lotemax®: 0.5% (2.5 mL, 5 mL, 10 mL, 15 mL)

General Dosage Range Ophthalmic: *Adults:* Ointment: Apply ~1/2 inch ribbon into affected eye(s) 4 times/day; Solution: Instill 1-2 drops into affected eye(s) 4 times/day

Administration

Other Shake suspension well before using.

Nursing Actions

Patient Education For use in eyes only. Shake suspension well before using. Do not let tip of applicator touch eye; do not contaminate tip of applicator (may cause eye infection, eye damage, or vision loss). Tilt head back, place medication in conjunctival sac, and close eyes. Apply finger pressure at corner of eye for 1 minute following application. May cause temporary sensitivity to bright light, blurring or stinging, changes in visual acuity, headache, runny nose, or sore throat. If improvement is not noted within 2 days, notify prescriber. Report persistent vision changes, signs of infection, swollen eyelids, or inflammation.

Loteprednol and Tobramycin

(loe te PRED nol & toe bra MYE sin)

Brand Names: U.S. Zylet®

Index Terms Loteprednol Etabonate and Tobramycin; Tobramycin and Loteprednol Etabonate

Pharmacologic Category Antibiotic/Corticosteroid, Ophthalmic

Pregnancy Risk Factor C

Lactation Excretion in breast milk unknown/use caution

Use Treatment of steroid-responsive ocular inflammatory conditions where either a superficial bacterial ocular infection or the risk of a superficial bacterial ocular infection exists

Available Dosage Forms

Suspension, ophthalmic [drops]:

Zylet®: Loteprednol 0.5% and tobramycin 0.3% (2.5 mL, 5 mL, 10 mL)

General Dosage Range Ophthalmic: *Children and Adults:* Instill 1-2 drops into the affected eye(s) every 4-6 hours

Administration

Other Contact lenses should not be worn during therapy. Shake well before using; Tilt head back, instill suspension in conjunctival sac and close eye(s). Do not touch dropper to eye. Apply light finger pressure on lacrimal sac for 1 minute following instillation.

Nursing Actions

Physical Assessment See individual agents.

Patient Education See individual agents.

Lovastatin (LOE va sta tin)

Brand Names: U.S. Altoprev®; Mevacor®

Index Terms Mevinolin; Monacolin K

Pharmacologic Category Antilipemic Agent, HMG-CoA Reductase Inhibitor

Medication Safety Issues

Sound-alike/look-alike issues:

Lovastatin may be confused with atorvastatin, Leustatin®, Livostin®, Lotensin®, nystatin, pitavastatin

Mevacor® may be confused with Benicar®, Lipitor®

International issues:

Lovacol [Chile and Finland] may be confused with Levatol brand name for penbutolol [U.S.]

Lovastin [Malaysia, Poland, and Singapore] may be confused with Livostin brand name for levocabastine [multiple international markets]

Mevacor [U.S., Canada, and multiple international markets} may be confused with Mivacron brand name for mivacurium [multiple international markets]

Pregnancy Risk Factor X

Lactation Excretion in breast milk unknown/contraindicated

Use

Adjunct to dietary therapy to decrease elevated serum total and LDL-cholesterol concentrations in primary hypercholesterolemia

Primary prevention of coronary artery disease (patients without symptomatic disease with average to moderately elevated total and LDL-cholesterol and below average HDL-cholesterol); slow progression of coronary atherosclerosis in patients with coronary heart disease and reduce the risk of myocardial infarction, unstable angina, and coronary revascularization procedures.

Adjunct to dietary therapy in adolescent patients (10-17 years of age, females >1 year postmenarche) with heterozygous familial hypercholesterolemia having LDL >189 mg/dL, **or** LDL >160 mg/dL with positive family history of premature cardiovascular disease (CVD), **or** LDL >160 mg/dL with the presence of at least two other CVD risk factors

Available Dosage Forms

Tablet, oral: 10 mg, 20 mg, 40 mg

Mevacor®: 20 mg, 40 mg

Tablet, extended release, oral:
Altoprev®: 20 mg, 40 mg, 60 mg

General Dosage Range Dosage adjustment recommended in patients with renal impairment or on concomitant therapy

Oral:

Extended release: *Adults:* Initial: 20 mg once daily; Maintenance: 20-60 mg once daily (maximum: 60 mg/day)

Immediate release:

Children 10-17 years: Initial: 10-20 mg once daily; Maintenance: 10-40 mg once daily (maximum: 40 mg/day)

Adults: Initial: 20 mg once daily; Maintenance: 20-80 mg once daily (maximum: 80 mg/day)

Administration

Oral Administer immediate release tablet with the evening meal. Administer extended release tablet at bedtime; do not crush or chew.

Nursing Actions

Physical Assessment Assess risk potential for interactions with other prescriptions or herbal products patient may be taking that may increase risk of myopathy or rhabdomyolysis. Teach proper diet and exercise program.

Patient Education Take with food at evening meal. Follow prescribed diet and exercise regimen. You will have periodic blood tests to assess effectiveness. Avoid excessive alcohol. Report unusual muscle cramping or weakness, yellowing of skin or eyes, easy bruising or bleeding, or unusual fatigue.

Lubiprostone (loo bi PROS tone)

Brand Names: U.S. Amitiza®

Index Terms RU 0211; SPI 0211

Pharmacologic Category Chloride Channel Activator; Gastrointestinal Agent, Miscellaneous

Pregnancy Risk Factor C

Lactation Excretion in breast milk unknown/not recommended

Use Treatment of chronic idiopathic constipation; treatment of irritable bowel syndrome with constipation in adult women

Mechanism of Action/Effect Increases intestinal fluid and intestinal motility

Contraindications Known or suspected mechanical bowel obstruction

Warnings/Precautions Symptoms of mechanical gastrointestinal obstruction should be evaluated before prescribing this medicine; use is contraindicated in patients with bowel obstruction. Avoid use in patients with severe diarrhea. Nausea may occur; administer with food to reduce symptoms. In long-term clinical studies for chronic idiopathic constipation, patients were allowed to reduce the dose to 24 mcg once daily if nausea was severe. Dyspnea, often described as chest tightness, has been observed with use, including postmarketing reports; generally occurs following the first dose with an acute onset (within 30-60 minutes) and resolves within a few hours; however, has been frequently reported with subsequent dosing. Dose adjustment is recommended in patients with moderate-to-severe hepatic impairment (Child Pugh class B or C). Not approved for use in males with irritable bowel syndrome with constipation.

Drug Interactions

Avoid Concomitant Use There are no known interactions where it is recommended to avoid concomitant use.

Decreased Effect There are no known significant interactions involving a decrease in effect.

Increased Effect/Toxicity There are no known significant interactions involving an increase in effect.

Adverse Reactions

>10%:

Central nervous system: Headache (3% to 11%)

Gastrointestinal: Nausea (7% to 29%; severe: 4%; dose related), diarrhea (7% to 12%; severe 2%)

1% to 10%:

Cardiovascular: Edema (3%), chest discomfort/pain (2%)

Central nervous system: Dizziness (3%), fatigue (2%)

Gastrointestinal: Abdominal pain (1% to 8%), abdominal distention (3% to 6%), flatulence (3% to 6%), vomiting (3%), loose stools (3%), dyspepsia (2%), xerostomia (1%)

Respiratory: Dyspnea (2% to 3%)

Available Dosage Forms

Capsule, softgel, oral:
Amitiza®: 8 mcg, 24 mcg

General Dosage Range Dosage adjustment recommended in hepatic impairment and in patients who develop toxicities

Oral:

Adults (females): 8 mcg twice daily **or** 24 mcg twice daily

Adults (males): 24 mcg twice daily

Administration

Oral Administer with food and water. Swallow whole; do not break or chew.

Stability

Storage Store at 25°C (77°F); excursions permitted to 15°C to 30°C (59°F to 86°F).

Dietary Considerations Take with food and water to decrease nausea.

Lurasidone (loo RAS i done)

Brand Names: U.S. Latuda®

Index Terms Lurasidone Hydrochloride; SM-13496

Pharmacologic Category Antipsychotic Agent, Atypical

Medication Safety Issues

Sound-alike/look-alike issues:

Latuda® may be confused with Lantus®

Pregnancy Risk Factor B

Lactation Excretion in breast milk unknown/not recommended

Use Treatment of schizophrenia

Mechanism of Action/Effect Atypical antipsychotic with high affinity for serotonin, dopamine, and moderate affinity for alpha$_2$-adrenergic receptors; no significant affinity for muscarinic or histamine receptors. Results in improvement of psychotic symptoms and reduction of extrapyramidal and antimuscarinic side effects as compared to typical antipsychotics.

Contraindications Hypersensitivity to lurasidone or any component of the formulation; concomitant use with potent CYP3A4 inhibitors (eg, ketoconazole) and inducers (eg, rifampin)

Warnings/Precautions [U.S. Boxed Warning]: Elderly patients with dementia-related psychosis treated with antipsychotics are at an increased risk of death compared to placebo. Most deaths appeared to be either cardiovascular (eg, heart failure, sudden death) or infectious (eg, pneumonia) in nature. Lurasidone is not approved for the treatment of dementia-related psychosis. An increased incidence of cerebrovascular effects (eg, transient ischemic attack, stroke), including fatalities, has been reported in placebo-controlled trials of antipsychotics for the unapproved use in elderly patients with dementia-related psychosis.

Leukopenia, neutropenia, and agranulocytosis (sometimes fatal) have been reported in clinical trials and postmarketing reports with antipsychotic use; presence of risk factors (eg, pre-existing low WBC or history of drug-induced leuko-/neutropenia) should prompt periodic blood count assessment. Discontinue therapy at first signs of blood dyscrasias or if absolute neutrophil count $<1000/mm^3$.

Low to moderately sedating, use with caution in disorders where CNS depression is a feature. Use with caution in Parkinson's disease. Caution in patients with predisposition to seizures. Use with caution in renal or hepatic dysfunction; dose reduction recommended in moderate-to-severe impairment. Esophageal dysmotility and aspiration have been associated with antipsychotic use; use with caution in patients at risk of aspiration pneumonia (ie, Alzheimer's disease). Use is associated with increased prolactin levels; clinical significance of hyperprolactinemia in patients with breast cancer or other prolactin-dependent tumors is unknown. May alter temperature regulation.

Use with caution in patients with severe cardiac disease, hemodynamic instability, prior myocardial infarction or ischemic heart disease. May cause orthostatic hypotension; use with caution in patients at risk of this effect (eg, concurrent medication use which may predispose to hypotension/bradycardia or presence of hypovolemia) or in those who would not tolerate transient hypotensive episodes. Antipsychotics may alter cardiac conduction; life-threatening arrhythmias have occurred with therapeutic doses of antipsychotics. Relative to other antipsychotics, lurasidone has minimal effects on the QT_c interval and therefore, risk for arrhythmias is low. Increases in total cholesterol and triglyceride concentrations have been observed with atypical antipsychotic use; during clinical trials of lurasidone, there were no significant changes in total cholesterol or triglycerides observed. Concurrent use with strong inhibitors/inducers of CYP3A4 is contraindicated; dosage adjustment is recommended with concurrent use of moderate CYP3A4 inhibitors (eg, diltiazem).

May cause extrapyramidal symptoms (EPS), including pseudoparkinsonism, acute dystonic reactions, akathisia, and tardive dyskinesia (potentially irreversible). Risk of tardive dyskinesia may be increased in elderly patients, particularly elderly women. Risk of dystonia (and probably other EPS) may be greater with increased doses, use of conventional antipsychotics, males, and younger patients. Use may be associated with neuroleptic malignant syndrome (NMS); monitor for mental status changes, fever, muscle rigidity and/or autonomic instability (risk may be increased in patients with Parkinson's disease or Lewy body dementia). May cause hyperglycemia; in some cases may be extreme and associated with ketoacidosis, hyperosmolar coma, or death. Use with caution in patients with diabetes or other disorders of glucose regulation; monitor for worsening of glucose control. Significant weight gain has been observed with antipsychotic therapy; incidence varies with product. Monitor waist circumference and BMI.

The possibility of a suicide attempt is inherent in psychotic illness or bipolar disorder; use caution in high-risk patients during initiation of therapy. Prescriptions should be written for the smallest quantity consistent with good patient care.

Drug Interactions

Avoid Concomitant Use

Avoid concomitant use of Lurasidone with any of the following: CYP3A4 Inducers (Strong); CYP3A4 Inhibitors (Strong); DOPamine; EPINEPHrine; EPINEPHrine (Systemic, Oral Inhalation); Metoclopramide; Pimozide

Decreased Effect

Lurasidone may decrease the levels/effects of: Amphetamines; Anti-Parkinson's Agents (Dopamine Agonist); Quinagolide

The levels/effects of Lurasidone may be decreased by: CYP3A4 Inducers (Strong); Deferasirox; Lithium formulations; Tocilizumab

Increased Effect/Toxicity

Lurasidone may increase the levels/effects of: Alcohol (Ethyl); ARIPiprazole; CNS Depressants; Disopyramide; Methotrimeprazine; Methylphenidate; Pimozide; Procainamide; QuiNIDine; Serotonin Modulators

The levels/effects of Lurasidone may be increased by: Acetylcholinesterase Inhibitors (Central); CYP3A4 Inhibitors (Moderate); CYP3A4 Inhibitors (Strong); Dasatinib; DOPamine; Droperidol; EPINEPHrine; EPINEPHrine (Systemic, Oral Inhalation); HydrOXYzine; Ivacaftor; Lithium formulations; MAO Inhibitors; Methotrimeprazine; Methylphenidate; Metoclopramide; Tetrabenazine

Nutritional/Ethanol Interactions

Ethanol: May increase CNS depression; monitor for increased effects with coadministration. Caution patients about effects.

Food: Administration with food (≥350 calories) increased C_{max} and AUC of lurasidone ~3 times and 2 times, respectively, compared to administration under fasting conditions. Lurasidone exposure was not affected by the fat content of the meal.

Adverse Reactions

10%:

Central nervous system: Somnolence (dose-related: 19% to 23%), akathisia (dose-related: 11% to 15%)

Endocrine & metabolic: Fasting glucose increased (10% to 14%)

Gastrointestinal: Nausea (12%)

Neuromuscular & skeletal: Extrapyramidal symptoms (24% to 26%), parkinsonism (11%)

1% to 10%:

Cardiovascular: Tachycardia

Central nervous system: Insomnia (8%), agitation (6%), anxiety (6%), dizziness (5%), dystonia (5%), fatigue (4%), restlessness (3%)

Dermatologic: Pruritus, rash

Endocrine & metabolic: Prolactin increased (≥5 x ULN: females: 8%; males: 2%)

Gastrointestinal: Dyspepsia (8%), vomiting (8%), weight gain (≥7% increase in baseline body weight: 6%), salivary hypersecretion (2%), abdominal pain, appetite decreased, diarrhea

Neuromuscular & skeletal: Back pain (4%), CPK increased

Ocular: Blurred vision

Renal: Creatinine increased (3%)

Available Dosage Forms

Tablet, oral:

Latuda®: 20 mg, 40 mg, 80 mg

General Dosage Range Dosage adjustment recommended in patients with hepatic or renal impairment or on concomitant therapy.

Oral: *Adults:* Initial: 40 mg once daily (maximum: 80 mg/day)

Administration

Oral Administer with food (≥350 calories).

Stability

Storage Store at controlled room temperature of 25°C (77°F).

Nursing Actions

Physical Assessment Monitor weight prior to treatment and periodically throughout. Be alert to the potential for orthostatic hypotension, especially during the titration phase. Initiate at lower doses and titrate to target dose. Taper dosage slowly when discontinuing.

Patient Education It may take several weeks to achieve desired results. Avoid alcohol. Maintain adequate hydration. If you have diabetes, you may experience increased blood sugars; monitor closely. You may experience excess sedation, drowsiness, problems sleeping, restlessness, dizziness, or blurred vision; dry mouth, nausea, or GI upset; postural hypotension; or urinary retention. Report persistent CNS effects; diaphoresis, chest pain, palpitations, rapid heartbeat, or severe dizziness; or worsening of condition.

Dietary Considerations Should be taken with food (≥350 calories).

Lutropin Alfa (LOO troe pin AL fa)

Brand Names: U.S. Luveris®

Index Terms r-hLH; Recombinant Human Luteinizing Hormone

Pharmacologic Category Gonadotropin; Ovulation Stimulator

Pregnancy Risk Factor X

Lactation Excretion in breast milk unknown/use caution

Use Stimulation of follicular development in infertile hypogonadotropic hypogonadal (HH) women with profound luteinizing hormone (LH) deficiency (<1.2 int. units/L); to be used in combination with follitropin alfa

Available Dosage Forms

Injection, powder for reconstitution:

Luveris®: 75 int. units

General Dosage Range SubQ: *Adults (females):* 75 int. units daily

Administration

Other SubQ: Administer on the stomach, a few inches above or below the navel. Do not shake solution; allow any bubbles to settle prior to administration.

Nursing Actions

Physical Assessment This medication should only be prescribed by a fertility specialist. For subcutaneous use only. Administer around navel area. Instruct patient in appropriate administration technique and disposal of used needles and syringes.

Patient Education For subcutaneous injection only. Follow administration schedule as directed by prescriber. You may experience headache, nausea, fatigue, constipation, or diarrhea. Report immediately abdominal pain/distension or persistent nausea.

Magnesium Chloride (mag NEE zhum KLOR ide)

Brand Names: U.S. Chloromag®; Mag 64™ [OTC]; Mag Delay [OTC]; Slow-Mag® [OTC]

Pharmacologic Category Electrolyte Supplement, Oral; Electrolyte Supplement, Parenteral; Magnesium Salt

Pregnancy Risk Factor C

Lactation Enters breast milk/compatible

Use Correction or prevention of hypomagnesemia; dietary supplement

Available Dosage Forms

Injection, solution: 200 mg/mL (50 mL)
Chloromag®: 200 mg/mL (50 mL)

Tablet, delayed release, enteric coated, oral:
Mag 64™ [OTC]: Elemental magnesium 64 mg
Mag Delay [OTC]: Elemental magnesium 64 mg

Tablet, enteric coated, oral:
Slow-Mag® [OTC]: Elemental magnesium 64 mg

General Dosage Range

I.V.:
Children <50 kg: 0.3-0.5 mEq/kg/day
Children >50 kg: 10-30 mEq/day
Adults: 8-24 mEq/day added to TPN

Oral: RDA (elemental magnesium):
Children: 80-240 mg/day
Adults: 360-410 mg/day

Magnesium Gluconate (mag NEE zhum GLOO koe nate)

Brand Names: U.S. Magonate® [OTC]; Magtrate® [OTC]; Mag®-G [OTC]

Pharmacologic Category Electrolyte Supplement, Oral; Magnesium Salt

Lactation Enters breast milk/compatible

Use Dietary supplement

Available Dosage Forms For available OTC formulations, consult specific product labeling.

General Dosage Range Oral: RDA (elemental magnesium):
Children 1-13 years: 80-240 mg/day
Children ≥14 years and Adults: 310-420 mg/day

Administration

Oral Administer on an empty stomach

Magnesium Sulfate (mag NEE zhum SUL fate)

Index Terms Epsom Salts; $MgSO_4$ (error-prone abbreviation)

Pharmacologic Category Anticonvulsant, Miscellaneous; Electrolyte Supplement, Parenteral; Magnesium Salt

Medication Safety Issues

Sound-alike/look-alike issues:

Magnesium sulfate may be confused with manganese sulfate, morphine sulfate

$MgSO_4$ is an error-prone abbreviation (mistaken as morphine sulfate)

High alert medication:

The Institute for Safe Medication Practices (ISMP) includes this medication (I.V. formulation) among its list of drugs which have a heightened risk of causing significant patient harm when used in error.

Pregnancy Risk Factor A/C (manufacturer dependent)

Lactation Enters breast milk/compatible

Use Treatment and prevention of hypomagnesemia; prevention and treatment of seizures in severe pre-eclampsia or eclampsia, pediatric acute nephritis; torsade de pointes; treatment of cardiac arrhythmias (VT/VF) caused by hypomagnesemia; soaking aid

Unlabeled Use Asthma exacerbation (life-threatening)

Available Dosage Forms

Infusion, premixed in D_5W: 10 mg/mL (100 mL)

Infusion, premixed in water for injection: 40 mg/mL (50 mL, 100 mL, 500 mL, 1000 mL); 80 mg/mL (50 mL)

Injection, solution: 500 mg/mL (5 mL, 10 mL, 20 mL, 25 mL, 50 mL)

Injection, solution [preservative free]: 500 mg/mL (2 mL, 5 mL, 10 mL, 20 mL, 50 mL)

Powder, oral/topical: USP: 100% (227 g, 454 g, 1810 g, 2720 g)

General Dosage Range

I.V.: *Children and Adults:* Dosage varies greatly depending on indication

Oral: RDA (elemental magnesium):
Children 1-13 years: 80-240 mg/day
Children ≥14 years and Adults: 310-420 mg/day

I.M.: *Adults:* Hypomagnesemia: 1-4 g/day in divided doses

Topical: *Adults:* Soaking aid: Dissolve 2 cupfuls of powder per gallon of warm water

Administration

I.M. A 25% or 50% concentration may be used for adults and dilution to a ≤20% solution is recommended for children

I.V. Magnesium should be diluted to a ≤20% solution for I.V. infusion and may be administered I.V. push, IVPB, or continuous I.V. infusion. When giving I.V. push, must dilute first and should not be given any faster than 150 mg/minute; may administer over 1-2 minutes in patients with persistent pulseless VT or VF with known hypomagnesemia (Dager, 2006). ACLS guidelines recommend administration over 15 minutes in patients with torsade de pointes (ACLS, 2010). In patients not in cardiac arrest, hypotension and asystole may occur with rapid administration.

Maximal rate of infusion: 2 g/hour to avoid hypotension; doses of 4 g/hour have been given in emergencies (eclampsia, seizures); optimally, should add magnesium to I.V. fluids, but bolus doses are also effective

Topical Dissolve 2 cups of powder per gallon of warm water to use as a soaking aid. To make a compress, dissolve 2 cups of powder per 2 cups of hot water and use a towel to apply as a wet dressing.

Nursing Actions

Physical Assessment When administered parenterally, monitor serum magnesium concentration, respiratory rate, deep tendon reflex, and renal function.

Patient Education Take in divided doses. Report diarrhea (>5 stools/day) or changes in mental function to prescriber.

Related Information

Compatibility of Drugs *on page 1264*

Mannitol (MAN i tole)

Brand Names: U.S. Aridol™; Osmitrol

Index Terms *D*-Mannitol

Pharmacologic Category Diagnostic Agent; Diuretic, Osmotic; Genitourinary Irrigant

Medication Safety Issues

Sound-alike/look-alike issues:

Osmitrol® may be confused with esmolol

Pregnancy Risk Factor C

Lactation Excretion in breast milk unknown/use caution

Use

Injection: Reduction of increased intracranial pressure associated with cerebral edema; reduction of increased intraocular pressure; promoting urinary excretion of toxic substances; genitourinary irrigant in transurethral prostatic resection or other transurethral surgical procedures

Note: Although FDA-labeled indications, the use of mannitol for the prevention of acute renal failure and/or promotion of diuresis is not routinely recommended (Kellum, 2008).

Genitourinary irrigation solution: Irrigation in transurethral prostatic resection or other transurethral surgical procedures

Powder for inhalation: Assessment of bronchial hyper-responsiveness

Unlabeled Use Improve renal transplant function

Available Dosage Forms

Injection, solution: 20% [200 mg/mL] (250 mL, 500 mL); 25% [250 mg/mL] (50 mL)

Osmitrol: 5% [50 mg/mL] (1000 mL); 10% [100 mg/mL] (500 mL); 15% [150 mg/mL] (500 mL); 20% [200 mg/mL] (250 mL, 500 mL)

Injection, solution [preservative free]: 25% [250 mg/mL] (50 mL)

Powder, for oral inhalation:

Aridol™: 0 mg (1s) [empty], 5 mg (1s), 10 mg (1s), 20 mg (1s), 40 mg (15s) (19s)

Solution, genitourinary irrigation: 5% [50 mg/mL] (2000 mL)

General Dosage Range

Inhalation: *Children ≥6 years and Adults:* 0-635 mg administered in a stepwise fashion until a positive response or the full dose has been administered (whichever comes first)

I.V.: *Adults:* Reduction of intraocular pressure: 1.5-2 g/kg

Transurethral: *Adults:* Use 5% urogenital solution as required for irrigation

Administration

I.V. Vesicant; avoid extravasation. Do not administer with blood. Crenation and agglutination of red blood cells may occur if administered with whole blood. Inspect for crystals prior to administration. If crystals present redissolve by warming solution. Use filter-type administration set for infusion solutions containing mannitol ≥20%. For cerebral edema or elevated ICP, administer over 20-30 minutes.

I.V. Detail pH: 4.5-7

Other

Inhalation (Aridol™): Administer using supplied single patient use inhaler; do not puncture capsule more than once; do not swallow capsules. A nose clip may be used if preferred. The patient should exhale completely, followed by a controlled rapid deep inspiration from the device; hold breath for 5 seconds and exhale through the mouth. Measure FEV_1 in duplicate 60 seconds after inhalation; repeat process until positive response or full dose (635 mg) has been administered.

Irrigation: Administer using only the appropriate transurethral urologic instrumentation.

Nursing Actions

Physical Assessment Adequate renal function should be present prior to administration. Monitor infusion site closely for extravasation; this is a vesicant. Monitor renal and cardiovascular status during infusion. Monitor for circulatory overload, CHF, rash, and water intoxication.

Patient Education Report immediately any nausea, dizziness, respiratory difficulty, chest pain, or pain at infusion site.

Related Information

Management of Drug Extravasations *on page 1269*

Maraviroc (mah RAV er rock)

Brand Names: U.S. Selzentry®

Index Terms UK-427,857

Pharmacologic Category Antiretroviral Agent, CCR5 Antagonist

Medication Guide Available Yes

Pregnancy Risk Factor B

Lactation Excretion in breast milk unknown/contraindicated

Breast-Feeding Considerations Maternal or infant antiretroviral therapy does not completely eliminate the risk of postnatal HIV transmission. In addition, multiclass-resistant virus has been detected in breast-feeding infants despite maternal therapy. Therefore, in the United States, where formula is accessible, affordable, safe, and sustainable, and the risk of infant mortality due to diarrhea and respiratory infections is low, complete avoidance of breast-feeding by HIV-infected women is recommended to decrease potential transmission of HIV (DHHS [perinatal], 2011).

Use Treatment of CCR5-tropic HIV-1 infection, in combination with other antiretroviral agents

Mechanism of Action/Effect Inhibits CCR5-tropic HIV-1 virus from entering into CD4 cells

Contraindications Patients with severe renal impairment (Cl_{cr} <30 mL/minute) or end-stage renal disease (ESRD) who are taking potent CYP3A4 inhibitors or inducers

Canadian labeling: Additional contraindications (not in U.S. labeling): Hypersensitivity to maraviroc or any component of the formulation

Warnings/Precautions [U.S. Boxed Warning] Possible drug-induced hepatotoxicity with allergic type features has been reported; hepatotoxicity (usually after 1 month of treatment) may be preceded by allergic type reactions (eg, pruritic rash, eosinophilia, fever or increased IgE) and/or hepatic adverse events (transaminase increases or signs/symptoms of hepatitis); some cases have been life-threatening; immediately evaluate patients with signs and symptoms of allergic reaction or hepatitis. Use with caution in patients with preexisting hepatic dysfunction or coinfection with HBV or HCV, however symptoms have occurred in the absence of preexisting hepatic conditions. Monitor hepatic function at baseline and as clinically indicated during treatment. Consider discontinuation in any patient with possible hepatitis or with elevated transaminases combined with systemic allergic events. Patients may develop immune reconstitution syndrome resulting in the occurrence of an inflammatory response to an indolent or residual opportunistic infection; further evaluation and treatment may be required. Monitor closely for signs/symptoms of developing infections; use associated with a small increase of certain upper respiratory tract infections and herpes virus infections during clinical trials. Use with caution in patients with cardiovascular disease or cardiac risk factors. During trials, a small increase in cardiovascular events (myocardial ischemia and/or infarction) occurred in treated patients compared to placebo, although a contributory relationship relative to therapy is unknown. Symptomatic postural hypotension has occurred; use caution in patients at risk for postural hypotension due to concomitant medication or history of condition. Adjust dose in patients with severe renal dysfunction if postural hypotension experienced.

Use caution in patients with mild-to-moderate hepatic impairment; maraviroc concentrations are increased; no dosage adjustment recommended. Maraviroc concentrations are further increased in patients with moderate hepatic impairment receiving concomitant strong CYP3A inhibitors; monitor closely for adverse events. Renal impairment may increase maraviroc concentrations. Use with caution in patients with mild-to-moderate renal impairment. Use with caution in patients taking strong CYP3A4/P-glycoprotein inhibitors and moderate or strong CYP3A4/P-glycoprotein inducers; may require dosage adjustments; avoid concurrent use in severe renal dysfunction (Cl_{cr} <30 mL/minute). Prior to therapy, tropism testing should be performed for presence of CCR5-tropic only virus HIV-1 infection. Therapy not recommended for use in patients with CXCR4- or dual/mixed tropic HIV-1 infection; efficacy not demonstrated in this population. In studies with treatment-naive patients, virologic failure and emergent lamivudine resistance was more common in maraviroc-treated patients compared to patients receiving efavirenz.

Drug Interactions

Avoid Concomitant Use

Avoid concomitant use of Maraviroc with any of the following: St Johns Wort

Decreased Effect

The levels/effects of Maraviroc may be decreased by: CYP3A4 Inducers (Strong); Deferasirox; St Johns Wort; Tocilizumab

Increased Effect/Toxicity

The levels/effects of Maraviroc may be increased by: CYP3A4 Inhibitors (Moderate); CYP3A4 Inhibitors (Strong); Dasatinib; Ivacaftor

Nutritional/Ethanol Interactions Herb/Nutraceutical: St. John's wort may decrease maraviroc concentrations leading to loss of therapeutic efficacy and potentially increased risk of resistance; concomitant use not recommended.

Adverse Reactions

>10%:

Central nervous system: Fever (13%)

Dermatologic: Rash (11%)

Respiratory: Upper respiratory tract infection (23%), cough (14%)

2% to 10%:

Cardiovascular: Vascular hypertensive disorder (3%)

Central nervous system: Dizziness (9%; including postural dizziness), insomnia (8%), anxiety (4%), consciousness disturbances (4%), depression (4%), pain (4%)

Dermatologic: Folliculitis (4%), pruritus (4%), skin neoplasms (benign; 3%), erythema (2%)

Endocrine & metabolic: Lipodystrophy (3%)

Gastrointestinal: Appetite disorders (8%), constipation (6%)

Genitourinary: Urinary tract/bladder symptoms (3% to 5%), genital warts (2%)

Hematologic: Neutropenia (grades 3/4: 4%)

Hepatic: Transaminases increased (grades 3/4: 3% to 5%), bilirubin increased (grades 3/4: 6%)

Neuromuscular & skeletal: Joint disorders (7%), paresthesia (5%), peripheral neuropathy (4%), sensory abnormality (4%), muscle pain (3%)

Ocular: Conjunctivitis (2%), infection/inflammation (2%)

Otic: Otitis media (2%)

Respiratory: Bronchitis (7%), sinusitis (7%), respiratory tract/sinus disorder (3% to 6%), breathing abnormality (4%)

Miscellaneous: Herpes infection (8%), sweat gland disturbances (5%), influenza (2%)

Available Dosage Forms

Tablet, oral:

Selzentry®: 150 mg, 300 mg

General Dosage Range Dosage adjustment recommended in patients with renal impairment or on concomitant therapy

Oral: *Children ≥16 years and Adults:* 300 mg twice daily

Administration

Oral Administer without regards to meals.

Stability

Storage Store at 25°C (77°F); excursions permitted to 15°C to 30°C (59°F to 86°F).

Nursing Actions

Physical Assessment Monitor for cardiotoxicity, hepatotoxicity, upper respiratory infections, hypotension, dizziness, insomnia, and rash. Teach patient proper timing of multiple medications.

Patient Education You will be provided with a medication guide with each prescription. This drug will not cure HIV, nor has it been found to reduce transmission of HIV; use appropriate precautions to prevent spread to other persons. This drug is prescribed as one part of a multidrug combination; take exactly as directed for full course of therapy. May be taken with or without food. Maintain adequate hydration unless advised by prescriber to restrict fluids. May cause dizziness, insomnia, constipation, or muscle or joint pain. Report skin rash, persistent muscle pain, unusual cough, fever, cold symptoms, abdominal pain, yellow eyes or skin, or fatigue.

Dietary Considerations May be taken without regards to meals.

Measles, Mumps, and Rubella Virus Vaccine (MEE zels, mumpz & roo BEL a VYE rus vak SEEN)

Brand Names: U.S. M-M-R® II

Index Terms MMR; Mumps, Measles and Rubella Vaccines; Rubella, Measles and Mumps Vaccines

Pharmacologic Category Vaccine, Live (Viral)

Medication Safety Issues

Sound-alike/look-alike issues:

MMR (measles, mumps and rubella virus vaccine) may be confused with MMRV (measles, mumps, rubella, and varicella) vaccine

Pregnancy Risk Factor C

Lactation

Measles/mumps: Excretion in breast milk unknown/use caution

Rubella: Enters breast milk/use caution

Use Measles, mumps, and rubella prophylaxis

The Advisory Committee on Immunization Practices (ACIP) recommends routine vaccination for the following:

- All children (first dose given at 12-15 months of age)
- Adults born 1957 or later (without evidence of immunity or documentation of vaccination).
- Adults at higher risk for exposure to and transmission of measles mumps and rubella should receive special consideration for vaccination, unless an acceptable evidence of immunity exists. This includes international travelers, persons attending colleges and other post-high school education, persons working in healthcare facilities.

Available Dosage Forms

Injection, powder for reconstitution [preservative free]:

M-M-R® II: Measles virus ≥1000 $TCID_{50}$, mumps virus ≥20,000 $TCID_{50}$, and rubella virus ≥1000 $TCID_{50}$

General Dosage Range SubQ:

Children ≥12 months: 0.5 mL

Adults: Born ≥1957 without evidence of immunity: 0.5 mL for 1 or 2 doses

Administration

I.V. Not for I.V. administration.

Other Administer SubQ in outer aspect of the upper arm in patients ≥12 months

Simultaneous administration of vaccines helps ensure the patients will be fully vaccinated by the appropriate age. Simultaneous administration of vaccines is defined as administering >1 vaccine on the same day at different anatomic sites. The use of licensed combination vaccines is generally preferred over separate injections of the equivalent components. Separate vaccines should not be combined in the same syringe unless indicated by product specific labeling. Separate needles and syringes should be used for each injection. The ACIP prefers each dose of a specific vaccine in a series come from the same manufacturer when possible. Adolescents and adults should be vaccinated while seated or lying down. In general, preterm infants should be vaccinated at the same chronological age as full-term infants (CDC, 2011).

Antipyretics have not been shown to prevent febrile seizures. Antipyretics may be used to treat fever or discomfort following vaccination (CDC, 2011). One study reported that routine prophylactic administration of acetaminophen to prevent fever prior to vaccination decreased the immune response of some vaccines; the clinical significance of this reduction in immune response has not been established (Prymula, 2009).

Nursing Actions

Physical Assessment U.S. federal law requires entry into the patient's medical record.

Related Information

Immunization Administration Recommendations *on page 1243*

Immunization Recommendations *on page 1248*

Measles, Mumps, Rubella, and Varicella Virus Vaccine

(MEE zels, mumpz, roo BEL a, & var i SEL a VYE rus vak SEEN)

Brand Names: U.S. ProQuad®

Index Terms MMR-V; MMRV; Mumps, Rubella, Varicella, and Measles Vaccine; Rubella, Varicella, Measles, and Mumps Vaccine; Varicella, Measles, Mumps, and Rubella Vaccine

Pharmacologic Category Vaccine, Live (Viral)

Pregnancy Risk Factor C

Lactation

Measles, mumps, varicella: Excretion in breast milk unknown/use caution

Rubella: Enters breast milk/use caution

Use To provide simultaneous active immunization against measles, mumps, rubella, and varicella

The Advisory Committee on Immunization Practices (ACIP) recommends routine vaccination against measles, mumps, rubella, and varicella in healthy children 12 months to 12 years of age. For children receiving their first dose at 12-47 months of age, either the MMRV combination vaccine or separate MMR and varicella vaccines can be used. (The ACIP prefers administration of separate MMR and varicella vaccines as the first dose in this age group unless the parent or caregiver expresses preference for the MMRV combination.) For children receiving the first dose at ≥48 months or their second dose at any age, use of MMRV is preferred.

Canadian labeling (not in U.S. labeling): MMRV combination vaccine is approved for use in healthy children 9 months to 6 years; may consider use in healthy children ≤12 years of age based upon prior experience with the separate component (live-attenuated MMR or live-attenuated varicella [OKA-strain]) vaccines.

Available Dosage Forms

Injection, powder for reconstitution [preservative free]:

ProQuad®: Measles virus ≥3.00 $\log_{10}$ $TCID_{50}$, mumps virus ≥4.30 $\log_{10}$ $TCID_{50}$, rubella virus ≥3.00 $\log_{10}$ $TCID_{50}$, and varicella virus ≥3.99 $\log_{10}$ PFU

General Dosage Range SubQ: *Children 12 months to 12 years:* 1 dose (0.5 mL)

Administration

Other Disinfectants (eg, alcohol) may inactivate the attenuated viruses in the vaccine. Allow disinfectant adequate time to evaporate from skin prior to administration.

U.S labeling: For SubQ injection only; inject in the outer aspect of the deltoid region of the upper arm or in the higher anterolateral area of the thigh. Administer immediately following reconstitution.

Canadian labeling: For SubQ or I.M. injection only; inject in the deltoid region of upper arm. Do not administer by I.M. injection in patients with bleeding disorders.

Note: The Canadian labeling states that Priorix-Tetra™ (MMRV) may be given simultaneously (at different injection sites) with the combination vaccine Infanrix-hexa™ (contains diphtheria-tetanus-acellular pertussis-hepatitis B-inactivated polio virus-*Haemophilus* influenzae type B [DTaP-HBV-IPV/Hib]) and with monovalent vaccines DTaP, Hib, IPV, HBV.

Simultaneous administration of vaccines helps ensure the patients will be fully vaccinated by the appropriate age. Simultaneous administration of vaccines is defined as administering >1 vaccine on the same day at different anatomic sites. The use of licensed combination vaccines is generally preferred over separate injections of the equivalent components. Separate vaccines should not be combined in the same syringe unless indicated by product specific labeling. Separate needles and syringes should be used for each injection. The ACIP prefers each dose of a specific vaccine in a series come from the same manufacturer when possible. Adolescents and adults should be vaccinated while seated or lying down. In general, preterm infants should be vaccinated at the same chronological age as full-term infants (CDC, 2011).

Antipyretics have not been shown to prevent febrile seizures. Antipyretics may be used to treat fever or discomfort following vaccination (CDC, 2011). One study reported that routine prophylactic administration of acetaminophen to prevent fever prior to vaccination decreased the immune response of some vaccines; the clinical significance of this reduction in immune response has not been established (Prymula, 2009).

Nursing Actions

Physical Assessment Assess hypersensitivity history and health status prior to administration. Treatment must be immediately available in event of anaphylactic or serious allergic reactions. U.S. federal law requires entry into the patient's medical record.

Patient Education Children who are moderately-to-severely ill should not get this vaccination until they have recovered. You may experience fever; mild pain, redness, or swelling at injection site; headache; mild gastrointestinal upset; irritability; mild rash; or upper respiratory tract infection. Report immediately any severe reaction at injection site, any chills or fever, persistent diarrhea, or severe rash.

Related Information

Immunization Administration Recommendations *on page 1243*

Immunization Recommendations *on page 1248*

Mebendazole (me BEN da zole)

Index Terms Vermox

Pharmacologic Category Anthelmintic

Medication Safety Issues

Sound-alike/look-alike issues:

Mebendazole may be confused with metroNIDAZOLE

Pregnancy Risk Factor C

Lactation Excretion in breast milk unknown/use caution

Use Treatment of *Enterobius vermicularis* (pinworms), *Trichuris trichiura* (whipworms), *Ascaris lumbricoides* (roundworms), and *Ancylostoma duodenale* or *Necator amiericanus* (hookworms)

Unlabeled Use Treatment of *Ancylostoma caninum* (eosinophilic enterocolitis), *Capillaria philippinensis* (capillariasis), *Giardia duodenalis* (giardiasis), *Mansonella perstans* (filariasis), visceral larva migrans (toxocariasis)

Available Dosage Forms

Tablet, chewable, oral: 100 mg

General Dosage Range Oral: *Children ≥2 years and Adults:* 100 mg as a single dose **or** twice daily

Administration

Oral Tablets may be chewed, swallowed whole, or crushed and mixed with food.

Nursing Actions

Physical Assessment Since worm infestations are easily transmitted, all persons sharing same household should be treated. Teach transmission prevention.

Patient Education Tablets may be chewed, swallowed whole, or crushed and mixed with food. Increase dietary intake of fruit juices. All family members and close friends should also be treated. To reduce possibility of reinfection, wash hands and scrub nails carefully with soap and hot water before handling food, before eating, and before and after toileting. Keep hands out of mouth. Disinfect toilet daily and launder bed linens, undergarments, and nightclothes daily with hot water and soap. Do not go barefoot and do not sit directly on grass or ground. May cause abdominal pain, nausea, vomiting, or hair loss (reversible). Report skin rash or itching, unusual fatigue or sore throat, unresolved diarrhea or vomiting, or CNS changes.

Meclizine (MEK li zeen)

Brand Names: U.S. Antivert®; Bonine® [OTC]; Dramamine® Less Drowsy Formula [OTC]; Medi-Meclizine [OTC]; Trav-L-Tabs® [OTC]

Index Terms Meclizine Hydrochloride; Meclozine Hydrochloride

Pharmacologic Category Antiemetic; Histamine H_1 Antagonist; Histamine H_1 Antagonist, First Generation; Piperazine Derivative

Medication Safety Issues

Sound-alike/look-alike issues:

Antivert® may be confused with Anzemet®, Axert®

Pregnancy Risk Factor B

Lactation Excretion in breast milk unknown/not recommended

Use Prevention and treatment of symptoms of motion sickness; management of vertigo with diseases affecting the vestibular system

Available Dosage Forms

Caplet, oral: 12.5 mg

Tablet, oral: 12.5 mg, 25 mg

Antivert®: 12.5 mg, 25 mg, 50 mg

Dramamine® Less Drowsy Formula [OTC]: 25 mg

Medi-Meclizine [OTC]: 25 mg

Trav-L-Tabs® [OTC]: 25 mg

Tablet, chewable, oral: 25 mg

Bonine® [OTC]: 25 mg

General Dosage Range Oral: *Children >12 years and Adults:* 12.5-50 mg 1 hour before travel, may repeat every 12-24 hours if needed **or** 25-100 mg/day in divided doses

Nursing Actions

Physical Assessment Observe safety precautions (eg, bed rails up, call bell at hand).

Patient Education Avoid alcohol. You may experience dizziness, drowsiness, blurred vision, dry mouth, constipation, or heat intolerance. Report CNS change (hallucination, confusion, nervousness), sudden or unusual weight gain, unresolved nausea or diarrhea, chest pain or palpitations, muscle pain, or changes in urinary pattern.

MedroxyPROGESTERone
(me DROKS ee proe JES te rone)

Brand Names: U.S. Depo-Provera®; Depo-Provera® Contraceptive; depo-subQ provera 104®; Provera®

Index Terms Acetoxymethylprogesterone; Medroxyprogesterone Acetate; Methylacetoxyprogesterone; MPA

Pharmacologic Category Contraceptive; Progestin

Medication Safety Issues

Sound-alike/look-alike issues:

Depo-Provera® may be confused with depo-subQ provera 104™

MedroxyPROGESTERone may be confused with hydroxyprogesterone caproate, methylPREDNISolone, methylTESTOSTERone

Provera® may be confused with Covera®, Femara®, Parlodel®, Premarin®, Proscar®, PROzac®

Administration issues:

The injection dosage form is available in different formulations. Carefully review prescriptions to assure the correct formulation and route of administration.

Pregnancy Risk Factor X

Lactation Enters breast milk

Breast-Feeding Considerations Composition, quality, and quantity of breast milk are not affected; adverse developmental and behavioral effects have not been noted following exposure of infant to MPA while breast-feeding. The manufacturer does not recommend the use of MPA tablets in breastfeeding mothers.

Use Secondary amenorrhea or abnormal uterine bleeding due to hormonal imbalance; reduction of endometrial hyperplasia in nonhysterectomized postmenopausal women receiving conjugated estrogens; prevention of pregnancy; management of endometriosis-associated pain; adjunctive therapy and palliative treatment of recurrent and metastatic endometrial carcinoma

Unlabeled Use Treatment of low-grade endometrial stromal sarcoma

Mechanism of Action/Effect Inhibits secretion of pituitary gonadotropins, which prevents follicular maturation and ovulation; causes endometrial thinning

Contraindications Hypersensitivity to medroxyprogesterone or any component of the formulation; history of or current thrombophlebitis or venous thromboembolic disorders (including DVT, PE); cerebral vascular disease; severe hepatic dysfunction or disease; carcinoma of the breast or other estrogen- or progesterone-dependent neoplasia; undiagnosed vaginal bleeding; missed abortion, diagnostic test for pregnancy, pregnancy

Warnings/Precautions [U.S. Boxed Warning]: Prolonged use of medroxyprogesterone contraceptive injection may result in a loss of bone mineral density (BMD). It is not known if use during adolescence or early adulthood will decrease peak bone mass accretion or increase the risk for osteoporotic fractures later in life. Loss is related to the duration of use, may not be completely reversible on discontinuation of the drug, and incidence is not significantly different between the SubQ and I.M. dosage forms. The impact on peak bone mass in adolescents should be weighed against the potential for unintended pregnancies in treatment decision. Consider alternative contraceptive methods in patients at risk for osteoporosis (eg, metabolic bone disease, family history of osteoporosis, chronic use of medications associated with osteoporosis such as corticosteroids). **[U.S. Boxed Warning]: Long-term use (ie, >2 years) should be limited to situations where other birth control methods are inadequate.** Consider other methods of birth control in women with (or at risk for) osteoporosis. **[U.S. Boxed Warning]: Inform patients that injectable contraceptives do not protect against HIV infection or other sexually-transmitted diseases.** When used for contraception, the possibility of ectopic pregnancy should be considered in patients with abdominal pain. Anaphylaxis or anaphylactoid reactions have been reported with use of the injection; medication for the treatment of hypersensitivity reactions should be available for immediate use.

[U.S. Boxed Warning]: Estrogens with or without progestin should not be used to prevent cardiovascular disease. Using data from the Women's Health Initiative (WHI) studies, an increased risk of deep vein thrombosis (DVT) and stroke has been reported with CE and an increased risk of DVT, stroke, pulmonary emboli (PE) and myocardial infarction (MI) has been reported with CE with MPA in postmenopausal women. Additional risk factors include diabetes mellitus, hypercholesterolemia, hypertension, SLE, obesity, tobacco use, and/or history of venous thromboembolism (VTE). Risk factors should be managed appropriately; discontinue use if adverse cardiovascular events occur or are suspected. If thrombosis develops with contraceptive treatment, discontinue treatment (unless no other acceptable contraceptive alternative). Whenever possible, progestins in combination with estrogens should be discontinued at least 4-6 weeks prior to and for 2 weeks following elective surgery associated with an increased risk of thromboembolism or during periods of prolonged immobilization.

[U.S. Boxed Warning]: Estrogens with or without progestin should not be used to prevent dementia. In the Women's Health Initiative Memory Study (WHIMS), an increased incidence of dementia was observed in women ≥65 years of age taking CE alone or in combination with MPA.

[U.S. Boxed Warning]: An increased risk of invasive breast cancer was observed in postmenopausal women using conjugated estrogens (CE) in combination with medroxyprogesterone acetate (MPA). An increase in abnormal mammogram findings has also been reported with estrogen alone or in combination with progestin therapy. Use is contraindicated in patients with known or suspected breast cancer. MPA is used to reduce the risk of endometrial hyperplasia in nonhysterectomized postmenopausal women receiving conjugated estrogens. The use of unopposed estrogen in women with an intact uterus is associated with an increased risk of endometrial cancer. The addition of a progestin to estrogen therapy may decrease the risk of endometrial hyperplasia, a precursor to endometrial cancer. Adequate diagnostic measures, including endometrial sampling if indicated, should be performed to rule out malignancy in postmenopausal women with undiagnosed abnormal vaginal bleeding. Estrogens may exacerbate endometriosis. Malignant transformation of residual endometrial implants has been reported posthysterectomy with unopposed estrogen therapy. Consider adding a progestin in women with residual endometriosis posthysterectomy. Postmenopausal estrogen therapy and combined estrogen/progesterone therapy may increase the risk of ovarian cancer; however, the absolute risk to an individual woman is small. Although results from various studies are not consistent, risk does not appear to be significantly associated with the duration, route, or dose of therapy. In one study, the risk decreased after 2 years following discontinuation of therapy (Mørch, 2009). Although the risk of ovarian cancer is rare, women who are at an increased risk (eg, family history) should be counseled about the association (NAMS, 2012).

[U.S. Boxed Warning]: Estrogens with or without progestin should be used for the shortest duration possible at the lowest effective dose consistent with treatment goals. Before prescribing estrogen therapy to postmenopausal women, the risks and benefits must be weighed for each patient. Women should be informed of these risks and benefits, as well as possible effects of progestin when added to estrogen therapy. Patients should be reevaluated as clinically appropriate to determine if treatment is still necessary. Available data related to treatment risks are from Women's Health Initiative (WHI) studies, which evaluated oral CE 0.625 mg with or without MPA 2.5 mg relative to placebo in postmenopausal women. Other combinations and dosage forms of estrogens and progestins were not studied. **Outcomes reported from clinical trials using CE with or without MPA should be assumed to be similar for other doses and other dosage forms of estrogens and progestins until comparable data becomes available.**

Discontinue pending examination in cases of sudden partial or complete vision loss, sudden onset of proptosis, diplopia, or migraine; discontinue permanently if papilledema or retinal vascular lesions are observed on examination. Use with caution in patients with diseases that may be exacerbated by fluid retention (including asthma, epilepsy, migraine, cardiac, or renal dysfunction). Contraceptive therapy with medroxyprogesterone commonly results in an average weight gain of ~2.5 kg after 1 year and ~3.7 kg after 2 years of treatment. Use caution with history of depression.

May have adverse effects on glucose tolerance; use caution in women with diabetes. MPA is extensively metabolized in the liver. Discontinue if jaundice develops or if acute or chronic hepatic disturbances occur. Use is contraindicated with severe hepatic disease. Unscheduled bleeding/spotting may occur. Presentation of irregular, unresolving vaginal bleeding following previously regular cycles warrants further evaluation including endometrial sampling, if indicated, to rule out malignancy. Not for use prior to menarche.

Drug Interactions

Avoid Concomitant Use

Avoid concomitant use of MedroxyPROGESTERone with any of the following: Axitinib; Griseofulvin

Decreased Effect

MedroxyPROGESTERone may decrease the levels/effects of: ARIPiprazole; Axitinib; Saxagliptin; Vitamin K Antagonists

The levels/effects of MedroxyPROGESTERone may be decreased by: Acitretin; Aminoglutethimide; Aprepitant; Artemether; Barbiturates; Bexarotene; Bexarotene (Systemic); Bile Acid Sequestrants; Bosentan; CarBAMazepine; Clobazam; CYP3A4 Inducers (Strong); Deferasirox; Felbamate; Fosaprepitant; Fosphenytoin; Griseofulvin; LamoTRIgine; Mycophenolate; Nevirapine; OXcarbazepine; Phenytoin; Prucalopride; Retinoic Acid Derivatives; Rifamycin Derivatives; St Johns Wort; Telaprevir; Tocilizumab; Topiramate

Increased Effect/Toxicity

MedroxyPROGESTERone may increase the levels/effects of: Benzodiazepines (metabolized by oxidation); Selegiline; Tranexamic Acid; Voriconazole

The levels/effects of MedroxyPROGESTERone may be increased by: Boceprevir; Conivaptan; Herbs (Progestogenic Properties); Voriconazole

Nutritional/Ethanol Interactions

Ethanol: Avoid ethanol (may increase risk of osteoporosis).

Food: Bioavailability of the oral tablet is increased when taken with food; half-life is unchanged.

Herb/Nutraceutical: St John's wort may diminish the therapeutic effect of progestin contraceptives (contraceptive failure is possible).

Adverse Reactions Adverse effects as reported with any dosage form; percent ranges presented are noted with the MPA I.M. contraceptive injection: >5%:

Central nervous system: Dizziness, headache, nervousness

Endocrine & metabolic: Libido decreased, menstrual irregularities (includes bleeding, amenorrhea, or both)
Gastrointestinal: Abdominal pain/discomfort, weight gain (>10 lbs at 24 months: 38%)

1% to 5%:

Cardiovascular: Edema
Central nervous system: Depression, fatigue, insomnia
Dermatologic: Acne, alopecia, rash
Endocrine & metabolic: Breast pain, hot flashes
Gastrointestinal: Bloating, nausea
Genitourinary: Dysmenorrhea, leukorrhea, vaginitis
Local: Injection site reaction (SubQ administration): Atrophy, induration, pain
Neuromuscular & skeletal: Arthralgia, backache, leg cramp, weakness

<1%, postmarketing, and/or case reports: Allergic reaction, anaphylaxis, anaphylactoid reactions, anemia, angioedema, anxiety, appetite changes, asthma, axillary swelling, blood dyscrasia, body odor, BMD loss, breast cancer, breast changes, cervical cancer, chest pain, chills, chloasma, cholestatic jaundice, deep vein thrombosis, diaphoresis, diarrhea, drowsiness, dry skin, dyspareunia, dyspnea, facial palsy, fainting, fever, galactorrhea, genitourinary infections, glucose tolerance decreased, hirsutism, hoarseness, jaundice, lack of return to fertility, lactation decreased, libido increased, melasma, nipple bleeding, oligomenorrhea, optic neuritis, osteoporosis, osteoporotic fractures, paralysis, paresthesia, pruritus, pulmonary embolus, rectal bleeding, retinal thrombosis, scleroderma, seizure, somnolence, syncope, tachycardia, thirst, thrombophlebitis, urticaria, uterine hyperplasia, vaginal cysts, varicose veins

In addition: Depo-Provera® aqueous suspension: Residual lump, sterile abscess, or skin discoloration at the injection

Available Dosage Forms

Injection, suspension: 150 mg/mL (1 mL)
Depo-Provera®: 400 mg/mL (2.5 mL)
Depo-Provera® Contraceptive: 150 mg/mL (1 mL)
depo-subQ provera 104®: 104 mg/0.65 mL (0.65 mL)

Tablet, oral: 2.5 mg, 5 mg, 10 mg
Provera®: 2.5 mg, 5 mg, 10 mg

General Dosage Range Dosage adjustment recommended in patients with hepatic impairment.

I.M.:
Adolescents and Adults: Contraception: 150 mg every 3 months
Adults: Endometrial cancer: 400-1000 mg/week

Oral: *Adolescents and Adults:* 5-10 mg once daily

SubQ: *Adolescents and Adults:* 104 mg every 3 months (every 12-14 weeks)

Administration

I.M. Depo-Provera® Contraceptive: Administer first dose during the first 5 days of menstrual period, or within the first 5 days postpartum if not breastfeeding, or at the sixth week postpartum if breastfeeding exclusively. Shake vigorously prior to administration. Administer by deep I.M. injection in the gluteal or deltoid muscle. When switching from combined hormonal contraceptives (estrogen plus progestin), the first injection should be on the day after the last active tablet or (at the latest) the day after the final inactive tablet. When switching from other contraceptive methods, ensure continuous contraceptive coverage.

Other SubQ: depo-subQ provera 104™: Administer first dose during the first 5 days of menstrual period, or at the sixth week postpartum if breastfeeding. Shake vigorously prior to administration. Administer by SubQ injection in the anterior thigh or abdomen; avoid boney areas and the umbilicus. Administer over 5-7 seconds. Do not rub the injection area. When switching from combined hormonal contraceptives (estrogen plus progestin), the first injection should be within 7 days after the last active pill, or removal of patch or ring. If switching from the I.M. to SubQ formulation, the next dose should be given within the prescribed dosing period for the I.M. injection to assure continuous coverage.

Stability

Storage Store at controlled room temperature.

Nursing Actions

Physical Assessment Instruct patient on appropriate dose scheduling.

Patient Education You may experience sensitivity to sunlight, dizziness, anxiety, depression, changes in appetite, hot flashes, or decreased libido or increased body hair (reversible when drug is discontinued). Maintain adequate hydration, unless instructed to restrict fluid intake. Report swelling of face, lips, or mouth; absent or altered menses; abdominal pain; vaginal itching, irritation, or discharge; heat, warmth, redness, or swelling of extremities; or sudden onset change in vision.

Dietary Considerations Ensure adequate calcium and vitamin D intake

Mefloquine (ME floe kwin)

Index Terms Mefloquine Hydrochloride

Pharmacologic Category Antimalarial Agent

Medication Guide Available Yes

Pregnancy Risk Factor B

Lactation Enters breast milk/use caution

Use Treatment of mild-to-moderate acute malarial infections (including treatment of chloroquine-resistant malaria) and prevention of malaria caused by *Plasmodium falciparum* or *P. vivax*

Note: Due to geographical resistance and cross-resistance, consult current CDC guidelines.

Unlabeled Use Treatment of uncomplicated, chloroquine-resistant *P. vivax* malaria

Available Dosage Forms

Tablet, oral: 250 mg

General Dosage Range Oral:

Children ≥6 months: Prophylaxis: 5 mg/kg/once weekly (maximum: 250 mg/dose); Treatment: 20-25 mg/kg/day in 2 divided doses (maximum: 1250 mg)

Adults: Prophylaxis: 250 mg once weekly; Treatment: 1250 mg (5 tablets) as a single dose

Administration

Oral Administer with food and with at least 8 oz of water. When used for malaria prophylaxis, dose should be taken once weekly on the same day each week. If vomiting occurs within 30 minutes after the dose, an additional full dose should be given; if it occurs within 30-60 minutes after dose, an additional half-dose should be given. Tablets may be crushed and suspended in a small amount of water, milk, or another beverage for persons unable to swallow tablets.

Nursing Actions

Physical Assessment Monitor for hypertension, cardiomyopathy, hyperglycemia, and hepatotoxicity on a regular basis throughout therapy. Monitor patient closely for any development of psychiatric symptoms (anxiety, paranoia, depression, hallucinations, and psychosis); may persist long after mefloquine has been discontinued. Advise patient about the importance of carrying medication guide and wallet provided when mefloquine is dispensed for malaria. Teach patient importance of adequate hydration.

Patient Education Take with food and at least 8 oz of water. Maintain adequate nutrition and hydration unless instructed to restrict fluid intake. Carry drug information card in wallet for as long as you are taking this drug. May cause dizziness, anxiety, loss of balance, nausea, vomiting, or decreased appetite. Report immediately any anxiety, confusion, agitation, restlessness, paranoia, depression, hallucinations, or suicide ideation.

Megestrol (me JES trole)

Brand Names: U.S. Megace®; Megace® ES

Index Terms 5071-1DL(6); Megestrol Acetate; NSC-71423

Pharmacologic Category Antineoplastic Agent, Hormone; Appetite Stimulant; Progestin

Medication Safety Issues

Sound-alike/look-alike issues:

Megace® may be confused with Reglan®

Megestrol may be confused with mesalamine

Pregnancy Risk Factor D (tablet) / X (suspension)

Lactation Enters breast milk/not recommended

Use Palliative treatment of breast and endometrial carcinoma; treatment of anorexia, cachexia, or unexplained significant weight loss in patients with AIDS

Available Dosage Forms

Suspension, oral: 40 mg/mL (10 mL, 20 mL, 237 mL, 240 mL, 473 mL, 480 mL)

Megace®: 40 mg/mL (240 mL)

Megace® ES: 125 mg/mL (150 mL)

Tablet, oral: 20 mg, 40 mg

General Dosage Range Oral:

Adults (females): Tablet: 40-320 mg/day in divided doses

Adults (males/females): Suspension: 400-800 mg/day [Megace®] **or** 625 mg/day [Megace® ES]

Administration

Oral Megestrol acetate (Megace®) oral suspension is compatible with water, orange juice, apple juice, or Sustacal H.C. for immediate consumption. Shake suspension well before use.

Nursing Actions

Physical Assessment Monitor for hypertension, CNS changes (confusion, insomnia), rash, changes in menses, gastrointestinal upset, jaundice, and thrombophlebitis regularly during therapy. Teach patient importance of adequate hydration.

Patient Education May cause sensitivity to sunlight, dizziness, anxiety, depression, change in appetite, decreased libido or increased body hair (reversible when drug is discontinued), or hot flashes. Report swelling of face, lips, or mouth; absent or altered menses; abdominal pain; vaginal itching, irritation, or discharge; heat, warmth, redness, or swelling of extremities; or sudden onset change in vision.

Meloxicam (mel OKS i kam)

Brand Names: U.S. Mobic®

Pharmacologic Category Nonsteroidal Anti-inflammatory Drug (NSAID), Oral

Medication Guide Available Yes

Pregnancy Risk Factor C /D ≥30 weeks gestation

Lactation Excretion in breast milk unknown/not recommended

Breast-Feeding Considerations It is not known whether meloxicam is excreted in human milk. Breast-feeding is not recommended by the manufacturer.

Use Relief of signs and symptoms of osteoarthritis, rheumatoid arthritis, and juvenile idiopathic arthritis (JIA)

Mechanism of Action/Effect Reversibly inhibits cyclooxygenase-1 and 2 (COX-1 and 2) enzymes, which results in decreased formation of prostaglandin precursors; has antipyretic, analgesic, and anti-inflammatory properties

Contraindications Hypersensitivity (eg, asthma, urticaria, allergic-type reactions) to meloxicam, aspirin, other NSAIDs, or any component of the formulation; perioperative pain in the setting of coronary artery bypass graft (CABG) surgery

Warnings/Precautions [U.S. Boxed Warning]: NSAIDs are associated with an increased risk of adverse cardiovascular thrombotic events, including MI and stroke. Risk may be increased with duration of use or pre-existing cardiovascular risk factors or disease. Carefully evaluate individual cardiovascular risk profiles prior to prescribing. May cause new-onset hypertension or worsening of existing hypertension. Use caution with fluid retention. Avoid use in heart failure. Concurrent administration of ibuprofen, and potentially other nonselective NSAIDs, may interfere with aspirin's cardioprotective effect. **[U.S. Boxed Warning]: Use is contraindicated for treatment of perioperative pain in the setting of coronary artery bypass graft (CABG) surgery.** Risk of MI and stroke may be increased with use within the first 10-14 days following CABG surgery.

Platelet adhesion and aggregation may be decreased; may prolong bleeding time; patients with coagulation disorders or who are receiving anticoagulants should be monitored closely. Anemia may occur; patients on long-term NSAID therapy should be monitored for anemia. Rarely, NSAID use may cause severe blood dyscrasias (eg, agranulocytosis, aplastic anemia, thrombocytopenia).

NSAID use may compromise existing renal function; dose-dependent decreases in prostaglandin synthesis may result from NSAID use, reducing renal blood flow which may cause renal decompensation. NSAID use may increase the risk for hyperkalemia. Patients with impaired renal function, dehydration, heart failure, liver dysfunction, those taking diuretics, and ACE inhibitors, and the elderly are at greater risk of renal toxicity and hyperkalemia. Rehydrate patient before starting therapy; monitor renal function closely. Not recommended for use in patients with advanced renal disease. Long-term NSAID use may result in renal papillary necrosis.

[U.S. Boxed Warning]: NSAIDs may increase risk of gastrointestinal irritation, inflammation, ulceration, bleeding, and perforation. These events may occur at any time during therapy and without warning. Use caution with a history of GI disease (bleeding or ulcers), concurrent therapy with aspirin, anticoagulants and/or corticosteroids, smoking, use of alcohol, the elderly or debilitated patients. When used concomitantly with ≤325 mg of aspirin, a substantial increase in the risk of gastrointestinal complications (eg, ulcer) occurs; concomitant gastroprotective therapy (eg, proton pump inhibitors) is recommended (Bhatt, 2008). Use the lowest effective dose for the shortest duration of time, consistent with individual patient goals, to reduce risk of cardiovascular or GI adverse events. Alternate therapies should be considered for patients at high risk.

NSAIDs may cause serious skin adverse events including exfoliative dermatitis, Stevens-Johnson syndrome (SJS) and toxic epidermal necrolysis (TEN); discontinue use at first sign of skin rash or hypersensitivity. Anaphylactoid reactions may occur, even without prior exposure; patients with "aspirin triad" (bronchial asthma, aspirin intolerance, rhinitis) may be at increased risk. Do not use in patients who experience bronchospasm, asthma, rhinitis, or urticaria with NSAID or aspirin therapy. Use caution in other forms of asthma.

Use with caution in patients with decreased hepatic function. Closely monitor patients with any abnormal LFT. Severe hepatic reactions (eg, fulminant hepatitis, liver failure) have occurred with NSAID use, rarely; discontinue if signs or symptoms of liver disease develop, or if systemic manifestations occur.

NSAIDS may cause drowsiness, dizziness, blurred vision and other neurologic effects which may impair physical or mental abilities; patients must be cautioned about performing tasks which require mental alertness (eg, operating machinery or driving). Discontinue use with blurred or diminished vision and perform ophthalmologic exam. Monitor vision with long-term therapy.

The elderly are at increased risk for adverse effects (especially peptic ulceration, CNS effects, renal toxicity) from NSAIDs even at low doses.

Oral suspension formulation may contain sorbitol. Concomitant use with sodium polystyrene sulfonate (Kayexalate®) may cause intestinal necrosis (including fatal cases); combined use should be avoided. Withhold for at least 4-6 half-lives prior to surgical or dental procedures.

Drug Interactions

Avoid Concomitant Use

Avoid concomitant use of Meloxicam with any of the following: Calcium Polystyrene Sulfonate; Floctafenine; Ketorolac; Ketorolac (Nasal); Ketorolac (Systemic); Sodium Polystyrene Sulfonate

Decreased Effect

Meloxicam may decrease the levels/effects of: ACE Inhibitors; Aliskiren; Angiotensin II Receptor Blockers; Antiplatelet Agents; Beta-Blockers; Eplerenone; HydrALAZINE; Loop Diuretics; Potassium-Sparing Diuretics; Salicylates; Selective Serotonin Reuptake Inhibitors; Thiazide Diuretics

The levels/effects of Meloxicam may be decreased by: Bile Acid Sequestrants; Nonsteroidal Anti-Inflammatory Agents; Salicylates; Tocilizumab

Increased Effect/Toxicity

Meloxicam may increase the levels/effects of: Aliskiren; Aminoglycosides; Anticoagulants; Antiplatelet Agents; Bisphosphonate Derivatives; Calcium Polystyrene Sulfonate; Collagenase (Systemic); CycloSPORINE; CycloSPORINE (Systemic); Deferasirox; Desmopressin; Digoxin; Drotrecogin Alfa (Activated); Eplerenone; Haloperidol; Ibritumomab; Lithium; Methotrexate; Nonsteroidal Anti-Inflammatory Agents; PEMEtrexed; Porfimer; Potassium-Sparing Diuretics; PRALAtrexate; Quinolone Antibiotics; Rivaroxaban; Salicylates; Sodium Polystyrene Sulfonate; Thrombolytic Agents; Tositumomab and Iodine I 131 Tositumomab; Vancomycin; Vitamin K Antagonists

The levels/effects of Meloxicam may be increased by: ACE Inhibitors; Angiotensin II Receptor Blockers; Antidepressants (Tricyclic, Tertiary Amine); Conivaptan; Corticosteroids (Systemic); CycloSPORINE; CycloSPORINE (Systemic); Dasatinib; Floctafenine; Glucosamine; Herbs (Anticoagulant/Antiplatelet Properties); Ketorolac; Ketorolac (Nasal); Ketorolac (Systemic); Nonsteroidal Anti-Inflammatory Agents; Omega-3-Acid Ethyl Esters; Pentosan Polysulfate Sodium; Pentoxifylline; Probenecid; Prostacyclin Analogues; Selective Serotonin Reuptake Inhibitors; Serotonin/Norepinephrine Reuptake Inhibitors; Sodium Phosphates; Treprostinil; Vitamin E; Voriconazole

Nutritional/Ethanol Interactions

Ethanol: Avoid ethanol (may enhance gastric mucosal irritation).

Herb/Nutraceutical: Avoid alfalfa, anise, bilberry, bladderwrack, bromelain, cat's claw, celery, chamomile, coleus, cordyceps, dong quai, evening primrose, fenugreek, feverfew, garlic, ginger, ginkgo biloba, ginseng (American, Panax, Siberian), grapeseed, green tea, guggul, horse chestnut seed, horseradish, licorice, prickly ash, red clover, reishi, SAMe (S-adenosylmethionine), sweet clover, turmeric, white willow (all have additional antiplatelet activity).

Adverse Reactions Percentages reported in adult patients; abdominal pain, diarrhea, fever, headache, pyrexia, and vomiting were reported more commonly in pediatric patients

2% to 10%:

Cardiovascular: Edema (≤5%)

Central nervous system: Headache (2% to 8%), pain (1% to 5%), dizziness (≤4%), insomnia (≤4%)

Dermatologic: Pruritus (≤2%), rash (≤3%)

Gastrointestinal: Dyspepsia (4% to 10%), diarrhea (2% to 8%), nausea (2% to 7%), abdominal pain (2% to 5%), constipation (≤3%), flatulence (≤3%), vomiting (≤3%)

Genitourinary: Urinary tract infection (≤7%), micturition (≤2%)

Hematologic: Anemia (≤4%)

Neuromuscular & skeletal: Arthralgia (≤5%), back pain (≤3%)

Respiratory: Upper respiratory infection (≤8%), cough (≤2%), pharyngitis (≤3%)

Miscellaneous: Flu-like syndrome (2% to 6%), falls (≤3%)

Available Dosage Forms

Suspension, oral: 7.5 mg/5 mL (100 mL)

Mobic®: 7.5 mg/5 mL (100 mL)

Tablet, oral: 7.5 mg, 15 mg

Mobic®: 7.5 mg, 15 mg

General Dosage Range Oral:

Children ≥2 years: 0.125 mg/kg/day (maximum: 7.5 mg/day)

Adults: Initial: 7.5 mg once daily; Maintenance: 7.5-15 mg once daily (maximum: 15 mg/day)

Administration

Oral May be administered with or without meals; take with food or milk to minimize gastrointestinal irritation. Oral suspension: Shake gently prior to use.

Stability

Storage Store at 25°C (77°F). Protect tablets from moisture.

Nursing Actions

Physical Assessment Monitor blood pressure at the beginning of therapy and periodically during use. Monitor for gastrointestinal effects and ototoxicity at beginning of therapy and periodically throughout.

Patient Education Take with food or milk to reduce GI distress. Avoid alcohol. You may experience anorexia, nausea, vomiting, heartburn, drowsiness, dizziness, nervousness, headache, or fluid retention; GI bleeding, ulceration, or perforation can occur with or without pain; discontinue medication and contact prescriber if persistent abdominal pain or cramping or blood in stool occurs. Report breathlessness, respiratory difficulty, or unusual cough; chest pain, rapid heartbeat, or palpitations; slurring of speech; unusual bruising/bleeding; blood in urine, stool, mouth, or vomitus; swollen extremities; skin blisters, rash, or itching; acute fatigue; jaundice; flu-like symptoms; or hearing changes (ringing in ears).

Dietary Considerations Should be taken with food or milk to minimize gastrointestinal irritation.

Melphalan (MEL fa lan)

Brand Names: U.S. Alkeran®

Index Terms L-PAM; L-Phenylalanine Mustard; L-Sarcolysin; Phenylalanine Mustard

Pharmacologic Category Antineoplastic Agent, Alkylating Agent

Medication Safety Issues

Sound-alike/look-alike issues:

Melphalan may be confused with Mephyton®, Myleran®

Alkeran® may be confused with Alferon®, Leukeran®, Myleran®

High alert medication:

This medication is in a class the Institute for Safe Medication Practices (ISMP) includes among its list of drug classes which have a heightened risk of causing significant patient harm when used in error.

Pregnancy Risk Factor D

Lactation Excretion in breast milk unknown/not recommended

Breast-Feeding Considerations According to the manufacturer, melphalan should not be administered if breast-feeding.

Use Palliative treatment of multiple myeloma and nonresectable epithelial ovarian carcinoma

Unlabeled Use Treatment of Hodgkin lymphoma, light chain amyloidosis; conditioning regimen for autologous hematopoietic stem cell transplantation in adults with hematologic disorders (eg, multiple myeloma) and autologous marrow or stem cell transplantation in pediatric neuroblastoma and Ewing's sarcoma

Mechanism of Action/Effect Alkylating agent which is a derivative of mechlorethamine that inhibits DNA and RNA synthesis via formation of carbonium ions; cross-links strands of DNA; acts on both resting and rapidly dividing tumor cells.

Contraindications Hypersensitivity to melphalan or any component of the formulation; patients whose disease was resistant to prior melphalan therapy

Warnings/Precautions [U.S. Boxed Warning]: Bone marrow suppression is common; may be severe and result in infection or bleeding; has been demonstrated more with the I.V. formulation (compared to oral); myelosuppression is dose-related. Monitor blood counts; may require treatment delay or dose modification for thrombocytopenia or neutropenia. Use with caution in patients with prior bone marrow suppression, impaired renal function (consider dose reduction), or who have received prior (or concurrent) chemotherapy or irradiation. Myelotoxicity is generally reversible, although irreversible bone marrow failure has been reported. In patients who are candidates for autologous transplantation, avoid melphalan-containing regimens prior to transplant (due to the effects on stem cell reserve). Signs of infection, such as fever and WBC rise, may not occur; lethargy and confusion may be more prominent signs of infection.

[U.S. Boxed Warning]: Hypersensitivity reactions (including anaphylaxis) have occurred in ~2% of patients receiving I.V. melphalan, usually after multiple treatment cycles. Discontinue infusion and treat symptomatically. Hypersensitivity may also occur (rarely) with oral melphalan. Do not readminister (oral or I.V.) in patients who experience hypersensitivity to melphalan.

Gastrointestinal toxicities, including nausea, vomiting, diarrhea and mucositis, are common. When administering high-dose melphalan in autologous transplantation, cryotherapy is recommended to prevent mucositis (Keefe, 2007). Abnormal liver function tests may occur; hepatitis and jaundice have also been reported; hepatic sinusoidal obstruction syndrome (SOS; formerly called veno-occlusive disease) has been reported with I.V. melphalan. Pulmonary fibrosis (some fatal) and interstitial pneumonitis have been observed with treatment. Dosage reduction is recommended with I.V. melphalan in patients with renal impairment; reduced initial doses may also be recommended with oral melphalan. Closely monitor patients with azotemia.

[U.S. Boxed Warning]: Produces chromosomal changes and is leukemogenic and potentially mutagenic; secondary malignancies (including acute myeloid leukemia, myeloproliferative disease, and carcinoma) have been reported reported (some patients were receiving combination chemotherapy or radiation therapy); the risk is increased with increased treatment duration and cumulative doses. Suppresses ovarian function and produces amenorrhea; may also cause testicular suppression.

Extravasation may cause local tissue damage; administration by slow injection into a fast running I.V. solution into an injection port or via a central line is recommended; do not administer directly into a peripheral vein. **[U.S. Boxed Warning]: Should be administered under the supervision of an experienced cancer chemotherapy physician.** Avoid vaccination with live vaccines during treatment if immunocompromised. Toxicity may be increased in elderly; start with lowest recommended adult doses.

Drug Interactions

Avoid Concomitant Use

Avoid concomitant use of Melphalan with any of the following: BCG; CloZAPine; Nalidixic Acid; Natalizumab; Pimecrolimus; Tacrolimus (Topical); Vaccines (Live)

Decreased Effect

Melphalan may decrease the levels/effects of: BCG; Cardiac Glycosides; Coccidioidin Skin Test; Sipuleucel-T; Vaccines (Inactivated); Vaccines (Live); Vitamin K Antagonists

The levels/effects of Melphalan may be decreased by: Echinacea

Increased Effect/Toxicity

Melphalan may increase the levels/effects of: Carmustine; CloZAPine; CycloSPORINE

CycloSPORINE (Systemic); Leflunomide; Natalizumab; Vaccines (Live); Vitamin K Antagonists

The levels/effects of Melphalan may be increased by: Denosumab; Nalidixic Acid; Pimecrolimus; Roflumilast; Tacrolimus (Topical); Trastuzumab

Nutritional/Ethanol Interactions

Ethanol: Avoid ethanol (due to GI irritation).

Food: Food interferes with oral absorption.

Adverse Reactions

>10%:

Gastrointestinal: Nausea/vomiting, diarrhea, oral ulceration

Hematologic: Myelosuppression, leukopenia (nadir: 14-21 days; recovery: 28-35 days), thrombocytopenia (nadir: 14-21 days; recovery: 28-35 days), anemia

Miscellaneous: Secondary malignancy (<2% to 20%; cumulative dose and duration dependent, includes acute myeloid leukemia, myeloproliferative syndrome, carcinoma)

1% to 10%: Miscellaneous: Hypersensitivity (I.V.: 2%; includes bronchospasm, dyspnea, edema, hypotension, pruritus, rash, tachycardia, urticaria)

Available Dosage Forms

Injection, powder for reconstitution: 50 mg

Alkeran®: 50 mg

Tablet, oral:

Alkeran®: 2 mg

General Dosage Range Dosage adjustment recommended in patients with renal impairment or who develop toxicities

I.V.: *Adults:* 16 mg/m^2 administered at 2-week intervals for 4 doses, then repeat at 4-week intervals

Oral: *Adults:* Dosage varies greatly depending on indication

Administration

Oral Administer on an empty stomach.

I.V. Due to limited stability, complete administration of I.V. dose should occur within 60 minutes of reconstitution. Infuse over 15-30 minutes. Extravasation may cause local tissue damage; administration by slow injection into a fast running I.V. solution into an injection port or via a central line is recommended; do not administer by direct injection into a peripheral vein.

I.V. Detail pH: 6.5-7.0

Stability

Reconstitution Use appropriate precautions for handling and disposal.

Injection: Stability is limited; must be prepared fresh. **The time between reconstitution/dilution and administration of parenteral melphalan must be kept to a minimum (manufacturer recommends <60 minutes) because reconstituted and diluted solutions are unstable.** Dissolve powder initially with 10 mL of supplied diluent to a concentration of 5 mg/mL; shake immediately and vigorously to dissolve. **Immediately** dilute dose in NS to a concentration of ≤0.45 mg/mL (manufacturer recommended concentration). Do not refrigerate solution; precipitation occurs. The manufacturer recommends administration within 60 minutes of reconstitution.

Storage

Tablet: Store in refrigerator at 2°C to 8°C (36°F to 46°F). Protect from light.

Injection: Store at room temperature of 15°C to 30°C (59°F to 86°F). Protect from light. Stability is limited; must be prepared fresh. A 5 mg/mL concentration is chemically and physically stable for ≤90 minutes when stored at room temperature, although the manufacturer recommends administration be completed within 60 minutes of reconstitution; **immediately** dilute dose in NS. Do not refrigerate solution; precipitation occurs.

Nursing Actions

Physical Assessment I.V.: Monitor infusion site carefully to prevent extravasation. Monitor for gastrointestinal upset, myelosuppression (leukopenia), diarrhea, and hypersensitivity reaction regularly during therapy.

Patient Education I.V.: Report immediately any burning, swelling, pain, or redness at infusion or injection site. Oral: Preferable to take oral doses on an empty stomach, 1 hour before or 2 hours after meals. Avoid excessive alcohol (may increase gastric irritation). Maintain adequate nutrition and adequate hydration, unless instructed to restrict fluid intake. You may be more susceptible to infection. May cause nausea, vomiting, hair loss (reversible), or easy bleeding or bruising. Report unusual lethargy, confusion, or fever; persistent or severe nausea or vomiting; diarrhea or abdominal pain; chest pain or palpitations; difficulty or pain on urination; unusual bruising/bleeding; or respiratory difficulty.

Dietary Considerations Should be taken on an empty stomach (1 hour prior to or 2 hours after meals).

Related Information

Management of Drug Extravasations *on page 1269*

Memantine (me MAN teen)

Brand Names: U.S. Namenda®

Index Terms Memantine Hydrochloride; Namenda XR

Pharmacologic Category N-Methyl-D-Aspartate Receptor Antagonist

Medication Safety Issues

Sound-alike/look-alike issues:

Memantine may be confused with mesalamine

Pregnancy Risk Factor B

Lactation Excretion in breast milk unknown/use caution

Use Treatment of moderate-to-severe dementia of the Alzheimer's type

Unlabeled Use Treatment of mild-to-moderate vascular dementia

Mechanism of Action/Effect Memantine reduces the decline in function in Alzheimer's disease; it has not been shown to prevent or slow neurodegeneration associated with this disease.

Contraindications Hypersensitivity to memantine or any component of the formulation

Warnings/Precautions Use with caution in patients with cardiovascular disease; an increased incidence of cardiac failure, angina, bradycardia, and hypertension (compared with placebo) was observed in clinical trials. Use caution with seizure disorders or severe hepatic impairment. Use with caution in moderate-to-severe renal impairment; dose adjustments may be required. Worsening of corneal condition has been observed in a clinical trial; periodic ophthalmic exams during use have been recommended (Canadian labeling). Clearance is significantly reduced by alkaline urine; use caution with medications, dietary changes, or patient conditions which may alter urine pH.

Drug Interactions

Avoid Concomitant Use There are no known interactions where it is recommended to avoid concomitant use.

Decreased Effect There are no known significant interactions involving a decrease in effect.

Increased Effect/Toxicity

Memantine may increase the levels/effects of: Trimethoprim

The levels/effects of Memantine may be increased by: Carbonic Anhydrase Inhibitors; Sodium Bicarbonate; Trimethoprim

Adverse Reactions 1% to 10%:

Cardiovascular: Hypertension (4%), hypotension (2%), cardiac failure, cerebrovascular accident, syncope, transient ischemic attack

Central nervous system: Dizziness (5% to 7%), confusion (6%), headache (6%), anxiety (4%), depression (3%), hallucinations (3%), pain (3%), somnolence (3%), fatigue (2%), aggressive reaction (1% to 2%), ataxia, vertigo

Dermatologic: Rash

Gastrointestinal: Constipation (3% to 5%), diarrhea (5%), weight gain (3%), vomiting (2% to 3%), abdominal pain (2%), weight loss

Genitourinary: Urinary incontinence (2%), micturition

Hematologic: Anemia

Hepatic: Alkaline phosphatase increased

Neuromuscular & skeletal: Back pain (3%), hypokinesia

Ocular: Cataract, conjunctivitis

Respiratory: Cough (4%), dyspnea (2%), pneumonia

Miscellaneous: Influenza (4%)

Product Availability

Namenda XR™: FDA approved in June 2010; anticipated availability is currently undetermined

Namenda XR™ is an extended release capsule (once-daily administration) approved for the treatment of moderate-to-severe dementia associated with Alzheimer's disease

Available Dosage Forms

Combination package, oral:

Namenda®: Tablet: 5 mg (28s) and Tablet: 10 mg (21s)

Solution, oral:

Namenda®: 2 mg/mL (360 mL)

Tablet, oral:

Namenda®: 5 mg, 10 mg

General Dosage Range Dosage adjustment recommended in patients with renal impairment

Oral: *Adults:* Immediate release: Initial: 5 mg once daily; Target: 20 mg/day in 2 divided doses; Extended release: Initial 7 mg once daily; Target: 28 mg/day

Administration

Oral Administer without regard to meals. Extended release capsules may be swallowed whole or entire contents of capsule may be sprinkled on applesauce and swallowed immediately. Do not chew, crush, or divide.

Stability

Storage Store at 25°C (77°C); excursions permitted to 15°C to 30°C (59°F to 86°F).

Nursing Actions

Physical Assessment Monitor for hypertension, CNS changes, rash, and constipation on a regular basis throughout therapy.

Patient Education Take with or without food. May cause hypertension or headache. Report increase or changes in CNS symptoms (confusion, hallucinations, fatigue, aggressive reaction), chest pain or palpitations, dizziness or fainting, difficulty breathing or tightness in chest, or rash.

Dietary Considerations May be taken without regard to meals.

Meningococcal Group C-CRM197 Conjugate Vaccine

(me NIN joe kok al groop see see ahr em wuhn nahyn tee sev uh KON joo gate vak SEEN)

Index Terms MenC-CRM197; MenCC

Pharmacologic Category Vaccine

Lactation Excretion in breast milk unknown/use caution

Use To provide active immunization against invasive meningococcal disease caused by *N. meningitidis* serogroup C, in children ≥2 months and adults

The National Advisory Committee on Immunization (NACI) recommendations for persons considered at an increased risk for meningococcal disease:

Chemoprophylaxis and immunoprophylaxis:

Selection of meningococcal vaccination to be based upon serogroup(s):

Individuals living in the same household or with close contact (eg, kissing, shared cigarettes, shared eating or drinking utensils) of infected patient

Employees and children of nursery schools or day care

Immunoprophylaxis: Selection of meningococcal vaccination to be based upon serogroup(s):

Adolescents and young adults

Laboratory workers routinely exposed to isolates of *N. meningitidis*

Military recruits

Persons traveling to or who reside in countries where *N. meningitidis* is hyperendemic or epidemic, particularly if contact with local population will be prolonged

Persons with terminal complement component deficiencies

Persons with anatomic or functional asplenia

Note: Use is also recommended during meningococcal outbreaks caused by serogroup C.

Chemoprophylaxis:

Healthcare workers with intensive unprotected contact with infected patients

Airline passengers sitting directly next to an infected patient for duration of at least 8 hours

See NACI guidelines for specific drug treatment at http://www.phac-aspc.gc.ca/naci-ccni

Product Availability Not available in U.S.

General Dosage Range I.M.:

Infants ≥2-12 months: 0.5 mL as a single dose for a total of 3 doses

Infants ≥4-11 months without prior vaccination: 0.5 mL as a single dose for a total of 2 doses

Children ≥1 year and Adults: 0.5 mL as a single dose

Administration

I.M. Administer by deep intramuscular injection only into the anterolateral thigh in infants and the deltoid area in older children, adolescents, and adults. Use separate injection sites if administering multiple vaccinations on the same day.

Acetaminophen may be used when needed to provide comfort; however, routine prophylactic administration of acetaminophen to prevent fever due to vaccine use is not recommended. There is evidence of a decreased immune response to some vaccines associated with acetaminophen administration; the clinical significance of this reduction in immune response has not been established.

I.V. Do not administer via I.V., SubQ, or I.D. routes.

Nursing Actions

Physical Assessment Use caution in immunocompromised patients, patients with bleeding disorders, or those taking anticoagulants. Anaphylactoid and/or hypersensitivity reactions may occur; treatment should be available for immediate use. All serious adverse reactions must be reported to the U.S. DHHS. U.S. federal law also requires entry into the patient's medical record.

Patient Education You may experience mild headache, fever or chills, nausea or vomiting, or unusual sleepiness. Report persistent pain, redness, or swelling at injection site.

Meningococcal (Groups A / C / Y and W-135) Diphtheria Conjugate Vaccine

(me NIN joe kok al groops aye, see, why & dubl yoo won thur tee fyve dif THEER ee a KON joo gate vak SEEN)

Brand Names: U.S. Menactra®; Menveo®

Index Terms MCV; MCV4; MenACWY-CRM (Menveo®); MenACWY-D (Menactra®); Meningococcal Conjugate Vaccine

Pharmacologic Category Vaccine, Inactivated (Bacterial)

Medication Safety Issues

Administration issue:

Menactra® (MCV4) should be administered by intramuscular (I.M.) injection only. Inadvertent subcutaneous (SubQ) administration has been reported; possibly due to confusion of this product with Menomune® (MPSV4), also a meningococcal polysaccharide vaccine, which is administered by the SubQ route.

Pregnancy Risk Factor B/C (manufacturer dependent)

Lactation Excretion in breast milk unknown/use caution

Use Provide active immunization of children and adults against invasive meningococcal disease caused by *N. meningitidis* serogroups A, C, Y, and W-135.

The Advisory Committee on Immunization Practices (ACIP) recommends routine vaccination of all persons at age 11 or 12 years of age, followed by a booster at age 16 years of age (CDC, 60 [3], 2011).

The ACIP also recommends vaccination for:

Children 9 through 23 months of age at increased risk for meningococcal disease (CDC, 60[40], 2011). Children at increased risk include:

- Children traveling to or who reside in countries where *N. meningitidis* is hyperendemic or epidemic
- Children with persistent complement component deficiencies (eg, C5-C9, properdin, factor H, or factor D)

Persons 2 through 55 years of age at increased risk for meningococcal disease (CDC, 60[3], 2011). Meningococcal conjugate vaccine (MCV4) is preferred for persons aged 2-55 years; meningococcal polysaccharide vaccine (MPSV4) is preferred in adults ≥56 years of age (CDC, 2005). Persons at increased risk include:

- Previously unvaccinated college freshmen living in dormitories
- Microbiologists routinely exposed to isolates of *N. meningitidis*
- Military recruits
- Persons traveling to or who reside in countries where *N. meningitidis* is hyperendemic or epidemic, particularly if contact with local population will be prolonged
- Persons with persistent complement component deficiencies (eg, C5-C9, properdin, factor H, or factor D)
- Persons with anatomic or functional asplenia

Use is also recommended during meningococcal outbreaks caused by vaccine preventable serogroups (all recommended age groups) (CDC, 2005; CDC, 60[40], 2011).

Available Dosage Forms

Injection, solution [preservative free]:

Menactra®: 4 mcg each of polysaccharide antigen groups A, C, Y, and W-135 [bound to diphtheria toxoid 48 mcg] per 0.5 mL

Menveo®: MenA oligosaccharide 10 mcg, MenC oligosaccharide 5 mcg, MenY oligosaccharide 5 mcg, and MenW-135 oligosaccharide 5 mcg [bound to CRM_{197} protein 32.7-64.1 mcg] per 0.5 mL

General Dosage Range I.M.:

Children 9-23 months (Menactra®):0.5 mL/dose given as a 2-dose series, 3 months apart

Children ≥2 years and Adults ≤55 years: 0.5 mL as a single dose

Administration

I.M. Administer by I.M. route, preferably into the upper deltoid region. Do not administer via I.V., SubQ or I.D. route. For patients at risk of hemorrhage, the ACIP recommends "it should be administered intramuscularly if, in the opinion of a physician familiar with the patient's bleeding risk, the vaccine can be administered by this route with reasonable safety. If the patient receives antihemophilia or other similar therapy, intramuscular vaccination can be scheduled shortly after such therapy is administered. A fine needle (23 gauge or smaller) can be used for the vaccination and firm pressure applied to the site (without rubbing) for at least 2 minutes. The patient or family should be instructed concerning the risk of hematoma from the injection." Patients on anticoagulant therapy should be considered to have the same bleeding risks and treated as those with clotting factor disorders (CDC, 60[2], 2011).

For I.M. administration only. Based on limited data, inadvertent SubQ administration provides a lower serologic response, however, the response is still considered to be protective. If inadvertently administered by the SubQ route, revaccination is not necessary.

Simultaneous administration of vaccines helps ensure the patients will be fully vaccinated by the appropriate age. Simultaneous administration of vaccines is defined as administering >1 vaccine on the same day at different anatomic sites. Separate vaccines should not be combined in the same syringe unless indicated by product specific labeling. Separate needles and syringes should be used for each injection. The ACIP prefers each dose of a specific vaccine in a series come from the same manufacturer when possible. Adolescents and adults should be vaccinated while seated or lying down. In general, preterm infants should be vaccinated at the same chronological age as full-term infants (CDC, 60[2], 2011).

Antipyretics have not been shown to prevent febrile seizures. Antipyretics may be used to treat fever or discomfort following vaccination (CDC 2011). One study reported that routine prophylactic administration of acetaminophen to prevent fever prior to vaccination decreased the immune response of some vaccines; the clinical significance of this reduction in immune response has not been established (Prymula, 2009).

I.V. Do not administer via I.V., SubQ or I.D. route

Other For I.M. administration only. Based on limited data, inadvertent SubQ administration provides a lower serologic response, however the response is still considered to be protective. If inadvertently administered by the SubQ route revaccination is not necessary.

Nursing Actions

Physical Assessment U.S. federal law require entry into the patient's medical record.

Instruct patient to report serious hypersensitivit reaction symptoms including respiratory distress hypotension, urticaria, upper airway swelling c symptoms of swelling (eg, dizziness or troubl breathing). Other side effects include pain, rec ness, tenderness, or swelling at injection sit along with headache or fever 1-2 days afte injection.

Patient Education Inform patient that this dru protects against serious bacterial infections, b patients may need a booster injection in 2- years. Instruct patient to report serious sympton of swelling, dizziness, or trouble breathing. Oth side effects include pain, redness, tenderness, swelling at injection site along with headache fever 1-2 days after injection.

Meningococcal Polysaccharide Vaccine (Groups A / C / Y and W-135)

(me NIN joe kok al pol i SAK a ride vak SEEN groops aye, see, why & dubl yoo won thur tee fyve)

Brand Names: U.S. Menomune®-A/C/Y/W-135

Index Terms Meningococcal Polysaccharide Vaccine; MPSV; MPSV4

Pharmacologic Category Vaccine, Inactivated (Bacterial)

Medication Safety Issues

Administration issue:

Menomune® (MPSV4) should be administered by subcutaneous (SubQ) injection. Menactra® (MCV4), also a meningococcal polysaccharide vaccine, is to be administered by intramuscular (I.M.) injection only.

Pregnancy Risk Factor C

Lactation Excretion in breast milk unknown/use caution

Use Provide active immunity to meningococcal serogroups contained in the vaccine

The Advisory Committee on Immunization Practices (ACIP) recommends routine vaccination for persons at increased risk for meningococcal disease. Meningococcal conjugate vaccine (MCV4) is preferred for persons aged 2-55 years; meningococcal polysaccharide vaccine (MPSV4) is preferred in adults ≥56 years of age (CDC, 2005).

Persons at increased risk include:

- Previously unvaccinated college freshmen living in dormitories
- Microbiologists routinely exposed to isolates of *N. meningitidis*
- Military recruits
- Persons traveling to or who reside in countries where *N. meningitidis* is hyperendemic or epidemic, particularly if contact with local population will be prolonged
- Persons with persistent complement component deficiencies (eg, C5-C9, properidin, factor H, or factor D)
- Persons with anatomic or functional asplenia
- Persons with HIV infection

Use is also recommended during meningococcal outbreaks caused by vaccine preventable serogroups.

Available Dosage Forms

Injection, powder for reconstitution [MPSV4]:

Menomune®-A/C/Y/W-135: 50 mcg each of polysaccharide antigen groups A, C, Y, and W-135 per 0.5 mL dose

General Dosage Range SubQ: *Children ≥2 years and Adults:* 0.5 mL as a single dose

Administration

Other Administer by SubQ injection to the deltoid region; do not administer intradermally, I.M., or I.V.

Simultaneous administration of vaccines helps ensure the patients will be fully vaccinated by the appropriate age. Simultaneous administration of vaccines is defined as administering ≥1 vaccine on the same day at different anatomic sites. Separate vaccines should not be combined in the same syringe unless indicated by product specific labeling. Separate needles and syringes should be used for each injection. The ACIP prefers each dose of a specific vaccine in a series come from the same manufacturer when possible. Adolescents and adults should be vaccinated while seated or lying down. In general, preterm infants should be vaccinated at the same chronological age as full-term infants (CDC, 2011).

Antipyretics have not been shown to prevent febrile seizures. Antipyretics may be used to treat fever or discomfort following vaccination (CDC, 2011). One study reported that routine prophylactic administration of acetaminophen to prevent fever prior to vaccination decreased the immune response of some vaccines; the clinical significance of this reduction in immune response has not been established (Prymula, 2009).

Nursing Actions

Physical Assessment U.S. federal law requires entry into the patient's medical record.

Related Information

Immunization Administration Recommendations *on page 1243*

Immunization Recommendations *on page 1248*

Menotropins

(men oh TROE pins)

Brand Names: U.S. Menopur®; Repronex®

Index Terms hMG; Human Menopausal Gonadotropin

Pharmacologic Category Gonadotropin; Ovulation Stimulator

Medication Safety Issues

Sound-alike/look-alike issues:

Repronex® may be confused with Regranex®

Pregnancy Risk Factor X

Lactation Excretion in breast milk unknown/use caution

Use Female:

In conjunction with hCG to induce ovulation and pregnancy in infertile females experiencing oligoanovulation or anovulation when the cause of anovulation is functional and not caused by primary ovarian failure (Repronex®)

Stimulation of multiple follicle development in ovulatory patients as part of an assisted reproductive technology (ART) (Menopur®, Repronex®)

Unlabeled Use Male: Stimulation of spermatogenesis in primary or secondary hypogonadotropic hypogonadism

Mechanism of Action/Effect Actions occur as a result of both follicle stimulating hormone (FSH) effects and luteinizing hormone (LH) effects; menotropins stimulate the development and maturation of the ovarian follicle (FSH), cause ovulation (LH), and stimulate the development of the corpus luteum (LH); in males it stimulates spermatogenesis (LH)

Contraindications Hypersensitivity to menotropins or any component of the formulation; primary ovarian failure as indicated by a high follicle-stimulating hormone (FSH) level; uncontrolled thyroid and adrenal dysfunction; abnormal bleeding of undetermined origin; intracranial lesion (ie, pituitary tumor); ovarian cyst or enlargement not due to polycystic ovary syndrome; infertility due to any cause other than anovulation (except candidates for *in vitro* fertilization); sex hormone-dependent tumors of the reproductive tract and accessory organs; pregnancy

Warnings/Precautions These medications should only be used by physicians who are thoroughly familiar with infertility problems and their management. Advise patient of frequency and potential hazards of multiple pregnancy. May cause ovarian hyperstimulation syndrome (OHSS); if severe, treatment should be discontinued and patient should be hospitalized (may become more severe if pregnancy occurs). Monitor for ovarian enlargement; to minimize the hazard of abnormal ovarian enlargement, use the lowest possible dose. Serious pulmonary conditions (atelectasis, acute respiratory distress syndrome) and arterial thromboembolism have been reported. Safety and efficacy have not been established in renal or hepatic impairment, or in pediatric and geriatric patients. Use may lead to multiple births. Products may contain lactose.

Drug Interactions

Avoid Concomitant Use There are no known interactions where it is recommended to avoid concomitant use.

Decreased Effect There are no known significant interactions involving a decrease in effect.

Increased Effect/Toxicity There are no known significant interactions involving an increase in effect.

Adverse Reactions Adverse effects may vary according to specific product, route, and/or dosage.

>10%:

Central nervous system: Headache (up to 34%)
Gastrointestinal: Abdominal pain (up to 18%), nausea (up to 12%)
Genitourinary: OHSS (up to 13%, dose related)
Local: Injection site reaction (4% to 12%)

1% to 10%:

Cardiovascular: Flushing
Central nervous system: Dizziness, malaise, migraine
Endocrine & metabolic: Breast tenderness, hot flashes, menstrual irregularities
Gastrointestinal: Abdominal cramping, abdominal fullness, constipation, diarrhea, enlarged abdomen, vomiting
Genitourinary: Ectopic pregnancy, ovarian disease, vaginal hemorrhage
Local: Injection site edema/pain
Neuromuscular & skeletal: Back pain
Respiratory: Cough increased, respiratory disorder
Miscellaneous: Infection, flu-like syndrome

Frequency not defined:

Cardiovascular: Stroke, tachycardia, thrombosis (venous or arterial)
Dermatologic: Angioedema, rash, urticaria
Genitourinary: Adnexal torsion, hemoperitoneum, ovarian enlargement
Neuromuscular & skeletal: Limb necrosis
Respiratory: Acute respiratory distress syndrome, atelectasis, dyspnea, embolism, laryngeal edema, pulmonary infarction, tachypnea
Miscellaneous: Allergic reaction, anaphylaxis

Available Dosage Forms

Injection, powder for reconstitution:

Menopur®, Repronex®: Follicle stimulating hormone activity 75 int. units and luteinizing hormone activity 75 int. units

General Dosage Range

I.M.: *Adults:* Repronex®: Initial: 150 int. units **or** 225 int. units daily (maximum: 450 int. units/day; 12 days of therapy)

SubQ: *Adults:* Menopur®: Initial: 225 int. units daily (maximum: 450 int. units/day; 20 days of therapy); Repronex®: Initial: 150 int. units **or** 225 int. units daily (maximum: 450 int. units/day; 12 days of therapy)

Administration

I.M. Repronex®: Administer deep in a large muscle.

Other SubQ:

Menopur®: Administer to alternating sites of the abdomen. When administration to the lower abdomen is not possible, the injection may be given into the thigh.

Repronex®: Administer to alternating sites of the lower abdomen.

Stability

Reconstitution After reconstitution inject immediately; discard any unused portion.

Storage Lyophilized powder may be refrigerated or stored at room temperature. Protect from light.

Nursing Actions

Physical Assessment Teach appropriate method for measuring basal body temperature to indicate ovulation. Stress importance of following prescriber's instructions for timing intercourse. If self-administered, teach appropriate injection technique and needle disposal.

Patient Education Self injection: Follow prescriber's recommended schedule for injections. You may experience headache, nausea, abdominal pain, flushing, dizziness, or menstrual irregularities. Report pain at injection site; enlarged breasts (male); respiratory difficulty; nosebleed acute abdominal discomfort; abdominal distention; fever; or warmth, swelling, weight gain, pain, or redness in calves.

Meperidine (me PER i deen)

Brand Names: U.S. Demerol®

Index Terms Isonipecaine Hydrochloride; Meperidine Hydrochloride; Pethidine Hydrochloride

Pharmacologic Category Analgesic, Opioid

Medication Safety Issues

Sound-alike/look-alike issues:

Meperidine may be confused with meprobamate

Demerol® may be confused with Demulen®, Desyrel, Dilaudid®, Pamelor™

High alert medication:

The Institute for Safe Medication Practices (ISMP) includes this medication among its list of drug classes which have a heightened risk of causing significant patient harm when used in error.

BEERS Criteria medication:

This drug may be inappropriate for use in geriatric patients (high severity risk).

Other safety concerns:

Avoid the use of meperidine for pain control, especially in elderly and renally-compromised patients because of the risk of neurotoxicity (American Pain Society, 2008; Institute for Safe Medication Practices [ISMP], 2007)

Pregnancy Risk Factor C

Lactation Enters breast milk/not recommended (AAP rates "compatible"; AAP 2001 update pending)

Use Management of moderate-to-severe pain; adjunct to anesthesia and preoperative sedation

Unlabeled Use Reduce postoperative shivering; reduce rigors from amphotericin B (conventional)

Controlled Substance C-II

Available Dosage Forms

Injection, solution: 10 mg/mL (30 mL, 50 mL, 60 mL); 25 mg/mL (1 mL); 50 mg/mL (1 mL); 100 mg/mL (1 mL)

Demerol®: 25 mg/mL (1 mL); 25 mg/0.5 mL (0.5 mL); 50 mg/mL (1 mL, 1.5 mL, 2 mL, 30 mL); 75 mg/mL (1 mL); 100 mg/mL (1 mL, 20 mL)

Solution, oral: 50 mg/5 mL (500 mL)

Tablet, oral: 50 mg, 100 mg

Demerol®: 50 mg, 100 mg

General Dosage Range Dosage adjustment recommended in patients with hepatic impairment

I.M., SubQ:

Children: 1.1-1.8 mg/kg/dose every 3-4 hours as needed (maximum: 50-150 mg/dose) **or** 1.1-2.2 mg/kg given 30-90 minutes before the beginning of anesthesia (maximum: 50-150 mg/dose)

Adults: 50-150 mg every 3-4 hours as needed **or** 50-150 mg given 30-90 minutes before the beginning of anesthesia **or** 50-100 mg when pain becomes regular; may repeat at every 1-3 hours

Elderly: Avoid use

Oral:

Children: 1.1-1.8 mg/kg/dose every 3-4 hours as needed (maximum: 50-150 mg/dose)

Adults: Initial: 50-150 mg every 3-4 hours as needed

Elderly: Avoid use

Administration

Oral Oral solution: Administer solution in 1/2 glass of water; undiluted solution may exert topical anesthetic effect on mucous membranes

I.V. Solution for injection: May be administered I.M., SubQ, or I.V.; I.V. push should be administered slowly using a diluted solution, use of a 10 mg/mL concentration has been recommended.

I.V. Detail pH: 3.5-6

Nursing Actions

Physical Assessment Monitor for effectiveness of pain relief. Monitor blood pressure, CNS and respiratory status, and degree of sedation at beginning of therapy and periodically thereafter. Assess patient's physical and/or psychological dependence. For inpatients, implement safety measures (eg, side rails up, call light within reach, instructions to call for assistance). Discontinue slowly after prolonged use.

Patient Education Drug may cause physical and/or psychological dependence. While using this medication, do not use alcohol and other prescription or OTC medications (especially sedatives, tranquilizers, antihistamines, or pain medications) without consulting prescriber. Maintain adequate hydration, unless instructed to restrict fluid intake. May cause hypotension, dizziness, drowsiness, impaired coordination, or blurred vision; loss of appetite, nausea, or vomiting; or constipation. Report chest pain, slow or rapid heartbeat, dizziness, or persistent headache; changes in mental status; seizures; changes in renal function; skin rash; or shortness of breath.

Mercaptopurine (mer kap toe PYOOR een)

Brand Names: U.S. Purinethol®

Index Terms 6-Mercaptopurine (error-prone abbreviation); 6-MP (error-prone abbreviation)

Pharmacologic Category Antineoplastic Agent, Antimetabolite; Antineoplastic Agent, Antimetabolite (Purine Analog); Immunosuppressant Agent

Medication Safety Issues

Sound-alike/look-alike issues:

Mercaptopurine may be confused with methotrexate

Purinethol® may be confused with propylthiouracil

High alert medication:

This medication is in a class the Institute for Safe Medication Practices (ISMP) includes among its list of drug classes which have a heightened risk of causing significant patient harm when used in error.

Other safety concerns:

To avoid potentially serious dosage errors, the terms "6-mercaptopurine" or "6-MP" should be avoided; use of these terms has been associated with sixfold overdosages.

Azathioprine is metabolized to mercaptopurine; concurrent use of these commercially-available products has resulted in profound myelosuppression.

Pregnancy Risk Factor D

Lactation Enters breast milk/not recommended

Breast-Feeding Considerations According to the manufacturer, the decision to continue or discontinue breast-feeding during therapy should take into account the risk of exposure to the infant and the benefits of treatment to the mother.

Use Maintenance treatment component of acute lymphoblastic leukemia (ALL)

Unlabeled Use Steroid-sparing agent for corticosteroid-dependent Crohn's disease (CD) and ulcerative colitis (UC); maintenance of remission in CD; fistulizing Crohn's disease; maintenance treatment in acute promyelocytic leukemia (APL); treatment component for non Hodgkin lymphoma (NHL), treatment of autoimmune hepatitis

Mechanism of Action/Effect Purine antagonist which inhibits DNA and RNA synthesis

Contraindications Hypersensitivity to mercaptopurine or any component of the formulation; patients whose disease showed prior resistance to mercaptopurine

Warnings/Precautions Hazardous agent - use appropriate precautions for handling and disposal.

Hepatotoxicity has been reported, including jaundice, ascites, hepatic necrosis (may be fatal), intrahepatic cholestasis, parenchymal cell necrosis, and/or hepatic encephalopathy; may be due to direct hepatic cell damage or hypersensitivity. While hepatotoxicity or hepatic injury may occur at any dose, dosages >2.5 mg/kg/day are associated with a higher incidence. Signs of jaundice generally appear early in treatment, after ~1-2 months (range: 1 week to 8 years) and may resolve following discontinuation; recurrence with rechallenge has been noted. Monitor liver function tests (monitor more frequently if used in combination with other hepatotoxic drugs or in patients with pre-existing hepatic impairment. Consider a reduced dose in patients with hepatic impairment. Withhold treatment for clinical signs of jaundice (hepatomegaly, anorexia, tenderness), deterioration in liver function tests, toxic hepatitis, or biliary stasis until hepatotoxicity is ruled out.

Dose-related leukopenia, thrombocytopenia, and anemia are common; however, may be indicative of disease progression. Hematologic toxicity may be delayed. Bone marrow may appear hypoplastic (could also appear normal). Monitor for bleeding (due to thrombocytopenia) or infection (due to neutropenia). Patients with homozygous genetic defect of thiopurine methyltransferase (TPMT) are more sensitive to myelosuppressive effects; generally associated with rapid myelosuppression. Significant mercaptopurine dose reductions wil be necessary (possibly with continued concomitan chemotherapy at normal doses). Patients who are heterozygous for TPMT defects will have inter mediate activity; may have increased toxicity (pri marily myelosuppression) although will generally tolerate normal mercaptopurine doses. Conside TPMT testing for severe toxicities/excessive mye losuppression. Patients on concurrent therapy with drugs which may inhibit TPMT (eg, olsalazine) o xanthine oxidase (eg, allopurinol) may be sensitive to myelosuppressive effects.

May increase the risk for secondary malignancies hepatic T-cell lymphoma (HTCL) has bee reported with mercaptopurine when used for th treatment of irritable bowel disease (an unlabele use). Because azathioprine is metabolized to me captopurine, concomitant use with azathioprin may result in profound myelosuppression an should be avoided. Mercaptopurine is immunosu pressive; the risk for infection is increased; com mon signs of infection, such as fever an leukocytosis may not occur; lethargy and confusio may be more prominent signs of infection. Immun response to vaccines may be diminished. Conside adjusting dosage in patients with renal impairmen To avoid potentially serious dosage errors, th terms "6-mercaptopurine" or "6-MP" should b avoided; use of these terms has been associate with sixfold overdosages.

Drug Interactions

Avoid Concomitant Use

Avoid concomitant use of Mercaptopurine w any of the following: AzaTHIOprine; BCG; CloZ Pine; Febuxostat; Natalizumab; Pimecrolimu Tacrolimus (Topical)

Decreased Effect

Mercaptopurine may decrease the levels/effec of: BCG; Coccidioidin Skin Test; Sipuleucel- Vaccines (Inactivated); Vitamin K Antagonists

The levels/effects of Mercaptopurine may decreased by: Echinacea

Increased Effect/Toxicity

Mercaptopurine may increase the levels/effects of: CloZAPine; Leflunomide; Natalizumab; Vaccines (Live); Vitamin K Antagonists

The levels/effects of Mercaptopurine may be increased by: 5-ASA Derivatives; Allopurinol; AzaTHIOprine; Denosumab; Febuxostat; Pimecrolimus; Roflumilast; Sulfamethoxazole; Tacrolimus (Topical); Trastuzumab; Trimethoprim

Nutritional/Ethanol Interactions Food: Absorption is variable with food. Management: Take on an empty stomach at the same time each day 1 hour before or 2 hours after a meal. Maintain adequate hydration, unless instructed to restrict fluid intake.

Adverse Reactions Frequency not defined.

Central nervous system: Drug fever

Dermatologic: Alopecia, hyperpigmentation, rash

Endocrine & metabolic: Hyperuricemia

Gastrointestinal: Anorexia, diarrhea, intestinal ulcers, mucositis/oral lesions (rare), nausea (minimal), pancreatitis, sprue-like symptoms, stomach pain, vomiting (minimal)

Genitourinary: Oligospermia

Hematologic: Myelosuppression (onset 7-10 days; nadir 14 days; recovery: 21 days); anemia, bleeding, granulocytopenia, leukopenia, marrow hypoplasia, thrombocytopenia

Hepatic: Hepatotoxicity, ascites, biliary stasis, hepatic damage/injury, hepatic encephalopathy, hepatic necrosis, hepatomegaly, intrahepatic cholestasis, jaundice, parenchymal cell necrosis, toxic hepatitis

Renal: Hyperuricosuria, renal toxicity

Miscellaneous: Hepatosplenic T cell lymphoma, immunosuppression, infection, secondary malignancy

Available Dosage Forms

Tablet, oral: 50 mg

Purinethol®: 50 mg

General Dosage Range Dosage adjustment recommended in patients with hepatic or renal impairment or on concomitant therapy

Oral: *Children and Adults:* Maintenance: 1.5-2.5 mg/kg/day

Administration

Oral Preferably on an empty stomach (1 hour before or 2 hours after meals)

For the treatment of ALL in children (Schmiegelow, 1997): Administration in the evening has demonstration superior outcome; administration with food did not significantly affect outcome.

Stability

Storage Store at room temperature of 15°C to 25°C (59°F to 77°F). Protect from moisture.

Nursing Actions

Physical Assessment Assess hepatic function; jaundice, ascites, and encephalopathy can occur some time following therapy. Monitor nutritional status and renal status. Monitor for dehydration, myelosuppression, anemia, and leukopenia on a regular basis. Teach patient importance of adequate hydration.

Patient Education Take daily dose at the same time each day. Preferable to take an on empty stomach, 1 hour before or 2 hours after meals. Maintain adequate hydration unless instructed to restrict fluid intake. You may be more susceptible to infection. May cause nausea, vomiting, diarrhea, loss of appetite, weakness or lethargy, mouth sores, or headache. Report signs of persistent fever, opportunistic infection (eg, fever, chills, sore throat, burning urination, fatigue), bleeding (eg, tarry stools, easy bruising), unresolved mouth sores, nausea or vomiting, swelling of extremities, respiratory difficulty, unusual weight gain, or changes in urinary pattern.

Dietary Considerations Should not be administered with meals.

Meropenem (mer oh PEN em)

Brand Names: U.S. Merrem® I.V.

Pharmacologic Category Antibiotic, Carbapenem

Medication Safety Issues

Sound-alike/look-alike issues:

Meropenem may be confused with ertapenem, imipenem, metroNIDAZOLE

Pregnancy Risk Factor B

Lactation Excretion in breast milk unknown/use caution

Breast-Feeding Considerations It is not known if meropenem is excreted in breast milk. The manufacturer recommends that caution be exercised when administering meropenem to breast-feeding women. Most penicillins and carbapenems are safe for use in breast-feeding. Nondose-related effects could include modification of bowel flora.

Use

Treatment of intra-abdominal infections (complicated appendicitis and peritonitis); treatment of bacterial meningitis in pediatric patients ≥3 months of age caused by *S. pneumoniae*, *H. influenzae*, and *N. meningitidis*; treatment of complicated skin and skin structure infections caused by susceptible organisms

Canadian labeling: Additional indications (not in U.S. labeling): Treatment of lower respiratory tract infections (community-acquired and nosocomial pneumonias), complicated urinary tract infections, gynecologic infections (excluding chlamydia), and septicemia; treatment of bacterial meningitis in adults caused by *S. pneumoniae*, *H. influenzae*, and *N. meningitidis* (use in adult meningitis based on pediatric data)

Unlabeled Use *Burkholderia pseudomallei* (melioidosis), febrile neutropenia, liver abscess, otitis externa

Mechanism of Action/Effect Inhibits cell wall synthesis in susceptible bacteria

Contraindications Hypersensitivity to meropenem, any component of the formulation, or other carbapenems (eg, doripenem, ertapenem, imipenem); patients who have experienced anaphylactic reactions to other beta-lactams

Warnings/Precautions Serious hypersensitivity reactions, including anaphylaxis, have been reported (some without a history of previous allergic reactions to beta-lactams). Carbapenems have been associated with CNS adverse effects, including confusional states and seizures (myoclonic); use caution with CNS disorders (eg, brain lesions and history of seizures) and adjust dose in renal impairment to avoid drug accumulation, which may increase seizure risk. Prolonged use may result in fungal or bacterial superinfection, including *C. difficile*-associated diarrhea (CDAD) and pseudomembranous colitis; CDAD has been observed >2 months postantibiotic treatment. Use with caution in patients with renal impairment; dosage adjustment required in patients with moderate-to-severe renal dysfunction. Thrombocytopenia has been reported in patients with renal dysfunction. Lower doses (based upon renal function) are often required in the elderly. May decrease divalproex sodium/valproic acid concentrations leading to breakthrough seizures; concomitant use not recommended. Alternative antimicrobial agents should be considered; if concurrent meropenem is necessary, consider additional antiseizure medication.

Drug Interactions

Avoid Concomitant Use

Avoid concomitant use of Meropenem with any of the following: BCG; Probenecid

Decreased Effect

Meropenem may decrease the levels/effects of: BCG; Divalproex; Typhoid Vaccine; Valproic Acid

Increased Effect/Toxicity

The levels/effects of Meropenem may be increased by: Probenecid

Adverse Reactions 1% to 10%:

Central nervous system: Headache (2% to 8%), pain (≤5%)

Dermatologic: Rash (2% to 3%, includes diaper-area moniliasis in infants), pruritus (1%)

Endocrine & metabolic: Hypoglycemia

Gastrointestinal: Diarrhea (4% to 7%), nausea/vomiting (1% to 8%), constipation (1% to 7%), oral moniliasis (up to 2% in pediatric patients), glossitis (1%)

Hematologic: Anemia (≤6%)

Local: Inflammation at the injection site (2%), phlebitis/thrombophlebitis (1%), injection site reaction (1%)

Respiratory: Apnea (1%), pharyngitis, pneumonia

Miscellaneous: Sepsis (2%), shock (1%)

Available Dosage Forms

Injection, powder for reconstitution: 500 mg, 1 g

Merrem® I.V.: 500 mg, 1 g

General Dosage Range Dosage adjustment recommended in patients with renal impairment

I.V.:

Children ≥3 months and <50 kg: 10-40 mg/kg every 8 hours (maximum: 2 g every 8 hours)

Children ≥50 kg and Adults: 500 mg to 2 g every 8 hours

Administration

I.V. Administer I.V. infusion over 15-30 minutes; I.V. bolus injection (5-20 mL) over 3-5 minutes

Extended infusion administration (unlabeled dosing): Administer over 3 hours (Crandon 2011; Dandekar, 2003). **Note:** Must consider meropenem's limited room temperature stability if using extended infusions

I.V. Detail pH: 7.3-8.3

Stability

Reconstitution Meropenem infusion vials may be reconstituted with SWFI or a compatible diluent (eg, NS). The 500 mg vials should be reconstituted with 10 mL, and 1 g vials with 20 mL. May be further diluted with compatible solutions for infusion. Consult detailed reference/product labeling for compatibility.

Storage Dry powder should be stored at controlled room temperature 20°C to 25°C (68°F to 77°F).

Injection reconstitution: Stability in vial when constituted (up to 50 mg/mL) with:

SWFI: Stable for up to 2 hours at controlled room temperature of 15°C to 25°C (59°F to 77°F) or for up to 12 hours under refrigeration.

Sodium chloride: Stable for up to 2 hours at controlled room temperature of 15°C to 25°C (59°F to 77°F) or for up to 18 hours under refrigeration.

Dextrose 5% injection: Stable for 1 hour at controlled room temperature of 15°C to 25°C (59°F to 77°F) or for 8 hours under refrigeration.

Infusion admixture (1-20 mg/mL): Solution stability when diluted in NS is 4 hours at controlled room temperature of 15°C to 25°C (59°F to 77°F) or 24 hours under refrigeration. Stability in D_5W is 1 hour at controlled room temperature of 15°C to 25°C (59°F to 77°F) or for 4 hours under refrigeration. For other diluents, see prescribing information.

Nursing Actions

Physical Assessment Results of culture and sensitivity tests and patient's allergy history should be assessed prior to beginning treatment. Infusion site should be monitored closely to prevent phlebitis/thrombophlebitis. Teach patient importance of adequate hydration.

Patient Education This medication can only be given by infusion. Report immediately any burning, pain, swelling, or redness at infusion site. Maintain adequate hydration unless instructed to restrict fluid intake. May cause nausea, vomiting, diarrhea, or headache. Report persistent distress, persistent diarrhea, mouth sores, respiratory difficulty, headache, or CNS changes (agitation, delirium).

Dietary Considerations Some products may contain sodium.

Mesalamine (me SAL a meen)

Brand Names: U.S. Apriso™; Asacol®; Asacol® HD; Canasa®; Lialda®; Pentasa®; Rowasa®; sfRowasa™

Index Terms 5-Aminosalicylic Acid; 5-ASA; Fisalamine; Mesalazine

Pharmacologic Category 5-Aminosalicylic Acid Derivative

Medication Safety Issues

Sound-alike/look-alike issues:

Mesalamine may be confused with mecamylamine, megestrol, memantine, metaxalone, methenamine

Apriso™ may be confused with Apri®

Asacol® may be confused with Ansaid®, Os-Cal®, Visicol®

Lialda® may be confused with Aldara®

Pentasa® may be confused with Pancrease®, Pangestyme®

Pregnancy Risk Factor B/C (product specific)

Lactation Enters breast milk/use caution

Breast-Feeding Considerations Adverse effects (diarrhea) in a nursing infant have been reported while the mother received rectal administration of mesalamine within 12 hours after the first dose. Low concentrations of the parent drug and higher concentrations of the N-acetyl metabolite of the parent drug have been detected in human breast milk.

Use

Oral:

Asacol®, Lialda®, Pentasa®: Treatment and maintenance of remission of mildly- to moderately-active ulcerative colitis

Apriso™: Maintenance of remission of ulcerative colitis

Asacol® HD: Treatment of moderately-active ulcerative colitis

Rectal: Treatment of active mild-to-moderate distal ulcerative colitis, proctosigmoiditis, or proctitis

Mechanism of Action/Effect Mesalamine (5-aminosalicylic acid) is the active component of sulfasalazine; the specific mechanism of action of mesalamine is unknown; however, it is thought that it modulates local chemical mediators of the inflammatory response, especially leukotrienes, and is also postulated to be a free radical scavenger or an inhibitor of tumor necrosis factor (TNF); action appears topical rather than systemic

Contraindications Hypersensitivity to mesalamine, aminosalicylates, salicylates, or any component of the formulation

Warnings/Precautions May cause an acute intolerance syndrome (cramping, acute abdominal pain, bloody diarrhea; sometimes fever, headache, rash); discontinue if this occurs. Use caution in patients with active peptic ulcers. Patients with pyloric stenosis may have prolonged gastric retention of tablets, delaying the release of mesalamine in the colon. Pericarditis or myocarditis should be considered in patients with chest pain; use with caution in patients predisposed to these conditions. Pancreatitis should be considered in patients with new abdominal discomfort. Symptomatic worsening of colitis/IBD may occur following initiation of therapy. Oligospermia (rare, reversible) has been reported in males. Use caution in patients with sulfasalazine hypersensitivity. Use caution in patients with impaired hepatic function; hepatic failure has been reported. Renal impairment (including minimal change nephropathy and acute/chronic interstitial nephritis) and rarely failure have been reported; use caution in patients with renal impairment. Use caution with other medications converted to mesalamine. Postmarketing reports suggest an increased incidence of blood dyscrasias in patients >65 years of age. In addition, elderly may have difficulty administering and retaining rectal suppositories or may have decreased renal function; use with caution and monitor.

Apriso™ contains phenylalanine. The Asacol® HD 800 mg tablet has not been shown to be bioequivalent to 2 Asacol® 400 mg tablets. Canasa® suppositories contain saturated vegetable fatty acid esters (contraindicated in patients with allergy to these components). Rowasa® enema contains potassium metabisulfite; may cause severe hypersensitivity reactions (ie, anaphylaxis) in patients with sulfite allergies.

Drug Interactions

Avoid Concomitant Use There are no known interactions where it is recommended to avoid concomitant use.

Decreased Effect

Mesalamine may decrease the levels/effects of: Cardiac Glycosides

The levels/effects of Mesalamine may be decreased by: Antacids; H2-Antagonists; Proton Pump Inhibitors

Increased Effect/Toxicity

Mesalamine may increase the levels/effects of: Heparin; Heparin (Low Molecular Weight); Thiopurine Analogs; Varicella Virus-Containing Vaccines

Adverse Reactions Adverse effects vary depending upon dosage form. Incidence usually on lower end with enema and suppository dosage forms.

>10%:

Central nervous system: Headache (2% to 35%), pain (≤14%)

Gastrointestinal: Abdominal pain (1% to 18%), eructation (16%), nausea (3% to 13%)

Respiratory: Pharyngitis (11%)

1% to 10%:

Cardiovascular: Chest pain (3%), peripheral edema (3%), vasodilation (≥2%)

Central nervous system: Dizziness (2% to 8%), fever (1% to 6%), chills (3%), malaise (2% to 3%), fatigue (<3%), vertigo (<3%), anxiety (≥2%), migraine (≥2%), nervousness (≥2%), insomnia (2%),

Dermatologic: Rash (1% to 6%), pruritus (1% to 3%), alopecia (<3%), acne (1% to 2%)

Endocrine & metabolic: Triglyceride increased (<3%)

Gastrointestinal: Diarrhea (2% to 8%), dyspepsia (1% to 6%), flatulence (1% to 6%), constipation (5%), vomiting (1% to 5%), colitis exacerbation (1% to 3%), rectal bleeding (<3%), abdominal distention (≥2%), gastroenteritis (≥2%), gastrointestinal bleeding (≥2%), stool abnormalities (≥2%), tenesmus (≥2%), rectal pain (1% to 2%), hemorrhoids (1%)

Genitourinary: Polyuria (≥2%)

Hematologic: Hematocrit/hemoglobin decreased (<3%)

Hepatic: Cholestatic hepatitis (<3%), transaminases increased (<3%), ALT increased (1%)

Local: Pain on insertion of enema tip (1%)

Neuromuscular & skeletal: Back pain (1% to 7%), arthralgia (≤5%), hypertonia (5%), myalgia (3%), paresthesia (≥2%), weakness (≥2%), arthritis (2%), leg/joint pain (2%)

Ocular: Vision abnormalities (≥2%), conjunctivitis (2%)

Otic: Tinnitus (<3%), ear pain (≥2%)

Renal: Creatinine clearance decreased (<3%), hematuria (<3%)

Respiratory: Nasopharyngitis (1% to 4%), dyspnea (<3%), bronchitis (≥2%), sinusitis (≥2%), cough (≤2%)

Miscellaneous: Flu-like syndrome (1% to 5%), infection (≥2%), diaphoresis (3%), intolerance syndrome (3%)

Available Dosage Forms

Capsule, controlled release, oral:
Pentasa®: 250 mg, 500 mg

Capsule, delayed and extended release, oral:
Apriso™: 0.375 g

Suppository, rectal:
Canasa®: 1000 mg (30s, 42s)

Suspension, rectal: 4 g/60 mL (7s, 28s)
Rowasa®: 4 g/60 mL (7s, 28s)
sfRowasa™: 4 g/60 mL (7s, 28s)

Tablet, delayed release, enteric coated, oral:
Asacol®: 400 mg
Asacol® HD: 800 mg
Lialda®: 1.2 g

General Dosage Range

Oral: *Adults:*
Capsule: Apriso™: 1.5 g once daily; Pentasa®: 1 g 4 times/day
Tablet: Asacol®: 800 mg 3 times/day or 1.6 g/da[y] in divided doses; Asacol® HD: 1.6 g 3 time[s/]day; Lialda®, Mezavant®: 2.4-4.8 g once daily

Rectal: *Adults:* Retention enema: 60 mL (4 g) [at] bedtime, retained overnight (~8 hours); Suppos[i]tory: Insert 1000 mg at bedtime

Administration

Oral Oral: Swallow capsules or tablets whole, d[o] not break, chew, or crush.

Capsules:

Apriso™: Administer with or without food; do n[ot] administer with antacids. The capsule shou[ld] be swallowed whole per the manufacturer['s] labeling; however, opening the capsule an[d] placing the contents (delayed release gra[n]ules) on food with a pH <6 is not expected [to] affect the release of mesalamine once ingeste[d] (data on file, Salix Pharmaceuticals Medic[al] Information). There is no safety/efficacy info[r]mation regarding this practice. The contents [of] the capsules should not be chewed or crushe[d].

Pentasa®: Administer with or without foo[d]. Although the manufacturer recommends swa[l]lowing the capsule whole, if a patient is unab[le] to swallow the capsule, some clinicians suppo[rt] opening the capsules and placing the conten[ts] (controlled-release beads) on yogurt or pean[ut] butter (Crohn's & Colitis Foundation of Ame[r]ica). There are currently no published da[ta] evaluating the safety/efficacy of this practic[e]. The contents of the capsules should not b[e] chewed or crushed.

Tablets:

Asacol®: Do not break outer coating.

Asacol® HD: Do not break outer coating; admi[n]ister with or without food.

Lialda®: Do not break outer coating; should b[e] administered once daily with a meal

Mezavant®: Do not break outer coating; shou[ld] be administered once daily with a meal

Other

Rectal enema: Shake bottle well. Retain enema for 8 hours or as long as practical.

Suppository: Remove foil wrapper; avoid exce[s]sive handling. Should be retained for at least 1-[3] hours to achieve maximum benefit.

Stability

Storage

Capsule:

Apriso™: Store at controlled room temperatu[re] of 20°C to 25°C (68°F to 77°F)

Pentasa®: Store at controlled room temperatu[re] of 15°C to 30°C (59°F to 86°F). Protect fro[m] light.

Enema: Store at controlled room temperatur[e]. Use promptly once foil wrap is removed. Co[n]tents may darken with time (do not use if da[rk] brown).

Suppository: Store below 25°C (below 77°F). Ma[y] store under refrigeration; do not freeze. Prote[ct] from direct heat, light, and humidity.

Tablet: Store at controlled room temperature:
Asacol®, Asacol® HD: 20°C to 25°C (68°F to 77°F)
Lialda®: 15°C to 30°C (59°F to 86°F)
Mezavant®: 15°C to 25°C (59°F to 77°F)

Nursing Actions

Physical Assessment Patient allergy history to salicylates should be assessed prior to beginning therapy. Monitor laboratory tests, therapeutic effectiveness, and adverse reactions (chest pain, CNS effects, gastrointestinal upset, exacerbation of colitis) on a regular basis throughout therapy. Teach patient proper use (according to formulation), possible side effects/appropriate interventions (eg, importance of adequate hydration), and adverse symptoms to report.

Patient Education Do not take any new prescriptions, OTC medications, or herbal products during therapy unless approved by prescriber. Take exactly as directed. Symptomatic exacerbation of colitis/IBD may occur when beginning treatment; this should resolve in a short time. May cause fatigue, dizziness, or insomnia (avoid driving or engaging in tasks requiring alertness until response to drug is known); mild gastrointestinal disturbance (eg, gas, constipation, nausea); back, joint, or muscle pain; or flu-like syndrome or cough (consult prescriber if persistent). Report immediately severe new abdominal pain or diarrhea; chest pain or rapid heartbeat; unusual pain (back, joint, muscle, or chest) or swelling of extremities; rash; ringing in ears or change in hearing; or other persistent adverse effects or lack of improvement.

Oral: Swallow tablets or capsules whole; do not break, crush, or chew. Notify prescriber if unable to swallow the medication. Notify prescriber if whole or partial tablets are repeatedly found in stool; should be taken with a meal.

Enema: Follow package insert direction for administering enema. Shake well before using; retain for 8 hours or as long as possible. May cause staining of clothing and undergarments. Do not use if solution is dark brown.

Suppository: Do not refrigerate; store at room temperature. After removing foil wrapper, insert high in rectum without excessive handling (warmth will melt suppository). Lubricating gel may be used if needed to assist insertion. Retain suppositories for at least 1-3 hours to achieve maximum benefit. May cause staining of clothing and undergarments.

Dietary Considerations Some products may contain phenylalanine.

Apriso™: Take with or without food; do not administer with antacids.

Asacol® HD: Take with or without food.

Canasa® rectal suppository contains saturated vegetable fatty acid esters.

Mesna (MES na)

Brand Names: U.S. Mesnex®

Index Terms Mercaptoethane Sulfonate; Sodium 2-Mercaptoethane Sulfonate

Pharmacologic Category Antidote; Uroprotectant

Pregnancy Risk Factor B

Lactation Excretion in breast milk unknown/not recommended

Use Preventative agent to reduce the incidence of ifosfamide-induced hemorrhagic cystitis

Unlabeled Use Preventative agent to reduce the incidence of cyclophosphamide-induced hemorrhagic cystitis with high-dose cyclophosphamide

Available Dosage Forms

Injection, solution: 100 mg/mL (10 mL)
Mesnex®: 100 mg/mL (10 mL)

Tablet, oral:
Mesnex®: 400 mg

General Dosage Range

I.V.: *Children and Adults:* 60% of the ifosfamide dose given in 3 divided doses

I.V., Oral: *Children and Adults:* 100% of the ifosfamide dose, given as 20% I.V., followed by 2 (40% each) doses orally

Administration

Oral Administer orally in tablet formulation or parenteral solution diluted in water, milk, juice, or carbonated beverages; patients who vomit within 2 hours after taking oral mesna should repeat the dose or receive I.V. mesna

I.V. Administer by short (15-30 minutes) infusion or continuous infusion (maintain continuous infusion for 12-24 after completion of ifosfamide infusion) (Hensley, 2008)

I.V. Detail pH: 6.5-8.5

Nursing Actions

Physical Assessment Assess frequently for hematuria/bladder hemorrhage. Hypersensitive reactions have been reported, ranging from mild hypersensitivity to systemic anaphylactic reactions. Monitor closely.

Patient Education This drug is given to help prevent side effects of other chemotherapeutic agents you are taking. Drink at least a quart of liquid each day. Report urine turning pink or red. You may experience a bad taste in your mouth, nausea, and/or vomiting with oral administration.

Metaxalone (me TAKS a lone)

Brand Names: U.S. Skelaxin®

Pharmacologic Category Skeletal Muscle Relaxant

Medication Safety Issues

Sound-alike/look-alike issues:

Metaxalone may be confused with mesalamine, metolazone

Skelaxin® may be confused with Robaxin®

Beers Criteria medication:

This drug may be inappropriate for use in geriatric patients (high severity risk).

Lactation Excretion in breast milk unknown/not recommended

Use Relief of discomfort associated with acute, painful musculoskeletal conditions

Mechanism of Action/Effect Precise mechanism has not been established; however, efficacy appears to result from disruption of the spasm-pain-spasm cycle, probably by a general CNS depressant effect. Does not have a direct effect on skeletal muscle.

Contraindications Hypersensitivity to metaxalone or any component of the formulation; significantly impaired hepatic or renal function, history of drug-induced hemolytic anemias or other anemias

Warnings/Precautions May cause CNS depression. CNS depressant effects may be augmented when used in conjunction with other depressants (eg, barbiturates, ethanol), when taken with food, or in the elderly. May impair mental and/or physical ability to perform hazardous tasks such as operating machinery or driving a motor vehicle. Use with caution in patients with impaired renal or hepatic function (contraindicated if significant impairment); routine monitoring of transaminases is recommended. An increase in bioavailability and half-life have been observed in female patients. This class of medication is poorly tolerated by the elderly due to anticholinergic effects, sedation, and weakness. Efficacy is questionable at dosages tolerated by elderly patients (Beers Criteria). Safety and efficacy have not been established in children ≤12 years of age.

Drug Interactions

Avoid Concomitant Use There are no known interactions where it is recommended to avoid concomitant use.

Decreased Effect

The levels/effects of Metaxalone may be decreased by: Cyproterone; Peginterferon Alfa-2b; Tocilizumab

Increased Effect/Toxicity

Metaxalone may increase the levels/effects of: Alcohol (Ethyl); CNS Depressants; Methotrimeprazine; Selective Serotonin Reuptake Inhibitors

The levels/effects of Metaxalone may be increased by: Conivaptan; Droperidol; HydrOXYzine; Methotrimeprazine

Nutritional/Ethanol Interactions

Ethanol: May increase CNS depression; monitor for increased effects with coadministration. Caution patients about effects.

Food: Bioavailability may be increased (may increase CNS depression).

Herb/Nutraceutical: Avoid valerian, St John's wort, kava kava, gotu kola (may increase CNS depression).

Adverse Reactions Frequency not defined.

Central nervous system: Dizziness, drowsiness, headache, irritability, nervousness

Dermatologic: Rash (with or without pruritus)

Gastrointestinal: Gastrointestinal upset, nausea, vomiting

Hematologic: Hemolytic anemia, leukopenia

Hepatic: Jaundice

Miscellaneous: Hypersensitivity (including rare anaphylactoid reactions)

Pharmacodynamics/Kinetics

Onset of Action ~1 hour

Duration of Action ~4-6 hours

Available Dosage Forms

Tablet, oral: 800 mg

Skelaxin®: 800 mg

General Dosage Range Oral: *Children >12 years and Adults:* 800 mg 3-4 times/day

Administration

Oral May be administered with or without food. However, serum concentrations may be increased when administered with food; clinical significance has not been established. Patients should be monitored.

Stability

Storage Store at controlled room temperature of 15°C to 30°C (59°F to 86°F).

Dietary Considerations Administration with food may increase serum concentrations.

MetFORMIN (met FOR min)

Brand Names: U.S. Fortamet®; Glucophage®; Glucophage® XR; Glumetza®; Riomet®

Index Terms Metformin Hydrochloride

Pharmacologic Category Antidiabetic Agent, Biguanide

Medication Safety Issues

Sound-alike/look-alike issues:

MetFORMIN may be confused with metroNIDAZOLE

Glucophage® may be confused with Glucotrol®, Glutofac®

International issues:

Dianben [Spain] may be confused with Diovan brand name for valsartan [U.S., Canada, and multiple international markets]

Pregnancy Risk Factor B

Lactation Enters breast milk/not recommended

Breast-Feeding Considerations Low amounts of metformin (generally ≤1% of the weight-adjusted maternal dose) are excreted into breast milk. Breast-feeding is not recommended by the manufacturer. Because breast milk concentrations of metformin stay relatively constant, avoiding nursing around peak plasma concentrations in the mother would not be helpful in reducing metformin exposure to the infant. Growth and development were not affected in infants born to mothers with PCOS and who took metformin while breast-feeding.

Use Management of type 2 diabetes mellitus (noninsulin dependent, NIDDM) when hyperglycemia cannot be managed with diet and exercise alone.

Unlabeled Use Gestational diabetes mellitus (GDM); polycystic ovary syndrome (PCOS); prevention of type 2 diabetes mellitus

Mechanism of Action/Effect Decreases hepatic glucose production, decreasing intestinal absorption of glucose and improves insulin sensitivity (increases peripheral glucose uptake and utilization)

Contraindications Hypersensitivity to metformin or any component of the formulation; renal disease or renal dysfunction (serum creatinine ≥1.5 mg/dL in males or ≥1.4 mg/dL in females) or abnormal creatinine clearance from any cause, including shock, acute myocardial infarction, or septicemia; acute or chronic metabolic acidosis with or without coma (including diabetic ketoacidosis)

Note: Temporarily discontinue in patients undergoing radiologic studies in which intravascular iodinated contrast media are utilized.

Warnings/Precautions [U.S. Boxed Warning]: Lactic acidosis is a rare, but potentially severe consequence of therapy with metformin. Lactic acidosis should be suspected in any patient with diabetes receiving metformin with evidence of acidosis but without evidence of ketoacidosis. Discontinue metformin in clinical situations predisposing to hypoxemia, including conditions such as cardiovascular collapse, respiratory failure, acute myocardial infarction, acute congestive heart failure, and septicemia. Use caution in patients with congestive heart failure requiring pharmacologic management, particularly in patients with unstable or acute CHF; risk of lactic acidosis may be increased secondary to hypoperfusion.

Metformin is substantially excreted by the kidney. The risk of accumulation and lactic acidosis increases with the degree of impairment of renal function. Patients with renal function below the limit of normal for their age should not receive metformin. In elderly patients, renal function should be monitored regularly; should not be initiated in patients ≥80 years of age unless normal renal function is confirmed. Use of concomitant medications that may affect renal function (ie, affect tubular secretion) may also affect metformin disposition. Metformin should be withheld in patients with dehydration and/or prerenal azotemia. Therapy should be suspended for any surgical procedures (resume only after normal oral intake resumed and normal renal function is verified). Therapy should be temporarily discontinued prior to or at the time of intravascular administration of iodinated contrast media (potential for acute alteration in renal function). Metformin should be withheld for 48 hours after the radiologic study and restarted only after renal function has been confirmed as normal. It may be necessary to discontinue metformin and administer insulin if the patient is exposed to stress (fever, trauma, infection, surgery).

Avoid use in patients with impaired liver function. Patient must be instructed to avoid excessive acute or chronic ethanol use; ethanol may potentiate metformin's effect on lactate metabolism. Administration of oral antidiabetic drugs has been reported to be associated with increased cardiovascular mortality; metformin does not appear to share this risk. Insoluble tablet shell of Glumetza® 1000 mg extended release tablet may remain intact and be visible in the stool. Other extended released tablets (Fortamet®, Glucophage® XR, Glumetza® 500 mg) may appear in the stool as a soft mass resembling the tablet.

Drug Interactions

Avoid Concomitant Use There are no known interactions where it is recommended to avoid concomitant use.

Decreased Effect

MetFORMIN may decrease the levels/effects of: Trospium

The levels/effects of MetFORMIN may be decreased by: Corticosteroids (Orally Inhaled); Corticosteroids (Systemic); Luteinizing Hormone-Releasing Hormone Analogs; Somatropin; Thiazide Diuretics

Increased Effect/Toxicity

MetFORMIN may increase the levels/effects of: Dofetilide

The levels/effects of MetFORMIN may be increased by: Carbonic Anhydrase Inhibitors; Cephalexin; Cimetidine; Glycopyrrolate; Iodinated Contrast Agents; Pegvisomant

Nutritional/Ethanol Interactions

Ethanol: Avoid or limit ethanol (incidence of lactic acidosis may be increased; may cause hypoglycemia).

Food: Food decreases the extent and slightly delays the absorption. May decrease absorption of vitamin B_{12} and/or folic acid.

Herb/Nutraceutical: Caution with chromium, garlic, gymnema (may cause hypoglycemia).

Adverse Reactions

>10%:

Gastrointestinal: Diarrhea (10% to 53%), nausea/vomiting (7% to 26%), flatulence (12%)

Neuromuscular & skeletal: Weakness (9%)

1% to 10%:

Cardiovascular: Chest discomfort, flushing, palpitation

Central nervous system: Headache (6%), chills, dizziness, lightheadedness
Dermatologic: Rash
Endocrine & metabolic: Hypoglycemia
Gastrointestinal: Indigestion (7%), abdominal discomfort (6%), abdominal distention, abnormal stools, constipation, dyspepsia/ heartburn, taste disorder
Neuromuscular & skeletal: Myalgia
Respiratory: Dyspnea, upper respiratory tract infection
Miscellaneous: Decreased vitamin B_{12} levels (7%), increased diaphoresis, flu-like syndrome, nail disorder

Pharmacodynamics/Kinetics

Onset of Action Within days; maximum effects up to 2 weeks

Available Dosage Forms

Solution, oral:
Riomet®: 100 mg/mL (118 mL, 473 mL)

Tablet, oral: 500 mg, 850 mg, 1000 mg
Glucophage®: 500 mg, 850 mg, 1000 mg

Tablet, extended release, oral: 500 mg, 750 mg
Fortamet®: 500 mg, 1000 mg
Glucophage® XR: 500 mg, 750 mg
Glumetza®: 500 mg, 1000 mg

General Dosage Range Oral:

Extended release: *Adults:* Initial: 500 mg once daily; Maintenance: Up to 2000-2500 mg/day (varies by product) in 1-2 divided doses

Immediate release:
Children 10-16 years: Initial: 500 mg twice daily; Maintenance: Up to 2000 mg/day in divided doses
Children >16 years and Adults: Initial: 500 mg twice daily **or** 850 mg once daily; Maintenance: Up to 2000 mg/day in 2 divided doses **or** 2550 mg/day in 3 divided doses

Administration

Oral Administer with a meal (to decrease GI upset).

Extended release: Swallow whole; do not crush, break, or chew. Administer once daily doses with the evening meal. Fortamet® should also be administered with a full glass of water.

Stability

Storage

Oral solution: Store at 15°C to 30°C (59°F to 86°F).

Tablets: Store at 20°C to 25°C (68°F to 77°F); excursion permitted to 15°C to 30°C (59°F to 86°F). Protect from light and moisture.

Nursing Actions

Physical Assessment Monitor for signs and symptoms of vitamin B_{12} and/or folic acid deficiency during therapy; supplementation may be required. Refer patient to diabetes educator for instruction if needed.

Patient Education Take with food to decrease GI upset. Do not chew or crush extended release tablets. Parts of extended-release tablets may be excreted in the stool (normal). Avoid alcohol; could cause severe reaction. Follow prescribed diet and lifestyle recommendations. You will be instructed in signs of hyper-/hypoglycemia by prescriber or diabetes educator. May cause weakness, nausea, vomiting, flatulence, or diarrhea. Report unusual weakness or fatigue, unusual muscle pain, persistent GI discomfort, dizziness or lightheadedness, unusual somnolence, poor glucose control, or chest discomfort.

Dietary Considerations Drug may cause GI upset; take with food (to decrease GI upset). Take at the same time(s) each day. Dietary modification based on ADA recommendations is a part of therapy. Monitor for signs and symptoms of vitamin B_{12} and/or folic acid deficiency; supplementation may be required.

Methadone (METH a done)

Brand Names: U.S. Dolophine®; Methadone Diskets®; Methadone Intensol™; Methadose®

Index Terms Methadone Hydrochloride

Pharmacologic Category Analgesic, Opioid

Medication Safety Issues

Sound-alike/look-alike issues:
Methadone may be confused with dexmethylphenidate, Mephyton®, methylphenidate, Metadate CD®, Metadate® ER, morphine

High alert medication:
The Institute for Safe Medication Practices (ISMP) includes this medication among its list of drug classes which have a heightened risk of causing significant patient harm when used in error.

Pregnancy Risk Factor C

Lactation Enters breast milk/not recommended (AAP rates "compatible"; AAP 2001 update pending)

Breast-Feeding Considerations Peak methadone levels appear in breast milk 4-5 hours after an oral dose. Methadone has been detected in the plasma of some breast-fed infants whose mothers are taking methadone. Use during breast-feeding is not recommended, and the manufacturer recommends that women on high dose methadone maintenance who already are breast-feeding be instructed to wean breast-feeding gradually to avoid neonatal abstinence syndrome. Sedation and respiratory depression have been reported in nursing infants.

Use Management of moderate-to-severe pain; detoxification and maintenance treatment of opioid addiction as part of an FDA-approved program

Mechanism of Action/Effect Binds to opiate receptors in the CNS, causing inhibition of ascending pain pathways, altering the perception of and response to pain; produces generalized CNS depression

Contraindications Hypersensitivity to methadone or any component of the formulation; respirator depression (in the absence of resuscitative equipment or in an unmonitored setting); acute bronchial asthma or hypercarbia; paralytic ileus; concurrent use of selegiline

Warnings/Precautions An opioid-containing analgesic regimen should be tailored to each patient's needs and based upon the type of pain being treated (acute versus chronic), the route of administration, degree of tolerance for opioids (naive versus chronic user), age, weight, and medical condition. The optimal analgesic dose varies widely among patients. Doses should be titrated to pain relief/prevention. Patients maintained on stable doses of methadone may need higher and/or more frequent doses in case of acute pain (eg, postoperative pain, physical trauma). Methadone is ineffective for the relief of anxiety.

[U.S. Boxed Warning]: May prolong the QT_c interval and increase risk for torsade de pointes. Patients should be informed of the potential arrhythmia risk, evaluated for any history of structural heart disease, arrhythmia, syncope, and for existence of potential drug interactions including drugs that possess QT_c interval-prolonging properties, promote hypokalemia, hypomagnesemia, or hypocalcemia, or reduce elimination of methadone (eg, CYP3A4 inhibitors). Obtain baseline ECG for all patients and risk stratify according to QT_c interval. Use with caution in patients at risk for QT_c prolongation, with medications known to prolong the QT_c interval, promote electrolyte depletion, or inhibit CYP3A4, or history of conduction abnormalities. QT_c interval prolongation and torsade de pointes may be associated with doses >100 mg/day, but have also been observed with lower doses. May cause severe hypotension; use caution with severe volume depletion or other conditions which may compromise maintenance of normal blood pressure. Use caution with cardiovascular disease or patients predisposed to dysrhythmias.

[U.S. Boxed Warning]: May cause respiratory depression. Use caution in patients with respiratory disease or pre-existing respiratory conditions (eg, severe obesity, asthma, COPD, sleep apnea, CNS depression). Because the respiratory effects last longer than the analgesic effects, slow titration is required. Use extreme caution during treatment initiation, dose titration and conversion from other opioid agonists. Incomplete cross tolerance may occur; patients tolerant to other mu opioid agonists may not be tolerant to methadone. Abrupt cessation may precipitate withdrawal symptoms.

May cause CNS depression, which may impair physical or mental abilities. Patients must be cautioned about performing tasks which require mental alertness (eg, operating machinery or driving). Effects with other sedative drugs or ethanol may be potentiated. Use with caution in patients with depression or suicidal tendencies, or in patients with a history of drug abuse. Tolerance or psychological and physical dependence may occur with prolonged use.

Use with caution in patients with head injury or increased intracranial pressure. May obscure diagnosis or clinical course of patients with acute abdominal conditions. Elderly may be more susceptible to adverse effects (eg, CNS, respiratory, gastrointestinal). Decrease initial dose and use caution in the elderly or debilitated; with hyper/hypothyroidism, morbid obesity, adrenal insufficiency, prostatic hyperplasia, or urethral stricture; or with severe renal or hepatic failure. Use with caution in patients with biliary tract dysfunction; acute pancreatitis may cause constriction of sphincter of Oddi. Safety and efficacy have not been established in children. **[U.S. Boxed Warning]: For oral administration only;** excipients to deter use by injection are contained in tablets.

[U.S. Boxed Warning]: When used for treatment of narcotic addiction: May only be dispensed by opioid treatment programs certified by the Substance Abuse and Mental Health Services Administration (SAMHSA) and certified by the designated state authority. Exceptions include inpatient treatment of other conditions and emergency period (not >3 days) while definitive substance abuse treatment is being sought.

Drug Interactions

Avoid Concomitant Use

Avoid concomitant use of Methadone with any of the following: Artemether; Conivaptan; Dronedarone; Lumefantrine; Nilotinib; Pimozide; QUEtiapine; QuiNINE; Tetrabenazine; Thioridazine; Toremifene; Vandetanib; Vemurafenib; Ziprasidone

Decreased Effect

Methadone may decrease the levels/effects of: Codeine; Didanosine; Pegvisomant; TraMADol

The levels/effects of Methadone may be decreased by: Ammonium Chloride; Barbiturates; Boceprevir; CarBAMazepine; CYP2B6 Inducers (Strong); CYP3A4 Inducers (Strong); Deferasirox; Etravirine; Fosphenytoin; Herbs (CYP3A4 Inducers); Mixed Agonist / Antagonist Opioids; Phenytoin; Protease Inhibitors; Reverse Transcriptase Inhibitors (Non-Nucleoside); Rifamycin Derivatives; Telaprevir; Tocilizumab

Increased Effect/Toxicity

Methadone may increase the levels/effects of: Alcohol (Ethyl); Alvimopan; ARIPiprazole; CNS Depressants; CYP2D6 Substrates; Desmopressin; Dronedarone; Fesoterodine; Nebivolol; Pimozide; QTc-Prolonging Agents; QuiNINE; Selective Serotonin Reuptake Inhibitors; Tamoxifen; Tetrabenazine; Thiazide Diuretics; Thioridazine; Toremifene; Vandetanib; Vemurafenib; Zidovudine; Ziprasidone

The levels/effects of Methadone may be increased by: Alfuzosin; Amphetamines; Antifungal Agents (Azole Derivatives, Systemic); Antipsychotic Agents (Phenothiazines); Artemether; Boceprevir; Chloroquine; Ciprofloxacin; Ciprofloxacin (Systemic); Conivaptan; CYP2B6 Inhibitors (Moderate); CYP2B6 Inhibitors (Strong); CYP3A4 Inhibitors (Moderate); CYP3A4 Inhibitors (Strong); Gadobutrol; HydrOXYzine; Indacaterol; Interferons (Alfa); Ivacaftor; Lumefantrine; MAO Inhibitors; Nilotinib; Quazepam; QUEtiapine; QuiNINE; Selective Serotonin Reuptake Inhibitors; Succinylcholine

Nutritional/Ethanol Interactions

Ethanol: Ethanol may increase CNS depression. Management: Avoid ethanol.

Food: Grapefruit/grapefruit juice may increase levels of methadone. Management: Avoid concurrent use of grapefruit juice.

Herb/Nutraceutical: St John's wort may decrease methadone levels and increase CNS depression; valerian, kava kava, and gotu kola may increase CNS depression. Management: Avoid St John's wort, valerian, kava kava, and gotu kola.

Adverse Reactions Frequency not defined. During prolonged administration, adverse effects may decrease over several weeks; however, constipation and sweating may persist.

Cardiovascular: Arrhythmia, bigeminal rhythms, bradycardia, cardiac arrest, cardiomyopathy, ECG changes, edema, extrasystoles, faintness, flushing, heart failure, hypotension, palpitation, peripheral vasodilation, phlebitis, orthostatic hypotension, QT interval prolonged, shock, syncope, tachycardia, torsade de pointes, T-wave inversion, ventricular fibrillation, ventricular tachycardia,

Central nervous system: Agitation, confusion, disorientation, dizziness, drowsiness, dysphoria, euphoria, hallucination, headache, insomnia, lightheadedness, sedation, seizure

Dermatologic: Hemorrhagic urticaria, pruritus, rash, urticaria

Endocrine & metabolic: Antidiuretic effect, amenorrhea, hypokalemia, hypomagnesemia, libido decreased

Gastrointestinal: Abdominal pain, anorexia, biliary tract spasm, constipation, glossitis, nausea, stomach cramps, vomiting, weight gain, xerostomia

Genitourinary: Impotence, urinary retention or hesitancy

Hematologic: Thrombocytopenia (reversible, reported in patients with chronic hepatitis)

Neuromuscular & skeletal: Weakness

Local: I.M./SubQ injection: Erythema, pain, swelling; I.V. injection: Hemorrhagic urticaria (rare), pruritus, urticaria, rash

Ocular: Miosis, visual disturbances

Respiratory: Pulmonary edema, respiratory depression, respiratory arrest

Miscellaneous: Death, diaphoresis, physical and psychological dependence

Pharmacodynamics/Kinetics

Onset of Action Oral: Analgesic: 0.5-1 hour; Parenteral: 10-20 minutes; Peak effect: Parenteral: 1-2 hours; Oral: Continuous dosing: 3-5 days

Duration of Action Analgesia: Oral: 4-8 hours, increases to 22-48 hours with repeated doses

Controlled Substance C-II

Available Dosage Forms

Injection, solution: 10 mg/mL (20 mL)

Solution, oral: 5 mg/5 mL (500 mL); 10 mg/5 mL (500 mL); 10 mg/mL (946 mL, 960 mL, 1000 mL, 1000s)

Methadone Intensol™: 10 mg/mL (30 mL)

Methadose®: 10 mg/mL (1000 mL)

Tablet, oral: 5 mg, 10 mg

Dolophine®: 5 mg, 10 mg

Tablet, dispersible, oral: 40 mg

Methadone Diskets®: 40 mg

Methadose®: 40 mg

General Dosage Range Dosage adjustment recommended in patients with renal impairment or who develop toxicities

I.M.:

Adults: Initial: 2.5 mg every 8-12 hours

Elderly: 2.5 mg every 8-12 hours

I.V., SubQ: *Adults:* Initial: 2.5 mg every 8-12 hours

Oral:

Adults: Detoxification: Initial: Up to 40 mg/day; Maintenance: 80-120 mg/day; Pain: 2.5-10 mg every 4-12 hours as needed

Elderly: 2.5 mg every 8-12 hours

Administration

Oral Oral dose for detoxification and maintenance may be administered in fruit juice or water. Dispersible tablet should not be chewed or swallowed; add to liquid and allow to dissolve before administering. May rinse if residual remains.

I.V. Detail pH: 4.5-6.5

Stability

Storage

Injection: Store at controlled room temperature of 15°C to 30°C (59°F to 86°F). Protect from light.

Oral concentrate, oral solution, tablet: Store at controlled room temperature of 15°C to 30°C (59°F to 86°F).

Nursing Actions

Physical Assessment Monitor for effectiveness of pain relief. Monitor QT_C, blood pressure, CNS and respiratory status, and degree of sedation at beginning of therapy and periodically thereafter. Assess patient's physical and/or psychological dependence. For inpatients, implement safety measures (eg, side rails up, call light within reach, instructions to call for assistance). Discontinue slowly after prolonged use.

Patient Education May cause physical and/or psychological dependence. While using this medication, do not use alcohol and other prescription or OTC medications (especially sedatives, tranquilizers, antihistamines, or pain medications) without consulting prescriber. Maintain adequate hydration, unless instructed to restrict fluid intake. May cause hypotension, dizziness, drowsiness, impaired coordination, or blurred vision; loss of appetite, nausea, or vomiting; or constipation. Report chest pain, slow or rapid heartbeat, dizziness, or persistent headache; confusion or respiratory difficulties; or severe constipation.

Methamphetamine (meth am FET a meen)

Brand Names: U.S. Desoxyn®

Index Terms Desoxyephedrine Hydrochloride; Methamphetamine Hydrochloride

Pharmacologic Category Anorexiant; Stimulant; Sympathomimetic

Medication Safety Issues

Sound-alike/look-alike issues:

Desoxyn® may be confused with digoxin

BEERS Criteria medication:

This drug may be inappropriate for use in geriatric patients (high severity risk).

Medication Guide Available Yes

Pregnancy Risk Factor C

Lactation Enters breast milk/contraindicated

Use Treatment of attention-deficit/hyperactivity disorder (ADHD); exogenous obesity (short-term adjunct)

Pharmacotherapy for weight loss is recommended only for obese patients with a body mass index ≥30 kg/m^2, or ≥27 kg/m^2 in the presence of other risk factors such as hypertension, diabetes, and/or dyslipidemia or a high waist circumference; therapy should be used in conjunction with a comprehensive weight management program.

Unlabeled Use Narcolepsy

Controlled Substance C-II

Available Dosage Forms

Tablet, oral: 5 mg

Desoxyn®: 5 mg

General Dosage Range Oral:

Children ≥6-11 years: Initial: 5 mg 1-2 times/day; Maintenance: 20-25 mg/day

Children ≥12 years and Adults: ADHD: Initial: 5 mg 1-2 times/day; Maintenance: 20-25 mg/day; Obesity: 5 mg before each meal

Nursing Actions

Physical Assessment Monitor vital signs at beginning of therapy and periodically during therapy.

Patient Education Report chest pain, difficulty breathing, fainting, and visual disturbances.

Methimazole (meth IM a zole)

Brand Names: U.S. Tapazole®

Index Terms Thiamazole

Pharmacologic Category Antithyroid Agent; Thioamide

Medication Safety Issues

Sound-alike/look-alike issues:

Methimazole may be confused with metolazone

Pregnancy Risk Factor D

Lactation Enters breast milk/contraindicated (per manufacturer's labeling) (AAP rates "compatible"; AAP 2001 update pending)

Use Treatment of hyperthyroidism; improve hyperthyroidism prior to thyroidectomy or radioactive iodine therapy

Unlabeled Use

Treatment of Graves' disease

Available Dosage Forms

Tablet, oral: 5 mg, 10 mg

Tapazole®: 5 mg, 10 mg

General Dosage Range Oral:

Children: Initial: 0.4 mg/kg/day in 3 divided doses; Maintenance: 0.2 mg/kg/day in 3 divided doses

Adults: Initial: 15-60 mg/day in 3 divided doses; Maintenance: 5-15 mg/day in 1-3 divided doses

Administration

Other Administer consistently in relation to meals every day. In thyrotoxic crisis, rectal administration has been described (Nabil, 1982).

Nursing Actions

Physical Assessment Monitor for improvement in hyperthyroid symptoms, rash, gastrointestinal upset, leucopenia, anemia, and arthralgia during therapy. Medication can lower blood counts leading to infections. Prolonged use may lead to hypothyroidism.

Patient Education Take at the same time each day, around-the-clock (eg, every 8 hours). This drug will need to be taken for an extended period to achieve appropriate results. Instruct patient that taking dose more frequently or in higher doses will not improve symptoms in a faster period. Medication must be taken as ordered by prescriber. May cause nausea, vomiting, abdominal pain, abnormal taste, dizziness, drowsiness, or unusual CNS stimulation. Inform patient to report any rash; fever; unusual bleeding or bruising; unresolved headache; yellowing of eyes or skin; changes in color of urine or feces; reddened, blistering, or peeling of skin; and unresolved malaise. Patients should not receive any live vaccines, such as MMR, BCG, or nasal influenza, while on medication.

Methocarbamol (meth oh KAR ba mole)

Brand Names: U.S. Robaxin®; Robaxin®-750

Pharmacologic Category Skeletal Muscle Relaxant

Medication Safety Issues

Sound-alike/look-alike issues:

Methocarbamol may be confused with mephobarbital

Robaxin® may be confused with ribavirin, Skelaxin®

International issues:

Robaxin [U.S., Canada, Great Britain, Greece, Spain] may be confused with Rubex brand name for ascorbic acid [Ireland]; doxorubicin [Brazil]

BEERS Criteria medication:

This drug may be inappropriate for use in geriatric patients (high severity risk).

Pregnancy Risk Factor C

Lactation Excretion in breast milk unknown/use caution

Use Adjunctive treatment of muscle spasm associated with acute painful musculoskeletal conditions (eg, tetanus)

Available Dosage Forms

Injection, solution:

Robaxin®: 100 mg/mL (10 mL)

Tablet, oral: 500 mg, 750 mg

Robaxin®: 500 mg

Robaxin®-750: 750 mg

General Dosage Range

I.M.: *Adults:* 1 g every 8 hours (maximum dose: 3 g/day for 3 consecutive days)

I.V.:

Children: 15 mg/kg/dose **or** 500 mg/m²/dose every 6 hours as needed (maximum dose: 1.8 g/m²/day for 3 consecutive days)

Adults: 1-3 g every 6 hours **or** 1 g every 8 hours (maximum dose: 3 g/day for 3 consecutive days)

Oral: *Children ≥16 years and Adults:* Initial: 1.5 g 4 times/day for 2-3 days (maximum: 8 g/day); Maintenance: 4-4.5 g/day in 3-6 divided doses

Administration

Oral Tablets may be crushed and mixed with food or liquid if needed.

I.M. A maximum of 5 mL can be administered into each gluteal region.

I.V. Maximum rate: 3 mL/minute; may be administered undiluted or mixed with 5% dextrose or 0.9% saline (1 vial/≤250 mL diluent). Monitor closely for extravasation. Administer I.V. while in recumbent position. Maintain position for at least 10-15 minutes following infusion.

Nursing Actions

Physical Assessment Assess allergies; packaging contains latex. Monitor I.V. site closely to prevent extravasation. Caution patient about sedation.

Patient Education Do not use alcohol. You may experience drowsiness, dizziness, or lightheadedness. Report excessive drowsiness.

Methotrexate (meth oh TREKS ate)

Brand Names: U.S. Rheumatrex®; Trexall™

Index Terms Amethopterin; Methotrexate Sodium; Methotrexatum; MTX (error-prone abbreviation)

Pharmacologic Category Antineoplastic Agent, Antimetabolite (Antifolate); Antirheumatic, Disease Modifying; Immunosuppressant Agent

Medication Safety Issues

Sound-alike/look-alike issues:

Methotrexate may be confused with mercaptopurine, methylPREDNISolone sodium succinate, metolazone, metroNIDAZOLE, mitoXANtrone, PRALAtrexate

High alert medication:

The Institute for Safe Medication Practices (ISMP) includes this medication among its list of drugs which have a heightened risk of causing significant patient harm when used in error.

Administration issues:

Errors have occurred (resulting in death) when methotrexate was administered as "daily" dose instead of the recommended "weekly" dose.

Intrathecal medication safety: The American Society of Clinical Oncology (ASCO)/Oncology Nursing Society (ONS) chemotherapy administration safety standards (Jacobson, 2009) encourage the following safety measures for intrathecal chemotherapy:

- Intrathecal medication should not be prepared during the preparation of any other agents
- After preparation, store in an isolated location or container clearly marked with a label identifying as "intrathecal" use only
- Delivery to the patient should only be with other medications intended for administration into the central nervous system

Other safety concerns:

MTX is an error-prone abbreviation (mistaken as mitoxantrone)

International issues:

Trexall [U.S.] may be confused with Trexol brand name for tamadol [Mexico]; Truxal brand name for chlorprothixene [multiple international markets]

Pregnancy Risk Factor X (psoriasis, rheumatoid arthritis)

Lactation Enters breast milk/contraindicated

Breast-Feeding Considerations Low amounts of methotrexate are excreted into breast milk. Due to the potential for serious adverse reactions in a breast-feeding infant, use is contraindicated in nursing mothers.

Use

Oncology-related uses: Treatment of trophoblastic neoplasms (gestational choriocarcinoma, chorioadenoma destruens and hydatidiform mole), acute lymphocytic leukemia (ALL), meningeal leukemia, breast cancer, head and neck cancer (epidermoid), cutaneous T-Cell lymphoma (advanced mycosis fungoides), lung cancer (squamous cell and small cell), advanced non-Hodgkin's lymphomas (NHL), osteosarcoma

Nononcology uses: Treatment of psoriasis (severe, recalcitrant, disabling) and severe rheumatoid arthritis (RA), including polyarticular-course juvenile idiopathic arthritis (JIA)

Unlabeled Use Treatment and maintenance of remission in Crohn's disease; ectopic pregnancy; dermatomyositis/polymyositis; bladder cancer, central nervous system tumors (including nonleukemic meningeal cancers), acute promyelocytic leukemia (maintenance treatment), soft tissue sarcoma (desmoid tumors); acute graft-versus-host disease (GVHD) prophylaxis; medical management of abortion; systemic lupus erythematosus; Takayasu arteritis

Mechanism of Action/Effect Methotrexate is a folate antimetabolite that inhibits DNA synthesis. Methotrexate irreversibly binds to dihydrofolate reductase, inhibiting the formation of reduced folates, and thymidylate synthetase, resulting in inhibition of purine and thymidylic acid synthesis. Methotrexate is cell cycle specific for the S phase of the cycle.

The MOA in the treatment of rheumatoid arthritis is unknown, but may affect immune function. In psoriasis, methotrexate is thought to target rapidly proliferating epithelial cells in the skin.

In Crohn's disease, it may have immune modulator and anti-inflammatory activity

Contraindications Hypersensitivity to methotrexate or any component of the formulation; breast-feeding

Additional contraindications for patients with psoriasis or rheumatoid arthritis: Pregnancy, alcoholism, alcoholic liver disease or other chronic liver disease, immunodeficiency syndrome (overt or laboratory evidence); pre-existing blood dyscrasias (eg, bone marrow hypoplasia, leukopenia, thrombocytopenia, significant anemia)

Warnings/Precautions Hazardous agent - use appropriate precautions for handling and disposal.

[U.S. Boxed Warning]: Methotrexate has been associated with acute (elevated transaminases) and potentially fatal chronic (fibrosis, cirrhosis) hepatotoxicity. Risk is related to cumulative dose and prolonged exposure. Monitor closely (with liver function tests, including serum albumin) for liver toxicities. Liver enzyme elevations may be noted, but may not be predictive of hepatic disease in long term treatment for psoriasis (but generally is predictive in rheumatoid arthritis [RA] treatment). With long-term use, liver biopsy may show histologic changes, fibrosis, or cirrhosis; periodic liver biopsy is recommended with long-term use for psoriasis patients with risk factors for hepatotoxicity and for persistent abnormal liver function tests in psoriasis patients without risk factors for hepatotoxicity and in RA patients; discontinue methotrexate with moderate-to-severe change in liver biopsy. Risk factors for hepatotoxicity include history of above moderate ethanol consumption, persistent abnormal liver chemistries, history of chronic liver disease (including hepatitis B or C), family history of inheritable liver disease, diabetes, obesity, hyperlipidemia, lack of folate supplementation during methotrexate therapy, and history of significant exposure to hepatotoxic drugs. Use caution with preexisting liver impairment; may require dosage reduction. Use caution when used with other hepatotoxic agents (azathioprine, retinoids, sulfasalazine). **[U.S. Boxed Warning]: Methotrexate elimination is reduced in patients with ascites;** may require dose reduction or discontinuation. Monitor closely for toxicity.

[U.S. Boxed Warning]: May cause renal damage leading to acute renal failure, especially with high-dose methotrexate; monitor renal function and methotrexate levels closely, maintain adequate hydration and urinary alkalinization. Use caution in osteosarcoma patients treated with high-dose methotrexate in combination with nephrotoxic chemotherapy (eg, cisplatin). **[U.S. Boxed Warning]: Methotrexate elimination is reduced in patients with renal impairment;** may require dose reduction or discontinuation; monitor closely for toxicity. **[U.S. Boxed Warning]: Tumor lysis syndrome may occur in patients with high tumor burden;** use appropriate prevention and treatment.

[U.S. Boxed Warning]: May cause potentially life-threatening pneumonitis (may occur at any time during therapy and at any dosage); monitor closely for pulmonary symptoms, particularly dry, nonproductive cough. Other potential symptoms include fever, dyspnea, hypoxemia, or pulmonary infiltrate. **[U.S. Boxed Warning]: Methotrexate elimination is reduced in patients with pleural effusions;** may require dose reduction or discontinuation. Monitor closely for toxicity.

[U.S. Boxed Warning]: Bone marrow suppression may occur, resulting in anemia, aplastic anemia, pancytopenia, leukopenia, neutropenia, and/or thrombocytopenia. Use caution in patients with pre-existing bone marrow suppression. Discontinue therapy in RA or psoriasis if a significant decrease in hematologic components is noted. **[U.S. Boxed Warning]: Use of low dose methotrexate has been associated with the development of malignant lymphomas;** may regress upon discontinuation of therapy; treat lymphoma appropriately if regression is not induced by cessation of methotrexate.

[U.S. Boxed Warning]: Diarrhea and ulcerative stomatitis may require interruption of therapy; death from hemorrhagic enteritis or intestinal perforation has been reported. Use with caution in patients with peptic ulcer disease, ulcerative colitis.

May cause neurotoxicity including seizures (usually in pediatric ALL patients), leukoencephalopathy (usually with concurrent cranial irradiation) and stroke-like encephalopathy (usually with high-dose regimens). Chemical arachnoiditis (headache, back pain, nuchal rigidity, fever), myelopathy and chronic leukoencephalopathy may result from intrathecal administration.

[U.S. Boxed Warning]: Any dose level or route of administration may cause severe and potentially fatal dermatologic reactions, including toxic epidermal necrolysis, Stevens-Johnson syndrome, exfoliative dermatitis, skin necrosis, and erythema multiforme. Radiation dermatitis and sunburn may be precipitated by methotrexate administration. Psoriatic lesions may be worsened by concomitant exposure to ultraviolet radiation.

[U.S. Boxed Warning]: Concomitant administration with NSAIDs may cause severe bone marrow suppression, aplastic anemia, and GI toxicity. Do not administer NSAIDs prior to or during high dose methotrexate therapy; may increase and prolong serum methotrexate levels. Doses used for psoriasis may still lead to unexpected toxicities; use caution when administering NSAIDs or salicylates with lower doses of methotrexate for RA. Methotrexate may increase the levels and effects of mercaptopurine; may require dosage adjustments. Vitamins containing folate may decrease response to systemic methotrexate; folate deficiency may increase methotrexate toxicity. **[U.S. Boxed Warning]: Concomitant methotrexate administration with radiotherapy may increase the risk of soft tissue necrosis and osteonecrosis.**

[U.S. Boxed Warnings]: Should be administered under the supervision of a physician experienced in the use of antimetabolite therapy; serious and fatal toxicities have occurred at all dose levels. Immune suppression may lead to potentially fatal opportunistic infections. For rheumatoid arthritis and psoriasis, immunosuppressive therapy should only be used when disease is active and less toxic, traditional therapy is ineffective. Methotrexate formulations and/or diluents containing preservatives should not be used for intrathecal or high-dose therapy. May cause fetal death or congenital abnormalities; do not use for psoriasis or RA treatment in pregnant women. May cause impairment of fertility, oligospermia, and menstrual dysfunction. Toxicity from methotrexate or any immunosuppressive is increased in the elderly. Methotrexate injection may contain benzyl alcohol and should not be used in neonates. Errors have occurred (some resulting in death) when methotrexate was administered as "daily" dose instead of an intended "weekly" dose.

When used for intrathecal administration, should not be prepared during the preparation of any other agents; after preparation, store intrathecal medications in an isolated location or container clearly marked with a label identifying as "intrathecal" use only; delivery of intrathecal medications to the patient should only be with other medications intended for administration into the central nervous system (Jacobson, 2009).

Drug Interactions

Avoid Concomitant Use

Avoid concomitant use of Methotrexate with any of the following: Acitretin; BCG; CloZAPine; Natalizumab; Pimecrolimus; Tacrolimus (Topical)

Decreased Effect

Methotrexate may decrease the levels/effects of: BCG; Cardiac Glycosides; Coccidioidin Skin Test; Loop Diuretics; Sapropterin; Sipuleucel-T; Vaccines (Inactivated); Vitamin K Antagonists

The levels/effects of Methotrexate may be decreased by: Bile Acid Sequestrants; Echinacea; P-glycoprotein/ABCB1 Inducers

Increased Effect/Toxicity

Methotrexate may increase the levels/effects of: CloZAPine; CycloSPORINE; CycloSPORINE (Systemic); Leflunomide; Loop Diuretics; Natalizumab; Theophylline Derivatives; Vaccines (Live); Vitamin K Antagonists

The levels/effects of Methotrexate may be increased by: Acitretin; Ciprofloxacin; Ciprofloxacin (Systemic); CycloSPORINE; CycloSPORINE (Systemic); Denosumab; Eltrombopag; Loop Diuretics; Nonsteroidal Anti-Inflammatory Agents; Penicillins; P-glycoprotein/ABCB1 Inhibitors; Pimecrolimus; Probenecid; Proton Pump Inhibitors; Roflumilast; Salicylates; SulfaSALAzine; Sulfonamide Derivatives; Tacrolimus (Topical); Trastuzumab; Trimethoprim

Nutritional/Ethanol Interactions

Ethanol: Ethanol may be associated with increased liver injury. Management: Avoid ethanol.

Food: Methotrexate peak serum levels may be decreased if taken with food. Milk-rich foods may decrease methotrexate absorption. Folate may decrease drug response.

Herb/Nutraceutical: Echinacea has immunostimulant properties. Management: Avoid echinacea.

Adverse Reactions Note: Adverse reactions vary by route and dosage. Hematologic and/or gastrointestinal toxicities may be common at dosages used in chemotherapy; these reactions are much less frequent when used at typical dosages for rheumatic diseases.

>10%:

Central nervous system (with I.T. administration or very high-dose therapy):

Arachnoiditis: Acute reaction manifested as severe headache, nuchal rigidity, vomiting, and fever; may be alleviated by reducing the dose

Subacute toxicity: 10% of patients treated with 12-15 mg of I.T. methotrexate may develop this in the second or third week of therapy; consists of motor paralysis of extremities, cranial nerve palsy, seizure, or coma. This has also been seen in pediatric cases receiving very high-dose I.V. methotrexate.

Demyelinating encephalopathy: Seen months or years after receiving methotrexate; usually in association with cranial irradiation or other systemic chemotherapy

Dermatologic: Reddening of skin

Endocrine & metabolic: Hyperuricemia, defective oogenesis or spermatogenesis

Gastrointestinal: Ulcerative stomatitis, glossitis, gingivitis, nausea, vomiting, diarrhea, anorexia, intestinal perforation, mucositis (dose dependent; appears in 3-7 days after therapy, resolving within 2 weeks)

Hematologic: Leukopenia, myelosuppression (nadir: 7-10 days), thrombocytopenia

Renal: Renal failure, azotemia, nephropathy

Respiratory: Pharyngitis

1% to 10%:

Cardiovascular: Vasculitis

Central nervous system: Dizziness, malaise, encephalopathy, seizure, fever, chills

Dermatologic: Alopecia, rash, photosensitivity, depigmentation or hyperpigmentation of skin

Endocrine & metabolic: Diabetes

Genitourinary: Cystitis

Hematologic: Hemorrhage

Hepatic: Cirrhosis and portal fibrosis have been associated with chronic methotrexate therapy; acute elevation of liver enzymes are common after high-dose methotrexate, and usually resolve within 10 days.

Neuromuscular & skeletal: Arthralgia

Ocular: Blurred vision

Renal: Renal dysfunction: Manifested by an abrupt rise in serum creatinine and BUN and a fall in urine output; more common with high-dose methotrexate, and may be due to precipitation of the drug.

Respiratory: Pneumonitis: Associated with fever, cough, and interstitial pulmonary infiltrates; treatment is to withhold methotrexate during the acute reaction; interstitial pneumonitis has been reported to occur with an incidence of 1% in patients with RA (dose 7.5-15 mg/week)

Pharmacodynamics/Kinetics

Onset of Action Antirheumatic: 3-6 weeks; additional improvement may continue longer than 12 weeks

Available Dosage Forms

Injection, powder for reconstitution: 1 g

Injection, solution: 25 mg/mL (2 mL, 10 mL)

Injection, solution [preservative free]: 25 mg/mL (2 mL, 4 mL, 8 mL, 10 mL, 20 mL, 40 mL, 100 mL)

Tablet, oral: 2.5 mg

Rheumatrex®: 2.5 mg

Trexall™: 5 mg, 7.5 mg, 10 mg, 15 mg

General Dosage Range Dosage adjustment recommended in patients with hepatic or renal impairment

I.M., oral:

Children: 5-30 mg/m² once weekly or every 2 weeks

Adults: Dosage varies greatly depending on indication

I.V.:

Children: 10-18,000 mg/m² bolus dosing or continuous infusion over 6-42 hours

Adults: Dosage varies greatly depending on indication

Intrathecal:

Children <1 year: 6 mg/dose

Children 1 year: 8 mg/dose

Children 2 years: 10 mg/dose

Children ≥3 years and Adults: 12 mg/dose

Administration

I.M. May be administered I.M.

I.V. May be administered I.V.; I.V. administration may be as slow push, short bolus infusion, or 24- to 42-hour continuous infusion

Specific dosing schemes vary, but high dose should be followed by leucovorin calcium to prevent toxicity; refer to Leucovorin Calcium monograph on page 679

Other May be administered I.T or SubQ.

Stability

Reconstitution Use appropriate precautions for handling and disposal. **Use preservative-free preparations for intrathecal or high-dose methotrexate administration.**

I.M., I.V., SubQ: Dilute powder with D_5W or NS to a concentration of ≤25 mg/mL (20 mg and 50 mg vials) and 50 mg/mL (1 g vial). May further dilute in D_5W or NS.

Intrathecal: Prepare intrathecal solutions with preservative-free NS, lactated Ringer's, or Elliot's B solution to a final volume of up to 12 mL (volume generally based on institution or practitioner preference). Intrathecal methotrexate concentrations may be institution specific or based on practitioner preference, generally ranging from a final concentration of 1 mg/mL (per prescribing information; Grossman, 1993; Lin, 2008) up to ~2-4 mg/mL (de Lemos, 2009; Glantz, 1999). For triple intrathecal therapy (methotrexate 12 mg/hydrocortisone 24 mg/cytarabine 36 mg), preparation to final volume of 12 mL is reported (Lin, 2008). Intrathecal medications should **NOT** be prepared during the preparation of any other agents.

Storage Store tablets and intact vials at room temperature (15°C to 25°C). Protect from light.

I.M., I.V., SubQ: Solution diluted in D_5W or NS is stable for 24 hours at room temperature (21°C to 25°C). Reconstituted solutions with a preservative may be stored under refrigeration for up to 3 months, and up to 4 weeks at room temperature.

Intrathecal: Intrathecal dilutions are preservative free and should be used as soon as possible after preparation. After preparation, store intrathecal medications (until use) in an isolated location or container clearly marked with a label identifying as "intrathecal" use only.

Nursing Actions

Physical Assessment Monitor frequently for pneumonitis (dry, nonproductive cough), gastrointestinal disturbance (ulcerative stomatitis, pain, intestinal perforation), dermatological reactions, and renal failure (decreased urine output).

Patient Education You will be more susceptible to infection. May cause sensitivity to sunlight, nausea, vomiting, drowsiness, dizziness, numbness, blurred vision, loss of hair (may be reversible), color change of skin, permanent sterility, or mouth sores. Report immediately any new skin rash, eruptions, redness, or peeling; respiratory difficulty, fever, or cough; rapid heartbeat or palpitations; black or tarry stools; fever; chills; unusual bleeding or bruising; persistent GI disturbances (abdominal pain, diarrhea, constipation); or pain on urination or change in urinary patterns. Oral: It is very important to maintain adequate nutrition and hydration. Avoid alcohol. Infusion/injection: Report immediately any redness, swelling, pain, or burning at infusion/injection site.

Dietary Considerations Some products may contain sodium.

Methoxsalen (Topical) (meth OKS a len)

Brand Names: U.S. Oxsoralen®

Index Terms Methoxypsoralen

Pharmacologic Category Psoralen

Pregnancy Risk Factor C

Lactation Excretion in breast milk unknown/not recommended

Use Repigmentation of idiopathic vitiligo

Available Dosage Forms

Lotion, topical:

Oxsoralen®: 1% (29.57 mL)

General Dosage Range Topical: *Children ≥12 years and Adults:* Lotion is applied by healthcare provider prior to UVA light exposure, usually no more than once weekly

Administration

Topical Hands and fingers of person applying the lotion should be protected to prevent possible photosensitization and/or burns.

Nursing Actions

Physical Assessment This drug is administered in conjunction with ultraviolet light or ultraviolet radiation therapy. Teach patient sunlight precautions.

Patient Education This medication is used in conjunction with specific ultraviolet treatment. Control exposure to direct sunlight as per prescriber's instructions. Consult prescriber immediately if burning, blistering, or skin irritation occur.

Methyldopa (meth il DOE pa)

Index Terms Aldomet; Methyldopate Hydrochloride

Pharmacologic Category Alpha$_2$-Adrenergic Agonist

Medication Safety Issues

Sound-alike/look-alike issues:

Methyldopa may be confused with L-dopa, levodopa

BEERS Criteria medication:

This drug may be inappropriate for use in geriatric patients (high severity risk).

Pregnancy Risk Factor B

Lactation Enters breast milk/use caution (AAP rates "compatible"; AAP 2001 update pending)

Use Management of moderate-to-severe hypertension

Available Dosage Forms

Injection, solution: 50 mg/mL (5 mL)

Tablet, oral: 250 mg, 500 mg

General Dosage Range Dosage adjustment recommended in patients with renal impairment

I.V.:

Children: 5-10 mg/kg/dose every 6-8 hours (maximum: 65 mg/kg/day; 3 g/day)

Adults: 250-500 mg every 6-8 hours (maximum: 1 g every 6 hours)

Oral:

Children: Initial: 10 mg/kg/day in 2-4 divided doses; Maintenance: Up to 65 mg/kg/day (maximum: 3 g/day)

Adults: Initial: 250 mg 2-3 times/day; Maintenance: 250-1000 mg/day in 2 divided doses (maximum: 3 g/day)

Elderly: Initial: 125 mg 1-2 times/day

Administration

I.V. Infuse over 30 minutes.

Nursing Actions

Physical Assessment Monitor for hypotension, bradycardia, or CNS changes on a regular basis

Patient Education Oral: Follow recommended diet and exercise program. Periodic laboratory tests may be required. This medication may cause altered color of urine (normal), drowsiness, dizziness, impaired judgment, postural hypotension, dry mouth, or nausea. Report altered CNS status (eg, nightmares, depression, anxiety, increased nervousness); sudden weight gain; unusual or persistent swelling of ankles, feet, or extremities; palpitations or rapid heartbeat; persistent weakness or fatigue; or unusual bleeding.

Methylergonovine (meth il er goe NOE veen)

Brand Names: U.S. Methergine®

Index Terms Methylergometrine Maleate; Methylergonovine Maleate

Pharmacologic Category Ergot Derivative

Medication Safety Issues

Sound-alike/look-alike issues:

Methergine® may be confused with Brethine

Methylergonovine and terbutaline parenteral dosage forms look similar. Due to their contrasting indications, use care when administering these agents.

Pregnancy Risk Factor C

Lactation Enters breast milk/use caution

Use Prevention and treatment of postpartum and postabortion hemorrhage caused by uterine atony or subinvolution

Available Dosage Forms

Injection, solution: 0.2 mg/mL (1 mL)

Methergine®: 0.2 mg/mL (1 mL)

Tablet, oral: 0.2 mg

Methergine®: 0.2 mg

General Dosage Range

I.M., I.V.: *Adults:* 0.2 mg after delivery; may repeat every 2-4 hours

Oral: *Adults:* 0.2 mg 3-4 times/day in the puerperium

Administration

I.V. Administer over ≥60 seconds. Should not be routinely administered I.V. because of possibility of inducing sudden hypertension and cerebrovascular accident.

I.V. Detail pH: 2.7-3.5

Nursing Actions

Physical Assessment Monitor blood pressure, CNS status, and vaginal bleeding on a regular basis. May cause nausea. Patient may require antiemetic.

Patient Education May cause nausea, vomiting, dizziness, or headache. Report immediately any chest pain or tightness; jaw, shoulder, or midback pain; difficulty breathing; headache; cold extremities; or severe abdominal cramping.

Methylnaltrexone (meth il nal TREKS one)

Brand Names: U.S. Relistor®

Index Terms Methylnaltrexone Bromide; N-methylnaltrexone Bromide

Pharmacologic Category Gastrointestinal Agent, Miscellaneous; Opioid Antagonist, Peripherally-Acting

Medication Safety Issues

Sound-alike/look-alike issues:

Methylnaltrexone may be confused with naltrexone

Pregnancy Risk Factor B

Lactation Excretion in breast milk unknown/use caution

Use Treatment of opioid-induced constipation in patients with advanced illness receiving palliative care with inadequate response to conventional laxative regimens

Mechanism of Action/Effect Peripherally-acting mu-opioid receptor antagonist which decreases opioid-induced constipation without affecting opioid analgesic effects or inducing opioid withdrawal symptom

Contraindications Known or suspected mechanical bowel obstruction

Canadian labeling: Additional contraindications (not in U.S. labeling): Hypersensitivity to methylnaltrexone or any component of the formulation

Warnings/Precautions Discontinue treatment for severe or persistent diarrhea. Gastrointestinal perforation of the colon, duodenum, and stomach has been reported (rarely) in patients with advanced illnesses associated with impaired structural integrity of the GI wall (eg, cancer, Ogilvie's syndrome, peptic ulcer). Use caution in patients with known or history of GI tract lesions; discontinue therapy if persistent, severe, or worsening abdominal symptoms occur. Use with caution in patients with renal impairment; dosage adjustment recommended for severe renal impairment (Cl_{cr} <30 mL/minute). Has not been studied in patients with end-stage renal impairment requiring dialysis. Discontinue methylnaltrexone if opioids are discontinued. Use has not been studied in patients with peritoneal catheters. Use beyond 4 months has not been studied.

Drug Interactions

Avoid Concomitant Use There are no known interactions where it is recommended to avoid concomitant use.

Decreased Effect

The levels/effects of Methylnaltrexone may be decreased by: Peginterferon Alfa-2b

Increased Effect/Toxicity There are no known significant interactions involving an increase in effect.

Adverse Reactions

>10%: Gastrointestinal: Abdominal pain (29%), flatulence (13%), nausea (12%)

1% to 10%:

Central nervous system: Dizziness (7%)

Dermatologic: Hyperhidrosis (7%)

Gastrointestinal: Diarrhea (6%)

Pharmacodynamics/Kinetics

Onset of Action Usually within 30-60 minutes (in responding patients)

Available Dosage Forms

Injection, solution:

Relistor®: 8 mg/0.4 mL (0.4 mL); 12 mg/0.6 mL (0.6 mL)

General Dosage Range Dosage adjustment recommended in patients with renal impairment

SubQ:

Adults <38 kg and >114 kg: 0.15 mg/kg (round dose up to nearest 0.1 mL of volume) every other day as needed (maximum: 1 dose/24 hours)

Adults 38 to <62 kg: 8 mg every other day as needed (maximum: 1 dose/24 hours)

Adults 62-114 kg: 12 mg every other day as needed (maximum: 1 dose/24 hours)

Administration

Other SubQ: Administer subcutaneously into upper arm, abdomen, or thigh. Rotate injection site. Do not use tender, bruised, red, or hard areas.

Stability

Storage Store intact vials and prefilled syringes at room temperature of 20°C to 25°C (68°F to 77°F); excursions permitted to 15°C to 30°C (59°F to 86°F); do not freeze. Protect from light. Solution withdrawn from the single-use vial is stable in a syringe for 24 hours at room temperature (protection from light during this 24 hours is not necessary).

Nursing Actions

Physical Assessment Contact prescriber if severe or persistent diarrhea occurs; may be discontinued. Must be discontinued if opioids are discontinued. Teach patient appropriate injection technique and syringe/needle disposal.

Patient Education This medication can only be administered via injection. If self-administered, follow instructions for injection and syringe/needle disposal. May cause dizziness. Report immediately any severe or persistent diarrhea or gastrointestinal upset (pain, nausea, vomiting).

Methylphenidate (meth il FEN i date)

Brand Names: U.S. Concerta®; Daytrana®; Metadate CD®; Metadate® ER; Methylin®; Methylin® ER [DSC]; Ritalin LA®; Ritalin-SR®; Ritalin®

Index Terms Methylphenidate Hydrochloride

Pharmacologic Category Central Nervous System Stimulant

Medication Safety Issues

Sound-alike/look-alike issues:

Metadate CD® may be confused with Metadate® ER

Metadate® ER may be confused with methadone

Methylphenidate may be confused with methadone

Ritalin® may be confused with Rifadin®, ritodrine

Ritalin LA® may be confused with Ritalin-SR®

Medication Guide Available Yes

Pregnancy Risk Factor C

Lactation Enters breast milk/use caution

Breast-Feeding Considerations Methylphenidate excretion into breast milk has been noted in case reports. In both cases, the authors calculated the relative infant dose to be ≤0.2% of the weight adjusted maternal dose. Adverse events were not noted in either infant, however, both were older (6 months of age and 11 months of age) and exposure was limited.

Use Treatment of attention-deficit/hyperactivity disorder (ADHD); symptomatic management of narcolepsy

Unlabeled Use Depression (especially elderly or medically ill)

Mechanism of Action/Effect Mild CNS stimulant; blocks the reuptake of norepinephrine and dopamine into presynaptic neurons; appears to stimulate the cerebral cortex and subcortical structures similar to amphetamines

Contraindications Hypersensitivity to methylphenidate, any component of the formulation, or idiosyncratic reactions to sympathomimetic amines; marked anxiety, tension, and agitation; glaucoma; use during or within 14 days following MAO inhibitor therapy; family history or diagnosis of Tourette's syndrome or tics

Metadate CD® and Metadate® ER: Additional contraindications: Severe hypertension, heart failure, arrhythmia, hyperthyroidism, recent MI or angina; concomitant use of halogenated anesthetics

Warnings/Precautions CNS stimulant use has been associated with serious cardiovascular events (eg, sudden death in children and adolescents; sudden death, stroke, and MI in adults) in patients with pre-existing structural cardiac abnormalities or other serious heart problems. These products should be avoided in patients with known serious structural cardiac abnormalities, cardiomyopathy, serious heart rhythm abnormalities, or other serious cardiac problems that could further increase their risk of sudden death. Patients should be carefully evaluated for cardiac disease prior to initiation of therapy. Use of stimulants can cause an increase in blood pressure (average 2-4 mm Hg) and increases in heart rate (average 3-6 bpm), although some patients may have larger than average increases. Use caution with hypertension, hyperthyroidism, or other cardiovascular conditions that might be exacerbated by increases in blood pressure or heart rate. Some products are contraindicated in patients with heart failure, arrhythmias, severe hypertension, hyperthyroidism, angina, or recent MI.

Has demonstrated value as part of a comprehensive treatment program for ADHD. Use with caution in patients with bipolar disorder (may induce mixed/manic episode). May exacerbate symptoms of behavior and thought disorder in psychotic patients; new-onset psychosis or mania may occur with stimulant use; observe for symptoms of aggression and/or hostility. Use caution with seizure disorders (may reduce seizure threshold). Use caution in patients with history of ethanol or drug abuse. May exacerbate symptoms of behavior and thought disorder in psychotic patients. **[U.S. Boxed Warning]: Potential for drug dependency exists - avoid abrupt discontinuation in patients who have received for prolonged periods.** Visual disturbances have been reported (rare). Not labeled for use in children <6 years of age. Use of stimulants has been associated with suppression of growth in children; monitor growth rate during treatment.

Concerta® should not be used in patients with esophageal motility disorders or pre-existing severe gastrointestinal narrowing (small bowel disease, short gut syndrome, history of peritonitis, cystic fibrosis, chronic intestinal pseudo-obstruction, Meckel's diverticulum). Metadate CD® contains sucrose; avoid administration in fructose intolerance, glucose-galactose malabsorption, or sucrase-isomaltase insufficiency. Metadate® ER contains lactose; avoid administration in hereditary galactose intolerance, Lapp lactase deficiency, or glucose-galactose malabsorption. Concomitant use with halogenated anesthetics is contraindicated; may cause sudden elevations in blood pressure; if surgery is planned, do not administer Metadate CD® or Metadate® ER on the day of surgery. Transdermal system may cause allergic contact sensitization, characterized by intense local reactions (edema, papules) that may spread beyond the patch site; sensitization may subsequently manifest systemically with other routes of methylphenidate administration; monitor closely. Avoid exposure of application site to any direct external heat sources (eg, hair dryers, heating pads, electric blankets); may increase the rate and extent of absorption and risk of overdose. Efficacy of transdermal methylphenidate therapy for >7 weeks has not been established.

Drug Interactions

Avoid Concomitant Use

Avoid concomitant use of Methylphenidate with any of the following: Inhalational Anesthetics; Iobenguane I 123; MAO Inhibitors

Decreased Effect

Methylphenidate may decrease the levels/effects of: Antihypertensives; Iobenguane I 123; Ioflupane I 123

Increased Effect/Toxicity

Methylphenidate may increase the levels/effects of: Anti-Parkinson's Agents (Dopamine Agonist); Antipsychotics; CloNIDine; Fosphenytoin; Inhalational Anesthetics; PHENobarbital; Phenytoin; Primidone; Sympathomimetics; Tricyclic Antidepressants; Vitamin K Antagonists

The levels/effects of Methylphenidate may be increased by: Antacids; Antipsychotics; Atomoxetine; Cannabinoids; H2-Antagonists; MAO Inhibitors; Proton Pump Inhibitors

Nutritional/Ethanol Interactions

Ethanol: Avoid ethanol (may cause CNS depression).

Food: Food may increase oral absorption; Concerta® formulation is not affected. Food delays early peak and high-fat meals increase C_{max} and AUC of Metadate CD® formulation.

Herb/Nutraceutical: Avoid ephedra (may cause hypertension or arrhythmias) and yohimbe (also has CNS stimulatory activity).

Adverse Reactions

All dosage forms: Frequency not defined:

Cardiovascular: Angina, cardiac arrhythmia, cerebral arteritis, cerebral hemorrhage, cerebral occlusion, cerebrovascular accidents, vasculitis, hyper-/hypotension, MI, murmur, palpitation, pulse increased/decreased, Raynaud's phenomenon, tachycardia

Central nervous system: Aggression, agitation, anger, anxiety, confusional state, depression, dizziness, drowsiness, fatigue, fever, headache, hypervigilance, insomnia, irritability, lethargy, mood alterations, nervousness, neuroleptic malignant syndrome (NMS) (rare), restlessness, stroke, tension, Tourette's syndrome (rare), toxic psychosis, tremor, vertigo

Dermatologic: Alopecia, erythema multiforme, exfoliative dermatitis, hyperhidrosis, rash, urticaria

Endocrine & metabolic: Dysmenorrhea, growth retardation, libido decreased

Gastrointestinal: Abdominal pain, anorexia, appetite decreased, bruxism, constipation, diarrhea, dyspepsia, nausea, vomiting, weight loss, xerostomia

Genitourinary: Erectile dysfunction

Hematologic: Anemia, leukopenia, pancytopenia, thrombocytopenic purpura, thrombocytopenia

Hepatic: Bilirubin increased, liver function tests abnormal, hepatic coma, transaminases increased

Neuromuscular & skeletal: Arthralgia, dyskinesia, muscle tightness, paresthesia

Ocular: Blurred vision, dry eyes, mydriasis, visual accommodation disturbance

Renal: Necrotizing vasculitis

Respiratory: Cough increased, dyspnea, pharyngitis, pharyngolaryngeal pain, rhinitis, sinusitis, upper respiratory tract infection

Miscellaneous: Accidental injury, hypersensitivity reactions

Transdermal system: Frequency of adverse events as reported in trials of 7-week duration. Incidence of some events higher with extended use.

>10%:

Central nervous system: Headache (≤15%; long-term use in children: 28%), insomnia (6% to 13%; long-term use in children: 30%), irritability (7% to 11%)

Gastrointestinal: Appetite decreased (26%), nausea (10% to 12%)

Miscellaneous: Viral infection (long-term use in children: 28%)

1% to 10%:

Cardiovascular: Tachycardia (≤1%)

Central nervous system: Tic (7%), dizziness (adolescents 6%), emotional instability (6%)

Gastrointestinal: Vomiting (3% to 10%), weight loss (6% to 9%), abdominal pain (5% to 7%), anorexia (5%; long-term use in children: 46%)

Local: Application site reaction

Respiratory: Nasal congestion (6%) nasopharyngitis (5%)

Postmarketing and/or case reports (limited to important or life-threatening): Allergic contact dermatitis/sensitization, anaphylaxis, angioedema, hallucinations, seizures

Pharmacodynamics/Kinetics

Onset of Action Peak effect:

Immediate release tablet: Cerebral stimulation: ~2 hours

Extended release capsule (Metadate CD®, Ritalin LA®): Biphasic; initial peak similar to immediate release product, followed by second rising portion (corresponding to extended release portion)

Sustained release tablet: 4-7 hours

Osmotic release tablet (Concerta®): Initial: 1-2 hours

Transdermal: ~2 hours; may be expedited by the application of external heat

Duration of Action Immediate release tablet: 3-6 hours; Sustained release tablet: 8 hours; Extended release tablet: Methylin® ER, Metadate® ER: 8 hours; Concerta®: 12 hours

Controlled Substance C-II

Available Dosage Forms

Capsule, extended release, oral: 20 mg, 30 mg, 40 mg

Metadate CD®: 10 mg, 20 mg, 30 mg, 40 mg, 50 mg, 60 mg

Ritalin LA®: 10 mg, 20 mg, 30 mg, 40 mg

Patch, transdermal:

Daytrana®: 10 mg/9 hours (30s); 15 mg/9 hours (30s); 20 mg/9 hours (30s); 30 mg/9 hours (30s)

Solution, oral: 5 mg/5 mL (500 mL); 10 mg/mL (500 mL)

Methylin®: 5 mg/5 mL (500 mL); 10 mg/5 mL (500 mL)

Tablet, oral: 5 mg, 10 mg, 20 mg

Ritalin®: 5 mg, 10 mg, 20 mg

Tablet, chewable, oral:

Methylin®: 2.5 mg, 5 mg, 10 mg

Tablet, extended release, oral: 10 mg, 18 mg, 20 mg, 27 mg, 36 mg, 54 mg

Concerta®: 18 mg, 27 mg, 36 mg, 54 mg

Metadate® ER: 20 mg

Tablet, sustained release, oral: 20 mg

Ritalin-SR®: 20 mg

General Dosage Range

Oral:

Immediate release:

Children ≥6 years: Initial: 5 mg twice daily; Maintenance: Increase by 5-10 mg/day at weekly intervals (maximum: 60 mg/day)

Adults: ADHD: Initial: 5 mg twice daily; Maintenance: Increase by 5-10 mg/day at weekly intervals (maximum: 60 mg/day); Narcolepsy: 10 mg 2-3 times/day (maximum: 60 mg/day)

Extended release:

Children 6-12 years: Concerta®: 18-54 mg once every morning (maximum: 54 mg/day); Metadate® ER, Methylin® ER, Ritalin® SR: Maximum: 60 mg/day; Metadate CD®, Ritalin LA®: Initial: 20 mg once daily (maximum: 60 mg/day)

Children 13-17 years and Adults: Concerta®: 18-72 mg once every morning (maximum: 72 mg/day); Metadate CD®, Ritalin LA®: Initial: 20 mg once daily (maximum: 60 mg/day)

Transdermal: *Children 6-17 years:* Initial: 10 mg patch once daily

Administration

Oral Do not crush or allow patient to chew sustained or extended release dosage form. To effectively avoid insomnia, dosing should be completed by noon.

Concerta®: Administer dose once daily in the morning. May be taken with or without food, but must be taken with water, milk, or juice.

Metadate CD®, Ritalin LA®: Capsules may be opened and the contents sprinkled onto a small amount (equal to 1 tablespoon) of cold applesauce. Swallow applesauce without chewing. Do not crush or chew capsule contents.

Methylin® chewable tablet: Administer with at least 8 ounces of water or other fluid.

Topical Transdermal (Daytrana™): Apply to clean, dry, non-oily, intact skin to the hip area, avoiding the waistline; do not premedicate the patch site with hydrocortisone or other solutions, creams, ointments, or emollients. Apply at the same time each day to alternating hips. Press firmly for 30 seconds to ensure proper adherence. Avoid exposure of application site to external heat source, which may increase the amount of drug absorbed. If difficulty is experienced when separating the patch from the liner or if any medication (sticky substance) remains on the liner after separation; discard that patch and apply a new patch. Do not use a patch that has been damaged or torn; do not cut patch. If patch should dislodge, may replace with new patch (to different site) but total wear time should not exceed 9 hours; do not reapply with dressings, tape, or common adhesives. Patch may be removed early if a shorter duration of effect is desired or if late day side effects occur. Wash hands with soap and water after handling. Avoid touching the sticky side of the patch. If patch removal is difficult, an oil-based product (eg, petroleum jelly, olive oil) may be applied to the patch edges to aid removal; never apply acetone-based products (eg, nail polish remover) to patch. Dispose of used patch by folding adhesive side onto itself, and discard in toilet or appropriate lidded container.

Stability

Storage

Capsule: *Extended release:* Store at 25°C (77°F); excursions permitted to 15°C to 30°C (59°F to 86°F). Protect from light.

Solution: Store at controlled room temperature of 20°C to 25°C (68°F to 77°F).

Tablet:

Chewable: Store at controlled room temperature of 20°C to 25°C (68°F to 77°F). Protect from light and moisture.

Extended and sustained release: Store at controlled room temperature of 20°C to 25°C (68°F to 77°F). Protect from light and moisture.

Immediate release: Store at controlled room temperature of 20°C to 25°C (68°F to 77°F). Protect from light and moisture.

Osmotic controlled release (Concerta®): Store at controlled room temperature of 25°C; excursions permitted to 15°C to 30°C (59°F to 86°F). Protect from humidity.

Transdermal system: Store at 25°C (77°F); excursions permitted to 15°C to 30°C (59°F to 86°F). Keep patches stored in protective pouch. Once tray is opened, use patches within 2 months; once an individual patch has been removed from the pouch and the protective liner removed, use immediately. Do not refrigerate or freeze.

Nursing Actions

Physical Assessment Assess for history of addiction; long-term use can result in dependence, abuse, or tolerance. Evaluate periodically for need for continued use. After long-term use, taper dosage slowly when discontinuing. Monitor growth pattern in children. Perform careful cardiovascular assessment prior to initiating therapy. Monitor vital signs at beginning of therapy and periodically throughout.

Patient Education Response may take some time. Do not crush or chew long-acting forms. Tablets and sustained release tablets should be taken 30-45 minutes before meals. Concerta® may be taken with or without food, but must be taken with water, milk, or juice. Metadate CD® and Ritalin LA® capsules may be opened and the contents sprinkled onto a small amount (equal to 1 tablespoon) of applesauce; swallow applesauce without chewing. Transdermal: Apply to clean, dry skin, immediately after removing from package. Firmly press in place and hold for 30 seconds. Avoid exposing application site to external heat sources. Total wear time should not exceed 9 hours. Avoid alcohol and caffeine. You may experience decreased appetite or weight loss, restlessness, impaired judgment, or dizziness, especially during early therapy. Report unresolved rapid heartbeat, chest pain, difficulty breathing, and fainting; excessive agitation or nervousness; insomnia, tremors, or dizziness; or skin rash.

Dietary Considerations Should be taken 30-45 minutes before meals. Concerta® is not affected by food. Some products may contain phenylalanine.

MethylPREDNISolone (meth il pred NIS oh lone)

Brand Names: U.S. A-Methapred®; Depo-Medrol®; Medrol®; Medrol® Dosepak™; Solu-MEDROL®

Index Terms 6-α-Methylprednisolone; A-Methapred; Medrol Dose Pack; Methylprednisolone Acetate; Methylprednisolone Sodium Succinate; Solumedrol

Pharmacologic Category Corticosteroid, Systemic

Medication Safety Issues

Sound-alike/look-alike issues:

MethylPREDNISolone may be confused with medroxyPROGESTERone, methotrexate, methylTESTOSTERone, predniSONE

Depo-Medrol® may be confused with Solu-Medrol®

Medrol® may be confused with Mebaral®

Solu-MEDROL® may be confused with salmeterol, Solu-CORTEF®

International issues:

Medrol [U.S., Canada, and multiple international markets] may be confused with Medral brand name for omeprazole [Mexico]

Lactation Enters breast milk/use caution

Breast-Feeding Considerations Low levels of methylprednisolone are excreted in breast milk

Use Primarily as an anti-inflammatory or immunosuppressant agent in the treatment of a variety of diseases including those of hematologic, allergic, inflammatory, neoplastic, and autoimmune origin. Prevention and treatment of graft-versus-host disease following allogeneic bone marrow transplantation.

Unlabeled Use Acute spinal cord injury

Mechanism of Action/Effect In a tissue-specific manner, corticosteroids regulate gene expression subsequent to binding specific intracellular receptors and translocation into the nucleus. Corticosteroids exert a wide array of physiologic effects, including modulation of carbohydrate, protein, and lipid metabolism, and maintenance of fluid and electrolyte homeostasis. Moreover, cardiovascular, immunologic, musculoskeletal, endocrine, and neurologic physiology are influenced by corticosteroids.

Contraindications Hypersensitivity to methylprednisolone or any component of the formulation; systemic fungal infection (except intra-articular injection in localized joint conditions); administration of live virus vaccines. methylprednisolone formulations containing benzyl alcohol preservative are contraindicated in premature infants; I.M. administration in idiopathic thrombocytopenia purpura; intrathecal administration

Warnings/Precautions Use with caution in patients with thyroid disease, hepatic impairment, renal impairment, cardiovascular disease, diabetes, glaucoma, cataracts, myasthenia gravis, patients at risk for osteoporosis, patients at risk for seizures, or GI diseases (diverticulitis, peptic ulcer, ulcerative colitis) due to perforation risk. Not recommended for the treatment of optic neuritis; may increase frequency of new episodes. Use caution following acute MI (corticosteroids have been associated with myocardial rupture). Cardiomegaly and congestive heart failure have been reported following concurrent use of amphotericin B and hydrocortisone for the management of fungal infections.

Because of the risk of adverse effects, systemic corticosteroids should be used cautiously in the elderly in the smallest possible effective dose for the shortest duration. May affect growth velocity; growth should be routinely monitored in pediatric patients. Withdraw therapy with gradual tapering of dose.

May cause hypercorticism or suppression of hypothalamic-pituitary-adrenal (HPA) axis, particularly in younger children or in patients receiving high doses for prolonged periods. HPA axis suppression may lead to adrenal crisis. Withdrawal and discontinuation of a corticosteroid should be done slowly and carefully. Particular care is required when patients are transferred from systemic corticosteroids to inhaled products due to possible adrenal insufficiency or withdrawal from steroids, including an increase in allergic symptoms. Patients receiving >20 mg per day of prednisone (or equivalent) may be most susceptible. Fatalities have occurred due to adrenal insufficiency in asthmatic patients during and after transfer from systemic corticosteroids to aerosol steroids; aerosol steroids do not provide the systemic steroid needed to treat patients having trauma, surgery, or infections.

Acute myopathy has been reported with high dose corticosteroids, usually in patients with neuromuscular transmission disorders; may involve ocular and/or respiratory muscles; monitor creatine kinase; recovery may be delayed. Corticosteroid use may cause psychiatric disturbances, including depression, euphoria, insomnia, mood swings, and personality changes. Pre-existing psychiatric conditions may be exacerbated by corticosteroid use. Prolonged use of corticosteroids may also increase the incidence of secondary infection, cause activation of latent infections, mask acute infection (including fungal infections), prolong or exacerbate viral or parasitic infections, or limit response to vaccines. Exposure to chickenpox or measles should be avoided; corticosteroids should not be used to treat ocular herpes simplex. Corticosteroids should not be used for cerebral malaria or viral hepatitis. Close observation is required in patients with latent tuberculosis and/or TB reactivity; restrict use in active TB (only in conjunction with antituberculosis treatment). Amebiasis should be ruled out in any patient with recent travel to tropic climates or unexplained diarrhea prior to initiation of corticosteroids. Prolonged treatment with corticosteroids has been associated with the development of Kaposi's sarcoma (case reports); discontinuation may result in clinical improvement.

High-dose corticosteroids should not be used to manage acute head injury. Rare cases of anaphylactoid reactions have been observed in patients receiving corticosteroids. Avoid injection or leakage into the dermis; dermal and/or subdermal skin depression may occur at the site of injection. Avoid deltoid muscle injection; subcutaneous atrophy may occur. Some dosage forms contain benzyl alcohol which has been associated with "gasping syndrome" in neonates.

Drug Interactions

Avoid Concomitant Use

Avoid concomitant use of MethylPREDNISolone with any of the following: Aldesleukin; BCG; Natalizumab; Pimecrolimus; Pimozide; Tacrolimus (Topical)

Decreased Effect

MethylPREDNISolone may decrease the levels/effects of: Aldesleukin; Antidiabetic Agents; BCG; Calcitriol; Coccidioidin Skin Test; Corticorelin; CycloSPORINE; CycloSPORINE (Systemic); Isoniazid; Salicylates; Sipuleucel-T; Telaprevir; Vaccines (Inactivated)

The levels/effects of MethylPREDNISolone may be decreased by: Aminoglutethimide; Antacids; Barbiturates; Bile Acid Sequestrants; CarBAMazepine; Echinacea; Fosphenytoin; Mitotane; Phenytoin; Primidone; Rifamycin Derivatives; Tocilizumab

Increased Effect/Toxicity

MethylPREDNISolone may increase the levels/effects of: Acetylcholinesterase Inhibitors; Amphotericin B; ARIPiprazole; CycloSPORINE; CycloSPORINE (Systemic); Deferasirox; Leflunomide; Loop Diuretics; Natalizumab; NSAID (COX-2 Inhibitor); NSAID (Nonselective); Pimozide; Thiazide Diuretics; Vaccines (Live); Warfarin

The levels/effects of MethylPREDNISolone may be increased by: Antifungal Agents (Azole Derivatives, Systemic); Aprepitant; Calcium Channel Blockers (Nondihydropyridine); CycloSPORINE; CycloSPORINE (Systemic); CYP3A4 Inhibitors (Strong); Denosumab; Estrogen Derivatives; Fluconazole; Fosaprepitant; Indacaterol; Macrolide Antibiotics; Neuromuscular-Blocking Agents (Nondepolarizing); Pimecrolimus; Quinolone Antibiotics; Roflumilast; Salicylates; Tacrolimus (Topical); Telaprevir; Trastuzumab

Nutritional/Ethanol Interactions

Ethanol: Ethanol may increase gastric mucosal irritation. Management: Avoid ethanol.

Food: Methylprednisolone interferes with calcium absorption. May cause GI upset. Management: Administer with food. Limit caffeine.

Herb/Nutraceutical: St John's wort may decrease methylprednisolone levels. Cat's claw and echinacea have immunostimulant properties. Management: Avoid St John's wort, cat's claw, and echinacea.

Adverse Reactions Frequency not defined.

Cardiovascular: Arrhythmias, bradycardia, cardiac arrest, cardiomegaly, circulatory collapse, congestive heart failure, edema, fat embolism, hypertension, hypertrophic cardiomyopathy in premature infants, myocardial rupture (post MI), syncope, tachycardia, thromboembolism, vasculitis

Central nervous system: Delirium, depression, emotional instability, euphoria, hallucinations, headache, intracranial pressure increased, insomnia, malaise, mood swings, nervousness, neuritis, personality changes, psychic disorders, pseudotumor cerebri (usually following discontinuation), seizure, vertigo

Dermatologic: Acne, allergic dermatitis, alopecia, dry scaly skin, ecchymoses, edema, erythema, hirsutism, hyper-/hypopigmentation, hypertrichosis, impaired wound healing, petechiae, rash, skin atrophy, sterile abscess, skin test reaction impaired, striae, urticaria

Endocrine & metabolic: Adrenal suppression, amenorrhea, carbohydrate intolerance increased, Cushing's syndrome, diabetes mellitus, fluid retention, glucose intolerance, growth suppression (children), hyperglycemia, hyperlipidemia, hypokalemia, hypokalemic alkalosis, menstrual irregularities, negative nitrogen balance, pituitary-adrenal axis suppression, protein catabolism, sodium and water retention

Gastrointestinal: Abdominal distention, appetite increased, bowel/bladder dysfunction (after intrathecal administration), gastrointestinal hemorrhage, gastrointestinal perforation, nausea, pancreatitis, peptic ulcer, perforation of the small and large intestine, ulcerative esophagitis, vomiting, weight gain

Hematologic: Leukocytosis (transient)

Hepatic: Hepatomegaly, transaminases increased

Local: Postinjection flare (intra-articular use), thrombophlebitis

Neuromuscular & skeletal: Arthralgia, arthropathy, aseptic necrosis (femoral and humoral heads), fractures, muscle mass loss, muscle weakness, myopathy (particularly in conjunction with neuromuscular disease or neuromuscular-blocking agents), neuropathy, osteoporosis, parasthesia, tendon rupture, vertebral compression fractures, weakness

Ocular: Cataracts, exophthalmoses, glaucoma, intraocular pressure increased

Renal: Glycosuria

Respiratory: Pulmonary edema

Miscellaneous: Abnormal fat disposition, anaphylactoid reaction, anaphylaxis, angioedema, avascular necrosis, diaphoresis, hiccups, hypersensitivity reactions, infections, secondary malignancy

Pharmacodynamics/Kinetics

Onset of Action Peak effect (route dependent): Oral: 1-2 hours; I.M.: 4-8 days; Intra-articular: 1 week; methylprednisolone sodium succinate is highly soluble and has a rapid effect by I.M. and I.V. routes

Duration of Action Route dependent: Oral: 30-36 hours; I.M.: 1-4 weeks; Intra-articular: 1-5 weeks; methylprednisolone acetate has a low solubility and has a sustained I.M. effect

Available Dosage Forms

Injection, powder for reconstitution: 40 mg, 125 mg, 500 mg, 1 g

A-Methapred®: 40 mg, 125 mg

Solu-MEDROL®: 500 mg, 1 g, 2 g

Injection, powder for reconstitution [preservative free]:

Solu-MEDROL®: 40 mg, 125 mg, 500 mg, 1 g

Injection, suspension: 40 mg/mL (1 mL, 5 mL, 10 mL); 80 mg/mL (1 mL, 5 mL)

Depo-Medrol®: 20 mg/mL (5 mL); 40 mg/mL (5 mL, 10 mL); 80 mg/mL (5 mL)

Injection, suspension [preservative free]:

Depo-Medrol®: 40 mg/mL (1 mL); 80 mg/mL (1 mL)

Tablet, oral: 4 mg, 8 mg, 16 mg, 32 mg

Medrol®: 2 mg, 4 mg, 8 mg, 16 mg, 32 mg

Medrol® Dosepak™: 4 mg

General Dosage Range

I.M.:

Acetate: *Adults:* 10-120 mg every 1-2 weeks

Sodium succinate:

Children: 0.5-1.7 mg/kg/day **or** 5-25 mg/m^2/day divided every 6-12 hours; "Pulse" therapy: 15-30 mg/kg/dose given once daily for 3 days

Adults: 10-80 mg once daily

I.V. (sodium succinate): *Children and Adults:* Dosage varies greatly by indication

Intra-articular (acetate): *Adults:* Administer every 1-5 weeks

Large joints (eg, knee, ankle): 20-80 mg

Medium joints (eg, elbow, wrist): 10-40 mg

Small joints: 4-10 mg

Intralesional (acetate): *Adults:* 20-60 mg every 1-5 weeks

Oral:

Children: 0.5-1.7 mg/kg/day **or** 5-25 mg/m²/day divided every 6-12 hours; "Pulse" therapy: 15-30 mg/kg/dose once daily for 3 days

Adults: 2-60 mg/day in 1-4 divided doses

Administration

Oral Administer with meals to decrease GI upset. Give daily dose in the morning to mimic normal peak blood levels.

I.V. Only sodium succinate formulation may be given I.V. Acetate salt should not be given I.V.

Parenteral: Methylprednisolone sodium succinate may be administered I.M. or I.V.; I.V. administration may be IVP over one to several minutes or IVPB or continuous I.V. infusion. Avoid injection or leakage into the dermis; dermal and/or subdermal skin depression may occur at the site of injection.

I.V.: Succinate:

Low dose: ≤1.8 mg/kg or ≤125 mg/dose: I.V. push over 3-15 minutes

Moderate dose: ≥2 mg/kg or 250 mg/dose: I.V. over 15-30 minutes

High dose: 15 mg/kg or ≥500 mg/dose: I.V. over ≥30 minutes

Doses >15 mg/kg or ≥1 g: Administer over 1 hour

Do **not** administer high-dose I.V. push; hypotension, cardiac arrhythmia, and sudden death have been reported in patients given high-dose methylprednisolone I.V. push (>0.5 g over <10 minutes). Intermittent infusion over 15-60 minutes; maximum concentration: I.V. push 125 mg/mL.

I.M.: Avoid injection into the deltoid muscle due to a high incidence of subcutaneous atrophy. Avoid injection or leakage into the dermis; dermal and/or subdermal skin depression may occur at the site of injection. Do not inject into areas that have evidence of acute local infection.

I.V. Detail pH: 7-8 (adjusted with sodium hydroxide)

Topical For external use only. Apply sparingly.

Stability

Reconstitution

Standard diluent (Solu-Medrol®): 40 mg/50 mL D_5W; 125 mg/50 mL D_5W.

Minimum volume (Solu-Medrol®): 50 mL D_5W.

Storage Intact vials of methylprednisolone sodium succinate should be stored at controlled room temperature of 20°C to 25°C (68°F to 77°F). Protect from light. Reconstituted solutions of methylprednisolone sodium succinate should be stored at room temperature of 20°C to 25°C (68°F to 77°F) and used within 48 hours. Stability of parenteral admixture at room temperature (25°C) and at refrigeration temperature (4°C) is 48 hours.

Nursing Actions

Physical Assessment Teach patients to report infection and adrenal suppression. Instruct patients with diabetes to monitor serum glucose levels closely; corticosteroids can alter glycemic response. Dose may need to be increased if patient is experiencing higher than normal levels of stress. When discontinuing, taper dose and frequency slowly.

Patient Education Maintain adequate nutritional intake; consult prescriber for possibility of special dietary instructions. If you have diabetes, monitor serum glucose closely and notify prescriber of any changes; this medication can alter glycemic response. Avoid alcohol. Inform prescriber if you are experiencing unusual stress; dosage may need to be adjusted. You will be susceptible to infection. You may experience insomnia or nervousness. Report increased pain, swelling, or redness in area being treated; excessive or sudden weight gain; swelling of extremities; muscle pain or weakness; change in menstrual pattern; vision changes; signs of hyperglycemia; signs of infection (eg, fever, chills, mouth sores, perianal itching, vaginal discharge); blackened stool; or worsening of condition.

Oral: Take with food or milk.

Intra-articular: Refrain from excessive use of joint following therapy, even if pain is gone.

Dietary Considerations Take with meals to decrease GI upset.; need diet rich in pyridoxine, vitamin C, vitamin D, folate, calcium, phosphorus, and protein.

Related Information

Compatibility of Drugs *on page 1264*

MethylTESTOSTERone

(meth il tes TOS te rone)

Brand Names: U.S. Android®; Methitest™; Testred®

Pharmacologic Category Androgen

Medication Safety Issues

Sound-alike/look-alike issues:

MethylTESTOSTERone may be confused with medroxyPROGESTERone, methylPREDNISolone

Beers Criteria medication:

This drug may be inappropriate for use in geriatric patients (high severity risk).

Pregnancy Risk Factor X

Lactation Excretion in breast milk unknown/not recommended

Use

Male: Hypogonadism; delayed puberty; impotence and climacteric symptoms

Female: Palliative treatment of metastatic breast cancer

Unlabeled Use Hypogonadism (male); delayed puberty (male)

Controlled Substance C-III

Available Dosage Forms

Capsule, oral:

Android®: 10 mg

Testred®: 10 mg

Tablet, oral:

Methitest™: 10 mg

General Dosage Range

Oral:

Adults (females): 50-200 mg/day

Adults (males): 10-50 mg/day

Nursing Actions

Physical Assessment Assess potential for interactions with other pharmacological agents patient may be taking (eg, effects of hypoglycemic agents may be increased). Monitor for virilism (male and female), edema, CNS changes (anxiety, depression), acne, baldness, GI irritation, leukopenia, and hepatic dysfunction frequently during therapy. Caution patients with diabetes; effects of hypoglycemic agents may be increased.

Patient Education If you have diabetes, monitor serum glucose closely and notify prescriber of changes; this medication can alter hypoglycemic requirements. May cause acne, growth of body hair, loss of libido, impotence, menstrual irregularity (usually reversible), nausea, or vomiting. Report changes in menstrual pattern, deepening of voice or unusual growth of body hair, gynecomastia or breast soreness, priapism, fluid retention (swelling of ankles, feet, or hands, respiratory difficulty, or sudden weight gain), change in color of urine or stool, yellowing of eyes or skin, unusual bruising or bleeding, or unusual fatigue or weakness.

Metoclopramide (met oh KLOE pra mide)

Brand Names: U.S. Metozolv™ ODT; Reglan®

Pharmacologic Category Antiemetic; Gastrointestinal Agent, Prokinetic

Medication Safety Issues

Sound-alike/look-alike issues:

Metoclopramide may be confused with metolazone, metoprolol, metroNIDAZOLE

Reglan® may be confused with Megace®, Regonol®, Renagel®

Medication Guide Available Yes

Pregnancy Risk Factor B

Lactation Enters breast milk/use caution

Breast-Feeding Considerations Enters breast milk; may increase milk production

Use

Oral: Symptomatic treatment of diabetic gastroparesis; gastroesophageal reflux

I.V., I.M.: Symptomatic treatment of diabetic gastroparesis; postpyloric placement of enteral feeding tubes; prevention and/or treatment of nausea and vomiting associated with chemotherapy, or post-surgery; to stimulate gastric emptying and intestinal transit of barium during radiological examination of the stomach/small intestine

Mechanism of Action/Effect Blocks dopamine receptors and (when given in higher doses) also blocks serotonin receptors in chemoreceptor trigger zone of the CNS; enhances the response to acetylcholine of tissue in upper GI tract causing enhanced motility and accelerated gastric emptying without stimulating gastric, biliary, or pancreatic secretions; increases lower esophageal sphincter tone

Contraindications Hypersensitivity to metoclopramide or any component of the formulation; GI obstruction, perforation or hemorrhage; pheochromocytoma; history of seizures or concomitant use of other agents likely to increase extrapyramidal reactions

Warnings/Precautions [U.S. Boxed Warning]: May cause tardive dyskinesia, which is often irreversible; duration of treatment and total cumulative dose are associated with an increased risk. Therapy durations >12 weeks should be avoided (except in rare cases following risk:benefit assessment). Risk appears to be increased in the elderly, women, and diabetics; however, it is not possible to predict which patients will develop tardive dyskinesia. Therapy should be discontinued in any patient if signs/symptoms of tardive dyskinesia appear.

May cause extrapyramidal symptoms, generally manifested as acute dystonic reactions within the initial 24-48 hours of use. Risk of these reactions is increased at higher doses, and in pediatric patients, and adults <30 years of age. Pseudoparkinsonism (eg, bradykinesia, tremor, rigidity) may also occur (usually within first 6 months of therapy) and is generally reversible following discontinuation. Use with caution or avoid in patients with Parkinson's disease. Use caution in the elderly; may have increased risk of tardive dyskinesia, particularly older women. Neuroleptic malignant syndrome (NMS) has been reported (rarely) with metoclopramide.

May cause transient increase in serum aldosterone; use caution in patients who are at risk of fluid overload (HF, cirrhosis). Use caution in patients with hypertension or following surgical anastomosis/closure. Use caution with a history of mental illness; has been associated with depression. Abrupt discontinuation may (rarely) result in withdrawal symptoms (dizziness, headache, nervousness). Use caution and adjust dose in renal impairment. Patients with NADH-cytochrome b5 reductase deficiency are at increased risk of methemoglobinemia and/or sulfhemoglobinemia. Neonates may have an increased risk of methemoglobinemia due to decreased levels of NADH-cytochrome b5 reductase deficiency and prolonged clearance of metoclopramide.

Drug Interactions

Avoid Concomitant Use

Avoid concomitant use of Metoclopramide with any of the following: Antipsychotics; Droperidol; Promethazine; Tetrabenazine

Decreased Effect

Metoclopramide may decrease the levels/effects of: Anti-Parkinson's Agents (Dopamine Agonist); Posaconazole; Quinagolide

The levels/effects of Metoclopramide may be decreased by: Cyproterone; Peginterferon Alfa-2b

Increased Effect/Toxicity

Metoclopramide may increase the levels/effects of: Antipsychotics; CycloSPORINE; CycloSPORINE (Systemic); Prilocaine; Promethazine; Selective Serotonin Reuptake Inhibitors; Tetrabenazine; Tricyclic Antidepressants; Venlafaxine

The levels/effects of Metoclopramide may be increased by: Droperidol; Serotonin Modulators

Nutritional/Ethanol Interactions Ethanol: Avoid ethanol (may increase CNS depression).

Adverse Reactions Frequency not always defined.

Cardiovascular: AV block, bradycardia, HF, fluid retention, flushing (following high I.V. doses), hyper-/hypotension, supraventricular tachycardia

Central nervous system: Drowsiness (~10% to 70%; dose related), acute dystonic reactions (<1% to 25%; dose and age related), fatigue (2% to 10%), lassitude (~10%), restlessness (~10%), headache (4% to 5%), dizziness (1% to 4%), somnolence (2% to 3%), akathisia, confusion, depression, hallucinations (rare), insomnia, neuroleptic malignant syndrome (rare), Parkinsonian-like symptoms, suicidal ideation, seizure, tardive dyskinesia

Dermatologic: Angioneurotic edema (rare), rash, urticaria

Endocrine & metabolic: Amenorrhea, galactorrhea, gynecomastia, hyperprolactinemia, impotence

Gastrointestinal: Nausea (4% to 6%), vomiting (1% to 2%), diarrhea

Hematologic: Agranulocytosis, leukopenia, neutropenia, porphyria

Hepatic: Hepatotoxicity (rare)

Ocular: Visual disturbance

Respiratory: Bronchospasm, laryngeal edema (rare), laryngospasm (rare)

Miscellaneous: Allergic reactions, methemoglobinemia, sulfhemoglobinemia

Pharmacodynamics/Kinetics

Onset of Action Oral: 30-60 minutes; I.V.: 1-3 minutes; I.M.: 10-15 minutes

Duration of Action Therapeutic: 1-2 hours, regardless of route

Available Dosage Forms

Injection, solution [preservative free]: 5 mg/mL (2 mL)

Reglan®: 5 mg/mL (2 mL, 10 mL, 30 mL)

Solution, oral: 5 mg/5 mL (0.9 mL, 10 mL, 473 mL)

Tablet, oral: 5 mg, 10 mg

Reglan®: 5 mg, 10 mg

Tablet, orally disintegrating, oral:

Metozolv™ ODT: 5 mg, 10 mg

General Dosage Range Dosage adjustment recommended in patients with renal impairment

I.M.: *Adults:* 10-20 mg as a single dose **or** 10 mg before each meal and at bedtime

I.V.:

Children <6 years: 0.1 mg/kg as a single dose

Children 6-14 years: 2.5-5 mg as a single dose

Children >14 years: 10 mg as a single dose

Adults: 10 mg before each meal and at bedtime **or** 1-2 mg/kg every 2-3 hours (maximum: 5 doses/day) **or** 10 mg as a single dose

Oral: *Adults:* 10-15 mg up to 4 times/day

Administration

Oral Orally-disintegrating tablets: Administer on an empty stomach at least 30 minutes prior to food. Do not remove from packaging until time of administration. If tablet breaks or crumbles while handling, discard and remove new tablet. Using dry hands, place tablet on tongue and allow to dissolve. Swallow with saliva.

I.M. May be administered I.M.

I.V. Injection solution may be given I.M., direct I.V. push, short infusion (15-30 minutes), or continuous infusion; lower doses (≤10 mg) of metoclopramide can be given I.V. push undiluted over 1-2 minutes; higher doses (>10 mg) to be diluted in 50 mL of compatible solution (preferably NS) and given IVPB over at least 15 minutes; continuous SubQ infusion and rectal administration have been reported. **Note:** Rapid I.V. administration may be associated with a transient (but intense) feeling of anxiety and restlessness, followed by drowsiness.

I.V. Detail pH: 3.0-6.5

Other Continuous SubQ infusion and rectal administration have been reported

Stability

Storage

Injection: Store intact vial at controlled room temperature; injection is photosensitive and should be protected from light during storage; parenteral admixtures in D_5W or NS are stable for at least 24 hours and do not require light protection if used within 24 hours.

Tablet: Store at controlled room temperature of 20°C to 25°C (68°F to 77°F).

Nursing Actions

Physical Assessment Monitor vital signs during intravenous administration. Inpatients should use safety measures to prevent falls (eg, side rails up, call light within reach) and caution patient to call for assistance with ambulation. Monitor for CNS changes (sedation, extrapyramidal effects, Parkinsonian-like reactions).

Patient Education Oral: Take 30 minutes prior to eating. Avoid alcohol; may increase adverse effects. May cause dizziness, drowsiness, insomnia, or blurred vision. Report persistent CNS changes (restlessness, anxiety, depression), spasticity or involuntary movements, unresolved diarrhea, or visual disturbances.

Metolazone (me TOLE a zone)

Brand Names: U.S. Zaroxolyn®

Pharmacologic Category Diuretic, Thiazide-Related

Medication Safety Issues

Sound-alike/look-alike issues:

Metolazone may be confused with metaxalone, methazolamide, methimazole, methotrexate, metoclopramide, metoprolol, minoxidil

Zaroxolyn® may be confused with Zarontin®

Pregnancy Risk Factor B

Lactation Enters breast milk/not recommended

Use Management of mild-to-moderate hypertension; treatment of edema in heart failure and nephrotic syndrome, impaired renal function

Mechanism of Action/Effect Inhibits sodium reabsorption in the distal tubules causing increased excretion of sodium and water, as well as, potassium and hydrogen ions

Contraindications Hypersensitivity to metolazone, any component of the formulation, other thiazides, and sulfonamide derivatives; anuria; hepatic coma; pregnancy (expert analysis)

Warnings/Precautions Electrolyte disturbances (hypokalemia, hypochloremic alkalosis, hyponatremia) can occur. Large or prolonged fluid and electrolyte losses may occur with concomitant furosemide administration. Use with caution in severe hepatic dysfunction; hepatic encephalopathy can be caused by electrolyte disturbances. Gout can be precipitate in certain patients with a history of gout, a familial predisposition to gout, or chronic renal failure. Cautious use in patients with prediabetes or diabetes; may see a change in glucose control. Can cause SLE exacerbation or activation. Use caution in severe renal impairment. Use with caution in patients with moderate or high cholesterol concentrations. Photosensitization may occur.

Chemical similarities are present among sulfonamides, sulfonylureas, carbonic anhydrase inhibitors, thiazides, and loop diuretics (except ethacrynic acid). Use in patients with thiazide or sulfonamide allergy is specifically contraindicated in product labeling, however, a risk of cross-reaction exists in patients with allergy to any of these compounds; avoid use when previous reaction has been severe. Discontinue if signs of hypersensitivity are noted.

Drug Interactions

Avoid Concomitant Use

Avoid concomitant use of Metolazone with any of the following: Dofetilide

Decreased Effect

Metolazone may decrease the levels/effects of: Antidiabetic Agents

The levels/effects of Metolazone may be decreased by: Bile Acid Sequestrants; Herbs (Hypertensive Properties); Methylphenidate; Nonsteroidal Anti-Inflammatory Agents; Yohimbine

Increased Effect/Toxicity

Metolazone may increase the levels/effects of: ACE Inhibitors; Allopurinol; Amifostine; Antihypertensives; Calcium Salts; CarBAMazepine; Dofetilide; Hypotensive Agents; Lithium; OXcarbazepine; Porfimer; RiTUXimab; Sodium Phosphates; Topiramate; Toremifene; Vitamin D Analogs

The levels/effects of Metolazone may be increased by: Alcohol (Ethyl); Alfuzosin; Analgesics (Opioid); Barbiturates; Beta2-Agonists; Corticosteroids (Orally Inhaled); Corticosteroids (Systemic); Herbs (Hypotensive Properties); Licorice; MAO Inhibitors; Pentoxifylline; Phosphodiesterase 5 Inhibitors; Prostacyclin Analogues

Nutritional/Ethanol Interactions

Ethanol: May potentiate hypotensive effect of metazolone.

Herb/Nutraceutical: Avoid herbs with *hypertensive* properties (bayberry, blue cohosh, cayenne, ephedra, ginger, ginseng [American], kola, licorice); may diminish the antihypertensive effect of metolazone. Avoid herbs with *hypotensive* properties (black cohosh, California poppy, coleus, golden seal, hawthorn, mistletoe, periwinkle, quinine, shepherd's purse); may enhance the hypotensive effect of metolazone.

Adverse Reactions Frequency not defined.

Cardiovascular: Chest pain/discomfort, necrotizing angiitis, orthostatic hypotension, palpitation, syncope, venous thrombosis, vertigo, volume depletion

Central nervous system: Chills, depression, dizziness, drowsiness, fatigue, headache, lightheadedness, restlessness

Dermatologic: Petechiae, photosensitivity, pruritus, purpura, rash, skin necrosis, Stevens-Johnson syndrome, toxic epidermal necrolysis, urticaria

Endocrine & metabolic: Gout attacks, hypercalcemia, hyperglycemia, hyperuricemia, hypochloremia, hypochloremic alkalosis, hypokalemia, hypomagnesemia, hyponatremia, hypophosphatemia

Gastrointestinal: Abdominal bloating, abdominal pain, anorexia, constipation, diarrhea, epigastric distress, nausea, pancreatitis, vomiting, xerostomia

Genitourinary: Impotence

Hematologic: Agranulocytosis, aplastic/hypoplastic anemia, hemoconcentration, leukopenia, thrombocytopenia

Hepatic: Cholestatic jaundice, hepatitis

Neuromuscular & skeletal: Joint pain, muscle cramps/spasm, neuropathy, paresthesia, weakness

Ocular: Blurred vision (transient)

Renal: BUN increased, glucosuria

Pharmacodynamics/Kinetics

Onset of Action Diuresis: ~60 minutes

Duration of Action ≥24 hours

Available Dosage Forms

Tablet, oral: 2.5 mg, 5 mg, 10 mg

Zaroxolyn®: 2.5 mg, 5 mg

General Dosage Range Oral: *Adults:* 2.5-20 mg every 24 hours

Administration

Oral May be taken with food or milk. Take early in day to avoid nocturia. Take the last dose of multiple doses no later than 6 PM unless instructed otherwise.

Nursing Actions

Physical Assessment Patient's renal status and allergy history (thiazides and sulfonamide derivatives) should be assessed prior to beginning therapy. Assess electrolytes and renal function. Monitor for hypersensitivity reactions, electrolyte imbalance, and hypotension.

Patient Education Take after breakfast. Include bananas or orange juice in daily diet, but do not take potassium supplements without advice of prescriber. Follow prescriber's instructions for diet and lifestyle changes. Weigh yourself weekly and report weight gain. May cause dizziness, weakness, nausea, or photosensitivity. Report chest pain or palpitations, dizziness, headache, pain, weakness, skin rash, excessive fatigue, or swelling of extremities.

Dietary Considerations Should be taken after breakfast; may require potassium supplementation

Metoprolol (me toe PROE lole)

Brand Names: U.S. Lopressor®; Toprol-XL®

Index Terms Metoprolol Succinate; Metoprolol Tartrate

Pharmacologic Category Antianginal Agent; Beta Blocker, Beta-1 Selective

Medication Safety Issues

Sound-alike/look-alike issues:

Lopressor® may be confused with Lyrica®

Metoprolol may be confused with metaproterenol, metoclopramide, metolazone, misoprostol

Metoprolol succinate may be confused with metoprolol tartrate

Toprol-XL® may be confused with TEGretol®, TEGretol®-XR, Topamax®

High alert medication:

The Institute for Safe Medication Practices (ISMP) includes this medication among its list of drugs which have a heightened risk of causing significant patient harm when used in error.

Administration issues:

Significant differences exist between oral and I.V. dosing. Use caution when converting from one route of administration to another.

Pregnancy Risk Factor C

Lactation Enters breast milk/use caution (AAP rates "compatible"; AAP 2001 update pending)

Breast-Feeding Considerations Small amounts of metoprolol can be detected in breast milk. The manufacturer recommends that caution be exercised when administering metoprolol to nursing women.

Use Treatment of angina pectoris, hypertension, or hemodynamically-stable acute myocardial infarction

Extended release: Treatment of angina pectoris or hypertension; to reduce mortality/hospitalization in patients with heart failure (stable NYHA Class II or III) already receiving ACE inhibitors, diuretics, and/or digoxin

Unlabeled Use Treatment of ventricular arrhythmias, atrial ectopy; migraine prophylaxis, essential tremor, aggressive behavior (not recommended for dementia-associated aggression); prevention of reinfarction and sudden death after myocardial infarction; prevention and treatment of atrial fibrillation and atrial flutter; multifocal atrial tachycardia; symptomatic treatment of hypertrophic obstructive cardiomyopathy; management of thyrotoxicosis

Mechanism of Action/Effect Due to inhibition of beta$_1$-receptors, metoprolol reduces myocardial contractility, heart rate, and blood pressure.

Contraindications

Hypersensitivity to metoprolol, any component of the formulation, or other beta-blockers

Note: Additional contraindications are formulation and/or indication specific.

Immediate release tablets/injectable formulation:

Hypertension and angina: Sinus bradycardia; second- and third-degree heart block; cardiogenic shock; overt heart failure; sick sinus syndrome (except in patients with a functioning artificial pacemaker); severe peripheral arterial disease; pheochromocytoma (without alpha blockade)

Myocardial infarction: Severe sinus bradycardia (heart rate <45 beats/minute); significant first-degree heart block (P-R interval ≥0.24 seconds); second- and third-degree heart block; systolic blood pressure <100 mm Hg; moderate-to-severe cardiac failure

Extended release tablet: Severe bradycardia, second- and third degree heart block; cardiogenic shock; decompensated heart failure; sick sinus syndrome (except in patients with a functioning artificial pacemaker)

Warnings/Precautions [U.S. Boxed Warning]: Beta-blocker therapy should not be withdrawn abruptly (particularly in patients with CAD), but gradually tapered over 1-2 weeks to avoid acute tachycardia, hypertension, and/or ischemia. Consider pre-existing conditions such as sick sinus syndrome before initiating. Metoprolol commonly produces mild first-degree heart block (P-R interval >0.2-0.24 sec). May also produce severe first- (P-R interval ≥0.26 sec), second-, or third-degree heart block. Patients with acute MI (especially right ventricular MI) have a high risk of developing heart block of varying degrees. If severe heart block occurs, metoprolol should be discontinued and measures to increase heart rate should be employed. Symptomatic hypotension may occur with use. May precipitate or aggravate symptoms of arterial insufficiency in patients with PVD and Raynaud's disease; use with caution and monitor for progression of arterial obstruction. Use caution with concurrent use of digoxin, verapamil, or diltiazem; bradycardia or heart block can occur; avoid concurrent I.V. use of both agents. Use with caution in patients receiving inhaled anesthetic agents known to depress myocardial contractility. Use with caution in patients receiving CYP2D6 inhibitors (eg, bupropion, chlorpromazine, cimetidine, diphenhydramine, hydroxychloroquine, fluoxetine, paroxetine, propafenone, propoxyphene, quinidine, ritonavir, terbinafine, thioridazine); concurrent use may increase metoprolol plasma concentrations.

In general, beta-blockers should be avoided in patients with bronchospastic disease. Metoprolol, with B_1 selectivity, should be used cautiously in bronchospastic disease with close monitoring. Use cautiously in patients with diabetes because it can mask prominent hypoglycemic symptoms. May mask signs of hyperthyroidism (eg, tachycardia); if hyperthyroidism is suspected, carefully manage and monitor; abrupt withdrawal may exacerbate symptoms of hyperthyroidism or precipitate thyroid storm. Alterations in thyroid function tests may be observed. Use caution with hepatic dysfunction. Use with caution in patients with myasthenia gravis or psychiatric disease (may cause CNS depression). Although perioperative beta-blocker therapy is recommended prior to elective surgery in selected patients, use of high-dose extended release metoprolol in patients naïve to beta-blocker therapy undergoing noncardiac surgery has been associated with bradycardia, hypotension, stroke, and death. Chronic beta-blocker therapy should not be routinely withdrawn prior to major surgery. Use of beta-blockers may unmask cardiac failure in patients without a history of dysfunction. Adequate alpha-blockade is required prior to use of any beta-blocker for patients with untreated pheochromocytoma. May induce or exacerbate psoriasis. Use caution with history of severe anaphylaxis to allergens; patients taking beta-blockers may become more sensitive to repeated allergen challenges. Treatment of anaphylaxis (eg, epinephrine) in patients taking beta-blockers may be ineffective or promote undesirable effects. Bradycardia may be observed more frequently in elderly patients (>65 years of age); dosage reductions may be necessary.

Extended release: Use with caution in patients with compensated heart failure; monitor for a worsening of heart failure.

Drug Interactions

Avoid Concomitant Use

Avoid concomitant use of Metoprolol with any of the following: Floctafenine; Methacholine

Decreased Effect

Metoprolol may decrease the levels/effects of: Beta2-Agonists; Theophylline Derivatives

The levels/effects of Metoprolol may be decreased by: Barbiturates; Herbs (Hypertensive Properties); Methylphenidate; Nonsteroidal Anti-Inflammatory Agents; Peginterferon Alfa-2b; Rifamycin Derivatives; Yohimbine

Increased Effect/Toxicity

Metoprolol may increase the levels/effects of: Alpha-/Beta-Agonists (Direct-Acting); Alpha1-Blockers; Alpha2-Agonists; Amifostine; Antihypertensives; Antipsychotic Agents (Phenothiazines); ARIPiprazole; Bupivacaine; Cardiac Glycosides; Cholinergic Agonists; Fingolimod; Hypotensive Agents; Insulin; Lidocaine; Lidocaine (Systemic); Lidocaine (Topical); Mepivacaine; Methacholine; Midodrine; RiTUXimab; Sulfonylureas

The levels/effects of Metoprolol may be increased by: Abiraterone Acetate; Acetylcholinesterase Inhibitors; Aminoquinolines (Antimalarial); Amiodarone; Anilidopiperidine Opioids; Antipsychotic Agents (Phenothiazines); Calcium Channel Blockers (Dihydropyridine); Calcium Channel Blockers (Nondihydropyridine); CYP2D6 Inhibitors (Moderate); CYP2D6 Inhibitors (Strong); Darunavir; Diazoxide; Dipyridamole; Disopyramide; Dronedarone; Floctafenine; Herbs (Hypotensive Properties); MAO Inhibitors; Pentoxifylline; Phosphodiesterase 5 Inhibitors; Propafenone; Prostacyclin Analogues; QuiNIDine; Reserpine; Selective Serotonin Reuptake Inhibitors

Nutritional/Ethanol Interactions

Food: Food increases absorption. Metoprolol serum levels may be increased if taken with food.

Management: Take immediate release tartrate tablets with food; succinate can be taken with or without food.

Herb/Nutraceutical: Some herbal medications may worsen hypertension (eg, licorice); others may increase the antihypertensive effect of metoprolol (eg, shepherd's purse). Management: Avoid bayberry, blue cohosh, cayenne, ephedra, ginger, ginseng (American), gotu kola, licorice, and yohimbe. Avoid black cohosh, California poppy, coleus, golden seal, hawthorn, mistletoe, periwinkle, quinine, and shepherd's purse.

Adverse Reactions Frequency may not be defined.

Cardiovascular: Hypotension (1% to 27%), bradycardia (2% to 16%), first-degree heart block (P-R interval ≥0.26 sec; 5%), arterial insufficiency (usually Raynaud type; 1%), chest pain (1%), CHF (1%), edema (peripheral; 1%), palpitation (1%), syncope (1%)

Central nervous system: Dizziness (2% to 10%), fatigue (1% to 10%), depression (5%), confusion, hallucinations, headache, insomnia, memory loss (short-term), nightmares, sleep disturbances, somnolence, vertigo

Dermatology: Pruritus (5%), rash (5%), photosensitivity, psoriasis exacerbated

Endocrine & metabolic: Libido decreased, Peyronie's disease (<1%), diabetes exacerbated

Gastrointestinal: Diarrhea (5%), constipation (1%), flatulence (1%), gastrointestinal pain (1%), heartburn (1%), nausea (1%), xerostomia (1%), vomiting

Hematologic: Claudication

Neuromuscular & skeletal: Musculoskeletal pain

Ocular: Blurred vision, visual disturbances

Otic: Tinnitus

Respiratory: Dyspnea (1% to 3%), bronchospasm (1%), wheezing (1%), rhinitis, shortness of breath

Miscellaneous: Cold extremities (1%)

Other events reported with beta-blockers: Catatonia, emotional lability, fever, hypersensitivity reactions, laryngospasm, nonthrombocytopenic purpura, respiratory distress, thrombocytopenic purpura

Pharmacodynamics/Kinetics

Onset of Action Peak effect: Oral: 1.5-4 hours; I.V.: 20 minutes (when infused over 10 minutes)

Duration of Action Oral: Immediate release: 10-20 hours, Extended release: ~24 hours; I.V.: 5-8 hours

Available Dosage Forms

Injection, solution: 1 mg/mL (5 mL)

Lopressor®: 1 mg/mL (5 mL)

Injection, solution [preservative free]: 1 mg/mL (5 mL)

Tablet, oral: 25 mg, 50 mg, 100 mg

Lopressor®: 50 mg, 100 mg

Tablet, extended release, oral: 25 mg, 50 mg, 100 mg, 200 mg

Toprol-XL®: 25 mg, 50 mg, 100 mg, 200 mg

General Dosage Range

I.V.: *Adults:* 1.25-5 mg every 6-12 hours (maximum: 15 mg every 3 hours) **or** 5 mg every 2 minutes for 3 doses (acute MI)

Oral:

Extended release:

Children ≥6 years: 1-2 mg/kg once daily (maximum: 2 mg/kg/day or 200 mg/day)

Adults: 12.5-200 mg/day (maximum: 400 mg/day)

Immediate release:

Children >1 year: 1-6 mg/kg/day divided twice daily (maximum: 200 mg/day)

Adults: 50-450 mg/day in 2-3 divided doses

Administration

Oral Extended release tablets may be divided in half; do not crush or chew.

I.V. I.V. dose is much smaller than oral dose. When administered acutely for cardiac treatment, monitor ECG and blood pressure; may administer by rapid infusion (I.V. push) over 1 minute. May also be administered by slow infusion (ie, 5-10 mg of metoprolol in 50 mL of fluid) over ~30-60 minutes during less urgent situations (eg, substitution for oral metoprolol).

I.V. Detail pH: 7.5

Stability

Storage

Injection: Store at 25°C (77°F); excursions permitted to 15°C to 30°C (59°F to 86°F). Protect from light.

Tablet: Store at 25°C (77°F); excursions permitted to 15°C to 30°C (59°F to 86°F). Protect from moisture.

Nursing Actions

Physical Assessment Monitor blood pressure and cardiac status. Monitor for fluid balance, heart failure symptoms, and postural hypotension. Taper dosage slowly when discontinuing. Report abdominal pain; unusual bleeding or bruising; or changes in color of urine or stool. Advise patients with diabetes to monitor glucose levels closely; beta-blockers may alter glucose tolerance.

Patient Education

I.V. use in emergency situations: Patient information is appropriate to patient condition.

Oral: Take pulse daily prior to medication and follow prescriber's instruction about holding medication. Do not skip doses. If you have diabetes, monitor serum sugar closely; drug may alter glucose tolerance or mask signs of hypoglycemia. May cause fatigue, dizziness, postural hypotension, or alteration in sexual performance (reversible). Report unresolved swelling of extremities, respiratory difficulty or new cough, unresolved fatigue, unusual weight gain, unresolved constipation, change in color of urine or stool, unusual bleeding or bruising, or unusual muscle weakness. Patient may notice an empty shell of medicine in toilet.

Dietary Considerations Regular tablets should be taken with food. Extended release tablets may be taken without regard to meals.

MetroNIDAZOLE (Systemic)

(met roe NYE da zole)

Brand Names: U.S. Flagyl®; Flagyl® 375; Flagyl® ER

Index Terms Metronidazole Hydrochloride

Pharmacologic Category Amebicide; Antibiotic, Miscellaneous; Antiprotozoal, Nitroimidazole

Medication Safety Issues

Sound-alike/look-alike issues:

MetroNIDAZOLE may be confused with mebendazole, meropenem, metFORMIN, methotrexate, metoclopramide, miconazole

Pregnancy Risk Factor B

Lactation Enters breast milk/not recommended (AAP rates "of concern"; AAP 2001 update pending)

Breast-Feeding Considerations Metronidazole and its active metabolite are measurable in the breast milk and infant plasma. Milk concentrations are similar to those in the maternal plasma and are highly variable. Peak concentrations of metronidazole in breast milk occur ~2-4 hours after the oral dose. In studies, the calculated relative infant doses have ranged from 0.13% to 36% of the weight-adjusted maternal dose. Use of metronidazole in a lactating patient is not recommended by the manufacturer. If metronidazole is given, breast-feeding should be withheld for 12-24 hours after the dose.

Use Treatment of susceptible anaerobic bacterial and protozoal infections in the following conditions: Amebiasis, symptomatic and asymptomatic trichomoniasis; skin and skin structure infections, bone and joint infections, CNS infections, endocarditis, gynecologic infections, intra-abdominal infections (as part of combination regimen), respiratory tract infections (lower), systemic anaerobic infections; treatment of antibiotic-associated pseudomembranous colitis (AAPC); as part of a multidrug regimen for *H. pylori* eradication to reduce the risk of duodenal ulcer recurrence; surgical prophylaxis (colorectal)

Unlabeled Use Crohn's disease

Mechanism of Action/Effect Inhibits DNA synthesis in susceptible organisms

Contraindications Hypersensitivity to metronidazole, nitroimidazole derivatives, or any component of the formulation; pregnancy (first trimester)

Warnings/Precautions Use with caution in patients with severe liver impairment due to potential accumulation, blood dyscrasias; history of seizures, CHF or other sodium-retaining states; reduce dosage in patients with severe liver impairment, CNS disease, and consider dosage reduction in longer-term therapy with severe renal failure (Cl_{cr} <10 mL/minute); if *H. pylori* is not eradicated in patients being treated with metronidazole in a regimen, it should be assumed that metronidazole-resistance has occurred and it should not again be used; aseptic meningitis, encephalopathy, seizures, and neuropathies have been reported especially with increased doses and chronic treatment; monitor and consider discontinuation of therapy if symptoms occur. **[U.S. Boxed Warning]: Possibly carcinogenic based on animal data.** Prolonged use may result in fungal or bacterial superinfection, including *C. difficile*-associated diarrhea (CDAD) and pseudomembranous colitis; CDAD has been observed >2 months postantibiotic treatment. The Infectious Disease Society of America (IDSA) recommends the use of oral metronidazole for initial treatment of mild-to-moderate *C. difficile* infection and the use of oral vancomycin for initial treatment of severe *C. difficile* infection with or without I.V. metronidazole depending on the presence of complications. May treat recurrent mild-to-moderate infection once with oral metronidazole; avoid use beyond first reoccurrence due to potential cumulative neurotoxicity (Cohen, 2010). Candidiasis infection (known or unknown) maybe more prominent during metronidazole treatment, antifungal treatment required. Disulfiram-like reactions to ethanol have been reported with oral metronidazole; avoid alcoholic beverages during therapy

Drug Interactions

Avoid Concomitant Use

Avoid concomitant use of MetroNIDAZOLE (Systemic) with any of the following: BCG; Pimozide; Tolvaptan

Decreased Effect

MetroNIDAZOLE (Systemic) may decrease the levels/effects of: BCG; Mycophenolate; Typhoid Vaccine

The levels/effects of MetroNIDAZOLE (Systemic) may be decreased by: Fosphenytoin; PHENobarbital; Phenytoin

Increased Effect/Toxicity

MetroNIDAZOLE (Systemic) may increase the levels/effects of: Alcohol (Ethyl); ARIPiprazole; Budesonide (Systemic, Oral Inhalation); Busulfan; Calcineurin Inhibitors; Colchicine; CYP3A4 Substrates; Eplerenone; Everolimus; FentaNYL; Fluorouracil; Fluorouracil (Systemic); Fosphenytoin; Halofantrine; Ivacaftor; Lurasidone; Phenytoin; Pimecrolimus; Pimozide; Propafenone; Ranolazine; Salmeterol; Saxagliptin; Tipranavir; Tolvaptan; Vilazodone; Vitamin K Antagonists; Zuclopenthixol

The levels/effects of MetroNIDAZOLE (Systemic) may be increased by: Disulfiram; Mebendazole

Nutritional/Ethanol Interactions

Ethanol: The manufacturer recommends to avoid all ethanol or any ethanol-containing drugs (may cause disulfiram-like reaction characterized by flushing, headache, nausea, vomiting, sweating, or tachycardia).

Food: Peak antibiotic serum concentration lowered and delayed, but total drug absorbed not affected.

Adverse Reactions Frequency not always defined.

Cardiovascular: Flattening of the T-wave, flushing, syncope

Central nervous system: Aseptic meningitis, ataxia, confusion, coordination impaired, depression, dizziness, encephalopathy, fever, headache, insomnia, irritability, seizure, vertigo

Dermatologic: Erythematous rash, pruritus, Stevens-Johnson syndrome, toxic epidermal necrolysis, urticaria

Endocrine & metabolic: Disulfiram-like reaction, dysmenorrhea

Gastrointestinal: Nausea (~12%), anorexia, abdominal cramping, constipation, diarrhea, epigastric distress, furry tongue, glossitis, pancreatitis (rare), proctitis, stomatitis, unusual/metallic taste, vomiting, xerostomia

Genitourinary: Cystitis, darkened urine (rare), dyspareunia, dysuria, incontinence, libido decreased, pelvic pressure, polyuria, vaginal dryness, vaginitis

Hematologic: Neutropenia (reversible), thrombocytopenia (reversible, rare)

Local: Thrombophlebitis

Neuromuscular & skeletal: Dysarthria, peripheral neuropathy, weakness

Ocular: Optic neuropathy

Respiratory: Nasal congestion, pharyngitis, rhinitis, sinusitis, pharyngitis

Miscellaneous: Flu-like syndrome, joint pains resembling serum sickness, moniliasis

Available Dosage Forms

Capsule, oral: 375 mg

Flagyl® 375: 375 mg

Infusion, premixed iso-osmotic sodium chloride solution: 500 mg (100 mL)

Tablet, oral: 250 mg, 500 mg

Flagyl®: 250 mg, 500 mg

Tablet, extended release, oral:

Flagyl® ER: 750 mg

General Dosage Range Dosage adjustment recommended in patients with hepatic or renal impairment

I.V.: *Adults:* 500 mg every 6-8 hours (maximum: 4 g/day)

Oral:

Extended release: *Adults:* 750 mg once daily

Regular release:

Infants and Children: 35-50 mg/kg/day divided every 8 hours

Adults: 250-750 mg every 6-12 hours (maximum: 4 g/day) **or** 2 g as a single dose

Administration

Oral May be taken with food to minimize stomach upset. Extended release tablets should be taken on an empty stomach (1 hour before or 2 hours after meals).

I.V. Infuse intravenously over 30-60 minutes. Avoid contact of drug solution with equipment containing aluminum.

I.V. Detail pH: 5-7 (ready to use); 0.5-2.0 (reconstituted); 6-7 (further dilution)

Stability

Reconstitution Standard diluent: 500 mg/100 mL NS.

Storage

Injection: Store at controlled room temperature of 15°C to 30°C (59°F to 8F°C). Protect from light. Keep in overwrap until ready to use. Product may be refrigerated but crystals may form. Crystals redissolve on warming to room temperature. Prolonged exposure to light will cause a darkening of the product. However, short-term exposure to normal room light does not adversely affect metronidazole stability. Direct sunlight should be avoided. Stability of parenteral admixture at room temperature (25°C); Out of overwrap stability: 30 days.

Tablets: Store at room temperature. Protect from light and moisture.

Nursing Actions

Physical Assessment Monitor for CNS, neuromuscular, and dermatologic reactions.

Patient Education May take with or without food. Take with food if medication causes upset stomach. Extended release tablets should be taken on an empty stomach. Avoid alcohol during therapy. With alcohol you may experience severe flushing, headache, nausea, vomiting, or chest and abdominal pain. May discolor urine (brown/black/dark). You may experience "metallic" taste disturbance, nausea, or vomiting. Report unresolved or severe fatigue; weakness; fever or chills; mouth or vaginal sores; numbness, tingling, or swelling of extremities; respiratory difficulty; or lack of improvement or worsening of condition.

Dietary Considerations Take on an empty stomach. Drug may cause GI upset; if GI upset occurs, take with food. Extended release tablets should be taken on an empty stomach (1 hour before or 2 hours after meals). Some products may contain sodium. The manufacturer recommends that ethanol be avoided during treatment and for 3 days after therapy is complete.

Related Information

Compatibility of Drugs *on page 1264*

Miconazole (Topical) (mi KON a zole)

Brand Names: U.S. 3M™ Cavilon™ Antifungal [OTC]; Aloe Vesta® Antifungal [OTC]; Baza® Antifungal [OTC]; Carrington® Antifungal [OTC]; Critic-Aid®

Clear AF [OTC]; DermaFungal [OTC]; Dermagran® AF [OTC]; DiabetAid® Antifungal Foot Bath [OTC]; Fungoid® [OTC]; Lotrimin AF® [OTC]; Micaderm® [OTC]; Micatin® [OTC]; Micro-Guard® [OTC]; Miranel AF™ [OTC]; Mitrazol® [OTC]; Monistat® 1 Day or Night [OTC]; Monistat® 1 [OTC]; Monistat® 3 [OTC]; Monistat® 7 [OTC]; Neosporin® AF [OTC]; Podactin Cream [OTC]; Secura® Antifungal Extra Thick [OTC]; Secura® Antifungal Greaseless [OTC]; Ting® Spray Powder [OTC]; Zeasorb®-AF [OTC]

Index Terms Miconazole Nitrate

Pharmacologic Category Antifungal Agent, Topical; Antifungal Agent, Vaginal

Medication Safety Issues

Sound-alike/look-alike issues:

Miconazole may be confused with metroNIDAZOLE, Micronase, Micronor®

Lotrimin® may be confused with Lotrisone®, Otrivin®

Micatin® may be confused with Miacalcin®

Lactation Excretion in breast milk unknown/use caution

Use Treatment of vulvovaginal candidiasis and a variety of skin and mucous membrane fungal infections

Available Dosage Forms For available OTC formulations, consult specific product labeling.

General Dosage Range

Intravaginal: *Children ≥12 years and Adults:* Insert 1 applicatorful or suppository (100 mg or 200 mg) once daily at bedtime **or** insert 1 suppository (1200 mg) as a single dose.

Topical: *Children and Adults:* Apply twice daily **or** dissolve 1 effervescent tablet in ~1 gallon of water and soak feet for 15-30 minutes

Nursing Actions

Physical Assessment Caution patients with diabetes to test serum glucose regularly; may inhibit the metabolism of oral sulfonylureas. Teach patient bleeding precautions.

Patient Education Some infections may require long periods of therapy. Report persistent burning, itching, or irritation to healthcare provider.

Topical: Wash and dry area before applying medication; apply thinly. Do not get in or near eyes.

Vaginal: Consult with healthcare provider if using for a vaginal yeast infection for the first time. Insert high in vagina. Refrain from intercourse during treatment. Condoms and diaphragms may not be effective during therapy. Do not use tampons, douches, spermicides, or other vaginal products during treatment. Deodorant-free pads or panty shields may be used to protect clothing during use.

Midazolam (MID aye zoe lam)

Index Terms Midazolam Hydrochloride; Versed

Pharmacologic Category Benzodiazepine

Medication Safety Issues

Sound-alike/look-alike issues:

Versed may be confused with VePesid, Vistaril®

High alert medication:

The Institute for Safe Medication Practices (ISMP) includes this medication among its list of drugs which have a heightened risk of causing significant patient harm when used in error.

Pregnancy Risk Factor D

Lactation Enters breast milk/use caution (AAP rates "of concern"; AAP 2001 update pending)

Breast-Feeding Considerations Midazolam and hydroxymidazolam can be detected in breast milk. Based on information from two women, 2-3 months postpartum, the half-life of midazolam in breast milk is ~1 hour. Milk concentrations were below the limit of detection (<5 nmol/L) 4 hours after a single maternal dose of midazolam 15 mg. Drowsiness, lethargy, or weight loss in nursing infants have been observed in case reports following maternal use of some benzodiazepines.

Use Preoperative sedation; moderate sedation prior to diagnostic or radiographic procedures; ICU sedation (continuous infusion); induction and maintenance of general anesthesia

Unlabeled Use Anxiety, status epilepticus, conscious sedation (intranasal route)

Mechanism of Action/Effect Binds to stereospecific benzodiazepine receptors on the postsynaptic GABA neuron at several sites within the central nervous system, including the limbic system, reticular formation. Enhancement of the inhibitory effect of GABA on neuronal excitability results by increased neuronal membrane permeability to chloride ions. This shift in chloride ions results in hyperpolarization (a less excitable state) and stabilization.

Contraindications Hypersensitivity to midazolam or any component of the formulation; intrathecal or epidural injection of parenteral forms containing preservatives (ie, benzyl alcohol); acute narrow-angle glaucoma; concurrent use of potent inhibitors of CYP3A4 (amprenavir, atazanavir, or ritonavir)

Warnings/Precautions [U.S. Boxed Warning]: May cause severe respiratory depression, respiratory arrest, or apnea. Use with extreme caution, particularly in noncritical care settings. Appropriate resuscitative equipment and qualified personnel must be available for administration and monitoring. Initial dosing must be cautiously titrated and individualized, particularly in elderly or debilitated patients, patients with hepatic impairment (including alcoholics), or in renal impairment, particularly if other CNS depressants (including opiates) are used concurrently. **[U.S. Boxed Warning]: Initial doses in elderly or debilitated patients should be conservative; as little as 1 mg, but not to exceed 2.5 mg.** Use with caution in patients with respiratory disease or impaired gag reflex. Use during upper airway procedures may increase risk of hypoventilation. Prolonged responses have been noted following extended administration by continuous infusion (possibly due to metabolite accumulation) or in the presence of drugs which inhibit midazolam metabolism.

Causes CNS depression (dose-related) resulting in sedation, dizziness, confusion, or ataxia which may impair physical and mental capabilities. Patients must be cautioned about performing tasks which require mental alertness (eg, operating machinery or driving). A minimum of 1 day should elapse after midazolam administration before attempting these tasks. Use with caution in patients receiving other CNS depressants or psychoactive agents. Effects with other sedative drugs or ethanol may be potentiated. Benzodiazepines have been associated with falls and traumatic injury and should be used with extreme caution in patients who are at risk of these events (especially the elderly).

May cause hypotension - hemodynamic events are more common in pediatric patients or patients with hemodynamic instability. Hypotension and/or respiratory depression may occur more frequently in patients who have received opioid analgesics. Use with caution in obese patients, chronic renal failure, and HF. Does not protect against increases in heart rate or blood pressure during intubation. Should not be used in shock, coma, or acute alcohol intoxication. **[U.S. Boxed Warning]: Do not administer by rapid I.V. injection in neonates; severe hypotension and seizures have been reported; risk may be increased with concomitant fentanyl use.**

Avoid intra-arterial administration or extravasation of parenteral formulation. Some parenteral dosage forms may contain benzyl alcohol which has been associated with "gasping syndrome" in neonates. Some formulations may contain cherry flavoring.

Midazolam causes anterograde amnesia. Paradoxical reactions, including hyperactive or aggressive behavior have been reported with benzodiazepines, particularly in adolescent/pediatric or psychiatric patients. Does not have analgesic, antidepressant, or antipsychotic properties.

Benzodiazepines have been associated with dependence and acute withdrawal symptoms on discontinuation or reduction in dose. Acute withdrawal, including seizures, may be precipitated after administration of flumazenil to patients receiving long-term benzodiazepine therapy.

Drug Interactions

Avoid Concomitant Use

Avoid concomitant use of Midazolam with any of the following: Boceprevir; Conivaptan; Efavirenz; OLANZapine; Pimozide; Protease Inhibitors; Telaprevir

Decreased Effect

The levels/effects of Midazolam may be decreased by: CarBAMazepine; CYP3A4 Inducers (Strong); Deferasirox; Ginkgo Biloba; Rifamycin Derivatives; St Johns Wort; Theophylline Derivatives; Tocilizumab; Yohimbine

Increased Effect/Toxicity

Midazolam may increase the levels/effects of: Alcohol (Ethyl); ARIPiprazole; CloZAPine; CNS Depressants; Fosphenytoin; Methotrimeprazine; Phenytoin; Pimozide; Propofol; Selective Serotonin Reuptake Inhibitors

The levels/effects of Midazolam may be increased by: Antifungal Agents (Azole Derivatives, Systemic); Aprepitant; Atorvastatin; Boceprevir; Calcium Channel Blockers (Nondihydropyridine); Cimetidine; Conivaptan; Contraceptives (Estrogens); Contraceptives (Progestins); CYP3A4 Inhibitors (Moderate); CYP3A4 Inhibitors (Strong); Dasatinib; Droperidol; Efavirenz; Fosaprepitant; Grapefruit Juice; HydrOXYzine; Isoniazid; Ivacaftor; Macrolide Antibiotics; Methotrimeprazine; OLANZapine; Propofol; Protease Inhibitors; Proton Pump Inhibitors; Selective Serotonin Reuptake Inhibitors; Telaprevir

Nutritional/Ethanol Interactions

Ethanol: Ethanol may increase CNS depression. Management: Avoid ethanol.

Food: Grapefruit juice may increase serum concentrations of midazolam. Management: Avoid concurrent use of grapefruit juice with oral midazolam.

Herb/Nutraceutical: St John's wort may decrease midazolam levels and increase CNS depression; valerian, kava kava, and gotu kola may increase CNS depression. Management: Avoid concurrent use with St John's wort, valerian, kava kava, and gotu kola.

Adverse Reactions As reported in adults unless otherwise noted:

>10%: Respiratory: Decreased tidal volume and/or respiratory rate decrease, apnea (3% children)

1% to 10%:

Cardiovascular: Hypotension (3% children)

Central nervous system: Drowsiness (1%), oversedation, headache (1%), seizure-like activity (1% children)

Gastrointestinal: Nausea (3%), vomiting (3%)

Local: Pain and local reactions at injection site (4% I.M., 5% I.V.; severity less than diazepam)

Neuromuscular & skeletal: Myoclonic jerks (preterm infants)

Ocular: Nystagmus (1% children)

Respiratory: Cough (1%)

Miscellaneous: Physical and psychological dependence with prolonged use, hiccups (4%, 1% children), paradoxical reaction (2% children)

Pharmacodynamics/Kinetics

Onset of Action I.M.: Sedation: ~15 minutes; I.V.: 3-5 minutes; Oral: 10-20 minutes; Intranasal: Children: 4-8 minutes (Lee-Kim, 2004); Peak effect: I.M.: 0.5-1 hour

Duration of Action I.M.: Up to 6 hours; Mean: 2 hours; Intranasal: Children: 18-41 minutes (Lee-Kim, 2004)

Controlled Substance C-IV

Available Dosage Forms

Injection, solution: 1 mg/mL (2 mL, 5 mL, 10 mL); 5 mg/mL (1 mL, 2 mL, 5 mL, 10 mL)

Injection, solution [preservative free]: 1 mg/mL (2 mL, 5 mL); 5 mg/mL (1 mL, 2 mL)

Syrup, oral: 2 mg/mL (2.5 mL, 118 mL)

General Dosage Range

I.M.:

Children: 0.05-0.15 mg/kg 30-60 minutes (maximum: 10 mg total)

Adults: 0.07-0.08 mg/kg 30-60 minutes; Usual dose: 5 mg

I.V.:

Infants <6 months: 0.05-0.2 mg/kg loading dose followed by 0.4-6 mcg/kg/minute infusion

Infants 6 months to Children 5 years: Initial: 0.05-0.1 mg/kg once (maximum: 6 mg or 0.6 mg/kg total) **or** 0.05-0.2 mg/kg loading dose followed by 0.4-6 mcg/kg/minute infusion

Children 6-12 years: 0.025-0.05 mg/kg once (maximum: 10 mg or 0.4 mg/kg total) **or** 0.05-0.2 mg/kg loading dose followed by 0.4-6 mcg/kg/minute infusion

Children 12-16 years: 0.02-0.2 mg/kg once (maximum: 10 mg total) **or** 0.05-0.2 mg/kg loading dose followed by 0.4-6 mcg/kg/minute infusion

Adults: Dosage varies greatly depending on indication

Oral:

Children <6 years: 0.25-0.5 mg/kg as single dose; may require as much as 1 mg/kg (maximum: 20 mg total)

Children 6-16 years: 0.25-0.5 mg/kg as a single dose (maximum: 20 mg total)

Administration

Oral Do not mix with any liquid (such as grapefruit juice) prior to administration.

I.M. Give deep I.M. into large muscle.

I.V. Administer by slow I.V. injection over at least 2-5 minutes at a concentration of 1-5 mg/mL or by I.V. infusion. Continuous infusions should be administered via an infusion pump.

I.V. Detail pH: 3 (adjusted)

Other Intranasal: **Note:** Due to the low pH of the solution, burning upon administration is likely to occur. Use of an atomizer, such as the MAD 300 Mucosal Atomizer which attaches to a tuberculin syringe, can reduce irritation. If possible, based upon dose to be administered, use higher concentration injectable solution to minimize volume administered intranasal. Smaller volume will reduce irritation and swallowing of administered dose. The maximum recommended dose volume (of the 5 mg/mL concentration) per nare is 1 mL. Using the 5 mg/mL injectable solution, draw up desired dose with a 1-3 mL needleless syringe; may attach a nasal mucosal atomization device prior to delivering dose. Deliver half of the total dose volume into the first nare using the atomizer device or by dripping slowly into nostril, then deliver the other half of the dose into the second nare.

Stability

Storage The manufacturer states that midazolam, at a final concentration of 0.5 mg/mL, is stable for up to 24 hours when diluted with D_5W or NS. A final concentration of 1 mg/mL in NS has been documented to be stable for up to 10 days (McMullen, 1995). Admixtures do not require protection from light for short-term storage.

Nursing Actions

Physical Assessment I.V.: Monitor cardiac and respiratory status continuously. Monitor I.V. infusion site carefully for extravasation. For inpatient use, institute safety measures. I.V./I.M.: Monitor closely following administration. Provide bedrest and assistance with ambulation for several hours.

Patient Education Avoid use of alcohol.

Dietary Considerations Avoid grapefruit juice with oral syrup.

Related Information

Compatibility of Drugs *on page 1264*

Midodrine (MI doe dreen)

Index Terms Midodrine Hydrochloride; ProAmatine

Pharmacologic Category $Alpha_1$ Agonist

Medication Safety Issues

Sound-alike/look-alike issues:

Midodrine may be confused with Midrin®, minoxidil

ProAmatine may be confused with protamine

Pregnancy Risk Factor C

Lactation Excretion in breast milk is unknown/use caution

Use Orphan drug: Treatment of symptomatic orthostatic hypotension

Unlabeled Use Management of urinary incontinence; vasovagal syncope; prevention of dialysis-induced hypotension

Available Dosage Forms

Tablet, oral: 2.5 mg, 5 mg, 10 mg

General Dosage Range Dosage adjustment recommended in patients with renal impairment

Oral: *Adults:* 10 mg 3 times/day (maximum: 40 mg/day)

Administration

Oral Doses may be given in approximately 3- to 4-hour intervals (eg, shortly before or upon rising in the morning, at midday, in the late afternoon not later than 6 PM). Avoid dosing after the evening meal or within 4 hours of bedtime. Continue therapy only in patients who appear to attain symptomatic improvement during initial treatment. Standing systolic blood pressure may be elevated 15-30 mm Hg at 1 hour after a 10 mg dose. Some effect may persist for 2-3 hours.

Nursing Actions

Physical Assessment Assess for reduction of hypotension and adverse reactions (eg, supine hypertension, urinary urgency/retention, rash) prior to treatment and periodically thereafter. Standing blood pressure may be elevated 1 hour after administration and remain slightly elevated 3-4 hours.

Patient Education Take when sitting upright. Do not take within 4 hours of bedtime or when lying down for any length of time. Follow instructions for checking blood pressure and pulse routinely (same time of day; for 1 week at least). May cause urinary urgency or retention, dizziness, drowsiness, or headache. Report skin rash, severe gastric upset or pain, or muscle weakness or pain.

Mifepristone (mi FE pris tone)

Brand Names: U.S. Mifeprex®

Index Terms RU-38486; RU-486

Pharmacologic Category Abortifacient; Antineoplastic Agent, Hormone Antagonist; Antiprogestin

Medication Safety Issues

Sound-alike/look-alike issues:

Mifeprex® may be confused with Mirapex®

Mifepristone may be confused with misoprostol

High alert medication:

The Institute for Safe Medication Practices (ISMP) includes this medication among its list of drug classes which have a heightened risk of causing significant patient harm when used in error.

Medication Guide Available Yes

Pregnancy Risk Factor X

Lactation Excretion in breast milk unknown/contraindicated

Use Medical termination of intrauterine pregnancy, through day 49 of pregnancy. Patients may need treatment with misoprostol and possibly surgery to complete therapy.

Unlabeled Use Treatment of unresectable meningioma; has been studied in the treatment of breast cancer, ovarian cancer, and adrenal cortical carcinoma

Product Availability

Korlym™: FDA approved February 2012; availability expected March 2012

Korlym™ is indicated to control hyperglycemia secondary to hypercortisolism in adult patients with endogenous Cushing's syndrome who have diabetes mellitus type 2 or glucose intolerance and have failed surgery or are not candidates for surgery; consult prescribing information for additional information

Available Dosage Forms

Tablet, oral:

Mifeprex®: 200 mg

General Dosage Range Oral: *Adults:* Day 1: 600 mg (three 200 mg tablets) as a single dose; Day 3: 400 mcg (two 200 mcg tablets) as a single dose if needed

Nursing Actions

Physical Assessment Monitor for excessive bleeding. Monitor vital signs.

Patient Education This medication is used to terminate pregnancy under 7 weeks. It must be administered under direction of a qualified physician. You will need follow-up visits as directed by your prescriber (approximately 3 days and 14 days after treatment). Surgical termination of pregnancy may be required if medication fails; there is a risk of fetal malformation if treatment fails. You may experience vaginal bleeding and cramping that is heavier than a normal menstrual period; report immediately if severe or persistent. You may experience nausea, vomiting, and diarrhea. It is possible to get pregnant before your next period. Once the pregnancy has proved to be ended, contraception should be started before having sexual intercourse.

Miglitol (MIG li tol)

Brand Names: U.S. Glyset®

Pharmacologic Category Antidiabetic Agent, Alpha-Glucosidase Inhibitor

Medication Safety Issues

Sound-alike/look-alike issues:

Glyset® may be confused with Cycloset®

Pregnancy Risk Factor B

Lactation Enters breast milk (small amounts)/not recommended

Use Type 2 diabetes mellitus (noninsulin-dependent, NIDDM):

Monotherapy as an adjunct to diet to improve glycemic control in patients with type 2 diabetes mellitus (noninsulin-dependent, NIDDM) whose hyperglycemia cannot be managed with diet alone

Combination therapy with a sulfonylurea when diet plus either miglitol or a sulfonylurea alone do not result in adequate glycemic control. The effect of miglitol to enhance glycemic control is additive to that of sulfonylureas when used in combination.

Available Dosage Forms

Tablet, oral:

Glyset®: 25 mg, 50 mg, 100 mg

General Dosage Range Oral: *Adults:* Initial: 25 mg 3 times/day; Maintenance: 25-100 mg 3 times/day (maximum: 300 mg/day)

Administration

Oral Should be taken orally at the start (with the first bite) of each main meal.

Nursing Actions

Physical Assessment Teach patient importance of adequate diabetic control.

Patient Education Take with the first bite of each main meal. Avoid alcohol. It is important to follow dietary and lifestyle recommendations of prescriber. You will be instructed in signs of hyper-/hypoglycemia. If combining this medication with other diabetic medication (eg, sulfonylureas, insulin), keep source of glucose in the form of dextrose (NOT table sugar, candy, or cookies) on hand in case hypoglycemia occurs. May cause mild side effects during first weeks of therapy (eg, bloating, flatulence, diarrhea, abdominal discomfort); these should diminish over time. Report severe or persistent side effects, fever, extended vomiting or flu, or change in color of urine or stool.

Milnacipran (mil NAY ci pran)

Brand Names: U.S. Savella®

Pharmacologic Category Antidepressant, Serotonin/Norepinephrine Reuptake Inhibitor

Medication Safety Issues

Sound-alike/look-alike issues:

Savella® may be confused with cevimeline, sevelamer

Medication Guide Available Yes

Pregnancy Risk Factor C

Lactation Excretion in breast milk unknown/not recommended

Breast-Feeding Considerations It is unknown if milnacipran is excreted in human milk. Breast-feeding is not recommended by the manufacturer.

Use Management of fibromyalgia

Mechanism of Action/Effect Inhibits norepinephrine and serotonin reuptake; improves symptoms associated with fibromyalgia

Contraindications Concomitant use or within 2 weeks of MAO inhibitors; uncontrolled narrow-angle glaucoma

Warnings/Precautions [U.S. Boxed Warning]: Milnacipran is a serotonin/norepinephrine reuptake inhibitor (SNRI) similar to SNRIs used to treat depression and other psychiatric disorders. **Antidepressants increase the risk of suicidal thinking and behavior in children, adolescents, and young adults (18-24 years of age) with major depressive disorder (MDD) and other psychiatric disorders**; consider risk prior to prescribing. Short-term studies did not show an increased risk in patients >24 years of age and showed a decreased risk in patients ≥65 years. Closely monitor for clinical worsening, suicidality, or unusual changes in behavior; the patient's family or caregiver should be instructed to closely observe the patient and communicate condition with healthcare provider. A medication guide should be dispensed with each prescription. **Milnacipran is not FDA approved for the treatment of major depressive disorder or for use in children.**

Suicide risks should be monitored in patients treated with SNRIs regardless of the indication. The possibility of a suicide attempt is inherent in major depression and may persist until remission occurs. Monitor for worsening of depression or suicidality, especially during initiation of therapy (generally first 1-2 months) or with dose increases or decreases. Use caution in high-risk patients. Worsening depression and severe abrupt suicidality that are not part of the presenting symptoms may require discontinuation or modification of drug therapy. The patient's family or caregiver should be alerted to monitor patients for the emergence of suicidality and associated behaviors (such as agitation, irritability, hostility, impulsivity, and hypomania) and call healthcare provider.

Patients with major depressive disorder were excluded from clinical trials evaluating milnacipran for fibromyalgia; however, mania has been reported in patients with mood disorders taking similar medications. May worsen psychosis in some patients or precipitate a shift to mania or hypomania in patients with bipolar disorder. Patients presenting with depressive symptoms should be screened for bipolar disorder. Monotherapy in patients with bipolar disorder should be avoided. **Milnacipran is not FDA approved for the treatment of bipolar depression.**

Serotonin syndrome and neuroleptic malignant syndrome (NMS)-like reactions have occurred with serotonin/norepinephrine reuptake inhibitors (SNRIs) and selective serotonin reuptake inhibitors (SSRIs) when used alone, and particularly when used in combination with serotonergic agents (eg, triptans) or antidopaminergic agents (eg, antipsychotics). Concurrent use with MAO inhibitors is contraindicated. May cause sustained increase in blood pressure or heart rate. Control pre-existing hypertension and cardiovascular disease prior to initiation of milnacipran. Use caution in patients with renal impairment; dose reduction required in severe renal impairment. Use caution in patients with hepatic impairment. Avoid ethanol use. May cause hyponatremia/SIADH (elderly at increased risk); volume depletion (diuretics may increase risk). Use cautiously in patients with a history of seizures. May impair platelet aggregation, resulting in bleeding. May cause increased urinary resistance. Use caution in patients with controlled narrow-angle glaucoma; use is contraindicated with uncontrolled narrow-angle glaucoma.

Abrupt discontinuation or dosage reduction after extended therapy may lead to agitation, dysphoria, anxiety, and other symptoms. When discontinuing therapy, dosage should be tapered gradually. If intolerable symptoms occur following a decrease in dosage or upon discontinuation of therapy, then resuming the previous dose with a more gradual taper should be considered.

Drug Interactions

Avoid Concomitant Use

Avoid concomitant use of Milnacipran with any of the following: Iobenguane I 123; MAO Inhibitors; Methylene Blue

Decreased Effect

Milnacipran may decrease the levels/effects of: Alpha2-Agonists; Iobenguane I 123; Ioflupane I 123

Increased Effect/Toxicity

Milnacipran may increase the levels/effects of: Alpha-/Beta-Agonists; Aspirin; Digoxin; Methylene Blue; Metoclopramide; NSAID (Nonselective); Serotonin Modulators; Vitamin K Antagonists

The levels/effects of Milnacipran may be increased by: Alcohol (Ethyl); Antipsychotics; ClomiPRAMINE; Linezolid; MAO Inhibitors

Nutritional/Ethanol Interactions

Ethanol: Ethanol may increase CNS depression. Management: Avoid ethanol.

Herb/Nutraceutical: Some herbal medications may increase risk of serotonin syndrome and/or excessive sedation. Management: Avoid valerian, St John's wort, SAMe, kava kava, and tryptophan.

Adverse Reactions

>10%:

Central nervous system: Headache (18%), insomnia (12%)

Endocrine & metabolic: Hot flashes (12%)

Gastrointestinal: Nausea (37%), constipation (16%)

1% to 10%:

Cardiovascular: Palpitation (7%), heart rate increased (6%), hypertension (5%), flushing (3%), blood pressure increased (3%), tachycardia (2%), peripheral edema (≥1%)

Central nervous system: Dizziness (10%), migraine (5%), chills (2%), tremor (2%), depression (≥1%), fatigue (≥1%), fever (≥1%), irritability (≥1%), somnolence (≥1%)

Dermatologic: Hyperhidrosis (9%), rash (3%)

Endocrine & metabolic: Hypercholesterolemia (≥1%)

Gastrointestinal: Vomiting (7%), xerostomia (5%), abdominal pain (3%), appetite decreased (2%), abdominal distension (≥1%), abnormal taste (≥1%), diarrhea (≥1%), dyspepsia (≥1%), flatulence (≥1%), gastroesophageal reflux disease (≥1%), weight changes (≥1%)

Genitourinary: Dysuria (≥2%), ejaculation disorder/failure (≥2%), erectile dysfunction (≥2%), libido decreased (≥2%), prostatitis (≥2%), scrotal pain (≥2%), testicular pain (≥2%), testicular swelling (≥2%), urethral pain (≥2%), urinary hesitation (≥2%), urinary retention (≥2%), urine flow decreased (≥2%), cystitis (≥1%), urinary tract infection (≥1%)

Neuromuscular & skeletal: Falling (≥1%)

Ocular: Blurred vision (2%)

Respiratory: Dyspnea (2%)

Miscellaneous: Night sweats (≥1%)

Available Dosage Forms

Combination package, oral:

Savella®: Tablet: 12.5 mg (5s), Tablet: 25 mg (8s), and Tablet: 50 mg (42s)

Tablet, oral:

Savella®: 12.5 mg, 25 mg, 50 mg, 100 mg

General Dosage Range Dosage adjustment recommended in patients with renal impairment

Oral: *Adults:* 50 mg twice daily (maximum dose: 200 mg/day)

Administration

Oral May be administered with or without food; food may improve tolerability.

Stability

Storage Store at 25°C (77°F); excursions permitted between 15°C to 30°C (59°F to 86°F).

Nursing Actions

Physical Assessment Monitor blood pressure and heart rate prior to initiating therapy and periodically throughout. Monitor for signs and symptoms of suicide ideation (eg, anxiety, depression, behavior changes). Taper dosage when discontinuing.

Patient Education Avoid use of alcohol. You may experience headaches, trouble sleeping, hot flashes, nausea, constipation, dizziness, increased perspiration, and dry mouth. Report unusual bleeding or bruising; blood in stool, vomitus, or urine; nosebleeds; bleeding gums; pain in joints or back; new or worsening depression; changes in mood; aggressive or violent behavior; panic attacks; or suicide ideation.

Dietary Considerations May be taken with or without food; food may improve tolerability.

Milrinone (MIL ri none)

Index Terms Milrinone Lactate

Pharmacologic Category Phosphodiesterase Enzyme Inhibitor

Medication Safety Issues

Sound-alike/look-alike issues:

Primacor® may be confused with Primaxin®

High alert medication:

The Institute for Safe Medication Practices (ISMP) includes this medication among its list of drugs which have a heightened risk of causing significant patient harm when used in error.

Pregnancy Risk Factor C

Lactation Excretion in breast milk unknown/use caution

Use Short-term I.V. therapy of acutely-decompensated heart failure

Unlabeled Use Inotropic therapy for patients unresponsive to other acute heart failure therapies (eg, dobutamine); outpatient inotropic therapy for heart transplant candidates; palliation of symptoms in end-stage heart failure patients who cannot otherwise be discharged from the hospital and are not transplant candidates

Mechanism of Action/Effect Phosphodiesterase inhibitor resulting in vasodilation

Contraindications Hypersensitivity to milrinone, inamrinone, or any component of the formulation; concurrent use of inamrinone

Warnings/Precautions Monitor closely for hypotension. Avoid in severe obstructive aortic or pulmonic valvular disease. Milrinone may aggravate outflow tract obstruction in hypertrophic subaortic stenosis. Supraventricular and ventricular arrhythmias have developed in high-risk patients. Ensure that ventricular rate controlled in atrial fibrillation/flutter prior to initiating milrinone. Not recommended for use in acute MI patients. Monitor and correct fluid and electrolyte problems. Adjust dose in renal dysfunction. Discontinue therapy if dose-related elevations in LFTs and clinical symptoms of hepatotoxicity occur.

Drug Interactions

Avoid Concomitant Use There are no known interactions where it is recommended to avoid concomitant use.

Decreased Effect There are no known significant interactions involving a decrease in effect.

Increased Effect/Toxicity There are no known significant interactions involving an increase in effect.

Adverse Reactions

>10%: Cardiovascular: Ventricular arrhythmia (ectopy 9%, NSVT 3%, sustained ventricular tachycardia 1%, ventricular fibrillation <1%)

1% to 10%:

Cardiovascular: Supraventricular arrhythmia (4%), hypotension (3%), angina/chest pain (1%)

Central nervous system: Headache (3%)

Pharmacodynamics/Kinetics

Onset of Action I.V.: 5-15 minutes

Available Dosage Forms

Infusion, premixed in D_5W: 200 mcg/mL (100 mL, 200 mL)

Injection, solution: 1 mg/mL (10 mL, 20 mL, 50 mL)

Injection, solution [preservative free]: 1 mg/mL (10 mL, 20 mL)

General Dosage Range Dosage adjustment recommended in patients with renal impairment

I.V.: *Adults:* Loading dose (optional): 50 mcg/kg; Maintenance: 0.375-0.75 mcg/kg/minute

Administration

I.V. Infuse via infusion pump.

I.V. Detail Injectable solution and premixed solution: pH: 3.2-4.0

Stability

Reconstitution Standard dilution: For a final concentration of 0.2 mg/mL: Dilute Primacor® 1 mg/mL (20 mL) with 80 mL diluent (final volume: 100 mL) of 1/2 NS, NS or D_5W. May also dilute 1 mg/mL (10 mL) with 40 mL diluent (final volume: 50 mL).

Storage Store at 15°C to 30°C (59°F to 86°F); avoid freezing. Stable at 0.2 mg/mL in 1/2NS, NS, or D_5W for 72 hours at room temperature in normal light.

Nursing Actions

Physical Assessment Monitor cardiac/hemodynamic status continuously during therapy and serum potassium at regular intervals. Monitor for fluid retention.

Patient Education This drug can only be given intravenously. Weigh daily and report weight gain. Report pain at infusion site; numbness, tingling, or swelling of extremities; or respiratory difficulty.

Minocycline (mi noe SYE kleen)

Brand Names: U.S. Dynacin®; Minocin®; Minocin® PAC; Solodyn®

Index Terms Minocycline Hydrochloride

Pharmacologic Category Antibiotic, Tetracycline Derivative

Medication Safety Issues

Sound-alike/look-alike issues:

Dynacin® may be confused with Dyazide®, DynaCirc®, Dynapen

Minocin® may be confused with Indocin®, Lincocin®, Minizide®, niacin

Pregnancy Risk Factor D

Lactation Enters breast milk/not recommended

Breast-Feeding Considerations Small amounts of minocycline are excreted in breast milk and therefore, breast-feeding is not recommended by the manufacturer. Minocycline absorption is not affected by dairy products. This may lead to increased absorption from maternal milk when compared to other tetracyclines which are bound by the calcium in the maternal milk. Nondose-related effects could include modification of bowel flora. There have been case reports of black discoloration of breast milk in women taking minocycline.

Use Treatment of susceptible bacterial infections of both gram-negative and gram-positive organisms; treatment of anthrax (inhalational, cutaneous, and gastrointestinal); moderate-to-severe acne; meningococcal (asymptomatic) carrier state; Rickettsial diseases (including Rocky Mountain spotted fever, Q fever); nongonococcal urethritis, gonorrhea; acute intestinal amebiasis; respiratory tract infection; skin/soft tissue infections; chlamydial infections

Extended release (Solodyn®): Only indicated for treatment of inflammatory lesions of non-nodular moderate-to-severe acne

Unlabeled Use Rheumatoid arthritis (patients with low disease activity of short duration); nocardiosis; alternative treatment for community-acquired MRSA infection

Mechanism of Action/Effect Inhibits bacterial protein synthesis by binding with the 30S and possibly the 50S ribosomal subunit(s) of susceptible bacteria; cell wall synthesis is not affected

Rheumatoid arthritis: The mechanism of action of minocycline in rheumatoid arthritis is not completely understood. It is thought to have antimicrobial, anti-inflammatory, immunomodulatory, and chondroprotective effects. More specifically, it is thought to be a potent inhibitor of metalloproteinases, which are active in rheumatoid arthritis joint destruction.

Contraindications Hypersensitivity to minocycline, other tetracyclines, or any component of the formulation; children <8 years of age

Warnings/Precautions May be associated with increases in BUN secondary to antianabolic effects; use caution in patients with renal impairment (Cl_{cr} <80 mL/minute). Hepatotoxicity has been reported; use caution in patients with hepatic insufficiency. Autoimmune syndromes (eg, lupus-like, hepatitis, and vasculitis) have been reported; discontinue if symptoms occur. CNS effects (lightheadedness, vertigo) may occur; patients must be cautioned about performing tasks which require mental alertness (eg, operating machinery or driving). Pseudotumor cerebri has been (rarely) reported with tetracycline use; usually resolves with discontinuation. May cause photosensitivity; discontinue if skin erythema occurs. Prolonged use may result in fungal or bacterial superinfection, including *C. difficile*-associated diarrhea (CDAD) and pseudomembranous colitis; CDAD has been observed >2 months postantibiotic treatment. May cause tissue hyperpigmentation, enamel hypoplasia, or permanent tooth discoloration; use of tetracyclines should be avoided during tooth development (children <8 years of age) unless other drugs are not likely to be effective or are contraindicated. Do not use during pregnancy. In addition to affecting tooth development, tetracycline use has been associated with retardation of skeletal development and reduced bone growth. Rash, along with eosinophilia, fever, and organ failure (Drug Rash with Eosinophilia and Systemic Symptoms [DRESS] syndrome) has been reported; discontinue treatment immediately if DRESS syndrome is suspected.

Drug Interactions

Avoid Concomitant Use

Avoid concomitant use of Minocycline with any of the following: BCG; Retinoic Acid Derivatives

Decreased Effect

Minocycline may decrease the levels/effects of: Atazanavir; BCG; Penicillins; Typhoid Vaccine

The levels/effects of Minocycline may be decreased by: Antacids; Bile Acid Sequestrants; Bismuth; Bismuth Subsalicylate; Calcium Salts; Iron Salts; Lanthanum; Magnesium Salts; Quinapril; Sucralfate; Zinc Salts

Increased Effect/Toxicity

Minocycline may increase the levels/effects of: Neuromuscular-Blocking Agents; Porfimer; Retinoic Acid Derivatives; Vitamin K Antagonists

Nutritional/Ethanol Interactions

Food: Minocycline serum concentrations are not significantly altered if taken with food or dairy products.

Herb/Nutraceutical: Avoid dong quai, St John's wort (may also cause photosensitization).

Adverse Reactions Frequency not defined.

Cardiovascular: Myocarditis, pericarditis, vasculitis

Central nervous system: Bulging fontanels, dizziness, fatigue, fever, headache, hypoesthesia, malaise, mood changes, paresthesia, pseudotumor cerebri, sedation, seizure, somnolence, vertigo

Dermatologic: Alopecia, angioedema, drug rash with eosinophilia and systemic symptoms (DRESS), erythema multiforme, erythema nodosum, erythematous rash, exfoliative dermatitis, hyperpigmentation of nails, maculopapular rash, photosensitivity, pigmentation of the skin and mucous membranes, pruritus, Stevens-Johnson syndrome, toxic epidermal necrolysis, urticaria

Endocrine & metabolic: Thyroid cancer, thyroid discoloration, thyroid dysfunction

Gastrointestinal: Anorexia, diarrhea, dyspepsia, dysphagia, enamel hypoplasia, enterocolitis, esophageal ulcerations, esophagitis, glossitis, inflammatory lesions (oral/anogenital), moniliasis, nausea, oral cavity discoloration, pancreatitis, pseudomembranous colitis, stomatitis, tooth discoloration, vomiting, xerostomia

Genitourinary: Balanitis, vulvovaginitis

Hematologic: Agranulocytosis, eosinophilia, hemolytic anemia, leukopenia, neutropenia, pancytopenia, thrombocytopenia

Hepatic: Autoimmune hepatitis, hepatic cholestasis, hepatic failure, hepatitis, hyperbilirubinemia, jaundice, liver enzyme increases

Local: Injection site reaction (I.V. administration)

Neuromuscular & skeletal: Arthralgia, arthritis, bone discoloration, joint stiffness, joint swelling, myalgia

Otic: Hearing loss, tinnitus

Renal: Acute renal failure, BUN increased, interstitial nephritis

Respiratory: Asthma, bronchospasm, cough, dyspnea, pneumonitis, pulmonary infiltrate (with eosinophilia)

Miscellaneous: Anaphylaxis, hypersensitivity, lupus erythematosus, lupus-like syndrome, serum sickness

Available Dosage Forms

Capsule, oral: 50 mg, 75 mg, 100 mg

Capsule, pellet filled, oral:

Minocin®: 50 mg, 100 mg

Minocin® PAC: 50 mg, 100 mg

Injection, powder for reconstitution:

Minocin®: 100 mg

Tablet, oral: 50 mg, 75 mg, 100 mg

Dynacin®: 50 mg, 75 mg, 100 mg

Tablet, extended release, oral: 45 mg, 90 mg, 135 mg

Solodyn®: 45 mg, 65 mg, 90 mg, 115 mg, 135 mg

General Dosage Range Dosage adjustment recommended in patients with renal impairment

I.V.:

Children >8 years: 4 mg/kg initially, followed by 2 mg/kg/dose every 12 hours (maximum: 400 mg/day)

Adults: 200 mg initially, followed by 100 mg every 12 hours (maximum: 400 mg/day)

Oral:

Children >8 years: 4 mg/kg initially, followed by 2 mg/kg/dose every 12 hours

Children ≥12 years: Solodyn®: 45-135 mg once daily (weight-based)

Adults: 200 mg initially, followed by 100 mg every 12 hours **or** 50-100 mg twice daily (acne); Solodyn®: 45-135 mg once daily (weight-based)

Administration

Oral May be administered with or without food. Administer with adequate fluid to decrease the risk of esophageal irritation and ulceration. Swallow pellet-filled capsule and extended release tablet whole; do not chew, crush, or split.

I.V. I.V.: Infuse slowly; avoid rapid administration. The manufacturer's labeling does not provide a recommended administration rate. The injectable route should be used only if the oral route is not feasible or adequate. Prolonged intravenous therapy may be associated with thrombophlebitis.

Stability

Reconstitution Injection: Reconstitute with 5 mL of sterile water for injection, and further dilute in 500-1000 mL of NS, D_5W, D_5NS, Ringer's injection, or LR.

Storage

Capsule (including pellet-filled), tablet: Store at 20°C to 25°C (68°F to 77°F); protect from heat. Protect from light and moisture.

Extended release tablet: Store at 15°C to 30°C (59°F to 86°F); protect from heat. Protect from light and moisture.

Injection: Store vials at 20°C to 25°C (68°F to 77°F) prior to reconstitution. Reconstituted solution is stable at room temperature for 24 hours. Final dilutions should be administered immediately.

Nursing Actions

Physical Assessment Results of culture and sensitivity tests and allergy history should be assessed before beginning therapy. Teach patient importance of adequate hydration.

Patient Education May cause photosensitivity reaction, nausea, fatigue, headache, dizziness, sedation, or diarrhea. Report rash or itching, unresolved nausea or diarrhea, change in urinary output (excess), and opportunistic infection (eg, fever, chills, sore throat, burning urination, fatigue).

I.V.: Report immediately any pain, burning, or swelling at infusion site or any signs of allergic reaction (eg, respiratory difficulty or swallowing, back pain, chest tightness, rash, hives, swelling of lips or mouth).

Oral: May be taken with or without food.

Dietary Considerations May be taken with or without food.

Mirtazapine (mir TAZ a peen)

Brand Names: U.S. Remeron SolTab®; Remeron®

Pharmacologic Category Antidepressant, Alpha-2 Antagonist

Medication Safety Issues

Sound-alike/look-alike issues:

Remeron® may be confused with Premarin®, ramelteon, Rozerem®, Zemuron®

International issues:

Avanza [Australia] may be confused with Albenza brand name for albendazole [U.S.]; Avandia brand name for rosiglitazone [U.S., Canada, and multiple international markets]

Remeron [U.S., Canada, and multiple international markets] may be confused with Reneuron which is a brand name for fluoxetine [Spain]

Medication Guide Available Yes

Pregnancy Risk Factor C

Lactation Excreted in breast milk/use caution

Breast-Feeding Considerations Mirtazapine and its active metabolite are found in breast milk, with higher levels in the hindmilk than foremilk. Adverse events have not been observed in nursing infants. The manufacturer recommends that caution be used if administered to a breast-feeding woman.

Use Treatment of depression

Unlabeled Use Post-traumatic stress disorder (PTSD)

Mechanism of Action/Effect Mirtazapine is a tetracyclic antidepressant that works by its central presynaptic alpha$_2$-adrenergic antagonist effects, which results in increased release of norepinephrine and serotonin. It is also a potent antagonist of 5-HT$_2$ and 5-HT$_3$ serotonin receptors and H1 histamine receptors and a moderate peripheral alpha$_1$-adrenergic and muscarinic antagonist; it does not inhibit the reuptake of norepinephrine or serotonin.

Contraindications Hypersensitivity to mirtazapine or any component of the formulation; use of MAO inhibitors within 14 days

Warnings/Precautions [U.S. Boxed Warning]: Antidepressants increase the risk of suicidal thinking and behavior in children, adolescents, and young adults (18-24 years of age) with major depressive disorder (MDD) and other psychiatric disorders; consider risk prior to prescribing. Short-term studies did not show an increased risk in patients >24 years of age and showed a decreased risk in patients ≥65 years. Closely monitor for clinical worsening, suicidality, or unusual changes in behavior; the patient's family or caregiver should be instructed to closely observe the patient and communicate condition with healthcare provider. A medication guide should be dispensed with each prescription. **Mirtazapine is not FDA approved for use in children.**

The possibility of a suicide attempt is inherent in major depression and may persist until remission occurs. Monitor for worsening of depression or suicidality, especially during initiation of therapy (generally first 1-2 months) or with dose increases or decreases. Use caution in high-risk patients. Worsening depression and severe abrupt suicidality that are not part of the presenting symptoms may require discontinuation or modification of drug therapy. The patient's family or caregiver should be alerted to monitor patients for the emergence of suicidality and associated behaviors (such as agitation, irritability, hostility, impulsivity, and hypomania) and call healthcare provider.

May worsen psychosis in some patients or precipitate a shift to mania or hypomania in patients with bipolar disorder. Patients presenting with depressive symptoms should be screened for bipolar disorder. Monotherapy in patients with bipolar disorder should be avoided. **Mirtazapine is not FDA approved for the treatment of bipolar depression.**

Patients should not discontinue treatment abruptly, unless significant life-threatening event, due to risk of withdrawal symptoms. A gradual reduction in the dose over several weeks is recommended.

Discontinue immediately if signs and symptoms of neutropenia/agranulocytosis occur. May cause sedation, resulting in impaired performance of tasks requiring alertness (eg, operating machinery or driving). Sedative effects may be additive with other CNS depressants and/or ethanol. The degree of sedation is moderate-high relative to other antidepressants. Conversely, may increase psychomotor restlessness within first few weeks of therapy. The risks of orthostatic hypotension or anticholinergic effects are low relative to other antidepressants. The incidence of sexual dysfunction with mirtazapine is generally lower than with SSRIs. Potential for severe reaction when used with MAO inhibitors; autonomic instability, coma, death, delirium, diaphoresis, hyperthermia, mental status changes/agitation, muscular rigidity, myoclonus, neuroleptic malignant syndrome features, and seizures may occur.

May increase appetite and stimulate weight gain. Weight gain of >7% of body weight reported in 7.5% of patients treated with mirtazapine compared to 0% for placebo; 8% of patients receiving mirtazapine discontinued treatment due to the weight gain. In an 8-week pediatric clinical trial, 49% of mirtazapine-treated patients had a weight gain of at least 7% (mean increase 4 kg) as compared to 5.7% of placebo-treated patients (mean increase 1 kg). May increase serum cholesterol and triglyceride levels.

Use caution in patients with a previous seizure disorder or condition predisposing to seizures such as brain damage, alcoholism, or concurrent therapy with other drugs which lower the seizure threshold. May cause hyponatremia.Use with caution in patients with hepatic or renal dysfunction and in elderly patients. Clinically significant transaminase elevations have been observed. SolTab® formulation contains phenylalanine.

Drug Interactions

Avoid Concomitant Use

Avoid concomitant use of Mirtazapine with any of the following: Conivaptan; MAO Inhibitors; Methylene Blue

Decreased Effect

Mirtazapine may decrease the levels/effects of: Alpha2-Agonists

The levels/effects of Mirtazapine may be decreased by: CYP1A2 Inducers (Strong); CYP3A4 Inducers (Strong); Cyproterone; Deferasirox; Peginterferon Alfa-2b; Tocilizumab

Increased Effect/Toxicity

Mirtazapine may increase the levels/effects of: Alcohol (Ethyl); CNS Depressants; Methylene Blue; Metoclopramide; Serotonin Modulators; Warfarin

The levels/effects of Mirtazapine may be increased by: Abiraterone Acetate; Antipsychotics; Conivaptan; CYP1A2 Inhibitors (Moderate); CYP1A2 Inhibitors (Strong); CYP2D6 Inhibitors (Moderate); CYP2D6 Inhibitors (Strong); CYP3A4 Inhibitors (Moderate); CYP3A4 Inhibitors (Strong); Darunavir; Dasatinib;

Deferasirox; HydrOXYzine; Ivacaftor; Linezolid; MAO Inhibitors

Nutritional/Ethanol Interactions

Ethanol: May increase CNS depression; monitor for increased effects with coadministration. Caution patients about effects.

Herb/Nutraceutical: Avoid St John's wort (may decrease mirtazapine levels). Avoid valerian, St John's wort, SAMe, kava kava (may increase CNS depression).

Adverse Reactions

>10%:

Central nervous system: Somnolence (54%)

Endocrine & metabolic: Increased cholesterol

Gastrointestinal: Constipation (13%), xerostomia (25%), increased appetite (17%), weight gain (12%; weight gain of >7% reported in 8% of adults, ≤49% of pediatric patients)

1% to 10%:

Cardiovascular: Hypertension, vasodilatation, peripheral edema (2%), edema (1%)

Central nervous system: Dizziness (7%), abnormal dreams (4%), abnormal thoughts (3%), confusion (2%), malaise

Endocrine & metabolic: Increased triglycerides

Gastrointestinal: Vomiting, anorexia, abdominal pain

Genitourinary: Urinary frequency (2%)

Hepatic: SGPT increased (≥3 times ULN: 2%)

Neuromuscular & skeletal: Myalgia (2%), back pain (2%), arthralgia, tremor (2%), weakness (8%)

Respiratory: Dyspnea (1%)

Miscellaneous: Flu-like syndrome (5%), thirst

Available Dosage Forms

Tablet, oral: 7.5 mg, 15 mg, 30 mg, 45 mg

Remeron®: 15 mg, 30 mg, 45 mg

Tablet, orally disintegrating, oral: 15 mg, 30 mg, 45 mg

Remeron SolTab®: 15 mg, 30 mg, 45 mg

General Dosage Range Oral: *Adults:* Initial: 15 mg nightly; Maintenance: 15-45 mg nightly

Administration

Oral SolTab®: Open blister pack and place tablet on the tongue. Do not split tablet. Tablet is formulated to dissolve on the tongue without water.

Stability

Storage Store at controlled room temperature of 25°C (77°F); excursions permitted to 15°C to 30°C (59°F to 86°F). Protect from light and moisture.

SolTab®: Protect from light and moisture. Use immediately upon opening tablet blister.

Nursing Actions

Physical Assessment Monitor therapeutic response (ie, mood, affect, mental status) at beginning of therapy and periodically throughout. Monitor for CNS depression/sedation. Monitor for clinical worsening and suicide ideation. Taper dosage slowly when discontinuing.

Patient Education It may take 2-3 weeks to achieve desired results. Take once-a-day dose at bedtime. Avoid alcohol. Maintain adequate hydration unless instructed to restrict fluid intake. You may experience drowsiness, dizziness, lightheadedness, nausea, vomiting, anorexia, dry mouth, or orthostatic hypotension. Report persistent insomnia, agitation, or confusion; suicide ideation; muscle cramping, tremors, weakness, or change in gait; breathlessness or respiratory difficulty; chest pain, palpitations, or rapid heartbeat; change in urinary pattern; vision changes or eye pain; yellowing of eyes or skin; pale stools/dark urine; or worsening of condition.

SolTab®: Tablet is formulated to dissolve on the tongue without water.

Dietary Considerations Some products may contain phenylalanine.

Misoprostol (mye soe PROST ole)

Brand Names: U.S. Cytotec®

Pharmacologic Category Prostaglandin

Medication Safety Issues

Sound-alike/look-alike issues:

Cytotec® may be confused with Cytoxan

Misoprostol may be confused with metoprolol, mifepristone

Pregnancy Risk Factor X

Lactation Enters breast milk/use caution

Use Prevention of NSAID-induced gastric ulcers; medical termination of pregnancy of ≤49 days (in conjunction with mifepristone)

Unlabeled Use Cervical ripening and labor induction (except in women with prior cesarean delivery or major uterine surgery); fat malabsorption in cystic fibrosis

Available Dosage Forms

Tablet, oral: 100 mcg, 200 mcg

Cytotec®: 100 mcg, 200 mcg

General Dosage Range Oral:

Adults: 100-200 mcg 4 times/day

Elderly: Initial: 100 mcg/day

Administration

Oral Incidence of diarrhea may be lessened by having patient take dose right after meals and avoiding magnesium-containing antacids. When used for the prevention of NSAID-induced ulcers, therapy is usually begun on the second or third day of the next normal menstrual period in women of childbearing potential.

Nursing Actions

Physical Assessment Teach appropriate diet and lifestyle if being used to prevent ulcers.

Patient Education Take with meals or after meals to prevent nausea, diarrhea, and flatulence. You may experience increased menstrual pain or cramping. Report abnormal menstrual periods, spotting (may occur even in postmenstrual women), or severe menstrual bleeding.

Mitotane (MYE toe tane)

Brand Names: U.S. Lysodren®

Index Terms Chloditan; Chlodithane; Khloditan; Mytotan; o,p'-DDD; Ortho,para-DDD

Pharmacologic Category Antineoplastic Agent, Miscellaneous

Medication Safety Issues

Sound-alike/look-alike issues:

Mitotane may be confused with mitoMYcin, mitoXANtrone

High alert medication:

The Institute for Safe Medication Practices (ISMP) includes this medication among its list of drug classes which have a heightened risk of causing significant patient harm when used in error.

Pregnancy Risk Factor C

Lactation Excretion in breast milk unknown/not recommended

Use Treatment of inoperable adrenocortical carcinoma

Unlabeled Use Treatment of Cushing's syndrome

Available Dosage Forms

Tablet, oral:

Lysodren®: 500 mg

General Dosage Range Dosage adjustment recommended in patients who develop toxicities

Oral: *Adults:* Initial: 2-6 g/day in divided doses; Maintenance: 9-10 g/day in 3-4 divided doses (maximum: 18 g/day)

Administration

Oral Administer in 3-4 divided doses/day. Do not crush tablets; wear gloves when handling; avoid exposure to crushed or broken tablets.

Nursing Actions

Physical Assessment Monitor for CNS changes, gastrointestinal upset, rash, and musculoskeletal weakness on a regular basis.

Patient Education Do not crush tablets or allow other people to handle crushed or broken tablets. Desired effects of this drug may not be seen for 2-3 months. Maintain adequate nutrition and hydration, unless instructed to restrict fluid intake. Avoid alcohol; may increase CNS depression. May cause dizziness, headache, confusion, nausea, vomiting, or loss of appetite. Report severe or persistent vomiting or diarrhea; CNS changes (depression, lethargy, dizziness); rash; or muscular twitching, tremor, numbness, or weakness.

Mitoxantrone (mye toe ZAN trone)

Brand Names: U.S. Novantrone® [DSC]

Index Terms CL-232315; DHAD; DHAQ; Dihydroxyanthracenedione; Dihydroxyanthracenedione Dihydrochloride; Mitoxantrone Dihydrochloride; Mitoxantrone HCl; Mitoxantrone Hydrochloride; Mitozantrone

Pharmacologic Category Antineoplastic Agent, Anthracenedione

Medication Safety Issues

Sound-alike/look-alike issues:

MitoXANtrone may be confused with methotrexate, mitoMYcin, mitotane, Mutamycin®

High alert medication:

This medication is in a class the Institute for Safe Medication Practices (ISMP) includes among its list of drug classes which have a heightened risk of causing significant patient harm when used in error.

Pregnancy Risk Factor D

Lactation Enters breast milk/not recommended

Breast-Feeding Considerations Mitoxantrone is excreted in human milk and significant concentrations (18 ng/mL) have been reported for 28 days after the last administration. Because of the potential for serious adverse reactions in infants from mitoxantrone, breast-feeding should be discontinued before starting treatment.

Use Treatment of acute nonlymphocytic leukemias (ANLL [includes myelogenous, promyelocytic, monocytic and erythroid leukemias]); advanced hormone-refractory prostate cancer; secondary progressive or relapsing-remitting multiple sclerosis (MS)

Unlabeled Use Treatment of Hodgkin's lymphoma, non-Hodgkin's lymphomas (NHL), acute lymphocytic leukemia (ALL), myelodysplastic syndrome, breast cancer, pediatric acute myelogenous leukemia (AML), pediatric acute promyelocytic leukemia (APL); part of a conditioning regimen for autologous hematopoietic stem cell transplantation (HSCT)

Mechanism of Action/Effect Related to the anthracyclines, mitoxantrone intercalates into DNA resulting in cross-links and strand breaks; also interferes with RNA and inhibits topoisomerase II; active throughout entire cell cycle (cell-cycle nonspecific)

Contraindications Hypersensitivity to mitoxantrone or any component of the formulation

Warnings/Precautions Hazardous agent - use appropriate precautions for handling and disposal.

[U.S. Boxed Warning]: Usually should not be administered if baseline neutrophil count <1500 cells/mm^3 (except for treatment of ANLL). Monitor blood counts and monitor for infection due to neutropenia. Treatment may lead to severe myelosuppression; unless the expected benefit outweighs the risk, use is generally not recommended in patients with pre-existing myelosuppression from prior chemotherapy.

[U.S. Boxed Warning]: May cause myocardial toxicity and potentially-fatal heart failure (HF); risk increases with cumulative dosing. Effects may occur during therapy or may be delayed (months or years after completion of therapy). Predisposing factors for mitoxantrone-induced

cardiotoxicity include prior anthracycline or anthracenedione therapy, prior cardiovascular disease, concomitant use of cardiotoxic drugs, and mediastinal/pericardial irradiation, although may also occur in patients without risk factors. Prior to therapy initiation, evaluate all patients for cardiac-related signs/symptoms, including history, physical exam, and ECG; and evaluate baseline left ventricular ejection fraction (LVEF) with echocardiogram or multigated radionuclide angiography (MUGA) or MRI. Not recommended for use in MS patients when LVEF <50%, or baseline LVEF below the lower limit of normal (LLN). Evaluate for cardiac signs/symptoms (by history, physical exam, and ECG) and evaluate LVEF (using same method as baseline LVEF) in MS patients prior to each dose and if signs/symptoms of HF develop. Use in MS should be limited to a cumulative dose of ≤140 mg/m^2, and discontinued if LVEF falls below LLN or a significant decrease in LVEF is observed; decreases in LVEF and HF have been observed in patients with MS who have received cumulative doses <100 mg/m^2. Patients with MS should undergo annual LVEF evaluation following discontinuation of therapy to monitor for delayed cardiotoxicity.

[U.S. Boxed Warnings]: For I.V. administration only, into a free-flowing I.V.; may cause severe local tissue damage if extravasation occurs; do not administer subcutaneously, intramuscularly, or intra-arterially. Do not administer intrathecally; may cause serious and permanent neurologic damage. Extravasation resulting in burning, erythema, pain, swelling and skin discoloration (blue) has been reported; extravasation may result in tissue necrosis and require debridement for skin graft. May cause urine, saliva, tears, and sweat to turn blue-green for 24 hours postinfusion. Whites of eyes may have blue-green tinge. **[U.S. Boxed Warning]: Treatment with mitoxantrone increases the risk of developing secondary acute myelogenous leukemia (AML) in patients with cancer and in patients with MS;** acute promyelocytic leukemia (APL) has also been observed. Symptoms of acute leukemia include excessive bruising, bleeding and recurrent infections. The risk for secondary leukemia is increased in patients who are heavily pretreated, with higher doses, and with combination chemotherapy.

[U.S. Boxed Warning]: Should be administered under the supervision of a physician experienced in cancer chemotherapy agents. Dosage should be reduced in patients with impaired hepatobiliary function (clearance is reduced); not for treatment of multiple sclerosis in patients with concurrent hepatic impairment. Not for treatment of primary progressive multiple sclerosis. Rapid lysis of tumor cells may lead to hyperuricemia.

Drug Interactions

Avoid Concomitant Use

Avoid concomitant use of MitoXANtrone with any of the following: BCG; CloZAPine; Natalizumab; Pimecrolimus; Pimozide; Tacrolimus (Topical); Vaccines (Live)

Decreased Effect

MitoXANtrone may decrease the levels/effects of: BCG; Coccidioidin Skin Test; Sipuleucel-T; Vaccines (Inactivated); Vaccines (Live)

The levels/effects of MitoXANtrone may be decreased by: Echinacea

Increased Effect/Toxicity

MitoXANtrone may increase the levels/effects of: ARIPiprazole; CloZAPine; Leflunomide; Natalizumab; Pimozide; Vaccines (Live)

The levels/effects of MitoXANtrone may be increased by: Denosumab; Pimecrolimus; Roflumilast; Tacrolimus (Topical); Trastuzumab

Nutritional/Ethanol Interactions Herb/Nutraceutical: Avoid echinacea (may diminish the immunosuppressant effect).

Adverse Reactions Includes events reported with any indication; incidence varies based on treatment, dose, and/or concomitant medications

>10%:

Cardiovascular: Edema (10% to 30%), arrhythmia (3% to 18%), cardiac function changes (≤18%), ECG changes (≤11%)

Central nervous system: Fever (6% to 78%), pain (8% to 41%), fatigue (≤39%), headache (6% to 13%)

Dermatologic: Alopecia (20% to 61%), nail bed changes (≤11%), petechiae/bruising (6% to 11%)

Endocrine & metabolic: Menstrual disorder (26% to 61%), amenorrhea (28% to 53%), hyperglycemia (10% to 31%)

Gastrointestinal: Nausea (26% to 76%), vomiting (6% to 72%), diarrhea (14% to 47%), mucositis (10% to 29%; onset: ≤1 week), stomatitis (8% to 29%; onset: ≤1 week), anorexia (22% to 25%), weight gain/loss (13% to 17%), constipation (10% to 16%), GI bleeding (2% to 16%), abdominal pain (9% to 15%), dyspepsia (5% to 14%)

Genitourinary: Urinary tract infection (7% to 32%), abnormal urine (5% to 11%)

Hematologic: Neutropenia (79% to 100%; onset: ≤3 weeks; grade 4: 23% to 54%), leukopenia (9% to 100%), lymphopenia (72% to 95%), anemia/hemoglobin decreased (5% to 75%) thrombocytopenia (33% to 39%; grades 3/4: 3% to 4%), neutropenic fever (≤11%)

Hepatic: Alkaline phosphatase increased (≤37%), transaminases increased (5% to 20%), GGT increased (3% to 15%)

Neuromuscular & skeletal: Weakness (≤24%)

Renal: BUN increased (≤22%), creatinine increased (≤13%), hematuria (≤11%)

Respiratory: Upper respiratory tract infection (7% to 53%), pharyngitis (≤19%), dyspnea (6% to 18%), cough (5% to 13%)
Miscellaneous: Infection (4% to 60%), sepsis (ANLL 31% to 34%), fungal infection (9% to 15%)

1% to 10%:
Cardiovascular: CHF (≤5%), ischemia (≤5%), LVEF decreased (≤5%), hypertension (≤4%)
Central nervous system: Chills (≤5%), anxiety (5%), depression (5%), seizure (2% to 4%)
Dermatologic: Cutaneous mycosis (≤10%), skin infection (≤5%)
Endocrine & metabolic: Hypocalcemia (10%), hypokalemia (7% to 10%), hyponatremia (9%), menorrhagia (7%)
Gastrointestinal: Aphthosis (≤10%)
Genitourinary: Impotence (≤7%), sterility (≤5%)
Hematologic: Granulocytopenia (6%), hemorrhage (5% to 6%), secondary acute leukemias (≤3%; includes AML, APL)
Hepatic: Jaundice (3% to 7%)
Neuromuscular & skeletal: Back pain (6% to 8%), myalgia (≤5%), arthralgia (≤5%)
Ocular: Conjunctivitis (≤5%), blurred vision (≤3%)
Renal: Renal failure (≤8%), proteinuria (≤6%)
Respiratory: Rhinitis (10%), pneumonia (≤9%), sinusitis (≤6%)
Miscellaneous: Systemic infection (≤10%), diaphoresis (≤9%)

Available Dosage Forms

Injection, solution [preservative free]: 2 mg/mL (10 mL, 12.5 mL, 15 mL)

General Dosage Range I.V.: *Adults:* 12 mg/m^2/day once daily for 2-3 days **or** 12-14 mg/m^2 every 3 weeks **or** 12 mg/m^2 every 3 months (multiple sclerosis; maximum lifetime cumulative dose: 140 mg/m^2)

Administration

I.V. Irritant (is considered a vesicant by some institutions). For I.V. administration only; do not administer intrathecally, subcutaneously, intramuscularly or intra-arterially. Must be diluted prior to use. Avoid extravasation; may cause severe local tissue damage if extravasation occurs. Usually administered as a short I.V. infusion over 5-15 minutes; do not infuse over less then 3 minutes.

High doses for bone marrow transplant (unlabeled use) are usually given as 3 divided doses over 1 hour each at 1-2 hour intervals on the same day (Oyan, 2006; Tarella, 2001).

I.V. Detail pH: 3-4.5

Stability

Reconstitution Dilute in at least 50 mL of NS or D_5W.

Storage Store intact vials at 15°C to 25°C (59°F to 77°F); do not freeze. Opened vials may be stored at room temperature for 7 days or under refrigeration for up to 14 days. Solutions diluted for administration are stable for 7 days at room temperature or under refrigeration, although the manufacturer recommends immediate use.

Nursing Actions

Physical Assessment Monitor infusion site closely to prevent extravasation, which may cause severe local tissue damage. Monitor for arrhythmia, hypersensitivity reactions, anemia, gastrointestinal upset, opportunistic infection, gout, and CHF (rales, dyspnea, edema) with each dose and throughout therapy. Caution patients with diabetes to monitor glucose levels closely; may cause hyperglycemia.

Patient Education This drug is only administered by infusion; report any redness, swelling, burning, or pain at infusion site. Maintain adequate nutrition and hydration unless instructed to restrict fluid intake. You will be more susceptible to infection. If you have diabetes, check your glucose levels closely; may cause hyperglycemia. May cause urine, saliva, tears, sweat, and whites of eyes to turn blue-green for 24 hours postinfusion (this is normal). May cause nausea, vomiting, GI upset, mouth sores, headache, dizziness, blurred vision, or loss of hair (may be reversible). Report chest pain or palpitations, rapid or erratic heartbeat, difficulty breathing or constant cough, swelling of extremities or sudden weight gain, persistent gastrointestinal response (nausea, vomiting, diarrhea, constipation, abdominal pain), signs of opportunistic infection (eg, fever, chills, sore throat, burning on urination), or changed or decreased urine output.

Related Information

Management of Drug Extravasations *on page 1269*

Modafinil (moe DAF i nil)

Brand Names: U.S. Provigil®

Pharmacologic Category Stimulant

Medication Guide Available Yes

Pregnancy Risk Factor C

Lactation Excretion in breast milk unknown/use caution

Use Improve wakefulness in patients with excessive daytime sleepiness associated with narcolepsy and shift work sleep disorder (SWSD); adjunctive therapy for obstructive sleep apnea/hypopnea syndrome (OSAHS)

Unlabeled Use Attention-deficit/hyperactivity disorder (ADHD); treatment of fatigue in MS and other disorders

Mechanism of Action/Effect The exact mechanism of action is unclear, it does not appear to alter the release of dopamine or norepinephrine, it may exert its stimulant effects by decreasing GABA-mediated neurotransmission, although this theory has not yet been fully evaluated; several studies also suggest that an intact central alpha-adrenergic system is required for modafinil's activity; the drug increases high-frequency alpha waves while decreasing both delta and theta wave activity, and these effects are consistent with generalized increases in mental alertness

Contraindications Hypersensitivity to modafinil, armodafinil, or any component of the formulation

Warnings/Precautions For use following complete evaluation of sleepiness and in conjunction with other standard treatments (eg, CPAP). The degree of sleepiness should be reassessed frequently; some patients may not return to a normal level of wakefulness. Use is not recommended with a history of angina, cardiac ischemia, recent history of myocardial infarction, left ventricular hypertrophy, or patients with mitral valve prolapse who have developed mitral valve prolapse syndrome with previous CNS stimulant use.

Serious and life-threatening rashes (including Stevens-Johnson syndrome and toxic epidermal necrolysis) have been reported with modafinil. Most cases have occurred within the first 5 weeks of therapy; however, rare cases have occurred after long-term use. No risk factors have been identified to predict occurrence or severity. Patients should be advised to discontinue at first sign of rash. The serious nature of these dermatologic adverse effects, as well reports of psychiatric events, resulted in the FDA's Pediatric Advisory Committee unanimously recommending that a specific warning against the use of modafinil in children be added to the manufacturer's labeling. Modafinil is not FDA-approved for use in pediatrics for any indication.

In addition, rare cases of multiorgan hypersensitivity reactions in association with modafinil use, and lone cases of angioedema and anaphylactoid reactions with armodafinil, have been reported. Signs and symptoms are diverse, reflecting the involvement of specific organs. Patients typically present with fever and rash associated with organ-system dysfunction. Patients should be advised to report any signs and symptoms related to these effects; discontinuation of therapy is recommended.

Caution should be exercised when modafinil is given to patients with a history of psychosis; may impair the ability to engage in potentially hazardous activities. Stimulants may unmask tics in individuals with coexisting Tourette's syndrome. Use caution with renal or hepatic impairment (dosage adjustment in severe hepatic dysfunction is recommended).

Drug Interactions

Avoid Concomitant Use

Avoid concomitant use of Modafinil with any of the following: Axitinib; Clopidogrel; Conivaptan; Iobenguane I 123; Pimozide

Decreased Effect

Modafinil may decrease the levels/effects of: ARIPiprazole; Axitinib; Clopidogrel; Contraceptives (Estrogens); CycloSPORINE; CycloSPORINE (Systemic); Iobenguane I 123; Saxagliptin

The levels/effects of Modafinil may be decreased by: CYP3A4 Inducers (Strong); Deferasirox; Herbs (CYP3A4 Inducers); Tocilizumab

Increased Effect/Toxicity

Modafinil may increase the levels/effects of: ARIPiprazole; Citalopram; CYP2C19 Substrates; Pimozide; Sympathomimetics

The levels/effects of Modafinil may be increased by: Atomoxetine; Cannabinoids; Conivaptan; CYP3A4 Inhibitors (Moderate); CYP3A4 Inhibitors (Strong); Dasatinib; Ivacaftor; Linezolid

Nutritional/Ethanol Interactions

Ethanol: Avoid or limit ethanol.

Food: Delays absorption, but does not affect bioavailability.

Adverse Reactions

>10%:

Central nervous system: Headache (34%, dose related)

Gastrointestinal: Nausea (11%)

1% to 10%:

Cardiovascular: Chest pain (3%), hypertension (3%), palpitation (2%), tachycardia (2%), vasodilation (2%), edema (1%)

Central nervous system: Nervousness (7%), dizziness (5%), anxiety (5%; dose related), insomnia (5%), depression (2%), somnolence (2%), chills (1%), agitation (1%), confusion (1%), emotional lability (1%), vertigo (1%)

Dermatologic: Rash (1%; includes some severe cases requiring hospitalization)

Gastrointestinal: Diarrhea (6%), dyspepsia (5%), xerostomia (4%), anorexia (4%), constipation (2%), flatulence (1%), mouth ulceration (1%), taste perversion (1%)

Genitourinary: Abnormal urine (1%), hematuria (1%), pyuria (1%)

Hematologic: Eosinophilia (1%)

Hepatic: LFTs abnormal (2%)

Neuromuscular & skeletal: Back pain (6%), paresthesia (2%), dyskinesia (1%), hyperkinesia (1%), hypertonia (1%), neck rigidity (1%), tremor (1%)

Ocular: Amblyopia (1%), eye pain (1%), vision abnormal (1%)

Respiratory: Rhinitis (7%), pharyngitis (4%), lung disorder (2%), asthma (1%), epistaxis (1%)

Miscellaneous: Flu-like syndrome (4%), thirst (1%), diaphoresis (1%), herpes simplex infection (1%)

Controlled Substance C-IV

Available Dosage Forms

Tablet, oral:

Provigil®: 100 mg, 200 mg

General Dosage Range Dosage adjustment recommended in patients with hepatic impairment.

Oral: *Adults:* 200 mg once daily (maximum: 400 mg/day)

Administration

Oral For the treatment of narcolepsy and obstructive sleep apnea/hypopnea syndrome (OSAHS), administer dose in the morning. For the treatment of shift work sleep disorder (SWSD), administer dose ~1 hour prior to start of work shift.

Stability

Storage Store at 20°C to 25°C (68°F to 77°F).

Nursing Actions

Physical Assessment Perform careful cardiovascular assessment prior to initiating therapy.

Patient Education Avoid alcohol or caffeine. You may experience headache, nervousness, dizziness, diarrhea, dry mouth, or loss of appetite. If you have diabetes, monitor glucose levels closely. Report chest pain or palpitations, respiratory difficulty, insomnia, agitation, depression, rash, or weight loss.

Moexipril (mo EKS i pril)

Brand Names: U.S. Univasc®

Index Terms Moexipril Hydrochloride

Pharmacologic Category Angiotensin-Converting Enzyme (ACE) Inhibitor

Medication Safety Issues

Sound-alike/look-alike issues:

Moexipril may be confused with Monopril®

Pregnancy Risk Factor D

Lactation Excretion in breast milk unknown/use caution

Breast-Feeding Considerations It is not known if moexipril is excreted into breast milk. The manufacturer recommends that caution be exercised when administering moexipril to nursing women.

Use Treatment of hypertension, alone or in combination with thiazide diuretics

Mechanism of Action/Effect Competitive inhibitor of angiotensin-converting enzyme (ACE); prevents conversion of angiotensin I to angiotensin II, a potent vasoconstrictor; results in lower levels of angiotensin II which causes an increase in plasma renin activity and a reduction in aldosterone secretion

Contraindications Hypersensitivity to moexipril or any component of the formulation; angioedema related to previous treatment with an ACE inhibitor

Warnings/Precautions Anaphylactic reactions may occur rarely with ACE inhibitors. At any time during treatment (especially following first dose) angioedema may occur rarely with ACE inhibitors; it may involve the head and neck (potentially compromising airway) or the intestine (presenting with abdominal pain). African-Americans and patients with idiopathic or hereditary angioedema may be at an increased risk. Prolonged frequent monitoring may be required especially if tongue, glottis, or larynx are involved as they are associated with airway obstruction. Patients with a history of airway surgery may have a higher risk of airway obstruction. Aggressive early and appropriate management is critical. Use in patients with previous angioedema associated with ACE inhibitor therapy is contraindicated. Severe anaphylactoid reactions may be seen during hemodialysis (eg, CVVHD) with high-flux dialysis membranes (eg, AN69), and rarely, during low density lipoprotein apheresis with dextran sulfate cellulose. Rare cases of anaphylactoid reactions have been reported in patients undergoing sensitization treatment with hymenoptera (bee, wasp) venom while receiving ACE inhibitors.

Symptomatic hypotension with or without syncope can occur with ACE inhibitors (usually with the first several doses); effects are most often observed in volume depleted patients; correct volume depletion prior to initiation; close monitoring of patient is required especially with initial dosing and dosing increases; blood pressure must be lowered at a rate appropriate for the patient's clinical condition. Initiation of therapy in patients with ischemic heart disease or cerebrovascular disease warrants close observation due to the potential consequences posed by falling blood pressure (eg, MI, stroke). Use with caution in hypertrophic cardiomyopathy with outflow tract obstruction, severe aortic stenosis, or before, during, or immediately after major surgery. **[U.S. Boxed Warning]: Drugs that act on the renin-angiotensin system can cause injury and death to the developing fetus. Discontinue as soon as possible once pregnancy is detected.**

Hyperkalemia may occur with ACE inhibitors; risk factors include renal dysfunction, diabetes mellitus, concomitant use of potassium-sparing diuretics, potassium supplements, and/or potassium-containing salts. Use cautiously, if at all, with these agents and monitor potassium closely. Cough may occur with ACE inhibitors. Other causes of cough should be considered (eg, pulmonary congestion in patients with heart failure) and excluded prior to discontinuation.

May be associated with deterioration of renal function and/or increases in serum creatinine, particularly in patients with low renal blood flow (eg, renal artery stenosis, heart failure) whose glomerular filtration rate (GFR) is dependent on efferent arteriolar vasoconstriction by angiotensin II; deterioration may result in oliguria, acute renal failure, and progressive azotemia. Small increases in serum creatinine may occur following initiation; consider discontinuation only in patients with progressive and/or significant deterioration in renal function. Use with caution in patients with unstented unilateral/bilateral renal artery stenosis. When unstented bilateral renal artery stenosis is present, use is generally avoided due to the elevated risk of deterioration in renal function unless possible benefits outweigh risks. Concurrent use of angiotensin receptor blockers may increase the risk of clinically-significant adverse events (eg, renal dysfunction, hyperkalemia).

Rare toxicities associated with ACE inhibitors include cholestatic jaundice (which may progress to fulminant hepatic necrosis), agranulocytosis, neutropenia, or leukopenia with myeloid hypoplasia. Patients with collagen vascular diseases (especially with concomitant renal impairment) or renal impairment alone may be at increased risk for hematologic toxicity; periodically monitor CBC with differential in these patients.

Drug Interactions

Avoid Concomitant Use There are no known interactions where it is recommended to avoid concomitant use.

Decreased Effect

The levels/effects of Moexipril may be decreased by: Antacids; Aprotinin; Herbs (Hypertensive Properties); Icatibant; Lanthanum; Methylphenidate; Nonsteroidal Anti-Inflammatory Agents; Salicylates; Yohimbine

Increased Effect/Toxicity

Moexipril may increase the levels/effects of: Allopurinol; Amifostine; Antihypertensives; AzaTHIOprine; CycloSPORINE; CycloSPORINE (Systemic); Ferric Gluconate; Gold Sodium Thiomalate; Hypotensive Agents; Iron Dextran Complex; Lithium; Nonsteroidal Anti-Inflammatory Agents; RiTUXimab; Sodium Phosphates

The levels/effects of Moexipril may be increased by: Alfuzosin; Angiotensin II Receptor Blockers; Diazoxide; DPP-IV Inhibitors; Eplerenone; Everolimus; Herbs (Hypotensive Properties); Loop Diuretics; MAO Inhibitors; Pentoxifylline; Phosphodiesterase 5 Inhibitors; Potassium Salts; Potassium-Sparing Diuretics; Prostacyclin Analogues; Sirolimus; Temsirolimus; Thiazide Diuretics; TiZANidine; Tolvaptan; Trimethoprim

Nutritional/Ethanol Interactions

Food: Food may delay and reduce peak serum levels. Potassium supplements and/or potassium-containing salts may cause or worsen hyperkalemia. Management: Take on an empty stomach 1 hour before or 2 hours after a meal. Consult prescriber before consuming a potassium-rich diet, potassium supplements, or salt substitutes.

Herb/Nutraceutical: Some herbal medications may worsen hypertension (eg, licorice); others may increase the antihypertensive effect of moexipril (eg, shepherd's purse). Management: Avoid bayberry, blue cohosh, cayenne, ephedra, ginger, ginseng (American), kola, licorice, and yohimbe. Avoid black cohosh, California poppy, coleus, golden seal, hawthorn, mistletoe, periwinkle, quinine, and shepherd's purse.

Adverse Reactions 1% to 10%:

Cardiovascular: Hypotension, peripheral edema

Central nervous system: Headache, dizziness, fatigue

Dermatologic: Flushing, rash

Endocrine & metabolic: Hyperkalemia, hyponatremia

Gastrointestinal: Diarrhea, nausea, heartburn

Genitourinary: Polyuria

Neuromuscular & skeletal: Myalgia

Renal: Reversible increases in creatinine or BUN

Respiratory: Cough, pharyngitis, upper respiratory infection, sinusitis

Pharmacodynamics/Kinetics

Onset of Action Peak effect: 1-2 hours

Duration of Action >24 hours

Available Dosage Forms

Tablet, oral: 7.5 mg, 15 mg

Univasc®: 7.5 mg, 15 mg

General Dosage Range Dosage adjustment recommended in patients with renal impairment

Oral: *Adults:* Initial: 3.75-7.5 mg once daily; Maintenance: 7.5-30 mg/day in 1 or 2 divided doses

Administration

Oral Administer on an empty stomach.

Nursing Actions

Physical Assessment Assess potential for interactions with other pharmacological agents or herbal products that may impact fluid balance or cardiac status. Patient should be monitored closely for anaphylactic reaction or angioedema which can occur at any time during treatment and may involve head and neck. Monitor blood pressure. Monitor for hypotension, rash, diarrhea, myalgia, and electrolyte imbalance regularly during therapy.

Patient Education Do not use potassium supplements or salt substitutes without consulting prescriber. Take first dose at bedtime. Take all doses on an empty stomach, 1 hour before or 2 hours after meals. This drug does not eliminate need for diet or exercise regimen as recommended by prescriber. May cause dizziness, fainting, lightheadedness, postural hypotension, nausea, vomiting, abdominal pain, dry mouth, or transient loss of appetite. Report immediately unusual swelling of mouth, tongue, face, or throat. Report respiratory difficulty or unusual cough, rash, excessive urination, chest pain or palpitations, mouth sores, fever or chills, numbness, or tingling or pain in muscles.

Dietary Considerations Take on an empty stomach.

Moexipril and Hydrochlorothiazide

(mo EKS i pril & hye droe klor oh THYE a zide)

Brand Names: U.S. Uniretic®

Index Terms Hydrochlorothiazide and Moexipril

Pharmacologic Category Angiotensin-Converting Enzyme (ACE) Inhibitor; Diuretic, Thiazide

Pregnancy Risk Factor D

Lactation Enters breast milk/use caution

Use Treatment of hypertension; not indicated for initial treatment of hypertension

Available Dosage Forms

Tablet, oral: 7.5/12.5: Moexipril 7.5 mg and hydrochlorothiazide 12.5; 15/12.5: Moexipril 15 mg and hydrochlorothiazide 12.5; 15/25: Moexipril 15 mg and hydrochlorothiazide 25

Uniretic®: 7.5/12.5: Moexipril 7.5 mg and hydrochlorothiazide 12.5 mg [scored]; 15/12.5: Moexipril 15 mg and hydrochlorothiazide 12.5 mg [scored]; 15/25: Moexipril 15 mg and hydrochlorothiazide 25 mg [scored]

General Dosage Range Oral: *Adults:* 7.5-30 mg of moexipril/day and ≤50 mg hydrochlorothiazide/day in a single or divided dose

Nursing Actions

Physical Assessment See individual agents.

Patient Education See individual agents.

Related Information

Hydrochlorothiazide *on page 570*
Moexipril *on page 788*

Mometasone (Oral Inhalation)

(moe MET a sone)

Brand Names: U.S. Asmanex® Twisthaler®

Index Terms Mometasone Furoate

Pharmacologic Category Corticosteroid, Inhalant (Oral)

Pregnancy Risk Factor C

Lactation Excretion in breast milk unknown/use caution

Breast-Feeding Considerations Systemic corticosteroids are excreted in human milk; however, information for mometasone is not available. The use of inhaled corticosteroids is not considered a contraindication to breast-feeding.

Use Maintenance treatment of asthma as prophylactic therapy

Mechanism of Action/Effect Blocks inflammation; reverses capillary permeability and release of inflammatory mediators (leukotrienes and prostaglandins); suppresses migration of polymorphonuclear leukocytes.

Contraindications Hypersensitivity to mometasone or any component of the formulation; hypersensitivity to milk proteins; primary treatment of status asthmaticus or acute bronchospasm

Warnings/Precautions May cause hypercorticism or suppression of hypothalamic-pituitary-adrenal (HPA) axis, particularly in younger children or in patients receiving high doses for prolonged periods. HPA axis suppression may lead to adrenal crisis. Withdrawal and discontinuation of a corticosteroid should be done slowly and carefully. Particular care is required when patients are transferred from systemic corticosteroids to inhaled products due to possible adrenal insufficiency or withdrawal from steroids, including an increase in allergic symptoms. Patients receiving >20 mg per day of prednisone (or equivalent) may be most susceptible. Fatalities have occurred due to adrenal insufficiency in asthmatic patients during and after transfer from systemic corticosteroids to aerosol steroids; aerosol steroids do not provide the systemic steroid needed to treat patients having trauma, surgery, or infections. When transferring to oral inhaler, previously-suppressed allergic conditions (rhinitis, conjunctivitis, eczema) may be unmasked.

Bronchospasm may occur with wheezing after inhalation; if this occurs, stop steroid and treat with a fast-acting bronchodilator. Supplemental steroids (oral or parenteral) may be needed during stress or severe asthma attacks. Not to be used in status asthmaticus or for the relief of acute bronchospasm. Corticosteroid use may cause psychiatric disturbances, including depression, euphoria, insomnia, mood swings, and personality changes. Pre-existing psychiatric conditions may be exacerbated by corticosteroid use. Prolonged use of corticosteroids may also increase the incidence of secondary infection, mask acute infection (including fungal infections), prolong or exacerbate viral infections, or limit response to vaccines. Exposure to chickenpox should be avoided; corticosteroids should not be used to treat ocular herpes simplex. Corticosteroids should not be used for cerebral malaria or viral hepatitis. Close observation is required in patients with latent tuberculosis and/or TB reactivity; restrict use in active TB (only in conjunction with antituberculosis treatment). Prolonged treatment with corticosteroids has been associated with the development of Kaposi's sarcoma (case reports); if noted, discontinuation of therapy should be considered. Local oropharyngeal *Candida* infections have been reported; if occurs treat appropriately while continuing mometasone therapy. Patients should be instructed to rinse mouth after each use.

Reactions including, anaphylaxis, angioedema, pruritus, and rash have been reported; if these symptoms occur discontinue use. Use with caution in patients with thyroid disease, hepatic impairment, renal impairment, cardiovascular disease, diabetes, glaucoma, cataracts, myasthenia gravis, patients with or who are at risk for osteoporosis, patients at risk for seizures, or GI diseases (diverticulitis, peptic ulcer, ulcerative colitis) due to perforation risk. Use caution following acute MI (corticosteroids have been associated with myocardial rupture). Because of the risk of adverse effects, systemic corticosteroids should be used cautiously in the elderly in the smallest possible effective dose for the shortest duration.

Orally-inhaled corticosteroids may cause a reduction in growth velocity in pediatric patients (~1 centimeter per year [range: 0.3-1.8 cm per year] and related to dose and duration of exposure). To minimize the systemic effects of orally-inhaled corticosteroids, each patient should be titrated to the lowest effective dose. Growth should be routinely monitored in pediatric patients. Prior to use, the dose and duration of treatment should be based on the risk versus benefit for each individual patient. In general, use the smallest effective dose for the shortest duration of time to minimize adverse events. A gradual tapering of dose may be required prior to discontinuing therapy. There have been reports of systemic corticosteroid withdrawal symptoms (eg, joint/muscle pain, lassitude, depression) when withdrawing inhalation therapy. May contain lactose; very rare anaphylactic reactions have been reported in patients with severe milk protein allergy.

Drug Interactions

Avoid Concomitant Use

Avoid concomitant use of Mometasone (Oral Inhalation) with any of the following: Aldesleukin

Decreased Effect

Mometasone (Oral Inhalation) may decrease the levels/effects of: Aldesleukin; Antidiabetic Agents; Corticorelin; Telaprevir

The levels/effects of Mometasone (Oral Inhalation) may be decreased by: Tocilizumab

Increased Effect/Toxicity

Mometasone (Oral Inhalation) may increase the levels/effects of: Amphotericin B; Deferasirox; Loop Diuretics; Thiazide Diuretics

The levels/effects of Mometasone (Oral Inhalation) may be increased by: CYP3A4 Inhibitors (Strong); Telaprevir

Adverse Reactions

>10%:

Central nervous system: Headache (17% to 22%), fatigue (1% to 13%), depression (11%)

Neuromuscular & skeletal: Musculoskeletal pain (4% to 22%), arthralgia (13%)

Respiratory: Sinusitis (5% to 22%), rhinitis (4% to 20%), upper respiratory infection (8% to 15%), pharyngitis (8% to 13%)

Miscellaneous: Oral candidiasis (4% to 22%)

1% to 10%:

Central nervous system: Fever (children 7%), pain (1% to <3%)

Dermatologic: Bruising (children 2%)

Gastrointestinal: Abdominal pain (2% to 6%), dyspepsia (3% to 5%), nausea (1% to 3%), vomiting (1% to ≤3%), anorexia (1% to <3%), dry throat (1% to <3%), gastroenteritis (1% to <3%)

Genitourinary: Dysmenorrhea (4% to 9%), urinary tract infection (children 2%)

Neuromuscular & skeletal: Back pain (3% to 6%), myalgia (2% to 3%)

Ocular: Ocular pressure increased (3%), cataracts (1%)

Otic: Earache (1% to <3%)

Respiratory: Sinus congestion (9%), dysphonia (1% to <3%), epistaxis (1% to <3%), nasal irritation (1% to <3%)

Miscellaneous: Flu-like syndrome (1% to <3%), infection (1% to <3%)

Available Dosage Forms

Powder, for oral inhalation:

Asmanex® Twisthaler®: 110 mcg (30 units); 220 mcg (14 units, 30 units, 60 units, 120 units)

General Dosage Range Inhalation:

Children 4-11 years: 110 mcg once daily (maximum: 110 mcg/day)

Children ≥12 years and Adults: 1-4 inhalations (220-880 mcg) in 1-2 divided doses (maximum: 880 mcg/day)

Administration

Inhalation Exhale fully prior to bringing the Twisthaler® up to the mouth. Place between lips and inhale quickly and deeply. Do not breathe out through the inhaler. Remove inhaler and hold breath for 10 seconds if possible. Rinse mouth after use.

Stability

Storage Store at 25°C (77°F); excursions permitted to 15°C to 30°C (59°F to 86°F). Discard when oral dose counter reads "00" (or 45 days after opening the foil pouch).

Nursing Actions

Physical Assessment Long-term use: Assess for glaucoma and cataracts periodically. Monitor growth in pediatric patients.

Patient Education Not a bronchodilator and not indicated for the acute relief of bronchospasm. May take 1-2 weeks before effects of medication are seen. Avoid exposure to chickenpox or measles. Consult prescriber immediately if exposure does occur. Discard inhaler 45 days after opening foil pouch or when dose counter reads "00." Rinse mouth after using. Keep the inhaler clean and dry.

Dietary Considerations Asmanex® Twisthaler® contains lactose.

Mometasone (Nasal) (moe MET a sone)

Brand Names: U.S. Nasonex®

Index Terms Mometasone Furoate

Pharmacologic Category Corticosteroid, Nasal

Pregnancy Risk Factor C

Lactation Excretion in breast milk unknown/use caution

Use Treatment of nasal symptoms of seasonal and perennial allergic rhinitis; prevention of nasal symptoms associated with seasonal allergic rhinitis; treatment of nasal polyps in adults

Canadian labeling: Additional use (not in U.S. labeling): Treatment of mild-to-moderate uncomplicated rhinosinusitis or as adjunctive treatment (with antimicrobials) in acute rhinosinusitis

Available Dosage Forms

Suspension, intranasal:

Nasonex®: 50 mcg/spray (17 g)

General Dosage Range Intranasal:

Children 2-11 years: 1 spray (50 mcg) in each nostril once daily

Children ≥12 years and Adults: 2 sprays (100 mcg) in each nostril once or twice daily

Administration

Inhalation Shake well prior to use. Prior to first use, prime pump by actuating 10 times or until fine spray appears; may store for a maximum of 1 week (U.S. labeling recommendations) or 2 weeks (Canadian labeling recommendations) without repriming; if unused for greater than recommended storage period, reprime by actuating 2 times or until fine spray appears. Spray should be administered once or twice daily, at a regular interval.

Nursing Actions

Physical Assessment Monitor growth with long-term use in pediatric patients.

Patient Education Gently blow your nose to clear nostrils prior to use. You may experience headache, cough, or nosebleed. Report unusual chest pain, gastrointestinal upset, muscle pain, flu-like symptoms, worsening of condition, or failure to improve.

Mometasone (Topical) (moe MET a sone)

Brand Names: U.S. Elocon®

Index Terms Mometasone Furoate

Pharmacologic Category Corticosteroid, Topical

Medication Safety Issues

Sound-alike/look-alike issues:

Elocon® lotion may be confused with ophthalmic solutions. Manufacturer's labeling emphasizes the product is **NOT** for use in the eyes.

Pregnancy Risk Factor C

Lactation Excretion in breast milk unknown/use caution

Use Relief of the inflammatory and pruritic manifestations of corticosteroid-responsive dermatoses (medium potency topical corticosteroid)

Available Dosage Forms

Cream, topical: 0.1% (15 g, 45 g)

Elocon®: 0.1% (15 g, 45 g)

Lotion, topical: 0.1% (30 mL, 60 mL)

Elocon®: 0.1% (30 mL, 60 mL)

Ointment, topical: 0.1% (15 g, 45 g)

Elocon®: 0.1% (15 g, 45 g)

General Dosage Range Topical:

Cream, ointment: *Children ≥2 years and Adults:* Apply a thin film to affected area once daily

Lotion: *Children ≥12 years and Adults:* Apply a few drops to affected area once daily

Administration

Topical Apply sparingly; avoid eyes, face, underarms, and groin. Do not wrap or bandage affected area.

Nursing Actions

Patient Education Do not use for eyes, mucous membranes, or open wounds. Before using, wash and dry area gently. Apply in a thin layer (cream, ointment) or a few drops (lotion) and rub in lightly. Apply light dressing (if necessary) to area being treated. Do not use occlusive dressing unless so advised by prescriber. Avoid prolonged or excessive use around sensitive tissues, underarms, genital, or rectal areas. Avoid exposing treated area to direct sunlight (severe sunburn may occur). Inform prescriber if condition worsens (redness, swelling, irritation, signs of infection, or open sores) or fails to improve.

Montelukast (mon te LOO kast)

Brand Names: U.S. Singulair®

Index Terms Montelukast Sodium

Pharmacologic Category Leukotriene-Receptor Antagonist

Medication Safety Issues

Sound-alike/look-alike issues:

Singulair® may be confused with SINEquan®

Pregnancy Risk Factor B

Lactation Excretion in breast milk unknown/use caution

Use Prophylaxis and chronic treatment of asthma; relief of symptoms of seasonal allergic rhinitis and perennial allergic rhinitis; prevention of exercise-induced bronchospasm

Unlabeled Use Acute asthma

Mechanism of Action/Effect Montelukast is a selective leukotriene receptor antagonist which inhibits cysteinyl leukotriene. Leukotrienes are responsible for edema and smooth muscle contraction that is felt to be associated with the signs and symptoms of asthma. Cysteinyl leukotrienes are also released following allergen exposure leading to symptoms associated with allergic rhinitis.

Contraindications Hypersensitivity to montelukast or any component of the formulation

Warnings/Precautions Montelukast is not FDA approved for use in the reversal of bronchospasm in acute asthma attacks, including status asthmaticus; some clinicians, however, support its use as adjunctive therapy (Camargo, 2003; Cylly, 2003; Ferreira, 2001; Harmancik 2006). Appropriate rescue medication should be available. Appropriate clinical monitoring and caution are recommended when systemic corticosteroid reduction is considered in patients receiving montelukast. Patients should be instructed to notify prescriber if behavioral changes occur. Inform phenylketonuric patients that the chewable tablet contains phenylalanine.

In rare cases, patients on therapy with montelukast may present with systemic eosinophilia, sometimes presenting with clinical features of vasculitis consistent with Churg-Strauss syndrome, a condition which is often treated with systemic corticosteroid therapy. Healthcare providers should be alert to eosinophilia, vasculitic rash, worsening pulmonary symptoms, cardiac complications, and/or neuropathy presenting in their patients. A causal association between montelukast and these underlying conditions has not been established. Montelukast will not interrupt bronchoconstrictor response to aspirin or other NSAIDs; aspirin sensitive asthmatics should continue to avoid these agents. Postmarketing reports of behavior changes (agitation, aggression, depression, insomnia) have been noted in children and adults.

Drug Interactions

Avoid Concomitant Use There are no known interactions where it is recommended to avoid concomitant use.

Decreased Effect

The levels/effects of Montelukast may be decreased by: CYP2C9 Inducers (Strong); CYP3A4 Inducers (Strong); Deferasirox; Herbs (CYP3A4 Inducers); Peginterferon Alfa-2b; Tocilizumab

Increased Effect/Toxicity

The levels/effects of Montelukast may be increased by: Conivaptan; CYP2C9 Inhibitors (Moderate); CYP2C9 Inhibitors (Strong)

Nutritional/Ethanol Interactions Herb/Nutraceutical: St John's wort may decrease montelukast levels.

Adverse Reactions Note: Percentages and adverse events as reported in adults: 1% to 10%:

Central nervous system: Headache (18%), dizziness (2%), fatigue (2%), fever (2%)

Dermatologic: Rash (2%)

Gastrointestinal: Dyspepsia (2%), dental pain (2%), gastroenteritis (2%)

Hepatic: AST increased (2%), ALT increased (≥1%)

Neuromuscular & skeletal: Weakness (2%)

Respiratory: Cough (≥1%), nasal congestion (2%), epistaxis (≥1%), sinusitis (≥1%), upper respiratory infection (≥1%)

Pharmacodynamics/Kinetics

Duration of Action >24 hours

Available Dosage Forms

Granules, oral:

Singulair®: 4 mg/packet (30s)

Tablet, oral:

Singulair®: 10 mg

Tablet, chewable, oral:

Singulair®: 4 mg, 5 mg

General Dosage Range Oral:

Children 6 months-5 years: 4 mg once daily

Children 6-14 years: 5 mg once daily

Children ≥15 years and Adults: 10 mg once daily **or** 10 mg 2 hours prior to exercise

Administration

Oral When treating asthma, administer dose in the evening. Patients with allergic rhinitis may individualize administration time (morning or evening). Patients with both asthma and allergic rhinitis should take their dose in the evening. Granules may be administered directly in the mouth or mixed with a spoonful of applesauce, carrots, rice, ice cream, baby formula, or breast milk; do not add to any other liquids or foods. Administer within 15 minutes of opening packet. May administer without regard to meals.

Stability

Storage Store at room temperature of 25°C (77°F); excursions permitted to 15°C to 30°C (59°F to 86°F).

Granules: Store in original package; use within 15 minutes of opening packet.

Nursing Actions

Physical Assessment Not for use in acute asthma attacks, including status asthmaticus. Monitor mental and mood status. Be alert to signs of depression, hallucinations, irritability, agitation, and suicide ideation.

Patient Education Do not stop other asthma medication unless advised by prescriber. Chewable tablet contains phenylalanine. Granules may be administered directly in the mouth or mixed with applesauce, carrots, rice, ice cream, baby formula, or breast milk (do not add to any other liquids); administer within 15 minutes of opening packet. You may experience mild headache, fatigue, or dizziness. Report skin rash or itching, abdominal pain or persistent GI upset, unusual cough or congestion, behavior and mood changes including depression and suicide ideation, feeling of numbness in arms or legs, flu-like illness, or worsening of asthmatic condition.

Dietary Considerations Some products may contain phenylalanine.

Morphine (Systemic) (MOR feen)

Brand Names: U.S. Astramorph®/PF; AVINza®; Duramorph; Infumorph 200; Infumorph 500; Kadian®; MS Contin®; Oramorph® SR

Index Terms MS (error-prone abbreviation and should not be used); MSO_4 (error-prone abbreviation and should not be used); Roxanol

Pharmacologic Category Analgesic, Opioid

Medication Safety Issues

Sound-alike/look-alike issues:

Morphine may be confused with HYDROmorphone, methadone

Morphine sulfate may be confused with magnesium sulfate

Kadian® may be confused with Kapidex [DSC]

MS Contin® may be confused with OxyCONTIN®

MSO_4 and MS are error-prone abbreviations (mistaken as magnesium sulfate)

AVINza® may be confused with Evista®, INVanz®

Roxanol may be confused with OxyFast®, Roxicet™, Roxicodone®

High alert medication:

The Institute for Safe Medication Practices (ISMP) includes this medication (I.V. formulation) among its list of drug classes which have a heightened risk of causing significant patient harm when used in error.

Other safety concerns:

Use care when prescribing and/or administering morphine solutions. These products are available in different concentrations. Always prescribe dosage in mg; **not** by volume (mL).

Use caution when selecting a morphine formulation for use in neurologic infusion pumps (eg, Medtronic delivery systems). The product should be appropriately labeled as "preservative-free" and suitable for intraspinal use via continuous infusion. In addition, the product should be formulated in a pH range that is compatible with the device operation specifications.

Significant differences exist between oral and I.V. dosing. Use caution when converting from one route of administration to another.

Medication Guide Available Yes

Pregnancy Risk Factor C

Lactation Enters breast milk/use caution (AAP rates "compatible"; AAP 2001 update pending)

Breast-Feeding Considerations Morphine concentrates in breast milk, with a milk to plasma AUC ratio of 2.5:1. Detectable serum levels of morphine can be found in infants following morphine administration to nursing mothers. Treatment of the mother with single doses of morphine is not expected to cause detrimental effects in nursing infants. Breast-feeding following chronic use or in neonates with hepatic or renal dysfunction may lead to higher levels of morphine in the infant and a risk of adverse effects.

Use Relief of moderate-to-severe acute and chronic pain; relief of pain of myocardial infarction; relief of dyspnea of acute left ventricular failure and pulmonary edema; preanesthetic medication

Infumorph®: Used in continuous microinfusion devices for intrathecal or epidural administration in treatment of intractable chronic pain

Controlled, extended, or sustained release products: Only intended/indicated for use when repeated doses for an extended period of time are required. The 100 mg and 200 mg tablets or capsules of Kadian®, MS Contin®, and morphine sulfate controlled-release tablets and the 60 mg, 90 mg, and 120 mg capsules of Avinza® should only be used in opioid-tolerant patients.

Mechanism of Action/Effect Binds to opiate receptors in the CNS, causing inhibition of ascending pain pathways, altering the perception of and response to pain; produces generalized CNS depression

Contraindications Note: Some contraindications are product specific. For details, please see detailed product prescribing information.

Hypersensitivity to morphine sulfate or any component of the formulation; severe respiratory depression (without resuscitative equipment); acute or severe asthma; known or suspected paralytic ileus; sustained release products are not recommended with gastrointestinal obstruction or in acute/postoperative pain. Oral solutions contraindicated in patients with heart failure due to chronic lung disease, cardiac arrhythmias, head injuries, brain tumors, acute alcoholism, deliriums tremens, seizure disorders, Injectable solution contraindicated during labor when a premature birth is anticipated. Some products contraindicated in patients with head injuries or increased intracranial pressure. MS Contin® and Kadian® contraindicated in patients with hypercarbia. Some immediate release formulations (tablets and solution) contraindicated in post biliary tract surgery, suspected surgical abdomen, surgical anastomosis, MAO inhibitor use (concurrent or within 14 days), general CNS depression.

Warnings/Precautions An opioid-containing analgesic regimen should be tailored to each patient's needs and based upon the type of pain being treated (acute versus chronic), the route of administration, degree of tolerance for opioids (naive versus chronic user), age, weight, and medical condition. The optimal analgesic dose varies widely among patients. Doses should be titrated to pain relief/prevention. When used as an epidural injection, monitor for delayed sedation. **[U.S. Boxed Warning]: Healthcare provider should be alert to problems of abuse, misuse, and diversion.**

May cause respiratory depression; use with caution in patients (particularly elderly or debilitated) with impaired respiratory function, morbid obesity, adrenal insufficiency, prostatic hyperplasia, urinary stricture, renal impairment, or severe hepatic dysfunction and in patients with hypersensitivity reactions to other phenanthrene derivative opioid agonists (codeine, hydrocodone, hydromorphone, levorphanol, oxycodone, oxymorphone). Use with caution in patients with biliary tract dysfunction; acute pancreatitis may cause constriction of sphincter of Oddi. Some preparations contain sulfites which may cause allergic reactions; infants <3 months of age are more susceptible to respiratory depression, use with caution and generally in reduced doses in this age group.

May cause CNS depression, which may impair physical or mental abilities; patients must be cautioned about performing tasks which require mental alertness (eg, operating machinery or driving). Effects may be potentiated when used with other sedative drugs or ethanol. May cause hypotension in patients with acute myocardial infarction, volume depletion, or concurrent drug therapy which may exaggerate vasodilation. Use with extreme caution in patients with head injury, intracranial lesions, or elevated intracranial pressure; exaggerated elevation of ICP may occur. May cause seizures if high doses are used; use with caution in patients with seizure disorders. Tolerance or drug dependence may result from extended use. Concurrent use of agonist/antagonist analgesics may precipitate withdrawal symptoms and/or reduced analgesic efficacy in patients following prolonged therapy with mu opioid agonists. Abrupt discontinuation following prolonged use may also lead to withdrawal symptoms. Elderly may be particularly susceptible to adverse effects of narcotics. May obscure diagnosis or clinical course of patients with acute abdominal conditions.

Extended or sustained-release formulations:

[U.S. Boxed Warning]: Extended or sustained release dosage forms should not be crushed or chewed. Controlled-, extended-, or sustained-release products are not intended for "as needed (PRN)" use. **MS Contin® 100 or 200 mg tablets and Kadian® 100 mg or 200 mg capsules are for use only in opioid-tolerant patients.** Avinza®, Kadian®, MS Contin®: **[U.S. Boxed Warning]: Indicated for the management of moderate-to-severe pain when around the clock pain control is needed for an extended time period.**

[U.S. Boxed Warning]: Avinza®: Do not administer with alcoholic beverages or ethanol-containing products, which may disrupt extended-release characteristic of product.

Highly concentrated oral solutions: [U.S. Boxed Warning]: Check doses carefully when using highly concentrated oral solutions.

Injections: Note: Products are designed for administration by specific routes (I.V., intrathecal, epidural). Use caution when prescribing, dispensing, or administering to use formulations only by intended route(s).

[U.S. Boxed Warning]: Duramorph®: Due to the risk of severe and/or sustained cardiopulmonary depressant effects of Duramorph® must be administered in a fully equipped and staffed environment. Naloxone injection should be immediately available. Patient should remain in this environment for at least 24 hours following the initial dose.

[U.S. Boxed Warning]: Intrathecal dosage is usually 1/10 that of epidural dosage.

Infumorph® solutions are **for use in microinfusion devices only**; not for I.V., I.M., or SubQ administration, or for single-dose administration.

When used as an epidural injection, monitor for delayed sedation.

Drug Interactions

Avoid Concomitant Use There are no known interactions where it is recommended to avoid concomitant use.

Decreased Effect

Morphine (Systemic) may decrease the levels/effects of: Pegvisomant

The levels/effects of Morphine (Systemic) may be decreased by: Ammonium Chloride; Mixed Agonist / Antagonist Opioids; Peginterferon Alfa-2b; Rifamycin Derivatives

Increased Effect/Toxicity

Morphine (Systemic) may increase the levels/effects of: Alcohol (Ethyl); Alvimopan; CNS Depressants; Desmopressin; Selective Serotonin Reuptake Inhibitors; Thiazide Diuretics

The levels/effects of Morphine (Systemic) may be increased by: Amphetamines; Antipsychotic Agents (Phenothiazines); Droperidol; HydrOXYzine; Succinylcholine

Nutritional/Ethanol Interactions

Ethanol: Alcoholic beverages or ethanol-containing products may disrupt extended-release formulation resulting in rapid release of entire morphine dose. Ethanol may also increase CNS depression. Management: Avoid alcohol.

Food: Administration of oral morphine solution with food may increase bioavailability (ie, a report of 34% increase in morphine AUC when morphine oral solution followed a high-fat meal). The bioavailability of Avinza®, Oramorph SR®, or Kadian® does not appear to be affected by food. Management: Take consistently with or without meals.

Herb/Nutraceutical: Gotu kola, valerian, and kava kava may increase CNS depression. Management: Avoid gotu kola, valerian, and kava kava.

Adverse Reactions Note: Individual patient differences are unpredictable, and percentage may differ in acute pain (surgical) treatment. Reactions may be dose, formulation, and/or route dependent.

Frequency not defined:

Cardiovascular: Circulatory depression, flushing, shock

Central nervous system: Dysphonia, physical and psychological dependence, sedation

Endocrine & metabolic: Antidiuretic hormone release, hypogonadism

Neuromuscular & skeletal: Bone mineral density decreased

>10%:

Cardiovascular: Bradycardia, hypotension

Central nervous system: Drowsiness (9% to 48%; tolerance usually develops to drowsiness with regular dosing for 1-2 weeks), dizziness (6% to 20%), fever (<3% to >10%), confusion, headache (following epidural or intrathecal use)

Dermatologic: Pruritus (may be dose related)

Gastrointestinal: Xerostomia (78%), constipation (9% to 40%; tolerance develops very slowly if at all), nausea (7% to 28%; tolerance usually develops to nausea and vomiting with chronic use), vomiting
Genitourinary: Urinary retention (16%; may be prolonged, up to 20 hours, following epidural or intrathecal use)
Hematologic: Anemia (following intrathecal use)
Local: Pain at injection site
Neuromuscular & skeletal: Weakness
Respiratory: Oxygen saturation decreased
Miscellaneous: Histamine release

1% to 10%:
Cardiovascular: Atrial fibrillation (<3%), chest pain (<3%), edema, hypertension, palpitation, peripheral edema, syncope, tachycardia, vasodilation
Central nervous system: Amnesia, agitation, anxiety, apathy, apprehension, ataxia, chills, coma, delirium, depression, dream abnormalities, euphoria, false sense of well being, hallucination, hypoesthesia, insomnia, lethargy, malaise, nervousness, restlessness, seizure, slurred speech, somnolence, vertigo
Dermatologic: Dry skin, rash, urticaria
Endocrine & metabolic: Gynecomastia (<3%), hypokalemia, hyponatremia, libido decreased
Gastrointestinal: Abdominal distension, abdominal pain, anorexia, biliary colic, diarrhea, dyspepsia, dysphagia, flatulence, gastroenteritis, GERD, GI irritation, paralytic ileus, rectal disorder, taste perversion, weight loss
Genitourinary: Bladder spasm, dysuria, ejaculation abnormal, impotence, urination decreased
Hematologic: Leukopenia (<3%), thrombocytopenia (<3%), hematocrit decreased
Hepatic: Liver function tests increased
Neuromuscular & skeletal: Arthralgia, back pain, bone pain, foot drop, gait abnormalities, paresthesia, rigors, skeletal muscle rigidity, tremor
Ocular: Amblyopia, conjunctivitis, eye pain, vision problems/disturbance
Renal: Oliguria
Respiratory: Asthma, atelectasis, dyspnea, hiccups, hypercapnia, hypoxia, pulmonary edema (noncardiogenic), respiratory depression, rhinitis
Miscellaneous: Diaphoresis, flu-like syndrome, infection, thirst, voice alteration, withdrawal syndrome

Pharmacodynamics/Kinetics

Onset of Action Patient dependent; dosing must be individualized: Oral (immediate release): ~30 minutes; I.V.: 5-10 minutes

Duration of Action Patient dependent; dosing must be individualized: Pain relief:
Immediate release formulations: 4 hours
Extended release capsule and tablet: 8-24 hours (formulation dependent)

Controlled Substance C-II

Available Dosage Forms

Capsule, extended release, oral: 10 mg, 20 mg, 30 mg, 50 mg, 60 mg, 80 mg, 100 mg, 200 mg
AVINza®: 30 mg, 45 mg, 60 mg, 75 mg, 90 mg, 120 mg
Kadian®: 10 mg, 20 mg, 30 mg, 50 mg, 60 mg, 80 mg, 100 mg, 200 mg

Injection, solution: 1 mg/mL (10 mL, 30 mL, 50 mL); 2 mg/mL (1 mL); 4 mg/mL (1 mL); 5 mg/mL (1 mL, 30 mL, 50 mL); 8 mg/mL (1 mL); 10 mg/mL (1 mL, 10 mL); 10 mg/0.7 mL (0.7 mL); 15 mg/mL (1 mL, 20 mL); 25 mg/mL (4 mL, 10 mL, 20 mL); 50 mg/mL (20 mL, 40 mL, 50 mL)

Injection, solution [preservative free]: 0.5 mg/mL (10 mL, 30 mL); 1 mg/mL (10 mL, 30 mL); 5 mg/mL (30 mL); 25 mg/mL (4 mL, 10 mL, 20 mL)
Astramorph®/PF: 0.5 mg/mL (2 mL, 10 mL); 1 mg/mL (2 mL, 10 mL)
Duramorph: 0.5 mg/mL (10 mL); 1 mg/mL (10 mL)
Infumorph 200: 10 mg/mL (20 mL)
Infumorph 500: 25 mg/mL (20 mL)

Solution, oral: 10 mg/5 mL (5 mL, 10 mL, 100 mL, 500 mL); 20 mg/5 mL (100 mL, 500 mL); 100 mg/5 mL (1 mL, 15 mL, 30 mL, 120 mL, 240 mL)

Suppository, rectal: 5 mg (12s); 10 mg (12s); 20 mg (12s); 30 mg (12s)

Tablet, oral: 15 mg, 30 mg

Tablet, controlled release, oral:
MS Contin®: 15 mg, 30 mg, 60 mg, 100 mg, 200 mg

Tablet, extended release, oral: 15 mg, 30 mg, 60 mg, 100 mg, 200 mg

Tablet, sustained release, oral:
Oramorph® SR: 15 mg, 30 mg, 60 mg, 100 mg

General Dosage Range Dosage adjustment recommended in patients with renal impairment

Epidural: *Adults:* 5 mg (Astromorph/PF™, Duramorph®) as a single dose **or** 1-6 mg bolus followed by 0.1-0.2 mg/hour (maximum: 10 mg/day) **or** continuous microinfusion (Infumorph®): Opioid-naive patients: 3.5-7.5 mg/day; Opioid-tolerant patients: 4.5-30 mg/day

I.M.:
Children >6 months and <50 kg: 0.1-0.2 mg/kg every 3-4 hours as needed
Adults: 5-20 mg every 4 hours as needed

I.T. (I.T. dose is usually 1/10 that of epidural dose):
Adults: Opioid-naive: 0.2-1 mg/dose as single dose or once daily; Opioid-tolerant: 1-10 mg/day

I.V.:
Children >6 months and <50 kg: 0.1-0.2 mg/kg every 3-4 hours as needed **or** 10-60 mcg/kg/**hour** as a continuous infusion
Adults: 2.5-5 mg every 3-4 hours **or** 0.8-10 mg/hour; Usual range: Up to 80 mg/hour
Adults (mechanically-ventilated): 0.7-10 mg every 1-2 hours as needed **or** 5-35 mg/hour infusion

Oral:

Controlled, extended or sustained release:

Adults:

Capsules: Established daily dose on prompt-release formulations administered in 1-2 divided doses (every 12 hours)

Tablets: Established daily dose on prompt-release formulations administered in divided doses every 8-12 hours

Immediate release:

Children >6 months and <50 kg: 0.15-0.3 mg/kg every 3-4 hours as needed

Adults: 10-30 mg every 4 hours as needed;

Note: Much higher doses may be necessary for chronic pain

PCA: *Adults:* Concentration: 1 mg/mL; Demand dose: 0.5-2.5 mg; Lockout interval: 5-10 minutes

Rectal: *Adults:* 10-20 mg every 3-4 hours

SubQ:

Adults: 5-20 mg every 3-4 hours as needed **or** 0.8-10 mg/hour (up to 80 mg/hour) as continuous infusion

Adults (mechanically-ventilated): 0.7-10 mg every 1-2 hours as needed **or** 5-35 mg/hour infusion

Administration

Oral Do not crush controlled release drug product, swallow whole. Kadian® and Avinza® can be opened and sprinkled on applesauce; do not crush or chew the beads. Contents of Kadian® capsules may be opened and sprinkled over 10 mL water and flushed through prewetted 16F gastrostomy tube; do not administer Kadian® through nasogastric tube.

I.V. When giving morphine I.V. push, it is best to first dilute with sterile water or NS for a final concentration of 1-2 mg/mL and then administer slowly.

I.V. Detail pH: 2.5-6.0

Other Use preservative-free solutions for intrathecal or epidural use.

Stability

Reconstitution Injection: Usual concentration for continuous I.V. infusion: 0.1-1 mg/mL in D_5W.

Storage

Capsule, sustained release (Avinza®, Kadian®): Store at 25°C (77°F); excursions permitted to 15°C to 30°C (59°F to 86°F). Protect from light and moisture.

Injection: Store at controlled room temperature of 20°C to 25°C (68°F to 77°F); do not freeze. Protect from light. Degradation depends on pH and presence of oxygen; relatively stable in pH ≤4; darkening of solutions indicate degradation.

Oral solution: Store at controlled room temperature of 25°C (68°F to 77°F); do not freeze.

Suppositories: Store at controlled room temperature 25°C (77°F). Protect from light.

Tablet, extended release: Store at controlled room temperature of 25°C (77°F).

Tablet, immediate release: Store at controlled room temperature of 25°C (77°F). Protect from moisture.

Nursing Actions

Physical Assessment Monitor for effectiveness of pain relief. Monitor blood pressure, CNS and respiratory status, and degree of sedation at beginning of therapy and periodically thereafter. Assess patient's physical and/or psychological dependence. For inpatients, implement safety measures (eg, side rails up, call light within reach, instructions to call for assistance). Discontinue slowly after prolonged use.

Patient Education Do not crush or chew controlled release tablet or capsule. May cause physical and/or psychological dependence. While using this medication, do not use alcohol (especially if using Avinza®) and other prescription or OTC medications (especially sedatives, tranquilizers, antihistamines, or pain medications) without consulting prescriber. Maintain adequate hydration, unless instructed to restrict fluid intake. May cause itching, hypotension, dizziness, drowsiness, impaired coordination, or blurred vision; loss of appetite, dry mouth, nausea, or vomiting; or constipation. Report chest pain, slow or rapid heartbeat, dizziness, or persistent headache; confusion or respiratory difficulties; or severe constipation.

Dietary Considerations Morphine may cause GI upset; take with food if GI upset occurs. Be consistent when taking morphine with or without meals.

Related Information

Compatibility of Drugs *on page 1264*

Morphine and Naltrexone

(MOR feen & nal TREKS one)

Brand Names: U.S. Embeda™

Index Terms Morphine Sulfate and Naltrexone Hydrochloride; MS (error-prone abbreviation and should not be used); MSO_4 (error-prone abbreviation and should not be used); Naltrexone and Morphine

Pharmacologic Category Analgesic, Opioid; Opioid Antagonist

Medication Safety Issues

Sound-alike/look-alike issues:

Morphine may be confused with HYDROmorphone

Morphine sulfate may be confused with magnesium sulfate

Naltrexone may be confused with methylnaltrexone, naloxone

MSO_4 and MS are error-prone abbreviations (mistaken as magnesium sulfate)

Medication Guide Available Yes

Pregnancy Risk Factor C

Lactation Enters breast milk/not recommended

Use Relief of moderate-to-severe pain when continual, around-the-clock therapy is needed for an extended period of time

Controlled Substance C-II

Available Dosage Forms

Capsule, extended release, oral:

Embeda™ 20/0.8: Morphine 20 mg and naltrexone 0.8 mg

Embeda™ 30/1.2: Morphine 30 mg and naltrexone 1.2 mg

Embeda™ 50/2: Morphine 50 mg and naltrexone 2 mg

Embeda™ 80/3.2: Morphine 80 mg and naltrexone 3.2 mg

Embeda™ 100/4: Morphine 100 mg and naltrexone 4 mg

General Dosage Range Oral: *Adults:* Initial: 20 mg/0.8 mg once or twice daily; Maintenance: Adjust based on individual patient requirement

Administration

Oral Capsule should be swallowed whole. Contents of the capsule may be sprinkled on applesauce (do not divide in separate doses) and swallowed immediately. Rinse mouth to ensure all contents have been swallowed. Do not crush, chew, or dissolve pellets in the capsule prior to swallowing. Not for nasogastric/gastric tube administration. First dose may be taken at the same time as the last dose of immediate release opioid medication.

Nursing Actions

Physical Assessment See individual agents.

Patient Education See individual agents.

Moxifloxacin (Systemic) (moxs i FLOKS a sin)

Brand Names: U.S. Avelox®; Avelox® ABC Pack; Avelox® I.V.

Index Terms Moxifloxacin Hydrochloride

Pharmacologic Category Antibiotic, Quinolone; Respiratory Fluoroquinolone

Medication Safety Issues

Sound-alike/look-alike issues:

Avelox® may be confused with Avonex®

Medication Guide Available Yes

Pregnancy Risk Factor C

Lactation Excretion in breast milk unknown/not recommended

Breast-Feeding Considerations It is not known if moxifloxacin is excreted into breast milk. Breast-feeding is not recommended by the manufacturer. Although there is no information on the use of moxifloxacin during breast-feeding, other quinolones are considered compatible. Nondose-related effects could include modification of bowel flora.

Use Treatment of mild-to-moderate community-acquired pneumonia, including multidrug-resistant *Streptococcus pneumoniae* (MDRSP); acute bacterial exacerbation of chronic bronchitis; acute bacterial sinusitis; complicated and uncomplicated skin and skin structure infections; complicated intra-abdominal infections

Unlabeled Use Treatment of *Legionella* pneumonia; treatment of mild-to-moderate community-acquired pneumonia (CAP), including multidrug-resistant *Streptococcus pneumoniae* (MDRSP) in adolescents with skeletal maturity

Mechanism of Action/Effect Moxifloxacin is a quinolone antibiotic with bactericidal activity against susceptible gram-negative and gram-positive microorganisms.

Contraindications Hypersensitivity to moxifloxacin, other quinolone antibiotics, or any component of the formulation

Warnings/Precautions [U.S. Boxed Warning]: There have been reports of tendon inflammation and/or rupture with quinolone antibiotics; risk may be increased with concurrent corticosteroids, organ transplant recipients, and in patients >60 years of age. Rupture of the Achilles tendon sometimes requiring surgical repair has been reported most frequently; but other tendon sites (eg, rotator cuff, biceps) have also been reported. Strenuous physical activity, rheumatoid arthritis, and renal impairment may be an independent risk factor for tendonitis. Discontinue at first sign of tendon inflammation or pain. Tendon rupture may occur even after discontinuation of therapy. Use with caution in patients with rheumatoid arthritis or renal impairment; may increase risk of tendon rupture.

Use with caution in patients with significant bradycardia or acute myocardial ischemia. Moxifloxacin causes a concentration-dependent QT prolongation. Do not exceed recommended dose or infusion rate. Avoid use with uncorrected hypokalemia, with other drugs that prolong the QT interval or induce bradycardia, or with class Ia or III antiarrhythmic agents. CNS effects may occur (tremor, restlessness, confusion, and very rarely hallucinations, increased intracranial pressure [including pseudotumor cerebri] or seizures). Use with caution in patients with known or suspected CNS disorder. Potential for seizures, although very rare, may be increased with concomitant NSAID therapy. Use with caution in individuals at risk of seizures. Use with caution in patients with mild, moderate, or severe hepatic impairment or liver cirrhosis; may increase the risk of QT prolongation. Fulminant hepatitis potentially leading to liver failure (including fatalities) has been reported with use. Use with caution in diabetes; glucose regulation may be altered.

Fluoroquinolones have been associated with the development of serious, and sometimes fatal, hypoglycemia, most often in elderly diabetics, but also in patients without diabetes. This occurred most frequently with gatifloxacin (no longer available systemically) but may occur at a lower frequency with other quinolones.

Severe hypersensitivity reactions, including anaphylaxis, have occurred with quinolone therapy. Reactions may present as typical allergic symptoms after a single dose, or may manifest as severe idiosyncratic dermatologic, vascular, pulmonary, renal, hepatic, and/or hematologic events, usually after multiple doses. Prompt discontinuation of drug should occur if skin rash or other symptoms arise. Avoid excessive sunlight and take precautions to limit exposure (eg, loose fitting clothing, sunscreen); may cause moderate-to-severe phototoxicity reactions. Discontinue use if photosensitivity occurs. Prolonged use may result in fungal or bacterial superinfection, including *C. difficile*-associated diarrhea (CDAD) and pseudomembranous colitis; CDAD has been observed >2 months postantibiotic treatment. **[U.S. Boxed Warning]: Quinolones may exacerbate myasthenia gravis; avoid use (rare, potentially life-threatening weakness of respiratory muscles may occur).** Peripheral neuropathy may rarely occur. Hemolytic reactions may (rarely) occur with quinolone use in patients with latent or actual G6PD deficiency. Adverse effects (eg, tendon rupture, QT changes) may be increased in the elderly. Some quinolones may exacerbate myasthenia gravis, use with caution (rare, potentially life-threatening weakness of respiratory muscles may occur). Safety and efficacy of systemically administered moxifloxacin (oral, intravenous) in patients <18 years of age have not been established.

Drug Interactions

Avoid Concomitant Use

Avoid concomitant use of Moxifloxacin (Systemic) with any of the following: Artemether; BCG; Dronedarone; Lumefantrine; Nilotinib; Pimozide; QUEtiapine; QuiNINE; Tetrabenazine; Thioridazine; Toremifene; Vandetanib; Vemurafenib; Ziprasidone

Decreased Effect

Moxifloxacin (Systemic) may decrease the levels/effects of: BCG; Mycophenolate; Sulfonylureas; Typhoid Vaccine

The levels/effects of Moxifloxacin (Systemic) may be decreased by: Antacids; Didanosine; Iron Salts; Lanthanum; Magnesium Salts; Quinapril; Sevelamer; Sucralfate; Zinc Salts

Increased Effect/Toxicity

Moxifloxacin (Systemic) may increase the levels/effects of: Corticosteroids (Systemic); Dronedarone; Pimozide; Porfimer; QTc-Prolonging Agents; QuiNINE; Sulfonylureas; Tetrabenazine; Thioridazine; Toremifene; Vandetanib; Varenicline; Vemurafenib; Vitamin K Antagonists; Ziprasidone

The levels/effects of Moxifloxacin (Systemic) may be increased by: Alfuzosin; Artemether; Chloroquine; Ciprofloxacin; Ciprofloxacin (Systemic); Gadobutrol; Indacaterol; Insulin; Lumefantrine; Nilotinib; Nonsteroidal Anti-Inflammatory Agents; Probenecid; QUEtiapine; QuiNINE

Nutritional/Ethanol Interactions Food: Absorption is not affected by administration with a high-fat meal or yogurt.

Adverse Reactions

2% to 10%:

Central nervous system: Dizziness (2%)

Endocrine & metabolic: Serum chloride increased (≥2%), serum ionized calcium increased (≥2%), serum glucose decreased (≥2%)

Gastrointestinal: Nausea (6%), diarrhea (5%), amylase decreased (≥2%)

Hematologic: Decreased serum levels of the following (≥2%): Basophils, eosinophils, hemoglobin, RBC, neutrophils; increased serum levels of the following (≥2%): MCH, neutrophils, WBC

Hepatic: Bilirubin decreased/increased (≥2%)

Renal: Serum albumin increased (≥2%)

Respiratory: PO_2 decreased (≥2%)

0.1% to <2%:

Cardiovascular: Cardiac arrhythmias, palpitation, QT_c prolongation, tachycardia, vasodilation

Central nervous system: Anxiety, headache, insomnia, malaise, nervousness, pain, somnolence, vertigo

Dermatologic: Pruritus, rash (maculopapular, purpuric, pustular), urticaria

Gastrointestinal: Abdominal pain, amylase increased, anorexia, constipation, dyspepsia, flatulence, glossitis, lactic dehydrogenase increased, stomatitis, taste perversion, vomiting, xerostomia

Genitourinary: Vaginal moniliasis, vaginitis

Hematologic: Eosinophilia, leukopenia, prothrombin time prolonged, increased INR, thrombocythemia

Hepatic: GGTP increased, liver function test abnormal

Local: Injection site reaction

Neuromuscular & skeletal: Arthralgia, myalgia, tremor, weakness

Respiratory: Pharyngitis, pneumonia, rhinitis, sinusitis

Miscellaneous: Allergic reaction, infection, diaphoresis, oral moniliasis

Available Dosage Forms

Infusion, premixed in sodium chloride 0.8% [preservative free]:

Avelox® I.V.: 400 mg (250 mL)

Tablet, oral:

Avelox®: 400 mg

Avelox® ABC Pack: 400 mg

General Dosage Range I.V., oral: *Adults:* 400 mg every 24 hours

Administration

I.V. Infuse over 60 minutes; do not infuse by rapid or bolus intravenous infusion

Stability

Storage Store at controlled room temperature of 25°C (77°F). Do not refrigerate infusion solution.

Nursing Actions

Physical Assessment Results of culture and sensitivity tests and patient's allergy history should be assessed before initiating therapy. Monitor patient closely; if an allergic reaction occurs (itching, urticaria, dyspnea or facial edema, loss of consciousness, tingling, cardiovascular collapse), drug should be discontinued immediately and prescriber notified. Monitor for hypersensitivity reactions, opportunistic infection, tendon rupture, and persistent diarrhea (*C. difficile*-associated colitis can occur post-treatment).

Patient Education If administered by infusion: Report immediately any redness, swelling, or pain at infusion site; any swelling of mouth, lips, tongue, or throat; chest pain or tightness; respiratory difficulty; back pain; itching; skin rash; tingling; tendon pain; dizziness; abnormal thinking; or anxiety. May cause dizziness, lightheadedness, confusion, nausea, or vomiting (request antiemetic from prescriber). Report any tendon pain, chest pain, or palpitations.

Oral: Do not take antacids 4 hours before or 8 hours after taking this medication. Maintain adequate hydration unless instructed to restrict fluid intake. Consult prescriber before having any vaccinations. May cause nausea, vomiting, taste perversion, headache, dizziness, insomnia, or anxiety. Avoid excessive sunlight and wear sunscreen during therapy. If you develop severe sunburn or sensitivity to sunlight, if tendon inflammation or pain occurs, or if you experience signs of an allergic reaction (eg, itching, urticaria, respiratory difficulty, facial edema or difficulty swallowing, loss of consciousness, tingling, chest pain, palpitations), discontinue use and contact prescriber immediately. Report persistent GI disturbances, CNS changes (eg, excessive sleepiness, agitation, tremors), skin rash, vision changes, respiratory difficulty, signs of opportunistic infection (eg, sore throat, chills, fever, burning, itching on urination, vaginal discharge, white plaques in mouth), persistent diarrhea (especially if it lasts after completing prescription); or worsening of condition.

Dietary Considerations May be taken without regard to meals. Take 4 hours before or 8 hours after multiple vitamins, antacids, or other products containing magnesium, aluminum, iron, or zinc.

Avelox® I.V. infusion (premixed in sodium chloride 0.8%) contains sodium 34.2 mEq (~787 mg)/ 250 mL.

Moxifloxacin (Ophthalmic)

(moxs i FLOKS a sin)

Brand Names: U.S. Moxeza™; Vigamox®

Index Terms Moxifloxacin Hydrochloride

Pharmacologic Category Antibiotic, Ophthalmic; Antibiotic, Quinolone

Medication Safety Issues

International issues:

Vigamox [U.S., Canada, and multiple international markets] may be confused with Fisamox brand name for amoxicillin [Australia]

Pregnancy Risk Factor C

Lactation Use caution

Use Treatment of bacterial conjunctivitis caused by susceptible organisms

Available Dosage Forms

Solution, ophthalmic:

Moxeza™: 0.5% (3 mL)

Vigamox®: 0.5% (3 mL)

General Dosage Range Ophthalmic:

Children ≥4 months and Adults: Moxeza™: Instill 1 drop into affected eye(s) 2 times/day

Children ≥1 year and Adults: Vigamox®: Instill 1 drop into affected eye(s) 3 times/day

Administration

Other For topical ophthalmic use only; avoid touching tip of applicator to eye or other surfaces.

Nursing Actions

Patient Education Wash hands before instilling solution. Sit or lie down to instill. Open eye, look at ceiling, and instill prescribed amount of solution as directed. Do not touch tip of applicator or let tip of applicator touch eye. Do not wear contact lenses during therapy. Temporary stinging, blurred vision, or dry eyes may occur. Report persistent pain, burning, excessive tearing, decreased visual acuity, swelling, itching, or worsening of condition.

Mycophenolate (mye koe FEN oh late)

Brand Names: U.S. CellCept®; Myfortic®

Index Terms MMF; MPA; Mycophenolate Mofetil; Mycophenolate Sodium; Mycophenolic Acid

Pharmacologic Category Immunosuppressant Agent

Medication Guide Available Yes

Pregnancy Risk Factor D

Lactation Excretion in breast milk unknown/not recommended

Breast-Feeding Considerations It is unknown if mycophenolate is excreted in human milk. Due to potentially serious adverse reactions, the decision to discontinue the drug or discontinue breast-feeding should be considered. Breast-feeding is not recommended during therapy or for 6 weeks after treatment is complete.

Use Prophylaxis of organ rejection concomitantly with cyclosporine and corticosteroids in patients receiving allogeneic renal (CellCept®, Myfortic®), cardiac (CellCept®), or hepatic (CellCept®) transplants

Unlabeled Use Treatment of rejection in liver transplant patients unable to tolerate tacrolimus or cyclosporine due to neurotoxicity; mild rejection in heart transplant patients; treatment of moderate-severe psoriasis; treatment of proliferative lupus nephritis; treatment of myasthenia gravis; prevention and treatment of graft-versus-host disease (GVHD)

Mechanism of Action/Effect Inhibition of purine synthesis of human lymphocytes and proliferation of human lymphocytes

Contraindications Hypersensitivity to mycophenolate mofetil, mycophenolic acid, mycophenolate sodium, or any component of the formulation; intravenous formulation is contraindicated in patients who are allergic to polysorbate 80

Warnings/Precautions Hazardous agent - use appropriate precautions for handling and disposal. **[U.S. Boxed Warning]: Risk for infection and development of lymphoma and skin malignancy is increased.** Opportunistic infections, sepsis, and/or fatal infections may occur with immunosuppressive therapy. Patients should be monitored appropriately. Instruct patients to limit exposure to sunlight/UV light and give supportive treatment should these conditions occur. Pure red cell aplasia (PRCA), progressive multifocal leukoencephalopathy (PML), or BK virus-associated nephropathy (BKVAN) may occur rarely, particularly in immunosuppressed patients or those receiving immunosuppressant therapy; monitor for signs of PRCA (anemia, fatigue, lethargy, pallor, dyspnea), PML (neurologic impairment, apathy, ataxia, cognitive deficiencies, confusion, and hemiparesis), or BKVAN (deterioration of renal function, renal graft loss); may require dosage reduction or discontinuation of therapy. Neutropenia (including severe neutropenia) may occur, requiring dose reduction or interruption of treatment (risk greater from day 31-180 post-transplant). Use caution with active peptic ulcer disease; may be associated with gastric or duodenal ulcers, GI bleeding and/or perforation. Use caution in renal impairment as toxicity may be increased; may require dosage adjustment in severe impairment.

[U.S. Boxed Warning]: Mycophenolate is associated with an increased risk of congenital malformations and spontaneous abortions when used during pregnancy. Females of childbearing potential should have a negative pregnancy test within 1 week prior to beginning therapy. Two reliable forms of contraception should be used beginning 4 weeks prior to, during, and for 6 weeks after therapy. Because mycophenolate mofetil has demonstrated teratogenic effects in rats and rabbits, tablets should not be crushed, and capsules should not be opened or crushed. Avoid inhalation or direct contact with skin or mucous membranes of the powder contained in the capsules and the powder for oral suspension. Caution should be exercised in the handling and preparation of solutions of intravenous mycophenolate. Avoid skin contact with the intravenous solution and reconstituted suspension. If such contact occurs, wash thoroughly with soap and water, rinse eyes with plain water.

Theoretically, use should be avoided in patients with the rare hereditary deficiency of hypoxanthine-guanine phosphoribosyltransferase (such as Lesch-Nyhan or Kelley-Seegmiller syndrome). Intravenous solutions should be given over at least 2 hours; never administer intravenous solution by rapid or bolus injection. **[U.S. Boxed Warning]: Should be administered under the supervision of a physician experienced in immunosuppressive therapy.**

Note: CellCept® and Myfortic® dosage forms should not be used interchangeably due to differences in absorption. Some dosage forms may contain phenylalanine.

Drug Interactions

Avoid Concomitant Use

Avoid concomitant use of Mycophenolate with any of the following: BCG; Cholestyramine Resin; Natalizumab; Pimecrolimus; Rifamycin Derivatives; Tacrolimus (Topical); Vaccines (Live)

Decreased Effect

Mycophenolate may decrease the levels/effects of: BCG; Coccidioidin Skin Test; Contraceptives (Estrogens); Contraceptives (Progestins); Sipuleucel-T; Vaccines (Inactivated); Vaccines (Live)

The levels/effects of Mycophenolate may be decreased by: Antacids; Cholestyramine Resin; CycloSPORINE; CycloSPORINE (Systemic); Echinacea; Magnesium Salts; MetroNIDAZOLE; MetroNIDAZOLE (Systemic); Penicillins; Proton Pump Inhibitors; Quinolone Antibiotics; Rifamycin Derivatives; Sevelamer

Increased Effect/Toxicity

Mycophenolate may increase the levels/effects of: Acyclovir-Valacyclovir; Ganciclovir-Valganciclovir; Leflunomide; Natalizumab; Vaccines (Live)

The levels/effects of Mycophenolate may be increased by: Acyclovir-Valacyclovir; Belatacept; Denosumab; Ganciclovir-Valganciclovir; Pimecrolimus; Probenecid; Roflumilast; Tacrolimus (Topical); Trastuzumab

Nutritional/Ethanol Interactions

Food: Food decreases C_{max} of MPA by 40% following CellCept® administration and 33% following Myfortic® use; the extent of absorption is not changed. Management: May be taken with food if necessary in stable patients; otherwise, take on an empty stomach to decrease variability.

Herb/Nutraceutical: Cat's claw and echinacea have immunostimulant properties. Management: Avoid cat's claw and echinacea.

Adverse Reactions Data for incidence >20% as reported in adults following oral dosing of

CellCept® alone in renal, cardiac, and hepatic allograft rejection studies. Profile in 3% to <20% range reflects use in combination with cyclosporine and corticosteroids. In general, lower doses used in renal rejection patients had less adverse effects than higher doses. Rates of adverse effects were similar for each indication, except for those unique to the specific organ involved. The type of adverse effects observed in pediatric patients was similar to those seen in adults; abdominal pain, anemia, diarrhea, fever, hypertension, infection, pharyngitis, respiratory tract infection, sepsis, and vomiting were seen in higher proportion; lymphoproliferative disorder was the only type of malignancy observed. Percentages of adverse reactions were similar in studies comparing CellCept® to Myfortic® in patients following renal transplant.

>20%:

- Cardiovascular: Hypertension (28% to 78%), hypotension (33%), peripheral edema (27% to 64%), edema (27% to 28%), chest pain (26%), tachycardia (20% to 22%)
- Central nervous system: Pain (31% to 76%), headache (16% to 54%), insomnia (41% to 52%), fever (21% to 52%), dizziness (29%), anxiety (28%)
- Dermatologic: Rash (22%)
- Endocrine & metabolic: Hyperglycemia (44% to 47%), hypercholesterolemia (41%), hypomagnesemia (39%), hypokalemia (32% to 37%), hypocalcemia (30%), hyperkalemia (22%)
- Gastrointestinal: Abdominal pain (25% to 63%), nausea (20% to 55%), diarrhea (31% to 51%), constipation (19% to 41%), vomiting (33% to 34%), anorexia (25%), dyspepsia (22%)
- Genitourinary: Urinary tract infection (37%)
- Hematologic: Leukopenia (23% to 46%), anemia (26% to 43%; hypochromic 25%), leukocytosis (22% to 41%), thrombocytopenia (24% to 38%)
- Hepatic: Liver function tests abnormal (25%), ascites (24%)
- Neuromuscular & skeletal: Back pain (35% to 47%), weakness (35% to 43%), tremor (24% to 34%), paresthesia (21%)
- Renal: Creatinine increased (39%), BUN increased (35%), kidney function abnormal (22% to 26%)
- Respiratory: Dyspnea (31% to 37%), respiratory tract infection (22% to 37%), pleural effusion (34%), cough (31%), lung disorder (22% to 30%), sinusitis (26%)
- Miscellaneous: Infection (18% to 27%), sepsis (27%), lactate dehydrogenase increased (23%), *Candida* (17% to 22%), herpes simplex (10% to 21%)

3% to <20%:

- Cardiovascular: Angina, arrhythmia, arterial thrombosis, atrial fibrillation, atrial flutter, bradycardia, cardiac arrest, cardiac failure, CHF, extrasystole, facial edema, hyper-/hypovolemia, pallor, palpitation, pericardial effusion, peripheral vascular disorder, postural hypotension, supraventricular extrasystoles, supraventricular tachycardia, syncope, thrombosis, vasodilation, vasospasm, venous pressure increased, ventricular extrasystole, ventricular tachycardia
- Central nervous system: Agitation, chills with fever, confusion, delirium, depression, emotional lability, hallucinations, hypoesthesia, malaise, nervousness, psychosis, seizure, somnolence, thinking abnormal, vertigo
- Dermatologic: Acne, alopecia, bruising, cellulitis, fungal dermatitis, hirsutism, petechia, pruritus, skin carcinoma, skin hypertrophy, skin ulcer, vesiculobullous rash
- Endocrine & metabolic: Acidosis, alkalosis, Cushing's syndrome, dehydration, diabetes mellitus, gout, hypercalcemia, hyper-hypophosphatemia, hyperlipemia, hyperuricemia, hypochloremia, hypoglycemia, hyponatremia, hypoproteinemia, hypothyroidism, parathyroid disorder
- Gastrointestinal: Abdomen enlarged, dysphagia, esophagitis, flatulence, gastritis, gastroenteritis, gastrointestinal hemorrhage, gastrointestinal moniliasis, gingivitis, gum hyperplasia, ileus, melena, mouth ulceration, oral moniliasis, stomach disorder, stomach ulcer, stomatitis, xerostomia, weight gain/loss
- Genitourinary: Impotence, nocturia, pelvic pain, prostatic disorder, scrotal edema, urinary frequency, urinary incontinence, urinary retention, urinary tract disorder
- Hematologic: Coagulation disorder, hemorrhage, neutropenia, pancytopenia, polycythemia, prothrombin time increased, thromboplastin time increased
- Hepatic: Alkaline phosphatase increased, bilirubinemia, cholangitis, cholestatic jaundice, GGT increased, hepatitis, jaundice, liver damage, transaminases increased
- Local: Abscess
- Neuromuscular & skeletal: Arthralgia, hypertonia, joint disorder, leg cramps, myalgia, myasthenia, neck pain, neuropathy, osteoporosis
- Ocular: Amblyopia, cataract, conjunctivitis, eye hemorrhage, lacrimation disorder, vision abnormal
- Otic: Deafness, ear disorder, ear pain, tinnitus
- Renal: Albuminuria, creatinine increased, dysuria, hematuria, hydronephrosis, oliguria, pyelonephritis, renal failure, renal tubular necrosis
- Respiratory: Apnea, asthma, atelectasis, bronchitis, epistaxis, hemoptysis, hiccup, hyperventilation, hypoxia, respiratory acidosis, pharyngitis, pneumonia, pneumothorax, pulmonary edema, pulmonary hypertension, respiratory moniliasis, rhinitis, sputum increased, voice alteration

Miscellaneous: *Candida* (mucocutaneous 16% to 18%), CMV viremia/syndrome (12% to 14%), CMV tissue invasive disease (6% to 12%), herpes zoster cutaneous disease (4% to 10%), cyst, diaphoresis, flu-like syndrome, healing abnormal, hernia, ileus infection, neoplasm, peritonitis, thirst

Pharmacodynamics/Kinetics

Onset of Action Peak effect: Correlation of toxicity or efficacy is still being developed, however, one study indicated that 12-hour AUCs >40 mcg/mL/hour were correlated with efficacy and decreased episodes of rejection

Available Dosage Forms

Capsule, oral: 250 mg
CellCept®: 250 mg

Injection, powder for reconstitution:
CellCept®: 500 mg

Powder for suspension, oral:
CellCept®: 200 mg/mL (175 mL)

Tablet, oral: 500 mg
CellCept®: 500 mg

Tablet, delayed release, oral:
Myfortic®: 180 mg, 360 mg

General Dosage Range Dosage adjustment recommended in patient with renal impairment and who develop toxicities

I.V.: *Adults:* 1-1.5 g twice daily

Oral:

Cellcept®:

Children (suspension): 600 mg/m^2/dose twice daily (maximum: 1 g twice daily)

Children with BSA 1.25-1.5 m^2: 750 mg capsule twice daily

Children with BSA >1.5 m^2: 1 g capsule or tablet twice daily

Adults: 1-1.5 g twice daily

Myfortic®:

Children with BSA 1.19-1.58 m^2: 540 mg twice daily (maximum: 1080 mg/day)

Children with BSA >1.58 m^2 and Adults: 720 mg twice daily (maximum: 1440 mg/day)

Administration

Oral Oral dosage formulations (tablet, capsule, suspension) should be administered on an empty stomach to avoid variability in MPA absorption. The oral solution may be administered via a nasogastric tube (minimum 8 French, 1.7 mm interior diameter); oral suspension should not be mixed with other medications. Delayed release tablets should not be crushed, cut, or chewed.

I.V. Intravenous solutions should be given over at least 2 hours. Do not administer intravenous solution by rapid or bolus injection.

I.V. Detail Reconstituted solution: pH 2.4-4.1

Stability

Reconstitution

Oral suspension: Should be constituted prior to dispensing to the patient and **not** mixed with any other medication. Add 47 mL of water to the bottle and shake well for ~1 minute. Add another 47 mL of water to the bottle and shake well for an additional minute. Final concentration is 200 mg/mL of mycophenolate mofetil.

I.V.: Reconstitute the contents of each vial with 14 mL of 5% dextrose injection; dilute the contents of a vial with 5% dextrose in water to a final concentration of 6 mg mycophenolate mofetil per mL. **Note:** Vial is vacuum-sealed; if a lack of vacuum is noted during preparation, the vial should not be used.

Storage

Capsules: Store at 25°C (77°F); excursions permitted to 15°C to 30°C (59°F to 86°F).

Tablets: Store at 25°C (77°F); excursions permitted to 15°C to 30°C (59°F to 86°F). Protect from moisture and light.

Oral suspension: Store powder for oral suspension at 25°C (77°F); excursions permitted to 15°C to 30°C (59°F to 86°F). Once reconstituted, the oral solution may be stored at room temperature or under refrigeration. Do not freeze. The mixed suspension is stable for 60 days.

Injection: Store intact vials and diluted solutions at 25°C (77°F); excursions permitted to 15°C to 30°C (59°F to 86°F). Begin infusion within 4 hours of reconstitution.

Nursing Actions

Physical Assessment Monitor blood pressure periodically while receiving this medication. Assess for peripheral edema and other signs of fluid retention. Patients with diabetes should monitor glucose levels closely (this medication may alter glucose levels). Monitor for signs of opportunistic infection (eg, persistent fever, malaise, sore throat, unusual bleeding or bruising). Patient is at risk for lymphoproliferative disease and certain other malignancies; monitor closely.

Patient Education Take oral formulations as directed, preferably 1 hour before or 2 hours after meals. Do not cut, chew, or crush delayed-release tablets. You will be susceptible to infection. You may be at increased risk for skin cancer. If you have diabetes, monitor glucose levels closely (drug may alter glucose levels). You may experience dizziness or trembling, trouble sleeping, nausea or vomiting, diarrhea, sores or white plaques in mouth, or muscle or back pain. Report chest pain; irregular or rapid heartbeat; acute headache or dizziness; swelling of extremities; unusual weight gain; symptoms of respiratory infection, cough, or respiratory difficulty; abdominal pain or unresolved GI effects; unusual weakness; fatigue, chills, or fever; unhealed sores or white plaques in mouth; irritation in genital area or unusual discharge; change in mental status, memory loss, or loss of coordination or clumsiness; weakness in legs; difficulty speaking or understanding what others say; or unusual bruising or bleeding.

Dietary Considerations Oral dosage formulations should be taken on an empty stomach to avoid variability in MPA absorption. However, in stable renal transplant patients, may be administered with food if necessary. Some products may contain phenylalanine.

Nabilone (NA bi lone)

Brand Names: U.S. Cesamet®

Pharmacologic Category Antiemetic

Pregnancy Risk Factor C

Lactation Excretion in breast milk unknown/not recommended

Use Treatment of refractory nausea and vomiting associated with cancer chemotherapy

Controlled Substance C-II

Available Dosage Forms

Capsule, oral:

Cesamet®: 1 mg

General Dosage Range Oral: *Adults:* 1-2 mg twice daily (maximum: 6 mg/day)

Administration

Oral Initial dose should be given 1-3 hours before chemotherapy; may be given 2-3 times a day during the entire chemotherapy course and for up to 48 hours after the last dose of chemotherapy; a dose of 1-2 mg the night before chemotherapy may be useful.

Nursing Actions

Physical Assessment Monitor for CNS changes and psychotic reactions (can persist for 3 days following discontinuation); this medicine may have properties similar to marijuana and has the potential for abuse or dependence.

Patient Education Avoid alcohol. May cause psychotic reaction, impaired coordination or judgment, faintness, dizziness, drowsiness, unsteadiness, sleep disturbance or visual disturbances, orthostatic hypotension, dry mouth, or decreased appetite. Report excessive or persistent CNS changes (euphoria, anxiety, depression, memory lapse, bizarre thought patterns, excitability, inability to control thoughts or behavior, fainting), respiratory difficulties, or rapid heartbeat.

Nabumetone (na BYOO me tone)

Index Terms Relafen

Pharmacologic Category Nonsteroidal Anti-inflammatory Drug (NSAID), Oral

Medication Guide Available Yes

Pregnancy Risk Factor C

Lactation Excretion in breast milk unknown/not recommended

Breast-Feeding Considerations It is not known if nabumetone or 6MNA are excreted into breast milk. Breast-feeding is not recommended by the manufacturer.

Use Management of osteoarthritis and rheumatoid arthritis

Unlabeled Use Moderate pain

Mechanism of Action/Effect Reversibly inhibits cyclooxygenase-1 and 2 (COX-1 and 2) enzymes, which results in decreased formation of prostaglandin precursors; has antipyretic, analgesic, and anti-inflammatory properties

Contraindications Hypersensitivity to nabumetone, aspirin, other NSAIDs, or any component of the formulation; perioperative pain in the setting of coronary artery bypass graft (CABG) surgery

Warnings/Precautions [U.S. Boxed Warning]: NSAIDs are associated with an increased risk of adverse cardiovascular thrombotic events, including MI and stroke. Risk may be increased with duration of use or pre-existing cardiovascular risk factors or disease. Carefully evaluate individual cardiovascular risk profiles prior to prescribing. May cause new-onset hypertension or worsening of existing hypertension. Use caution with fluid retention. Avoid use in heart failure. Concurrent administration of ibuprofen, and potentially other nonselective NSAIDs, may interfere with aspirin's cardioprotective effect. **[U.S. Boxed Warning]: Use is contraindicated for treatment of perioperative pain in the setting of coronary artery bypass graft (CABG) surgery.** Risk of MI and stroke may be increased with use following CABG surgery.

Platelet adhesion and aggregation may be decreased; may prolong bleeding time; patients with coagulation disorders or who are receiving anticoagulants should be monitored closely. Anemia may occur; patients on long-term NSAID therapy should be monitored for anemia. Rarely, NSAID use may cause severe blood dyscrasias (eg, agranulocytosis, aplastic anemia, thrombocytopenia).

NSAID use may compromise existing renal function; dose-dependent decreases in prostaglandin synthesis may result from NSAID use, reducing renal blood flow which may cause renal decompensation. NSAID use may increase the risk for hyperkalemia. Patients with impaired renal function, dehydration, heart failure, liver dysfunction, those taking diuretics, and ACE inhibitors, and the elderly are at greater risk of renal toxicity and hyperkalemia. Rehydrate patient before starting therapy; monitor renal function closely. Not recommended for use in patients with advanced renal disease. Long-term NSAID use may result in renal papillary necrosis.

[U.S. Boxed Warning]: NSAIDs may increase risk of gastrointestinal irritation, inflammation, ulceration, bleeding, and perforation. These events may occur at any time during therapy and without warning. Use caution with a history of GI disease (bleeding or ulcers), concurrent therapy with aspirin, anticoagulants and/or corticosteroids, smoking, use of alcohol, the elderly or debilitated patients. When used concomitantly with ≤325 mg of aspirin, a substantial increase in the risk of gastrointestinal complications (eg, ulcer) occurs; concomitant gastroprotective therapy (eg, proton pump inhibitors) is recommended (Bhatt, 2008).

Use the lowest effective dose for the shortest duration of time, consistent with individual patient goals, to reduce risk of cardiovascular or GI adverse events. Alternate therapies should be considered for patients at high risk.

NSAIDs may cause serious skin adverse events including exfoliative dermatitis, Stevens-Johnson syndrome (SJS) and toxic epidermal necrolysis (TEN); discontinue use at first sign of skin rash or hypersensitivity. Anaphylactoid reactions may occur, even without prior exposure; patients with "aspirin triad" (bronchial asthma, aspirin intolerance, rhinitis) may be at increased risk. Do not use in patients who experience bronchospasm, asthma, rhinitis, or urticaria with NSAID or aspirin therapy. Use caution in other forms of asthma.

Use with caution in patients with decreased hepatic function. Closely monitor patients with any abnormal LFT. Severe hepatic reactions (eg, fulminant hepatitis, liver failure) have occurred with NSAID use, rarely; discontinue if signs or symptoms of liver disease develop, or if systemic manifestations occur.

NSAIDS may cause drowsiness, dizziness, blurred vision and other neurologic effects which may impair physical or mental abilities; patients must be cautioned about performing tasks which require mental alertness (eg, operating machinery or driving). Discontinue use with blurred or diminished vision and perform ophthalmologic exam. Monitor vision with long-term therapy.

The elderly are at increased risk for adverse effects (especially peptic ulceration, CNS effects, renal toxicity) from NSAIDs even at low doses.

Withhold for at least 4-6 half-lives prior to surgical or dental procedures. May cause photosensitivity reactions.

Drug Interactions

Avoid Concomitant Use

Avoid concomitant use of Nabumetone with any of the following: Floctafenine; Ketorolac; Ketorolac (Nasal); Ketorolac (Systemic)

Decreased Effect

Nabumetone may decrease the levels/effects of: ACE Inhibitors; Aliskiren; Angiotensin II Receptor Blockers; Antiplatelet Agents; Beta-Blockers; Eplerenone; HydrALAZINE; Loop Diuretics; Potassium-Sparing Diuretics; Salicylates; Selective Serotonin Reuptake Inhibitors; Thiazide Diuretics

The levels/effects of Nabumetone may be decreased by: Bile Acid Sequestrants; Nonsteroidal Anti-Inflammatory Agents; Salicylates

Increased Effect/Toxicity

Nabumetone may increase the levels/effects of: Aliskiren; Aminoglycosides; Anticoagulants; Antiplatelet Agents; Bisphosphonate Derivatives; Collagenase (Systemic); CycloSPORINE; CycloSPORINE (Systemic); Deferasirox; Desmopressin; Digoxin; Drotrecogin Alfa (Activated); Eplerenone; Haloperidol; Ibritumomab; Lithium; Methotrexate; Nonsteroidal Anti-Inflammatory Agents; PEMEtrexed; Porfimer; Potassium-Sparing Diuretics; PRALAtrexate; Quinolone Antibiotics; Rivaroxaban; Salicylates; Thrombolytic Agents; Tositumomab and Iodine I 131 Tositumomab; Vancomycin; Vitamin K Antagonists

The levels/effects of Nabumetone may be increased by: ACE Inhibitors; Angiotensin II Receptor Blockers; Antidepressants (Tricyclic, Tertiary Amine); Corticosteroids (Systemic); CycloSPORINE; CycloSPORINE (Systemic); Dasatinib; Floctafenine; Glucosamine; Herbs (Anticoagulant/Antiplatelet Properties); Ketorolac; Ketorolac (Nasal); Ketorolac (Systemic); Nonsteroidal Anti-Inflammatory Agents; Omega-3-Acid Ethyl Esters; Pentosan Polysulfate Sodium; Pentoxifylline; Probenecid; Prostacyclin Analogues; Selective Serotonin Reuptake Inhibitors; Serotonin/Norepinephrine Reuptake Inhibitors; Sodium Phosphates; Treprostinil; Vitamin E

Nutritional/Ethanol Interactions

Ethanol: Avoid ethanol (may enhance gastric mucosal irritation).

Food: Nabumetone peak serum concentrations may be increased if taken with food or dairy products.

Herb/Nutraceutical: Avoid alfalfa, anise, bilberry, bladderwrack, bromelain, cat's claw, celery, chamomile, coleus, cordyceps, dong quai, evening primrose, fenugreek, feverfew, garlic, ginger, ginkgo biloba, ginseng (American, Panax, Siberian), grapeseed, green tea, guggul, horse chestnut seed, horseradish, licorice, prickly ash, red clover, reishi, SAMe (S-adenosylmethionine), sweet clover, turmeric, white willow (all have additional antiplatelet activity).

Adverse Reactions

>10%: Gastrointestinal: Diarrhea (14%), dyspepsia (13%), abdominal pain (12%)

1% to 10%:

Cardiovascular: Edema (3% to 9%)

Central nervous system: Dizziness (3% to 9%), headache (3% to 9%), fatigue (1% to 3%), insomnia (1% to 3%), nervousness (1% to 3%), somnolence (1% to 3%)

Dermatologic: Pruritus (3% to 9%), rash (3% to 9%)

Gastrointestinal: Constipation (3% to 9%), flatulence (3% to 9%), guaiac positive (3% to 9%), nausea (3% to 9%), gastritis (1% to 3%), stomatitis (1% to 3%), vomiting (1% to 3%), xerostomia (1% to 3%)

Otic: Tinnitus

Miscellaneous: Diaphoresis (1% to 3%)

Pharmacodynamics/Kinetics

Onset of Action Several days

Available Dosage Forms

Tablet, oral: 500 mg, 750 mg

General Dosage Range Dosage adjustment recommended in patients with renal impairment

Oral: *Adults:* 1000 mg/day in 1-2 divided doses (maximum: 2000 mg/day)

Nursing Actions

Physical Assessment Monitor blood pressure at the beginning of therapy and periodically during use. Monitor for GI effects, hepatotoxicity, and ototoxicity at beginning of therapy and periodically throughout. Schedule ophthalmic evaluations for patients who develop eye complaints during long-term NSAID therapy.

Patient Education Do not crush tablets. Take with food or milk to reduce GI distress. Do not use alcohol. You may experience drowsiness, dizziness, nervousness, headache, anorexia, nausea, vomiting, heartburn, or fluid retention; GI bleeding, ulceration, or perforation can occur with or without pain; discontinue medication and contact prescriber if persistent abdominal pain or cramping or blood in stool occurs. Report respiratory difficulty or unusual cough; chest pain, rapid heartbeat, or palpitations; bruising/bleeding; blood in urine, stool, mouth, or vomitus; swollen extremities; skin rash or itching; or hearing changes (ringing in ears).

Nadolol (NAY doe lol)

Brand Names: U.S. Corgard®

Pharmacologic Category Antianginal Agent; Beta Blocker, Nonselective

Medication Safety Issues

Sound-alike/look-alike issues:

Corgard® may be confused with Cognex®, Coreg®

International issues:

Nadolol may be confused with Mandol brand name for cefamandole [Belgium, Netherlands, New Zealand, Russia]

Pregnancy Risk Factor C

Lactation Enters breast milk/use caution consider risk:benefit (AAP rates "compatible"; AAP 2001 update pending)

Use Treatment of hypertension and angina pectoris; prophylaxis of migraine headaches

Unlabeled Use Primary and secondary prophylaxis of variceal hemorrhage; management of thyrotoxicosis

Available Dosage Forms

Tablet, oral: 20 mg, 40 mg, 80 mg

Corgard®: 20 mg, 40 mg, 80 mg

General Dosage Range Dosage adjustment recommended in patients with renal impairment

Oral:

Adults: Initial: 40 mg once daily; Maintenance: 40-320 mg once daily

Elderly: Initial: 20 mg once daily; Maintenance: 20-240 mg once daily

Administration

Oral May be administered without regard to meals.

Nursing Actions

Physical Assessment Assess blood pressure and heart rate prior to and following first dose, any change in dosage, and periodically thereafter. Monitor or advise patient to monitor weight, fluid balance (I & O), and signs of CHF (edema, new cough or dyspnea, unresolved fatigue). Monitor serum glucose levels of patients with diabetes since beta-blockers may alter glucose tolerance.

Patient Education Check pulse daily prior to taking medication. If pulse is <50, hold medication and consult prescriber. May cause dizziness, fatigue, blurred vision, difficulty breathing, wheezing, or constipation. If you have diabetes, monitor serum glucose closely (the drug may mask symptoms of hypoglycemia). Report swelling in feet or legs, respiratory difficulty or persistent cough, unresolved fatigue, or unusual weight gain. Use caution with concurrent usage of over-the-counter NSAIDs or cough or cold products.

Nafarelin (naf a REL in)

Brand Names: U.S. Synarel®

Index Terms Nafarelin Acetate

Pharmacologic Category Gonadotropin Releasing Hormone Agonist

Medication Safety Issues

Sound-alike/look-alike issues:

Nafarelin may be confused with Anafranil®, enalapril

Pregnancy Risk Factor X

Lactation Excretion in breast milk unknown/contraindicated

Use Treatment of endometriosis, including pain and reduction of lesions; treatment of central precocious puberty (CPP; gonadotropin-dependent precocious puberty) in children of both sexes

Available Dosage Forms

Solution, intranasal:

Synarel®: 2 mg/mL (8 mL)

General Dosage Range Nasal:

Children: 2 sprays (400 mcg) into each nostril twice daily; may increase to 3 sprays (600 mcg) into alternating nostrils 3 times/day

Adults: 1 spray (200 mcg) in 1-2 nostrils twice daily

Administration

Inhalation Nasal spray: Do not use topical nasal decongestant for at least 2 hours after nafarelin use. Allow ~30 seconds to elapse between sprays. Sneezing during or immediately after dosing should be avoided (may decrease drug absorption).

Nursing Actions

Physical Assessment For treatment of precocious puberty. Teach patient or caregiver correct timing and administration of nasal spray.

Patient Education Endometriosis: You will begin this treatment between days 2-4 of your regular menstrual cycle. Use daily at the same time (arising and bedtime) and rotate nostrils. Maintain regular follow-up schedule. May cause hot flashes, flushing, or redness; decreased or increased libido; emotional lability; weight gain; decreased breast size; or hirsutism. Report any breakthrough bleeding or continuing menstruation or musculoskeletal pain. Do not use a nasal decongestant within 2 hours after nafarelin.

Nafcillin (naf SIL in)

Index Terms Ethoxynaphthamido Penicillin Sodium; Nafcillin Sodium; Nallpen; Sodium Nafcillin

Pharmacologic Category Antibiotic, Penicillin

Pregnancy Risk Factor B

Lactation Enters breast milk/use caution

Use Treatment of infections such as osteomyelitis, septicemia, endocarditis, and CNS infections caused by susceptible strains of staphylococci species

Available Dosage Forms

Infusion, premixed iso-osmotic dextrose solution: 1 g (50 mL); 2 g (100 mL)

Injection, powder for reconstitution: 1 g, 2 g, 10 g

General Dosage Range

I.M.:

Children: 25 mg/kg twice daily

Adults: 500 mg every 4-6 hours

I.V.:

Children: 50-200 mg/kg/day in divided every 4-6 hours (maximum: 12 g/day)

Adults: 500-2000 mg every 4-6 hours

Administration

I.M. Rotate injection sites.

I.V. Vesicant. Administer around-the-clock to promote less variation in peak and trough serum levels. Infuse over 30-60 minutes.

I.V. Detail Extravasation management: Use cold packs.

Hyaluronidase: Add 1 mL NS to 150 unit vial to make 150 units/mL of concentration; mix 0.1 mL of above with 0.9 mL NS in 1 mL syringe to make final concentration = 15 units/mL.

pH: 6.0-8.5

Nursing Actions

Physical Assessment Assess results of culture and sensitivity tests and allergy history prior to starting therapy. Injection site must be monitored closely to prevent extravasation. Monitor for hypersensitivity and opportunistic infection (eg, fever, chills, unhealed sores, white plaques in mouth or vagina, purulent vaginal discharge).

Patient Education This medication can only be administered by infusion or injection. Report immediately any redness, swelling, burning, or pain at injection/infusion site; respiratory difficulty or swallowing; chest pain; persistent diarrhea; or rash. May cause nausea or opportunistic infection (eg, fever, chills, sore throat, burning urination). Report persistent side effects or if condition does not respond to treatment.

Related Information

Management of Drug Extravasations *on page 1269*

Nalbuphine (NAL byoo feen)

Index Terms Nalbuphine Hydrochloride; Nubain

Pharmacologic Category Analgesic, Opioid; Analgesic, Opioid Partial Agonist

Medication Safety Issues

Sound-alike/look-alike issues:

Nubain may be confused with Navane®, Nebcin

High alert medication:

The Institute for Safe Medication Practices (ISMP) includes this medication among its list of drug classes which have a heightened risk of causing significant patient harm when used in error.

Pregnancy Risk Factor C

Lactation Enters breast milk/use caution

Use Relief of moderate-to-severe pain; preoperative analgesia, postoperative and surgical anesthesia, and obstetrical analgesia during labor and delivery

Unlabeled Use Opioid-induced pruritus

Mechanism of Action/Effect Binds to opiate receptors in the CNS, causing inhibition of ascending pain pathways, altering the perception of and response to pain; produces generalized CNS depression

Contraindications Hypersensitivity to nalbuphine or any component of the formulation

Warnings/Precautions Use caution in CNS depression. Sedation and psychomotor impairment are likely, and are additive with other CNS depressants or ethanol. May cause respiratory depression. Ambulatory patients must be cautioned about performing tasks which require mental alertness (eg, operating machinery or driving). Effects may be potentiated when used with other sedative drugs or ethanol. Use with caution in patients with recent myocardial infarction, biliary tract impairment, morbid obesity, thyroid dysfunction, head trauma, or increased intracranial pressure. Use caution in patients with prostatic hyperplasia and/or urinary stricture, adrenal insufficiency, decreased hepatic or renal function. Use with caution in patients with pre-existing respiratory compromise (hypoxia and/or hypercapnia), COPD or other obstructive pulmonary disease; critical respiratory depression may occur, even at therapeutic dosages. May cause hypotension; use with caution in patients with hypovolemia, cardiovascular disease (including acute MI), or drugs which may exaggerate hypotensive effects (including phenothiazines or general anesthetics). May obscure diagnosis or clinical course of patients with acute abdominal conditions. May result in tolerance and/or drug dependence with chronic use; use with caution in patients with a history of drug dependence. Abrupt discontinuation following prolonged use may lead to withdrawal symptoms. May precipitate withdrawal symptoms in patients following prolonged therapy with mu opioid agonists. Use with caution in pregnancy (close neonatal monitoring required when used in labor and delivery). Use with caution in the elderly and debilitated patients; may be more sensitive to adverse effects. Safety and efficacy in children have not been established.

Drug Interactions

Avoid Concomitant Use There are no known interactions where it is recommended to avoid concomitant use.

Decreased Effect

Nalbuphine may decrease the levels/effects of: Analgesics (Opioid); Pegvisomant

The levels/effects of Nalbuphine may be decreased by: Ammonium Chloride; Mixed Agonist / Antagonist Opioids

Increased Effect/Toxicity

Nalbuphine may increase the levels/effects of: Alcohol (Ethyl); Alvimopan; CNS Depressants; Desmopressin; Selective Serotonin Reuptake Inhibitors; Thiazide Diuretics

The levels/effects of Nalbuphine may be increased by: Amphetamines; Antipsychotic Agents (Phenothiazines); Droperidol; HydrOXYzine; Succinylcholine

Nutritional/Ethanol Interactions

Ethanol: May increase CNS depression; monitor for increased effects with coadministration. Caution patients about effects.

Herb/Nutraceutical: Avoid valerian, St John's wort, kava kava, gotu kola (may increase CNS depression).

Adverse Reactions

>10%: Central nervous system: Sedation (36%)

1% to 10%:

Central nervous system: Dizziness (5%), headache (3%)

Gastrointestinal: Nausea/vomiting (6%), xerostomia (4%)

Miscellaneous: Clamminess (9%)

Pharmacodynamics/Kinetics

Onset of Action Peak effect: SubQ, I.M.: <15 minutes; I.V.: 2-3 minutes

Available Dosage Forms

Injection, solution: 10 mg/mL (10 mL); 20 mg/mL (10 mL)

Injection, solution [preservative free]: 10 mg/mL (1 mL); 20 mg/mL (1 mL)

General Dosage Range

I.M., SubQ: *Adults:* 10 mg/70 kg every 3-6 hours (maximum: 20 mg/dose; 160 mg/day)

I.V.: *Adults:* 10 mg/70 kg every 3-6 hours (maximum: 20 mg/dose; 160 mg/day) **or** 0.3-3 mg/kg over 10-15 minutes, then 0.25-0.5 mg/kg as required for anesthesia **or** 2.5-5 mg (1-2 doses)

Administration

I.V. Detail pH: 3.5-3.7 (adjusted)

Stability

Storage Store at room temperature of 15°C to 30°C (59°F to 86°F). Protect from light.

Nursing Actions

Physical Assessment Monitor for effectiveness of pain relief. Monitor blood pressure, CNS and respiratory status, and degree of sedation at beginning of therapy and periodically thereafter. For inpatients, implement safety measures (eg, side rails up, call light within reach, instructions to call for assistance). Assess patient's physical and/or psychological dependence. Discontinue slowly after prolonged use.

Patient Education May cause physical and/or psychological dependence. While using this medication, do not use alcohol and other prescription or OTC medications (especially sedatives, tranquilizers, antihistamines, or pain medications) without consulting prescriber. Maintain adequate hydration, unless instructed to restrict fluid intake. May cause hypotension, dizziness, drowsiness, impaired coordination, or blurred vision; loss of appetite, nausea, or vomiting; or constipation. Report chest pain, slow or rapid heartbeat, dizziness, or persistent headache; confusion or respiratory difficulties; or severe constipation.

Naloxone (nal OKS one)

Index Terms *N*-allylnoroxymorphine Hydrochloride; Naloxone Hydrochloride; Narcan

Pharmacologic Category Antidote; Opioid Antagonist

Medication Safety Issues

Sound-alike/look-alike issues:

Naloxone may be confused with Lanoxin®, naltrexone

Narcan may be confused with Marcaine®, Norcuron®

International issues:

Narcan [multiple international markets] may be confused with Marcen brand name for ketazolam [Spain]

Pregnancy Risk Factor C

Lactation Excretion in breast milk unknown/not recommended

Breast-Feeding Considerations No data reported. Since naloxone is used for opiate reversal the concern should be on opiate drug levels in a breast-feeding mother and transfer to the infant rather than naloxone exposure. The safest approach would be **not** to breast-feed.

Use Complete or partial reversal of opioid drug effects, including respiratory depression; management of known or suspected opioid overdose; diagnosis of suspected opioid dependence or acute opioid overdose

Unlabeled Use Opioid-induced pruritus

Mechanism of Action/Effect Pure opioid antagonist that competes and displaces narcotics at opioid receptor sites

Contraindications Hypersensitivity to naloxone or any component of the formulation

Warnings/Precautions Due to an association between naloxone and acute pulmonary edema, use with caution in patients with cardiovascular disease or in patients receiving medications with potential adverse cardiovascular effects (eg, hypotension, pulmonary edema, or arrhythmias). Administration of naloxone causes the release of catecholamines; may precipitate acute withdrawal or unmask pain in those who regularly take opioids. Excessive dosages should be avoided after use of opiates in surgery. Abrupt postoperative reversal may result in nausea, vomiting, sweating, tachycardia, hypertension, seizures, and other cardiovascular events (including pulmonary edema and arrhythmias). May precipitate withdrawal symptoms in patients addicted to opiates, including pain, hypertension, sweating, agitation, irritability; in neonates: shrill cry, failure to feed; carefully titrate dose to reverse hypoventilation; do not fully awaken patient or reverse analgesic effect (postoperative patient). Use caution in patients with history of seizures; avoid use in treatment of meperidine-induced seizures. Recurrence of respiratory depression is possible if the opioid involved is long-acting; observe patients until there is no reasonable risk of recurrent respiratory depression.

Drug Interactions

Avoid Concomitant Use There are no known interactions where it is recommended to avoid concomitant use.

Decreased Effect There are no known significant interactions involving a decrease in effect.

Increased Effect/Toxicity There are no known significant interactions involving an increase in effect.

Adverse Reactions Adverse reactions are related to reversing dependency and precipitating withdrawal. Withdrawal symptoms are the result of sympathetic excess. Adverse events occur secondarily to reversal (withdrawal) of narcotic analgesia and sedation.

Central nervous system: Narcotic withdrawal

Pharmacodynamics/Kinetics

Onset of Action Endotracheal, I.M., SubQ: 2-5 minutes; Intranasal: ~8-13 minutes (Kelley, 2005; Robertson, 2009); I.V.: ~2 minutes

Duration of Action Depending on route of administration, ~30-120 minutes; I.V. has a shorter duration of action than I.M. administration; since naloxone's action is shorter than that of most opioids, repeated doses are usually needed

Available Dosage Forms

Injection, solution: 0.4 mg/mL (1 mL, 10 mL)

Injection, solution [preservative free]: 0.4 mg/mL (1 mL); 1 mg/mL (2 mL)

General Dosage Range I.M., I.V., SubQ, intratracheal:

Birth (including premature infants) to 5 years or ≤20 kg: 0.01 mg/kg **or** 0.1 mg/kg (maximum dose: 2 mg) every 2-3 minutes as needed

Children >5 years or >20 kg: 0.01 mg/kg **or** 2 mg/dose, if no response repeat every 2-3 minutes as needed

Adults: 0.1-2 mg every 2-3 minutes as needed (maximum: 10 mg)

Administration

I.M. May administer I.M. if unable to obtain I.V. access.

I.V.

I.V. push: Administer over 30 seconds as undiluted preparation **or** (unlabeled) administer as diluted preparation slow I.V. push by diluting 0.4 mg (1 mL) ampul with 9 mL of normal saline for a total volume of 10 mL to achieve a concentration of 0.04 mg/mL

I.V. continuous infusion: Dilute to 4 mcg/mL in D_5W or normal saline

Other

Endotracheal (unlabeled route): There is only anecdotal support for this route of administration. May require a slightly higher dose than used in other routes. Dilute to 1-2 mL with normal saline; flush with 5 cc of saline and then administer 5 ventilations

Intranasal (unlabeled route): Administer total dose equally divided into each nostril using a mucosal atomizer device (MAD) (ACLS, 2010; Kelly, 2005; Robertson, 2009)

SubQ: May administer SubQ if unable to obtain I.V. access

Stability

Reconstitution Stable in 0.9% sodium chloride and D_5W at 4 mcg/mL for 24 hours.

Storage Store at 25°C (77°F). Protect from light.

Nursing Actions

Physical Assessment Assess patient for opioid dependency. Monitor vital signs and cardiorespiratory status continuously during infusion; maintain patent airway.

Patient Education Report respiratory difficulty, palpitations, or tremors.

Naltrexone (nal TREKS one)

Brand Names: U.S. ReVia®; Vivitrol®

Index Terms Naltrexone Hydrochloride

Pharmacologic Category Antidote; Opioid Antagonist

Medication Safety Issues

Sound-alike/look-alike issues:

Naltrexone may be confused with methylnaltrexone, naloxone

ReVia® may be confused with Revatio®, Revex®

Administration issues:

Vivitrol®: For intramuscular (I.M.) gluteal injection only

Medication Guide Available Yes

Pregnancy Risk Factor C

Lactation Enters breast milk/not recommended

Use Treatment of ethanol dependence; prevention of relapse in opioid dependent patients, following opioid detoxification

Mechanism of Action/Effect Naltrexone (a pure opioid antagonist) is a cyclopropyl derivative of oxymorphone similar in structure to naloxone and nalorphine (a morphine derivative); it acts as a competitive antagonist at opioid receptor sites, showing the highest affinity for mu receptors.

Contraindications Hypersensitivity to naltrexone or any component of the formulation; narcotic dependence or current use of opioid analgesics; acute opioid withdrawal; failure to pass naloxone challenge or positive urine screen for opioids; acute hepatitis; liver failure

Warnings/Precautions

[U.S. Boxed Warning]: Dose-related hepatocellular injury is possible; the margin of separation between the apparent safe and hepatotoxic doses appears to be ≤ fivefold. Discontinue therapy if signs/symptoms of acute hepatitis develop. Therapy may precipitate withdrawal symptoms in patients addicted to opiates; patients should be opioid-free for a minimum of 7-10 days; use naloxone challenge test to confirm patient is opioid-free prior to therapy if there is any suspicion since urinary opioid screen may not be sufficient proof. Use of naltrexone does not eliminate or diminish withdrawal symptoms. Patients who had been treated with naltrexone may respond to lower opioid doses than previously used. This could result in potentially life-threatening opioid intoxication. Patients should be aware that they may be more sensitive to lower doses of opioids after naltrexone treatment is discontinued, after a missed dose, or near the end of the dosing interval. Warn patients that any attempt to overcome opioid blockade during naltrexone therapy, could potentially lead to fatal opioid overdose; the opioid competitive receptor blockade produced by naltrexone is potentially surmountable in the presence of large amounts of opioids. In naltrexone-treated patients requiring emergency pain management, consider alternatives to opioid therapy (eg, regional analgesia, nonopioid analgesics, general anesthesia). If opioid therapy is required for pain therapy, patients should be under the direct care of a trained anesthesia provider.

Suicidal thoughts and depression have been reported in both alcohol- and opioid-dependent patients; monitor closely. Hypersensitivity, including anaphylaxis, has been reported. Cases of eosinophilic pneumonia have been reported and should be considered in patients presenting with progressive hypoxia and dyspnea. Use with caution in patients with a history of bleeding disorders (including thrombocytopenia) and/or patients on anticoagulant therapy; bleeding/hematoma may occur from I.M. administration. Serious injection site reactions (eg, cellulitis, induration, hematoma, abscess, necrosis) have been reported with use, including severe cases requiring surgical debridement. Females appear to be at a higher risk. Patients should report any injection site pain, swelling, bruising, pruritus, or redness that does not improve (or worsens). For I.M. use only in the gluteal muscle; do **not** administer I.V., SubQ, or into fatty tissue; incorrect administration may increase the risk of injection site reactions. Use with caution in patients with hepatic or renal impairment; not studied in moderate-to-severe renal impairment or in severe hepatic impairment. Use is contraindicated in patients with acute hepatitis or hepatic failure. Vehicle used in the injectable naltrexone formulation (polylactide-co-glycolide microspheres) has rarely been associated with retinal artery occlusion in patients with abnormal arteriovenous anastomosis following injection of other drug products that also use the polylactide-co-glycolide microspheres vehicle.

Drug Interactions

Avoid Concomitant Use There are no known interactions where it is recommended to avoid concomitant use.

Decreased Effect There are no known significant interactions involving a decrease in effect.

Increased Effect/Toxicity There are no known significant interactions involving an increase in effect.

Adverse Reactions Combined reporting of adverse events from oral and injectable formulations:

>10%:

Cardiovascular: Syncope (13%)

Central nervous system: Headache (3% to 25%), insomnia (3% to 14%), dizziness (4% to 13%), anxiety (2% to 12%), nervousness (4% to >10%)
Gastrointestinal: Nausea (10% to 33%), vomiting (3% to 14%), appetite decreased (14%), diarrhea (13%), abdominal pain (11%), abdominal cramping
Hepatic: ALT increased (13%)
Local: Injection site reaction (≤69%; includes bruising, induration, nodules, pain, pruritus, swelling, tenderness)
Neuromuscular & skeletal: Arthralgia (12%), CPK increased (11% to 39%)
Respiratory: Pharyngitis (7% to 11%)

1% to 10%:
Cardiovascular: Hypertension (5%)
Central nervous system: Suicidal thoughts (≤10%), depression (8%), somnolence (2% to 4%), fatigue (4%), chills, energy increased, feeling down, irritability
Dermatologic: Rash (6%)
Endocrine & metabolic: Polydipsia
Gastrointestinal: Dry mouth (5%), toothache (4%)
Genitourinary: Delayed ejaculation, impotency
Hepatic: AST increased (2% to 10%), GGT increased (7%)
Neuromuscular & skeletal: Muscle cramps (8%), back pain (6%)
Miscellaneous: Influenza (5%)

Pharmacodynamics/Kinetics

Duration of Action Oral: 50 mg: 24 hours; 100 mg: 48 hours; 150 mg: 72 hours; I.M.: 4 weeks

Available Dosage Forms

Injection, microspheres for suspension, extended release:
Vivitrol®: 380 mg

Tablet, oral: 50 mg
ReVia®: 50 mg

General Dosage Range

I.M.: *Adults:* 380 mg once every 4 weeks
Oral: *Adults:* 25-50 mg once daily

Administration

Oral May be administered with or without food. Administration with food or after meals may minimize adverse gastrointestinal effects. Advise patient not to self-administer opiates while receiving naltrexone therapy.

I.M. Vivitrol®: Administer I.M. into the upper outer quadrant of the gluteal area; must inject dose using one of the provided needles for administration. Use either the 1.5-inch 20-gauge needle or the 2-inch 20-gauge needle (for patients with a larger amount of subcutaneous tissue overlying the gluteal muscle). Avoid inadvertent injection into a blood vessel; do not administer I.V., SubQ, or into fatty tissue (the risk of serious injection site reaction is increased if given incorrectly as a SubQ injection or into fatty tissue instead of the gluteal muscle). Injection should alternate between the 2 buttocks. Do not substitute any components of the dose-pack.

Stability

Reconstitution Injection: Prior to reconstitution, allow drug vial and provided diluent to reach room temperature (~45 minutes). Using the provided 1-inch *preparation* needle, reconstitute with 3.4 mL of the diluent and allow to dissolve by vigorously shaking the vial for ~1 minute. Mixed suspension will be milky white, free of clumps, and will move freely down the walls of the vial. Immediately after suspension, withdraw 4.2 mL of the suspension using the same preparation needle.

Prior to administration, replace the preparation needle with the appropriate size provided *administration* needle (1.5-inch Terumo® needle or 2-inch Needle-Pro® needle). Prior to injection, remove any air bubbles and push on the plunger until 4 mL of the suspension remains in the syringe. Following reconstitution of the suspension, administer immediately.

Storage

Injection: Store unopened kit at 2°C to 8°C (36°F to 46°F). Kit may be kept at room temperature of ≤25°C (77°F) for ≤7 days prior to use; do not freeze. Following reconstitution of the suspension, administer immediately.

Tablet: Store at room temperature. Protect from light.

Nursing Actions

Physical Assessment Do not use until patient has been opioid-free for 7-10 days. Assess carefully for several days following start of therapy for narcotic withdrawal symptoms or severe adverse reactions. Monitor injection site for reaction. Use non-narcotic analgesics for pain. Monitor for suicide ideation.

Patient Education This medication will help you achieve abstinence from opiates if taken as directed. Do not use opiates. This medication can also help treat alcohol dependence. Carry documentation to alert medical personnel you are taking medication in the event of an emergency. You may experience drowsiness, dizziness, or blurred vision; trouble sleeping; or nausea or vomiting. Report yellowing of skin or eyes; change in color of stool or urine; suicide ideation; increased perspiration or chills; acute headache; palpitations; severe dizziness; or injection site pain, swelling, or unresolved redness.

Naproxen (na PROKS en)

Brand Names: U.S. Aleve® [OTC]; Anaprox®; Anaprox® DS; EC-Naprosyn®; Mediproxen [OTC]; Midol® Extended Relief [OTC]; Naprelan®; Naprosyn®; Pamprin® Maximum Strength All Day Relief [OTC]

Index Terms Naproxen Sodium

Pharmacologic Category Nonsteroidal Anti-inflammatory Drug (NSAID), Oral

Medication Safety Issues

Sound-alike/look-alike issues:

Naproxen may be confused with Natacyn®, Nebcin

Anaprox® may be confused with Anaspaz®, Avapro®

Naprelan® may be confused with Naprosyn®

Naprosyn® may be confused with Natacyn®, Nebcin

Beers Criteria medication:

This drug may be inappropriate for use in geriatric patients (high severity risk).

International issues:

Flogen [Mexico] may be confused with Flovent brand name for fluticasone [U.S., Canada]

Flogen [Mexico] may be confused with Floxin brand name for flunarizine [Thailand], norfloxacin [South Africa], ofloxacin [U.S., Canada], and perfloxacin [Philippines]

Medication Guide Available Yes

Pregnancy Risk Factor C

Lactation Enters breast milk/not recommended (AAP rates "compatible"; AAP 2001 update pending)

Use Management of ankylosing spondylitis, osteoarthritis, and rheumatoid disorders (including juvenile idiopathic arthritis [JIA]); acute gout; mild-to-moderate pain; tendonitis, bursitis; dysmenorrhea; fever

Available Dosage Forms

Caplet, oral: 220 mg

Aleve® [OTC]: 220 mg

Midol® Extended Relief [OTC]: 220 mg

Pamprin® Maximum Strength All Day Relief [OTC]: 220 mg

Capsule, liquid gel, oral:

Aleve® [OTC]: 220 mg

Combination package, oral:

Naprelan®: Day 1-3: Tablet, controlled release: 825 mg [equivalent to naproxen base 750 mg] (6s) [contains sodium 75 mg] and Day 4-10: Tablet, controlled release: 550 mg [equivalent to naproxen base 500 mg] (14s) [contains sodium 50 mg]

Gelcap, oral:

Aleve® [OTC]: 220 mg

Suspension, oral: 125 mg/5 mL (500 mL)

Naprosyn®: 125 mg/5 mL (473 mL)

Tablet, oral: 220 mg, 250 mg, 275 mg, 375 mg, 500 mg, 550 mg

Aleve® [OTC]: 220 mg

Anaprox®: 275 mg

Anaprox® DS: 550 mg

Mediproxen [OTC]: 220 mg

Naprosyn®: 250 mg, 375 mg, 500 mg

Tablet, controlled release, oral:

Naprelan®: 412.5 mg, 550 mg, 825 mg

Tablet, delayed release, enteric coated, oral: 375 mg, 500 mg

EC-Naprosyn®: 375 mg, 500 mg

General Dosage Range Oral:

Children >2-11 years: 10 mg/kg/day in 2 divided doses (maximum: 10 mg/kg/day)

Children ≥12 years: 10 mg/kg/day in 2 divided doses (maximum: 10 mg/kg/day) **or** 200 mg every 8-12 hours (maximum: 600 mg/day)

Adults: Initial: 200-750 mg as a single dose; Maintenance: 200-500 mg every 6-12 hours (maximum: 1500 mg/day)

Administration

Oral Administer with food, milk, or antacids to decrease GI adverse effects

Suspension: Shake suspension well before administration.

Tablet, extended release: Swallow tablet whole; do not break, crush, or chew.

Nursing Actions

Physical Assessment Monitor blood pressure at the beginning of therapy and periodically during use. Monitor for GI effects, hepatotoxicity, and ototoxicity at beginning of therapy and periodically throughout. Schedule ophthalmic evaluations for patients who develop eye complaints during long-term NSAID therapy.

Patient Education Do not crush tablets. Take with food or milk to reduce GI distress. Do not use alcohol. You may experience drowsiness, dizziness, lightheadedness, headache, anorexia, nausea, vomiting, heartburn, or fluid retention; GI bleeding, ulceration, or perforation can occur with or without pain; discontinue medication and contact prescriber if persistent abdominal pain or cramping or blood in stool occurs. Report breathlessness, respiratory difficulty, or unusual cough; chest pain, rapid heartbeat, or palpitations; bruising/bleeding; blood in urine, stool, mouth, or vomitus; swollen extremities; skin rash; changes in eyesight (double vision, color changes, blurred vision) or hearing; or ringing in ears.

Naproxen and Esomeprazole

(na PROKS en & es oh ME pray zol)

Brand Names: U.S. Vimovo™

Index Terms Esomeprazole and Naproxen

Pharmacologic Category Nonsteroidal Anti-inflammatory Drug (NSAID), Oral; Proton Pump Inhibitor; Substituted Benzimidazole

Medication Safety Issues

Sound-alike/look-alike issues:

Vimovo™ may be confused with Vimpat®

Medication Guide Available Yes

Pregnancy Risk Factor C; Naproxen: D/3rd trimester)

Lactation Enters breast milk/not recommended

Use Reduction of the risk of NSAID-associated gastric ulcers in patients at risk of developing gastric ulcers who require an NSAID for the treatment of rheumatoid arthritis, osteoarthritis, and ankylosing spondylitis

Available Dosage Forms

Tablet, variable release, oral:

Vimovo™: Naproxen [delayed release] 375 mg and esomeprazole [immediate release] 20 mg, Naproxen [delayed release] 500 mg and esomeprazole [immediate release] 20 mg

General Dosage Range Oral: *Adults:* 1 tablet (naproxen 375-500 mg/esomeprazole 20 mg) twice daily; Maximum daily dose of esomeprazole: 40 mg/day

Administration

Oral Administer dose at least 30 minutes prior to meals. Tablets should be swallowed whole; do not chew, crush, dissolve, or split tablet.

Nursing Actions

Physical Assessment See individual agents.

Patient Education See individual agents.

Related Information

Esomeprazole *on page 421*

Naproxen *on page 811*

Naratriptan (NAR a trip tan)

Brand Names: U.S. Amerge®

Index Terms Naratriptan Hydrochloride

Pharmacologic Category Antimigraine Agent; Serotonin 5-$HT_{1B, 1D}$ Receptor Agonist

Medication Safety Issues

Sound-alike/look-alike issues:

Amerge® may be confused with Altace®, Amaryl®

Pregnancy Risk Factor C

Lactation Excretion in breast milk unknown/use caution

Use Treatment of acute migraine headache with or without aura

Mechanism of Action/Effect Selective agonist for serotonin receptor in cranial arteries; causes vasoconstriction and relief of migraine

Contraindications Hypersensitivity to naratriptan or any component of the formulation; cerebrovascular, peripheral vascular disease (ischemic bowel disease), ischemic heart disease (angina pectoris, history of myocardial infarction, or proven silent ischemia); or in patients with symptoms consistent with ischemic heart disease, coronary artery vasospasm, or Prinzmetal's angina; uncontrolled hypertension or patients who have received within 24 hours another 5-HT agonist (sumatriptan, zolmitriptan) or ergotamine-containing product; patients with known risk factors associated with coronary artery disease; patients with severe hepatic (Child-Pugh grade C) or renal disease (Cl_{cr} <15 mL/minute); do not administer naratriptan to patients with hemiplegic or basilar migraine

Warnings/Precautions Use only if there is a clear diagnosis of migraine. Dosage reduction is required in mild-to-moderate hepatic impairment and moderate renal impairment; use is contraindicated in patients with severe hepatic or renal impairment. Do not give to patients with risk factors for CAD until a cardiovascular evaluation has been performed; if evaluation is satisfactory, the healthcare provider should administer the first dose (consider ECG monitoring) and cardiovascular status should be periodically re-evaluated. Cardiac events (coronary artery vasospasm, transient ischemia, myocardial infarction, ventricular tachycardia/fibrillation, cardiac arrest, and death), cerebral/subarachnoid hemorrhage, stroke, peripheral vascular ischemia, and colonic ischemia have been reported with 5-HT_1 agonist administration. Patients who experience sensations of chest pain/pressure/tightness or symptoms suggestive of angina following dosing should be evaluated for coronary artery disease or Prinzmetal's angina before receiving additional doses; if dosing is resumed and similar symptoms recur, monitor with ECG. Significant elevation in blood pressure, including hypertensive crisis, has also been reported on rare occasions in patients with and without a history of hypertension. Only indicated for the acute treatment of migraine; not indicated for migraine prophylaxis, or for the treatment of cluster headache, hemiplegic or basilar migraine. If a patient does not respond to the first dose, the diagnosis of migraine should be reconsidered; rule out underlying neurologic disease in patients with atypical headache and in patients with no prior history of migraine.

Symptoms of agitation, confusion, hallucinations, hyper-reflexia, myoclonus, shivering, and tachycardia may occur with concomitant proserotonergic drugs (ie, SSRIs/SNRIs or triptans) or agents which reduce naratriptan's metabolism. Concurrent use of serotonin precursors (eg, tryptophan) is not recommended. If concomitant administration with SSRIs is warranted, monitor closely, especially at initiation and with dose increases.

Drug Interactions

Avoid Concomitant Use

Avoid concomitant use of Naratriptan with any of the following: Ergot Derivatives

Decreased Effect There are no known significant interactions involving a decrease in effect.

Increased Effect/Toxicity

Naratriptan may increase the levels/effects of: Ergot Derivatives; Metoclopramide; Serotonin Modulators

The levels/effects of Naratriptan may be increased by: Antipsychotics; Ergot Derivatives

Adverse Reactions 1% to 10%:

Central nervous system: Pain/pressure (2% to 4%), malaise/fatigue (2%), dizziness (1% to 2%), drowsiness (1% to 2%), vertigo (1%)

Gastrointestinal: Nausea (4% to 5%), hyposalivation (1%), vomiting (1%)
Neuromuscular & skeletal: Paresthesia (1% to 2%)
Ocular: Photophobia (1%)
Miscellaneous: Ear/nose/throat infection (1%), pressure/tightness/heaviness sensations (1%), warm/cold temperature sensations (1%)

Pharmacodynamics/Kinetics

Onset of Action ~1-2 hours (Bomhof, 1999; Tfelt-Hansen, 2000)

Available Dosage Forms

Tablet, oral: 1 mg, 2.5 mg
Amerge®: 1 mg, 2.5 mg

General Dosage Range Dosage adjustment recommended in patients with hepatic or renal impairment

Oral: *Adults:* 1-2.5 mg, may repeat after 4 hours (maximum: 5 mg/day)

Administration

Oral Do **not** crush or chew tablet; swallow whole with water.

Stability

Storage Store at 20°C to 25°C (68°F to 77°F).

Nursing Actions

Physical Assessment Assess potential for interactions with ergot-containing drugs and SSRIs patient may be taking. Monitor closely, especially after the first dose. Monitor for drowsiness, nausea/vomiting, paresthesias, hypertension, and cardiac events. Teach patient proper use (treatment of acute migraine).

Patient Education Do not crush or chew tablet; swallow whole with water. This drug is to be used to reduce your migraine, not to prevent or reduce the number of attacks. If headache returns or is not fully resolved, the dose may be repeated after 4 hours. If you have no relief with first dose, do not take a second dose without consulting prescriber. **Do not exceed 5 mg in 24 hours. Do not take within 24 hours of any other migraine medication without first consulting prescriber.** May cause dizziness, fatigue, drowsiness, nausea, or vomiting. Report immediately any chest pain, palpitations, or rapid heartbeat; tightness in throat or neck; or rash, itching, or hives.

Natalizumab (na ta LIZ u mab)

Brand Names: U.S. Tysabri®

Index Terms AN100226; Anti-4 Alpha Integrin; IgG4-Kappa Monoclonal Antibody

Pharmacologic Category Gastrointestinal Agent, Miscellaneous; Monoclonal Antibody, Selective Adhesion-Molecule Inhibitor

Medication Guide Available Yes

Pregnancy Risk Factor C

Lactation Excretion in breast milk unknown/not recommended

Use Monotherapy for the treatment of relapsing forms of multiple sclerosis; treatment of moderately- to severely-active Crohn's disease

Canada labeling: Treatment of relapsing forms of multiple sclerosis

Available Dosage Forms

Injection, solution [preservative free]:
Tysabri®: 300 mg/15 mL (15 mL)

General Dosage Range I.V.: *Adults:* 300 mg every 4 weeks

Administration

I.V. Solution may be warmed to room temperature prior to administration. Diluted solution should be infused over 1 hour; do not administer by I.V. bolus or push. Patients should be closely monitored for signs and symptoms of hypersensitivity during the infusion and for at least 1 hour after the infusion is complete. The infusion should be discontinued if a reaction occurs, and treatment of the reaction should be instituted. Following infusion, flush line with NS.

I.V. Detail pH: 6.1

Nursing Actions

Physical Assessment Monitor patient closely for infusion-related reactions (eg, urticaria, dizziness, fever, rash, rigors, pruritus, nausea, flushing, hypotension, dyspnea, chest pain) during and for 1 hour following infusion. If hypersensitivity reaction occurs, promptly discontinue infusion and notify prescriber. Monitor for hepatotoxicity; opportunistic infection (including herpes), nausea or vomiting, excessive fatigue, depression, anxiety, cognitive changes, suicidal ideation, vision changes, tremors, or rash.

Patient Education This drug can only be administered by intravenous infusion. You will be monitored closely during and following infusion. Report immediately any skin rash; dizziness; nausea; flushing; difficulty breathing; chest pain or tightness; redness, swelling, or pain at infusion site; signs of urinary tract infection (itching, pain, discharge); dark urine or altered frequency of urination; lower respiratory infection (cough, difficulty breathing, chest tightness); unusual sores or unhealed sores; chest discomfort or pain; back pain; unusual depression or anxiety; changes in speech or movement; vision changes; or worsening symptoms. Following infusion, you may experience headache, joint pain, or unusual fatigue.

Nateglinide (na te GLYE nide)

Brand Names: U.S. Starlix®

Pharmacologic Category Antidiabetic Agent, Meglitinide Derivative

Medication Safety Issues

High alert medication:

The Institute for Safe Medication Practices (ISMP) includes this medication among its list of drug classes which have a heightened risk of causing significant patient harm when used in error.

Pregnancy Risk Factor C

Lactation Excretion in breast milk unknown/not recommended

Breast-Feeding Considerations It is not known if nateglinide is excreted in breast milk. Breast-feeding is not recommended by the manufacturer.

Use Management of type 2 diabetes mellitus (noninsulin dependent, NIDDM) as monotherapy when hyperglycemia cannot be managed by diet and exercise alone; in combination with metformin or a thiazolidinedione to lower blood glucose in patients whose hyperglycemia cannot be controlled by exercise, diet, or a single agent alone

Mechanism of Action/Effect Increases insulin release from pancreatic beta cells; decreases postprandial hyperglycemia; not a sulfonylurea

Contraindications Hypersensitivity to nateglinide or any component of the formulation; diabetic ketoacidosis, with or without coma (treat with insulin); type 1 diabetes mellitus (insulin dependent, IDDM)

Warnings/Precautions Use with caution in patients with moderate-to-severe hepatic impairment. Use caution in severe renal dysfunction, elderly, malnourished, or patients with adrenal/pituitary dysfunction; may be more susceptible to glucose-lowering effects. All oral hypoglycemic agents are capable of producing hypoglycemia. Proper patient selection, dosage, and instructions to the patients are important to avoid hypoglycemic episodes. It may be necessary to discontinue nateglinide and administer insulin if the patient is exposed to stress (ie, fever, trauma, infection, surgery). Indicated for adjunctive therapy with metformin; not to be used as a substitute for metformin monotherapy. Combination treatment with sulfonylureas is not recommended (no additional benefit). Patients not adequately controlled on oral agents which stimulate insulin release (eg, glyburide) should not be switched to nateglinide or have nateglinide added to therapy.

Drug Interactions

Avoid Concomitant Use

Avoid concomitant use of Nateglinide with any of the following: Conivaptan

Decreased Effect

The levels/effects of Nateglinide may be decreased by: Corticosteroids (Orally Inhaled); Corticosteroids (Systemic); CYP2C9 Inducers (Strong); CYP3A4 Inducers (Strong); Deferasirox; Herbs (CYP3A4 Inducers); Luteinizing Hormone-Releasing Hormone Analogs; Peginterferon Alfa-2b; Somatropin; Thiazide Diuretics; Tocilizumab

Increased Effect/Toxicity

Nateglinide may increase the levels/effects of: Hypoglycemic Agents

The levels/effects of Nateglinide may be increased by: Conivaptan; CYP2C9 Inhibitors (Moderate); CYP2C9 Inhibitors (Strong); CYP3A4 Inhibitors (Moderate); CYP3A4 Inhibitors (Strong); Dasatinib; Eltrombopag; Herbs (Hypoglycemic Properties); Ivacaftor; Pegvisomant

Nutritional/Ethanol Interactions

Ethanol: Avoid ethanol (increased risk of hypoglycemia).

Food: Rate of absorption is decreased and time to T_{max} is delayed when taken with food. Food does not affect AUC. Multiple peak plasma concentrations may be observed if fasting. Not affected by composition of meal.

Herb/Nutraceutical: Avoid alfalfa, aloe, bilberry, bitter melon, burdock, celery, damiana, fenugreek, garcinia, garlic, ginger, ginseng (American), gymnema, marshmallow, and stinging nettle (may enhance the hypoglycemic effects of antidiabetic agents). St. John's wort may decrease the levels/effect of nateglinide.

Adverse Reactions As reported with nateglinide monotherapy:

>10%: Respiratory: Upper respiratory infection (11%)

1% to 10%:

- Central nervous system: Dizziness (4%)
- Endocrine & metabolic: Hypoglycemia (2%), uric acid increased
- Gastrointestinal: Diarrhea (3%), weight gain
- Neuromuscular & skeletal: Back pain, (4%), arthropathy (3%)
- Respiratory: Bronchitis (3%), cough (2%)
- Miscellaneous: Flu-like syndrome (4%)

Pharmacodynamics/Kinetics

Onset of Action Insulin secretion: ~20 minutes; Peak effect: 1 hour

Duration of Action 4 hours

Available Dosage Forms

Tablet, oral: 60 mg, 120 mg

Starlix®: 60 mg, 120 mg

General Dosage Range Oral: *Adults:* 60-120 mg 3 times/day

Stability

Storage Store at 25°C (77°F).

Nursing Actions

Physical Assessment Teach patient importance of proper administration.

Patient Education Take 1-30 minutes before a meal. If you skip a meal, skip a dose for that meal. Follow dietary and lifestyle recommendations of provider. You will be instructed in signs of hyper-/hypoglycemia by prescriber or diabetic educator; be alert for adverse hypoglycemia (tachycardia, profuse perspiration, tingling of lips and tongue, seizures, or change in sensorium) and follow prescriber's instructions for intervention. Note that unusual strenuous exercise, excessive alcohol intake, or acute reduction in caloric intake may increase risk of hypoglycemia. Persistent nausea or vomiting, or severely decreased dietary intake may increase risk of hyperglycemia. May cause mild side effects during first weeks of therapy (dizziness, weight gain, mild muscle aches or pain, or flu-like symptoms); if these do not diminish, notify prescriber. Report signs of respiratory infection.

Dietary Considerations Nateglinide should be taken 1-30 minutes prior to meals. Scheduled dose should not be taken if meal is missed. Dietary modification based on ADA recommendations is a part of therapy. Decreases blood glucose concentration. Hypoglycemia may occur. Must be able to recognize symptoms of hypoglycemia (palpitations, sweaty palms, lightheadedness).

Nebivolol (ne BIV oh lole)

Brand Names: U.S. Bystolic®

Index Terms Nebivolol Hydrochloride

Pharmacologic Category Beta Blocker, Beta-1 Selective

Pregnancy Risk Factor C

Lactation Excretion in breast milk unknown/not recommended

Use Treatment of hypertension, alone or in combination with other agents

Unlabeled Use Heart failure

Available Dosage Forms

Tablet, oral:

Bystolic®: 2.5 mg, 5 mg, 10 mg, 20 mg

General Dosage Range Dosage adjustment recommended in patients with hepatic or renal impairment

Oral: *Adults:* Initial: 5 mg once daily; Maintenance: 5-40 mg once daily

Administration

Oral May be administered with or without food.

Nursing Actions

Physical Assessment Monitor therapeutic response, especially pulse rate and blood pressure, prior to initiation and periodically thereafter. Taper dosage slowly when discontinuing. Advise patients with diabetes to monitor glucose levels closely; beta-blockers may alter glucose tolerance.

Patient Education If you have diabetes, monitor serum sugar closely; drug may alter glucose tolerance or mask signs of hypoglycemia. May cause postural hypotension. Use caution when climbing stairs or changing position. Report signs of fluid retention (unusual weight gain, swelling of the extremities), shortness of breath, or chest pain.

Nedocromil (ne doe KROE mil)

Brand Names: U.S. Alocril®

Index Terms Nedocromil Sodium

Pharmacologic Category Mast Cell Stabilizer

Pregnancy Risk Factor B

Lactation Excretion in breast milk unknown/use caution

Use Treatment of itching associated with allergic conjunctivitis

Mechanism of Action/Effect Inhibits the activation of and mediator release from a variety of inflammatory cell types associated with hypersensitivity reactions including eosinophils, neutrophils, macrophages, mast cells, monocytes, and platelets; it inhibits the release of histamine, leukotrienes, and slow-reacting substance of anaphylaxis.

Contraindications Hypersensitivity to nedocromil or any component of the formulation

Warnings/Precautions Ophthalmic solution contains benzalkonium chloride, which may be absorbed by contact lenses; users of contact lenses should not wear them during periods of symptomatic allergic conjunctivitis.

Drug Interactions

Avoid Concomitant Use There are no known interactions where it is recommended to avoid concomitant use.

Decreased Effect There are no known significant interactions involving a decrease in effect.

Increased Effect/Toxicity There are no known significant interactions involving an increase in effect.

Adverse Reactions

>10%:

Central nervous system: Headache (40%)

Gastrointestinal: Unpleasant taste

Ocular: Burning, irritation, stinging

Respiratory: Nasal congestion

1% to 10%:

Ocular: Conjunctivitis, eye redness, photophobia

Respiratory: Asthma, rhinitis

Available Dosage Forms

Solution, ophthalmic:

Alocril®: 2% (5 mL)

General Dosage Range

Ophthalmic: *Children ≥3 years and Adults:* 1-2 drops in each eye twice daily

Administration

Other For ophthalmic use only; do not allow tip of container to touch eye, surrounding structures, fingers, or other surfaces to avoid bacterial contamination.

Stability

Storage Store at 2°C to 25°C (36°F to 77°F).

Nursing Actions

Patient Education Do not wear contact lenses with allergic conjunctivitis. For the eye only. Open eyes, look up, and pull lower lid down. Squeeze medicine into lower eyelid and close eye. Do not touch bottle tip to eye, eyelid, or other skin.

Nefazodone (nef AY zoe done)

Index Terms Nefazodone Hydrochloride; Serzone

Pharmacologic Category Antidepressant, Serotonin Reuptake Inhibitor/Antagonist

Medication Safety Issues

Sound-alike/look-alike issues:

Serzone® may be confused with selegiline, SEROquel®, sertraline

Medication Guide Available Yes

Pregnancy Risk Factor C

Lactation Enters breast milk/use caution

Use Treatment of depression

Unlabeled Use Post-traumatic stress disorder (PTSD)

Available Dosage Forms

Tablet, oral: 50 mg, 100 mg, 150 mg, 200 mg, 250 mg

General Dosage Range Oral:

Adults: Initial: 200 mg/day in 2 divided doses; Maintenance: 300-600 mg/day in 2 divided doses

Elderly: Initial: 50 mg twice daily; Maintenance: 200-400 mg/day in 2 divided doses

Administration

Oral Dosing after meals may decrease lightheadedness and postural hypotension, but may also decrease absorption and therefore effectiveness.

Nursing Actions

Physical Assessment Monitor therapeutic response (eg, mental status, mood). Monitor for clinical worsening and suicide ideation. Taper dosage slowly when discontinuing.

Patient Education It may take 2-3 weeks to achieve desired results. Avoid alcohol. Maintain adequate hydration unless instructed to restrict fluid intake. You may experience drowsiness, dizziness, lightheadedness, nausea, vomiting, or orthostatic hypotension. Report persistent insomnia or excessive daytime sedation; suicide ideation; muscle cramping, tremors, weakness, tiredness, or change in gait; chest pain, palpitations, or rapid heartbeat; vision changes or eye pain; respiratory difficulty or breathlessness; malaise, loss of appetite, GI complaints, abdominal pain, or blood in stool; yellowing of skin or eyes (jaundice); or worsening of condition.

Nelfinavir (nel FIN a veer)

Brand Names: U.S. Viracept®

Index Terms NFV

Pharmacologic Category Antiretroviral Agent, Protease Inhibitor

Medication Safety Issues

Sound-alike/look-alike issues:

Nelfinavir may be confused with nevirapine

Viracept® may be confused with Viramune®, Viramune® XR™

Pregnancy Risk Factor B

Lactation Excretion in breast milk unknown/contraindicated

Breast-Feeding Considerations Maternal or infant antiretroviral therapy does not completely eliminate the risk of postnatal HIV transmission. In addition, multiclass-resistant virus has been detected in breast-feeding infants despite maternal therapy. Therefore, in the United States, where formula is accessible, affordable, safe, and sustainable, and the risk of infant mortality due to diarrhea and respiratory infections is low, complete avoidance of breast-feeding by HIV-infected women is recommended to decrease potential transmission of HIV (DHHS [perinatal], 2011).

Use In combination with other antiretroviral therapy in the treatment of HIV infection

Mechanism of Action/Effect Blocks the site of HIV-1 protease activity, resulting in the formation of immature, noninfectious viral particles.

Contraindications Hypersensitivity to nelfinavir or any component of the formulation; concurrent therapy with alfuzosin, amiodarone, ergot derivatives, midazolam, pimozide, quinidine, sildenafil (when used for pulmonary artery hypertension [eg, Revatio®]), triazolam

Warnings/Precautions Use with caution in patients taking strong CYP3A4 inhibitors, moderate or strong CYP3A4 inducers and major CYP3A4 substrates and if coadministered with QT-prolonging drugs that are metabolized by CYP3A (see Drug Interactions); consider alternative agents that avoid or lessen the potential for CYP-mediated interactions. Not recommended for use with rifampin, St John's wort, lovastatin, simvastatin, phosphodiesterase-5 (PDE-5) inhibitors, or proton pump inhibitors (based on omeprazole data). Do not coadminister colchicine in patient with renal or hepatic impairment; avoid concurrent use with salmeterol.

Use caution with hepatic impairment; use not recommended with moderate-to-severe impairment. Warn patients that redistribution of body fat can occur. New-onset diabetes mellitus, exacerbation of diabetes, and hyperglycemia have been reported in HIV-infected patients receiving protease inhibitors. Use with caution in patients with hemophilia A or B; increased bleeding during protease inhibitor therapy has been reported. Immune reconstitution syndrome has been reported; may require additional evaluation and treatment. The oral powder contains phenylalanine. Safety and efficacy have not been established in children <2 years of age.

Drug Interactions

Avoid Concomitant Use

Avoid concomitant use of Nelfinavir with any of the following: Alfuzosin; Amiodarone; Axitinib; Cisapride; Conivaptan; Crizotinib; Dronedarone; Eplerenone; Ergot Derivatives; Everolimus; Fluticasone (Oral Inhalation); Halofantrine; Lapatinib; Lovastatin; Lurasidone; Midazolam; Nilotinib; Nisoldipine; Pimozide; Proton Pump Inhibitors; QuiNIDine; Ranolazine; Rifampin; Rivaroxaban; RomiDEPsin; Salmeterol; Silodosin; Simvastatin; St Johns Wort; Tamsulosin; Ticagrelor; Tolvaptan; Topotecan; Toremifene; Triazolam

Decreased Effect

Nelfinavir may decrease the levels/effects of: Abacavir; Boceprevir; Clarithromycin; Contraceptives (Estrogens); Delavirdine; Divalproex; Etravirine; Lopinavir; Meperidine; Methadone; Phenytoin; Prasugrel; Theophylline Derivatives; Ticagrelor; Valproic Acid; Warfarin; Zidovudine

The levels/effects of Nelfinavir may be decreased by: Antacids; Boceprevir; Bosentan; CarBAMazepine; CYP2C19 Inducers (Strong); CYP3A4 Inducers (Strong); Deferasirox; Efavirenz; Fosphenytoin; Garlic; H2-Antagonists; Nevirapine; Peginterferon Alfa-2b; P-glycoprotein/ABCB1 Inducers; Proton Pump Inhibitors; Rifabutin; Rifampin; St Johns Wort; Tenofovir; Tocilizumab

Increased Effect/Toxicity

Nelfinavir may increase the levels/effects of: Alfuzosin; Almotriptan; Alosetron; ALPRAZolam; Amiodarone; Antifungal Agents (Azole Derivatives, Systemic); ARIPiprazole; Axitinib; Azithromycin; Azithromycin (Systemic); Bortezomib; Bosentan; Brentuximab Vedotin; Brinzolamide; Budesonide (Nasal); Budesonide (Systemic, Oral Inhalation); Calcium Channel Blockers (Dihydropyridine); Calcium Channel Blockers (Nondihydropyridine); CarBAMazepine; Ciclesonide; Cisapride; Clarithromycin; Colchicine; Conivaptan; Corticosteroids (Orally Inhaled); Crizotinib; CycloSPORINE; CycloSPORINE (Systemic); CYP3A4 Substrates; Dabigatran Etexilate; Dienogest; Digoxin; Dronedarone; Dutasteride; Enfuvirtide; Eplerenone; Ergot Derivatives; Everolimus; FentaNYL; Fesoterodine; Fluticasone (Nasal); Fluticasone (Oral Inhalation); Fusidic Acid; GuanFACINE; Halofantrine; HMG-CoA Reductase Inhibitors; Iloperidone; Ivacaftor; Ixabepilone; Lapatinib; Lovastatin; Lumefantrine; Lurasidone; Maraviroc; Meperidine; MethylPREDNISolone; Midazolam; Nefazodone; Nilotinib; Nisoldipine; Paricalcitol; Pazopanib; P-glycoprotein/ABCB1 Substrates; Pimecrolimus; Pimozide; Propafenone; Protease Inhibitors; Prucalopride; QuiNIDine; Ranolazine; Rifabutin; Rivaroxaban; RomiDEPsin; Ruxolitinib; Salmeterol; Saxagliptin; Sildenafil; Silodosin; Simvastatin; Sirolimus; SORAfenib; Tacrolimus; Tacrolimus (Systemic); Tacrolimus (Topical); Tadalafil; Tamsulosin; Temsirolimus; Tenofovir; Ticagrelor; Tolterodine; Tolvaptan; Topotecan; Toremifene; TraZODone; Triazolam; Tricyclic Antidepressants; Vardenafil; Vemurafenib; Vilazodone; Warfarin; Zuclopenthixol

The levels/effects of Nelfinavir may be increased by: Antifungal Agents (Azole Derivatives, Systemic); Clarithromycin; CycloSPORINE; CycloSPORINE (Systemic); Delavirdine; Efavirenz; Enfuvirtide; Etravirine; Fusidic Acid; Lopinavir; P-glycoprotein/ABCB1 Inhibitors

Nutritional/Ethanol Interactions

Food: Nelfinavir taken with food increases plasma concentration time curve (AUC) by two- to three-fold. Do not administer with acidic food or juice (orange juice, apple juice, or applesauce) since the combination may have a bitter taste.

Herb/Nutraceutical: St John's wort may decrease the levels/effects of protease inhibitors; concurrent use should probably be avoided.

Adverse Reactions Data presented on experience in adults, unless otherwise noted.

>10%: Gastrointestinal: Diarrhea (14% to 20%; children: 39% to 47%)

2% to 10%:

- Dermatologic: Rash (1% to 3%)
- Gastrointestinal: Nausea (3% to 7%), flatulence (1% to 5%)
- Hematologic: Lymphocytes decreased (1% to 6%), neutrophils decreased (1% to 5%)

Available Dosage Forms

Tablet, oral:

Viracept®: 250 mg, 625 mg

General Dosage Range Oral:

Children 2-13 years: 45-55 mg/kg twice daily **or** 25-35 mg/kg 3 times/day (maximum: 2500 mg/day)

Adults: 750 mg 3 times/day **or** 1250 mg twice daily

Administration

Oral

Oral powder: Administer with a meal. Mix powder in a small amount of water, milk, formula, soy milk, soy formula, pudding, ice cream, or dietary supplement. Do not reconstitute the oral powder in its original container. Be sure entire contents is consumed to receive full dose. Do not use acidic food/juice to dilute due to bitter taste. Once mixed, solution should be used immediately, but may be stored for up to 6 hours if refrigerated.

Tablets: Administer with a meal. If unable to swallow tablets, may dissolve tablets in a small amount of water; mix cloudy liquid well and consume immediately. Rinse glass with water to ensure receiving full dose. Tablets may also be crushed and mixed with pudding.

Stability

Storage Store at room temperature of 15°C to 30°C (59°F to 86°F). Oral powder (or dissolved tablets) diluted in nonacidic liquid is stable for 6 hours under refrigeration.

Nursing Actions

Physical Assessment Monitor for adherence to regimen. Monitor for gastrointestinal disturbance (nausea or diarrhea) that can lead to dehydration and weight loss. Caution patients to monitor glucose levels closely; may cause hyperglycemia or new-onset diabetes. Teach patient proper timing of multiple medications.

Patient Education This is not a cure for HIV, nor has it been found to reduce transmission of HIV; use appropriate precautions to prevent spread to other people. Take with food. Mix powder with water, formula, or dairy products. Maintain adequate hydration unless instructed to restrict fluid intake. This medication will be prescribed with a combination of other medications; time these medications as directed by prescriber. You may be advised to check your glucose levels; this drug can cause hyperglycemia. Frequent blood tests may be required. May cause body changes due to redistribution of body fat, facial atrophy, or breast enlargement (normal effects of drug); diarrhea; or nausea.

Dietary Considerations Should be taken as scheduled with a meal. Some products may contain phenylalanine.

Nepafenac (ne pa FEN ak)

Brand Names: U.S. Nevanac®

Pharmacologic Category Nonsteroidal Anti-inflammatory Drug (NSAID), Ophthalmic

Pregnancy Risk Factor C/D (3rd trimester)

Lactation Excretion in breast milk unknown/use caution

Use Treatment of pain and inflammation associated with cataract surgery

Available Dosage Forms

Suspension, ophthalmic:

Nevanac®: 0.1% (3 mL)

General Dosage Range Ophthalmic: *Children ≥10 years and Adults:* Instill 1 drop into affected eye(s) 3 times/day

Administration

Other

Ophthalmic: Shake well prior to use. May be used with other eye drops; wait at least 5 minutes between application of each medication. For topical ophthalmic use only; avoid touching tip of applicator to eye, fingers, or other surfaces.

Nursing Actions

Patient Education Wash hands before instilling. Sit or lie down to instill. Open eye, look at the ceiling, and instill prescribed amount. Close eye and roll eye in all directions. Apply gentle pressure to inner corner of eye for 1-2 minutes after instillation. Do not wear soft contract lenses while using this medication.

Nesiritide (ni SIR i tide)

Brand Names: U.S. Natrecor®

Index Terms B-type Natriuretic Peptide (Human); hBNP; Natriuretic Peptide

Pharmacologic Category Natriuretic Peptide, B-Type, Human

Medication Safety Issues

High alert medication:

The Institute for Safe Medication Practices (ISMP) includes this medication among its list of drugs which have a heightened risk of causing significant patient harm when used in error.

International issues:

Natrecor [U.S., Canada, Argentina, Venezuela] may be confused with Nitrocor brand name for nitroglycerin [Italy, Russia, Venezuela]

Pregnancy Risk Factor C

Lactation Excretion in breast milk unknown/use caution

Use Treatment of acutely decompensated heart failure (HF) with dyspnea at rest or with minimal activity

Mechanism of Action/Effect Binds to cell surface receptors in vasculature, resulting in smooth muscle cell relaxation. Has been shown to produce dose-dependent reductions in pulmonary capillary wedge pressure (PCWP) and systemic arterial pressure providing symptomatic improvements (dyspnea decreased) for several days.

Contraindications Hypersensitivity to natriuretic peptide or any component of the formulation; cardiogenic shock (when used as primary therapy); hypotension (systolic blood pressure <90 mm Hg)

Warnings/Precautions May cause hypotension; administer in clinical situations when blood pressure may be closely monitored. Use caution in patients systolic blood pressure <100 mm Hg (contraindicated if <90 mm Hg); more likely to experience hypotension. Effects may be additive with other agents capable of causing hypotension. Hypotensive effects may last for several hours.

Should not be used in patients with low cardiac filling pressures, or in patients with conditions which depend on venous return including significant valvular stenosis, restrictive or obstructive cardiomyopathy, constrictive pericarditis, and pericardial tamponade. May be associated with development of azotemia; use caution in patients with renal impairment or in patients where renal perfusion is dependent on renin-angiotensin-aldosterone system; avoid initiation at doses higher than recommended.

Monitor for allergic or anaphylactic reactions. Use caution with prolonged infusions; limited experience with infusions >48 hours.

Drug Interactions

Avoid Concomitant Use There are no known interactions where it is recommended to avoid concomitant use.

Decreased Effect There are no known significant interactions involving a decrease in effect.

Increased Effect/Toxicity

Nesiritide may increase the levels/effects of: Hypotensive Agents

Nutritional/Ethanol Interactions Herb/Nutraceutical: Avoid bayberry, blue cohosh, cayenne, ephedra, ginger, ginseng (American), kola, and licorice (may increase blood pressure). Avoid black cohosh, California poppy, coleus, golden seal, hawthorn, mistletoe, periwinkle, quinine, and shepherd's purse (may enhance decreased blood pressure).

Adverse Reactions Note: Frequencies cited below were recorded in VMAC trial at dosages similar to approved labeling. Higher frequencies have been observed in trials using higher dosages of nesiritide. The percentages marked with an asterisk (*) indicate frequency less than or equal to placebo or other standard therapy.

>10%:

Cardiovascular: Hypotension (total: 11%; symptomatic: 4% at recommended dose, up to 17% at higher doses)

Renal: Increased serum creatinine (28% with >0.5 mg/dL increase over baseline)

1% to 10%:

Cardiovascular: Ventricular tachycardia (3%)*, ventricular extrasystoles (3%)*, angina (2%)*, bradycardia (1%), tachycardia, atrial fibrillation, AV node conduction abnormalities

Central nervous system: Headache (8%)*, dizziness (3%), insomnia (2%)*, anxiety (3%), confusion, fever, paresthesia, somnolence, tremor

Dermatologic: Pruritus, rash

Gastrointestinal: Nausea (4%)*, abdominal pain (1%)*, vomiting (1%)*

Hematologic: Anemia

Local: Injection site reaction, catheter pain

Neuromuscular & skeletal: Back pain (4%), leg cramps

Ocular: Amblyopia

Respiratory: Apnea, cough increased, hemoptysis

Miscellaneous: Diaphoresis

Postmarketing and/or case reports: Hypersensitivity reactions (rare)

Pharmacodynamics/Kinetics

Onset of Action 15 minutes (60% of 3-hour effect achieved)

Duration of Action >60 minutes (up to several hours) for systolic blood pressure; hemodynamic effects persist longer than serum half-life would predict

Available Dosage Forms

Injection, powder for reconstitution:

Natrecor®: 1.5 mg

General Dosage Range I.V.: *Adults:* Bolus: 2 mcg/kg; Infusion: Initial: 0.01 mcg/kg/minute (maximum: 0.03 mcg/kg/minute)

Administration

I.V. Do not administer through a heparin-coated catheter (concurrent administration of heparin via a separate catheter is acceptable, per manufacturer).

I.V. Detail Prime I.V. tubing with 5 mL of infusion prior to connection with vascular access port and prior to administering bolus or starting the infusion. Withdraw bolus from the prepared infusion bag and administer over 60 seconds. Begin infusion immediately following administration of the bolus.

Stability

Reconstitution Reconstitute 1.5 mg vial with 5 mL of diluent removed from a prepefilled 250 mL plastic I.V. bag (compatible with D_5W, $D_5{}^1/_2NS$, $D_5{}^1/_4NS$, NS). Do not shake vial to dissolve (roll gently). Withdraw entire contents of vial and add to 250 mL I.V. bag. Invert several times to mix. Resultant concentration of solution is ~6 mcg/mL.

Storage Vials may be stored below 25°C (77°F); do not freeze. Protect from light. Following reconstitution, vials are stable at 2°C to 25°C (36°F to 77°F) for up to 24 hours. Use reconstituted solution within 24 hours.

Nursing Actions

Physical Assessment Monitor blood pressure and cardiac function before, at frequent intervals during, and for 24 hours following infusion (hemodynamic monitoring with larger doses). Assess renal function and monitor for hypersensitivity reaction on a regular basis during therapy.

Patient Education This medication can only be administered by infusion; you will be monitored closely during and following infusion. Report immediately any pain, burning, swelling at infusion site, or any signs of allergic reaction (eg, respiratory or swallowing difficulty, back pain, chest tightness, rash, hives, swelling of lips or mouth). Remain in bed until advised otherwise; call for assistance with turning or changing position. Report any chest pain, respiratory difficulty, persistent dizziness, or swelling of extremities.

Related Information

Compatibility of Drugs *on page 1264*

Nevirapine (ne VYE ra peen)

Brand Names: U.S. Viramune®; Viramune® XR™

Index Terms NVP

Pharmacologic Category Antiretroviral Agent, Reverse Transcriptase Inhibitor (Non-nucleoside)

Medication Safety Issues

Sound-alike/look-alike issues:

Nevirapine may be confused with nelfinavir

Viramune®, Viramune® XR™ may be confused with Viracept®

Medication Guide Available Yes
Pregnancy Risk Factor B
Lactation Enters breast milk/contraindicated
Breast-Feeding Considerations Although breast-feeding is not recommended, nevirapine is excreted into breast milk and measurable in the serum of nursing infants. Maternal or infant antiretroviral therapy does not completely eliminate the risk of postnatal HIV transmission. In addition, multiclass resistant virus has been detected in breast-feeding infants despite maternal therapy. Therefore, in the United States, where formula is accessible, affordable, safe, and sustainable, and the risk of infant mortality due to diarrhea and respiratory infections is low, complete avoidance of breast-feeding by HIV-infected women is recommended to decrease potential transmission of HIV (DHHS [perinatal], 2011).
Use In combination therapy with other antiretroviral agents for the treatment of HIV-1
Mechanism of Action/Effect Blocks the RNA-dependent DNA polymerase activity
Contraindications Moderate-to-severe hepatic impairment (Child-Pugh class B or C); use in occupational or nonoccupational postexposure prophylaxis (PEP) regimens
Warnings/Precautions [U.S. Boxed Warning]: Severe hepatotoxic reactions may occur (fulminant and cholestatic hepatitis, hepatic necrosis) and, in some cases, have resulted in hepatic failure and death. The greatest risk of these reactions is within the initial 6 weeks of treatment. Patients with a history of chronic hepatitis (B or C) or increased baseline transaminase levels may be at increased risk of hepatotoxic reactions. Female gender and patients with increased $CD4^+$-cell counts may be at substantially greater risk of hepatic events (often associated with rash). Therapy in antiretroviral naive patients should not be started with elevated $CD4^+$-cell counts unless the benefit of therapy outweighs the risk of serious hepatotoxicity (adult/postpubertal females: $CD4^+$-cell counts >250 cells/mm^3; adult males: $CD4^+$-cell counts >400 cells/mm^3). Use with caution in patients with pre-existing dysfunction; monitor closely for drug-induced hepatotoxicity; contraindicated in patients with moderate-to-severe impairment (Child-Pugh class B or C).

[U.S. Boxed Warning]: Severe life-threatening skin reactions (eg, Stevens-Johnson syndrome, toxic epidermal necrolysis, hypersensitivity reactions with rash and organ dysfunction), including fatal cases, have occurred. The greatest risk of these reactions is within the initial 6 weeks of treatment; intensive monitoring is required during the initial 18 weeks of therapy to detect potentially life-threatening dermatologic, hypersensitivity, and hepatic reactions. Risk is greatest in African-Americans, Asian, or Hispanic race/ethnicity or in females. A 14-day lead-in dosing period with immediate release formulation must be initiated to decrease the incidence of adverse effects. The lead-in dosing can be extended up to 28 days if necessary, but an alternative regimen is necessary if >28 days is required. If a severe dermatologic or hypersensitivity reaction occurs, or if signs and symptoms of hepatitis occur, nevirapine should be permanently discontinued. These events may include a severe rash, or a rash associated with fever, blisters, oral lesions, conjunctivitis, facial edema, muscle or joint aches, transaminase elevations, general malaise, hepatitis, eosinophilia, granulocytopenia, lymphadenopathy, or renal dysfunction. Coadministration of prednisone during the first 6 weeks of therapy increases incidence and severity of rash; concomitant prednisone is not recommended to prevent rash.

May cause redistribution of fat (eg, buffalo hump, peripheral wasting with increased abdominal girth, cushingoid appearance). Patients may develop immune reconstitution syndrome resulting in the occurrence of an inflammatory response to an indolent or residual opportunistic infection; further evaluation and treatment may be required. Rhabdomyolysis has been observed in conjunction with skin and/or hepatic adverse events during postmarketing surveillance. Termination of therapy is warranted with evidence of severe skin or liver toxicity.

Use with caution in patients taking strong CYP3A4 inhibitors, moderate or strong CYP3A4 inducers and major CYP3A4 substrates (see Drug Interactions); consider alternative agents that avoid or lessen the potential for CYP-mediated interactions. Concurrent use of St John's wort or efavirenz is not recommended; may decrease the therapeutic efficacy (St John's wort) or increase adverse effects (efavirenz).

Nevirapine-based initial regimens should not be used in children <3 years of age if previously exposed to nevirapine during prevention of maternal-to-child transmission of HIV due to increased risk of resistance and treatment failure. Protease inhibitor-based initial regimens preferred in this population.

Due to rapid emergence of resistance, nevirapine should not be used as monotherapy or the only agent added to a failing regimen for the treatment of HIV. Consider alteration of antiretroviral therapies if disease progression occurs while patients are receiving nevirapine. Use care when timing discontinuation of regimens containing nevirapine; levels are sustained after levels of other medications decrease, leading to nevirapine resistance. Cross-resistance may be conferred to other non-nucleoside reverse transcriptase inhibitors (DHHS, 2011).

Drug Interactions

Avoid Concomitant Use

Avoid concomitant use of Nevirapine with any of the following: Atazanavir; Axitinib; Bortezomib; Crizotinib; Dronedarone; Efavirenz; Etravirine; Everolimus; Itraconazole; Ketoconazole (Systemic); Lapatinib; Lurasidone; Nilotinib; Nisoldipine; Pazopanib; Pimozide; Praziquantel; Ranolazine; Rilpivirine; Rivaroxaban; Roflumilast; RomiDEPsin; SORAfenib; St Johns Wort; Ticagrelor; Tolvaptan; Toremifene; Vandetanib

Decreased Effect

Nevirapine may decrease the levels/effects of: ARIPiprazole; Atazanavir; Axitinib; Boceprevir; Bortezomib; Brentuximab Vedotin; Caspofungin; Clarithromycin; Contraceptives (Estrogens); Contraceptives (Progestins); Crizotinib; CYP2B6 Substrates; CYP3A4 Substrates; Dasatinib; Dronedarone; Efavirenz; Etravirine; Everolimus; Exemestane; Fosamprenavir; Gefitinib; GuanFACINE; Imatinib; Indinavir; Itraconazole; Ixabepilone; Ketoconazole (Systemic); Lapatinib; Linagliptin; Lopinavir; Lurasidone; Maraviroc; Methadone; Nelfinavir; NIFEdipine; Nilotinib; Nisoldipine; Pazopanib; Praziquantel; Ranolazine; Rifabutin; Rilpivirine; Rivaroxaban; Roflumilast; RomiDEPsin; Saquinavir; Saxagliptin; SORAfenib; SUNItinib; Tadalafil; Ticagrelor; Tolvaptan; Toremifene; Ulipristal; Vandetanib; Vemurafenib; Voriconazole; Zuclopenthixol

The levels/effects of Nevirapine may be decreased by: CYP3A4 Inducers (Strong); Deferasirox; Peginterferon Alfa-2b; Rifabutin; Rifampin; St Johns Wort; Tocilizumab

Increased Effect/Toxicity

Nevirapine may increase the levels/effects of: ARIPiprazole; Clarithromycin; Efavirenz; Etravirine; PACLitaxel; Pimozide; Rifabutin; Rilpivirine

The levels/effects of Nevirapine may be increased by: Atazanavir; Clarithromycin; Conivaptan; Efavirenz; Fluconazole; Voriconazole

Nutritional/Ethanol Interactions Herb/Nutraceutical: Nevirapine serum concentration may be decreased by St John's wort; avoid concurrent use.

Adverse Reactions Note: Potentially life-threatening nevirapine-associated adverse effects may present with the following symptoms: Abrupt onset of flu-like symptoms, abdominal pain, jaundice, or fever with or without rash; may progress to hepatic failure with encephalopathy. Skin rash is present in ~50% of cases.

Percentages of adverse effects vary by clinical trial and may vary by formulation; incidences reported below are based on immediate release formulation:

>10%:

Dermatologic: Rash (grade 1/2: 13%; grade 3/4: 2%)

Hepatic: ALT >250 units/L (5% to 14%); symptomatic hepatic events (4%, range: up to 11%)

1% to 10%:

Central nervous system: Headache (1% to 4%), fatigue (≤5%)

Gastrointestinal: Nausea (<1% to 9%), abdominal pain (≤2%), diarrhea (≤2%)

Hematologic: Neutropenia (4%)

Hepatic: AST >250 units/L (4% to 8%)

Available Dosage Forms

Suspension, oral:

Viramune®: 50 mg/5 mL (240 mL)

Tablet, oral:

Viramune®: 200 mg

Tablet, extended release, oral:

Viramune® XR™: 400 mg

General Dosage Range Dosage adjustment recommended in patients with renal impairment

Oral, immediate release:

Infants and Children <8 years: Initial: 150-200 mg/m²/dose once daily (maximum: 200 mg/day); Maintenance: 150-200 mg/m²/dose twice daily (maximum: 400 mg/day)

Children ≥8 years: Initial: 120-150 mg/m²/dose once daily (maximum: 200 mg/day); Maintenance: 120-150 mg/m²/dose twice daily (maximum: 400 mg/day)

Adolescents and Adults: Initial: 200 mg once daily; Maintenance: 200 mg twice daily

Oral, extended release: *Adults:* Maintenance: 400 mg once daily

Administration

Oral May be administered with or without food. May be administered with an antacid or didanosine. Shake suspension gently prior to administration; the use of an oral dosing syringe is recommended, especially if the dose is ≤5 mL; if using a dosing cup, after administration, rinse cup with water and also administer rinse. Extended release tablets must be swallowed whole and not crushed, chewed, or divided.

Stability

Storage Store at 25°C (77°F); excursion permitted to 15°C to 30°C (59°F to 86°F).

Nursing Actions

Physical Assessment Assess LFTs at baseline and frequently during therapy. Monitor patient closely for any signs of hypersensitivity during 14 days of lead-in dosing. Monitor regularly and frequently during initial 18 weeks of therapy for symptoms of hypersensitivity/dermatologic reactions (which may include severe rash, rash with fever, blisters, oral lesions, conjunctivitis, facial edema, muscle or joint aches, general malaise, jaundice, hepatitis, or renal dysfunction). Assess adherence to therapy.

Patient Education You will be provided with an FDA-approved medication guide with your prescription; read this guide carefully. This is not a cure for HIV, nor has it been found to reduce transmission of HIV; use appropriate precautions to prevent spread to other persons. Shake suspension gently prior to use. Frequent blood tests may be required. If rash, blisters, or facial edema develops, stop medicine and contact prescriber immediately. Report any change in urinary pattern, dark urine or light stool, easy bleeding, unusual fatigue, flu-like symptoms, or abdominal pain.

Niacin (NYE a sin)

Brand Names: U.S. Niacin-Time® [OTC]; Niacor®; Niaspan®; Slo-Niacin® [OTC]

Index Terms Nicotinic Acid; Vitamin B_3

Pharmacologic Category Antilipemic Agent, Miscellaneous; Vitamin, Water Soluble

Medication Safety Issues

Sound-alike/look-alike issues:

Niacin may be confused with Minocin®, Niaspan®

Pregnancy Risk Factor A/C (dose exceeding RDA recommendation)

Lactation Enters breast milk/consider risk:benefit

Breast-Feeding Considerations Niacin is excreted in human breast milk. Because lipid-lowering doses of niacin may cause serious adverse reactions in nursing infants, a decision should be made whether to discontinue nursing or discontinue the drug, taking into account the importance of the drug to the mother.

Use Treatment of dyslipidemias (Fredrickson types IIa and IIb or primary hypercholesterolemia) as mono- or adjunctive therapy; to lower the risk of recurrent MI in patients with a history of MI and hyperlipidemia; to slow progression or promote regression of coronary artery disease; treatment of hypertriglyceridemia in patients at risk of pancreatitis

Unlabeled Use Treatment of pellagra; dietary supplement

Mechanism of Action/Effect Component of two coenzymes which is necessary for tissue respiration, lipid metabolism, and glycogenolysis; inhibits the synthesis of very low density lipoproteins (VLDL) and low density lipoproteins (LDL); may also increase the rate of chylomicron triglyceride removal from plasma.

Contraindications Hypersensitivity to niacin, niacinamide, or any component of the formulation; active hepatic disease or significant or unexplained persistent elevations in hepatic transaminases; active peptic ulcer; arterial hemorrhage

Warnings/Precautions Use with caution in patients with unstable angina or MI, diabetes (may interfere with glucose control), renal disease, active gallbladder disease (can exacerbate), gout, or with anticoagulants (may slightly increase prothrombin time). Use with caution in patients with a past history of hepatic impairment and/or who consume substantial amounts of ethanol; contraindicated with active liver disease or unexplained persistent transaminase elevation. Rare cases of rhabdomyolysis have occurred during concomitant use with HMG-CoA reductase inhibitors. With concurrent use or if symptoms suggestive of myopathy occur, monitor creatine phosphokinase (CPK) and potassium; use with caution in patients with renal impairment, inadequately treated hypothyroidism, patients with diabetes or the elderly; risk for myopathy and rhabdomyolysis may be increased.

Immediate and extended or sustained release products are not interchangeable. Cases of severe hepatotoxicity have occurred when immediate release (crystalline) niacin products have been substituted with sustained-release (modified release, timed-release) niacin products at equivalent doses. Patients should be initiated with low doses (eg, 500 mg at bedtime) with titration to achieve desired response. Flushing and pruritus, common adverse effects of niacin, may be attenuated with a gradual increase in dose, and/or by taking aspirin (adults: 325 mg) or an NSAID 30-60 minutes before dosing. Compliance is enhanced with twice-daily dosing (extended-release product excluded). Prior to initiation, secondary causes for hypercholesterolemia (eg, poorly controlled diabetes mellitus, hypothyroidism) should be excluded; management with diet and other nonpharmacologic measures (eg, exercise or weight reduction) should be attempted prior to initiation. Use has not been evaluated in Fredrickson type I or III dyslipidemias.

Drug Interactions

Avoid Concomitant Use There are no known interactions where it is recommended to avoid concomitant use.

Decreased Effect

The levels/effects of Niacin may be decreased by: Bile Acid Sequestrants

Increased Effect/Toxicity

Niacin may increase the levels/effects of: HMG-CoA Reductase Inhibitors

Nutritional/Ethanol Interactions Ethanol: Avoid heavy use; avoid use around niacin dose.

Adverse Reactions Frequency not defined.

Cardiovascular: Arrhythmias, atrial fibrillation, edema, flushing, hypotension, orthostasis, palpitation, syncope (rare), tachycardia

Central nervous system: Chills, dizziness, headache, insomnia, migraine, nervousness, pain

Dermatologic: Acanthosis nigricans, burning skin, dry skin, hyperpigmentation, maculopapular rash, pruritus, rash, skin discoloration, urticaria

Endocrine & metabolic: Glucose tolerance decreased, gout, phosphorous levels decreased, hyperuricemia

Gastrointestinal: Abdominal pain, amylase increased, diarrhea, dyspepsia, eructation, flatulence, nausea, peptic ulcers, vomiting

Hematologic: Platelet counts decreased

Hepatic: Hepatic necrosis (rare), hepatitis, jaundice, transaminases increased (dose-related), prothrombin time increased, total bilirubin increased

Neuromuscular & skeletal: CPK increased, leg cramps, myalgia, myasthenia, myopathy (with concurrent HMG-CoA reductase inhibitor), paresthesia, rhabdomyolysis (with concurrent HMG-CoA reductase inhibitor; rare), weakness

Ocular: Blurred vision, cystoid macular edema, toxic amblyopia

Respiratory: Cough, dyspnea

Miscellaneous: Diaphoresis, hypersensitivity reactions (rare; includes anaphylaxis, angioedema, laryngismus, vesiculobullous rash), LDH increased

Available Dosage Forms

Caplet, timed release, oral: 500 mg

Capsule, oral: 50 mg, 250 mg

Capsule, extended release, oral: 250 mg, 500 mg

Capsule, timed release, oral: 250 mg, 400 mg, 500 mg

Tablet, oral: 50 mg, 100 mg, 250 mg, 500 mg

Niacor®: 500 mg

Tablet, controlled release, oral:

Slo-Niacin® [OTC]: 250 mg, 500 mg, 750 mg

Tablet, extended release, oral:

Niaspan®: 500 mg, 750 mg, 1000 mg

Tablet, timed release, oral: 250 mg, 500 mg, 750 mg, 1000 mg

Niacin-Time® [OTC]: 500 mg

General Dosage Range Oral:

Extended release: *Adults:* 500 mg to 2 g once daily

Regular release: *Adults:* 100-250 mg/day in 1-2 divided doses **or** 1.5-6 g/day in 2-3 divided doses (maximum dose: 6 g/day in 3 divided doses)

Sustained release: *Adults:* Usual: 1-2 g/day

Administration

Oral Administer with food.

Niaspan®: Administer at bedtime. Tablet strengths are not interchangeable. When switching from immediate release tablet, initiate Niaspan® at lower dose and titrate. If therapy is interrupted for an extended period, dose should be retitrated. Long-acting forms should not be crushed, broken, or chewed. Do not substitute long-acting forms for immediate release ones.

Stability

Storage

Niaspan®: Store at room temperature of 20°C to 25°C (68°F to 77°F).

Niacor®: Store at controlled room temperature of 15°C to 30°C (59°F to 86°F).

Nursing Actions

Patient Education Take with food to reduce incidence of GI upset. Do not crush sustained release capsules. You may experience flushing, sensation of heat, or headache; these reactions may be decreased by increasing dose slowly or by taking aspirin 30-60 minutes prior to taking niacin. Avoid alcohol to minimize flushing. Taking at bedtime, after a low-fat snack, is also recommended. You may experience dizziness or lightheadedness. Report persistent GI disturbance or changes in color of urine or stool.

Dietary Considerations Should be taken with meal; low-fat meal if treating hyperlipidemia. Avoid hot drinks around the time of niacin dose.

Niacin and Simvastatin

(NYE a sin & sim va STAT in)

Brand Names: U.S. Simcor®

Index Terms Simvastatin and Niacin

Pharmacologic Category Antilipemic Agent, HMG-CoA Reductase Inhibitor; Antilipemic Agent, Miscellaneous

Pregnancy Risk Factor X

Lactation Excretion in breast milk unknown/contraindicated

Use Reduce total cholesterol, LDL, Apo B, non-HDL, TG, and/or increase HDL in patients with primary hypercholesterolemia, mixed dyslipidemia, or hypertriglyceridemia in combination with standard cholesterol-lowering diet when simvastatin or niacin monotherapy is inadequate

Available Dosage Forms

Tablet, variable release, oral:

Simcor®: 500/20: Niacin 500 mg [extended release] and simvastatin 20 mg [immediate release]; 500/40: Niacin 500 mg [extended release] and simvastatin 40 mg [immediate release]; 750/20: Niacin 750 mg [extended release] and simvastatin 20 mg [immediate release]; 1000/20: Niacin 1000 mg [extended release] and simvastatin 20 mg [immediate release]; 1000/40: Niacin 1000 mg [extended release] and simvastatin 40 mg [immediate release]

General Dosage Range Oral: *Adults:* Niacin 500-2000 mg/simvastatin 20-40 mg once daily

Administration

Oral Tablets must be swallowed whole; do not crush or chew. Administer with a low-fat snack at bedtime.

Nursing Actions

Physical Assessment See individual agents.

Patient Education See individual agents.

Related Information

Niacin *on page 823*

Simvastatin *on page 1037*

NiCARdipine

(nye KAR de peen)

Brand Names: U.S. Cardene® I.V.; Cardene® SR

Index Terms Nicardipine Hydrochloride

Pharmacologic Category Antianginal Agent; Calcium Channel Blocker; Calcium Channel Blocker, Dihydropyridine

Medication Safety Issues

Sound-alike/look-alike issues:

NiCARdipine may be confused with niacinamide, NIFEdipine, niMODipine

Cardene® may be confused with Cardizem®, Cardura®, codeine

Administration issues:

Significant differences exist between oral and I.V. dosing. Use caution when converting from one route of administration to another.

International issues:

Cardene [U.S., Great Britain, Netherlands] may be confused with Cardem brand name for celiprolol [Spain]; Cardin brand name for simvastatin [Poland]

Pregnancy Risk Factor C

Lactation Enters breast milk

Breast-Feeding Considerations Nicardipine is minimally excreted into breast milk. In one study, peak milk concentrations ranged from 1.9-18.8 mcg/mL following oral maternal doses of 40-150 mg/day. The estimated exposure to the breast-feeding infant was calculated to be 0.073% of the weight-adjusted maternal oral dose or 0.14% of the weight-adjusted maternal I.V. dose.

Use Chronic stable angina (immediate-release product only); management of hypertension (immediate and sustained release products); parenteral only for short-term use when oral treatment is not feasible

Unlabeled Use Congestive heart failure, control of blood pressure in acute ischemic stroke and spontaneous intracranial hemorrhage, postoperative hypertension associated with carotid endarterectomy, perioperative hypertension, prevention of migraine headaches, subarachnoid hemorrhage associated cerebral vasospasm

Mechanism of Action/Effect Inhibits calcium ion from entering the "slow channels" or select voltage-sensitive areas of vascular smooth muscle and myocardium during depolarization, producing a relaxation of coronary vascular smooth muscle and coronary vasodilation; increases myocardial oxygen delivery in patients with vasospastic angina

Contraindications Hypersensitivity to nicardipine or any component of the formulation; advanced aortic stenosis

Warnings/Precautions Symptomatic hypotension with or without syncope can rarely occur; blood pressure must be lowered at a rate appropriate for the patient's clinical condition. Close monitoring of blood pressure and heart rate is required. Reflex tachycardia may occur resulting in angina and/or MI in patients with obstructive coronary disease especially in the absence of concurrent beta blockade. The most common side effect is peripheral edema (dose-dependent); occurs within 2-3 weeks of starting therapy. Use with caution in CAD (can cause increase in angina), HF (can worsen heart failure symptoms), aortic stenosis (may reduce coronary perfusion resulting in ischemia; use is contraindicated in patients with advanced aortic stenosis), and hypertrophic cardiomyopathy with outflow tract obstruction. To minimize infusion site reactions, peripheral infusion sites (for I.V. therapy) should be changed every 12 hours; use of small peripheral veins should be avoided. Titrate I.V. dose cautiously in patients with HF, renal or hepatic dysfunction. Use the I.V. form cautiously in patients with portal hypertension (can cause increase in hepatic pressure gradient). Initiate at the low end of the dosage range in the elderly.

Drug Interactions

Avoid Concomitant Use

Avoid concomitant use of NiCARdipine with any of the following: Alfuzosin; Axitinib; Conivaptan; Crizotinib; Dronedarone; Eplerenone; Everolimus; Fluticasone (Oral Inhalation); Halofantrine; Lapatinib; Lovastatin; Lurasidone; Nilotinib; Nisoldipine; Pimozide; Ranolazine; Rivaroxaban; RomiDEPsin; Salmeterol; Silodosin; Simvastatin; Tamsulosin; Thioridazine; Ticagrelor; Tolvaptan; Topotecan; Toremifene

Decreased Effect

NiCARdipine may decrease the levels/effects of: Clopidogrel; Codeine; Prasugrel; QuiNIDine; Ticagrelor; TraMADol

The levels/effects of NiCARdipine may be decreased by: Barbiturates; Calcium Salts; CarBAMazepine; CYP3A4 Inducers (Strong); Cyproterone; Deferasirox; Herbs (Hypertensive Properties); Methylphenidate; Nafcillin; Peginterferon Alfa-2b; P-glycoprotein/ABCB1 Inducers; Rifamycin Derivatives; Tocilizumab; Yohimbine

Increased Effect/Toxicity

NiCARdipine may increase the levels/effects of: Alfuzosin; Almotriptan; Alosetron; Amifostine; Antihypertensives; ARIPiprazole; Axitinib; Beta-Blockers; Bortezomib; Brentuximab Vedotin; Brinzolamide; Budesonide (Nasal); Budesonide (Systemic, Oral Inhalation); Calcium Channel Blockers (Nondihydropyridine); Ciclesonide; Citalopram; Colchicine; Conivaptan; Corticosteroids (Orally Inhaled); Crizotinib; CYP2C19 Substrates; CYP2C9 Substrates; CYP2D6 Substrates; CYP3A4 Substrates; Dabigatran Etexilate; Diclofenac; Dienogest; Dronedarone; Dutasteride; Eplerenone; Everolimus; FentaNYL; Fesoterodine; Fluticasone (Nasal); Fluticasone (Oral Inhalation); Fosphenytoin; GuanFACINE; Halofantrine; Hypotensive Agents; Iloperidone; Ivacaftor; Ixabepilone; Lapatinib; Lovastatin; Lumefantrine; Lurasidone; Magnesium Salts; Maraviroc; MethylPREDNISolone; Neuromuscular-Blocking Agents (Nondepolarizing); Nilotinib; Nisoldipine; Nitroprusside; Paricalcitol; Pazopanib; P-glycoprotein/ABCB1 Substrates; Phenytoin; Pimecrolimus; Pimozide; Propafenone; Prucalopride; QuiNIDine; Ranolazine; RiTUXimab; Rivaroxaban; RomiDEPsin; Ruxolitinib; Salmeterol; Saxagliptin; Sildenafil; Silodosin;

Simvastatin; SORAfenib; Tacrolimus; Tacrolimus (Systemic); Tadalafil; Tamsulosin; Thioridazine; Ticagrelor; Tolterodine; Tolvaptan; Topotecan; Toremifene; Vardenafil; Vemurafenib; Vilazodone; Zuclopenthixol

The levels/effects of NiCARdipine may be increased by: Alpha1-Blockers; Antifungal Agents (Azole Derivatives, Systemic); Calcium Channel Blockers (Nondihydropyridine); CycloSPORINE; CycloSPORINE (Systemic); CYP3A4 Inhibitors (Moderate); CYP3A4 Inhibitors (Strong); Dasatinib; Diazoxide; Fluconazole; Grapefruit Juice; Herbs (Hypotensive Properties); Macrolide Antibiotics; Magnesium Salts; MAO Inhibitors; Pentoxifylline; P-glycoprotein/ABCB1 Inhibitors; Prostacyclin Analogues; Protease Inhibitors; QuiNIDine

Nutritional/Ethanol Interactions

Ethanol: Ethanol may increase CNS depression. Management: Avoid ethanol.

Food: Nicardipine average peak concentrations may be decreased if taken with food. Serum concentrations/toxicity of nicardipine may be increased by grapefruit juice. Management: Avoid grapefruit juice.

Herb/Nutraceutical: St John's wort may decrease levels. Some herbal medications may worsen hypertension (eg, licorice); others may increase the antihypertensive effect of nicardipine (eg, shepherd's purse). Management: Avoid St John's wort. Avoid bayberry, blue cohosh, cayenne, ephedra, ginger, ginseng (American), kola, licorice, and yohimbe. Avoid black cohosh, California poppy, coleus, golden seal, hawthorn, mistletoe, periwinkle, quinine, and shepherd's purse.

Adverse Reactions 1% to 10%:

Cardiovascular: Cardiovascular: Flushing (6% to 10%), peripheral edema (dose related; 6% to 8%), hypotension (I.V. 6%), increased angina (dose related; 6%), palpitation (3% to 4%), tachycardia (1% to 4%), vasodilation (1% to 5%), chest pain (I.V. 1%), ECG abnormal (I.V. 1%), extrasystoles (I.V. 1%), hemopericardium (I.V. 1%), hypertension (I.V. 1%), orthostasis (1%), supraventricular tachycardia (I.V. 1%), syncope (1%), ventricular extrasystoles (I.V. 1%), ventricular tachycardia (I.V. 1%)

Central nervous system: Headache (6% to 15%), dizziness (1% to 7%), hypoesthesia (1%), intracranial hemorrhage (1%) pain (1%), somnolence (1%)

Dermatologic: Rash (1%)

Endocrine & metabolic: Hypokalemia (I.V. 1%)

Gastrointestinal: Nausea (2% to 5%), vomiting (I.V. 5%), dyspepsia (oral 2%), abdominal pain (I.V. 1%), dry mouth (1%)

Genitourinary: Polyuria (1%)

Local: Injection site pain (I.V. 1%), injection site reaction (I.V. 1%)

Neuromuscular & skeletal: Weakness (1% to 6%), myalgia (1%), paresthesia (1%)

Renal: Hematuria (1%)

Respiratory: Dyspnea (1%)

Miscellaneous: Diaphoresis (1%)

Pharmacodynamics/Kinetics

Onset of Action Oral: 0.5-2 hours; I.V.: 10 minutes; Hypotension: ~20 minutes

Duration of Action I.V.: ≤8 hours; Oral: Immediate release capsules: ≤8 hours, Sustained release capsules: 8-12 hours

Available Dosage Forms

Capsule, oral: 20 mg, 30 mg

Capsule, sustained release, oral:

Cardene® SR: 30 mg, 45 mg, 60 mg

Infusion, premixed iso-osmotic dextrose solution:

Cardene® I.V.: 20 mg (200 mL); 40 mg (200 mL)

Infusion, premixed iso-osmotic sodium chloride solution:

Cardene® I.V.: 20 mg (200 mL); 40 mg (200 mL)

Injection, solution: 2.5 mg/mL (10 mL)

Cardene® I.V.: 2.5 mg/mL (10 mL)

General Dosage Range Dosage adjustment recommended in patients with hepatic or renal impairment

I.V.: *Adults:* Initial: 5 mg/hour; Maintenance: 3-15 mg/hour

Oral:

Immediate release: *Adults:* Initial: 20 mg 3 times/day; Maintenance: 20-40 mg 3 times/day

Sustained release: *Adults:* Initial: 30 mg twice daily; Maintenance: Up to 60 mg twice daily

Administration

Oral The total daily dose of immediate-release product may not automatically be equivalent to the daily sustained-release dose; use caution in converting. Do not chew or crush the sustained release formulation, swallow whole. Do not open or cut capsules.

I.V.

Vials must be diluted before use. Administer as a slow continuous infusion at a concentration of 0.1 mg/mL or 0.2 mg/mL. Concentrations of 0.5 mg/mL may be administered via a central line only.

Premixed bags: No further dilution needed. For single use only, discard any unused portion. Use only if solution is clear; the manufacturer recommends not to admix or run in the same line as other medications.

I.V. Detail Avoid extravasation.

pH: Vial: 3.5; Premixed bag: 3.7-4.7

Stability

Reconstitution I.V.: Vial: Dilute 25 mg vial with 240 mL of compatible solution to provide a 250 mL total volume solution and a final concentration of 0.1 mg/mL.

Storage

I.V.:

Premixed bags: Store at controlled room temperature of 20°C to 25°C (68°F to 77°F). Protect from light and excessive heat. Do not freeze.

Vials: Store at controlled room temperature of 20°C to 25°C (68°F to 77°F). Protect from light. Diluted solution (0.1 mg/mL) is stable at room temperature for 24 hours in glass or PVC containers. Stability has also been demonstrated at room temperature at concentrations up to 0.5 mg/mL in PVC containers for 24 hours or in glass containers for up to 7 days (Baaske, 1996).

Oral (Cardene®, Cardene SR®): Store at 15°C to 30°C (59°F to 86°F). Protect from light. Freezing does not affect stability.

Nursing Actions

Physical Assessment Infusion site must be monitored closely to prevent extravasation; peripheral infusion sites should be changed every 12 hours. Evaluate cardiac status and blood pressure and monitor for rash, hypotension, bradycardia, confusion, and nausea when starting, adjusting dose, or discontinuing. Teach patient orthostatic precautions.

Patient Education This medication may be administered by intravenous infusion; report immediately any swelling, redness, burning, or pain at infusion site. Oral: Do not crush or chew sustained release forms; swallow whole. Take with nonfatty food. Avoid caffeine and alcohol. Consult prescriber before increasing exercise routine. May cause orthostatic hypotension, gum pain or swelling, dizziness, and constipation. Report chest pain or pressure, palpitations, severe constipation, swelling of extremities, or respiratory difficulty.

Dietary Considerations Avoid grapefruit juice.

Nicotine (nik oh TEEN)

Brand Names: U.S. Commit® [OTC]; NicoDerm® CQ® [OTC]; Nicorelief [OTC]; Nicorette® [OTC]; Nicotrol® Inhaler; Nicotrol® NS; Thrive™ [OTC]

Index Terms Habitrol; Nicotine Patch

Pharmacologic Category Smoking Cessation Aid

Medication Safety Issues

Sound-alike/look-alike issues:

NicoDerm® may be confused with Nitroderm

Nicorette® may be confused with Nordette®

Other safety concerns:

Transdermal patch may contain conducting metal (eg, aluminum); remove patch prior to MRI.

Pregnancy Risk Factor D (nasal)

Lactation Excretion in breast milk unknown/use caution

Use Treatment to aid smoking cessation for the relief of nicotine withdrawal symptoms (including nicotine craving)

Unlabeled Use Management of ulcerative colitis (transdermal)

Available Dosage Forms

Gum, chewing, oral: 2 mg (20s, 40s, 50s, 100s, 108s, 110s); 4 mg (20s, 40s, 48s, 50s, 100s, 108s, 110s)

Nicorelief [OTC]: 2 mg (50s, 110s); 4 mg (50s, 110s)

Nicorette® [OTC]: 2 mg (40s, 48s, 50s, 100s, 108s, 110s, 168s, 170s, 192s, 200s, 216s); 4 mg (40s, 48s, 50s, 100s, 108s, 110s, 168s, 170s, 192s, 200s, 216s)

Thrive™ [OTC]: 2 mg (40s); 4 mg (40s)

Lozenge, oral:

Commit® [OTC]: 2 mg (48s, 72s); 4 mg (48s, 72s)

Nicorette® [OTC]: 4 mg (50s)

Oral inhalation system, for oral inhalation:

Nicotrol® Inhaler: 10 mg (10 mL)

Patch, transdermal: 7 mg/24 hours (7s, 14s, 30s); 14 mg/24 hours (7s, 14s, 30s); 21 mg/24 hours (7s, 14s, 30s)

NicoDerm® CQ® [OTC]: 7 mg/24 hours (14s); 14 mg/24 hours (14s); 21 mg/24 hours (7s, 14s)

Solution, intranasal:

Nicotrol® NS: 10 mg/mL (10 mL)

General Dosage Range Dosage adjustment recommended for transdermal route in patients on concomitant therapy

Inhalation:

Nasal: *Adults:* 1-2 sprays/hour (maximum: 10 sprays/hour; 80 sprays/day)

Oral: *Adults:* Usually 6 to 16 cartridges per day; best effect was achieved by frequent continuous puffing (20 minutes)

Oral: *Adults:* 2 mg or 4 mg every 1-2 hours (weeks 1-6); every 2-4 hours (weeks 7-9); and every 4-8 hours (weeks 10-12) (maximum: 24 pieces gum/day; 20 lozenges/day)

Transdermal:

Patients smoking >10 cigarettes/day: Begin with **step 1** (21 mg/day) for 6 weeks, followed by **step 2** (14 mg/day) for 2 weeks; finish with **step 3** (7 mg/day) for 2 weeks

Patients smoking ≤10 cigarettes/day: Begin with **step 2** (14 mg/day) for 6 weeks, followed by **step 3** (7 mg/day) for 2 weeks

Administration

Oral

Gum: Should be chewed slowly to avoid jaw ache and to maximize benefit. Chew slowly until it tingles, then park gum between cheek and gum until tingle is gone; repeat process until most of tingle is gone (~30 minutes).

Lozenge: Should not be chewed or swallowed; allow to dissolve slowly (~20-30 minutes)

Inhalation

Nasal spray: Prime pump prior to first use (pump 6-8 times until fine spray appears) or if it has not been used for 24 hours (pump 1-2 times). Blow nose prior to use. Tilt head back slightly and insert tip of bottle into nostril. Breathe through mouth and spray once in each nostril. Do not sniff, swallow, or inhale through the nose during administration. After administration, wait 2-3 minutes before blowing nose.

Oral inhalant: Insert cartridge into inhaler and push hard until it pops into place. Replace mouthpiece and twist the top and bottom so that markings do not line up. Inhale deeply into the back of the throat or puff in short breaths. Nicotine in cartridge is used up after about 20 minutes of active puffing.

Topical Do not cut patch; causes rapid evaporation, rendering the patch useless.

Nursing Actions

Physical Assessment Monitor cardiac status and vital signs prior to, when beginning, and periodically during therapy.

Patient Education Do not smoke, chew tobacco, use snuff, nicotine gum, or any other form of nicotine.

Gum: Chew slowly for 30 minutes. Discard chewed gum away from access by children.

Lozenge: Allow to dissolve slowly in the mouth. Do not chew or swallow lozenge whole. Avoid food or drink 15 minutes prior to, during, or after lozenge.

Transdermal patch: Do not cut patches or wear more than one patch at a time. Remove backing from patch and press immediately on skin. Hold for 10 seconds. Apply to clean, dry skin in different site each day. Do not touch eyes; wash hands after application. You may experience vivid dreams and sleep disturbances, dizziness, lightheadedness, vomiting, or GI upset. Report persistent vomiting, diarrhea, chills, sweating, chest pain or palpitations, or burning or redness at application site. Remove patch while having MRI scan; can cause burns.

Spray: Blow nose gently before use. Use 1-2 sprays/hour; do not exceed 5 doses (10 sprays) per hour. Excessive use can result in severe (even life-threatening) reactions. You may experience temporary stinging or burning after spray.

NIFEdipine (nye FED i peen)

Brand Names: U.S. Adalat® CC; Afeditab® CR; Nifediac CC®; Nifedical XL®; Procardia XL®; Procardia®

Pharmacologic Category Antianginal Agent; Calcium Channel Blocker; Calcium Channel Blocker, Dihydropyridine

Medication Safety Issues

Sound-alike/look-alike issues:

NIFEdipine may be confused with niCARdipine, niMODipine, nisoldipine

Procardia XL® may be confused with Cartia XT®

Beers Criteria medication:

This drug may be inappropriate for use in geriatric patients (high severity risk).

International issues:

Depin [India] may be confused with Depen brand name for penicillamine [U.S.]; Depon brand name for acetaminophen [Greece]; Dipen brand name for diltiazem [Greece]

Nipin [Italy and Singapore] may be confused with Nipent brand name for pentostatin [U.S., Canada, and multiple international markets]

Pregnancy Risk Factor C

Lactation Enters breast milk/not recommended (AAP considers "compatible"; AAP 2001 update pending)

Use Management of chronic stable or vasospastic angina; treatment of hypertension (sustained release products only)

Unlabeled Use Management of pulmonary hypertension, preterm labor, and Raynaud's phenomenon; prevention and treatment of high altitude pulmonary edema

Available Dosage Forms

Capsule, softgel, oral: 10 mg, 20 mg

Procardia®: 10 mg

Tablet, extended release, oral: 30 mg, 60 mg, 90 mg

Adalat® CC: 30 mg, 60 mg, 90 mg

Afeditab® CR: 30 mg, 60 mg

Nifediac CC®: 30 mg, 60 mg, 90 mg

Nifedical XL®: 30 mg, 60 mg

Procardia XL®: 30 mg, 60 mg, 90 mg

General Dosage Range Oral:

Immediate release: *Adults:* Initial: 10 mg 3-4 times/day (maximum: 180 mg/day)

Extended release: *Adults:* Initial: 30 mg once daily; Maintenance: 30-60 mg once daily (maximum: 120-180 mg/day)

Administration

Oral

Immediate release: In general, may be administered with or without food.

Extended release: Tablets should be swallowed whole; do not crush, split, or chew.

Adalat® CC, Afeditab® CR, Nifediac CC®: Administer on an empty stomach (per manufacturer). Other extended release products may not have this recommendation; consult product labeling.

Nursing Actions

Physical Assessment Monitor for hypotension, peripheral edema, and constipation when starting, adjusting dose, or discontinuing. Teach patient orthostatic precautions.

Patient Education Do not crush or chew sustained release forms; swallow whole. Avoid grapefruit and grapefruit juice. When used to manage angina, consult prescriber before increasing exercise routine. May cause dizziness, gum pain and swelling, flushing, difficulties in balance, fatigue, or constipation. Notify prescriber of chest pain or palpitations, swelling of extremities, respiratory difficulty, rash, severe headache, or severe constipation.

Nilotinib (nye LOE ti nib)

Brand Names: U.S. Tasigna®

Index Terms AMN107; Nilotinib Hydrochloride Monohydrate

Pharmacologic Category Antineoplastic Agent, Tyrosine Kinase Inhibitor

Medication Safety Issues

Sound-alike/look-alike issues:

Nilotinib may be confused with dasatinib, imatinib, nilutamide, SUNItinib, vandetanib

High alert medication:

This medication is in a class the Institute for Safe Medication Practices (ISMP) includes among its list of drug classes which have a heightened risk of causing significant patient harm when used in error.

Medication Guide Available Yes

Pregnancy Risk Factor D

Lactation Excretion in breast milk unknown/not recommended

Breast-Feeding Considerations Due to the potential for serious adverse effects in the nursing infant, breast-feeding is not recommended.

Use Treatment of newly-diagnosed Philadelphia chromosome-positive chronic myelogenous leukemia (Ph+ CML) in chronic phase; treatment of chronic and accelerated phase Ph+ CML (refractory or intolerant to prior therapy, including imatinib)

Mechanism of Action/Effect Selective tyrosine kinase inhibitor that inhibits leukemic cell proliferation.

Contraindications Use in patients with hypokalemia, hypomagnesemia, or long QT syndrome

Canadian labeling: Additional contraindication (not in U.S. labeling): Hypersensitivity to nilotinib or any component of the formulation

Warnings/Precautions **[U.S. Boxed Warning]: May prolong the QT interval; sudden deaths have been reported. Use in patients with hypokalemia, hypomagnesemia, or long QT syndrome is contraindicated. Correct electrolyte imbalance prior to initiating therapy. Monitor ECG and QT_c (baseline, at 7 days, with dose change, and periodically). Avoid the use of QT-prolonging agents and strong CYP3A4 inhibitors.** Concurrent use with other drugs which may prolong QT interval may increase the risk of potentially-fatal arrhythmias. Concurrent use with CYP3A4 inhibitors/inducers is not recommended; dosage reductions are recommended if concurrent use with CYP3A4 inhibitors cannot be avoided. Sudden deaths appear to be related to dose-dependent ventricular repolarization abnormalities. Prolonged QT interval may result in torsade de pointes, which may cause syncope, seizure, and/or death. Patients with uncontrolled or significant cardiovascular disease were excluded from studies.

[U.S. Boxed Warning]: Use with caution in patients with hepatic impairment; dosage reduction recommended. Nilotinib metabolism is primarily hepatic; carefully monitor for QT prolongation. May cause hepatotoxicity, including dose-limiting elevations in bilirubin, transaminases, and alkaline phosphatase; monitor liver function.

Reversible myelosuppression, including grades 3 and 4 thrombocytopenia, neutropenia, and anemia may occur; may require dose reductions and/or treatment delay. **[U.S. Boxed Warning]: Administer on an empty stomach, at least 1 hour before and 2 hours after food;** administration with food may prolong the QT_c. Use with caution in patients with a history of pancreatitis, may cause dose-limiting elevations of serum lipase and amylase; monitor. Consider alternative therapy or a dosage increase (with frequent monitoring) in patients with total gastrectomy. Capsules contain lactose; do not use with galactose intolerance, severe lactase deficiency, or glucose-galactose malabsorption syndromes. Safety and efficacy have not been established in children.

Drug Interactions

Avoid Concomitant Use

Avoid concomitant use of Nilotinib with any of the following: Artemether; BCG; CloZAPine; CYP3A4 Inducers (Strong); CYP3A4 Inhibitors (Strong); Dronedarone; Lumefantrine; Natalizumab; Pimecrolimus; Pimozide; QTc-Prolonging Agents; QUEtiapine; QuiNINE; Silodosin; Tacrolimus (Topical); Tetrabenazine; Thioridazine; Topotecan; Toremifene; Vaccines (Live); Vandetanib; Vemurafenib; Ziprasidone

Decreased Effect

Nilotinib may decrease the levels/effects of: BCG; Cardiac Glycosides; Coccidioidin Skin Test; Codeine; Sipuleucel-T; TraMADol; Vaccines (Inactivated); Vaccines (Live); Vitamin K Antagonists

The levels/effects of Nilotinib may be decreased by: CYP3A4 Inducers (Strong); Deferasirox; Echinacea; Herbs (CYP3A4 Inducers); Tocilizumab

Increased Effect/Toxicity

Nilotinib may increase the levels/effects of: ARIPiprazole; CloZAPine; Colchicine; CYP2C8 Substrates; CYP2C9 Substrates; CYP2D6 Substrates; Dabigatran Etexilate; Dronedarone; Everolimus; Fesoterodine; Leflunomide;

Natalizumab; Nebivolol; P-glycoprotein/ABCB1 Substrates; Pimozide; Prucalopride; QTc-Prolonging Agents; QuiNINE; Rivaroxaban; Silodosin; Tamoxifen; Tetrabenazine; Thioridazine; Topotecan; Toremifene; Vaccines (Live); Vandetanib; Vemurafenib; Vitamin K Antagonists; Ziprasidone

The levels/effects of Nilotinib may be increased by: Alfuzosin; Artemether; Chloroquine; Ciprofloxacin; Ciprofloxacin (Systemic); CYP3A4 Inhibitors (Moderate); CYP3A4 Inhibitors (Strong); Denosumab; Gadobutrol; Indacaterol; Ivacaftor; Lumefantrine; Pimecrolimus; QUEtiapine; QuiNINE; Roflumilast; Tacrolimus (Topical); Trastuzumab

Nutritional/Ethanol Interactions

Food: Grapefruit juice may result in increased concentrations of nilotinib and potentiate QT prolongation. Management: Avoid grapefruit juice.

Herb/Nutraceutical: St John's wort may decrease nilotinib levels. Administration with grapefruit juice may result in increased concentrations of nilotinib and potentiate QT prolongation. Management: Avoid St John's wort and grapefruit juice.

Adverse Reactions

>10%:

Cardiovascular: Peripheral edema (8% to 11%)

Central nervous system: Headache (21% to 31%), fatigue (16% to 28%), fever (10% to 24%)

Dermatologic: Rash (28% to 36%), pruritus (19% to 29%)

Endocrine & metabolic: Hyperglycemia (grades 3/4: 4% to 11%)

Gastrointestinal: Nausea (18% to 31%), diarrhea (14% to 22%), constipation (15% to 21%), vomiting (9% to 21%), lipase increased (grades 3/4: 7% to 17%), abdominal pain (11% to 15%)

Hematologic: Neutropenia (grades 3/4: 12% to 37%; median duration: 15 days), thrombocytopenia (grade 3/4: 10% to 37%; median duration: 22 days), anemia (grades 3/4: 4% to 23%)

Neuromuscular & skeletal: Arthralgia (15% to 18%), limb pain (9% to 16%), myalgia (14%), weakness (11% to 14%), muscle spasm (10% to 14%), bone pain (11% to 13%), back pain (10% to 12%)

Respiratory: Cough (12% to 17%), nasopharyngitis (11% to 19%), upper respiratory tract infection (≤13%), dyspnea (8% to 11%)

1% to 10%:

Cardiovascular: Angina, arrhythmia (including AV block, atrial fibrillation, bradycardia, cardiac flutter, and extrasystoles), chest pain, flushing, hypertension, palpitation, pericardial effusion, QT interval prolonged

Central nervous system: Depression, dizziness, dysphonia, hypoesthesia, insomnia, pain, vertigo

Dermatologic: Acne, alopecia, bruising, dry skin, dermatitis, eczema, erythema, folliculitis, hyperhidrosis, skin papilloma, urticaria

Endocrine & metabolic: Hypophosphatemia (grades 3/4: 5% to 10%), hypokalemia (grades 3/4: ≤5%), hyperkalemia (grades 3/4: 2% to 4%), hypocalcemia (grades 3/4: ≤4%), hyponatremia (grades 3/4: ≤3%), albumin decreased (grades 3/4: ≤1%), diabetes mellitus, hypercalcemia, hypercholesterolemia, hyperlipidemia, hyperphosphatemia, hypomagnesemia

Gastrointestinal: Abdominal discomfort, amylase increased, anorexia, dyspepsia, flatulence, pancreatitis

Genitourinary: Pollakuria

Hematologic: Lymphopenia, neutropenic fever, pancytopenia

Hepatic: Hyperbilirubinemia (grades 3/4: 4% to 10%), ALT increased (grades 3/4: 2% to 4%), alkaline phosphatase increased (grades 3/4: ≤3%), AST increased (grades 3/4: 1%), GGT increased

Neuromuscular & skeletal: Musculoskeletal pain, paresthesia

Ocular: Conjunctivitis, dry eye, eye hemorrhage, eyelid edema, periorbital edema, pruritus

Respiratory: Dyspnea (exertional), epistaxis, pleural effusion (≤1%), pneumonia

Miscellaneous: Night sweats

Available Dosage Forms

Capsule, oral:

Tasigna®: 150 mg, 200 mg

General Dosage Range Dosage adjustment recommended in patients with hepatic impairment, on concomitant therapy, or who develop toxicities

Oral: *Adults:* 300-400 mg twice daily

Administration

Oral Administer twice daily doses ~12 hours apart. Swallow capsules whole with water. Administer on an empty stomach, at least 1 hour before or 2 hours after food.

Stability

Storage Store at 25°C (77°F); excursions permitted to 15°C to 30°C (59°F to 86°F).

Nursing Actions

Physical Assessment Monitor for myelosuppression, cardiac changes, gastrointestinal disturbance, and hyperglycemia. Monitor pulmonary status.

Patient Education Take on an empty stomach, 1 hour before or 2 hours after a meal. Avoid grapefruit or grapefruit juice while taking this medication. Maintain adequate hydration unless instructed to restrict fluid intake. You may be required to have regularly scheduled laboratory tests while on this medication. You will be more susceptible to infection. You may experience diarrhea; constipation; insomnia or fatigue; nausea, vomiting, stomach pain, or dyspepsia; or unusual pain or weakness in joints, muscles, or bones. Report chest pain, rapid heart beat, or palpitations; swelling or unusual weight gain; unusual cough, respiratory difficulty, or wheezing; easy bruising; or unusual bleeding.

Dietary Considerations The bioavailability of nilotinib is increased with food. Take on an empty stomach, at least 1 hour before or 2 hours after food. Avoid grapefruit juice.

Nilutamide (ni LOO ta mide)

Brand Names: U.S. Nilandron®

Index Terms RU-23908

Pharmacologic Category Antiandrogen; Antineoplastic Agent, Antiandrogen

Medication Safety Issues

Sound-alike/look-alike issues:

Nilutamide may be confused with nilotinib

Pregnancy Risk Factor C

Use Treatment of metastatic prostate cancer (in combination with surgical castration)

Available Dosage Forms

Tablet, oral:

Nilandron®: 150 mg

General Dosage Range Oral: *Adults:* Initial: 300 mg once daily; Maintenance: 150 mg once daily

Administration

Oral Administer without regard to meals.

Nursing Actions

Physical Assessment Teach patient orthostatic precautions.

Patient Education Avoid alcohol while taking this medication; may cause intolerance. Periodic laboratory tests are necessary while taking this medication. May cause loss of light or dark accommodation, dizziness, confusion, blurred vision, nausea, anorexia, hot flashes, gynecomastia, decreased libido, impotence, or sexual dysfunction (consult prescriber). Report any decreased respiratory function (eg, dyspnea, increased cough), unexplained fever, or difficulty or painful voiding or blood in urine.

NiMODipine (nye MOE di peen)

Pharmacologic Category Calcium Channel Blocker; Calcium Channel Blocker, Dihydropyridine

Medication Safety Issues

Sound-alike/look-alike issues:

NiMODipine may be confused with niCARdipine, NIFEdipine, nisoldipine

Administration issues:

For oral administration only. For patients unable to swallow a capsule, the drug should be dispensed in an oral syringe (preferably amber in color) labeled **"WARNING: For ORAL use only"** or **"Not for I.V. use."** Nimodipine has inadvertently been administered I.V. when withdrawn from capsules into a syringe for subsequent nasogastric tube administration. Severe cardiovascular adverse events, including fatalities, have resulted. Employ precautions against such an event.

Pregnancy Risk Factor C

Lactation Enters breast milk/not recommended

Use Vasospasm following subarachnoid hemorrhage from ruptured intracranial aneurysms

Unlabeled Use Prevention of migraines (inconsistent data)

Mechanism of Action/Effect Nimodipine shares the pharmacology of other calcium channel blockers; animal studies indicate that nimodipine has a greater effect on cerebral arterials than other arterials; inhibits calcium ion from entering the "slow channels" or select voltage sensitive areas of vascular smooth muscle and myocardium during depolarization

Contraindications Hypersensitivity to nimodipine or any component of the formulation

Warnings/Precautions Increased angina and/or MI has occurred with initiation or dosage titration of calcium channel blockers. The most common side effect is peripheral edema; occurs within 2-3 weeks of starting therapy. Reflex tachycardia may occur with use. Symptomatic hypotension with or without syncope can rarely occur; blood pressure must be lowered at a rate appropriate for the patient's clinical condition. Use caution in hepatic impairment. Intestinal pseudo-obstruction and ileus have been reported during the use of nimodipine. Use caution in patients with decreased GI motility of a history of bowel obstruction. Use caution when treating patients with hypertrophic cardiomyopathy.

[U.S. Boxed Warning]: Nimodipine has inadvertently been administered I.V. when withdrawn from capsules into a syringe for subsequent nasogastric administration. Severe cardiovascular adverse events, including fatalities, have resulted; precautions (eg, adequate labeling, use of oral syringes) should be employed against such an event.

Drug Interactions

Avoid Concomitant Use

Avoid concomitant use of NiMODipine with any of the following: Conivaptan; Grapefruit Juice

Decreased Effect

NiMODipine may decrease the levels/effects of: Clopidogrel; QuiNIDine

The levels/effects of NiMODipine may be decreased by: Barbiturates; Calcium Salts; CarBAMazepine; CYP3A4 Inducers (Strong); Deferasirox; Herbs (CYP3A4 Inducers); Herbs (Hypertensive Properties); Methylphenidate; Nafcillin; Rifamycin Derivatives; Tocilizumab; Yohimbine

Increased Effect/Toxicity

NiMODipine may increase the levels/effects of: Amifostine; Antihypertensives; Beta-Blockers; Calcium Channel Blockers (Nondihydropyridine); Fosphenytoin; Hypotensive Agents; Magnesium Salts; Neuromuscular-Blocking Agents (Nondepolarizing); Nitroprusside; Phenytoin; QuiNIDine; RiTUXimab; Tacrolimus; Tacrolimus (Systemic)

The levels/effects of NiMODipine may be increased by: Alpha1-Blockers; Antifungal Agents (Azole Derivatives, Systemic); Calcium Channel Blockers (Nondihydropyridine); Cimetidine; Conivaptan; CycloSPORINE; CycloSPORINE (Systemic); CYP3A4 Inhibitors (Moderate); CYP3A4 Inhibitors (Strong); Dasatinib; Diazoxide; Fluconazole; FLUoxetine; Grapefruit Juice; Herbs (Hypotensive Properties); Ivacaftor; Macrolide Antibiotics; Magnesium Salts; MAO Inhibitors; Pentoxifylline; Phosphodiesterase 5 Inhibitors; Prostacyclin Analogues; Protease Inhibitors; QuiNIDine

Nutritional/Ethanol Interactions

Food: Nimodipine has shown a 1.5-fold increase in bioavailability when taken with grapefruit juice. Management: Avoid concurrent use of grapefruit juice and nimodipine.

Herb/Nutraceutical: St John's wort may decrease levels. Dong quai has estrogenic activity. Some herbal medications may worsen hypertension (eg, ephedra); garlic may increase antihypertensive effects of nimodipine. Management: Avoid dong quai if using for hypertension. Avoid St John's wort, ephedra, yohimbe, ginseng, and garlic.

Adverse Reactions 1% to 10%:

Cardiovascular: Reductions in systemic blood pressure (1% to 8%)

Central nervous system: Headache (1% to 4%)

Dermatologic: Rash (1% to 2%)

Gastrointestinal: Diarrhea (2% to 4%), abdominal discomfort (2%)

Available Dosage Forms

Capsule, liquid filled, oral: 30 mg

Capsule, softgel, oral: 30 mg

General Dosage Range Dosage adjustment recommended in patients with hepatic impairment

Oral: *Adults:* 60 mg every 4 hours

Administration

Oral For oral administration ONLY. Life-threatening adverse events have occurred when administered parenterally. Administer on an empty stomach.

Nasogastric (NG) tube administration: If the capsules cannot be swallowed, the liquid may be removed by making a hole in each end of the capsule with an 18-gauge needle and extracting the contents into a syringe; transfer these contents into an oral syringe (amber-colored oral syringe preferred). It is strongly recommended that preparation be done in the pharmacy. Label oral syringe with **"WARNING: For ORAL use only"** or **"Not for I.V. use."** Follow with a flush of 30 mL NS.

Nursing Actions

Physical Assessment Assess blood pressure and cardiac status. Monitor for rash, hypotension, constipation, and peripheral edema when starting or adjusting dose and periodically during therapy.

Patient Education May cause orthostatic hypotension, headache, or constipation. Report chest pain, palpitations, severe constipation, ankle swelling, or respiratory difficulty.

Nisoldipine (nye SOL di peen)

Brand Names: U.S. Sular®

Pharmacologic Category Calcium Channel Blocker; Calcium Channel Blocker, Dihydropyridine

Medication Safety Issues

Sound-alike/look-alike issues:

Nisoldipine may be confused with NIFEdipine, niMODipine

Pregnancy Risk Factor C

Lactation Excretion in breast milk unknown/not recommended

Use Management of hypertension, alone or in combination with other antihypertensive agents

Mechanism of Action/Effect As a dihydropyridine calcium channel blocker, structurally similar to nifedipine, nisoldipine impedes the movement of calcium ions into vascular smooth muscle and cardiac muscle. Dihydropyridines are potent vasodilators and are not as likely to suppress cardiac contractility and slow cardiac conduction as other calcium antagonists such as verapamil and diltiazem; nisoldipine is 5-10 times as potent a vasodilator as nifedipine.

Contraindications Hypersensitivity to nisoldipine, any component of the formulation, or other dihydropyridine calcium channel blockers

Warnings/Precautions With initiation or dosage titration of dihydropyridine calcium channel blockers, reflex tachycardia may occur resulting in angina and/or MI in patients with obstructive coronary disease especially in the absence of concurrent beta-blockade. Use with caution in patients with severe aortic stenosis, HF, and hypertrophic cardiomyopathy with outflow tract obstruction. Use with caution in hepatic impairment; lower starting dose required. The most common side effect is peripheral edema; occurs within 2-3 weeks of starting therapy. Symptomatic hypotension with or without syncope can rarely occur; blood pressure must be lowered at a rate appropriate for the patient's clinical condition. Some dosage forms contain tartrazine, which may cause allergic reactions in certain individuals (eg, aspirin hypersensitivity). Use with caution in patients >65 years of age; lower starting dose recommended.

Drug Interactions

Avoid Concomitant Use

Avoid concomitant use of Nisoldipine with any of the following: CYP3A4 Inducers (Strong); CYP3A4 Inhibitors (Strong); Grapefruit Juice; Pimozide

Decreased Effect

Nisoldipine may decrease the levels/effects of: Clopidogrel

The levels/effects of Nisoldipine may be decreased by: Barbiturates; Calcium Salts; CarBAMazepine; CYP3A4 Inducers (Strong); Deferasirox; Herbs (CYP3A4 Inducers); Herbs (Hypertensive Properties); Methylphenidate; Nafcillin; Rifamycin Derivatives; Tocilizumab; Yohimbine

Increased Effect/Toxicity

Nisoldipine may increase the levels/effects of: Amifostine; Antihypertensives; ARIPiprazole; Beta-Blockers; Calcium Channel Blockers (Nondihydropyridine); Fosphenytoin; Hypotensive Agents; Magnesium Salts; Neuromuscular-Blocking Agents (Nondepolarizing); Nitroprusside; Phenytoin; Pimozide; RiTUXimab; Tacrolimus; Tacrolimus (Systemic)

The levels/effects of Nisoldipine may be increased by: Alpha1-Blockers; Antifungal Agents (Azole Derivatives, Systemic); Calcium Channel Blockers (Nondihydropyridine); Cimetidine; CycloSPORINE; CycloSPORINE (Systemic); CYP3A4 Inhibitors (Moderate); CYP3A4 Inhibitors (Strong); Dasatinib; Diazoxide; Fluconazole; Grapefruit Juice; Herbs (Hypotensive Properties); Ivacaftor; Macrolide Antibiotics; Magnesium Salts; MAO Inhibitors; Pentoxifylline; Phosphodiesterase 5 Inhibitors; Prostacyclin Analogues; Protease Inhibitors

Nutritional/Ethanol Interactions

Food: Peak concentrations of nisoldipine may be significantly increased if taken with high-lipid foods; however, total exposure (AUC) may be reduced. Grapefruit juice has been shown to significantly increase the bioavailability of nisoldipine. Management: Take on an empty stomach 1 hour before or 2 hours after a meal. Avoid a high-fat diet. Avoid grapefruit products before and after dosing.

Herb/Nutraceutical: St John's wort may decrease nisoldipine levels. Some herbal medications may worsen hypertension (eg, licorice); others may increase the antihypertensive effect of nisoldipine (eg, shepherd's purse). Management: Avoid St John's wort. Avoid bayberry, blue cohosh, cayenne, ephedra, ginger, ginseng (American), kola, licorice, and yohimbe. Avoid black cohosh, California poppy, coleus, golden seal, hawthorn, mistletoe, periwinkle, quinine, and shepherd's purse.

Adverse Reactions

>10%:

Cardiovascular: Peripheral edema (dose related; 7% to 29%)

Central nervous system: Headache (22%)

1% to 10%:

Cardiovascular: Vasodilation (4%), palpitation (3%), angina exacerbation (2%), chest pain (2%)

Central nervous system: Dizziness (3% to 10%)

Dermatologic: Rash (2%)

Gastrointestinal: Nausea (2%)

Respiratory: Pharyngitis (5%), sinusitis (3%)

Pharmacodynamics/Kinetics

Duration of Action >24 hours

Available Dosage Forms

Tablet, extended release, oral: 8.5 mg, 17 mg, 20 mg, 25.5 mg, 30 mg, 34 mg, 40 mg

Sular®: 8.5 mg, 17 mg, 25.5 mg, 34 mg

General Dosage Range Dosage adjustment recommended in patients with hepatic impairment

Oral:

Adults:

Sular® (Geomatrix® delivery system): Initial: 17 mg once daily; Maintenance: 17-34 mg once daily (maximum: 34 mg/day)

Nisoldipine extended-release (original formulation): Initial: 20 mg once daily; Maintenance: 10-40 mg once daily (maximum: 60 mg/day)

Elderly: Sular® (Geomatrix® delivery system): Initial: 8.5 mg once daily; Nisoldipine extended-release (original formulation): Initial: 10 mg once daily

Administration

Oral Administer at the same time each day to ensure minimal fluctuation of serum levels. Avoid high-fat diet. Administer on an empty stomach (1 hour before or 2 hours after a meal). Swallow whole; do not crush, break, split, or chew.

Stability

Storage Store at controlled room temperature of 20°C to 25°C (68°F to 77°F). Protect from light; protect from moisture.

Nursing Actions

Physical Assessment Assess cardiac status and blood pressure. Monitor for chest pain, dyspnea, edema, rash, and constipation when starting or adjusting dose and periodically during therapy. Dose should be tapered gradually when discontinuing.

Patient Education Do not crush or chew tablets; swallow whole. Take on an empty stomach (1 hour before or 2 hours after a meal). This drug does not replace diet and other exercise recommendations of prescriber. May cause orthostatic hypotension, headache, dizziness, or constipation. Report weight gain or swelling of extremities, chest pain, palpitations, persistent dizziness, respiratory difficulty, rash, or fatigue.

Dietary Considerations Take on an empty stomach (1 hour before or 2 hours after a meal). Avoid grapefruit juice before and after dosing. Avoid grapefuit juice; avoid high-fat diet.

Nitazoxanide (nye ta ZOX a nide)

Brand Names: U.S. Alinia®

Index Terms NTZ

Pharmacologic Category Antiprotozoal

Pregnancy Risk Factor B

Lactation Excretion in breast milk unknown/use caution

Use Treatment of diarrhea caused by *Cryptosporidium parvum* or *Giardia lamblia*

Unlabeled Use Alternative treatment for *Clostridium difficile*-associated diarrhea (CDAD)

Mechanism of Action/Effect Nitazoxanide is rapidly metabolized to the active metabolite tizoxanide *in vivo*. Nitazoxanide and its metabolite inhibit the growth of sporozoites and oocysts of *Cryptosporidium parvum* and trophozoites of *Giardia lamblia*.

Contraindications Hypersensitivity to nitazoxanide or any component of the formulation

Warnings/Precautions Use caution with renal or hepatic impairment. Safety and efficacy have not been established with HIV infection, immunodeficiency, or in children <1 year of age (suspension) and <12 years of age (tablet).

Drug Interactions

Avoid Concomitant Use There are no known interactions where it is recommended to avoid concomitant use.

Decreased Effect There are no known significant interactions involving a decrease in effect.

Increased Effect/Toxicity There are no known significant interactions involving an increase in effect.

Nutritional/Ethanol Interactions Food: Food increases AUC. Management: Take with food.

Adverse Reactions Rates of adverse effects were similar to those reported with placebo.

1% to 10%:

Central nervous system: Headache (1% to 3%)

Gastrointestinal: Abdominal pain (7% to 8%), diarrhea (2% to 4%), nausea (3%), vomiting (1%)

Available Dosage Forms

Powder for suspension, oral:

Alinia®: 100 mg/5 mL (60 mL)

Tablet, oral:

Alinia®: 500 mg

General Dosage Range Oral:

Children 1-3 years: 100 mg every 12 hours

Children 4-11 years: 200 mg every 12 hours

Children ≥12 years and Adults: 500 mg every 12 hours

Administration

Oral Administer with food. Shake suspension well prior to administration.

Stability

Reconstitution For preparation at time of dispensing, add 48 mL incrementally to 60 mL bottle; shake vigorously. Resulting suspension is 20 mg/mL (100 mg per 5 mL).

Storage

Suspension: Prior to and following reconstitution, store at room temperature of 15°C to 30°C (59°F to 86°F). Following reconstitution, discard unused portion of suspension after 7 days.

Tablet: Store at room temperature.

Nursing Actions

Patient Education Administer with food. May cause headache, abdominal pain, diarrhea, or vomiting. If severe or persistent, contact prescriber.

Dietary Considerations Should be taken with food.

Nitrofurantoin (nye troe fyoor AN toyn)

Brand Names: U.S. Furadantin®; Macrobid®; Macrodantin®

Pharmacologic Category Antibiotic, Miscellaneous

Medication Safety Issues

Sound alike/look alike issues:

Macrobid® may be confused with microK®, Nitro-Bid®

Nitrofurantoin may be confused with Neurontin®, nitroglycerin

BEERS Criteria medication:

This drug may be inappropriate for use in geriatric patients (high severity risk).

Pregnancy Risk Factor B (contraindicated at term)

Lactation Enters breast milk/not recommended (infants <1 month); AAP rates "compatible" (AAP 2001 update pending)

Use Prevention and treatment of urinary tract infections caused by susceptible strains of *E. coli*, *S. aureus*, *Enterococcus*, *Klebsiella*, and *Enterobacter*

Available Dosage Forms

Capsule, oral: 50 mg, 100 mg

Macrobid®: 100 mg

Macrodantin®: 25 mg, 50 mg, 100 mg

Suspension, oral: 25 mg/5 mL (230 mL)

Furadantin®: 25 mg/5 mL (230 mL)

General Dosage Range Oral:

Children >1 month: Furadantin®, Macrodantin®: 5-7 mg/kg/day divided every 6 hours (maximum: 400 mg/day) **or** 1-2 mg/kg/day divided every 12-24 hours (maximum: 100 mg/day)

Children >12 years: Macrobid®: 100 mg twice daily

Adults: Furadantin®, Macrodantin®: 50-100 mg every 6 hours **or** once daily; Macrobid®: 100 mg twice daily

Administration

Oral Administer with meals to improve absorption and decrease adverse effects; suspension may be mixed with water, milk, fruit juice, or infant formula. Shake suspension well before use.

Nursing Actions

Physical Assessment Allergy history and renal status should be assessed prior to beginning therapy.

Patient Education Take with food. Suspension may be mixed with water, milk, fruit juice, or infant formula. Shake suspension well before use. Maintain adequate hydration unless instructed to restrict fluid intake. May cause nausea, vomiting, or diarrhea. Report immediately any rash; swelling of face, tongue, mouth, or throat; or chest tightness. Report if condition being treated worsens or does not improve by the time prescription is completed.

Nitroglycerin (nye troe GLI ser in)

Brand Names: U.S. Minitran™; Nitro-Bid®; Nitro-Dur®; Nitro-Time®; Nitrolingual®; NitroMist®; Nitrostat®; Rectiv™

Index Terms Glyceryl Trinitrate; Nitroglycerol; NTG; Tridil

Pharmacologic Category Antianginal Agent; Vasodilator

Medication Safety Issues

Sound-alike/look-alike issues:

Nitroglycerin may be confused with nitrofurantoin, nitroprusside

Nitro-Bid® may be confused with Macrobid®

Nitroderm may be confused with NicoDerm®

Nitrol may be confused with Nizoral®

Nitrostat® may be confused with Nilstat, nystatin

Other safety concerns:

Transdermal patch may contain conducting metal (eg, aluminum); remove patch prior to MRI.

International issues:

Nitrocor [Italy, Russia, and Venezuela] may be confused with Natrecor brand name for nesiritide [U.S., Canada, and multiple international markets]; Nutracort brand name for hydrocortisone in the [U.S. and multiple international markets]; Nitro-Dur [U.S., Canada, and multiple international markets]

Pregnancy Risk Factor C

Lactation Excretion in breast milk unknown/use caution

Use Treatment or prevention of angina pectoris

Intravenous (I.V.) administration: Treatment or prevention of angina pectoris; acute decompensated heart failure (especially when associated with acute myocardial infarction); perioperative hypertension (especially during cardiovascular surgery); induction of intraoperative hypotension

Intra-anal administration (Rectiv™ ointment): Treatment of moderate-to-severe pain associated with chronic anal fissure

Unlabeled Use Short-term management of pulmonary hypertension (I.V.); esophageal spastic disorders; uterine relaxation

Mechanism of Action/Effect Relaxes smooth muscle, producing a vasodilator effect on the peripheral veins and arteries with more prominent effects on the veins. Primarily reduces cardiac oxygen demand by decreasing preload (left ventricular end-diastolic pressure); may modestly reduce afterload; dilates coronary arteries and improves collateral flow to ischemic regions. For use in rectal fissures, intra-anal administration results in decreased sphincter tone and intra-anal pressure.

Contraindications Hypersensitivity to organic nitrates or any component of the formulation (includes adhesives for transdermal product); concurrent use with phosphodiesterase-5 (PDE-5) inhibitors (sildenafil, tadalafil, or vardenafil); increased intracranial pressure; severe anemia

Additional contraindications for I.V. product: Constrictive pericarditis; pericardial tamponade; restrictive cardiomyopathy

Note: According to the 2010 American Heart Association guidelines for the treatment of acute coronary syndromes, nitrates are considered contraindicated in the following conditions: Hypotension (SBP <90 mm Hg or ≥30 mm Hg below baseline), extreme bradycardia (<50 bpm), tachycardia in the absence of heart failure (>100 bpm), and right ventricular infarction (O'Connor, 2010).

Warnings/Precautions Severe hypotension can occur. Use with caution in volume depletion, moderate hypotension, and extreme caution with inferior wall MI and suspected right ventricular involvement. Use considered contraindicated in patients with severe hypotension (SBP <90 mm Hg or ≥30 mm Hg below baseline), extreme bradycardia (<50 bpm), and right ventricular MI (O'Connor, 2010).

Paradoxical bradycardia and increased angina pectoris can accompany hypotension. Orthostatic hypotension can also occur. Ethanol can accentuate this. Tolerance does develop to nitrates and appropriate dosing is needed to minimize this (drug-free interval). Avoid use of long-acting agents in acute MI or acute HF; cannot easily reverse effects. Nitrates may aggravate angina caused by hypertrophic cardiomyopathy. Nitroglycerin may precipitate or aggravate increased intracranial pressure and subsequently may worsen clinical outcomes in patients with neurologic injury (eg, intracranial hemorrhage, traumatic brain injury). Nitroglycerin transdermal patches may contain conducting metal (eg, aluminum); remove patch prior to MRI. Avoid concurrent use with PDE-5 inhibitors. When nitrate administration becomes medically necessary, may administer nitrates only if 24 hours have elapsed after use of sildenafil or vardenafil (48 hours after tadalafil use) (Trujillo, 2007).

Use caution when treating rectal anal fissures with nitroglycerin ointment formulation in patients with suspected or known significant cardiovascular disorders (eg, cardiomyopathies, heart failure, acute MI); intra-anal nitroglycerin administration may decrease systolic blood pressure and decrease arterial vascular resistance.

Drug Interactions

Avoid Concomitant Use

Avoid concomitant use of Nitroglycerin with any of the following: Ergot Derivatives; Phosphodiesterase 5 Inhibitors

Decreased Effect

Nitroglycerin may decrease the levels/effects of: Alteplase; Heparin

The levels/effects of Nitroglycerin may be decreased by: Ergot Derivatives

Increased Effect/Toxicity

Nitroglycerin may increase the levels/effects of: Ergot Derivatives; Hypotensive Agents; Prilocaine; Rosiglitazone

The levels/effects of Nitroglycerin may be increased by: Alfuzosin; Phosphodiesterase 5 Inhibitors

Nutritional/Ethanol Interactions

Ethanol: Avoid ethanol (may increase the hypotensive effects of nitroglycerin). Monitor.

Herb/Nutraceutical: Avoid bayberry, blue cohosh, cayenne, ephedra, ginger, ginseng (American), kola, licorice (may worsen hypertension). Avoid black cohosh, California poppy, coleus, golden seal, hawthorn, mistletoe, periwinkle, quinine, shepherd's purse (may cause hypotension).

Adverse Reactions

Frequency not defined.

Cardiovascular: Flushing, hypotension, peripheral edema, postural hypotension, syncope, tachycardia

Central nervous system: Headache (common), dizziness, lightheadedness

Gastrointestinal: Nausea, vomiting, xerostomia

Neuromuscular & skeletal: Paresthesia, weakness

Respiratory: Dyspnea, pharyngitis, rhinitis

Miscellaneous: Diaphoresis

Pharmacodynamics/Kinetics

Onset of Action Sublingual tablet: 1-3 minutes; Translingual spray: Similar to sublingual tablet; Extended release: ~60 minutes; Topical: 15-30 minutes; Transdermal: ~30 minutes; I.V.: Immediate

Peak effect: Sublingual tablet: 5 minutes; Translingual spray: 4-10 minutes; Extended release: 2.5-4 hours; Topical: ~60 minutes; Transdermal: 120 minutes; I.V.: Immediate

Duration of Action Sublingual tablet: At least 25 minutes; Translingual spray: Similar to sublingual tablet; Extended release: 4-8 hours (Gibbons, 2002); Topical: 7 hours; Transdermal: 10-12 hours; I.V.: 3-5 minutes

Available Dosage Forms

Aerosol, spray, translingual:

NitroMist®: 0.4 mg/spray (8.5 g)

Capsule, extended release, oral: 2.5 mg, 6.5 mg, 9 mg

Nitro-Time®: 2.5 mg, 6.5 mg, 9 mg

Infusion, premixed in D_5W: 25 mg (250 mL); 50 mg (250 mL, 500 mL); 100 mg (250 mL)

Injection, solution: 5 mg/mL (5 mL, 10 mL)

Ointment, rectal:

Rectiv™: 0.4% (30 g)

Ointment, topical:

Nitro-Bid®: 2% (1 g, 30 g, 60 g)

Patch, transdermal: 0.1 mg/hr (30s); 0.2 mg/hr (30s); 0.4 mg/hr (30s); 0.6 mg/hr (30s)

Minitran™: 0.1 mg/hr (30s); 0.2 mg/hr (30s); 0.4 mg/hr (30s); 0.6 mg/hr (30s)

Nitro-Dur®: 0.1 mg/hr (30s); 0.2 mg/hr (30s); 0.3 mg/hr (30s); 0.4 mg/hr (30s); 0.6 mg/hr (30s); 0.8 mg/hr (30s)

Solution, translingual: 0.4 mg/spray (4.9 g, 12 g)

Nitrolingual®: 0.4 mg/spray (4.9 g, 12 g)

Tablet, sublingual:

Nitrostat®: 0.3 mg, 0.4 mg, 0.6 mg

General Dosage Range

I.V.: *Adults:* Initial: 5 mcg/minute; Maintenance: 20-200 mcg/minute (maximum: 400 mcg/minute)

Intra-anal: *Adults:* 1 inch every 12 hours

Oral: *Adults:* 2.5-6.5 mg 3-4 times/day; Maintenance: Up to 26 mg 4 times/day

Sublingual: *Adults:* 0.3-0.6 mg every 5 minutes for maximum of 3 doses in 15 minutes **or** 5-10 minutes prior to activities which may provoke an attack

Topical: *Adults:*

Ointment: Apply 0.5" to 2" every 6 hours with a daily nitrate-free interval of ~10-12 hours

Patch: Initial: 0.2-0.4 mg/hour for 12-14 hours/day; Maintenance: 0.2-0.8 mg/hour for 12-14 hours

Translingual: *Adults:* 1-2 sprays under tongue every 3-5 minutes for maximum of 3 doses in 15 minutes **or** 5-10 minutes prior to activities which may provoke an attack

Administration

Oral

Oral (extended release capsule): Swallow whole. Do not chew, break, or crush. Take with a full glass of water.

Sublingual: Do not crush sublingual product (tablet). Place under tongue and allow to dissolve.

Translingual spray: Do not shake container. Prior to initial use, the pump must be primed by spraying 5 times (Nitrolingual®) or 10 times (Nitromist®) into the air. Priming sprays should be directed away from patient and others. Release spray onto or under tongue. Close mouth after administration. Do not rinse the mouth for at least 5-10 minutes. The end of the pump should be covered by the fluid in the bottle. If pump is unused for 6 weeks, a single priming spray (Nitrolingual®) or 2 priming sprays (Nitromist®) should be completed.

I.V. Prepare in glass bottles, EXCEL® or PAB® containers. Adsorption occurs to soft plastic (eg, PVC); use administration sets intended for nitroglycerin.

I.V. Detail Nitroglycerin can be absorbed by plastic (eg, PVC) tubing or containers. Infusion pump may not infuse accurately with different tubing. Be alert to potential for unregulated flow.

pH: 3.0-6.5

Topical

Topical ointment: Wash hands prior to and after use. Application site should be clean, dry, and hair-free. Apply to chest or back with the applicator or dose-measuring paper. Spread in a thin layer over a 2.25 x 3.5 inch area. Do not rub into skin. Tape applicator into place.

Topical patch, transdermal: Application site should be clean, dry and hair-free. Remove patch after 12-14 hours. Rotate patch sites.

Other Intra-anal ointment: Using a finger covering (eg, plastic wrap, surgical glove, finger cot), place finger beside 1 inch measuring guide on the box and squeeze ointment the length of the measuring line directly onto covered finger. Insert ointment into the anal canal using the covered finger up to first finger joint (do not insert further than the first finger joint) and apply ointment around the side of the anal canal. If intra-anal application is too painful, may apply the ointment to the outside of the anus. Wash hands following application.

Stability

Reconstitution

Standard diluent: 50 mg/250 mL D_5W; 50 mg/500 mL D_5W.

Minimum volume: 100 mg/250 mL D_5W; concentration should not exceed 400 mcg/mL.

Storage

I.V. solution: Doses should be made in glass bottles, EXCEL® or PAB® containers. Adsorption occurs to soft plastic (eg, PVC). Nitroglycerin diluted in D_5W or NS in glass containers is physically and chemically stable for 48 hours at room temperature and 7 days under refrigeration. In D_5W or NS in EXCEL®/PAB® containers it is physically and chemically stable for 24 hours at room temperature. Premixed bottles are stable according to the manufacturer's expiration dating.

Store sublingual tablets, topical ointment, and rectal ointment in tightly closed containers at 20°C to 25°C (68°F to 77°F); slow release capsules at 20°C to 25°C (68°F to 77°F); translingual spray and transdermal patch at 15°C to 30°C (59°F to 86°F).

Nursing Actions

Physical Assessment Assess cardiac status and monitor for hypotension and GI disturbances. Teach patient importance of drug-free intervals.

Patient Education Keep medication in original container, tightly closed. If anginal chest pain is unresolved in 15 minutes, seek emergency medical help at once. Daily use may cause dizziness, headache, and GI disturbances. Report severe headache, persistent dizziness, loss of consciousness, or any rash. Do not use within 4 hours of medications used for erectile dysfunction.

Oral: Do not chew or swallow sublingual tablets; allow to dissolve under tongue. Sit down before using sublingual or buccal tablet or spray form. Do not chew or crush capsules; swallow with water.

Spray: Spray directly on mucous membranes; do not inhale.

Topical: Spread prescribed amount thinly on applicator; rotate application sites.

Transdermal: Place on hair-free area of skin and rotate sites (usually, patches will be removed for a period each day). Remove patch while having MRI scan; can cause burns.

Intra-anal: Apply to inside of anal canal; if too painful, may apply to outside of anus.

Related Information

Compatibility of Drugs *on page 1264*

Management of Drug Extravasations *on page 1269*

Nitroprusside (nye troe PRUS ide)

Brand Names: U.S. Nitropress®

Index Terms Nitroprusside Sodium; Sodium Nitroferricyanide; Sodium Nitroprusside

Pharmacologic Category Vasodilator

Medication Safety Issues

Sound-alike/look-alike issues:

Nitroprusside may be confused with nitroglycerin

High alert medication:

The Institute for Safe Medication Practices (ISMP) includes this medication among its list of drugs which have a heightened risk of causing significant patient harm when used in error.

Pregnancy Risk Factor C

Lactation Excretion in breast milk unknown/not recommended

Use Management of hypertensive crises; acute decompensated heart failure (HF); used for controlled hypotension to reduce bleeding during surgery

Mechanism of Action/Effect Causes peripheral vasodilation by direct action on venous and arteriolar smooth muscle, thus reducing peripheral resistance; will increase cardiac output by decreasing afterload; reduces aortal and left ventricular impedance

Contraindications Treatment of compensatory hypertension (aortic coarctation, arteriovenous shunting); to produce controlled hypotension during surgery in patients with known inadequate cerebral circulation or in moribund patients requiring emergency surgery; high output heart failure associated with reduced systemic vascular resistance (eg, septic shock); congenital optic atrophy or tobacco amblyopia

Warnings/Precautions [U.S. Boxed Warning] Excessive hypotension resulting in compromised perfusion of vital organs may occur; continuous blood pressure monitoring by experienced personnel is required. Except when used briefly or at low (<2 mcg/kg/minute) infusion rates, nitroprusside gives rise to large cyanide quantities. Do not use the maximum dose for more than 10 minutes; if blood pressure is not controlled by the maximum rate after 10 minutes, discontinue infusion. Monitor for cyanide toxicity via acid-base balance and venous oxygen concentration; however, clinicians should note that these indicators may not always reliably indicate cyanide toxicity. When nitroprusside is used for controlled hypotension during surgery, correct pre-existing anemia and hypovolemia prior to use when possible. Use with extreme caution in patients with elevated intracranial pressure (head trauma, cerebral hemorrhage), severe renal impairment, hepatic failure, hypothyroidism. Use the lowest end of the dosage range with renal impairment. Cyanide toxicity may occur in patients with decreased liver function. Thiocyanate toxicity occurs in patients with renal impairment or those on prolonged infusions. **[U.S. Boxed Warning]: Solution must be further diluted with 5% dextrose in water. Do not administer by direct injection.**

Drug Interactions

Avoid Concomitant Use There are no known interactions where it is recommended to avoid concomitant use.

Decreased Effect

The levels/effects of Nitroprusside may be decreased by: Herbs (Hypertensive Properties); Methylphenidate; Yohimbine

Increased Effect/Toxicity

Nitroprusside may increase the levels/effects of: Amifostine; Antihypertensives; Hypotensive Agents; Prilocaine; RiTUXimab

The levels/effects of Nitroprusside may be increased by: Alfuzosin; Calcium Channel Blockers; Diazoxide; Herbs (Hypotensive Properties); MAO Inhibitors; Pentoxifylline; Phosphodiesterase 5 Inhibitors; Prostacyclin Analogues

Adverse Reactions Frequency not defined.

Cardiovascular: Bradycardia, ECG changes, flushing, hypotension (excessive), palpitation, substernal distress, tachycardia

Central nervous system: Apprehension, dizziness, headache, intracranial pressure increased, restlessness

Dermatologic: Rash

Endocrine & metabolic: Metabolic acidosis (secondary to cyanide toxicity), hypothyroidism

Gastrointestinal: Abdominal pain, ileus, nausea, retching, vomiting

Hematologic: Methemoglobinemia, platelet aggregation decreased

Local: Injection site irritation

Neuromuscular & skeletal: Hyperreflexia (secondary to thiocyanate toxicity), muscle twitching

Ocular: Miosis (secondary to thiocyanate toxicity)

Otic: Tinnitus (secondary to thiocyanate toxicity)

Respiratory: Hyperoxemia (secondary to cyanide toxicity)

Miscellaneous: Cyanide toxicity, diaphoresis, thiocyanate toxicity

Pharmacodynamics/Kinetics

Onset of Action Hypotensive effect: <2 minutes

Duration of Action Hypotensive effect: 1-10 minutes

Available Dosage Forms

Injection, solution:

Nitropress®: 25 mg/mL (2 mL)

General Dosage Range I.V.: *Children and Adults:* Initial: 0.3 mcg/kg/minute; Usual dose: 3 mcg/kg/minute (maximum: 10 mcg/kg/minute)

Administration

I.V. I.V. infusion only; infusion pump required. Must be diluted with D5W (preferred), LR, or NS prior to administration; not for direct injection. Due to potential for excessive hypotension, continuously monitor patient's blood pressure during therapy.

I.V. Detail pH: 3.5-6.0

Stability

Reconstitution

Prior to administration, nitroprusside sodium should be further diluted by diluting 50 mg in 250-1000 mL of D_5W.

Use only clear solutions; solutions of nitroprusside exhibit a color described as brownish, brown, brownish-pink, light orange, and straw. Solutions are highly sensitive to light. Exposure to light causes decomposition, resulting in a highly colored solution of orange, dark brown or blue. **A blue color indicates almost complete decomposition.** Do not use discolored solutions (eg, blue, green, red) or solutions in which particulate matter is visible.

Prepared solutions should be wrapped with aluminum foil or other opaque material to protect from light (do as soon as possible).

Storage Store the intact vial at 20°C to 25°C (68°F to 77°F). Protect from light.

Stability of parenteral admixture at room temperature (25°C) and at refrigeration temperature (4°C) is 24 hours.

Nursing Actions

Physical Assessment Monitor infusion site closely to prevent extravasation. Monitor patient blood pressure continuously. Assess acid/base balance (metabolic acidosis is early sign of cyanide toxicity). Monitor for disorientation, hypoxia, and muscular twitching.

Patient Education This drug can only be given I.V. You will be monitored at all times during infusion. Promptly report any pain/burning at site of infusion.

Related Information

Compatibility of Drugs *on page 1264*

Nizatidine (ni ZA ti deen)

Brand Names: U.S. Axid®

Pharmacologic Category Histamine H_2 Antagonist

Medication Safety Issues

Sound-alike/look-alike issues:

Axid® may be confused with Ansaid®

International issues:

Tazac [Australia] may be confused with Tazact brand name for piperacillin/tazobactam [India]; Tiazac brand name for diltiazem [U.S., Canada]

Pregnancy Risk Factor B

Lactation Enters breast milk/consider risk:benefit

Use Treatment and maintenance of duodenal ulcer; treatment of benign gastric ulcer; treatment of gastroesophageal reflux disease (GERD)

Unlabeled Use Part of a multidrug regimen for *H. pylori* eradication to reduce the risk of duodenal ulcer recurrence

Available Dosage Forms

Capsule, oral: 150 mg, 300 mg

Solution, oral: 15 mg/mL (473 mL)

Axid®: 15 mg/mL (480 mL)

General Dosage Range Dosage adjustment recommended in patients with renal impairment

Oral:

Children ≥12 years: 150 mg twice daily

Adults: 300 mg/day in 1-2 divided doses **or** 75 mg twice daily (OTC dosing)

Nursing Actions

Patient Education May cause drowsiness. Report fever, sore throat, tarry stools, CNS changes, or muscle or joint pain.

Norepinephrine (nor ep i NEF rin)

Brand Names: U.S. Levophed®

Index Terms Levarterenol Bitartrate; Noradrenaline; Noradrenaline Acid Tartrate; Norepinephrine Bitartrate

Pharmacologic Category Alpha/Beta Agonist

Medication Safety Issues

Sound-alike/look-alike issues:

Levophed® may be confused with levofloxacin

High alert medication:

The Institute for Safe Medication Practices (ISMP) includes this medication among its list of drugs which have a heightened risk of causing significant patient harm when used in error.

Pregnancy Risk Factor C

Lactation Excretion in breast milk unknown/use caution

Use Treatment of shock which persists after adequate fluid volume replacement; severe hypotension

Mechanism of Action/Effect Stimulates $beta_1$-adrenergic receptors and alpha-adrenergic receptors causing increased contractility and heart rate as well as vasoconstriction, thereby increasing systemic blood pressure and coronary blood flow; clinically, alpha effects (vasoconstriction) are greater than beta effects (inotropic and chronotropic effects)

Contraindications Hypersensitivity to norepinephrine, bisulfites (contains metabisulfite), or any component of the formulation; hypotension from hypovolemia except as an emergency measure to maintain coronary and cerebral perfusion until volume could be replaced; mesenteric or peripheral vascular thrombosis unless it is a lifesaving procedure; during anesthesia with cyclopropane (not available in U.S.) or halothane (not available in U.S.) anesthesia (risk of ventricular arrhythmias)

Warnings/Precautions Assure adequate circulatory volume to minimize need for vasoconstrictors. Avoid hypertension; monitor blood pressure closely and adjust infusion rate. Use with extreme caution in patients taking MAO-Inhibitors. Avoid extravasation; infuse into a large vein if possible. Avoid infusion into leg veins. Watch I.V. site closely. **[U.S. Boxed Warning]: If extravasation occurs, infiltrate the area with diluted phentolamine (5-10 mg in 10-15 mL of saline) with a fine hypodermic needle. Phentolamine should be administered as soon as possible after extravasation is noted.** Product may contain sodium metasulfite.

Drug Interactions

Avoid Concomitant Use

Avoid concomitant use of Norepinephrine with any of the following: Ergot Derivatives; Inhalational Anesthetics; Iobenguane I 123

Decreased Effect

Norepinephrine may decrease the levels/effects of: Benzylpenicilloyl Polylysine; Iobenguane I 123; Ioflupane I 123

The levels/effects of Norepinephrine may be decreased by: Spironolactone

Increased Effect/Toxicity

Norepinephrine may increase the levels/effects of: Bromocriptine; Sympathomimetics

The levels/effects of Norepinephrine may be increased by: Antacids; Atomoxetine; Beta-Blockers; Cannabinoids; Carbonic Anhydrase Inhibitors; COMT Inhibitors; Ergot Derivatives; Inhalational Anesthetics; MAO Inhibitors; Serotonin/Norepinephrine Reuptake Inhibitors; Tricyclic Antidepressants

Adverse Reactions Frequency not defined.

Cardiovascular: Arrhythmias, bradycardia, peripheral (digital) ischemia

Central nervous system: Anxiety, headache (transient)

Local: Skin necrosis (with extravasation)

Respiratory: Dyspnea, respiratory difficulty

Pharmacodynamics/Kinetics

Onset of Action I.V.: Very rapid-acting

Duration of Action Vasopressor: 1-2 minutes

Available Dosage Forms

Injection, solution: 1 mg/mL (4 mL)

Levophed®: 1 mg/mL (4 mL)

General Dosage Range I.V.:

Children: Initial: 0.05-0.1 mcg/kg/minute; Maintenance: Titrate to desired effect (maximum: 2 mcg/kg/minute)

Adults: Initial: 8-12 mcg/minute; Maintenance: Titrate to desired effect (usual maintenance range: 2-4 mcg/minute)

Administration

I.V. Administer as a continuous infusion with the use of an infusion pump. Dilute prior to use. Administration via central line recommended; may cause severe ischemic necrosis if extravasated. Do not administer sodium bicarbonate (or any alkaline solution) through an I.V. line containing norepinephrine; inactivation of norepinephrine may occur.

Stability

Reconstitution Dilute with D_5W, D_5NS, or NS; dilution in NS is not recommended by the manufacturer; however, stability in NS has been demonstrated (Tremblay, 2008).

Storage Readily oxidized. Protect from light. Do not use if brown coloration. Stability of parenteral admixture at room temperature (25°C) is 24 hours.

Nursing Actions

Physical Assessment Monitor blood pressure and cardiac status, CNS status, skin temperature, and color during and following infusion. Monitor fluid status (I & O). Assess infusion site frequently for extravasation. Blanching along vein pathway is a preliminary sign of extravasation.

Patient Education This drug is used in emergency situations. Patient information is based on patient condition.

Related Information

Compatibility of Drugs *on page 1264*

Management of Drug Extravasations *on page 1269*

Norethindrone (nor ETH in drone)

Brand Names: U.S. Aygestin®; Camila®; Errin®; Heather; Jolivette®; Nor-QD®; Nora-BE®; Ortho Micronor®

Index Terms Norethindrone Acetate; Norethisterone

Pharmacologic Category Contraceptive; Progestin

Medication Safety Issues

Sound-alike/look-alike issues:

Micronor® may be confused with miconazole, Micronase

Pregnancy Risk Factor X

Lactation Enters breast milk/use caution

Use Treatment of amenorrhea; abnormal uterine bleeding; endometriosis; prevention of pregnancy

Available Dosage Forms

Tablet, oral: 0.35 mg, 5 mg

Aygestin®: 5 mg

Camila®: 0.35 mg

Errin®: 0.35 mg

Heather: 0.35 mg

Jolivette®: 0.35 mg

Nor-QD®: 0.35 mg

Nora-BE®: 0.35 mg

Ortho Micronor®: 0.35 mg

General Dosage Range Oral:

Norethindrone: *Children (postmenarche) and Adults:* 0.35 mg every day

Norethindrone acetate: *Adolescents and Adults:* 2.5-15 mg once daily for 5-14 days of menstrual cycle

Administration

Oral Administer at the same time each day. When used for the prevention of pregnancy, a back up method of contraception should be used for 48 hours if dose is missed or taken ≥3 hours late.

Nursing Actions

Physical Assessment Teach appropriate administration schedule. Schedule physical exam with reference to the breasts and pelvis, including a Papanicolaou smear. Exam may be deferred if appropriate; pregnancy should be ruled out prior to use. Monitor patient closely for loss of vision, sudden onset of proptosis, diplopia, migraine, blood pressure, signs and symptoms of thromboembolic disorders, signs or symptoms of depression, glycemic control in diabetics, and lipid profiles in patients being treated for hyperlipidemias. Adequate diagnostic measures, including endometrial sampling, if indicated, should be performed to rule out malignancy in all cases of undiagnosed abnormal vaginal bleeding. Emphasize need for regular breast self-exam and necessity of annual physical check-up with long-term use.

Patient Education Take according to prescribed schedule. Follow instructions for regular self-breast exam. You may experience dizziness or lightheadedness. Limit intake of caffeine. Avoid high-dose vitamin C. If you have diabetes, monitor blood glucose closely. You may experience photosensitivity, loss of hair (reversible), swelling of hands or feet, or weight gain or loss. Report sudden severe headache or vomiting; disturbances of vision or speech; sudden blindness;

numbness or weakness in an extremity; chest pain; calf pain; respiratory difficulty; weight gain; depression or acute fatigue; or unusual bleeding, spotting, or changes in menstrual flow.

Norethindrone and Mestranol

(nor eth IN drone & MES tra nole)

Brand Names: U.S. Necon® 1/50; Norinyl® 1+50

Index Terms Mestranol and Norethindrone; Ortho Novum 1/50

Pharmacologic Category Contraceptive; Estrogen and Progestin Combination

Medication Safety Issues

Sound-alike/look-alike issues:

Norinyl® may be confused with Nardil®

Pregnancy Risk Factor X

Lactation Enters breast milk/not recommended

Use Prevention of pregnancy

Unlabeled Use Treatment of hypermenorrhea (menorrhagia); pain associated with endometriosis; dysmenorrhea; dysfunctional uterine bleeding

Available Dosage Forms

Tablet, monophasic formulations:

Necon® 1/50: Norethindrone 1 mg and mestranol 0.05 mg [21 light blue tablets and 7 white inactive tablets] (28s)

Norinyl® 1+50: Norethindrone 1 mg and mestranol 0.05 mg [21 white tablets and 7 orange inactive tablets] (28s)

General Dosage Range Oral:

21-tablet package: *Children (menarche) and Adults:* 1 tablet daily for 21 days, followed by 7 days off

28-tablet package: *Children (menarche) and Adults:* 1 tablet daily

Administration

Oral Administer at the same time each day. Administer at bedtime to minimize occurrence of adverse effects.

Nursing Actions

Physical Assessment See individual agents.

Patient Education See individual agents.

Related Information

Norethindrone *on page 840*

Nortriptyline

(nor TRIP ti leen)

Brand Names: U.S. Pamelor™

Index Terms Nortriptyline Hydrochloride

Pharmacologic Category Antidepressant, Tricyclic (Secondary Amine)

Medication Safety Issues

Sound-alike/look-alike issues:

Aventyl® HCl may be confused with Bentyl®

Nortriptyline may be confused with amitriptyline, desipramine, Norpramin®

Pamelor™ may be confused with Demerol®, Tambocor™

Medication Guide Available Yes

Lactation Enters breast milk/not recommended (AAP rates "of concern"; AAP 2001 update pending)

Use Treatment of symptoms of depression

Unlabeled Use Chronic pain (including neuropathic pain), myofascial pain, burning mouth sydrome, anxiety disorders, attention-deficit/hyperactivity disorder (ADHD); enuresis; adjunctive therapy for smoking cessation

Available Dosage Forms

Capsule, oral: 10 mg, 25 mg, 50 mg, 75 mg

Pamelor™: 10 mg, 25 mg, 50 mg, 75 mg

Solution, oral: 10 mg/5 mL (473 mL)

General Dosage Range Oral:

Adults: 25 mg 3-4 times/day (maximum: 150 mg/day)

Elderly: Initial: 10-25 mg once daily; Maintenance: 75 mg/day in 1-2 divided doses

Nursing Actions

Physical Assessment Assess for suicidal tendencies before beginning therapy. Assess therapeutic response (mental status, mood, affect). Monitor for suicide ideation at beginning of therapy and periodically throughout. Dosage should be tapered slowly when discontinuing. Caution patients with diabetes to monitor glucose levels closely; may increase or decrease serum glucose levels.

Patient Education Take once-a-day dose at bedtime. Do not increase dose or frequency; may take 2-3 weeks to achieve desired results. Avoid alcohol. Maintain adequate hydration unless instructed to restrict fluid intake. May cause drowsiness, lightheadedness, impaired coordination, dizziness, blurred vision, nausea, vomiting, loss of appetite, disturbed taste, constipation, urinary retention, postural hypotension, altered sexual drive or ability (reversible), or photosensitivity. Report chest pain, palpitations, or rapid heartbeat; persistent adverse CNS effects (eg, suicide ideation, nervousness, restlessness, insomnia, anxiety, excitation, headache, agitation, impaired coordination, changes in cognition); muscle cramping, weakness, tremors, or rigidity; blurred vision or eye pain; breast enlargement or swelling; yellowing of skin or eyes; or worsening of condition.

Related Information

Peak and Trough Guidelines *on page 1276*

Nystatin (Oral)

(nye STAT in)

Pharmacologic Category Antifungal Agent, Oral Nonabsorbed

Medication Safety Issues

Sound-alike/look-alike issues:

Nystatin may be confused with HMG-CoA reductase inhibitors (also known as "statins"; eg, atorvastatin, fluvastatin, lovastatin, pitavastatin, pravastatin, rosuvastatin, simvastatin), Nitro-stat®

Pregnancy Risk Factor C

Lactation Excretion in breast milk unknown/use caution

Use Treatment of susceptible cutaneous, mucocutaneous, and oral cavity fungal infections normally caused by the *Candida* species

Available Dosage Forms

Powder, for prescription compounding: 50 million units (10 g); 150 million units (30 g); 500 million units (100 g)

Suspension, oral: 100,000 units/mL (5 mL, 60 mL, 240 mL, 473 mL, 480 mL, 3785 mL)

Tablet, oral: 500,000 units

General Dosage Range Oral:

Premature infants: 100,000 units 4 times/day

Infants: 200,000 units 4 times/day

Children: 400,000-600,000 units 4 times/day

Adults: 400,000-1,000,000 units/day in 3-4 divided doses

Administration

Oral Suspension: Shake well before using. Should be swished about the mouth and retained in the mouth for as long as possible (several minutes) before swallowing. For neonates and infants, paint nystatin suspension into recesses of the mouth.

Nursing Actions

Patient Education Maintain adequate hydration unless instructed to restrict fluid intake. Do not allow medication to come in contact with eyes. Report persistent nausea, vomiting, diarrhea, or if condition being treated worsens or does not improve.

Oral tablet: Swallow whole; do not crush or chew.

Oral suspension: Shake well before using. Remove dentures; clean mouth (do not replace dentures until after using medications). Swish suspension in mouth for several minutes before swallowing.

Nystatin (Topical) (nye STAT in)

Brand Names: U.S. Nyamyc®; Nystop®; Pedi-Dri®; Pediaderm™ AF

Pharmacologic Category Antifungal Agent, Topical; Antifungal Agent, Vaginal

Medication Safety Issues

Sound-alike/look-alike issues:

Nystatin may be confused with HMG-CoA reductase inhibitors (also known as "statins"; eg, atorvastatin, fluvastatin, lovastatin, pitavastatin, pravastatin, rosuvastatin, simvastatin), Nitro-stat®

Pregnancy Risk Factor A (vaginal)/C (topical)

Lactation Excretion in breast milk unknown/not recommended

Use Treatment of susceptible cutaneous and mucocutaneous fungal infections normally caused by the *Candida* species

Available Dosage Forms

Cream, topical: 100,000 units/g (15 g, 30 g)

Pediaderm™ AF: 100,000 units/g (30 g)

Ointment, topical: 100,000 units/g (15 g, 30 g)

Powder, topical: 100,000 units/g (15 g, 30 g, 60 g)

Nyamyc®: 100,000 units/g (15 g, 30 g, 60 g)

Nystop®: 100,000 units/g (15 g, 30 g, 60 g)

Pedi-Dri®: 100,000 units/g (56.7 g)

Tablet, vaginal: 100,000 units

General Dosage Range

Intravaginal: *Adults:* Insert 1 vaginal tablet/day at bedtime

Topical: *Children and Adults:* Apply 2-3 times/day to affected areas

Nursing Actions

Physical Assessment Determine that cause of infection is fungal. Avoid skin contact when applying.

Patient Education Do not allow medication to come in contact with eyes. Report if condition being treated worsens or does not improve.

Topical: Wash and dry area before applying (do not reuse towels without washing, apply clean clothing after use). Report unresolved burning, redness, or swelling in treated areas.

Vaginal tablet: Wash hands before using. Lie down to insert high into vagina at bedtime.

Nystatin and Triamcinolone

(nye STAT in & trye am SIN oh lone)

Index Terms Triamcinolone and Nystatin

Pharmacologic Category Antifungal Agent, Topical; Corticosteroid, Topical

Pregnancy Risk Factor C

Lactation Excretion in breast milk unknown

Use Treatment of cutaneous candidiasis

Available Dosage Forms

Cream: Nystatin 100,000 units and triamcinolone 0.1% (15 g, 30 g, 60 g)

Ointment: Nystatin 100,000 units and triamcinolone 0.1% (15 g, 30 g, 60 g)

General Dosage Range

Topical:

Children: Apply sparingly 2-4 times/day

Adults: Apply sparingly 2-4 times/day

Administration

Topical External use only; do not use on open wounds. Apply sparingly to occlusive dressings; should not be used in the presence of open or weeping lesions.

Nursing Actions

Physical Assessment See individual agents.

Patient Education See individual agents.

Related Information

Nystatin (Topical) *on page 842*

Triamcinolone (Topical) *on page 1151*

Octreotide (ok TREE oh tide)

Brand Names: U.S. SandoSTATIN LAR®; SandoSTATIN®

Index Terms Longastatin; Octreotide Acetate

Pharmacologic Category Antidiarrheal; Antidote; Somatostatin Analog

Medication Safety Issues

Sound-alike/look-alike issues:

SandoSTATIN® may be confused with SandIMMUNE®, SandoSTATIN LAR®, sargramostim, simvastatin

Pregnancy Risk Factor B

Lactation Excretion in breast milk unknown/use caution

Use Control of symptoms (diarrhea and flushing) in patients with metastatic carcinoid tumors; treatment of watery diarrhea associated with vasoactive intestinal peptide-secreting tumors (VIPomas); treatment of acromegaly

Unlabeled Use Treatment of AIDS-associated diarrhea (including *Cryptosporidiosis*), chemotherapy-induced diarrhea, graft-versus-host disease (GVHD) associated diarrhea, postgastrectomy dumping syndrome; control of bleeding of esophageal varices; second-line treatment for thymic malignancies; Cushing's syndrome (ectopic); insulinomas; small bowel fistulas; islet cell tumors; Zollinger-Ellison syndrome; congenital hyperinsulinism; hypothalamic obesity; treatment of hypoglycemia secondary to sulfonylurea poisoning; treatment of malignant bowel obstruction

Available Dosage Forms

Injection, microspheres for suspension:

SandoSTATIN LAR®: 10 mg, 20 mg, 30 mg

Injection, solution: 100 mcg/mL (1 mL); 200 mcg/mL (5 mL); 1000 mcg/mL (5 mL)

SandoSTATIN®: 200 mcg/mL (5 mL); 1000 mcg/mL (5 mL)

Injection, solution [preservative free]: 50 mcg/mL (1 mL); 100 mcg/mL (1 mL); 200 mcg/mL (5 mL); 500 mcg/mL (1 mL)

SandoSTATIN®: 50 mcg/mL (1 mL); 100 mcg/mL (1 mL); 500 mcg/mL (1 mL)

General Dosage Range Dosage adjustment recommended in patients with hepatic or renal impairment

I.M.: *Adults:* Depot: 20 mg every 4 weeks (maximum: 40 mg every 2 weeks)

I.V., SubQ: *Adults:* 50-1500 mcg/day in 2-4 divided doses

Administration

I.M. Depot formulation: Administer I.M. intragluteal (avoid deltoid administration); alternate gluteal injection sites to avoid irritation. **Do not** administer Sandostatin LAR® intravenously or subcutaneously; must be administered immediately after mixing.

I.V. Regular injection only (not suspension): I.V. administration may be I.V. push (undiluted over 3 minutes), intermittent I.V. infusion (over 15-30 minutes), or continuous I.V. infusion (unlabeled route).

I.V. Detail Do not use if solution contains particles or is discolored.

pH: Solution: ~4.2

Other SubQ: Use the concentration with smallest volume to deliver dose to reduce injection site pain. Rotate injection site; may bring to room temperature prior to injection.

Nursing Actions

Physical Assessment May effect response to insulin or sulfonylureas and/or response to cardiovascular medications. Monitor for hyperglycemia, hypothyroidism, bradycardia, chest pain, GI disturbances, CNS changes, and dyspnea. Caution patients with diabetes to monitor serum glucose closely; may affect response to insulin or sulfonylureas. Teach patient appropriate injection technique and syringe/needle disposal.

Patient Education If self-administered, follow instructions for injection and syringe/needle disposal. Schedule injections between meals to decrease GI effects. Consult prescriber about appropriate diet. If you have diabetes, monitor serum glucose closely and notify prescriber of significant changes (this drug may alter the effects of insulin or sulfonylureas). May cause skin flushing, nausea, vomiting, dizziness, fatigue, drowsiness, or joint or muscle pain. Report unusual weight gain; swelling of extremities; respiratory difficulty; acute or persistent GI distress (eg, diarrhea, vomiting, constipation, abdominal pain); muscle weakness or tremors or loss of motor function; chest pain or palpitations; blurred vision; depression; or redness, swelling, burning, or pain at injection site.

Ofatumumab (oh fa TOOM yoo mab)

Brand Names: U.S. Arzerra™

Index Terms HuMax-CD20

Pharmacologic Category Antineoplastic Agent, Monoclonal Antibody; Monoclonal Antibody

Medication Safety Issues

Sound-alike/look-alike issues:

Ofatumumab may be confused with omalizumab

High alert medication:

This medication is in a class the Institute for Safe Medication Practices (ISMP) includes among its list of drug classes which have a heightened risk of causing significant patient harm when used in error.

Pregnancy Risk Factor C

Lactation Excretion in breast milk unknown/use caution

Use Treatment of refractory chronic lymphocytic leukemia (CLL)

Available Dosage Forms

Injection, solution [preservative free]:

Arzerra™: 20 mg/mL (5 mL, 50 mL)

General Dosage Range Dosage adjustment recommended in patients who develop toxicities

I.V.: *Adults:* 300 mg week 1, followed 1 week later by 2000 mg once weekly for 7 doses (doses 2-8), followed 4 weeks later by 2000 mg once every 4 weeks for 4 doses (doses 9-12; for a total of 12 doses)

Administration

I.V. Do not administer I.V. push or as a bolus. Premedicate with acetaminophen, an antihistamine and a corticosteroid 30-120 minutes prior to administration. Administer with an in-line filter (supplied) and polyvinyl chloride (PVC) administration sets. Do not mix with or infuse with other medications. Flush line before and after infusion with NS. Begin infusion within 12 hours of preparation. The final concentration of dose 1 is 0.3 mg/mL and final concentration of doses 2-12 is 2 mg/mL.

Premedication: Premedicate with oral acetaminophen (1000 mg), an oral or I.V. antihistamine (eg, cetirizine 10 mg orally or equivalent), and an I.V. corticosteroid. Full dose corticosteroid is recommended for doses 1, 2, and 9; in the absence of infusion reaction ≥grade 3, may gradually reduce corticosteroid dose for doses 3-8; administer full or half corticosteroid dose with doses 10-12 if ≥grade 3 did not occur with dose 9.

Doses 1 and 2: Initiate infusion at 12 mL/hour for 30 minutes, if tolerated (no infusion reaction) increase to 25 mL/hour for 30 minutes, if tolerated, increase to 50 mL/hour for 30 minutes, if tolerated, increase to 100 mL/hour for 30 minutes, if tolerated, increase to 200 mL/hour for duration of infusion.

Doses 3-12: Initiate infusion at 25 mL/hour for 30 minutes, if tolerated (no infusion reaction) increase to 50 mL/hour for 30 minutes, if tolerated, increase to 100 mL/hour for 30 minutes, if tolerated, increase to 200 mL/hour for 30 minutes, if tolerated, increase to 400 mL/hour for remainder of infusion.

I.V. Detail pH: 6.5; may contain a small amount of visible transparent or white, amorphous ofatumumab particles

Nursing Actions

Physical Assessment Premedication may be ordered. Monitor patient very closely for infusion reactions; appropriate treatment for hypersensitivity reactions should be available.

Patient Education You will be closely monitored during infusion. Report immediately any pain, burning, or swelling at infusion site; sudden chest pain or palpitations; difficulty breathing or swallowing; or chills. Between infusions, maintain adequate nutrition and hydration unless instructed to restrict fluid intake. You will need frequent laboratory tests during course of therapy. You will be more susceptible to infection. You may experience some nausea or vomiting. Report unresolved GI problems, persistent fever, chills, muscle pain, skin rash, unusual bleeding or bruising, signs of infection (mouth sores, sore throat, white plaques in mouth or perianal area, burning on urination), swelling of extremities, respiratory difficulty, chest pain, or palpitations.

Ofloxacin (Ophthalmic) (oh FLOKS a sin)

Brand Names: U.S. Ocuflox®

Pharmacologic Category Antibiotic, Ophthalmic; Antibiotic, Quinolone

Medication Safety Issues

Sound-alike/look-alike issues:

Ocuflox® may be confused with Occlusal™-HP, Ocufen®

Pregnancy Risk Factor C

Lactation Enters breast milk/not recommended (AAP rates "compatible"; AAP 2001 update pending)

Use Treatment of superficial ocular infections involving the conjunctiva or cornea due to strains of susceptible organisms

Available Dosage Forms

Solution, ophthalmic: 0.3% (5 mL, 10 mL)

Ocuflox®: 0.3% (5 mL)

General Dosage Range Ophthalmic: *Children >1 year and Adults:* Initial: 1-2 drops every 30 minutes to 4 hours; Maintenance: 1-2 drops every 4-6 hours

Administration

Other For ophthalmic use only; avoid touching tip of applicator to eye or other surfaces.

Nursing Actions

Physical Assessment Instruct patient to report allergic reaction and tendon pain.

Patient Education Wash hands before instilling solution. Sit or lie down to instill. Open eye, look at ceiling, and instill prescribed amount of solution as directed. Close eye, roll eye in all directions, and apply gentle pressure to inner corner of eye. Do not touch tip of applicator or let tip of applicator touch eye (may cause eye infection, eye damage, or vision loss). Do not wear contact lenses during therapy. Temporary stinging, blurred vision, dry eyes, or a bad taste in your mouth may occur after installation. Report persistent pain, burning, excessive tearing, decreased visual acuity, swelling, itching, or worsening of condition.

Ofloxacin (Otic) (oh FLOKS a sin)

Index Terms Floxin Otic Singles

Pharmacologic Category Antibiotic, Quinolone

Medication Safety Issues

Sound-alike/look-alike issues:

Floxin may be confused with Flexeril®

International issues:

Floxin: Brand name for ofloxacin [U.S., Canada], but also the brand name for flunarizine [Thailand], norfloxacin [South Africa], and perfloxacin [Philippines]

Floxin [U.S., Canada] may be confused with Flexin brand name for diclofenac [Argentina], cyclobenzaprine [Chile], and orphenadrine [Israel]; Flogen brand name for naproxen [Mexico]

Pregnancy Risk Factor C

Lactation Enters breast milk/not recommended (AAP rates "compatible"; AAP 2001 update pending)

Use Otitis externa, chronic suppurative otitis media, acute otitis media

Available Dosage Forms

Solution, otic: 0.3% (5 mL, 10 mL)

General Dosage Range

Otic:

Children <6 months: Dosage not established

Children ≥6 months to 12 years: 5 drops daily

Children >12 years: 10 drops once or twice daily

Adults: 10 drops once or twice daily

Administration

Other Prior to use, warm solution by holding container in hands for 1-2 minutes. Patient should lie down with affected ear upward and medication instilled. Pump tragus 4 times to ensure penetration of medication. Patient should remain in this position for 5 minutes.

Nursing Actions

Patient Education Wash hands before and after applying drops. Warm solution by holding container in hands for a few minutes. Lie with affected ear up and instill prescribed number of drops into ear. Remain on side with ear up for 5 minutes.

OLANZapine (oh LAN za peen)

Brand Names: U.S. ZyPREXA®; ZyPREXA® IntraMuscular; ZyPREXA® Relprevv™; ZyPREXA® Zydis®

Index Terms LY170053; Olanzapine Pamoate; Zyprexa Zydis

Pharmacologic Category Antimanic Agent; Antipsychotic Agent, Atypical

Medication Safety Issues

Sound-alike/look-alike issues:

OLANZapine may be confused with olsalazine, QUEtiapine

ZyPREXA® may be confused with CeleXA®, Reprexain™, Zestril®, ZyrTEC®

ZyPREXA® Zydis® may be confused with Zelapar®, zolpidem

ZyPREXA® Relprevv™ may be confused with ZyPREXA® IntraMuscular

Medication Guide Available Yes

Pregnancy Risk Factor C

Lactation Enters breast milk/not recommended

Breast-Feeding Considerations At steady-state concentrations, it is estimated that a breast-fed infant may be exposed to ~2% of the maternal dose.

Use

Oral: Treatment of the manifestations of schizophrenia; treatment of acute or mixed mania episodes associated with bipolar I disorder (as monotherapy or in combination with lithium or valproate); maintenance treatment of bipolar disorder; in combination with fluoxetine for treatment-resistant or bipolar I depression

I.M., extended-release (Zyprexa® Relprevv™): Treatment of schizophrenia

I.M., short-acting (Zyprexa® IntraMuscular): Treatment of acute agitation associated with schizophrenia and bipolar I mania

Unlabeled Use Treatment of psychosis/schizophrenia in children; chronic pain; prevention of chemotherapy-associated delayed nausea or vomiting; psychosis/agitation related to Alzheimer's dementia; acute treatment of delirium

Mechanism of Action/Effect The efficacy of olanzapine in schizophrenia and bipolar disorder is thought to be mediated through combined antagonism of dopamine and serotonin type 2 receptor sites.

Contraindications There are no contraindications listed in the manufacturer's labeling.

Canadian labeling: Hypersensitivity to olanzapine or any component of the formulation

Warnings/Precautions [U.S. Boxed Warning]: Elderly patients with dementia-related psychosis treated with antipsychotics are at an increased risk of death compared to placebo. Most deaths appeared to be either cardiovascular (eg, heart failure, sudden death) or infectious (eg, pneumonia) in nature. In addition, an increased incidence of cerebrovascular effects (eg, transient ischemic attack, stroke) has been reported in studies of placebo-controlled trials of olanzapine in elderly patients with dementia-related psychosis. Olanzapine is not approved for the treatment of dementia-related psychosis.

Moderate to highly sedating, use with caution in disorders where CNS depression is a feature; patients must be cautioned about performing tasks which require mental alertness (eg, operating machinery or driving). Use caution in patients with cardiac disease. Use with caution in Parkinson's disease, predisposition to seizures, or severe hepatic or renal disease. Life-threatening arrhythmias have occurred with therapeutic doses of some neuroleptics. May induce orthostatic hypotension; use caution with history of cardiovascular disease, hemodynamic instability, prior myocardial infarction, or ischemic heart disease. Increases in cholesterol and triglycerides have been noted. Use with caution in patients with pre-existing abnormal lipid profile. Esophageal dysmotility and aspiration have been associated with antipsychotic use; use with caution in patients at risk of aspiration pneumonia. May increase prolactin levels; clinical significance of hyperprolactinemia in patients with breast cancer or other prolactin-dependent tumors is unknown. Significant weight gain (>7% of baseline weight) may occur; monitor waist circumference and BMI. Impaired core body temperature regulation may occur; caution with strenuous exercise, heat exposure, dehydration, and concomitant medication possessing anticholinergic effects.

Leukopenia, neutropenia, and agranulocytosis (sometimes fatal) have been reported in clinical trials and postmarketing reports with antipsychotic use; presence of risk factors (eg, pre-existing low WBC or history of drug-induced leuko-/neutropenia) should prompt periodic blood count assessment. Discontinue therapy at first signs of blood dyscrasias or if absolute neutrophil count $<1000/mm^3$.

May cause anticholinergic effects; use with caution in patients with decreased gastrointestinal motility, urinary retention, BPH, xerostomia, or narrow-angle glaucoma. Relative to other neuroleptics, olanzapine has a moderate potency of cholinergic blockade. May cause extrapyramidal symptoms (EPS), although risk of these reactions is lower relative to other neuroleptics. Risk of dystonia (and probably other EPS) may be greater with increased doses, use of conventional antipsychotics, males, and younger patients. May be associated with neuroleptic malignant syndrome (NMS). May cause extreme and life-threatening hyperglycemia; use with caution in patients with diabetes or other disorders of glucose regulation; monitor. Olanzapine levels may be lower in patients who smoke; the manufacturer does not require dosage adjustments, although dosage adjustments may be considered. Use in adolescent patients ≥13 years of age may result in increased weight gain and sedation, as well as greater increases in LDL cholesterol, total cholesterol, triglycerides, prolactin, and liver transaminase levels when compared to adults. Adolescent patients should be maintained on the lowest dose necessary.

The possibility of a suicide attempt is inherent in psychotic illness or bipolar disorder; use caution in high-risk patients during initiation of therapy. Prescriptions should be written for the smallest quantity consistent with good patient care.

There are two Zyprexa® formulations for intramuscular injection: Zyprexa® Relprevv™ is an extended-release formulation and Zyprexa® IntraMuscular is short-acting:

Extended-release I.M. injection (Zyprexa® Relprevv™): Monitor for post injection delirium/sedation syndrome; patients should be continuously watched (≥3 hours) for symptoms of olanzapine overdose. Only available through a restricted drug distribution program.

Short-acting I.M. injection (Zyprexa® IntraMuscular): Patients should remain recumbent if drowsy/dizzy until hypotension, bradycardia, and/or hypoventilation have been ruled out. Concurrent use of I.M./I.V. benzodiazepines is not recommended (fatalities have been reported, though causality not determined).

Drug Interactions

Avoid Concomitant Use

Avoid concomitant use of OLANZapine with any of the following: Benzodiazepines; Metoclopramide; Pimozide

Decreased Effect

OLANZapine may decrease the levels/effects of: Amphetamines; Anti-Parkinson's Agents (Dopamine Agonist); Quinagolide

The levels/effects of OLANZapine may be decreased by: CYP1A2 Inducers (Strong); Cyproterone; Lithium formulations; Peginterferon Alfa-2b

Increased Effect/Toxicity

OLANZapine may increase the levels/effects of: Alcohol (Ethyl); Anticholinergics; ARIPiprazole; Benzodiazepines; CNS Depressants; Methotrimeprazine; Methylphenidate; Pimozide; Serotonin Modulators

The levels/effects of OLANZapine may be increased by: Abiraterone Acetate; Acetylcholinesterase Inhibitors (Central); CYP1A2 Inhibitors (Moderate); CYP1A2 Inhibitors (Strong); Deferasirox; Droperidol; FluvoxaMINE; HydrOXYzine; LamoTRIgine; Lithium formulations; Methotrimeprazine; Methylphenidate; Metoclopramide; Pramlintide; Tetrabenazine

Nutritional/Ethanol Interactions

Ethanol: May increase CNS depression; monitor for increased effects with coadministration. Caution patients about effects.

Herb/Nutraceutical: Avoid dong quai, St John's wort (may also cause photosensitization). Avoid kava kava, gotu kola, valerian, St John's wort (may increase CNS depression).

Adverse Reactions

Oral: Unless otherwise noted, adverse events are reported for placebo-controlled trials in adult patients on monotherapy:

>10%:

Central nervous system: Somnolence (dose dependent; 20% to 39%; adolescents 39% to 48%), extrapyramidal symptoms (dose dependent; ≤32%), dizziness (11% to 18%), headache (adolescents 17%), fatigue (adolescents 3% to 14%), insomnia (12%)

Endocrine & metabolic: Prolactin increased (30%; adolescents 47%)

Gastrointestinal: Weight gain (5% to 6%, has been reported as high as 40%; adolescents 29% to 31%), appetite increased (3% to 6%; adolescents 17% to 29%), xerostomia (dose dependent; 3% to 22%), constipation (9% to 11%), dyspepsia (7% to 11%)

Hepatic: ALT increased ≥3 x ULN (adolescents 12%; adults 5%)

Neuromuscular & skeletal: Weakness (dose dependent; 8% to 20%)

Miscellaneous: Accidental injury (12%)

1% to 10%:

Cardiovascular: Chest pain, hypertension, peripheral edema, postural hypotension, tachycardia

Central nervous system: Fever, personality changes, restlessness (adolescents)

Dermatologic: Bruising

Endocrine & metabolic: Breast-related events ([adolescents] discharge, enlargement, galactorrhea, gynecomastia, lactation disorder); menstrual-related events (amenorrhea, hypomenorrhea, menstruation delayed, oligomenorrhea); sexual function-related events (anorgasmia, ejaculation delayed, erectile dysfunction, changes in libido, abnormal orgasm, sexual dysfunction)

Gastrointestinal: Abdominal pain (adolescents), diarrhea (adolescents), flatulence, nausea (dose dependent), vomiting

Genitourinary: Incontinence, UTI

Hepatic: Hepatic enzymes increased

Neuromuscular & skeletal: Abnormal gait, akathisia, articulation impairment, back pain, falling, hypertonia, joint/extremity pain, muscle stiffness (adolescents), tremor (dose dependent)

Ocular: Amblyopia

Respiratory: Cough, epistaxis (adolescents), pharyngitis, respiratory tract infection (adolescents), rhinitis, sinusitis (adolescents)

Injection: Unless otherwise noted, adverse events are reported for placebo-controlled trials in adult patients on extended-release I.M. injection (Zyprexa® Relprevv™). Also refer to adverse reactions noted with oral therapy.

>10%: Central nervous system: Headache (13% to 18%), sedation (8% to 13%)

1% to 10%:

Cardiovascular: Hypertension, hypotension (short-acting), postural hypotension (short-acting), QT prolongation

Central nervous system: Abnormal dreams, abnormal thinking, auditory hallucination, dizziness, dysarthria, extrapyramidal symptoms, fatigue, fever, pain, restlessness, somnolence

Dermatologic: Acne

Gastrointestinal: Abdominal pain, appetite increased, diarrhea, flatulence, nausea, vomiting, weight gain, xerostomia

Genitourinary: Vaginal discharge

Hepatic: Liver enzymes increased

Local: Injection site pain

Neuromuscular & skeletal: Arthralgia, back pain, muscle spasms, stiffness, tremor, weakness (short-acting)

Otic: Ear pain

Respiratory: Cough, nasal congestion, nasopharyngitis, pharyngolaryngeal pain, sneezing, upper respiratory tract infection

Miscellaneous: Toothache, tooth infection, viral infection

<1%, postmarketing, and/or case reports (limited to important or life-threatening): CPK increased, post-injection delirium/sedation syndrome, syncope (short-acting)

Available Dosage Forms

Injection, powder for reconstitution:

ZyPREXA® IntraMuscular: 10 mg

Injection, powder for suspension, extended release:

ZyPREXA® Relprevv™: 210 mg, 300 mg, 405 mg

Tablet, oral: 2.5 mg, 5 mg, 7.5 mg, 10 mg, 15 mg, 20 mg

ZyPREXA®: 2.5 mg, 5 mg, 7.5 mg, 10 mg, 15 mg, 20 mg

Tablet, orally disintegrating, oral: 5 mg, 10 mg, 15 mg, 20 mg

ZyPREXA® Zydis®: 5 mg, 10 mg, 15 mg, 20 mg

General Dosage Range

I.M.: *Adults:*

Extended release: 150-300 mg every 2 weeks **or** 300-405 mg every 4 weeks (maximum: 300 mg every 2 weeks; 405 mg every 4 weeks)

Short-acting: Initial: 10 mg/dose; 2-4 hours between doses (maximum: 30 mg/day)

Oral:

Adolescents ≥13 years: Initial: 2.5-5 mg once daily; dosing range: 2.5-20 mg/day

Adults: Initial: 5-15 mg once daily; Maintenance: 5-20 mg once daily

Elderly: Initial: 2.5-5 mg/day

Administration

Oral

Tablet: May be administered without regard to meals.

Orally-disintegrating tablet: Remove from foil blister by peeling back (do not push tablet through the foil). Place tablet in mouth immediately upon removal. Tablet dissolves rapidly in saliva and may be swallowed with or without liquid. May be administered with or without food/meals.

I.M.

Short-acting I.M. injection: **For I.M. administration only**; do not administer injection intravenously or subcutaneously; inject slowly, deep into muscle. If dizziness and/or drowsiness are noted, patient should remain recumbent until examination indicates postural hypotension and/or bradycardia are not a problem.

Extended-release I.M. injection: **For I.M. gluteal injection only**; do not administer I.V. or subcutaneously. After needle insertion into muscle, aspirate to verify that no blood appears. Do not massage injection site. Use diluent, syringes, and needles provided in convenience kit; obtain a new kit if aspiration of blood occurs.

Stability

Reconstitution

Injection, extended-release: Dilute as directed to final concentration of 150 mg/mL. Shake vigorously to mix; will form yellow, opaque suspension. Following reconstitution, suspension may be stored at room temperature and used within 24 hours. Shake vigorously to resuspend prior to administration. Use immediately once suspension is in syringe. Suspension may be irritating to skin; wear gloves during reconstitution.

Injection, short-acting: Reconstitute 10 mg vial with 2.1 mL SWFI. Resulting solution is ~5 mg/mL. Use immediately (within 1 hour) following reconstitution. Discard any unused portion.

Storage

Injection, extended-release: Store at 20°C to 25°C (68°F to 77°F); excursions permitted to 15°C to 30°C (59°F to 86°F).

Injection, short-acting: Store at 20°C to 25°C (68°F to 77°F); excursions permitted to 15°C to 30°C (59°F to 86°F); do not freeze. Protect from light.

Tablet and orally-disintegrating tablet: Store at 20°C to 25°C (68°F to 77°F); excursions permitted to 15°C to 30°C (59°F to 86°F). Protect from light and moisture.

Nursing Actions

Physical Assessment Initiate at lower doses. Taper dosage slowly when discontinuing. Instruct patients with diabetes to monitor blood glucose levels closely; may cause hyperglycemia. Assess for extrapyramidal symptoms, suicide ideation, sedation, CNS changes, and neuroleptic malignant syndrome prior to treatment and periodically throughout. Monitor weight prior to initiating therapy and at least monthly. If Zyprexa® Relprevv™ is administered, monitor closely for at least 3 hours for symptoms of oversedation and/or delirium.

Patient Education It may take 2-3 weeks to achieve desired results. Avoid alcohol. Maintain adequate hydration. If you have diabetes, you may experience increased blood sugars; monitor closely. If you have glaucoma, periodic ophthalmic exams are recommended. You may experience excess drowsiness, restlessness, weakness, dizziness, or blurred vision; postural hypotension; constipation; heartburn; dry mouth; or weight gain. Report persistent CNS effects (eg, trembling fingers, altered gait or balance, excessive sedation, seizures, unusual movements, anxiety, abnormal thoughts, confusion, personality changes); suicide ideation; unresolved constipation or GI effects; vision changes; respiratory difficulty; unusual cough; or worsening of condition.

Orally-disintegrating tablet: Remove from foil blister by peeling back; do not push tablet through the foil. Place tablet in mouth immediately upon removal. Tablet dissolves rapidly in saliva and may be swallowed with or without liquid.

Dietary Considerations Tablets may be taken without regard to meals. Some products may contain phenylalanine.

Olanzapine and Fluoxetine

(oh LAN za peen & floo OKS e teen)

Brand Names: U.S. Symbyax®

Index Terms Fluoxetine and Olanzapine; Olanzapine and Fluoxetine Hydrochloride

Pharmacologic Category Antidepressant, Selective Serotonin Reuptake Inhibitor; Antipsychotic Agent, Atypical

Medication Safety Issues

Sound-alike/look-alike issues:

Symbyax® may be confused with Cymbalta®

Medication Guide Available Yes

Pregnancy Risk Factor C

Lactation Enters breast milk/not recommended

Use Treatment of depressive episodes associated with bipolar I disorder; treatment-resistant depression (unresponsive to 2 trials of different antidepressants in the current episode)

Available Dosage Forms

Capsule, oral:

Symbyax®:

3/25: Olanzapine 3 mg and fluoxetine 25 mg

6/25: Olanzapine 6 mg and fluoxetine 25 mg

6/50: Olanzapine 6 mg and fluoxetine 50 mg

12/25: Olanzapine 12 mg and fluoxetine 25 mg

12/50: Olanzapine 12 mg and fluoxetine 50 mg

General Dosage Range Dosage adjustment recommended in patients with hepatic impairment

Oral:

Adults: Initial: Olanzapine 6 mg and fluoxetine 25 mg once daily; Maintenance: Olanzapine 6-12 mg and fluoxetine 25-50 mg once daily

Elderly >65 years: Initial: Olanzapine 3-6 mg and fluoxetine 25 mg once daily

Administration

Oral Capsules should be taken once daily in the evening. May be taken without regard to meals.

Nursing Actions

Physical Assessment See individual agents.

Patient Education See individual agents.

Related Information
FLUoxetine *on page 495*
OLANZapine *on page 845*

Olmesartan (ole me SAR tan)

Brand Names: U.S. Benicar®

Index Terms Olmesartan Medoxomil

Pharmacologic Category Angiotensin II Receptor Blocker

Medication Safety Issues

Sound-alike/look-alike issues:
Benicar® may be confused with Mevacor®

Pregnancy Risk Factor C (1st trimester); D (2nd and 3rd trimesters)

Lactation Excretion in breast milk unknown/not recommended

Use Treatment of hypertension with or without concurrent use of other antihypertensive agents

Mechanism of Action/Effect As a selective and competitive, nonpeptide angiotensin II receptor antagonist, olmesartan blocks the vasoconstrictor and aldosterone-secreting effects of angiotensin II. Olmesartan increases urinary flow rate and in addition to being natriuretic and kaliuretic, increases excretion of chloride, magnesium, uric acid, calcium, and phosphate.

Contraindications There are no contraindications listed in the manufacturer's labeling.

Warnings/Precautions [U.S. Boxed Warning]: Drugs that act on the renin-angiotensin system can cause injury and death to the developing fetus. Discontinue as soon as possible once pregnancy is detected. May cause hyperkalemia; avoid potassium supplementation unless specifically required by healthcare provider. Avoid use or use a smaller dose in patients who are volume depleted; correct depletion first. May be associated with deterioration of renal function and/or increases in serum creatinine, particularly in patients with low renal blood flow (eg, renal artery stenosis, heart failure) whose glomerular filtration rate (GFR) is dependent on efferent arteriolar vasoconstriction by angiotensin II. Use with caution in unstented unilateral/bilateral renal artery stenosis. When unstented bilateral renal artery stenosis is present, use is generally avoided due to the elevated risk of deterioration in renal function unless possible benefits outweigh risks. Use with caution with preexisting renal insufficiency; significant aortic/mitral stenosis. Concurrent use of ACE inhibitors may increase the risk of clinically-significant adverse events (eg, renal dysfunction, hyperkalemia).

Drug Interactions

Avoid Concomitant Use There are no known interactions where it is recommended to avoid concomitant use.

Decreased Effect

The levels/effects of Olmesartan may be decreased by: Herbs (Hypertensive Properties); Methylphenidate; Nonsteroidal Anti-Inflammatory Agents; Yohimbine

Increased Effect/Toxicity

Olmesartan may increase the levels/effects of: ACE Inhibitors; Amifostine; Antihypertensives; Hypotensive Agents; Lithium; Nonsteroidal Anti-Inflammatory Agents; Potassium-Sparing Diuretics; RiTUXimab; Sodium Phosphates

The levels/effects of Olmesartan may be increased by: Alfuzosin; Diazoxide; Eltrombopag; Eplerenone; Herbs (Hypotensive Properties); MAO Inhibitors; Pentoxifylline; Phosphodiesterase 5 Inhibitors; Potassium Salts; Prostacyclin Analogues; Tolvaptan; Trimethoprim

Nutritional/Ethanol Interactions

Food: Does not affect olmesartan bioavailability. Potassium supplements and/or potassium-containing salts may cause or worsen hyperkalemia. Management: Consult prescriber before consuming a potassium-rich diet, potassium supplements, or salt substitutes.

Herb/Nutraceutical: Some herbal medications may worsen hypertension (eg, licorice); others may increase the antihypertensive effect of olmesartan (eg, shepherd's purse). Management: Avoid bayberry, blue cohosh, cayenne, ephedra, ginger, ginseng (American), kola, licorice, and yohimbe. Avoid black cohosh, California poppy, coleus, golden seal, hawthorn, mistletoe, periwinkle, quinine, and shepherd's purse.

Adverse Reactions 1% to 10%:

Central nervous system: Dizziness (3%), headache

Endocrine & metabolic: Hyperglycemia, hypertriglyceridemia

Gastrointestinal: Diarrhea

Neuromuscular & skeletal: Back pain, CPK increased

Renal: Hematuria

Respiratory: Bronchitis, pharyngitis, rhinitis, sinusitis

Miscellaneous: Flu-like syndrome

Available Dosage Forms

Tablet, oral:

Benicar®: 5 mg, 20 mg, 40 mg

General Dosage Range Oral:

Children 6-16 years:

20 kg to <35 kg: Initial: 10 mg once daily (maximum: 20 mg once daily)

≥35 kg: Initial: 20 mg once daily (maximum: 40 mg once daily)

Adolescents >16 years and Adults: Initial: 20 mg once daily; Maintenance: 20-40 mg once daily

Elderly: Initial: 5-20 mg once daily

Administration

Oral May be administered with or without food.

Stability

Storage Store at 20°C to 25°C (68°F to 77°F).

Nursing Actions

Physical Assessment Monitor blood pressure. Monitor for tachycardia, hypotension, diarrhea, and bronchitis on a regular basis throughout therapy. Instruct patients with diabetes to monitor glucose levels closely (may cause hyperglycemia).

Patient Education Do not use potassium supplement or salt substitutes without consulting prescriber. May be taken with or without food. This drug does not eliminate the need for diet or exercise regimen as recommended by prescriber. If you have diabetes, check glucose levels closely (drug may alter glucose levels). May cause headache or dizziness, diarrhea, or back or joint pain. Report chest pain or palpitations, unrelieved headache, or flu-like symptoms or upper respiratory infection.

Dietary Considerations May be taken with or without food.

Olmesartan and Hydrochlorothiazide

(ole me SAR tan & hye droe klor oh THYE a zide)

Brand Names: U.S. Benicar HCT®

Index Terms Hydrochlorothiazide and Olmesartan Medoxomil; Olmesartan Medoxomil and Hydrochlorothiazide

Pharmacologic Category Angiotensin II Receptor Blocker; Diuretic, Thiazide

Pregnancy Risk Factor D

Lactation Enters breast milk/contraindicated

Use Treatment of hypertension (not recommended for initial treatment)

Available Dosage Forms

Tablet:

Benicar HCT®: 20/12.5: Olmesartan 20 mg and hydrochlorothiazide 12.5 mg; 40/12.5: Olmesartan 40 mg and hydrochlorothiazide 12.5 mg; 40/25: Olmesartan 40 mg and hydrochlorothiazide 25 mg

General Dosage Range Oral: *Adults:* Olmesartan 20-40 mg and hydrochlorothiazide 12.5-25 mg once daily (maximum: 25 mg/day [hydrochlorothiazide]; 40 mg/day [olmesartan])

Nursing Actions

Physical Assessment See individual agents.

Patient Education See individual agents.

Related Information

Hydrochlorothiazide *on page 570*
Olmesartan *on page 849*

Olopatadine (Nasal)

(oh la PAT a deen)

Brand Names: U.S. Patanase®

Index Terms Olopatadine Hydrochloride

Pharmacologic Category Histamine H_1 Antagonist; Histamine H_1 Antagonist, Second Generation; Piperidine Derivative

Pregnancy Risk Factor C

Lactation Excretion in breast milk unknown/use caution

Use Treatment of the symptoms of seasonal allergic rhinitis

Available Dosage Forms

Solution, intranasal:

Patanase®: 0.6% (30.5 g)

General Dosage Range Intranasal: *Children ≥12 years and Adults:* 2 sprays into each nostril twice daily

Administration

Inhalation For intranasal use only. Before initial use of the nasal spray, the delivery system should be primed with 5 sprays or until a fine mist appears. If 7 or more days have elapsed since last use, the delivery system should be reprimed with 2 sprays or until a fine mist appears. Blow nose to clear nostrils. Keep head tilted downward when spraying. Insert applicator into nostril, keeping bottle upright, and close off the other nostril. Breathe in through nose. While inhaling, press pump to release spray. Alternate sprays between nostrils. After each use, wipe the spray tip with a clean tissue or cloth.

Nursing Actions

Physical Assessment Assess nasal mucosa periodically for ulceration.

Patient Education May cause drowsiness or bitter taste. Avoid alcohol use. Report ulcers or discomfort in nose.

Olopatadine (Ophthalmic)

(oh la PAT a deen)

Brand Names: U.S. Pataday™; Patanol®

Index Terms Olopatadine Hydrochloride

Pharmacologic Category Histamine H_1 Antagonist; Histamine H_1 Antagonist, Second Generation; Piperidine Derivative

Medication Safety Issues

Sound-alike/look-alike issues:

Patanol® may be confused with Platinol

International issues:

Patanol [U.S., Canada, and multiple international markets] may be confused with Bétanol brand name for metipranolol [Monaco]

Pregnancy Risk Factor C

Lactation Excretion in breast milk unknown/use caution

Use Treatment of the signs and symptoms of allergic conjunctivitis

Available Dosage Forms

Solution, ophthalmic:

Pataday™: 0.2% (2.5 mL)

Patanol®: 0.1% (5 mL)

General Dosage Range Ophthalmic: *Children ≥3 years and Adults:* Patanol®: Instill 1 drop into affected eye(s) twice daily; Pataday™: Instill 1 drop into affected eye(s) once daily

Administration

Other For topical ophthalmic use only. After instilling drops, wait at least 10 minutes before inserting contact lenses. Do not insert contacts if eyes are red.

Nursing Actions

Patient Education For use in eyes only. Do not let tip of applicator touch eye; do not contaminate tip of applicator (may cause eye infection, eye damage, or vision loss). Do not wear contact lenses if eyes are red. Can cause cold-like symptoms and headache.

Olsalazine (ole SAL a zeen)

Brand Names: U.S. Dipentum®

Index Terms Olsalazine Sodium

Pharmacologic Category 5-Aminosalicylic Acid Derivative

Medication Safety Issues

Sound-alike/look-alike issues:

Olsalazine may be confused with OLANZapine

Dipentum® may be confused with Dilantin®

Pregnancy Risk Factor C

Lactation Enters breast milk/not recommended

Use Maintenance of remission of ulcerative colitis in patients intolerant to sulfasalazine

Available Dosage Forms

Capsule, oral:

Dipentum®: 250 mg

General Dosage Range Oral: *Adults:* 1 g/day in 2 divided doses

Administration

Oral Administer with food in evenly divided doses.

Nursing Actions

Physical Assessment Assess allergy history before initiating therapy (salicylates, sulfasalazine, or mesalamine). Monitor for reduction of clinical signs of ulcerative colitis. Monitor for diarrhea.

Patient Education Take with meals, in evenly divided doses. May cause flu-like symptoms or muscle pain, diarrhea, nausea, or loss of appetite. Report persistent diarrhea or abdominal cramping, or skin rash or itching.

Omalizumab (oh mah lye ZOO mab)

Brand Names: U.S. Xolair®

Index Terms rhuMAb-E25

Pharmacologic Category Monoclonal Antibody, Anti-Asthmatic

Medication Safety Issues

Sound-alike/look-alike issues:

Omalizumab may be confused with ofatumumab

Medication Guide Available Yes

Pregnancy Risk Factor B

Lactation Excretion in breast milk unknown/use caution

Breast-Feeding Considerations IgG is excreted in human milk and excretion of omalizumab is expected. Effects to nursing infant are not known; use with caution.

Use Treatment of moderate-to-severe, persistent allergic asthma not adequately controlled with inhaled corticosteroids

Mechanism of Action/Effect Blocks the binding of IgE to mast cells and basophils, decreasing the allergic response, corticosteroid usage, and asthma exacerbations.

Contraindications Hypersensitivity to omalizumab or any component of the formulation; acute bronchospasm, status asthmaticus

Warnings/Precautions [U.S. Boxed Warning]: Anaphylaxis, including delayed-onset anaphylaxis, has been reported following administration; reactions usually occur within 2 hours of administration, but may occur up to 24 hours and in some cases >1 year after initiation of regular treatment. Patients should receive treatment only under direct medical supervision and be observed for a minimum of 2 hours following administration; appropriate medications for the treatment of anaphylactic reactions should be available. Hypersensitivity reactions may occur following any dose, even during chronic therapy; discontinue therapy following any severe reaction.

For use in patients with a documented reactivity to a perennial aeroallergen and with symptoms uncontrolled using inhaled corticosteroids; not used to control acute asthma symptoms. Dosing is based on pretreatment IgE serum levels and body weight. IgE levels remain elevated up to 1 year following treatment, therefore, levels taken during treatment cannot be used as a dosage guide. Corticosteroid therapy should be tapered gradually, do not discontinue abruptly. Malignant neoplasms have been reported with use in short-term studies; impact of long-term use is not known. Use caution with and monitor patients at risk for parasitic (helminth) infections (risk of infection may be increased). Safety and efficacy in children <12 years of age have not been established.

Drug Interactions

Avoid Concomitant Use

Avoid concomitant use of Omalizumab with any of the following: BCG; Natalizumab; Pimecrolimus; Tacrolimus (Topical); Vaccines (Live)

Decreased Effect

Omalizumab may decrease the levels/effects of: BCG; Coccidioidin Skin Test; Sipuleucel-T; Vaccines (Inactivated); Vaccines (Live)

The levels/effects of Omalizumab may be decreased by: Echinacea

Increased Effect/Toxicity

Omalizumab may increase the levels/effects of: Leflunomide; Natalizumab; Vaccines (Live)

The levels/effects of Omalizumab may be increased by: Denosumab; Pimecrolimus; Roflumilast; Tacrolimus (Topical); Trastuzumab

Adverse Reactions

>10%:

Central nervous system: Headache (15%)

Local: Injection site reaction (45%; placebo 43%; severe 12%). Most reactions occurred within 1 hour, lasted <8 days, and decreased in frequency with additional dosing.

Respiratory: Upper respiratory tract infection (20%), sinusitis (16%), pharyngitis (11%)

Miscellaneous: Viral infection (23%)

1% to 10%:

Central nervous system: Pain (7%), fatigue (3%), dizziness (3%)

Dermatologic: Dermatitis (2%), pruritus (2%)

Neuromuscular & skeletal: Arthralgia (8%), leg pain (4%), arm pain (2%), fracture (2%)

Otic: Earache (2%)

Available Dosage Forms

Injection, powder for reconstitution:

Xolair®: 150 mg

General Dosage Range SubQ:

IgE ≥30-100 int. units/mL:

Children ≥12 years and Adults 30-90 kg: 150 mg every 4 weeks

Children ≥12 years and Adults >90-150 kg: 300 mg every 4 weeks

IgE >100-200 int. units/mL:

Children ≥12 years and Adults 30-90 kg: 300 mg every 4 weeks

Children ≥12 years and Adults >90-150 kg: 225 mg every 2 weeks

IgE >200-300 int. units/mL:

Children ≥12 years and Adults 30-60 kg: 300 mg every 4 weeks

Children ≥12 years and Adults >60-90 kg: 225 mg every 2 weeks

Children ≥12 years and Adults >90-150 kg: 300 mg every 2 weeks

IgE >300-400 int. units/mL:

Children ≥12 years and Adults 30-70 kg: 225 mg every 2 weeks

Children ≥12 years and Adults >70-90 kg: 300 mg every 2 weeks

IgE >400-500 int. units/mL:

Children ≥12 years and Adults 30-70 kg: 300 mg every 2 weeks

Children ≥12 years and Adults >70-90 kg: 375 mg every 2 weeks

IgE >500-600 int. units/mL:

Children ≥12 years and Adults 30-60 kg: 300 mg every 2 weeks

Children ≥12 years and Adults >60-70 kg: 375 mg every 2 weeks

IgE >600-700 int. units/mL: *Children ≥12 years and Adults 30-60 kg:* 375 mg every 2 weeks

Administration

Other For SubQ injection only; doses >150 mg should divided over more than one site. Injections may take 5-10 seconds to administer. Administer only under direct medical supervision and observe patient for a minimum of 2 hours following administration of any dose given.

Stability

Reconstitution Prepare using SWFI, USP only; add SWFI 1.4 mL to upright vial and swirl gently for 5-10 seconds every 5 minutes until dissolved; may take >20 minutes to dissolve completely. Resulting solution is 150 mg/1.2 mL. Do not use if powder takes >40 minutes to dissolve.

Storage Prior to reconstitution, store under refrigeration at 2°C to 8°C (36°F to 46°F); product may be shipped at room temperature. Following reconstitution, protect from direct sunlight. May be stored for up to 8 hours if refrigerated or 4 hours if stored at room temperature.

Nursing Actions

Physical Assessment For SubQ use only. Evaluate pulmonary function tests at baseline and as necessary with treatment. Anaphylactic reactions have been reported within 2-24 hours of initial dose; monitor patient for a minimum of 2 hours following injection; appropriate medications for the treatment of hypersensitivity reactions should be available. Monitor for hypersensitivity reaction, upper respiratory tract infection, viral infection, dermatitis, and arthralgia at beginning of and periodically during therapy.

Patient Education This medication is administered by injection and you will be closely monitored for some time following injection. Report immediately any sign of allergic response (redness, swelling, pain or itching at injection site; chest pain or tightness; difficulty breathing or swallowing; swelling of mouth or tongue; skin rash). If allergic response occurs, follow prescriber's directions for contacting emergency treatment immediately. May cause headache; dizziness; or joint, bone, or ear pain. Report unusual or increased respiratory difficulty, signs of infection, or skin rash.

Omega-3-Acid Ethyl Esters

(oh MEG a three AS id ETH il ES ters)

Brand Names: U.S. Lovaza®

Index Terms Ethyl Esters of Omega-3 Fatty Acids; Fish Oil; Omega 3; P-OM3

Pharmacologic Category Antilipemic Agent, Miscellaneous

Medication Safety Issues

Sound-alike/look-alike issues:

Lovaza® may be confused with LORazepam

International issues:

Omacor [multiple international markets] may be confused with Amicar brand name for aminocaproic acid [U.S.]

Other safety concerns:

The Institute for Safe Medication Practices (ISMP) reported a case of a foam plastic cup dissolving after contact with the liquid contents from a Lovaza® capsule. ISMP is requesting the manufacturer to add warnings to its labeling and that healthcare providers add Lovaza® to their list of medications to not crush.

Pregnancy Risk Factor C

Lactation Excretion in breast milk unknown/use caution

Use Lovaza®: Adjunct to diet therapy in the treatment of hypertriglyceridemia (≥500 mg/dL)

Note: A number of OTC formulations containing omega-3 fatty acids are marketed as nutritional supplements; these do not have FDA-approved indications and may not contain the same amounts of the active ingredient.

Unlabeled Use Lovaza®: Treatment of IgA nephropathy

Available Dosage Forms

Capsule, liquid gel, oral:

Lovaza®: 1 g

General Dosage Range Oral: *Adults:* 4 g/day in 1-2 divided doses

Administration

Oral May be administered with or without food. Administer whole, do not crush.

Nursing Actions

Physical Assessment Do not use if allergic to fish. Encourage diet and exercise along with use of this medication.

Patient Education Do not use if allergic to fish. This medication should be used in addition to diet and exercise. Avoid alcohol use; significant use may increase triglycerides. You may experience flu-like syndrome, fever, burping, or an upset stomach.

Omeprazole (oh MEP ra zole)

Brand Names: U.S. First®-Omeprazole; PriLOSEC OTC® [OTC]; PriLOSEC®

Index Terms Omeprazole Magnesium

Pharmacologic Category Proton Pump Inhibitor; Substituted Benzimidazole

Medication Safety Issues

Sound-alike/look-alike issues:

Omeprazole may be confused with aripiprazole, fomepizole

PriLOSEC® may be confused with Plendil®, Prevacid®, predniSONE, prilocaine, Prinivil®, Proventil®, PROzac®

International issues:

Losec [multiple international markets] may be confused with Lasix brand name for furosemide [U.S., Canada, and multiple international markets]

Medral [Mexico] may be confused with Medrol brand name for methylprednisolone [U.S., Canada, and multiple international markets]

Norpramin: Brand name for omeprazole [Spain], but also the brand name for desipramine [U.S., Canada] and enalapril/hydrochlorothiazide [Portugal]

Pregnancy Risk Factor C

Lactation Enters breast milk/not recommended

Breast-Feeding Considerations Following administration of omeprazole 20 mg, peak concentrations detected in the breast milk were <7% of the maternal serum concentration.

Use Short-term (4-8 weeks) treatment of active duodenal ulcer disease or active benign gastric ulcer; treatment of heartburn and other symptoms associated with gastroesophageal reflux disease (GERD); short-term (4-8 weeks) treatment of endoscopically-diagnosed erosive esophagitis; maintenance healing of erosive esophagitis; long-term treatment of pathological hypersecretory conditions; as part of a multidrug regimen for *H. pylori* eradication to reduce the risk of duodenal ulcer recurrence

OTC labeling: Short-term treatment of frequent, uncomplicated heartburn occurring ≥2 days/week

Unlabeled Use Healing NSAID-induced ulcers; prevention of NSAID-induced ulcer; stress-ulcer prophylaxis in the critically-ill

Mechanism of Action/Effect Proton pump inhibitor; suppresses gastric basal and stimulated acid secretion by inhibiting the parietal cell H+/K+ ATP pump

Contraindications Hypersensitivity to omeprazole, substituted benzimidazoles (eg, esomeprazole, lansoprazole), or any component of the formulation

Warnings/Precautions Use of proton pump inhibitors (PPIs) may increase the risk of gastrointestinal infections (eg, *Salmonella, Campylobacter*). Relief of symptoms does not preclude the presence of a gastric malignancy. Atrophic gastritis (by biopsy) has been noted with long-term omeprazole therapy. In long-term (2-year) studies in rats, omeprazole produced a dose-related increase in gastric carcinoid tumors. While available endoscopic evaluations and histologic examinations of biopsy specimens from human stomachs have not detected a risk from short-term exposure to omeprazole, further human data on the effect of sustained hypochlorhydria and hypergastrinemia are needed to rule out the possibility of an increased risk for the development of tumors in humans receiving long-term therapy.

PPIs may diminish the therapeutic effect of clopidogrel, thought to be due to reduced formation of the active metabolite of clopidogrel. The manufacturer of clopidogrel recommends either avoidance of omeprazole (even when scheduled 12 hours apart) or use of a PPI with less potent CYP2C19 inhibition (eg, pantoprazole). Others have recommended the continued use of PPIs, regardless of the degree of inhibition, in patients with a history of GI bleeding or multiple risk factors for GI bleeding who are also receiving clopidogrel since no evidence has established clinically meaningful differences in outcome; however, a clinically-significant interaction cannot be excluded in those who are poor metabolizers of clopidogrel (Abraham, 2010; Levine, 2011). Avoid concurrent use of CYP3A4 and 2C19 inducers (eg, St John's wort, rifampin) as omeprazole's efficacy may be reduced.

Increased incidence of osteoporosis-related bone fractures of the hip, spine, or wrist may occur with PPI therapy. Patients on high-dose (multiple daily doses)or long-term (≥1 year) therapy should be monitored. Use the lowest effective dose for the shortest duration of time, use vitamin D and calcium supplementation, and follow appropriate guidelines to reduce risk of fractures in patients at risk.

Hypomagnesemia, reported rarely, usually with prolonged PPI use of >3 months (most cases >1 year of therapy); may be symptomatic or asymptomatic; severe cases may cause tetany, seizures, and cardiac arrhythmias. Consider obtaining serum magnesium concentrations prior to beginning long-term therapy, especially if taking concomitant digoxin, diuretics, or other drugs known to cause hypomagnesemia; and periodically thereafter. Hypomagnesemia may be corrected by magnesium supplementation, although discontinuation of omeprazole may be necessary; magnesium levels typically return to normal within 1 week of stopping. Serum chromogranin A levels may be increased if assessed while patient on omeprazole; may lead to diagnostic errors related to neuroendocrine tumors.

Decreased *H. pylori* eradication rates have been observed with short-term (≤7 days) combination therapy. The American College of Gastroenterology recommends 10-14 days of therapy (triple or quadruple) for eradication of *H. pylori* (Chey, 2007). Bioavailability may be increased in Asian populations and patients with hepatic dysfunction; consider dosage reductions, especially for maintenance healing of erosive esophagitis. Bioavailability may be increased in the elderly. When used for self-medication (OTC), do not use for >14 days.

Drug Interactions

Avoid Concomitant Use

Avoid concomitant use of Omeprazole with any of the following: Clopidogrel; Delavirdine; Erlotinib; Nelfinavir; Pimozide; Posaconazole; Rifampin; Rilpivirine; St Johns Wort

Decreased Effect

Omeprazole may decrease the levels/effects of: Atazanavir; Bisphosphonate Derivatives; Cefditoren; Clopidogrel; CloZAPine; Dabigatran Etexilate; Dasatinib; Delavirdine; Erlotinib; Gefitinib; Indinavir; Iron Salts; Itraconazole; Ketoconazole; Ketoconazole (Systemic); Mesalamine; Mycophenolate; Nelfinavir; Posaconazole; Rilpivirine; Vismodegib

The levels/effects of Omeprazole may be decreased by: CYP2C19 Inducers (Strong); Peginterferon Alfa-2b; Rifampin; St Johns Wort; Tipranavir; Tocilizumab

Increased Effect/Toxicity

Omeprazole may increase the levels/effects of: Amphetamines; ARIPiprazole; Benzodiazepines (metabolized by oxidation); Carvedilol; Cilostazol; Citalopram; CloZAPine; CycloSPORINE; CycloSPORINE (Systemic); CYP2C19 Substrates; CYP2C9 Substrates; Dexmethylphenidate; Fosphenytoin; Methotrexate; Methylphenidate; Phenytoin; Pimozide; Raltegravir; Saquinavir; Tacrolimus; Tacrolimus (Systemic); Vitamin K Antagonists; Voriconazole

The levels/effects of Omeprazole may be increased by: Conivaptan; Fluconazole; Ketoconazole; Ketoconazole (Systemic)

Nutritional/Ethanol Interactions

Ethanol: Avoid ethanol (may cause gastric mucosal irritation).

Food: Food delays absorption.

Herb/Nutraceutical: Avoid use of St John's wort (may decrease efficacy of omeprazole).

Adverse Reactions 1% to 10%:

Central nervous system: Headache (7%), dizziness (2%)

Dermatologic: Rash (2%)

Gastrointestinal: Abdominal pain (5%), diarrhea (4%), nausea (4%), vomiting (3%), flatulence (3%), acid regurgitation (2%), constipation (2%)

Neuromuscular & skeletal: Back pain (1%), weakness (1%)

Respiratory: Upper respiratory infection (2%), cough (1%)

Pharmacodynamics/Kinetics

Onset of Action Antisecretory: ~1 hour; Peak effect: Within 2 hours

Duration of Action Up to 72 hours; 50% of maximum effect at 24 hours; after stopping treatment, secretory activity gradually returns over 3-5 days

Available Dosage Forms

Capsule, delayed release, oral: 10 mg, 20 mg, 40 mg

PriLOSEC®: 10 mg, 20 mg, 40 mg

Granules for suspension, delayed release, oral:

PriLOSEC®: 2.5 mg/packet (30s); 10 mg/packet (30s)

Powder for suspension, oral:

First®-Omeprazole: 2 mg/mL (90 mL, 150 mL, 300 mL)

Tablet, delayed release, oral: 20 mg

PriLOSEC OTC® [OTC]: 20 mg

General Dosage Range Oral:

Children 1-16 years and 5 kg to <10 kg: 5 mg once daily

Children 1-16 years and 10 kg to <20 kg: 10 mg once daily

Children 1-16 years and ≥20 kg: 20 mg once daily

Adults: 20-40 mg/day (may be given in 2 divided doses); doses up to 360 mg/day [pathological hypersecretory syndrome]

Administration

Oral Best if administered before breakfast.

Capsule: Should be swallowed whole; do not chew or crush. Delayed release capsule may be opened and contents added to 1 tablespoon of applesauce (use immediately after adding to applesauce); mixture should not be chewed or warmed.

Oral suspension: Following reconstitution, the suspension should be left to thicken for 2-3 minutes and administered within 30 minutes. If any material remains after administration, add more water, stir, and administer immediately.

Tablet: Should be swallowed whole; do not crush or chew.

Other Nasogastric/orogastric (NG/OG) tube administration:

Capsule: When using capsules to extemporaneously prepare a solution for NG/OG administration, the manufacturers of Prilosec® recommend the use of an acidic juice for preparation and administration. Alternative methods have been described as follows:

NG/OG tube administration for the prevention of stress-related mucosal damage in ventilated, critically-ill patients:

Study 1 (Phillips, 1996): Pour the contents of one or two 20 mg omeprazole delayed release capsules (depending on the dose) into a syringe (after removing plunger); withdraw 10-20 mL of an 8.4% sodium bicarbonate solution into the syringe; allow 30 minutes for the enteric-coated omeprazole granules to break down. Shake the resulting milky substance prior to administration. Flush the NG tube with 5-10 mL of water and clamp for at least 1 hour.

Study 2 (Balaban, 1997): Open the omeprazole delayed release capsule (20 mg or 40 mg), then pour the intact granules into a container holding 30 mL of water. Pour one-third to one-half of the granules into a 30 mL syringe (with the plunger removed) attached to a nasogastric tube (NG). Replace the plunger with 1 cm of air between the granules and the plunger top while the plunger is depressed. Repeat this process until all the granules are flushed, then flush a final 15 mL of water through the tube.

Oral suspension: Following reconstitution in a catheter-tipped syringe, shake the suspension well and leave to thicken for 2-3 minutes. Administer within 30 minutes of reconstitution. Use an NG tube or gastric tube that is a size 6 French or larger; flush the syringe and tube with water.

Stability

Reconstitution Granules for oral suspension: For oral administration, empty the contents of the 2.5 mg packet into 5 mL of water (10 mg packet into 15 mL of water); stir. For NG administration, add 5 mL of water into a catheter-tipped syringe, and then add the contents of a 2.5 mg packet (15 mL water for the 10 mg packet); shake. **Note:** Regardless of the route of administration, the suspension should be left to thicken for 2-3 minutes prior to administration.

Storage

Capsules, tablets: Store at 15°C to 30°C (59°F to 86°F). Protect from light and moisture.

Granules for oral suspension: Store at 25°C (77°F); excursions permitted to 15°C to 30°C (59°F to 86°F).

Nursing Actions

Physical Assessment Optimize prevention of fractures in patients with osteoporosis.

Patient Education Take before eating. Do not crush or chew capsules. Delayed release capsule may be opened and contents added to applesauce. Avoid alcohol. You may experience anorexia; small frequent meals may help to maintain adequate nutrition. Report severe headache, unresolved severe diarrhea, or abdominal pain.

Dietary Considerations Should be taken on an empty stomach; best if taken before breakfast.

Omeprazole and Sodium Bicarbonate

(oh ME pray zol & SOW dee um bye KAR bun ate)

Brand Names: U.S. Zegerid OTC™ [OTC]; Zegerid®

Index Terms Sodium Bicarbonate and Omeprazole

Pharmacologic Category Proton Pump Inhibitor; Substituted Benzimidazole

Medication Safety Issues

Sound-alike/look-alike issues:

Zegerid® may be confused with Zestril®

Pregnancy Risk Factor C

Lactation Enters breast milk/not recommended

Use Short-term (4-8 weeks) treatment of active duodenal ulcer or active benign gastric ulcer; treatment of heartburn and other symptoms associated with gastroesophageal reflux disease (GERD); short-term (4-8 weeks) treatment of endoscopically-diagnosed erosive esophagitis; maintenance healing of erosive esophagitis; reduction of risk of upper gastrointestinal bleeding in critically-ill patients

OTC labeling: Short-term (2 weeks) treatment of frequent (2 days/week), uncomplicated heartburn

Available Dosage Forms

Capsule, oral: Omeprazole 20 mg [immediate release] and sodium bicarbonate 1100 mg; omeprazole 40 mg [immediate release] and sodium bicarbonate 1100 mg

Zegerid®: Omeprazole 20 mg [immediate release] and sodium bicarbonate 1100 mg

Zegerid®: Omeprazole 40 mg [immediate release] and sodium bicarbonate 1100 mg

Zegerid OTC™ [OTC]: Omeprazole 20 mg [immediate release] and sodium bicarbonate 1100 mg

Powder for suspension, oral:

Zegerid®: Omeprazole 20 mg and sodium bicarbonate 1680 mg per packet

Zegerid®: Omeprazole 40 mg and sodium bicarbonate 1680 mg per packet

General Dosage Range Oral: *Adults:* 20-40 mg/day in 1-2 divided doses

Administration

Oral Note: Both strengths of Zegerid® capsule and powder for oral suspension have identical sodium bicarbonate content, respectively. Do not substitute two 20 mg capsules/packets for one 40 mg dose.

Capsule: Should be swallowed whole with water (do not use other liquids); do not chew or crush. Capsules should **not** be opened, sprinkled on food, or administered via NG. Best if taken at least 1 hour before breakfast.

Powder for oral suspension: Administer 1 hour before a meal. Mix with 15-30 mL of water; stir well and drink immediately. Rinse cup with water and drink. Do not use other liquids or sprinkle on food.

Other Nasogastric/orogastric tube: Powder for oral suspension: Mix well with 20 mL of water (do not use other liquids) and administer immediately; flush tube with an additional 20 mL of water. Suspend enteral feeding for 3 hours before and 1 hour after administering.

Nursing Actions

Physical Assessment See individual agents.

Patient Education See individual agents.

Ondansetron (on DAN se tron)

Brand Names: U.S. Zofran®; Zofran® ODT; Zuplenz®

Index Terms GR38032R; Ondansetron Hydrochloride; Zuplenz®

Pharmacologic Category Antiemetic; Selective 5-HT_3 Receptor Antagonist

Medication Safety Issues

Sound-alike/look-alike issues:

Ondansetron may be confused with dolasetron, granisetron, palonosetron

Zofran® may be confused with Zantac®, Zosyn®

Pregnancy Risk Factor B

Lactation Excretion in breast milk unknown/use caution

Use Prevention of nausea and vomiting associated with moderately- to highly-emetogenic cancer chemotherapy; radiotherapy; prevention of postoperative nausea and vomiting (PONV); treatment of PONV if no prophylactic dose of ondansetron received

Unlabeled Use Hyperemesis gravidarum; breakthrough treatment of nausea and vomiting associated with chemotherapy

Mechanism of Action/Effect Selective 5-HT_3 receptor antagonist, blocking serotonin, both peripherally on vagal nerve terminals and centrally in the chemoreceptor trigger zone

Contraindications Hypersensitivity to ondansetron, other selective 5-HT_3 antagonists, or any component of the formulation; concomitant use of apomorphine

Warnings/Precautions Ondansetron should be used on a scheduled basis, not on an "as needed" (PRN) basis, since data support the use of this drug only in the prevention of nausea and vomiting (due to antineoplastic therapy) and not in the rescue of nausea and vomiting. Ondansetron should only be used in the first 24-48 hours of chemotherapy. Data do not support any increased efficacy of ondansetron in delayed nausea and vomiting. Does not stimulate gastric or intestinal peristalsis; may mask progressive ileus and/or gastric distension. Use with caution in patients allergic to other 5-HT_3 receptor antagonists; cross-reactivity has been reported.

Use with caution in patients with congenital long QT syndrome or other risk factors for QT prolongation (eg, medications known to prolong QT interval, electrolyte abnormalities, and cumulative high-dose anthracycline therapy). 5-HT_3 antagonists have been associated with a number of dose-dependent increases in ECG intervals (eg, PR, QRS duration, QT/QT_c, JT), usually occurring 1-2 hours after I.V. administration. In general, these changes are not clinically relevant, however, when used in conjunction with other agents that prolong these intervals, arrhythmia may occur. When used with agents that prolong the QT interval (eg, Class I and III antiarrhythmics), clinically relevant QT interval prolongation may occur resulting in torsade de pointes. I.V. formulations of 5-HT_3 antagonists have more association with ECG interval changes, compared to oral formulations. Dose recommendations provided for patients with severe hepatic impairment (Child-Pugh class C); use with caution in mild-moderate hepatic impairment; clearance is decreased and half-life increased in hepatic impairment.

Orally-disintegrating tablets contain phenylalanine.

Drug Interactions

Avoid Concomitant Use

Avoid concomitant use of Ondansetron with any of the following: Apomorphine; Artemether; Dronedarone; Lumefantrine; Nilotinib; Pimozide; QUEtiapine; QuiNINE; Tetrabenazine; Thioridazine; Toremifene; Vandetanib; Vemurafenib; Ziprasidone

Decreased Effect

The levels/effects of Ondansetron may be decreased by: CYP3A4 Inducers (Strong); Cyproterone; Deferasirox; Peginterferon Alfa-2b; P-glycoprotein/ABCB1 Inducers; Rifamycin Derivatives; Tocilizumab

Increased Effect/Toxicity

Ondansetron may increase the levels/effects of: Apomorphine; ARIPiprazole; Dronedarone; Pimozide; QTc-Prolonging Agents; QuiNINE; Tetrabenazine; Thioridazine; Toremifene; Vandetanib; Vemurafenib; Ziprasidone

The levels/effects of Ondansetron may be increased by: Alfuzosin; Artemether; Chloroquine; Ciprofloxacin; Ciprofloxacin (Systemic); Conivaptan; Gadobutrol; Indacaterol; Lumefantrine; Nilotinib; P-glycoprotein/ABCB1 Inhibitors; QUEtiapine; QuiNINE

Nutritional/Ethanol Interactions

Food: Tablet: Food slightly increases the extent of absorption.

Herb/Nutraceutical: St John's wort may decrease ondansetron levels.

Adverse Reactions **Note:** Percentages reported in adult patients.

>10%:

Central nervous system: Headache (9% to 27%), malaise/fatigue (9% to 13%)

Gastrointestinal: Constipation (6% to 11%)

1% to 10%:

Central nervous system: Drowsiness (8%), fever (2% to 8%), dizziness (4% to 7%), anxiety (6%), cold sensation (2%)

Dermatologic: Pruritus (2% to 5%), rash (1%)

Gastrointestinal: Diarrhea (2% to 7%)

Genitourinary: Gynecological disorder (7%), urinary retention (5%)

Hepatic: ALT increased (1% to 5%), AST increased (1% to 5%)

Local: Injection site reaction (4%; pain, redness, burning)

Neuromuscular & skeletal: Paresthesia (2%)

Respiratory: Hypoxia (9%)

Pharmacodynamics/Kinetics

Onset of Action ~30 minutes

Available Dosage Forms

Film, soluble, oral:

Zuplenz®: 4 mg (10s); 8 mg (10s)

Infusion, premixed in D_5W [preservative free]: 32 mg (50 mL)

Zofran®: 32 mg (50 mL)

Infusion, premixed in NS [preservative free]: 32 mg (50 mL)

Injection, solution: 2 mg/mL (2 mL, 20 mL)

Zofran®: 2 mg/mL (20 mL)

Injection, solution [preservative free]: 2 mg/mL (2 mL)

Solution, oral: 4 mg/5 mL (5 mL, 50 mL)

Zofran®: 4 mg/5 mL (50 mL)

Tablet, oral: 4 mg, 8 mg

Zofran®: 4 mg, 8 mg

Tablet, orally disintegrating, oral: 4 mg, 8 mg

Zofran® ODT: 4 mg, 8 mg

General Dosage Range Dosage adjustment recommended in patients with hepatic impairment

I.M.: *Adults:* 4 mg as a single dose

I.V.:

Infants 1-6 months: 0.1 mg/kg as a single dose

Children 6 months to 12 years and ≤40 kg: 0.1-0.45 mg/kg as a single dose **or** 0.15 mg/kg/dose for 3 doses

Children 6 months to 12 years and >40 kg and Children >12 years to 18 years: 0.45 mg/kg **or** 4 mg as a single dose **or** 0.15 mg/kg/dose for 3 doses

Adults: Dosage varies greatly depending on indication

Oral:

Children 4-11 years: 4 mg for 3 doses, then 4 mg every 8 hours for 1-2 days

Children ≥12 years: 24 mg as a single dose **or** 8 mg every 8-12 hours

Adults: 8-24 mg as a single dose **or** 8 mg every 8-12 hours

Administration

Oral Oral dosage forms should be given 30 minutes prior to chemotherapy; 1-2 hours before radiotherapy; 1 hour prior to the induction of anesthesia.

Orally-disintegrating tablets: Do not remove from blister until needed. Peel backing off the blister, do not push tablet through. Using dry hands, place tablet on tongue and allow to dissolve. Swallow with saliva.

Oral soluble film: Do not remove from pouch until immediately before use. Using dry hands, place film on top of tongue and allow to dissolve (4-20 seconds). Swallow with or without liquid. If using more than one film, each film should be allowed to dissolve completely before administering the next film.

I.M. Should be given undiluted.

I.V.

IVPB: Dilute in 50 mL D_5W or NS. Infuse over 15-30 minutes; 24-hour continuous infusions have been reported, but are rarely used.

Chemotherapy-induced nausea and vomiting: Give first dose 30 minutes prior to beginning chemotherapy.

I.V. push: Prevention of postoperative nausea and vomiting: Single doses may be administered I.V. injection over 2-5 minutes as undiluted solution.

I.V. Detail pH: 3-4

Stability

Reconstitution Prior to I.V. infusion, dilute in 50 mL D_5W or NS.

Storage

Oral soluble film: Store between 20°C and 25°C (68°F and 77°F). Store pouches in cartons; keep film in individual pouch until ready to use.

Oral solution: Store between 15°C and 30°C (59°F and 86°F). Protect from light.

Premixed bag: Store between 2°C and 30°C (36°F and 86°F). Protect from light.

Tablet: Store between 2°C and 30°C (36°F and 86°F).

Vial: Store between 2°C and 30°C (36°F and 86°F). Protect from light. Stable when mixed in D_5W or NS for 48 hours at room temperature.

Nursing Actions

Physical Assessment Allergy history to selective 5-HT_3 receptor antagonists should be assessed prior to administering. Assess other drugs patient may be taking that may prolong QT interval. I.V.: Follow infusion specifics. Oral and I.V. doses have different schedules and should not be administered on "PRN" basis.

Patient Education This drug is given to prevent nausea and vomiting. Zuplenz (oral film): Place film on top of tongue and allow to dissolve. May swallow with or without liquid. Allow one film to dissolve before using another. If this medication is given by intravenous infusion you will be monitored during infusion. Report immediately any chest pain, respiratory difficulty, or pain or itching at infusion site. May cause headache, drowsiness, or dizziness. Report chest pain or palpitations, persistent headache, excessive drowsiness, fever, constipation, or diarrhea. Orally-disintegrating tablets: Using dry hands, place tablet on tongue and allow to dissolve. Swallow with saliva.

Dietary Considerations Take without regard to meals. Some products may contain phenylalanine.

Opium Tincture (OH pee um TING chur)

Index Terms Deodorized Tincture of Opium (error-prone synonym); DTO (error-prone abbreviation); Opium Tincture, Deodorized; Tincture of Opium

Pharmacologic Category Analgesic, Opioid; Antidiarrheal

Medication Safety Issues

Sound-alike/look-alike issues:

Opium tincture may be confused with camphorated tincture of opium (paregoric)

High alert medication:

The Institute for Safe Medication Practices (ISMP) includes this medication among its list of drugs which have a heightened risk of causing significant patient harm when used in error.

Administration issues:

Use care when prescribing opium tincture; opium tincture is 25 times more concentrated than paregoric, each undiluted mL of opium tincture contains the equivalent of morphine 10 mg/mL.

If opium tincture is used in neonates, a 25-fold dilution should be prepared (final concentration: 0.4 mg/mL morphine). Of note, paregoric (which contains the equivalent of morphine 0.4 mg/mL) is **not** recommended for use in neonates due to the high alcohol content (~45%) and the presence of other additives; as an alternative to the use of diluted opium tincture or paregoric, ISMP recommends using a diluted preservative free injectable morphine solution orally.

Although historically opium tincture is dosed as mL/kg, the preferred dosing units are **mg**/kg (Levine, 2001). ISMP suggests hospitals evaluate the need for this product at their institution.

Other safety concerns:

DTO is an error-prone abbreviation and should never be used as an abbreviation for opium tincture (also known as *Deodorized* Tincture of Opium) due to potential for being mistaken as *Diluted* Tincture of Opium

Pregnancy Risk Factor C

Lactation Enters breast milk/use caution

Use Treatment of diarrhea in adults

Controlled Substance C-II

Available Dosage Forms

Tincture, oral: Anhydrous morphine 10 mg/mL (118 mL, 473 mL)

General Dosage Range

Oral: Opium tincture 10% contains morphine 10 mg/mL. Use caution in ordering, dispensing, and/or administering. The following doses are expressed in **mg** (milligram) dosing units of morphine.

Adults: Usual: 6 **mg** of undiluted opium tincture (10 mg/mL) 4 times daily

Administration

Oral May administer with food to decrease GI upset.

Nursing Actions

Physical Assessment If being used to control diarrhea, monitor stools. Monitor for effectiveness. Monitor blood pressure, CNS and respiratory status, and degree of sedation at beginning of therapy and periodically thereafter. Assess patient's physical and/or psychological dependence. For inpatients, implement safety measures (eg, side rails up, call light within reach, instructions to call for assistance). Discontinue slowly after prolonged use.

Patient Education May cause physical and/or psychological dependence. While using this medication, do not use alcohol and other prescription or OTC medications (especially sedatives, tranquilizers, antihistamines, or pain medications) without consulting prescriber. Maintain adequate hydration. May cause hypotension, dizziness, drowsiness, impaired coordination, blurred vision, or dry mouth. Report chest pain, slow or rapid heartbeat, dizziness, or persistent headache; confusion or respiratory difficulties; or severe constipation.

Orlistat (OR li stat)

Brand Names: U.S. Alli® [OTC]; Xenical®

Pharmacologic Category Lipase Inhibitor

Medication Safety Issues

Sound-alike/look-alike issues:

Xenical® may be confused with Xeloda®

Pregnancy Risk Factor X

Lactation Excretion in breast milk unknown/use caution

Breast-Feeding Considerations Weight-loss therapy is generally not recommended for lactating women. Weight-loss programs which include physical activity and nutrition components should be discussed at the 6-week postpartum visit (ADA, 2009; IOM, 2009).

Use Management of obesity, including weight loss and weight management, when used in conjunction with a reduced-calorie and low-fat diet; reduce the risk of weight regain after prior weight loss; indicated for obese patients with an initial body mass index (BMI) ≥30 kg/m² or ≥27 kg/m² in the presence of other risk factors (eg, diabetes, dyslipidemia, hypertension)

Mechanism of Action/Effect Inhibits gastric and pancreatic lipases, thus inhibiting the absorption of dietary fats (by 30% at doses of 120 mg 3 times/day)

Contraindications Hypersensitivity to orlistat or any component of the formulation; chronic malabsorption syndrome or cholestasis; pregnancy

Warnings/Precautions Prior to use other causes for obesity (eg, hypothyroidism) should be ruled out. Cases of severe liver injury (some fatal) with hepatocellular necrosis or acute hepatic failure have been reported (rare); liver transplantation has been required in some patients. Patients should be instructed to report any symptoms of hepatic dysfunction (eg, anorexia, pruritus, jaundice, dark urine, light colored stools, right upper quadrant pain); discontinue orlistat and obtain liver function test immediately if symptoms occur. Advise patients to adhere to dietary guidelines; if taken with a diet high in fat (>30% total daily calories from fat) gastrointestinal adverse events may increase. Distribute daily fat intake over 3 main meals. If taken with any 1 meal very high in fat, the possibility of gastrointestinal effects increases. Counsel patients to take a multivitamin supplement that contains fat-soluble vitamins ≥2 hours before or after orlistat administration to ensure adequate nutrition; orlistat has been shown to reduce the absorption of some fat-soluble vitamins and beta-carotene. Increased levels of urinary oxalate following treatment may occur in some patients; monitor renal function in patients at risk for renal failure; use with caution in patients with a history of hyperoxaluria or calcium oxalate nephrolithiasis. Orlistat may decrease cyclosporine plasma concentrations; administer cyclosporine ≥3 hours before or after orlistat and monitor frequently. The potential exists for misuse in inappropriate patient populations (eg, patients with anorexia nervosa or bulimia) similar to any weight loss agent. In general, substantial weight loss may increase the risk of cholelithiasis.

Self-medication (OTC use): Prior to use, patients should contact their healthcare provider if they have ever had kidney stones, gall bladder disease, or pancreatitis. Patients taking medications for diabetes or thyroid disease, anticoagulants, or other weight-loss products should consult their healthcare provider or pharmacist. Patients who have had an organ transplant should not use orlistat. If severe and/or continuous abdominal pain, itching, yellowing of the eyes or skin, dark urine, or loss of appetite occurs, use should be discontinued and healthcare provider consulted.

Drug Interactions

Avoid Concomitant Use There are no known interactions where it is recommended to avoid concomitant use.

Decreased Effect

Orlistat may decrease the levels/effects of: Amiodarone; CycloSPORINE; CycloSPORINE (Systemic); Levothyroxine; Paricalcitol; Propafenone; Vitamin D Analogs; Vitamins (Fat Soluble)

Increased Effect/Toxicity

Orlistat may increase the levels/effects of: Warfarin

Nutritional/Ethanol Interactions Fat-soluble vitamins: Absorption of vitamins A, D, E, and K may be decreased by orlistat. A multivitamin containing the fat-soluble vitamins (A, D, E, and K) should be administered once daily at least 2 hours before or after orlistat.

Adverse Reactions Note: The frequency of most adverse reactions (especially gastrointestinal effects) decreases over time.

>10%:

Central nervous system: Headache (≤31%)

Gastrointestinal: Oily spotting (4% to 27%), abdominal pain/discomfort (≤26%), flatus with discharge (2% to 24%), fecal urgency (3% to 22%), fatty/oily stool (6% to 20%), oily evacuation (2% to 12%), defecation increased (3% to 11%)

Neuromuscular & skeletal: Back pain (≤14%)

Respiratory: Upper respiratory infection (26% to 38%)

Miscellaneous: Influenza (≤40%)

1% to 10%:

Cardiovascular: Pedal edema (≤3%)

Central nervous system: Fatigue (3% to 7%), anxiety (3% to 5%), sleep disorder (≤4%)

Dermatologic: Dry skin (≤2%)

Endocrine & metabolic: Menstrual irregularities (≤10%)

Gastrointestinal: Nausea (4% to 8%), fecal incontinence (2% to 8%), infectious diarrhea (≤5%), rectal pain/discomfort (3% to 5%), tooth disorder (3% to 4%), gingival disorder (2% to 4%)

Genitourinary: Urinary tract infection (6% to 8%), vaginitis (3% to 4%)

Neuromuscular & skeletal: Myalgia (≤4%)

Otic: Otitis (3% to 4%)

Respiratory: Lower respiratory infection (≤8%)

Pharmacodynamics/Kinetics

Onset of Action 24-48 hours

Duration of Action 48-72 hours

Available Dosage Forms

Capsule, oral:

Alli® [OTC]: 60 mg

Xenical®: 120 mg

General Dosage Range Oral:

Children ≥12 years and Adults: Xenical®: 120 mg 3 times/day

Adults: Alli™ (OTC labeling): 60 mg 3 times/day

Administration

Oral Administer during or up to 1 hour after each main meal containing fat.

Stability

Storage Store at 25°C (77°F); excursions permitted to 15°C to 30°C (59°F to 86°F).

Nursing Actions

Patient Education Maintain prescribed diet (ideally a low-fat diet; high-fat meals may result in GI distress), exercise regimen, and vitamin supplements as prescribed. You may experience dizziness, lightheadedness, or increased flatus and fecal urgency (this may lessen with continued use). Report persistent back, muscle, or joint pain; signs of respiratory tract infection or flu-like symptoms; skin rash or irritation; severe fatigue; fever; yellowing of skin or eyes; brown urine; abdominal pain; or persistent nausea or vomiting.

Dietary Considerations Multivitamin supplements that contain fat-soluble vitamins should be taken once daily at least 2 hours before or after the administration of orlistat (ie, bedtime). Gastrointestinal effects of orlistat may increase if taken with any one meal very high in fat. Distribute daily intake of carbohydrates, fat (~30% of daily calories), and protein over three main meals.

Orphenadrine (or FEN a dreen)

Brand Names: U.S. Norflex™

Index Terms Orphenadrine Citrate

Pharmacologic Category Skeletal Muscle Relaxant

Medication Safety Issues

Sound-alike/look-alike issues:

Norflex™ may be confused with norfloxacin, Noroxin®

BEERS Criteria medication:

This drug may be inappropriate for use in geriatric patients (high severity risk).

International issues:

Flexin: Brand name for orphenadrine [Israel] but is also the brand name for cyclobenzaprine [Chile] and diclofenac [Argentina]

Flexin [Israel] may be confused with Floxin which is a brand name for flunarizine [Thailand], norfloxacin [South Africa], ofloxacin [U.S., Canada], and perfloxacin [Philippines]

Pregnancy Risk Factor C

Lactation Excretion in breast milk unknown/use caution

Use Treatment of muscle spasm associated with acute painful musculoskeletal conditions

Available Dosage Forms

Injection, solution: 30 mg/mL (2 mL)

Norflex™: 30 mg/mL (2 mL)

Injection, solution [preservative free]: 30 mg/mL (2 mL)

Tablet, extended release, oral: 100 mg

General Dosage Range

I.M., I.V.: *Adults:* 60 mg every 12 hours

Oral: *Adults:* 100 mg twice daily

Administration

Oral Do not crush sustained release drug product.

Nursing Actions

Physical Assessment Do not discontinue abruptly if patient using chronically; taper dosage slowly.

Patient Education Do not chew or crush extended release tablets. Do not use alcohol. You may experience drowsiness, dizziness, or lightheadedness. Report excessive drowsiness.

Oseltamivir (oh sel TAM i vir)

Brand Names: U.S. Tamiflu®

Pharmacologic Category Antiviral Agent; Neuraminidase Inhibitor

Medication Safety Issues

Sound-alike/look-alike issues:

Tamiflu® may be confused with Tambocor™, Thera-Flu®

Other safety concerns:

Oseltamivir (Tamiflu®) oral suspension is packaged with an oral syringe. When dispensing commercially prepared oseltamivir oral suspension, verify the intended concentration to be dispensed and the correct dose, dosing instructions, and oral dosing device provided for the patient. Oseltamivir oral suspension is available in a 6 mg/mL concentration. The previous concentration (12 mg/mL) has been discontinued, but may be still be on the market until product expires. The 6 mg/mL concentration is packaged with an oral syringe calibrated in **milliliters** up to a total of 10 mL. The previous, discontinued concentration (12 mg/mL) was packaged with an oral syringe calibrated in mg (30 mg, 45 mg, and 60 mg graduations). **When the oral syringe is dispensed, instructions to the patient should be provided based on these units of measure (ie, mL or mg). Do NOT dispense an oral syringe with units of measure in milligrams when providing oseltamivir suspension for children <1 year of age** instead supply an oral syringe capable of measuring mL doses. Patients should always be provided with a measuring device calibrated the same way as their labeled instructions.

When commercially-prepared oseltamivir oral suspension is not available, an extemporaneously prepared suspension may be compounded to provide a 6 mg/mL concentration (to match the preferred, currently manufactured commercially available oral suspension concentration).

Pregnancy Risk Factor C

Lactation Enters breast milk/not recommended

Breast-Feeding Considerations Small amounts of oseltamivir and oseltamivir carboxylate have been detected in breast milk. Breast-feeding is not recommended by the manufacturer. According to the CDC, breast-feeding while taking oseltamivir can be continued. The CDC recommends that women infected with the influenza virus follow general precautions (eg, frequent hand washing) to decrease viral transmission to the child. Mothers with influenza-like illnesses at delivery should consider avoiding close contact with the infant until they have received 48 hours of antiviral medication, fever has resolved, and cough and secretions can be controlled. These measures may help decrease (but not eliminate) the risk of transmitting influenza to the newborn. During this time, breast milk can be expressed and bottle-fed to the infant by another person who is well. Protective measures, such as wearing a face mask, changing into a clean gown or clothing, and strict hand hygiene should be continued by the mother for ≥7 days after the onset of symptoms or until symptom-free for 24 hours. Infant care should be performed by a noninfected person when possible (consult current CDC guidelines). Influenza may cause serious illness in postpartum women and prompt evaluation for febrile respiratory illnesses is recommended.

Use Treatment of uncomplicated acute illness due to influenza (A or B) infection in children ≥1 year of age and adults who have been symptomatic for no more than 2 days; prophylaxis against influenza (A or B) infection in children ≥1 year of age and adults

The Advisory Committee on Immunization Practices (ACIP) recommends that **treatment** be considered for the following:

- Persons with severe, complicated or progressive illness
- Hospitalized persons
- Persons at higher risk for influenza complications:
  - Children <2 years of age (highest risk in children <6 months of age)
  - Adults ≥65 years of age
  - Persons with chronic disorders of the pulmonary (including asthma) or cardiovascular systems (except hypertension)
  - Persons with chronic metabolic diseases (including diabetes mellitus), hepatic disease, renal dysfunction, hematologic disorders (including sickle cell disease), or immunosuppression (including immunosuppression caused by medications or HIV)
  - Persons with neurologic/neuromuscular conditions (including conditions such as spinal cord injuries, seizure disorders, cerebral palsy, stroke, mental retardation, moderate to severe developmental delay, or muscular dystrophy) which may compromise respiratory function, the handling of respiratory secretions, or that can increase the risk of aspiration
  - Pregnant or postpartum women (≤2 weeks after delivery)
  - Persons <19 years of age on long-term aspirin therapy
  - American Indians and Alaskan Natives
  - Persons who are morbidly obese (BMI ≥40)
  - Residents of nursing homes or other chronic care facilities
- Use may also be considered for previously healthy, nonhigh-risk outpatients with confirmed or suspected influenza based on clinical judgment when treatment can be started within 48 hours of illness onset.

The ACIP recommends that **prophylaxis** be considered for the following:

- Postexposure prophylaxis may be considered for family or close contacts of suspected or confirmed cases, who are at higher risk of influenza complications, and who have not been vaccinated against the circulating strain at the time of the exposure.

- Postexposure prophylaxis may be considered for unvaccinated healthcare workers who had occupational exposure without protective equipment.
- Pre-exposure prophylaxis should only be used for persons at very high risk of influenza complications who cannot be otherwise protected at times of high risk for exposure.
- Prophylaxis should also be administered to all eligible residents of institutions that house patients at high risk when needed to control outbreaks.

The ACIP recommends that treatment and prophylaxis be given to children <1 year of age when indicated.

Mechanism of Action/Effect Thought to inhibit influenza virus by altering virus particle aggregation and release

Contraindications Hypersensitivity to oseltamivir or any component of the formulation

Warnings/Precautions Oseltamivir is not a substitute for the influenza virus vaccine. It has not been shown to prevent primary or concomitant bacterial infections that may occur with influenza virus. Use caution with renal impairment; dosage adjustment is required for creatinine clearance <30 mL/minute. Safety and efficacy for use in patients with chronic cardiac and/or kidney disease, severe hepatic impairment, or for treatment or prophylaxis in immunocompromised patients have not been established. Rare but severe hypersensitivity reactions (anaphylaxis, severe dermatologic reactions) have been associated with use. Rare occurrences of neuropsychiatric events (including confusion, delirium, hallucinations, and/or self-injury) have been reported from postmarketing surveillance (primarily in pediatric patients); direct causation is difficult to establish (influenza infection may also be associated with behavioral and neurologic changes). Monitor closely for signs of any unusual behavior.

Antiviral treatment should begin within 48 hours of symptom onset. However, the CDC recommends that treatment may still be beneficial and should be started in hospitalized patients with severe, complicated or progressive illness if >48 hours. Nonhospitalized persons who are not at high risk for developing severe or complicated illness and who have a mild disease are not likely to benefit if treatment is started >48 hours after symptom onset. Nonhospitalized persons who are already beginning to recover do not need treatment.

Drug Interactions

Avoid Concomitant Use There are no known interactions where it is recommended to avoid concomitant use.

Decreased Effect

Oseltamivir may decrease the levels/effects of: Influenza Virus Vaccine (Live/Attenuated)

Increased Effect/Toxicity

The levels/effects of Oseltamivir may be increased by: Probenecid

Adverse Reactions

>10%: Gastrointestinal: Vomiting (2% to 15%)

1% to 10%:

Gastrointestinal: Nausea (4% to 10%), abdominal pain (2% to 5%), diarrhea (1% to 3%)

Ocular: Conjunctivitis (1%)

Respiratory: Epistaxis (1%)

Available Dosage Forms

Capsule, oral:

Tamiflu®: 30 mg, 45 mg, 75 mg

Powder for suspension, oral:

Tamiflu®: 6 mg/mL (60 mL)

General Dosage Range Dosage adjustment recommended in patients with renal impairment

Oral:

Children <1 year: 3 mg/kg/dose once daily

Children 1-12 years and ≤15 kg: 30 mg once or twice daily

Children 1-12 years and >15 to ≤23 kg: 45 mg once or twice daily

Children 1-12 years and >23 to ≤40 kg: 60 mg once or twice daily

Children 1-12 years and >40 kg, Children ≥13 years, and Adults: 75 mg once or twice daily

Administration

Oral May be administered without regard to meals; take with food to improve tolerance. Capsules may be opened and mixed with sweetened liquid (eg, chocolate syrup).

Other Mechanically-ventilated critically-ill patients: May administer via naso- or orogastric (NG/OG) tube. For a 150 mg dose, dissolve powder from two 75 mg capsules in 20 mL of sterile water and inject down the NG/OG tube; follow with a 10 mL sterile water flush (Taylor, 2008).

Stability

Reconstitution Oral suspension:

New concentration (6 mg/mL): Reconstitute with 55 mL of water to a final concentration of 6 mg/mL (to make 60 mL total suspension).

Discontinued concentration (12 mg/mL): Reconstitute with 23 mL of water to a final concentration of 12 mg/mL (to make 25 mL total suspension).

Storage

Capsules: Store at 25°C (77°F); excursions permitted to 15°C to 30°C (59°F to 86°F).

Oral suspension: Store powder for suspension at 25°C (77°F); excursions permitted to 15°C to 30°C (59°F to 86°F). Once reconstituted, store suspension under refrigeration at 2°C to 8°C (36°F to 46°F); do not freeze. Use within 10 days of preparation if stored at room temperature or within 17 days of preparation if stored under refrigeration.

Nursing Actions

Physical Assessment Recommendations for antiviral susceptibility and effectiveness may change. Validate with the CDC recommendations for use prior to prescribing.

Patient Education This is not a substitute for the flu shot. Must be taken within 2 days of contact with an infected individual or onset of flu symptoms (eg, fever, cough, headache, fatigue, muscular weakness, and sore throat). You may experience dizziness, nausea, vomiting, loose stools, headache, or feeling tired and weak. Report hallucinations, unusual behavior, or inability to think clearly.

Dietary Considerations Take without regard to meals; take with food to improve tolerance.

Oxaliplatin (ox AL i pla tin)

Brand Names: U.S. Eloxatin®

Index Terms Diaminocyclohexane Oxalatoplatinum; L-OHP; Oxalatoplatin; Oxalatoplatinum

Pharmacologic Category Antineoplastic Agent, Alkylating Agent; Antineoplastic Agent, Platinum Analog

Medication Safety Issues

Sound-alike/look-alike issues:

Oxaliplatin may be confused with Aloxi®, carboplatin, cisplatin

High alert medication:

The Institute for Safe Medication Practices (ISMP) includes this medication among its list of drug classes which have a heightened risk of causing significant patient harm when used in error.

Pregnancy Risk Factor D

Lactation Excretion in breast milk unknown/not recommended

Breast-Feeding Considerations Due to the potential for serious adverse reactions in the nursing infant, breast-feeding is not recommended.

Use Treatment of stage III colon cancer (adjuvant) and advanced colorectal cancer

Unlabeled Use Treatment of esophageal cancer, gastric cancer, hepatobiliary cancer, non-Hodgkin's lymphoma, ovarian cancer, pancreatic cancer, testicular cancer

Mechanism of Action/Effect Oxaliplatin, a platinum derivative, is an alkylating agent. Following intracellular hydrolysis, the platinum compound binds to DNA forming cross-links which inhibit DNA replication and transcription, resulting in cell death. Cytotoxicity is cell-cycle nonspecific.

Contraindications Hypersensitivity to oxaliplatin, other platinum-containing compounds, or any component of the formulation

Canadian labeling: Additional contraindications (not in U.S. labeling): Pregnancy, breast-feeding; severe renal impairment (Cl_{cr} <30 mL/minute)

Warnings/Precautions Hazardous agent - use appropriate precautions for handling and disposal. **[U.S. Boxed Warning]: Anaphylactic/anaphylactoid reactions may occur within minutes of oxaliplatin administration; symptoms may be managed with epinephrine, corticosteroids, and antihistamines.** Grade 3 or 4 hypersensitivity has been observed. Allergic reactions may occur with any cycle and may include bronchospasm (rare), erythema, hypotension (rare), pruritus, rash, and/or urticaria.

Two different types of peripheral sensory neuropathy may occur: First, an acute (within first 2 days), reversible (resolves within 14 days), with primarily peripheral symptoms that are often exacerbated by cold (may include pharyngolaryngeal dysesthesia); may recur with subsequent doses; avoid mucositis prophylaxis with ice chips during oxaliplatin infusion. Secondly, a more persistent (>14 days) presentation that often interferes with daily activities (eg, writing, buttoning, swallowing), these symptoms may improve in some patients upon discontinuing treatment.

May cause pulmonary fibrosis; withhold treatment for unexplained pulmonary symptoms (eg, crackles, dyspnea, nonproductive cough, pulmonary infiltrates) until interstitial lung disease or pulmonary fibrosis are excluded. Hepatotoxicity (including rare cases of hepatitis and hepatic failure) has been reported. Liver biopsy has revealed peliosis, nodular regenerative hyperplasia, sinusoidal alterations, perisinusoidal fibrosis, and veno-occlusive lesions; the presence of hepatic vascular disorders (including veno-occlusive disease) should be considered, especially in individuals developing portal hypertension or who present with increased liver function tests. Use caution with renal dysfunction; increased toxicity may occur. When administered as sequential infusions, taxane derivatives (docetaxel, paclitaxel) should be administered before platinum derivatives (carboplatin, cisplatin, oxaliplatin) to limit myelosuppression and enhance efficacy. Concomitant use with 5-FU may increase risk for adverse hematologic or GI effects. Elderly patients are more sensitive to some adverse events including diarrhea, dehydration, hypokalemia, leukopenia, fatigue and syncope. Safety and efficacy in children have not been established.

Drug Interactions

Avoid Concomitant Use

Avoid concomitant use of Oxaliplatin with any of the following: BCG; CloZAPine; Natalizumab; Pimecrolimus; Tacrolimus (Topical); Vaccines (Live)

Decreased Effect

Oxaliplatin may decrease the levels/effects of: BCG; Cardiac Glycosides; Coccidioidin Skin Test; Sipuleucel-T; Vaccines (Inactivated); Vaccines (Live); Vitamin K Antagonists

The levels/effects of Oxaliplatin may be decreased by: Echinacea

Increased Effect/Toxicity

Oxaliplatin may increase the levels/effects of: CloZAPine; Leflunomide; Natalizumab; Taxane Derivatives; Topotecan; Vaccines (Live); Vitamin K Antagonists

The levels/effects of Oxaliplatin may be increased by: Denosumab; Pimecrolimus; Roflumilast; Tacrolimus (Topical); Trastuzumab

Adverse Reactions Percentages reported with monotherapy.

>10%:

Central nervous system: Fatigue (61%), fever (25%), pain (14%), headache (13%), insomnia (11%)

Gastrointestinal: Nausea (64%), diarrhea (46%), vomiting (37%), abdominal pain (31%), constipation (31%), anorexia (20%), stomatitis (14%)

Hematologic: Anemia (64%; grades 3/4: 1%), thrombocytopenia (30%; grades 3/4: 3%), leukopenia (13%)

Hepatic: AST increased (54%; grades 3/4: 4%), ALT increased (36%; grades 3/4: 1%), total bilirubin increased (13%; grades 3/4: 5%)

Neuromuscular & skeletal: Peripheral neuropathy (may be dose limiting; 76%; acute 65%; grades 3/4: 5%; persistent 43%; grades 3/4: 3%), back pain (11%)

Respiratory: Dyspnea (13%), cough (11%)

1% to 10%:

Cardiovascular: Edema (10%), chest pain (5%), peripheral edema (5%), flushing (3%), thromboembolism (2%)

Central nervous system: Dizziness (7%)

Dermatologic: Rash (5%), alopecia (3%), hand-foot syndrome (1%)

Endocrine & metabolic: Dehydration (5%), hypokalemia (3%)

Gastrointestinal: Dyspepsia (7%), taste perversion (5%), flatulence (3%), mucositis (2%), gastroesophageal reflux (1%), dysphagia (acute 1% to 2%)

Genitourinary: Dysuria (1%)

Hematologic: Neutropenia (7%)

Local: Injection site reaction (9%; redness/swelling/pain)

Neuromuscular & skeletal: Rigors (9%), arthralgia (7%)

Ocular: Abnormal lacrimation (1%)

Renal: Serum creatinine increased (5% to 10%)

Respiratory: URI (7%), rhinitis (6%), epistaxis (2%), pharyngitis (2%), pharyngolaryngeal dysesthesia (grades 3/4: 1% to 2%)

Miscellaneous: Allergic reactions (3%); hypersensitivity (includes urticaria, pruritus, facial flushing, shortness of breath, bronchospasm, diaphoresis, hypotension, syncope: grades 3/4: 2% to 3%); hiccup (2%)

Available Dosage Forms

Injection, solution [preservative free]:

Eloxatin®: 5 mg/mL (10 mL, 20 mL, 40 mL)

General Dosage Range Dosage adjustment recommended in patients who develop toxicities

I.V.: *Adults:* 85 mg/m^2 every 2 weeks

Administration

I.V. Administer as I.V. infusion over 2-6 hours. Flush infusion line with D_5W prior to administration of any concomitant medication. Patients should receive an antiemetic premedication regimen. Avoid mucositis prophylaxis with ice chips during oxaliplatin infusion (may exacerbate acute neurological symptoms).

Stability

Reconstitution Do not prepare using a chloride-containing solution such as NaCl due to rapid conversion to monochloroplatinum, dichloroplatinum, and diaquoplatinum; all highly reactive in sodium chloride (Takimoto, 2007). Use appropriate precautions for handling and disposal. Do not use needles or administration sets containing aluminum during preparation.

Aqueous solution: Dilution with D_5W (250 or 500 mL) is required prior to administration.

Lyophilized powder [CAN; not available in U.S.]: Use only water for injection or D_5W to reconstitute powder. To obtain final concentration of 5 mg/mL add 10 mL of diluent to 50 mg vial or 20 mL diluent to 100 mg vial. Gently swirl vial to dissolve powder. Dilution with D_5W (250 or 500 mL) is required prior to administration. Discard unused portion of vial.

Storage Store intact vials at room temperature of 25°C (77°F); excursions permitted to 15°C to 30°C (59°F to 86°F); do not freeze. Protect concentrated solution from light (store in original outer carton). According to the manufacturer, solutions diluted for infusion are stable up to 6 hours at room temperature of 20°C to 25°C (68°F to 77°F) or up to 24 hours under refrigeration at 2°C to 8°C (36°F to 46°F). Oxaliplatin solution diluted with D_5W to a final concentration of 0.7 mg/mL (polyolefin container) has been shown to retain >90% of its original concentration for up to 30 days when stored at room temperature or refrigerated; artificial light did not affect the concentration (Andre, 2007). As this study did not examine sterility, refrigeration would be preferred to limit microbial growth. Solutions diluted for infusion do not require protection from light.

Nursing Actions

Physical Assessment Patient must be observed closely for anaphylactic-like reactions (can occur within minutes of administration; appropriate medications for the treatment of hypersensitivity reactions should be available). Monitor for pulmonary and hepatic toxicity, neuropathy (acute or persistent), GI disturbance, anemia, chest pain, and thromboembolism during and between each infusion.

Patient Education This medication can only be administered by infusion; you will be monitored closely during and following infusion. Report immediately any pain, burning, or swelling at infusion site or any signs of allergic reaction (eg, respiratory difficulty, difficulty swallowing, back pain, chest tightness, rash, hives, swelling of lips or mouth). It is important that you maintain adequate nutrition and hydration, unless instructed to restrict fluid intake. You may be more susceptible to infection. You may experience temporary numbness, pain, tingling, or loss of sensation in hands, feet, or throat (cold will exacerbate these effects; remain warm, cover skin before exposure to cold, and avoid cold drinks or the use of ice); if this condition persists or is severe contact prescriber. May cause fatigue, headache, insomnia, nausea, vomiting, loss of appetite, taste perversion, mouth sores, diarrhea, constipation, or loss of hair (reversible). Report chest pain or palpitations; swelling, pain, or hot areas in legs; unusual fatigue; unusual bruising or bleeding; cough, sore throat, or respiratory difficulty; or muscle cramps or twitching.

Related Information

Management of Drug Extravasations *on page 1269*

Oxaprozin (oks a PROE zin)

Brand Names: U.S. Daypro®

Pharmacologic Category Nonsteroidal Anti-inflammatory Drug (NSAID), Oral

Medication Safety Issues

Sound-alike/look-alike issues:

Oxaprozin may be confused with oxazepam

BEERS Criteria medication:

This drug may be inappropriate for use in geriatric patients (high severity risk).

Medication Guide Available Yes

Pregnancy Risk Factor C

Lactation Excretion in breast milk unknown/not recommended

Use Acute and long-term use in the management of signs and symptoms of osteoarthritis and rheumatoid arthritis; juvenile idiopathic arthritis (JIA)

Available Dosage Forms

Caplet, oral:

Daypro®: 600 mg

Tablet, oral: 600 mg

General Dosage Range Dosage adjustment recommended in patients with renal impairment

Oral:

Children 6-16 years and 22-31 kg: 600 mg once daily

Children 6-16 years and 32-54 kg: 900 mg once daily

Children 6-16 years and ≥55 kg: 1200 mg once daily

Adults: 600-1800 mg once daily (maximum: 1200 mg/day [<50 kg]; 1800 mg/day or 26 mg/kg/day (whichever lower) [>50 kg])

Nursing Actions

Physical Assessment Monitor blood pressure at the beginning of therapy and periodically during use. Monitor for GI effects, hepatotoxicity, and ototoxicity at beginning of therapy and periodically throughout. Schedule ophthalmic evaluations for patients who develop eye complaints during long-term NSAID therapy.

Patient Education Do not crush tablets. Take with food or milk to reduce GI distress. Do not use alcohol. You may experience drowsiness, dizziness, nervousness, anorexia, nausea, vomiting, or heartburn; GI bleeding, ulceration, or perforation can occur with or without pain. Discontinue medication and contact prescriber if persistent abdominal pain, cramping, or blood in stool occurs. Report vaginal bleeding; respiratory difficulty or unusual cough; chest pain, rapid heartbeat, or palpitations; bruising or bleeding (blood in urine, mouth, or vomitus); swollen extremities; skin rash or itching; or swelling of face, lips, tongue, or throat.

Oxazepam (oks A ze pam)

Index Terms Serax

Pharmacologic Category Benzodiazepine

Medication Safety Issues

Sound-alike/look-alike issues:

Oxazepam may be confused with oxaprozin, quazepam

Serax may be confused with Eurax®, Urex, Zyr-TEC®

BEERS Criteria medication:

This drug may be inappropriate for use in geriatric patients (high severity risk).

International issues:

Murelax [Australia] may be confused with MiraLax brand name for polyethylene glycol 3350 [U.S.]

Use Treatment of anxiety; management of ethanol withdrawal

Unlabeled Use Anticonvulsant in management of simple partial seizures; hypnotic

Controlled Substance C-IV

Available Dosage Forms

Capsule, oral: 10 mg, 15 mg, 30 mg

General Dosage Range Oral:

Adults: 10-30 mg 3-4 times/day

Elderly: Initial: 10 mg 2-3 times/day; Maintenance: 30-45 mg/day

Administration

Oral Administer orally in divided doses.

Nursing Actions

Physical Assessment Assess for history of addiction; long-term use can result in dependence, abuse, or tolerance; periodically evaluate need for continued use. For inpatient use, institute safety measures to prevent falls. Monitor for oversedation, dizziness, confusion, or ataxia which may impair physical and mental capabilities.

Patient Education Drug may cause physical and/or psychological dependence. Do not use alcohol. Maintain adequate hydration unless instructed to restrict fluid intake. You may experience drowsiness, lightheadedness, impaired coordination, dizziness, blurred vision, nausea, vomiting, dry mouth, or constipation. Report persistent CNS effects (eg, confusion, depression, suicide ideation, increased sedation, excitation, headache, agitation, insomnia or nightmares, dizziness, fatigue, impaired coordination, changes in personality, or changes in cognition) or worsening of condition.

OXcarbazepine (ox car BAZ e peen)

Brand Names: U.S. Trileptal®

Index Terms GP 47680; OCBZ

Pharmacologic Category Anticonvulsant, Miscellaneous

Medication Safety Issues

Sound-alike/look-alike issues:

OXcarbazepine may be confused with carBAMazepine

Trileptal® may be confused with TriLipix®

Medication Guide Available Yes

Pregnancy Risk Factor C

Lactation Enters breast milk/not recommended

Breast-Feeding Considerations Oxcarbazepine and the active 10-hydroxy metabolite (MHD) are found in breast milk (small amounts). According to the manufacturer, the decision to continue or discontinue breast-feeding during therapy should take into account the risk of exposure to the infant and the benefits of treatment to the mother.

Use Monotherapy or adjunctive therapy in the treatment of partial seizures in adults and children ≥4 years of age with epilepsy; adjunctive therapy in the treatment of partial seizures in children ≥2 years of age with epilepsy

Unlabeled Use Bipolar disorder; treatment of neuropathic pain

Mechanism of Action/Effect Precise mechanism of action has not been determined. Believed to prevent the spread of seizures by decreasing propagation of synaptic impulses.

Contraindications Hypersensitivity to oxcarbazepine or any component of the formulation

Warnings/Precautions Antiepileptics are associated with an increased risk of suicidal behavior/thoughts with use (regardless of indication); patients should be monitored for signs/symptoms of depression, suicidal tendencies, and other unusual behavior changes during therapy and instructed to inform their healthcare provider immediately if symptoms occur.

Clinically-significant hyponatremia (serum sodium <125 mmol/L) may develop during oxcarbazepine use. Rare cases of anaphylaxis and angioedema have been reported, even after initial dosing; permanently discontinue should symptoms occur. Use caution in patients with previous hypersensitivity to carbamazepine (cross-sensitivity occurs in 25% to 30%). Potentially serious, sometimes fatal, dermatologic reactions (eg, Stevens-Johnson, toxic epidermal necrolysis) and multiorgan hypersensitivity reactions have been reported in adults and children; monitor for signs and symptoms of skin reactions and possible disparate manifestations associated with lymphatic, hepatic, renal, and/or hematologic organ systems; discontinuation and conversion to alternate therapy may be required. As with all antiepileptic drugs, oxcarbazepine should be withdrawn gradually to minimize the potential of increased seizure frequency. Use of oxcarbazepine has been associated with CNS-related adverse events, most significant of these were cognitive symptoms including psychomotor slowing, difficulty with concentration, speech or language problems, somnolence or fatigue, and coordination abnormalities, including ataxia and gait disturbances. Effects with other sedative drugs or ethanol may be potentiated. Single-dose studies show that half-life of the primary active metabolite is prolonged 3-4 fold and AUC is doubled in patients with Cl_{cr} <30 mL/minute; dose adjustment required in these patients. May reduce the efficacy of oral contraceptives (nonhormonal contraceptive measures are recommended). Agranulocytosis, leukopenia, and pancytopenia have been reported with use (rare). Discontinuation and conversion to alternate therapy may be required.

Drug Interactions

Avoid Concomitant Use

Avoid concomitant use of OXcarbazepine with any of the following: Axitinib; Bortezomib; Crizotinib; Dronedarone; Everolimus; Lapatinib; Lurasidone; Nilotinib; Nisoldipine; Pazopanib; Praziquantel; Ranolazine; Rilpivirine; Rivaroxaban; Roflumilast; RomiDEPsin; Selegiline; SORAfenib; Ticagrelor; Tolvaptan; Toremifene; Vandetanib

Decreased Effect

OXcarbazepine may decrease the levels/effects of: ARIPiprazole; Axitinib; Boceprevir; Bortezomib; Brentuximab Vedotin; Clarithromycin; Contraceptives (Estrogens); Contraceptives (Progestins); Crizotinib; CYP3A4 Substrates; Dasatinib; Dronedarone; Everolimus; Exemestane; Gefitinib; GuanFACINE; Imatinib; Ixabepilone; Lapatinib; Linagliptin; Lurasidone; Maraviroc; NIFEdipine; Nilotinib; Nisoldipine;

Pazopanib; Praziquantel; Ranolazine; Rilpivirine; Rivaroxaban; Roflumilast; RomiDEPsin; Saxagliptin; SORAfenib; SUNItinib; Tadalafil; Ticagrelor; Tolvaptan; Toremifene; Ulipristal; Vandetanib; Vemurafenib; Zuclopenthixol

The levels/effects of OXcarbazepine may be decreased by: Divalproex; Fosphenytoin; PHENobarbital; Phenytoin; Valproic Acid

Increased Effect/Toxicity

OXcarbazepine may increase the levels/effects of: Clarithromycin; Fosphenytoin; Phenytoin; Selegiline

The levels/effects of OXcarbazepine may be increased by: Clarithromycin; Thiazide Diuretics

Nutritional/Ethanol Interactions

Ethanol: Avoid ethanol (may increase CNS depression).

Herb/Nutraceutical: St John's wort may decrease oxcarbazepine levels. Avoid evening primrose (seizure threshold decreased). Avoid valerian, St John's wort, kava kava, gotu kola.

Adverse Reactions As reported in adults with doses of up to 2400 mg/day (includes patients on monotherapy, adjunctive therapy, and those not previously on AEDs); incidence in children was similar.

>10%:

Central nervous system: Dizziness (22% to 49%), somnolence (20% to 36%), headache (13% to 32%), ataxia (5% to 31%), fatigue (12% to 15%), vertigo (6% to 15%)

Gastrointestinal: Vomiting (7% to 36%), nausea (15% to 29%), abdominal pain (10% to 13%)

Neuromuscular & skeletal: Abnormal gait (5% to 17%), tremor (3% to 16%)

Ocular: Diplopia (14% to 40%), nystagmus (7% to 26%), abnormal vision (4% to 14%)

1% to 10%:

Cardiovascular: Hypotension (≤2%), leg edema (1% to 2%)

Central nervous system: Nervousness (2% to 5%), amnesia (4%), abnormal thinking (≤4%), insomnia (2% to 4%), fever (3%), speech disorder (1% to 3%), abnormal feelings (≤2%), EEG abnormalities (≤2%), agitation (1% to 2%), confusion (1% to 2%)

Dermatologic: Rash (4%), acne (1% to 2%)

Endocrine & metabolic: Hyponatremia (1% to 3%)

Gastrointestinal: Diarrhea (5% to 7%), dyspepsia (5% to 6%), constipation (2% to 6%), taste perversion (5%), xerostomia (3%), gastritis (1% to 2%), weight gain (1% to 2%)

Genitourinary: Micturition (2%)

Neuromuscular & skeletal: Weakness (3% to 6%), back pain (4%), falling down (4%), abnormal coordination (1% to 4%), dysmetria (1% to 3%), sprains/strains (≤2%), muscle weakness (1% to 2%)

Ocular: Abnormal accommodation (≤2%)

Respiratory: Upper respiratory tract infection (7%), rhinitis (2% to 5%), chest infection (4%), epistaxis (4%), sinusitis (4%)

Available Dosage Forms

Suspension, oral: 300 mg/5 mL (250 mL)

Trileptal®: 300 mg/5 mL (250 mL)

Tablet, oral: 150 mg, 300 mg, 600 mg

Trileptal®: 150 mg, 300 mg, 600 mg

General Dosage Range Dosage adjustment recommended in patients with renal impairment

Oral:

Children 2-3 years and <20 kg: Initial: 8-20 mg/kg/day (maximum: 600 mg/day) in 2 divided doses; Maintenance: maximum of 60 mg/kg/day in 2 divided doses

Children 2-3 years and ≥20 kg: Initial: 8-10 mg/kg/day (maximum: 600 mg/day) in 2 divided doses; Maintenance: maximum of 60 mg/kg/day in 2 divided doses

Children 4-16 years and <25 kg: Initial: 8-10 mg/kg/day (maximum: 600 mg/day) in 2 divided doses; Maintenance: up to 900 mg/day

Children 4-16 years and 25-30 kg: Initial: 8-10 mg/kg/day (maximum: 600 mg/day) in 2 divided doses; Maintenance: up to 1200 mg/day

Children 4-16 years and 31-45 kg: Initial: 8-10 mg/kg/day (maximum: 600 mg/day) in 2 divided doses; Maintenance: up to 1500 mg/day

Children 4-16 years and 46-55 kg: Initial: 8-10 mg/kg/day (maximum: 600 mg/day) in 2 divided doses; Maintenance: up to 1800 mg/day

Children 4-16 years and >56 kg: Initial: 8-10 mg/kg/day (maximum: 600 mg/day) in 2 divided doses; Maintenance: up to 2100 mg/day

Children >16 years and Adults: Initial: 300 mg twice daily; Maintenance: 1200-2400 mg/day in 2 divided doses (maximum: 2400 mg/day)

Administration

Oral All dosing should be administered twice daily.

Suspension: Prior to using for the first time, firmly insert the plastic adapter provided with the bottle. Cover adapter with child-resistant cap when not in use. Shake bottle for at least 10 seconds, remove child-resistant cap, and insert the oral dosing syringe provided to withdraw appropriate dose. Dose may be taken directly from oral syringe or may be mixed in a small glass of water immediately prior to swallowing. Rinse syringe with warm water after use and allow to dry thoroughly. Discard any unused portion after 7 weeks of first opening bottle.

Stability

Storage Store tablets and suspension at 25°C (77°F). Use suspension within 7 weeks of first opening container.

Nursing Actions

Physical Assessment Determine absence of any allergic reactions to other anticonvulsants (carbamazepine). Monitor therapeutic effectiveness (seizure activity, frequency, duration, type). Monitor for sedation, CNS changes, visual changes, and skin reactions. Dosage should be tapered when discontinuing to reduce risk of increased seizures. Teach patient safety and seizure precautions.

Patient Education While using the medication, do not use alcohol. Maintain adequate hydration unless instructed to restrict fluid intake. You may experience drowsiness, dizziness, blurred vision, nausea, or vomiting. Report CNS changes, increase in seizure frequency or severity, mentation changes, suicide ideation, depression, changes in cognition or memory, persistent fever, acute fatigue, weakness, insomnia, muscle cramping, weakness, abdominal pain, rash or skin irritations, unusual bruising or bleeding (mouth, urine, stool), or swelling of extremities.

Dietary Considerations May be taken without regard to meals.

Oxybutynin (oks i BYOO ti nin)

Brand Names: U.S. Ditropan XL®; Gelnique®; Oxytrol®

Index Terms Anturol®; Ditropan; Oxybutynin Chloride

Pharmacologic Category Antispasmodic Agent, Urinary

Medication Safety Issues

Sound-alike/look-alike issues:

Oxybutynin may be confused with OxyCONTIN®

Ditropan may be confused with Detrol®, diazepam, Diprivan®, dithranol

Beers Criteria medication:

This drug may be inappropriate for use in geriatric patients (high severity risk).

Other safety concerns:

Transdermal patch may contain conducting metal (eg, aluminum); remove patch prior to MRI.

Pregnancy Risk Factor B

Lactation Excretion in breast milk unknown/use caution

Breast-Feeding Considerations Suppression of lactation has been reported.

Use Antispasmodic for neurogenic bladder (urgency, frequency, leakage, urge incontinence, dysuria); extended release formulation also indicated for treatment of symptoms associated with detrusor overactivity due to a neurological condition (eg, spina bifida)

Mechanism of Action/Effect Direct antispasmodic effect on smooth muscle, also inhibits the action of acetylcholine on smooth muscle (exhibits 1/5 the anticholinergic activity of atropine, but is 4-10 times the antispasmodic activity); does not block effects at skeletal muscle or at autonomic ganglia; increases bladder capacity, decreases uninhibited contractions, and delays desire to void, therefore, decreases urgency and frequency

Contraindications Hypersensitivity to oxybutynin or any component of the formulation; patients with or at risk for uncontrolled narrow-angle glaucoma, urinary retention, gastric retention or conditions with severely decreased GI motility

Warnings/Precautions Cases of angioedema have been reported with oral oxybutynin; some cases have occurred after a single dose. Discontinue immediately if develops. Use with caution in patients with bladder outflow obstruction, angle-closure glaucoma (treated), hyperthyroidism, reflux esophagitis (including concurrent therapy with oral bisphosphonates or drugs which may increase the risk of esophagitis), heart disease, hepatic or renal disease, prostatic hyperplasia, autonomic neuropathy, ulcerative colitis (may cause ileus and toxic megacolon), hypertension, hiatal hernia, myasthenia gravis, dementia, ulcerative colitis, or intestinal atony. May increase the risk of heat prostration. May cause anticholinergic effects (agitation, confusion, hallucinations, somnolence) which may require dose reduction or discontinuation of therapy. May cause CNS depression, which may impair physical or mental abilities; patients must be cautioned about performing tasks which require mental alertness (eg, operating machinery or driving).

This class of medication is poorly tolerated by the elderly due to anticholinergic effects, sedation, and weakness. Efficacy is questionable at dosages tolerated by elderly patients. Oxybutynin extended-release is considered an exception. (Beers Criteria).

The extended release formulation consists of drug within a nondeformable matrix; following drug release/absorption, the matrix/shell is expelled in the stool. The use of nondeformable products in patients with known stricture/narrowing of the GI tract has been associated with symptoms of obstruction. Transdermal patch may contain conducting metal (eg, aluminum); remove patch prior to MRI. When using the topical gel, cover treatment area with clothing after gel has dried to minimize transferring medication to others. Discontinue gel if skin irritation occurs. Gel contains ethanol; do not expose to open flame or smoking until gel has dried.

Drug Interactions

Avoid Concomitant Use

Avoid concomitant use of Oxybutynin with any of the following: Pimozide

Decreased Effect

Oxybutynin may decrease the levels/effects of: Acetylcholinesterase Inhibitors (Central); Secretin

The levels/effects of Oxybutynin may be decreased by: Acetylcholinesterase Inhibitors (Central); Tocilizumab

Increased Effect/Toxicity

Oxybutynin may increase the levels/effects of: AbobotulinumtoxinA; Anticholinergics; ARIPiprazole; Cannabinoids; OnabotulinumtoxinA; Pimozide; Potassium Chloride; RimabotulinumtoxinB

The levels/effects of Oxybutynin may be increased by: Conivaptan; Pramlintide

Nutritional/Ethanol Interactions Ethanol: Use ethanol with caution (may increase CNS depression and toxicity). Watch for sedation.

Adverse Reactions

Oral:

>10%:

Central nervous system: Dizziness (4% to 17%), somnolence (2% to 14%)

Gastrointestinal: Xerostomia (29% to 71%; dose related), constipation (7% to 15%), nausea (2% to 12%)

5% to 10%:

Central nervous system: Headache (6% to 10%), pain (1% to 7%), nervousness (1% to 7%), insomnia (1% to 6%)

Gastrointestinal: Diarrhea (1% to 9%), dyspepsia (5% to 7%)

Genitourinary: Urinary hesitation (9%), urinary tract infection (5% to 7%), urinary retention (6%)

Neuromuscular & skeletal: Weakness (3% to 7%)

Ocular: Blurred vision (1% to 10%), dry eyes (3% to 6%)

Respiratory: Rhinitis (2% to 6%)

Topical gel:

1% to 10%:

Central nervous system: Dizziness (2% to 3%), fatigue (2%), headache (2%)

Dermatologic: Pruritus (1%)

Gastrointestinal: Xerostomia (7% to 8%), gastroenteritis (2%), constipation (1%)

Genitourinary: Urinary tract infection (7%)

Local: Application site reaction (5%; includes anesthesia, dermatitis, erythema, irritation, pain, papules, pruritus)

Respiratory: Nasopharyngitis (3%)

Transdermal:

>10%: Local: Application site reaction (17%), pruritus (14%)

1% to 10%:

Gastrointestinal: Xerostomia (4% to 10%), diarrhea (3%), constipation (3%)

Genitourinary: Dysuria (2%)

Local: Erythema (6% to 8%), vesicles (3%), rash (3%)

Ocular: Vision changes (3%)

Pharmacodynamics/Kinetics

Onset of Action Onset of action: Oral: 30-60 minutes; Peak effect: 3-6 hours

Duration of Action 6-10 hours (up to 24 hours for extended release oral formulation)

Product Availability Anturol® 3% gel: FDA approved December 2011; availability is currently undetermined. Consult prescribing information for additional information.

Available Dosage Forms

Gel, topical:

Gelnique®: 10% (1 g)

Patch, transdermal:

Oxytrol®: 3.9 mg/24 hours (8s)

Syrup, oral: 5 mg/5 mL (5 mL, 473 mL, 480 mL)

Tablet, oral: 5 mg

Tablet, extended release, oral: 5 mg, 10 mg, 15 mg

Ditropan XL®: 5 mg, 10 mg, 15 mg

General Dosage Range

Oral:

Extended release:

Children >6 years: 5 mg once daily (maximum: 20 mg/day)

Adults: Initial: 5-10 mg once daily; Maintenance: 5-30 mg once daily (maximum: 30 mg/day)

Regular release:

Children >5 years: 5 mg 2-3 times/day (maximum: 15 mg/day)

Adults: 5 mg 2-4 times/day (maximum: 20 mg/day)

Elderly: 2.5 mg 2-3 times/day

Topical gel: *Adults:* Apply contents of 1 sachet (100 mg/g) once daily

Transdermal: *Adults:* Apply one 3.9 mg/day patch twice weekly

Administration

Oral Administer without regard to meals. Extended release tablets must be swallowed whole with liquid; do not crush, divide, or chew; take at approximately the same time each day.

Topical Topical gel: For topical use only. Apply to clean, dry, intact skin on abdomen, thighs, or upper arms/shoulders. Rotate site; do not apply to same site on consecutive days. Wash hands after use. Cover treated area with clothing after gel has dried to prevent transfer of medication to others. Do not bathe, shower, or swim until 1 hour after gel applied.

Other Transdermal: Apply to clean, dry skin on abdomen, hip, or buttock. Select a new site for each new system (avoid reapplication to same site within 7 days).

Stability

Storage

Immediate release: Store at controlled room temperature of 15°C to 30°C (59°F to 86°F). Protect syrup from light.

Extended release: Store at 25°C (77°F); excursions permitted to 15°C to 30°C (59°F to 86°F). Protect from moisture and humidity.

Gel sachet, transdermal patch: Store at 25°C (77°F); excursions permitted to 15°C to 30°C (59°F to 86°F). Protect from moisture and humidity. Keel gel away from open flame. Keep patch in sealed pouch. Throw away used sachets or patches where children and pets cannot reach.

Nursing Actions

Physical Assessment Assess voiding pattern, incontinent episodes, frequency, urgency, distention, and urinary retention prior to beginning therapy and periodically throughout.

Patient Education Swallow extended-release tablets whole; do not chew or crush. You may experience dizziness, lightheadedness, drowsiness, dry mouth or changes in appetite, constipation, decreased sexual ability (reversible with discontinuance of drug), or decreased sweating. Use alcohol with caution; may increase drowsiness. Report rapid heartbeat, palpitations, or chest pain; difficulty voiding; or vision changes.

Gel: Apply to dry, intact skin. Rotate application sites. Wash hands immediately after applying. Keep dry for 1 hour after application.

Dietary Considerations Food causes a slight delay in the absorption of the oral solution and bioavailability is increased by ~25%. Absorption of the extended release tablet is not affected by food. May be taken without regard to meals.

OxyCODONE (oks i KOE done)

Brand Names: U.S. Oxecta™; OxyCONTIN®; Roxicodone®

Index Terms Dihydrohydroxycodeinone; Oxecta™; Oxycodone Hydrochloride

Pharmacologic Category Analgesic, Opioid

Medication Safety Issues

Sound-alike/look-alike issues:

OxyCODONE may be confused with HYDROcodone, OxyCONTIN®, oxymorphone

OxyCONTIN® may be confused with MS Contin®, oxybutynin

OxyFast® may be confused with Roxanol

Roxicodone® may be confused with Roxanol

High alert medication:

The Institute for Safe Medication Practices (ISMP) includes this medication among its list of drug classes which have a heightened risk of causing significant patient harm when used in error.

Medication Guide Available Yes

Pregnancy Risk Factor B

Lactation Enters breast milk/not recommended

Breast-Feeding Considerations Sedation and/or respiratory depression may occur in the infant; symptoms of opioid withdrawal may occur following the cessation of breast-feeding.

Use Management of moderate-to-severe pain, normally used in combination with nonopioid analgesics

OxyContin® is indicated for around-the-clock management of moderate-to-severe pain when an analgesic is needed for an extended period of time.

Mechanism of Action/Effect Binds to opiate receptors in the CNS, causing inhibition of ascending pain pathways, altering the perception of and response to pain; produces generalized CNS depression

Contraindications Hypersensitivity to oxycodone or any component of the formulation; significant respiratory depression; hypercarbia; acute or severe bronchial asthma; paralytic ileus (known or suspected)

Warnings/Precautions May cause CNS depression, which may impair physical or mental abilities; patients must be cautioned about performing tasks which require mental alertness (eg, operating machinery or driving). Effects may be potentiated when used with other sedative drugs or ethanol. Use with caution in patients with hypersensitivity reactions to other phenanthrene derivative opioid agonists (morphine, hydrocodone, hydromorphone, levorphanol, oxymorphone), respiratory diseases including asthma, emphysema, or COPD. Use with caution in pancreatitis or biliary tract disease, acute alcoholism (including delirium tremens), morbid obesity, adrenocortical insufficiency, history of seizure disorders, CNS depression/coma, kyphoscoliosis (or other skeletal disorder which may alter respiratory function), hypothyroidism (including myxedema), prostatic hyperplasia, urethral stricture, and toxic psychosis. May obscure diagnosis or clinical course of patients with acute abdominal conditions.

Use with caution in the elderly, debilitated, and hepatic or renal function. Hemodynamic effects (hypotension, orthostasis) may be exaggerated in patients with hypovolemia, concurrent vasodilating drugs, or in patients with head injury. Respiratory depressant effects and capacity to elevate CSF pressure may be exaggerated in presence of head injury, other intracranial lesion, or pre-existing intracranial pressure.

[U.S. Boxed Warning]: Concomitant use with CYP3A4 inhibitors may result in increased effects and potentially fatal respiratory depression. Concurrent use of agonist/antagonist analgesics may precipitate withdrawal symptoms and/or reduced analgesic efficacy in patients following prolonged therapy with mu opioid agonists. Abrupt discontinuation following prolonged use may also lead to withdrawal symptoms. **[U.S. Boxed Warning]: Healthcare provider should be alert to problems of abuse, misuse, and diversion.** Tolerance or drug dependence may result from extended use. Patients should be assessed for risk of abuse or addition prior to therapy and all patients should be monitored for signs of misuse, abuse, and addiction.

Controlled-release formulations: [U.S. Boxed Warning]: OxyContin® is not intended for use as an "as needed" analgesic or for immediately-postoperative pain management (should be used postoperatively only if the patient has received it prior to surgery or if severe, persistent pain is anticipated). **[U.S. Boxed Warning]: Do NOT crush, break, or chew controlled-release tablets**; 60 mg and 80 mg strengths, a single dose >40 mg, or a total dose of >80 mg/day are for use only in opioid-tolerant patients. Tablets may be difficult to swallow and could become lodged in throat; patients with swallowing difficulties may be at increased risk. Cases of intestinal obstruction or diverticulitis exacerbation have also been reported, including cases requiring medical intervention to remove the tablet; patients with an underlying GI disease (eg, esophageal cancer, colon cancer) may be at increased risk.

Highly-concentrated oral solutions: [U.S. Boxed Warning]: Concentrated oral solutions (20 mg/mL) should only be used in opioid tolerant patients (taking ≥30 mg/day of oxycodone or equivalent for ≥1 week); orders should be clearly written to include the intended dose (in mg vs mL) and the intended product concentration to be dispensed.

Drug Interactions

Avoid Concomitant Use

Avoid concomitant use of OxyCODONE with any of the following: Conivaptan

Decreased Effect

OxyCODONE may decrease the levels/effects of: Pegvisomant

The levels/effects of OxyCODONE may be decreased by: Ammonium Chloride; CYP3A4 Inducers (Strong); Deferasirox; Mixed Agonist / Antagonist Opioids; Rifampin; St Johns Wort; Tocilizumab

Increased Effect/Toxicity

OxyCODONE may increase the levels/effects of: Alcohol (Ethyl); Alvimopan; CNS Depressants; Desmopressin; Selective Serotonin Reuptake Inhibitors; Thiazide Diuretics

The levels/effects of OxyCODONE may be increased by: Amphetamines; Antipsychotic Agents (Phenothiazines); Conivaptan; CYP3A4 Inhibitors (Moderate); CYP3A4 Inhibitors (Strong); Dasatinib; Droperidol; HydrOXYzine; Ivacaftor; Succinylcholine; Voriconazole

Nutritional/Ethanol Interactions

Ethanol: May increase CNS depression; monitor for increased effects with coadministration. Caution patients about effects.

Herb/Nutraceutical: Avoid valerian, St John's wort, kava kava, gotu kola (may increase CNS depression).

Adverse Reactions Note: Percentages as reported with OxyContin®

>10%:

Central nervous system: Somnolence (23%), dizziness (13%)

Dermatologic: Pruritus (13%)

Gastrointestinal: Constipation (23%), nausea (23%), vomiting (12%)

1% to 10%:

Cardiovascular: Postural hypotension (1% to 5%)

Central nervous system: Headache (7%), abnormal dreams (1% to 5%), anxiety (1% to 5%), chills (1% to 5%), confusion (1% to 5%), dysphoria (1% to 5%), euphoria (1% to 5%), fever (1% to 5%), insomnia (1% to 5%), nervousness (1% to 5%), thought abnormalities (1% to 5%)

Dermatologic: Rash (1% to 5%)

Gastrointestinal: Xerostomia (6%), abdominal pain (1% to 5%), anorexia (1% to 5%), diarrhea (1% to 5%), dyspepsia (1% to 5%), gastritis (1% to 5%)

Neuromuscular & skeletal: Weakness (6%), twitching (1% to 5%)

Respiratory: Dyspnea (1% to 5%), hiccups (1% to 5%)

Miscellaneous: Diaphoresis (5%)

Pharmacodynamics/Kinetics

Onset of Action Pain relief: Immediate release: 10-15 minutes; Peak effect: Immediate release: 0.5-1 hour

Duration of Action Immediate release: 3-6 hours; Controlled release: ≤12 hours

Controlled Substance C-II

Available Dosage Forms

Capsule, oral: 5 mg

Solution, oral: 20 mg/mL (30 mL)

Tablet, oral: 5 mg, 10 mg, 15 mg, 20 mg, 30 mg

Oxecta™: 5 mg, 7.5 mg

Roxicodone®: 5 mg, 15 mg, 30 mg

Tablet, controlled release, oral:

OxyCONTIN®: 10 mg, 15 mg, 20 mg, 30 mg, 40 mg, 60 mg, 80 mg

General Dosage Range Dosage adjustment recommended in patients with hepatic impairment or on concomitant therapy

Oral:

Controlled release: *Adults:* 10-160 mg every 12 hours

Immediate release: *Adults:* 5-20 mg every 4-6 hours as needed

Administration

Oral

Controlled release: Do not moisten, crush, break, or chew controlled release tablets. Controlled release tablets are not indicated for rectal administration; increased risk of adverse events due to better rectal absorption. Controlled release tablets should be administered one at a time and each followed with water immediately after placing in the mouth.

Immediate release (Oxecta™): Must be swallowed whole with enough water to ensure complete swallowing immediately after placing in the mouth. The tablet should not be wet prior to placing in the mouth. Do not crush, chew, or dissolve the tablets. Do not administer via feeding tubes (eg, gastric, NG) due to potential for obstruction. The formulation uses technology designed to discourage common methods of tampering to prevent misuse/abuse.

Appropriate laxatives should be administered to avoid the constipating side effects associated with use. Antiemetics may be needed for persistent nausea.

Stability

Storage Store at 25°C (77°F); excursions permitted between 15°C to 30°C (59°F to 86°F). Protect from light.

Nursing Actions

Physical Assessment Monitor for effectiveness of pain relief. Monitor blood pressure, CNS and respiratory status, and degree of sedation at beginning of therapy and periodically thereafter. Assess patient's physical and/or psychological dependence. For inpatients, implement safety measures (eg, side rails up, call light within reach, instructions to call for assistance). Discontinue slowly after prolonged use.

Patient Education May cause physical and/or psychological dependence. Do not moisten, crush, or chew controlled release tablets. While using this medication, do not use alcohol and other prescription or OTC medications (especially sedatives, tranquilizers, antihistamines, or pain medications) without consulting prescriber. Maintain adequate hydration unless instructed to restrict fluid intake. Increase in fiber or stool softeners if okay with prescriber. May cause hypotension, dizziness, drowsiness, impaired coordination, or blurred vision; nausea, vomiting, or dry mouth; or constipation. The wax matrix from controlled release tablets may appear in stool. Report chest pain, slow or rapid heartbeat, dizziness, or persistent headache; confusion or respiratory difficulties; or severe constipation.

Dietary Considerations Instruct patient to avoid high-fat meals when taking some products (food has no effect on the reformulated OxyContin®).

Oxycodone and Acetaminophen

(oks i KOE done & a seet a MIN oh fen)

Brand Names: U.S. Endocet®; Percocet®; Primlev™; Roxicet™; Roxicet™ 5/500; Tylox®

Index Terms Acetaminophen and Oxycodone

Pharmacologic Category Analgesic, Opioid

Medication Safety Issues

Sound-alike/look-alike issues:

Endocet® may be confused with Indocid®

Percocet® may be confused with Fioricet®, Percodan®

Roxicet™ may be confused with Roxanol

Tylox® may be confused with Trimox, Tylenol®, Xanax®

High alert medication:

The Institute for Safe Medication Practices (ISMP) includes this medication among its list of drug classes which have a heightened risk of causing significant patient harm when used in error.

Other safety concerns:

Duplicate therapy issues: This product contains acetaminophen, which may be a component of other combination products. Do not exceed the maximum recommended daily dose of acetaminophen.

Pregnancy Risk Factor C

Lactation Enters breast milk/use caution

Use Management of moderate-to-severe pain

Controlled Substance C-II

Available Dosage Forms

Caplet: Oxycodone 5 mg and acetaminophen 500 mg

Roxicet™ 5/500: Oxycodone 5 mg and acetaminophen 500 mg

Capsule: Oxycodone 5 mg and acetaminophen 500 mg

Tylox®: Oxycodone 5 mg and acetaminophen 500 mg

Solution, oral: Oxycodone 5 mg and acetaminophen 325 mg per 5 mL

Roxicet™: Oxycodone 5 mg and acetaminophen 325 mg per 5 mL

Tablet:

Generics:

Oxycodone 2.5 mg and acetaminophen 325 mg

Oxycodone 5 mg and acetaminophen 325 mg

Oxycodone 7.5 mg and acetaminophen 325 mg

Oxycodone 7.5 mg and acetaminophen 500 mg

Oxycodone 10 mg and acetaminophen 325 mg

Oxycodone 10 mg and acetaminophen 650 mg

Brands:

Endocet®:

5/325 [scored]: Oxycodone 5 mg and acetaminophen 325 mg

7.5/325: Oxycodone 7.5 mg and acetaminophen 325 mg

7.5/500: Oxycodone 7.5 mg and acetaminophen 500 mg

10/325: Oxycodone 10 mg and acetaminophen 325 mg

10/650: Oxycodone 10 mg and acetaminophen 650 mg

Percocet®:

2.5/325: Oxycodone 2.5 mg and acetaminophen 325 mg

5/325 [scored]: Oxycodone 5 mg and acetaminophen 325 mg

7.5/325: Oxycodone 7.5 mg and acetaminophen 325 mg

7.5/500: Oxycodone 7.5 mg and acetaminophen 500 mg

10/325: Oxycodone 10 mg and acetaminophen 325 mg

10/650: Oxycodone 10 mg and acetaminophen 650 mg

Primlev™:

5/300: Oxycodone 5 mg and acetaminophen 300 mg

7.5/300: Oxycodone 7.5 mg and acetaminophen 300 mg

10/300: Oxycodone 10 mg and acetaminophen 300 mg

Roxicet™ [scored]: Oxycodone 5 mg and acetaminophen 325 mg

General Dosage Range Dosage adjustment recommended in patients with hepatic impairment

Oral:

Acetaminophen:

Children <45 kg: 10-15 mg/kg every 4-6 hours as needed (maximum: 90 mg/kg/day)

Children ≥45 kg: 10-15 mg/kg every 4-6 hours (maximum: 4 g/day)

Adults: 325-650 mg every 4-6 hours (maximum: 4 g/day)

Oxycodone:

Children: 0.05-0.3 mg/kg every 4-6 hours as needed

Adults: 2.5-30 mg/dose every 4-6 hours as needed

Elderly: Initial: 2.5-5 mg every 6 hours as needed

Nursing Actions

Physical Assessment See individual agents.

Patient Education See individual agents.

Related Information

Acetaminophen *on page 23*

OxyCODONE *on page 870*

Oxycodone and Ibuprofen

(oks i KOE done & eye byoo PROE fen)

Index Terms Ibuprofen and Oxycodone

Pharmacologic Category Analgesic, Opioid; Nonsteroidal Anti-inflammatory Drug (NSAID), Oral

Medication Safety Issues

High alert medication:

The Institute for Safe Medication Practices (ISMP) includes this medication among its list of drug classes which have a heightened risk of causing significant patient harm when used in error.

Medication Guide Available Yes

Pregnancy Risk Factor C/D ≥30 weeks gestation

Lactation Enters breast milk/not recommended

Use Short-term (≤7 days) management of acute, moderate-to-severe pain

Controlled Substance C-II

Available Dosage Forms

Tablet: Oxycodone 5 mg and ibuprofen 400 mg

General Dosage Range Oral: *Adults:* 1 tablet as needed (maximum: 4 tablets/day; 7 days)

Administration

Oral Administer without regard to meals.

Nursing Actions

Physical Assessment See individual agents.

Patient Education See individual agents.

Oxymorphone (oks i MOR fone)

Brand Names: U.S. Opana®; Opana® ER

Index Terms Oxymorphone Hydrochloride

Pharmacologic Category Analgesic, Opioid

Medication Safety Issues

Sound-alike/look-alike issues:

Oxymorphone may be confused with oxycodone, oxymetholone

High alert medication:

The Institute for Safe Medication Practices (ISMP) includes this medication among its list of drug classes which have a heightened risk of causing significant patient harm when used in error.

Medication Guide Available Yes

Pregnancy Risk Factor C

Lactation Excretion in breast milk unknown/use caution

Breast-Feeding Considerations Some opioids can be found in breast milk. Withdrawal symptoms may be observed in breast-feeding infants when opioid analgesics are discontinued.

Use

Parenteral: Management of moderate-to-severe acute pain; relief of anxiety in patients with dyspnea associated with pulmonary edema secondary to acute left ventricular failure

Oral, regular release: Management of moderate-to-severe acute pain

Oral, extended release: Management of moderate-to-severe pain in patients requiring around-the-clock opioid treatment for an extended period of time

Mechanism of Action/Effect Oxymorphone hydrochloride is a potent narcotic analgesic with uses similar to those of morphine. The drug is a semisynthetic derivative of morphine (phenanthrene derivative) and is closely related to hydromorphone chemically (Dilaudid®).

Contraindications Hypersensitivity to oxymorphone, other morphine analogs (phenanthrene derivatives), or any component of the formulation; paralytic ileus (known or suspected); moderate-to-severe hepatic impairment; severe respiratory depression (unless in monitored setting with resuscitative equipment); acute/severe bronchial asthma; hypercarbia

Note: Injection formulation is also contraindicated in the treatment of upper airway obstruction and pulmonary edema due to a chemical respiratory irritant.

Warnings/Precautions An opioid-containing analgesic regimen should be tailored to each patient's needs and based upon the type of pain being treated (acute versus chronic), the route of administration, degree of tolerance for opioids (naive versus chronic user), age, weight, and medical condition. The optimal analgesic dose varies widely among patients. Doses should be titrated to pain relief/prevention.

May cause CNS depression, which may impair physical or mental abilities; patients must be cautioned about performing tasks which require mental alertness (eg, operating machinery or driving). Effects may be potentiated when used with other sedative drugs or ethanol. Use not recommended within 14 days of MAO inhibitors. Use with caution in patients with hypersensitivity reactions to other phenanthrene-derivative opioid agonists (codeine, hydrocodone, hydromorphone, levorphanol, oxycodone). May cause respiratory depression. Use extreme caution in patients with COPD or other chronic respiratory conditions characterized by hypoxia, hypercapnia, or diminished respiratory reserve (myxedema, cor pulmonale, kyphoscoliosis, obstructive sleep apnea, severe obesity). Use with caution in patients (particularly elderly or debilitated) with impaired respiratory function, adrenal disease, morbid obesity, seizure disorders, toxic psychosis, thyroid dysfunction, prostatic hyperplasia, or renal impairment. Use caution in mild hepatic dysfunction; use is contraindicated in moderate-to-severe hepatic impairment. Use only with extreme caution (if at all) in patients with head injury or increased intracranial pressure (ICP); potential to elevate ICP and/or blunt papillary response may be greatly exaggerated in these patients. Use with caution in biliary tract disease or acute pancreatitis (may cause constriction of sphincter of Oddi). May obscure diagnosis or clinical course of patients with acute abdominal conditions.

Oxymorphone shares the toxic potential of opiate agonists and usual precautions of opiate agonist therapy should be observed; may cause hypotension in patients with acute myocardial infarction, volume depletion, or concurrent drug therapy which may exaggerate vasodilation. The elderly may be particularly susceptible to adverse effects of narcotics.

[U.S. Boxed Warning]: Healthcare provider should be alert to problems of abuse, misuse, and diversion. Tolerance or drug dependence may result from extended use. Use caution in patients with a history of drug dependence or abuse. Abrupt discontinuation may precipitate withdrawal syndrome.

Extended release formulation:

[U.S. Boxed Warnings]: Opana® ER is an extended release oral formulation of oxymorphone and is not suitable for use as an "as needed" analgesic. Tablets should not be broken, chewed, dissolved, or crushed; tablets should be swallowed whole. Opana® ER is intended for use in long-term, continuous management of moderate-to-severe chronic pain. It is not indicated for use in the immediate postoperative period (12-24 hours). **[U.S. Boxed Warning]: The coingestion of ethanol or ethanol-containing medications with Opana® ER may result in accelerated release of drug from the dosage form, abruptly increasing plasma levels, which may have fatal consequences.**

Drug Interactions

Avoid Concomitant Use

Avoid concomitant use of Oxymorphone with any of the following: MAO Inhibitors

Decreased Effect

Oxymorphone may decrease the levels/effects of: Pegvisomant

The levels/effects of Oxymorphone may be decreased by: Ammonium Chloride; Mixed Agonist / Antagonist Opioids

Increased Effect/Toxicity

Oxymorphone may increase the levels/effects of: Alcohol (Ethyl); Alvimopan; CNS Depressants; Desmopressin; MAO Inhibitors; Selective Serotonin Reuptake Inhibitors; Thiazide Diuretics

The levels/effects of Oxymorphone may be increased by: Amphetamines; Antipsychotic Agents (Phenothiazines); Droperidol; HydrOXYzine; Succinylcholine

Nutritional/Ethanol Interactions

Ethanol: Ethanol ingestion with extended-release tablets is specifically contraindicated due to possible accelerated release and potentially fatal overdose. Ethanol may also increase CNS depression; monitor for increased effects with coadministration. Caution patients about effects.

Food: When taken orally with a high-fat meal, peak concentration is 38% to 50% greater. Both immediate-release and extended-release tablets should be taken 1 hour before or 2 hours after eating.

Herb/Nutraceutical: Avoid valerian, St John's wort, kava kava, gotu kola (may increase CNS depression).

Adverse Reactions Incidence usually on higher end with extended release tablet.

>10%:

Central nervous system: Somnolence (9% to 19%), dizziness (7% to 18%), fever (1% to 14%), headache (7% to 12%)

Dermatologic: Pruritus (8% to 15%)

Gastrointestinal: Nausea (19% to 33%), constipation (4% to 28%), vomiting (9% to 16%)

1% to 10%:

Cardiovascular: Hypotension (<10%), tachycardia (<10%), edema (<10%), flushing (<10%), hypertension (<10%)

Central nervous system: Anxiety (1% to <10%), sedation (1% to <10%), depression (<10%), disorientation (<10%), lethargy (<10%), nervousness (<10%), restlessness (<10%), fatigue (≤4%), insomnia (≤4%), confusion (3%)

Endocrine & metabolic: Dehydration (<10%)

Gastrointestinal: Abdominal distension (<10%), flatulence (1% to <10%), xerostomia (1% to <10%), dyspepsia (<10%), weight loss (<10%), diarrhea (≤4%), abdominal pain (≤3%), appetite decreased (≤3%)

Neuromuscular & skeletal: Weakness (<10%)

Ocular: Blurred vision (<10%)

Respiratory: Hypoxia (<10%), dyspnea (<10%)

Miscellaneous: Diaphoresis (1% to <10%)

Pharmacodynamics/Kinetics

Onset of Action Parenteral: 5-10 minutes

Duration of Action Analgesic: Parenteral: 3-6 hours

Controlled Substance C-II

Available Dosage Forms

Injection, solution:

Opana®: 1 mg/mL (1 mL)

Tablet, oral: 5 mg, 10 mg

Opana®: 5 mg, 10 mg

Tablet, extended release, oral: 7.5 mg, 15 mg

Opana® ER: 5 mg, 10 mg, 20 mg, 30 mg, 40 mg

General Dosage Range Dosage adjustment recommended in patients with hepatic or renal impairment

I.M., SubQ: *Adults:* Initial: 0.5 mg; Maintenance: 1-1.5 mg every 4-6 hours as needed

I.V.: *Adults:* Initial: 0.5 mg

Oral:

Extended release: *Adults (opioid-naive):* Initial: 5 mg every 12 hours; Maintenance: Titrate upward with 5-10 mg every 12 hours at 3-7 day intervals until desired response

Immediate release: *Adults (opioid-naive):* Initial: 5-20 mg every 4-6 hours; Maintenance: Titrate upward to desired response

Administration

Oral Administer immediate release and extended release tablets 1 hour before or 2 hours after eating. Opana® ER tablet should be swallowed; do not break, crush, or chew.

I.V. Detail pH: 2.7-4.5

Stability

Storage Injection solution, tablet: Store at 25°C (77°F); excursions permitted to 15°C to 30°C (59°F to 86°F). Protect injection from light.

Nursing Actions

Physical Assessment If used to control diarrhea, monitor stools. Monitor for effectiveness of pain relief. Monitor blood pressure, CNS and respiratory status, and degree of sedation at beginning of therapy and periodically thereafter. Assess patient's physical and/or psychological dependence. For inpatients, implement safety measures (eg, side rails up, call light within reach, instructions to call for assistance). Discontinue slowly after prolonged use.

Patient Education May cause physical and/or psychological dependence. Do not break, chew, dissolve, or crush extended release tablets. Swallow whole. While using this medication, do not use alcohol and other prescription or OTC medications (especially sedatives, tranquilizers, antihistamines, or pain medications) without consulting prescriber. Maintain adequate hydration, unless instructed to restrict fluid intake. May cause hypotension, dizziness, drowsiness, impaired coordination, or blurred vision; nausea, vomiting, or dry mouth; or constipation. Report chest pain, slow or rapid heartbeat, dizziness, or persistent headache; confusion or respiratory difficulties; or severe constipation.

Dietary Considerations Immediate release and extended release tablets should be taken 1 hour before or 2 hours after eating.

Oxytocin (oks i TOE sin)

Brand Names: U.S. Pitocin®

Index Terms Pit

Pharmacologic Category Oxytocic Agent

Medication Safety Issues

High alert medication:

The Institute for Safe Medication Practices (ISMP) includes this medication among its list of drugs which have a heightened risk of causing significant patient harm when used in error.

Pregnancy Risk Factor C (manufacturer specific)

Lactation Excretion in breast milk unknown/use caution

Breast-Feeding Considerations Endogenous levels of oxytocin naturally increase during breast-feeding.

Use Induction of labor in patients with a medical indication; stimulation or reinforcement of labor; adjunctive therapy in management of abortion; to produce uterine contractions during the third stage of labor; control of postpartum bleeding

Mechanism of Action/Effect Oxytocin stimulates uterine contraction by activating G-protein-coupled receptors that trigger increases in intracellular calcium levels in uterine myofibrils. Oxytocin also increases local prostaglandin production, further stimulating uterine contraction.

Contraindications Hypersensitivity to oxytocin or any component of the formulation; significant cephalopelvic disproportion; unfavorable fetal positions; fetal distress when delivery is not imminent; hypertonic or hyperactive uterus; contraindicated vaginal delivery (invasive cervical cancer, active genital herpes, prolapse of the cord, cord presentation, total placenta previa, or vasa previa); obstetrical emergencies where surgical intervention is favored; where adequate uterine activity fails to achieve satisfactory progress

Warnings/Precautions Hazardous agent - use appropriate precautions for handling and disposal. **[U.S. Boxed Warning]: To be used for medical rather than elective induction of labor.** Medical indications for labor induction may include Rh problems, maternal diabetes, preeclampsia at or near term, when delivery is in the best interest of mother or fetus, or premature rupture of membranes when delivery is indicated. Use is generally not recommended in the following conditions: Fetal distress, hydramnios, partial placenta previa, prematurity, borderline cephalopelvic disproportion, or conditions where there is a predisposition for uterine rupture. May produce antidiuretic effect (ie, water intoxication). Severe water intoxication with convulsions, coma, and death is associated with a slow oxytocin infusion over 24 hours. High doses or hypersensitivity to oxytocin may cause uterine hypertonicity, spasm, tetanic contraction, or rupture of the uterus. Intravenous preparations should be administered by adequately trained individuals familiar with its use and able to identify complications.

Drug Interactions

Avoid Concomitant Use There are no known interactions where it is recommended to avoid concomitant use.

Decreased Effect There are no known significant interactions involving a decrease in effect.

Increased Effect/Toxicity

The levels/effects of Oxytocin may be increased by: Dinoprostone; Misoprostol

Adverse Reactions Frequency not defined.

Fetus or neonate:

Cardiovascular: Arrhythmias (including premature ventricular contractions), bradycardia

Central nervous system: Brain or CNS damage (permanent), neonatal seizure

Hepatic: Neonatal jaundice

Ocular: Neonatal retinal hemorrhage

Miscellaneous: Fetal death, low Apgar score (5 minute)

Mother:

Cardiovascular: Arrhythmias (including premature ventricular contractions), hypertensive episodes

Gastrointestinal: Nausea, vomiting

Genitourinary: Pelvic hematoma, postpartum hemorrhage, uterine hypertonicity, tetanic contraction of the uterus, uterine rupture, uterine spasm

Hematologic: Afibrinogenemia (fatal)

Miscellaneous: Anaphylactic reaction, subarachnoid hemorrhage; severe water intoxication with convulsions, coma, and death is associated with a slow oxytocin infusion over 24 hours

Pharmacodynamics/Kinetics

Onset of Action Uterine contractions: I.M.: 3-5 minutes; I.V.: ~1 minute

Duration of Action I.M.: 2-3 hour; I.V.: 1 hour

Available Dosage Forms

Injection, solution: 10 units/mL (1 mL, 10 mL, 30 mL)

Pitocin®: 10 units/mL (1 mL, 10 mL)

General Dosage Range

I.M.: *Adults:* Total dose of 10 units after delivery of the placenta

I.V.: *Adults:* Dosage varies greatly depending on indication

Administration

I.V. An infusion pump is required for administration.

Stability

Reconstitution I.V.:

Induction or stimulation of labor: Add oxytocin 10 units to NS or LR 1000 mL to yield a solution containing oxytocin 10 milliunits/mL. Rotate solution to mix.

Postpartum uterine bleeding: Add oxytocin 10-40 units to running I.V. infusion; maximum: 40 units/1000 mL.

Adjunctive management of abortion: Add oxytocin 10 units to 500 mL of a physiologic saline solution or D_5W.

Storage Store at 20°C to 25°C (68°F to 77°F); excursions permitted to 15°C to 30°C (59°F to 86°F); do not freeze.

Nursing Actions

Physical Assessment Monitor blood pressure, fluid intake and output, and labor closely if using oxytocin for induction; fetal monitoring is strongly recommended.

Paclitaxel (pac li TAKS el)

Index Terms Conventional Paclitaxel; Paclitaxel (Conventional); Taxol

Pharmacologic Category Antineoplastic Agent, Antimicrotubular; Antineoplastic Agent, Natural Source (Plant) Derivative; Antineoplastic Agent, Taxane Derivative

Medication Safety Issues

Sound-alike/look-alike issues:

PACLitaxel may be confused with DOCEtaxel, PARoxetine, Paxil®

PACLitaxel (conventional) may be confused with PACLitaxel (protein-bound)

Taxol® may be confused with Abraxane®, Paxil®, Taxotere®

High alert medication:

This medication is in a class the Institute for Safe Medication Practices (ISMP) includes among its list of drug classes which have a heightened risk of causing significant patient harm when used in error.

Pregnancy Risk Factor D

Lactation Excretion in breast milk unknown/contraindicated

Use Treatment of breast, nonsmall cell lung, and ovarian cancers; treatment of AIDS-related Kaposi's sarcoma (KS)

Unlabeled Use Treatment of bladder, cervical, small cell lung, and head and neck cancers; treatment of (unknown primary) adenocarcinoma

Available Dosage Forms

Injection, solution: 6 mg/mL (5 mL, 16.7 mL, 25 mL, 50 mL)

General Dosage Range Dosage adjustment recommended in patients with hepatic impairment or who develop toxicities

I.V.: *Adults:* Dosage varies greatly depending on indication

Administration

I.V. Infuse over 1-96 hours. When administered as sequential infusions, taxane derivatives should be administered before platinum derivatives (cisplatin, carboplatin) to limit myelosuppression and to enhance efficacy.

Premedication with dexamethasone (20 mg orally or I.V. at 12 and 6 hours **or** 14 and 7 hours before the dose; reduce to 10 mg with advanced HIV disease), diphenhydramine (50 mg I.V. 30-60 minutes prior to the dose), and cimetidine 300 mg, famotidine 20 mg, or ranitidine 50 mg (I.V. 30-60 minutes prior to the dose) is recommended.

Administer I.V. infusion over 1-24 hours; infuse through a 0.22 micron in-line filter and nonsorbing administration set.

I.V. Detail pH: 4.4-5.6

Other Intraperitoneal: 1- to 2-hour infusion

Nursing Actions

Physical Assessment Monitor infusion site closely to avoid extravasation. Monitor for hypersensitivity reaction, cardiovascular abnormalities, sensory neuropathy, myelosuppression, and GI irritation prior to, during, and between each infusion.

Patient Education This drug is only administered by intravenous infusion; you will be monitored closely during and following infusions. Immediately report burning, pain, or swelling at infusion site; unusual chest pain or tightness, rapid heartbeat, or palpitations; difficulty breathing; difficulty swallowing; or nausea or vomiting during infusion. You will be more susceptible to infection. It is important that you maintain adequate nutrition and fluid intake unless instructed to restrict fluid intake. May cause nausea, vomiting, sore mouth, loss of hair (will grow back after therapy), or diarrhea (if persistent, consult prescriber). Report chest pain, palpitations, or swelling of extremities; difficult breathing; pain or decreased sensation in extremities; unusual signs of weakness, fatigue, or lethargy; or persistent gastrointestinal disturbances.

Related Information

Management of Drug Extravasations *on page 1269*

Paclitaxel (Protein Bound)

(pac li TAKS el PROE teen bownd)

Brand Names: U.S. Abraxane®

Index Terms ABI-007; Albumin-Bound Paclitaxel; Albumin-Stabilized Nanoparticle Paclitaxel; nab-Paclitaxel; Nanoparticle Albumin-Bound Paclitaxel; Paclitaxel, Albumin-Bound; Protein-Bound Paclitaxel

Pharmacologic Category Antineoplastic Agent, Antimicrotubular; Antineoplastic Agent, Natural Source (Plant) Derivative; Antineoplastic Agent, Taxane Derivative

Medication Safety Issues

Sound-alike/look-alike issues:

PACLitaxel may be confused with DOCEtaxel

PACLitaxel (protein bound) may be confused with PACLitaxel (conventional)

Abraxane® may be confused with Paxil®, Taxol®, Taxotere®

High alert medication:

This medication is in a class the Institute for Safe Medication Practices (ISMP) includes among its list of drug classes which have a heightened risk of causing significant patient harm when used in error.

Pregnancy Risk Factor D

Lactation Excretion in breast milk unknown/not recommended

Use Treatment of refractory (metastatic) or relapsed (within 6 months of adjuvant therapy) breast cancer

Unlabeled Use Treatment of advanced nonsmall cell lung cancer (NSCLC)

Available Dosage Forms

Injection, powder for reconstitution:

Abraxane®: 100 mg

General Dosage Range Dosage adjustment recommended in patients with hepatic impairment or who develop toxicities

I.V.: *Adults:* 260 mg/m^2 every 3 weeks

Administration

I.V. Administer over 30 minutes. Do not use an in-line filter. Monitor infusion site; avoid extravasation. When given on a weekly (unlabeled) schedule, infusions were administered over ~30 minutes (Gradishar, 2009; Rizvi, 2008).

Nursing Actions

Physical Assessment Paclitaxel (protein bound) is not interchangeable with paclitaxel. Monitor for cardiovascular abnormalities, sensory neuropathy (numbness, tingling, burning pain), myelosuppression (anemia, opportunistic infection), and GI irritation (nausea, vomiting, mucositis, stomatitis) prior to, during, and between each infusion.

Patient Education This drug can only be administered by intravenous infusion; you will be monitored closely during and following infusions.

Immediately report any burning, pain, or swelling at infusion site; any unusual chest pain or tightness, rapid heartbeat or palpitations; difficulty breathing; difficulty swallowing; or nausea or vomiting. You will be more susceptible to infection. It is important that you maintain adequate nutrition and fluid intake unless instructed to restrict fluid intake. May cause nausea, vomiting, mouth sores, diarrhea, or loss of hair (will grow back after therapy). Report chest pain, palpitations, swelling of extremities; difficult breathing; pain or decreased sensation in extremities; unusual sign of weakness, fatigue, lethargy, or persistent gastrointestinal disturbances (nausea, vomiting, diarrhea).

Related Information

Management of Drug Extravasations *on page 1269*

Paliperidone (pal ee PER i done)

Brand Names: U.S. Invega®; Invega® Sustenna®

Index Terms 9-hydroxy-risperidone; 9-OH-risperidone; Paliperidone Palmitate

Pharmacologic Category Antipsychotic Agent, Atypical

Pregnancy Risk Factor C

Lactation Enters breast milk/not recommended

Use

Oral: Acute and maintenance treatment of schizophrenia; acute treatment of schizoaffective disorder (monotherapy or adjunctive therapy to mood stabilizers and/or antidepressants)

Injection: Acute and maintenance treatment of schizophrenia

Unlabeled Use Psychosis/agitation related to Alzheimer's dementia

Mechanism of Action/Effect Paliperidone is the primary active metabolite of risperidone. Mixed central serotonergic and dopaminergic antagonism is thought to improve negative symptoms of psychoses and reduce the incidence of extrapyramidal side effects.

Contraindications Hypersensitivity to paliperidone, risperidone, or any component of the formulation

Warnings/Precautions [U.S. Boxed Warning]: Elderly patients with dementia-related psychosis treated with antipsychotics are at an increased risk of death compared to placebo. Most deaths appeared to be either cardiovascular (eg, heart failure, sudden death) or infectious (eg, pneumonia) in nature. In addition, an increased incidence of cerebrovascular adverse effects (eg, transient ischemic attack, cerebrovascular accidents) has been reported in studies of placebo-controlled trials of risperidone (paliperidone is the primary active metabolite of risperidone) in elderly patients with dementia-related psychosis. Paliperidone is not approved for the treatment of dementia-related psychosis.

Compared with risperidone, paliperidone is low to moderately sedating; use with caution in disorders where CNS depression is a feature. Use caution in patients with predisposition to seizures. Use with caution in renal dysfunction; dose reduction recommended. Esophageal dysmotility and aspiration have been associated with antipsychotic use; use with caution in patients at risk of aspiration pneumonia (eg, Alzheimer's disease).

Leukopenia, neutropenia, and agranulocytosis (sometimes fatal) have been reported in clinical trials and postmarketing reports with antipsychotic use; presence of risk factors (eg, pre-existing low WBC or history of drug-induced leuko-/neutropenia) should prompt periodic blood count assessment. Discontinue therapy at first signs of blood dyscrasias or if absolute neutrophil count $<1000/mm^3$.

Paliperidone is associated with increased prolactin levels; clinical significance of hyperprolactinemia in patients with breast cancer or other prolactin-dependent tumors is unknown. May alter temperature regulation. May mask toxicity of other drugs or conditions (eg intestinal obstruction, Reyes syndrome, brain tumor) due to antiemetic effects. Priapism has been reported rarely with use.

May cause orthostasis and syncope. Use with caution in patients with cardiovascular diseases (eg, heart failure, history of myocardial infarction or ischemia, cerebrovascular disease, conduction abnormalities). Use caution in patients receiving medications for hypertension (orthostatic effects may be exacerbated) or in patients with hypovolemia or dehydration. May alter cardiac conduction; life-threatening arrhythmias have occurred with therapeutic doses of neuroleptics. Avoid use in combination with QT_c-prolonging drugs. Avoid use in patients with congenital long QT syndrome and in patients with history of cardiac arrhythmia.

May cause extrapyramidal symptoms (EPS), including pseudoparkinsonism, acute dystonic reactions, akathisia, and tardive dyskinesia (risk of these reactions is low relative to other neuroleptics, and is dose dependent). Risk of dystonia (and probably other EPS) may be greater with increased doses, use of conventional antipsychotics, males, and younger patients. Risk of neuroleptic malignant syndrome (NMS) may be increased in patients with Parkinson's disease or Lewy body dementia; monitor for symptoms of confusion, obtundation, postural instability and extrapyramidal symptoms. May cause hyperglycemia; in some cases may be extreme and associated with ketoacidosis, hyperosmolar coma, or death. Use with caution in patients with diabetes (or risk factors) or other disorders of glucose regulation; monitor for worsening of glucose control. Significant weight gain has been observed with antipsychotic therapy; incidence varies with product. Monitor waist circumference and BMI. May cause lipid abnormalities (LDL and triglycerides increased; HDL decreased).

The possibility of a suicide attempt is inherent in psychotic illness or bipolar disorder; use caution in high-risk patients during initiation of therapy. Prescriptions should be written for the smallest quantity consistent with good patient care.

The tablet formulation consists of drug within a nonabsorbable shell that is expelled and may be visible in the stool. Use is not recommended in patients with pre-existing severe gastrointestinal narrowing disorders. Patients with upper GI tract alterations in transit time may have increased or decreased bioavailability of paliperidone. Do not use in patients unable to swallow the tablet whole.

Drug Interactions

Avoid Concomitant Use

Avoid concomitant use of Paliperidone with any of the following: Metoclopramide

Decreased Effect

Paliperidone may decrease the levels/effects of: Amphetamines; Anti-Parkinson's Agents (Dopamine Agonist); Quinagolide

The levels/effects of Paliperidone may be decreased by: CarBAMazepine; Lithium formulations; P-glycoprotein/ABCB1 Inducers

Increased Effect/Toxicity

Paliperidone may increase the levels/effects of: Alcohol (Ethyl); CNS Depressants; Methotrimeprazine; Methylphenidate; Serotonin Modulators

The levels/effects of Paliperidone may be increased by: Acetylcholinesterase Inhibitors (Central); Divalproex; Droperidol; HydrOXYzine; Itraconazole; Lithium formulations; Methotrimeprazine; Methylphenidate; Metoclopramide; P-glycoprotein/ABCB1 Inhibitors; RisperiDONE; Tetrabenazine; Valproic Acid

Nutritional/Ethanol Interactions

Ethanol: May increase CNS depression; monitor for increased effects with coadministration. Caution patients about effects.

Herb/Nutraceutical: Avoid kava kava, gotu kola, valerian, St John's wort (may increase CNS depression).

Adverse Reactions Unless otherwise noted, frequency of adverse effects is reported for the oral/I.M. formulation in adults.

>10%:

Cardiovascular: Tachycardia (1% to 14%)

Central nervous system: EPS (≤26%; dose dependent), insomnia (10% to 15%), headache (6% to 15%), parkinsonism (3% to 14%; dose dependent), somnolence (adolescents 9% to 26%; adults 1% to 12%; dose dependent)

Neuromuscular & skeletal: Tremor (2% to 12%)

3% to 10%:

Cardiovascular: Orthostatic hypotension (1% to 4%; dose dependent), bundle branch block (≤3%)

Central nervous system: Agitation (4% to 10%), akathisia (adolescents 4% to 17%; adults 1% to 10%; dose dependent), anxiety (adolescents ≤9%; adults 3% to 8%), dizziness (1% to 6%), dystonia (1% to 5%; dose dependent), dysarthria (1% to 4%; dose dependent), fatigue (adolescents ≤4%), sleep disorder (≤3%), lethargy (adolescents ≤3%)

Endocrine & metabolic: Amenorrhea (adolescents ≤6%), galactorrhea (adolescents ≤4%), gynecomastia (adolescents ≤3%)

Gastrointestinal: Weight gain (1% to 9%; dose dependent), nausea (2% to 8%), dyspepsia (5% to 6%), vomiting (adolescents ≤11%; adults 2% to 5%), constipation (1% to 5%), salivation increased (adolescents ≤6%; adults ≤4%; dose dependent), appetite increased (2% to 3%), toothache (1% to 3%), abdominal pain (≤3%), diarrhea (≤3%), xerostomia (≤3%); tongue swelling (adolescents ≤3%), tongue paralysis (adolescents ≤3%)

Local: I.M. formulation: Injection site reaction (≤10%)

Neuromuscular & skeletal: Hyperkinesia (2% to 10% dose dependent), dyskinesia (1% to 9%), weakness (≤4%), myalgia (≤4% dose dependent), back pain (1% to 3%), extremity pain (≤3%)

Ocular: Blurred vision (adolescents ≤3%)

Respiratory: Nasopharyngitis (≤5%; dose dependent), upper respiratory tract infection (1% to 4%), cough (≤3%; dose dependent), rhinitis (1% to 3%; dose dependent)

Available Dosage Forms

Injection, suspension, extended release:

Invega® Sustenna®: 39 mg/0.25 mL (0.25 mL); 78 mg/0.5 mL (0.5 mL); 117 mg/0.75 mL (0.75 mL); 156 mg/mL (1 mL); 234 mg/1.5 mL (1.5 mL)

Tablet, extended release, oral:

Invega®: 1.5 mg, 3 mg, 6 mg, 9 mg

General Dosage Range Dosage adjustment recommended in patients with renal impairment

I.M.: *Adults:* Initial: 234 mg, then 156 mg 1 week later; Maintenance: 39-234 mg/month

Oral: *Adolescents 12-17 years and Adults:* 3-12 mg once daily (maximum: 12 mg/day)

Administration

Oral Administer in the morning without regard to meals. Extended release tablets should be swallowed whole with liquids; do not crush, chew, or divide.

I.M. Invega® Sustenna™ should be administered by I.M. route only as a single injection (do not divide); do not administer I.V. or subcutaneously. Avoid inadvertent injection into vasculature. Prior to injection, shake syringe for at least 10 seconds to ensure a homogenous suspension. The 2 initial injections should be administered in the deltoid muscle using a 1 1/2 inch, 22-gauge needle for patients ≥90 kg, and a 1 inch, 23-gauge needle for patients <90 kg. The 2 initial deltoid intramuscular injections help attain therapeutic concentrations rapidly. Alternate deltoid injections (right and left deltoid muscle). The second dose may be administered 2 days before or after the weekly timepoint. Monthly maintenance doses can be administered in either the deltoid or gluteal muscle. Administer injections in the gluteal muscle using a 1 1/2 inch, 22-gauge needle in the upper-outer quadrant of the gluteal area. Alternate gluteal injections (right and left gluteal muscle). The monthly maintenance dose may be administered 7 days before or after the monthly timepoint.

I.V. Do not administer I.V. or SubQ.

Stability

Storage Store at controlled room temperature of ≤25°C (77°F); excursions permitted to 15°C to 30°C (59°F to 86°F). Protect tablets from moisture.

Nursing Actions

Physical Assessment Monitor laboratory tests prior to treatment, at 3 months, and annually. Assess closely for suicide ideation prior to treatment, when changing dose, and at regular intervals. Instruct patients with diabetes to monitor serum glucose closely; may seriously affect glucose control. Monitor for suicide ideation, cardiovascular changes, extrapyramidal effects, and CNS changes.

Patient Education Do not chew, crush, or break tablet; swallow whole with liquids. It may take several weeks to achieve desired results. Avoid alcohol. Maintain adequate hydration. If you have diabetes, monitor blood sugars closely; may alter glucose control (notify prescriber of any change in glucose control). This medication comes in a nonabsorbable shell; after release of the drug, the shell is expelled and may be visible in stool (this is normal). May cause headache, dizziness, restlessness, anxiety, or blurred vision; orthostatic hypotension; or mild nausea, heartburn, abdominal pain, or sore mouth. Report immediately chest pain or rapid or irregular heart beat; muscle or bone pain, tremors, rigidity, or spasms; twitching of extremities or unusual movements; altered gait or loss of balance; CNS changes (persistent or unusual anxiety, nervousness, abnormal thought, confusion, fatigue, suicide ideation); or weight gain.

Dietary Considerations May be taken without regard to meals.

Palonosetron (pal oh NOE se tron)

Brand Names: U.S. Aloxi®

Index Terms Palonosetron Hydrochloride; RS-25259; RS-25259-197

Pharmacologic Category Antiemetic; Selective 5-HT_3 Receptor Antagonist

Medication Safety Issues

Sound-alike/look-alike issues:

Aloxi® may be confused with Eloxatin®, oxaliplatin

Palonosetron may be confused with dolasetron, granisetron, ondansetron

Pregnancy Risk Factor B

Lactation Excretion in breast milk unknown/not recommended

Breast-Feeding Considerations The extent to which palonosetron is excreted in breast milk, if at all, is unknown. Due to the potential for adverse effects in the nursing infant, breast-feeding is not recommended.

Use Prevention of chemotherapy-associated nausea and vomiting; indicated for prevention of acute (highly-emetogenic therapy) as well as acute and delayed (moderately-emetogenic therapy) nausea and vomiting; prevention of postoperative nausea and vomiting (PONV)

Mechanism of Action/Effect Selective 5-HT_3 receptor antagonist, blocking serotonin, both on vagal nerve terminals in the periphery and centrally in the chemoreceptor trigger zone

Contraindications Hypersensitivity to palonosetron or any component of the formulation

Warnings/Precautions Hypersensitivity has been observed rarely with I.V. palonosetron. Use caution in patients allergic to other 5-HT_3 receptor antagonists; cross-reactivity is possible. Some selective 5-HT_3 receptor antagonists have been associated with dose-dependent increases in ECG intervals (eg, PR, QRS duration, QT/QT_c, JT), usually occurring 1-2 hours after I.V. administration. In general, these changes are not clinically relevant, however, when these agents are used in conjunction with other agents that prolong these intervals, arrhythmia may occur. When used with agents that prolong the QT interval (eg, Class I and III antiarrhythmics), clinically relevant QT interval prolongation could result in torsade de pointes. A number of trials have shown that 5-HT_3 antagonists produce QT interval prolongation to variable degrees. Use with caution in patients at risk of QT prolongation and/or ventricular arrhythmia. Reduction in heart rate may also occur with the 5-HT_3 antagonists. Use with caution in patients with congenital long QT syndrome or other risk factors for QT prolongation (eg, medications known to prolong QT interval, electrolyte abnormalities, and cumulative high dose anthracycline therapy).

Not intended for treatment of nausea and vomiting or for chronic continuous therapy. **For chemotherapy, should be used on a scheduled basis, not on an "as needed" (PRN) basis,** since data support the use of this drug only in the prevention of nausea and vomiting (due to antineoplastic therapy) and not in the rescue of nausea and vomiting. For PONV, may use for low expectation of PONV if it is essential to avoid nausea and vomiting in the postoperative period; use is not recommended if there is little expectation of nausea and vomiting.

Drug Interactions

Avoid Concomitant Use

Avoid concomitant use of Palonosetron with any of the following: Apomorphine

Decreased Effect

The levels/effects of Palonosetron may be decreased by: Cyproterone; Peginterferon Alfa-2b; Tocilizumab

Increased Effect/Toxicity

Palonosetron may increase the levels/effects of: Apomorphine

The levels/effects of Palonosetron may be increased by: Conivaptan

Adverse Reactions Adverse events may vary according to indication.

1% to 10%:

Cardiovascular: QT prolongation (chemotherapy-associated <1%; PONV 1% to 5%), bradycardia (chemotherapy-associated 1%; PONV 4%), hypotension (≤1%), sinus bradycardia (≤1%), tachycardia (nonsustained) (≤1%)

Central nervous system: Headache (chemotherapy-associated 5% to 9%; PONV 3%), anxiety (1%), dizziness (≤1%)

Dermatologic: Pruritus (≤1%)

Endocrine & metabolic: Hyperkalemia (1%)

Gastrointestinal: Constipation (2% to 5%), diarrhea (≤1%), flatulence (≤1%)

Genitourinary: Urinary retention (≤1%)

Hepatic: ALT increased (≤1%; transient), AST increased (≤1%; transient)

Neuromuscular & skeletal: Weakness (1%)

Available Dosage Forms

Injection, solution:

Aloxi®: 0.05 mg/mL (1.5 mL, 5 mL)

General Dosage Range I.V.: *Adults:* 0.25 mg **or** 0.075 mg as a single dose

Administration

I.V. Flush I.V. line with NS prior to and following administration.

Chemotherapy-associated nausea and vomiting: Infuse over 30 seconds, 30 minutes prior to the start of chemotherapy

PONV: Infuse over 10 seconds immediately prior to anesthesia induction

I.V. Detail pH: 4.5-5.5

Stability

Storage Store intact vials at room temperature of 20°C to 25°C (68°F to 77°F); excursions permitted to 15°C to 30°C (59°F to 86°F); do not freeze. Protect from light. Solutions of 5 mcg/mL and 30 mcg/mL in NS, D_5W, $D_5\frac{1}{2}NS$, and D_5LR injection are stable for 48 hours at room temperature and 14 days under refrigeration (Trissel, 2004).

Nursing Actions

Physical Assessment Allergy history to selective 5-HT_3 receptor antagonists should be assessed prior to administering. Assess other drugs patient may be taking that may prolong QT interval. To be used on a scheduled basis for prevention of nausea and vomiting associated with cancer chemotherapy and postoperative nausea and vomiting; not recommended for treatment of existing chemotherapy-induced emesis. I.V.: Follow infusion specifics.

Patient Education This drug is given to prevent nausea and vomiting. If this medication is administered I.V., you will be monitored during infusion; report immediately any chest pain, respiratory difficulty, or pain or itching at infusion site. May cause headache, drowsiness, or dizziness. Report chest pain or palpitations, persistent headache, excessive drowsiness, fever, constipation, or diarrhea.

Pamidronate (pa mi DROE nate)

Brand Names: U.S. Aredia®

Index Terms Pamidronate Disodium

Pharmacologic Category Antidote; Bisphosphonate Derivative

Medication Safety Issues

Sound-alike/look-alike issues:

Aredia® may be confused with Adriamycin®

Pamidronate may be confused with papaverine

Pregnancy Risk Factor D

Lactation Excretion in breast milk unknown/use caution

Use Treatment of moderate or severe hypercalcemia associated with malignancy (in conjunction with adequate hydration) with or without bone metastases; treatment of osteolytic bone lesions associated with multiple myeloma or metastatic breast cancer; moderate-to-severe Paget's disease of bone

Unlabeled Use Treatment of osteogenesis imperfecta; treatment of symptomatic bone metastases of thyroid cancer; prevention of bone loss associated with androgen deprivation treatment in prostate cancer

Mechanism of Action/Effect A bisphosphonate which inhibits bone resorption via actions on osteoclasts and/or on osteoclast precursors. Does not appear to produce any significant effects on renal tubular calcium handling and is poorly absorbed following oral administration (high oral doses have been reported effective); therefore, I.V. therapy is preferred.

Contraindications Hypersensitivity to pamidronate, other bisphosphonates, or any component of the formulation

Warnings/Precautions Osteonecrosis of the jaw (ONJ) has been reported in patients receiving bisphosphonates. Risk factors include invasive dental procedures (eg, tooth extraction, dental implants, boney surgery); a diagnosis of cancer, with concomitant chemotherapy, radiotherapy, or corticosteroids; poor oral hygiene, ill-fitting dentures; and comorbid disorders (anemia, coagulopathy, infection, pre-existing dental disease). Most reported cases occurred after I.V. bisphosphonate therapy; however, cases have been reported following oral therapy. A dental exam and preventative dentistry should be performed prior to placing patients with risk factors on chronic bisphosphonate therapy. The manufacturer's labeling states that discontinuing bisphosphonates in patients requiring invasive dental procedures reduces the risk of ONJ. However, other experts suggest that there is no evidence that discontinuing therapy reduces the risk of developing ONJ (Assael, 2009). The benefit/risk must be assessed by the treating physician and/or dentist/surgeon prior to any invasive dental procedure. Patients developing ONJ while on bisphosphonates should receive care by an oral surgeon.

Infrequently, severe (and occasionally debilitating) musculoskeletal (bone, joint, and/or muscle) pain have been reported during bisphosphonate treatment. The onset of pain ranged from a single day to several months. Consider discontinuing therapy in patients who experience severe symptoms; symptoms usually resolve upon discontinuation. Some patients experienced recurrence when rechallenged with same drug or another bisphosphonate; avoid use in patients with a history of these symptoms in association with bisphosphonate therapy.

Initial or single doses have been associated with renal deterioration, progressing to renal failure and dialysis. Withhold pamidronate treatment (until renal function returns to baseline) in patients with evidence of renal deterioration. Glomerulosclerosis (focal segmental) with or without nephrotic syndrome has also been reported. Longer infusion times (>2 hours) may reduce the risk for renal toxicity, especially in patients with pre-existing renal insufficiency. Single pamidronate doses should not exceed 90 mg. Patients with serum creatinine >3 mg/dL were not studied in clinical trials; limited data are available in patients with Cl_{cr} <30 mL/minute. Evaluate serum creatinine prior to each treatment. For the treatment of bone metastases, use is not recommended in patients with severe renal impairment; for renal impairment in indications other than bone metastases, use clinical judgment to determine if benefits outweigh potential risks.

Use has been associated with asymptomatic electrolyte abnormalities (including hypophosphatemia, hypokalemia, hypomagnesemia, and hypocalcemia). Rare cases of symptomatic hypocalcemia, including tetany have been reported. Patients with a history of thyroid surgery may have relative hypoparathyroidism; predisposing them to pamidronate-related hypocalcemia. Patients with pre-existing anemia, leukopenia, or thrombocytopenia should be closely monitored during the first 2 weeks of treatment.

According to the American Society of Clinical Oncology (ASCO) guidelines for bisphosphonates in multiple myeloma, treatment with pamidronate is not recommended for asymptomatic (smoldering) or indolent myeloma or with solitary plasmacytoma (Kyle, 2007). The National Comprehensive Cancer Network® (NCCN) multiple myeloma guidelines (v.1.2011) also do not recommend pamidronate use in stage 1 or smoldering disease, unless part of a clinical trial.

Adequate hydration is required during treatment (urine output ~2 L/day); avoid overhydration, especially in patients with heart failure. Vein irritation and thrombophlebitis may occur with infusions. Women of childbearing potential should be advised to use effective contraception and avoid becoming pregnant during therapy.

Drug Interactions

Avoid Concomitant Use There are no known interactions where it is recommended to avoid concomitant use.

Decreased Effect

The levels/effects of Pamidronate may be decreased by: Proton Pump Inhibitors

Increased Effect/Toxicity

Pamidronate may increase the levels/effects of: Deferasirox; Phosphate Supplements

The levels/effects of Pamidronate may be increased by: Aminoglycosides; Nonsteroidal Anti-Inflammatory Agents; Thalidomide

Adverse Reactions Note: Actual percentages may vary by indication; treatment for multiple myeloma is associated with higher percentage.

>10%:

Central nervous system: Fever (18% to 39%; transient), fatigue (≤37%), headache (≤26%), insomnia (≤22%)

Endocrine & metabolic: Hypophosphatemia (≤18%), hypokalemia (4% to 18%), hypomagnesemia (4% to 12%), hypocalcemia (≤12%)

Gastrointestinal: Nausea (≤54%), vomiting (≤36%), anorexia (≤26%), abdominal pain (≤23%), dyspepsia (≤23%)

Genitourinary: Urinary tract infection (≤19%)

Hematologic: Anemia (≤43%), granulocytopenia (≤20%)

Local: Infusion site reaction (≤18%; includes induration, pain, redness and swelling)

Neuromuscular & skeletal: Myalgia (≤26%), weakness (≤22%), arthralgia (≤14%), osteonecrosis of the jaw (cancer patients: 1% to 11%)

Renal: Serum creatinine increased (≤19%)

Respiratory: Dyspnea (≤30%), cough (≤26%), upper respiratory tract infection (≤24%), sinusitis (≤16%), pleural effusion (≤11%)

1% to 10%:

Cardiovascular: Atrial fibrillation (≤6%), hypertension (≤6%), syncope (≤6%), tachycardia (≤6%), atrial flutter (≤1%), cardiac failure (≤1%), edema (≤1%)

Central nervous system: Somnolence (≤6%), psychosis (≤4%), seizure (≤2%)

Endocrine & metabolic: Hypothyroidism (≤6%)

Gastrointestinal: Constipation (≤6%), gastrointestinal hemorrhage (≤6%), diarrhea (≤1%), stomatitis (≤1%)

Hematologic: Leukopenia (≤4%), neutropenia (≤1%), thrombocytopenia (≤1%)

Neuromuscular & skeletal: Back pain, bone pain

Renal: Uremia (≤4%)

Respiratory: Rales (≤6%), rhinitis (≤6%)

Miscellaneous: Moniliasis (≤6%)

Pharmacodynamics/Kinetics

Onset of Action 24-48 hours; Peak effect: Maximum: 5-7 days

Available Dosage Forms

Injection, powder for reconstitution: 30 mg, 90 mg

Aredia®: 30 mg

Injection, solution: 3 mg/mL (10 mL); 6 mg/mL (10 mL); 9 mg/mL (10 mL)

Injection, solution [preservative free]: 3 mg/mL (10 mL); 9 mg/mL (10 mL)

General Dosage Range Dosage adjustment recommended in patients with renal impairment

I.V.: *Adults:* 60-90 mg as a single dose, may repeat every 3-4 weeks **or** 30 mg daily for 3 consecutive days

Administration

I.V. Infusion rate varies by indication. Longer infusion times (>2 hours) may reduce the risk for renal toxicity, especially in patients with pre-existing renal insufficiency. The manufacturer recommends infusing over 2-24 hours for hypercalcemia of malignancy; over 2 hours for osteolytic bone lesions with metastatic breast cancer; and over 4 hours for Paget's disease and for osteolytic bone lesions with multiple myeloma. The ASCO guidelines for bisphosphonate use in multiple myeloma recommend infusing pamidronate over at least 2 hours; if therapy is withheld due to renal toxicity, infuse over at least 4 hours upon reintroduction of treatment after renal recovery.

I.V. Detail pH: 6-7.4

Stability

Reconstitution Powder for injection: Reconstitute by adding 10 mL of SWFI to each vial of lyophilized pamidronate disodium powder, the resulting solution will be 30 mg/10 mL or 90 mg/10 mL.

Pamidronate may be further diluted in 250-1000 mL of 0.45% or 0.9% sodium chloride or 5% dextrose. (The manufacturer recommends dilution in 1000 mL for hypercalcemia of malignancy, 500 mL for Paget's disease and bone metastases of myeloma, and 250 mL for bone metastases of breast cancer.)

Storage

Powder for reconstitution: Store below 30°C (86°F). The reconstituted solution is stable for 24 hours stored under refrigeration at 2°C to 8°C (36°F to 46°F).

Solution for injection: Store at 20°C to 25°C (68°F to 77°F).

Pamidronate solution for infusion is stable at room temperature for up to 24 hours.

Nursing Actions

Physical Assessment A thorough oral exam should be done prior to initiating any therapy. Patients need to be instructed on maintaining good oral hygiene throughout treatment. It is important to know that if a patient is undergoing chemotherapy, radiation therapy, or a combination of both, they are at a higher risk for osteonecrosis of the jaw.

Patient Education Patients should be aware that a dental exam and any needed dental work should be completed before starting this medication. Patients need to understand the importance of good oral hygiene throughout treatment, especially if they are receiving chemotherapy, radiation therapy, or both. Report persistent muscle or bone pain or pain in mouth, jaws, or teeth.

Dietary Considerations Multiple myeloma or metastatic bone lesions from solid tumors or Paget's disease: Take adequate daily calcium and vitamin D supplement (if patient is not hypercalcemic).

Pancrelipase (pan kre LYE pase)

Brand Names: U.S. Creon®; Pancreaze™; Pancrelipase™; Zenpep®

Index Terms Amylase, Lipase, and Protease; Lipancreatin; Lipase, Protease, and Amylase; Pancreatic Enzymes; Protease, Lipase, and Amylase

Pharmacologic Category Enzyme

Medication Safety Issues

Sound-alike/look-alike issues:

Pancrelipase may be confused with pancreatin

Medication Guide Available Yes

Pregnancy Risk Factor C

Lactation Excretion in breast milk unknown/use caution

Use Treatment of exocrine pancreatic insufficiency (EPI) due to conditions such as cystic fibrosis (Creon®, Pancreaze™, Zenpep®); chronic pancreatitis (Creon®); or pancreatectomy (Creon®)

Product Availability

Ultresa™: FDA approved March 2012; anticipated availability currently undetermined. Consult prescribing information for additional information.

Viokace™: FDA approved March 2012; anticipated availability currently undetermined. Consult prescribing information for additional information.

Available Dosage Forms

Capsule, delayed release, enteric coated beads [porcine derived]:

Pancrelipase™: Lipase 5000 units, protease 17,000 units, and amylase 27,000 units

Zenpep®: Lipase 3000 units, protease 10,000 units, and amylase 16,000 units

Zenpep®: Lipase 5000 units, protease 17,000 units, and amylase 27,000 units

Zenpep®: Lipase 10,000 units, protease 34,000 units, and amylase 55,000 units

Zenpep®: Lipase 15,000 units, protease 51,000 units, and amylase 82,000 units

Zenpep®: Lipase 20,000 units, protease 68,000 units, and amylase 109,000 units

Zenpep®: Lipase 25,000 units, protease 85,000 units, and amylase 136,000 units

Capsule, delayed release, enteric coated microspheres [new formulation; porcine derived]:

Creon®: Lipase 3000 units, protease 9500 units, and amylase 15,000 units

Creon®: Lipase 6000 units, protease 19,000 units, and amylase 30,000 units

Creon®: Lipase 12000 units, protease 38,000 units, and amylase 60,000 units

Creon®: Lipase 24,000 units, protease 76,000 units, and amylase 120,000 units

Capsule, delayed release, enteric coated microtablets [porcine derived]:

Pancreaze™: Lipase 4200 units, protease 10,000 units, and amylase 17,500 units

Pancreaze™: Lipase 10,500 units, protease 25,000 units, and amylase 43,750 units

Pancreaze™: Lipase 16,800 units, protease 40,000 units, and amylase 70,000 units

Pancreaze™: Lipase 21,000 units, protease 37,000 units, and amylase 61,000 units

General Dosage Range Oral:

Children ≤1 year: Lipase 2000-4000 units per 120 mL of formula or breast milk

Children >1 and <4 years: Lipase 1000-2500 units/kg/meal; Maximum dose: Lipase 10,000 units/kg/day **or** lipase 4000 units/g of fat per day

Children ≥4 years and Adults: Lipase 500-2500 units/kg/meal **or** lipase 72,000 units/meal (while consuming ≥100 g of fat per day); Maximum dose: Lipase 10,000 units/kg/day **or** lipase 4000 units/g of fat per day

Administration

Oral Administer with meals or snacks and swallow whole with a generous amount of liquid. Do not crush or chew; retention in the mouth before swallowing may cause mucosal irritation and stomatitis. If necessary, capsules may also be opened and contents added to a small amount of an acidic food (pH ≤4.5), such as applesauce. The food should be at room temperature and swallowed immediately after mixing. The contents of the capsule should not be crushed or chewed. Follow with water or juice to ensure complete ingestion and that no medication remains in the mouth.

When administering to infants <1 year of age, do not mix with breast milk or infant formula. Open capsule and place the contents directly into the mouth or mix with a small amount of acidic soft food (pH ≤4.5), such as applesauce or other acidic commercially prepared baby food (pears or bananas) at room temperature. Administer immediately after mixing (or within 15 minutes of mixing using Pancreaze™). Follow with infant formula or breast milk to ensure complete ingestion and that no medication remains in the mouth.

Creon®: Capsules contain enteric coated spheres which are 0.71-1.6 mm in diameter

Pancreaze™: Capsules contain enteric coated microtablets which are ~2 mm in diameter

Zenpep®: Capsules contain enteric coated beads which are 1.8-2.5 mm in diameter

Other Administration via gastrostomy (G) tube: An *in vitro* study demonstrated that Creon® delayed-release capsules sprinkled onto a small amount of baby food (pH<4.5; applesauce or bananas manufactured by both Gerber and Beech-Nut) stirred gently and after 15 minutes was administered through the following G-tubes without significant loss of lipase activity: Kimberly-Clark MIC Bolus® size 18 Fr, Kimberly-Clark MIC-KEY® size 16 Fr, Bard® Tri-Funnel size 18 Fr, and Bard® Button size 18 Fr (Shlieout, 2011).

Nursing Actions

Physical Assessment Dosing and administration depend on purpose for use and formulation (available products are not interchangeable).

Patient Education Take right before or with foods, and swallow whole with a generous amount of liquid. Dairy products may have a high pH and should not be taken together with this medication. Do not crush or chew the contents of the capsules. Delayed-release capsules containing enteric-coated microspheres or microtablets may be opened and the contents sprinkled on soft food; do not chew. Report unusual rash, persistent GI upset, or respiratory difficulty.

Pancuronium (pan kyoo ROE nee um)

Index Terms Pancuronium Bromide; Pavulon [DSC]

Pharmacologic Category Neuromuscular Blocker Agent, Nondepolarizing

Medication Safety Issues

High alert medication:

The Institute for Safe Medication Practices (ISMP) includes this medication among its list of drugs which have a heightened risk of causing significant patient harm when used in error.

Other safety concerns:

United States Pharmacopeia (USP) 2006: The Interdisciplinary Safe Medication Use Expert Committee of the USP has recommended the following:

- Hospitals, clinics, and other practice sites should institute special safeguards in the storage, labeling, and use of these agents and should include these safeguards in staff orientation and competency training.
- Healthcare professionals should be on high alert (especially vigilant) whenever a neuromuscular-blocking agent (NMBA) is stocked, ordered, prepared, or administered.

Pregnancy Risk Factor C

Use Facilitation of endotracheal intubation and relaxation of skeletal muscles during surgery; facilitation of mechanical ventilation in ICU patients; does not relieve pain or produce sedation

Available Dosage Forms

Injection, solution: 1 mg/mL (10 mL)

General Dosage Range Dosage adjustment recommended in patients with renal impairment

I.V.: *Children >1 month and Adults:*

ICU paralysis: 0.06-0.1 mg/kg bolus followed by 1-2 mcg/kg/minute infusion **or** 0.1-0.2 mg/kg every 1-3 hours

Surgery: Intubation: Initial: 0.06-1 mg/kg **or** 0.05 mg/kg after succinylcholine; Maintenance: 0.01 mg/kg administered 60-100 minutes after initial dose and then every 25-60 minutes

Administration

I.V. May be administered undiluted by rapid I.V. injection.

I.V. Detail pH: 4 (adjusted)

Nursing Actions

Physical Assessment Ventilatory support must be instituted and maintained until adequate respiratory muscle function and/or airway protection are assured. This drug is not an anesthetic or analgesic; pain must be treated with other agents. Continuous monitoring of vital signs, cardiac status, respiratory status, and degree of neuromuscular block (objective assessment with peripheral external nerve stimulator) is mandatory until full muscle tone has returned. It may take longer for return of muscle tone in obese or elderly patients or patients with renal or hepatic disease, myasthenia gravis, myopathy, other neuromuscular disease, dehydration, electrolyte imbalance, or severe acid/base imbalance.

Long-term use: Monitor level of neuromuscular blockade, skeletal muscle movement, and respiratory effort. Reposition patient and provide appropriate skin care, mouth care, and care of patient's eyes every 2-3 hours while sedated. Provide appropriate emotional and sensory support (auditory and environmental).

Patient Education Patient will usually be unconscious prior to administration. Reassurance of constant monitoring and emotional support to reduce fear and anxiety should precede and follow administration. Following return of muscle tone, do not attempt to change position or rise from bed without assistance.

Panitumumab (pan i TOOM yoo mab)

Brand Names: U.S. Vectibix®

Index Terms ABX-EGF; MOAB ABX-EGF; Monoclonal Antibody ABX-EGF; rHuMAb-EGFr

Pharmacologic Category Antineoplastic Agent, Monoclonal Antibody; Epidermal Growth Factor Receptor (EGFR) Inhibitor

Pregnancy Risk Factor C

Lactation Excretion in breast milk unknown/not recommended

Use Monotherapy in treatment of refractory metastatic colorectal cancer

Note: Subset analyses (retrospective) in metastatic colorectal cancer trials have not shown a benefit with EGFR inhibitor treatment in patients whose tumors have codon 12 or 13 *KRAS* mutations; use is not recommended in these patients.

Available Dosage Forms

Injection, solution [preservative free]:

Vectibix®: 20 mg/mL (5 mL, 20 mL)

General Dosage Range Dosage adjustment recommended in patients who develop toxicities

I.V.: *Adults:* 6 mg/kg every 2 weeks

Administration

I.V. Doses ≤1000 mg, infuse over 1 hour; doses >1000 mg, infuse over 90 minutes; reduce infusion rate by 50% for mild-to-moderate infusion reactions (grades 1 and 2); discontinue for severe infusion reactions (grades 3 and 4). Administer through a low protein-binding 0.2 or 0.22 micrometer in-line filter. Flush with NS before and after infusion.

I.V. Detail pH: 5.6-6; may contain a small amount of visible transparent or white, amorphous panitumumab particles

Nursing Actions

Physical Assessment Monitor patient closely during and following infusion for infusion reaction; appropriate medical support for the management of infusion reactions should be readily available. Monitor for severe skin reactions (may necessitate dose reduction), peripheral edema, and gastrointestinal upset (pain, nausea, diarrhea, constipation, vomiting) at each infusion and throughout therapy.

Patient Education This medication can only be administered by infusion; you will be closely monitored. Report immediately unusual back or abdominal pain; acute headache; difficulty breathing or chest tightness; difficulty swallowing; itching or rash; or redness, swelling, or pain at infusion site. Maintain adequate nutrition and hydration, unless instructed to restrict fluid intake. You may experience nausea, vomiting, diarrhea, or constipation. Report immediately any skin rash, redness, or infection; any unusual swelling of extremities or weight gain; unremitting abdominal pain, vomiting, diarrhea, or constipation; any changes in vision; or unusual infection (respiratory or wound).

Pantoprazole (pan TOE pra zole)

Brand Names: U.S. Protonix®; Protonix® I.V.

Pharmacologic Category Proton Pump Inhibitor; Substituted Benzimidazole

Medication Safety Issues

Sound-alike/look-alike issues:

Pantoprazole may be confused with ARIPiprazole

Protonix® may be confused with Lotronex®, Lovenox®, protamine

Administration issues:

Vials containing Protonix® I.V. for injection are not recommended for use with spiked I.V. system adaptors. Nurses and pharmacists have reported breakage of the glass vials during attempts to connect spiked I.V. system adaptors, which may potentially result in injury to healthcare professionals.

International issues:

Protonix [U.S., Canada] may be confused with Pretanix brand name for indapamide [Hungary]

Pregnancy Risk Factor B

Lactation Enters breast milk/not recommended

Breast-Feeding Considerations Not recommended due to carcinogenicity in animal studies.

Use

Oral: Treatment and maintenance of healing of erosive esophagitis associated with GERD; reduction in relapse rates of daytime and nighttime heartburn symptoms in GERD; hypersecretory disorders associated with Zollinger-Ellison syndrome or other GI hypersecretory disorders

I.V.: Short-term treatment (7-10 days) of patients with gastroesophageal reflux disease (GERD) and a history of erosive esophagitis; hypersecretory disorders associated with Zollinger-Ellison syndrome or other neoplastic disorders

Unlabeled Use Peptic ulcer disease, active ulcer bleeding (parenteral formulation); adjunct treatment with antibiotics for *Helicobacter pylori* eradication; stress-ulcer prophylaxis in the critically-ill

Mechanism of Action/Effect Suppresses gastric acid secretion by inhibiting the parietal cell H^+/K^+ ATP pump

Contraindications Hypersensitivity to pantoprazole, substituted benzamidazoles (eg, esomeprazole, lansoprazole, omeprazole, rabeprazole), or any component of the formulation

Canadian labeling: Additional contraindication (not in U.S. labeling): Concomitant use with atazanavir

Warnings/Precautions Use of proton pump inhibitors (PPIs) may increase the risk of gastrointestinal infections (eg, *Salmonella, Campylobacter*). Relief of symptoms does not preclude the presence of a gastric malignancy. Long-term pantoprazole therapy (especially in patients who were *H. pylori* positive) has caused biopsy-proven atrophic gastritis. No reports of enterochromaffin-like (ECL) cell carcinoids, dysplasia, or neoplasia such as those seen in rodent studies have occurred in humans. Not indicated for maintenance therapy; safety and efficacy for use beyond 16 weeks have not been established. Prolonged treatment (typically >3 years) may lead to vitamin B_{12} malabsorption and subsequent deficiency. Intravenous preparation contains edetate sodium (EDTA); use caution in patients who are at risk for zinc deficiency if other EDTA-containing solutions are coadministered. Decreased *H. pylori* eradication rates have been observed with short-term (≤7 days) combination therapy. The American College of Gastroenterology recommends 10-14 days of therapy (triple or quadruple) for eradication of *H. pylori* (Chey, 2007).

PPIs may diminish the therapeutic effect of clopidogrel, thought to be due to reduced formation of the active metabolite of clopidogrel. Of the PPIs, pantoprazole has the lowest degree of CYP2C19 inhibition. Therefore, the manufacturer of clopidogrel prefers pantoprazole if concomitant use of a PPI is necessary. Others have recommended the continued use of PPIs, regardless of the degree of inhibition, in patients with a history of GI bleeding or multiple risk factors for GI bleeding who are also receiving clopidogrel since no evidence has established clinically meaningful differences in outcome; however, a clinically-significant interaction cannot be excluded in those who are poor metabolizers of clopidogrel (Abraham, 2010; Levine, 2011).

Increased incidence of osteoporosis-related bone fractures of the hip, spine, or wrist may occur with PPI therapy. Patients on high-dose or long-term therapy should be monitored. Use the lowest effective dose for the shortest duration of time, use vitamin D and calcium supplementation, and follow appropriate guidelines to reduce risk of fractures in patients at risk.

Hypomagnesemia, reported rarely, usually with prolonged PPI use of >3 months (most cases >1 year of therapy); may be symptomatic or asymptomatic; severe cases may cause tetany, seizures, and cardiac arrhythmias. Consider obtaining serum magnesium concentrations prior to beginning long-term therapy, especially if taking concomitant digoxin, diuretics, or other drugs known to cause hypomagnesemia; and periodically thereafter. Hypomagnesemia may be corrected by magnesium supplementation, although discontinuation of pantoprazole may be necessary; magnesium levels typically return to normal within 1 week of stopping.

Drug Interactions

Avoid Concomitant Use

Avoid concomitant use of Pantoprazole with any of the following: Delavirdine; Erlotinib; Nelfinavir; Posaconazole; Rilpivirine

Decreased Effect

Pantoprazole may decrease the levels/effects of: Atazanavir; Bisphosphonate Derivatives; Cefditoren; Clopidogrel; Dabigatran Etexilate; Dasatinib; Delavirdine; Erlotinib; Gefitinib; Indinavir; Iron Salts; Itraconazole; Ketoconazole; Ketoconazole (Systemic); Mesalamine; Mycophenolate; Nelfinavir; Posaconazole; Rilpivirine; Vismodegib

The levels/effects of Pantoprazole may be decreased by: CYP2C19 Inducers (Strong); Peginterferon Alfa-2b; Tipranavir; Tocilizumab

Increased Effect/Toxicity

Pantoprazole may increase the levels/effects of: Amphetamines; Citalopram; CYP2C19 Substrates; Dexmethylphenidate; Methotrexate; Methylphenidate; Raltegravir; Saquinavir; Topotecan; Voriconazole

The levels/effects of Pantoprazole may be increased by: Conivaptan; Fluconazole; Ketoconazole; Ketoconazole (Systemic)

Nutritional/Ethanol Interactions

Ethanol: Avoid ethanol (may cause gastric mucosal irritation).

Herb/Nutraceutical: Prolonged treatment (typically >3 years) may lead to vitamin B_{12} malabsorption and subsequent deficiency.

Adverse Reactions 1% to 10%:

Cardiovascular: Chest pain

Central nervous system: Headache (2% to 9%), insomnia (≤1%), anxiety, dizziness, migraine, pain

Dermatologic: Rash (≤2%)

Endocrine & metabolic: Hyperglycemia (≤1%), hyperlipidemia

Gastrointestinal: Diarrhea (2% to 6%), flatulence (2% to 4%), abdominal pain (1% to 4%), nausea (≤2%), vomiting (≤2%), eructation (≤1%), constipation, dyspepsia, gastroenteritis, rectal disorder

Genitourinary: Urinary frequency, UTI

Hepatic: Liver function tests abnormal (≤2%)

Local: Injection site reaction (includes thrombophlebitis and abscess)

Neuromuscular & skeletal: Arthralgia, back pain, hypertonia, neck pain, weakness

Respiratory: Bronchitis, cough, dyspnea, pharyngitis, rhinitis, sinusitis, upper respiratory tract infection

Miscellaneous: Flu syndrome, infection

Available Dosage Forms

Granules for suspension, delayed release, enteric coated, oral:

Protonix®: 40 mg/packet (30s)

Injection, powder for reconstitution:

Protonix® I.V.: 40 mg

Tablet, delayed release, oral: 20 mg, 40 mg

Protonix®: 20 mg, 40 mg

General Dosage Range

I.V.: *Adults:* Erosive gastritis: 40 mg once daily; Hypersecretory disorders: 160-240 mg/day in divided doses

Oral: *Adults:* 20-40 mg once or twice daily (maximum: 240 mg/day normally reserved for treatment of hypersecretory conditions)

Administration

Oral

Tablet: Should be swallowed whole, do not crush or chew. Best if taken before breakfast.

Delayed-release oral suspension: Should only be administered in apple juice or applesauce and taken ~30 minutes before a meal. Do not administer with any other liquid (eg, water) or foods.

Oral administration in **applesauce**: Sprinkle intact granules on 1 tablespoon of applesauce and swallow within 10 minutes of preparation.

Oral administration in **apple juice**: Empty intact granules into 5 mL of apple juice, stir for 5 seconds, and swallow immediately after preparation. Rinse container once or twice with apple juice and swallow immediately.

Nasogastric tube administration: Separate the plunger from the barrel of a 60 mL catheter tip syringe and connect to a ≥16 French nasogastric tube. Holding the syringe attached to the tubing as high as possible, empty the contents of the packet into barrel of the syringe, add 10 mL of apple juice and gently tap/shake the barrel of the syringe to help empty the syringe. Add an additional 10 mL of apple juice and gently tap/shake the barrel to help rinse. Repeat rinse with at least 2-10 mL aliquots of apple juice. No granules should remain in the syringe.

I.V. Flush I.V. line before and after administration. In-line filter not required.

2-minute infusion: The volume of reconstituted solution (4 mg/mL) to be injected may be administered intravenously over at least 2 minutes.

15-minute infusion: Infuse over 15 minutes at a rate not to exceed 7 mL/minute (3 mg/minute).

Stability

Reconstitution Reconstitute with 10 mL NS (final concentration 4 mg/mL). Reconstituted solution may be given intravenously (over 2 minutes) or may be added to 100 mL D_5W, NS, or LR (for 15-minute infusion).

Storage

Oral: Store tablet and oral suspension at controlled room temperature of 20°C to 25°C (68°F to 77°F).

I.V.: Prior to reconstitution, store at controlled room temperature of 20°C to 25°C (68°F to 77°F). Protect from light. When reconstituted, solution is stable up to 96 hours at room temperature (Johnson, 2005). The preparation should be stored at 3°C to 5°C (37°F to 41°F) if it is stored beyond 48 hours to minimize discoloration. If further diluting in 100 mL of D_5W, LR, or NS, dilute within 6 hours of reconstitution. Diluted solution is stable at room temperature for up to 24 hours from the time of initial reconstitution; protection from light is not required.

Nursing Actions

Physical Assessment Monitor for rebleeding.

Patient Education Take at similar time each day. Swallow tablet whole (do not crush or chew). Avoid alcohol. You may experience headache, vomiting, or diarrhea. Report persistent abdominal discomfort; chest pain; persistent headache; unresolved diarrhea; excessive fatigue; increased muscle, joint, or body pain; or changes in urinary pattern.

Dietary Considerations

Oral: May be taken with or without food; best if taken before breakfast.

I.V.: Due to EDTA in preparation, zinc supplementation may be needed in patients prone to zinc deficiency.

Related Information

Compatibility of Drugs *on page 1264*

Papillomavirus (Types 6, 11, 16, 18) Vaccine (Human, Recombinant)

(pap ih LO ma VYE rus typs six e LEV en SIX teen AYE teen vak SEEN YU man ree KOM be nant)

Brand Names: U.S. Gardasil®

Index Terms HPV Vaccine; HPV4; Human Papillomavirus Vaccine; Papillomavirus Vaccine, Recombinant; Quadrivalent Human Papillomavirus Vaccine

Pharmacologic Category Vaccine, Inactivated (Viral)

Medication Safety Issues

Sound-alike/look-alike issues:

Papillomavirus vaccine types 6, 11, 16, 18 (Gardasil®) may be confused with Papillomavirus vaccine types 16, 18 (Cervarix®)

Pregnancy Risk Factor B

Lactation Excretion in breast milk unknown/use caution

Use

U.S. labeling:

Females ≥9 years and ≤26 years of age: Prevention of cervical, vulvar, vaginal, and anal cancer caused by HPV types 16 and 18; genital warts caused by HPV types 6 and 11; cervical adenocarcinoma *in situ*, and vulvar, vaginal, cervical, or anal intraepithelial neoplasia caused by HPV types 6, 11, 16, and 18

Males ≥9 years and ≤26 years of age: Prevention of genital warts caused by human papillomavirus (HPV) types 6 and 11; anal cancer caused by HPV types 16 and 18, and anal intraepithelial neoplasia caused by HPV types 6, 11, 16, and 18

Canadian labeling:

Females ≥9 years and ≤26 years of age: Prevention of anal cancer caused by HPV types 16 and 18; anal intraepithelial neoplasia caused by HPV types 6, 11, 16, and 18

Females ≥9 years and ≤45 years of age: Prevention of cervical, vulvar, and vaginal cancer caused by HPV types 16 and 18; genital warts caused by HPV types 6 and 11; cervical adenocarcinoma *in situ*, vulvar, vaginal, or cervical intraepithelial neoplasia caused by HPV types 6, 11, 16, and 18

Males ≥9 years and ≤26 years of age: Prevention of anal cancer caused by HPV types 16 and 18; anal intraepithelial neoplasia caused by HPV types 6, 11, 16, and 18; genital warts caused by HPV types 6 and 11

The Advisory Committee on Immunization Practices (ACIP) recommends routine vaccination for females and males 11-12 years of age; catch-up vaccination is recommended for females 13-26 years of age and males 13-21 years of age. Males 22-26 years may also be vaccinated. The ACIP also recommends routine vaccination for men who have sex with men (MSM) through 26 years of age (CDC, 59[20], 2010; CDC, 60[50], 2011). Vaccination is also recommended for immunocompromised persons or MSM through 26 years of age who were not previously vaccinated when they were younger. Although not specifically recommended for their profession, health care providers within the recommended age groups should also receive the HPV vaccine (CDC, 61[4], 2012).

Available Dosage Forms

Injection, suspension [preservative free]:

Gardasil®: HPV 6 L1 protein 20 mcg, HPV 11 L1 protein 40 mcg, HPV 16 L1 protein 40 mcg, and HPV 18 L1 protein 20 mcg per 0.5 mL (0.5 mL)

General Dosage Range I.M.: *Children ≥9 years and Adults ≤26 years:* 0.5 mL initial dose, followed by 0.5 mL 2 and 6 months later

Administration

I.M. Shake suspension well before use. Inject the entire dose I.M. into the deltoid region of the upper arm or higher anterolateral thigh area. Observe for syncope for 15 minutes following administration. If the vaccine series is interrupted and only one dose was given, administer the second dose as soon as possible and give the third dose ≥12 weeks later. If the vaccine series is interrupted and the first two doses were given, administer the third dose as soon as possible. The HPV vaccine series should be completed with the same product whenever possible.

For patients at risk of hemorrhage following intramuscular injection, the ACIP recommends "it should be administered intramuscularly if, in the opinion of the physician familiar with the patients bleeding risk, the vaccine can be administered by this route with reasonable safety. If the patient receives antihemophilia or other similar therapy, intramuscular vaccination can be scheduled shortly after such therapy is administered. A fine needle (23 gauge or smaller) can be used for the vaccination and firm pressure applied to the site (without rubbing) for at least 2 minutes. The patient should be instructed concerning the risk of hematoma from the injection." Patients on anticoagulant therapy should be considered to have the same bleeding risks and treated as those with clotting factor disorders (CDC, 2011).

Simultaneous administration of vaccines helps ensure the patients will be fully vaccinated by the appropriate age. Simultaneous administration of vaccines is defined as administering >1 vaccine on the same day at different anatomic sites. Separate vaccines should not be combined in the same syringe unless indicated by product specific labeling. Separate needles and syringes should be used for each injection. The ACIP prefers each dose of a specific vaccine in a series come from the same manufacturer when possible. Adolescents and adults should be vaccinated while seated or lying down. In general, preterm infants should be vaccinated at the same chronological age as full-term infants (CDC, 2011).

Antipyretics have not been shown to prevent febrile seizures. Antipyretics may be used to treat fever or discomfort following vaccination (CDC, 2011). One study reported that routine prophylactic administration of acetaminophen to prevent fever prior to vaccination decreased the immune response of some vaccines; the clinical significance of this reduction in immune response has not been established (Prymula, 2009).

Nursing Actions

Physical Assessment Treatment for anaphylactic/anaphylactoid reaction should be available during vaccine use; if there is a hypersensitivity response after receiving a dose of Gardasil®, patient should not receive further doses. All patients should be informed that the vaccine is not a treatment for active disease and is not a substitute for regular, routine cervical screening. All serious adverse reactions must be reported to the U.S. DHHS. U.S. federal law also requires entry into the patient's medical record.

Patient Education This vaccine is not a treatment for active disease and does not substitute for regular, routine cervical cancer screening. Three doses will be required for effective immunity; consult prescriber for appropriate schedule of vaccinations. May cause fever, headache, or dizziness. May cause some redness, pain, or swelling at injection site; consult prescriber if excessive or persistent. Notify prescriber immediately of any allergic reaction (eg, difficulty breathing; rash; difficulty swallowing; or swelling of hands, feet, face, or lips).

Papillomavirus (Types 16, 18) Vaccine (Human, Recombinant)

(pap ih LO ma VYE rus typs SIX teen AYE teen vak SEEN YU man ree KOM be nant)

Brand Names: U.S. Cervarix®

Index Terms Bivalent Human Papillomavirus Vaccine; GSK-580299; HPV 16/18 L1 VLP/AS04 VAC; HPV Vaccine; HPV2; Human Papillomavirus Vaccine; Papillomavirus Vaccine, Recombinant

Pharmacologic Category Vaccine, Inactivated (Viral)

Medication Safety Issues

Sound-alike/look-alike issues:

Papillomavirus vaccine types 16, 18 (Cervarix®) may be confused with Papillomavirus vaccine types 6, 11, 16, 18 (Gardasil®)

Cervarix® may be confused with Cerebyx®, CeleBREX®

Pregnancy Risk Factor B

Lactation Excretion in breast milk unknown/use caution

Use Females 9 through 25 years of age: Prevention of cervical cancer, cervical adenocarcinoma *in situ*, and cervical intraepithelial neoplasia caused by human papillomavirus (HPV) types 16, 18

The Advisory Committee on Immunization Practices (ACIP) recommends routine vaccination for females 11-12 years of age; catch-up vaccination is recommended for females 13-25 years of age (CDC, 59[20], 2010). Vaccination is also recommended for immunocompromised females through 26 years of age who were not previously vaccinated when they were younger. Although not specifically recommended for their profession, female health care providers within the recommended age groups should also receive the HPV vaccine (CDC, 61[4], 2012).

Available Dosage Forms

Injection, suspension [preservative free]:

Cervarix®: HPV 16 L1 protein 20 mcg and HPV 18 L1 protein 20 mcg per 0.5 mL (0.5 mL)

General Dosage Range I.M.: *Children ≥9 years and Adults ≤25 years (females):* 0.5 mL initial dose, followed by 0.5 mL 1 and 6 months later

Administration

I.M. Shake well prior to use. Do not use if discolored or if containing particulate matter, or if vial or syringe is cracked. Inject I.M. into the deltoid region of the upper arm. Do not administer I.V., SubQ, or intradermally.

For patients at risk of hemorrhage following intramuscular injection, the ACIP recommends "it should be administered intramuscularly if, in the opinion of the physician familiar with the patients bleeding risk, the vaccine can be administered by this route with reasonable safety. If the patient receives antihemophilia or other similar therapy, intramuscular vaccination can be scheduled shortly after such therapy is administered. A fine needle (23 gauge or smaller) can be used for the vaccination and firm pressure applied to the site (without rubbing) for at least 2 minutes. The patient should be instructed concerning the risk of hematoma from the injection." Patients on anticoagulant therapy should be considered to have the same bleeding risks and treated as those with clotting factor disorders (CDC, 2011).

Simultaneous administration of vaccines helps ensure the patients will be fully vaccinated by the appropriate age. Simultaneous administration of vaccines is defined as administering >1 vaccine on the same day at different anatomic sites. Separate vaccines should not be combined in the same syringe unless indicated by product specific labeling. Separate needles and syringes should be used for each injection. The ACIP prefers each dose of a specific vaccine in a series come from the same manufacturer when possible. Adolescents and adults should be vaccinated while seated or lying down. In general, preterm infants should be vaccinated at the same chronological age as full-term infants (CDC, 2011).

Antipyretics have not been shown to prevent febrile seizures. Antipyretics may be used to treat fever or discomfort following vaccination (CDC, 2011). One study reported that routine prophylactic administration of acetaminophen to prevent fever prior to vaccination decreased the immune response of some vaccines; the clinical significance of this reduction in immune response has not been established (Prymula, 2009).

Nursing Actions

Physical Assessment Have emergency treatment for anaphylactoid or hypersensitivity reaction available. Syncope following administration may occur. If latex sensitive, be advised that packaging may contain latex. Emphasize necessity to complete all 3 doses for maximum efficacy. All serious adverse reactions must be reported to the U.S. DHHS. U.S. federal law also requires entry into the patient's medical record.

Patient Education This vaccine is not a substitute for routine cervical cancer screening. It is important for you to receive all 3 doses for maximum benefit. This medication does not protect against disease from HPV already exposed to through sexual activity. You may experience fatigue; headache; abdominal pain; nausea, vomiting, or diarrhea; flu-like symptoms; fever; muscle or joint pain; and redness and tenderness at injection site. Notify prescriber immediately of any allergic reaction (eg, difficulty breathing; rash; difficulty swallowing; or swelling of hands, feet, face, or lips).

Paregoric (par e GOR ik)

Index Terms Camphorated Tincture of Opium (error-prone synonym)

Pharmacologic Category Analgesic, Opioid

Medication Safety Issues

Sound-alike/look-alike issues:

Camphorated tincture of opium is an error-prone synonym (mistaken as opium tincture)

Paregoric may be confused with Percogesic®

High alert medication:

The Institute for Safe Medication Practices (ISMP) includes this medication among its list of drug classes which have a heightened risk of causing significant patient harm when used in error.

Administration issues:

Use care when prescribing opium tincture; each mL contains the equivalent of morphine 10 mg; paregoric contains the equivalent of morphine 0.4 mg/mL

Pregnancy Risk Factor B/D (prolonged use or high doses)

Lactation Enters breast milk/use caution

Use Treatment of diarrhea or relief of pain

Controlled Substance C-III

Available Dosage Forms

Liquid, oral: Morphine equivalent 2 mg/5 mL (473 mL)

General Dosage Range Oral:

Children: 0.25-0.5 mL/kg 1-4 times/day

Adults: 5-10 mL 1-4 times/day

Nursing Actions

Physical Assessment If used to control diarrhea, monitor stools. Monitor for excessive sedation, respiratory depression, or hypotension. For inpatients, implement safety measures (eg, side rails up, call light within reach, patient instructions to call for assistance). Assess patient's physical and/or psychological dependence. Discontinue slowly after prolonged use

Patient Education May cause dependence with prolonged or excessive use. Avoid alcohol or any other prescription and OTC medications that may cause sedation (eg, sleeping medications, some cough/cold remedies, antihistamines). You may experience drowsiness, dizziness, impaired judgment, or postural hypotension. You may experience nausea, loss of appetite, or constipation. Report unresolved nausea, vomiting, respiratory difficulty (shortness of breath or decreased respirations), chest pain, or palpitations.

Paricalcitol (pah ri KAL si tole)

Brand Names: U.S. Zemplar®

Pharmacologic Category Vitamin D Analog

Medication Safety Issues

Sound alike/look alike issues:

Paricalcitol may be confused with calcitriol

Zemplar® may be confused with zaleplon, Zelapar®, zolpidem, ZyPREXA® Zydis®

Pregnancy Risk Factor C

Lactation Excretion in breast milk unknown/not recommended

Use

I.V.: Prevention and treatment of secondary hyperparathyroidism associated with stage 5 chronic kidney disease (CKD)

Oral: Prevention and treatment of secondary hyperparathyroidism associated with stage 3 and 4 CKD and stage 5 CKD patients on hemodialysis or peritoneal dialysis

Available Dosage Forms

Capsule, soft gelatin, oral:

Zemplar®: 1 mcg, 2 mcg, 4 mcg

Injection, solution:

Zemplar®: 2 mcg/mL (1 mL); 5 mcg/mL (1 mL, 2 mL)

General Dosage Range Dosage adjustment recommended in patients with renal impairment

I.V.: *Children ≥5 years and Adults:* 0.04-0.24 mcg/kg (2.8-16.8 mcg) every other day during dialysis

Oral: *Adults:* 1-2 mcg/day **or** 2-4 mcg 3 times/week

Administration

Oral May be administered with or without food. With the 3 times/week dosing schedule, doses should not be given more frequently than every other day.

I.V. Administered as a bolus dose at anytime during dialysis. Doses should not be administered more often than every other day.

Nursing Actions

Physical Assessment Instruct patient on dietary requirements.

Patient Education Adhere to diet as recommended (do not take any other vitamin D-related compounds while taking paricalcitol). You may experience nausea, vomiting, lightheadedness, or dizziness. Report gastric disturbances, bone pain, irritability, muscular twitching, or weakness.

PARoxetine (pa ROKS e teen)

Brand Names: U.S. Paxil CR®; Paxil®; Pexeva®

Index Terms Paroxetine Hydrochloride; Paroxetine Mesylate

Pharmacologic Category Antidepressant, Selective Serotonin Reuptake Inhibitor

Medication Safety Issues

Sound-alike/look-alike issues:

PARoxetine may be confused with FLUoxetine, PACLitaxel, piroxicam, pyridoxine

Paxil® may be confused with Doxil®, PACLitaxel, Plavix®, PROzac®, Taxol®

Medication Guide Available Yes

Pregnancy Risk Factor D

Lactation Enters breast milk/use caution (AAP rates "of concern"; AAP 2001 update pending)

Breast-Feeding Considerations Paroxetine is excreted in breast milk and concentrations in the hindmilk are higher than in foremilk. Paroxetine has not been detected in the serum of nursing infants and adverse events have not been reported. The manufacturer recommends that caution be exercised when administering paroxetine to nursing women.

The long-term effects on development and behavior have not been studied; therefore, one should prescribe paroxetine to a mother who is breastfeeding only when the benefits outweigh the potential risks.

Use Treatment of major depressive disorder (MDD); treatment of panic disorder with or without agoraphobia; obsessive-compulsive disorder (OCD); social anxiety disorder (social phobia); generalized anxiety disorder (GAD); post-traumatic stress disorder (PTSD); premenstrual dysphoric disorder (PMDD)

Unlabeled Use May be useful in eating disorders, impulse control disorders; vasomotor symptoms of menopause; treatment of obsessive-compulsive disorder (OCD) in children; treatment of mild dementia-associated agitation in nonpsychotic patients

Mechanism of Action/Effect Paroxetine is a selective serotonin reuptake inhibitor, chemically unrelated to tricyclic, tetracyclic, or other antidepressants; presumably, the inhibition of serotonin reuptake from brain synapse stimulated serotonin activity in the brain

Contraindications Hypersensitivity to paroxetine or any component of the formulation; use with or within 14 days of MAO inhibitors intended to treat depression; concurrent use with reversible MAO inhibitors (eg, linezolid, methylene blue); concurrent use with thioridazine or pimozide

Warnings/Precautions Hazardous agent - use appropriate precautions for handling and disposal. **[U.S. Boxed Warning]: Antidepressants increase the risk of suicidal thinking and behavior in children, adolescents, and young adults (18-24 years of age) with major depressive disorder (MDD) and other psychiatric disorders;** consider risk prior to prescribing. Short-term studies did not show an increased risk in patients >24 years of age and showed a decreased risk in patients ≥65 years. Closely monitor patients for clinical worsening, suicidality, or unusual changes in behavior, particularly during the initial 1-2 months of therapy or during periods of dosage adjustments (increases or decreases); the patient's family or caregiver should be instructed to closely observe the patient and communicate condition with healthcare provider. A medication guide concerning the use of antidepressants should be dispensed with each prescription. **Paroxetine is not FDA approved for use in children.**

The possibility of a suicide attempt is inherent in major depression and may persist until remission occurs. Patients treated with antidepressants (for any indication) should be observed for clinical worsening and suicidality, especially during the initial few months of a course of drug therapy, or at times of dose changes, either increases or decreases. Use caution in high-risk patients. Worsening depression and severe abrupt suicidality that are not part of the presenting symptoms may require discontinuation or modification of drug therapy. The patient's family or caregiver should be alerted to monitor patients for the emergence of suicidality and associated behaviors (such as agitation, irritability, hostility, impulsivity, and hypomania) and call healthcare provider.

May worsen psychosis in some patients or precipitate a shift to mania or hypomania in patients with bipolar disorder. Patients presenting with depressive symptoms should be screened for bipolar disorder. Monotherapy in patients with bipolar disorder should be avoided. **Paroxetine is not FDA approved for the treatment of bipolar depression.**

Serotonin syndrome and neuroleptic malignant syndrome (NMS)-like reactions have occurred with serotonin/norepinephrine reuptake inhibitors (SNRIs) and selective serotonin reuptake inhibitors (SSRIs) when used alone, and particularly when used in combination with serotonergic agents (eg, triptans) or antidopaminergic agents (eg, antipsychotics). Concurrent use with MAO inhibitors, including reversible MAO inhibitors (eg, linezolid, methylene blue) is contraindicated. If the administration of linezolid or methylene blue cannot be avoided, paroxetine should be discontinued prior to administration of the reversible MAO inhibitor. Monitor for symptoms of serotonin syndrome/NMS-like reactions for 2 weeks or 24 hours after the last dose of the reversible MAO inhibitor (whichever comes first). Paroxetine may then be resumed 24 hours after the last dose of linezolid or methylene blue.

Paroxetine may increase the risks associated with electroconvulsive therapy. Has a low potential to impair cognitive or motor performance - use caution when operating hazardous machinery or driving. Symptoms of agitation and/or restlessness may occur during initial few weeks of therapy. Low potential for sedation or anticholinergic effects relative to cyclic antidepressants.

Use caution in patients with a previous seizure disorder or condition predisposing to seizures such as brain damage, alcoholism, or concurrent therapy with other drugs which lower the seizure threshold. Use with caution in patients with hepatic dysfunction and in elderly patients. May cause hyponatremia/SIADH (elderly at increased risk); volume depletion (diuretics may increase risk). Use caution with concomitant use of NSAIDs, ASA, or other drugs that affect coagulation; the risk of bleeding may be potentiated. Concurrent use with tamoxifen may decrease the efficacy of tamoxifen; consider an alternative antidepressant with little or no CYP2D6 inhibition when using tamoxifen for the treatment or prevention of breast cancer. Use with caution in patients with renal insufficiency or other concurrent illness (due to limited experience); dose reduction recommended with severe renal impairment. May cause or exacerbate sexual dysfunction. Use caution in patients with narrow-angle glaucoma. Avoid use in the first trimester of pregnancy.

Upon discontinuation of paroxetine therapy, gradually taper dose and monitor for discontinuation symptoms (eg, dizziness, dysphoric mood, irritability, agitation, confusion, paresthesias). If intolerable symptoms occur following a decrease in dosage or upon discontinuation of therapy, then resuming the previous dose with a more gradual taper should be considered.

Drug Interactions

Avoid Concomitant Use

Avoid concomitant use of PARoxetine with any of the following: Iobenguane I 123; MAO Inhibitors; Methylene Blue; Pimozide; Tamoxifen; Tryptophan

Decreased Effect

PARoxetine may decrease the levels/effects of: Aprepitant; Fosaprepitant; Iobenguane I 123; Ioflupane I 123

The levels/effects of PARoxetine may be decreased by: Aprepitant; CarBAMazepine; Cyproheptadine; Darunavir; Fosamprenavir; Fosaprepitant; NSAID (COX-2 Inhibitor); NSAID (Nonselective); Peginterferon Alfa-2b

Increased Effect/Toxicity

PARoxetine may increase the levels/effects of: Alpha-/Beta-Blockers; Anticoagulants; Antidepressants (Serotonin Reuptake Inhibitor/Antagonist); Antiplatelet Agents; Aspirin; Atomoxetine; Beta-Blockers; BusPIRone; CarBAMazepine; CloZAPine; Collagenase (Systemic); CYP2B6 Substrates; CYP2D6 Substrates; Desmopressin; Dextromethorphan; Drotrecogin Alfa (Activated); DULoxetine; Fesoterodine; Galantamine; Ibritumomab; Lithium; Methadone; Methylene Blue; Metoclopramide; Mexiletine; NSAID (COX-2 Inhibitor); NSAID (Nonselective); Pimozide; Propafenone; RisperiDONE; Rivaroxaban; Salicylates; Serotonin Modulators; Tamoxifen; Tetrabenazine; Thrombolytic Agents; Tositumomab and Iodine I 131 Tositumomab; TraMADol; Tricyclic Antidepressants; Vitamin K Antagonists

The levels/effects of PARoxetine may be increased by: Abiraterone Acetate; Alcohol (Ethyl); Analgesics (Opioid); Antipsychotics; Asenapine; BusPIRone; Cimetidine; CNS Depressants; CYP2D6 Inhibitors (Moderate); CYP2D6 Inhibitors (Strong); Dasatinib; Glucosamine; Herbs (Anticoagulant/Antiplatelet Properties); Linezolid; MAO Inhibitors; Metoclopramide; Omega-3-Acid Ethyl Esters; Pentosan Polysulfate Sodium; Pentoxifylline; Pravastatin; Prostacyclin Analogues; TraMADol; Tryptophan; Vitamin E

Nutritional/Ethanol Interactions

Ethanol: May increase CNS depression; monitor for increased effects with coadministration. Caution patients about effects.

Food: Peak concentration is increased, but bioavailability is not significantly altered by food.

Herb/Nutraceutical: Avoid valerian, St John's wort, SAMe, kava kava.

Adverse Reactions Frequency varies by dose and indication. Adverse reactions reported as a composite of all indications.

>10%:

Central nervous system: Somnolence (15% to 24%), insomnia (11% to 24%), headache (17% to 18%), dizziness (6% to 14%)

Endocrine & metabolic: Libido decreased (3% to 15%)

Gastrointestinal: Nausea (19% to 26%), xerostomia (9% to 18%), constipation (5% to 16%), diarrhea (9% to 12%)

Genitourinary: Ejaculatory disturbances (13% to 28%)

Neuromuscular & skeletal: Weakness (12% to 22%), tremor (4% to 11%)

Miscellaneous: Diaphoresis (5% to 14%)

1% to 10%:

Cardiovascular: Vasodilation (2% to 4%), chest pain (3%), palpitation (2% to 3%), hypertension (≥1%), tachycardia (≥1%)

Central nervous system: Nervousness (4% to 9%), anxiety (5%), agitation (3% to 5%), abnormal dreams (3% to 4%), concentration impaired (3% to 4%), yawning (2% to 4%), depersonalization (≤3%), amnesia (2%), chills (2%), emotional lability (≥1%), vertigo (≥1%), confusion (1%)

Dermatologic: Rash (2% to 3%), pruritus (≥1%)

Endocrine & metabolic: Orgasmic disturbance (2% to 9%), dysmenorrhea (5%)

Gastrointestinal: Appetite decreased (5% to 9%), dyspepsia (2% to 5%), flatulence (4%), abdominal pain (4%), appetite increased (2% to 4%), vomiting (2% to 3%), taste perversion (2%), weight gain (≥1%)

Genitourinary: Genital disorder (male 10%; female 2% to 9%), impotence (2% to 9%), urinary frequency (2% to 3%), urinary tract infection (2%)

Neuromuscular & skeletal: Paresthesia (4%), myalgia (2% to 4%), back pain (3%), myoclonus (2% to 3%), myopathy (2%), myasthenia (1%), arthralgia (≥1%)

Ocular: Blurred vision (4%), abnormal vision (2% to 4%)

Otic: Tinnitus (≥1%)

Respiratory: Respiratory disorder (≤7%), pharyngitis (4%), sinusitis (≤4%), rhinitis (3%)

Miscellaneous: Infection (5% to 6%)

Pharmacodynamics/Kinetics

Onset of Action Depression: The onset of action is within a week, however, individual response varies greatly and full response may not be seen until 8-12 weeks after initiation of treatment.

Available Dosage Forms

Suspension, oral:

Paxil®: 10 mg/5 mL (250 mL)

Tablet, oral: 10 mg, 20 mg, 30 mg, 40 mg

Paxil®: 10 mg, 20 mg, 30 mg, 40 mg

Pexeva®: 10 mg, 20 mg, 30 mg, 40 mg

Tablet, controlled release, enteric coated, oral: 12.5 mg, 25 mg, 37.5 mg

Paxil CR®: 12.5 mg, 25 mg, 37.5 mg

Tablet, extended release, enteric coated, oral: 12.5 mg, 25 mg

General Dosage Range Dosage adjustment recommended in patients with hepatic or renal impairment

Oral:

Controlled release:

Adults: Initial: 12.5-25 mg once daily; Maintenance: 12.5-75 mg once daily (maximum: 75 mg/day)

Elderly: Initial: 12.5 mg once daily; Maintenance: 12.5-50 mg/day (maximum: 50 mg/day)

Immediate release:

Adults: Initial: 10-20 mg once daily; Maintenance: 10-60 mg once daily (maximum: 60 mg/day)

Elderly: Initial: 10 mg once daily; Maintenance: 10-40 mg once daily (maximum: 40 mg/day)

Administration

Oral May be administered without regard to meals, preferably in the morning. Do not crush, break, or chew controlled release tablets.

Stability

Storage

Suspension: Store at ≤25°C (≤77°F).

Tablets:

Paxil®: Store at 15°C to 30°C (59°F to 86°F).

Paxil CR®: Store at ≤25°C (≤77°F).

Pexeva®: Store at 25°C (77°F); excursions permitted to 15°C to 30°C (59°F to 86°F).

Nursing Actions

Physical Assessment Monitor for clinical worsening and suicide ideation. Taper dosage slowly when discontinuing.

Patient Education It may take 2-3 weeks to achieve desired results. Take in the morning to reduce the incidence of insomnia (may be taken with or without food). Do not crush, break, or chew controlled release (Paxil CR®) tablets. Avoid alcohol. Maintain adequate hydration unless instructed to restrict fluid intake. You may experience drowsiness, dizziness, lightheadedness, nausea, vomiting, anorexia, dry mouth, or orthostatic hypotension. Report persistent insomnia or excessive daytime sedation; tremors or weakness; chest pain, palpitations, or rapid heartbeat; vision changes; abnormal bleeding; change in affect or thought processes or abnormal dreams; worsening of condition; or suicide ideation.

Dietary Considerations May be taken without regard to meals.

Pazopanib (paz OH pa nib)

Brand Names: U.S. Votrient™

Index Terms GW786034; Pazopanib Hydrochloride

Pharmacologic Category Antineoplastic Agent, Tyrosine Kinase Inhibitor; Vascular Endothelial Growth Factor (VEGF) Inhibitor

Medication Safety Issues

Sound-alike/look-alike issues:

Pazopanib may be confused with axitinib, SUNItinib, vandetanib

Votrient™ may be confused with vorinostat

High alert medication:

This medication is in a class the Institute for Safe Medication Practices (ISMP) includes among its list of drug classes which have a heightened risk of causing significant patient harm when used in error.

Medication Guide Available Yes

Pregnancy Risk Factor D

Lactation Excretion in breast milk unknown/not recommended

Use Treatment of advanced renal cell cancer (RCC)

Unlabeled Use Treatment of advanced, differentiated thyroid cancer; treatment of some histologic types of refractory metastatic soft tissue sarcomas

Available Dosage Forms

Tablet, oral:

Votrient™: 200 mg

General Dosage Range Dosage adjustment recommended in patients with hepatic impairment, on concomitant therapy, or who develop toxicities

Oral: *Adults:* 800 mg once daily

Administration

Oral Administer on an empty stomach, 1 hour before or 2 hours after a meal. Do not crush tablet. If a dose is missed, do not take if <12 hours until the next dose.

Nursing Actions

Physical Assessment Monitor for hypertension, gastrointestinal perforation, diarrhea, hyper-/hypoglycemia, and cardiac changes; dose adjustments may be necessary.

Patient Education Take 1 hour before or 2 hours after food; do not crush. Avoid grapefruit juice. Maintain adequate nutrition and hydration, unless instructed to restrict fluid intake. May cause fatigue, anemia, low blood cell counts, headache, loose stools, upset stomach, high blood pressure, blood sugar changes (high or low), belly pain, and change in color of hair. Liver damage can rarely occur. Report to prescriber persistent gastrointestinal changes, including diarrhea, abdominal pain, nausea, or vomiting; black, tarry, or bloody stools; loss of appetite; dark-colored urine; yellowing of eyes or skin; chest pain or palpitations; difficulty breathing; or signs of infection (fever ≥100.5°F [38°C], sore throat, sinus pain, cough, mouth sores, burning on urination, increased sputum or change in color of sputum; wounds that will not heal; or anal itching or pain); severe dizziness or loss of consciousness; neurological changes (weakness on one side of the body, aphasia, loss of balance, blurred vision, or tiredness); or any unusual bruising or bleeding.

Pegaspargase (peg AS par jase)

Brand Names: U.S. Oncaspar®

Index Terms L-asparaginase with Polyethylene Glycol; PEG-ASP; PEG-asparaginase; PEG-L-asparaginase; PEGLA; Polyethylene Glycol-L-asparaginase

Pharmacologic Category Antineoplastic Agent, Miscellaneous; Enzyme

Medication Safety Issues

Sound-alike/look-alike issues:

Oncaspar® may be confused with Elspar®

Pegaspargase may be confused with asparaginase

High alert medication:

The Institute for Safe Medication Practices (ISMP) includes this medication among its list of drugs which have a heightened risk of causing significant patient harm when used in error.

Pregnancy Risk Factor C

Lactation Excretion in breast milk unknown/not recommended

Breast-Feeding Considerations Due to the potential for serious adverse reactions in the nursing infant, breast-feeding is not recommended.

Use Treatment of acute lymphocytic leukemia (ALL); treatment of ALL with previous hypersensitivity to native L-asparaginase

Mechanism of Action/Effect Pegaspargase is a modified version of asparaginase. Leukemic cells, especially lymphoblasts, require exogenous asparagine; normal cells can synthesize asparagine. Asparaginase contains L-asparaginase amidohydrolase type EC-2 which inhibits protein synthesis by deaminating asparagine to aspartic acid and ammonia in the plasma and extracellular fluid and therefore deprives tumor cells of the amino acid for protein synthesis. Asparaginase is cycle-specific for the G_1 phase of the cell cycle.

Contraindications History of serious allergic reactions to pegaspargase; history of any of the following with prior L-asparaginase treatment: pancreatitis, serious hemorrhagic events, serious thrombosis

Warnings/Precautions Hazardous agent - use appropriate precautions for handling and disposal. Serious allergic reactions may occur; discontinue in patients with serious allergic reaction. Observe patients for at least 1 hour after administration; immediate treatment for hypersensitivity reactions should be available during administration. Pegaspargase is indicated for use in patients who have had hypersensitivity reactions to native L-asparaginase; however, in one study, 32% of patients with a history of allergic reaction to *E. coli* asparaginase products also experienced allergic reaction to pegaspargase.

Serious thrombotic events, including sagittal sinus thrombosis may occur; discontinue with serious thrombotic event. Pancreatitis may occur; promptly evaluate patients with abdominal pain; discontinue if pancreatitis occurs during treatment. May cause glucose intolerance; irreversible in some cases; use with caution in patients with hyperglycemia, or diabetes. Coagulopathy has been reported; monitor coagulation parameters; severe or symptomatic coagulopathy may require treatment with fresh-frozen plasma; use with caution in patients with underlying coagulopathy. Reversible hepatotoxicity (hyperbilirubinemia and liver enzyme elevation) may occur; use with caution in patients with hepatic dysfunction or concomitant hepatotoxic medications. Use cautiously in patients with previous hematologic complications from asparaginase.

Drug Interactions

Avoid Concomitant Use

Avoid concomitant use of Pegaspargase with any of the following: BCG; Natalizumab; Pimecrolimus; Tacrolimus (Topical); Vaccines (Live)

Decreased Effect

Pegaspargase may decrease the levels/effects of: BCG; Coccidioidin Skin Test; Sipuleucel-T; Vaccines (Inactivated); Vaccines (Live)

The levels/effects of Pegaspargase may be decreased by: Echinacea; Pegloticase

Increased Effect/Toxicity

Pegaspargase may increase the levels/effects of: Leflunomide; Natalizumab; Vaccines (Live)

The levels/effects of Pegaspargase may be increased by: Denosumab; Pimecrolimus; Roflumilast; Tacrolimus (Topical); Trastuzumab

Adverse Reactions

>5%:

Cardiovascular: Edema

Central nervous system: Fever, malaise

Dermatologic: Rash

Gastrointestinal: Nausea, vomiting

Hematologic: Coagulopathy (7%; grades 3/4: 2%)

Hepatic: Transaminases increased (11%; grades 3/4: 3%)

Miscellaneous: Allergic reactions (including bronchospasm, chills, dyspnea, edema, erythema, hypotension, rash, swelling, urticaria; no prior asparaginase hypersensitivity: 1% to 10%; grades 3/4: 2%; prior asparaginase hypersensitivity: 32%; grades 3/4: 8%)

1% to 5%:

Cardiovascular: Hypotension, peripheral edema, tachycardia, thrombosis (4%)

Central nervous system: Chills, CNS thrombosis (2% to 4%; grades 3/4: 3%), CNS hemorrhage (2%), headache, seizure

Dermatologic: Lip edema, urticaria

Endocrine & metabolic: Hyperglycemia (3% to 5%; grades 3/4: ≤5%), hyperuricemia, hypoglycemia, hypoproteinemia

Gastrointestinal: Abdominal pain, anorexia, diarrhea, pancreatitis (1% to 2%; grades 3/4: 2%)

Hematologic: Anticoagulant effect decreased, disseminated intravascular coagulation (DIC), fibrinogen decreased, hemolytic anemia, leukopenia, pancytopenia, thrombocytopenia, thromboplastin increased, myelosuppression

Hepatic: Liver function tests abnormal (grades 3/4: 5%), hyperbilirubinemia (grades 3/4: 2%), jaundice

Local: Injection site hypersensitivity, pain or reaction

Neuromuscular & skeletal: Arthralgia, limb pain, myalgia, paresthesia

Respiratory: Dyspnea

Miscellaneous: Anaphylactic reactions, night sweats

Pharmacodynamics/Kinetics

Onset of Action

Asparagine depletion: I.M.: Within 4 days

Duration of Action Asparagine depletion: I.M.: ~21 days; I.V. (in asparaginase naive adults): 2-4 weeks

Available Dosage Forms

Injection, solution [preservative free]:

Oncaspar®: 750 int. units/mL (5 mL)

General Dosage Range I.M., I.V.: *Children and Adults:* 2500 units/m² every 14 days

Administration

I.M. Must only be administered as a deep intramuscular injection into a large muscle. Do not exceed 2 mL per injection site; use multiple injection sites for I.M. injection volume >2 mL.

I.V. Administer over 1-2 hours through a running I.V. infusion line; **do not administer I.V. push.**

I.V. Detail Have available appropriate agents for maintenance of an adequate airway and treatment of a hypersensitivity reaction (antihistamine, epinephrine, oxygen, I.V. corticosteroids). Be prepared to treat anaphylaxis at each administration.

pH: 7.3

Stability

Reconstitution I.V.: Dilute in 100 mL NS or D_5W.

Storage Refrigerate unused vials at 2°C to 8°C (36°F to 46°F); do not freeze. Do not shake; protect from light. Discard vial if previously frozen, stored at room temperature for >48 hours, excessively shaken/agitated, or if cloudy, discolored, or if precipitate is present. If not used immediately, solutions for infusion should be refrigerated at 2°C to 8°C (36°F to 46°F) and used within 48 hours (including administration time).

Nursing Actions

Physical Assessment Monitor patient during and for at least 1 hour following administration; treatment for anaphylactic reactions should be available. Monitor for GI disturbance, thrombotic events, pancreatitis, depression of clotting factors, glucose intolerance, and hypotension.

Patient Education This drug is given by infusion or injection; report immediately any redness, swelling, burning, or pain at infusion/injection site or any signs of allergic reaction (eg, respiratory difficulty or swallowing, chest tightness, rash, hives, swelling of lips or mouth, palpitations or rapid heartbeat). Maintain adequate nutrition and hydration, unless instructed to restrict fluid intake. You may be more susceptible to infection. If you have diabetes, check your glucose levels closely and notify prescriber of significant changes; this medication can affect glucose control and diabetic medications may need to be adjusted. May cause nausea, vomiting, loss of appetite, mouth sores, dizziness, fatigue, drowsiness, syncope, or blurred vision. Report immediately any abdominal pain, unusual bruising or bleeding (nose bleeds, bleeding gums, black tarry stools, blood in urine or stool, pinpoint red spots on your skin), persistent nausea or vomiting, and edema (eg, swelling of extremities, sudden weight gain).

Peginterferon Alfa-2a

(peg in ter FEER on AL fa too aye)

Brand Names: U.S. Pegasys®

Index Terms Interferon Alfa-2a (PEG Conjugate); Pegylated Interferon Alfa-2a

Pharmacologic Category Interferon

Medication Guide Available Yes

Pregnancy Risk Factor C / X in combination with ribavirin

Lactation Excretion in breast milk unknown/not recommended

Breast-Feeding Considerations Breast milk samples obtained from a lactating mother prior to and after administration of interferon alfa-2b showed that interferon alfa is present in breast milk and administration of the medication did not significantly affect endogenous levels. Breast-feeding is not linked to the spread of hepatitis C virus; however, if nipples are cracked or bleeding, breast-feeding is not recommended. Mothers coinfected with HIV are discouraged from breast-feeding to decrease potential transmission of HIV.

Use Treatment of chronic hepatitis C (CHC), alone or in combination with ribavirin, in patients with compensated liver disease and not previously treated with alfa interferons (includes patients with histological evidence of cirrhosis [Child-Pugh class A] and patients with clinically-stable HIV disease); treatment of patients with HBeAg-positive and HBeAg-negative chronic hepatitis B with compensated liver disease and evidence of viral replication and liver inflammation

Mechanism of Action/Effect Alpha interferons are a family of proteins, produced by nucleated cells that have antiviral, antiproliferative, and immune-regulating activity. There are 16 known subtypes of alpha interferons. Interferons interact with cells through high affinity cell surface receptors. Following activation, multiple effects can be detected including induction of gene transcription. Interferons inhibit cellular growth, alter the state of cellular differentiation, interfere with oncogene expression, alter cell surface antigen expression, increase phagocytic activity of macrophages, and augment cytotoxicity of lymphocytes for target cells.

Contraindications Hypersensitivity to polyethylene glycol (PEG), interferon alfa, or any component of the formulation; autoimmune hepatitis; decompensated liver disease in cirrhotic patients (Child-Pugh score >6); decompensated liver disease (Child-Pugh score ≥6, class B and C) in CHC coinfected with HIV; neonates and infants

Warnings/Precautions Hazardous agent: Use appropriate precautions for handling and disposal.

[U.S. Boxed Warning]: May cause or aggravate fatal or life-threatening autoimmune disorders, neuropsychiatric symptoms (including depression and/or suicidal thoughts/behaviors), ischemic and/or infectious disorders; discontinue treatment for persistent severe or worsening symptoms.

Neuropsychiatric disorders: Severe psychiatric adverse effects (including depression, suicidal ideation, and suicide attempt) may occur in patients with or without a prior history of psychiatric disorder. Avoid use in severe psychiatric disorders; use with extreme caution in patients with a history of depression. Patients who experience dizziness, confusion, somnolence or fatigue should use caution when performing tasks which require mental alertness (eg, operating machinery or driving).

Bone marrow suppression: May cause myelosuppression (including neutropenia, thrombocytopenia, lymphopenia, aplastic anemia). Use caution with baseline neutrophil count <1500/mm^3, platelet count <90,000/mm^3 or hemoglobin <10 g/dL. Discontinue therapy (at least temporarily) if ANC <500/mm^3 or platelet count <25,000/mm^3. Use with caution in patients with an increased risk for severe anemia (eg, spherocytosis, history of GI bleeding).

Hepatic disease: Hepatic decompensation and death have been associated with the use of alpha interferons including Pegasys®, in cirrhotic chronic hepatitis C patients; patients coinfected with HIV and receiving highly active antiretroviral therapy have shown an increased risk. Monitor hepatic function; discontinue if decompensation occurs (Child-Pugh score >6) in monoinfected patients and (Child-Pugh score ≥6, class B and C) in patients coinfected with HIV. In hepatitis B patients, flares (transient and potentially severe increases in serum ALT) may occur during or after treatment; more frequent monitoring of LFTs and a dose reduction are recommended. Discontinue if ALT elevation continues despite dose reduction or if increased bilirubin or hepatic decompensation occur.

Gastrointestinal disorders: Gastrointestinal hemorrhage, ulcerative and hemorrhagic/ischemic colitis have been observed with interferon alfa treatment; may be severe and/or life-threatening; discontinue if symptoms of colitis (eg, abdominal pain, bloody diarrhea, and/or fever) develop. Discontinue therapy if known or suspected pancreatitis develops.

Dermatologic disorders: Serious cutaneous reactions, including vesiculobullous eruptions, Stevens-Johnson syndrome and exfoliative dermatitis, have been reported (rarely) with use, with or without ribavirin therapy; discontinue with signs or symptoms of severe skin reactions.

Ophthalmic disease: Discontinue if new or worsening ophthalmologic disorders occur including retinal hemorrhages, cotton wool spots, retinal detachment (serous), and retinal artery or vein obstruction; visual exams are recommended in these instances, at the initiation of therapy, and periodically during therapy.

Pulmonary disorders: May cause or aggravate dyspnea, pulmonary infiltrates, pneumonia, bronchiolitis obliterans, interstitial pneumonia, and sarcoidosis, resulting in potentially fatal respiratory failure may occur with treatment; may recur upon rechallenge with interferons. Discontinue with unexplained pulmonary infiltrates or evidence of impaired pulmonary function. Use caution in patients with a history of pulmonary disease.

Endocrine disorders: Use with caution in patients with diabetes mellitus; hyper- or hypoglycemia have been reported which may require adjustments in medications. Use with caution in patients with pre-existing thyroid disease; thyroid disorders (hyper- or hypothyroidism) or exacerbations have been reported.

Severe acute hypersensitivity reactions have occurred rarely; prompt discontinuation is advised. Commonly associated with flu-like symptoms, including fever; rule out other causes/infection with persistent or high fever. Serious and severe infections (bacterial, viral and fungal) have been reported with treatment. Use with caution in patients with renal dysfunction (Cl_{cr} <30 mL/minute); monitor for signs/symptoms of toxicity (dosage adjustment required if toxicity occurs). Use with caution in patients with pulmonary dysfunction, prior cardiovascular disease, or autoimmune disease. Use with caution in the elderly. **Due to differences in dosage, patients should not change brands of interferon without the concurrence of their healthcare provider.** Safety and efficacy have not been established in patients who have failed other alpha interferon therapy, have received organ transplants, have been coinfected with HBV **and** HCV or HIV, have been coinfected with HCV **and** HBV or HIV with a CD4$^+$ cell count <100 cells/microL, or been treated for >48 weeks.

[U.S. Boxed Warning]: Combination treatment with ribavirin may cause birth defects and/or fetal mortality (avoid pregnancy in females and female partners of male patients); hemolytic anemia (which may worsen cardiac disease), genotoxicity, mutagenicity, and may possibly be carcinogenic.

Drug Interactions

Avoid Concomitant Use

Avoid concomitant use of Peginterferon Alfa-2a with any of the following: CloZAPine; Telbivudine

Decreased Effect

The levels/effects of Peginterferon Alfa-2a may be decreased by: Pegloticase

Increased Effect/Toxicity

Peginterferon Alfa-2a may increase the levels/effects of: Aldesleukin; CloZAPine; Methadone; Ribavirin; Telbivudine; Theophylline Derivatives; Zidovudine

Nutritional/Ethanol Interactions Ethanol: Avoid use in patients with hepatitis C virus.

Adverse Reactions Note: Percentages are reported for peginterferon alfa-2a in chronic hepatitis C (CHC) patients. Other percentages indicated as "with ribavirin" or "in HIV/CHC" are those which significantly exceed incidence reported for peginterferon monotherapy in CHC patients.

>10%:

Central nervous system: Headache (54%), fatigue (56%), fever (37%; 41% with ribavirin; 54% in hepatitis B), insomnia (19%; 30% with ribavirin), depression (18%), dizziness (16%), irritability/anxiety/nervousness (19%; 33% with ribavirin), pain (11%)

Dermatologic: Alopecia (23%; 28% with ribavirin), pruritus (12%; 19% with ribavirin), dermatitis (16% with ribavirin)

Gastrointestinal: Nausea/vomiting (24%), anorexia (17%; 24% with ribavirin), diarrhea (16%), weight loss (16% in HIV/CHC), abdominal pain (15%)

Hematologic: Neutropenia (21%; 27% with ribavirin; 40% in HIV/CHC), lymphopenia (14% with ribavirin), anemia (11% with ribavirin; 14% in HIV/CHC)

Hepatic: ALT increases 5-10 x ULN during treatment (25% to 27% in hepatitis B); ALT increases >10 x ULN during treatment (12% to 18% in hepatitis B); ALT increases 5-10 x ULN after treatment (13% to 16% in hepatitis B); ALT increases >10 x ULN after treatment (7% to 12% in hepatitis B)

Local: Injection site reaction (22%)

Neuromuscular & skeletal: Weakness (56%; 65% with ribavirin), myalgia (37%), rigors (35%; 25% to 27% in hepatitis B), arthralgia (28%)

Respiratory: Dyspnea (13% with ribavirin)

1% to 10%:

Central nervous system: Concentration impaired (8%), memory impaired (5%), mood alteration (3%; 9% in HIV/CHC)

Dermatologic: Dermatitis (8%), rash (5%), dry skin (4%; 10% with ribavirin), eczema (1%; 5% with ribavirin)

Endocrine & metabolic: Hypothyroidism (3% to 4%), hyperthyroidism (≤1%)

Gastrointestinal: Xerostomia (6%), dyspepsia (<1%; 6% with ribavirin), weight loss (4%; 10% with ribavirin)

Hematologic: Thrombocytopenia (5%; 8% in HIV/CHC), lymphopenia (3%), anemia (2%)

Hepatic: Hepatic decompensation (2% in CHC/HIV)

Neuromuscular & skeletal: Back pain (9%)

Ocular: Blurred vision (4%)

Respiratory: Cough (4%; 10% with ribavirin), dyspnea (4%), exertional dyspnea (4% with ribavirin)

Miscellaneous: Diaphoresis (6%), bacterial infection (3%; 5% in HIV/CHC)

Available Dosage Forms

Injection, solution:

Pegasys®: 180 mcg/mL (1 mL); 180 mcg/0.5 mL (0.5 mL)

General Dosage Range Dosage adjustment recommended in patients with hepatic or renal impairment or who develop toxicities

SubQ: *Adults:* 180 mcg once weekly

Administration

Other SubQ: Administer in the abdomen or thigh. Rotate injection site. Do not use if solution contains particulate matter or is discolored. Discard unused solution. Administration should be done on the same day and at approximately the same time each week.

Stability

Storage Store in refrigerator at 2°C to 8°C (36°F to 46°F). Do not freeze or shake. Protect from light. The following stability information has also been reported:

Intact vial: May be stored at room temperature for up to 14 days (Cohen, 2007).

Prefilled syringe: May be stored at room temperature for up to 6 days (Cohen, 2007).

Nursing Actions

Physical Assessment Evaluate for depression and other psychiatric symptoms before and during therapy. Patients may need baseline eye examination; patients with cardiac disease require baseline echocardiogram. Teach patient appropriate injection technique and syringe/needle disposal.

Patient Education This medication must be given by injection; follow instructions for injection and syringe/needle disposal. Avoid alcohol. You will need laboratory tests and ophthalmic exams prior to and during therapy. May cause headache; insomnia; dizziness; loss of hair (will grow back after therapy); nausea or anorexia; diarrhea; weakness or fatigue; flu-like symptoms; or muscle, skeletal, or joint pain. Report any persistent nausea, vomiting, or abdominal pain; severe depression or suicide ideation; skin rash; pain, redness, or swelling at injection site; signs of infection; unusual bleeding or bruising; changes in vision; or chest pain, palpitations, or respiratory difficulty.

Dietary Considerations Avoid ethanol use in patients with hepatitis C virus.

Pegloticase (peg LOE ti kase)

Brand Names: U.S. Krystexxa™

Index Terms PEG-Uricase; Pegylated Urate Oxidase; Polyethylene Glycol-Conjugated Uricase; Recombinant Urate Oxidase, Pegylated; Urate Oxidase, Pegylated

Pharmacologic Category Enzyme; Enzyme, Urate-Oxidase (Recombinant)

Medication Guide Available Yes

Pregnancy Risk Factor C

Lactation Excretion in breast milk unknown/not recommended

Breast-Feeding Considerations Due to the potential for serious adverse reactions in the nursing infant, breast-feeding is not recommended.

Use Treatment of chronic gout refractory to conventional therapy

Mechanism of Action/Effect Converts uric acid to allantoin (an inactive and water soluble metabolite of uric acid) which lowers serum uric acid concentrations; it does not inhibit the formation of uric acid

Contraindications Glucose-6-phosphate dehydrogenase (G6PD) deficiency

Warnings/Precautions [U.S. Boxed Warning]: Anaphylaxis and infusion reactions have been reported during and after administration; patients should be closely monitored during infusion and for an appropriate period of time after the infusion. Therapy should be administered in a healthcare facility by skilled medical personnel prepared for the immediate treatment of anaphylaxis. All patients should be premedicated with antihistamines and corticosteroids. Anaphylaxis may occur at any time during treatment (including the initial dose). **Reactions generally occur within 2 hours of administration; however, delayed hypersensitivity reactions have also been reported.** Infusion reactions are varied; symptoms range from chest pain, pruritus/urticaria, or dyspnea to a clinical presentation of anaphylaxis (eg, hemodynamic instability, perioral or lingual edema). If a less severe (nonanaphylactic) infusion reaction occurs, the infusion may be slowed, or stopped and restarted at a slower rate, at the physician's discretion. **Risk of an infusion reaction is increased in patients whose uric acid is >6 mg/dL; therefore, monitor serum uric acid concentrations prior to infusion and consider discontinuing treatment if concentrations exceed 6 mg/dL, particularly in the event of 2 consecutive concentrations >6 mg/dL.**

Therapy with antihyperuricemic agents commonly results in gout flare, particularly upon initiation due to rapid lowering of urate concentrations; gout flare-ups during treatment do not warrant discontinuation of therapy. Gout flare prophylaxis is recommended, using nonsteroidal anti-inflammatory agents (NSAID) or colchicines, unless contraindicated, beginning ≥1 week before initiation of pegloticase and continuing for at least 6 months. Exacerbation of heart failure has been observed in clinical trials; use caution in patients with preexisting heart failure. Due to the risk for hemolysis and methemoglobinemia, pegloticase is contraindicated in patients with G6PD deficiency. Patients at higher risk for G6PD deficiency (eg, African, Mediterranean) should be screened prior to therapy. Therapy is not appropriate for the treatment of asymptomatic hyperuricemia. Potential for immunogenicity exists with the use of therapeutic proteins. Antipegloticase antibodies and antiPEG antibodies commonly occurred during clinical trials in pegloticase-treated patients. High antipegloticase antibody titers were associated with failure to maintain uric acid normalization and were also associated with a higher incidence of infusion reactions. Due to potential for immunogenicity, closely monitor patients who reinitiate therapy after discontinuing treatment for >4 weeks; patients may be at increased risk for anaphylaxis and infusion reactions.

Drug Interactions

Avoid Concomitant Use There are no known interactions where it is recommended to avoid concomitant use.

Decreased Effect

Pegloticase may decrease the levels/effects of: Certolizumab Pegol; Pegademase Bovine; Pegaptanib; Pegaspargase; Pegfilgrastim; Peginterferon Alfa-2a; Peginterferon Alfa-2b; Pegvisomant

Increased Effect/Toxicity There are no known significant interactions involving an increase in effect.

Adverse Reactions

>10%:

Dermatologic: Bruising (11%), urticaria (11%)

Gastrointestinal: Nausea (12%)

Miscellaneous: Antibody formation (antipegloticase antibodies: 92%; antiPEG antibodies: 42%), gout flare (74% within the first 3 months), infusion reactions (26%)

1% to 10%:

Cardiovascular: Chest pain (6% to 10%)

Dermatologic: Erythema (10%), pruritus (10%)

Gastrointestinal: Constipation (6%), vomiting (5%)

Respiratory: Dyspnea (7%), nasopharyngitis (7%)

Miscellaneous: Anaphylaxis (≤7%)

Frequency not defined: Anemia, diarrhea, headache, muscle spasms, nephrolithiasis

Pharmacodynamics/Kinetics

Onset of Action ~24 hours following the first dose, serum uric acid concentrations decreased

Duration of Action >300 hours (12.5 days)

Available Dosage Forms

Injection, solution:

Krystexxa™: Uricase protein 8 mg/mL (2 mL)

General Dosage Range I.V.: *Adults:* 8 mg every 2 weeks

Administration

I.V. Administer diluted solution by I.V. infusion over ≥120 minutes via gravity feed or an infusion pump or syringe-type pump. Do **not** administer by I.V. push or bolus. Administer in a healthcare setting by healthcare providers prepared to manage potential anaphylaxis. Monitor closely for infusion reactions during infusion and for an appropriate period of time after the infusion (anaphylaxis has been reported within 2 hours of the infusion). In the event or a less severe infusion reaction, infusion may be slowed, or stopped and restarted at a slower rate, based on the discretion of the physician.

Stability

Reconstitution To prepare solution for administration, withdraw 1 mL (8 mg) and add to a 250 mL bag of NS or 1/2NS; invert bag several times to mix thoroughly (do **not** shake). Do not use vial if particulate matter is present or if solution is discolored (solution should be a clear and colorless). After withdrawal, discard any unused portion of the product remaining in the vial.

Storage Prior to use, vials must be stored in the carton to protect from light and kept under refrigeration between 2°C to 8°C (36° to 46°F) at all times. Do **not** shake or freeze.

Diluted solution may be stored up to 4 hours at 2°C to 8°C (36°F to 46°F). Diluted solution is also stable for 4 hours at room temperature of 20°C to 25°C (68°F to 77°F); however, refrigeration is preferred. The diluted solution should be protected from light, not frozen, and used within 4 hours of dilution. Prior to administration, allow the diluted solution to reach room temperature; do not warm to room temperature using any form of artificial heating such as a microwave or warm water bath.

Pegvisomant (peg VI soe mant)

Brand Names: U.S. Somavert®

Index Terms B2036-PEG

Pharmacologic Category Growth Hormone Receptor Antagonist

Pregnancy Risk Factor B

Lactation Excretion in breast milk unknown/use caution

Use Treatment of acromegaly in patients resistant to or unable to tolerate other therapies

Available Dosage Forms

Injection, powder for reconstitution:

Somavert®: 10 mg, 15 mg, 20 mg

General Dosage Range SubQ: *Adults:* Initial loading dose: 40 mg; Maintenance: 10-30 mg/day (maximum: 30 mg/day)

Administration

Other For SubQ administration only; to minimize the risk for lipohypertrophy, rotate injection site daily; may administer in upper arm, thigh, abdomen, or buttocks; do not rub injection site. The manufacturer recommends the initial dose be administered under the supervision of prescribing healthcare provider.

Nursing Actions

Physical Assessment First dose should be administered under supervision of prescriber. Teach patient proper storage, reconstitution, injection technique, site rotation, and disposal of syringes/needles.

Patient Education This medication may only be administered by injection. Report immediately any redness, swelling, or itching at injection site. May cause diarrhea, nausea, or allergic response (eg, chest pain, respiratory difficulty, skin rash).

Pemetrexed (pem e TREKS ed)

Brand Names: U.S. Alimta®

Index Terms LY231514; Pemetrexed Disodium

Pharmacologic Category Antineoplastic Agent, Antimetabolite; Antineoplastic Agent, Antimetabolite (Antifolate)

Medication Safety Issues

Sound-alike/look-alike issues:

PEMEtrexed may be confused with methotrexate, PRALAtrexate

High alert medication:

This medication is in a class the Institute for Safe Medication Practices (ISMP) includes among its list of drug classes which have a heightened risk of causing significant patient harm when used in error.

Pregnancy Risk Factor D

Lactation Excretion in breast milk unknown/not recommended

Breast-Feeding Considerations According to the manufacturer, the decision to continue or discontinue breast-feeding during therapy should take into account the risk of exposure to the infant and the benefits of treatment to the mother.

Use Treatment of unresectable malignant pleural mesothelioma (in combination with cisplatin); treatment of locally advanced or metastatic **non**squamous nonsmall cell lung cancer (NSCLC; as initial treatment in combination with cisplatin, as single-agent maintenance treatment after 4 cycles of initial platinum-based double therapy, and single-agent treatment after prior chemotherapy)

Note: Not indicated for the treatment of **squamous** cell NSCLC

Unlabeled Use Treatment of bladder cancer (metastatic), cervical cancer (recurrent or metastatic), ovarian cancer (recurrent or persistent), thymic malignancies; treatment of malignant pleural mesothelioma (either as a single agent or in combination with carboplatin)

Mechanism of Action/Effect Disrupts folate-dependent metabolic processes essential for cell replication.

Contraindications Severe hypersensitivity to pemetrexed or any component of the formulation

Canadian labeling (additional contraindications; not in U.S. labeling): Concomitant yellow fever vaccine

Warnings/Precautions Hazardous agent - use appropriate precautions for handling and disposal. Hypersensitivity (including anaphylaxis) has been reported with use. May cause bone marrow suppression (anemia, neutropenia, thrombocytopenia and/or pancytopenia); may require dose reductions in subsequent cycles. Prophylactic folic acid and vitamin B_{12} supplements are necessary to reduce hematologic and gastrointestinal toxicity and infection; initiate supplementation 1 week before the first dose of pemetrexed. Pretreatment with corticosteroids (dexamethasone or equivalent) reduces the incidence and severity of cutaneous reactions. Rarely, Stevens-Johnson syndrome and toxic epidermal necrolysis have been reported. Although the effect of third space fluid is not fully defined, studies have determined pemetrexed concentrations in patients with mild-to-moderate ascites/pleural effusions were similar to concentrations in trials of patients without third space fluid accumulation. Drainage of fluid from ascites/effusions may be considered, but is not likely necessary. Use caution with hepatic dysfunction not due to metastases; may require dose adjustment. Interstitial pneumonitis with respiratory insufficiency has been observed with use; interrupt therapy and evaluate promptly with progressive dyspnea and cough.

The manufacturer does not recommend use in patients with Cl_{cr} <45 mL/minute. Decreased renal function results in increased toxicity. Use caution in patients receiving concurrent nephrotoxins; may result in delayed pemetrexed clearance. NSAIDs may reduce the clearance of pemetrexed. In patients with Cl_{cr} 45-79 mL/minute, interruption of NSAID therapy may be necessary prior to, during, and immediately after pemetrexed therapy. Not indicated for use in patients with squamous cell NSCLC.

Drug Interactions

Avoid Concomitant Use

Avoid concomitant use of PEMEtrexed with any of the following: BCG; CloZAPine; Natalizumab; Pimecrolimus; Tacrolimus (Topical); Vaccines (Live)

Decreased Effect

PEMEtrexed may decrease the levels/effects of: BCG; Coccidioidin Skin Test; Sipuleucel-T; Vaccines (Inactivated); Vaccines (Live)

The levels/effects of PEMEtrexed may be decreased by: Echinacea

Increased Effect/Toxicity

PEMEtrexed may increase the levels/effects of: CloZAPine; Leflunomide; Natalizumab; Vaccines (Live)

The levels/effects of PEMEtrexed may be increased by: Denosumab; NSAID (Nonselective); Pimecrolimus; Roflumilast; Tacrolimus (Topical); Trastuzumab

Nutritional/Ethanol Interactions Lower ANC nadirs occur in patients with elevated baseline cystathionine or homocysteine concentrations. Levels of these substances can be reduced by folic acid and vitamin B_{12} supplementation.

Adverse Reactions Note: Reported for single-agent therapy in patients who received folate and B_{12} supplementation.

>10%:

Central nervous system: Fatigue (25% to 34%; dose-limiting)

Dermatologic: Rash/desquamation (10% to 14%)

Gastrointestinal: Nausea (19% to 31%), anorexia (19% to 22%), vomiting (9% to 16%), stomatitis (7% to 15%), diarrhea (5% to 13%)

Hematologic: Anemia (15% to 19%; grades 3/4: 3% to 4%), leukopenia (6% to 12%; grades 3/4: 2% to 4%), neutropenia (6% to 11%; grades 3/4: 3% to 5%; dose-limiting; nadir: 8-10 days; recovery: 4-8 days after nadir)

Respiratory: Pharyngitis (15%)

1% to 10%:

Cardiovascular: Edema (1% to 5%)

Central nervous system: Fever (1% to 8%)

Dermatologic: Pruritus (1% to 7%), alopecia (1% to 6%), erythema multiforme (≤5%)

Gastrointestinal: Constipation (1% to 6%), weight loss (1%), abdominal pain (≤5%)

Hematologic: Thrombocytopenia (1% to 8%; grades 3/4: 2%; dose-limiting), febrile neutropenia (grades 3/4: 2%)

Hepatic: ALT increased (8% to 10%; grades 3/4: ≤2%), AST increased (7% to 8%; grades 3/4: ≤1%)

Neuromuscular & skeletal: Sensory neuropathy (≤9%), motor neuropathy (≤5%)

Ocular: Conjunctivitis (≤5%), lacrimation increased (≤5%)

Renal: Creatinine increased/creatinine clearance decreased (1% to 5%)

Miscellaneous: Allergic reaction/hypersensitivity (≤5%), infection (≤5%), sepsis (1%)

Pharmacodynamics/Kinetics

Duration of Action V_{dss}: 16.1 L

Available Dosage Forms

Injection, powder for reconstitution:

Alimta®: 100 mg, 500 mg

General Dosage Range Dosage adjustment recommended in patients with hepatic impairment, on concomitant therapy, or who develop toxicities

I.V.: *Adults:* 500 mg/m^2 on day 1 of each 21-day cycle

Administration

I.V. Infuse over 10 minutes.

I.V. Detail pH: 6.6-7.8

Stability

Reconstitution Reconstitute with NS (preservative free); add 4.2 mL to the 100 mg vial and 20 mL to the 500 mg vial, resulting in a 25 mg/mL concentration. Gently swirl. Solution may be colorless to green-yellow. Further dilute in 100 mL NS for infusion; may also dilute in D_5W (Zhang, 2006), although the manufacturer recommends NS. Use appropriate precautions for handling and disposal.

Storage Store intact vials at room temperature of 25°C (77°F); excursions permitted to 15°C to 30°C (59°F to 86°F). Reconstituted solution in NS and infusion solutions (in D_5W or NS) are stable for 24 hours when refrigerated at 2°C to 8°C (36°F to 46°F) or stored at room temperature of 15°C to 30°C (59°F to 86°F). Concentrations at 25 mg/mL are stable in polypropylene syringes for 2 days at room temperature (23°C) (Zhang, 2005).

Nursing Actions

Physical Assessment Pre- and post-treatment medication may be prescribed (eg, oral folic acid and vitamin B_{12} 1 week [injection] before first dose). Corticosteroids may be ordered to reduce cutaneous reactions. Monitor for CNS changes, GI upset (nausea, vomiting, diarrhea, constipation), anemia, neuropathy, rash, and infection.

Patient Education This medication is only administered intravenously. Report immediately any burning, pain, itching, or redness at infusion site or any sudden feelings of anxiety, difficulty breathing, chest discomfort, or back pain. It is important that you maintain adequate nutrition and hydration, unless instructed to restrict fluid intake. Maintain regularly scheduled dietary supplements (vitamin B_{12} and folic acid) as prescribed. May cause severe nausea, vomiting, constipation, diarrhea, or mouth sores. Report immediately any chest pain, swelling of extremities, unusual weight gain, rash, tingling or loss of sensation in extremities, difficulty breathing, fever, chills, or unusual or persistent fatigue.

Dietary Considerations Initiate folic acid supplementation 1 week before first dose of pemetrexed, continue for full course of therapy, and for 21 days after last dose. Institute vitamin B_{12} 1 week before the first dose; administer every 9 weeks thereafter.

Penicillin G Benzathine

(pen i SIL in jee BENZ a theen)

Brand Names: U.S. Bicillin® L-A

Index Terms Benzathine Benzylpenicillin; Benzathine Penicillin G; Benzylpenicillin Benzathine

Pharmacologic Category Antibiotic, Penicillin

Medication Safety Issues

Sound-alike/look-alike issues:

Penicillin may be confused with penicillamine

Bicillin® may be confused with Wycillin®

Administration issues:

Penicillin G benzathine may only be administered by deep intramuscular injection; intravenous administration of penicillin G benzathine has been associated with cardiopulmonary arrest and death.

Other safety concerns:

Bicillin® C-R (penicillin G benzathine and penicillin G procaine) may be confused with Bicillin® L-A (penicillin G benzathine). Penicillin G benzathine is the only product currently approved for the treatment of syphilis. Administration of penicillin G benzathine and penicillin G procaine combination instead of Bicillin® L-A may result in inadequate treatment response.

Pregnancy Risk Factor B

Lactation Enters breast milk/use caution

Use Active against some gram-positive organisms, few gram-negative organisms such as *Neisseria gonorrhoeae*, and some anaerobes and spirochetes; used in the treatment of syphilis; used only for the treatment of mild to moderately-severe upper respiratory tract infections caused by organisms susceptible to low concentrations of penicillin G or for prophylaxis of infections caused by these organisms; primary and secondary prevention of rheumatic fever

Available Dosage Forms

Injection, suspension:

Bicillin® L-A: 600,000 units/mL (1 mL, 2 mL, 4 mL)

General Dosage Range I.M.:

Children ≤27 kg: 600,000 units/dose

Children >27 kg: 1.2 million units/dose

Adults: 1.2-2.4 million units as a single dose

Administration

I.M. Warm to room temperature before administration to lessen the pain associated with injection. Administer by deep I.M. injection in the upper outer quadrant of the buttock; in children <2 years of age, I.M. injections should be made into the midlateral muscle of the thigh, not the gluteal region. Do not inject near an artery or a nerve; permanent neurological damage or gangrene may result. When doses are repeated, rotate the injection site. **Do not administer I.V., intra-arterially, or SubQ.**

Nursing Actions

Physical Assessment Results of culture and sensitivity tests and patient's allergy history should be assessed prior to starting therapy. Monitor for hypersensitivity reactions and opportunistic infection.

Patient Education This drug can only be given by injection. Report immediately any redness, swelling, burning, or pain at injection site or any signs of allergic reaction (eg, respiratory difficulty or swallowing, chest tightness, rash, hives, swelling of lips or mouth). Maintain adequate hydration unless instructed to restrict fluid intake. If being treated for sexually-transmitted disease, partner will also need to be treated. May cause confusion or drowsiness. Report persistent adverse effects or signs of opportunistic infection (eg, fever, chills, diarrhea, unhealed sores, white plaques in mouth or vagina, purulent vaginal discharge).

Penicillin G (Parenteral/Aqueous)

(pen i SIL in jee pa REN ter al AYE kwee us)

Brand Names: U.S. Pfizerpen®

Index Terms Benzylpenicillin Potassium; Benzylpenicillin Sodium; Crystalline Penicillin; Penicillin G Potassium; Penicillin G Sodium

Pharmacologic Category Antibiotic, Penicillin

Medication Safety Issues

Sound-alike/look-alike issues:

Penicillin may be confused with penicillamine

Pregnancy Risk Factor B

Lactation Enters breast milk/compatible

Breast-Feeding Considerations Very small amounts of penicillin G transfer into breast milk. Peak milk concentrations occur at approximately 1 hour after an IM dose and are higher if multiple doses are given. The manufacturer recommends that caution be exercised when administering penicillin to nursing women. Nondose-related effects could include modification of bowel flora and allergic sensitization.

Use Treatment of infections (including sepsis, pneumonia, pericarditis, endocarditis, meningitis, anthrax) caused by susceptible organisms; active against some gram-positive organisms, generally not *Staphylococcus aureus*; some gram-negative organisms such as *Neisseria gonorrhoeae*, and some anaerobes and spirochetes

Mechanism of Action/Effect Interferes with bacterial cell wall synthesis during active multiplication, causing cell wall death and resultant bactericidal activity against susceptible bacteria

Contraindications Hypersensitivity to penicillin or any component of the formulation

Warnings/Precautions Avoid intra-arterial administration or injection into or near major peripheral nerves or blood vessels since such injections may cause severe and/or permanent neurovascular damage; use with caution in patients with renal impairment (dosage reduction required), concomitant renal and hepatic impairment (further dosage adjustment may be required), pre-existing seizure disorders, or with a history of hypersensitivity to cephalosporins. Prolonged use may result in fungal or bacterial superinfection, including *C. difficile*-associated diarrhea (CDAD) and pseudomembranous colitis; CDAD has been observed >2 months postantibiotic treatment. Serious and occasionally severe or fatal hypersensitivity (anaphylactoid) reactions have been reported in patients on penicillin therapy, especially with a history of beta-lactam hypersensitivity, history of sensitivity to multiple allergens, or previous IgE-mediated reactions (eg, anaphylaxis, angioedema, urticaria). Use with caution in asthmatic patients. Extended duration of therapy or use associated with high serum concentrations may be associated with an increased risk for some adverse reactions. Neonates may have decreased renal clearance of penicillin and require frequent dosage adjustments depending on age. Product contains sodium and potassium; high doses of I.V. therapy may alter serum levels.

Drug Interactions

Avoid Concomitant Use

Avoid concomitant use of Penicillin G (Parenteral/Aqueous) with any of the following: BCG

Decreased Effect

Penicillin G (Parenteral/Aqueous) may decrease the levels/effects of: BCG; Mycophenolate; Typhoid Vaccine

The levels/effects of Penicillin G (Parenteral/Aqueous) may be decreased by: Fusidic Acid; Tetracycline Derivatives

Increased Effect/Toxicity

Penicillin G (Parenteral/Aqueous) may increase the levels/effects of: Methotrexate; Vitamin K Antagonists

The levels/effects of Penicillin G (Parenteral/Aqueous) may be increased by: Probenecid

Adverse Reactions Frequency not defined.

Central nervous system: Coma (high doses), hyper-reflexia (high doses), seizures (high doses)

Dermatologic: Contact dermatitis, rash

Endocrine & metabolic: Electrolyte imbalance (high doses)

Gastrointestinal: Pseudomembranous colitis

Hematologic: Neutropenia, positive Coombs' hemolytic anemia (rare, high doses)

Local: Injection site reaction, phlebitis, thrombophlebitis

Neuromuscular & skeletal: Myoclonus (high doses)

Renal: Acute interstitial nephritis (high doses), renal tubular damage (high doses)

Miscellaneous: Anaphylaxis, hypersensitivity reactions (immediate and delayed), Jarisch-Herxheimer reaction, serum sickness

Available Dosage Forms

Infusion, premixed iso-osmotic dextrose solution: 1 million units (50 mL); 2 million units (50 mL); 3 million units (50 mL)

Injection, powder for reconstitution: 5 million units, 20 million units

Pfizerpen®: 5 million units, 20 million units

General Dosage Range Dosage adjustment recommended in patients with renal impairment

I.M., I.V.:

Infants ≥1 month and Children: 100,000-400,000 units/kg/day in divided doses every 4-6 hours (maximum: 24 million units/day)

Adults: 2-30 million units/day in divided doses every 4-6 hours

Administration

I.M. Administer I.M. by deep injection in the upper outer quadrant of the buttock. Administer injection around-the-clock to promote less variation in peak and trough levels. **Note:** The 20 million unit dosage form may be administered by continuous I.V. infusion only.

I.V. Usually administered by intermittent infusion. In some centers, large doses may be administered by continuous I.V. infusion. **Note:** The 20 million unit dosage form may be administered by continuous I.V. infusion only.

Intermittent I.V.: May be dissolved in small amounts of SWFI, NS, D_5W and administered peripherally as a 50,000-100,000 unit/mL solution. In fluid-restricted patients, 146,000 units/mL in SW results in a maximum recommended osmolality for peripheral infusion. Infuse over 15-30 minutes.

Continuous I.V. infusion: Determine the volume of fluid and rate of its administration required by the patient in a 24-hour period. Add the appropriate daily dosage of penicillin to this fluid. For example, if the daily dose is 10 million units and 2 L of fluid/day is required, add 5 million units to 1 L and adjust the rate of flow so the liter will be infused over 12 hours (83 mL/hour). Repeat steps (5 million units/L at 83 mL/hour) for the remaining 12 hours.

I.V. Detail pH: 6-7.5

Stability

Reconstitution

Intermittent I.V.: 5 million unit vial: Add 8.2 mL for a final concentration of 500,000 units/mL; add 3.2 mL for a final concentration of 1,000,000 units/mL. Dilute further to 50,000-145,000 units/mL prior to infusion.

Continuous I.V. infusion: 20 million unit vial: Add 11.5 mL for a final concentration of 1,000,000 units/mL. Dilute further in 1-2 L of infusion solution and administer over a 24-hour period.

Storage

Penicillin G potassium powder for injection should be stored below 86°F (30°C). Following reconstitution, solution may be stored for up to 7 days under refrigeration. Premixed bags for infusion should be stored in the freezer (-20°C to -4°F); frozen bags may be thawed at room temperature or in refrigerator. Once thawed, solution is stable for 14 days if stored in refrigerator or for 24 hours when stored at room temperature. Do not refreeze once thawed.

Penicillin G sodium powder for injection should be stored at controlled room temperature. Reconstituted solution may be stored under refrigeration for up to 3 days.

Nursing Actions

Physical Assessment Results of culture and sensitivity tests and patient's allergy history should be assessed prior to starting therapy. Avoid intravascular or intra-arterial administration or injection into or near major peripheral nerves or blood vessels; may cause severe and/or permanent neurovascular damage. Monitor for hypersensitivity reactions, opportunistic infection (fever, chills, unhealed sores, white plaques in mouth or vagina, purulent vaginal discharge), CNS changes, and thrombophlebitis.

Patient Education This drug can only be given by injection or infusion. Report immediately any redness, swelling, burning, or pain at infusion site or any signs of allergic reaction (eg, respiratory or swallowing difficulty, chest tightness, rash, hives, swelling of lips or mouth). Maintain adequate hydration unless instructed to restrict fluid intake. If being treated for sexually-transmitted disease, partner will also need to be treated. May cause confusion or drowsiness. Report signs of opportunistic infection (eg, fever, chills, diarrhea, unhealed sores, white plaques in mouth or vagina, purulent vaginal discharge).

Dietary Considerations Some products may contain potassium and/or sodium.

Penicillin G Procaine

(pen i SIL in jee PROE kane)

Index Terms APPG; Aqueous Procaine Penicillin G; Procaine Benzylpenicillin; Procaine Penicillin G; Wycillin [DSC]

Pharmacologic Category Antibiotic, Penicillin

Medication Safety Issues

Sound-alike/look-alike issues:

Penicillin G procaine may be confused with penicillin V potassium

Wycillin® may be confused with Bicillin®

Pregnancy Risk Factor B

Lactation Enters breast milk/compatible

Use Treatment of moderately-severe infections due to *Treponema pallidum* and other penicillin G-sensitive microorganisms that are susceptible to low, but prolonged serum penicillin concentrations; anthrax due to *Bacillus anthracis* (postexposure) to reduce the incidence or progression of disease following exposure to aerolized *Bacillus anthracis*

Available Dosage Forms

Injection, suspension: 600,000 units/mL (1 mL, 2 mL)

General Dosage Range Dosage adjustment recommended in patients with renal impairment

I.M.:

Children: 25,000-50,000 units/kg/day in divided doses 1-2 times/day (maximum: 4.8 million units/day)

Adults: 0.6-4.8 million units/day in divided doses every 12-24 hours

Administration

I.M. Procaine suspension is for deep I.M. injection only. Rotate the injection site. Do not inject in gluteal muscle in children <2 years of age. Avoid I.V., intravascular, or intra-arterial administration of penicillin G procaine since severe and/or permanent neurovascular damage may occur.

Nursing Actions

Physical Assessment Results of culture and sensitivity tests and patient's allergy history should be assessed prior to starting therapy. Avoid intravascular or intra-arterial administration or injection into or near major peripheral nerves or blood vessels; may cause severe and/or permanent neurovascular damage. Monitor for hypersensitivity reactions, opportunistic infection (fever, chills, unhealed sores, white plaques in mouth or vagina, purulent vaginal discharge), CNS changes, and thrombophlebitis.

Patient Education This drug can only be given by injection. Report immediately any redness, swelling, burning, or pain at injection site or any signs of allergic reaction (eg, respiratory or swallowing difficulty, chest tightness, rash, hives, swelling of lips or mouth). Maintain adequate hydration unless instructed to restrict fluid intake. If being treated for sexually-transmitted disease, partner will also need to be treated. May cause confusion or drowsiness. Report signs of opportunistic infection (eg, fever, chills, diarrhea, unhealed sores, white plaques in mouth or vagina, purulent vaginal discharge).

Penicillin V Potassium

(pen i SIL in vee poe TASS ee um)

Index Terms Pen VK; Phenoxymethyl Penicillin

Pharmacologic Category Antibiotic, Penicillin

Medication Safety Issues

Sound-alike/look-alike issues:

Penicillin V procaine may be confused with penicillin G potassium

Pregnancy Risk Factor B

Lactation Enters breast milk/compatible

Breast-Feeding Considerations Penicillins are excreted in breast milk. The manufacturer recommends that caution be exercised when administering penicillin to nursing women. Nondose-related effects could include modification of bowel flora and allergic sensitization.

Use Treatment of infections caused by susceptible organisms involving the respiratory tract, otitis media, sinusitis, skin, and urinary tract; prophylaxis in rheumatic fever

Mechanism of Action/Effect Inhibits bacterial cell wall synthesis by binding to one or more of the penicillin-binding proteins (PBPs); which in turn inhibits the final transpeptidation step of peptidoglycan synthesis in bacterial cell walls, thus inhibiting cell wall biosynthesis. Bacteria eventually lyse due to ongoing activity of cell wall autolytic enzymes (autolysins and murein hydrolases) while cell wall assembly is arrested.

Contraindications Hypersensitivity to penicillin or any component of the formulation

Warnings/Precautions Use with caution in patients with severe renal impairment (modify dosage) or history of seizures. Serious and occasionally severe or fatal hypersensitivity (anaphylactoid) reactions have been reported in patients on penicillin therapy, especially with a history of beta-lactam hypersensitivity, history of sensitivity to multiple allergens, or previous IgE-mediated reactions (eg, anaphylaxis, angioedema, urticaria). Use with caution in asthmatic patients. Extended duration of therapy or use associated with high serum concentrations may be associated with an increased risk for some adverse reactions. Prolonged use may result in fungal or bacterial superinfection, including *C. difficile*-associated diarrhea (CDAD) and pseudomembranous colitis; CDAD has been observed >2 months postantibiotic treatment.

Drug Interactions

Avoid Concomitant Use

Avoid concomitant use of Penicillin V Potassium with any of the following: BCG

Decreased Effect

Penicillin V Potassium may decrease the levels/effects of: BCG; Mycophenolate; Typhoid Vaccine

The levels/effects of Penicillin V Potassium may be decreased by: Fusidic Acid; Tetracycline Derivatives

Increased Effect/Toxicity

Penicillin V Potassium may increase the levels/effects of: Methotrexate; Vitamin K Antagonists

The levels/effects of Penicillin V Potassium may be increased by: Probenecid

Nutritional/Ethanol Interactions Food: Decreases drug absorption rate; decreases drug serum concentration. Management: Take on an empty stomach 1 hour before or 2 hours after meals around-the-clock to promote less variation in peak and trough serum levels.

Adverse Reactions >10%: Gastrointestinal: Mild diarrhea, vomiting, nausea, oral candidiasis

Available Dosage Forms

Powder for solution, oral: 125 mg/5 mL (100 mL, 200 mL); 250 mg/5 mL (100 mL, 200 mL)

Tablet, oral: 250 mg, 500 mg

General Dosage Range Dosage adjustment recommended in patients with renal impairment

Oral:

Children <12 years: 25-50 mg/kg/day divided every 6-8 hours (maximum: 3 g/day)

Children ≥12 years and Adults: 125-500 mg every 6-8 hours

Administration

Oral Administer around-the-clock to promote less variation in peak and trough serum levels. Take on an empty stomach 1 hour before or 2 hours after meals, to enhance absorption, take until gone, do not skip doses.

I.V. Detail pH: 6.0-8.5

Stability

Storage Refrigerate suspension after reconstitution; discard after 14 days.

Nursing Actions

Physical Assessment Results of culture and sensitivity tests and patient's allergy history should be assessed prior to starting therapy. Monitor for hypersensitivity reactions and opportunistic infection (fever, chills, unhealed sores, white plaques in mouth or vagina, purulent vaginal discharge, fatigue).

Patient Education Take at intervals around-the-clock, preferably on an empty stomach (1 hour before or 2 hours after a meal). Maintain adequate hydration unless instructed to restrict fluid intake. May cause nausea, vomiting, or diarrhea. Report signs of opportunistic infection (eg, fever, chills, diarrhea, unhealed sores, white plaques in mouth or vagina, purulent vaginal discharge) or signs of hypersensitivity reaction (rash, hives, itching, swelling of lips, tongue, mouth, or throat).

Dietary Considerations Take on an empty stomach 1 hour before or 2 hours after meals.

Pentamidine (pen TAM i deen)

Brand Names: U.S. Nebupent®; Pentam® 300

Index Terms Pentamidine Isethionate

Pharmacologic Category Antifungal Agent; Antiprotozoal

Pregnancy Risk Factor C

Lactation Excretion in breast milk unknown/not recommended

Use

I.M., I.V.: Treatment of pneumonia caused by *Pneumocystis jirovecii* pneumonia (PCP)

Inhalation: Prevention of PCP in high-risk, HIV-infected patients either with a history of PCP or with a CD4+ count ≤200/mm^3

Unlabeled Use Prevention of PCP in nonHIV-infected patients; treatment of African trypanosomiasis, cutaneous leishmaniasis, and amebic meningoencephalitis

Available Dosage Forms

Injection, powder for reconstitution:

Pentam® 300: 300 mg

Powder for solution, for nebulization:

Nebupent®: 300 mg

General Dosage Range Dosage adjustment recommended in patients with renal impairment

I.M.: *Children >4 months and Adults:* 4 mg/kg once daily for 14-21 days

I.V.:

Children >4 months and Adults: 4 mg/kg once daily for 14-21 days

Inhalation: *Children >16 years and Adults:* 300 mg/dose every 4 weeks

Administration

I.M. Administer deep I.M. Do not use NS as a diluent.

I.V. Do not use NS as an initial diluent. Infuse slowly over 60-120 minutes. Avoid extravasation; assess catheter position before and during infusion.

I.V. Detail pH: 5.4 (sterile water); 4.09-4.38 (D_5W)

Inhalation Deliver via Respirgard® II nebulizer until nebulizer is emptied (30-45 minutes). Administer at a flow rate of 5-7 L/minute from a 40-50 pound-per-square inch (PSI) oxygen or air source. A 40-50 PSI air compressor can be used alternatively, with a set flow rate at 5-7 L/minute or a set pressure of 22-25 PSI. Air compressors <20 PSI should not be used. Use appropriate precautions to minimize exposure to healthcare personnel; refer to individual institutional policy.

Nursing Actions

Physical Assessment I.V., I.M.: Patients should be lying down. Blood pressure, cardiac status, and respiratory function should be monitored closely during administration and several times thereafter until blood pressure is stable. Monitor for hypotension, rash, confusion, hallucinations, hypoglycemia, dyspnea, and cough. If self-administered, teach patient proper use of nebulizer.

Patient Education Inhalant drug must be prepared and used with a nebulizer exactly as directed and as often as prescribed. Frequent blood tests and blood pressure checks may be required while using this drug. PCP pneumonia may still occur despite use of this medication. Maintain adequate hydration unless instructed to restrict fluid intake. Avoid excessive alcohol (may exacerbate adverse effects). If you have diabetes, monitor glucose levels closely and frequently. May cause hypotension, metallic taste, nausea, vomiting, or anorexia. Report chest pain or irregular heartbeat; unusual confusion or hallucinations; rash; or unusual wheezing, coughing, or respiratory difficulty.

Pentazocine and Naloxone
(pen TAZ oh seen & nal OKS one)

Index Terms Naloxone Hydrochloride and Pentazocine; Pentazocine Hydrochloride and Naloxone Hydrochloride; Talwin NX

Pharmacologic Category Analgesic, Opioid; Analgesic, Opioid Partial Agonist

Medication Safety Issues

High alert medication:

The Institute for Safe Medication Practices (ISMP) includes this medication among its list of drug classes which have a heightened risk of causing significant patient harm when used in error.

Pregnancy Risk Factor C

Lactation Pentazocine enters breast milk/use caution

Use Relief of moderate-to-severe pain; indicated for oral use only

Controlled Substance C-IV

Available Dosage Forms

Tablet: Pentazocine 50 mg and naloxone 0.5 mg

General Dosage Range Dosage adjustment recommended in patients with renal impairment

Oral: *Children ≥12 years and Adults:* Based upon pentazocine: 50-100 mg every 3-4 hours (maximum: 600 mg/day)

Nursing Actions

Physical Assessment See individual agents.

Patient Education See individual agents.

Related Information

Naloxone *on page 808*

Pentosan Polysulfate Sodium

(PEN toe san pol i SUL fate SOW dee um)

Brand Names: U.S. Elmiron®

Index Terms PPS

Pharmacologic Category Analgesic, Urinary

Medication Safety Issues

Sound-alike/look-alike issues:

Pentosan may be confused with pentostatin

Elmiron® may be confused with Imuran®

Pregnancy Risk Factor B

Lactation Excretion in breast milk unknown/use caution

Use Relief of bladder pain or discomfort due to interstitial cystitis

Available Dosage Forms

Capsule, oral:

Elmiron®: 100 mg

General Dosage Range Oral: *Children ≥16 years and Adults:* 100 mg 3 times/day

Administration

Oral Should be administered with water 1 hour before or 2 hours after meals.

Pentoxifylline (pen toks IF i lin)

Brand Names: U.S. TRENtal®

Index Terms Oxpentifylline

Pharmacologic Category Blood Viscosity Reducer Agent

Medication Safety Issues

Sound-alike/look-alike issues:

Pentoxifylline may be confused with tamoxifen

TRENtal® may be confused with Bentyl®, TEGretol®, Trandate®

Pregnancy Risk Factor C

Lactation Enters breast milk/not recommended

Use Treatment of intermittent claudication on the basis of chronic occlusive arterial disease of the limbs; may improve function and symptoms, but not intended to replace more definitive therapy

Note: The American College of Chest Physicians discourages the use of pentoxifylline for the treatment of intermittent claudication refractory to exercise therapy (and smoking cessation) (Guyatt, 2012).

Unlabeled Use Severe alcoholic liver disease; venous leg ulcers (with compression therapy)

Available Dosage Forms

Tablet, controlled release, oral:

TRENtal®: 400 mg

Tablet, extended release, oral: 400 mg

General Dosage Range Dosage adjustment recommended in patients with renal impairment

Oral: *Adults:* 400 mg 2-3 times/day

Administration

Oral Tablets should be swallowed whole; do not chew, break, or crush. May be administered with food.

Nursing Actions

Physical Assessment Monitor ability to increase walking distance without discomfort.

Patient Education This may relieve pain of claudication, but additional therapy may be recommended. May cause dizziness, heartburn, nausea, or vomiting. Report chest pain; swelling of lips, mouth, or tongue; persistent headache; respiratory difficulty; rash; or unrelieved nausea or vomiting.

Perindopril Erbumine

(per IN doe pril er BYOO meen)

Brand Names: U.S. Aceon®

Pharmacologic Category Angiotensin-Converting Enzyme (ACE) Inhibitor

Pregnancy Risk Factor D

Lactation Excretion in breast milk unknown/use caution

Use Treatment of hypertension; reduction of cardiovascular mortality or nonfatal myocardial infarction in patients with stable coronary artery disease

Canadian labeling: Additional use (unlabeled use in U.S.): Treatment of mild-moderate (NYHA I-III) heart failure

Unlabeled Use To delay the progression of nephropathy and reduce risks of cardiovascular events in hypertensive patients with type 1 or 2 diabetes mellitus

Available Dosage Forms

Tablet, oral: 2 mg, 4 mg, 8 mg

Aceon®: 2 mg, 4 mg, 8 mg

General Dosage Range Dosage adjustment recommended in patients with renal impairment

Oral: *Adults:* Initial: 2-4 mg once daily; Maintenance: 4-8 mg/day in 1-2 divided doses (maximum: 16 mg/day)

Administration

Oral

Administer prior to a meal.

Nursing Actions

Physical Assessment Monitor first dose carefully (hypotension can occur, especially with first dose; angioedema can occur at any time during treatment, especially following first dose). Monitor BP (standing and sitting), cardiac status, and fluid balance at beginning of therapy, when adjusting dose, and periodically throughout.

Patient Education Take first dose at bedtime. Do not take potassium supplements or salt substitutes containing potassium without consulting prescriber. This drug does not eliminate need for diet or exercise regimen as recommended by prescriber. May cause increased cough (if persistent or bothersome, contact prescriber), headache, postural hypotension, dizziness, nausea, vomiting, or diarrhea. Report chest pain, respiratory difficulty or persistent cough, painful muscles or joints, rash, or ringing in ears.

Perphenazine (per FEN a zeen)

Index Terms Trilafon
Pharmacologic Category Antiemetic; Antipsychotic Agent, Typical, Phenothiazine
Medication Safety Issues
Sound-alike/look-alike issues:
Trilafon may be confused with Tri-Levlen®
Use Treatment of schizophrenia; severe nausea and vomiting
Unlabeled Use Psychosis; psychosis/agitation related to Alzheimer's dementia (risks vs benefits)
Available Dosage Forms
Tablet, oral: 2 mg, 4 mg, 8 mg, 16 mg
General Dosage Range Oral: *Adults:* 4-16 mg 2-4 times/day (maximum: 64 mg/day)
Administration
Oral May be administered without regard to meals.
Nursing Actions
Physical Assessment Monitor blood pressure and therapeutic response (mental status, mood, affect) at beginning of therapy and periodically throughout. Monitor for orthostatic hypotension, anticholinergic response, extrapyramidal symptoms, and pigmentary retinopathy.
Patient Education It may take 2-3 weeks to achieve desired results. Avoid alcohol. Maintain adequate hydration unless instructed to restrict fluid intake. You may experience excess drowsiness, restlessness, dizziness, blurred vision, dry mouth, nausea, vomiting, constipation, postural hypotension, urinary retention, photosensitivity, or decreased perspiration. Report persistent CNS effects (eg, trembling fingers, altered gait or balance, excessive sedation, seizures, unusual movements, anxiety, confusion); chest pain, palpitations, or rapid heartbeat; severe dizziness; unresolved urinary retention; change in libido or ejaculatory difficulty; vision changes; skin rash or yellowing of skin; respiratory difficulty; or worsening of condition.

Phenazopyridine (fen az oh PEER i deen)

Brand Names: U.S. AZO Standard® Maximum Strength [OTC]; AZO Standard® [OTC]; Azo-Gesic™ [OTC]; Baridium [OTC]; Pyridium®; ReAzo [OTC]; UTI Relief® [OTC]
Index Terms Phenazopyridine Hydrochloride; Phenylazo Diamino Pyridine Hydrochloride
Pharmacologic Category Analgesic, Urinary
Medication Safety Issues
Sound-alike/look-alike issues:
Phenazopyridine may be confused with phenoxybenzamine
Pyridium® may be confused with Dyrenium®, Perdiem®, pyridoxine, pyrithione
Pregnancy Risk Factor B
Lactation Excretion in breast milk unknown/not recommended
Use Symptomatic relief of urinary burning, itching, frequency, and urgency in association with urinary tract infection or following urologic procedures
Available Dosage Forms
Tablet, oral: 100 mg, 200 mg
AZO Standard® [OTC]: 95 mg
AZO Standard® Maximum Strength [OTC]: 97.5 mg
Azo-Gesic™ [OTC]: 95 mg
Baridium [OTC]: 97.2 mg
Pyridium®: 100 mg, 200 mg
ReAzo [OTC]: 95 mg
UTI Relief® [OTC]: 97.2 mg
General Dosage Range Dosage adjustment recommended in patients with renal impairment
Oral:
Children: 12 mg/kg/day in 3 divided doses
Adults: 100-200 mg 3 times/day
Administration
Oral Administer after meals.
Nursing Actions
Physical Assessment Instruct patients with diabetes to use serum glucose monitoring (phenazopyridine may interfere with certain urine testing reagents).
Patient Education May discolor urine (orange/yellow); this is normal, but will also stain fabric. If you have diabetes, use serum glucose tests; this medication may interfere with accuracy of urine testing. Report persistent headache, dizziness, or stomach cramping.

Phenelzine (FEN el zeen)

Brand Names: U.S. Nardil®
Index Terms Phenelzine Sulfate
Pharmacologic Category Antidepressant, Monoamine Oxidase Inhibitor
Medication Safety Issues
Sound-alike/look-alike issues:
Phenelzine may be confused with phenytoin
Nardil® may be confused with Norinyl®
Medication Guide Available Yes
Pregnancy Risk Factor C
Lactation Excretion in breast milk unknown/not recommended
Use Symptomatic treatment of atypical, nonendogenous, or neurotic depression
Available Dosage Forms
Tablet, oral: 15 mg
Nardil®: 15 mg
General Dosage Range Oral: *Adults:* Initial: 45 mg/day in 3 divided doses; Maintenance: 15-90 mg/day in 1-3 divided doses

Nursing Actions

Physical Assessment Monitor blood pressure, mental status, mood, affect, and suicide ideation. Observe for clinical worsening, suicidality, and unusual behavior changes, especially during the initial few months of therapy or during dosage changes. Patients with diabetes should monitor serum glucose closely (phenelzine may lower glucose level). Instruct patient to follow a tyramine-free diet.

Patient Education It may take 2-3 weeks to achieve desired results. Avoid alcohol. Avoid tyramine-containing foods. Maintain adequate hydration unless instructed to restrict fluid intake. You may experience postural hypotension, drowsiness, lightheadedness, dizziness, anorexia, dry mouth, constipation, or diarrhea. If you have diabetes, monitor serum glucose closely (Nardil® may effect glucose levels). Report persistent insomnia; chest pain, palpitations, irregular or rapid heartbeat, or swelling of extremities; muscle cramping, tremors, or altered gait; blurred vision or eye pain; yellowing of eyes or skin; pale stools/dark urine; suicide ideation; or worsening of condition.

PHENobarbital (fee noe BAR bi tal)

Index Terms Luminal Sodium; Phenobarbital Sodium; Phenobarbitone; Phenylethylmalonylurea

Pharmacologic Category Anticonvulsant, Barbiturate; Barbiturate

Medication Safety Issues

Sound-alike/look-alike issues:

PHENobarbital may be confused with PENTobarbital, Phenergan®, phenytoin

Pregnancy Risk Factor B/D (manufacturer dependent)

Lactation Enters breast milk/use caution (AAP recommends use "with caution"; AAP 2001 update pending)

Use Management of generalized tonic-clonic (grand mal), status epilepticus, and partial seizures; sedative/hypnotic

Note: Use to treat insomnia is not recommended (Schutte-Rodin, 2008)

Unlabeled Use Prevention and treatment of neonatal hyperbilirubinemia and lowering of bilirubin in chronic cholestasis; neonatal seizures

Controlled Substance C-IV

Available Dosage Forms

Elixir, oral: 20 mg/5 mL (5 mL, 7.5 mL, 15 mL, 473 mL)

Injection, solution: 65 mg/mL (1 mL); 130 mg/mL (1 mL)

Tablet, oral: 15 mg, 30 mg, 60 mg, 100 mg

General Dosage Range Dosage adjustment recommended in patients with renal impairment

I.M.:

Children: 3-5 mg/kg at bedtime or 1-3 mg/kg 1-1.5 hours before procedure

Adults: Dosage varies greatly depending on indication

I.V.:

Infants: Loading dose: 10-20 mg/kg in a single or divided dose; Maintenance: 5-8 mg/kg/day in 1-2 divided doses

Children: Loading dose: 15-20 mg/kg in a single or divided dose; Maintenance: Dosage varies greatly depending on indication

Adults: Loading dose: 10-20 mg/kg; may repeat dose in 20-minute intervals as needed (maximum total dose: 30 mg/kg); Maintenance: Dosage varies greatly depending on indication

Oral:

Infants: 5-8 mg/kg/day in 1-2 divided doses

Children and Adults: Dosage varies greatly depending on indication

Administration

I.M. Inject deep into muscle. Do not exceed 5 mL per injection site due to potential for tissue irritation.

I.V. Avoid rapid I.V. administration >60 mg/minute in adults and >30 mg/minute in children. Avoid extravasation. Intra-arterial injection is contraindicated. Avoid subcutaneous administration.

I.V. Detail Parenteral solutions are highly alkaline.

pH: 9.2-10.2

Nursing Actions

Physical Assessment Assess for history of addiction or suicide ideation; long-term use can result in dependence, abuse, or tolerance. **I.V.:** Keep patient under observation (vital signs, neurologic, cardiac, and respiratory status); use safety precautions.

Patient Education I.V.: Patient instructions and information are determined by patient condition and therapeutic purpose. Oral: Drug may cause physical and/or psychological dependence. While using this medication, do not use alcohol and other prescription or OTC medications (especially pain medications, sedatives, antihistamines, or hypnotics) without consulting prescriber. Maintain adequate hydration unless instructed to restrict fluid intake. You may experience drowsiness, dizziness, blurred vision, nausea, vomiting, loss of appetite, or constipation. Report skin rash or irritation, CNS changes (confusion, depression, increased sedation, suicide ideation, excitation, headache, insomnia, or nightmares), respiratory difficulty or shortness of breath, changes in urinary pattern or menstrual pattern, muscle weakness or tremors, or difficulty swallowing or feeling of tightness in throat.

Related Information

Peak and Trough Guidelines *on page 1276*

Phentolamine (fen TOLE a meen)

Brand Names: U.S. OraVerse™

Index Terms Phentolamine Mesylate; Regitine [DSC]

Pharmacologic Category Alpha$_1$ Blocker

Medication Safety Issues

Sound-alike/look-alike issues:

Phentolamine may be confused with phentermine, Ventolin®

Pregnancy Risk Factor C

Lactation Excretion in breast milk unknown/use caution

Use Diagnosis of pheochromocytoma and treatment of hypertension associated with pheochromocytoma or other forms of hypertension caused by excess sympathomimetic amines; treatment of dermal necrosis after extravasation of drugs with alpha-adrenergic effects (ie, dopamine, epinephrine, norepinephrine, phenylephrine)

OraVerse™: Reversal of soft tissue anesthesia and the associated functional deficits resulting from a local dental anesthetic containing a vasoconstrictor

Unlabeled Use Treatment of pralidoxime-induced hypertension

Available Dosage Forms

Injection, powder for reconstitution: 5 mg

Injection, solution [preservative free]:

OraVerse™: 0.4 mg/1.7 mL (1.7 mL)

General Dosage Range

I.M., I.V.:

Children: 0.05-0.1 mg/kg/dose as a single dose 1-2 hours before procedure, repeat as needed every 2-4 hours (maximum: 5 mg/dose)

Adults: 5 mg as a single dose 1-2 hours before procedure, may repeat as needed every 2-4 hours **or** 5-20 mg (hypertensive crisis)

Submucosal injection:

Children 15-30 kg and <12 years: 0.2 mg (maximum)

Children >30 kg and <12 years: 0.4 mg (maximum)

Children >30 kg and ≥12 years and Adults: 0.2 mg to 0.8 mg (depending on number of cartridges of anesthesia)

SubQ: *Children and Adults:* Infiltrate area with a small amount (eg, 1 mL) of solution (made by diluting 5-10 mg in 10 mL of NS) within 12 hours of extravasation; in general, do not exceed 0.1-0.2 mg/kg (5 mg total); typically doses of ≤5 mg are effective

Administration

I.V.

Vasoconstrictor (alpha-adrenergic agonist) extravasation: Infiltrate the area of extravasation with multiple small injections using only 27- or 30-gauge needles and changing the needle between each skin entry. Be careful not to cause so much swelling of the extremity or digit that a compartment syndrome occurs. If infiltration is severe, may also need to consult vascular surgeon.

Pheochromocytoma: Inject each 5 mg over 1 minute.

I.V. Detail pH: 4.5-6.5

Nursing Actions

Physical Assessment When used to prevent tissue necrosis after extravasation, monitor effectiveness of treatment closely.

Patient Education This medication can only be administered by infusion or by subQ injection. Assist patient with ambulation if used to manage pheochromocytoma. Report immediately any pain at infusion/injection site. May cause orthostatic hypotension. Report dizziness, rapid heartbeat, feelings of weakness, or nausea/vomiting.

Phenylephrine (Systemic) (fen il EF rin)

Brand Names: U.S. LuSonal™ [DSC]; Medi-First® Sinus Decongestant [OTC]; Medi-Phenyl [OTC]; PediaCare® Children's Decongestant [OTC]; Sudafed PE® Children's [OTC]; Sudafed PE® Congestion [OTC]; Sudafed PE™ Nasal Decongestant [OTC]; Sudogest™ PE [OTC]; Triaminic Thin Strips® Children's Cold with Stuffy Nose [OTC]

Index Terms Phenylephrine Hydrochloride

Pharmacologic Category Alpha-Adrenergic Agonist

Medication Safety Issues

Sound-alike/look-alike issues:

Sudafed PE® may be confused with Sudafed®

High alert medication:

The Institute for Safe Medication Practices (ISMP) includes this medication among its list of drugs which have a heightened risk of causing significant patient harm when used in error.

Pregnancy Risk Factor C

Lactation Excretion in breast milk unknown/use caution

Breast-Feeding Considerations It is not known if phenylephrine is excreted into breast milk. The manufacturer recommends that caution be exercised when administering phenylephrine to nursing women.

Use Treatment of hypotension, vascular failure in shock; as a vasoconstrictor in regional analgesia; supraventricular tachycardia (**Note:** Not for routine use in treatment of supraventricular tachycardias); as a decongestant [OTC]

Mechanism of Action/Effect Potent, direct-acting alpha-adrenergic agonist with virtually no beta-adrenergic activity; produces systemic arterial vasoconstriction

Contraindications Hypersensitivity to phenylephrine or any component of the formulation

Injection: Severe hypertension; ventricular tachycardia

Oral: Use with or within 14 days of MAO inhibitor therapy

Warnings/Precautions Some products contain sulfites which may cause allergic reactions in susceptible individuals. Use with extreme caution in patients taking MAO inhibitors.

Intravenous: Use with caution in the elderly, patients with hyperthyroidism, bradycardia, partial heart block, myocardial disease, or severe CAD. Avoid or use with extreme caution in patients with heart failure or cardiogenic shock; increased systemic vascular resistance may significantly reduce cardiac output. Assure adequate circulatory volume to minimize need for vasoconstrictors. Avoid use in patients with hypertension (contraindicated in severe hypertension); monitor blood pressure closely and adjust infusion rate. Avoid extravasation; infuse into a large vein if possible. Avoid infusion into leg veins. Watch I.V. site closely. If extravasation occurs, infiltrate the area subcutaneously with diluted phentolamine (5-10 mg in 10 mL of saline) with a fine hypodermic needle. **Phentolamine should be administered as soon as possible after extravasation is noted. [U.S. Boxed Warning]: Should be administered by adequately trained individuals familiar with its use.**

Oral: When used for self-medication (OTC), use caution with asthma, bowel obstruction/narrowing, hyperthyroidism, diabetes mellitus, cardiovascular disease, ischemic heart disease, hypertension, increased intraocular pressure, prostatic hyperplasia or in the elderly. Notify healthcare provider if symptoms do not improve within 7 days or are accompanied by fever. Discontinue and contact healthcare provider if nervousness, dizziness, or sleeplessness occur.

Drug Interactions

Avoid Concomitant Use

Avoid concomitant use of Phenylephrine (Systemic) with any of the following: Ergot Derivatives; Iobenguane I 123; MAO Inhibitors

Decreased Effect

Phenylephrine (Systemic) may decrease the levels/effects of: Benzylpenicilloyl Polylysine; FentaNYL; Iobenguane I 123

Increased Effect/Toxicity

Phenylephrine (Systemic) may increase the levels/effects of: Sympathomimetics

The levels/effects of Phenylephrine (Systemic) may be increased by: Atomoxetine; Cannabinoids; Ergot Derivatives; MAO Inhibitors; Tricyclic Antidepressants

Nutritional/Ethanol Interactions Herb/Nutraceutical: Avoid ephedra, yohimbe (may cause CNS stimulation).

Adverse Reactions Frequency not defined.

Injection:

Cardiovascular: Arrhythmia (rare), decreased cardiac output, hypertension, pallor, precordial pain or discomfort, reflex bradycardia, severe peripheral and visceral vasoconstriction

Central nervous system: Anxiety, dizziness, excitability, giddiness, headache, insomnia, nervousness, restlessness

Endocrine & metabolic: Metabolic acidosis

Gastrointestinal: Gastric irritation, nausea

Local: I.V.: Extravasation which may lead to necrosis and sloughing of surrounding tissue, blanching of skin

Neuromuscular & skeletal: Paresthesia, pilomotor response, tremor, weakness

Renal: Decreased renal perfusion, reduced urine output

Respiratory: Respiratory distress

Miscellaneous: Hypersensitivity reactions (including rash, urticaria, leukopenia, agranulocytosis, thrombocytopenia)

Oral: Central nervous system: Anxiety, dizziness, excitability, giddiness, headache, insomnia, nervousness, restlessness

Pharmacodynamics/Kinetics

Onset of Action

Blood pressure increase/vasoconstriction: I.M., SubQ: 10-15 minutes; I.V.: Immediate

Nasal decongestant: Oral: 15-30 minutes (Kollar, 2007)

Duration of Action

Blood pressure increase/vasoconstriction: I.M.: 1-2 hours; I.V.: ~15-20 minutes; SubQ: 50 minutes

Nasal decongestant: Oral: ≤4 hours (Kollar, 2007)

Available Dosage Forms

Injection, solution: 1% [10 mg/mL] (1 mL, 2 mL, 5 mL, 10 mL)

Liquid, oral:

PediaCare® Children's Decongestant [OTC]: 2.5 mg/5 mL (118 mL)

Sudafed PE® Children's [OTC]: 2.5 mg/5 mL (118 mL)

Strip, orally disintegrating, oral:

Triaminic Thin Strips® Children's Cold with Stuffy Nose [OTC]: 2.5 mg (14s)

Tablet, oral: 10 mg

Medi-First® Sinus Decongestant [OTC]: 10 mg

Medi-Phenyl [OTC]: 5 mg

Sudafed PE® Congestion [OTC]: 10 mg

Sudafed PE™ Nasal Decongestant [OTC]: 10 mg

Sudogest™ PE [OTC]: 10 mg

General Dosage Range

I.V.:

Children: Bolus: 5-20 mcg/kg/dose every 10-15 minutes as needed; Infusion: 0.1-0.5 mcg/kg/minute

Adults: Bolus: 100-500 mcg/dose every 10-15 minutes as needed (maximum: 500 mcg); Infusion: Initial: 100-180 mcg/minute

Oral:

Children 4 to <6 years: 2.5 mg every 4 hours as needed (maximum: 15 mg/24 hours)

Children 6 to <12 years: 5 mg every 4 hours as needed (maximum: 30 mg/24 hours)

Children ≥12 years and Adults: 10 mg every 4 hours as needed (maximum: 60 mg/24 hours)

Administration

I.V. Detail May cause necrosis or sloughing tissue if extravasation occurs during I.V. administration or SubQ administration.

Extravasation management: Use phentolamine as antidote; mix 5-10 mg with 10 mL of NS. Inject a small amount of this dilution subcutaneously into extravasated area. Blanching should reverse immediately. Monitor site. If blanching should recur, additional injections of phentolamine may be needed.

pH: 3.0-6.5

Stability

Reconstitution Solution for injection:

I.V. infusion: Usual concentration: 10 mg in 500 mL NS or D_5W. May also dilute 50 mg in 500 mL NS or 100 mg in 500 mL NS; both concentrations are stable for at least 14 days at room temperature of 25°C (77°F) (Gupta, 2004). Dilution of 1250 mg in 500 mL NS retained potency for at least 24 hours at 22°C (Weber, 1970).

I.V. injection: May dilute with SWFI to a concentration of 1 mg/mL.

Stability in syringes (Kiser, 2007): Concentration of 0.1 mg/mL in NS (polypropylene syringes) is stable for at least 30 days at -20°C (-4°F), 3°C to 5°C (37°F to 41°F), or 23°C to 25°C (73.4°F to 77°F).

Storage

Solution for injection: Store vials at controlled room temperature of 15°C to 25°C (59°F to 77°F). Protect from light. Do not use solution if brown or contains a precipitate.

Oral: Store at controlled room temperature of 15°C to 25°C (59°F to 77°F). Protect from light.

Nursing Actions

Physical Assessment Parenteral: Monitor arterial blood gases, vital signs, and adverse reactions; monitor infusion site frequently for patency. If extravasation should occur, implement extravasation management immediately; can cause tissue sloughing.

Patient Education Oral: You may experience headache, trouble sleeping, nervousness, or dizziness.

Dietary Considerations Some products may contain phenylalanine and/or sodium.

Related Information

Management of Drug Extravasations *on page 1269*

Phenylephrine (Nasal) (fen il EF rin)

Brand Names: U.S. 4 Way® Fast Acting [OTC]; 4 Way® Menthol [OTC]; Little Noses® Decongestant [OTC]; Neo-Synephrine® Extra Strength [OTC]; Neo-Synephrine® Mild Formula [OTC]; Neo-Synephrine® Regular Strength [OTC]; Rhinall® [OTC]; Vicks® Sinex® VapoSpray™ 4 Hour Decongestant [OTC]

Index Terms Phenylephrine Hydrochloride

Pharmacologic Category Alpha-Adrenergic Agonist; Decongestant

Medication Safety Issues

Sound-alike/look-alike issues:

Neo-Synephrine® (phenylephrine, nasal) may be confused with Neo-Synephrine® (oxymetazoline)

Use For OTC use as symptomatic relief of nasal and nasopharyngeal mucosal congestion

Available Dosage Forms

Solution, intranasal:

4 Way® Fast Acting [OTC]: 1% (15 mL, 30 mL, 37 mL)

4 Way® Menthol [OTC]: 1% (15 mL, 30 mL)

Little Noses® Decongestant [OTC]: 0.125% (15 mL)

Neo-Synephrine® Extra Strength [OTC]: 1% (15 mL)

Neo-Synephrine® Mild Formula [OTC]: 0.25% (15 mL)

Neo-Synephrine® Regular Strength [OTC]: 0.5% (15 mL)

Rhinall® [OTC]: 0.25% (30 mL, 40 mL)

Vicks® Sinex® VapoSpray™ 4 Hour Decongestant [OTC]: 0.5% (15 mL)

General Dosage Range Intranasal:

Children 2-6 years: 0.125% solution: Instill 1 drop in each nostril every 2-4 hours as needed for ≤3 days

Children 6-12 years: 0.25% solution: Instill 2-3 sprays in each nostril every 4 hours as needed for ≤3 days

Children >12 years: 0.25% to 0.5% solution: Instill 2-3 sprays or 2-3 drops in each nostril every 4 hours as needed for ≤3 days

Adults: 0.25% to 1% solution: Instill 2-3 sprays or 2-3 drops in each nostril every 4 hours as needed for ≤3 days

Nursing Actions

Physical Assessment Ensure patient is not using chronically; may cause rebound congestion when discontinued.

Patient Education Do not use for more than 3 days in a row. Blow nose before use. Tilt head back and instill recommended dose of drops or spray. Do not blow nose for 5-10 minutes. You may experience transient stinging or burning. You may experience headache, trouble sleeping, nervousness, or dizziness.

Phenylephrine (Ophthalmic) (fen il EF rin)

Brand Names: U.S. AK-Dilate™; Altafrin; Mydfrin®; Neofrin; OcuNefrin™ [OTC] [DSC]

Index Terms Phenylephrine Hydrochloride

Pharmacologic Category Alpha-Adrenergic Agonist; Ophthalmic Agent, Antiglaucoma; Ophthalmic Agent, Mydriatic

Medication Safety Issues

Sound-alike/look-alike issues:

Mydfrin® may be confused with Midrin®

Pregnancy Risk Factor C

Lactation Excretion in breast milk unknown/use caution

Use Used as a mydriatic in ophthalmic procedures and treatment of wide-angle glaucoma; OTC use as symptomatic relief of redness of the eye due to irritation

Available Dosage Forms

Solution, ophthalmic: 2.5% (2 mL, 3 mL, 5 mL, 15 mL)

AK-Dilate™: 2.5% (2 mL, 15 mL); 10% (5 mL)

Altafrin: 2.5% (15 mL); 10% (5 mL)

Mydfrin®: 2.5% (3 mL, 5 mL)

Neofrin: 2.5% (15 mL); 10% (5 mL)

General Dosage Range Ophthalmic:

Infants <1 year: Instill 1 drop of 2.5% solution 15-30 minutes before procedures

Children ≥1 year and Adults: Instill 1 drop of 2.5% or 10% solution; may repeat in 10-60 minutes as needed **or** 1-2 drops of 0.12% solution up to 4 times/day [OTC dosing] (maximum: 72 hours)

Nursing Actions

Physical Assessment Systemic absorption from ophthalmic instillation is minimal, so there are no specific monitoring recommendations to identify adverse events.

Patient Education Do not let tip of applicator touch eye; do not contaminate tip of applicator (may cause eye infection, eye damage, or vision loss). Open eye, look at ceiling, and instill prescribed amount of solution. Close eye and roll eye in all directions, and apply gentle pressure to inner corner of eye for 1-2 minutes after instillation. Temporary stinging or blurred vision may occur. Report persistent pain, burning, double vision, or if condition worsens.

Phenytoin (FEN i toyn)

Brand Names: U.S. Dilantin-125®; Dilantin®; Phenytek®

Index Terms Diphenylhydantoin; DPH; Phenytoin Sodium; Phenytoin Sodium, Extended; Phenytoin Sodium, Prompt

Pharmacologic Category Anticonvulsant, Hydantoin

Medication Safety Issues

Sound-alike/look-alike issues:

Phenytoin may be confused with phenelzine, phentermine, PHENobarbital

Dilantin® may be confused with Dilaudid®, diltiazem, Dipentum®

High alert medication:

The Institute for Safe Medication Practices (ISMP) includes this medication (I.V. formulation) among its list of drug classes which have a heightened risk of causing significant patient harm when used in error.

International issues:

Dilantin [U.S., Canada, and multiple international markets] may be confused with Dolantine brand name for pethidine [Belgium]

Medication Guide Available Yes

Pregnancy Risk Factor D

Lactation Enters breast milk/not recommended (AAP rates "compatible"; AAP 2001 update pending)

Breast-Feeding Considerations Phenytoin is excreted in breast milk; however, the amount to which the infant is exposed is considered small. The manufacturers of phenytoin do not recommend breast-feeding during therapy. Women should be counseled of the possible risks and benefits associated with breast-feeding while on phenytoin.

Use Management of generalized tonic-clonic (grand mal), complex partial seizures; prevention of seizures following head trauma/neurosurgery

Mechanism of Action/Effect Stabilizes neuronal membranes and decreases seizure activity by increasing efflux or decreasing influx of sodium ions across cell membranes in the motor cortex during generation of nerve impulses; prolongs effective refractory period and suppresses ventricular pacemaker automaticity, shortens action potential in the heart

Contraindications Hypersensitivity to phenytoin, other hydantoins, or any component of the formulation; pregnancy

Warnings/Precautions Antiepileptics are associated with an increased risk of suicidal behavior/thoughts with use (regardless of indication); patients should be monitored for signs/symptoms of depression, suicidal tendencies, and other unusual behavior changes during therapy and instructed to inform their healthcare provider immediately if symptoms occur.

[U.S. Boxed Warning]: Phenytoin must be administered slowly. Intravenous administration should not exceed 50 mg/minute in adult patients. In neonates, intravenous administration rate should not exceed 1-3 mg/kg/minute (most clinicians use a lower maximum rate of infusion in neonates of 0.5-1 mg/kg/minute). Hypotension may occur with rapid administration. I.V. form may cause skin necrosis at I.V. site; avoid I.V.

administration in small veins; may increase frequency of petit mal seizures; use with caution in patients with porphyria; discontinue if rash or lymphadenopathy occurs; a spectrum of hematologic effects have been reported with use (eg, neutropenia, leukopenia, thrombocytopenia, pancytopenia, and anemias); use with caution in patients with hepatic dysfunction, sinus bradycardia, S-A block, or AV block; use with caution in elderly or debilitated patients, or in any condition associated with low serum albumin levels, which will increase the free fraction of phenytoin in the serum and, therefore, the pharmacologic response. Sedation, confusional states, or cerebellar dysfunction (loss of motor coordination) may occur at higher total serum concentrations, or at lower total serum concentrations when the free fraction of phenytoin is increased. Effects with other sedative drugs or ethanol may be potentiated. Abrupt withdrawal may precipitate status epilepticus. Severe reactions, including toxic epidermal necrolysis and Stevens-Johnson syndromes, although rarely reported, have resulted in fatalities; drug should be discontinued if there are any signs of rash. Patients of Asian descent with the variant *HLA-B*1502* may be at an increased risk of developing Stevens-Johnson syndrome and/or toxic epidermal necrolysis.

Drug Interactions

Avoid Concomitant Use

Avoid concomitant use of Phenytoin with any of the following: Axitinib; Boceprevir; Bortezomib; Crizotinib; Darunavir; Delavirdine; Dronedarone; Etravirine; Everolimus; Lapatinib; Lurasidone; Nilotinib; Pazopanib; Praziquantel; Ranolazine; Rilpivirine; Rivaroxaban; Roflumilast; RomiDEPsin; SORAfenib; Telaprevir; Ticagrelor; Tolvaptan; Toremifene; Vandetanib

Decreased Effect

Phenytoin may decrease the levels/effects of: Acetaminophen; Amiodarone; Antifungal Agents (Azole Derivatives, Systemic); ARIPiprazole; Axitinib; Boceprevir; Bortezomib; Brentuximab Vedotin; Busulfan; CarBAMazepine; Caspofungin; Chloramphenicol; Clarithromycin; CloZAPine; Contraceptives (Estrogens); Contraceptives (Progestins); Crizotinib; CycloSPORINE; CycloSPORINE (Systemic); CYP2B6 Substrates; CYP2C19 Substrates; CYP2C8 Substrates; CYP2C9 Substrates; CYP3A4 Substrates; Darunavir; Dasatinib; Deferasirox; Delavirdine; Diclofenac; Disopyramide; Divalproex; Doxycycline; Dronedarone; Efavirenz; Ethosuximide; Etoposide; Etoposide Phosphate; Etravirine; Everolimus; Exemestane; Felbamate; Flunarizine; Gefitinib; GuanFACINE; HMG-CoA Reductase Inhibitors; Imatinib; Irinotecan; Ixabepilone; Lacosamide; LamoTRIgine; Lapatinib; Levodopa; Linagliptin; Loop Diuretics; Lopinavir; Lurasidone; Maraviroc; Mebendazole; Meperidine; Methadone; MethylPREDNISolone; MetroNIDAZOLE; MetroNIDAZOLE (Systemic); Metyrapone; Mexiletine; Nilotinib; OXcarbazepine; Pazopanib; Praziquantel; PrednisoLONE; PrednisoLONE (Systemic); PredniSONE; Primidone; QUEtiapine; QuiNIDine; QuiNINE; Ranolazine; Rilpivirine; Ritonavir; Rivaroxaban; Roflumilast; RomiDEPsin; Rufinamide; Saxagliptin; Sertraline; Sirolimus; SORAfenib; SUNItinib; Tacrolimus; Tacrolimus (Systemic); Tadalafil; Telaprevir; Temsirolimus; Teniposide; Theophylline Derivatives; Thyroid Products; Ticagrelor; Tipranavir; Tolvaptan; Topiramate; Toremifene; TraZODone; Treprostinil; Ulipristal; Valproic Acid; Vandetanib; Vecuronium; Vemurafenib; Zonisamide; Zuclopenthixol

The levels/effects of Phenytoin may be decreased by: Alcohol (Ethyl); Amphetamines; Antacids; Barbiturates; CarBAMazepine; Ciprofloxacin; Ciprofloxacin (Systemic); CISplatin; Colesevelam; CYP2C19 Inducers (Strong); CYP2C9 Inducers (Strong); Diazoxide; Divalproex; Folic Acid; Fosamprenavir; Ketorolac; Ketorolac (Nasal); Ketorolac (Systemic); Leucovorin Calcium-Levoleucovorin; Levomefolate; Lopinavir; Mefloquine; Methylfolate; Nelfinavir; Peginterferon Alfa-2b; Pyridoxine; Rifamycin Derivatives; Ritonavir; Telaprevir; Theophylline Derivatives; Tipranavir; Tocilizumab; Valproic Acid; Vigabatrin

Increased Effect/Toxicity

Phenytoin may increase the levels/effects of: Barbiturates; Clarithromycin; CNS Depressants; Fosamprenavir; Lithium; Methotrimeprazine; Prilocaine; Selective Serotonin Reuptake Inhibitors; Vecuronium; Vitamin K Antagonists

The levels/effects of Phenytoin may be increased by: Alcohol (Ethyl); Allopurinol; Amiodarone; Antifungal Agents (Azole Derivatives, Systemic); Benzodiazepines; Calcium Channel Blockers; Capecitabine; CarBAMazepine; Carbonic Anhydrase Inhibitors; CeFAZolin; Chloramphenicol; Cimetidine; Clarithromycin; Conivaptan; CYP2C19 Inhibitors (Moderate); CYP2C19 Inhibitors (Strong); CYP2C9 Inhibitors (Moderate); CYP2C9 Inhibitors (Strong); Delavirdine; Dexmethylphenidate; Disulfiram; Droperidol; Efavirenz; Ethosuximide; Felbamate; Floxuridine; Fluconazole; Fluorouracil; Fluorouracil (Systemic); Fluorouracil (Topical); FLUoxetine; FluvoxaMINE; Halothane; HydrOXYzine; Isoniazid; Methotrimeprazine; Methylphenidate; MetroNIDAZOLE; MetroNIDAZOLE (Systemic); OXcarbazepine; Proton Pump Inhibitors; Rufinamide; Sertraline; Sulfonamide Derivatives; Tacrolimus; Tacrolimus (Systemic); Telaprevir; Ticlopidine; Topiramate; TraZODone; Trimethoprim; Vitamin K Antagonists

Nutritional/Ethanol Interactions

Ethanol:

Acute use: Ethanol inhibits metabolism of phenytoin and may also increase CNS depression.

Management: Avoid or limit ethanol. Caution patients about effects.

Chronic use: Ethanol stimulates metabolism of phenytoin. Management: Avoid or limit ethanol.

Food: Phenytoin serum concentrations may be altered if taken with food. If taken with enteral nutrition, phenytoin serum concentrations may be decreased. Tube feedings decrease bioavailability. Phenytoin may decrease calcium, folic acid, and vitamin D levels. Supplementing folic acid may lower the seizure threshold. Management: Hold tube feedings 1-2 hours before and 1-2 hours after phenytoin administration. Do not supplement folic acid. Consider vitamin D supplementation. Take preferably on an empty stomach.

Herb/Nutraceutical: Evening primrose may decrease the seizure threshold; other herbal medications may increase CNS depression. Management: Avoid evening primrose, valerian, St John's wort, kava kava, and gotu kola.

Adverse Reactions I.V. effects: Hypotension, bradycardia, cardiac arrhythmia, cardiovascular collapse (especially with rapid I.V. use), venous irritation and pain, thrombophlebitis

Effects not related to plasma phenytoin concentrations: Hypertrichosis, gingival hypertrophy, thickening of facial features, carbohydrate intolerance, folic acid deficiency, peripheral neuropathy, vitamin D deficiency, osteomalacia, systemic lupus erythematosus

Concentration-related effects: Nystagmus, blurred vision, diplopia, ataxia, slurred speech, dizziness, drowsiness, lethargy, coma, rash, fever, nausea, vomiting, gum tenderness, confusion, mood changes, folic acid depletion, osteomalacia, hyperglycemia

Related to elevated concentrations:

>20 mcg/mL: Far lateral nystagmus

>30 mcg/mL: 45° lateral gaze nystagmus and ataxia

>40 mcg/mL: Decreased mentation

>100 mcg/mL: Death

Cardiovascular: Hypotension, bradycardia, cardiac arrhythmia, cardiovascular collapse

Central nervous system: Psychiatric changes, slurred speech, dizziness, drowsiness, headache, insomnia

Dermatologic: Rash

Gastrointestinal: Constipation, nausea, vomiting, gingival hyperplasia, enlargement of lips

Hematologic: Leukopenia, thrombocytopenia, agranulocytosis

Hepatic: Hepatitis

Local: Thrombophlebitis

Neuromuscular & skeletal: Tremor, peripheral neuropathy, paresthesia

Ocular: Diplopia, nystagmus, blurred vision

Rarely seen effects: Blood dyscrasias, coarsening of facial features, dyskinesias, hepatitis, hypertrichosis, lymphadenopathy, lymphoma, pseudolymphoma, SLE-like syndrome, Stevens-Johnson syndrome, toxic epidermal necrolysis, venous irritation and pain

Pharmacodynamics/Kinetics

Onset of Action I.V.: ~0.5-1 hour

Available Dosage Forms

Capsule, extended release, oral: 100 mg, 200 mg, 300 mg

Dilantin®: 30 mg, 100 mg

Phenytek®: 200 mg, 300 mg

Injection, solution: 50 mg/mL (2 mL, 5 mL)

Suspension, oral: 100 mg/4 mL (4 mL); 125 mg/5 mL (237 mL, 240 mL)

Dilantin-125®: 125 mg/5 mL (240 mL)

Tablet, chewable, oral:

Dilantin®: 50 mg

General Dosage Range

I.V.:

Children 6 months to 3 years: Loading dose: 15-20 mg/kg in a single or divided dose; Maintenance: 5-10 mg/kg/day in 2 divided doses

Children 4-6 years: Loading dose: 15-20 mg/kg in a single or divided dose; Maintenance: 5-9 mg/kg/day in 2 divided doses

Children 7-9 years: Loading dose: 15-20 mg/kg in a single or divided dose; Maintenance: 5-8 mg/kg/day in 2 divided doses

Children 10-16 years: Loading dose: 15-20 mg/kg in a single or divided dose; Maintenance: 5-7 mg/kg/day in 2 divided doses

Adolescents >16 years and Adults: Loading dose: 10-25 mg/kg in a single or divided dose; Maintenance: 300 mg/day **or** 5-6 mg/kg/day in 3 divided doses

Oral:

Children: Loading dose: 15-20 mg/kg in divided doses; Maintenance: 4-8 mg/kg/day in divided doses

Adults: Loading dose: 15-20 mg/kg in 3 divided doses every 2-4 hours; Maintenance: 300 mg/day in 1-3 divided doses **or** 5-6 mg/kg/day in 1-3 divided doses **or** 100 mg every 6-8 hours (range: 200-1200 mg/day)

Administration

Oral Suspension: Shake well prior to use. Absorption is impaired when phenytoin suspension is given concurrently to patients who are receiving continuous nasogastric feedings. A method to resolve this interaction is to divide the daily dose of phenytoin and withhold the administration of nutritional supplements for 1-2 hours before and after each phenytoin dose.

I.M. Avoid this route (manufacturer recommends I.M. administration) due to severe risk of local tissue destruction and necrosis; use **fos**phenytoin if I.M. administration necessary (Boucher, 1996; Meek, 1999).

I.V. Vesicant. Fosphenytoin may be considered for loading in patients who are in status epilepticus, hemodynamically unstable, or develop hypotension/bradycardia with I.V. administration of phenytoin. Although, phenytoin may be administered by direct I.V. injection, it is preferable that phenytoin be administered via infusion pump either undiluted or diluted in normal saline as an I.V. piggyback (IVPB) to prevent exceeding the maximum infusion rate (monitor closely for extravasation during infusion). The maximum rate of I.V. administration is 50 mg/minute in adults. Highly sensitive patients (eg, elderly, patients with preexisting cardiovascular conditions) should receive phenytoin more slowly (eg, 20 mg/minute) (Meek, 1999). In neonates, the manufacturer recommends a maximum rate of 1-3 mg/kg/minute; however, a lower maximum rate of 0.5-1 mg/kg/minute is used clinically (Sankar, 2010; Shields, 1989). An in-line 0.22-5 micron filter is recommended for IVPB solutions due to the high potential for precipitation of the solution. Avoid extravasation. Following I.V. administration, NS should be injected through the same needle or I.V. catheter to prevent irritation.

I.V. Detail An in-line 0.22-5 micron filter is recommended for IVPB solutions due to the high potential for precipitation of the solution. Avoid extravasation. Following I.V. administration, NS should be injected through the same needle or I.V. catheter to prevent irritation.

pH: 10.0-12.3

Other SubQ administration is not recommended because of the possibility of local tissue damage (due to high pH).

Stability

Reconstitution I.V.: Further dilution of the solution for I.V. infusion is controversial and no consensus exists as to the optimal concentration and length of stability. Stability is concentration and pH dependent. Based on limited clinical consensus, NS or LR are recommended diluents; dilutions of 1-10 mg/mL have been used and should be administered as soon as possible after preparation (some recommend to discard if not used within 4 hours). Do not refrigerate.

Storage

Capsule, tablet: Store at controlled room temperature. Protect from light and moisture.

Oral suspension: Store at room temperature of 20°C to 25°C (68°F to 77°F); do not freeze. Protect from light.

Solution for injection: Store at room temperature of 15°C to 30°C (59°F to 86°F). Use only clear solutions free of precipitate and haziness; slightly yellow solutions may be used. Precipitation may occur if solution is refrigerated and may dissolve at room temperature.

Nursing Actions

Physical Assessment When oral phenytoin is discontinued, dose should be tapered gradually; abrupt discontinuance can cause status epilepticus. **I.V.:** Monitor blood pressure. Monitor infusion site closely to prevent extravasation. Monitor patient closely for adverse results (eg, cardiorespiratory, CNS status, suicide ideation).

Patient Education Take preferably on an empty stomach. Do not crush, break, or chew extended release capsules. Shake liquid suspension well before using. Follow recommended diet, avoid alcohol, and maintain adequate hydration unless instructed to restrict fluid intake. May cause gum or mouth soreness, drowsiness, dizziness, nervousness, headache, nausea, or vomiting. Report chest pain, irregular heartbeat, or palpitations; slurred speech, unsteady gait, coordination difficulties, suicide ideation, or change in mentation; skin rash; unresolved nausea, vomiting, or constipation; swollen glands; swollen, sore, or bleeding gums; unusual bruising or bleeding; acute persistent fatigue; or vision changes.

Dietary Considerations

Folic acid: Phenytoin may decrease mucosal uptake of folic acid; to avoid folic acid deficiency and megaloblastic anemia, some clinicians recommend giving patients on anticonvulsants prophylactic doses of folic acid and cyanocobalamin. However, folate supplementation may increase seizures in some patients (dose dependent). Discuss with healthcare provider prior to using any supplements.

Calcium: Hypocalcemia has been reported in patients taking prolonged high-dose therapy with an anticonvulsant. Some clinicians have given an additional 4000 units/week of vitamin D (especially in those receiving poor nutrition and getting no sun exposure) to prevent hypocalcemia.

Vitamin D: Phenytoin interferes with vitamin D metabolism and osteomalacia may result; may need to supplement with vitamin D

Tube feedings: Tube feedings decrease phenytoin absorption. To avoid decreased serum levels with continuous NG feeds, hold feedings for 1-2 hours prior to and 1-2 hours after phenytoin administration, if possible. There is a variety of opinions on how to administer phenytoin with enteral feedings. Be **consistent** throughout therapy.

Injection may contain sodium.

Related Information

Management of Drug Extravasations *on page 1269*

Peak and Trough Guidelines *on page 1276*

Phytonadione (fye toe na DYE one)

Brand Names: U.S. Mephyton®

Index Terms Methylphytyl Napthoquinone; Phylloquinone; Phytomenadione; Vitamin K_1

Pharmacologic Category Vitamin, Fat Soluble

Medication Safety Issues

Sound-alike/look-alike issues:

Mephyton® may be confused with melphalan, methadone

Pregnancy Risk Factor C

Lactation Enters breast milk/use caution (AAP rates "compatible"; AAP 2001 update pending)

Use Prevention and treatment of hypoprothrombinemia caused by coumarin derivative-induced or other drug-induced vitamin K deficiency, hypoprothrombinemia caused by malabsorption or inability to synthesize vitamin K; hemorrhagic disease of the newborn

Unlabeled Use Treatment of hypoprothrombinemia caused by anticoagulant rodenticides

Mechanism of Action/Effect Promotes liver synthesis of clotting factors (II, VII, IX, X); however, the exact mechanism as to this stimulation is unknown. Menadiol is a water soluble form of vitamin K; phytonadione has a more rapid and prolonged effect than menadione; menadiol sodium diphosphate (K_4) is half as potent as menadione (K_3).

Contraindications Hypersensitivity to phytonadione or any component of the formulation

Warnings/Precautions [U.S. Boxed Warning]: Severe reactions resembling hypersensitivity (eg, anaphylaxis) reactions have occurred rarely during or immediately after I.V. administration. Allergic reactions have also occurred with I.M. and SubQ injections; oral administration is the safest. In obstructive jaundice or with biliary fistulas concurrent administration of bile salts is necessary. Manufacturers recommend the SubQ route over other parenteral routes. SubQ is less predictable when compared to the oral route. The American College of Chest Physicians recommends the I.V. route in patients with serious or life-threatening bleeding secondary to warfarin. The I.V. route should be restricted to emergency situations where oral phytonadione cannot be used. Efficacy is delayed regardless of route of administration; patient management may require other treatments in the interim. Administer a dose that will quickly lower the INR into a safe range without causing resistance to warfarin. High phytonadione doses may lead to warfarin resistance for at least one week. Use caution in newborns especially premature infants; hemolysis, jaundice and hyperbilirubinemia have been reported with larger than recommended doses. Some dosage forms contain benzyl alcohol which has been associated with "gasping syndrome" in premature infants. In liver disease, if initial doses do not reverse coagulopathy then higher doses are unlikely to have any effect. Ineffective in hereditary hypoprothrombinemia. Use caution with renal dysfunction (including premature infants). Injectable products may contain aluminum; may result in toxic levels following prolonged administration. Product may contain polysorbate 80.

Drug Interactions

Avoid Concomitant Use There are no known interactions where it is recommended to avoid concomitant use.

Decreased Effect

Phytonadione may decrease the levels/effects of: Vitamin K Antagonists

The levels/effects of Phytonadione may be decreased by: Mineral Oil; Orlistat

Increased Effect/Toxicity There are no known significant interactions involving an increase in effect.

Adverse Reactions Parenteral administration: Frequency not defined.

Cardiovascular: Cyanosis, flushing, hypotension

Central nervous system: Dizziness

Dermatologic: Scleroderma-like lesions

Endocrine & metabolic: Hyperbilirubinemia (newborn; greater than recommended doses)

Gastrointestinal: Abnormal taste

Local: Injection site reactions

Respiratory: Dyspnea

Miscellaneous: Anaphylactoid reactions, diaphoresis, hypersensitivity reactions

Pharmacodynamics/Kinetics

Onset of Action

Onset of action: Increased coagulation factors: Oral: 6-10 hours; I.V.: 1-2 hours

Peak effect: INR values return to normal: Oral: 24-48 hours; I.V.: 12-14 hours

Available Dosage Forms

Injection, aqueous colloidal: 1 mg/0.5 mL (0.5 mL); 10 mg/mL (1 mL)

Injection, aqueous colloidal [preservative free]: 1 mg/0.5 mL (0.5 mL)

Tablet, oral: 100 mcg

Mephyton®: 5 mg

General Dosage Range

I.M.:

Newborns: Prophylaxis: 0.5-1 mg within 1 hour of birth; Treatment: 1 mg/dose/day

Adults: Initial: 2.5-25 mg/dose (usual: 5-10 mg; maximum: 50 mg)

I.V.: *Adults:* Initial: 2.5-25 mg/dose (usual: 5-10 mg; maximum: 50 mg)

Oral:

Children 1-3 years: RDA: 30 mcg/day

Children 4-8 years: RDA: 55 mcg/day

Children 9-13 years: RDA: 60 mcg/day

Children 14-18 years: RDA: 75 mcg/day

Adults: Initial: 2.5-25 mg/dose (usual: 5-10 mg; maximum: 50 mg)

SubQ:

Newborns: 1 mg/dose/day

Adults: Initial: 2.5-25 mg/dose (usual: 5-10 mg; maximum: 50 mg)

Administration

Oral The parenteral formulation may also be used for small oral doses (eg, 1 mg) or situations in which tablets cannot be swallowed (Crowther, 2000; O'Connor, 1986).

I.V. Infuse slowly; rate of infusion should not exceed 1 mg/minute (3 mg/m²/minute in children and infants). The injectable route should be used only if the oral route is not feasible or there is a greater urgency to reverse anticoagulation.

I.V. Detail pH: 3.5-7.0

Stability

Reconstitution Dilute injection solution in preservative-free NS, D_5W, or D_5NS.

Storage

Injection: Store at 15°C to 30°C (59°F to 86°F).

Note: Store Hospira product at 20°C to 25°C (68°F to 77°F).

Oral: Store tablets at 15°C to 30°C (59°F to 86°F). Protect from light.

Nursing Actions

Physical Assessment Note dosing specifics according to use. Monitor degree of bleeding.

Patient Education Oral: Consult prescriber for recommended diet. Report bleeding gums; blood in urine, stool, or vomitus; unusual bruising or bleeding; or abdominal cramping.

Pimozide (PI moe zide)

Brand Names: U.S. Orap®

Pharmacologic Category Antipsychotic Agent, Typical

Pregnancy Risk Factor C

Lactation Excretion in breast milk unknown/not recommended

Use Suppression of severe motor and phonic tics in patients with Tourette's disorder who have failed to respond satisfactorily to standard treatment

Unlabeled Use Psychosis; reported use in individuals with delusions focused on physical symptoms (ie, preoccupation with parasitic infestation); Huntington's chorea

Available Dosage Forms

Tablet, oral:

Orap®: 1 mg, 2 mg

General Dosage Range Dosage adjustment recommended in patients who develop toxicities or those with a CYP2D6 poor metabolizer status.

Oral:

Children 2-12 years: Initial: 0.05 mg/kg once daily (preferably bedtime); Maintenance: 2-4 mg once daily (maximum: 10 mg/day [0.2 mg/kg/day])

Children >12 years and Adults: Initial: 1-2 mg in divided doses (maximum: 10 mg/day [0.2 mg/kg/day])

Nursing Actions

Physical Assessment Review ophthalmic exam and monitor blood pressure at beginning of therapy and periodically throughout. Monitor for endocrine changes, extrapyramidal symptoms, and neuroleptic malignant syndrome. Conduct ECG at baseline and periodically during therapy (especially during dosage adjustment).

Patient Education It may take 2-3 weeks to achieve desired results. Avoid alcohol. Maintain adequate hydration unless instructed to restrict fluid intake. You may experience excess drowsiness, restlessness, dizziness, blurred vision, constipation, dry mouth, or anorexia. Report persistent CNS effects (eg, trembling fingers, altered gait or balance, excessive sedation, seizures, unusual muscle or facial movements, anxiety, abnormal thoughts, confusion, personality changes), unresolved constipation or GI effects, breast swelling (male and female) or decreased sexual ability, vision changes, respiratory difficulty, unusual cough or flu-like symptoms, or worsening of condition.

Pindolol (PIN doe lole)

Pharmacologic Category Beta Blocker With Intrinsic Sympathomimetic Activity

Medication Safety Issues

Sound-alike/look-alike issues:

Pindolol may be confused with Parlodel®, Plendil®

Visken® may be confused with Visine®, Viskazide®

Pregnancy Risk Factor B

Lactation Enters breast milk/not recommended

Use Treatment of hypertension, alone or in combination with other agents

Unlabeled Use Potential augmenting agent for antidepressants; ventricular arrhythmias/tachycardia, antipsychotic-induced akathisia, situational anxiety; aggressive behavior associated with dementia

Available Dosage Forms

Tablet, oral: 5 mg, 10 mg

General Dosage Range Dosage adjustment recommended in patients with hepatic impairment

Oral:

Adults: Initial: 5 mg twice daily; Maintenance: 10-40 mg twice daily (maximum: 60 mg/day)

Elderly: Initial: 5 mg once daily

Administration

Oral May be administered without regard to meals.

Pioglitazone (pye oh GLI ta zone)

Brand Names: U.S. Actos®

Pharmacologic Category Antidiabetic Agent, Thiazolidinedione

Medication Safety Issues

Sound-alike/look-alike issues:

Actos® may be confused with Actidose®, Actonel®

International issues:

Tiazac: Brand name for piogitazone [Chile], but also the brand name for diltiazem [U.S, Canada]

Medication Guide Available Yes

Pregnancy Risk Factor C

Lactation Excretion in breast milk unknown/not recommended

Use

Type 2 diabetes mellitus (noninsulin dependent, NIDDM), monotherapy: Adjunct to diet and exercise, to improve glycemic control

Type 2 diabetes mellitus (noninsulin dependent, NIDDM), combination therapy with sulfonylurea, metformin, or insulin: When diet, exercise, and a single agent alone does not result in adequate glycemic control

Available Dosage Forms

Tablet, oral:

Actos®: 15 mg, 30 mg, 45 mg

General Dosage Range Oral: *Adults:* Initial: 15-30 mg once daily; Maintenance: 15-45 mg once daily (maximum: 45 mg/day)

Administration

Oral May be administered without regard to meals.

Nursing Actions

Physical Assessment Monitor for signs of heart failure (weight gain, edema, dyspnea). Teach risks of hyperglycemia. Refer patient to a diabetic educator, if available.

Patient Education May be taken without regard to meals. Avoid or use caution with alcohol while taking this medication. If dose is missed, take as soon as possible. If dose is missed completely one day, do not double dose the next day. Follow dietary, exercise, and glucose monitoring instructions of prescriber (more frequent monitoring may be advised in periods of stress, trauma, surgery, increased exercise). Report respiratory infection, unusual weight gain, aggravation of hyper-/hypoglycemic condition, unusual swelling of extremities, shortness of breath, fatigue, yellowing of skin or eyes, dark urine, pale stool, nausea/vomiting, abdominal pain, or muscle pain.

Pioglitazone and Glimepiride

(pye oh GLI ta zone & GLYE me pye ride)

Brand Names: U.S. Duetact™

Index Terms Glimepiride and Pioglitazone; Glimepiride and Pioglitazone Hydrochloride

Pharmacologic Category Antidiabetic Agent, Sulfonylurea; Antidiabetic Agent, Thiazolidinedione; Hypoglycemic Agent, Oral

Medication Safety Issues

High alert medication:

The Institute for Safe Medication Practices (ISMP) includes this medication among its list of drugs which have a heightened risk of causing significant patient harm when used in error.

Medication Guide Available Yes

Pregnancy Risk Factor C

Lactation Excretion in breast milk unknown/not recommended

Use Management of type 2 diabetes mellitus (noninsulin dependent, NIDDM) as an adjunct to diet and exercise

Available Dosage Forms

Tablet:

Duetact™: 30 mg/2 mg: Pioglitazone 30 mg and glimepiride 2 mg; 30 mg/4 mg: Pioglitazone 30 mg and glimepiride 4 mg

General Dosage Range Dosage adjustment recommended in patients with renal impairment

Oral:

Adults:

Patients inadequately controlled on **glimepiride** alone: Initial dose: Pioglitazone 30 mg and glimepiride 2-4 mg once daily (maximum: 45 mg/day [pioglitazone]; 8 mg/day [glimepiride])

Patients inadequately controlled on **pioglitazone** alone: Initial dose: Pioglitazone 30 mg and glimepiride 2 mg once daily (maximum: 45 mg/day [pioglitazone]; 8 mg/day [glimepiride])

Elderly: Initial: Glimepiride 1 mg/day prior to initiating Duetact™

Administration

Oral Administer once daily with the first main meal of the day. To avoid hypoglycemia, patients without oral intake may need to have the dose held.

Nursing Actions

Physical Assessment See individual agents.

Patient Education See individual agents.

Pioglitazone and Metformin

(pye oh GLI ta zone & met FOR min)

Brand Names: U.S. Actoplus Met®; Actoplus Met® XR

Index Terms Metformin Hydrochloride and Pioglitazone Hydrochloride

Pharmacologic Category Antidiabetic Agent, Biguanide; Antidiabetic Agent, Thiazolidinedione

Medication Guide Available Yes

Pregnancy Risk Factor C

Lactation

Metformin: Enters breast milk/not recommended

Pioglitazone: Excretion in breast milk unknown/not recommended

Breast-Feeding Considerations See individual agents.

Use Management of type 2 diabetes mellitus (noninsulin dependent, NIDDM)

Mechanism of Action/Effect

Pioglitazone is a thiazolidinedione antidiabetic agent that lowers blood glucose by improving target cell response to insulin, without increasing pancreatic insulin secretion. It has a mechanism of action that is dependent on the presence of insulin for activity.

Metformin decreases hepatic glucose production, decreasing intestinal absorption of glucose, and improves insulin sensitivity (increases peripheral glucose uptake and utilization).

Contraindications Hypersensitivity to pioglitazone, metformin, or any component of the formulation; NYHA Class III/IV heart failure (initiation of therapy); renal disease or renal dysfunction (serum creatinine ≥1.5 mg/dL in males or ≥1.4 mg/dL in females, or abnormal creatinine clearance which may also result from conditions such as cardiovascular collapse, acute myocardial infarction, and septicemia); acute or chronic metabolic acidosis with or without coma (including diabetic ketoacidosis); concurrent iodinated radiocontrast adminstration (manufacturer recommends temporary discontinuation of metformin)

Warnings/Precautions [U.S. Boxed Warning]: Lactic acidosis is a rare, but potentially severe consequence of therapy with metformin. Lactic acidosis should be suspected in any patient with diabetes receiving metformin with evidence of acidosis but without evidence of ketoacidosis. Discontinue metformin in clinical situations predisposing to hypoxemia, including conditions such as cardiovascular collapse, respiratory failure, acute myocardial infarction, acute congestive heart failure, and septicemia.

Metformin is substantially excreted by the kidney. The risk of accumulation and lactic acidosis increases with the degree of impairment of renal function. Patients with renal function below the limit of normal for their age should not receive metformin. In elderly patients, renal function should be monitored regularly; should not be used in any patient ≥80 years of age unless normal renal function is confirmed. Use of concomitant medications that may affect renal function (ie, affect tubular secretion) may also affect metformin disposition. Metformin should be withheld in patients with dehydration and/or prerenal azotemia. Metformin therapy should be temporarily discontinued prior to or at the time of intravascular administration of iodinated contrast media (potential for acute alteration in renal function). Metformin should be withheld for 48 hours after the radiologic study and restarted only after renal function has been confirmed as normal.

[U.S. Boxed Warning]: Thiazolidinediones, including pioglitazone, may cause or exacerbate heart failure; closely monitor for signs and symptoms of heart failure (eg, rapid weight gain, dyspnea, edema), particularly after initiation or dose increases. Not recommended for use in any patient with symptomatic heart failure; initiation of therapy is contraindicated in patients with NYHA class III or IV heart failure. If used in patients with NYHA class II (systolic) heart failure, initiate at lowest dosage and monitor closely. In addition metformin should be used with caution in patients with heart failure requiring pharmacologic management, particularly in unstable or acute heart failure due to risk of lactic acidosis secondary to hypoperfusion. Use with caution in patients with edema; may increase plasma volume and/or cause fluid retention. Dose reduction or discontinuation is recommended if heart failure suspected. Dose-related weight gain observed with pioglitazone use; mechanism unknown but likely associated with fluid retention and fat accumulation.

Avoid metformin use in patients with impaired liver function due to potential for lactic acidosis. Use pioglitazone with caution in patients with elevated transaminases (AST or ALT); do not initiate in patients with active liver disease of ALT >2.5 times the upper limit of normal at baseline. During therapy, if ALT >3 times the upper limit of normal, reevaluate promptly and discontinue if elevation persists or if jaundice occurs at any time during use. Idiosyncratic hepatotoxicity has been reported with another thiazolidinedione agent (troglitazone); avoid use in patients who previously experienced jaundice during troglitazone therapy. Monitoring should include periodic determinations of liver function. Instruct patients to avoid excessive acute or chronic ethanol use; ethanol may potentiate metformin's effect on lactate metabolism.

Mechanism of pioglitazone requires the presence of insulin; therefore, use in type 1 diabetes (insulin dependent, IDDM) or diabetic ketoacidosis is not recommended. It may be necessary to discontinue metformin and administer insulin if the patient is exposed to stress (fever, trauma, infection, surgery). Increased incidence of bone fractures in females treated with pioglitazone; majority of fractures occurred in the lower limb and distal upper limb. Consider risk of fracture prior to initiation and during use. Pioglitazone may decrease hemoglobin/hematocrit; effects may be related to increased plasma volume. Metformin may impair vitamin B_{12} absorption; monitor for anemia. Use pioglitazone with caution in premenopausal, anovulatory women; may result in a resumption of ovulation, increasing the risk of pregnancy. Use pioglitazone with caution in patients with pre-existing macular edema or diabetic retinopathy; postmarketing events of new-onset or worsening diabetic macular edema with decreased visual acuity have been reported.

Drug Interactions

Avoid Concomitant Use

Avoid concomitant use of Pioglitazone and Metformin with any of the following: Axitinib

Decreased Effect

Pioglitazone and Metformin may decrease the levels/effects of: ARIPiprazole; Axitinib; Saxagliptin; Trospium

The levels/effects of Pioglitazone and Metformin may be decreased by: Bile Acid Sequestrants; Corticosteroids (Orally Inhaled); Corticosteroids (Systemic); CYP2C8 Inducers (Strong); Luteinizing Hormone-Releasing Hormone Analogs; Rifampin; Somatropin; Thiazide Diuretics; Tocilizumab

Increased Effect/Toxicity

Pioglitazone and Metformin may increase the levels/effects of: CYP2C8 Substrates; Dofetilide; Hypoglycemic Agents

The levels/effects of Pioglitazone and Metformin may be increased by: Carbonic Anhydrase Inhibitors; Cephalexin; Cimetidine; Conivaptan; CYP2C8 Inhibitors (Moderate); CYP2C8 Inhibitors (Strong); Deferasirox; Gemfibrozil; Glycopyrrolate; Herbs (Hypoglycemic Properties); Insulin; Iodinated Contrast Agents; Pegvisomant; Pregabalin; Trimethoprim

Nutritional/Ethanol Interactions See individual agents.

Adverse Reactions Also see individual agents. Percentages of adverse effects as reported with the combination product.

>10%:

Cardiovascular: Edema (lower limb, 3% to 11%)

Respiratory: Upper respiratory infection (12% to 16%)

1% to 10%:

Central nervous system: Headache (2% to 6%), dizziness (5%)

Endocrine & metabolic: Weight gain (3% to 7%)

Gastrointestinal: Diarrhea (5% to 6%), nausea (4% to 6%)

Genitourinary: Urinary tract infection (5% to 6%)

Hematologic: Anemia (≤2%)

Respiratory: Sinusitis (4% to 5%)

Available Dosage Forms

Tablet, oral:

Actoplus Met®: 15/500: Pioglitazone 15 mg and metformin 500 mg; 15/850: Pioglitazone 15 mg and metformin 850 mg

Tablet, variable release, oral:

Actoplus Met® XR: 15/1000: Pioglitazone 15 mg and metformin 1000 mg; 30/1000: Pioglitazone 30 mg and metformin 1000 mg

General Dosage Range Oral: *Adults:*

Immediate release tablet: Pioglitazone 15-45 mg/day and metformin 500-2550 mg/day (maximum: 45 mg/day [pioglitazone]; 2550 mg/day [metformin])

Variable release tablet: Pioglitazone 15-45 mg/day and metformin 1000-2000 mg/day (maximum: 45 mg/day [pioglitazone]; 2000 mg/day [metformin])

Administration

Oral

Immediate release formulation: Administer with meals.

Variable release formulation: Administer with the evening meal. Tablets should be swallowed whole; do not crush, split, or chew. Inactive tablet ingredients may be eliminated in the feces as a soft mass that resembles the orginal tablet.

Stability

Storage Store at 25°C (77°F); excursions permitted to 15°C to 30°C (59°F to 86°F). Protect from moisture and humidity

Nursing Actions

Physical Assessment See individual agents.

Patient Education See individual agents.

Dietary Considerations Immediate release tablets should be administered with meals. Variable release tablets should be administered with the evening meal. Avoid ethanol. Dietary modification based on ADA recommendations is a part of therapy. Monitor for signs and symptoms of vitamin B_{12} and/or folic acid deficiency; supplementation may be required.

Piperacillin and Tazobactam

(pi PER a sil in & ta zoe BAK tam)

Brand Names: U.S. Zosyn®

Index Terms Piperacillin and Tazobactam Sodium; Piperacillin Sodium and Tazobactam Sodium; Tazobactam and Piperacillin

Pharmacologic Category Antibiotic, Penicillin

Medication Safety Issues

Sound-alike/look-alike issues:

Zosyn® may be confused with Zofran®, Zyvox®

International issues:

Tazact [India] may be confused with Tazac brand name for nizatidine [Australia]; Tiazac brand name for diltiazem [U.S., Canada]

Pregnancy Risk Factor B

Lactation Enters breast milk/use caution

Breast-Feeding Considerations Low concentrations of piperacillin are excreted in breast milk; information for tazobactam is not available. The manufacturer recommends that caution be exercised when administering piperacillin/tazobactam to nursing women. Other penicillins are considered safe for use during breast-feeding. Nondose-related effects could include modification of bowel flora. When given alone in the early postpartum period, some pharmacokinetic parameters of piperacillin may be altered.

Use Treatment of moderate-to-severe infections caused by susceptible organisms, including infections of the lower respiratory tract (community-acquired pneumonia, nosocomial pneumonia); uncomplicated and complicated skin and skin structures (including diabetic foot infections); gynecologic (endometritis, pelvic inflammatory disease); and intra-abdominal infections (appendicitis with rupture/abscess, peritonitis). Tazobactam expands activity of piperacillin to include beta-lactamase producing strains of *S. aureus*, *H. influenzae*, *E. coli*, *Bacteroides* spp, and other gram-positive and gram-negative aerobic and anaerobic bacteria.

Unlabeled Use Treatment of moderate-to-severe infections caused by susceptible organisms, including urinary tract infections, bone and joint infections, septicemia, endocarditis, and cystic fibrosis exacerbations

Mechanism of Action/Effect Piperacillin interferes with bacterial cell wall synthesis during active multiplication, causing cell wall death and resultant bactericidal activity against susceptible bacteria. Piperacillin exhibits time-dependent killing. Tazobactam prevents degradation of piperacillin by binding to the active side on beta-lactamase; tazobactam inhibits many beta-lactamases, including staphylococcal penicillinase and Richmond-Sykes types 2, 3, 4, and 5, including extended spectrum enzymes; it has only limited activity against class 1 beta-lactamases other than class 1C types.

Contraindications Hypersensitivity to penicillins, cephalosporins, beta-lactamase inhibitors, or any component of the formulation

Warnings/Precautions Serious and occasionally severe or fatal hypersensitivity (anaphylactic/anaphylactoid) reactions have been reported in patients on penicillin therapy, especially with a history of beta-lactam hypersensitivity, history of sensitivity to multiple allergens, or previous IgE-mediated reactions (eg, anaphylaxis, angioedema, urticaria). Bleeding disorders have been observed, particularly in patients with renal impairment; discontinue if thrombocytopenia or bleeding occurs. Due to sodium load and to the adverse effects of high serum concentrations of penicillins, dosage modification is required in patients with impaired or underdeveloped renal function; use with caution in patients with seizures or in patients with history of beta-lactam allergy; associated with an increased incidence of rash and fever in cystic fibrosis patients. Use may result in fungal or bacterial superinfection, including *C. difficile*-associated diarrhea (CDAD) and pseudomembranous colitis; CDAD has been observed >2 months postantibiotic treatment.

Drug Interactions

Avoid Concomitant Use

Avoid concomitant use of Piperacillin and Tazobactam with any of the following: BCG

Decreased Effect

Piperacillin and Tazobactam may decrease the levels/effects of: Aminoglycosides; BCG; Mycophenolate; Typhoid Vaccine

The levels/effects of Piperacillin and Tazobactam may be decreased by: Fusidic Acid; Tetracycline Derivatives

Increased Effect/Toxicity

Piperacillin and Tazobactam may increase the levels/effects of: Methotrexate; Vitamin K Antagonists

The levels/effects of Piperacillin and Tazobactam may be increased by: Probenecid

Adverse Reactions

>10%: Gastrointestinal: Diarrhea (7% to 11%)

1% to 10%:

Cardiovascular: Hypertension (2%), chest pain (1%), edema (1%)

Central nervous system: Insomnia (7%), headache (8%), fever (2% to 5%), agitation (2%), pain (2%), anxiety (1% to 2%), dizziness (1% to 2%)

Dermatologic: Rash (4%), pruritus (3%)

Gastrointestinal: Constipation (1% to 8%), nausea (7%), vomiting (3% to 4%), dyspepsia (3%), stool changes (2%), abdominal pain (1% to 2%)

Hepatic: AST increased (1%)

Local: Local reaction (3%), phlebitis (1%)

Respiratory: Pharyngitis (2%), dyspnea (1%), rhinitis (1%)

Miscellaneous: Moniliasis (2%), sepsis (2%), infection (2%)

Available Dosage Forms 8:1 ratio of piperacillin sodium/tazobactam sodium

Infusion [premixed iso-osmotic solution, frozen]:

Zosyn®:

2.25 g: Piperacillin 2 g and tazobactam 0.25 g (50 mL)

3.375 g: Piperacillin 3 g and tazobactam 0.375 g (50 mL)

4.5 g: Piperacillin 4 g and tazobactam 0.5 g (100 mL)

Injection, powder for reconstitution: 2.25 g: Piperacillin 2 g and tazobactam 0.25 g; 3.375 g: Piperacillin 3 g and tazobactam 0.375 g; 4.5 g: Piperacillin 4 g and tazobactam 0.5 g; 40.5 g: Piperacillin 36 g and tazobactam 4.5 g

Zosyn®:

2.25 g: Piperacillin 2 g and tazobactam 0.25 g

3.375 g: Piperacillin 3 g and tazobactam 0.375 g

4.5 g: Piperacillin 4 g and tazobactam 0.5 g

40.5 g: Piperacillin 36 g and tazobactam 4.5 g

General Dosage Range Dosage adjustment recommended in patients with renal impairment

I.V.:

Children 2-8 months: 80 mg/kg every 8 hours

Children ≥9 months and ≤40 kg: 100 mg/kg every 8 hours

Children >40 kg: 4.5 g every 8 hours **or** 3.375 g every 6 hours

Adults: 3.375 g every 6 hours **or** 4.5 g every 6-8 hours (maximum: 18 g/day)

Administration

I.V. Administer by I.V. infusion over 30 minutes. For extended infusion administration (unlabeled dosing), administer over 3-4 hours (Kim 2007; Shea, 2009).

Some penicillins (eg, carbenicillin, ticarcillin, and piperacillin) have been shown to inactivate aminoglycosides *in vitro*. This has been observed to a greater extent with tobramycin and gentamicin, while amikacin has shown greater stability against inactivation. Concurrent use of these agents may pose a risk of reduced antibacterial efficacy *in vivo*, particularly in the setting of profound renal impairment. However, definitive clinical evidence is lacking. If combination penicillin/aminoglycoside therapy is desired in a patient with renal dysfunction, separation of doses (if feasible), and routine monitoring of aminoglycoside levels, CBC, and clinical response should be considered. **Note:** Reformulated Zosyn® containing EDTA (applies only to specific concentrations and diluents and varies by product; consult manufacturer's labeling) has been shown to be compatible *in vitro* for Y-site infusion with amikacin and gentamicin, but not compatible with tobramycin.

Stability

Reconstitution Reconstitute with 5 mL of diluent per 1 g of piperacillin and then further dilute.

Storage

Vials: Store at controlled room temperature of 20°C to 25°C (68°F to 77°F). Use single-dose vials immediately after reconstitution (discard unused portions after 24 hours at room temperature and 48 hours if refrigerated). After reconstitution, vials or solution are stable in NS or D_5W for 24 hours at room temperature and 48 hours (vials) or 7 days (solution) when refrigerated.

Premixed solution: Store frozen at -20°C (-4°F). Thawed solution is stable for 24 hours at room temperature or 14 days under refrigeration; do not refreeze.

Nursing Actions

Physical Assessment Assess results of culture and sensitivity tests and patient's allergy history prior to starting therapy. Use with caution in presence of renal impairment. Monitor for hypersensitivity reactions and opportunistic infection (eg, fever, chills, unhealed sores, white plaques in mouth or vagina, purulent vaginal discharge, fatigue).

Patient Education Common side effects include nausea, vomiting, diarrhea, and headache. Report signs of opportunistic infection (eg, fever, chills, diarrhea, unhealed sores, white plaques in mouth or vagina, purulent vaginal discharge) or signs of hypersensitivity reaction (eg, rash; hives; itching; swelling of lips, tongue, mouth, or throat).

Dietary Considerations Some products may contain sodium.

Related Information

Compatibility of Drugs *on page 1264*

Piroxicam (peer OKS i kam)

Brand Names: U.S. Feldene®

Pharmacologic Category Nonsteroidal Anti-inflammatory Drug (NSAID), Oral

Medication Safety Issues

Sound-alike/look-alike issues:

Feldene® may be confused with FLUoxetine

Piroxicam may be confused with PARoxetine

BEERS Criteria medication:

This drug may be inappropriate for use in geriatric patients (high severity risk).

International issues:

Flogene [Brazil] may be confused with Flogen brand name for naproxen [Mexico]; Florone brand name for diflorasone [Germany, Greece]; Flovent brand name for fluticasone [U.S., Canada]

Medication Guide Available Yes

Pregnancy Risk Factor C

Lactation Enters breast milk/not recommended (AAP rates "compatible"; AAP 2001 update pending)

Use Symptomatic treatment of acute and chronic rheumatoid arthritis and osteoarthritis

Canadian labeling: Additional use (not in U.S. labeling): Symptomatic treatment of ankylosing spondylitis

Available Dosage Forms

Capsule, oral: 10 mg, 20 mg

Feldene®: 10 mg, 20 mg

General Dosage Range Dosage adjustment recommended in patients with hepatic impairment

Oral: *Adults:* 10-20 mg/day in 1-2 divided doses (maximum: 20 mg/day)

Administration

Oral May administer with food or milk to decrease GI upset.

Nursing Actions

Physical Assessment Monitor blood pressure at the beginning of therapy and periodically during use. Monitor for GI effects, hepatotoxicity, and ototoxicity at beginning of therapy and periodically throughout. Schedule ophthalmic evaluations for patients who develop eye complaints during long-term NSAID therapy.

Patient Education Take with food or milk to reduce GI distress. Do not use alcohol. You may experience drowsiness, dizziness, nervousness, anorexia, nausea, vomiting, flatulence, heartburn, or fluid retention; GI bleeding, ulceration, or perforation can occur with or without pain; discontinue medication and contact prescriber if persistent abdominal pain or cramping or blood in stool occurs. Report unusual swelling of extremities or unusual weight gain; breathlessness, respiratory difficulty, or unusual cough; chest pain, rapid heartbeat, or palpitations; bruising/bleeding; blood in urine, stool, mouth, or vomitus; unusual fatigue; skin rash; or ringing in ears.

Pitavastatin (pi TA va sta tin)

Brand Names: U.S. Livalo®

Index Terms Pitavastatin Calcium

Pharmacologic Category Antilipemic Agent, HMG-CoA Reductase Inhibitor

Medication Safety Issues

Sound-alike/look-alike issues:

Pitavastatin may be confused with atorvastatin, fluvastatin, lovastatin, nystatin, pravastatin, rosuvastatin, simvastatin

Pregnancy Risk Factor X

Lactation Excretion in breast milk unknown/contraindicated

Use Adjunct to dietary therapy to reduce elevations in total cholesterol (TC), LDL-C, apolipoprotein B (Apo B), and triglycerides (TG), and to increase low HDL-C in patients with primary hyperlipidemia and mixed dyslipidemia

Mechanism of Action/Effect Inhibitor of 3-hydroxy-3-methylglutaryl coenzyme A (HMG-CoA) reductase, the rate-limiting enzyme in cholesterol synthesis (reduces the production of mevalonic acid from HMG-CoA); this then results in a compensatory increase in the expression of LDL receptors on hepatocyte membranes and a stimulation of LDL catabolism

Contraindications Hypersensitivity to pitavastatin or any component of the formulation; active liver disease including unexplained persistent elevations of hepatic transaminases; concurrent use with cyclosporine; pregnancy; breast-feeding

Warnings/Precautions Secondary causes of hyperlipidemia should be ruled out prior to therapy. Pitavastatin has not been studied when the primary lipid abnormality is chylomicron elevation (Fredrickson types I and V) or in familial dysbetalipoproteinemia (Fredrickson type III). May cause hepatic dysfunction; in all patients, liver function must be monitored prior to initiation of therapy; repeat LFTs if clinically indicated thereafter; routine periodic monitoring of liver enzymes is not necessary. Use with caution in patients who consume large amounts of ethanol or have a history of liver disease; use is contraindicated in patients with active liver disease or unexplained persistent elevations of serum transaminases. If serious hepatotoxicity with clinical symptoms and/or hyperbilirubinemia or jaundice occurs during treatment, interrupt therapy. If an alternate etiology is not identified, do not restart pitavastatin.

Myopathy and rhabdomyolysis with acute renal failure have occurred with use. Risk is dose related and is increased with concurrent use of lipid-lowering agents which may cause rhabdomyolysis (fibric acid derivatives or niacin at doses ≥1 g/day) or during concurrent use with erythromycin or protease inhibitors. Use caution in patients with renal impairment, inadequately treated hypothyroidism, and those taking other drugs associated with myopathy (eg, colchicine); these patients are predisposed to myopathy. Monitor closely if used with other drugs associated with myopathy. Weigh the risk versus benefit when combining any of these drugs with pitavastatin. The manufacturer recommends temporary discontinuation for elective major surgery, acute medical or surgical conditions, or in any patient experiencing an acute or serious condition predisposing to renal failure (eg, sepsis, hypotension, trauma, uncontrolled seizures). However, based upon current evidence, HMG-CoA reductase inhibitor therapy should be continued in the perioperative period unless risk outweighs cardioprotective benefit. Patients should be instructed to report unexplained muscle pain, tenderness, weakness, or brown urine. Concurrent use with cyclosporine is contraindicated. Ensure patient is on the lowest effective pitavastatin dose. Use with caution in elderly patients, as these patients are predisposed to myopathy. Increases in Hb A_{1c} and fasting blood glucose have been reported with HMG-CoA reductase inhibitors; however, the benefits of statin therapy far outweigh the risk of dysglycemia.

Drug Interactions

Avoid Concomitant Use

Avoid concomitant use of Pitavastatin with any of the following: CycloSPORINE; CycloSPORINE (Systemic); Red Yeast Rice

Decreased Effect

Pitavastatin may decrease the levels/effects of: Lanthanum

The levels/effects of Pitavastatin may be decreased by: Antacids; Bosentan; St Johns Wort

Increased Effect/Toxicity

Pitavastatin may increase the levels/effects of: DAPTOmycin; Trabectedin; Vitamin K Antagonists

The levels/effects of Pitavastatin may be increased by: Atazanavir; Colchicine; CycloSPORINE; CycloSPORINE (Systemic); Danazol; Eltrombopag; Fenofibrate; Fenofibric Acid; Gemfibrozil; Macrolide Antibiotics; Niacin; Niacinamide; Protease Inhibitors; Red Yeast Rice; Rifamycin Derivatives; Sildenafil

Nutritional/Ethanol Interactions

Ethanol: Avoid excessive ethanol consumption (due to potential hepatic effects).

Food: Red yeast rice contains an estimated 2.4 mg lovastatin per 600 mg rice.

Adverse Reactions

2% to 10%:

Gastrointestinal: Constipation (2% to 4%), diarrhea (2% to 3%)

Neuromuscular & skeletal: Back pain (1% to 4%), myalgia (2% to 3%), pain in extremities (1% to 2%)

Additional class-related events or case reports (not necessarily reported with pitavastatin therapy): Cataracts, cirrhosis, dermatomyositis, eosinophilia, extraocular muscle movement impaired, fulminant hepatic necrosis, gynecomastia, hypersensitivity syndrome (symptoms may include anaphylaxis, angioedema, arthralgia, erythema multiforme, eosinophilia, hemolytic anemia, interstitial lung disease, lupus syndrome, photosensitivity, polymyalgia rheumatica, positive ANA, purpura, Stevens-Johnson syndrome, toxic epidermal necrolysis, urticaria, vasculitis), ophthalmoplegia, peripheral nerve palsy, rhabdomyolysis, renal failure (secondary to rhabdomyolysis), thyroid dysfunction, tremor, vertigo

Available Dosage Forms

Tablet, oral:

Livalo®: 1 mg, 2 mg, 4 mg

General Dosage Range Dosage adjustment recommended in patients with renal impairment or on concomitant therapy

Oral: *Adults:* Initial: 2 mg once daily; Maintenance: 2-4 mg once daily (maximum: 4 mg/day)

Administration

Oral May be administered with or without food; may take without regard to time of day.

Stability

Storage Store at controlled room temperature of 15°C to 30°C (59°F to 86°F). Protect from light.

Nursing Actions

Physical Assessment Assess risk potential for interactions with other prescriptions or herbal products patient may be taking that may increase risk of myopathy or rhabdomyolysis. Teach proper diet and exercise regimen.

Patient Education Take with or without food. Follow prescribed diet and exercise regimen. You will have periodic blood tests to assess effectiveness. Avoid excessive alcohol. Report unusual muscle cramping or weakness, yellowing of skin or eyes, easy bruising or bleeding, or unusual fatigue.

Dietary Considerations May be taken with or without food; may take without regard to time of day. Red yeast rice contains an estimated 2.4 mg lovastatin per 600 mg rice.

Plerixafor (pler IX a fore)

Brand Names: U.S. Mozobil™

Index Terms AMD3100; LM3100

Pharmacologic Category Hematopoietic Stem Cell Mobilizer

Pregnancy Risk Factor D

Lactation Excretion in breast milk unknown/not recommended

Use Mobilization of hematopoietic stem cells (HSC) for collection and subsequent autologous transplantation (in combination with filgrastim) in patients with non-Hodgkin's lymphoma (NHL) and multiple myeloma (MM)

Available Dosage Forms

Injection, solution [preservative free]:

Mozobil™: 20 mg/mL (1.2 mL)

General Dosage Range Dosage adjustment recommended in patients with renal impairment

SubQ: *Adults:* 0.24 mg/kg/day (maximum dose: 40 mg/day)

Administration

I.V. Detail pH: 6-7.5

Other Administer subcutaneously, ~11 hours prior to initiation of apheresis. In some clinical trials, plerixafor administration began in the evening prior to apheresis. (filgrastim was begun on day 1, plerixafor initiated in the evening on day 4 and apheresis in the morning on day 5; with filgrastim, plerixafor and apheresis then continued daily until sufficient cell collection for autologous transplant.)

Nursing Actions

Physical Assessment Teach patient appropriate injection techniques and syringe/needle disposal.

Patient Education This medication is administered via injection. Local injection site reactions, such as redness, inflammation, irritation, and itching, are not unusual. Contact prescriber if injection site reaction is severe. You may experience dizziness, nausea, diarrhea, gas, headache, muscle pain, problems sleeping, and fatigue. Report persistent abdominal pain to prescriber.

Pneumococcal Conjugate Vaccine (7-Valent)

(noo moe KOK al KON ju gate vak SEEN, seven vay lent)

Brand Names: U.S. Prevnar®

Index Terms Diphtheria CRM_{197} Protein; PCV; PCV-7; PCV7; Pneumococcal 7-Valent Conjugate Vaccine

Pharmacologic Category Vaccine, Inactivated (Bacterial)

Medication Safety Issues

Sound-alike/look-alike issues:

Pneumococcal 7-Valent Conjugate Vaccine (Prevnar®) may be confused with Pneumococcal 13-Valent Conjugate Vaccine (Prevnar 13™) or with Pneumococcal 23-Valent Polysaccharide Vaccine (Pneumovax® 23)

Pregnancy Risk Factor C

Lactation Excretion in breast milk unknown/not recommended

Use Note: In March 2010, the Advisory Committee on Immunization Practices (ACIP) released recommendations that pneumococcal 13-valent conjugate vaccine (PCV13; Prevnar 13™) replace pneumococcal 7-valent conjugate vaccine (PCV7; Prevnar®) for all doses for immunization of all children 2-59 months of age. Refer to the Pneumococcal Conjugate Vaccine (13-Valent) monograph for additional information.

Immunization of infants and toddlers against *Streptococcus pneumoniae* infection caused by serotypes included in the vaccine

Immunization of infants and toddlers against otitis media caused by serotypes included in the vaccine

The Advisory Committee on Immunization Practices (ACIP) recommends pneumococcal conjugate vaccine (PCV) for routine vaccination of all children 2-59 months and children 60-71 months with underlying medical conditions. PCV13 should be used to complete the vaccination of children who received ≥1 dose of PCV7.

Available Dosage Forms

Injection, suspension:

Prevnar®: 2 mcg of each capsular saccharide for serotypes 4, 9V, 14, 18C, 19F, and 23F, and 4 mcg of serotype 6B per 0.5 mL (0.5 mL)

General Dosage Range I.M.: *Infants 2-6 months:* 0.5 mL at approximately 2-month intervals for 3 consecutive doses, followed by a fourth dose of 0.5 mL at 12-15 months of age

Administration

I.M. Shake well prior to use. Administer I.M. (deltoid muscle for toddlers and young children or lateral midthigh in infants). Do not inject I.V.; avoid intradermal route.

For patients at risk of hemorrhage following intramuscular injection, the ACIP recommends "it should be administered intramuscularly if, in the opinion of the physician familiar with the patients bleeding risk, the vaccine can be administered by this route with reasonable safety. If the patient receives antihemophilia or other similar therapy, intramuscular vaccination can be scheduled shortly after such therapy is administered. A fine needle (23 gauge or smaller) can be used for the vaccination and firm pressure applied to the site (without rubbing) for at least 2 minutes. The patient should be instructed concerning the risk of hematoma from the injection." Patients on anticoagulant therapy should be considered to have the same bleeding risks and treated as those with clotting factor disorders (CDC, 2011).

Antipyretics have not been shown to prevent febrile seizures. Antipyretics may be used to treat fever or discomfort following vaccination (CDC, 2011). One study reported that routine prophylactic administration of acetaminophen to prevent fever prior to vaccination decreased the immune response of some vaccines; the clinical significance of this reduction in immune response has not been established (Prymula, 2009).

Simultaneous administration of vaccines helps ensure the patients will be fully vaccinated by the appropriate age. Simultaneous administration of vaccines is defined as administering >1 vaccine on the same day at different anatomic sites. Separate vaccines should not be combined in the same syringe unless indicated by product specific labeling. Separate needles and syringes should be used for each injection. The ACIP prefers each dose of a specific vaccine in a series come from the same manufacturer when possible. Adolescents and adults should be vaccinated while seated or lying down. In general, preterm infants should be vaccinated at the same chronological age as full-term infants (CDC, 2011).

Nursing Actions

Physical Assessment U.S. federal law requires entry into the patient's medical record.

Related Information

Immunization Administration Recommendations *on page 1243*

Immunization Recommendations *on page 1248*

Pneumococcal Conjugate Vaccine (13-Valent)

(noo moe KOK al KON ju gate vak SEEN, thur TEEN vay lent)

Brand Names: U.S. Prevnar 13™

Index Terms Diphtheria CRM_{197} Protein; PCV-13; PCV13; PCV13-CRM(197); Pneumococcal 13-Valent Conjugate Vaccine

Pharmacologic Category Vaccine, Inactivated (Bacterial)

Medication Safety Issues

Sound-alike/look-alike issues:

Pneumococcal 13-Valent Conjugate Vaccine (Prevnar 13™) may be confused with Pneumococcal 7-Valent Conjugate Vaccine (Prevnar®) or with Pneumococcal 23-Valent Polysaccharide Vaccine (Pneumovax® 23)

Pregnancy Risk Factor B

Lactation Excretion in breast milk unknown/use caution

Use

Immunization of infants and children against *Streptococcus pneumoniae* infection caused by serotypes included in the vaccine

Immunization of infants and children against otitis media caused by *Streptococcus pneumoniae* serotypes 4, 6B, 9V, 14, 18C, 19F, and 23F

Immunization of adults ≥50 years against pneumococcal pneumonia and invasive disease caused by *Streptococcus pneumoniae* serotypes included in the vaccine

The Advisory Committee on Immunization Practices (ACIP) recommends routine vaccination for the following:

All children age 2-59 months

Children 60-71 months with underlying medical conditions including: Cochlear implants, functional or anatomic asplenia (includes sickle cell disease and other hemoglobinopathies, congenital or acquired asplenia, or splenic dysfunction); immunocompromising conditions (includes HIV infection, congenital immunodeficiencies [excluding chronic granulomatous disease], chronic renal failure, nephrotic syndrome, diseases associated with immunosuppressive or radiation therapy, solid organ transplant); chronic illnesses (cardiac disease, cerebrospinal fluid leaks, diabetes mellitus, pulmonary disease [excluding asthma unless on high dose oral corticosteroids])

Children who received ≥1 dose of PCV7

Children 6-18 years of age at increased risk for invasive pneumococcal disease due to anatomic or functional asplenia (including sickle cell disease), HIV infection or other immunocompromising conditions, cochlear implant, or cerebrospinal fluid leaks (regardless of prior receipt of PCV7 or PPSV23). Routine use is not recommended for healthy children ≥5 years of age.

Available Dosage Forms

Injection, suspension:

Prevnar 13™: 2 mcg of each capsular saccharide for serotypes 1, 3, 4, 5, 6A, 7F, 9V, 14, 18C, 19A, 19F, and 23F, and 4 mcg of serotype 6B [bound to diphtheria CRM_{197} protein ~34 mcg] per 0.5 mL (0.5 mL)

General Dosage Range I.M.:

Infants 2-6 months: 0.5 mL at approximately 2-month intervals for 3 consecutive doses, followed by a fourth dose of 0.5 mL at 12-15 months of age

Infants 7-11 months (previously unvaccinated): 0.5 mL for a total of 3 doses, 2 doses at least 4 weeks apart, followed by a third dose at 12-15 months (at least 2 months after second dose)

Children 12-23 months (previously unvaccinated) and Children 24-71 months (previously unvaccinated) with underlying conditions: 0.5 mL for a total of 2 doses, separated by at least 2 months

Healthy Children 24-59 months (previously unvaccinated) and Children 6-18 years at high risk for invasive pneumococcal disease: 0.5 mL as a single dose

Children 14 months-71 months (previously completing vaccination with PCV7): 0.5 mL supplemental dose

Adults ≥50 years: 0.5 mL as a single dose

Administration

I.M. Shake well prior to use. Do not use if a homogenous white suspension does not form. Administer I.M. (deltoid muscle for toddlers, young children, and adults or lateral midthigh in infants). Do not inject I.V. or SubQ; avoid intradermal route. Concurrent administration of PCV13 and PPV23 has not been studied and is not recommended (CDC, 2010).

For patients at risk of hemorrhage following intramuscular injection, the ACIP recommends "it should be administered intramuscularly if, in the opinion of the physician familiar with the patients bleeding risk, the vaccine can be administered by this route with reasonable safety. If the patient receives antihemophilia or other similar therapy, intramuscular vaccination can be scheduled shortly after such therapy is administered. A fine needle (23 gauge or smaller) can be used for the vaccination and firm pressure applied to the site (without rubbing) for at least 2 minutes. The patient should be instructed concerning the risk of hematoma from the injection." Patients on anticoagulant therapy should be considered to have the same bleeding risks and treated as those with clotting factor disorders (CDC, 2011).

Antipyretics have not been shown to prevent febrile seizures. Antipyretics may be used to treat fever or discomfort following vaccination (CDC, 2011). One study reported that routine prophylactic administration of acetaminophen to prevent fever prior to vaccination decreased the immune response of some vaccines; the clinical significance of this reduction in immune response has not been established (Prymula, 2009).

Simultaneous administration of vaccines helps ensure the patients will be fully vaccinated by the appropriate age. Simultaneous administration of vaccines is defined as administering >1 vaccine on the same day at different anatomic sites. Separate vaccines should not be combined in the same syringe unless indicated by product specific labeling. Separate needles and syringes should be used for each injection. The ACIP prefers each dose of a specific vaccine in a series come from the same manufacturer when possible. Adolescents and adults should be vaccinated while seated or lying down. In general, preterm infants should be vaccinated at the same chronological age as full-term infants (CDC, 2011).

Nursing Actions

Physical Assessment U.S. federal law requires entry into the patient's medical record.

Patient Education Common side effects may include irritability, fussiness, drowsiness, temporary loss of appetite, irritation or swelling where shot is given, and mild fever. Have parent call prescriber if child has high fever, behavior changes, difficulty breathing, hoarseness, wheezing, hives, paleness, weakness, fast heartbeat, or dizziness.

Related Information

Immunization Administration Recommendations *on page 1243*

Immunization Recommendations *on page 1248*

Pneumococcal Polysaccharide Vaccine (Polyvalent)

(noo moe KOK al pol i SAK a ride vak SEEN, pol i VAY lent)

Brand Names: U.S. Pneumovax® 23

Index Terms 23-Valent Pneumococcal Polysaccharide Vaccine; 23PS; PPSV; PPSV23; PPV23

Pharmacologic Category Vaccine, Inactivated (Bacterial)

Medication Safety Issues

Sound-alike/look-alike issues:

Pneumococcal 23-Valent Polysaccharide Vaccine (Pneumovax® 23) may be confused with Pneumococcal 7-Valent Conjugate Vaccine (Prevnar®) or with Pneumococcal 13-Valent Conjugate Vaccine (Prevnar 13™)

Pregnancy Risk Factor C

Lactation Excretion in breast milk unknown/use caution

Use Immunization against pneumococcal disease caused by serotypes included in the vaccine. Routine vaccination is recommended for persons ≥50 years of age and persons ≥2 years in certain situations.

The Advisory Committee on Immunization Practices (ACIP) recommends routine vaccination for the following (CDC, 59[34], 2010; CDC, 59[11], 2010):

Patients ≥65 years of age without a history of vaccination (CDC, 61[4], 2012)

Patients 2-18 years of age with certain high-risk condition(s):

- Chronic heart disease (particularly cyanotic congenital heart disease and cardiac failure)
- Chronic lung disease (including asthma if treated with high-dose oral corticosteroids)

Patients 2-64 years of age with certain high-risk condition(s):

- Diabetes mellitus
- Cochlear implants
- Cerebrospinal fluid leaks
- Functional or anatomic asplenia (including sickle cell disease and other hemoglobinopathies, splenic dysfunction, or splenectomy)
- Immunocompromising conditions including congenital immunodeficiency (includes B- or T-lymphocyte deficiency, complement deficiencies, and phagocytic disorders [excluding chronic granulomatous disease]); HIV infection; leukemia, lymphoma, Hodgkin's disease, multiple myeloma, generalized malignancy; chronic renal failure, nephrotic syndrome; patients requiring treatment with immunosuppressive therapy, including chemotherapy, long-term systemic corticosteroids, or radiation therapy; patients who have received a solid organ transplant

Patients 19-64 years of age with certain high-risk condition(s):

- Chronic heart disease (including heart failure and cardiomyopathy, and excluding hypertension)
- Chronic lung disease (including COPD, emphysema, and asthma)
- Persons who smoke cigarettes
- Alcoholism
- Chronic liver disease (including cirrhosis)
- Residents of nursing homes or long term care facilities (CDC, 61[4], 2012)

Routine vaccination is not recommended for Alaska Natives or American Indian persons unless they have underlying conditions which are indications for vaccination; in special situations, vaccination may be recommended when living in an area at increased risk of invasive pneumococcal disease.

Available Dosage Forms

Injection, solution:

Pneumovax® 23: 25 mcg each of 23 capsular polysaccharide isolates/0.5 mL (0.5 mL, 2.5 mL)

General Dosage Range I.M., SubQ: *Children ≥2 years and Adults:* 0.5 mL

Administration

I.M. Do not inject I.V.; avoid intradermal administration (may cause severe local reactions); administer SubQ or I.M. (deltoid muscle or lateral midthigh)

For patients at risk of hemorrhage following intramuscular injection, the ACIP recommends "it should be administered intramuscularly if, in the opinion of the physician familiar with the patients bleeding risk, the vaccine can be administered by this route with reasonable safety. If the patient receives antihemophilia or other similar therapy, intramuscular vaccination can be scheduled shortly after such therapy is administered. A fine needle (23 gauge or smaller) can be used for the vaccination and firm pressure applied to the site (without rubbing) for at least 2 minutes. The patient should be instructed concerning the risk of hematoma from the injection." Patients on anticoagulant therapy should be considered to have the same bleeding risks and treated as those with clotting factor disorders (CDC, 2011).

Antipyretics have not been shown to prevent febrile seizures. Antipyretics may be used to treat fever or discomfort following vaccination (CDC, 2011). One study reported that routine prophylactic administration of acetaminophen to prevent fever prior to vaccination decreased the immune response of some vaccines; the clinical significance of this reduction in immune response has not been established (Prymula, 2009).

Simultaneous administration of vaccines helps ensure the patients will be fully vaccinated by the appropriate age. Simultaneous administration of vaccines is defined as administering >1 vaccine on the same day at different anatomic sites. Separate vaccines should not be combined in the same syringe unless indicated by product specific labeling. Separate needles and syringes should be used for each injection. The ACIP prefers each dose of a specific vaccine in a series come from the same manufacturer when possible. Adolescents and adults should be vaccinated while seated or lying down. In general, preterm infants should be vaccinated at the same chronological age as full-term infants (CDC, 2011).

Other Do not inject I.V., avoid intradermal administration (may cause severe local reactions); administer SubQ or I.M. (deltoid muscle or lateral midthigh).

Nursing Actions

Physical Assessment U.S. federal law requires entry into the patient's medical record.

Related Information

Immunization Administration Recommendations *on page 1243*

Immunization Recommendations *on page 1248*

Poliovirus Vaccine (Inactivated)

(POE lee oh VYE rus vak SEEN, in ak ti VAY ted)

Brand Names: U.S. IPOL®

Index Terms Enhanced-Potency Inactivated Poliovirus Vaccine; IPV; Polio Vaccine; Salk Vaccine

Pharmacologic Category Vaccine, Inactivated (Viral)

Medication Safety Issues

Administration issues:

Poliovirus vaccine (inactivated) may be confused with tuberculin products. Medication errors have occurred when poliovirus vaccine (IPV) has been inadvertently administered instead of tuberculin skin tests (PPD). These products are refrigerated and often stored in close proximity to each other.

Pregnancy Risk Factor C

Lactation Excretion into breast milk unknown/use caution

Use Active immunization against poliomyelitis caused by poliovirus types 1, 2 and 3. **Note:** Combination products containing polio vaccine are also available and may be preferred in certain age groups if recipients are likely to be susceptible to the agents contained within each vaccine.

The Advisory Committee on Immunization Practices (ACIP) recommends routine vaccination for the following:

- All children (first dose given at 2 months of age)

Routine immunization of adults in the United States is generally not recommended. Adults with previous wild poliovirus disease, who have never been immunized, or those who are incompletely immunized may receive inactivated poliovirus vaccine if they fall into one of the following categories:

- Travelers to regions or countries where poliomyelitis is endemic or epidemic
- Healthcare workers in close contact with patients who may be excreting poliovirus
- Laboratory workers handling specimens that may contain poliovirus
- Members of communities or specific population groups with diseases caused by wild poliovirus
- Incompletely vaccinated or unvaccinated adults in a household or with other close contact with children receiving oral poliovirus (may be at increased risk of vaccine associated paralytic poliomyelitis)

Available Dosage Forms

Injection, suspension:

IPOL®: Type 1 poliovirus 40 D-antigen units, type 2 poliovirus 8 D-antigen units, and type 3 poliovirus 32 D-antigen units per 0.5 mL (0.5 mL, 5 mL)

General Dosage Range I.M., SubQ:

Children: Primary immunization: Administer three 0.5 mL doses at 2, 4, and 6-18 months of age; do not administer more frequently than 4 weeks apart (preferably given more than 8 weeks apart). Booster dose: 0.5 mL at 4-6 years of age; Minimum interval between booster and previous dose is 6 months.

Adults (previously unvaccinated): Two 0.5 mL doses administered at 1- to 2-month intervals followed by a third dose 6-12 months later.

Administration

I.M. Administer to midlateral aspect of the thigh in infants and small children. Administer in the deltoid area to adults or older children.

I.V. Do not administer I.V.

Other SubQ: Administer to midlateral aspect of the thigh in infants and small children. Administer in the deltoid area to adults or older children.

Simultaneous administration of vaccines helps ensure the patients will be fully vaccinated by the appropriate age. Simultaneous administration of vaccines is defined as administering >1 vaccine on the same day at different anatomic sites. The use of licensed combination vaccines is generally preferred over separate injections of the equivalent components. Separate vaccines should not be combined in the same syringe unless indicated by product specific labeling. Separate needles and syringes should be used for each injection. The ACIP prefers each dose of a specific vaccine in a series come from the same manufacturer when possible. Adolescents and adults should be vaccinated while seated or lying down. In general, preterm infants should be vaccinated at the same chronological age as full-term infants (CDC, 2011).

Antipyretics have not been shown to prevent febrile seizures. Antipyretics may be used to treat fever or discomfort following vaccination (CDC, 2011). One study reported that routine prophylactic administration of acetaminophen to prevent fever prior to vaccination decreased the immune response of some vaccines; the clinical significance of this reduction in immune response has not been established (Prymula, 2009).

Nursing Actions

Physical Assessment All serious adverse reactions must be reported to the U.S. DHHS. U.S. federal law also requires entry into the patient's medical record.

Patient Education Inform healthcare provider if you have an allergy to neomycin, streptomycin, or polymyxin B. Contact healthcare provider immediately if you develop a high fever, unusual behavior, or a rash.

Related Information

Immunization Administration Recommendations *on page 1243*

Immunization Recommendations *on page 1248*

Polyethylene Glycol-Electrolyte Solution

(pol i ETH i leen GLY kol ee LEK troe lite soe LOO shun)

Brand Names: U.S. Colyte®; GaviLyte™-C; GaviLyte™-G; GaviLyte™-N; GoLYTELY®; MoviPrep®; NuLYTELY®; TriLyte®

Index Terms Electrolyte Lavage Solution

Pharmacologic Category Laxative, Osmotic

Medication Safety Issues

Sound-alike/look-alike issues:

GoLYTELY® may be confused with NuLYTELY®

TriLyte® may be confused with TriLipix®

Medication Guide Available Yes

Pregnancy Risk Factor C

Lactation Excretion in breast milk unknown/use caution

Use Bowel cleansing prior to GI examination

Unlabeled Use Whole bowel irrigation (WBI) in the following toxic ingestions: Packets of illicit drugs (body packers, body stuffers), potentially toxic sustained-release or enteric-coated agents, substantial amounts of iron (AACT, 2004)

Available Dosage Forms

Powder, for solution, oral: PEG 3350 240 g, sodium sulfate 22.72 g, sodium bicarbonate 6.72 g, sodium chloride 5.84 g, and potassium 2.98 g (4000 mL); PEG 3350 236 g, sodium sulfate 22.74 g, sodium bicarbonate 6.74 g, sodium chloride 5.86 g, and potassium chloride 2.97 g (4000 mL); PEG 3350 240 g, sodium bicarbonate 5.72 g, sodium chloride 11.2 g, and potassium chloride 1.48 g (4000 mL)

Colyte®: PEG 3350 227.1 g, sodium sulfate 21.5 g, sodium bicarbonate 6.36 g, sodium chloride 5.53 g, and potassium chloride 2.82 g (3785 mL)

Colyte®: PEG 3350 240 g, sodium sulfate 22.72 g, sodium bicarbonate 6.72 g, sodium chloride 5.84 g, and potassium 2.98 g (4000 mL)

GaviLyte™-C: PEG 3350 240 g, sodium sulfate 22.72 g, sodium bicarbonate 6.72 g, sodium chloride 5.84 g, and potassium chloride 2.98 g (4000 mL)

GaviLyte™-G: PEG 3350 236 g, sodium sulfate 22.74 g, sodium bicarbonate 6.74 g, sodium chloride 5.86 g, and potassium chloride 2.97 g (4000 mL)

GaviLyte™-N: PEG 3350 420 g, sodium bicarbonate 5.72 g, sodium chloride 11.2 g, and potassium chloride 1.48 g (4000 mL)

GoLYTELY®: PEG 3350 227.1 g, sodium sulfate 21.5 g, sodium bicarbonate 6.36 g, sodium chloride 5.53 g, and potassium 2.82 g per packet (1s)

GoLYTELY®: PEG 3350 236 g, sodium sulfate 22.74 g, sodium bicarbonate 6.74 g, sodium chloride 5.86 g, and potassium 2.97 g (4000 mL)

MoviPrep®: Pouch A: PEG 3350 100g, sodium sulfate 7.5 g, sodium chloride 2.69 g, potassium chloride 1.015 g; Pouch B: Ascorbic acid 4.7 g, sodium ascorbate 5.9 g

NuLYTELY®: PEG 3350 420 g, sodium bicarbonate 5.72 g, sodium chloride 11.2 g, and potassium 1.48 g

TriLyte®: PEG 3350 420 g, sodium bicarbonate 5.72 g, sodium chloride 11.2 g, and potassium 1.48 g

General Dosage Range

Nasogastric tube:

Children ≥6 months: 25 mL/kg/hour until rectal effluent is clear

Adults: 20-30 mL/minute (1.2-1.8 L/hour) until rectal effluent is clear

Oral:

Children ≥6 months: (GaviLyte™-N, NuLYTELY®, TriLyte®): 25 mL/kg/hour (some studies have used up to 40 mL/kg/hour) for 4-10 hours until rectal effluent is clear (maximum total dose: 4 L)

Adults: CoLyte®, GaviLyte™-C, GaviLyte™-G, GaviLyte™-N, GoLYTELY®, NuLYTELY®, TriLyte®: 240 mL (8 oz) every 10 minutes, until 4 L are consumed or the rectal effluent is clear; MoviPrep®: 240 mL (8 oz) every 15 minutes until 1 L consumed; repeat 1 time

Administration

Oral Rapid drinking of each portion is preferred to drinking small amounts continuously. Do not add flavorings, unless provided by the manufacturer, as additional ingredients before use. Chilled solution often more palatable. Oral medications should not be administered within 1 hour of start of therapy.

Nursing Actions

Patient Education For bowel cleansing prior to GI exam, take every 10 minutes until recommended amount is consumed or the rectal effluent is clear. Rapid drinking of each portion is preferred to drinking small amounts continuously. The first bowel movement should occur approximately 1 hour after the start of administration. May cause abdominal bloating and distention before bowel starts to move. If severe discomfort or distention occurs, stop drinking temporarily or drink each portion at longer intervals until these symptoms disappear. Continue drinking until the watery stool is clear and free of solid matter.

Polyethylene Glycol-Electrolyte Solution and Bisacodyl

(pol i ETH i leen GLY kol ee LEK troe lite soe LOO shun & bis a KOE dil)

Brand Names: U.S. HalfLytely® and Bisacodyl

Index Terms Bisacodyl and Polyethylene Glycol-Electrolyte Solution; Electrolyte Lavage Solution

Pharmacologic Category Laxative, Bowel Evacuant; Laxative, Stimulant

Medication Guide Available Yes

Pregnancy Risk Factor C

Lactation Excretion in breast milk unknown/use caution

Use Bowel cleansing prior to colonoscopy

Available Dosage Forms

Kit [each kit contains]:

HalfLytely® and Bisacodyl:

Powder for solution, oral (HalfLytely®): PEG 3350 210 g, sodium bicarbonate 2.86 g, sodium chloride 5.6 g, potassium chloride 0.74 g (2000 mL) [contains 4 flavor packs (each 1 g) cherry, lemon-lime, orange, pineapple flavors]

Tablet, delayed release (Bisacodyl): 5 mg (1s)

General Dosage Range Oral: *Adults:* 5 mg of bisacodyl as a single dose, after bowel movement or 6 hours (whichever occurs first) initiate 8 ounces of polyethylene glycol-electrolyte solution every 10 minutes until 2 L are consumed

Administration

Oral Administer bisacodyl tablet with water; do not chew or crush tablet. Do not take antacids within 1 hour of taking bisacodyl. Rapidly drinking the polyethylene glycol-electrolyte solution is preferred to drinking small amount continuously. If severe bloating, distention, or abdominal pain occurs, administration should be slowed or temporarily discontinued until symptoms resolve.

Nursing Actions

Patient Education See individual agents.

Posaconazole (poe sa KON a zole)

Brand Names: U.S. Noxafil®

Index Terms SCH 56592

Pharmacologic Category Antifungal Agent, Oral

Medication Safety Issues

Sound-alike/look-alike issues:

Noxafil® may be confused with minoxidil

International issues:

Noxafil [U.S. and multiple international markets] may be confused with Noxidil brand name for minoxidil [Thailand]

Pregnancy Risk Factor C

Lactation Excretion in breast milk unknown/not recommended

Breast-Feeding Considerations Excretion in breast milk has not been investigated; use only if the benefit to the mother justifies potential risk to the fetus.

Use Prophylaxis of invasive *Aspergillus* and *Candida* infections in severely-immunocompromised patients [eg, hematopoietic stem cell transplant (HSCT) recipients with graft-versus-host disease (GVHD) or those with prolonged neutropenia secondary to chemotherapy for hematologic malignancies]; treatment of oropharyngeal candidiasis (including patients refractory to itraconazole and/or fluconazole)

Unlabeled Use Salvage therapy of refractory or relapsed invasive fungal infections; mucormycosis; pulmonary infection (nonimmunosuppressed)

Mechanism of Action/Effect Interferes with fungal cytochrome P450 (latosterol-14α-demethylase) activity, decreasing ergosterol synthesis (principal sterol in fungal cell membrane) and inhibiting fungal cell membrane formation.

Contraindications Hypersensitivity to posaconazole, other azole antifungals, or any component of the formulation; coadministration of cisapride, ergot alkaloids, pimozide, quinidine, simvastatin, or sirolimus

Warnings/Precautions Hepatic dysfunction has occurred, ranging from reversible mild/moderate increases of ALT, AST, alkaline phosphatase, total bilirubin, and/or clinical hepatitis to severe reactions (cholestasis, hepatic failure including death). Consider discontinuation of therapy in patients who develop clinical evidence of liver disease that may be secondary to posaconazole. Use caution in patients with an increased risk of arrhythmia (long QT syndrome, concurrent QT_c-prolonging drugs, hypokalemia). Correct electrolyte abnormalities (eg, potassium, magnesium, and calcium) before initiating therapy. Concurrent use with cyclosporine or tacrolimus may significantly increase cyclosporine/tacrolimus concentrations and may result in rare serious adverse events (eg, nephrotoxicity, leukoencephalopathy, and death); dose reduction and close monitoring are recommended with initiation of posaconazole therapy. Concurrent use with midazolam may increase midazolam concentrations and potentiate midazolam-related adverse effects.

Use caution in hypersensitivity with other azole antifungal agents; cross-reaction may occur, but has not been established. Consider alternative therapy or closely monitor for breakthrough fungal infections in patients receiving drugs that decrease absorption or increase the metabolism of posaconazole or in any patient unable to eat or tolerate an oral liquid nutritional supplement. Use caution in severe renal impairment or GI disturbances; monitor for breakthrough fungal infections.

Drug Interactions

Avoid Concomitant Use

Avoid concomitant use of Posaconazole with any of the following: Alfuzosin; Axitinib; Cisapride; Conivaptan; Crizotinib; Dofetilide; Dronedarone; Efavirenz; Eplerenone; Ergot Derivatives; Everolimus; Fluticasone (Oral Inhalation); Halofantrine; Lapatinib; Lovastatin; Lurasidone; Nilotinib; Nisoldipine; Pimozide; Proton Pump Inhibitors; QuiNIDine; Ranolazine; Rivaroxaban; RomiDEPsin; Salmeterol; Silodosin; Simvastatin; Sirolimus; Tamsulosin; Ticagrelor; Tolvaptan; Toremifene

Decreased Effect

Posaconazole may decrease the levels/effects of: Amphotericin B; Prasugrel; Saccharomyces boulardii; Ticagrelor

The levels/effects of Posaconazole may be decreased by: Didanosine; Efavirenz; Etravirine; Fosamprenavir; Fosphenytoin; H2-Antagonists; Metoclopramide; Phenytoin; Proton Pump Inhibitors; Rifamycin Derivatives; Sucralfate

Increased Effect/Toxicity

Posaconazole may increase the levels/effects of: Alfentanil; Alfuzosin; Almotriptan; Alosetron; Antineoplastic Agents (Vinca Alkaloids); Aprepitant; ARIPiprazole; Axitinib; Benzodiazepines (metabolized by oxidation); Boceprevir; Bortezomib; Bosentan; Brentuximab Vedotin; Brinzolamide; Budesonide (Nasal); Budesonide (Systemic, Oral Inhalation); BusPIRone; Busulfan; Calcium Channel Blockers; CarBAMazepine; Cardiac Glycosides; Ciclesonide; Cilostazol; Cinacalcet; Cisapride; Colchicine; Conivaptan; Corticosteroids (Orally Inhaled); Corticosteroids (Systemic); Crizotinib; CycloSPORINE; CycloSPORINE (Systemic); CYP3A4 Substrates; Dienogest; DOCEtaxel; Dofetilide; Dronedarone; Dutasteride; Eletriptan; Eplerenone; Ergot Derivatives; Erlotinib; Eszopiclone; Etravirine; Everolimus; FentaNYL; Fesoterodine; Fluticasone (Nasal); Fluticasone (Oral Inhalation); Fosamprenavir; Fosaprepitant; Fosphenytoin; Gefitinib; GlipiZIDE; GuanFACINE; Halofantrine; HMG-CoA Reductase Inhibitors; Iloperidone; Imatinib; Irinotecan; Ivacaftor; Ixabepilone; Lapatinib; Losartan; Lovastatin; Lumefantrine; Lurasidone; Macrolide Antibiotics; Maraviroc; Methadone; MethylPREDNISolone; Nilotinib; Nisoldipine; Paricalcitol; Pazopanib; Phenytoin; Phosphodiesterase 5 Inhibitors; Pimecrolimus; Pimozide; Propafenone; Protease Inhibitors; QuiNIDine; Ramelteon; Ranolazine; Repaglinide; Rifamycin Derivatives; Rivaroxaban; RomiDEPsin; Ruxolitinib; Salmeterol; Saxagliptin; Sildenafil; Silodosin; Simvastatin; Sirolimus; Solifenacin; SORAfenib; SUNItinib; Tacrolimus; Tacrolimus (Systemic); Tacrolimus (Topical); Tadalafil; Tamsulosin; Telaprevir; Temsirolimus; Ticagrelor; Tolterodine; Tolvaptan; Toremifene; Vardenafil; Vemurafenib; Vilazodone; Vitamin K Antagonists; Ziprasidone; Zolpidem; Zuclopenthixol

The levels/effects of Posaconazole may be increased by: Boceprevir; Etravirine; Grapefruit Juice; Macrolide Antibiotics; Protease Inhibitors; Tacrolimus; Telaprevir

Nutritional/Ethanol Interactions Food: Bioavailability increased ~3 times when posaconazole is administered with a nonfat meal or an oral liquid nutritional supplement; increased ~4 times when administered with a high-fat meal. Grapefruit juice may decrease the levels/effects of posaconazole. Management: Must be administered with or within 20 minutes of a full meal or an oral liquid nutritional supplement, or may be administered with an acidic carbonated beverage (eg, ginger ale). Consider alternative antifungal therapy in patients with inadequate oral intake or severe diarrhea/vomiting. Avoid concurrent use of grapefruit juice.

Adverse Reactions Note: Percentages reflect data from use in comparator trials with multiple concomitant conditions and medications; some adverse reactions may be due to underlying condition(s).

>10%:

Cardiovascular: Hypertension (18%), edema (9% to 15%), hypotension (14%), tachycardia (12%)

Central nervous system: Fever (6% to 45%), headache (8% to 28%), fatigue (3% to 17%), insomnia (1% to 17%), dizziness (11%), pain (1% to 11%)

Endocrine & metabolic: Hypokalemia (≤30%), hypomagnesemia (18%), dehydration (1% to 11%), hyperglycemia (11%)

Gastrointestinal: Diarrhea (10% to 42%), nausea (9% to 38%), vomiting (7% to 29%), abdominal pain (5% to 27%), constipation (21%), anorexia (2% to 19%), mucositis (17%), weight loss (1% to 14%), oral candidiasis (1% to 12%)

Hematologic: Thrombocytopenia (29%), anemia (2% to 25%), neutropenia (4% to 23%), neutropenic fever (20%)

Hepatic: ALT increased (6% to 17%)

Neuromuscular & skeletal: Rigors (≤20%), musculoskeletal pain (16%), weakness (2% to 13%), arthralgia (11%)

Respiratory: Cough (3% to 25%), dyspnea (1% to 20%), epistaxis (14%), pharyngitis (12%)

Miscellaneous: Bacteremia (18%), herpes simplex (3% to 15%), CMV infection (14%)

1% to 10%:

Central nervous system: Anxiety (9%)

Endocrine & metabolic: Hypocalcemia (9%)

Gastrointestinal: Dyspepsia (10%)

Genitourinary: Vaginal hemorrhage (10%)

Hepatic: Hyperbilirubinemia (7% to 10%), AST increased (3% to 4%), alkaline phosphatase increased (1% to 3%)

Neuromuscular & skeletal: Back pain (10%)

Respiratory: Pneumonia (3% to 10%), upper respiratory infection (7%)
Miscellaneous: Diaphoresis (2% to 10%)

Available Dosage Forms

Suspension, oral:
Noxafil®: 40 mg/mL (123 mL)

General Dosage Range Oral: *Children ≥13 years and Adults:* 100-800 mg/day; doses >100 mg/day are given in 2-3 divided doses

Administration

Oral Shake well before use. Must be administered during or within 20 minutes following a full meal or an oral liquid nutritional supplement; alternatively, posaconazole may be administered with an acidic carbonated beverage (eg, ginger ale). In patients able to swallow, administer oral suspension using dosing spoon provided by the manufacturer; spoon should be rinsed clean with water after each use and before storage.

Stability

Storage Store at 25°C (77°F); excursions permitted to 15°C to 30°C (59°F to 86°F). Do not freeze.

Nursing Actions

Physical Assessment Monitor for gastrointestinal disturbance, vision changes, hepatic toxicity (increased liver enzymes, jaundice), and CNS changes on a regular basis during therapy.

Patient Education Take preferably during or immediately after a full meal or liquid nutritional supplement (can alternatively be taken with an acidic carbonated beverage, such as ginger ale). Take full course of medication; fungal infections may take weeks or months of therapy. Maintain adequate hydration unless instructed to restrict fluid intake. You may experience nausea, vomiting, abdominal pain, loss of appetite, constipation, headache, dizziness, blurred vision, or insomnia. Report immediately chest pain or palpitations, unusual muscle pain or weakness, severe diarrhea or vomiting, urinary pattern changes, yellowing of skin or eyes, or changes in color of stool or urine.

Dietary Considerations Give during or within 20 minutes following a full meal or liquid nutritional supplement; alternatively, posaconazole may be administered with an acidic carbonated beverage (eg, ginger ale). Consider alternative antifungal therapy in patients with inadequate oral intake or severe diarrhea/vomiting; if alternative therapy is not an option, closely monitoring for breakthrough fungal infections. Adequate posaconazole absorption from GI tract and subsequent plasma concentrations are dependent on food for efficacy. Lower average plasma concentrations have been associated with an increased risk of treatment failure.

Potassium Bicarbonate

(poe TASS ee um bye KAR bun ate)

Brand Names: U.S. K-Effervescent

Pharmacologic Category Electrolyte Supplement, Oral

Pregnancy Risk Factor C

Use Potassium deficiency, hypokalemia

Available Dosage Forms

Tablet for solution, oral: Potassium 25 mEq
K-Effervescent: Potassium 25 mEq

General Dosage Range Oral:
Children: 1-4 mEq/kg/day
Adults: 25 mEq 2-4 times/day

Potassium Bicarbonate and Potassium Chloride

(poe TASS ee um bye KAR bun ate & poe TASS ee um KLOR ide)

Index Terms K-Lyte/Cl; Potassium Bicarbonate and Potassium Chloride (Effervescent)

Pharmacologic Category Electrolyte Supplement, Oral

Pregnancy Risk Factor C

Lactation Enters breast milk/compatible

Use Treatment or prevention of hypokalemia

Available Dosage Forms

Tablet for solution, oral [effervescent]: Potassium chloride 25 mEq

General Dosage Range

Oral:
Children: 1-4 mEq/kg/day in divided doses
Adults: Prevention: 16-24 mEq/day in 2-4 divided doses; Treatment: 40-100 mEq/day in 2-4 divided doses

Administration

Oral Administer with meals; solution should be sipped slowly, over 5-10 minutes

Nursing Actions

Physical Assessment See individual agents.

Patient Education See individual agents.

Related Information

Potassium Bicarbonate *on page 933*
Potassium Chloride *on page 934*

Potassium Bicarbonate and Potassium Citrate

(poe TASS ee um bye KAR bun ate & poe TASS ee um SIT rate)

Brand Names: U.S. Effer-K®; Klor-Con®/EF

Index Terms Potassium Bicarbonate and Potassium Citrate (Effervescent)

Pharmacologic Category Electrolyte Supplement, Oral

Medication Safety Issues

Sound-alike/look-alike issues:
Klor-Con® may be confused with Klaron®

Pregnancy Risk Factor C

Use Treatment or prevention of hypokalemia

Available Dosage Forms

Tablet for solution, oral [effervescent]:
Effer-K®: Potassium 10 mEq; potassium 20 mEq; potassium 25 mEq
Klor-Con®/EF: Potassium 25 mEq

General Dosage Range

Oral:

Children: 1-4 mEq/kg/day in divided doses

Adults: Prevention: 16-24 mEq/day in 2-4 divided doses; Treatment: 40-100 mEq/day in 2-4 divided doses

Nursing Actions

Physical Assessment See individual agents.

Patient Education See individual agents.

Related Information

Potassium Bicarbonate *on page 933*

Potassium Citrate *on page 935*

Potassium Chloride (poe TASS ee um KLOR ide)

Brand Names: U.S. Epiklor™; Epiklor™/25; K-Tab®; Kaon-CL® 10; Klor-Con®; Klor-Con® 10; Klor-Con® 8; Klor-Con® M10; Klor-Con® M15; Klor-Con® M20; Klor-Con®/25; microK®; microK® 10

Index Terms KCl; Kdur

Pharmacologic Category Electrolyte Supplement, Oral; Electrolyte Supplement, Parenteral

Medication Safety Issues

Sound-alike/look-alike issues:

Kaon-Cl-10® may be confused with kaolin

KCl may be confused with HCl

Klor-Con® may be confused with Klaron®

microK® may be confused with Macrobid®, Micronase

High alert medication:

The Institute for Safe Medication Practices (ISMP) includes this medication (I.V. formulation) among its list of drugs which have a heightened risk of causing significant patient harm when used in error.

Other safety concerns:

Per JCAHO recommendations, concentrated electrolyte solutions should not be available in patient care areas.

Consider special storage requirements for intravenous potassium salts; I.V. potassium salts have been administered IVP in error, leading to fatal outcomes.

Pregnancy Risk Factor C

Lactation Enters breast milk/not recommended

Breast-Feeding Considerations Potassium is excreted into breast milk (IOM, 2004). The normal content of potassium in human milk is ~13 mEq/L. Supplementation (that does not cause maternal hyperkalemia) would not be expected to affect normal concentrations.

Use Treatment or prevention of hypokalemia

Contraindications Hypersensitivity to any component of the formulation; hyperkalemia. In addition, solid oral dosage forms are contraindicated in patients in whom there is a structural, pathological, and/or pharmacologic cause for delay or arrest in passage through the GI tract.

Warnings/Precautions Close monitoring of serum potassium concentrations is needed to avoid hyperkalemia. Use with caution in patients with renal impairment, cardiac disease, acid/base disorders, or potassium-altering conditions/disorders. Use with caution in digitalized patients or patients receiving concomitant medications or therapies that increase potassium (eg, ACEI, potassium-sparing diuretics, potassium containing salt substitutes). Do **NOT** administer undiluted or I.V. push; inappropriate parenteral administration may be fatal. Always administer potassium further diluted; refer to appropriate dilution and administration rate recommendations. Pain and phlebitis may occur during parenteral infusion requiring a decrease in infusion rate or potassium concentration. Avoid administering potassium diluted in dextrose solutions during initial therapy; potential for transient decreases in serum potassium due to intracellular shift of potassium from dextrose-stimulated insulin release. May cause GI upset (eg, nausea, vomiting, diarrhea, abdominal pain, discomfort) and lead to GI ulceration, bleeding, perforation, and/or obstruction. Oral liquid preparations (not solid) should be used in patients with esophageal compression or delayed gastric emptying.

Drug Interactions

Avoid Concomitant Use

Avoid concomitant use of Potassium Chloride with any of the following: Glycopyrrolate

Decreased Effect There are no known significant interactions involving a decrease in effect.

Increased Effect/Toxicity

Potassium Chloride may increase the levels/effects of: ACE Inhibitors; Angiotensin II Receptor Blockers; Potassium-Sparing Diuretics

The levels/effects of Potassium Chloride may be increased by: Anticholinergic Agents; Eplerenone; Glycopyrrolate

Adverse Reactions Frequency not defined.

Dermatologic: Rash

Endocrine & metabolic: Hyperkalemia

Gastrointestinal: Abdominal pain/discomfort, diarrhea, flatulence, GI bleeding (oral), GI obstruction (oral), GI perforation (oral), nausea, vomiting

Available Dosage Forms

Capsule, extended release, microencapsulated, oral: 8 mEq, 10 mEq

microK®: 8 mEq

microK® 10: 10 mEq

Infusion, premixed in 1/2 NS: 20 mEq (1000 mL)

Infusion, premixed in D_5 1/2 NS: 10 mEq (500 mL, 1000 mL); 20 mEq (1000 mL); 30 mEq (1000 mL); 40 mEq (1000 mL)

Infusion, premixed in D_5 1/3 NS: 20 mEq (1000 mL)

Infusion, premixed in D_5 1/4 NS: 5 mEq (250 mL); 10 mEq (500 mL, 1000 mL); 20 mEq (1000 mL); 40 mEq (1000 mL)

Infusion, premixed in D_5LR: 20 mEq (1000 mL)

Infusion, premixed in D_5NS: 20 mEq (1000 mL); 40 mEq (1000 mL)

Infusion, premixed in D_5W: 20 mEq (500 mL, 1000 mL); 40 mEq (1000 mL)

Infusion, premixed in NS: 20 mEq (1000 mL); 40 mEq (1000 mL)

Infusion, premixed in water for injection: 10 mEq (50 mL, 100 mL); 20 mEq (50 mL, 100 mL); 30 mEq (100 mL); 40 mEq (100 mL)

Injection, solution: 2 mEq/mL (5 mL, 10 mL, 15 mL, 20 mL, 30 mL, 250 mL, 500 mL)

Injection, solution [preservative free]: 2 mEq/mL (5 mL, 10 mL, 15 mL, 20 mL)

Powder for solution, oral:
Epiklor™: 20 mEq/packet (30s, 100s)
Epiklor™/25: 25 mEq/packet (30s, 100s)
Klor-Con®: 20 mEq/packet (30s, 100s)
Klor-Con®/25: 25 mEq/packet (30s, 100s)

Solution, oral: 20 mEq/15 mL (15 mL, 30 mL, 473 mL, 480 mL); 40 mEq/15 mL (15 mL, 473 mL)

Tablet, extended release, oral: 10 mEq

Tablet, extended release, microencapsulated, oral: 8 mEq, 10 mEq, 20 mEq
Klor-Con® M10: 10 mEq
Klor-Con® M15: 15 mEq
Klor-Con® M20: 20 mEq

Tablet, extended release, wax matrix, oral: 8 mEq, 10 mEq
K-Tab®: 10 mEq
Kaon-CL® 10: 10 mEq
Klor-Con® 8: 8 mEq
Klor-Con® 10: 10 mEq

General Dosage Range

I.V.:

Children: Initial: 0.5-1 mEq/kg/dose (maximum dose: 40 mEq); repeat as needed based on lab values

Adults: Intermittent infusion: ≤10 mEq/hour; repeat as needed based on lab values (maximum: 200 mEq/day)

Oral:

Children: 1-2 mEq/kg/day in 1-2 divided doses or as needed based on lab values

Adults: Initial: 6-10 mEq/dose (maximum: 40 mEq/dose); Maintenance: 40-100 mEq/day in divided doses or as needed based on lab values

Administration

Oral Oral dosage forms should be taken with meals and a full glass of water or other liquid to minimize the risk of GI irritation. Prescribing information for the various oral preparations recommend that no more than 20 mEq or 25 mEq should be given as single dose.

Capsule: MicroK®: Swallow whole, do not chew. Capsules may also be opened and contents sprinkled on a spoonful of applesauce or pudding and should be swallowed immediately without chewing.

Powder: Klor-Con®: Dissolve one packet in 4-5 ounces of water or other beverage prior to administration.

Tablet:
K-Tab®, Kaon-Cl®, Klor-Con®: Swallow tablets whole; do not crush, chew, or suck on tablet.
Klor-Con® M: Swallow tablets whole; do not crush, chew, or suck on tablet. Tablet may also be broken in half and each half swallowed separately; the whole tablet may be dissolved in ~4 ounces of water (allow ~2 minutes to dissolve, stir well and drink immediately)

I.V. Potassium must be diluted prior to parenteral administration. Do not administer I.V. push. In general, the dose, concentration of infusion and rate of administration may be dependent on patient condition and specific institution policy. Some clinicians recommend that the maximum concentration for peripheral infusion is 10 mEq/100 mL and maximum rate of administration for peripheral infusion is 10 mEq/hour. ECG monitoring is recommended for peripheral or central infusions >10 mEq/hour in adults. Concentrations and rates of infusion may be greater with central line administration. Some clinicians recommend that the maximum concentration for central infusion is 20-40 mEq/100 mL and maximum rate of administration for central infusion is 40 mEq/hour.

Stability

Storage

Capsule: MicroK®: Store between 20°C to 25°C (68°F to 77°F).

Powder for oral solution: Klor-Con®: Store at room temperature of 15°C to 30°C (59°F to 86°F).

Solution for injection: Store at room temperature; do not freeze. Use only clear solutions. Use admixtures within 24 hours.

Tablet: K-Tab®: Store below 30°C (86°F).

Nursing Actions

Physical Assessment Monitor infusion site closely.

Patient Education Long-acting and wax matrix tablets should be swallowed whole; do not crush or chew. Powder must be dissolved in water before use. Liquid can be diluted or dissolved in water or juice. Take with food to avoid GI irritation and upset. Report abdominal pain, nausea, or vomiting.

Dietary Considerations Administer with plenty of fluid to decrease stomach irritation and discomfort. Some dietary sources of potassium include leafy green vegetables (eg, spinach, cabbage), tomatoes, cucumbers, zucchini, fruits (eg, apples, oranges, and bananas), root vegetables (eg, carrots, radishes), beans, and peas.

Related Information

Compatibility of Drugs *on page 1264*
Management of Drug Extravasations *on page 1269*

Potassium Citrate (poe TASS ee um SIT rate)

Brand Names: U.S. Urocit®-K

Pharmacologic Category Alkalinizing Agent, Oral

Medication Safety Issues

Sound-alike/look-alike issues:

Urocit®-K may be confused with Urised

Pregnancy Risk Factor C

Lactation Excreted in breast milk/not recommended

Use Prevention of uric acid nephrolithiasis; prevention of calcium renal stones in patients with hypocitraturia; urinary alkalinizer when sodium citrate is contraindicated

Available Dosage Forms

Tablet, extended release, oral: 540 mg, 1080 mg

Urocit®-K: 540 mg, 1080 mg, 1620 mg

General Dosage Range Oral: *Adults:*

Immediate release: 10-20 mEq 3 times/day or 15 mEq 4 times/day (maximum: 100 mEq/day)

Extended release: 15-30 mEq 2 times/day or 10-20 mEq 3 times/day (maximum: 100 mEq/day)

Administration

Oral Administer with meals or bedtime snack (or within 30 minutes after). Swallow tablets whole with a full glass of water.

Nursing Actions

Physical Assessment Assess kidney function prior to treatment. Monitor cardiac status and serum potassium prior to treatment and at regular intervals.

Patient Education Swallow tablet whole with full glass of water with (or within 30 minutes after) meals or a bedtime snack (do not take on an empty stomach). Take any antacids 2 hours before or after potassium. Consult prescriber about advisability of increasing dietary potassium. Report unresolved nausea or vomiting, chest pain or palpitations, persistent abdominal pain, feelings of weakness, dizziness, acute muscle weakness, or cramping.

Potassium Iodide (poe TASS ee um EYE oh dide)

Brand Names: U.S. iOSAT™ [OTC]; SSKI®; ThyroSafe® [OTC]; Thyroshield® [OTC]

Index Terms KI

Pharmacologic Category Antithyroid Agent; Expectorant

Medication Safety Issues

Sound-alike/look-alike issues:

Potassium iodide products, including saturated solution of potassium iodide (SSKI®) may be confused with potassium iodide and iodine (Strong Iodide Solution or Lugol's solution)

Pregnancy Risk Factor D

Lactation Enters breast milk/use caution (AAP rates "compatible"; AAP 2001 update pending)

Use Expectorant for the symptomatic treatment of chronic pulmonary diseases complicated by mucous; block thyroidal uptake of radioactive isotopes of iodine in a radiation emergency

Unlabeled Use Lymphocutaneous and cutaneous sporotrichosis; reduce thyroid vascularity prior to thyroidectomy; management of thyrotoxic crisis; block thyroidal uptake of radioactive isotopes of iodine after therapeutic or diagnostic exposure to radioactive iodine

Available Dosage Forms

Solution, oral:

SSKI®: 1 g/mL (30 mL, 237 mL)

Thyroshield® [OTC]: 65 mg/mL (30 mL)

Tablet, oral:

iOSAT™ [OTC]: 130 mg

ThyroSafe® [OTC]: 65 mg

General Dosage Range Oral:

Infants 1-12 months and Children 1-3 years: Iosat™, ThyroSafe®, ThyroShield®: 32.5 mg once daily

Children 3-18 years: Iosat™, ThyroSafe®, ThyroShield®: 65-130 mg once daily

Adults: Iosat™, ThyroSafe®, ThyroShield®: 130 mg once daily; SSKI®: 300-600 mg (6-12 drops) 3-4 times/day

Administration

Oral SSKI®: Dilute in a glassful of water, fruit juice, or milk. Take with food to decrease gastric irritation.

Nursing Actions

Patient Education SSKI®: Dilute in water, fruit juice, or milk and take with meals to reduce gastric irritation. May cause metallic taste, nausea, or vomiting; soreness of teeth, gums, or glands; fever, headache, or sore joints; or confusion or tiredness. Discontinue and report if you experience any swelling of lips, mouth, or tongue; difficulty swallowing; chest pain or irregular heartbeat; unusual muscle weakness; eye irritation or eyelid swelling; or skin rash.

Potassium Iodide and Iodine

(poe TASS ee um EYE oh dide & EYE oh dine)

Index Terms Iodine and Potassium Iodide; Lugol's Solution; Strong Iodine Solution

Pharmacologic Category Antithyroid Agent

Medication Safety Issues

Sound-alike/look-alike issues:

Potassium iodide and iodine (Strong Iodide Solution or Lugol's solution) may be confused with potassium iodide products, including saturated solution of potassium iodide (SSKI®)

Pregnancy Risk Factor D (potassium iodide)

Lactation Enters breast milk/use caution (AAP rates "compatible"; AAP 2001 update pending)

Use Topical antiseptic

Unlabeled Use Reduce thyroid vascularity prior to thyroidectomy and management of thyrotoxic crisis; block thyroidal uptake of radioactive isotopes of iodine in a radiation emergency or after therapeutic/diagnostic use of radioactive iodine

Available Dosage Forms

Solution, oral: Potassium iodide 100 mg/mL and iodine 50 mg/mL (473 mL)

Solution, topical: Potassium iodide 100 mg/mL and iodine 50 mg/mL (8 mL)

General Dosage Range Oral:

Children: 4-8 drops 3 times/day

Adults: Dosing varies greatly depending on indication

Nursing Actions

Patient Education See individual agents.

Potassium Phosphate

(poe TASS ee um FOS fate)

Brand Names: U.S. Neutra-Phos®-K [OTC] [DSC]

Index Terms Phosphate, Potassium

Pharmacologic Category Electrolyte Supplement, Parenteral

Medication Safety Issues

High alert medication:

The Institute for Safe Medication Practices (ISMP) includes this medication (I.V. formulation) among its list of drugs which have a heightened risk of causing significant patient harm when used in error.

Other safety concerns:

Per JCAHO recommendations, concentrated electrolyte solutions should not be available in patient care areas.

Consider special storage requirements for intravenous potassium salts; I.V. potassium salts have been administered IVP in error, leading to fatal outcomes.

Safe Prescribing: Because inorganic phosphate exists as monobasic and dibasic anions, with the mixture of valences dependent on pH, ordering by mEq amounts is unreliable and may lead to large dosing errors. In addition, I.V. phosphate is available in the sodium and potassium salt; therefore, the content of these cations must be considered when ordering phosphate. The most reliable method of ordering I.V. phosphate is by millimoles, then specifying the potassium or sodium salt. For example, an order for 15 mmol of phosphate as potassium phosphate in one liter of normal saline.

Pregnancy Risk Factor C

Breast-Feeding Considerations Phosphorus, sodium, and potassium are normal constituents of human milk.

Use Treatment and prevention of hypophosphatemia; **Note:** The concomitant amount of potassium must be calculated into the total electrolyte content. For each 1 mmol of phosphate, ~1.5 mEq of potassium will be administered. Therefore, if ordering 30 mmol of potassium phosphate, the patient will receive ~45 mEq of potassium.

Contraindications Hyperphosphatemia, hyperkalemia, hypocalcemia, hypomagnesemia, renal failure (oral product)

Warnings/Precautions Close monitoring of serum potassium concentrations is needed to avoid hyperkalemia. Use with caution in patients with renal insufficiency, cardiac disease, metabolic alkalosis. Use with caution in digitalized patients and patients receiving concomitant potassium-altering therapies. Parenteral potassium may cause pain and phlebitis, requiring a decrease in infusion rate or potassium concentration. Solutions for injection may contain aluminum; toxic levels may occur following prolonged administration in premature neonates or patients with renal impairment.

Drug Interactions

Avoid Concomitant Use There are no known interactions where it is recommended to avoid concomitant use.

Decreased Effect There are no known significant interactions involving a decrease in effect.

Increased Effect/Toxicity

Potassium Phosphate may increase the levels/effects of: ACE Inhibitors; Angiotensin II Receptor Blockers; Potassium-Sparing Diuretics

The levels/effects of Potassium Phosphate may be increased by: Bisphosphonate Derivatives; Eplerenone

Nutritional/Ethanol Interactions Food: Avoid administering with oxalate (berries, nuts, chocolate, beans, celery, tomato) or phytate-containing foods (bran, whole wheat).

Adverse Reactions Frequency not defined.

Cardiovascular: Arrhythmia, bradycardia, chest pain, ECG changes, edema, heart block, hypotension

Central nervous system: Listlessness, mental confusion, tetany (with large doses of phosphate)

Endocrine & metabolic: Hyperkalemia

Gastrointestinal: Diarrhea, nausea, stomach pain, vomiting

Genitourinary: Urine output decreased

Local: Phlebitis

Neuromuscular & skeletal: Paralysis, paresthesia, weakness

Renal: Acute renal failure

Respiratory: Dyspnea

Available Dosage Forms

Injection, solution: Potassium 4.4 mEq and phosphorus 3 mmol per mL (5 mL, 15 mL, 50 mL)

General Dosage Range

I.V.:

Children: 0.08-1 mmol phosphate/kg **or** Parenteral nutrition Infusion: 0.5-2 mmol/kg/24 hours

Adults: 0.08-1 mmol phosphate/kg **or** Parenteral nutrition: Infusion: 20-40 mmol/24 hours

Administration

I.V. Injection must be diluted in appropriate I.V. solution and volume prior to administration. In general, the dose, concentration of infusion, and rate of administration may be dependent on patient condition and specific institution policy.

Must consider administration precautions for phosphate and potassium when prescribing.

For adult patients with severe symptomatic hypophosphatemia (ie, <1.5 mg/dL), may administer at rates up to 15 mmol phosphate/hour (this rate will deliver potassium at 22.5 mEq/hour) (Rosen, 1995, Charron, 2003). Potassium infusion rates >10 mEq/hour should be administered via central line (minimizes burning and phlebitis). ECG monitoring is recommended for potassium infusions >10 mEq/hour in adults or >0.5 mEq/kg/hour in children. In patients with renal dysfunction and/or less severe hypophosphatemia, slower administration rates (eg, over 4-6 hours) or oral repletion is recommended.

Intermittent infusion doses of potassium phosphate are typically prepared in 100-250 mL of NS or D_5W (usual phosphate concentration range: 0.15 - 0.6 mmol/mL) (Charron, 2003; Rosen, 1995). Suggested maximum concentrations:

Peripheral line administration: 6.7 mmoL potassium phosphate/100 mL (10 mEq potassium/100 mL)

Central line administration: 26.8 mmoL potassium phosphate/100 mL (40 mEq potassium/100 mL)

Stability

Storage Store at room temperature; do not freeze. Use only clear solutions. Up to 10-15 mEq of calcium may be added per liter before precipitate may occur.

Stability of parenteral admixture at room temperature (25°C) is 24 hours.

Phosphate salts may precipitate when mixed with calcium salts. Solubility is improved in amino acid parenteral nutrition solutions. Check with a pharmacist to determine compatibility.

Related Information

Compatibility of Drugs *on page 1264*

Potassium Phosphate and Sodium Phosphate

(poe TASS ee um FOS fate & SOW dee um FOS fate)

Brand Names: U.S. K-Phos® MF; K-Phos® Neutral; K-Phos® No. 2; Phos-NaK; Phospha 250™ Neutral

Index Terms Neutra-Phos; Sodium Phosphate and Potassium Phosphate

Pharmacologic Category Electrolyte Supplement, Oral

Medication Safety Issues

Sound-alike/look-alike issues:

K-Phos® Neutral may be confused with Neutra-Phos-K®

Pregnancy Risk Factor C

Use Treatment of conditions associated with excessive renal phosphate loss or inadequate GI absorption of phosphate; to acidify the urine to lower calcium concentrations; to increase the antibacterial activity of methenamine; reduce odor and rash caused by ammonia in urine

Available Dosage Forms

Powder for solution, oral:

Phos-NaK: Dibasic potassium phosphate, monobasic potassium phosphate, dibasic sodium phosphate, and monobasic sodium phosphate per packet (100s)

Tablet, oral:

K-Phos® MF: Potassium phosphate 155 mg and sodium phosphate 350 mg

K-Phos® Neutral: Monobasic potassium phosphate 155 mg, dibasic sodium phosphate 852 mg, and monobasic sodium phosphate 130 mg

K-Phos® No. 2: Potassium phosphate 305 mg and sodium phosphate 700 mg

Phospha 250™ Neutral: Monobasic potassium phosphate 155 mg, dibasic sodium phosphate 852 mg, and monobasic sodium phosphate 130 mg

General Dosage Range Oral: *Children ≥4 years and Adults:* Elemental phosphorus 250 mg 4 times/day after meals and at bedtime

Administration

Oral Administer with food to reduce risk of diarrhea.

Powder: Phos-NaK: Contents of 1 packet should be diluted in 75 mL water before administration. Following dilution of powder, solution may be chilled to increase palatability.

Tablet: Should be taken with a full glass of water.

Nursing Actions

Patient Education See individual agents.

Related Information

Potassium Phosphate *on page 937*

Pralatrexate (pral a TREX ate)

Brand Names: U.S. Folotyn®

Index Terms PDX

Pharmacologic Category Antineoplastic Agent, Antimetabolite (Antifolate)

Medication Safety Issues

Sound-alike/look-alike issues:

PRALAtrexate may be confused with methotrexate, PEMEtrexed, raltitrexed

Folotyn® may be confused with Focalin®

High alert medication:

This medication is in a class the Institute for Safe Medication Practices (ISMP) includes among its list of drug classes which have a heightened risk of causing significant patient harm when used in error.

Pregnancy Risk Factor D

Lactation Excretion in breast milk unknown/not recommended

Use Treatment of relapsed or refractory peripheral T-cell lymphoma (PTCL)

Unlabeled Use Treatment of relapsed or refractory cutaneous T-cell lymphoma (CTCL)

Available Dosage Forms

Injection, solution [preservative free]:

Folotyn®: 20 mg/mL (1 mL, 2 mL)

General Dosage Range Dosage adjustment recommended in patients who develop toxicities

I.V.: *Adults:* 30 mg/m^2 once weekly for 6 weeks of a 7-week treatment cycle

Administration

I.V. Administer I.V. push over 3-5 minutes into the line of a free-flowing normal saline I.V.

I.V. Detail pH: 7.5-8.5

Nursing Actions

Physical Assessment Drugs with significant renal clearance may affect the levels/effects of pralatrexate. Monitor for mucositis, gastrointestinal disturbance, and renal or hepatic impairment.

Patient Education This drug is administered intravenously; report immediately any redness, swelling, pain, or burning at infusion/injection site. It is very important to maintain adequate nutrition and hydration, unless instructed to restrict fluid intake. You will be more susceptible to infection. May cause nausea, vomiting, fatigue or weakness, mouth sores, or limb or back pain. Report persistent or increasing gastrointestinal upset, mouth sores, rapid heartbeat or palpitations, black or tarry stools, fever, chills, unusual bleeding or bruising, shortness of breath, pain on urination, or change in urinary patterns.

Pramipexole (pra mi PEKS ole)

Brand Names: U.S. Mirapex®; Mirapex® ER®

Index Terms Pramipexole Dihydrochloride Monohydrate

Pharmacologic Category Anti-Parkinson's Agent, Dopamine Agonist

Medication Safety Issues

Sound-alike/look-alike issues:

Mirapex® may be confused with Hiprex®, Mifeprex®, MiraLax®

Pregnancy Risk Factor C

Lactation Excretion in breast milk unknown/not recommended

Breast-Feeding Considerations Prolactin secretion may be inhibited.

Use

Immediate release: Treatment of the signs and symptoms of idiopathic Parkinson's disease; treatment of moderate-to-severe primary Restless Legs Syndrome (RLS)

Extended release: Treatment of the signs and symptoms of idiopathic Parkinson's disease

Unlabeled Use Treatment of depression; treatment of fibromyalgia

Mechanism of Action/Effect Pramipexole is a nonergot dopamine agonist with specificity for the D_2 subfamily dopamine receptor, and has also been shown to bind to D_3 and D_4 receptors. By binding to these receptors, it is thought that pramipexole can stimulate dopamine activity on the nerves of the striatum and substantia nigra.

Contraindications Hypersensitivity to pramipexole or any component of the formulation

Warnings/Precautions Caution should be taken in patients with renal insufficiency; dose adjustment necessary. May cause or exacerbate dyskinesias; use caution in patients with pre-existing dyskinesias. May cause orthostatic hypotension; Parkinson's disease patients appear to have an impaired capacity to respond to a postural challenge. Use with caution in patients at risk of hypotension or where transient hypotensive episodes would be poorly tolerated. Parkinson's patients being treated with dopaminergic agonists ordinarily require careful monitoring for signs and symptoms of postural hypotension, especially during dose escalation. May cause hallucinations.

Dopamine agonists have been associated with compulsive behaviors and/or loss of impulse control, which has manifested as pathological gambling, libido increases (hypersexuality), and/or binge eating. Causality has not been established, and controversy exists as to whether this phenomenon is related to the underlying disease, prior behaviors/addictions and/or drug therapy. Dose reduction or discontinuation of therapy has been reported to reverse these behaviors in some, but not all cases. Risk for melanoma development is increased in Parkinson's disease patients; drug causation or factors contributing to risk have not been established. Patients should be monitored closely and periodic skin examinations should be performed.

Taper gradually over a period of 1 week when discontinuing therapy; dopaminergic agents have been associated with a syndrome resembling neuroleptic malignant syndrome on abrupt withdrawal or significant dosage reduction after long-term use. Ergot-derived dopamine agonists have been associated with fibrotic complications (eg, retroperitoneal fibrosis, pleural thickening, and pulmonary infiltrates). Although pramipexole is not an ergot, there have been postmarketing reports of possible fibrotic complications with pramipexole; monitor closely for signs and symptoms of fibrosis.

Pramipexole has been associated with somnolence, particularly at higher dosages (>1.5 mg/day). In addition, patients have been reported to fall asleep during activities of daily living, including driving, while taking this medication. Whether these patients exhibited somnolence prior to these events is not clear. Patients should be advised of this issue and factors which may increase risk (sleep disorders, other sedating medications, or concomitant medications which increase pramipexole concentrations) and instructed to report daytime somnolence or sleepiness to the prescriber. Patients should use caution in performing activities which require alertness (driving or operating machinery), and to avoid other medications which may cause CNS depression, including ethanol. Use caution in the elderly as they may be more sensitive to these adverse drug reactions.

Pathologic degenerative changes were observed in the retinas of albino rats during studies with this agent, but were not observed in the retinas of albino mice or in other species. The significance of these data for humans remains uncertain. Augmentation (earlier onset of symptoms in the evening/afternoon, increase and/or spread of symptoms to other extremities) or rebound (shifting of symptoms to early morning hours) may occur in some RLS patients.

Drug Interactions

Avoid Concomitant Use There are no known interactions where it is recommended to avoid concomitant use.

Decreased Effect

Pramipexole may decrease the levels/effects of: Antipsychotics (Typical)

The levels/effects of Pramipexole may be decreased by: Antipsychotics (Atypical); Metoclopramide

Increased Effect/Toxicity

Pramipexole may increase the levels/effects of: Alcohol (Ethyl); CNS Depressants; Selective Serotonin Reuptake Inhibitors

The levels/effects of Pramipexole may be increased by: Antipsychotics (Typical); Cimetidine; HydrOXYzine; MAO Inhibitors; Methylphenidate

Nutritional/Ethanol Interactions

Ethanol: May increase CNS depression; monitor for increased effects with coadministration. Caution patients about effects.

Food: Food intake does not affect the extent of drug absorption although the time to maximal plasma concentration is delayed when taken with a meal.

Herb/Nutraceutical: Avoid valerian, St John's wort, SAMe, kava kava (may increase risk of serotonin syndrome and/or excessive sedation).

Adverse Reactions

Parkinson's disease: Actual frequency may be dependent on dose and/or formulation:

>10%:

Cardiovascular: Postural hypotension (dose related; ≤53%)

Central nervous system: Somnolence (dose related; 9% to 36%), extrapyramidal syndrome (28%), insomnia (4% to 27%), dizziness (2% to 26%), hallucinations (5% to 17%), abnormal dreams (11%), headache (4% to 7%)

Gastrointestinal: Nausea (dose related; 11% to 28%), constipation (dose related; 6% to 14%)

Neuromuscular & skeletal: Dyskinesia (17% to 47%), weakness (1% to 14%)

1% to 10%:

Cardiovascular: Edema (2% to 8%), chest pain (3%)

Central nervous system: Confusion (4% to 10%), dystonia (2% to 8%), fatigue (6%), amnesia (dose related; 4% to 6%), sudden onset of sleep (3% to 6%), vertigo (2% to 4%), hypesthesia (3%), abnormal thinking (2% to 3%), akathisia (2% to 3%), malaise (2% to 3%), paranoia (2%), sleep disorder (1% to 3%), depression (≤2%), delusions (1%), fever (1%), myoclonus (1%)

Endocrine & metabolic: Libido decreased (1%)

Gastrointestinal: Xerostomia (4% to 7%), anorexia (1% to 5%), vomiting (4%), abdominal discomfort/pain (1% to 4%), dyspepsia (3%), appetite increased (2% to 3%), dysphagia (2%), weight loss (2%), salivary hypersecretion (≤2%), diarrhea (1% to 2%)

Genitourinary: Urinary frequency (6%), urinary tract infection (4%), impotence (2%), urinary incontinence (2%)

Neuromuscular & skeletal: Gait abnormalities (7%), hypertonia (7%), muscle spasm (3% to 5%), falls (4%), arthritis (3%), tremor (3%), back pain (2% to 3%), bursitis (2%), muscle twitching (2%), balance abnormalities (≤2%), CPK increased (1%), myasthenia (1%)

Ocular: Accommodation abnormalities (4%), vision abnormalities (3%), diplopia (1%)

Respiratory: Dyspnea (4%), cough (3%), rhinitis (3%), pneumonia (2%)

Restless legs syndrome: Actual frequency may be dependent on dose:

>10%:

Central nervous system: Headache (16%), insomnia (9% to 13%), abnormal dreams (1% to 8%), somnolence (6%)

Gastrointestinal: Nausea (11% to 27%), constipation (4%)

1% to 10%:

Central nervous system: Fatigue (3% to 9%)

Gastrointestinal: Diarrhea (1% to 7%), xerostomia (3%)

Neuromuscular & skeletal: Extremity pain (3% to 7%)

Respiratory: Nasal congestion (≤6%)

Miscellaneous: Influenza (1% to 7%)

Available Dosage Forms

Tablet, oral: 0.125 mg, 0.25 mg, 0.5 mg, 0.75 mg, 1 mg, 1.5 mg

Mirapex®: 0.125 mg, 0.25 mg, 0.5 mg, 0.75 mg, 1 mg, 1.5 mg

Tablet, extended release, oral:
Mirapex® ER®: 0.375 mg, 0.75 mg, 1.5 mg, 2.25 mg, 3 mg, 3.75 mg, 4.5 mg

General Dosage Range Dosage adjustment recommended in patients with renal impairment

Oral: Immediate release: *Adults:* Initial: 0.375 mg/day given in 3 divided doses **or** 0.125 mg once daily before bedtime; Maintenance: 1.5-4.5 mg/day in 3 divided doses **or** 0.125-0.5 mg/day

Oral: Extended release: *Adults:* Initial: 0.375-4.5 mg once daily

Administration

Oral Doses should be titrated gradually in all patients to avoid the onset of intolerable side effects. The dosage should be increased to achieve a maximum therapeutic effect, balanced against the side effects of dyskinesia, hallucinations, somnolence, and dry mouth. May be administered with or without food; may be administered with food to decrease nausea. Extended release tablets should be swallowed whole and not chewed, crushed, or divided.

Stability

Storage Store at 25°C (77°F); excursions permitted to 15°C to 30°C (59°F to 86°F). Protect from light and high humidity.

Nursing Actions

Physical Assessment Monitor blood pressure. Assess degree of somnolence.

Patient Education Avoid alcohol. May cause drowsiness and extreme sedation or somnolence, loss of impulse control (possibly manifested as pathological gambling, libido increases, and/or binge eating), postural hypotension, weakness, headache, nausea, abnormal dreams, dry mouth, nausea, hallucinations, new or increased occurrence of involuntary purposeless movements, constipation, or urinary frequency. Report to prescriber hallucinations, suicide ideation, changes in the appearance of skin moles or other unusual skin changes, or difficulty performing or controlling voluntary movements.

Dietary Considerations May be taken with or without food. May be taken with food to decrease nausea.

Pramlintide (PRAM lin tide)

Brand Names: U.S. SymlinPen®; Symlin® [DSC]

Index Terms Pramlintide Acetate

Pharmacologic Category Amylinomimetic; Antidiabetic Agent

Medication Safety Issues

High alert medication:

The Institute for Safe Medication Practices (ISMP) includes this medication among its list of drug classes which have a heightened risk of causing significant patient harm when used in error.

Administration issues:

Use caution when drawing up doses from the vial (concentration 600 micrograms (mcg)/mL). Manufacturer recommended dosing ranges from 15 mcg to 120 mcg, which corresponds to injectable volumes of 0.025 mL to 0.2 mL. Patients and healthcare providers should exercise caution when administering this product to avoid inadvertent calculation of the dose based on "units," which could result in a sixfold overdose.

Medication Guide Available Yes

Pregnancy Risk Factor C

Lactation Excretion in breast milk unknown/use caution

Breast-Feeding Considerations It is not known if pramlintide is present in breast milk. The manufacturer recommends that pramlintide be used in nursing women only when the potential benefit to the mother outweighs the possible risk to the infant.

Use

Adjunctive treatment with mealtime insulin in type 1 diabetes mellitus (insulin dependent, IDDM) patients who have failed to achieve desired glucose control despite optimal insulin therapy

Adjunctive treatment with mealtime insulin in type 2 diabetes mellitus (noninsulin dependent, NIDDM) patients who have failed to achieve desired glucose control despite optimal insulin therapy, with or without concurrent sulfonylurea and/or metformin

Mechanism of Action/Effect Human amylin analog which, in conjunction with insulin, reduces postprandial glucose

Contraindications Hypersensitivity to pramlintide or any component of the formulation; confirmed diagnosis of gastroparesis; hypoglycemia unawareness

Warnings/Precautions [U.S. Boxed Warning]: Coadministration with insulin may induce severe hypoglycemia (usually within 3 hours following administration); coadministration with insulin therapy is an approved indication but does require an initial dosage reduction of insulin and frequent pre and post blood glucose monitoring to reduce risk of severe hypoglycemia. Concurrent use of other glucose-lowering agents may increase risk of hypoglycemia. Avoid use in patients with poor compliance with their insulin regimen and/or blood glucose monitoring. Do not use in patients with Hb A_{1c} levels >9% or recent, recurrent episodes of hypoglycemia; obtain detailed history of glucose control (eg, Hb A_{1c}, incidence of hypoglycemia, glucose monitoring, and medication compliance) and body weight before initiating therapy.

Use caution in patients with visual or dexterity impairment. Use caution when driving or operating heavy machinery until effects on blood sugar are known. Use caution with certain antihypertensive agents (eg, beta-adrenergic blockers) or neuropathic conditions which may mask signs/symptoms of hypoglycemia. Use caution in patients with history of nausea; avoid use in patients with conditions or concurrent medications likely to impair gastric motility (eg, anticholinergics); do not use in patients requiring medication(s) to stimulate gastric emptying.

Drug Interactions

Avoid Concomitant Use There are no known interactions where it is recommended to avoid concomitant use.

Decreased Effect There are no known significant interactions involving a decrease in effect.

Increased Effect/Toxicity

Pramlintide may increase the levels/effects of: Anticholinergics

Nutritional/Ethanol Interactions

Ethanol: Use caution with ethanol (may increase hypoglycemia).

Herb/Nutraceutical: Use caution with garlic, chromium, gymnema (may increase hypoglycemia).

Adverse Reactions

>10%:

Central nervous system: Headache (5% to 13%)

Gastrointestinal: Nausea (28% to 48%), vomiting (7% to 11%), anorexia (≤17%)

Endocrine & metabolic: Severe hypoglycemia (type 1 diabetes ≤17%)

Miscellaneous: Inflicted injury (8% to 14%)

1% to 10%:

Central nervous system: Fatigue (3% to 7%), dizziness (2% to 6%)

Endocrine & metabolic: Severe hypoglycemia (type 2 diabetes ≤8%)

Gastrointestinal: Abdominal pain (2% to 8%)

Respiratory: Pharyngitis (3% to 5%), cough (2% to 6%)

Neuromuscular & skeletal: Arthralgia (2% to 7%)

Miscellaneous: Allergic reaction (≤6%)

Pharmacodynamics/Kinetics

Duration of Action 3 hours

Available Dosage Forms

Injection, solution:

SymlinPen®: 1000 mcg/mL (1.5 mL, 2.7 mL)

General Dosage Range SubQ: *Adults:*

Type 1 diabetes mellitus (insulin dependent, IDDM): Initial: 15 mcg immediately prior to meals; Target dose: 30-60 mcg prior to meals

Type 2 diabetes mellitus (noninsulin dependent, NIDDM): Initial: 60 mcg immediately prior to meals; after 3-7 days increase to 120 mcg prior to meals

Administration

Other Do not mix with other insulins; administer subcutaneously into abdominal or thigh areas at sites distinct from concomitant insulin injections (do not administer into arm due to variable absorption); rotate injection sites frequently. Allow solution to reach room temperature before administering; may reduce injection site reactions. For oral medications in which a rapid onset of action is desired, administer 1 hour before, or 2 hours after pramlintide, if possible. When using the pen-injector, do not transfer drug to a syringe; dosing errors could occur.

Stability

Storage Store unopened vials at 2°C to 8°C (36°F to 46°F); do not freeze. Opened vials may be kept refrigerated or at room temperature ≤30°C (≤86°F). Discard opened vial after 30 days. Protect from light.

Nursing Actions

Physical Assessment Monitor for hypoglycemia. Teach patient appropriate injection techniques and syringe/needle disposal.

Patient Education This medication is used to control diabetes; it is not a cure. It is imperative to follow other components of prescribed treatment (eg, diet and exercise regimen). This medication cannot be mixed with insulin. Use a different syringe for each medication. If you experience hypoglycemic reaction, contact prescriber immediately. Always carry quick source of sugar with you. Monitor glucose levels as directed by prescriber. You may experience nausea, headache, fatigue, or dizziness. Report unresolved nausea or vomiting and hypoglycemic reactions.

Dietary Considerations Dietary modification based on ADA recommendations is a part of therapy; pramlintide to be administered prior to major meals consisting of ≥250 Kcal or ≥30 g carbohydrates

Prasugrel (PRA soo grel)

Brand Names: U.S. Effient®

Index Terms CS-747; LY-640315; Prasugrel Hydrochloride

Pharmacologic Category Antiplatelet Agent; Antiplatelet Agent, Thienopyridine

Medication Safety Issues

Sound-alike/look-alike issues:

Prasugrel may be confused with pravastatin, propranolol

Medication Guide Available Yes

Pregnancy Risk Factor B

Lactation Excretion in breast milk unknown/consider risk:benefit

Use Reduces rate of thrombotic cardiovascular events (eg, stent thrombosis) in patients who are to be managed with percutaneous coronary intervention (PCI) for unstable angina, non-ST-segment elevation MI, or ST-elevation MI (STEMI)

Mechanism of Action/Effect Irreversibly blocks platelet activation and aggregation

Contraindications Hypersensitivity (eg, anaphylaxis) to prasugrel or any component of the formulation; active pathological bleeding such as peptic ulcer disease (PUD) or intracranial hemorrhage; history of transient ischemic attack (TIA) or stroke

Warnings/Precautions [U.S. Boxed Warning]: May cause significant or fatal bleeding. Use is contraindicated in patients with active pathological bleeding or history of TIA or stroke. Use with caution in patients who may be at risk of increased bleeding, including patients with active PUD, recent or recurrent GI bleeding, severe hepatic impairment, trauma, or surgery. Additional risk factors include body weight <60 kg, CABG or other surgical procedure, concomitant use of medications that increase risk of bleeding.

[U.S. Boxed Warning]: In patients ≥75 years of age, use is not recommended due to increased risk of fatal and intracranial bleeding and uncertain benefit; use may be considered in high-risk situations (eg, patients with diabetes or history of MI). **[U.S. Boxed Warning]: Do not initiate therapy in patients likely to undergo urgent CABG surgery; when possible, discontinue ≥7 days prior to any surgery; increased risk of bleeding.** When urgent CABG is necessary, the ACCF/AHA CABG guidelines suggest that it may be reasonable to perform surgery within 7 days of discontinuing prasugrel (Hillis, 2011).

Because of structural similarities, cross-reactivity is possible among the thienopyridines (clopidogrel, prasugrel, and ticlopidine); use with caution or avoid in patients with previous thienopyridine hypersensitivity. Use of prasugrel is contraindicated in patients with hypersensitivity (eg, anaphylaxis) to prasugrel. If necessary, discontinue therapy for active bleeding, elective surgery, stroke, or TIA; reinitiate therapy as soon as possible unless patient suffers stroke or TIA where subsequent use is contraindicated. If possible, manage bleeding without discontinuing prasugrel. Use caution in concurrent treatment with oral anticoagulants (eg, warfarin), NSAIDs, or fibrinolytic agents; bleeding risk is increased. Use with caution in patients with severe liver impairment or end-stage renal disease (experience is limited). Cases of thrombotic thrombocytopenic purpura (TTP) (usually occurring within the first 2 weeks of therapy), resulting in some fatalities, have been reported with prasugrel; urgent plasmapheresis is required. In patients <60 kg, risk of bleeding increased; consider lower maintenance dose.

Drug Interactions

Avoid Concomitant Use There are no known interactions where it is recommended to avoid concomitant use.

Decreased Effect

The levels/effects of Prasugrel may be decreased by: CYP3A4 Inhibitors (Strong); Nonsteroidal Anti-Inflammatory Agents; Ranitidine; Rifampin; Tocilizumab

Increased Effect/Toxicity

Prasugrel may increase the levels/effects of: Anticoagulants; Antiplatelet Agents; Collagenase (Systemic); Drotrecogin Alfa (Activated); Ibritumomab; Rivaroxaban; Salicylates; Thrombolytic Agents; Tositumomab and Iodine I 131 Tositumomab

The levels/effects of Prasugrel may be increased by: Dasatinib; Glucosamine; Herbs (Anticoagulant/Antiplatelet Properties); Nonsteroidal Anti-Inflammatory Agents; Omega-3-Acid Ethyl Esters; Pentosan Polysulfate Sodium; Pentoxifylline; Prostacyclin Analogues; Vitamin E

Adverse Reactions As with all drugs which may affect hemostasis, bleeding is associated with prasugrel. Hemorrhage may occur at virtually any site. Risk is dependent on multiple variables, including patient susceptibility and concurrent use of multiple agents which alter hemostasis.

2% to 10%:

Cardiovascular: Hypertension (8%), hypotension (4%), atrial fibrillation (3%), bradycardia (3%), noncardiac chest pain (3%), peripheral edema (3%)

Central nervous system: Headache (6%), dizziness (4%), fatigue (4%), fever (3%), extremity pain (3%)

Dermatologic: Rash (3%)

Endocrine & metabolic: Hypercholesterolemia/hyperlipidemia (7%)

Gastrointestinal: Nausea (5%), diarrhea (2%), gastrointestinal hemorrhage (2%)

Hematologic: Leukopenia (3%), anemia (2%)

Neuromuscular & skeletal: Back pain (5%)

Respiratory: Epistaxis (6%), dyspnea (5%), cough (4%)

Pharmacodynamics/Kinetics

Onset of Action Inhibition of platelet aggregation (IPA): Dose dependent: 60 mg loading dose: <30 minutes; median time to reach 20% IPA: 30 minutes (Brandt, 2007)

Peak effect: Time to maximal IPA: Dose-dependent: **Note:** Degree of IPA based on adenosine diphosphate (ADP) concentration used during light aggregometry: 60 mg loading dose: Occurs 4 hours post administration; mean IPA (ADP 5 μmol/L): 78.8%: mean IPA (ADP 20 micromole/L): 84.1%

Duration of Action Duration of effect: >3 days; platelet aggregation gradually returns to baseline values over 5-9 days after discontinuation; reflective of new platelet production

Available Dosage Forms

Tablet, oral:

Effient®: 5 mg, 10 mg

General Dosage Range Oral: *Adults:* Loading dose: 60 mg; Maintenance dose: 10 mg once daily (in combination with aspirin 81-325 mg/day)

Administration

Oral Administer without regard to meals.

Stability

Storage Store at 25°C (77°F); excursions permitted to 15°C to 30°C (59°F to 86°F).

Nursing Actions

Physical Assessment Due to the effect on platelets, there is an increased risk of bleeding and prasugrel should be held 5-10 days prior to surgery or dental procedures; assess risk of temporarily discontinuing clopidogrel in patients with recently placed cardiac stents. Monitor for enhanced bleeding effects if used concurrently with warfarin.

Patient Education Patients should inform their prescriber of a history of hemophilia, blood clots, or GI bleed. Instruct patients on increased risk of bruising and bleeding with prasugrel. Patients need to inform their prescriber if they develop gum or nose bleeding; coughing up blood; unusual or heavy menstrual cycles; or bloody or dark, tarry stools. In addition, patients should call for help immediately if experiencing chest or jaw pain, shortness of breath, sweating or weakness, slurred speech, confusion, or vision changes.

Dietary Considerations May be taken without regard to meals.

Pravastatin (prav a STAT in)

Brand Names: U.S. Pravachol®

Index Terms Pravastatin Sodium

Pharmacologic Category Antilipemic Agent, HMG-CoA Reductase Inhibitor

Medication Safety Issues

Sound-alike/look-alike issues:

Pravachol® may be confused with atorvastatin, Prevacid®, Prinivil®, propranolol

Pravastatin may be confused with nystatin, pitavastatin, prasugrel

Pregnancy Risk Factor X

Lactation Enters breast milk/contraindicated

Use Use with dietary therapy for the following:

Primary prevention of coronary events: In hypercholesterolemic patients without established coronary heart disease to reduce cardiovascular morbidity (myocardial infarction, coronary revascularization procedures) and mortality.

Secondary prevention of cardiovascular events in patients with established coronary heart disease: To slow the progression of coronary atherosclerosis; to reduce cardiovascular morbidity (myocardial infarction, coronary vascular procedures) and to reduce mortality; to reduce the risk of stroke and transient ischemic attacks

Hyperlipidemias: Reduce elevations in total cholesterol, LDL-C, apolipoprotein B, and triglycerides (elevations of 1 or more components are present in Fredrickson type IIa, IIb, III, and IV hyperlipidemias)

Heterozygous familial hypercholesterolemia (HeFH): In pediatric patients, 8-18 years of age, with HeFH having LDL-C ≥190 mg/dL **or** LDL ≥160 mg/dL with positive family history of premature cardiovascular disease (CVD) or 2 or more CVD risk factors in the pediatric patient

Mechanism of Action/Effect Pravastatin is a competitive inhibitor of 3-hydroxy-3-methylglutaryl coenzyme A (HMG-CoA) reductase, which is the rate-limiting enzyme involved in *de novo* cholesterol synthesis.

Contraindications Hypersensitivity to pravastatin or any component of the formulation; active liver disease; unexplained persistent elevations of serum transaminases; pregnancy; breast-feeding

Warnings/Precautions Secondary causes of hyperlipidemia should be ruled out prior to therapy. Liver function must be monitored by periodic laboratory assessment. Rhabdomyolysis with acute renal failure has occurred. Risk may be increased with concurrent use of other drugs which may cause rhabdomyolysis (including colchicine, gemfibrozil, fibric acid derivatives, or niacin at doses ≥1 g/day). Discontinue in any patient in which CPK levels are markedly elevated (>10 times ULN) or if myopathy is suspected/diagnosed. The manufacturer recommends temporary discontinuation for elective major surgery, acute medical or surgical conditions, or in any patient experiencing an acute or serious condition predisposing to renal failure (eg, sepsis, hypotension, trauma, uncontrolled seizures). However, based upon current evidence, HMG-CoA reductase inhibitor therapy should be continued in the perioperative period unless risk outweighs cardioprotective benefit. Use with caution in patients with advanced age, these patients are predisposed to myopathy. Use caution in patients with previous liver disease or heavy ethanol use. If serious hepatotoxicity with clinical symptoms and/or hyperbilirubinemia or jaundice occurs during treatment, interrupt therapy. If an alternate etiology is not identified, do not restart pravastatin. Liver enzyme tests should be obtained at baseline and as clinically indicated; routine periodic monitoring of liver enzymes is not necessary. Increases in Hb A_{1c} and fasting blood glucose have been reported with HMG-CoA reductase inhibitors; however, the benefits of statin therapy far outweigh the risk of dysglycemia. Treatment in patients <8 years of age is not recommended.

Drug Interactions

Avoid Concomitant Use

Avoid concomitant use of Pravastatin with any of the following: Pimozide; Red Yeast Rice

Decreased Effect

Pravastatin may decrease the levels/effects of: Lanthanum

The levels/effects of Pravastatin may be decreased by: Antacids; Bile Acid Sequestrants;

Efavirenz; Fosphenytoin; P-glycoprotein/ABCB1 Inducers; Phenytoin; Rifamycin Derivatives; Tocilizumab

Increased Effect/Toxicity

Pravastatin may increase the levels/effects of: ARIPiprazole; DAPTOmycin; PARoxetine; Pimozide; Trabectedin; Vitamin K Antagonists

The levels/effects of Pravastatin may be increased by: Antifungal Agents (Azole Derivatives, Systemic); Colchicine; Conivaptan; CycloSPORINE; CycloSPORINE (Systemic); Eltrombopag; Fenofibrate; Fenofibric Acid; Gemfibrozil; Niacin; Niacinamide; P-glycoprotein/ABCB1 Inhibitors; Protease Inhibitors; Red Yeast Rice

Nutritional/Ethanol Interactions

Ethanol: Consumption of large amounts of ethanol may increase the risk of liver damage with HMG-CoA reductase inhibitors.

Food: Red yeast rice contains an estimated 2.4 mg lovastatin per 600 mg rice.

Herb/Nutraceutical: St John's wort may decrease pravastatin levels.

Adverse Reactions As reported in short-term trials; safety and tolerability with long-term use were similar to placebo

1% to 10%:

Cardiovascular: Chest pain (4%)

Central nervous system: Headache (2% to 6%), fatigue (4%), dizziness (1% to 3%)

Dermatologic: Rash (4%)

Gastrointestinal: Nausea/vomiting (7%), diarrhea (6%), heartburn (3%)

Hepatic: Transaminases increased (>3x normal on two occasions: 1%)

Neuromuscular & skeletal: Myalgia (2%)

Respiratory: Cough (3%)

Miscellaneous: Influenza (2%)

Additional class-related events or case reports (not necessarily reported with pravastatin therapy): Angioedema, blood glucose increased, cataracts, depression, diabetes mellitus (new onset), dyspnea, eosinophilia, erectile dysfunction, facial paresis, glycosylated hemoglobin (Hb A_{1c}) increased, hypersensitivity reaction, impaired extraocular muscle movement, impotence, interstitial lung disease, leukopenia, malaise, memory loss, ophthalmoplegia, paresthesia, peripheral neuropathy, photosensitivity, psychic disturbance, skin discoloration, thrombocytopenia, thyroid dysfunction, toxic epidermal necrolysis, transaminases increased, vomiting

Pharmacodynamics/Kinetics

Onset of Action Several days; Peak effect: 4 weeks

Available Dosage Forms

Tablet, oral: 10 mg, 20 mg, 40 mg, 80 mg

Pravachol®: 10 mg, 20 mg, 40 mg, 80 mg

General Dosage Range Dosage adjustment recommended in patients with hepatic or renal impairment or on concomitant therapy

Oral:

Children 8-13 years: 20 mg once daily

Children 14-18 years: 40 mg once daily

Adults: Initial: 10-40 mg once daily; Maintenance: 10-80 mg once daily (maximum: 80 mg/day)

Administration

Oral May be administered without regard to meals.

Stability

Storage Store at 25°C (77°F); excursions permitted to 15°C to 30°C (59°F to 86°F). Protect from moisture and light.

Nursing Actions

Physical Assessment Assess risk potential for interactions with other prescriptions or herbal products patient may be taking that may increase risk of myopathy or rhabdomyolysis. Teach proper diet and exercise regimen.

Patient Education Take at same time each day, with or without food. Follow prescribed cholesterol-lowering diet and exercise regimen. Avoid excess alcohol. You will have periodic blood tests to assess effectiveness. Avoid excessive alcohol. Report unusual muscle cramping or weakness, yellowing of skin or eyes, easy bruising or bleeding, or unusual fatigue.

Dietary Considerations May be taken without regard to meals. Before initiation of therapy, patients should be placed on a standard cholesterol-lowering diet for 6 weeks and the diet should be continued during drug therapy. Red yeast rice contains an estimated 2.4 mg lovastatin per 600 mg rice.

PrednisoLONE (Systemic)

(pred NISS oh lone)

Brand Names: U.S. Flo-Pred™; Millipred™; Millipred™ DP; Orapred ODT®; Orapred®; Pediapred®; Veripred™ 20

Index Terms Prednisolone Sodium Phosphate

Pharmacologic Category Corticosteroid, Systemic

Medication Safety Issues

Sound-alike/look-alike issues:

PrednisoLONE may be confused with predniSONE

Pediapred® may be confused with Pediazole®

Prelone® may be confused with PROzac®

Pregnancy Risk Factor C/D (Flo-Pred™)

Lactation Enters breast milk/use caution (AAP rates "compatible"; AAP 2001 update pending)

Breast-Feeding Considerations Prednisolone is excreted into breast milk with peak concentrations occurring ~1 hour after the maternal dose. The milk/plasma ratio was found to be 0.2 with doses ≥30 mg/day and 0.1 with doses <30 mg/day. Following a maternal dose of prednisolone 80 mg/day, a breast-feeding infant would ingest <0.1% of the dose.

Use Treatment of endocrine disorders, rheumatic disorders, collagen diseases, allergic states, respiratory diseases, hematologic disorders, neoplastic diseases, edematous states, and gastrointestinal diseases; resolution of acute exacerbations of multiple sclerosis; management of fulminating or disseminated tuberculosis and trichinosis; acute or chronic solid organ rejection

Mechanism of Action/Effect Decreases inflammation by suppression of migration of polymorphonuclear leukocytes and reversal of increased capillary permeability; suppresses the immune system by reducing activity and volume of the lymphatic system

Contraindications Hypersensitivity to prednisolone or any component of the formulation; acute superficial herpes simplex keratitis; live or attenuated virus vaccines (with immunosuppressive doses of corticosteroids); systemic fungal infections; varicella

Warnings/Precautions May cause hypercorticism or suppression of hypothalamic-pituitary-adrenal (HPA) axis, particularly in younger children or in patients receiving high doses for prolonged periods. HPA axis suppression may lead to adrenal crisis. Withdrawal and discontinuation of a corticosteroid should be done slowly and carefully. Particular care is required when patients are transferred from systemic corticosteroids to inhaled products due to possible adrenal insufficiency or withdrawal from steroids, including an increase in allergic symptoms. Patients receiving >20 mg per day of prednisone (or equivalent) may be most susceptible. Fatalities have occurred due to adrenal insufficiency in asthmatic patients during and after transfer from systemic corticosteroids to aerosol steroids; aerosol steroids do **not** provide the systemic steroid needed to treat patients having trauma, surgery, or infections.

Acute myopathy has been reported with high dose corticosteroids, usually in patients with neuromuscular transmission disorders; may involve ocular and/or respiratory muscles; monitor creatine kinase; recovery may be delayed. Corticosteroid use may cause psychiatric disturbances, including depression, euphoria, insomnia, mood swings, and personality changes. Pre-existing psychiatric conditions may be exacerbated by corticosteroid use. Prolonged use of corticosteroids may also increase the incidence of secondary infection, mask acute infection (including fungal infections), prolong or exacerbate viral infections, or limit response to vaccines. Exposure to chickenpox should be avoided; corticosteroids should not be used to treat ocular herpes simplex. Corticosteroids should not be used for cerebral malaria or viral hepatitis. Close observation is required in patients with latent tuberculosis and/or TB reactivity; restrict use in active TB (only in conjunction with antituberculosis treatment). Prolonged use of corticosteroids may result in glaucoma; cataract formation may occur. Prolonged treatment with corticosteroids has been associated with the development of Kaposi's sarcoma (case reports); if noted, discontinuation of therapy should be considered.

Use with caution in patients with thyroid disease, hepatic impairment, renal impairment, cardiovascular disease, diabetes, glaucoma, cataracts, myasthenia gravis, patients at risk for osteoporosis, patients at risk for seizures, or GI diseases (diverticulitis, peptic ulcer, ulcerative colitis) due to perforation risk. Use caution following acute MI (corticosteroids have been associated with myocardial rupture). Because of the risk of adverse effects, systemic corticosteroids should be used cautiously in the elderly in the smallest possible effective dose for the shortest duration. Withdraw therapy with gradual tapering of dose. May affect growth velocity; growth should be routinely monitored in pediatric patients.

Drug Interactions

Avoid Concomitant Use

Avoid concomitant use of PrednisoLONE (Systemic) with any of the following: Aldesleukin; BCG; Natalizumab; Pimecrolimus; Pimozide; Tacrolimus (Topical)

Decreased Effect

PrednisoLONE (Systemic) may decrease the levels/effects of: Aldesleukin; Antidiabetic Agents; BCG; Calcitriol; Coccidioidin Skin Test; Corticorelin; CycloSPORINE; CycloSPORINE (Systemic); Isoniazid; Salicylates; Sipuleucel-T; Telaprevir; Vaccines (Inactivated)

The levels/effects of PrednisoLONE (Systemic) may be decreased by: Aminoglutethimide; Antacids; Barbiturates; Bile Acid Sequestrants; Echinacea; Fosphenytoin; Mitotane; Phenytoin; Primidone; Rifamycin Derivatives; Tocilizumab

Increased Effect/Toxicity

PrednisoLONE (Systemic) may increase the levels/effects of: Acetylcholinesterase Inhibitors; Amphotericin B; ARIPiprazole; CycloSPORINE; CycloSPORINE (Systemic); Deferasirox; Leflunomide; Loop Diuretics; Natalizumab; NSAID (COX-2 Inhibitor); NSAID (Nonselective); Pimozide; Thiazide Diuretics; Vaccines (Live); Warfarin

The levels/effects of PrednisoLONE (Systemic) may be increased by: Antifungal Agents (Azole Derivatives, Systemic); Aprepitant; Calcium Channel Blockers (Nondihydropyridine);

Conivaptan; CycloSPORINE; CycloSPORINE (Systemic); Denosumab; Estrogen Derivatives; Fluconazole; Fosaprepitant; Indacaterol; Macrolide Antibiotics; Neuromuscular-Blocking Agents (Nondepolarizing); Pimecrolimus; Quinolone Antibiotics; Roflumilast; Salicylates; Tacrolimus (Topical); Telaprevir; Trastuzumab

Nutritional/Ethanol Interactions

Ethanol: Avoid ethanol (may increase gastric mucosal irritation).

Food: Prednisolone interferes with calcium absorption. Limit caffeine.

Herb/Nutraceutical: St John's wort may decrease prednisolone levels. Avoid cat's claw, echinacea (have immunostimulant properties).

Adverse Reactions Frequency not defined.

Cardiovascular: Cardiomyopathy, CHF, edema, facial edema, hypertension

Central nervous system: Headache, insomnia, malaise, nervousness, pseudotumor cerebri, psychic disorders, seizure, vertigo

Dermatologic: Bruising, facial erythema, hirsutism, petechiae, skin test reaction suppression, thin fragile skin, urticaria

Endocrine & metabolic: Carbohydrate tolerance decreased, Cushing's syndrome, diabetes mellitus, growth suppression, hyperglycemia, hypernatremia, hypokalemia, hypokalemic alkalosis, menstrual irregularities, negative nitrogen balance, pituitary adrenal axis suppression

Gastrointestinal: Abdominal distention, increased appetite, indigestion, nausea, pancreatitis, peptic ulcer, ulcerative esophagitis, weight gain

Hepatic: LFTs increased (usually reversible)

Neuromuscular & skeletal: Arthralgia, aseptic necrosis (humeral/femoral heads), fractures, muscle mass decreased, muscle weakness, osteoporosis, steroid myopathy, tendon rupture, weakness

Ocular: Cataracts, exophthalmus, eyelid edema, glaucoma, intraocular pressure increased, irritation

Respiratory: Epistaxis

Miscellaneous: Diaphoresis increased, impaired wound healing

Pharmacodynamics/Kinetics

Duration of Action 18-36 hours

Available Dosage Forms

Solution, oral: 5 mg/5 mL (5 mL, 10 mL, 20 mL, 118 mL, 120 mL); 15 mg/5 mL (237 mL, 240 mL, 473 mL, 480 mL)

Millipred™: 10 mg/5 mL (237 mL)

Orapred®: 15 mg/5 mL (20 mL, 237 mL)

Pediapred®: 5 mg/5 mL (120 mL)

Veripred™ 20: 20 mg/5 mL (237 mL)

Suspension, oral:

Flo-Pred™: 15 mg/5 mL (52 mL)

Tablet, oral:

Millipred™: 5 mg

Millipred™ DP: 5 mg

Tablet, orally disintegrating, oral:

Orapred ODT®: 10 mg, 15 mg, 30 mg

General Dosage Range Oral:

Children: Dosage varies greatly depending on indication

Adults: 5-60 mg/day **or** 200 mg/day for 1 week followed by 80 mg every other day for 1 month

Administration

Oral Administer oral formulation with food or milk to decrease GI effects.

Flo-Pred™: Administer using the provided calibrated syringe (supplied by manufacturer) to accurately measure the dose. Syringe should be washed prior to next use.

Orapred ODT®: Do not break or use partial tablet. Remove tablet from blister pack just prior to use. May swallow whole or allow to dissolve on tongue.

Stability

Storage

Flo-Pred™: Store at 20°C to 25°C (68°F to 77°F). Flo-Pred™ should be dispensed in the original container (to avoid loss of formulation during transfer).

Millipred™: Store at 20°C to 25°C (68°F to 77°F).

Orapred ODT®: Store at 20°C to 25°C (68°F to 77°F) in blister pack. Protect from moisture.

Orapred®, Veripred™ 20: 2°C to 8°C (36°F to 46°F).

Pediapred®: 4°C to 25°C (39°F to 77°F); may be refrigerated.

Nursing Actions

Physical Assessment Teach patients to report infection and adrenal suppression. Instruct patients with diabetes to monitor serum glucose levels closely; corticosteroids can alter glycemic response. Dose may need to be increased if patient is experiencing higher than normal levels of stress. When discontinuing, taper dose and frequency slowly.

Patient Education Avoid alcohol. Prescriber may recommend increased dietary vitamins, minerals, or iron. If you have diabetes, monitor glucose levels closely (antidiabetic medication may need to be adjusted). Inform prescriber if you are experiencing greater-than-normal levels of stress (medication may need adjustment). This medication may cause GI upset (oral medication should be taken with meals to reduce GI upset). You may be more susceptible to infection. Report promptly excessive nervousness or sleep disturbances, any signs of infection (sore throat, unhealed injuries), excessive growth of body hair or loss of skin color, vision changes, weight gain, swelling of face or extremities, muscle weakness, change in color of stools (black or tarry) or persistent abdominal pain, or worsening of condition or failure to improve.

Dietary Considerations Should be taken after meals or with food or milk to decrease GI effects; increase dietary intake of pyridoxine, vitamin C, vitamin D, folate, calcium, and phosphorus.

PrednisoLONE (Ophthalmic)

(pred NISS oh lone)

Brand Names: U.S. Omnipred™; Pred Forte®; Pred Mild®

Index Terms Econopred; Prednisolone Acetate, Ophthalmic; Prednisolone Sodium Phosphate, Ophthalmic

Pharmacologic Category Corticosteroid, Ophthalmic

Medication Safety Issues

Sound-alike/look-alike issues:

PrednisoLONE may be confused with predniSONE

Pregnancy Risk Factor C

Use Treatment of palpebral and bulbar conjunctivitis; corneal injury from chemical, radiation, thermal burns, or foreign body penetration; steroid-responsive inflammatory ophthalmic diseases

Available Dosage Forms

Solution, ophthalmic: 1% (5 mL, 10 mL, 15 mL)

Suspension, ophthalmic: 1% (5 mL, 10 mL, 15 mL)

Omnipred™: 1% (5 mL, 10 mL)

Pred Forte®: 1% (1 mL, 5 mL, 10 mL, 15 mL)

Pred Mild®: 0.12% (5 mL, 10 mL)

General Dosage Range Ophthalmic: *Children and Adults:* Initial: Instill 1-2 drops into conjunctival sac every hour during day, every 2 hours at night; Maintenance: 1 drop every 4 hours

Nursing Actions

Patient Education For ophthalmic use only. Wash hands before using. Tilt head back and look upward. Put drops inside lower eyelid. Close eye and roll eyeball in all directions. Do not blink for 1/2 minute. Apply gentle pressure to inner corner of eye for 30 seconds. Do not use any other eye preparation for at least 5 minutes. Do not let tip of applicator touch eye; do not contaminate tip of applicator (may cause eye infection, eye damage, or vision loss). Wear sunglasses when in sunlight; you may be more sensitive to bright light. Inform prescriber if condition worsens or fails to improve or if you experience eye pain or disturbances of vision.

PredniSONE

(PRED ni sone)

Brand Names: U.S. PredniSONE Intensol™

Index Terms Deltacortisone; Deltadehydrocortisone

Pharmacologic Category Corticosteroid, Systemic

Medication Safety Issues

Sound-alike/look-alike issues:

PredniSONE may be confused with methylPREDNISolone, Pramosone®, prazosin, prednisoLONE, PriLOSEC®, primidone, promethazine

Lactation Enters breast milk/AAP rates "compatible" (AAP 2001 update pending)

Breast-Feeding Considerations Prednisone and its metabolite prednisolone are found in low concentrations in breast milk. Peak milk concentrations of both were found ~2 hours after the maternal dose in one case report. In a study which included 6 mother/infant pairs, adverse events were not observed in nursing infants (maternal prednisone dose not provided).

Use Treatment of a variety of diseases, including:

Allergic states (including adjunctive treatment of anaphylaxis)

Autoimmune disorders (including systemic lupus erythematosus [SLE])

Collagen diseases

Dermatologic conditions/diseases

Edematous states (including nephrotic syndrome)

Endocrine disorders

Gastrointestinal diseases

Hematologic disorders (including idiopathic thrombocytopenia purpura [ITP])

Multiple sclerosis exacerbations

Neoplastic diseases

Ophthalmic diseases

Respiratory diseases (including acute asthma exacerbation)

Rheumatic disorders (including rheumatoid arthritis)

Trichinosis with neurologic or myocardial involvement

Tuberculous meningitis

Unlabeled Use Adjunctive therapy for *Pneumocystis jirovecii* (formerly *carinii*) pneumonia (PCP); autoimmune hepatitis; adjunctive therapy for pain management in immunocompetent patients with herpes zoster; tuberculosis (severe, paradoxical reactions); Takayasu arteritis; giant cell arteritis; Grave's ophthalmopathy prophylaxis; subacute thyroiditis; thyrotoxicosis (type II amiodarone-induced)

Mechanism of Action/Effect Decreases inflammation by suppression of migration of polymorphonuclear leukocytes and reversal of increased capillary permeability; suppresses the immune system by reducing activity and volume of the lymphatic system; suppresses adrenal function at high doses

Contraindications Hypersensitivity to any component of the formulation; systemic fungal infections; administration of live or live attenuated vaccines with immunosuppressive doses of prednisone

Warnings/Precautions May cause hypercorticism or suppression of hypothalamic-pituitary-adrenal (HPA) axis, particularly in younger children or in patients receiving high doses for prolonged periods. HPA axis suppression may lead to adrenal crisis. Withdrawal and discontinuation of a corticosteroid should be done slowly and carefully. Particular care is required when patients are transferred from systemic corticosteroids to inhaled products due to possible adrenal insufficiency or withdrawal from steroids, including an increase in allergic symptoms. Patients receiving >20 mg per day of prednisone (or equivalent) may be most susceptible. Fatalities have occurred due to adrenal insufficiency in asthmatic patients during and after transfer from systemic corticosteroids to aerosol steroids; aerosol steroids do **not** provide the systemic steroid needed to treat patients having trauma, surgery, or infections.

Acute myopathy has been reported with high dose corticosteroids, usually in patients with neuromuscular transmission disorders; may involve ocular and/or respiratory muscles; monitor creatine kinase; recovery may be delayed. Prolonged use of corticosteroids may increase the incidence of secondary infection, mask acute infection (including fungal infections), prolong or exacerbate viral infections, or limit response to vaccines. Exposure to chickenpox should be avoided. Corticosteroids should not be used to treat ocular herpes simplex or cerebral malaria. Close observation is required in patients with latent tuberculosis and/or TB reactivity; restrict use in active TB (only in conjunction with antituberculosis treatment). Prolonged treatment with corticosteroids has been associated with the development of Kaposi's sarcoma (case reports); if noted, discontinuation of therapy should be considered. Prolonged use may cause posterior subcapsular cataracts, glaucoma (with possible nerve damage) and may increase the risk for ocular infections. Corticosteroid use may cause psychiatric disturbances, including depression, euphoria, insomnia, mood swings, and personality changes. Pre-existing psychiatric conditions may be exacerbated by corticosteroid use.

Use with caution in patients with HF, diabetes, GI diseases (diverticulitis, peptic ulcer, ulcerative colitis; due to risk of perforation), hepatic impairment, myasthenia gravis, MI, patients with or who are at risk for osteoporosis, seizure disorders or thyroid disease. May affect growth velocity; growth should be routinely monitored in pediatric patients.

Prior to use, the dose and duration of treatment should be based on the risk versus benefit for each individual patient. In general, use the smallest effective dose for the shortest duration of time to minimize adverse events. A gradual tapering of dose may be required prior to discontinuing therapy.

Drug Interactions

Avoid Concomitant Use

Avoid concomitant use of PredniSONE with any of the following: Aldesleukin; Axitinib; BCG; Natalizumab; Pimecrolimus; Tacrolimus (Topical)

Decreased Effect

PredniSONE may decrease the levels/effects of: Aldesleukin; Antidiabetic Agents; ARIPiprazole; Axitinib; BCG; Calcitriol; Coccidioidin Skin Test; Corticorelin; CycloSPORINE; CycloSPORINE (Systemic); Isoniazid; Salicylates; Sipuleucel-T; Telaprevir; Vaccines (Inactivated)

The levels/effects of PredniSONE may be decreased by: Aminoglutethimide; Antacids; Barbiturates; Bile Acid Sequestrants; Echinacea; Fosphenytoin; Mitotane; Phenytoin; Primidone; Rifamycin Derivatives; Somatropin; Tesamorelin; Tocilizumab

Increased Effect/Toxicity

PredniSONE may increase the levels/effects of: Acetylcholinesterase Inhibitors; Amphotericin B; CycloSPORINE; CycloSPORINE (Systemic); Deferasirox; Leflunomide; Loop Diuretics; Natalizumab; NSAID (COX-2 Inhibitor); NSAID (Nonselective); Thiazide Diuretics; Vaccines (Live); Warfarin

The levels/effects of PredniSONE may be increased by: Antifungal Agents (Azole Derivatives, Systemic); Aprepitant; Calcium Channel Blockers (Nondihydropyridine); Conivaptan; CycloSPORINE; CycloSPORINE (Systemic); Denosumab; Estrogen Derivatives; Fluconazole; Fosaprepitant; Indacaterol; Macrolide Antibiotics; Neuromuscular-Blocking Agents (Nondepolarizing); Pimecrolimus; Quinolone Antibiotics; Ritonavir; Roflumilast; Salicylates; Tacrolimus (Topical); Telaprevir; Trastuzumab

Nutritional/Ethanol Interactions

Ethanol: Avoid ethanol (may increase gastric mucosal irritation)

Food: Prednisone interferes with calcium absorption. Limit caffeine.

Herb/Nutraceutical: St John's wort may decrease prednisone levels. Avoid cat's claw, echinacea (have immunostimulant properties).

Adverse Reactions Frequency not defined.

Cardiovascular: Congestive heart failure (in susceptible patients), hypertension

Central nervous system: Emotional instability, headache, intracranial pressure increased (with papilledema), psychic derangements (including euphoria, insomnia, mood swings, personality changes, severe depression), seizure, vertigo

Dermatologic: Bruising, facial erythema, petechiae, thin fragile skin, urticaria, wound healing impaired

Endocrine & metabolic: Adrenocortical and pituitary unresponsiveness (in times of stress), carbohydrate intolerance, Cushing's syndrome, diabetes mellitus, fluid retention, growth suppression (in children), hypokalemic alkalosis, hypothyroidism enhanced, menstrual irregularities, negative nitrogen balance due to protein catabolism, potassium loss, sodium retention

Gastrointestinal: Abdominal distension, pancreatitis, peptic ulcer (with possible perforation and hemorrhage), ulcerative esophagitis
Hepatic: ALT increased, AST increased, alkaline phosphatase increased
Neuromuscular & skeletal: Aseptic necrosis of femoral and humeral heads, muscle mass loss, muscle weakness, osteoporosis, pathologic fracture of long bones, steroid myopathy, tendon rupture (particularly Achilles tendon), vertebral compression fractures
Ocular: Exophthalmos, glaucoma, intraocular pressure increased, posterior subcapsular cataracts
Miscellaneous: Allergic reactions, anaphylactic reactions, diaphoresis, hypersensitivity reactions, infections, Kaposi's sarcoma

Available Dosage Forms

Solution, oral: 1 mg/mL (5 mL, 120 mL, 500 mL)
PredniSONE Intensol™: 5 mg/mL (30 mL)
Tablet, oral: 1 mg, 2.5 mg, 5 mg, 10 mg, 20 mg, 50 mg

General Dosage Range Oral: *Children:* Initial: 5-60 mg/day

Administration

Oral Administer with food to decrease GI upset.

Nursing Actions

Physical Assessment Teach patient to report opportunistic infection and adrenal suppression. Instruct patients with diabetes to monitor serum glucose levels closely; corticosteroids can alter glucose tolerance. Monitor growth with long-term use in pediatric patients. Dose may need to be increased if patient is experiencing higher than normal levels of stress. When discontinuing, taper dose and frequency slowly.

Patient Education Take with or after meals. Avoid alcohol. Maintain adequate nutrition; consult prescriber for possibility of special dietary recommendations. If you have diabetes, monitor serum glucose closely and notify prescriber of changes; this medication can alter glycemic response. Notify prescriber if you are experiencing higher than normal levels of stress; medication may need adjustment. Periodic ophthalmic examinations will be necessary. Patient will be susceptible to infection and may experience insomnia or nervousness. Report weakness, change in menstrual pattern, vision changes, signs of hyperglycemia, signs of infection (eg, fever, chills, mouth sores, perianal itching, vaginal discharge), or worsening of condition. Long-term use of prednisone can lead to thinning skin, easy bruising, redistribution of body fat, and increase in acne or hair growth. Instruct patients to not receive live vaccines while taking this medication for long periods or in high doses.

Dietary Considerations Should be taken after meals or with food or milk; may require increased dietary intake of pyridoxine, vitamin C, vitamin D, folate, calcium, and phosphorus; may require decreased dietary intake of sodium

Pregabalin (pre GAB a lin)

Brand Names: U.S. Lyrica®

Index Terms CI-1008; S-(+)-3-isobutylgaba

Pharmacologic Category Analgesic, Miscellaneous; Anticonvulsant, Miscellaneous

Medication Safety Issues

Sound-alike/look-alike issues:
Lyrica® may be confused with Lopressor®

Medication Guide Available Yes

Pregnancy Risk Factor C

Lactation Excretion in breast milk unknown/not recommended

Use Management of pain associated with diabetic peripheral neuropathy; management of postherpetic neuralgia; adjunctive therapy for partial-onset seizure disorder in adults; management of fibromyalgia

Mechanism of Action/Effect Decreases symptoms of painful peripheral neuropathies and, as adjunctive therapy in partial seizures, decreases the frequency of seizures

Contraindications Hypersensitivity to pregabalin or any component of the formulation

Warnings/Precautions Antiepileptics are associated with an increased risk of suicidal behavior/thoughts with use (regardless of indication); patients should be monitored for signs/symptoms of depression, suicidal tendencies, and other unusual behavior changes during therapy and instructed to inform their healthcare provider immediately if symptoms occur.

Angioedema has been reported; may be life threatening; use with caution in patients with a history of angioedema episodes. Concurrent use with other drugs known to cause angioedema (eg, ACE inhibitors) may increase risk. Hypersensitivity reactions, including skin redness, blistering, hives, rash, dyspnea and wheezing have been reported; discontinue treatment of hypersensitivity occurs. May cause CNS depression and/or dizziness, which may impair physical or mental abilities. Patients must be cautioned about performing tasks which require mental alertness (eg, operating machinery or driving). Effects with other sedative drugs or ethanol may be potentiated. Visual disturbances (blurred vision, decreased acuity and visual field changes) have been associated with pregabalin therapy; patients should be instructed to notify their physician if these effects are noted.

Pregabalin has been associated with increases in CPK and rare cases of rhabdomyolysis. Patients should be instructed to notify their prescriber if unexplained muscle pain, tenderness, or weakness, particularly if fever and/or malaise are associated with these symptoms. Use may be associated with weight gain and peripheral edema; use caution in patients with congestive heart failure, hypertension, or diabetes. Effect on weight gain/edema may be additive to thiazolidinedione antidiabetic agent; particularly in patients with prior cardiovascular disease. May decrease platelet count or prolong PR interval.

Has been noted to be tumorigenic (increased incidence of hemangiosarcoma) in animal studies; significance of these findings in humans is unknown. Pregabalin has been associated with discontinuation symptoms following abrupt cessation, and increases in seizure frequency (when used as an antiepileptic) may occur. Should not be discontinued abruptly; dosage tapering over at least 1 week is recommended. Use caution in renal impairment; dosage adjustment required.

Drug Interactions

Avoid Concomitant Use There are no known interactions where it is recommended to avoid concomitant use.

Decreased Effect

The levels/effects of Pregabalin may be decreased by: Ketorolac; Ketorolac (Nasal); Ketorolac (Systemic); Mefloquine

Increased Effect/Toxicity

Pregabalin may increase the levels/effects of: Alcohol (Ethyl); Antidiabetic Agents (Thiazolidinedione); CNS Depressants; Methotrimeprazine; Selective Serotonin Reuptake Inhibitors

The levels/effects of Pregabalin may be increased by: Droperidol; HydrOXYzine; Methotrimeprazine

Nutritional/Ethanol Interactions

Ethanol: May increase CNS depression; monitor for increased effects with coadministration. Caution patients about effects.

Herb/Nutraceutical: Avoid valerian, St John's wort, kava kava, gotu kola (may increase CNS depression).

Adverse Reactions Note: Frequency of adverse effects may be influenced by dose or concurrent therapy. In add-on trials in epilepsy, frequency of CNS and visual adverse effects were higher than those reported in pain management trials. Range noted below is inclusive of all trials.

>10%:

Cardiovascular: Peripheral edema (up to 16%)

Central nervous system: Dizziness (8% to 45%), somnolence (4% to 28%), ataxia (up to 20%), headache (up to 14%)

Gastrointestinal: Weight gain (up to 16%), xerostomia (1% to 15%)

Neuromuscular & skeletal: Tremor (up to 11%)

Ocular: Blurred vision (1% to 12%), diplopia (up to 12%)

Miscellaneous: Infection (up to 14%), accidental injury (2% to 11%)

1% to 10%:

Cardiovascular: Chest pain (up to 4%), edema (up to 6%)

Central nervous system: Neuropathy (up to 9%), thinking abnormal (up to 9%), fatigue (up to 8%), confusion (up to 7%), euphoria (up to 7%), speech disorder (up to 7%), attention disturbance (up to 6%), incoordination (up to 6%), amnesia (up to 6%), pain (up to 5%), memory impaired (up to 4%), vertigo (up to 4%), feeling abnormal (up to 3%), hypoesthesia (up to 3%), anxiety (up to 2%), depression (up to 2%), disorientation (up to 2%), lethargy (up to 2%), fever (≥1%), depersonalization (≥1%), hypertonia (≥1%), stupor (≥1%), nervousness (up to 1%)

Dermatologic: Facial edema (up to 3%), bruising (≥1%), pruritus (≥1%)

Endocrine & metabolic: Fluid retention (up to 3%), hypoglycemia (up to 3%), libido decreased (≥1%)

Gastrointestinal: Constipation (up to 10%), appetite increased (up to 7%), flatulence (up to 3%), vomiting (up to 3%), abdominal distension (up to 2%), abdominal pain (≥1%), gastroenteritis (≥1%)

Genitourinary: Incontinence (up to 2%), anorgasmia (≥1%), impotence (≥1%), urinary frequency (≥1%)

Hematologic: Thrombocytopenia (3%)

Neuromuscular & skeletal: Balance disorder (up to 9%), abnormal gait (up to 8%), weakness (up to 7%), arthralgia (up to 6%), twitching (up to 5%), back pain (up to 4%), muscle spasm (up to 4%), myoclonus (up to 4%), paresthesia (>2%), CPK increased (2%), leg cramps (≥1%), myalgia (≥1%), myasthenia (up to 1%)

Ocular: Visual abnormalities (up to 5%), visual field defect (≥2%), eye disorder (up to 2%), nystagmus (>2%), conjunctivitis (≥1%)

Otic: Otitis media (≥1%), tinnitus (≥1%)

Respiratory: Sinusitis (up to 7%), dyspnea (up to 3%), bronchitis (up to 3%), pharyngolaryngeal pain (up to 3%)

Miscellaneous: Flu-like syndrome (up to 2%), allergic reaction (≥1%)

Pharmacodynamics/Kinetics

Onset of Action Pain management: Effects may be noted as early as the first week of therapy

Product Availability Lyrica® oral solution: FDA approved December 2009; anticipated availability is currently undetermined

Controlled Substance C-V

Available Dosage Forms

Capsule, oral:

Lyrica®: 25 mg, 50 mg, 75 mg, 100 mg, 150 mg, 200 mg, 225 mg, 300 mg

General Dosage Range Dosage adjustment recommended in patients with renal impairment

Oral: *Adults:* Initial: 150 mg/day in 2-3 divided doses; Maintenance: 150-600 mg/day in 2-3 divided doses (maximum: 600 mg/day)

Administration

Oral May be administered with or without food.

Stability

Storage Store at 15°C to 30°C (59°F to 86°F).

Nursing Actions

Physical Assessment Monitor weight. Assess for signs of fluid retention. Taper dosage over at least one week when discontinuing.

Patient Education Avoid alcohol; may increase drowsiness/CNS depression. Taper dosage slowly when discontinuing. Maintain adequate hydration unless instructed to restrict fluid intake by prescriber. May cause CNS depression and/or dizziness, headache, weight gain, or fluid retention. Report immediately any visual disturbances, suicide ideation, or depression. Report unexplained muscle pain, tenderness, or weakness, especially if accompanied by unexplained fever and malaise, dizziness, confusion or abnormal thinking, shortness of breath, weight gain, swelling of extremities, problems with coordination, tremor, facial swelling, excessively dry mouth, and excessive drowsiness.

Dietary Considerations May be taken with or without food.

Primidone (PRI mi done)

Brand Names: U.S. Mysoline®

Index Terms Desoxyphenobarbital; Primaclone

Pharmacologic Category Anticonvulsant, Miscellaneous; Barbiturate

Medication Safety Issues

Sound-alike/look-alike issues:

Primidone may be confused with predniSONE, primaquine, pyridoxine

Medication Guide Available Yes

Lactation Enters breast milk/not recommended (AAP recommends use "with caution"; AAP 2001 update pending)

Use Management of grand mal, psychomotor, and focal seizures

Unlabeled Use Benign familial tremor (essential tremor)

Available Dosage Forms

Tablet, oral: 50 mg, 250 mg

Mysoline®: 50 mg, 250 mg

General Dosage Range Dosage adjustment recommended in patients with renal impairment

Oral:

Children <8 years: Initial: 50 mg once daily at bedtime; Maintenance: 375-750 mg/day (10-25 mg/kg/day) in 3-4 divided doses

Children ≥8 years and Adults: Initial: 100-125 mg/day at bedtime; Maintenance: 750-1500 mg/day in 3-4 divided doses (maximum: 2 g/day)

Nursing Actions

Physical Assessment Monitor for signs and symptoms of depression or suicide ideation. Monitor therapeutic response (seizure activity, force, type, duration) at beginning of therapy and periodically throughout. Teach patient safety and seizure precautions.

Patient Education While using this medication, do not use alcohol. Maintain adequate hydration unless instructed to restrict fluid intake. You may experience drowsiness, dizziness, blurred vision, nausea, vomiting, loss of appetite, or impotence (reversible). Wear identification of epileptic status and medications. Report behavioral or CNS changes (confusion, depression, increased sedation, excitation, headache, insomnia, or lethargy), suicide ideation, muscle weakness or tremors, unusual bruising or bleeding (mouth, urine, stool), or worsening of seizure activity or loss of seizure control.

Related Information

Peak and Trough Guidelines *on page 1276*

Probenecid (proe BEN e sid)

Index Terms Benemid [DSC]

Pharmacologic Category Uricosuric Agent

Medication Safety Issues

Sound-alike/look-alike issues:

Probenecid may be confused with Procanbid

Lactation Enters breast milk; based on a single case report, very small amounts of probenecid have been detected in breast milk

Use Treatment of hyperuricemia associated with gout or gouty arthritis; prolongation and elevation of beta-lactam plasma levels (eg, uncomplicated gonococcal infection)

Unlabeled Use Prolongation and elevation of beta-lactam plasma levels (eg, neurosyphilis, pelvic inflammatory disease)

Available Dosage Forms

Tablet, oral: 500 mg

General Dosage Range Avoid use if Cl_{cr} <30 mL/minute.

Oral:

Children 2-14 years: Prolong penicillin serum levels: Initial: 25 mg/kg then 40 mg/kg/day given 4 times/day (maximum: 500 mg/dose)

Children >50 kg and Adults:

Gonorrhea, PID: 1 g as a single dose

Gout: Initial: 250 mg twice daily (maximum: 2 g/day)

Neurosyphilis: 500 mg 4 times/day for 10-14 days

Prolong PCN levels: 500 mg 4 times/day

Administration

Oral Administer with food or antacids to minimize GI effects.

Nursing Actions

Physical Assessment Monitor frequency and severity of gouty attacks.

Patient Education Do not start during a gout flare. May take 6-12 months to reduce gouty attacks (attacks may increase in frequency and severity for first few months of therapy). After starting therapy, continue medication if a flare occurs. Take with food. Maintain adequate hydration. You may experience dizziness, nausea, vomiting, headache, flushing, or loss of appetite. Report to prescriber skin rash, signs of infection (a fever of ≥100.5°F [38°C], chills, severe sore throat, ear or sinus pain, cough, increased sputum or change in color of sputum, pain with passing urine, mouth sores, wounds that will not heal, or anal itching), blood in urine, abdominal or back pain (kidney stone), extreme tiredness or weakness, or easy bruising or bleeding.

Procainamide (pro KANE a mide)

Index Terms PCA (error-prone abbreviation); Procainamide Hydrochloride; Procaine Amide Hydrochloride; Procanbid; Pronestyl

Pharmacologic Category Antiarrhythmic Agent, Class Ia

Medication Safety Issues

Sound-alike/look-alike issues:

Procanbid may be confused with probenecid, Procan SR®

Pronestyl may be confused with Ponstel®

High alert medication:

The Institute for Safe Medication Practices (ISMP) includes this medication among its list of drugs which have a heightened risk of causing significant patient harm when used in error.

Administration issues:

Procainamide hydrochloride is available in 10 mL vials of 100 mg/mL and in 2 mL vials with 500 mg/mL. Note that **BOTH** vials contain 1 gram of drug; confusing the strengths can lead to massive overdoses or underdoses.

Other safety concerns:

PCA is an error-prone abbreviation (mistaken as patient controlled analgesia)

Pregnancy Risk Factor C

Lactation Enters breast milk/not recommended (AAP rates "compatible"; AAP 2001 update pending)

Use

Intravenous: Treatment of life-threatening ventricular arrhythmias

Oral (Canadian labeling; not available in U.S.): Treatment of supraventricular arrhythmias. **Note:** In the treatment of atrial fibrillation, use only when preferred treatment is ineffective or cannot be used. Use in paroxysmal atrial tachycardia when reflex stimulation or other measures are ineffective.

Unlabeled Use

Paroxysmal supraventricular tachycardia (PSVT); prevent recurrence of ventricular tachycardia; symptomatic premature ventricular contractions

ACLS guidelines: I.V.: Treatment of the following arrhythmias in patients with preserved left ventricular function: Stable monomorphic VT; pre-excited atrial fibrillation; stable wide complex regular tachycardia (likely VT)

PALS guidelines: I.V.: Tachycardia with pulses and poor perfusion (probable SVT [unresponsive to vagal maneuvers and adenosine or synchronized cardioversion]; probable VT [unresponsive to synchronized cardioversion or adenosine])

Available Dosage Forms

Injection, solution: 100 mg/mL (10 mL); 500 mg/mL (2 mL)

General Dosage Range Dosage adjustment recommended in patients with hepatic or renal impairment

I.M.:

Children: 20-30 mg/kg/day divided every 4-6 hours (maximum: 4 g/day)

Adults: 50 mg/kg/day divided every 3-6 hours **or** 0.5-1 g every 4-8 hours

I.V.:

Children: Loading dose: 3-6 mg/kg/dose over 5 minutes (maximum: 100 mg/dose), may repeat every 5-10 minutes to maximum of 15 mg/kg/load; Infusion: 20-80 mcg/kg/minute (maximum: 2 g/day)

Adults: Loading dose: 15-18 mg/kg administered as slow infusion over 25-30 minutes **or** 100 mg/dose at a rate not to exceed 50 mg/minute repeated every 5 minutes as needed (maximum total dose: 1 g); Infusion: 1-4 mg/minute

Administration

Oral Do **not** crush or chew sustained release drug products (not available in the U.S.).

I.V. Must dilute prior to I.V. administration. Loading dose: Maximum rate: 50 mg/minute

I.V. Detail pH: 4-6

Nursing Actions

Physical Assessment I.V. requires use of infusion pump and continuous cardiac and hemodynamic monitoring. Monitor cardiac status at beginning of therapy, when titrating dosage, and on a regular basis. Monitor QT_c, QRS, and PR intervals.

Patient Education Oral: Avoid alcohol. You will need regular cardiac checkups and blood tests while taking this medication. You may experience dizziness, lightheadedness, visual changes, loss of appetite, headaches, or diarrhea (if persistent consult prescriber). Report chest pain, palpitation, or erratic heartbeat; increased weight or swelling of hands or feet; shortness of breath; acute diarrhea; or unusual fatigue and tiredness.

Related Information

Peak and Trough Guidelines *on page 1276*

Procarbazine (proe KAR ba zeen)

Brand Names: U.S. Matulane®

Index Terms Benzmethyzin; N-Methylhydrazine; Procarbazine Hydrochloride

Pharmacologic Category Antineoplastic Agent, Alkylating Agent

Medication Safety Issues

Sound-alike/look-alike issues:

Procarbazine may be confused with dacarbazine

High alert medication:

The Institute for Safe Medication Practices (ISMP) includes this medication among its list of drugs which have a heightened risk of causing significant patient harm when used in error.

Pregnancy Risk Factor D

Lactation Excretion in breast milk unknown/not recommended

Use Treatment of Hodgkin's disease

Unlabeled Use Treatment of non-Hodgkin's lymphoma, brain tumors

Mechanism of Action/Effect Mechanism of action is not clear, methylating of nucleic acids; inhibits DNA, RNA, and protein synthesis; may damage DNA directly and suppresses mitosis; metabolic activation required by host

Contraindications Hypersensitivity to procarbazine or any component of the formulation; pre-existing bone marrow aplasia; ethanol ingestion; pregnancy

Warnings/Precautions Hazardous agent - use appropriate precautions for handling and disposal. Use with caution in patients with pre-existing renal or hepatic impairment. Procarbazine possesses MAO inhibitor activity and has potential for severe drug and food interactions; follow MAO-I diet. Avoid ethanol consumption, may cause disulfiram-like reaction. May cause hemolysis and/or presence of Heinz inclusion bodies in erythrocytes. Bone marrow depression may occur 2-8 weeks after treatment initiation. Allow ≥1 month interval between radiation therapy or myelosuppressive chemotherapy and initiation of treatment. Withhold treatment for CNS toxicity, leukopenia (WBC <4000/mm^3), thrombocytopenia (platelets <100,000/mm^3), hypersensitivity, stomatitis, diarrhea, or hemorrhage. Procarbazine is a carcinogen which may cause acute leukemia. May cause infertility. **[U.S. Boxed Warning]: Should be administered under the supervision of an experienced cancer chemotherapy physician.**

Drug Interactions

Avoid Concomitant Use

Avoid concomitant use of Procarbazine with any of the following: Alpha-/Beta-Agonists (Indirect-Acting); Alpha1-Agonists; Alpha2-Agonists (Ophthalmic); Amphetamines; Anilidopiperidine Opioids; Antidepressants (Serotonin Reuptake Inhibitor/Antagonist); Atomoxetine; BCG; Bezafibrate; Buprenorphine; BuPROPion; BusPIRone; CarBAMazepine; CloZAPine; Cyclobenzaprine; Dexmethylphenidate; Dextromethorphan; Diethylpropion; HYDROmorphone; Linezolid; Maprotiline; Meperidine; Methyldopa; Methylene Blue; Methylphenidate; Mirtazapine; Natalizumab; Oxymorphone; Pimecrolimus; Pizotifen; Selective Serotonin Reuptake Inhibitors; Serotonin 5-HT1D Receptor Agonists; Serotonin/Norepinephrine Reuptake Inhibitors; Tacrolimus (Topical); Tapentadol; Tetrabenazine; Tetrahydrozoline; Tetrahydrozoline (Nasal); Tricyclic Antidepressants; Tryptophan; Vaccines (Live)

Decreased Effect

Procarbazine may decrease the levels/effects of: BCG; Cardiac Glycosides; Coccidioidin Skin Test; Sipuleucel-T; Vaccines (Inactivated); Vaccines (Live); Vitamin K Antagonists

The levels/effects of Procarbazine may be decreased by: Echinacea

Increased Effect/Toxicity

Procarbazine may increase the levels/effects of: Alpha-/Beta-Agonists (Direct-Acting); Alpha-/Beta-Agonists (Indirect-Acting); Alpha1-Agonists; Alpha2-Agonists (Ophthalmic); Amphetamines; Antidepressants (Serotonin Reuptake Inhibitor/Antagonist); Antihypertensives; Atomoxetine; Beta2-Agonists; Bezafibrate; BuPROPion; CloZAPine; Dexmethylphenidate; Dextromethorphan; Diethylpropion; Doxapram; HYDROmorphone; Leflunomide; Linezolid; Lithium; Meperidine; Methadone; Methyldopa; Methylene Blue; Methylphenidate; Metoclopramide; Mirtazapine; Natalizumab; Orthostatic Hypotension Producing Agents; Pizotifen; Reserpine; Selective Serotonin Reuptake Inhibitors; Serotonin 5-HT1D Receptor Agonists; Serotonin Modulators; Serotonin/Norepinephrine Reuptake Inhibitors; Tetrahydrozoline; Tetrahydrozoline (Nasal); Tricyclic Antidepressants; Vaccines (Live); Vitamin K Antagonists

The levels/effects of Procarbazine may be increased by: Altretamine; Anilidopiperidine Opioids; Antipsychotics; Buprenorphine; BusPIRone; CarBAMazepine; COMT Inhibitors; Cyclobenzaprine; Denosumab; Levodopa; MAO Inhibitors; Maprotiline; Oxymorphone; Pimecrolimus; Roflumilast; Tacrolimus (Topical); Tapentadol; Tetrabenazine; TraMADol; Trastuzumab; Tryptophan

Nutritional/Ethanol Interactions

Ethanol: Ethanol may enhance the adverse/toxic effects of procarbazine or cause a disulfiram reaction. Management: Avoid ethanol.

Food: Concurrent ingestion of foods rich in tyramine may cause sudden and severe high blood pressure (hypertensive crisis or serotonin syndrome). Management: Avoid tyramine-containing foods (aged or matured cheese, air-dried or cured meats including sausages and salamis; fava or broad bean pods, tap/draft beers, Marmite concentrate, sauerkraut, soy sauce, and other soybean condiments). Food's freshness is also an important concern; improperly stored or spoiled food can create an environment in which tyramine concentrations may increase.

Herb/Nutraceutical: Supplements containing caffeine, tyrosine, tryptophan, or phenylalanine may increase the risk of severe side effects (eg, hypertensive reactions, serotonin syndrome). Echinacea may diminish the therapeutic effect of immunosuppressants. Management: Avoid supplements containing caffeine, tyrosine, tryptophan, or phenylalanine. Consider avoiding echinacea.

Adverse Reactions Most frequencies not defined.

Cardiovascular: Edema, flushing, hypotension, syncope, tachycardia

Central nervous system: Apprehension, ataxia, chills, coma, confusion, depression, dizziness, drowsiness, fatigue, fever, hallucination, headache, insomnia, lethargy, nervousness, nightmares, pain, seizure, slurred speech

Dermatologic: Alopecia, dermatitis, hyperpigmentation, petechiae, pruritus, purpura, rash, urticaria

Endocrine & metabolic: Gynecomastia (in prepubertal and early pubertal males)

Hematologic: Eosinophilia; hemolysis (in patients with G6PD deficiency); hemolytic anemia; myelosuppression (leukopenia, anemia, thrombocytopenia); pancytopenia

Gastrointestinal: Abdominal pain, anorexia, constipation, diarrhea, dysphagia, hematemesis, melena; nausea and vomiting ([60% to 90%], increasing the dose in a stepwise fashion over several days may minimize); stomatitis, xerostomia

Genitourinary: Azoospermia (reported with combination chemotherapy), hematuria, nocturia, polyuria, reproductive dysfunction (>10%)

Hepatic: Hepatic dysfunction, jaundice

Neuromuscular & skeletal: Arthralgia, falling, foot drop, myalgia, neuropathy, paresthesia, reflex diminished, tremor, unsteadiness, weakness

Ocular: Diplopia, inability to focus, nystagmus, papilledema, photophobia, retinal hemorrhage

Otic: Hearing loss

Respiratory: Cough, epistaxis, hemoptysis, hoarseness, pleural effusion, pneumonitis, pulmonary toxicity (<1%)

Miscellaneous: Allergic reaction, diaphoresis, herpes, infection, secondary malignancies (2% to 15%; reported with combination therapy)

Available Dosage Forms

Capsule, oral:

Matulane®: 50 mg

General Dosage Range Dosage adjustment recommended in patients with hepatic impairment

Oral:

Children: 100 mg/m^2/day for 14 days and repeated every 4 weeks

Adults: Initial: 2-4 mg/kg/day in single or divided doses for 7 days, then increase dose to 4-6 mg/kg/day; Maintenance: 1-2 mg/kg/day

Administration

Oral May be given as a single daily dose or in 2-3 divided doses.

Stability

Storage Protect from light.

Nursing Actions

Physical Assessment Use of CNS depressants increases risk of adverse reactions. Emetic potential is high; antiemetic is generally required. Monitor for neurotoxicity, nausea and vomiting, pneumonitis, arthralgia, and paresthesia. Instruct patient about dietary and alcohol cautions (procarbazine has some MAO inhibitory effects; can result in life-threatening hypertension with ingestion of tyramine-containing food; alcohol may cause disulfiram-like reaction).

Patient Education Avoid alcohol; may cause acute disulfiram reaction (headache, respiratory difficulties, nausea, vomiting, sweating, thirst, hypotension, and flushing). Avoid tyramine-containing foods; could cause serious hypertensive effects. Maintain adequate hydration unless instructed to restrict fluid intake. You will be more sensitive to infection. May cause considerable nausea or vomiting, mental depression, nervousness, insomnia, nightmares, dizziness, confusion, lethargy, rash, hair loss or hyperpigmentation (reversible), loss of libido, sterility, or amenorrhea. Report persistent fever, chills, or sore throat; unusual bleeding, blood in urine, stool (black stool), or vomitus; unresolved depression; mania; hallucinations; nightmares; disorientation; seizures; chest pain or palpitations; respiratory difficulty; or vision changes.

Dietary Considerations Avoid tyramine-containing foods/beverages. Some examples include aged or matured cheese, air-dried or cured meats (including sausages and salamis), fava or broad bean pods, tap/draft beers, Marmite concentrate, sauerkraut, soy sauce and other soybean condiments.

Prochlorperazine (proe klor PER a zeen)

Brand Names: U.S. Compro®

Index Terms Chlormeprazine; Compazine; Prochlorperazine Edisylate; Prochlorperazine Maleate

Pharmacologic Category Antiemetic; Antipsychotic Agent, Typical, Phenothiazine

Medication Safety Issues

Sound-alike/look-alike issues:

Prochlorperazine may be confused with chlorproMAZINE

Compazine may be confused with Copaxone®, Coumadin®

Other safety concerns:

CPZ (occasional abbreviation for Compazine) is an error-prone abbreviation (mistaken as chlorpromazine)

Lactation Excretion in breast milk unknown/use caution

Use Management of nausea and vomiting; psychotic disorders, including schizophrenia and anxiety

Unlabeled Use Behavioral syndromes in dementia; psychosis/agitation related to Alzheimer's dementia

Available Dosage Forms

Injection, solution: 5 mg/mL (2 mL, 10 mL)

Suppository, rectal: 25 mg (12s)

Compro®: 25 mg (12s)

Tablet, oral: 5 mg, 10 mg

General Dosage Range

I.M.:

Children ≥2 years and ≥9 kg: 0.13 mg/kg/dose; change to oral as soon as possible

Adults:

Antiemetic: 5-10 mg every 3-4 hours **or** 5-10 mg as a single dose with surgery, may repeat (maximum: 40 mg/day)

Antipsychotic: Initial: 10-20 mg every 1-4 hours to gain control (more than 3-4 doses are rarely needed); Maintenance: 10-20 mg every 4-6 hours

I.V.: *Adults:* 2.5-10 mg every 3-4 hours as needed (maximum: 40 mg/day) **or** 5-10 mg as a single dose with surgery, may repeat

Oral, rectal:

Children ≥2 years and ≥9 kg: Antiemetic:

>9 kg: 0.4 mg/kg/day in 3-4 divided doses

9-13 kg: 2.5 mg every 12-24 hours as needed (maximum: 7.5 mg/day)

13.1-17 kg: 2.5 mg every 8-12 hours as needed (maximum: 10 mg/day)

17.1-37 kg: 2.5 mg every 8 hours or 5 mg every 12 hours as needed (maximum: 15 mg/day)

Children 2-12 years: Antipsychotic: Initial: 2.5 mg 2-3 times/day; Maintenance: Increase as needed to maximum of 20 mg/day for 2-5 years and 25 mg/day for 6-12 years

Adults:

Antiemetic: 5-10 mg 3-4 times/day (maximum: 40 mg/day)

Antipsychotic: Initial: 5-10 mg 3-4 times/day; Maintenance: Up to 150 mg/day

Nonpsychotic anxiety: 15-20 mg/day in divided doses; do not give doses >20 mg/day or for longer than 12 weeks

Administration

I.M. Inject by deep IM into outer quadrant of buttocks.

I.V. Administer slow I.V. at a rate not exceeding 5 mg/minute. To reduce the risk of hypotension, patients receiving I.V. prochlorperazine must remain lying down and be observed for at least 30 minutes following administration

I.V. Detail Do not dilute with any diluent containing parabens as a preservative. Avoid skin contact with injection solution, contact dermatitis has occurred. I.V. may be administered IVP or IVPB.

pH: 4.2-6.2

Nursing Actions

Physical Assessment For I.V., continuously monitor blood pressure and heart rate during administration. Monitor blood pressure and heart rate, fluid balance (I & O ratio), and for dehydration. Monitor for seizures, especially with known seizure disorder. Monitor for excessive sedation, neuromuscular malignant syndrome, autonomic instability (eg, anticholinergic effects, such as flushing, excessive sweating, constipation, urinary retention), and extrapyramidal symptoms (eg, tardive dyskinesia, akathisia, pseudoparkinsonism).

Patient Education Avoid alcohol. You may experience appetite changes. Maintain adequate hydration unless instructed to restrict fluid intake. May cause dizziness, tremors, or visual disturbance (especially during early therapy). Do not change position rapidly(rise slowly). May cause photosensitivity reaction. Report immediately any changes in gait or muscular tremors. Report unresolved changes in voiding or elimination (constipation or diarrhea), acute dizziness or unresolved sedation, vision changes, palpitations, yellowing of skin or eyes, or changes in color of urine or stool (pink or red brown urine is expected).

Related Information

Compatibility of Drugs *on page 1264*

Progesterone (proe JES ter one)

Brand Names: U.S. Crinone®; Endometrin®; First™-Progesterone VGS 100; First™-Progesterone VGS 200; First™-Progesterone VGS 25; First™-Progesterone VGS 400; First™-Progesterone VGS 50; Prometrium®

Index Terms Pregnenedione; Progestin

Pharmacologic Category Progestin

Pregnancy Risk Factor B (Prometrium®, per manufacturer); none established for vaginal gel, vaginal tablet, or injection

Lactation Enters breast milk/use caution (AAP rates "compatible"; AAP 2001 update pending)

Use

Oral: Prevention of endometrial hyperplasia in nonhysterectomized, postmenopausal women who are receiving conjugated estrogen tablets; secondary amenorrhea

I.M.: Amenorrhea; abnormal uterine bleeding due to hormonal imbalance

Intravaginal gel: Part of assisted reproductive technology (ART) for infertile women with progesterone deficiency; secondary amenorrhea

Vaginal tablet: Part of ART for infertile women with progesterone deficiency

Available Dosage Forms

Capsule, oral: 100 mg, 200 mg

Prometrium®: 100 mg, 200 mg

Gel, vaginal:

Crinone®: 4% (1.45 g); 8% (1.45 g)

Injection, oil: 50 mg/mL (10 mL)

Suppository, vaginal:
First™-Progesterone VGS 25: 25 mg (30s)
First™-Progesterone VGS 50: 50 mg (30s)
First™-Progesterone VGS 100: 100 mg (30s)
First™-Progesterone VGS 200: 200 mg (30s)
First™-Progesterone VGS 400: 400 mg (30s)

Tablet, vaginal:
Endometrin®: 100 mg

General Dosage Range

I.M.: *Adults (females):* 5-10 mg/day for 6 doses

Intravaginal: *Adults (females):*
ART: 90 mg (8% gel) once or twice daily or 100 mg (vaginal tablet) 2-3 times/day
Secondary amenorrhea: 45 mg (4% gel) every other day, may increase to 90 mg (8% gel) every other day if needed (maximum: 6 doses)

Oral: *Adults (females):*
Amenorrhea: 400 mg once daily in the evening for 10 days
Endometrial hyperplasia prevention: 200 mg once daily in the evening for 12 days sequentially per 28-day cycle

Administration

Oral Oral capsule: For patients who experience difficulty swallowing the capsules, taking with a full glass of water in the standing position may be beneficial.

I.M. Administer deep I.M. only

Other

Vaginal gel: (A small amount of gel will remain in the applicator following insertion): Administer into the vagina directly from sealed applicator. Remove applicator from wrapper; holding applicator by thickest end, shake down to move contents to thin end; while holding applicator by flat section of thick end, twist off tab; gently insert into vagina and squeeze thick end of applicator.

For use at altitudes above 2500 feet: Remove applicator from wrapper; hold applicator on both sides of bubble in the thick end; using a lancet, make a single puncture in the bubble to relieve air pressure; holding applicator by thickest end, shake down to move contents to thin end; while holding applicator by flat section of thick end, twist off tab; gently insert into vagina and squeeze thick end of applicator.

Vaginal tablet: Insert tablet in vagina using disposable applicator provided.

Nursing Actions

Physical Assessment Assess blood pressure, mammogram, and results of Pap smears and pregnancy tests before beginning treatment and at least annually. Teach patient importance of annual physicals, Pap smears, and vision assessment.

Patient Education Inform prescriber if you are allergic to peanut or palm oil. Take at bedtime to minimize side effects. It is important that you have an annual physical assessment, Pap smear, and vision assessment while taking this medication and that you perform monthly self-breast exams. May cause temporary dizziness or drowsiness, headache, joint pain, nausea and/or vomiting, mood swings, or irritability. Report immediately warmth, swelling, or redness in calves; shortness of breath; chest pain; sudden loss or change in vision; breast mass; blurred vision; confusion; or depression.

Vaginal gel: A small amount of gel will remain in the applicator following insertion. Administer into the vagina directly from applicator.

Promethazine (proe METH a zeen)

Brand Names: U.S. Phenadoz®; Phenergan®; Promethegan™

Index Terms Promethazine Hydrochloride

Pharmacologic Category Antiemetic; Histamine H_1 Antagonist; Histamine H_1 Antagonist, First Generation; Phenothiazine Derivative

Medication Safety Issues

Sound-alike/look-alike issues:
Promethazine may be confused with chlorproMAZINE, predniSONE
Phenergan® may be confused with PHENobarbital, Phrenilin®, Theragran

High alert medication:
The Institute for Safe Medication Practices (ISMP) includes this medication (I.V. formulation) among its list of drugs which have a heightened risk of causing significant patient harm when used in error.

Beers Criteria medication:
This drug may be inappropriate for use in geriatric patients (high severity risk).

Administration issues:
To prevent or minimize tissue damage during I.V. administration, the Institute for Safe Medication Practices (ISMP) has the following recommendations:
- Limit concentration available to the 25 mg/mL product
- Consider limiting initial doses to 6.25-12.5 mg
- Further dilute the 25 mg/mL strength into 10-20 mL NS
- Administer through a large bore vein (not hand or wrist)
- Administer via running I.V. line at port farthest from patient's vein
- Consider administering over 10-15 minutes
- Instruct patients to report immediately signs of pain or burning

International issues:
Sominex: Brand name for promethazine in Great Britain, but also is a brand name for diphenhydrAMINE in the U.S.

Pregnancy Risk Factor C

Lactation Excretion in breast milk unknown/not recommended

Use Symptomatic treatment of various allergic conditions; antiemetic; motion sickness; sedative; adjunct to postoperative analgesia and anesthesia

Available Dosage Forms

Injection, solution: 25 mg/mL (1 mL, 10 mL); 50 mg/mL (1 mL)

Phenergan®: 25 mg/mL (1 mL); 50 mg/mL (1 mL)

Suppository, rectal: 12.5 mg (12s); 25 mg (12s)

Phenadoz®: 12.5 mg (12s); 25 mg (12s)

Promethegan™: 12.5 mg (12s); 25 mg (12s); 50 mg (12s)

Syrup, oral: 6.25 mg/5 mL (118 mL, 473 mL)

Tablet, oral: 12.5 mg, 25 mg, 50 mg

General Dosage Range

I.M., I.V.:

Children ≥2 years: 0.25-1 mg/kg 4-6 times/day as needed (maximum: 25 mg/dose; sedation: 50 mg/dose)

Adults: 12.5-75 mg/dose as a single dose **or** 12.5-50 mg every 4-6 hours as needed

Oral, rectal:

Children ≥2 years:

Allergic reactions: 0.1 mg/kg every 6 hours (maximum: 12.5 mg) during the day and 0.5 mg/kg (maximum: 25 mg/dose) at bedtime as needed

Antiemetic: 0.25-1 mg/kg 4-6 times/day as needed (maximum: 25 mg/dose)

Motion sickness: 0.5 mg/kg 30 minutes to 1 hour before departure, then every 12 hours as needed (maximum: 25 mg twice daily)

Sedation: 0.5-1 mg/kg every 6 hours as needed (maximum: 50 mg/dose)

Adults: 6.25-25 mg every 4-8 hours as needed **or** 12.5-50 mg as a single dose **or** 25 mg 30-60 minutes before departure, then every 12 hours as needed

Administration

I.M. Preferred route of administration; administer into deep muscle

I.V. I.V. administration is **not** the preferred route; severe tissue damage may occur. Solution for injection should be administered in a maximum concentration of 25 mg/mL (more dilute solutions are recommended). Administer via running I.V. line at port farthest from patient's vein, or through a large bore vein (not hand or wrist). Consider administering over 10-15 minutes (maximum: 25 mg/minute). Discontinue immediately if burning or pain occurs with administration.

I.V. Detail Rapid I.V. administration may produce a transient fall in blood pressure.

pH: 4.0-5.5

Other Not for SubQ or intra-arterial administration.

Nursing Actions

Physical Assessment I.M. is the preferred route of administration. I.V.: Infusion site must be monitored closely; severe tissue damage may result. Do not give SubQ or intra-arterially; necrotic lesions may occur. Monitor for sedation, bradycardia, akathisia, delirium, extrapyramidal symptoms, dermatitis, gastrointestinal upset, urinary retention, blurred vision, and respiratory depression. May be sedating and impair physical or mental abilities; use and teach sedation safety measures (eg, side rails up, call light within reach).

Patient Education I.V.: Report immediately any pain or burning at infusion/injection site. Oral/suppository: Avoid alcohol; may increase CNS depression. May cause dizziness, drowsiness, blurred vision, orthostatic hypotension, photosensitivity, nausea, dry mouth, or appetite disturbances. Report unresolved nausea or diarrhea, palpitations, dizziness, excess/persistent sedation, changes in urination, sore throat, or respiratory difficulty.

Related Information

Compatibility of Drugs *on page 1264*

Management of Drug Extravasations *on page 1269*

Propafenone (pro PAF en one)

Brand Names: U.S. Rythmol®; Rythmol® SR

Index Terms Propafenone Hydrochloride

Pharmacologic Category Antiarrhythmic Agent, Class Ic

Pregnancy Risk Factor C

Lactation Enters breast milk/not recommended

Use Treatment of life-threatening ventricular arrhythmias; treatment of paroxysmal atrial fibrillation/flutter (PAF) or paroxysmal supraventricular tachycardia (PSVT) in patients with disabling symptoms and without structural heart disease

Extended release capsule: Prolong the time to recurrence of symptomatic atrial fibrillation in patients without structural heart disease

Unlabeled Use Cardioversion of recent-onset atrial fibrillation (single dose); supraventricular tachycardia in patients with Wolff-Parkinson-White syndrome

Available Dosage Forms

Capsule, extended release, oral: 225 mg, 325 mg, 425 mg

Rythmol® SR: 225 mg, 325 mg, 425 mg

Tablet, oral: 150 mg, 225 mg, 300 mg

Rythmol®: 150 mg, 225 mg

General Dosage Range Dosage adjustment recommended in patients with hepatic impairment

Oral:

Extended release: *Adults:* Initial: 225 mg every 12 hours; Maintenance: 225-425 mg every 12 hours

Immediate release: *Adults:* Initial: 150 mg every 8 hours; Maintenance: 150-300 mg every 8 hours

Administration

Oral Capsules should be swallowed whole; do not crush or chew; may be taken without regard to meals.

Nursing Actions

Physical Assessment Correct electrolyte abnormalities prior to and throughout use. May cause new or worsened arrhythmias.

Patient Education You will need regular cardiac checkups. You may experience dizziness, drowsiness, insomnia, or blurred vision; abnormal taste, nausea, vomiting, or loss of appetite; headache; or muscle or joint pain. Report unusual weight gain, swelling of extremities, or respiratory difficulty. Report immediately or seek emergency help if you experience chest pain; palpitations; or increased, decreased, or erratic heartbeat.

Propranolol (proe PRAN oh lole)

Brand Names: U.S. Inderal® LA; InnoPran XL®

Index Terms Propranolol Hydrochloride

Pharmacologic Category Antianginal Agent; Antiarrhythmic Agent, Class II; Beta-Adrenergic Blocker, Nonselective

Medication Safety Issues

Sound-alike/look-alike issues:

Propranolol may be confused with prasugrel, Pravachol®, Propulsid®

Inderal® may be confused with Adderall®, Enduron, Imdur®, Imuran®, Inderide, Isordil®, Toradol®

High alert medication:

The Institute for Safe Medication Practices (ISMP) includes this medication among its list of drugs which have a heightened risk of causing significant patient harm when used in error.

Administration issues:

Significant differences exist between oral and I.V. dosing. Use caution when converting from one route of administration to another.

International issues:

Inderal [Canada and multiple international markets] and Inderal LA [U.S.] may be confused with Indiaral brand name for loperamide [France]

Pregnancy Risk Factor C

Lactation Enters breast milk/use caution (AAP rates "compatible"; AAP 2001 update pending)

Use Management of hypertension; angina pectoris; pheochromocytoma; essential tremor; supraventricular arrhythmias (such as atrial fibrillation and flutter, AV nodal re-entrant tachycardias), ventricular tachycardias (catecholamine-induced arrhythmias, digoxin toxicity); prevention of myocardial infarction; migraine headache prophylaxis; symptomatic treatment of hypertrophic subaortic stenosis (hypertrophic obstructive cardiomyopathy)

Unlabeled Use Tremor due to Parkinson's disease; aggressive behavior (not recommended for dementia-associated aggression), anxiety, schizophrenia; antipsychotic-induced akathisia; primary and secondary prophylaxis of variceal hemorrhage; acute panic; thyrotoxicosis; tetralogy of Fallot (TOF) hypercyanotic spells

Available Dosage Forms

Capsule, extended release, oral: 60 mg, 80 mg, 120 mg, 160 mg

InnoPran XL®: 80 mg, 120 mg

Capsule, sustained release, oral:

Inderal® LA: 60 mg, 80 mg, 120 mg, 160 mg

Injection, solution: 1 mg/mL (1 mL)

Injection, solution [preservative free]: 1 mg/mL (1 mL)

Solution, oral: 4 mg/mL (500 mL); 8 mg/mL (500 mL)

Tablet, oral: 10 mg, 20 mg, 40 mg, 60 mg, 80 mg

General Dosage Range

I.V.: *Adults:* 1-3 mg, repeat every 2-5 minutes up to a total of 5 mg **or** 0.1 mg/kg divided into 3 equal doses given at 2- to 3-minute intervals; may repeat total dose in 2 minutes if needed

Oral:

Extended release: *Adults:* Initial: 80 mg once daily; Maintenance: 60-320 mg once daily (maximum: 640 mg/day)

Regular release: *Adults:* 30-320 mg/day in 2-4 divided doses (maximum: 640 mg/day)

Administration

Oral Do not crush long-acting forms.

I.V. I.V. dose is much smaller than oral dose. When administered acutely for cardiac treatment, monitor ECG and blood pressure. May administer by rapid infusion (I.V. push) at a rate of 1 mg/minute or by slow infusion over ~30 minutes. Necessary monitoring for surgical patients who are unable to take oral beta-blockers (prolonged ileus) has not been defined. Some institutions require monitoring of baseline and postinfusion heart rate and blood pressure when a patient's response to beta-blockade has not been characterized (ie, the patient's initial dose or following a change in dose). Consult individual institutional policies and procedures.

I.V. Detail pH: 2.8-3.5

Nursing Actions

Physical Assessment I.V. infusion usually requires hemodynamic monitoring; consult institution protocols. When discontinuing, drug must be tapered gradually over 2 weeks to avoid acute tachycardia, hypertension, and/or ischemia. Caution patients with diabetes to monitor blood glucose levels closely; beta-blockers can mask hypoglycemic symptoms.

Patient Education If administered by infusion, report immediately any pain, redness, or swelling at infusion site; palpitations or chest pain; dizziness; or difficulty breathing. **Oral:** If you have diabetes, monitor blood sugars carefully; beta-blockers may mask hypoglycemic symptoms. Do not crush or chew long-acting forms; swallow whole. Report to your prescriber symptoms of orthostatic hypotension, dizziness, drowsiness, or blurred vision. May cause nausea, vomiting, clay-colored stool, or stomach discomfort. Report chest pain or palpitations; persistent dizziness or lethargy; any CNS symptoms (amnesia, change in cognition, confusion, depression, hallucinations, insomnia, vivid dreams); discolored skin or rash; difficulty breathing or wheezing; or weakness, pain, or loss of sensation in extremities.

Propranolol and Hydrochlorothiazide

(proe PRAN oh lole & hye droe klor oh THYE a zide)

Index Terms Hydrochlorothiazide and Propranolol; Inderide

Pharmacologic Category Beta Blocker, Nonselective; Diuretic, Thiazide

Medication Safety Issues

Sound-alike/look-alike issues:

Inderide may be confused with Inderal®

Pregnancy Risk Factor C

Lactation Enters breast milk/use caution

Use Management of hypertension

Available Dosage Forms

Tablet: Propranolol 40 mg and hydrochlorothiazide 25 mg; propranolol 80 mg and hydrochlorothiazide 25 mg

General Dosage Range Oral: *Adults:* Propranolol 80-160 mg/day and hydrochlorothiazide 12.5-50 mg/day in 2 divided doses

Nursing Actions

Physical Assessment See individual agents.

Patient Education See individual agents.

Related Information

Hydrochlorothiazide *on page 570*

Propranolol *on page 959*

Propylthiouracil (proe pil thye oh YOOR a sil)

Index Terms PTU (error-prone abbreviation)

Pharmacologic Category Antithyroid Agent; Thioamide

Medication Safety Issues

Sound-alike/look-alike issues:

Propylthiouracil may be confused with Purinethol®

PTU is an error-prone abbreviation (mistaken as mercaptopurine [Purinethol®; 6-MP])

Medication Guide Available Yes

Pregnancy Risk Factor D

Lactation Enters breast milk/AAP rates "compatible" (AAP 2001 update pending)

Use Adjunctive therapy in patients intolerant of methimazole to ameliorate hyperthyroidism symptoms in preparation for surgical treatment or radioactive iodine therapy; treatment of hyperthyroidism in patients intolerant of methimazole and not candidates for surgical/radiotherapy

Unlabeled Use Management of Graves' disease, thyrotoxic crisis, or thyroid storm

Available Dosage Forms

Tablet, oral: 50 mg

General Dosage Range Oral:

Children 6-10 years: 50-150 mg/day

Children >10 years: 150-300 mg/day

Adults: Initial: 300-900 mg/day in 3 divided doses; Maintenance: 100-150 mg/day

Administration

Oral Administer at the same time in relation to meals each day, either always with meals or always between meals.

Nursing Actions

Physical Assessment Monitor for rash, goiter, nausea, vomiting, leucopenia, agranulocytosis, anemia, jaundice, arthralgia, and CNS stimulation or depression.

Patient Education Take at the same time each day at around-the-clock intervals; take at the same time in relation to meals, either always with meals or always between meals. This drug may need to be taken for an extended period to achieve appropriate results and you may need periodic blood tests to assess effectiveness of therapy. Blood counts will be monitored to evaluate for risk of bleeding and infection. May cause nausea or vomiting; constipation; or dizziness or drowsiness. Report rash, skin eruptions, or loss of hair; fever; unusual bleeding or bruising; unusual weight gain; unresolved headache or fever; yellowing of eyes or skin; changes in color of urine or feces; or joint or muscle pain or weakness.

Protamine (PROE ta meen)

Index Terms Protamine Sulfate

Pharmacologic Category Antidote

Medication Safety Issues

Sound-alike/look-alike issues:

Protamine may be confused with ProAmatine, Protonix®, Protopam®

Pregnancy Risk Factor C

Lactation Excretion in breast milk unknown/use caution

Use Treatment of heparin overdosage; neutralize heparin during surgery or dialysis procedures

Unlabeled Use Treatment of low molecular weight heparin (LMWH) overdose

Available Dosage Forms

Injection, solution [preservative free]: 10 mg/mL (5 mL, 25 mL)

General Dosage Range I.V.: *Children and Adults:* 1 mg of protamine neutralizes 90 USP units of heparin (lung) and 115 USP units of heparin (intestinal) (maximum dose: 50 mg)

Administration

I.V. For I.V. use only. Administer slow IVP (50 mg over 10 minutes). Rapid I.V. infusion causes hypotension. Inject without further dilution over 1-3 minutes; maximum of 50 mg in any 10-minute period.

I.V. Detail pH: 6-7

Nursing Actions

Physical Assessment Monitor closely for hemodynamic changes.

Patient Education Report any respiratory difficulty, rash or flushing, feeling of warmth, tingling or numbness, dizziness, or disorientation.

Pseudoephedrine (soo doe e FED rin)

Brand Names: U.S. Children's Nasal Decongestant [OTC]; Contac® Cold + Flu Maximum Strength Non-Drowsy [OTC]; Genaphed™ [OTC] [DSC]; Oranyl [OTC]; Silfedrine Children's [OTC]; Sudafed® 12 Hour [OTC]; Sudafed® 24 Hour [OTC]; Sudafed® Children's [OTC]; Sudafed® Maximum Strength Nasal Decongestant [OTC]; Sudo-Tab® [OTC]; SudoGest 12 Hour [OTC]; SudoGest Children's [OTC]; SudoGest [OTC]

Index Terms *d*-Isoephedrine Hydrochloride; Pseudoephedrine Hydrochloride; Pseudoephedrine Sulfate; Sudafed

Pharmacologic Category Alpha/Beta Agonist; Decongestant

Medication Safety Issues

Sound-alike/look-alike issues:

Sudafed® may be confused with sotalol, Sudafed PE®, Sufenta®

Lactation Enters breast milk (AAP rates "compatible"; AAP 2001 update pending)

Use Temporary symptomatic relief of nasal congestion due to common cold, upper respiratory allergies, and sinusitis; also promotes nasal or sinus drainage

Available Dosage Forms For available OTC formulations, consult specific product labeling.

General Dosage Range Oral:

Immediate release:

Children 4-5 years: 15 mg every 4-6 hours (maximum: 60 mg/day)

Children 6-12 years: 30 mg every 4-6 hours (maximum: 120 mg/day)

Adults: 60 mg every 4-6 hours (maximum: 240 mg/day)

Extended release: *Adults:* 120 mg every 12 hours or 240 mg every 24 hours (maximum: 240 mg/day)

Administration

Oral Do not crush extended release drug product, swallow whole. May administer with or without food. Sudafed® 24 Hour tablet may not completely dissolve and appear in stool

Nursing Actions

Physical Assessment Monitor relief of congestion. Monitor for cardiac and CNS changes prior to treatment and throughout.

Patient Education Do not chew or crush extended release forms. Maintain adequate hydration unless instructed to restrict fluid intake. You may experience nervousness, insomnia, dizziness, or drowsiness. Report persistent CNS changes (dizziness, tremor, or agitation), respiratory difficulty, chest pain, palpitations, rapid heartbeat; muscle tremor, or lack of improvement or worsening of condition.

Pyrazinamide (peer a ZIN a mide)

Index Terms Pyrazinoic Acid Amide

Pharmacologic Category Antitubercular Agent

Pregnancy Risk Factor C

Lactation Enters breast milk/use caution

Use Adjunctive treatment of tuberculosis in combination with other antituberculosis agents

Available Dosage Forms

Tablet, oral: 500 mg

General Dosage Range Dosage adjustment recommended in patients with renal impairment

Oral:

Children: 15-30 mg/kg once daily (maximum: 2 g/day) **or** 50 mg/kg/dose twice weekly (maximum: 2 g/dose)

Adults 40-55 kg: 1000 mg once daily **or** 2000 mg twice weekly **or** 1500 mg 3 times/week

Adults 56-75 kg: 1500 mg once daily **or** 3000 mg twice weekly **or** 2500 mg 3 times/week

Adults 76-90 kg: 2000 mg once daily (maximum dose regardless of weight) **or** 4000 mg twice weekly (maximum dose regardless of weight) **or** 3000 mg 3 times/week (maximum dose regardless of weight)

Nursing Actions

Physical Assessment Assess patient history for use cautions and evaluate any history of alcohol intake prior to beginning treatment. Monitor chest x-ray regularly.

Patient Education You will need regular medical follow-up and laboratory tests while taking this medication. May cause nausea or loss of appetite. Report change in color of urine, pale stools, easy bruising or bleeding, blood in urine or difficulty urinating, yellowing of skin or eyes, extreme joint pain, unusual fever, or unresolved nausea or vomiting.

Pyrethrins and Piperonyl Butoxide

(pye RE thrins & pi PER oh nil byo TOKS ide)

Brand Names: U.S. A-200® Lice Treatment Kit [OTC]; A-200® Maximum Strength [OTC]; Licide® [OTC]; Pronto® Complete Lice Removal System [OTC]; Pronto® Plus Lice Killing Mousse Plus Vitamin E [OTC]; Pronto® Plus Lice Killing Mousse Shampoo Plus Natural Extracts and Oils [OTC]; Pronto® Plus Warm Oil Treatment and Conditioner [OTC]; RID® Maximum Strength [OTC]

Index Terms Piperonyl Butoxide and Pyrethrins

Pharmacologic Category Antiparasitic Agent, Topical; Pediculocide; Shampoo, Pediculocide

Pregnancy Risk Factor C

Use Treatment of *Pediculus humanus* infestations (head lice, body lice, pubic lice, and their eggs)

Available Dosage Forms

Kit:

A-200® Lice Treatment Kit [OTC]:

Shampoo: Pyrethrins 0.33% and piperonyl butoxide 4% (120 mL)

Solution: Permethrin 0.5% (180 mL)

Pronto® Complete Lice Removal System [OTC]:

Shampoo: Pyrethrins 0.33% and piperonyl butoxide 4% (60 mL)

Solution, topical: Benzalkonium chloride 0.1% (60 mL)

Oil, topical:

Pronto® Plus Warm Oil Treatment and Conditioner [OTC]: Pyrethrins 0.33% and piperonyl butoxide 4% (36 mL)

Shampoo:

A-200® Maximum Strength [OTC]: Pyrethrins 0.33% and piperonyl butoxide 4% (60 mL, 120 mL)

Licide® [OTC], Pronto® Plus Lice Killing Mousse Shampoo Plus Vitamin E [OTC]: Pyrethrins 0.33% and piperonyl butoxide 4% (120 mL)

Pronto® Plus Lice Killing Mousse Shampoo Plus Natural Extracts and Oils [OTC]: Pyrethrins 0.33% and piperonyl butoxide 4% (60 mL)

Pronto® Plus Lice Killing Mousse Shampoo Plus Vitamin E [OTC]: Pyrethrins 0.33% and piperonyl butoxide 4% (120 mL)

RID® Maximum Strength [OTC]: Pyrethrins 0.33% and piperonyl butoxide 4% (60 mL, 120 mL, 180 mL, 240 mL)

General Dosage Range Topical: *Children and Adults:* Apply to infested area, keep on for 10 minutes, wash, and rinse; may repeat once in a 24-hour period and then again in 7-10 days

Administration

Topical For external use only. Avoid touching eyes, mouth, or other mucous membranes.

Pyridostigmine (peer id oh STIG meen)

Brand Names: U.S. Mestinon®; Mestinon® Timespan®; Regonol®

Index Terms Pyridostigmine Bromide

Pharmacologic Category Acetylcholinesterase Inhibitor

Medication Safety Issues

Sound-alike/look-alike issues:

Pyridostigmine may be confused with physostigmine

Regonol® may be confused with Reglan®, Renagel®

Pregnancy Risk Factor B

Lactation Enters breast milk/compatible

Use Symptomatic treatment of myasthenia gravis; antagonism of nondepolarizing neuromuscular blockers

Military use: Pretreatment for Soman nerve gas exposure

Available Dosage Forms

Injection, solution:

Regonol®: 5 mg/mL (2 mL)

Syrup, oral:

Mestinon®: 60 mg/5 mL (480 mL)

Tablet, oral: 60 mg

Mestinon®: 60 mg

Tablet, sustained release, oral:

Mestinon® Timespan®: 180 mg

General Dosage Range

I.M.:

Children: 0.05-0.15 mg/kg/dose

Adults: ~1/30th of oral dose

I.V.:

Children: 0.05-0.25 mg/kg/dose

Adults: IVP: ~1/30th of oral dose **or** 0.1-0.25 mg/kg/dose (usual: 10-20 mg); Infusion: 2 mg/hour with gradual titration in increments of 0.5-1 mg/hour (maximum: 4 mg/hour)

Oral:

Immediate release:

Children: 7 mg/kg/day divided into 5-6 doses

Adults: 60-1500 mg/day in 5-6 divided doses (usual: 600 mg/day)

Sustained release: *Adults:* 180-540 mg once or twice daily (doses separated by at least 6 hours)

Administration

Oral Do **not** crush sustained release tablet.

I.V. Detail pH: 5

Nursing Actions

Physical Assessment When used to reverse neuromuscular block (anesthesia or excessive acetylcholine), monitor patient safety until full return of neuromuscular functioning. Assess bladder and sphincter adequacy prior to treatment. Monitor for cholinergic crisis: DUMBELS - **d**iarrhea, **u**rination, **m**iosis, **b**ronchospasm/bradycardia, **e**xcitability, **l**acrimation, and **s**alivation/ excessive sweating.

Patient Education This drug will not cure myasthenia gravis, but may help reduce symptoms. Take extended release tablets at bedtime; do not chew or crush extended release tablets. May cause dizziness, drowsiness, or hypotension; vomiting or loss of appetite; or diarrhea. Report persistent abdominal discomfort; significantly increased salivation, sweating, tearing, or urination; flushed skin; chest pain or palpitations; acute headache; unresolved diarrhea; excessive fatigue, insomnia, dizziness, or depression; increased muscle, joint, or body pain; vision changes or blurred vision; or shortness of breath or wheezing.

Pyridoxine (peer i DOKS een)

Brand Names: U.S. Aminoxin® [OTC]; Pyri-500 [OTC]

Index Terms B6; B_6; Pyridoxine Hydrochloride; Vitamin B_6

Pharmacologic Category Vitamin, Water Soluble

Medication Safety Issues

Sound-alike/look-alike issues:

Pyridoxine may be confused with paroxetine, pralidoxime, Pyridium®

International issues:

Doxal [Brazil] may be confused with Doxil brand name for DOXOrubicin [U.S.]

Doxal: Brand name for pyridoxine/thiamine combination [Brazil], but also the brand name for doxepin [Finland]

Pregnancy Risk Factor A

Lactation Enters breast milk/compatible (AAP rates "compatible"; AAP 2001 update pending)

Use Prevention and treatment of vitamin B_6 deficiency, pyridoxine-dependent seizures in infants

Unlabeled Use Treatment and prophylaxis of neurological toxicities (ie, seizures, coma) associated with isoniazid, hydrazine, and Gyromitrin-containing mushroom (false morel) overdose/toxicity

Available Dosage Forms

Capsule, oral: 50 mg, 250 mg

Aminoxin® [OTC]: 20 mg

Injection, solution: 100 mg/mL (1 mL)

Liquid, oral: 200 mg/5 mL (120 mL)

Tablet, oral: 25 mg, 50 mg, 100 mg, 250 mg, 500 mg

Tablet, sustained release, oral:

Pyri-500 [OTC]: 500 mg

General Dosage Range

I.M., I.V., SubQ: *Infants:* Deficiency: 10-100 mg

Oral:

Infants: Deficiency: 2-100 mg/day

Children: Deficiency: 1.5-25 mg/day; Neuritis: Prophylaxis: 1-2 mg/kg/day; Treatment: 10-50 mg/day

Adults: Deficiency: 10-20 mg/day; Neuritis: Prophylaxis: 25-100 mg/day; Treatment: 100-200 mg/day

Administration

I.M. Burning may occur at the injection site after I.M. or SubQ administration.

I.V. Seizures have occurred following I.V. administration of very large doses.

Isoniazid toxicity (unlabeled use): Initial doses should be administered at a rate of 0.5-1 g/minute. If the parenteral formulation is not available, anecdotal reports suggest that pyridoxine tablets may be crushed and made into a slurry and given at the same dose orally or via nasogastric (NG) tube (Boyer, 2006). Oral administration is not recommended for acutely poisoned patients with seizure activity.

I.V. Detail pH: 2.0-3.8

Nursing Actions

Physical Assessment Provide patient appropriate dietary instructions.

Patient Education Do not exceed recommended intake of dietary B_6. You may experience burning or pain at injection site; notify prescriber if this persists.

QUEtiapine (kwe TYE a peen)

Brand Names: U.S. SEROquel XR®; SEROquel®

Index Terms Quetiapine Fumarate

Pharmacologic Category Antipsychotic Agent, Atypical

Medication Safety Issues

Sound-alike/look-alike issues:

QUEtiapine may be confused with OLANZapine

SEROquel® may be confused with Serzone, SINEquan®

Medication Guide Available Yes

Pregnancy Risk Factor C

Lactation Enters breast milk/not recommended

Breast-Feeding Considerations Based on information from 8 mother/infant pairs, concentrations of quetiapine in breast milk have been reported as 0-170 µg/L. The estimated exposure to the breast-feeding infant would be up to 1 mg/kg/day (relative infant dose up to 0.43% based on a weight adjusted maternal dose of 400 mg/day).

Use Treatment of schizophrenia; treatment of acute manic or mixed episodes associated with bipolar I disorder (as monotherapy or in combination with lithium or divalproex); maintenance treatment of bipolar I disorder (in combination with lithium or divalproex); treatment of acute depressive episodes associated with bipolar disorder; adjunctive treatment of major depressive disorder

Unlabeled Use Autism; delirium in the critically-ill patient; psychosis/agitation related to Alzheimer's dementia

Mechanism of Action/Effect Quetiapine is a dibenzothiazepine atypical antipsychotic. It has been proposed that this drug's antipsychotic activity is mediated through a combination of dopamine type 2 and serotonin type 2 antagonism.

Antagonism at receptors other than dopamine and 5-HT_2 with similar receptor affinities may explain some of the other effects of quetiapine. The drug's antagonism of histamine H_1-receptors may explain the somnolence observed. The drug's antagonism of adrenergic $alpha_1$-receptors may explain the orthostatic hypotension observed.

Contraindications There are no contraindications listed in manufacturers labeling.

Canadian labeling: Hypersensitivity to quetiapine or any component of the formulation

Warnings/Precautions [U.S. Boxed Warning]: Antidepressants increase the risk of suicidal thinking and behavior in children, adolescents, and young adults (18-24 years of age) with major depressive disorder (MDD) and other psychiatric disorders; consider risk prior to prescribing. Short-term studies did not show an increased risk in patients >24 years of age and showed a decreased risk in patients ≥65 years.

Closely monitor all patients for clinical worsening, suicidality, or unusual changes in behavior; particularly during the initial 1-2 months of therapy or during periods of dosage adjustments (increased or decreases); the patient's family or caregiver should be instructed to closely observe the patient and communicate condition with healthcare provider. A medication guide concerning the use of antidepressants should be dispensed with each prescription.

[U.S. Boxed Warning]: Elderly patients with dementia-related psychosis treated with antipsychotics are at an increased risk of death compared to placebo. Most deaths appeared to be either cardiovascular (eg, heart failure, sudden death) or infectious (eg, pneumonia) in nature. Quetiapine is not approved for the treatment of dementia-related psychosis.

Leukopenia, neutropenia, and agranulocytosis (sometimes fatal) have been reported in clinical trials and postmarketing reports with antipsychotic use; presence of risk factors (eg, pre-existing low WBC or history of drug-induced leuko-/neutropenia) should prompt periodic blood count assessment. Discontinue therapy at first signs of blood dyscrasias or if absolute neutrophil count <1000/mm^3.

May be sedating, use with caution in disorders where CNS depression is a feature. Use with caution in Parkinson's disease. May induce orthostatic hypotension associated with dizziness, tachycardia, and, in some cases, syncope, especially during the initial dose titration period. Should be used with particular caution in patients with known cardiovascular disease (history of MI or ischemic heart disease, heart failure, or conduction abnormalities), cerebrovascular disease, or conditions that predispose to hypotension. Use has been associated with QT prolongation; postmarketing reports have occurred in patients with concomitant illness, quetiapine overdose, or who were receiving concomitant therapy known to affect QT interval or cause electrolyte imbalance. Esophageal dysmotility and aspiration have been associated with antipsychotic use; use with caution in patients at risk of aspiration pneumonia (eg, Alzheimer's disease). May cause dose-related decreases in thyroid levels, including cases requiring thyroid replacement therapy. Development of cataracts has been observed in animal studies; lens changes have been observed in humans during long-term treatment. Lens examination on initiation of therapy and every 6 months thereafter is recommended.

Due to anticholinergic effects, use with caution in patients with decreased gastrointestinal motility, urinary retention, BPH, xerostomia, visual problems, and narrow-angle glaucoma. Relative to other antipsychotics, quetiapine has a moderate potency of cholinergic blockade. May cause extrapyramidal symptoms (EPS), pseudoparkinsonism, and/or tardive dyskinesia. Risk of dystonia (and probably other EPS) may be greater with increased doses, use of conventional antipsychotics, males, and younger patients. Impaired core body temperature regulation may occur; caution with strenuous exercise, heat exposure, dehydration, and concomitant medication possessing anticholinergic effects. Neuroleptic malignant syndrome (NMS) is a potentially fatal symptom complex that has been reported in association with administration of antipsychotic drugs. Clinical manifestations of NMS are hyperpyrexia, muscle rigidity, altered mental status, and evidence of autonomic instability (irregular pulse or blood pressure, tachycardia, diaphoresis, and cardiac dysrhythmia). Management of NMS should include immediate discontinuation of antipsychotic drugs and other drugs not essential to concurrent therapy, intensive symptomatic treatment and medication monitoring, and treatment of any concomitant medical problems for which specific treatment are available.

Use caution in patients with a history of seizures. May cause decreases in total free thyroxine, elevations of liver enzymes, cholesterol levels, and/or triglyceride increases. Rare cases of priapism have been reported. May increase prolactin levels; clinical significance of hyperprolactinemia in patients with breast cancer or other prolactin-dependent tumors is unknown.

May cause hyperglycemia; in some cases may be extreme and associated with ketoacidosis, hyperosmolar coma, or death. Use with caution in patients with diabetes or other disorders of glucose regulation; monitor for worsening of glucose control. Significant weight gain has been observed with antipsychotic therapy; incidence varies with product. Monitor waist circumference and BMI. Patients using immediate release tablets may be switched to extended release tablets at the same total daily dose taken once daily. Dosage adjustments may be necessary based on response and tolerability. May cause withdrawal symptoms (rare) with abrupt cessation; gradually taper dose during discontinuation.

Drug Interactions

Avoid Concomitant Use

Avoid concomitant use of QUEtiapine with any of the following: Artemether; Conivaptan; Dronedarone; Lumefantrine; Metoclopramide; Nilotinib; Pimozide; QTc-Prolonging Agents; QuiNINE; Tetrabenazine; Thioridazine; Toremifene; Vandetanib; Vemurafenib; Ziprasidone

Decreased Effect

QUEtiapine may decrease the levels/effects of: Amphetamines; Anti-Parkinson's Agents (Dopamine Agonist); Quinagolide

The levels/effects of QUEtiapine may be decreased by: CYP3A4 Inducers (Strong); Deferasirox; Fosphenytoin; Lithium formulations; Peginterferon Alfa-2b; Phenytoin; Tocilizumab

Increased Effect/Toxicity

QUEtiapine may increase the levels/effects of: Alcohol (Ethyl); Anticholinergics; CNS Depressants; Dronedarone; Methylphenidate; Pimozide; QTc-Prolonging Agents; QuiNINE; Serotonin Modulators; Tetrabenazine; Thioridazine; Toremifene; Vandetanib; Vemurafenib; Ziprasidone

The levels/effects of QUEtiapine may be increased by: Acetylcholinesterase Inhibitors (Central); Alfuzosin; Artemether; Chloroquine; Ciprofloxacin; Ciprofloxacin (Systemic); Conivaptan; CYP3A4 Inhibitors (Moderate); CYP3A4 Inhibitors (Strong); Gadobutrol; HydrOXYzine; Indacaterol; Ivacaftor; Lithium formulations; Lumefantrine; Methylphenidate; Metoclopramide; Nilotinib; Pramlintide; QuiNINE; Tetrabenazine

Nutritional/Ethanol Interactions

Ethanol: May increase CNS depression; monitor for increased effects with coadministration. Caution patients about effects.

Food: In healthy volunteers, administration of quetiapine (immediate release) with food resulted in an increase in the peak serum concentration and AUC by 25% and 15%, respectively, compared to the fasting state. Administration of the extended release formulation with a high-fat meal (~800-1000 calories) resulted in an increase in peak serum concentration by 44% to 52% and AUC by 20% to 22% for the 50 mg and 300 mg tablets; administration with a light meal (≤300 calories) had no significant effect on the C_{max} or AUC.

Herb/Nutraceutical: St John's wort may decrease quetiapine levels. Avoid valerian, St John's wort, kava kava, gotu kola (may increase CNS depression).

Adverse Reactions Actual frequency may be dependent upon dose and/or indication. Unless otherwise noted, frequency of adverse effects is reported for adult patients; spectrum and incidence of adverse effects similar in children (with significant exceptions noted).

>10%:

Cardiovascular: Diastolic blood pressure increased (children and adolescents, 41%), systolic blood pressure increased (children and adolescents, 15%)

Central nervous system: Somnolence (18% to 57%), headache (7% to 21%), agitation (5% to 20%), dizziness (1% to 18%), fatigue (3% to 14%), extrapyramidal symptoms (1% to 13%)

Endocrine & metabolic: Triglycerides increased (≥200 mg/dL, 8% to 22%), HDL cholesterol decreased (≤40 mg/dL, 6% to 19%), total cholesterol increased (≥240 mg/dL, 7% to 18%), LDL cholesterol increased (≥160 mg/dL, 4% to 17%), hyperglycemia (≥200 mg/dL post glucose challenge or fasting glucose ≥126 mg/dL, 2% to 12%)

Gastrointestinal: Xerostomia (9% to 44%), weight gain (dose related; 3% to 23%), appetite increased (2% to 12%), constipation (6% to 11%)

1% to 10%:

Cardiovascular: Orthostatic hypotension (2% to 7%; children and adolescents <1%), tachycardia (1% to 6%), syncope (<5%), palpitation (4%), peripheral edema (4%), hypotension (3%), hypertension (1% to 2%)

Central nervous system: Insomnia (9%), akathisia (≤8%), pain (1% to 7%), dystonia (≤6%), lethargy (1% to 5%), tardive dyskinesia (<5%), anxiety (2% to 4%), irritability (1% to 4%), parkinsonism (≤4%), abnormal dreams (2% to 3%), depression (1% to 3%), hypersomnia (1% to 3%), abnormal thinking (2%), ataxia (2%), attention disturbance (2%), coordination impaired (2%), disorientation (2%), hypoesthesia (2%), mental impairment (2%), migraine (2%), sluggishness (2%), vertigo (2%), confusion (1% to 2%), restlessness (1% to 2%), fever (1% to 2%), chills (1%)

Dermatologic: Rash (4%), hyperhidrosis (2%)

Endocrine & metabolic: Hyperprolactinemia (4%), libido decreased (≤2%), hypothyroidism (≤2%), female lactation (1%)

Gastrointestinal: Nausea (7% to 8%), abdominal pain (dose related; 4% to 7%), dyspepsia (dose related; 2% to 7%), vomiting (1% to 6%), drooling (<5%), gastroenteritis (2% to 4%), toothache (2% to 3%), appetite decreased (2%), dysphagia (2%), flatulence (2%), GERD (2%), anorexia (≥1%), abnormal taste (1%), abdominal distension (≤1%)

Genitourinary: Pollakiuria (2%), urinary tract infection (2%), impotence (1%)

Hematologic: Neutropenia (≤2%), leukopenia (≥1%), hemorrhage (1%)

Hepatic: Transaminases increased (1% to 6%), GGT increased (1%)

Neuromuscular & skeletal: Weakness (2% to 10%), tremor (2% to 8%), back pain (3% to 5%), dysarthria (1% to 5%), hypertonia (4%), twitching (4%), dyskinesia (≤4%), arthralgia (1% to 4%), paresthesia (3%), muscle spasm (1% to 3%), limb pain (2%), myalgia (2%), neck pain (2%), neck rigidity (1%)

Ocular: Blurred vision (1% to 4%), amblyopia (2% to 3%)

Otic: Ear pain (1% to 2%)

Respiratory: Pharyngitis (4% to 6%), nasal congestion (5%), rhinitis (3% to 4%), upper respiratory tract infection (2% to 3%), sinus congestion (2%), sinus headache (2%), sinusitis (2%), cough (3%), dyspnea (≥1%), dry throat (1%)

Miscellaneous: Diaphoresis (2%), restless legs syndrome (2%), flu-like syndrome (1% to 2%), lymphadenopathy (1%)

Available Dosage Forms

Tablet, oral:

SEROquel®: 25 mg, 50 mg, 100 mg, 200 mg, 300 mg, 400 mg

Tablet, extended release, oral:

SEROquel XR®: 50 mg, 150 mg, 200 mg, 300 mg, 400 mg

General Dosage Range Dosage adjustment recommended in patients with hepatic impairment

Oral:

Immediate release:

Children ≥10 years: Initial: 25 mg twice daily; Maintenance: Titrate to 50-800 mg/day

Adults: Initial: 25-50 mg twice daily; Maintenance: 150-800 mg/day in 2-3 divided doses

Elderly: Initial: 25 mg/day

Extended release:

Adults: Initial: 50-300 mg once daily; Maintenance: Titrate to 150-800 mg/day

Elderly: Initial: 50 mg/day

Administration

Oral

Immediate release tablet: May be administered with or without food.

Extended release tablet: Administer without food or with a light meal (≤300 calories), preferably in the evening. Swallow tablet whole; do not break, crush, or chew.

Other Nasogastric/enteral tube (unlabeled route): Hold tube feeds for 30 minutes before administration; flush with 25 mL of sterile water. Crush dose using immediate-release formulation, mix in 10 mL water and administer via NG/enteral tube; follow with a 50 mL flush of sterile water (Devlin, 2010).

Stability

Storage Store at controlled room temperature of 25°C (77°F); excursions permitted to 15°C to 30°C (59°F to 86°F).

Nursing Actions

Physical Assessment Monitor CNS responses, orthostatic hypotension, and seizure threshold. Assess mental status for depression and suicide ideation and observe for abnormal involuntary movements. Evaluate for cataracts before initiating treatment and every 6 months during chronic treatment. Monitor weight prior to initiating therapy and at least monthly.

Patient Education It may take 2-3 weeks to achieve desired results. Avoid alcohol. Maintain adequate hydration. If you have diabetes, you may experience increased blood sugars; monitor closely. Avoid overeating and/or dehydration. You may experience excess drowsiness, restlessness, dizziness, urinary retention, or blurred vision; mouth sores, dry mouth, or GI upset; weight gain; constipation; or postural hypotension. Report persistent CNS effects (eg, somnolence, agitation, insomnia), anormal involuntary movements, suicide ideation, severe dizziness, vision changes, respiratory difficulty, muscle stiffness, high fever, or worsening of condition.

Dietary Considerations Immediate-release tablet may be taken without regard to meals. Extended release tablet should be taken without food or with a light meal (≤300 calories).

Quinapril (KWIN a pril)

Brand Names: U.S. Accupril®

Index Terms Quinapril Hydrochloride

Pharmacologic Category Angiotensin-Converting Enzyme (ACE) Inhibitor

Medication Safety Issues

Sound-alike/look-alike issues:

Accupril® may be confused with Accolate®, Accutane®, AcipHex®, Monopril®

International issues:

Accupril [U.S., Canada] may be confused with Acepril which is a brand name for captopril [Great Britain]; enalapril [Hungary, Switzerland]; lisinopril [Malaysia]

Pregnancy Risk Factor D

Lactation Enters breast milk/use caution

Breast-Feeding Considerations Quinapril is excreted in breast milk. The manufacturer recommends that caution be exercised when administering quinapril to nursing women.

Use Treatment of hypertension; treatment of heart failure

Unlabeled Use Treatment of left ventricular dysfunction after myocardial infarction; pediatric hypertension; to delay the progression of nephropathy and reduce risks of cardiovascular events in hypertensive patients with type 1 or 2 diabetes mellitus

Mechanism of Action/Effect Competitive inhibitor of angiotensin-converting enzyme (ACE); prevents conversion of angiotensin I to angiotensin II, a potent vasoconstrictor; results in lower levels of angiotensin II which causes an increase in plasma renin activity and a reduction in aldosterone secretion

Contraindications Hypersensitivity to quinapril or any component of the formulation; angioedema related to previous treatment with an ACE inhibitor

Warnings/Precautions Anaphylactic reactions may occur rarely with ACE inhibitors. At any time during treatment (especially following first dose) angioedema may occur rarely with ACE inhibitors; it may involve the head and neck (potentially compromising airway) or the intestine (presenting with abdominal pain). African-Americans and patients with idiopathic or hereditary angioedema may be at an increased risk. Prolonged frequent monitoring may be required especially if tongue, glottis, or larynx are involved as they are associated with airway obstruction. Patients with a history of airway surgery may have a higher risk of airway obstruction. Aggressive early and appropriate management is critical. Use in patients with previous angioedema associated with ACE inhibitor therapy is contraindicated. Severe anaphylactoid reactions may be seen during hemodialysis (eg, CVVHD) with high-flux dialysis membranes (eg, AN69), and rarely, during low density lipoprotein apheresis with dextran sulfate cellulose. Rare cases of anaphylactoid reactions have been reported in patients undergoing sensitization treatment with hymenoptera (bee, wasp) venom while receiving ACE inhibitors.

Symptomatic hypotension with or without syncope can occur with ACE inhibitors (usually with the first several doses); effects are most often observed in volume-depleted patients; close monitoring of patient is required especially with initial dosing and dosing increases; blood pressure must be lowered at a rate appropriate for the patient's clinical condition. Initiation of therapy in patients with ischemic heart disease or cerebrovascular disease warrants close observation due to the potential consequences posed by falling blood pressure (eg, MI, stroke). Use with caution in hypertrophic cardiomyopathy with outflow tract obstruction, severe aortic stenosis, or before, during, or immediately after major surgery. **[U.S. Boxed Warning]: Drugs that act on the renin-angiotensin system can cause injury and death to the developing fetus. Discontinue as soon as possible once pregnancy is detected.**

Hyperkalemia may occur with ACE inhibitors; risk factors include renal dysfunction, diabetes mellitus, concomitant use of potassium-sparing diuretics, potassium supplements, and/or potassium-containing salts. Use cautiously, if at all, with these agents and monitor potassium closely. Cough may occur with ACE inhibitors. Other causes of cough should be considered (eg, pulmonary congestion in patients with heart failure) and excluded prior to discontinuation.

May be associated with deterioration of renal function and/or increases in serum creatinine, particularly in patients with low renal blood flow (eg, renal artery stenosis, heart failure) whose glomerular filtration rate (GFR) is dependent on efferent arteriolar vasoconstriction by angiotensin II; deterioration may result in oliguria, acute renal failure, and progressive azotemia. Small increases in serum creatinine may occur following initiation; consider discontinuation only in patients with progressive and/or significant deterioration in renal function. Use with caution in patients with unstented unilateral/bilateral renal artery stenosis. When unstented bilateral renal artery stenosis is present, use is generally avoided due to the elevated risk of deterioration in renal function unless possible benefits outweigh risks. Concurrent use of angiotensin receptor blockers may increase the risk of clinically-significant adverse events (eg, renal dysfunction, hyperkalemia).

Rare toxicities associated with ACE inhibitors include cholestatic jaundice (which may progress to fulminant hepatic necrosis), agranulocytosis, neutropenia, or leukopenia with myeloid hypoplasia. Patients with collagen vascular diseases (especially with concomitant renal impairment) or renal impairment alone may be at increased risk for hematologic toxicity; periodically monitor CBC with differential in these patients.

Drug Interactions

Avoid Concomitant Use There are no known interactions where it is recommended to avoid concomitant use.

Decreased Effect

Quinapril may decrease the levels/effects of: Quinolone Antibiotics; Tetracycline Derivatives

The levels/effects of Quinapril may be decreased by: Antacids; Aprotinin; Herbs (Hypertensive Properties); Icatibant; Lanthanum; Methylphenidate; Nonsteroidal Anti-Inflammatory Agents; Salicylates; Yohimbine

Increased Effect/Toxicity

Quinapril may increase the levels/effects of: Allopurinol; Amifostine; Antihypertensives; AzaTHIOprine; CycloSPORINE; CycloSPORINE (Systemic); Ferric Gluconate; Gold Sodium Thiomalate; Hypotensive Agents; Iron Dextran Complex; Lithium; Nonsteroidal Anti-Inflammatory Agents; RiTUXimab; Sodium Phosphates

The levels/effects of Quinapril may be increased by: Alfuzosin; Angiotensin II Receptor Blockers; Diazoxide; DPP-IV Inhibitors; Eplerenone; Everolimus; Herbs (Hypotensive Properties); Loop Diuretics; MAO Inhibitors; Pentoxifylline; Phosphodiesterase 5 Inhibitors; Potassium Salts; Potassium-Sparing Diuretics; Prostacyclin Analogues; Sirolimus; Temsirolimus; Thiazide Diuretics; TiZANidine; Tolvaptan; Trimethoprim

Nutritional/Ethanol Interactions

Food: Potassium supplements and/or potassium-containing salts may cause or worsen hyperkalemia. Management: Consult prescriber before consuming a potassium-rich diet, potassium supplements, or salt substitutes.

Herb/Nutraceutical: Some herbal medications may worsen hypertension (eg, licorice); others may increase the antihypertensive effects of quinapril (eg, shepherd's purse). Management: Avoid bayberry, blue cohosh, cayenne, ephedra, ginger, ginseng (American), kola, licorice, and yohimbe. Avoid black cohosh, California poppy, coleus, golden seal, hawthorn, mistletoe, periwinkle, quinine, and shepherd's purse.

Adverse Reactions Note: Frequency ranges include data from hypertension and heart failure trials. Higher rates of adverse reactions have generally been noted in patients with CHF. However, the frequency of adverse effects associated with placebo is also increased in this population.

1% to 10%:

Cardiovascular: Hypotension (3%), chest pain (2%), first-dose hypotension (up to 3%)

Central nervous system: Dizziness (4% to 8%), headache (2% to 6%), fatigue (3%)

Dermatologic: Rash (1%)

Endocrine & metabolic: Hyperkalemia (2%)

Gastrointestinal: Vomiting/nausea (1% to 2%), diarrhea (2%)

Neuromuscular & skeletal: Myalgias (2% to 5%), back pain (1%)

Renal: BUN/serum creatinine increased (2%, transient elevations may occur with a higher frequency), worsening of renal function (in patients with bilateral renal artery stenosis or hypovolemia)

Respiratory: Upper respiratory symptoms, cough (2% to 4%; up to 13% in some studies), dyspnea (2%)

Pharmacodynamics/Kinetics

Onset of Action 1 hour

Duration of Action 24 hours

Available Dosage Forms

Tablet, oral: 5 mg, 10 mg, 20 mg, 40 mg

Accupril®: 5 mg, 10 mg, 20 mg, 40 mg

General Dosage Range Dosage adjustment recommended in patients with renal impairment

Oral:

Adults: Initial: 5-20 mg/day in 1-2 divided doses; Maintenance: 10-40 mg/day in 1-2 divided doses

Elderly: Initial: 2.5-5 mg/day

Stability

Reconstitution To prepare solution for oral administration, mix prior to administration and use within 10 minutes.

Storage Store at room temperature.

Nursing Actions

Physical Assessment Assess potential for interactions with other pharmacological agents or herbal products that may impact fluid balance or cardiac status. Monitor blood pressure carefully (hypotension or angioedema can occur at any time during treatment, especially following first dose). Monitor cardiac status and blood pressure. Monitor for hypovolemia, angioedema, and postural hypotension on a regular basis during therapy.

Patient Education Take first dose at bedtime or when sitting down (hypotension may occur). This drug does not eliminate need for diet or exercise regimen as recommended by prescriber. May cause increased cough (if persistent or bothersome, contact prescriber), postural hypotension, headache, dizziness, nausea, vomiting, or muscle or back pain. Immediately report swelling of face, mouth, lips, tongue, or throat; chest pain or respiratory difficulty; persistent cough; persistent pain in muscles, joints, or back; or skin rash.

Quinapril and Hydrochlorothiazide

(KWIN a pril & hye droe klor oh THYE a zide)

Brand Names: U.S. Accuretic®

Index Terms Hydrochlorothiazide and Quinapril; Quinaretic

Pharmacologic Category Angiotensin-Converting Enzyme (ACE) Inhibitor; Diuretic, Thiazide

Pregnancy Risk Factor D

Lactation Enters breast milk/use caution

Use Treatment of hypertension (not for initial therapy)

Available Dosage Forms

Tablet, oral: 10/12.5: Quinapril 10 mg and hydrochlorothiazide 12.5 mg; 20/12.5: Quinapril 20 mg and hydrochlorothiazide 12.5 mg; 20/25: Quinapril 20 mg and hydrochlorothiazide 25 mg

Accuretic®: 10/12.5: Quinapril 10 mg and hydrochlorothiazide 12.5 mg; 20/12.5: Quinapril 20 mg and hydrochlorothiazide 12.5 mg; 20/25: Quinapril 20 mg and hydrochlorothiazide 25 mg

General Dosage Range Oral: *Adults:* Initial: 10-20 mg quinapril and 12.5 mg hydrochlorothiazide once daily; Maintenance: 5-40 mg quinapril and 6.25-25 mg hydrochlorothiazide once daily

Nursing Actions

Physical Assessment See individual agents.

Patient Education See individual agents.

Related Information

Hydrochlorothiazide *on page 570*

Quinapril *on page 966*

QuiNIDine (KWIN i deen)

Index Terms Quinidine Gluconate; Quinidine Polygalacturonate; Quinidine Sulfate

Pharmacologic Category Antiarrhythmic Agent, Class Ia; Antimalarial Agent

Medication Safety Issues

Sound-alike/look-alike issues:

QuiNIDine may be confused with cloNIDine, quiNINE

High alert medication:

The Institute for Safe Medication Practices (ISMP) includes this medication (I.V. formulation) among its list of drug classes which have a heightened risk of causing significant patient harm when used in error.

Pregnancy Risk Factor C

Lactation Enters breast milk/not recommended (AAP rates "compatible"; AAP 2001 update pending)

Use

Quinidine gluconate and sulfate salts: Conversion and prevention of relapse into atrial fibrillation and/or flutter; suppression of ventricular arrhythmias. **Note:** Due to proarrhythmic effects, use should be reserved for life-threatening arrhythmias. Moreover, the use of quinidine has largely been replaced by more effective/safer antiarrhythmic agents and/or nonpharmacologic therapies (eg, radiofrequency ablation).

Quinidine gluconate (I.V. formulation): Conversion of atrial fibrillation/flutter and ventricular tachycardia. **Note:** The use of I.V. quinidine gluconate for these indications has been replaced by more effective/safer antiarrhythmic agents (eg, amiodarone and procainamide).

Quinidine gluconate (I.V. formulation) and quinidine sulfate: Treatment of malaria (*Plasmodium falciparum*)

Unlabeled Use Paroxysmal supraventricular tachycardia, paroxysmal AV junctional rhythm, and symptomatic atrial or ventricular premature contractions; short QT syndrome; Brugada syndrome

Available Dosage Forms

Injection, solution: 80 mg/mL (10 mL)

Tablet, oral: 200 mg, 300 mg

Tablet, extended release, oral: 300 mg, 324 mg

General Dosage Range Dosages expressed in terms of the salt. Dosage adjustment recommended in patients with renal impairment.

I.V.: Quinidine gluconate: *Children and Adults:* 10 mg/kg bolus followed by 0.02 mg/kg/minute **or** 24 mg/kg bolus followed by 12 mg/kg every 8 hours

Oral:

Immediate release: Quinidine sulfate: *Adults:* Initial: 200-400 mg/dose every 6 hours

Extended release:

Quinidine gluconate: *Adults:* Initial: 324 mg every 8-12 hours

Quinidine sulfate: *Adults:* Initial: 300 mg every 8-12 hours

Administration

Oral Do not crush, chew, or break sustained release dosage forms. Give around-the-clock to promote less variation in peak and trough serum levels. Some preparations of quinidine gluconate extended release tablets may be split in half to facilitate dosage titration; tablets are not scored.

I.V. Minimize use of PVC tubing to enhance bioavailability; shorter tubing lengths are recommended by the manufacturer

I.V. Detail pH: 5.5-7.0 (injection)

Nursing Actions

Physical Assessment I.V. requires use of infusion pump and continuous cardiac and hemodynamic monitoring. Monitor cardiac status at beginning of therapy, when titrating dosage, and on a regular basis. Quinidine has a low toxic: therapeutic ratio and overdose may easily produce severe and life-threatening reactions.

Patient Education Take around-the-clock. Do not crush, chew, or break sustained release dosage forms. Do not take with grapefruit juice. You will need regular cardiac checkups and blood tests while taking this medication. You may experience dizziness, drowsiness, visual changes, abnormal taste, nausea, vomiting, loss of appetite, headaches, or diarrhea (if persistent consult prescriber). Report chest pain, palpitation, or erratic heartbeat; respiratory difficulty or wheezing; CNS changes (confusion, delirium, fever, consistent dizziness); skin rash; sense of fullness or ringing in ears; or vision changes.

Related Information

Peak and Trough Guidelines *on page 1276*

QuiNINE (KWYE nine)

Brand Names: U.S. Qualaquin®

Index Terms Quinine Sulfate

Pharmacologic Category Antimalarial Agent

Medication Safety Issues

Sound-alike/look-alike issues:

QuiNINE may be confused with quiNIDine

Medication Guide Available Yes

Pregnancy Risk Factor C

Lactation Enters breast milk/use caution (AAP rate "compatible"; AAP 2001 update pending)

Use In conjunction with other antimalarial agents, treatment of uncomplicated chloroquine-resistant *P. falciparum* malaria

Unlabeled Use Treatment of *Babesia microti* infection in conjunction with clindamycin; treatment of uncomplicated chloroquine-resistant *P. vivax* malaria (in conjunction with other antimalarial agents)

Available Dosage Forms

Capsule, oral:

Qualaquin®: 324 mg

General Dosage Range Dosage adjustment recommended in patients with renal impairment

Oral:

Children: 30 mg/kg/day divided every 8 hours

Adults: 648 mg every 8 hours

Administration

Oral Avoid use of aluminum- or magnesium-containing antacids because of drug absorption problems. Swallow dose whole to avoid bitter taste. May be administered with food.

Nursing Actions

Physical Assessment Allergy history should be assessed prior to beginning therapy.

Patient Education Take with 8 oz of water, with or without food. You will need to return for follow-up blood tests. May cause severe headache, nausea, vomiting, or diarrhea. Report any vision changes (blurring, night-blindness, double vision, etc) or ringing in ears. Seek emergency help for chest pain, respiratory difficulty, seizures, or bleeding.

Quinupristin and Dalfopristin

(kwi NYOO pris tin & dal FOE pris tin)

Brand Names: U.S. Synercid®

Index Terms Dalfopristin and Quinupristin; Pristinamycin; RP-59500

Pharmacologic Category Antibiotic, Streptogramin

Pregnancy Risk Factor B

Lactation Excretion in breast milk unknown/use caution

Use Treatment of complicated skin and skin structure infections caused by methicillin-susceptible *Staphylococcus aureus* or *Streptococcus pyogenes*

Unlabeled Use Treatment of persistent MRSA bacteremia associated with vancomycin failure

Available Dosage Forms

Injection, powder for reconstitution:

Synercid®: 500 mg: Quinupristin 150 mg and dalfopristin 350 mg

General Dosage Range I.V.: *Children ≥12 years and Adults:* 7.5 mg/kg every 12 hours

Administration

I.V. Line should be flushed with 5% dextrose in water prior to and following administration. Infusion should be completed over 60 minutes (toxicity may be increased with shorter infusion). If severe venous irritation occurs following peripheral administration of quinupristin/dalfopristin diluted in 250 mL 5% dextrose in water, consideration should be given to increasing the infusion volume to 500 mL or 750 mL, changing the infusion site, or infusing by a peripherally-inserted central catheter (PICC) or a central venous catheter.

Nursing Actions

Physical Assessment Infusion site must be closely monitored. Monitor for arthralgia, headache, rash, hyperglycemia, opportunistic infection (fever, chills, sore throat, burning urination, fatigue), pseudomembranous colitis, hyperbilirubinemia, dyspnea, and ataxia.

Patient Education This drug can only be administered by intravenous infusion. Report immediately any pain, irritation, redness, burning, or swelling at infusion site. Report headache; rash; nausea; vomiting; diarrhea; pain; heat or swelling in muscle areas, especially in lower extremities; respiratory difficulty, tremors; or difficulty speaking.

Rabeprazole

(ra BEP ra zole)

Brand Names: U.S. AcipHex®

Index Terms Pariprazole

Pharmacologic Category Proton Pump Inhibitor; Substituted Benzimidazole

Medication Safety Issues

Sound-alike/look-alike issues:

AcipHex® may be confused with Acephen™, Accupril®, Aricept®, pHisoHex®

RABEprazole may be confused with ARIPiprazole, donepezil, lansoprazole, omeprazole, raloxifene

Pregnancy Risk Factor B

Lactation Excretion in breast milk unknown/not recommended

Use Short-term (4-8 weeks) treatment and maintenance of erosive or ulcerative gastroesophageal reflux disease (GERD); symptomatic GERD; short-term (up to 4 weeks) treatment of duodenal ulcers; long-term treatment of pathological hypersecretory conditions, including Zollinger-Ellison syndrome; *H. pylori* eradication (in combination therapy)

Canadian labeling: Additional uses (not in U.S. labeling): Treatment of nonerosive reflux disease (NERD); treatment of gastric ulcers

Unlabeled Use Maintenance of duodenal ulcer

Mechanism of Action/Effect Prevents gastric acid secretion

Contraindications Hypersensitivity to rabeprazole, substituted benzimidazoles (ie, esomeprazole, lansoprazole, omeprazole, pantoprazole), or any component of the formulation

Warnings/Precautions Use of proton pump inhibitors (PPIs) may increase the risk of gastrointestinal infections (eg, *Salmonella, Campylobacter*). Use caution in severe hepatic impairment. Relief of symptoms with rabeprazole does not preclude the presence of a gastric malignancy. Decreased *H. pylori* eradication rates have been observed with short-term (≤7 days) combination therapy. The American College of Gastroenterology recommends 10-14 days of therapy (triple or quadruple) for eradication of *H. pylori* (Chey, 2007).

PPIs may diminish the therapeutic effect of clopidogrel, thought to be due to reduced formation of the active metabolite of clopidogrel. The manufacturer of clopidogrel recommends either avoidance of omeprazole or use of a PPI with less potent CYP2C19 inhibition (eg, pantoprazole); given the potency of CYP2C19 inhibitory activity, avoidance of rabeprazole would appear prudent. Others have recommended the continued use of PPIs, regardless of the degree of inhibition, in patients with a history of GI bleeding or multiple risk factors for GI bleeding who are also receiving clopidogrel since no evidence has established clinically meaningful differences in outcome; however, a clinically-significant interaction cannot be excluded in those who are poor metabolizers of clopidogrel (Abraham, 2010; Levine, 2011).

Increased incidence of osteoporosis-related bone fractures of the hip, spine, or wrist may occur with PPI therapy. Patients on high-dose (multiple daily doses) or long-term therapy (≥1 year) should be monitored. Use the lowest effective dose for the shortest duration of time, use vitamin D and calcium supplementation, and follow appropriate guidelines to reduce risk of fractures in patients at risk.

Hypomagnesemia, reported rarely, usually with prolonged PPI use of >3 months (most cases >1 year of therapy); may be symptomatic or asymptomatic; severe cases may cause tetany, seizures, and cardiac arrhythmias. Consider obtaining serum magnesium concentrations prior to beginning long-term therapy, especially if taking concomitant digoxin, diuretics, or other drugs known to cause hypomagnesemia; and periodically thereafter. Hypomagnesemia may be corrected by magnesium supplementation, although discontinuation of rabeprazole may be necessary; magnesium levels typically return to normal within 1 week of stopping.

Drug Interactions

Avoid Concomitant Use

Avoid concomitant use of RABEprazole with any of the following: Delavirdine; Erlotinib; Nelfinavir; Pimozide; Posaconazole; Rilpivirine

Decreased Effect

RABEprazole may decrease the levels/effects of: Atazanavir; Bisphosphonate Derivatives; Cefditoren; Clopidogrel; Dabigatran Etexilate; Dasatinib; Delavirdine; Erlotinib; Gefitinib; Indinavir; Iron Salts; Itraconazole; Ketoconazole; Ketoconazole (Systemic); Mesalamine; Mycophenolate; Nelfinavir; Posaconazole; Rilpivirine; Vismodegib

The levels/effects of RABEprazole may be decreased by: CYP2C19 Inducers (Strong); CYP3A4 Inducers (Strong); Deferasirox; Herbs (CYP3A4 Inducers); Tipranavir; Tocilizumab

Increased Effect/Toxicity

RABEprazole may increase the levels/effects of: Amphetamines; ARIPiprazole; Citalopram; CYP2C19 Substrates; CYP2C8 Substrates; Dexmethylphenidate; Methotrexate; Methylphenidate; Pimozide; Raltegravir; Saquinavir; Tacrolimus; Tacrolimus (Systemic); Voriconazole

The levels/effects of RABEprazole may be increased by: Conivaptan; Fluconazole; Ketoconazole; Ketoconazole (Systemic)

Nutritional/Ethanol Interactions

Ethanol: Avoid ethanol (may cause gastric mucosal irritation).

Food: High-fat meals may delay absorption, but C_{max} and AUC are not altered.

Herb/Nutraceutical: St John's wort may increase the metabolism and thus decrease the levels/effects of rabeprazole.

Adverse Reactions 1% to 10%:

Central nervous system: Pain (3%), headache (2% to 5%)

Gastrointestinal: Diarrhea (3%), flatulence (3%), constipation (2%), nausea (2%)

Respiratory: Pharyngitis (3%)

Miscellaneous: Infection (2%)

Pharmacodynamics/Kinetics

Onset of Action Within 1 hour

Duration of Action 24 hours

Available Dosage Forms

Tablet, delayed release, enteric coated, oral:

AcipHex®: 20 mg

General Dosage Range Oral:

Children ≥12 years: 20 mg/day

Adults: 10-20 mg once to twice daily **or** 60 mg once daily

Administration

Oral May be administered without regard to meals; best if taken before breakfast. Do not crush, split, or chew tablet. May be administered with an antacid.

Stability

Storage Store at 25°C (77°F). Protect from moisture.

Nursing Actions

Physical Assessment Assess those medications requiring acid environment for absorption. Monitor reduction in symptoms.

Patient Education Swallow whole; do not crush, split, or chew. Follow recommended diet and activity instructions. Avoid alcohol. You may experience headache, diarrhea, or gas. Report persistent abdominal pain or headaches.

Dietary Considerations May be taken without regard to meals; best if taken before breakfast.

Rabies Vaccine (RAY beez vak SEEN)

Brand Names: U.S. Imovax® Rabies; RabAvert®

Index Terms HDCV; Human Diploid Cell Cultures Rabies Vaccine; PCEC; Purified Chick Embryo Cell

Pharmacologic Category Vaccine, Inactivated (Viral)

Pregnancy Risk Factor C

Lactation Excretion in breast milk unknown

Use Pre-exposure and postexposure vaccination against rabies

The Advisory Committee on Immunization Practices (ACIP) recommends a primary course of prophylactic immunization (pre-exposure vaccination) for the following:

- Persons with continuous risk of infection, including rabies research laboratory and biologics production workers
- Persons with frequent risk of infection in areas where rabies is enzootic, including rabies diagnostic laboratory workers, cavers, veterinarians and their staff, and animal control and wildlife workers; persons who frequently handle bats

- Persons with infrequent risk of infection, including veterinarians and animal control staff with terrestrial animals in areas where rabies infection is rare, veterinary students, and travelers visiting areas where rabies is enzootic and immediate access to medical care and biologicals is limited

The ACIP recommends the use of postexposure vaccination for a particular person be assessed by the severity and likelihood versus the actual risk of acquiring rabies. Consideration should include the type of exposure, epidemiology of rabies in the area, species of the animal, circumstances of the incident, and the availability of the exposing animal for observation or rabies testing. Postexposure vaccination is used in both previously vaccinated and previously unvaccinated individuals.

Available Dosage Forms

Injection, powder for reconstitution [preservative free]:

Imovax® Rabies: ≥ 2.5 int. units

RabAvert®: ≥ 2.5 int. units

General Dosage Range I.M.: *Children and Adults:* 1 mL

Administration

I.M. For I.M. administration only; this rabies vaccine product must not be administered intradermally; in adults and children, administer I.M. injections in the deltoid muscle, not the gluteal; for younger children, use the outer aspect of the thigh. Postexposure prophylaxis should begin with immediate cleansing of wounds with soap and water; if available, a virucidal agent (eg povidone-iodine solution) should be used to irrigate the wounds.

For patients at risk of hemorrhage following intramuscular injection, the ACIP recommends "it should be administered intramuscularly if, in the opinion of the physician familiar with the patients bleeding risk, the vaccine can be administered by this route with reasonable safety. If the patient receives antihemophilia or other similar therapy, intramuscular vaccination can be scheduled shortly after such therapy is administered. A fine needle (23 gauge or smaller) can be used for the vaccination and firm pressure applied to the site (without rubbing) for at least 2 minutes. The patient should be instructed concerning the risk of hematoma from the injection." Patients on anticoagulant therapy should be considered to have the same bleeding risks and treated as those with clotting factor disorders (CDC, 2011).

Simultaneous administration of vaccines helps ensure the patients will be fully vaccinated by the appropriate age. Simultaneous administration of vaccines is defined as administering >1 vaccine on the same day at different anatomic sites. The use of licensed combination vaccines is generally preferred over separate injections of the equivalent components. Separate vaccines should not be combined in the same syringe unless indicated by product specific labeling. Separate needles and syringes should be used for each injection. The ACIP prefers each dose of a specific vaccine in a series come from the same manufacturer when possible. Adolescents and adults should be vaccinated while seated or lying down. In general, preterm infants should be vaccinated at the same chronological age as full-term infants (CDC, 2011).

Antipyretics have not been shown to prevent febrile seizures. Antipyretics may be used to treat fever or discomfort following vaccination (CDC, 2011). One study reported that routine prophylactic administration of acetaminophen to prevent fever prior to vaccination decreased the immune response of some vaccines; the clinical significance of this reduction in immune response has not been established (Prymula, 2009).

Nursing Actions

Physical Assessment All serious adverse reactions must be reported to the U.S. DHHS. U.S. federal law also requires entry into the patient's medical record.

Patient Education Common reactions include pain, irritation, swelling, and itching at the site of administration. Contact healthcare provider if you develop a high fever or signs of an allergic reaction.

Related Information

Immunization Administration Recommendations *on page 1243*

Immunization Recommendations *on page 1248*

Raloxifene (ral OKS i feen)

Brand Names: U.S. Evista®

Index Terms Keoxifene Hydrochloride; Raloxifene Hydrochloride

Pharmacologic Category Selective Estrogen Receptor Modulator (SERM)

Medication Safety Issues

Sound-alike/look-alike issues:

Evista® may be confused with AVINza®, Eovist®

Medication Guide Available Yes

Pregnancy Risk Factor X

Lactation Excretion in breast milk unknown/contraindicated

Use Prevention and treatment of osteoporosis in postmenopausal women; risk reduction for invasive breast cancer in postmenopausal women with osteoporosis and in postmenopausal women with high risk for invasive breast cancer

Mechanism of Action/Effect A selective estrogen receptor modulator (SERM), meaning that it affects some of the same receptors that estrogen does, but not all, and in some instances, it antagonizes or blocks estrogen; it acts like estrogen to prevent bone loss and has the potential to block some estrogen effects in the breast uterine cancer tissues. Raloxifene decreases bone resorption, increasing bone mineral density and decreasing fracture incidence.

Contraindications History of or current venous thromboembolic disorders (including DVT, PE, and retinal vein thrombosis); pregnancy or women who could become pregnant; breast-feeding

Warnings/Precautions Hazardous agent - use appropriate precautions for handling and disposal. **[U.S. Boxed Warning]: May increase the risk for DVT or PE; use contraindicated in patients with history of or current venous thromboembolic disorders.** Use with caution in patients at high risk for venous thromboembolism; the risk for DVT and PE are higher in the first 4 months of treatment. Discontinue at least 72 hours prior to and during prolonged immobilization (postoperative recovery or prolonged bedrest). **[U.S. Boxed Warning]: The risk of death due to stroke may be increased in women with coronary heart disease or in women at risk for coronary events**; use with caution in patients with cardiovascular disease. Not be used for the prevention of cardiovascular disease. Use caution with moderate-to-severe renal dysfunction, hepatic impairment, unexplained uterine bleeding, and in women with a history of elevated triglycerides in response to treatment with oral estrogens (or estrogen/progestin). Safety with concomitant estrogen therapy has not been established. Safety and efficacy in premenopausal women or men have not been established. Not indicated for treatment of invasive breast cancer, to reduce the risk of recurrence of invasive breast cancer or to reduce the risk of noninvasive breast cancer. The efficacy (for breast cancer risk reduction) in women with inherited BRCA1 and BRCA1 mutations has not been established.

Drug Interactions

Avoid Concomitant Use There are no known interactions where it is recommended to avoid concomitant use.

Decreased Effect

Raloxifene may decrease the levels/effects of: Levothyroxine

The levels/effects of Raloxifene may be decreased by: Bile Acid Sequestrants

Increased Effect/Toxicity There are no known significant interactions involving an increase in effect.

Nutritional/Ethanol Interactions Ethanol: Avoid ethanol (may increase risk of osteoporosis).

Adverse Reactions Note: Raloxifene has been associated with increased risk of thromboembolism (DVT, PE) and superficial thrombophlebitis; risk is similar to reported risk of HRT

>10%:

Cardiovascular: Peripheral edema (3% to 14%)

Endocrine & metabolic: Hot flashes (8% to 29%)

Neuromuscular & skeletal: Arthralgia (11% to 16%), leg cramps/muscle spasm (6% to 12%)

Miscellaneous: Flu syndrome (14% to 15%), infection (11%)

1% to 10%:

Cardiovascular: Chest pain (3%), venous thromboembolism (1% to 2%)

Central nervous system: Insomnia (6%)

Dermatologic: Rash (6%)

Endocrine & metabolic: Breast pain (4%)

Gastrointestinal: Weight gain (9%), abdominal pain (7%), vomiting (5%), flatulence (2% to 3%), cholelithiasis (≤3%), gastroenteritis (≤3%)

Genitourinary: Vaginal bleeding (6%), leukorrhea (3%), urinary tract disorder (3%), uterine disorder (3%), vaginal hemorrhage (3%), endometrial disorder (≤3%)

Neuromuscular & skeletal: Myalgia (8%), tendon disorder (4%)

Respiratory: Bronchitis (10%), sinusitis (10%), pharyngitis (8%), pneumonia (3%), laryngitis (≤2%)

Miscellaneous: Diaphoresis (3%)

Pharmacodynamics/Kinetics

Onset of Action 8 weeks

Available Dosage Forms

Tablet, oral:

Evista®: 60 mg

General Dosage Range Oral: *Adults (females):* 60 mg/day

Administration

Oral May be administered without regard to meals

Stability

Storage Store at controlled room temperature of 20°C to 25°C (68°F to 77°F); excursions permitted to 15°C to 30°C (59°F to 86°F).

Nursing Actions

Physical Assessment Evaluate lipid profile and BMD. Monitor for DVT, PE, chest pain, migraine, and rash on a regular basis during therapy.

Patient Education Avoid excessive use of alcohol (ethanol may increase risk of osteoporosis). May be taken at similar time each day without regard to meals. Additional vitamin and mineral supplements (vitamin D, calcium) may be recommended by your prescriber. May cause nausea, vomiting, diarrhea, or joint pain. Report immediately any pain, redness, warmth, or swelling in leg; sudden chest pain; respiratory difficulty; or sudden change in vision. Report acute migraine, weight gain, urinary infection, or vaginal burning or itching.

Dietary Considerations May be taken without regard to meals. Osteoporosis prevention or treatment: Ensure adequate calcium and vitamin D intake; postmenopausal women should consume ~1500 mg/day of elemental calcium and 400-800 int. units/day of vitamin D.

Raltegravir (ral TEG ra vir)

Brand Names: U.S. Isentress®

Index Terms MK-0518

Pharmacologic Category Antiretroviral Agent, Integrase Inhibitor

Pregnancy Risk Factor C

Lactation Excretion in breast milk unknown/contraindicated

Breast-Feeding Considerations Maternal or infant antiretroviral therapy does not completely eliminate the risk of postnatal HIV transmission. In addition, multiclass-resistant virus has been detected in breast-feeding infants despite maternal therapy. Therefore, in the United States, where formula is accessible, affordable, safe, and sustainable, and the risk of infant mortality due to diarrhea and respiratory infections is low, complete avoidance of breast-feeding by HIV-infected women is recommended to decrease potential transmission of HIV (DHHS [perinatal], 2011).

Use Treatment of HIV-1 infection in combination with other antiretroviral agents

Mechanism of Action/Effect Inhibits the integration of viral DNA into host DNA, thereby blocking subsequent viral replication.

Contraindications There are no contraindications listed in the manufacturer's labeling.

Canadian labeling: Hypersensitivity to raltegravir or any other component of the formulation

Warnings/Precautions Patients may develop immune reconstitution syndrome resulting in the occurrence of an inflammatory response to an indolent or residual opportunistic infection; further evaluation and treatment may be required. Severe, life-threatening or fatal cases of Stevens-Johnson syndrome and toxic epidermal necrolysis have been reported. Hypersensitivity reactions (rash [may occur with fever, fatigue, malaise, conjunctivitis, or other constitutional symptoms], organ dysfunction and/or hepatic failure) have also been reported. Discontinue immediately if a severe skin reaction or hypersensitivity symptoms develop. Monitor liver transaminases and start supportive therapy. Myopathy and rhabdomyolysis have been reported; use caution in patients with risk factors for CK elevations and/or skeletal muscle abnormalities. Use caution with medications known to induce (eg, rifampin) or inhibit (eg, atazanavir) UGT1A1 glucuronidation, as serum levels/therapeutic effects may be reduced or increased, respectively. Avoid use as a boosted PI replacement in antiretroviral experienced patients with documented resistance to nucleoside reverse transcriptase inhibitors. Chewable tablet contains phenylalanine.

Drug Interactions

Avoid Concomitant Use There are no known interactions where it is recommended to avoid concomitant use.

Decreased Effect

Raltegravir may decrease the levels/effects of: Fosamprenavir

The levels/effects of Raltegravir may be decreased by: Efavirenz; Fosamprenavir; Rifampin; Tipranavir

Increased Effect/Toxicity

The levels/effects of Raltegravir may be increased by: Proton Pump Inhibitors

Nutritional/Ethanol Interactions

Food: Variable absorption depending upon meal type (low- vs high-fat meal) and dosage form; raltegravir was administered without regard to meals in clinical trials.

Herb/Nutraceutical: Avoid St John's wort (may decrease the levels/effects of raltegravir).

Adverse Reactions 2% to 10%:

Central nervous system: Insomnia (4%), headache (2%)

Endocrine & metabolic: Glucose increased (126-250 mg/dL: 3% to 10%; 251-500 mg/dL: 2% to 3%)

Gastrointestinal: Lipase increased (1.6-3 x ULN: 5%; 3.1-5 x ULN: 2%), amylase increased (1.6-2 x ULN: 2%; 2.1-5 x ULN: 4%)

Hematologic: Absolute neutrophil count decreased (grade 2: 3% to 4%; grade 3: 2% to 3%), platelets decreased (grade 2: 2% to 3%)

Hepatic: AST increased (2.6-5 x ULN: 4% to 9%, 5.1-10 x ULN: 2% to 4%), hyperbilirubinemia (1.6-2.5 x ULN: 4% to 6%; 2.6-5 x ULN: 1% to 3%), ALT increased (2.6-5 x ULN: 6% to 9%; 5.1-10 x ULN: 4% to 6%), alkaline phosphatase increased (2.6-5 x ULN: 1% to 2%)

Note: Incidence of liver function abnormalities higher with hepatitis B and/or C coinfection.

Neuromuscular & skeletal: Creatine kinase increased (6.0-9.9 x ULN: 2%; 10-19.9 x ULN: 4%; ≥20 x ULN: 3%)

Product Availability Isentress® chewable tablets (25 mg, 100 mg): FDA approved December 2011; availability anticipated mid-2012

Available Dosage Forms

Tablet, oral:

Isentress®: 400 mg

General Dosage Range Dosage adjustment recommended in patients on concomitant therapy

Oral:

Children 2 to <6 years: Chewable tablet: Weight-based dosing: 75-300 mg twice daily

Children 6 to <12 years: Chewable tablet: Weight-based dosing: 75-300 mg twice daily; if ≥25 kg, refer to weight-based dosing or adult dosing

Adolescents ≥12 years and Adults: Film-coated tablet: 400 mg twice daily

Administration

Oral May be administered without regard to meals; however, clinically insignificant variability in absorption exists depending on meal type.

Stability

Storage

Chewable tablet: Store in the original package with the bottle tightly closed, at room temperature of 20°C to 25°C (68°F to 77°F); excursions permitted to 15°C to 30°C (59°F to 86°F). Keep the desiccant in the bottle to protect from moisture.

Film-coated tablet: Store at room temperature of 20°C to 25°C (68°F to 77°F); excursions permitted to 15°C to 30°C (59°F to 86°F).

Nursing Actions

Physical Assessment Monitor for muscle pain and tenderness, changes in cholesterol, and signs and symptoms of depression.

Patient Education This drug will not cure HIV, nor has it been found to reduce the transmission of HIV; use appropriate precautions to prevent spread of the disease. This drug may be prescribed as one part of a multidrug combination; take exactly as directed for full course of therapy. If you miss a dose, take it as soon as you remember; do not double doses. You may be more susceptible to infection. May cause dizziness, headache, fatigue, nausea, vomiting, diarrhea. Report signs of infection (unusual fever or chills, white plaques in mouth, vaginal itching or foul-smelling vaginal discharge, unusual cough, congestion, or unhealed wounds) or muscle pain, tenderness, or weakness.

Dietary Considerations May be taken without regard to meals. Some products may contain phenylalanine.

Ramelteon (ra MEL tee on)

Brand Names: U.S. Rozerem®

Index Terms TAK-375

Pharmacologic Category Hypnotic, Nonbenzodiazepine

Medication Safety Issues

Sound-alike/look-alike issues:

Ramelteon may be confused with Remeron®

Rozerem® may be confused with Razadyne®, Remeron®

Medication Guide Available Yes

Pregnancy Risk Factor C

Lactation Excretion in breast milk unknown/use caution

Use Treatment of insomnia characterized by difficulty with sleep onset

Mechanism of Action/Effect Activates melatonin receptors within an area of the CNS controlling circadian rhythms and sleep-wake cycle.

Contraindications History of angioedema with previous ramelteon therapy (do not rechallenge); concurrent use with fluvoxamine

Warnings/Precautions Symptomatic treatment of insomnia should be initiated only after careful evaluation of potential causes of sleep disturbance. Failure of sleep disturbance to resolve after a reasonable period of treatment may indicate psychiatric and/or medical illness. Because of the rapid onset of action, administer immediately prior to bedtime or after the patient has gone to bed and is having difficulty falling asleep. Hypnotics/sedatives have been associated with abnormal thinking and behavior changes including decreased inhibition, aggression, bizarre behavior, agitation, hallucinations, and depersonalization. These changes may occur unpredictably and may indicate previously unrecognized psychiatric disorders; evaluate appropriately. Postmarketing studies have indicated that the use of hypnotic/sedative agents (including ramelteon) for sleep has been associated with hypersensitivity reactions including anaphylaxis as well as angioedema. Do not rechallenge patients who have developed angioedema with ramelteon therapy. An increased risk for hazardous sleep-related activities such as sleep-driving; cooking and eating food, and making phone calls while asleep have also been noted. Use caution with pre-existing depression or other psychiatric conditions. Caution when using with other CNS depressants; avoid engaging in hazardous activities or activities requiring mental alertness. Not recommended for use in patients with severe sleep apnea or COPD. Use caution with moderate hepatic impairment; not recommended in patients with severe impairment. May cause disturbances of hormonal regulation. Use caution when administered concomitantly with strong CYP1A2 inhibitors.

Drug Interactions

Avoid Concomitant Use

Avoid concomitant use of Ramelteon with any of the following: FluvoxaMINE

Decreased Effect

The levels/effects of Ramelteon may be decreased by: Cyproterone; Rifamycin Derivatives; Tocilizumab

Increased Effect/Toxicity

Ramelteon may increase the levels/effects of: Alcohol (Ethyl); CNS Depressants; Methotrimeprazine; Selective Serotonin Reuptake Inhibitors

The levels/effects of Ramelteon may be increased by: Abiraterone Acetate; Antifungal Agents (Azole Derivatives, Systemic); Conivaptan; CYP1A2 Inhibitors (Moderate); CYP1A2 Inhibitors (Strong); Deferasirox; Droperidol; Fluconazole; FluvoxaMINE; HydrOXYzine; Methotrimeprazine

Nutritional/Ethanol Interactions

Ethanol: May increase CNS depression. Management: Avoid or limit ethanol.

Food: Taking with high-fat meal delays T_{max} and increases AUC (~31%). Management: Do not take with a high-fat meal.

Herb/Nutraceutical: Some herbal medications may increase CNS depression. Management: Avoid valerian, St John's wort, kava kava, and gotu kola.

Adverse Reactions 1% to 10%:

Central nervous system: Dizziness (4% to 5%), somnolence (3% to 5%), fatigue (3% to 4%), insomnia worsened (3%), depression (2%)

Endocrine & metabolic: Serum cortisol decreased (1%)

Gastrointestinal: Nausea (3%), taste perversion (2%)

Neuromuscular & skeletal: Myalgia (2%), arthralgia (2%)

Respiratory: Upper respiratory infection (3%)

Miscellaneous: Influenza (1%)

Pharmacodynamics/Kinetics

Onset of Action 30 minutes

Available Dosage Forms

Tablet, oral:

Rozerem®: 8 mg

General Dosage Range Oral: *Adults:* 8 mg at bedtime

Administration

Oral Do not administer with a high-fat meal. Swallow tablet whole; do not break.

Stability

Storage Store at 25°C (77°F); excursions permitted to 15°C to 30°C (59°F to 86°F). Protect from moisture.

Nursing Actions

Physical Assessment Monitor for CNS changes, abnormal thinking, and behavior changes.

Patient Education Take approximately 30 minutes before desiring to go to sleep. Avoid alcohol and other CNS depressants. You may experience dizziness, lightheadedness, or headache. Avoid meal high in fat prior to taking this medication. Report abnormal thinking or behavior; unusual swelling, especially on face or neck; or respiratory difficulty.

Dietary Considerations Do not take with high-fat meal.

Ramipril (RA mi pril)

Brand Names: U.S. Altace®

Pharmacologic Category Angiotensin-Converting Enzyme (ACE) Inhibitor

Medication Safety Issues

Sound-alike/look-alike issues:

Ramipril may be confused with enalapril, Monopril®

Altace® may be confused with Altace® HCT, alteplase, Amaryl®, Amerge®, Artane

Pregnancy Risk Factor D

Lactation Excretion in breast milk unknown/not recommended

Breast-Feeding Considerations Ramipril and its metabolites were not detected in breast milk following a single oral dose of 10 mg. It is not known if multiple doses will produce detectable levels. Breast-feeding is not recommended by the manufacturer.

Use Treatment of hypertension, alone or in combination with thiazide diuretics; treatment of left ventricular dysfunction after MI; to reduce risk of MI, stroke, and death in patients at increased risk for these events

Unlabeled Use Treatment of heart failure; to delay the progression of nephropathy and reduce risks of cardiovascular events in hypertensive patients with type 1 or 2 diabetes mellitus

Mechanism of Action/Effect Ramipril is an ACE inhibitor which prevents the formation of angiotensin II from angiotensin I and exhibits pharmacologic effects that are similar to captopril. Ramipril must undergo conversion in the liver to its biologically active metabolite, ramiprilat. The pharmacodynamic effects of ramipril result from the high-affinity, competitive, reversible binding of ramiprilat to angiotensin-converting enzyme thus preventing the formation of the potent vasoconstrictor angiotensin II.

Contraindications Hypersensitivity to ramipril or any component of the formulation; prior hypersensitivity (including angioedema) to ACE inhibitors

Warnings/Precautions Anaphylactic reactions may occur rarely with ACE inhibitors. At any time during treatment (especially following first dose) angioedema may occur rarely with ACE inhibitors; it may involve the head and neck (potentially compromising airway) or the intestine (presenting with abdominal pain). African-Americans and patients with idiopathic or hereditary angioedema may be at an increased risk. Prolonged frequent monitoring may be required especially if tongue, glottis, or larynx are involved as they are associated with airway obstruction. Patients with a history of airway surgery may have a higher risk of airway obstruction. Aggressive early and appropriate management is critical. Use in patients with previous angioedema associated with ACE inhibitor therapy is contraindicated. Severe anaphylactoid reactions may be seen during hemodialysis (eg, CVVHD) with high-flux dialysis membranes (eg, AN69), and rarely, during low density lipoprotein apheresis with dextran sulfate cellulose. Rare cases of anaphylactoid reactions have been reported in patients undergoing sensitization treatment with hymenoptera (bee, wasp) venom while receiving ACE inhibitors.

Symptomatic hypotension with or without syncope can occur with ACE inhibitors (usually with the first several doses); effects are most often observed in volume-depleted patients; close monitoring of patient is required especially with initial dosing and dosing increases; blood pressure must be lowered at a rate appropriate for the patient's clinical condition. Initiation of therapy in patients with ischemic heart disease or cerebrovascular disease warrants close observation due to the potential consequences posed by falling blood pressure (eg, MI, stroke). Use with caution in hypertrophic cardiomyopathy with outflow tract obstruction, severe aortic stenosis, or before, during, or immediately after major surgery. **[U.S. Boxed Warning]: Drugs that act on the renin-angiotensin system can cause injury and death to the developing fetus. Discontinue as soon as possible once pregnancy is detected.**

Hyperkalemia may occur with ACE inhibitors; risk factors include renal dysfunction, diabetes mellitus, concomitant use of potassium-sparing diuretics, potassium supplements, and/or potassium containing salts. Use cautiously, if at all, with these agents and monitor potassium closely. Cough may occur with ACE inhibitors. Other causes of cough should be considered (eg, pulmonary congestion in patients with heart failure) and excluded prior to discontinuation.

May be associated with deterioration of renal function and/or increases in serum creatinine, particularly in patients with low renal blood flow (eg, renal artery stenosis, heart failure) whose glomerular filtration rate (GFR) is dependent on efferent arteriolar vasoconstriction by angiotensin II; deterioration may result in oliguria, acute renal failure, and progressive azotemia. Small increases in serum creatinine may occur following initiation; consider discontinuation only in patients with progressive and/or significant deterioration in renal function. Use with caution in patients with unstented unilateral/bilateral renal artery stenosis. When unstented bilateral renal artery stenosis is present, use is generally avoided due to the elevated risk of deterioration in renal function unless possible benefits outweigh risks. Concurrent use of angiotensin receptor blockers may increase the risk of clinically-significant adverse events (eg, renal dysfunction, hyperkalemia). Concurrent use with telmisartan is not recommended.

Rare toxicities associated with ACE inhibitors include cholestatic jaundice (which may progress to fulminant hepatic necrosis), agranulocytosis, neutropenia, or leukopenia with myeloid hypoplasia. Patients with collagen vascular diseases (especially with concomitant renal impairment) or renal impairment alone may be at increased risk for hematologic toxicity; periodically monitor CBC with differential in these patients.

Drug Interactions

Avoid Concomitant Use There are no known interactions where it is recommended to avoid concomitant use.

Decreased Effect

The levels/effects of Ramipril may be decreased by: Aprotinin; Herbs (Hypertensive Properties); Icatibant; Lanthanum; Methylphenidate; Nonsteroidal Anti-Inflammatory Agents; Salicylates; Yohimbine

Increased Effect/Toxicity

Ramipril may increase the levels/effects of: Allopurinol; Amifostine; Antihypertensives; AzaTHIOprine; CycloSPORINE; CycloSPORINE (Systemic); Ferric Gluconate; Gold Sodium Thiomalate; Hypotensive Agents; Iron Dextran Complex; Lithium; Nonsteroidal Anti-Inflammatory Agents; RiTUXimab; Sodium Phosphates

The levels/effects of Ramipril may be increased by: Alfuzosin; Angiotensin II Receptor Blockers; Diazoxide; DPP-IV Inhibitors; Eplerenone; Everolimus; Herbs (Hypotensive Properties); Loop Diuretics; MAO Inhibitors; Pentoxifylline; Phosphodiesterase 5 Inhibitors; Potassium Salts; Potassium-Sparing Diuretics; Prostacyclin Analogues; Sirolimus; Telmisartan; Temsirolimus; Thiazide Diuretics; TiZANidine; Tolvaptan; Trimethoprim

Nutritional/Ethanol Interactions Herb/Nutraceutical: Avoid bayberry, blue cohosh, cayenne, ephedra, ginger, ginseng (American), kola, licorice (may worsen hypertension). Avoid black cohosh, California poppy, coleus, golden seal, hawthorn, mistletoe, periwinkle, quinine, shepherd's purse (may have increased antihypertensive effect).

Adverse Reactions Note: Frequency ranges include data from hypertension and heart failure trials. Higher rates of adverse reactions have generally been noted in patients with CHF. However, the frequency of adverse effects associated with placebo is also increased in this population.

>10%: Respiratory: Cough increased (7% to 12%)

1% to 10%:

- Cardiovascular: Hypotension (11%), angina (up to 3%), postural hypotension (2%), syncope (up to 2%)
- Central nervous system: Headache (1% to 5%), dizziness (2% to 4%), fatigue (2%), vertigo (up to 2%)
- Endocrine & metabolic: Hyperkalemia (1% to 10%)
- Gastrointestinal: Nausea/vomiting (1% to 2%)
- Neuromuscular & skeletal: Chest pain (noncardiac) (1%)
- Renal: Renal dysfunction (1%), serum creatinine increased (1% to 2%), BUN increased (<1% to 3%); transient increases of creatinine and/or BUN may occur more frequently
- Respiratory: Cough (estimated 1% to 10%)

Worsening of renal function may occur in patients with bilateral renal artery stenosis or in hypovolemia. In addition, a syndrome which may include fever, myalgia, arthralgia, interstitial nephritis, vasculitis, rash, eosinophilia and positive ANA, and elevated ESR has been reported with ACE inhibitors. Risk of pancreatitis and agranulocytosis may be increased in patients with collagen vascular disease or renal impairment.

Pharmacodynamics/Kinetics

Onset of Action 1-2 hours

Duration of Action 24 hours

Available Dosage Forms

Capsule, oral: 1.25 mg, 2.5 mg, 5 mg, 10 mg

Altace®: 1.25 mg, 2.5 mg, 5 mg, 10 mg

General Dosage Range Dosage adjustment recommended in patients with renal impairment

Oral: *Adults:* 2.5-20 mg/day (maximum: 20 mg/day)

Administration

Oral Capsule is usually swallowed whole, but contents may be mixed in water, apple juice, or applesauce.

Stability

Storage Store at controlled room temperature.

Nursing Actions

Physical Assessment Assess potential for interactions with other pharmacological agents or herbal products that may impact fluid balance or cardiac status. Monitor first dose carefully (hypotension or angioedema can occur at any time during treatment, especially following first dose). Monitor blood pressure and cardiac status. Monitor for cough, renal dysfunction, nausea/vomiting, hypovolemia, angioedema, and postural hypotension on a regular basis during therapy.

Patient Education Take first dose at bedtime or when sitting down (hypotension may occur). This drug does not eliminate need for diet or exercise regimen as recommended by prescriber. May cause increased cough (if persistent or bothersome, contact prescriber), headache, postural hypotension, dizziness, nausea, or vomiting. Immediately report swelling of face, mouth, lips, tongue or throat; chest pain or irregular heartbeat. Report respiratory difficulty or persistent cough or persistent pain in muscles, joints, or back.

Ranitidine (ra NI ti deen)

Brand Names: U.S. Zantac 150® [OTC]; Zantac 75® [OTC]; Zantac®; Zantac® EFFERdose®

Index Terms Ranitidine Hydrochloride

Pharmacologic Category Histamine H_2 Antagonist

Medication Safety Issues

Sound-alike/look-alike issues:

Ranitidine may be confused with amantadine, rimantadine

Zantac® may be confused with Xanax®, Zarontin®, Zofran®, ZyrTEC®

Pregnancy Risk Factor B

Lactation Enters breast milk/use caution

Breast-Feeding Considerations Ranitidine is excreted into breast milk. The manufacturer recommends that caution be exercised when administering ranitidine to nursing women. Peak milk concentrations of ranitidine occur ~5.5 hours after the dose (case report).

Use

Zantac®: Short-term and maintenance therapy of duodenal ulcer, gastric ulcer, gastroesophageal reflux disease (GERD), active benign ulcer, erosive esophagitis, and pathological hypersecretory conditions; as part of a multidrug regimen for *H. pylori* eradication to reduce the risk of duodenal ulcer recurrence

Zantac 75® [OTC]: Relief of heartburn, acid indigestion, and sour stomach

Unlabeled Use Recurrent postoperative ulcer, upper GI bleeding, prevention of acid-aspiration pneumonitis during surgery, and prevention of stress-induced ulcers

Mechanism of Action/Effect Competitive inhibition of histamine at H_2-receptors, gastric acid secretion, gastric volume and hydrogen ion concentration are reduced

Contraindications Hypersensitivity to ranitidine or any component of the formulation

Warnings/Precautions Ranitidine has been associated with confusional states (rare). Use with caution in patients with hepatic impairment; use with caution in renal impairment, dosage modification required. Avoid use in patients with history of acute porphyria (may precipitate attacks); long-term therapy may be associated with vitamin B_{12} deficiency. Symptoms of GI distress may be associated with a variety of conditions; symptomatic response to H_2 antagonists does not rule out the potential for significant pathology (eg, malignancy). EFFERdose® formulation contains phenylalanine.

Drug Interactions

Avoid Concomitant Use

Avoid concomitant use of Ranitidine with any of the following: Delavirdine

Decreased Effect

Ranitidine may decrease the levels/effects of: Atazanavir; Cefditoren; Cefpodoxime; Cefuroxime; Dasatinib; Delavirdine; Erlotinib; Fosamprenavir; Gefitinib; Indinavir; Iron Salts; Itraconazole; Ketoconazole; Ketoconazole (Systemic); Mesalamine; Nelfinavir; Posaconazole; Prasugrel; Rilpivirine; Vismodegib

The levels/effects of Ranitidine may be decreased by: Cyproterone; Peginterferon Alfa-2b; P-glycoprotein/ABCB1 Inducers

Increased Effect/Toxicity

Ranitidine may increase the levels/effects of: ARIPiprazole; Dexmethylphenidate; Methylphenidate; Procainamide; Saquinavir; Sulfonylureas; Varenicline; Warfarin

The levels/effects of Ranitidine may be increased by: P-glycoprotein/ABCB1 Inhibitors

Nutritional/Ethanol Interactions

Ethanol: Avoid ethanol (may cause gastric mucosal irritation).

Food: Does not interfere with absorption of ranitidine.

Adverse Reactions Frequency not defined.

Cardiovascular: Asystole, atrioventricular block, bradycardia (with rapid I.V. administration), premature ventricular beats, tachycardia, vasculitis
Central nervous system: Agitation, dizziness, depression, hallucinations, headache, insomnia, malaise, mental confusion, somnolence, vertigo
Dermatologic: Alopecia, erythema multiforme, rash
Endocrine & metabolic: Prolactin levels increased
Gastrointestinal: Abdominal discomfort/pain, constipation, diarrhea, nausea, pancreatitis, vomiting
Hematologic: Acquired immune hemolytic anemia, acute porphyritic attack, agranulocytosis, aplastic anemia, granulocytopenia, leukopenia, pancytopenia, thrombocytopenia
Hepatic: Cholestatic hepatitis, hepatic failure, hepatitis, jaundice
Local: Transient pain, burning or itching at the injection site
Neuromuscular & skeletal: Arthralgia, involuntary motor disturbance, myalgia
Ocular: Blurred vision
Renal: Acute interstitial nephritis, serum creatinine increased
Respiratory: Pneumonia (causal relationship not established)
Miscellaneous: Anaphylaxis, angioneurotic edema, hypersensitivity reactions (eg, bronchospasm, fever, eosinophilia)

Available Dosage Forms

Capsule, oral: 150 mg, 300 mg

Infusion, premixed in 1/2 NS [preservative free]:
Zantac®: 50 mg (50 mL)

Injection, solution: 25 mg/mL (2 mL, 6 mL, 40 mL)
Zantac®: 25 mg/mL (2 mL, 6 mL, 40 mL)

Syrup, oral: 15 mg/mL (5 mL, 10 mL, 120 mL, 473 mL, 474 mL, 480 mL)
Zantac®: 15 mg/mL (480 mL)

Tablet, oral: 75 mg, 150 mg, 300 mg
Zantac 150® [OTC]: 150 mg
Zantac 75® [OTC]: 75 mg
Zantac®: 150 mg, 300 mg

Tablet for solution, oral:
Zantac® EFFERdose®: 25 mg

General Dosage Range Dosage adjustment recommended in patients with renal impairment

I.M.: *Children >16 years and Adults:* 50 mg every 6-8 hours

I.V.:

Children 1 month to 16 years: 2-4 mg/kg/day divided every 6-8 hours (maximum: 200 mg/day) **or** 1 mg/kg/dose for one dose followed by infusion of 0.08-0.17 mg/kg/hour

Children >16 years and Adults: 50 mg every 6-8 hours **or** Infusion: 6.25 mg/hour **or** 1-2.5 mg/kg/hour

Oral:

Children 1 month to 11 years: 2-4 mg/kg/dose once or twice daily **or** 5-10 mg/kg/day in 2 divided doses (maximum: 300 mg/day)

Children ≥12 to 16 years: 2-4 mg/kg once or twice daily **or** 5-10 mg/kg/day in 2 divided doses (maximum: 300 mg/day); OTC dosing: 75 mg 30-60 minutes before eating or drinking (maximum: 150 mg/day)

Children >16 years and Adults: 150 mg 1-4 times/day **or** 300 mg once daily; OTC dosing: 75 mg 30-60 minutes before eating or drinking (maximum: 150 mg/day)

Administration

Oral EFFERdose®: Should not be chewed, swallowed whole, or dissolved on tongue: 25 mg tablet: Dissolve in at least 5 mL of water; wait until completely dissolved before administering

I.M. No dilution is needed

I.V.

I.V. push: Ranitidine (usually 50 mg) should be diluted to a total of 20 mL (or a concentration not exceeding 2.5 mg/mL) with NS or D_5W and administered over at least 5 minutes or a maximum rate of 10 mg/minute.

Intermittent I.V. infusion: Dilute to a maximum concentration of 0.5 mg/mL; administer over 15-20 minutes

Continuous I.V. infusion: Dilute to a maximum concentration of 2.5 mg/mL. Titrate dosage based on gastric pH.

I.V. Detail I.V. must be diluted; may be administered I.V. push, intermittent I.V. infusion, or continuous I.V. infusion

pH: 6.7-7.3

Stability

Reconstitution Vials can be mixed with NS or D_5W.

Intermittent bolus injection, continuous infusion: Dilute to maximum of 2.5 mg/mL.

Intermittent infusion: Dilute to maximum of 0.5 mg/mL.

Storage

Injection: Vials: Store between 4°C to 25°C (39°F to 77°F); excursion permitted to 30°C (86°F). Protect from light. Solution is a clear, colorless to yellow solution; slight darkening does not affect potency. Vials mixed with NS or D_5W are stable for 48 hours at room temperature.

Premixed bag: Store between 2°C to 25°C (36°F to 77°F). Protect from light.

EFFERdose® formulations: Store between 2°C to 30°C (36°F to 86°F).

Syrup: Store between 4°C to 25°C (39°F to 77°F). Protect from light.

Tablets: Store in dry place, between 15°C to 30°C (59°F to 86°F). Protect from light.

Nursing Actions

Physical Assessment Monitor for CNS changes (depression, hallucinations, confusion, malaise), rash, and GI disturbance.

Patient Education May take several days before you notice relief. Avoid excessive alcohol. May cause drowsiness, dizziness, or fatigue. Report immediately skin rash, CNS changes (mental confusion, hallucinations, somnolence), or unusual persistent weakness or lethargy.

Dietary Considerations Some products may contain phenylalanine and/or sodium. Oral dosage forms may be taken with or without food.

Related Information

Compatibility of Drugs *on page 1264*

Ranolazine (ra NOE la zeen)

Brand Names: U.S. Ranexa®

Pharmacologic Category Antianginal Agent; Cardiovascular Agent, Miscellaneous

Medication Safety Issues

Sound-alike/look-alike issues:

Ranexa® may be confused with CeleXA®

Pregnancy Risk Factor C

Lactation Excretion in breast milk unknown/not recommended

Breast-Feeding Considerations Due to the potential for serious adverse reactions in the nursing infant, breast-feeding is not recommended.

Use Treatment of chronic angina

Mechanism of Action/Effect May increase myocardial relaxation during myocardial ischemia and improve energy supply during ischemia.

Contraindications Hepatic cirrhosis; concurrent strong CYP3A inhibitors; concurrent CYP3A inducers

Warnings/Precautions Ranolazine does not relieve acute angina attacks. Has been shown to prolong QT interval in a dose/plasma concentration-related manner; assess risk versus benefit of use in patients with potential for prolonged QT including a family history. Hepatically-impaired patients may have a more significant increase in QT interval. Use is contraindicated in patients with cirrhosis (Child-Pugh class ≥A). Use caution in patients ≥75 years of age; they may experience more adverse events. Use caution and monitor blood pressure in patients with renal dysfunction; has not been evaluated in patients requiring dialysis.

Ranolazine is a substrate for and a moderate inhibitor of P-glycoprotein. Inhibitors of P-glycoprotein may increase serum concentrations of ranolazine. Ranolazine may increase serum concentrations of substrates for P-glycoprotein (eg, digoxin). Ranolazine is primarily metabolized by CYP3A; use is contraindicated with inducers and strong inhibitors of CYP3A. Ranolazine has potential to prolong the QT-interval; use caution when administered concomitantly with QT-prolonging drugs. Use caution when administering ranolazine to patients with a history of malignant neoplasms or adenomatous polyps.

Drug Interactions

Avoid Concomitant Use

Avoid concomitant use of Ranolazine with any of the following: Antifungal Agents (Azole Derivatives, Systemic); Artemether; CYP3A4 Inducers (Strong); CYP3A4 Inhibitors (Strong); Dronedarone; Lumefantrine; Nilotinib; Pimozide; QUEtiapine; QuiNINE; Rifampin; Silodosin; St Johns Wort; Tetrabenazine; Thioridazine; Topotecan; Toremifene; Vandetanib; Vemurafenib; Ziprasidone

Decreased Effect

The levels/effects of Ranolazine may be decreased by: CYP3A4 Inducers (Strong); Deferasirox; Peginterferon Alfa-2b; P-glycoprotein/ABCB1 Inducers; Rifampin; St Johns Wort; Tocilizumab

Increased Effect/Toxicity

Ranolazine may increase the levels/effects of: ARIPiprazole; Colchicine; Dabigatran Etexilate; Digoxin; Dronedarone; Everolimus; Lovastatin; P-glycoprotein/ABCB1 Substrates; Pimozide; Prucalopride; QTc-Prolonging Agents; QuiNINE; Rivaroxaban; Silodosin; Simvastatin; Tacrolimus; Tacrolimus (Systemic); Tetrabenazine; Thioridazine; Topotecan; Toremifene; Vandetanib; Vemurafenib; Ziprasidone

The levels/effects of Ranolazine may be increased by: Alfuzosin; Antifungal Agents (Azole Derivatives, Systemic); Artemether; Calcium Channel Blockers (Nondihydropyridine); Chloroquine; Ciprofloxacin; Ciprofloxacin (Systemic); CYP3A4 Inhibitors (Moderate); CYP3A4 Inhibitors (Strong); Gadobutrol; Indacaterol; Lumefantrine; Nilotinib; P-glycoprotein/ABCB1 Inhibitors; QUEtiapine; QuiNINE

Nutritional/Ethanol Interactions

Food: Grapefruit, grapefruit juice, or grapefruit-containing products may increase the serum concentration of ranolazine. Management: Avoid grapefruit-containing products or dose adjustment of ranolazine may be required.

Herb/Nutraceutical: St John's wort may decrease the serum concentration of ranolazine. Management: Avoid St John's wort.

Adverse Reactions >0.5% to 10%:

Cardiovascular: Bradycardia (≤4%), hypotension (≤4%), orthostatic hypotension (≤4%), palpitation (≤4%), peripheral edema (≤4%), QT_c prolongation (>500 msec: ≤1%)

Central nervous system: Headache (≤6%), dizziness (1% to 6%), confusion (≤4%), vasovagal attacks (≤4%), vertigo (≤4%)

Dermatologic: Hyperhidrosis (≤4%)

Gastrointestinal: Constipation (≤9%), abdominal pain (≤4%), anorexia (≤4%), dyspepsia (≤4%), nausea (≤4%; dose related), vomiting (≤4%), xerostomia (≤4%)

Neuromuscular: Weakness (≤4%)

Ocular: Blurred vision (≤4%)

Otic: Tinnitus (≤4%)
Renal: Hematuria (≤4%)
Respiratory: Dyspnea (≤4%)

Available Dosage Forms

Tablet, extended release, oral:
Ranexa®: 500 mg, 1000 mg

General Dosage Range Dosage adjustment recommended in patients on concomitant therapy

Oral: *Adults:* Initial: 500 mg twice daily; Maintenance: 500-1000 mg twice daily (maximum: 2000 mg/day)

Administration

Oral May be taken with or without meals. Swallow tablet whole; do not crush, break, or chew.

Stability

Storage Store at 25°C (77°F); excursions permitted to 15°C to 30°C (59°F to 86°F).

Nursing Actions

Physical Assessment Check QT_c if ECG obtained. Stress that this medication is not intended to treat an acute angina episode. Instruct patient in appropriate measures to take if an acute episode occurs.

Patient Education This medication is not intended to treat an acute angina episode. Follow instructions provided by prescriber for acute management. Swallow tablets whole; do not crush, break, or chew the tablets. You may experience dizziness or constipation. Report palpitations, dizziness, or passing out. Educate patient about how to prevent constipation.

Dietary Considerations May be taken without regard to meals. Limit the use of grapefuit juice.

Rasagiline (ra SA ji leen)

Brand Names: U.S. Azilect®

Index Terms AGN 1135; Rasagiline Mesylate; TVP-1012

Pharmacologic Category Anti-Parkinson's Agent, MAO Type B Inhibitor

Medication Safety Issues

Sound-alike/look-alike issues:
Azilect® may be confused with Aricept®

Pregnancy Risk Factor C

Lactation Excretion in breast milk unknown/use caution

Breast-Feeding Considerations Animal studies have shown rasagiline is capable of inhibiting prolactin secretion.

Use Treatment of idiopathic Parkinson's disease (initial monotherapy or as adjunct to levodopa)

Mechanism of Action/Effect Rasagiline selectively inhibits MAO-B which enhances brain dopamine levels, thus reducing symptomatic motor deficits.

Contraindications Concomitant use of cyclobenzaprine, dextromethorphan, methadone, propoxyphene, St John's wort, or tramadol; concomitant use of meperidine or an MAO inhibitor (including selective MAO-B inhibitors) within 14 days of rasagiline

Warnings/Precautions Hazardous agent - use appropriate precautions for handling and disposal.

Cardiovascular system: May cause orthostatic hypotension, particularly in combination with levodopa; use with caution in patients with hypotension or patients who would not tolerate transient hypotensive episodes (cardiovascular or cerebrovascular disease); orthostasis is usually most problematic during first 2 months of therapy and tends to abate thereafter. Due to the potential for hemodynamic instability, patients should not undergo elective surgery requiring general anesthesia and should avoid local anesthesia containing sympathomimetic vasoconstrictors within 14 days of discontinuing rasagiline. If surgery is required, benzodiazepines, mivacurium, fentanyl, morphine or codeine may be used cautiously. In patients taking recommended doses of rasagiline, dietary restriction of most tyramine-containing products is not necessary; however, certain foods (eg, aged cheeses) may contain high amounts (>150 mg) of tyramine and could lead to hypertensive crisis. Avoid concomitant use with foods high in tyramine.

Central nervous system: Serotonin syndrome (SS)/neuroleptic malignant syndrome (NMS)-like reactions may occur rarely, particularly when used at doses exceeding recommendations or when used in combination with an antidepressant (eg, SSRI, SNRI, TCA). May cause hallucinations; signs of severe CNS toxicity (some fatal), including hyperpyrexia, hyperthermia, rigidity, altered mental status, seizure and coma have been reported with selective and nonselective MAO inhibitor use in combination with antidepressants. Do not use within 5 weeks of fluoxetine discontinuation; do not initiate tricyclic, SSRI, or SNRI therapy within 2 weeks of discontinuing rasagiline. Addition to levodopa therapy may result in exacerbation of dyskinesias, requiring a reduction in levodopa dosage.

Dermatologic: Risk of melanoma may be increased with rasagiline, although increased risk has been associated with Parkinson's disease itself; patients should have regular and frequent skin examinations.

Organ dysfunction: Use caution in mild hepatic impairment; dose reduction recommended. Do not use with moderate-to-severe hepatic impairment.

Drug Interactions

Avoid Concomitant Use

Avoid concomitant use of Rasagiline with any of the following: Alpha-/Beta-Agonists (Indirect-Acting); Alpha1-Agonists; Alpha2-Agonists (Ophthalmic); Amphetamines; Anilidopiperidine Opioids; Antidepressants (Serotonin Reuptake Inhibitor/ Antagonist); Atomoxetine; Bezafibrate;

Buprenorphine; BuPROPion; BusPIRone; CarBAMazepine; Cyclobenzaprine; Dexmethylphenidate; Dextromethorphan; Diethylpropion; HYDROmorphone; Linezolid; Maprotiline; Meperidine; Methyldopa; Methylene Blue; Methylphenidate; Mirtazapine; Oxymorphone; Pizotifen; Selective Serotonin Reuptake Inhibitors; Serotonin 5-HT1D Receptor Agonists; Serotonin/Norepinephrine Reuptake Inhibitors; Tapentadol; Tetrabenazine; Tetrahydrozoline; Tetrahydrozoline (Nasal); Tricyclic Antidepressants; Tryptophan

Decreased Effect

The levels/effects of Rasagiline may be decreased by: CYP1A2 Inducers (Strong); Cyproterone

Increased Effect/Toxicity

Rasagiline may increase the levels/effects of: Alpha-/Beta-Agonists (Direct-Acting); Alpha-/Beta-Agonists (Indirect-Acting); Alpha1-Agonists; Alpha2-Agonists (Ophthalmic); Amphetamines; Antidepressants (Serotonin Reuptake Inhibitor/Antagonist); Antihypertensives; Atomoxetine; Beta2-Agonists; Bezafibrate; BuPROPion; Dexmethylphenidate; Dextromethorphan; Diethylpropion; Doxapram; HYDROmorphone; Linezolid; Lithium; Meperidine; Methadone; Methyldopa; Methylene Blue; Methylphenidate; Metoclopramide; Mirtazapine; Orthostatic Hypotension Producing Agents; Pizotifen; Reserpine; Selective Serotonin Reuptake Inhibitors; Serotonin 5-HT1D Receptor Agonists; Serotonin Modulators; Serotonin/Norepinephrine Reuptake Inhibitors; Tetrahydrozoline; Tetrahydrozoline (Nasal); Tricyclic Antidepressants

The levels/effects of Rasagiline may be increased by: Abiraterone Acetate; Altretamine; Anilidopiperidine Opioids; Antipsychotics; Buprenorphine; BusPIRone; CarBAMazepine; COMT Inhibitors; Cyclobenzaprine; CYP1A2 Inhibitors (Moderate); CYP1A2 Inhibitors (Strong); Deferasirox; Levodopa; MAO Inhibitors; Maprotiline; Oxymorphone; Tapentadol; Tetrabenazine; TraMADol; Tryptophan

Nutritional/Ethanol Interactions

Ethanol: Management: Avoid ethanol.

Food: Concurrent ingestion of foods rich in tyramine may cause sudden and severe high blood pressure (hypertensive crisis). Management: Avoid foods containing high amounts (>150 mg) of tyramine (aged or matured cheese, air-dried or cured meats including sausages and salamis; fava or broad bean pods, tap/draft beers, Marmite concentrate, sauerkraut, soy sauce, and other soybean condiments). Food's freshness is also an important concern; improperly stored or spoiled food can create an environment in which tyramine concentrations may increase. Avoid these foods during and for 2 weeks after discontinuation of medication.

Herb/Nutraceutical: Some herbal medications may cause excessive sedation; others may increase the risk of serotonin syndrome or hypertensive reactions. Management: Avoid valerian, St John's wort, SAMe, and kava kava; avoid supplements containing caffeine, tyrosine, tryptophan, or phenylalanine.

Adverse Reactions Unless otherwise noted, the following adverse reactions are as reported for monotherapy. Spectrum of adverse events was generally similar with adjunctive (levodopa) therapy, though the incidence tended to be higher.

>10%:

- Cardiovascular: Postural hypotension (6% to 13% adjunct therapy, dose dependent)
- Central nervous system: Dyskinesia (18% adjunct therapy), headache (14%)
- Gastrointestinal: Nausea (10% to 12% adjunct therapy)

1% to 10%:

- Cardiovascular: Angina, bundle branch block, chest pain, syncope
- Central nervous system: Depression (5%), hallucinations (4% to 5% adjunct therapy), fever (3%), malaise (2%), vertigo (2%), anxiety, dizziness
- Dermatologic: Bruising (2%), alopecia, skin carcinoma, vesiculobullous rash
- Endocrine & metabolic: Impotence, libido decreased
- Gastrointestinal: Constipation (4% to 9% adjunct therapy), weight loss (2% to 9% adjunct therapy; dose dependent), dyspepsia (7%), xerostomia (2% to 6% adjunct therapy; dose dependent), gastroenteritis (3%), anorexia, diarrhea, gastrointestinal hemorrhage, vomiting
- Genitourinary: Hematuria, urinary incontinence
- Hematologic: Leukopenia
- Hepatic: Liver function tests increased
- Neuromuscular & skeletal: Arthralgia (7%), neck pain (2%), arthritis (2%), paresthesia (2%), abnormal gait, hyperkinesias, hypertonia, neuropathy, tremor, weakness
- Ocular: Conjunctivitis (3%)
- Renal: Albuminuria
- Respiratory: Rhinitis (3%), asthma, cough increased
- Miscellaneous: Fall (5%), flu-like syndrome (5%), allergic reaction

Pharmacodynamics/Kinetics

Onset of Action Therapeutic: Within 1 hour

Duration of Action ~1 week (irreversible inhibition); may require ~14-40 days for complete restoration of (brain) MAO-B activity

Available Dosage Forms

Tablet, oral:

Azilect®: 0.5 mg, 1 mg

General Dosage Range Dosage adjustment recommended in patients with hepatic impairment or on concomitant therapy

Oral: *Adults:* 0.5-1 mg once daily

Administration

Oral Administer without regard to meals.

Stability

Storage Store at 25°C (77°F); excursions permitted to 15°C to 30°C (59°F to 86°F).

Nursing Actions

Physical Assessment Monitor blood pressure. Be alert to suicide ideation. Patient should be cautioned against eating foods high in tyramine.

Patient Education May be prescribed in conjunction with levodopa/carbidopa. Therapeutic effects may take several weeks or months to achieve and you may need frequent monitoring during first weeks of therapy. Take with meals if GI upset occurs. Take at the same time each day. Avoid tyramine-containing foods during treatment and for two weeks after the medication had been stopped. Maintain adequate hydration unless instructed to restrict fluid intake. Do not use alcohol. You may experience drowsiness, dizziness, confusion, vision changes, orthostatic hypotension, constipation, runny nose or flu-like symptoms, nausea, vomiting, loss of appetite, or stomach discomfort. You are at an increased risk of melanoma. Have skin monitored by a qualified professional. Report any skin changes or suspicious areas. Report unresolved constipation or vomiting; chest pain, palpitations, irregular heartbeat; CNS changes (hallucination, loss of memory, seizures, acute headache, nervousness, suicide ideation, etc); painful or difficult urination; increased muscle spasticity, rigidity, or involuntary movements; skin rash; or significant worsening of condition.

Dietary Considerations May be taken without regard to meals. Avoid products containing high amounts of tyramine (>150 mg), such as aged cheeses (eg, Stilton cheese). Restriction of tyramine-containing products with lower amounts (<150 mg) of tyramine is not necessary in patients taking recommended doses. Some examples of tyramine-containing products include aged or matured cheese, air-dried or cured meats (including sausages and salamis), fava or broad bean pods, tap/draft beers, Marmite concentrate, sauerkraut, soy sauce and other soybean condiments. Food's freshness is also an important concern; improperly stored or spoiled food can create an environment where tyramine concentrations may increase.

Rasburicase (ras BYOOR i kayse)

Brand Names: U.S. Elitek®

Index Terms Recombinant Urate Oxidase; Urate Oxidase

Pharmacologic Category Enzyme; Enzyme, Urate-Oxidase (Recombinant)

Pregnancy Risk Factor C

Lactation Excretion in breast milk unknown/not recommended

Use Initial management of uric acid levels in patients with leukemia, lymphoma, and solid tumor malignancies receiving chemotherapy expected to result in tumor lysis and elevation of plasma uric acid

Available Dosage Forms

Injection, powder for reconstitution:

Elitek®: 1.5 mg, 7.5 mg

General Dosage Range I.V.: *Children and Adults:* 0.2 mg/kg once daily

Administration

I.V. I.V. infusion over 30 minutes; do **not** administer as a bolus infusion. Do **not** filter during infusion. If not possible to administer through a separate line, I.V. line should be flushed with at least 15 mL saline prior to and following rasburicase infusion. May begin chemotherapy 4 hours after the initiation of rasburicase (Coiffier, 2008).

Nursing Actions

Physical Assessment Monitor patient closely for hypersensitivity reaction.

Patient Education This medication can only be administered by infusion; you will be monitored closely during and following infusion. Report immediately any swelling or any signs of allergic reaction (eg, respiratory difficulty or swallowing, back pain, chest tightness, rash, hives, swelling of lips or mouth). Report severe headache, persistent gastrointestinal upset (nausea, vomiting, or abdominal pain), respiratory difficulty, or swelling of extremities.

Repaglinide (re PAG li nide)

Brand Names: U.S. Prandin®

Pharmacologic Category Antidiabetic Agent, Meglitinide Derivative

Medication Safety Issues

Sound-alike/look-alike issues:

Prandin® may be confused with Avandia®

High alert medication:

The Institute for Safe Medication Practices (ISMP) includes this medication among its list of drug classes which have a heightened risk of causing significant patient harm when used in error.

Pregnancy Risk Factor C

Lactation Excretion in breast milk unknown/not recommended

Breast-Feeding Considerations It is not known if repaglinide is excreted in breast milk. Breast-feeding is not recommended by the manufacturer.

Use Management of type 2 diabetes mellitus (noninsulin dependent, NIDDM) as an adjunct to diet and exercise; may be used in combination with metformin or thiazolidinediones

Mechanism of Action/Effect Nonsulfonylurea hypoglycemic agent of the meglitinide class (the nonsulfonylurea moiety of glyburide) used in the management of type 2 diabetes mellitus; stimulates insulin release from the pancreatic beta cells. Repaglinide-induced insulin release is glucose-dependent.

Contraindications Hypersensitivity to repaglinide or any component of the formulation; diabetic ketoacidosis, with or without coma; type 1 diabetes (insulin dependent, IDDM); concurrent gemfibrozil therapy

Warnings/Precautions Use with caution in patients with hepatic impairment. Use caution in severe renal dysfunction, elderly, malnourished, or patients with adrenal/pituitary dysfunction; may be more susceptible to glucose-lowering effects. May cause hypoglycemia; appropriate patient selection, dosage, and patient education are important to avoid hypoglycemic episodes. It may be necessary to discontinue repaglinide and administer insulin if the patient is exposed to stress (fever, trauma, infection, surgery). Theoretically, repaglinide may increase cardiovascular events as observed in some studies using sulfonylureas, but there are no long-term studies assessing this concern. Not indicated for use in combination with NPH insulin as there have been case reports of myocardial ischemia; further evaluation required to assess the safety of this combination.

Drug Interactions

Avoid Concomitant Use

Avoid concomitant use of Repaglinide with any of the following: Conivaptan; Gemfibrozil

Decreased Effect

The levels/effects of Repaglinide may be decreased by: Corticosteroids (Orally Inhaled); Corticosteroids (Systemic); CYP2C8 Inducers (Strong); CYP3A4 Inducers (Strong); Deferasirox; Herbs (CYP3A4 Inducers); Luteinizing Hormone-Releasing Hormone Analogs; Rifamycin Derivatives; Somatropin; Thiazide Diuretics; Tocilizumab

Increased Effect/Toxicity

Repaglinide may increase the levels/effects of: Hypoglycemic Agents

The levels/effects of Repaglinide may be increased by: Antifungal Agents (Azole Derivatives, Systemic); Conivaptan; CycloSPORINE; CycloSPORINE (Systemic); CYP2C8 Inhibitors (Moderate); CYP2C8 Inhibitors (Strong); CYP3A4 Inhibitors (Moderate); CYP3A4 Inhibitors (Strong); Dasatinib; Deferasirox; Eltrombopag; Gemfibrozil; Herbs (Hypoglycemic Properties); Ivacaftor; Macrolide Antibiotics; Pegvisomant; Trimethoprim

Nutritional/Ethanol Interactions

Ethanol: Ethanol may increase risk of hypoglycemia. Management: Avoid ethanol.

Food: When given with food, the AUC of repaglinide is decreased. Taking medication without eating may cause hypoglycemia. Management: Administer 15-30 minutes prior to a meal. If a meal is skipped, skip dose for that meal.

Herb/Nutraceutical: St John's wort may decrease the levels/effect of repaglinide. Other herbal medications may enhance the hypoglycemic effects of repaglinide. Management: Avoid St John's wort, alfalfa, aloe, bilberry, bitter melon, burdock, celery, damiana, fenugreek, garcinia, garlic, ginger, ginseng (American), gymnema, marshmallow, and stinging nettle.

Adverse Reactions

>10%:

Central nervous system: Headache (9% to 11%)

Endocrine & metabolic: Hypoglycemia (16% to 31%)

Respiratory: Upper respiratory tract infection (10% to 16%)

1% to 10%:

Cardiovascular: Ischemia (4%), chest pain (2% to 3%)

Gastrointestinal: Diarrhea (4% to 5%), constipation (2% to 3%)

Genitourinary: Urinary tract infection (2% to 3%)

Neuromuscular & skeletal: Back pain (5% to 6%), arthralgia (3% to 6%)

Respiratory: Sinusitis (3% to 6%), bronchitis (2% to 6%)

Miscellaneous: Allergy (1% to 2%)

Pharmacodynamics/Kinetics

Onset of Action Single dose: Increased insulin levels: ~15-60 minutes

Duration of Action 4-6 hours

Available Dosage Forms

Tablet, oral:

Prandin®: 0.5 mg, 1 mg, 2 mg

General Dosage Range Dosage adjustment recommended in patients with renal impairment

Oral: *Adults:* Initial: 0.5-2 mg before each meal; Maintenance: 0.5-4 mg before each meal (maximum: 16 mg/day)

Administration

Oral Administer 15 minutes before meals; however, time may vary from immediately preceding a meal to as long as 30 minutes before a meal. If the patient misses a meal or is unable to take anything by mouth, repaglinide should not be administered to avoid hypoglycemia. Patients consuming extra meals should be instructed to add a dose for the extra meal.

Stability

Storage Do not store above 25°C (77°F). Protect from moisture.

Nursing Actions

Physical Assessment Instruct patient to treat signs of hypoglycemia and report them to health care provider.

Patient Education Take 3-4 times a day 15-30 minutes prior to a meal. If you skip a meal, skip a dose for that meal. Follow dietary and lifestyle directions of prescriber or diabetic educator. Avoid alcohol. You will be instructed in signs of hyper-/hypoglycemia by prescriber or diabetic educator; be alert for adverse hypoglycemia (lightheadedness, tachycardia or palpitations, sweaty palms or profuse perspiration, yawning, tingling of lips and tongue, seizures, or change in sensorium) and follow prescriber's instructions for intervention. May cause headache or mild GI effects during first weeks of therapy (nausea, vomiting, diarrhea, constipation, heartburn); if these do not diminish, consult prescriber for approved medication. Report chest pain, respiratory difficulty or symptoms of upper respiratory infection, urinary tract infection (burning or itching on urination), or muscle or back pain.

Dietary Considerations Take repaglinide 15-30 minutes before meals. Individualized medical nutrition therapy (MNT) based on ADA recommendations is an integral part of therapy. May cause hypoglycemia. Must be able to recognize symptoms of hypoglycemia (palpitations, tachycardia, sweaty palms, diaphoresis, lightheadedness).

Repaglinide and Metformin

(re PAG li nide & met FOR min)

Brand Names: U.S. PrandiMet®

Index Terms Metformin and Repaglinide; Repaglinide and Metformin Hydrochloride

Pharmacologic Category Antidiabetic Agent, Biguanide; Antidiabetic Agent, Meglitinide Derivative; Hypoglycemic Agent, Oral

Medication Safety Issues

Sound-alike/look-alike issues:

PrandiMet® may be confused with Avandamet®, Prandin®

High alert medication:

The Institute for Safe Medication Practices (ISMP) includes this medication among its list of drug classes which have a heightened risk of causing significant patient harm when used in error.

Pregnancy Risk Factor C

Lactation

Metformin: Enters breast milk/not recommended

Repaglinide: Excretion in breast milk unknown/not recommended

Use Management of type 2 diabetes mellitus (noninsulin dependent, NIDDM), as an adjunct to diet and exercise, in patients currently receiving or not adequately controlled on metformin and/or a meglitinide

Available Dosage Forms

Tablet:

PrandiMet®: 1/500: Repaglinide 1 mg and metformin hydrochloride 500 mg; 2/500: Repaglinide 2 mg and metformin hydrochloride 500 mg

General Dosage Range Oral: *Adults:* Repaglinide 1-2 mg and metformin 500 mg 2-3 times daily with meals (maximum single dose: 4 mg/dose [repaglinide], 1000 mg/dose [metformin]; maximum daily dose: 10 mg/day [repaglinide], 2500 mg/day [metformin])

Administration

Oral Administer 15-30 minutes before meals to avoid risk of hypoglycemia/GI upset; if a meal skipped or patient is unable to take anything by mouth, do not administer dose.

Nursing Actions

Physical Assessment See individual agents.

Patient Education See individual agents.

Related Information

MetFORMIN *on page 746*

Repaglinide *on page 983*

Reteplase

(RE ta plase)

Brand Names: U.S. Retavase® Half-Kit; Retavase® Kit

Index Terms r-PA; Recombinant Plasminogen Activator

Pharmacologic Category Thrombolytic Agent

Medication Safety Issues

High alert medication:

The Institute for Safe Medication Practices (ISMP) includes this medication (I.V.) among its list of drugs which have a heightened risk of causing significant patient harm when used in error.

Pregnancy Risk Factor C

Lactation Excretion in breast milk unknown/use caution

Use Management of ST-elevation myocardial infarction (STEMI); improvement of ventricular function; reduction of the incidence of CHF and the reduction of mortality following AMI

Recommended criteria for treatment: STEMI: Chest pain ≥20 minutes duration, onset of chest pain within 12 hours of treatment (or within prior 12-24 hours in patients with continuing ischemic symptoms), and ST-segment elevation >0.1 mV in at least two contiguous precordial leads or two adjacent limb leads on ECG or new or presumably new left bundle branch block (LBBB)

Mechanism of Action/Effect Reteplase initiates local fibrinolysis by binding to fibrin in a thrombus (clot) and converting entrapped plasminogen to plasmin. Dissolution of thrombus occluding a coronary artery restores perfusion to ischemic myocardium. Reteplase is manufactured by recombinant DNA technology using *E. coli*.

Contraindications Hypersensitivity to reteplase or any component of the formulation; active internal bleeding; history of cerebrovascular accident; recent intracranial or intraspinal surgery or trauma; intracranial neoplasm, arteriovenous malformations, or aneurysm; known bleeding diathesis; severe uncontrolled hypertension

Warnings/Precautions Concurrent heparin anticoagulation can contribute to bleeding; careful attention to all potential bleeding sites. I.M. injections and nonessential handling of the patient should be avoided. Venipunctures should be performed carefully and only when necessary. If arterial puncture is necessary, use an upper extremity vessel that can be manually compressed. If serious bleeding occurs then the infusion of anistreplase and heparin should be stopped.

For the following conditions the risk of bleeding is higher with use of reteplase and should be weighed against the benefits of therapy: recent major surgery (eg, CABG, obstetrical delivery, organ biopsy, previous puncture of noncompressible vessels), cerebrovascular disease, recent gastrointestinal or genitourinary bleeding, recent trauma including CPR, hypertension (systolic BP >180 mm Hg and/or diastolic BP >110 mm Hg), high likelihood of left heart thrombus (eg, mitral stenosis with atrial fibrillation), acute pericarditis, subacute bacterial endocarditis, hemostatic defects including ones caused by severe renal or hepatic dysfunction, significant hepatic dysfunction, pregnancy, diabetic hemorrhagic retinopathy or other hemorrhagic ophthalmic conditions, septic thrombophlebitis or occluded AV cannula at seriously infected site, advanced age (eg, >75 years), patients receiving oral anticoagulants, any other condition in which bleeding constitutes a significant hazard or would be particularly difficult to manage because of location.

Coronary thrombolysis may result in reperfusion arrhythmias. Follow standard MI management. Rare anaphylactic reactions can occur. Safety and efficacy in pediatric patients have not been established.

Drug Interactions

Avoid Concomitant Use There are no known interactions where it is recommended to avoid concomitant use.

Decreased Effect

The levels/effects of Reteplase may be decreased by: Aprotinin

Increased Effect/Toxicity

Reteplase may increase the levels/effects of: Anticoagulants; Drotrecogin Alfa (Activated)

The levels/effects of Reteplase may be increased by: Antiplatelet Agents; Herbs (Anticoagulant/Antiplatelet Properties); Nonsteroidal Anti-Inflammatory Agents; Salicylates

Adverse Reactions Bleeding is the most frequent adverse effect associated with reteplase. Heparin and aspirin have been administered concurrently with reteplase in clinical trials. The incidence of adverse events is a reflection of these combined therapies, and are comparable with comparison thrombolytics.

>10%: Local: Injection site bleeding (4.6% to 48.6%)

1% to 10%:

Gastrointestinal: Bleeding (1.8% to 9.0%)

Genitourinary: Bleeding (0.9% to 9.5%)

Hematologic: Anemia (0.9% to 2.6%)

Other adverse effects noted are frequently associated with MI (and therefore may or may not be attributable to Retavase®) and include arrhythmia, hypotension, cardiogenic shock, pulmonary edema, cardiac arrest, reinfarction, pericarditis, tamponade, thrombosis, and embolism.

Pharmacodynamics/Kinetics

Onset of Action Thrombolysis: 30-90 minutes

Available Dosage Forms

Injection, powder for reconstitution [preservative free]:

Retavase® Half-Kit: 10.4 units

Retavase® Kit: 10.4 units

General Dosage Range I.V.: *Adults:* 10 units; repeat after 30 minutes

Administration

I.V. Infuse over 2 minutes.

I.V. Detail No other medications should be added to the injection solution.

Stability

Reconstitution Reteplase should be reconstituted using the diluent, syringe, needle, and dispensing pin provided with each kit.

Storage Dosage kits should be stored at 2°C to 25°C (36°F to 77°F) and remain sealed until use in order to protect from light.

Nursing Actions

Physical Assessment Use caution when there is significant risk of bleeding. Monitor patient closely for bleeding during and following treatment. Monitor infusion site, neurological status (eg, intracranial hemorrhage), vital signs, and ECG. Maintain bleeding precautions; avoid I.M. injections, venipunctures (unless absolutely necessary), and nonessential handling of the patient. If arterial puncture is necessary, use an upper extremity vessel that can be manually compressed.

Patient Education This medication can only be administered by infusion; you will be monitored closely during and after treatment. You will have a tendency to bleed easily; use caution to prevent injury. Follow instructions for strict bedrest to reduce the risk of injury. If bleeding occurs, report immediately and apply pressure to bleeding spot until bleeding stops completely. Report unusual pain (acute headache, joint pain, chest pain); unusual bruising or bleeding; blood in urine, stool, or vomitus; bleeding gums; vision changes; or change in mentation.

Rh_o(D) Immune Globulin

(ar aych oh (dee) i MYUN GLOB yoo lin)

Brand Names: U.S. HyperRHO™ S/D Full Dose; HyperRHO™ S/D Mini-Dose; MICRhoGAM® UF Plus; RhoGAM® UF Plus; Rhophylac®; WinRho® SDF

Index Terms RhIG; Rho(D) Immune Globulin (Human); RhoIGIV; RhoIVIM

Pharmacologic Category Blood Product Derivative; Immune Globulin

Pregnancy Risk Factor C

Lactation Does not enter breast milk

Use

Suppression of Rh isoimmunization: Use in the following situations when an Rh_o(D)-negative individual is exposed to Rh_o(D)-positive blood: During delivery of an Rh_o(D)-positive infant; abortion; amniocentesis; chorionic villus sampling; ruptured tubal pregnancy; abdominal trauma; hydatidiform mole; transplacental hemorrhage. Used when the mother is Rh_o(D)-negative, the father of the child is either Rh_o(D)-positive or Rh_o(D)-unknown, or the baby is either Rh_o(D)-positive or Rh_o(D)-unknown.

Transfusion: Suppression of Rh isoimmunization in Rh_o(D)-negative individuals transfused with Rh_o(D) antigen-positive RBCs or blood components containing Rh_o(D) antigen-positive RBCs

Treatment of idiopathic thrombocytopenic purpura (ITP): Used intravenously in the following nonsplenectomized Rh_o(D)-positive individuals: Children with acute or chronic ITP, adults with chronic ITP, and children and adults with ITP secondary to HIV infection

Available Dosage Forms

Injection, solution [preservative free]:

HyperRHO™ S/D Full Dose: ≥300 mcg/mL (1 mL)

HyperRHO™ S/D Mini-Dose: ≥50 mcg/0.17 mL (0.17 mL)

MICRhoGAM® UF Plus: ~50 mcg/0.75 mL (0.75 mL)

RhoGAM® UF Plus: ~300 mcg/0.75 mL (0.75 mL)

Rhophylac®: ≥300 mcg/2 mL (2 mL)

WinRho® SDF: 300 mcg/~1.3 mL (1.3 mL); 3000 mcg/~13 mL (13 mL); 500 mcg/~2.2 mL (2.2 mL); 1000 mcg/~4.4 mL (4.4 mL)

General Dosage Range I.M., I.V.: *Children and Adults:* Dosage varies greatly depending on indication

Administration

I.M. Administer into the deltoid muscle of the upper arm or anterolateral aspect of the upper thigh. Avoid gluteal region due to risk of sciatic nerve injury. If large doses (>5 mL) are needed, administration in divided doses at different sites is recommended. **Note:** Do not administer I.M. Rh_o(D) immune globulin for ITP.

I.V.

WinRho® SDF: Infuse over at least 3-5 minutes; do not administer with other medications

Rhophylac®: ITP: Infuse at 2 mL per 15-60 seconds

I.V. Detail Note: If preparing dose using liquid formulation, withdraw the entire contents of the vial to ensure accurate calculation of the dosage requirement.

Nursing Actions

Physical Assessment Monitor blood pressure; may cause hyper-/hypotension. Be alert to the possibility of anaphylaxis. Assess for signs and symptoms of intravascular hemolysis (IVH) in patients with ITP, anemia, renal insufficiency, back pain, shaking, chills, discolored urine, or hematuria; observe patient for side effects for 8 hours following administration.

Patient Education Do not have live virus vaccinations within 6 months of receiving this medication. This medication can only be administered by injection or infusion; report immediately any difficulty breathing; rapid heartbeat; chills; back rash; pain; redness, swelling, or pain at injection site; discolored urine or blood in the urine; decreased urine output; sudden weight gain; or swelling of extremities. You may experience headache, sleepiness, or dizziness.

Ribavirin (rye ba VYE rin)

Brand Names: U.S. Copegus®; Rebetol®; Ribasphere®; Ribasphere® RibaPak®; Virazole®

Index Terms RTCA; Tribavirin

Pharmacologic Category Antiviral Agent

Medication Safety Issues

Sound-alike/look-alike issues:

Ribavirin may be confused with riboflavin, rifampin, Robaxin®

Medication Guide Available Yes

Pregnancy Risk Factor X

Lactation Excretion in breast milk unknown/not recommended

Use

Inhalation: Treatment of hospitalized infants and young children with respiratory syncytial virus (RSV) infections; specially indicated for treatment of severe lower respiratory tract RSV infections in patients with an underlying compromising condition (prematurity, cardiopulmonary disease, or immunosuppression)

Oral capsule:

In combination with interferon alfa-2b (Intron® A) injection for the treatment of chronic hepatitis C in patients with compensated liver disease who have relapsed after alpha interferon therapy or were previously untreated with alpha interferons

In combination with peginterferon alfa-2b (PEG-Intron®) injection for the treatment of chronic hepatitis C in patients with compensated liver disease who were previously untreated with alpha interferons

Oral solution: In combination with interferon alfa 2b (Intron® A) injection for the treatment of chronic hepatitis C in patients with compensated liver disease who were previously untreated with alpha interferons or patients who have relapsed after alpha interferon therapy

Oral tablet: In combination with peginterferon alfa-2a (Pegasys®) injection for the treatment of chronic hepatitis C in patients with compensated liver disease who were previously untreated with alpha interferons (includes patients with histological evidence of cirrhosis [Child-Pugh class A] and patients with clinically-stable HIV disease)

Unlabeled Use

Inhalation: Treatment for RSV in adult hematopoietic stem cell or heart/lung transplant recipients

Used in other viral infections including influenza A and B and adenovirus

Mechanism of Action/Effect Inhibits viral protein synthesis

Contraindications Hypersensitivity to ribavirin or any component of the formulation; women of childbearing age who will not use contraception reliably; pregnancy

Additional contraindications for oral formulation: Male partners of pregnant women; hemoglobinopathies (eg, thalassemia major, sickle cell anemia); patients with autoimmune hepatitis; ribavirin tablets are contraindicated in patients with hepatic decompensation (Child-Pugh class B and C); concomitant use of didanosine

Additional contraindication for Ribasphere® capsules and Rebetrol® capsules/solution: Patients with a Cl_{cr} <50 mL/minute

Refer to individual monographs for Interferon Alfa-2b (Intron® A) and Peginterferon Alfa-2a (Pegasys®) for additional contraindication information.

Warnings/Precautions Oral: **[U.S. Boxed Warning]: Significant teratogenic effects have been observed in all animal studies.** A negative pregnancy test is required before initiation and monthly thereafter. Avoid pregnancy in female patients and female partners of male patients, during therapy, and for at least 6 months after treatment; two forms of contraception should be used. Safety and efficacy have not been established in patients who have failed other alfa interferon therapy, received organ transplants, or been coinfected with hepatitis B or HIV (Copegus® may be used in HIV coinfected patients unless CD4+ cell count is <100 cells/microL). Oral products should not be used for HIV infection, adenovirus, RSV, or influenza infections.

[U.S. Boxed Warning]: Monotherapy not effective for chronic hepatitis C infection. Severe psychiatric events have occurred including depression and suicidal behavior during combination therapy. Avoid use in patients with a psychiatric history; discontinue if severe psychiatric symptoms occur. Acute hypersensitivity reactions (eg, anaphylaxis, angioedema, bronchoconstriction, and urticaria) have been observed (rarely) with ribavirin and alfa interferon combination therapy. Severe cutaneous reactions, including Stevens-Johnson syndrome and exfoliative dermatitis have been reported (rarely) with ribavirin and alfa interferon combination therapy; discontinue with signs or symptoms of severe skin reactions. Use with caution in patients with renal impairment; dosage adjustment or discontinuation may be required. Elderly patients are more susceptible to adverse effects; use caution.

[U.S. Boxed Warning]: Hemolytic anemia is the primary toxicity of oral therapy; usually occurring within 1-2 weeks of therapy initiation; observed in ~10% to 13% of patients when alfa interferons were combined with ribavirin. Assess cardiac disease before initiation. Anemia may worsen underlying cardiac disease; avoid use in patients with significant/unstable cardiac disease. If deterioration in cardiovascular status occurs, discontinue therapy. Patients with renal dysfunction and/or those >50 years of age should be carefully assessed for development of anemia. Pancytopenia and bone marrow suppression have been reported with the combination of ribavirin, interferon, and azathioprine. Use caution in pulmonary disease; pulmonary symptoms have been associated with administration. Discontinue therapy if evidence of hepatic decompensation (Child-Pugh score ≥6) is observed. Use caution in patients with sarcoidosis (exacerbation reported). Dental and periodontal disorders have been reported with ribavirin and interferon therapy; patients should be instructed to brush teeth twice daily and have regular dental exams. Serious ophthalmologic disorders have occurred with combination therapy. All patients require an eye exam at baseline; those with pre-existing ophthalmologic disorders (eg, diabetic or hypertensive retinopathy) require periodic follow up. In combination with peginterferon alfa-2b, ribavirin may cause a reduction in growth velocity in pediatric patients during treatment and for about 6 months post-treatment.

Inhalation: **[U.S. Boxed Warning]: Use with caution in patients requiring assisted ventilation because precipitation of the drug in the respiratory equipment may interfere with safe and effective patient ventilation; sudden deterioration of respiratory function has been observed;** monitor carefully in patients with COPD and asthma for deterioration of respiratory function.

Ribavirin is potentially mutagenic, tumor-promoting, and gonadotoxic. Although anemia has not been reported with inhalation therapy, consider monitoring for anemia 1-2 weeks post-treatment. Pregnant healthcare workers may consider unnecessary occupational exposure; ribavirin has been detected in healthcare workers' urine. Healthcare professionals or family members who are pregnant (or may become pregnant) should be counseled about potential risks of exposure and counseled about risk reduction strategies. Hazardous agent - use appropriate precautions for handling and disposal.

Drug Interactions

Avoid Concomitant Use

Avoid concomitant use of Ribavirin with any of the following: Didanosine

Decreased Effect

Ribavirin may decrease the levels/effects of: Influenza Virus Vaccine (Live/Attenuated)

Increased Effect/Toxicity

Ribavirin may increase the levels/effects of: AzaTHIOprine; Didanosine; Reverse Transcriptase Inhibitors (Nucleoside)

The levels/effects of Ribavirin may be increased by: Interferons (Alfa); Zidovudine

Nutritional/Ethanol Interactions Food: Oral: High-fat meal increases the AUC and C_{max}. Management: Capsule (in combination with peginterferon alfa-2b) and tablet should be administered with food. Other dosage forms and combinations should be taken consistently in regards to food.

Adverse Reactions

Inhalation:

1% to 10%:

Central nervous system: Fatigue, headache, insomnia

Gastrointestinal: Nausea, anorexia

Hematologic: Anemia

<1%: Hypotension, cardiac arrest, digitalis toxicity, conjunctivitis, mild bronchospasm, worsening of respiratory function, apnea

Note: Incidence of adverse effects (approximate) in healthcare workers: Headache (51%); conjunctivitis (32%); rhinitis, nausea, rash, dizziness, pharyngitis, and lacrimation (10% to 20%); bronchospasm and/or chest pain (case reports in individuals with underlying airway disease)

Oral (all adverse reactions are documented while receiving combination therapy with alfa interferons; percentages as reported in adults); asterisked (*) percentages are those similar to interferon therapy alone:

>10%:

Central nervous system: Fatigue (60% to 70%)*, headache (43% to 66%)*, fever (32% to 55%)*, insomnia (26% to 41%), depression (20% to 36%)*, irritability (23% to 33%), dizziness (14% to 26%), impaired concentration (10% to 21%)*, emotional lability (7% to 12%)*

Dermatologic: Alopecia (27% to 36%), pruritus (13% to 29%), rash (5% to 28%), dry skin (10% to 24%), dermatitis (≤16%)

Endocrine and metabolic: Hyperuricemia (33% to 38%)

Gastrointestinal: Nausea (25% to 47%), anorexia (21% to 32%), weight decrease (10% to 29%), vomiting (9% to 25%)*, diarrhea (10% to 22%), dyspepsia (6% to 16%), abdominal pain (8% to 13%), xerostomia (≤12%), RUQ pain (≤12%)

Hematologic: Leukopenia (6% to 45%), neutropenia (8% to 42%; grade 4: 2% to 11%; 40% with HIV coinfection), hemoglobin decreased (11% to 35%), anemia (11% to 17%), thrombocytopenia (<1% to 15%), lymphopenia (12% to 14%), hemolytic anemia (10% to 13%)

Hepatic: Bilirubin increase (10% to 32%)

Neuromuscular & skeletal: Myalgia (40% to 64%)*, rigors (25% to 48%), arthralgia (22% to 34%)*, musculoskeletal pain (19% to 28%)

Respiratory: Dyspnea (13% to 26%), cough (7% to 23%), pharyngitis (≤13%), sinusitis (≤12%)*

Miscellaneous: Flu-like syndrome (13% to 18%)*, viral infection (≤12%), diaphoresis (≤11%)

1% to 10%:

Cardiovascular: Chest pain (5% to 9%)*, flushing (≤4%)

Central nervous system: Pain (≤10%), mood alteration (≤6%; 9% with HIV coinfection), agitation (5% to 8%), nervousness (6%)*, memory impairment (≤6%), malaise (≤6%), suicidal ideation (adolescents: 2%; adults: 1%)

Dermatologic: Eczema (4% to 5%)

Endocrine & metabolic: Menstrual disorder (≤7%), hypothyroidism (≤5%)

Gastrointestinal: Taste perversion (4% to 9%), constipation (5%)

Hepatic: Hepatomegaly (4%), transaminases increased (1% to 3%), hepatic decompensation (2% with HIV coinfection)

Neuromuscular & skeletal: Weakness (9% to 10%), back pain (5%)

Ocular: Blurred vision (≤6%), conjunctivitis (≤5%)

Respiratory: Rhinitis (≤8%), exertional dyspnea (≤7%)

Miscellaneous: Fungal infection (≤6%), bacterial infection (3% to 5%)

Note: Incidence of anorexia, headache, fever, suicidal ideation, and vomiting are higher in children.

Available Dosage Forms

Capsule, oral: 200 mg

Rebetol®: 200 mg

Ribasphere®: 200 mg

Combination package, oral:

Ribasphere® RibaPak®: Tablet: 400 mg (7s) [medium blue tablets] and Tablet: 600 mg (7s) [dark blue tablets] (14s, 56s)

Powder for solution, for nebulization:

Virazole®: 6 g

Solution, oral:
Rebetol®: 40 mg/mL (100 mL)
Tablet, oral: 200 mg
Copegus®: 200 mg
Ribasphere®: 200 mg, 400 mg, 600 mg
Ribasphere® RibaPak®: 400 mg, 600 mg

General Dosage Range Dosage adjustment recommended in patients with renal impairment and in patients who develop toxicities.

Inhalation: *Children:* 20 mg/mL (6 g in 300 mL) solution; continuous: 12-18 hours/day

Oral:
Children ≥3 years and ≤25 kg: 15 mg/kg/day in 2 divided doses
Children ≥3 years and 26-36 kg: 400 mg/day in 2 divided doses
Children ≥3 years and 37-49 kg: 600 mg/day in 2 divided doses
Children ≥3 years and 50-61 kg: 800 mg/day in 2 divided doses
Children ≥3 years and >61 kg to <75 kg: 1000 mg/day in 2 divided doses
Adults ≤75 kg: 800-1000 mg/day in 2 divided doses
Adults >75 kg: 800-1200 mg/day in 2 divided doses

Administration

Oral Administer concurrently with interferon alfa injection. Capsule should not be opened, crushed, chewed, or broken. Capsules are not for use in children <5 years of age. Use oral solution for children 3-5 years, those ≤25 kg, or those who cannot swallow capsules.

Capsule, in combination with interferon alfa-2b: May be administered with or without food, but always in a consistent manner in regard to food intake.

Capsule, in combination with peginterferon alfa-2b: Administer with food.

Solution, in combination with interferon alfa-2b: May be administered with or without food, but always in a consistent manner in regard to food intake.

Tablet: Should be administered with food.

Inhalation Ribavirin should be administered in well-ventilated rooms (at least 6 air changes/hour). In mechanically-ventilated patients, ribavirin can potentially be deposited in the ventilator delivery system depending on temperature, humidity, and electrostatic forces; this deposition can lead to malfunction or obstruction of the expiratory valve, resulting in inadvertently high positive end-expiratory pressures. The use of one-way valves in the inspiratory lines, a breathing circuit filter in the expiratory line, and frequent monitoring and filter replacement have been effective in preventing these problems. Solutions in SPAG-2 unit should be discarded at least every 24 hours and when the liquid level is low before adding newly reconstituted solution. Should not be mixed with other aerosolized medication.

Stability

Reconstitution Inhalation: Do not use any water containing an antimicrobial agent to reconstitute drug. Reconstituted solution is stable for 24 hours at room temperature.

Storage
Inhalation: Store vials in a dry place at 15°C to 30°C (59°F to 86°F).
Oral: Store at controlled room temperature of 25°C (77°F). Solution may also be refrigerated at 2°C to 8°C (36°F to 46°F).

Nursing Actions

Physical Assessment Note specific cautions for healthcare professionals' exposure risks with inhalation formulation. Monitor weight on a regular basis throughout therapy. Monitor for headache; fatigue; irritability; impaired concentration; nausea, vomiting, or anorexia; anemia; or deterioration of hepatic, respiratory, or cardiac status on a regular basis.

Patient Education For oral administration, take capsules with food and solution with or without food. Do not allow pregnant women or women of childbearing age to come in any contact with this medication. If prescribed in conjunction with other medications, maintain schedule as directed. Maintain adequate hydration, unless instructed to restrict fluid intake. You will need regular blood tests while taking this drug. You may experience increased susceptibility to infection. May cause dental or periodontal disorders. You may be required to have regular ophthalmic exams during therapy. May cause confusion, dizziness, insomnia, impaired concentration, emotional liability, headache, nausea, vomiting, anorexia, extreme fatigue, diarrhea, loss of hair (reversible), or dermatitis. Report chest pain or palpitations; unusual cough or difficulty breathing; rash; signs of infection (fever, chills, unusual bleeding or bruising, infection, or unhealed sores or white plaques in mouth); tingling, weakness, or pain in extremities; CNS changes (suicide ideation, fatigue, insomnia, irritability, depression, impaired concentration); or changes in vision.

Dietary Considerations When used in combination with interferon alfa-2b, capsules and solution may be taken with or without food, but always in a consistent manner in regard to food intake (ie always take with food or always take on an empty stomach). When used in combination with peginterferon alfa-2b, capsules should be taken with food. Tablets should be taken with food.

Rifabutin (rif a BYOO tin)

Brand Names: U.S. Mycobutin®

Index Terms Ansamycin

Pharmacologic Category Antibiotic, Miscellaneous; Antitubercular Agent

Medication Safety Issues

Sound-alike/look-alike issues:

Rifabutin may be confused with rifampin

Pregnancy Risk Factor B

Lactation Excretion in breast milk unknown/not recommended

Use Prevention of disseminated *Mycobacterium avium* complex (MAC) in patients with advanced HIV infection

Unlabeled Use Utilized in multidrug regimens for treatment of MAC; alternative to rifampin as prophylaxis for latent tuberculosis infection (LTBI) or part of multidrug regimen for treatment active tuberculosis infection

Mechanism of Action/Effect Inhibits DNA-dependent RNA polymerase at the beta subunit which prevents chain initiation

Contraindications Hypersensitivity to rifabutin, any other rifamycins, or any component of the formulation

Warnings/Precautions Rifabutin must not be administered for MAC prophylaxis to patients with active tuberculosis since its use may lead to the development of tuberculosis that is resistant to both rifabutin and rifampin. May be associated with neutropenia and/or thrombocytopenia (rarely). Dosage reduction recommended in severe impairment (Cl_{cr} <30 mL/minute). Prolonged use may result in fungal or bacterial superinfection, including *C. difficile*-associated diarrhea (CDAD) and pseudomembranous colitis; CDAD has been observed >2 months postantibiotic treatment. May cause brown/orange discoloration of urine, feces, saliva, sweat, tears, and skin. Remove soft contact lenses during therapy since permanent staining may occur.

Drug Interactions

Avoid Concomitant Use

Avoid concomitant use of Rifabutin with any of the following: Axitinib; BCG; Boceprevir; Bortezomib; Crizotinib; Dronedarone; Everolimus; Lapatinib; Lurasidone; Mycophenolate; Nilotinib; Pazopanib; Praziquantel; Ranolazine; Rilpivirine; Rivaroxaban; Roflumilast; RomiDEPsin; SORAfenib; Telaprevir; Ticagrelor; Tolvaptan; Toremifene; Vandetanib; Voriconazole

Decreased Effect

Rifabutin may decrease the levels/effects of: Alfentanil; Amiodarone; Angiotensin II Receptor Blockers; Antiemetics (5HT3 Antagonists); Antifungal Agents (Azole Derivatives, Systemic); Aprepitant; ARIPiprazole; Atovaquone; Axitinib; Barbiturates; BCG; Benzodiazepines (metabolized by oxidation); Boceprevir; Bortezomib; Brentuximab Vedotin; BusPIRone; Calcium Channel Blockers; Contraceptives (Estrogens); Contraceptives (Progestins); Corticosteroids (Systemic); Crizotinib; CycloSPORINE; CycloSPORINE (Systemic); CYP3A4 Substrates; Dapsone; Dapsone (Systemic); Dasatinib; Delavirdine; Disopyramide; Dronedarone; Efavirenz; Etravirine; Everolimus; Exemestane; FentaNYL; Fluconazole; Fosphenytoin; Gefitinib; GuanFACINE; HMG-CoA Reductase Inhibitors; Imatinib; Indinavir; Ixabepilone; Lapatinib; Linagliptin; Lurasidone; Maraviroc; Morphine (Systemic); Morphine Sulfate; Mycophenolate; Nelfinavir; Nevirapine; Nilotinib; Pazopanib; Phenytoin; Praziquantel; Propafenone; QuiNIDine; Ramelteon; Ranolazine; Repaglinide; Rilpivirine; Rivaroxaban; Roflumilast; RomiDEPsin; Saxagliptin; SORAfenib; SUNItinib; Tacrolimus; Tacrolimus (Systemic); Tadalafil; Tamoxifen; Telaprevir; Temsirolimus; Terbinafine (Systemic); Ticagrelor; Tolvaptan; Toremifene; Typhoid Vaccine; Ulipristal; Vandetanib; Vemurafenib; Vitamin K Antagonists; Voriconazole; Zaleplon; Zolpidem; Zuclopenthixol

The levels/effects of Rifabutin may be decreased by: CYP3A4 Inducers (Strong); Cyproterone; Deferasirox; Efavirenz; Herbs (CYP3A4 Inducers); Nevirapine; Tocilizumab

Increased Effect/Toxicity

Rifabutin may increase the levels/effects of: Clopidogrel; Darunavir; Fosamprenavir; Isoniazid; Lopinavir; Pitavastatin

The levels/effects of Rifabutin may be increased by: Antifungal Agents (Azole Derivatives, Systemic); Atazanavir; Boceprevir; Conivaptan; Darunavir; Delavirdine; Fluconazole; Fosamprenavir; Indinavir; Lopinavir; Macrolide Antibiotics; Nelfinavir; Nevirapine; Ritonavir; Saquinavir; Telaprevir; Tipranavir; Voriconazole

Nutritional/Ethanol Interactions Food: High-fat meal may decrease the rate but not the extent of absorption.

Adverse Reactions

>10%:

Dermatologic: Rash (11%)

Genitourinary: Discoloration of urine (30%)

Hematologic: Neutropenia (25%), leukopenia (17%)

1% to 10%:

Central nervous system: Headache (3%), fever (2%)

Gastrointestinal: Nausea (3% to 6%), abdominal pain (4%), dyspepsia (3%), eructation (3%), taste perversion (3%), vomiting (3%), flatulence (2%)

Hematologic: Thrombocytopenia (5%)

Hepatic: ALT increased (7% to 9%; incidence less than placebo), AST increased (7% to 9%; incidence less than placebo)

Neuromuscular & skeletal: Myalgia (2%)

Available Dosage Forms

Capsule, oral:

Mycobutin®: 150 mg

General Dosage Range Dosage adjustment recommended in patients with renal impairment or on concomitant therapy

Oral:
Children <6 years: 5 mg/kg once daily
Children ≥6 years and Adults: 300 mg once daily

Administration

Oral May be taken with meals to minimize nausea or vomiting.

Stability

Storage Store at 25°C (77°F); excursions permitted to 15°C to 30°C (59°F to 86°F).

Nursing Actions

Physical Assessment Monitor for anemia, neutropenia, GI disturbance, and rash.

Patient Education Will discolor urine, stool, saliva, tears, sweat, and other body fluids a red-brown color; this is normal. Stains on clothing or contact lenses are permanent. May cause headache, vomiting, loss of appetite, or taste perversion. Report skin rash, persistent vomiting or diarrhea, or persistent muscle pain.

Dietary Considerations May be taken with meals.

Rifampin (rif AM pin)

Brand Names: U.S. Rifadin®

Index Terms Rifampicin

Pharmacologic Category Antibiotic, Miscellaneous; Antitubercular Agent

Medication Safety Issues

Sound-alike/look-alike issues:
Rifadin® may be confused with Rifater®, Ritalin®
Rifampin may be confused with ribavirin, rifabutin, Rifamate®, rifapentine, rifaximin

Pregnancy Risk Factor C

Lactation Enters breast milk/not recommended (AAP rates "compatible"; AAP 2001 update pending)

Breast-Feeding Considerations The manufacturer does not recommend breast-feeding due to tumorigenicity observed in animal studies; however, the CDC does not consider rifampin a contraindication to breast-feeding.

Use Management of active tuberculosis in combination with other agents; elimination of meningococci from the nasopharynx in asymptomatic carriers

Unlabeled Use Prophylaxis of *Haemophilus influenzae* type b infection; *Legionella* pneumonia; used in combination with other anti-infectives in the treatment of staphylococcal infections; treatment of *M. leprae* infections

Mechanism of Action/Effect Inhibits bacterial RNA synthesis by binding to the beta subunit of DNA-dependent RNA polymerase, blocking RNA transcription

Contraindications Hypersensitivity to rifampin, any rifamycins, or any component of the formulation; concurrent use of amprenavir, saquinavir/ritonavir (possibly other protease inhibitors)

Warnings/Precautions Use with caution and modify dosage in patients with liver impairment; observe for hyperbilirubinemia; discontinue therapy if this in conjunction with clinical symptoms or any signs of significant hepatocellular damage develop. Use with caution in patients receiving concurrent medications associated with hepatotoxicity. Use with caution in patients with a history of alcoholism (even if ethanol consumption is discontinued during therapy). Since rifampin since rifampin has enzyme-inducing properties, porphyria exacerbation is possible; use with caution in patients with porphyria; do not use for meningococcal disease, only for short-term treatment of asymptomatic carrier states

Regimens of >600 mg once or twice weekly have been associated with a high incidence of adverse reactions including a flu-like syndrome, hypersensitivity, thrombocytopenia, leukopenia, and anemia. Urine, feces, saliva, sweat, tears, and CSF may be discolored to red/orange; remove soft contact lenses during therapy since permanent staining may occur. Do not administer I.V. form via I.M. or SubQ routes; restart infusion at another site if extravasation occurs. Prolonged use may result in fungal or bacterial superinfection, including *C. difficile*-associated diarrhea (CDAD) and pseudomembranous colitis; CDAD has been observed >2 months postantibiotic treatment. Monitor for compliance in patients on intermittent therapy.

Drug Interactions

Avoid Concomitant Use

Avoid concomitant use of Rifampin with any of the following: Atazanavir; Axitinib; BCG; Boceprevir; Bortezomib; Dabigatran Etexilate; Darunavir; Esomeprazole; Etravirine; Fosamprenavir; Indinavir; Lopinavir; Lurasidone; Mycophenolate; Nelfinavir; Omeprazole; Praziquantel; QuiNINE; Ranolazine; Rilpivirine; Ritonavir; Roflumilast; Saquinavir; SORAfenib; Telaprevir; Ticagrelor; Tipranavir; Toremifene; Voriconazole

Decreased Effect

Rifampin may decrease the levels/effects of: Alfentanil; Amiodarone; Angiotensin II Receptor Blockers; Antidiabetic Agents (Thiazolidinedione); Antiemetics (5HT3 Antagonists); Antifungal Agents (Azole Derivatives, Systemic); Aprepitant; ARIPiprazole; Atazanavir; Atovaquone; Axitinib; Barbiturates; BCG; Bendamustine; Benzodiazepines (metabolized by oxidation); Beta-Blockers; Boceprevir; Bortezomib; Brentuximab Vedotin; BusPIRone; Calcium Channel Blockers; Caspofungin; Chloramphenicol; Contraceptives (Estrogens); Contraceptives (Progestins); Corticosteroids (Systemic); CycloSPORINE; CycloSPORINE (Systemic); CYP1A2 Substrates; CYP2A6 Substrates; CYP2B6 Substrates; CYP2C19 Substrates; CYP2C8 Substrates; CYP2C9 Substrates; CYP3A4 Substrates; Dabigatran Etexilate; Dapsone; Dapsone (Systemic); Darunavir; Dasatinib; Deferasirox; Delavirdine; Diclofenac; Disopyramide; Divalproex; Efavirenz;

Erlotinib; Esomeprazole; Etravirine; Exemestane; FentaNYL; Fexofenadine; Fluconazole; Fosamprenavir; Fosaprepitant; Fosphenytoin; Gefitinib; GuanFACINE; HMG-CoA Reductase Inhibitors; Imatinib; Indinavir; Ixabepilone; LamoTRIgine; Linagliptin; Lopinavir; Lurasidone; Maraviroc; Methadone; Morphine (Systemic); Morphine Sulfate; Mycophenolate; Nelfinavir; Nevirapine; Omeprazole; OxyCODONE; P-glycoprotein/ABCB1 Substrates; Phenytoin; Prasugrel; Praziquantel; Propafenone; QuiNIDine; QuiNINE; Raltegravir; Ramelteon; Ranolazine; Repaglinide; Rilpivirine; Ritonavir; Roflumilast; Saquinavir; Sirolimus; SORAfenib; Sulfonylureas; Tacrolimus; Tacrolimus (Systemic); Tadalafil; Tamoxifen; Telaprevir; Temsirolimus; Terbinafine; Terbinafine (Systemic); Thyroid Products; Ticagrelor; Tipranavir; Toremifene; Treprostinil; Typhoid Vaccine; Ulipristal; Valproic Acid; Vitamin K Antagonists; Voriconazole; Zaleplon; Zidovudine; Zolpidem; Zuclopenthixol

The levels/effects of Rifampin may be decreased by: P-glycoprotein/ABCB1 Inducers

Increased Effect/Toxicity

Rifampin may increase the levels/effects of: Clopidogrel; Isoniazid; Leflunomide; Lopinavir; Pitavastatin; Saquinavir

The levels/effects of Rifampin may be increased by: Antifungal Agents (Azole Derivatives, Systemic); Delavirdine; Eltrombopag; Fluconazole; Macrolide Antibiotics; P-glycoprotein/ABCB1 Inhibitors; Pyrazinamide; Voriconazole

Nutritional/Ethanol Interactions

Ethanol: Avoid ethanol (may increase risk of hepatotoxicity).

Food: Food decreases the extent of absorption; rifampin concentrations may be decreased if taken with food.

Herb/Nutraceutical: St John's wort may decrease rifampin levels.

Adverse Reactions

1% to 10%:

Dermatologic: Rash (1% to 5%)

Gastrointestinal (1% to 2%): Anorexia, cramps, diarrhea, epigastric distress, flatulence, heartburn, nausea, pseudomembranous colitis, pancreatitis, vomiting

Hepatic: LFTs increased (up to 14%)

Frequency not defined:

Cardiovascular: Edema, flushing

Central nervous system: Ataxia, behavioral changes, concentration impaired, confusion, dizziness, drowsiness, fatigue, fever, headache, numbness, psychosis

Dermatologic: Pemphigoid reaction, pruritus, urticaria

Endocrine & metabolic: Adrenal insufficiency, menstrual disorders

Hematologic: Agranulocytosis (rare), DIC, eosinophilia, hemoglobin decreased, hemolysis, hemolytic anemia, leukopenia, thrombocytopenia (especially with high-dose therapy)

Hepatic: Hepatitis (rare), jaundice

Neuromuscular & skeletal: Myalgia, osteomalacia, weakness

Ocular: Exudative conjunctivitis, visual changes

Renal: Acute renal failure, BUN increased, hemoglobinuria, hematuria, interstitial nephritis, uric acid increased

Miscellaneous: Flu-like syndrome

Pharmacodynamics/Kinetics

Duration of Action ≤24 hours

Available Dosage Forms

Capsule, oral: 150 mg, 300 mg

Rifadin®: 150 mg, 300 mg

Injection, powder for reconstitution: 600 mg

Rifadin®: 600 mg

General Dosage Range I.V., oral:

Children <12 years: 10-20 mg/kg/day in 1-2 divided doses **or** 10-20 mg/kg twice weekly (maximum: 600 mg/day)

Children ≥12 years and Adults: 10 mg/kg/day **or** 10 mg/kg 2-3 times/week **or** 600 mg every 12-24 hours

Administration

Oral Administer on an empty stomach with a glass of water (ie, 1 hour prior to, or 2 hours after meals or antacids) to increase total absorption (food may delay and reduce the amount of rifampin absorbed). The compounded oral suspension must be shaken well before using. May mix contents of capsule with applesauce or jelly.

I.M. Do not administer I.M. or SubQ

I.V. Administer I.V. preparation by slow I.V. infusion over 30 minutes to 3 hours at a final concentration not to exceed 6 mg/mL.

I.V. Detail Avoid extravasation.

pH: 7.8-8.8

Stability

Reconstitution Reconstitute powder for injection with SWFI. Prior to injection, dilute in appropriate volume of compatible diluent (eg, 100 mL D_5W).

Storage Rifampin powder is reddish brown. Intact vials should be stored at room temperature and protected from excessive heat and light. Reconstituted vials are stable for 24 hours at room temperature.

Stability of parenteral admixture at room temperature (25°C) is 4 hours for D_5W and 24 hours for NS.

Nursing Actions

Physical Assessment Concurrent use with rifampin may decrease levels/effects of multiple other drugs. Infusion site must be monitored to prevent extravasation. Monitor chest x-ray. Monitor for hypersensitivity reactions, hepatotoxicity, CNS changes, hematologic changes, visual disturbances, and gastrointestinal upset on a regular basis during therapy. Monitor patient compliance with treatment regimen.

Patient Education Rifampin may be prescribed in conjunction with other antibiotics; maintain dosing schedule as directed. Take rifampin on an empty stomach, 1 hour before or 2 hours after meals. Keep appointments for scheduled laboratory tests and chest x-rays. This medication will discolor urine, stool, saliva, tears, sweat, and other body fluids a red-brown color. Stains on contact lenses and clothing are permanent. Report persistent vomiting, diarrhea, rash, fever, chills, flu-like symptoms, or unusual bruising or bleeding.

Dietary Considerations Rifampin should be taken on an empty stomach.

Rifampin and Isoniazid

(rif AM pin & eye soe NYE a zid)

Brand Names: U.S. IsonaRif™; Rifamate®

Index Terms Isoniazid and Rifampin

Pharmacologic Category Antibiotic, Miscellaneous

Medication Safety Issues

Sound-alike/look-alike issues:

Rifamate® may be confused with rifampin

Pregnancy Risk Factor C

Lactation Enters breast milk/compatible

Use Management of active tuberculosis; see individual agents for additional information

Available Dosage Forms

Capsule, oral:

IsonaRif™, Rifamate®: Rifampin 300 mg and isoniazid 150 mg

General Dosage Range Oral: *Adults:* 2 capsules (rifampin 300 mg/isoniazid 150 mg/capsule) once daily

Nursing Actions

Physical Assessment See individual agents.

Patient Education See individual agents.

Related Information

Isoniazid *on page* 646

Rifampin *on page* 992

Rilonacept

(ri LON a sept)

Brand Names: U.S. Arcalyst™

Pharmacologic Category Interleukin-1 Inhibitor

Pregnancy Risk Factor C

Lactation Excretion in breast milk unknown/use caution

Use Treatment of cryopyrin-associated periodic syndromes (CAPS) including familial cold autoinflammatory syndrome (FCAS) and Muckle-Wells syndrome (MWS)

Available Dosage Forms

Injection, powder for reconstitution:

Arcalyst™: 220 mg

General Dosage Range SubQ:

Children ≥12 years: Loading dose 4.4 mg/kg (maximum dose: 320 mg); Maintenance dose: 2.2 mg/kg once weekly (maximum dose: 160 mg)

Adults: Loading dose: 320 mg; Maintenance dose: 160 mg once weekly

Administration

Other SubQ: Rotate injection sites (thigh, abdomen, upper arm); injections should never be made at sites that are bruised, red, tender, or hard

Nursing Actions

Physical Assessment Evaluate for signs and symptoms of infection. This drug should not be used when active or chronic infections are present. Immunization should be given prior to initiating therapy. Teach patient appropriate injection techniques and syringe/needle disposal.

Patient Education You may experience redness, pain, itching, or swelling at the site of injection. This typically lasts 1-2 days. Do not receive any immunizations unless approved by prescriber. You may be susceptible to infections. Report signs of infection immediately.

Rilpivirine

(ril pi VIR een)

Brand Names: U.S. Edurant™

Index Terms TMC278

Pharmacologic Category Antiretroviral Agent, Reverse Transcriptase Inhibitor (Non-nucleoside)

Pregnancy Risk Factor B

Lactation Excretion in breast milk unknown/contraindicated

Breast-Feeding Considerations Maternal or infant antiretroviral therapy does not completely eliminate the risk of postnatal HIV transmission. In addition, multiclass-resistant virus has been detected in breast-feeding infants despite maternal therapy. Therefore, in the United States, where formula is accessible, affordable, safe, and sustainable, and the risk of infant mortality due to diarrhea and respiratory infections is low, complete avoidance of breast-feeding by HIV-infected women is recommended to decrease potential transmission of HIV (DHHS [perinatal], 2011).

Use Treatment of HIV-1 infections in combination with at least two other antiretroviral agents

Mechanism of Action/Effect As a non-nucleoside reverse transcriptase inhibitor, rilpivirine has activity against HIV-1 by binding to reverse transcriptase. It consequently blocks the RNA-dependent and DNA-dependent DNA polymerase activities, including HIV-1 replication. It does not require intracellular phosphorylation for antiviral activity.

Contraindications Concurrent use of carbamazepine, dexamethasone (>1 dose), oxcarbazepine, phenobarbital, phenytoin, proton pump inhibitors (PPIs), rifabutin, rifampin, rifapentine, or St John's wort

Warnings/Precautions Not for use in treatment-experienced patients. May cause depressive disorders (depression, depressed mood, dysphoria, mood changes, negative thoughts, suicide attempts, or suicidal ideation); monitor for changes and need for intervention. May cause redistribution of fat (eg, buffalo hump, peripheral wasting with increased abdominal girth, cushingoid appearance). Patients may develop immune reconstitution syndrome resulting in the occurrence of an inflammatory response to an indolent or residual opportunistic infection; further evaluation and treatment may be required.

Use with caution in patients taking major CYP3A4 (see Drug Interactions) inducers or drugs that increase gastric pH. Use caution with drugs known to prolong the QT_c interval.

Drug Interactions

Avoid Concomitant Use

Avoid concomitant use of Rilpivirine with any of the following: CarBAMazepine; Conivaptan; Dexamethasone; Dexamethasone (Systemic); Etravirine; Fosphenytoin; OXcarbazepine; PHENobarbital; Phenytoin; Primidone; Proton Pump Inhibitors; Reverse Transcriptase Inhibitors (Non-Nucleoside); Rifamycin Derivatives; St Johns Wort

Decreased Effect

Rilpivirine may decrease the levels/effects of: Dexamethasone; Didanosine; Etravirine; Ketoconazole; Ketoconazole (Systemic); Methadone

The levels/effects of Rilpivirine may be decreased by: Antacids; CarBAMazepine; CYP3A4 Inducers (Strong); Deferasirox; Dexamethasone (Systemic); Didanosine; Fosphenytoin; H2-Antagonists; OXcarbazepine; PHENobarbital; Phenytoin; Primidone; Proton Pump Inhibitors; Reverse Transcriptase Inhibitors (Non-Nucleoside); Rifamycin Derivatives; St Johns Wort; Tocilizumab

Increased Effect/Toxicity

Rilpivirine may increase the levels/effects of: Etravirine; PACLitaxel

The levels/effects of Rilpivirine may be increased by: Conivaptan; CYP3A4 Inhibitors (Moderate); CYP3A4 Inhibitors (Strong); Darunavir; Dasatinib; Ivacaftor; Ketoconazole; Ketoconazole (Systemic); Lopinavir; Reverse Transcriptase Inhibitors (Non-Nucleoside)

Nutritional/Ethanol Interactions

Food: Absorption increased by ~40% when taken with a normal to high-caloric meal. Management: Administer with a normal- to high-calorie meal. Administration with a protein supplement drink alone does not increase absorption.

Herb/Nutraceutical: St John's wort may decrease the levels/effects of rilpivirine. Management: Avoid St John's wort; concurrent use is contraindicated.

Adverse Reactions 2% to 10%:

Central nervous system: Depressive disorders (depression, depressed mood, dysphoria, mood changes, negative thoughts, suicide attempts, suicidal ideation) (4% to 8%; grades 3/4: 1%), headache (3%), insomnia (3%)

Dermatologic: Rash (3%)

Endocrine & metabolic: Cholesterol increased (200-300 mg/dL: 19%; >300 mg/dL: <1%), LDL increased (130-190 mg/dL: 17%; >191 mg/dL: <1%), triglycerides increased (500-750 mg/dL: 2%; >750 mg/dL: <1%)

Hepatic: ALT increased (≤5 x ULN: 19%; >5 x ULN: <1%), AST increased (≤5 x ULN: 15%; >5 x ULN: ~2%), bilirubin increased (≤2.5 x ULN: 7%; >2.5 x ULN: <1%)

Renal: Creatinine increased (≤1.8 x ULN: ~5%)

Available Dosage Forms

Tablet, oral:

Edurant™: 25 mg

General Dosage Range Oral: *Adults:* 25 mg once daily

Administration

Oral Administer with a normal- to high-calorie meal. Taking with a protein supplement drink alone does not increase absorption.

Stability

Storage Store at 25°C (77°F); excursions permitted to 15°C to 30°C (59°F to 86°F). Keep in original container; protect from light.

Nursing Actions

Physical Assessment This is not a cure for HIV. Monitor closely for mood changes, depression, or suicide tendencies, as this requires immediate medical attention. Review patient's medications, as proton pump inhibitors or H_2 blockers reduce the absorption of the drug, resulting in decreased effectiveness. Rilpivirine should be used with caution in liver impairment. Patients with an impaired immune system (eg, HIV patients) need to be monitored for symptoms of infection, which may include fever, chills, cough, wheezing, and shortness of breath.

Patient Education Instruct patient that rilpivirine should be taken once a day with a meal. If patients are on a proton pump inhibitor, such as omeprazole, or H_2 blocker (famotidine/ranitidine), they should space the medications apart as directed to avoid decreased effectiveness. Please inform prescriber of heart, liver, and hepatitis B or C history. Patients and their families should be aware of mood changes, depression, or suicidal tendencies, as these require immediate medical attention.

Dietary Considerations Take with a normal- to high-calorie meal. Taking with a protein supplement drink alone does not increase absorption.

Riluzole (RIL yoo zole)

Brand Names: U.S. Rilutek®

Index Terms 2-Amino-6-Trifluoromethoxy-benzothiazole; RP-54274

Pharmacologic Category Glutamate Inhibitor

Pregnancy Risk Factor C

Lactation Excretion in breast milk unknown/not recommended

Use Treatment of amyotrophic lateral sclerosis (ALS); riluzole can extend survival or time to tracheostomy

Mechanism of Action/Effect Mechanism of action is not known. Pharmacologic properties include inhibitory effect on glutamate release, inactivation of voltage-dependent sodium channels; and ability to interfere with intracellular events that follow transmitter binding at excitatory amino acid receptors

Contraindications Severe hypersensitivity reactions to riluzole or any component of the formulation

Warnings/Precautions Among 4000 patients given riluzole for ALS, there were 3 cases of marked neutropenia (ANC <500/mm^3), all seen within the first 2 months of treatment. Interstitial lung disease (primarily hypersensitivity pneumonitis) has occurred, requires prompt evaluation and possible discontinuation. Use with caution in patients with concomitant renal insufficiency. Use with caution in patients with current evidence or history of abnormal liver function; do not administer if baseline liver function tests are elevated. May cause elevations in transaminases (usually transient). May cause elevations in transaminases (usually transient) within first 3 months of therapy; discontinue if ALT levels are ≥5 times upper limit of normal or if jaundice develops. The elderly or female patients may have decreased clearance of riluzole; use with caution. May cause dizziness or somnolence; caution should be used performing tasks which require alertness (operating machinery or driving).

Drug Interactions

Avoid Concomitant Use There are no known interactions where it is recommended to avoid concomitant use.

Decreased Effect

The levels/effects of Riluzole may be decreased by: CYP1A2 Inducers (Strong); Cyproterone

Increased Effect/Toxicity There are no known significant interactions involving an increase in effect.

Nutritional/Ethanol Interactions

Ethanol: Avoid ethanol (due to CNS depression and possible risk of liver toxicity).

Food: A high-fat meal decreases absorption of riluzole (decreasing AUC by 20% and peak blood levels by 45%). Charbroiled food may increase riluzole elimination.

Adverse Reactions

>10%:

Gastrointestinal: Nausea (16%)

Neuromuscular & skeletal: Weakness (19%)

1% to 10%:

Cardiovascular: Hypertension (5%), peripheral edema (3%), tachycardia (3%)

Central nervous system: Dizziness (4%), somnolence (2%), vertigo (2%), malaise (1%)

Dermatologic: Pruritus (4%), eczema (2%), exfoliative dermatitis (1%)

Gastrointestinal: Abdominal pain (5%), vomiting (4%), flatulence (3%), oral moniliasis (1%), stomatitis (1%), tooth caries (1%)

Genitourinary: Urinary tract infection (3%), dysuria (1%)

Hepatic: Liver function tests increased (8% >3 x ULN; 2% >5 x ULN)

Neuromuscular & skeletal: Arthralgia (4%), paresthesia (circumoral; 2%), tremor (1%)

Respiratory: Lung function decreased (10%), cough increased (3%)

Available Dosage Forms

Tablet, oral:

Rilutek®: 50 mg

General Dosage Range Oral: *Adults:* 50 mg every 12 hours

Administration

Oral Administer at the same time each day, at least 1 hour before or 2 hours after a meal.

Stability

Storage Store at 20°C to 25°C (68°F to 77°F). Protect from bright light.

Nursing Actions

Patient Education This drug will not cure or stop disease, but it may slow progression. Take at the same time each day, preferably on an empty stomach, 1 hour before or 2 hours after meals. Avoid alcohol. You may experience increased spasticity, dizziness, sleepiness, nausea, vomiting, or anorexia. Report fever; severe vomiting, diarrhea, or constipation; change in color of urine or stool; yellowing of skin or eyes; acute back pain or muscle pain; or worsening of condition.

Dietary Considerations Take at least 1 hour before or 2 hours after a meal.

Rimantadine (ri MAN ta deen)

Brand Names: U.S. Flumadine®

Index Terms Rimantadine Hydrochloride

Pharmacologic Category Antiviral Agent; Antiviral Agent, Adamantane

Medication Safety Issues

Sound-alike/look-alike issues:

Rimantadine may be confused with amantadine ranitidine, Rimactane

Flumadine® may be confused with fludarabine flunisolide, flutamide

Pregnancy Risk Factor C

Lactation Excretion in breast milk unknown/ not recommended

Breast-Feeding Considerations Do not use in nursing mothers due to potential adverse effect in infants. The CDC recommends that women infected with the influenza virus follow general precautions (eg, frequent hand washing) to decrease viral transmission to the child. Mothers with influenza-like illnesses at delivery should consider avoiding close contact with the infant until they have received 48 hours of antiviral medication, fever has resolved, and cough and secretions can be controlled. These measures may help decrease (but not eliminate) the risk of transmitting influenza to the newborn during breast-feeding. During this time, breast milk can be expressed and bottle-fed to the infant by another person who is not infected. Protective measures, such as wearing a face mask, changing into a clean gown or clothing, and strict hand hygiene should be continued by the mother for ≥7 days after the onset of symptoms or until symptom-free for 24 hours. Infant care should be performed by a noninfected person when possible (consult current CDC guidelines).

Use Prophylaxis (adults and children >1 year of age) and treatment (adults) of influenza A viral infection (per manufacturer labeling; also refer to current ACIP guidelines for recommendations during current flu season)

Note: In certain circumstances, the ACIP recommends use of rimantadine in combination with oseltamivir for the treatment or prophylaxis of influenza A infection when resistance to oseltamivir is suspected.

Mechanism of Action/Effect Exerts its inhibitory effect on three antigenic subtypes of influenza A virus (H1N1, H2N2, H3N2) early in the viral replicative cycle, possibly inhibiting the uncoating process; it has no activity against influenza B virus and is two- to eightfold more active than amantadine

Contraindications Hypersensitivity to drugs of the adamantine class, including rimantadine and amantadine, or any component of the formulation

Warnings/Precautions Use with caution in patients with renal and hepatic dysfunction; avoid use, if possible, in patients with uncontrolled psychosis or severe psychoneurosis. An increase in seizure incidence may occur in patients with seizure disorders; discontinue drug if seizures occur; resistance may develop during treatment; viruses exhibit cross-resistance between amantadine and rimantadine. Due to increased resistance, the ACIP has recommended that rimantadine and amantadine no longer be used for the treatment or prophylaxis of influenza A in the United States until susceptibility has been re-established; consult current guidelines. Rimantadine is not effective in the prevention or treatment of influenza B virus infections. The elderly are at higher risk for CNS (eg, dizziness, headache, weakness) and gastrointestinal (eg, nausea/vomiting, abdominal pain) adverse events; dosage adjustment is recommended in elderly patients >65 years of age.

Drug Interactions

Avoid Concomitant Use There are no known interactions where it is recommended to avoid concomitant use.

Decreased Effect

Rimantadine may decrease the levels/effects of: Influenza Virus Vaccine (Live/Attenuated)

Increased Effect/Toxicity

The levels/effects of Rimantadine may be increased by: MAO Inhibitors

Nutritional/Ethanol Interactions Food: Food does not affect rate or extent of absorption

Adverse Reactions 1% to 10%:

Central nervous system: Insomnia (2% to 3%), concentration impaired (≤2%), dizziness (1% to 2%), nervousness (1% to 2%), fatigue (1%), headache (1%)

Gastrointestinal: Nausea (3%), anorexia (2%), vomiting (2%), xerostomia (2%), abdominal pain (1%)

Neuromuscular & skeletal: Weakness (1%)

Pharmacodynamics/Kinetics

Onset of Action Antiviral activity: No data exist establishing a correlation between plasma concentration and antiviral effect

Available Dosage Forms

Tablet, oral: 100 mg

Flumadine®: 100 mg

General Dosage Range Dosage adjustment recommended in patients with hepatic or renal impairment

Oral:

Children 1-9 years: 5 mg/kg/day in 1-2 divided doses (maximum: 150 mg/day)

Children ≥10 years and <40 kg: 5 mg/kg/day in 2 divided doses

Children ≥10 years and Adults: 100 mg twice daily

Elderly: 100 mg daily

Administration

Oral Initiation of rimantadine within 48 hours of the onset of influenza A illness halves the duration of illness and significantly reduces the duration of viral shedding and increased peripheral airways resistance. Continue therapy for 5-7 days after symptoms begin; discontinue as soon as clinically warranted to reduce the emergence of antiviral drug resistant viruses

Stability

Storage Store at 25°C (77°F); excursions permitted to 15°C to 30°C (59°F to 86°F).

Nursing Actions

Physical Assessment Recommendations for antiviral susceptibility and effectiveness may change. Validate with the CDC recommendations for use prior to prescribing. Monitor for hypotension, CNS changes (confusion, anxiety, agitation), gastrointestinal upset, and anticholinergic effects (dry mouth, urinary retention, mydriases).

Patient Education May cause dizziness, insomnia, fatigue, nervousness, or gastrointestinal upset. Report rash, palpitations, severe nausea or vomiting, or persistent CNS changes (eg, confusion, insomnia, anxiety, restlessness, irritability, hallucinations).

Risedronate (ris ED roe nate)

Brand Names: U.S. Actonel®; Atelvia™

Index Terms Risedronate Sodium

Pharmacologic Category Bisphosphonate Derivative

Medication Safety Issues

Sound-alike/look-alike issues:

Actonel® may be confused with Actos®

Risedronate may be confused with alendronate

Medication Guide Available Yes

Pregnancy Risk Factor C

Lactation Excretion in breast milk unknown/not recommended

Breast-Feeding Considerations The manufacturer recommends discontinuing nursing or discontinuing risedronate.

Use

Actonel®: Treatment of Paget's disease of the bone; treatment and prevention of glucocorticoid-induced osteoporosis; treatment and prevention of osteoporosis in postmenopausal women; treatment of osteoporosis in men

Atelvia™: Treatment of osteoporosis in postmenopausal women

Mechanism of Action/Effect A bisphosphonate which inhibits bone resorption via actions on osteoclasts or on osteoclast precursors; decreases the rate of bone resorption, leading to an indirect increase in bone mineral density. In Paget's disease, characterized by disordered resorption and formation of bone, inhibition of resorption leads to an indirect decrease in bone formation; but the newly-formed bone has a more normal architecture.

Contraindications Hypersensitivity to risedronate, bisphosphonates, or any component of the formulation; hypocalcemia; inability to stand or sit upright for at least 30 minutes; abnormalities of the esophagus which delay esophageal emptying, such as stricture or achalasia

Warnings/Precautions Bisphosphonates may cause upper gastrointestinal disorders such as dysphagia, esophagitis, esophageal ulcer, and gastric ulcer; risk increases in patients unable to comply with dosing instructions. Use with caution in patients with dysphagia, esophageal disease, gastritis, duodenitis, or ulcers (may worsen underlying condition). Discontinue if new or worsening symptoms occur. Use caution in patients with renal impairment (not recommended in patients with a Cl_{cr} <30 mL/minute). Hypocalcemia must be corrected before therapy initiation with risedronate. Ensure adequate calcium and vitamin D intake, especially for patients with Paget's disease in whom the pretreatment rate of bone turnover may be greatly elevated.

Bisphosphonate therapy has been associated with osteonecrosis, primarily of the jaw. Risk factors for osteonecrosis of the jaw (ONJ) include invasive dental procedures (eg, tooth extraction, dental implants, boney surgery); a diagnosis of cancer, with concomitant chemotherapy or corticosteroids; poor oral hygiene, ill-fitting dentures; and comorbid disorders (anemia, coagulopathy, infection, preexisting dental disease). Most reported cases occurred after I.V. bisphosphonate therapy; however, cases have been reported following oral therapy. A dental exam and preventative dentistry should be performed prior to placing patients with risk factors on chronic bisphosphonate therapy. The manufacturer's labeling states that discontinuing bisphosphonates in patients requiring invasive dental procedures may reduce the risk of ONJ. However, other experts suggest that there is no evidence that discontinuing therapy reduces the risk of developing ONJ (Assael, 2009). The benefit/risk must be assessed by the treating physician and/or dentist/surgeon prior to any invasive dental procedure. Patients developing ONJ while on bisphosphonates should receive care by an oral surgeon.

Atypical femur fractures have been reported in patients receiving bisphosphonates for treatment/prevention of osteoporosis. The fractures include subtrochanteric femur (bone just below the hip joint) and diaphyseal femur (long segment of the thigh bone). Some patients experience prodromal pain weeks or months before the fracture occurs. It is unclear if bisphosphonate therapy is the cause for these fractures, although the majority have been reported in patients taking bisphosphonates. Patients receiving long-term (>3-5 years) therapy may be at an increased risk. Discontinue bisphosphonate therapy in patients who develop a femoral shaft fracture.

Infrequently, severe (and occasionally debilitating) bone, joint, and/or muscle pain have been reported during bisphosphonate treatment. The onset of pain ranged from a single day to several months. Consider discontinuing therapy in patients who experience severe symptoms; symptoms usually resolve upon discontinuation. Some patients experienced recurrence when rechallenged with same drug or another bisphosphonate; avoid use in patients with a history of these symptoms in association with bisphosphonate therapy.

When using for glucocorticoid-induced osteoporosis, evaluate sex steroid hormonal status prior to treatment initiation; consider appropriate hormone replacement if necessary. Not approved for use in pediatric patients with osteogenesis imperfecta due to lack of efficacy in reducing the risk of fracture.

Drug Interactions

Avoid Concomitant Use There are no known interactions where it is recommended to avoid concomitant use.

Decreased Effect

The levels/effects of Risedronate may be decreased by: Antacids; Calcium Salts; Iron Salts; Magnesium Salts; Proton Pump Inhibitors

Increased Effect/Toxicity

Risedronate may increase the levels/effects of: Deferasirox; Phosphate Supplements

The levels/effects of Risedronate may be increased by: Aminoglycosides; Nonsteroidal Anti-Inflammatory Agents

Nutritional/Ethanol Interactions

Ethanol: Avoid ethanol (may increase risk of osteoporosis).

Food: Food reduces absorption (similar to other bisphosphonates); mean oral bioavailability is decreased when given with food.

Adverse Reactions Frequency may vary with product, dose, and indication.

>10%:

Cardiovascular: Hypertension (11%)

Central nervous system: Headache (3% to 18%)

Dermatologic: Rash (8% to 12%)

Endocrine & metabolic: Serum PTH levels increased (transient; <30%)

Gastrointestinal: Diarrhea (5% to 20%), nausea (4% to 13%), constipation (3% to 13%), abdominal pain (2% to 12%), dyspepsia (4% to 11%)

Genitourinary: Urinary tract infection (11%)

Neuromuscular & skeletal: Arthralgia (7% to 33%), back pain (6% to 28%)

Miscellaneous: Infection (≤31%)

1% to 10%:

Cardiovascular: Peripheral edema (8%), chest pain (5% to 7%), arrhythmia (2%)

Central nervous system: Depression (7%), dizziness (3% to 7%)

Endocrine & metabolic: Hypocalcemia (≤5%), hypophosphatemia (<3%)

Gastrointestinal: Vomiting (2% to 5%), gastritis (3%), duodenitis (≤1%), glossitis (≤1%)

Genitourinary: Prostatic hyperplasia (5%; benign), nephrolithiasis (3%)

Neuromuscular & skeletal: Joint disorder (7%), myalgia (2% to 7%), neck pain (5%), muscle spasm (1% to 2%)

Ocular: Cataract (7%)

Respiratory: Bronchitis (3% to 10%), pharyngitis (6%), rhinitis (6%), dyspnea (4%)

Miscellaneous: Flu-like syndrome (10%), acute phase reaction (≤8%; includes fever, influenza-like illness)

Pharmacodynamics/Kinetics

Onset of Action May require weeks

Available Dosage Forms

Tablet, oral:

Actonel®: 5 mg, 30 mg, 35 mg, 150 mg

Tablet, delayed release, oral:

Atelvia™: 35 mg

General Dosage Range Oral: *Adults:* 5 mg or 30 mg once daily **or** 35 mg once weekly **or** 150 mg once a month

Administration

Oral Note: Avoid administration of oral calcium supplements, antacids, magnesium supplements/laxatives, and iron preparations within 30 minutes of risedronate administration.

Immediate release tablet: Risedronate immediate release tablets must be taken on an empty stomach with a full glass (6-8 oz) of **plain water** (not mineral water) at least 30 minutes before any food, drink, or other medications orally to avoid interference with absorption. Patient must remain sitting upright or standing for at least 30 minutes after taking (to reduce esophageal irritation). Tablet should be swallowed whole; do not crush or chew.

Delayed release tablet: Risedronate delayed release tablets must be taken with at least 4 oz of **plain water** (not mineral water) immediately **after** breakfast. Patient must remain sitting upright or standing for at least 30 minutes after taking (to reduce esophageal irritation). Tablet should be swallowed whole; do not cut, split, crush, or chew.

Stability

Storage Store at room temperature of 20°C to 25°C (68°F to 77°F).

Nursing Actions

Physical Assessment Monitor for immediate or long-term musculoskeletal pain. Patients at risk for osteonecrosis of the jaw (eg, chemotherapy, corticosteroids, poor oral hygiene) should have dental exams; necessary preventive dentistry should be done before beginning bisphosphonate therapy. Teach patient specific administration directions. Instruct patient in lifestyle and dietary changes.

Patient Education Stay in upright sitting or standing position for 30 minutes following administration to reduce potential for esophageal irritation. Take immediate release tablets with a full glass (6-8 oz) of water on an empty stomach at least 30 minutes before eating or taking anything else. Take delayed release tablets with at least 4 ounces of water immediately after breakfast. Do not cut, crush, or chew tablets. Certain dental procedures should be avoided if possible while you are taking this medication. You may experience temporary nausea or vomiting, diarrhea, or bone pain. Report persistent muscle or bone pain; leg cramps; muscle twitching; unusual fever; seizures; difficulty breathing; rash; bloody stool; or pain in mouth, jaws, or teeth.

Dietary Considerations Ensure adequate calcium and vitamin D intake. Take immediate release tablet with at least 6 oz of **plain water** (not mineral water) ≥30 minutes before the first food or drink of the day other than water. Take delayed release tablet with at least 4 ounces of **plain water** immediately **after** breakfast.

Risperidone (ris PER i done)

Brand Names: U.S. RisperDAL®; RisperDAL® Consta®; RisperDAL® M-Tab®

Index Terms Risperdal M-Tab

Pharmacologic Category Antimanic Agent; Antipsychotic Agent, Atypical

Medication Safety Issues

Sound-alike/look-alike issues:

RisperiDONE may be confused with reserpine, rOPINIRole

RisperDAL® may be confused with lisinopril, reserpine, Restoril™

Pregnancy Risk Factor C

Lactation Enters breast milk/not recommended

Breast-Feeding Considerations Risperidone and its metabolite are excreted in breast milk; it is recommended that women not breast-feed during therapy or for 12 weeks after the last injection if using Risperdal® Consta®.

Use

Oral: Treatment of schizophrenia; treatment of acute mania or mixed episodes associated with bipolar I disorder (as monotherapy in children or adults, or in combination with lithium or valproate in adults); treatment of irritability/aggression associated with autistic disorder

Injection: Treatment of schizophrenia; maintenance treatment of bipolar I disorder in adults as monotherapy or in combination with lithium or valproate

Unlabeled Use Treatment of Tourette's syndrome; psychosis/agitation related to Alzheimer's dementia; post-traumatic stress disorder (PTSD)

Mechanism of Action/Effect Risperidone is a benzisoxazole atypical antipsychotic with affinity for dopamine and serotonin. Results in improvement of psychotic symptoms and reduction of extrapyramidal side effects.

Contraindications Hypersensitivity to risperidone or any component of the formulation

Warnings/Precautions Hazardous agent - use appropriate precautions for handling and disposal. **[U.S. Boxed Warning]: Elderly patients with dementia-related psychosis treated with antipsychotics are at an increased risk of death compared to placebo.** Most deaths appeared to be either cardiovascular (eg, heart failure, sudden death) or infectious (eg, pneumonia) in nature. In addition, an increased incidence of cerebrovascular effects (eg, transient ischemic attack, cerebrovascular accidents) has been reported in studies of placebo-controlled trials of risperidone in elderly patients with dementia-related psychosis. Risperidone is not approved for the treatment of dementia-related psychosis.

Leukopenia, neutropenia, and agranulocytosis (sometimes fatal) have been reported in clinical trials and postmarketing reports with antipsychotic use; presence of risk factors (eg, pre-existing low WBC or history of drug-induced leuko-/neutropenia) should prompt periodic blood count assessment. Discontinue therapy at first signs of blood dyscrasias or if absolute neutrophil count <1000/mm^3.

Low to moderately sedating, use with caution in disorders where CNS depression is a feature. Use with caution in Parkinson's disease. Caution in patients with predisposition to seizures. Use with caution in renal or hepatic dysfunction; dose reduction recommended. Esophageal dysmotility and aspiration have been associated with antipsychotic use; use with caution in patients at risk of aspiration pneumonia (ie, Alzheimer's disease). Use is associated with increased prolactin levels; clinical significance of hyperprolactinemia in patients with breast cancer or other prolactin-dependent tumors is unknown. May alter temperature regulation. May mask toxicity of other drugs or conditions (eg intestinal obstruction, Reyes syndrome, brain tumor) due to antiemetic effects. Neutropenia has been reported with antipsychotic use, including fatal cases of agranulocytosis. Pre-existing myelosuppression (disease or drug-induced) increases risk and these patients should have frequent CBC monitoring; decreased blood counts in absence of other causative factors should prompt discontinuation of therapy.

Use with caution in patients with cardiovascular diseases (eg, heart failure, history of myocardial infarction or ischemia, cerebrovascular disease, conduction abnormalities). May cause orthostatic hypotension; use with caution in patients at risk of this effect (eg, concurrent medication use which may predispose to hypotension/bradycardia or presence of hypovolemia) or in those who would not tolerate transient hypotensive episodes. May alter cardiac conduction (low risk relative to other neuroleptics); life-threatening arrhythmias have occurred with therapeutic doses of neuroleptics.

May cause anticholinergic effects (confusion, agitation, constipation, xerostomia, blurred vision, urinary retention); therefore, they should be used with caution in patients with decreased gastrointestinal motility, urinary retention, BPH, xerostomia, or visual problems (including narrow-angle glaucoma)

Relative to other neuroleptics, risperidone has a low potency of cholinergic blockade.

May cause extrapyramidal symptoms (EPS), including pseudoparkinsonism, acute dystonic reactions, akathisia, and tardive dyskinesia (risk of these reactions is low relative to other neuroleptics, and is dose dependent). Risk of dystonia (and probably other EPS) may be greater with increased doses, use of conventional antipsychotics, males, and younger patients. Risk of neuroleptic malignant syndrome (NMS) may be increased in patients with Parkinson's disease or Lewy body dementia; monitor for symptoms of confusion, obtundation, postural instability and extrapyramidal symptoms. May cause hyperglycemia; in some cases may be extreme and associated with ketoacidosis, hyperosmolar coma, or death. Use with caution in patients with diabetes or other disorders of glucose regulation; monitor for worsening of glucose control. Significant weight gain has been observed with antipsychotic therapy; incidence varies with product. Monitor waist circumference and BMI. Rare cases of priapism have been reported.

The possibility of a suicide attempt is inherent in psychotic illness or bipolar disorder; use caution in high-risk patients during initiation of therapy. Prescriptions should be written for the smallest quantity consistent with good patient care. Long-term effects on growth or sexual maturation have not been evaluated. Vehicle used in injectable (polylactide-co-glycolide microspheres) has rarely been associated with retinal artery occlusion in patients with abnormal arteriovenous anastomosis.

Drug Interactions

Avoid Concomitant Use

Avoid concomitant use of RisperiDONE with any of the following: Artemether; Dronedarone; Lumefantrine; Metoclopramide; Nilotinib; Pimozide; QUEtiapine; QuiNINE; Tetrabenazine; Thioridazine; Toremifene; Vandetanib; Vemurafenib; Ziprasidone

Decreased Effect

RisperiDONE may decrease the levels/effects of: Amphetamines; Anti-Parkinson's Agents (Dopamine Agonist); Quinagolide

The levels/effects of RisperiDONE may be decreased by: CarBAMazepine; Lithium formulations; Peginterferon Alfa-2b; Tocilizumab

Increased Effect/Toxicity

RisperiDONE may increase the levels/effects of: Alcohol (Ethyl); Anticholinergics; ARIPiprazole; CNS Depressants; Dronedarone; Methylphenidate; Paliperidone; Pimozide; QTc-Prolonging Agents; QuiNINE; Serotonin Modulators; Tetrabenazine; Thioridazine; Toremifene; Vandetanib; Vemurafenib; Ziprasidone

The levels/effects of RisperiDONE may be increased by: Abiraterone Acetate; Acetylcholinesterase Inhibitors (Central); Alfuzosin; Artemether; Chloroquine; Ciprofloxacin; Ciprofloxacin (Systemic); Conivaptan; CYP2D6 Inhibitors (Moderate); CYP2D6 Inhibitors (Strong); Darunavir; Divalproex; Gadobutrol; HydrOXYzine; Indacaterol; Lithium formulations; Loop Diuretics; Lumefantrine; Methylphenidate; Metoclopramide; Nilotinib; Pramlintide; QUEtiapine; QuiNINE; Selective Serotonin Reuptake Inhibitors; Tetrabenazine; Valproic Acid; Verapamil

Nutritional/Ethanol Interactions

Ethanol: Ethanol may increase CNS depression. Management: Limit or avoid ethanol.

Food: Oral solution is not compatible with beverages containing tannin or pectinate (cola or tea). Management: Administer oral solution with water, coffee, orange juice, or low-fat milk.

Herb/Nutraceutical: Some herbal medications may increase CNS depression. Management: Avoid kava kava, gotu kola, valerian, and St John's wort.

Adverse Reactions The frequency of adverse effects is reported as absolute percentages and is not based upon net frequencies as compared to placebo. Actual frequency may be dependent upon dose and/or indication. Events are reported from placebo-controlled studies. Unless otherwise noted, frequency of adverse effects is reported for the oral formulation in adults.

>10%:

Central nervous system: Somnolence (children 12% to 67%; adults 5% to 14%; I.M. injection 5% to 6%), fatigue (children 18% to 42%; adults 1% to 3%), headache (I.M. injection 15% to 21%), fever (children 20%; adults 1% to 2%), dystonia (children 9% to 18%; adults 5% to 11%), anxiety (children ≤16%; adults 2% to 16%), dizziness (children 7% to 16%; adults 4% to 10%), Parkinsonism (children 2% to 16%; adults 12% to 20%)

Dermatologic: Rash (children ≤11%; adults 2% to 4%)

Gastrointestinal: Appetite increased (children 4% to 49%), weight gain (≥7% kg increase from baseline: children 33%; adults 9% to 21%), vomiting (children 10% to 25%), salivation increased (children ≤22%; adults 1% to 3%), constipation (children 21%; adults 8% to 9%), abdominal pain (children 15% to 18%; adults 3% to 4%), nausea (children 8% to 16%; adults 4% to 9%), dyspepsia (children 5% to 16%; adults 4% to 10%), xerostomia (children 13%; adults ≤4%)

Genitourinary: Urinary incontinence (children 5% to 22%; adults <2%)

Neuromuscular & skeletal: Tremor (adults 6%; children 10% to 12%)

Respiratory: Rhinitis (children 13% to 36%; adults 7% to 11%), upper respiratory infection (children 34%; adults 2% to 3%), cough (children 34%; adults 3%)

1% to 10%:

Cardiovascular: Tachycardia (children ≤7%; adults 1% to 5%), hypertension (I.M. injection 3%), chest pain (1% to 3%), creatine phosphokinase increased (≤2%), postural hypotension (≤2%), arrhythmia (≤1%), edema (≤1%), hypotension (≤1%), syncope (≤1%)

Central nervous system: Akathisia (children ≤10%; adults 5% to 9%), automatism (children 7%), confusion (children 5%)

Dermatologic: Seborrhea (up to 2%), acne (1%)

Endocrine & metabolic: Lactation nonpuerperal (children 2% to 5%; adults 1%), ejaculation failure (≤1%)

Gastrointestinal: Diarrhea (children 7% to 8%; adults ≤3%), anorexia (children 8%; adults ≤2%), toothache (I.M. injection 1% to 3%)

Genitourinary: Urinary tract infection (≤3%)

Hematologic: Neutropenia (I.M. injection <2%), anemia (I.M. injection <2%; oral ≤1%)

Hepatic: Transaminases increased (I.M. injection ≥1%; oral 1%)

Neuromuscular & skeletal: Dyskinesia (children 7%; adults 1%), arthralgia (2% to 3%), back pain (2% to 3%), myalgia (≤2%), weakness (1%)

Ocular: Abnormal vision (children 4% to 7%; adults 1% to 3%), blurred vision (I.M. injection 2% to 3%)

Otic: Earache (1%)

Respiratory: Dyspnea (children 2% to 5%; adults 2%), epistaxis (≤2%)

Available Dosage Forms

Injection, microspheres for reconstitution, extended release:

RisperDAL® Consta®: 12.5 mg, 25 mg, 37.5 mg, 50 mg

Solution, oral: 1 mg/mL (30 mL)

RisperDAL®: 1 mg/mL (30 mL)

Tablet, oral: 0.25 mg, 0.5 mg, 1 mg, 2 mg, 3 mg, 4 mg

RisperDAL®: 0.25 mg, 0.5 mg, 1 mg, 2 mg, 3 mg, 4 mg

Tablet, orally disintegrating, oral: 0.25 mg, 0.5 mg, 1 mg, 2 mg, 3 mg, 4 mg

RisperDAL® M-Tab®: 0.5 mg, 1 mg, 2 mg, 3 mg, 4 mg

General Dosage Range Dosage adjustment recommended in patients with hepatic or renal impairment

I.M.:

Adults: 25 mg every 2 weeks (range: 12.5-50 mg every 2 weeks; maximum: 50 mg every 2 weeks)

Elderly: 12.5-25 mg every 2 weeks

Oral:

Children ≥5 years: Autism: Initial: 0.25 mg/day (<20 kg) or 0.5 mg/day (≥20 kg); Maximum dose: 1 mg/day (<20 kg) or 2.5 mg/day (≥20 kg) (3 mg/day in children >45 kg)

Children 10-17 years: Bipolar disorder: Initial: 0.5 mg once daily; Recommended target dose: 2.5 mg/day; dosing range 0.5-6 mg/day

Children: 13-17 years: Schizophrenia: Initial: 0.5 mg once daily; Recommended target dose: 3 mg/day; dosing range 1-6 mg/day

Adults: Initial: 2-3 mg/day in 1-2 divided doses; Maintenance: 1-8 mg/day in 1-2 divided doses

Elderly: Initial: 0.5 mg twice daily

Administration

Oral

Oral: May be administered without regard to meals.

Oral solution can be administered directly from the provided pipette or may be mixed with water, coffee, orange juice, or low-fat milk, but is **not compatible** with cola or tea.

In children or adolescents experiencing somnolence, half the daily dose may be administered twice daily **or** the once-daily dose may be administered at bedtime.

Risperdal® M-Tab® should not be removed from blister pack until administered. Using dry hands, place immediately on tongue. Tablet will dissolve within seconds, and may be swallowed with or without liquid. Do not split or chew.

I.M. Risperdal® Consta® should be administered I.M. into either the deltoid muscle or the upper outer quadrant of the gluteal area. Avoid inadvertent injection into vasculature. Injection should alternate between the two arms or buttocks. Do not combine two different dosage strengths into one single administration. Do not substitute any components of the dose-pack; administer with needle provided (1-inch needle for deltoid administration or 2-inch needle for gluteal administration).

Stability

Reconstitution Risperdal® Consta®: Bring to room temperature prior to reconstitution. Reconstitute with provided diluent only. Shake vigorously to mix; will form thick, milky suspension. Following reconstitution, store at room temperature and use within 6 hours. Suspension settles in ~2 minutes; shake vigorously to resuspend prior to administration.

Storage

Injection: Risperdal® Consta®: Store in refrigerator at 2°C to 8°C (36°F to 46°F) and protect from light. May be stored at room temperature of 25°C (77°F) for up to 7 days prior to administration. Following reconstitution, store at room temperature and use within 6 hours. Suspension settles in ~2 minutes; shake vigorously to resuspend prior to administration.

Oral solution, tablet: Store at 15°C to 25°C (59°F to 77°F). Protect from light and moisture. Keep orally-disintegrating tablets sealed in foil pouch until ready to use. Do not freeze solution.

Nursing Actions

Physical Assessment Review ophthalmic exam and monitor mental status, mood, affect, CNS responses, anticholinergic and extrapyramidal symptoms, and orthostatic hypotension prior to treatment and periodically throughout. Monitor weight prior to initiating therapy and at least monthly. Be alert to the possibility of suicide ideation.

Patient Education It may take several weeks to achieve desired results. Dilute solution with water, milk, or orange juice; do not dilute with beverages containing tannin or pectinate (eg, colas, tea). Avoid alcohol. Maintain adequate hydration. If you have diabetes, you may experience increased blood sugars; monitor closely. You may experience excess sedation, drowsiness, restlessness, dizziness, or blurred vision; dry mouth, nausea, or GI upset; postural hypotension; or urinary retention (void before taking medication). Report persistent CNS effects (eg, trembling fingers, altered gait or balance, excessive sedation, seizures, unusual muscle or skeletal movements, anxiety, abnormal thoughts [especially suicide ideation], confusion, personality changes); chest pain, palpitations, irregular or rapid heartbeat, or severe dizziness; signs of infection or fever; altered menstrual pattern or sexual dysfunction; pain or difficulty on urination; vision changes; skin rash or yellowing of skin; respiratory difficulty; or worsening of condition.

Dietary Considerations May be taken without regard to meals. Some products may contain phenylalanine.

Ritonavir (ri TOE na veer)

Brand Names: U.S. Norvir®

Pharmacologic Category Antiretroviral Agent, Protease Inhibitor

Medication Safety Issues

Sound-alike/look-alike issues:

Ritonavir may be confused with Retrovir®

Norvir® may be confused with Norvasc®

Pregnancy Risk Factor B

Lactation Excretion in breast milk unknown/not recommended

Breast-Feeding Considerations Maternal or infant antiretroviral therapy does not completely eliminate the risk of postnatal HIV transmission. In addition, multiclass-resistant virus has been detected in breast-feeding infants despite maternal therapy. Therefore, in the United States, where formula is accessible, affordable, safe, and sustainable, and the risk of infant mortality due to diarrhea and respiratory infections is low, complete avoidance of breast-feeding by HIV-infected women is recommended to decrease potential transmission of HIV (DHHS [perinatal], 2011).

Use Treatment of HIV infection; should always be used as part of a multidrug regimen (at least three antiretroviral agents); may be used as a pharmacokinetic "booster" for other protease inhibitors

Mechanism of Action/Effect Blocks the site of HIV-1 protease activity, resulting in the formation of immature, noninfectious viral particles.

Contraindications Hypersensitivity to ritonavir or any component of the formulation; concurrent alfuzosin, amiodarone, bepridil, cisapride, dihydroergotamine, ergonovine, ergotamine, flecainide, lovastatin, methylergonovine, midazolam (oral), pimozide, propafenone, quinidine, sildenafil (when used for the treatment of pulmonary arterial hypertension [eg, Revatio®]), simvastatin, St John's wort, triazolam, and voriconazole (when ritonavir ≥800 mg/day)

Warnings/Precautions [U.S. Boxed Warning]: Ritonavir may interact with many medications, resulting in potentially serious and/or life-threatening adverse events. Use with caution in patients taking strong CYP3A4 inhibitors, moderate or strong CYP3A4 inducers and major CYP3A4 substrates (see Drug Interactions); consider alternative agents that avoid or lessen the potential for CYP-mediated interactions. Concomitant use with fluticasone, salmeterol, or high-dose or long-term use of meperidine is not recommended. Do not coadminister colchicine in patient with renal or hepatic impairment

Pancreatitis has been observed; use with caution in patients with increased triglycerides; monitor serum lipase and amylase and for gastrointestinal symptoms. Increases in total cholesterol and triglycerides have been reported; screening should be done prior to therapy and periodically throughout treatment.

Protease inhibitors have been associated with a variety of hypersensitivity events (some severe), including rash, anaphylaxis (rare), angioedema, bronchospasm, erythema multiforme, toxic epidermal necrolysis, and/or Stevens-Johnson syndrome (rare). It is generally recommended to discontinue treatment if severe rash or moderate symptoms accompanied by other systemic symptoms occur. Use with caution in patients with cardiomyopathy, ischemic heart disease, pre-existing conduction abnormalities, or structural heart disease; may be at increased risk of conduction abnormalities (eg, second- or third-degree AV block). Ritonavir has been associated with AV block due to prolongation of PR interval; use caution with drugs that prolong the PR interval. Use with caution in patients with hemophilia A or B; increased bleeding during protease inhibitor therapy has been reported. Changes in glucose tolerance, hyperglycemia, exacerbation of diabetes, DKA, and new-onset diabetes mellitus have been reported in patients receiving protease inhibitors. May be associated with fat redistribution (buffalo hump, increased abdominal girth, breast engorgement, facial atrophy, and dyslipidemia). Immune reconstitution syndrome may develop resulting in the occurrence of an inflammatory response to an indolent or residual opportunistic infection; further evaluation and treatment may be required. May cause hepatitis or exacerbate pre-existing hepatic dysfunction; use with caution in patients with hepatitis B or C and in hepatic disease. Norvir® tablets are **not** bioequivalent to Norvir® capsules. Gastrointestinal side effects (eg, nausea, vomiting, abdominal pain, diarrhea) or paresthesias may be more common when patients are switching from the capsule to the tablet formulation due to a higher C_{max} (26% increase) observed with the tablet formulation compared to the capsule. These side effects should decrease as therapy is continued. Safety and efficacy have not been established in children <1 month of age.

Drug Interactions

Avoid Concomitant Use

Avoid concomitant use of Ritonavir with any of the following: Alfuzosin; Amiodarone; Axitinib; Cisapride; Conivaptan; Crizotinib; Disulfiram; Dronedarone; Eplerenone; Ergot Derivatives; Etravirine; Everolimus; Flecainide; Fluticasone (Nasal); Fluticasone (Oral Inhalation); Halofantrine; Lapatinib; Lovastatin; Lurasidone; Midazolam; Nilotinib; Nisoldipine; Pimozide; Propafenone; QuiNIDine; QuiNINE; Ranolazine; Rifampin; Rivaroxaban; RomiDEPsin; Salmeterol; Silodosin; Simvastatin; St Johns Wort; Tamsulosin; Thioridazine; Ticagrelor; Tolvaptan; Topotecan; Toremifene; Triazolam; Voriconazole

Decreased Effect

Ritonavir may decrease the levels/effects of: Abacavir; Atovaquone; Boceprevir; BuPROPion; Clarithromycin; Codeine; Contraceptives (Estrogens); Deferasirox; Delavirdine; Divalproex; Etravirine; Fosphenytoin; LamoTRIgine; Meperidine; Methadone; Phenytoin; Prasugrel; Telaprevir; Theophylline Derivatives; Ticagrelor; TraMADol; Valproic Acid; Voriconazole; Warfarin; Zidovudine

The levels/effects of Ritonavir may be decreased by: Antacids; Boceprevir; CarBAMazepine; CYP3A4 Inducers (Strong); Cyproterone; Efavirenz; Fosphenytoin; Garlic; Peginterferon Alfa-2b; P-glycoprotein/ABCB1 Inducers; Phenytoin; Rifampin; St Johns Wort; Tenofovir; Tocilizumab

Increased Effect/Toxicity

Ritonavir may increase the levels/effects of: Alfuzosin; Almotriptan; Alosetron; ALPRAZolam; Amiodarone; Antifungal Agents (Azole Derivatives, Systemic); ARIPiprazole; Atomoxetine; Axitinib; Bortezomib; Bosentan; Brentuximab Vedotin; Brinzolamide; Budesonide (Nasal); Budesonide (Systemic, Oral Inhalation); Calcium Channel Blockers (Dihydropyridine); Calcium Channel Blockers (Nondihydropyridine); CarBAMazepine; Ciclesonide; Cisapride; Clarithromycin; Clorazepate; Colchicine; Conivaptan; Corticosteroids (Orally Inhaled); Crizotinib; CycloSPORINE; CycloSPORINE (Systemic); CYP2C8 Substrates; CYP2D6 Substrates; CYP3A4 Substrates; Dabigatran Etexilate; Diazepam; Dienogest; Digoxin; Dronabinol; Dronedarone; Dutasteride; Enfuvirtide; Eplerenone; Ergot Derivatives; Estazolam; Everolimus; FentaNYL; Fesoterodine; Flecainide; Flurazepam; Fluticasone (Nasal); Fluticasone (Oral Inhalation); Fusidic Acid; GuanFACINE; Halofantrine; HMG-CoA Reductase Inhibitors; Iloperidone; Ivacaftor; Ixabepilone; Lapatinib; Linagliptin; Lovastatin; Lumefantrine; Lurasidone; Maraviroc; Meperidine; MethylPREDNISolone; Midazolam; Nebivolol; Nefazodone; Nilotinib; Nisoldipine; Paricalcitol; Pazopanib; P-glycoprotein/ABCB1 Substrates; Pimecrolimus; Pimozide; PrednisoLONE; PredniSONE; Propafenone; Protease Inhibitors; Prucalopride; QuiNIDine; QuiNINE; Ranolazine; Rifabutin; Rivaroxaban; RomiDEPsin; Ruxolitinib; Salmeterol; Saxagliptin; Sildenafil; Silodosin; Simvastatin; Sirolimus; SORAfenib; Tacrolimus; Tacrolimus (Systemic); Tacrolimus (Topical); Tadalafil; Tamsulosin; Telaprevir; Temsirolimus; Tenofovir; Tetrabenazine; Thioridazine; Ticagrelor; Tolterodine; Tolvaptan; Topotecan; Toremifene; TraZODone; Treprostinil; Triazolam; Tricyclic Antidepressants; Vardenafil; Vemurafenib; Vilazodone; VinBLAStine; VinCRIStine; Zuclopenthixol

The levels/effects of Ritonavir may be increased by: Antifungal Agents (Azole Derivatives, Systemic); Clarithromycin; CycloSPORINE; CycloSPORINE (Systemic); Delavirdine; Disulfiram; Efavirenz; Enfuvirtide; Fusidic Acid; MetroNIDAZOLE (Topical); P-glycoprotein/ABCB1 Inhibitors; QuiNINE

Nutritional/Ethanol Interactions

Food: Food enhances absorption. Management: Take with food. Maintain adequate hydration, unless instructed to restrict fluid intake.

Herb/Nutraceutical: St John's wort may decrease ritonavir serum levels. Garlic may decrease the serum concentration of ritonavir. Management: Avoid St John's wort; concurrent use is contraindicated. Garlic supplementation is not recommended.

Adverse Reactions Percentages as reported for combined experiences in both treatment-naive and experienced adults:

>10%:

Endocrine & metabolic: Hypercholesterolemia (>240 mg/dL: 37% to 45%), triglycerides increased (>800 mg/dL: 17% to 34%; >1500 mg/dL: 1% to 13%)

Gastrointestinal: Nausea (26% to 30%), diarrhea (15% to 23%), vomiting (14% to 17%), taste perversion (7% to 11%)

Hepatic: GGT increased (5% to 20%)

Neuromuscular & skeletal: Weakness (10% to 15%), creatine phosphokinase increased (9% to 12%)

2% to 10%:

Cardiovascular: Vasodilation (2%), syncope (1% to 2%)

Central nervous system: Headache (6% to 7%), fever (1% to 5%), dizziness (3% to 4%), insomnia (2% to 3%), somnolence (2% to 3%), depression (2%), anxiety (up to 2%), malaise (1% to 2%)

Dermatologic: Rash (up to 4%)

Endocrine & metabolic: Uric acid increased (up to 4%)

Gastrointestinal: Abdominal pain (6% to 8%), anorexia (2% to 8%), dyspepsia (up to 6%), local throat irritation (2% to 3%), flatulence (1% to 2%)

Hepatic: Transaminases increased (6% to 10%)

Neuromuscular & skeletal: Paresthesia (3% to 7%), arthralgia (up to 2%), myalgia (2%)

Respiratory: Pharyngitis (≤1% to 3%)

Miscellaneous: Diaphoresis (2% to 3%)

Available Dosage Forms

Capsule, soft gelatin, oral:

Norvir®: 100 mg

Solution, oral:

Norvir®: 80 mg/mL (240 mL)

Tablet, oral:

Norvir®: 100 mg

General Dosage Range Dosage adjustment recommended in patients on concurrent therapy

Oral:

Children >1 month: Initial: 250 mg/m² twice daily; Maintenance: 350-400 mg/m² twice daily (maximum dose: 1200 mg/day)

Adults: 300-600 mg twice daily (maximum: 1200 mg/day)

Administration

Oral Administer capsules or oral solution with or without food (DHHS, 2011). Food improves tolerability. Liquid formulations usually have an unpleasant taste. Consider mixing it with chocolate milk or a liquid nutritional supplement. Whenever possible, administer oral solution with calibrated dosing syringe. Shake liquid well before use. Tablets should be administered with food and swallowed whole; do not chew, break, or crush.

Stability

Storage

Capsule: Store under refrigeration at 2°C to 8°C (36°F to 46°F); may be left out at room temperature of <25°C (<77°F) if used within 30 days. Protect from light. Avoid exposure to excessive heat.

Solution: Store at room temperature at 20°C to 25°C (68°F to 77°F); do not refrigerate. Avoid exposure to excessive heat.

Tablet: Store at room temperature at 20°C to 25°C (68°F to 77°F); excursions permitted to 15°C to 30°C (59°F to 86°F); avoid exposure to excessive heat. Exposure to high humidity outside of the original container (or a USP equivalent container) for >2 weeks is not recommended.

Nursing Actions

Physical Assessment Monitor for adherence to regimen. Monitor for gastrointestinal disturbance (nausea, vomiting, diarrhea) that can lead to dehydration and weight loss, hyperlipidemia and redistribution of body fat, rash, CNS effects (malaise, insomnia, abnormal thinking), and electrolyte imbalance. Teach patient proper timing of multiple medications and drugs that should not be used concurrently. Instruct patient on glucose testing (protease inhibitors may cause hyperglycemia; exacerbation or new-onset diabetes).

Patient Education This is not a cure for HIV, nor has it been found to reduce transmission of HIV; use appropriate precautions to prevent spread to other persons. Take with meals. Mix liquid formulation with chocolate milk or liquid nutritional supplement. Maintain adequate hydration, unless instructed to restrict fluid intake. Frequent blood tests may be required. You may be advised to check your glucose levels (this drug can cause exacerbation or new-onset diabetes). May cause body changes due to redistribution of body fat, facial atrophy, or breast enlargement (normal effects of drug). May cause dizziness, insomnia, abnormal thinking, nausea, vomiting, taste perversion, muscle weakness, or headache. Inform prescriber if you experience muscle numbness or tingling; unresolved persistent vomiting, diarrhea, or abdominal pain; respiratory difficulty or chest pain; unusual skin rash; or change in color of stool or urine.

Dietary Considerations Should be taken with food. Oral solution contains 43% ethanol by volume.

RITUXimab (ri TUK si mab)

Brand Names: U.S. Rituxan®

Index Terms Anti-CD20 Monoclonal Antibody; C2B8 Monoclonal Antibody; IDEC-C2B8

Pharmacologic Category Antineoplastic Agent, Monoclonal Antibody; Antirheumatic Miscellaneous; Monoclonal Antibody

Medication Safety Issues

Sound-alike/look-alike issues:

Rituxan® may be confused with Remicade®

RiTUXimab may be confused with brentuximab, bevacizumab, inFLIXimab, ruxolitinib

High alert medication:

The medication is in a class the Institute for Safe Medication Practices (ISMP) includes among its list of drug classes which have a heightened risk of causing significant patient harm when used in error.

Administration issues:

The rituximab dose for rheumatoid arthritis is a flat dose (1000 mg) and is not based on body surface area (BSA).

Medication Guide Available Yes

Pregnancy Risk Factor C

Lactation Excretion in breast milk unknown/not recommended

Breast-Feeding Considerations It is not known if rituximab is excreted in human milk. However, human IgG is excreted in breast milk, and therefore, rituximab may also be excreted in milk. The manufacturer recommends discontinuing breast-feeding until circulating levels of rituximab are no longer detectable.

Use

Treatment of CD20-positive non-Hodgkin's lymphomas (NHL):

Relapsed or refractory, low-grade or follicular B-cell NHL (as a single agent)

Follicular B-cell NHL, previously untreated (in combination with first-line chemotherapy, and as single-agent maintenance therapy if response to first-line rituximab with chemotherapy)

Nonprogressing, low-grade B-cell NHL (as a single agent after first-line CVP treatment)

Diffuse large B-cell NHL, previously untreated (in combination with CHOP chemotherapy [or other anthracycline-based regimen])

Treatment of CD20-positive chronic lymphocytic leukemia (CLL) (in combination with fludarabine and cyclophosphamide)

Treatment of moderately- to severely-active rheumatoid arthritis (in combination with methotrexate) in adult patients with inadequate response to one or more TNF antagonists

Treatment of Wegener's granulomatosis (WG) (in combination with glucocorticoids)

Treatment of microscopic polyangiitis (MPA) (in combination with glucocorticoids)

Unlabeled Use Treatment of Burkitt's lymphoma, central nervous system lymphoma, Hodgkin's lymphoma (lymphocyte predominant); mucosal associated lymphoid tissue (MALT) lymphoma (gastric and nongastric), splenic marginal zone lymphoma; Waldenström's macroglobulinemia (WM); post-transplant lymphoproliferative disorder (PTLD); autoimmune hemolytic anemia (AIHA) in children; chronic immune thrombocytopenic purpura (ITP); refractory pemphigus vulgaris; treatment of steroid-refractory chronic graft-versus-host disease (GVHD)

Mechanism of Action/Effect Binds to the CD20 antigen on B-lymphocytes and recruits immune effector functions to mediate B-cell lysis *in vitro*. The antibody induces cell death in the DHL-4 human B-cell lymphoma line.

Contraindications There are no contraindications listed in the FDA-approved manufacturer's labeling.

Canadian labeling (not in U.S. labeling): Type 1 hypersensitivity or anaphylactic reaction to murine proteins, Chinese Hamster Ovary (CHO) cell proteins, or any component of the formulation; patients who have or have had progressive multifocal leukoencephalopathy (PML)

Warnings/Precautions [U.S. Boxed Warning]: Severe (occasionally fatal) infusion-related reactions have been reported, usually with the first infusion; fatalities have been reported within 24 hours of infusion; monitor closely during infusion; discontinue with grades 3 or 4 infusion reactions. Reactions usually occur within 30-120 minutes and may include hypotension, angioedema, bronchospasm, hypoxia, urticaria, and in more severe cases pulmonary infiltrates, acute respiratory distress syndrome, myocardial infarction, ventricular fibrillation, cardiogenic shock and/or anaphylaxis. Risk factors associated with fatal outcomes include chronic lymphocytic leukemia, female gender, mantle cell lymphoma, or pulmonary infiltrates. Closely monitor patients with a history of prior cardiopulmonary reactions or with pre-existing cardiac or pulmonary conditions and patients with high numbers of circulating malignant cells (>25,000/mm^3). Prior to infusion, premedicate patients with acetaminophen and an antihistamine (and methylprednisolone for patients with RA). Discontinue infusion for severe reactions; treatment is symptomatic. Medications for the treatment of hypersensitivity reactions (eg, bronchodilators, epinephrine, antihistamines, corticosteroids) should be available for immediate use. Discontinue infusion for serious or life-threatening cardiac arrhythmias; subsequent doses should include cardiac monitoring during and after the infusion. Mild-to-moderate infusion-related reactions (eg, chills, fever, rigors) occur frequently and are typically managed through slowing or interrupting the infusion. Infusion may be resumed at a 50% infusion rate reduction upon resolution of symptoms. Due to the potential for hypotension, consider withholding antihypertensives 12 hours prior to treatment.

[U.S. Boxed Warning]: Progressive multifocal leukoencephalopathy (PML) due to JC virus infection has been reported with rituximab use; may be fatal. Cases were reported in patients with hematologic malignancies receiving rituximab either with combination chemotherapy, or with hematopoietic stem cell transplant. Cases were also reported in patients receiving rituximab for autoimmune diseases who had received prior or concurrent immunosuppressant therapy. Onset may be delayed, although most cases were diagnosed within 12 months of the last rituximab dose. A retrospective analysis of patients (n=57) diagnosed with PML following rituximab therapy, found a median of 16 months (following rituximab initiation), 5.5 months (following last rituximab dose), and 6 rituximab doses preceded PML diagnosis. Clinical findings included confusion/disorientation, motor weakness/hemiparesis, altered vision/speech, and poor motor coordination with symptoms progressing over weeks to months (Carson, 2009). Promptly evaluate any patient presenting with neurological changes; consider neurology consultation, brain MRI and lumbar puncture for suspected PML. Discontinue rituximab in patients who develop PML; consider reduction/discontinuation of concurrent chemotherapy or immunosuppressants. Avoid use if severe active infection is present. Serious and potentially fatal bacterial, fungal, and either new or reactivated viral infections may occur during treatment, and up to 1 year after completing rituximab. Associated new or reactivated viral infections have included cytomegalovirus, herpes simplex virus, parvovirus B19, varicella zoster virus, West Nile virus, and hepatitis B and C. Rarely, reactivation of hepatitis B (with fulminant hepatitis, hepatic failure, and death) has been reported in association with rituximab; median time to hepatitis diagnosis was ~4 months after initiation of therapy and 1 month following last dose; screen high-risk patients prior to therapy initiation; monitor for several months following completion of therapy. Discontinue rituximab (and concomitant chemotherapy) in patients who develop viral hepatitis and initiate antiviral therapy. Discontinue rituximab in patients who develop other serious infections and initiate appropriate anti-infective treatment.

[U.S. Boxed Warning]: Tumor lysis syndrome leading to acute renal failure requiring dialysis may occur 12-24 hours following the first dose when used as a single agent in the treatment of NHL. Hyperkalemia, hypocalcemia, hyperuricemia, and/or hyperphosphatemia may occur. Administer prophylaxis (allopurinol, hydration) in patients at high risk (high numbers of circulating malignant cells ≥25,000/mm^3 or high tumor burden). May cause fatal renal toxicity in patients with hematologic malignancies. Patients who received combination therapy with cisplatin and rituximab for NHL experienced renal toxicity during clinical trials; this combination is not an approved treatment regimen. Monitor for signs of renal failure; discontinue rituximab with increasing serum creatinine or oliguria. Correct electrolyte abnormalities; monitor hydration status.

[U.S. Boxed Warning]: Severe and sometimes fatal mucocutaneous reactions (lichenoid dermatitis, paraneoplastic pemphigus, Stevens-Johnson syndrome, toxic epidermal necrolysis and vesiculobullous dermatitis) have been reported, occurring from 1-13 weeks following exposure. Discontinue in patients experiencing severe mucocutaneous skin reactions; the safety of re-exposure following mucocutaneous reactions has not been evaluated. Use caution with preexisting cardiac or pulmonary disease, or prior cardiopulmonary events. Rheumatoid arthritis patients are at increased risk for cardiovascular events; monitor closely during and after each infusion. Elderly patients are at higher risk for cardiac (supraventricular arrhythmia) and pulmonary adverse events (pneumonia, pneumonitis). Abdominal pain, bowel obstruction, and perforation (rarely fatal) have been reported with an average onset of symptoms of ~6 days (range: 1-77 days); complaints of abdominal pain should be evaluated, especially if early in the treatment course. Live vaccines should not be given concurrently with rituximab; there is no data available concerning secondary transmission of live vaccines with or following rituximab treatment. RA patients should be brought up to date with nonlive immunizations (following current guidelines) at least 4 weeks before initiating therapy; evaluate risks of therapy delay versus benefit (of nonlive vaccines) for NHL patients. Safety and efficacy of rituximab in combination with biologic agents or disease-modifying antirheumatic drugs (DMARD) other than methotrexate have not been established. Rituximab is not recommended for use in RA patients who have not had prior inadequate response to TNF antagonists. Safety and efficacy of retreatment for RA have not been established. The safety of concomitant immunosuppressants other than corticosteroids has not been evaluated in patients with Wegener's granulomatosis (WG) or microscopic polyangiitis (MPA) after rituximab-induced B-cell depletion. There are only limited data on subsequent courses of rituximab for WG or MPA; safety and efficacy of retreatment has not been established.

Drug Interactions

Avoid Concomitant Use

Avoid concomitant use of RiTUXimab with any of the following: BCG; Belimumab; Certolizumab Pegol; CloZAPine; Natalizumab; Pimecrolimus; Tacrolimus (Topical); Vaccines (Live)

Decreased Effect

RiTUXimab may decrease the levels/effects of: BCG; Coccidioidin Skin Test; Sipuleucel-T; Vaccines (Inactivated); Vaccines (Live)

The levels/effects of RiTUXimab may be decreased by: Echinacea

Increased Effect/Toxicity

RiTUXimab may increase the levels/effects of: Belimumab; Certolizumab Pegol; CloZAPine; Hypoglycemic Agents; Leflunomide; Natalizumab; Vaccines (Live)

The levels/effects of RiTUXimab may be increased by: Abciximab; Antihypertensives; Denosumab; Herbs (Hypoglycemic Properties); Pimecrolimus; Roflumilast; Tacrolimus (Topical); Trastuzumab

Nutritional/Ethanol Interactions Herb/Nutraceutical: Avoid echinacea (may diminish the therapeutic effect of immunosuppressants). Avoid hypoglycemic herbs, including alfalfa, aloe, bilberry, bitter melon, burdock, celery, damiana, fenugreek, garcinia, garlic, ginger, ginseng (American), gymnema, marshmallow, and stinging nettle (may enhance the hypoglycemic effect of rituximab).

Adverse Reactions Note: Patients treated with rituximab for rheumatoid arthritis (RA) may experience fewer adverse reactions.

>10%:

Cardiovascular: Peripheral edema (8% to 16%), hypertension (6% to 12%)

Central nervous system: Fever (5% to 53%), fatigue (13% to 39%), chills (3% to 33%), headache (17% to 19%), insomnia (≤14%), pain (12%)

Dermatologic: Rash (10% to 17%; grades 3/4: 1%), pruritus (5% to 17%), angioedema (11%; grades 3/4: 1%)

Gastrointestinal: Nausea (8% to 23%), diarrhea (10% to 17%), abdominal pain (2% to 14%), weight gain (11%)

Hematologic: Cytopenias (grades 3/4: ≤48%; may be prolonged), lymphopenia (48%; grades 3/4: 40%; median duration 14 days), anemia (8% to 35%; grades 3/4: 3%), leukopenia (NHL: 14%; grades 3/4: 4%; CLL: grades 3/4: 23%; WG/MPA: 10%), neutropenia (NHL: 14%; grades 3/4: 4% to 6%; median duration 13 days; CLL: grades 3/4: 30% to 49%), neutropenic fever (CLL: grades 3/4: 9% to 15%), thrombocytopenia (12%; grades 3/4: 2% to 11%)

Hepatic: ALT increased (≤13%)

Neuromuscular & skeletal: Neuropathy (≤30%), weakness (2% to 26%), muscle spasm (≤17%), arthralgia (6% to 13%)

Respiratory: Cough (13%), rhinitis (3% to 12%), epistaxis (≤11%)

Miscellaneous: Infusion-related reactions (lymphoma: first dose 77%; decreases with subsequent infusions; may include angioedema, bronchospasm, chills, dizziness, fever, headache, hyper-/hypotension, myalgia, nausea, pruritus, rash, rigors, urticaria, and vomiting; reactions reported are lower [first infusion: 32%] in RA; CLL: 59%; grades 3/4: 7% to 9%; WG/MPA: 12%); infection (19% to 62%; grades 3/4: 4%; bacterial: 19%; viral 10%; fungal: 1%), human antichimeric antibody (HACA) positive (1% to 23%), night sweats (15%)

1% to 10%:

Cardiovascular: Hypotension (10%; grades 3/4: 2%), flushing (5%)

Central nervous system: Dizziness (10%), anxiety (2% to 5%), migraine (RA: 2%)

Dermatologic: Urticaria (2% to 8%)

Endocrine & metabolic: Hyperglycemia (9%)

Gastrointestinal: Vomiting (10%), dyspepsia (RA: 3%)

Neuromuscular & skeletal: Back pain (10%), myalgia (10%), paresthesia (2%)

Respiratory: Dyspnea (≤10%), throat irritation (2% to 9%), bronchospasm (8%), dyspnea (7%), upper respiratory tract infection (RA: 7%), sinusitis (6%)

Miscellaneous: LDH increased (7%)

Pharmacodynamics/Kinetics

Duration of Action Detectable in serum 3-6 months after completion of treatment; B-cell recovery begins ~6 months following completion of treatment; median B-cell levels return to normal by 12 months following completion of treatment

Available Dosage Forms

Injection, solution [preservative free]:

Rituxan®: 10 mg/mL (10 mL, 50 mL)

General Dosage Range I.V.: *Adults:* Dosage varies greatly depending on indication

Administration

I.V. Do **not** administer I.V. push or bolus.

Initial infusion: Start rate of 50 mg/hour; if there is no reaction, increase the rate by 50 mg/hour increments every 30 minutes, to a maximum rate of 400 mg/hour.

Subsequent infusions: If patient did not tolerate initial infusion follow initial infusion guidelines. If patient tolerated initial infusion, start at 100 mg/hour; if there is no reaction, increase the rate by 100 mg/hour increments every 30 minutes, to a maximum rate of 400 mg/hour.

Note: If a reaction occurs, slow or stop the infusion. If the reaction abates, restart infusion at 50% of the previous rate.

In patients with NHL who are receiving a corticosteroid as part of their combination chemotherapy regimen and after tolerance has been established at the recommended infusion rate in cycle 1, a rapid infusion rate has been used beginning with cycle 2. The daily corticosteroid, acetaminophen, and diphenhydramine are administered prior to treatment, then the rituximab dose is administered over 90 minutes, with 20% of the dose administered in the first 30 minutes and the remaining 80% is given over 60 minutes (Sehn, 2007).

I.V. Detail Discontinue infusions in the event of serious or life-threatening cardiac arrhythmias.

pH: 6.5

Stability

Reconstitution Withdraw necessary amount of rituximab and dilute to a final concentration of 1-4 mg/mL with 0.9% sodium chloride or 5% dextrose in water. Gently invert the bag to mix the solution. Do not shake.

Storage Store vials under refrigeration at 2°C to 8°C (36°F to 46°F); do not freeze. Do not shake. Protect vials from direct sunlight. Solutions for infusion are stable at 2°C to 8°C (36°F to 46°F) for 24 hours and at room temperature for an additional 24 hours.

Nursing Actions

Physical Assessment Premedication may be ordered. Monitor patient closely for chills, fever, rigors, dizziness, angioedema, respiratory distress, myalgia, nausea, pruritus, rash, and vomiting during and following each infusion. Emergency equipment and medications (epinephrine, antihistamines, corticosteroids) should be immediately available during infusion. In the event of severe infusion reaction, infusion should be stopped and prescriber notified immediately. Monitor patient closely for abdominal pain (bowel obstruction and perforation), hyper-/hypotension, CNS changes, hyper-/hypoglycemia, and rash after each dose and following discontinuation of therapy. Bowel obstruction and perforation can occur early in therapy; acute tumor lysis syndrome leading to acute renal failure can occur 12-24 hours after first dose; severe mucocutaneous reactions can occur from 1-13 weeks following treatment; and new or reactivated serious viral infection may occur up to one year following discontinuation of therapy.

Patient Education This medication is only administered by infusion. You may experience a reaction during the infusion of this medication, including high fever, chills, respiratory difficulty, or congestion. You will be closely monitored and comfort measures provided. Maintain adequate hydration during entire course of therapy, unless instructed to restrict fluid intake. You will be susceptible to infection. If you have diabetes, monitor glucose levels closely; this medication may impact glucose control. May cause dizziness, trembling, nausea, vomiting, loss of appetite, diarrhea, or bone or muscle pain. Report immediately any unusual abdominal pain; skin rash or redness; persistent dizziness; swelling of extremities; unusual weight gain; respiratory difficulty; chest pain or tightness; symptoms of respiratory infection (wheezing, bronchospasms, or difficulty breathing); unresolved GI disturbance (nausea, vomiting); opportunistic infection (sore or irritated throat, unusual and persistent fatigue, chills, fever, unhealed sores, white plaques in mouth or genital area, unusual bruising or bleeding); CNS changes (confusion, agitation, insomnia); pain, tingling, or loss of sensation in extremities; or loss of coordination.

Rivastigmine (ri va STIG meen)

Brand Names: U.S. Exelon®

Index Terms ENA 713; Rivastigmine Tartrate; SDZ ENA 713

Pharmacologic Category Acetylcholinesterase Inhibitor (Central)

Pregnancy Risk Factor B

Lactation Excretion in breast milk unknown/use caution

Use Treatment of mild-to-moderate dementia associated with Alzheimer's disease or Parkinson's disease

Unlabeled Use Severe dementia associated with Alzheimer's disease; Lewy body dementia

Mechanism of Action/Effect A deficiency of cortical acetylcholine is thought to account for some of the symptoms of Alzheimer's disease and the dementia of Parkinson's disease; rivastigmine increases acetylcholine in the central nervous system through reversible inhibition of its hydrolysis by cholinesterase

Contraindications Hypersensitivity to rivastigmine, other carbamate derivatives (eg, neostigmine, pyridostigmine, physostigmine), or any component of the formulation

Warnings/Precautions Significant nausea, vomiting, anorexia, and weight loss are associated with use; occurs more frequently in women and during the titration phase. Nausea and/or vomiting may be severe, particularly at doses higher than recommended. Monitor weight during therapy. Therapy should be initiated at lowest dose and titrated; if treatment is interrupted for more than several days, reinstate at the lowest daily dose. Cholinesterase inhibitors may have vagotonic effects which may cause bradycardia and/or heart block with or without a history of cardiac disease. Alzheimer's treatment guidelines consider bradycardia to be a relative contraindication for use of centrally-active cholinesterase inhibitors. Post-market cases of overdose (including a few fatalities) have been reported in association with medication errors/improper use of rivastigmine transdermal patches. No more than 1 patch should be applied daily and existing patch must be removed prior to applying new patch.

Use caution in patients with a history of peptic ulcer disease or concurrent NSAID use. Use caution in patients undergoing anesthesia who will receive succinylcholine-type muscle relaxation, patients with sick-sinus syndrome, bradycardia or supraventricular conduction conditions, urinary obstruction, seizure disorders, or pulmonary conditions such as asthma or COPD. Use caution in patients with low body weight (<50 kg) due to increased risk of adverse reactions.

Drug Interactions

Avoid Concomitant Use There are no known interactions where it is recommended to avoid concomitant use.

Decreased Effect

Rivastigmine may decrease the levels/effects of: Anticholinergics; Neuromuscular-Blocking Agents (Nondepolarizing)

The levels/effects of Rivastigmine may be decreased by: Anticholinergics; Dipyridamole

Increased Effect/Toxicity

Rivastigmine may increase the levels/effects of: Antipsychotics; Beta-Blockers; Cholinergic Agonists; Succinylcholine

The levels/effects of Rivastigmine may be increased by: Corticosteroids (Systemic)

Nutritional/Ethanol Interactions

Smoking: Nicotine increases the clearance of rivastigmine by 23%.

Ethanol: Avoid ethanol (due to risk of sedation; may increase GI irritation).

Food: Food delays absorption by 90 minutes, lowers C_{max} by 30% and increases AUC by 30%.

Herb/Nutraceutical: Avoid ginkgo biloba (may increase cholinergic effects).

Adverse Reactions Note: Many concentration-related effects are reported at a lower frequency by transdermal route.

>10%:

Central nervous system: Dizziness (2% to 21%), headache (3% to 17%)

Gastrointestinal: Nausea (7% to 47%), vomiting (6% to 31%), diarrhea (5% to 19%), anorexia (3% to 17%), abdominal pain (1% to 13%)

1% to 10%:

Cardiovascular: Syncope (3%), hypertension (3%)

Central nervous system: Fatigue (2% to 9%), insomnia (1% to 9%), confusion (8%), depression (4% to 6%), anxiety (2% to 5%), malaise (5%), somnolence (4% to 5%), hallucinations (4%), aggressiveness (3%), parkinsonism symptoms worsening (2% to 3%), vertigo (≤2%)

Gastrointestinal: Dyspepsia (9%), constipation (5%), flatulence (4%), weight loss (3% to 8%), eructation (2%), dehydration (2%)

Genitourinary: Urinary tract infection (1% to 7%)

Neuromuscular & skeletal: Weakness (2% to 6%), tremor (1%; up to 10% in Parkinson's patients)

Respiratory: Rhinitis (4%)

Miscellaneous: Diaphoresis (4%), flu-like syndrome (3%)

Pharmacodynamics/Kinetics

Duration of Action Anticholinesterase activity (CSF): ~10 hours (6 mg oral dose)

Available Dosage Forms

Capsule, oral: 1.5 mg, 3 mg, 4.5 mg, 6 mg

Exelon®: 1.5 mg, 3 mg, 4.5 mg, 6 mg

Patch, transdermal:

Exelon®: 4.6 mg/24 hours (30s); 9.5 mg/24 hours (30s)

Solution, oral:

Exelon®: 2 mg/mL (120 mL)

General Dosage Range

Oral: *Adults:* Initial: 1.5 mg twice daily; Maintenance: 1.5-6 mg twice daily (maximum: 12 mg/day)

Transdermal patch: *Adults:* Initial: 4.6 mg/24 hours; Maintenance: 9.5 mg/24 hours (maximum dose: 9.5 mg/24 hours)

Administration

Oral Should be administered with meals (breakfast or dinner). Capsule should be swallowed whole. Liquid form is available for patients who cannot swallow capsules (can be swallowed directly from syringe or mixed with water, soda, or cold fruit juice). Stir well and drink within 4 hours of mixing.

Topical Transdermal patch: Apply transdermal patch to upper or lower back (alternatively, may apply to upper arm or chest). Avoid reapplication to same spot of skin for 14 days (may rotate sections of back, for example). Do not apply to red, irritated, or broken skin. Avoid areas of recent application of lotion or powder. After removal, fold patch to press adhesive surfaces together, and discard. Avoid eye contact; wash hands after handling patch. Replace patch every 24 hours. Avoid exposing the patch to external sources of heat (eg, sauna, excessive light) for prolonged periods of time. No more than 1 patch should be applied daily and existing patch must be removed prior to applying new patch.

Stability

Storage

Oral: Store at 15°C to 30°C (59°F to 86°F); do not freeze. Store solution in an upright position.

Transdermal patch: Store at 15°C to 30°C (59°F to 86°F). Patches should be kept in sealed pouch until use.

Nursing Actions

Physical Assessment Assess bladder and sphincter adequacy prior to treatment. Monitor weight and for cholinergic crisis: DUMBELS - **d**iarrhea, **u**rination, **m**iosis, **b**ronchospasm/bradycardia, **e**xcitability, **l**acrimation, and **s**alivation/excessive sweating prior to treatment and regularly throughout. Assess cognitive function at periodic intervals.

Patient Education This drug is not a cure for Alzheimer's disease, but it may reduce the symptoms. Swallow capsule whole with meals (do not crush or chew). Liquid can be swallowed directly from syringe or mixed with water, soda, or cold fruit juice; stir well and drink within 4 hours of mixing. Apply transdermal patch to skin free from redness or irritation. Rotate sites; do not apply to same site within 14 days. No more than 1 patch should be applied daily and existing patch must be removed prior to applying new patch. Avoid alcohol. May cause dizziness, drowsiness, or postural hypotension; vomiting or loss of appetite; diarrhea; constipation; or urinary frequency. Report persistent abdominal discomfort, diarrhea, or constipation; significantly increased salivation, sweating, tearing, or urination; chest pain or palpitations; acute headache; CNS changes (eg, excessive fatigue, agitation, insomnia, dizziness, confusion, aggressiveness, depression);

increased muscle, joint, or body pain; vision changes or blurred vision; shortness of breath, coughing, or wheezing; or skin rash.

Dietary Considerations Capsules should be taken with meals.

Rizatriptan (rye za TRIP tan)

Brand Names: U.S. Maxalt-MLT®; Maxalt®

Index Terms MK462

Pharmacologic Category Antimigraine Agent; Serotonin 5-$HT_{1B,\ 1D}$ Receptor Agonist

Pregnancy Risk Factor C

Lactation Excretion in breast milk unknown/use caution

Use Acute treatment of migraine with or without aura

Mechanism of Action/Effect Selective agonist for serotonin receptor in cranial arteries; causes vasoconstriction and relief of migraine

Contraindications Hypersensitivity to rizatriptan or any component of the formulation; documented ischemic heart disease or Prinzmetal's angina; uncontrolled hypertension; basilar or hemiplegic migraine; during or within 2 weeks of MAO inhibitors; during or within 24 hours of treatment with another 5-HT_1 agonist, or an ergot-containing or ergot-type medication (eg, methysergide, dihydroergotamine)

Warnings/Precautions Only indicated for treatment of acute migraine; if a patient does not respond to the first dose, the diagnosis of migraine should be reconsidered. Coronary artery vasospasm, transient ischemia, myocardial infarction, ventricular tachycardia/fibrillation, cardiac arrest, and death have been reported with 5-HT_1 agonist administration. Patients who experience sensations of chest pain/pressure/tightness or symptoms suggestive of angina following dosing should be evaluated for coronary artery disease or Prinzmetal's angina before receiving additional doses; if dosing is resumed and similar symptoms recur, monitor with ECG. Should not be given to patients who have risk factors for CAD (eg, hypertension, hypercholesterolemia, smoker, obesity, diabetes, strong family history of CAD, menopause, male >40 years of age) without adequate cardiac evaluation. Patients with suspected CAD should have cardiovascular evaluation to rule out CAD before considering use; if cardiovascular evaluation is "satisfactory," first dose should be given in the healthcare provider's office (consider ECG monitoring). Periodic evaluation of cardiovascular status should be done in all patients. Significant elevation in blood pressure, including hypertensive crisis, has also been reported on rare occasions in patients with and without a history of hypertension. Cerebral/subarachnoid hemorrhage, stroke, peripheral vascular ischemia, and colonic ischemia have been reported with 5-HT_1 agonist administration.

Use with caution in elderly or patients with hepatic or renal impairment (including dialysis patients). Symptoms of agitation, confusion, hallucinations, hyper-reflexia, myoclonus, shivering, and tachycardia may occur with concomitant proserotonergic drugs (eg, SSRIs/SNRIs or triptans) or agents which reduce rizatriptan's metabolism. Concurrent use of serotonin precursors (eg, tryptophan) is not recommended. If concomitant administration with SSRIs is warranted, monitor closely, especially at initiation and with dose increases. Maxalt-MLT® tablets contain phenylalanine.

Drug Interactions

Avoid Concomitant Use

Avoid concomitant use of Rizatriptan with any of the following: Ergot Derivatives; MAO Inhibitors

Decreased Effect There are no known significant interactions involving a decrease in effect.

Increased Effect/Toxicity

Rizatriptan may increase the levels/effects of: Ergot Derivatives; Metoclopramide; Serotonin Modulators

The levels/effects of Rizatriptan may be increased by: Antipsychotics; Ergot Derivatives; MAO Inhibitors; Propranolol

Nutritional/Ethanol Interactions Food: Food delays absorption.

Adverse Reactions

>10%:

Central nervous system: Fatigue (adults 7% to 30%, dose related; children >1%)

Gastrointestinal: Xerostomia (<5% to 13%)

1% to 10%:

Cardiovascular: Chest pain (<2% to 5%), flushing (>1%), palpitation (>1%), systolic/diastolic blood pressure increases (5-10 mm Hg)

Central nervous system: Dizziness (9%), somnolence (8%), headache (≤2%), euphoria (>1%), hypoesthesia (>1%), drowsiness

Dermatologic: Skin flushing

Endocrine & metabolic: Growth hormone increased (mild), hot flashes

Gastrointestinal: Nausea (3%), diarrhea (>1%), vomiting (>1%), abdominal pain

Neuromuscular & skeletal: Weakness (4% to 7%), paresthesia (3% to 4%); myalgia (3%); neck, throat, and jaw pain/tightness/pressure (≤2%), tremor (>1%)

Respiratory: Dyspnea (>1%)

Miscellaneous: Feeling of heaviness (<1% to 2%)

Pharmacodynamics/Kinetics

Onset of Action ~30 minutes

Duration of Action 14-16 hours

Available Dosage Forms

Tablet, oral:

Maxalt®: 5 mg, 10 mg

Tablet, orally disintegrating, oral:

Maxalt-MLT®: 5 mg, 10 mg

General Dosage Range Oral: *Adults:* 5-10 mg once, repeat if needed (maximum: 30 mg/day)

Stability

Storage Store in blister pack until administration.

Nursing Actions

Physical Assessment For use only with clear diagnosis of migraine. Presence of or risk for coronary disease should be assessed prior to beginning therapy. Monitor for hypertension, cardiac events, drowsiness, nausea/vomiting, chest pain, and palpitations. Teach patient proper use (treatment of acute migraine).

Patient Education This drug is to be used to reduce your migraine, not to prevent or reduce the number of attacks. For orally-disintegrating tablets (Maxalt-MLT®), do not open blister pack before using. Open with dry hands, place on tongue, and allow to dissolve (dissolved tablet will be swallowed with saliva). Do not crush, break, or chew. If first dose brings relief, second dose may be taken anytime after 2 hours if migraine returns. Do not take more than two doses without consulting prescriber. May cause dizziness, drowsiness, dry mouth, skin flushing or hot flashes, mild abdominal discomfort, nausea, or vomiting. Report immediately any chest pain, palpitations, or irregular heartbeat; severe dizziness, acute headache, stiff or painful neck or facial swelling; muscle weakness or pain; changes in mental acuity; blurred vision or eye pain; or excessive perspiration or urination.

Dietary Considerations Some products may contain phenylalanine.

Roflumilast (roe FLUE mi last)

Brand Names: U.S. Daliresp®

Pharmacologic Category Phosphodiesterase-4 Enzyme Inhibitor

Medication Guide Available Yes

Pregnancy Risk Factor C

Breast-Feeding Considerations Roflumilast and/or its metabolites are excreted into the breast milk of lactating rats. Excretion into human breast milk is likely. Avoid use while breast-feeding.

Use Adjunct to bronchodilator therapy in the maintenance treatment of severe chronic obstructive pulmonary disease (COPD) associated with chronic bronchitis

Mechanism of Action/Effect Roflumilast and its active metabolite selectively inhibit phosphodiesterase-4 (PDE4) leading to an accumulation of cyclic AMP (cAMP) within inflammatory and structural cells important in the development of COPD. Inflammation, pulmonary remodeling, and mucociliary malfunction are decreased.

Contraindications Moderate or severe hepatic impairment (Child-Pugh class B or C)

Canadian labeling: Additional contraindication (not in U.S. labeling): Hypersensitivity to roflumilast or any component of the formulation

Warnings/Precautions Not indicated for relieving acute bronchospasms or for use as monotherapy of COPD; use only as adjunctive therapy to bronchodilator therapy. Neuropsychiatric effects (eg, anxiety, depression) have been reported with use; rarely, suicidal behavior/ ideation and completed suicide were reported. Avoid use in patients with a history of depression with suicidal behavior/ideations; instruct patients/caregivers to report psychiatric symptoms and consider discontinuation of therapy in such patients. Systemic exposure may be increased in patients with mild hepatic impairment; use in moderate-to-severe impairment is contraindicated.

May cause weight loss and/or diarrhea (sometimes severe); weight loss usually observed within 6 months of initiating therapy and diarrhea within 4 weeks. Instruct patients to monitor weight regularly. Avoid initiation of therapy or discontinue therapy with unexplained/pronounced weight loss.

Drug Interactions

Avoid Concomitant Use

Avoid concomitant use of Roflumilast with any of the following: CYP3A4 Inducers (Strong); Rifampin

Decreased Effect

The levels/effects of Roflumilast may be decreased by: CYP3A4 Inducers (Strong); Cyproterone; Deferasirox; Herbs (CYP3A4 Inducers); Rifampin

Increased Effect/Toxicity

Roflumilast may increase the levels/effects of: Immunosuppressants

The levels/effects of Roflumilast may be increased by: Cimetidine; Ciprofloxacin; Conivaptan; FluvoxaMINE

Adverse Reactions

2% to 10%:

Central nervous system: Headache (4%), dizziness (2%), insomnia (2%)

Gastrointestinal: Diarrhea (10%), weight loss (8%; 7%: >10% loss), nausea (5%), appetite decreased (2%)

Neuromuscular & skeletal: Back pain (3%)

Miscellaneous: Influenza (3%)

Available Dosage Forms

Tablet, oral:

Daliresp®: 500 mcg

General Dosage Range Oral: *Adults:* 500 mcg once daily

Administration

Oral Administer without regard to meals.

Stability

Storage Store at 20°C to 25°C (68°F to 77°F), excursions permitted from 15°C to 30°C (59°F to 86°F).

Nursing Actions

Physical Assessment This drug reduces inflammation in the lungs, which helps to slow progression of COPD. It is not a bronchodilator and therefore is not to be used for treatment of acute bronchospasms. This drug can cause depression, thoughts of suicide, or mood swings. Instruct patient and family to be aware of behavior or mood changes. If patient has moderate-to-severe liver damage, roflumilast is not indicated. Monitor patient's weight, as rapid weight loss is a serious side effect.

Patient Education Instruct patient that this drug is to be used for long-term use; patient needs to carry their rescue inhaler for bronchospasms. Dizziness may be worsened with alcohol intake. Instruct patients that drug may cause depression or suicidal tendencies. Inform patient of symptoms to be aware of, such as difficulty sleeping, mood swings, depression, or weight loss. Call the prescriber if patient develops tremors, painful urination, chest tightness, or swelling around the face or mouth.

Dietary Considerations May be given with or without food.

Ropinirole (roe PIN i role)

Brand Names: U.S. Requip®; Requip® XL™

Index Terms Ropinirole Hydrochloride

Pharmacologic Category Anti-Parkinson's Agent, Dopamine Agonist

Medication Safety Issues

Sound-alike/look-alike issues:

Requip® may be confused with Reglan®

ROPINIRole may be confused with RisperDAL®, risperiDONE, ropivacaine

Pregnancy Risk Factor C

Lactation Excretion in breast milk unknown/not recommended

Breast-Feeding Considerations Ropinirole inhibits prolactin secretion in humans and may potentially inhibit lactation. It is not known if ropinirole is excreted into breast milk. Due to the potential for serious adverse reactions, a decision should be made whether to discontinue nursing or discontinue the drug, taking into account the importance of the drug to the mother.

Use Treatment of idiopathic Parkinson's disease; in patients with early Parkinson's disease who were not receiving concomitant levodopa therapy as well as in patients with advanced disease on concomitant levodopa; treatment of moderate-to-severe primary Restless Legs Syndrome (RLS)

Contraindications Hypersensitivity to ropinirole or any component of the formulation

Warnings/Precautions Syncope, sometimes associated with bradycardia, was observed in association with ropinirole in both early Parkinson's disease (without levodopa) patients and advanced Parkinson's disease (with levodopa) patients. Dopamine agonists appear to impair the systemic regulation of blood pressure resulting in postural hypotension, especially during dose escalation. Parkinson's disease patients appear to have an impaired capacity to respond to a postural challenge; use with caution in patients at risk of hypotension (ie, those receiving antihypertensive or antiarrhythmic drugs) or where transient hypotensive episodes would be poorly tolerated (cardiovascular disease or cerebrovascular disease). Parkinson's patients being treated with dopaminergic agonists ordinarily require careful monitoring for signs and symptoms of postural hypotension, especially during dose escalation, and should be informed of this risk.

May cause hallucinations (dose dependent); risk may be increased in the elderly. Use with caution in patients with pre-existing dyskinesia, hepatic or severe renal dysfunction (use in patients with severe renal impairment and who are not undergoing regular hemodialysis is not recommended in the Canadian labeling). Avoid use in patients with a major psychotic disorder; may exacerbate psychosis.

Patients treated with ropinirole have reported falling asleep while engaging in activities of daily living; this has been reported to occur without significant warning signs. Monitor for daytime somnolence or pre-existing sleep disorder; caution with concomitant sedating medication; discontinue if significant daytime sleepiness or episodes of falling asleep occur. Patients must be cautioned about performing tasks which require mental alertness (eg, operating machinery or driving). Use with caution in patients receiving other CNS depressants or psychoactive agents. Effects with other sedative drugs or ethanol may be potentiated.

Dopamine agonists have been associated with compulsive behaviors and/or loss of impulse control, which has manifested as pathological gambling, libido increases (hypersexuality), and/or binge eating. Causality has not been established, and controversy exists as to whether this phenomenon is related to the underlying disease, prior behaviors/addictions and/or drug therapy. Dose reduction or discontinuation of therapy has been reported to reverse these behaviors in some, but not all cases. Risk for melanoma development is increased in Parkinson's disease patients; drug causation or factors contributing to risk have not been established. Patients should be monitored closely and periodic skin examinations should be performed.

Some patients treated for RLS may experience worsening of symptoms in the early morning hours (rebound) or an increase and/or spread of daytime symptoms (augmentation); clinical management of these phenomena has not been evaluated in controlled clinical trials. Pathologic degenerative changes were observed in the retinas of albino rats during studies with this agent, but were not observed in the retinas of albino mice or in other species. The significance of these data for humans remains uncertain.

Other dopaminergic agents have been associated with a syndrome resembling neuroleptic malignant syndrome on withdrawal or significant dosage reduction after long-term use. Risk of fibrotic complications (eg, pleural effusion/fibrosis, interstitial lung disease) and melanoma has been reported in patients receiving ropinirole; drug causation has not been established.

Drug Interactions

Avoid Concomitant Use There are no known interactions where it is recommended to avoid concomitant use.

Decreased Effect

ROPINIRole may decrease the levels/effects of: Antipsychotics (Typical)

The levels/effects of ROPINIRole may be decreased by: Antipsychotics (Atypical); CYP1A2 Inducers (Strong); Cyproterone; Metoclopramide; Tocilizumab

Increased Effect/Toxicity

The levels/effects of ROPINIRole may be increased by: Abiraterone Acetate; Antipsychotics (Typical); Ciprofloxacin; Ciprofloxacin (Systemic); Conivaptan; CYP1A2 Inhibitors (Moderate); CYP1A2 Inhibitors (Strong); Deferasirox; Estrogen Derivatives; MAO Inhibitors; Methylphenidate

Nutritional/Ethanol Interactions

Ethanol: Avoid ethanol (may increase CNS depression).

Herb/Nutraceutical: Avoid kava kava, gotu kola, valerian, St John's wort (may increase CNS depression).

Adverse Reactions

Data inclusive of trials in early Parkinson's disease (without levodopa) and Restless Legs Syndrome:

>10%:

Cardiovascular: Syncope (1% to 12%)

Central nervous system: Somnolence (11% to 40%), dizziness (6% to 40%), fatigue (8% to 11%)

Gastrointestinal: Nausea (immediate release: 40% to 60%; extended release: 19%), vomiting (11% to 12%)

Miscellaneous: Viral infection (11%)

1% to 10%:

Cardiovascular: Dependent/leg edema (2% to 7%), orthostasis (1% to 6%), hypertension (5%), chest pain (4%), flushing (3%), palpitation (3%), peripheral ischemia (2% to 3%), atrial fibrillation (2%), extrasystoles (2%), hypotension (2%), tachycardia (2%)

Central nervous system: Pain (3% to 8%), headache (extended release: 6%), confusion (5%), hallucinations (up to 5%; dose related), hypoesthesia (4%), amnesia (3%), malaise (3%), yawning (3%), concentration impaired (2%), vertigo (2%)

Dermatologic: Hyperhidrosis (3%)

Gastrointestinal: Dyspepsia (4% to 10%), abdominal pain (3% to 7%), constipation (≥5%), xerostomia (3% to 5%), diarrhea (5%), anorexia (4%), flatulence (3%)

Genitourinary: Urinary tract infection (5%), impotence (3%)

Hepatic: Alkaline phosphatase increased (3%)

Neuromuscular & skeletal: Weakness (6%), arthralgia (4%), muscle cramps (3%), paresthesia (3%), hyperkinesia (2%)

Ocular: Abnormal vision (6%), xerophthalmia (2%)

Respiratory: Pharyngitis (6% to 9%), rhinitis (4%), sinusitis (4%), bronchitis (3%), dyspnea (3%), influenza (3%), cough (3%), nasal congestion (2%)

Miscellaneous: Diaphoresis increased (3% to 6%)

Advanced Parkinson's disease (with levodopa):

>10%:

Central nervous system: Dizziness (immediate release: 26%; extended-release: 8%), somnolence (immediate release: 20%, extended release: 7%), headache (17%)

Gastrointestinal: Nausea (immediate release: 30%; extended-release: 11%)

Neuromuscular & skeletal: Dyskinesias (immediate release: 34%; extended-release: 13%; dose related)

1% to 10%:

Cardiovascular: Hypotension (2% to 5%; including orthostatic), peripheral edema (4%), syncope (3%), hypertension (3%; dose related)

Central nervous system: Hallucinations (7% to 10%; dose related), confusion (9%), anxiety (2% to 6%), amnesia (5%), nervousness (5%), pain (5%), vertigo (4%), abnormal dreaming (3%), paresis (3%), aggravated parkinsonism, insomnia

Gastrointestinal: Abdominal pain (6% to 9%), vomiting (7%), constipation (4% to 6%), diarrhea (3% to 5%), xerostomia (2% to 5%), dysphagia (2%), flatulence (2%), salivation increased (2%), weight loss (2%)

Genitourinary: Urinary tract infection (6%), pyuria (2%), urinary incontinence (2%)

Hematologic: Anemia (2%)

Neuromuscular & skeletal: Falls (2% to 10%; dose related), arthralgia (7%), tremor (6%), hypokinesia (5%), paresthesia (5%), arthritis (3%), back pain (3%)

Ocular: Diplopia (2%)

Respiratory: Upper respiratory tract infection (9%), dyspnea (3%)

Miscellaneous: Injury, diaphoresis increased (7%), viral infection, increased drug level (7%)

Other adverse effects (all phase 2/3 trials for Parkinson's disease and Restless Leg Syndrome): ≥1%: Asthma, BUN increased, depression, gastroenteritis, gastrointestinal reflux, irritability, migraine, muscle spasm, myalgia, neck pain, neuralgia, osteoarthritis, pharyngolaryngeal pain, rash, rigors, sleep disorder, tendonitis

Available Dosage Forms

Tablet, oral: 0.25 mg, 0.5 mg, 1 mg, 2 mg, 3 mg, 4 mg, 5 mg

Requip®: 0.25 mg, 0.5 mg, 1 mg, 2 mg, 3 mg, 4 mg, 5 mg

Tablet, extended release, oral:

Requip® XL™: 2 mg, 4 mg, 6 mg, 8 mg, 12 mg

General Dosage Range Oral: *Adults:*

Parkinson's:

Immediate release: Initial: 0.25 mg 3 times/day; Maintenance: 0.75-24 mg/day in 3 divided doses

Extended release: Initial: 2 mg once daily; Maintenance: 2-24 mg once daily (maximum: 24 mg/day)

Restless legs: Immediate release: Initial: 0.25 mg prior to bedtime; Maintenance: 0.25-4 mg prior to bedtime

Administration

Oral May be administered without regard to meals; taking with food may reduce nausea. Swallow extended-release tablet whole; do not crush, split, or chew.

Stability

Storage Store at controlled room temperature of 20°C to 25°C (68°F to 77°F). Protect from light.

Nursing Actions

Physical Assessment Monitor blood pressure periodically. Monitor for CNS depression/somnolence.

Patient Education Take without regard to food. Avoid alcohol. May cause dizziness; sudden, overwhelming sleepiness; postural hypotension; loss of impulse control (possibly manifested as pathological gambling, libido increases, and/or binge eating); nausea; vomiting; lack of appetite; or mouth sores. Report unusual and persistent sleepiness, chest pain or palpitations, CNS changes (confusion, hallucinations, amnesia, abnormal dreaming, insomnia), suicide ideation, skeletal weakness or increased random tremors or movements, gait changes or difficulty walking, signs of urinary tract or respiratory infection (pain or burning on urination, pus or blood in urine, or unusual cough and chest tightness), changes in the appearance of skin moles, or other unusual skin changes.

Dietary Considerations May be taken without regard to meals; taking with food may reduce nausea.

Rosiglitazone (roh si GLI ta zone)

Brand Names: U.S. Avandia®

Pharmacologic Category Antidiabetic Agent, Thiazolidinedione

Medication Safety Issues

Sound-alike/look-alike issues:

Avandia® may be confused with Avalide®, Coumadin®, Prandin®

International issues:

Avandia [U.S., Canada, and multiple international markets] may be confused with Avanza brand name for mirtazapine [Australia]

Medication Guide Available Yes

Pregnancy Risk Factor C

Lactation Excretion in breast milk unknown/not recommended

Breast-Feeding Considerations It is not known if rosiglitazone is excreted in breast milk. Breast-feeding is not recommended by the manufacturer.

Use Type 2 diabetes mellitus (noninsulin dependent, NIDDM):

Monotherapy: Improve glycemic control as an adjunct to diet and exercise

Note: Canadian labeling approves use as monotherapy only when metformin is contraindicated or not tolerated.

Combination therapy: **Note:** Use when diet, exercise, and a single agent do not result in adequate glycemic control.

U.S. labeling: In combination with a sulfonylurea, metformin, or sulfonylurea plus metformin

Canadian labeling: In combination with metformin; in combination with a sulfonylurea only when metformin use is contraindicated or not tolerated

Mechanism of Action/Effect Thiazolidinedione antidiabetic agent that lowers blood glucose by improving target cell response to insulin, without increasing pancreatic insulin secretion. It has a mechanism of action that is dependent on the presence of insulin for activity.

Contraindications NYHA Class III/IV heart failure (initiation of therapy)

Canadian labeling: Hypersensitivity to rosiglitazone or any component of the formulation; any stage of heart failure (eg, NYHA Class I, II, III, IV); serious hepatic impairment; pregnancy

Warnings/Precautions [U.S. Boxed Warning]: Thiazolidinediones, including rosiglitazone, may cause or exacerbate congestive heart failure; closely monitor for signs/symptoms of congestive heart failure (eg, rapid weight gain, dyspnea, edema), particularly after initiation or dose increases. Not recommended for use in any patient with symptomatic heart failure. In the U.S., initiation of therapy is contraindicated in patients with NYHA class III or IV heart failure; in Canada use is contraindicated in patients with any stage of heart failure (NYHA Class I, II, III, IV). Use with caution in patients with edema; may increase plasma volume and/or cause fluid retention, leading to heart failure. Dose-related weight gain observed with use; mechanism unknown but likely associated with fluid retention and fat accumulation. Use may also be associated with an increased risk of angina and MI. Use caution in patients at risk for cardiovascular events and monitor closely. Discontinue if any deterioration in cardiac status occurs.

[U.S. Boxed Warning]: Due to cardiovascular risks, rosiglitazone-containing medications are only available through the Avandia-Rosiglitazone Medicines Access Program™. Patients and prescribers must be registered with and meet conditions of the program. Call 1-800-282-6342 or visit www.avandia.com for more information.

Should not be used in diabetic ketoacidosis. Mechanism requires the presence of insulin; therefore, use in type 1 diabetes (insulin dependent, IDDM) is not recommended. Combination therapy with other hypoglycemic agents may increase risk for hypoglycemic events; dose reduction with the concomitant agent may be warranted. Concomitant use with nitrates is not recommended due to increased risk of myocardial ischemia. Avoid use with insulin due to an increased risk of edema, congestive heart failure, and myocardial ischemic events.

Use with caution in patients with elevated transaminases (AST or ALT); do not initiate in patients with active liver disease or ALT >2.5 times ULN at baseline; evaluate patients with ALT ≤2.5 times ULN at baseline or during therapy for cause of enzyme elevation; during therapy, if ALT >3 times ULN, reevaluate levels promptly and discontinue if elevation persists or if jaundice occurs at any time during use. Idiosyncratic hepatotoxicity has been reported with another thiazolidinedione agent (troglitazone); avoid use in patients who previously experienced jaundice during troglitazone therapy. Monitoring should include periodic determinations of liver function. Increased incidence of bone fractures in females treated with rosiglitazone observed during analysis of long-term trial; majority of fractures occurred in the upper arm, hand, and foot (differing from the hip or spine fractures usually associated with postmenopausal osteoporosis). May decrease hemoglobin/hematocrit and/or WBC count (slight); effects may be related to increased plasma volume and/or dose related; use with caution in patients with anemia.

Rosiglitazone has been associated with new onset and/or worsening of macular edema in patients with diabetes. Rosiglitazone should be used with caution in patients with a pre-existing macular edema or diabetic retinopathy. Discontinuation of rosiglitazone should be considered in any patient who reports visual deterioration. In addition, ophthalmological consultation should be initiated in these patients. Use with caution in premenopausal, anovulatory women; may result in resumption of ovulation, increasing the risk of pregnancy. Safety and efficacy in pediatric patients have not been established.

Additional Canadian warnings (not included in U.S. labeling): If glycemic control is inadequate, rosiglitazone may be added to metformin or a sulfonylurea (if metformin use is contraindicated or not tolerated); use of triple therapy (rosiglitazone in combination with both metformin and a sulfonylurea) is not indicated due to increased risks of heart failure and fluid retention.

Drug Interactions

Avoid Concomitant Use There are no known interactions where it is recommended to avoid concomitant use.

Decreased Effect

The levels/effects of Rosiglitazone may be decreased by: Bile Acid Sequestrants; Corticosteroids (Orally Inhaled); Corticosteroids (Systemic); CYP2C8 Inducers (Strong); Luteinizing Hormone-Releasing Hormone Analogs; Rifampin; Somatropin; Thiazide Diuretics

Increased Effect/Toxicity

Rosiglitazone may increase the levels/effects of: CYP2C8 Substrates; Hypoglycemic Agents

The levels/effects of Rosiglitazone may be increased by: CYP2C8 Inhibitors (Moderate); CYP2C8 Inhibitors (Strong); Deferasirox; Gemfibrozil; Herbs (Hypoglycemic Properties); Insulin; Pegvisomant; Pregabalin; Trimethoprim; Vasodilators (Organic Nitrates)

Nutritional/Ethanol Interactions

Ethanol: Avoid ethanol (may cause hypoglycemia).

Food: Peak concentrations are lower by 28% and delayed when administered with food, but these effects are not believed to be clinically significant.

Herb/Nutraceutical: Avoid alfalfa, aloe, bilberry, bitter melon, burdock, celery, damiana, fenugreek, garcinia, garlic, ginger, ginseng (American), gymnema, marshmallow, stinging nettle (may cause hypoglycemia).

Adverse Reactions Note: The rate of certain adverse reactions (eg, anemia, edema, hypoglycemia) may be higher with some combination therapies.

>10%: Endocrine & metabolic: HDL-cholesterol increased, LDL-cholesterol increased, total cholesterol increased, weight gain

1% to 10%:

Cardiovascular: Edema (5%), hypertension (4%); heart failure/CHF (up to 2% to 3% in patients receiving insulin; incidence likely higher in patients with pre-existing HF; myocardial ischemia (3%; incidence likely higher in patients with preexisting CAD)

Central nervous system: Headache (6%)

Endocrine & metabolic: Hypoglycemia (1% to 3%; combination therapy with insulin: 12% to 14%)

Gastrointestinal: Diarrhea (3%)
Hematologic: Anemia (2%)
Neuromuscular & skeletal: Fractures (up to 9%; incidence greater in females; usually upper arm, hand, or foot), arthralgia (5%), back pain (4% to 5%)
Respiratory: Upper respiratory tract infection (4% to 10%), nasopharyngitis (6%)
Miscellaneous: Injury (8%)

Pharmacodynamics/Kinetics

Onset of Action Delayed; Maximum effect: Up to 12 weeks

Available Dosage Forms

Tablet, oral:
Avandia®: 2 mg, 4 mg, 8 mg

General Dosage Range Oral: *Adults:* Initial: 4 mg/day in 1-2 divided doses; Maintenance: 4-8 mg/day in 1-2 divided doses

Administration

Oral May be administered without regard to meals.

Stability

Storage Store at 15°C to 30°C (59°F to 86°F). Protect from light.

Nursing Actions

Physical Assessment Monitor laboratory results closely. Assess for signs of fluid retention and heart failure. Monitor weight. Monitor response to therapy closely until response is stable. Advise women using oral contraceptives about need for alternative method of contraception. Teach risks of hyperglycemia, its symptoms, treatment, and predisposing conditions. Refer patient to a diabetic educator, if possible.

Patient Education May be taken without regard to meals. If dose is missed at the usual meal, take it with next meal. Do not double dose if daily dose is missed completely. Monitor serum glucose as recommended by prescriber. More frequent monitoring is required during periods of stress, trauma, surgery, pregnancy, increased activity, or exercise. Avoid alcohol. Report chest pain, rapid heartbeat or palpitations, abdominal pain, fever, rash, hypoglycemia reactions, yellowing of skin or eyes, dark urine or light stool, unusual fatigue, or nausea/vomiting. Report unusually rapid weight gain; swelling of ankles, legs, or abdomen; or weakness or shortness of breath.

Dietary Considerations Management of type 2 diabetes mellitus (noninsulin dependent, NIDDM) should include diet control. May be taken without regard to meals.

Rosiglitazone and Glimepiride

(roh si GLI ta zone & GLYE me pye ride)

Brand Names: U.S. Avandaryl®

Index Terms Glimepiride and Rosiglitazone Maleate

Pharmacologic Category Antidiabetic Agent, Sulfonylurea; Antidiabetic Agent, Thiazolidinedione

Medication Safety Issues

High alert medication:
The Institute for Safe Medication Practices (ISMP) includes this medication among its list of drugs which have a heightened risk of causing significant patient harm when used in error.

Medication Guide Available Yes

Pregnancy Risk Factor C

Lactation Excretion in breast milk unknown/not recommended

Use Management of type 2 diabetes mellitus (non-insulin dependent, NIDDM) as an adjunct to diet and exercise

Available Dosage Forms

Tablet:
Avandaryl®: 4 mg/1 mg: Rosiglitazone 4 mg and glimepiride 1 mg; 4 mg/2 mg: Rosiglitazone 4 mg and glimepiride 2 mg; 4 mg/4 mg: Rosiglitazone 4 mg and glimepiride 4 mg; 8 mg/2 mg: Rosiglitazone 8 mg and glimepiride 2 mg; 8 mg/4 mg: Rosiglitazone 8 mg and glimepiride 4 mg

General Dosage Range Dosage adjustment recommended in patients with hepatic or renal impairment

Oral:
Adults: Initial: Rosiglitazone 4 mg and glimepiride 1-2 mg once daily; Maintenance: Rosiglitazone 4-8 mg and glimepiride 1-4 mg once daily
Elderly: Initial: Rosiglitazone 4 mg and glimepiride 1 mg once daily

Administration

Oral Should be administered with the first meal of the day.

Nursing Actions

Physical Assessment See individual agents.

Patient Education See individual agents.

Related Information

Glimepiride *on page 542*
Rosiglitazone *on page 1015*

Rosiglitazone and Metformin

(roh si GLI ta zone & met FOR min)

Brand Names: U.S. Avandamet®

Index Terms Metformin and Rosiglitazone; Metformin Hydrochloride and Rosiglitazone Maleate; Rosiglitazone Maleate and Metformin Hydrochloride

Pharmacologic Category Antidiabetic Agent, Biguanide; Antidiabetic Agent, Thiazolidinedione

Medication Safety Issues

Sound-alike/look-alike issues:
Avandamet® may be confused with Anzemet®

Medication Guide Available Yes

Pregnancy Risk Factor C

Lactation
Rosiglitazone: Excretion in breast milk unknown/not recommended
Metformin: Enters breast milk/not recommended

Use Management of type 2 diabetes mellitus (non-insulin dependent, NIDDM) as an adjunct to diet and exercise in patients where dual rosiglitazone and metformin therapy is appropriate

Available Dosage Forms

Tablet:

Avandamet®: 2/500: Rosiglitazone 2 mg and metformin 500 mg; 4/500: Rosiglitazone 4 mg and metformin 500 mg; 2/1000: Rosiglitazone 2 mg and metformin 1000 mg; 4/1000: Rosiglitazone 4 mg and metformin 1000 mg

General Dosage Range Oral: *Adults:* Initial: Rosiglitazone 2 mg and metformin 500 mg once or twice daily; may increase by 2 mg/500 mg per day after 4 weeks (maximum: rosiglitazone 8 mg/day; metformin 2000 mg/day)

Administration

Oral Administer with meals. Patients who are NPO may need to have their dose held to avoid hypoglycemia.

Nursing Actions

Physical Assessment See individual agents.

Patient Education See individual agents.

Related Information

MetFORMIN *on page 746*

Rosiglitazone *on page 1015*

Rosuvastatin (roe soo va STAT in)

Brand Names: U.S. Crestor®

Index Terms Rosuvastatin Calcium

Pharmacologic Category Antilipemic Agent, HMG-CoA Reductase Inhibitor

Medication Safety Issues

Sound-alike/look-alike issues:

Rosuvastatin may be confused with atorvastatin, nystatin, pitavastatin

Pregnancy Risk Factor X

Lactation Excretion in breast milk unknown/contraindicated

Use

Treatment of dyslipidemias:

Used with dietary therapy for hyperlipidemias to reduce elevations in total cholesterol (TC), LDL-C, apolipoprotein B, nonHDL-C, and triglycerides (TG) in patients with primary hypercholesterolemia (elevations of 1 or more components are present in Fredrickson type IIa, IIb, and IV hyperlipidemias); increase HDL-C; treatment of primary dysbetalipoproteinemia (Fredrickson type III hyperlipidemia); treatment of homozygous familial hypercholesterolemia (FH); to slow progression of atherosclerosis as an adjunct to diet to lower TC and LDL-C

Heterozygous familial hypercholesterolemia (HeFH): In adolescent patients (10-17 years of age, females >1 year postmenarche) with HeFH having LDL-C >190 mg/dL or LDL >160 mg/dL with positive family history of premature cardiovascular disease (CVD), or ≥2 other CVD risk factors.

Primary prevention of cardiovascular disease: To reduce the risk of stroke, myocardial infarction, or arterial revascularization procedures in patients without clinically evident coronary heart disease or lipid abnormalities but with all of the following: 1) an increased risk of cardiovascular disease based on age ≥50 years old in men and ≥60 years old in women, 2) hsCRP ≥2 mg/L, and 3) the presence of at least one additional cardiovascular disease risk factor such as hypertension, low HDL-C, smoking, or a family history of premature coronary heart disease.

Secondary prevention of cardiovascular disease: To slow progression of atherosclerosis

Mechanism of Action/Effect Inhibitor of 3-hydroxy-3-methylglutaryl coenzyme A (HMG-CoA) reductase, the rate limiting enzyme in cholesterol synthesis (reduces the production of mevalonic acid from HMG-CoA); lowers TC, LDL-C, TG and improves HDL:LDL ratio

Contraindications Hypersensitivity to rosuvastatin or any component of the formulation; active liver disease; unexplained persistent elevations of serum transaminases (>3 times ULN); pregnancy; breast-feeding

Canadian labeling: Additional contraindications (not in U.S. labeling): Concomitant administration of cyclosporine; use of 40 mg dose in Asian patients, patients with predisposing risk factors for myopathy/rhabdomyolysis (eg, hereditary muscle disorders, history of myotoxicity with other HMG-CoA reductase inhibitors, concomitant use with fibrates or niacin, severe hepatic impairment, severe renal impairment [Cl_{cr} <30 mL/minute/1.73 m^2], hypothyroidism, alcohol abuse)

Warnings/Precautions Secondary causes of hyperlipidemia should be ruled out prior to therapy. Rosuvastatin has not been studied when the primary lipid abnormality is chylomicron elevation (Fredrickson types I and V). Liver enzyme tests should be obtained at baseline and as clinically indicated; routine periodic monitoring of liver enzymes is not necessary. Use with caution in patients who consume large amounts of ethanol or have a history of liver disease; use is contraindicated with active liver disease or unexplained transaminase elevations. Hematuria (microscopic) and proteinuria have been observed; more commonly reported in patients receiving rosuvastatin 40 mg daily, but typically transient and not associated with a decrease in renal function. Consider dosage reduction if unexplained hematuria and proteinuria persists. HMG-CoA reductase inhibitors may cause rhabdomyolysis with acute renal failure and/or myopathy. Discontinue in any patient in which CPK levels are markedly elevated (>10 times ULN) or if myopathy is suspected/diagnosed. This risk is dose-related and is increased with concurrent use of other lipid-lowering medications (fibric acid derivatives or niacin doses ≥1 g/day), other interacting drugs, drugs associated with myopathy (eg, colchicine), age ≥65 years, female gender, certain subgroups of Asian ancestry, uncontrolled hypothyroidism, and renal dysfunction. Dose reductions may be necessary.

The manufacturer recommends temporary discontinuation for elective major surgery, acute medical or surgical conditions, or in any patient experiencing an acute or serious condition predisposing to renal failure (eg, sepsis, hypotension, trauma, uncontrolled seizures). However, based upon current evidence, HMG-CoA reductase inhibitor therapy should be continued in the perioperative period unless risk outweighs cardioprotective benefit. Patients should be instructed to report unexplained muscle pain, tenderness, weakness, or brown urine; in Canada, concomitant use with cyclosporine or niacin is contraindicated, and rosuvastatin at a dose of 40 mg/day in Asian patients is contraindicated. Small increases in Hb A_{1c} (mean: ~0.1%) and fasting blood glucose have been reported with rosuvastatin; however, the benefits of statin therapy far outweigh the risk of dysglycemia.

Drug Interactions

Avoid Concomitant Use

Avoid concomitant use of Rosuvastatin with any of the following: Red Yeast Rice

Decreased Effect

Rosuvastatin may decrease the levels/effects of: Lanthanum

The levels/effects of Rosuvastatin may be decreased by: Antacids; Tocilizumab

Increased Effect/Toxicity

Rosuvastatin may increase the levels/effects of: DAPTOmycin; Trabectedin; Vitamin K Antagonists

The levels/effects of Rosuvastatin may be increased by: Amiodarone; Colchicine; Conivaptan; CycloSPORINE; CycloSPORINE (Systemic); Eltrombopag; Fenofibrate; Fenofibric Acid; Gemfibrozil; Niacin; Niacinamide; Protease Inhibitors; Red Yeast Rice

Nutritional/Ethanol Interactions

Ethanol: Avoid excessive ethanol consumption (due to potential hepatic effects).

Food: Red yeast rice contains an estimated 2.4 mg lovastatin per 600 mg rice.

Adverse Reactions

>10%: Neuromuscular & skeletal: Myalgia (3% to 13%)

2% to 10%:

Central nervous system: Headache (6%), dizziness (4%)

Gastrointestinal: Nausea (3%), abdominal pain (2%), constipation (2%)

Hepatic: ALT increased (2%; >3 times ULN)

Neuromuscular & skeletal: Arthralgia (4% to 10%), CPK increased (3%; >10 x ULN: Children 3%), weakness (3%)

Adverse reactions reported with other HMG-CoA reductase inhibitors (not necessarily reported with rosuvastatin therapy) include a hypersensitivity syndrome (symptoms may include anaphylaxis, angioedema, arthralgia, erythema multiforme, eosinophilia, hemolytic anemia, interstitial lung disease, lupus syndrome, photosensitivity, polymyalgia rheumatica, positive ANA, purpura, Stevens-Johnson syndrome, toxic epidermal necrolysis, urticaria, vasculitis)

Pharmacodynamics/Kinetics

Onset of Action Within 1 week; maximal at 4 weeks

Available Dosage Forms

Tablet, oral:

Crestor®: 5 mg, 10 mg, 20 mg, 40 mg

General Dosage Range Dosage adjustment recommended in patients with renal impairment, on concomitant therapy, or who develop toxicities

Oral:

Children 10-17 years (females >1 year postmenarche): Initial: 5-20 mg once daily (maximum: 20 mg/day)

Adults: Initial: 5-20 mg once daily; Maintenance: 5-40 mg once daily (maximum: 40 mg/day)

Administration

Oral May be administered with or without food. May be taken at any time of the day.

Stability

Storage Store between 20°C and 25°C (68°F to 77°F). Protect from moisture.

Nursing Actions

Physical Assessment Assess risk potential for interactions with other prescriptions or herbal products patient may be taking that may increase risk of myopathy or rhabdomyolysis. Assess cholesterol profile prior to treatment and at regular intervals. Assess LFT prior to initiating therapy and recheck when clinically indicated. Teach proper diet and exercise regimen.

Patient Education Take at same time each day, with or without food. Follow prescribed cholesterol-lowering diet and exercise regimen. You will have periodic blood tests to assess effectiveness. Avoid excessive alcohol. Report unusual muscle cramping or weakness, yellowing of skin or eyes, easy bruising or bleeding, or unusual fatigue.

Dietary Considerations May be taken with or without food. Red yeast rice contains an estimated 2.4 mg lovastatin per 600 mg rice.

Rotavirus Vaccine (ROE ta vye rus vak SEEN)

Brand Names: U.S. Rotarix®; RotaTeq®

Index Terms Human Rotavirus Vaccine, Attenuated (HRV); Pentavalent Human-Bovine

Reassortant Rotavirus Vaccine (PRV); Rotavirus Vaccine, Pentavalent; RV1 (Rotarix®); RV5 (RotaTeq®)

Pharmacologic Category Vaccine, Live (Viral)

Pregnancy Risk Factor C

Use Prevention of rotavirus gastroenteritis in infants and children

The Advisory Committee on Immunization Practices (ACIP) recommends routine vaccination of all infants.

Available Dosage Forms

Powder, for suspension, oral [preservative free; human derived]:

Rotarix®: G1P[8] ≥10^6 $CCID_{50}$ per 1 mL

Suspension, oral [preservative free]:

RotaTeq®: G1 ≥2.2 x 10^6 infectious units, G2 ≥2.8 x 10^6 infectious units, G3 ≥2.2 x 10^6 infectious units, G4 ≥2 x 10^6 infectious units, and P1A [8] ≥2.3 x 10^6 infectious units per 2 mL (2 mL)

General Dosage Range Oral:

Infants 6-24 weeks: Rotarix®: A total of two 1 mL doses administered at 2 and 4 months of age

Infants 6-32 weeks: RotaTeq®: A total of three 2 mL doses given at 2, 4, and 6 months of age

Administration

Oral

Rotarix®: Using oral applicator, administer contents into infant's inner cheek. Dispose of applicator and vaccine vial in biologic waste container.

RotaTeq®: Gently squeeze dose from ready-to-use dosing tube into infant's inner cheek. After use, dispose of the empty tube and cap in a biologic waste container.

Note: A single dose of the rotavirus vaccine should not be readministered to an infant who regurgitates, spits out, or vomits the vaccine during administration. Any remaining dose(s) should be administered on schedule (CDC, 2009).

Simultaneous administration of vaccines helps ensure the patients will be fully vaccinated by the appropriate age. Simultaneous administration of vaccines is defined as administering >1 vaccine on the same day at different anatomic sites. Separate vaccines should not be combined in the same syringe unless indicated by product specific labeling. The ACIP prefers each dose of a specific vaccine in a series come from the same manufacturer when possible. In general, preterm infants should be vaccinated at the same chronological age as full-term infants (CDC, 2011).

Antipyretics have not been shown to prevent febrile seizures. Antipyretics may be used to treat fever or discomfort following vaccination (CDC, 2011). One study reported that routine prophylactic administration of acetaminophen to prevent fever prior to vaccination decreased the immune response of some vaccines; the clinical significance of this reduction in immune response has not been established (Prymula, 2009).

Nursing Actions

Physical Assessment Have treatment for anaphylactoid or hypersensitivity reaction available. If latex sensitive, be advised that packaging may contain latex. Consider deferring administration in patients with moderate or severe acute illness (with or without fever); may administer to patients with mild acute illness (with or without fever). U.S. federal law requires entry into the patient's medical record.

Patient Education May experience fever, irritability, diarrhea, vomiting, and otitis media. Acetaminophen may be helpful. Notify prescriber if symptoms persist.

Related Information

Immunization Administration Recommendations *on page 1243*

Immunization Recommendations *on page 1248*

Rufinamide (roo FIN a mide)

Brand Names: U.S. Banzel®

Index Terms CGP 33101; E 2080; RUF 331; Xilep

Pharmacologic Category Anticonvulsant, Triazole Derivative

Medication Guide Available Yes

Pregnancy Risk Factor C

Lactation Excretion in breast milk unknown/not recommended

Use Adjunctive therapy in the treatment of generalized seizures of Lennox-Gastaut syndrome

Available Dosage Forms

Suspension, oral:

Banzel®: 40 mg/mL (460 mL)

Tablet, oral:

Banzel®: 200 mg, 400 mg

General Dosage Range Oral:

Children ≥4 years: Initial: 10 mg/kg/day in 2 equally divided doses (maximum: 45 mg/kg/day or 3200 mg/day)

Adults: Initial: 400-800 mg/day in 2 equally divided doses (maximum: 3200 mg/day)

Administration

Oral Administer with food. Tablets may be swallowed whole, split in half, or crushed. Oral suspension should be administered using the provided adapter and oral syringe; shake well before every administration.

Nursing Actions

Physical Assessment Monitor for signs and symptoms of suicide ideation (eg, anxiety, depression, unusual mood or behavior changes).

Patient Education Take with food. Avoid alcohol. You may experience drowsiness or dizziness. May cause headache, fatigue, nausea, or vomiting. Report suicide ideation, depression, rash (especially if accompanied by fever), problems with vision, tremors, or problems with gait.

Ruxolitinib (rux oh LI ti nib)

Brand Names: U.S. Jakafi™

Index Terms INCB 18424; INCB018424; Jakafi™; Ruxolitinib Phosphate

Pharmacologic Category Antineoplastic Agent, Janus Associated Kinase Inhibitor; Antineoplastic Agent, Tyrosine Kinase Inhibitor; Janus Associated Kinase Inhibitor

Medication Safety Issues

Sound-alike/look-alike issues:

Ruxolitinib may be confused with riTUXimab

Pregnancy Risk Factor C

Lactation Excretion in breast milk unknown/ not recommended

Use Treatment of intermediate or high-risk myelofibrosis, including primary myelofibrosis, post-polycythemia vera (post-PV) myelofibrosis and post-essential thrombocythemia (post-ET) myelofibrosis

Available Dosage Forms

Tablet, oral:

Jakafi™: 5 mg, 10 mg, 15 mg, 20 mg, 25 mg

General Dosage Range Dosage adjustment recommended in patients with hepatic impairment, renal impairment, on concomitant therapy, or who develop toxicities.

Oral: *Adults:* 15-20 mg twice daily; maximum dose: 25 mg twice daily

Administration

Oral May be administered orally with or without food. If a dose is missed, return to the usual dosing schedule and do **not** administer an additional dose.

If unable to ingest tablets, may administer through a nasogastric (NG) tube (≥8 Fr): Suspend tablet in ~40 mL water and stir for ~10 minutes and administer (within 6 hours after dispersion) with appropriate syringe; rinse NG tube with ~75 mL water (effect of enteral tube feeding on ruxolitinib exposure has not been evaluated)

Nursing Actions

Physical Assessment Assess for viral, fungal, or bacterial infections. Ongoing infections should be resolved prior to therapy. Instruct patient to report shortness of breath, painful skin rash, or blisters.

Patient Education Do not use if pregnant or breast-feeding. Instruct patient to avoid people with active infections or colds. Instruct patient to keep appointments for blood work. Common side effects include dizziness, headache, or weight gain. Patients need to report any signs of infection including fever, chills, cough, and shortness of breath; burning or blood with urination. Other serious side effects to report include skin rash or painful blisters.

Salmeterol (sal ME te role)

Brand Names: U.S. Serevent® Diskus®

Index Terms Salmeterol Xinafoate

Pharmacologic Category $Beta_2$ Agonist; $Beta_2$-Adrenergic Agonist, Long-Acting

Medication Safety Issues

Sound-alike/look-alike issues:

Salmeterol may be confused with Salbutamol, Solu-Medrol®

Serevent® may be confused with Atrovent®, Combivent®, sertraline, Sinemet®, Spiriva®, Zoloft®

Medication Guide Available Yes

Pregnancy Risk Factor C

Lactation Enters breast milk/use caution

Use Maintenance treatment of asthma and prevention of bronchospasm (as concomitant therapy) in patients with reversible obstructive airway disease, including patients with symptoms of nocturnal asthma; prevention of exercise-induced bronchospasm (monotherapy may be indicated in patients without persistent asthma); maintenance treatment of bronchospasm associated with COPD

Mechanism of Action/Effect Relaxes bronchial smooth muscle by selective action on $beta_2$-receptors with little effect on heart rate; salmeterol acts locally in the lung.

Contraindications Hypersensitivity to salmeterol or any component of the formulation (milk proteins); monotherapy in the treatment of asthma (ie, use without a concomitant long-term asthma control medication, such as an inhaled corticosteroid); status asthmaticus or other acute episodes of asthma or COPD

Warnings/Precautions

Asthma treatment: [U.S. Boxed Warning]: Long-acting $beta_2$-agonists (LABAs) increase the risk of asthma-related deaths. Salmeterol should only be used in asthma patients as adjuvant therapy in patients who are currently receiving but are not adequately controlled on a long-term asthma control medication (ie, an inhaled corticosteroid). Monotherapy with an LABA is contraindicated in the treatment of asthma. In a large, randomized, placebo-controlled U.S. clinical trial (SMART, 2006), salmeterol was associated with an increase in asthma-related deaths (when added to usual asthma therapy); risk is considered a class effect among all LABAs. Data are not available to determine if the addition of an inhaled corticosteroid lessens this increased risk of death associated with LABA use. Assess patients at regular intervals once asthma control is maintained on combination therapy to determine if step-down therapy is appropriate and the LABA can be discontinued (without loss of asthma control), and the patient can be maintained on an inhaled corticosteroid. LABAs are not appropriate in patients whose asthma is adequately controlled on low- or medium-dose inhaled corticosteroids. Do **not** use for acute bronchospasm. Short-acting $beta_2$-agonist (eg, albuterol) should be used for acute symptoms and symptoms occurring between treatments. Do **not** initiate in patients with significantly worsening or acutely deteriorating asthma; reports of severe (sometimes fatal) respiratory events have been reported when salmeterol has been initiated in this situation. Corticosteroids should not be stopped or reduced when salmeterol is initiated. During initiation, watch for signs of worsening asthma. Patients must be instructed to use short-acting beta$_2$-agonists (eg, albuterol) for acute asthmatic or COPD symptoms and to seek medical attention in cases where acute symptoms are not relieved or a previous level of response is diminished. The need to increase frequency of use of short-acting beta$_2$-agonist may indicate deterioration of asthma, and treatment must not be delayed. Because LABAs may disguise poorly controlled persistent asthma, frequent or chronic use of LABAs for exercise-induced bronchospasm is discouraged by the NIH Asthma Guidelines (NIH, 2007). Salmeterol should not be used more than twice daily; do not use with other long-acting beta$_2$-agonists. **[U.S. Boxed Warning]: LABAs may increase the risk of asthma-related hospitalization in pediatric and adolescent patients.** In general, a combination product containing a LABA and an inhaled corticosteroid is preferred in patients <18 years of age to ensure compliance.

COPD treatment: Appropriate use: Do **not** use for acute episodes of COPD. Do **not** initiate in patients with significantly worsening or acutely deteriorating COPD. Data are not available to determine if LABA use increases the risk of death in patients with COPD.

Concurrent diseases: Use caution in patients with cardiovascular disease (eg, arrhythmia, hypertension, or HF), seizure disorders, diabetes, hyperthyroidism, hepatic impairment, or hypokalemia. Beta-agonists may cause elevation in blood pressure, heart rate, CNS stimulation/excitation, increased risk of arrhythmia, increase serum glucose, or decrease serum potassium.

Adverse events: Immediate hypersensitivity reactions (urticaria, angioedema, rash, bronchospasm) have been reported. There have been reports of laryngeal spasm, irritation, swelling (stridor, choking) with use. Salmeterol should not be used more than twice daily; do not exceed recommended dose; do not use with other long-acting beta$_2$-agonists; serious adverse events have been associated with excessive use of inhaled sympathomimetics. Rarely, paradoxical bronchospasm may occur with use of inhaled bronchodilating agents; this should be distinguished from inadequate response. Use with strong CYP3A4 inhibitors (see Drug Interactions) is not recommended due to potential for an increased risk of cardiovascular events. Powder for oral inhalation contains lactose; very rare anaphylactic reactions have been reported in patients with severe milk protein allergy.

Drug Interactions

Avoid Concomitant Use

Avoid concomitant use of Salmeterol with any of the following: Beta-Blockers (Nonselective); CYP3A4 Inhibitors (Strong); Iobenguane I 123; Telaprevir

Decreased Effect

Salmeterol may decrease the levels/effects of: Iobenguane I 123

The levels/effects of Salmeterol may be decreased by: Alpha-/Beta-Blockers; Beta-Blockers (Beta1 Selective); Beta-Blockers (Nonselective); Betahistine; Tocilizumab

Increased Effect/Toxicity

Salmeterol may increase the levels/effects of: Loop Diuretics; Sympathomimetics; Thiazide Diuretics

The levels/effects of Salmeterol may be increased by: Atomoxetine; Cannabinoids; CYP3A4 Inhibitors (Moderate); CYP3A4 Inhibitors (Strong); Dasatinib; Ivacaftor; MAO Inhibitors; Telaprevir; Tricyclic Antidepressants

Adverse Reactions

>10%:

Central nervous system: Headache (13% to 17%)
Neuromuscular & skeletal: Pain (1% to 12%)

1% to 10%:

Cardiovascular: Hypertension (4%), edema (1% to 3%), pallor
Central nervous system: Dizziness (4%), sleep disturbance (1% to 3%), fever (1% to 3%), anxiety (1% to 3%), migraine (1% to 3%)
Dermatologic: Rash (1% to 4%), contact dermatitis (1% to 3%), eczema (1% to 3%), urticaria (3%), photodermatitis (1% to 2%)
Endocrine & metabolic: Hyperglycemia (1% to 3%)
Gastrointestinal: Throat irritation (7%), nausea (1% to 3%), dyspepsia (1% to 3%), dental pain (1% to 3%), gastrointestinal infection (1% to 3%), oropharyngeal candidiasis (1% to 3%), xerostomia (1% to 3%)
Hepatic: Liver enzymes increased
Neuromuscular & skeletal: Muscular cramps/spasm (3%), articular rheumatism (1% to 3%), arthralgia (1% to 3%), joint pain (1% to 3%), muscular stiffness (1% to 3%), paresthesia (1% to 3%), rigidity (1% to 3%)
Ocular: Keratitis/conjunctivitis (1% to 3%)
Respiratory: Nasal congestion (4% to 9%), tracheitis/bronchitis (7%), pharyngitis (≤6%), cough (5%), influenza (5%), viral respiratory tract infection (5%), sinusitis (4% to 5%), rhinitis (4% to 5%), asthma (3% to 4%)

Pharmacodynamics/Kinetics

Onset of Action Asthma: 30-48 minutes, COPD: 2 hours; Peak effect: Asthma: 3 hours, COPD: 2-5 hours

Duration of Action 12 hours

Available Dosage Forms

Powder, for oral inhalation:

Serevent® Diskus®: 50 mcg (28s, 60s)

General Dosage Range Inhalation: *Children ≥4 years and Adults:* 1 inhalation (50 mcg) twice daily

Administration

Inhalation Not to be used for the relief of acute attacks. Not for use with a spacer device. Administer with Diskus® in a level, horizontal position. Do not wash mouthpiece; Diskus® should be kept dry. Discard device 6 weeks after removal from foil pouch or when the dose counter reads "0" (whichever comes first).

Stability

Storage Inhalation powder (Serevent® Diskus®): Store at controlled room temperature 20°C to 25°C (68°F to 77°F) in a dry place away from direct heat or sunlight. Stable for 6 weeks after removal from foil pouch.

Nursing Actions

Physical Assessment Not for use to relieve acute asthmatic attacks. Monitor for increased use of short-acting beta$_2$-agonist inhalers; may be marker of a deteriorating asthma condition. For inpatient care, monitor vital signs and lung sounds prior to and periodically during therapy.

Patient Education This medication is not to be used as a rescue treatment for acute asthmatic symptoms. You may experience headache, nervousness, dizziness, fatigue, dry mouth, or stomach upset. Report immediately any swelling of face, tongue, or throat; rash; or difficulty swallowing or choking. Report unresolved GI upset; dizziness or fatigue; vision changes; chest pain, rapid heartbeat, or palpitations; insomnia; nervousness or hyperactivity; or muscle cramping or tremors.

Dietary Considerations Some products may contain lactose; very rare anaphylactic reactions have been reported in patients with severe milk protein allergy.

Saquinavir (sa KWIN a veer)

Brand Names: U.S. Invirase®

Index Terms Saquinavir Mesylate; SQV

Pharmacologic Category Antiretroviral Agent, Protease Inhibitor

Medication Safety Issues

Sound-alike/look-alike issues:

Saquinavir may be confused with SINEquan®

Medication Guide Available Yes

Pregnancy Risk Factor B

Lactation Excretion in breast milk unknown/contraindicated

Breast-Feeding Considerations Maternal or infant antiretroviral therapy does not completely eliminate the risk of postnatal HIV transmission. In addition, multiclass-resistant virus has been detected in breast-feeding infants despite maternal therapy. Therefore, in the United States, where formula is accessible, affordable, safe, and sustainable, and the risk of infant mortality due to diarrhea and respiratory infections is low, complete avoidance of breast-feeding by HIV-infected women is recommended to decrease potential transmission of HIV (DHHS [perinatal], 2011).

Use Treatment of HIV infection; used in combination with at least two other antiretroviral agents

Mechanism of Action/Effect Blocks the site of HIV-1 protease activity, resulting in the formation of immature, noninfectious viral particles.

Contraindications Hypersensitivity to saquinavir or any component of the formulation; congenital or acquired QT prolongation, refractory hypokalemia or hypomagnesemia, concomitant use of other medications that both increase saquinavir plasma concentrations and prolong the QT interval; complete AV block (without implanted ventricular pacemaker) or patients at high risk of complete AV block; severe hepatic impairment; coadministration of saquinavir/ritonavir with alfuzosin, amiodarone, bepridil, cisapride, dofetilide, ergot derivatives, flecainide, lidocaine (systemic), lovastatin, midazolam (oral), pimozide, propafenone, quinidine, rifampin, sildenafil (when used for pulmonary artery hypertension [eg, Revatio®]),simvastatin, trazodone, or triazolam

Warnings/Precautions Use caution in patients with hepatic insufficiency. May exacerbate preexisting hepatic dysfunction; use with caution in patients with hepatitis B or C and in cirrhosis. May be associated with fat redistribution (buffalo hump, increased abdominal girth, breast engorgement, facial atrophy). Use caution in hemophilia. May increase cholesterol and/or triglycerides. Changes in glucose tolerance, hyperglycemia, exacerbation of diabetes, DKA, and new-onset diabetes mellitus have been reported in patients receiving protease inhibitors.

Altered cardiac conduction: Saquinavir/ritonavir prolongs the QT interval, potentially leading to torsade de pointes, and prolongs the PR interval, potentially leading to heart block. An ECG should be performed for all patients prior to starting saquinavir/ritonavir therapy; do not initiate therapy in patients with a baseline QT interval >450 msec. If baseline QT interval <450 msec, may initiate therapy but a subsequent ECG is recommended after ~3-4 days of therapy. If subsequent QT interval is >480 msec or is prolonged over baseline by >20 msec, therapy should be discontinued. Patients who may be at increased risk for QT- or PR-interval prolongation include those with heart failure, bradyarrhythmias, hepatic impairment, electrolyte abnormalities, ischemic heart disease, cardiomyopathy, structural heart disease, or those with preexisting cardiac conduction abnormalities; ECG monitoring is recommended for these patients. ▶

Use with caution in patients taking strong CYP3A4 inhibitors, moderate or strong CYP3A4 inducers and major CYP3A4 substrates (see Drug Interactions); consider alternative agents that avoid or lessen the potential for CYP-mediated interactions. St John's wort, lovastatin, and simvastatin should not be used concurrently with saquinavir/ritonavir. A listing of medications that should not be used is available with each bottle and patients should be provided with this information. Do not coadminister colchicine in patient with renal or hepatic impairment; avoid concurrent use with salmeterol. Patients may develop immune reconstitution syndrome resulting in the occurrence of an inflammatory response to an indolent or residual opportunistic infection; further evaluation and treatment may be required. Invirase® may be used only if combined with ritonavir. Safety and efficacy have not been established in children ≤16 years of age.

Drug Interactions

Avoid Concomitant Use

Avoid concomitant use of Saquinavir with any of the following: Alfuzosin; Amiodarone; Artemether; Axitinib; Bepridil [Off Market]; Cisapride; Conivaptan; Crizotinib; Darunavir; Dofetilide; Dronedarone; Eplerenone; Ergot Derivatives; Everolimus; Flecainide; Fluticasone (Oral Inhalation); Halofantrine; Lapatinib; Lidocaine (Systemic); Lovastatin; Lumefantrine; Lurasidone; Midazolam; Nilotinib; Nisoldipine; Pimozide; Propafenone; QUEtiapine; QuiNIDine; QuiNINE; Ranolazine; Rifampin; Rivaroxaban; RomiDEPsin; Salmeterol; Silodosin; Simvastatin; St Johns Wort; Tamsulosin; Tetrabenazine; Thioridazine; Ticagrelor; Tolvaptan; Topotecan; Toremifene; TraZODone; Triazolam; Vandetanib; Vemurafenib; Ziprasidone

Decreased Effect

Saquinavir may decrease the levels/effects of: Abacavir; Boceprevir; Clarithromycin; Contraceptives (Estrogens); Darunavir; Delavirdine; Divalproex; Etravirine; Meperidine; Methadone; Prasugrel; Theophylline Derivatives; Ticagrelor; Valproic Acid; Zidovudine

The levels/effects of Saquinavir may be decreased by: Antacids; Boceprevir; CarBAMazepine; CYP3A4 Inducers (Strong); Deferasirox; Efavirenz; Garlic; Nevirapine; Peginterferon Alfa-2b; P-glycoprotein/ABCB1 Inducers; Rifampin; St Johns Wort; Tocilizumab

Increased Effect/Toxicity

Saquinavir may increase the levels/effects of: Alfuzosin; Almotriptan; Alosetron; ALPRAZolam; Amiodarone; Antifungal Agents (Azole Derivatives, Systemic); ARIPiprazole; Axitinib; Bepridil [Off Market]; Bortezomib; Brentuximab Vedotin; Brinzolamide; Budesonide (Nasal); Budesonide (Systemic, Oral Inhalation); Calcium Channel Blockers (Dihydropyridine); Calcium Channel Blockers (Nondihydropyridine); CarBAMazepine; Ciclesonide; Cisapride; Clarithromycin; Clorazepate; Colchicine; Conivaptan; Corticosteroids (Orally Inhaled); Crizotinib; CycloSPORINE; CycloSPORINE (Systemic); CYP3A4 Substrates; Dabigatran Etexilate; Diazepam; Dienogest; Digoxin; Dofetilide; Dronedarone; Dutasteride; Enfuvirtide; Eplerenone; Ergot Derivatives; Everolimus; FentaNYL; Fesoterodine; Flecainide; Flurazepam; Fluticasone (Nasal); Fluticasone (Oral Inhalation); Fusidic Acid; GuanFACINE; Halofantrine; HMG-CoA Reductase Inhibitors; Iloperidone; Ivacaftor; Ixabepilone; Lapatinib; Lidocaine (Systemic); Lovastatin; Lumefantrine; Lurasidone; Maraviroc; Meperidine; MethylPREDNISolone; Midazolam; Nefazodone; Nilotinib; Nisoldipine; Paricalcitol; Pazopanib; P-glycoprotein/ABCB1 Substrates; Pimecrolimus; Pimozide; Propafenone; Protease Inhibitors; Prucalopride; QTc-Prolonging Agents; QuiNIDine; QuiNINE; Ranolazine; Rifabutin; Rivaroxaban; RomiDEPsin; Ruxolitinib; Salmeterol; Saxagliptin; Sildenafil; Silodosin; Simvastatin; Sirolimus; SORAfenib; Tacrolimus; Tacrolimus (Systemic); Tacrolimus (Topical); Tadalafil; Tamsulosin; Temsirolimus; Tetrabenazine; Thioridazine; Ticagrelor; Tolterodine; Tolvaptan; Topotecan; Toremifene; TraZODone; Triazolam; Tricyclic Antidepressants; Vandetanib; Vardenafil; Vemurafenib; Vilazodone; Warfarin; Ziprasidone; Zuclopenthixol

The levels/effects of Saquinavir may be increased by: Alfuzosin; Antifungal Agents (Azole Derivatives, Systemic); Artemether; Bepridil [Off Market]; Chloroquine; Ciprofloxacin; Ciprofloxacin (Systemic); Clarithromycin; CycloSPORINE; CycloSPORINE (Systemic); Delavirdine; Efavirenz; Enfuvirtide; Etravirine; Fusidic Acid; Gadobutrol; H2-Antagonists; Indacaterol; Lumefantrine; Nilotinib; P-glycoprotein/ABCB1 Inhibitors; Proton Pump Inhibitors; QUEtiapine; QuiNINE; Rifampin

Nutritional/Ethanol Interactions

Food: A high-fat meal maximizes bioavailability. Saquinavir levels may increase if taken with grapefruit juice. Management: Administer within 2 hours of a full meal.

Herb/Nutraceutical: Saquinavir serum concentrations may be decreased by St John's wort and garlic capsules. Management: Avoid St John's wort. Avoid garlic supplementation; especially if saquinavir is the only protease inhibitor being used.

Adverse Reactions

Incidence data shown for saquinavir soft gel capsule formulation (no longer available) in combination with ritonavir.

10%: Gastrointestinal: Nausea (11%)

1% to 10%:

Cardiovascular: Chest pain

Central nervous system: Fatigue (6%), fever (3%), anxiety, depression, headache, insomnia, pain

Dermatologic: Pruritus (3%), rash (3%), dry lips/skin (2%), eczema (2%), verruca

Endocrine & metabolic: Lipodystrophy (5%), hyperglycemia (3%), hypoglycemia, hyperkalemia, libido disorder, serum amylase increased

Gastrointestinal: Diarrhea (8%), vomiting (7%), abdominal pain (6%), constipation (2%), abdominal discomfort, appetite decreased, buccal mucosa ulceration, dyspepsia, flatulence, taste alteration

Hepatic: AST increased, ALT increased, bilirubin increased

Neuromuscular & skeletal: Back pain (2%), CPK increased, paresthesia, weakness

Renal: Creatinine kinase increased

Respiratory: Pneumonia (5%), bronchitis (3%), sinusitis (3%)

Miscellaneous: Influenza (3%)

Incidence not currently defined (limited to significant reactions; reported for hard or soft gel capsule with/without ritonavir)

Cardiovascular: Cyanosis, heart valve disorder (including murmur), hyper-/hypotension, peripheral vasoconstriction, prolonged QT interval, prolonged PR interval, syncope, thrombophlebitis

Central nervous system: Agitation, amnesia, ataxia, confusion, hallucination, hyper-/hyporeflexia, myelopolyradiculoneuritis, neuropathies, poliomyelitis, progressive multifocal encephalopathy, psychosis, seizures, somnolence, speech disorder, suicide attempt

Dermatologic: Alopecia, bullous eruption, dermatitis, erythema, maculopapular rash, photosensitivity, Stevens-Johnson syndrome, skin ulceration, urticaria

Endocrine & metabolic: Dehydration, diabetes, electrolyte changes, TSH increased

Gastrointestinal: Ascites, colic, dysphagia, esophagitis, bloody stools, gastritis, intestinal obstruction, hemorrhage (rectal), pancreatitis, stomatitis

Genitourinary: impotence, prostate enlarged, hematuria, UTI

Hematologic; Acute myeloblastic leukemia, anemia (including hemolytic), leukopenia, neutropenia, pancytopenia, splenomegaly, thrombocytopenia

Hepatic: Alkaline phosphatase increased, GGT increased, hepatitis, hepatomegaly, hepatosplenomegaly, jaundice, liver disease exacerbation

Neuromuscular & skeletal: Arthritis, LDH increased

Ocular: Blepharitis, visual disturbance

Otic: Otitis, hearing decreased, tinnitus

Renal: Nephrolithiasis, renal calculus

Respiratory: Dyspnea, hemoptysis, pharyngitis, upper respiratory tract infection

Miscellaneous: Infections (bacterial, fungal, viral)

Available Dosage Forms

Capsule, oral:

Invirase®: 200 mg

Tablet, oral:

Invirase®: 500 mg

General Dosage Range Dosage adjustment recommended in patients on concomitant therapy

Oral: *Children >16 years and Adults*: 1000 mg twice daily

Administration

Oral Administer within 2 hours after a full meal. When used with ritonavir, saquinavir and ritonavir should be administered at the same time.

Stability

Storage Invirase®: Store at room temperature.

Nursing Actions

Physical Assessment Monitor for adherence to regimen. Monitor for gastrointestinal disturbance (nausea, vomiting, diarrhea) that can lead to dehydration and weight loss, hyperlipidemia and redistribution of body fat, rash, CNS effects (malaise, insomnia, abnormal thinking), and electrolyte imbalance at regular intervals during therapy. Teach patient proper timing of multiple medications. Instruct patient on glucose testing (protease inhibitors may cause hyperglycemia, exacerbation or new-onset diabetes).

Patient Education This is not a cure for HIV, nor has it been found to reduce transmission of HIV; use appropriate precautions to prevent spread to other persons. Maintain adequate hydration unless instructed to restrict fluid intake. Frequent blood tests may be required. You may be advised to check your glucose levels (this drug can cause exacerbation or new-onset diabetes). May cause body changes due to redistribution of body fat, facial atrophy, or breast enlargement (normal effects of drug). May cause dizziness, insomnia, abnormal thinking, nausea, vomiting, taste perversion, muscle weakness, headache, or insomnia. Inform prescriber if you experience muscle numbness or tingling; unresolved persistent vomiting, diarrhea, or abdominal pain; respiratory difficulty or chest pain; unusual skin rash; or change in color of stool or urine.

Dietary Considerations Take within 2 hours of a meal. Invirase® capsules contain lactose (not expected to induce symptoms of intolerance).

Sargramostim (sar GRAM oh stim)

Brand Names: U.S. Leukine®

Index Terms GM-CSF; Granulocyte-Macrophage Colony Stimulating Factor; NSC-613795; rhuGM-CSF

Pharmacologic Category Colony Stimulating Factor

Medication Safety Issues

Sound-alike/look-alike issues:

Leukine® may be confused with Leukeran®, leucovorin

Pregnancy Risk Factor C

Lactation Excretion in breast milk unknown/use caution

Use

Acute myelogenous leukemia (AML) following induction chemotherapy in older adults (≥55 years of age) to shorten time to neutrophil recovery and to reduce the incidence of severe and life-threatening infections and infections resulting in death

Bone marrow transplant (allogeneic or autologous) failure or engraftment delay

Myeloid reconstitution after allogeneic bone marrow transplantation

Myeloid reconstitution after autologous bone marrow transplantation: Non-Hodgkin's lymphoma (NHL), acute lymphoblastic leukemia (ALL), Hodgkin's lymphoma

Peripheral stem cell transplantation: Mobilization and myeloid reconstitution following autologous peripheral stem cell transplantation

Mechanism of Action/Effect Stimulates proliferation, differentiation and functional activity of neutrophils, eosinophils, monocytes, and macrophages.

Contraindications Hypersensitivity to sargramostim, yeast-derived products, or any component of the formulation; concurrent (24 hours preceding/following) myelosuppressive chemotherapy or radiation therapy; patients with excessive (≥10%) leukemic myeloid blasts in bone marrow or peripheral blood

Warnings/Precautions Simultaneous administration, or administration 24 hours preceding/following cytotoxic chemotherapy or radiotherapy is not recommended. Use with caution in patients with pre-existing cardiac problems or HF; supraventricular arrhythmias have been reported in patients with history of arrhythmias. Edema, capillary leak syndrome, pleural and/or pericardial effusion have been reported; use with caution in patients with pre-existing fluid retention; may worsen. Use with caution in patients with hepatic or renal impairment; monitor hepatic and/or renal function in patients with history of hepatic or renal dysfunction. Elevations in bilirubin, transaminases, and serum creatinine have been observed with use. Dyspnea may occur; monitor respiratory symptoms during and following infusion; use with caution in patients with hypoxia or pulmonary infiltrates.

With rapid increase in blood counts (ANC >20,000/mm^3, WBC >50,000/mm^3, or platelets >500,000/mm^3); decrease dose by 50% or discontinue drug (counts will fall to normal within 3-7 days after discontinuing drug). May potentially act as a growth factor for any tumor type, particularly myeloid malignancies; caution should be exercised when using in any malignancy with myeloid characteristics; tumors of nonhematopoietic origin may have surface receptors for sargramostim. Discontinue use if disease progression occurs during treatment.

There is a "first-dose effect" (refer to Adverse Reactions for details) which is seen (rarely) with the first dose of a cycle and does not usually occur with subsequent doses within that cycle. Anaphylaxis or other serious allergic reactions have been reported; discontinue immediately if occur. Solution contains benzyl alcohol; do not use in premature infants or neonates.

Drug Interactions

Avoid Concomitant Use There are no known interactions where it is recommended to avoid concomitant use.

Decreased Effect There are no known significant interactions involving a decrease in effect.

Increased Effect/Toxicity

Sargramostim may increase the levels/effects of: Bleomycin

Adverse Reactions

>10%:

Cardiovascular: Hypertension (34%), pericardial effusion (4% to 25%), edema (13% to 25%), chest pain (15%), peripheral edema (11%), tachycardia (11%)

Central nervous system: Fever (81%), malaise (57%), headache (26%), chills (25%), anxiety (11%), insomnia (11%)

Dermatologic: Rash (44%), pruritus (23%)

Endocrine & metabolic: Hyperglycemia (25%), hypercholesterolemia (17%), hypomagnesemia (15%)

Gastrointestinal: Diarrhea (≤89%), nausea (58% to 70%), vomiting (46% to 70%), abdominal pain (38%), weight loss (37%), anorexia (13%), hematemesis (13%), dysphagia (11%), gastrointestinal hemorrhage (11%)

Genitourinary: Urinary tract disorder (14%)

Hepatic: Hyperbilirubinemia (30%)

Neuromuscular & skeletal: Weakness (66%), bone pain (21%), arthralgia (11% to 21%) myalgia (18%)

Ocular: Eye hemorrhage (11%)

Renal: BUN increased (23%), serum creatinine increased (15%)

Respiratory: Pharyngitis (23%), epistaxis (17%), dyspnea (15%)

1% to 10%: Respiratory: Pleural effusion (1%)

Pharmacodynamics/Kinetics

Onset of Action Increase in WBC: 7-14 days

Duration of Action WBCs return to baseline within 1 week of discontinuing drug

Available Dosage Forms

Injection, powder for reconstitution:

Leukine®: 250 mcg

Injection, solution:

Leukine®: 500 mcg/mL (1 mL)

General Dosage Range

I.V.: *Children and Adults:* Infusion: 250 mcg/m^2/day (maximum: 500 mcg/m^2/day)

SubQ: *Children and Adults:* 250 mcg/m^2 once daily

Administration

I.V. Can premedicate with analgesics and antipyretics (eg, acetaminophen) to control adverse events (eg, fever, chills, myalgia, etc); control bone pain with non-narcotic analgesics I.V. infusion should be over 2-24 hours; incompatible with dextrose-containing solutions. An in-line membrane filter should **NOT** be used for intravenous administration.

I.V. Detail pH: 7.1-7.7

Other Administer by SubQ (undiluted). Do not shake solution. When administering GM-CSF subcutaneously, rotate injection sites.

Stability

Reconstitution

Powder for injection: May be reconstituted with preservative free SWFI or bacteriostatic water for injection (with benzyl alcohol 0.9%). Gently swirl to reconstitute; do not shake.

Sargramostim may also be further diluted in 25-50 mL NS to a concentration ≥10 mcg/mL for I.V. infusion administration.

If the final concentration of sargramostim is <10 mcg/mL, 1 mg of human albumin/1 mL of NS (eg, 1 mL of 5% human albumin/50 mL of NS) should be added.

Storage Store at 2°C to 8°C (36°F to 46°F); do not freeze. Do not shake.

Solution for injection: May be stored for up to 20 days at 2°C to 8°C (36°F to 46°F) once the vial has been entered. Discard remaining solution after 20 days.

Powder for injection: Preparations made with SWFI should be administered as soon as possible, and discarded within 6 hours of reconstitution. Preparations made with bacteriostatic water may be stored for up to 20 days at 2°C to 8°C (36°F to 46°F).

I.V. infusion administration: Preparations diluted with NS are stable for 48 hours at room temperature and refrigeration.

Nursing Actions

Physical Assessment Patient must be monitored closely during and following infusion for respiratory symptoms and "first-dose effect" (hypotension, tachycardia, flushing, and syncope with the first dose of a cycle). Monitor for respiratory symptoms, fluid balance (I and O), rash, hypotension, tachycardia, GI disturbance (diarrhea, stomatitis, mucositis), myalgia, and bone pain.

Patient Education This medication can only be administered by infusion or injection. Report immediately any redness, swelling, pain, or burning at infusion/injection site; difficulty breathing; or chest pain. You will require frequent blood tests during treatment. You may experience bone, joint, or muscle pain; nausea, vomiting, or loss of appetite; hair loss (reversible); diarrhea; headache; dizziness; or insomnia. At any time during treatment, report chest pain or palpitations, signs or symptoms of edema (eg, swollen extremities, difficulty breathing, rapid weight gain), onset of severe headache, acute back or chest pain, muscular tremors, or seizure activity.

Saxagliptin and Metformin

(sax a GLIP tin & met FOR min)

Brand Names: U.S. Kombiglyze™ XR

Index Terms Metformin and Saxagliptin; Metformin Hydrochloride and Saxagliptin; Saxagliptin and Metformin Hydrochloride

Pharmacologic Category Antidiabetic Agent, Biguanide; Antidiabetic Agent, Dipeptidyl Peptidase IV (DPP-IV) Inhibitor

Medication Safety Issues

Sound-alike/look-alike issues:

Saxagliptin and Metformin may be confused with sitaGLIPtin and Metformin

Medication Guide Available Yes

Pregnancy Risk Factor B

Lactation

Saxagliptin: Excretion in breast milk unknown/use caution

Metformin: Enters breast milk/not recommended

Use Management of type 2 diabetes mellitus (noninsulin dependent, NIDDM) as an adjunct to diet and exercise when treatment with both saxagliptin and metformin is appropriate

Available Dosage Forms

Tablet, variable release, oral:

Kombiglyze™ XR 2.5/1000: Saxagliptin 2.5 mg [immediate release] and metformin hydrochloride 1000 mg [extended release]; 5/500: Saxagliptin 5 mg [immediate release] and metformin hydrochloride 500 mg [extended release]; 5/1000: Saxagliptin 5 mg [immediate release] and metformin hydrochloride 1000 mg [extended release]

General Dosage Range Dosage adjustment recommended in patients on concomitant therapy

Oral: *Adults:* Saxagliptin 2.5-5 mg and metformin 500-2000 mg once daily (maximum: 5 mg/day [saxagliptin], 2000 mg/day [metformin])

Administration

Oral Administer once daily with the evening meal. Swallow whole; do not crush, cut, or chew tablets.

Nursing Actions

Physical Assessment See individual agents.

Patient Education See individual agents.

Scopolamine (Systemic) (skoe POL a mee)

Brand Names: U.S. Transderm Scōp®

Index Terms Hyoscine Butylbromide; Scopolamine Base; Scopolamine Butylbromide; Scopolamine Hydrobromide

Pharmacologic Category Anticholinergic Agent

Medication Safety Issues

Other safety concerns:

Transdermal patch may contain conducting metal (eg, aluminum); remove patch prior to MRI.

Pregnancy Risk Factor C

Lactation Enters breast milk/use caution (AAP rates "compatible"; AAP 2001 update pending)

Use

Scopolamine base: Transdermal: Prevention of nausea/vomiting associated with motion sickness and recovery from anesthesia and surgery

Scopolamine hydrobromide: Injection: Preoperative medication to produce amnesia, sedation, tranquilization, antiemetic effects, and decrease salivary and respiratory secretions

Scopolamine butylbromide [not available in the U.S.]: Oral/injection: Treatment of smooth muscle spasm of the genitourinary or gastrointestinal tract; injection may also be used prior to radiological/diagnostic procedures to prevent spasm

Unlabeled Use Scopolamine base: Transdermal: Breakthrough treatment of nausea and vomiting associated with chemotherapy

Available Dosage Forms

Injection, solution: 0.4 mg/mL (1 mL)

Patch, transdermal:

Transderm Scōp®: 1.5 mg (4s, 10s, 24s)

General Dosage Range

I.M., I.V., SubQ:

Children 6 months to 3 years: 0.1-0.15 mg

Children 3-6 years: 0.2-0.3 mg

Adults: 0.3-0.65 mg (single dose) **or** 0.6 mg 3-4 times/day

Transdermal: *Adults:* Apply 1 patch every 3 days as needed

Administration

Oral Tablet should be swallowed whole and taken with a full glass of water.

I.M. Butylbromide: Intramuscular injections should be administered 10-15 minutes prior to radiological/diagnostic procedures.

I.V.

Butylbromide: No dilution is necessary prior to injection; inject at a rate of 1 mL/minute

Hydrobromide: Dilute with an equal volume of sterile water and administer by direct I.V.; inject over 2-3 minutes

I.V. Detail Hydrobromide: pH: 3.5-6.5

Topical Transdermal: Apply to hairless area of skin behind the ear. Wash hands before and after applying the disc to avoid drug contact with eyes. Topical patch is programmed to deliver 1 mg over 3 days. Once applied, do not remove the patch for 3 full days (motion sickness). When used postoperatively for nausea/vomiting, the patch should be removed 24 hours after surgery. If patch becomes displaced, discard and apply a new patch.

Other Butylbromide or hydrobromide: May administer by subcutaneous injection.

Nursing Actions

Physical Assessment When used preoperatively, safety precautions should be observed and patient should be advised about blurred vision.

Patient Education May cause drowsiness, confusion, impaired judgment, vision changes, dry mouth, nausea, vomiting, orthostatic hypotension, constipation, increased sensitivity to heat and decreased perspiration, or decreased milk if breast-feeding. If dry mouth is experienced, have patients suck on hard or sugarless candy or ice chips. Report hot, dry, flushed skin; blurred vision or vision changes; difficulty swallowing; chest pain, palpitations, or rapid heartbeat; painful or difficult urination; increased confusion, depression, or loss of memory; rapid or difficult respirations; muscle weakness or tremors; or eye pain.

Transdermal: Apply patch behind ear the day before traveling. Wash hands before and after applying and avoid contact with the eyes. Do not remove for 3 days. Patch may contain metal; remove prior to MRI; can cause burns.

Selegiline (se LE ji leen)

Brand Names: U.S. Eldepryl®; Emsam®; Zelapar®

Index Terms Deprenyl; L-Deprenyl; Selegiline Hydrochloride

Pharmacologic Category Anti-Parkinson's Agent, MAO Type B Inhibitor; Antidepressant, Monoamine Oxidase Inhibitor

Medication Safety Issues

Sound-alike/look-alike issues:

Selegiline may be confused with Salagen®, sertraline, Serzone, Stelazine

Eldepryl® may be confused with Elavil®, enalapril

Zelapar® may be confused with zaleplon, Zemplar®, zolpidem, ZyPREXA® Zydis®

Medication Guide Available Yes

Pregnancy Risk Factor C

Lactation Excretion in breast milk unknown/use caution

Use Adjunct in the management of parkinsonian patients in which levodopa/carbidopa therapy is deteriorating (oral products); treatment of major depressive disorder (transdermal product)

Unlabeled Use Early Parkinson's disease; attention-deficit/hyperactivity disorder (ADHD)

Mechanism of Action/Effect At lower oral doses (capsule/tablet ≤10 mg/day; orally disintegrating tablet <2.5 mg/day), selegiline is a selective monoamine oxidase (MAO) type B inhibitor, which increases dopaminergic synaptic activity thus reducing symptoms of Parkinsonism. At higher oral doses or administered transdermally in recommended doses, selegiline nonselectively inhibits both MAO-B and MAO-A which blocks catabolism of other centrally-active biogenic amine neurotransmitters leading to improved mood

Contraindications Hypersensitivity to selegiline or any component of the formulation; concomitant use of meperidine

Orally disintegrating tablet: Additional contraindications: Concomitant use of dextromethorphan, methadone, propoxyphene, tramadol, oral selegiline, other MAO inhibitors

Transdermal: Additional contraindications: Pheochromocytoma; concomitant use of bupropion, selective or dual serotonin reuptake inhibitors (including SSRIs and SNRIs), tricyclic antidepressants, tramadol, propoxyphene, methadone, dextromethorphan, St. John's wort, mirtazapine, cyclobenzaprine, oral selegiline and other MAO inhibitors; carbamazepine, and oxcarbazepine; elective surgery requiring general anesthesia, local anesthesia containing sympathomimetic vasoconstrictors; sympathomimetics (and related compounds); foods high in tyramine content; supplements containing tyrosine, phenylalanine, tryptophan, or caffeine

Warnings/Precautions

Oral: MAO-B selective inhibition should not pose a problem with tyramine-containing products as long as the typical oral doses are employed, however, rare reactions have been reported. Increased risk of nonselective MAO inhibition occurs with oral capsule/tablet doses >10 mg/day or orally disintegrating tablet doses >2.5 mg/day. Use of oral selegiline with tricyclic antidepressants and SSRIs has also been associated with rare reactions and should generally be avoided. Addition to levodopa therapy may result in exacerbation of levodopa adverse effects, requiring a reduction in levodopa dosage. Dopaminergic agents used for Parkinson's disease or restless legs syndrome have been associated with compulsive behaviors and/or loss of impulse control, which has manifested as pathological gambling, libido increases (hypersexuality), and/or binge eating. Causality has not been established, and controversy exists as to whether this phenomenon is related to the underlying disease, prior behaviors/addictions and/or drug therapy. Dose reduction or discontinuation of therapy has been reported to reverse these behaviors in some, but not all cases. Use caution in patients with hepatic or renal impairment. Incidence of orthostatic hypotension may be increased in older adults and when titrating to the 2.5 mg dosage in patients taking the orally disintegrating tablet. Risk for melanoma development is increased in Parkinson's disease patients; drug causation or factors contributing to risk have not been established. Patients should be monitored closely and periodic skin examinations should be performed. Orally disintegrating tablet may cause oral mucosa edema, irritation, pain, ulceration and/or swallowing pain. Do not use orally disintegrating tablet concurrently with other selegiline products; wait at least 14 days from discontinuation before initiating treatment with another selegiline dosage form. Some products may contain phenylalanine.

Transdermal: Nonselective MAO inhibition occurs with transdermal delivery and is necessary for antidepressant efficacy. Hypertensive crisis as a result of ingesting tyramine-rich foods is always a concern with nonselective MAO inhibition. Although transdermal delivery minimizes inhibition of MAO-A in the gut, there is limited data with higher transdermal doses; dietary modifications are recommended with doses >6 mg/24 hours.

Transdermal patch: May cause orthostatic hypotension; use with caution in patients at risk of this effect or in those who would not tolerate transient hypotensive episodes (cerebrovascular disease, cardiovascular disease, hypovolemia, or concurrent medication use which may predispose to hypotension/bradycardia). Discontinue transdermal product at least 10 days prior to elective surgery. May contain conducting metal (eg, aluminum); remove patch prior to MRI. Avoid exposure of application site and surrounding area to direct external heat sources.

Transdermal: **[U.S. Boxed Warning]: Antidepressants increase the risk of suicidal thinking and behavior in children, adolescents, and young adults (18-24 years of age) with major depressive disorder (MDD) and other psychiatric disorders;** consider risk prior to prescribing. Short-term studies did not show an increased risk in patients >24 years of age and showed a decreased risk in patients ≥65 years. Closely monitor patients for worsening of depression, suicidality and/or associated behaviors, particularly during the initial 1-2 months of therapy or during periods of dosage adjustments (increases or decreases); the patient's family or caregiver should be instructed to closely observe the patient and communicate condition with healthcare provider. A medication guide concerning the use of antidepressants should be dispensed with each prescription. **Transdermal selegiline is not FDA approved for use in children <12 years of age.**

Transdermal: The possibility of a suicide attempt is inherit in major depression and may persist until remission occurs. Patients treated with antidepressants (for any indication) should be observed for clinical worsening and suicidality, especially during the initial few months of a course of drug therapy, or at times of dose changes, either increases or decreases. Use caution in high-risk patients. Worsening depression and severe abrupt suicidality that are not part of the presenting symptoms may require discontinuation or modification of drug therapy. Use caution in high-risk patients during initiation of therapy. The patient's family or caregiver should be alerted to monitor patients for the emergence of suicidality and associated behaviors ▶

(such as agitation, irritability, hostility, and hypomania) and call healthcare provider.

Transdermal selegiline may worsen psychosis in some patients or precipitate a shift to mania or hypomania in patients with bipolar disorder. Monotherapy in patients with bipolar disorder should be avoided. Patients presenting with depressive symptoms should be screened for bipolar disorder. **Selegiline is not FDA approved for the treatment of bipolar depression.**

Drug Interactions

Avoid Concomitant Use

Avoid concomitant use of Selegiline with any of the following: Alpha-/Beta-Agonists (Indirect-Acting); Alpha1-Agonists; Alpha2-Agonists (Ophthalmic); Amphetamines; Anilidopiperidine Opioids; Antidepressants (Serotonin Reuptake Inhibitor/Antagonist); Atomoxetine; Bezafibrate; Buprenorphine; BuPROPion; BusPIRone; CarBAMazepine; Cyclobenzaprine; Dexmethylphenidate; Dextromethorphan; Diethylpropion; HYDROmorphone; Linezolid; Maprotiline; Meperidine; Methyldopa; Methylene Blue; Methylphenidate; Mirtazapine; OXcarbazepine; Oxymorphone; Pizotifen; Selective Serotonin Reuptake Inhibitors; Serotonin 5-HT1D Receptor Agonists; Serotonin/Norepinephrine Reuptake Inhibitors; Tapentadol; Tetrabenazine; Tetrahydrozoline; Tetrahydrozoline (Nasal); Tricyclic Antidepressants; Tryptophan

Decreased Effect

Selegiline may decrease the levels/effects of: Ioflupane I 123

The levels/effects of Selegiline may be decreased by: CYP2B6 Inducers (Strong); Cyproterone; Peginterferon Alfa-2b; Tocilizumab

Increased Effect/Toxicity

Selegiline may increase the levels/effects of: Alpha-/Beta-Agonists (Direct-Acting); Alpha-/Beta-Agonists (Indirect-Acting); Alpha1-Agonists; Alpha2-Agonists (Ophthalmic); Amphetamines; Antidepressants (Serotonin Reuptake Inhibitor/Antagonist); Antihypertensives; Atomoxetine; Beta2-Agonists; Bezafibrate; BuPROPion; Dexmethylphenidate; Dextromethorphan; Diethylpropion; Doxapram; HYDROmorphone; Linezolid; Lithium; Meperidine; Methadone; Methyldopa; Methylene Blue; Methylphenidate; Metoclopramide; Mirtazapine; Orthostatic Hypotension Producing Agents; Pizotifen; Reserpine; Selective Serotonin Reuptake Inhibitors; Serotonin 5-HT1D Receptor Agonists; Serotonin Modulators; Serotonin/Norepinephrine Reuptake Inhibitors; Tetrahydrozoline; Tetrahydrozoline (Nasal); Tricyclic Antidepressants

The levels/effects of Selegiline may be increased by: Altretamine; Anilidopiperidine Opioids; Antipsychotics; Buprenorphine; BusPIRone; CarBAMazepine; COMT Inhibitors; Conivaptan; Contraceptives (Estrogens); Contraceptives (Progestins); Cyclobenzaprine; CYP2B6 Inhibitors (Moderate); CYP2B6 Inhibitors (Strong); Levodopa; MAO Inhibitors; Maprotiline; OXcarbazepine; Oxymorphone; Quazepam; Tapentadol; Tetrabenazine; TraMADol; Tryptophan

Nutritional/Ethanol Interactions

Ethanol: Ethanol may enhance the adverse/toxic effects of selegiline. Beverages containing tyramine (eg, hearty red wine and beer) may increase toxic effects. Management: Avoid ethanol and beverages containing tyramine.

Food: Concurrent ingestion of foods rich in tyramine, dopamine, tyrosine, phenylalanine, tryptophan, or caffeine may cause sudden and severe high blood pressure (hypertensive crisis or serotonin syndrome). Management: Avoid tyramine-containing foods (aged or matured cheese, air-dried or cured meats including sausages and salamis; fava or broad bean pods, tap/draft beers, Marmite concentrate, sauerkraut, soy sauce, and other soybean condiments). Food's freshness is also an important concern; improperly stored or spoiled food can create an environment in which tyramine concentrations may increase. Avoid foods containing dopamine, tyrosine, phenylalanine, tryptophan, or caffeine.

Herb/Nutraceutical: Kava kava, valerian, St John's wort, and SAMe may increase risk of serotonin syndrome and/or excessive sedation. Supplements containing caffeine, tyrosine, tryptophan, or phenylalanine may increase the risk of severe side effects like hypertensive reactions or serotonin syndrome. Management: Avoid kava kava, valerian, St John's wort, SAMe, and supplements containing caffeine, tyrosine, tryptophan, or phenylalanine.

Adverse Reactions Unless otherwise noted, the percentage of adverse events is reported for the transdermal patch (**Note:** ODT = orally disintegrating tablet, Oral = capsule/tablet)

>10%:

- Central nervous system: Headache (18%; ODT 7%; oral 4%), insomnia (12%; ODT 7%), dizziness (oral 14%; ODT 11%)
- Gastrointestinal: Nausea (oral 20%; ODT 11%)
- Local: Application site reaction (24%)

1% to 10%:

- Cardiovascular: Hypotension (including postural 3% to 10%), palpitation (oral 2%), chest pain (≥1%; ODT 2%), hypertension (≥1%; ODT 3%), peripheral edema (≥1%)
- Central nervous system: Pain (ODT 8%; oral 2%), hallucinations (oral 6%; ODT 4%), confusion (oral 6%; ODT 4%), vivid dreams (oral 4%), ataxia (ODT 3%), somnolence (ODT 3%), lethargy (oral 2%), agitation (≥1%), amnesia (≥1%), paresthesia (≥1%), thinking abnormal (≥1%), depression (<1%; ODT 2%)
- Dermatologic: Rash (4%), bruising (≥1%; ODT 2%), pruritus (≥1%), acne (≥1%)

Endocrine & metabolic: Weight loss (5%; oral 2%), hypokalemia (ODT 2%), sexual side effects (≤1%)

Gastrointestinal: Diarrhea (9%; ODT 2%; oral 2%), xerostomia (8%; oral 6%; ODT 4%), stomatitis (ODT 5%), abdominal pain (oral 8%), dyspepsia (4%; ODT 5%), dysphagia (ODT 2%), dental caries (ODT 2%), constipation (≥1%; ODT 4%), flatulence (≥1%; ODT 2%), anorexia (≥1%), gastroenteritis (≥1%), taste perversion (≥1%; ODT 2%), vomiting (≥1%; ODT 3%)

Genitourinary: Urinary retention (oral 2%), dysmenorrhea (≥1%), metrorrhagia (≥1%), UTI (≥1%), urinary frequency (≥1%)

Neuromuscular & skeletal: Dyskinesia (ODT 6%), back pain (ODT 5%; oral 2%), ataxia (<1%; ODT 3%), leg cramps (ODT 3%; oral 2%), myalgia (≥1%; ODT 3%), neck pain (≥1%), tremor (<1%; ODT 3%)

Otic: Tinnitus (≥1%)

Respiratory: Rhinitis (ODT 7%), pharyngitis (3%; ODT 4%), sinusitis (3%), cough (≥1%), bronchitis (≥1%), dyspnea (<1%; ODT 3%)

Miscellaneous: Diaphoresis (≥1%)

Pharmacodynamics/Kinetics

Onset of Action Therapeutic: Oral: Within 1 hour

Duration of Action Oral: 24-72 hours

Available Dosage Forms

Capsule, oral: 5 mg

Eldepryl®: 5 mg

Patch, transdermal:

Emsam®: 6 mg/24 hours (30s); 9 mg/24 hours (30s); 12 mg/24 hours (30s)

Tablet, oral: 5 mg

Tablet, orally disintegrating, oral:

Zelapar®: 1.25 mg

General Dosage Range

Oral:

Capsule/Tablet: *Adults:* 5 mg twice daily

Disintegrating tablet: *Adults:* Initial: 1.25 mg daily; Maintenance: 1.25-2.5 mg daily (maximum: 2.5 mg daily)

Transdermal:

Adults: Initial: 6 mg once daily; Maintenance: 6-12 mg once daily (maximum: 12 mg/day)

Elderly: 6 mg once daily

Administration

Oral Orally disintegrating tablet (Zelapar®): Take in morning before breakfast; place on top of tongue and allow to dissolve. Avoid food or liquid 5 minutes before and after administration.

Topical Transdermal (Emsam®): Apply to clean, dry, intact skin to the upper torso (below the neck and above the waist), upper thigh, or outer surface of the upper arm. Avoid exposure of application site to external heat source, which may increase the amount of drug absorbed. Apply at the same time each day and rotate application sites. Wash hands with soap and water after handling. Avoid touching the sticky side of the patch.

Stability

Storage

Capsule, tablet, transdermal: Store at 20°C to 25°C (68°F to 77°F). Store patch in sealed pouch and apply immediately after removal.

Orally disintegrating tablet: Store at controlled room temperature 25°C (77°F); excursions permitted to 15°C to 30°C (59°F to 86°F). Use within 3 months of opening pouch and immediately after opening individual blister.

Nursing Actions

Physical Assessment Monitor therapeutic response (eg, mental status, involuntary movements) at beginning of therapy and periodically throughout. Monitor blood pressure. Be alert to suicide ideation. Patient should be cautioned against eating foods high in tyramine. Discontinue transdermal product at least 10 days prior to elective surgery. Taper dose when discontinuing.

Patient Education May be prescribed in conjunction with levodopa/carbidopa. Therapeutic effects may take several weeks or months to achieve and you may need frequent monitoring during first weeks of therapy. Take oral capsule/tablet with meals if GI upset occurs. Do not take food or liquid for 5 minutes before or after administering orally disintegrating tablets. Do not swallow orally disintegrating tablet; allow to dissolve on tongue. Take at the same time each day. Avoid tyramine-containing foods (low potential for reaction) with oral products. Maintain adequate hydration unless instructed to restrict fluid intake. Do not use alcohol. You may experience drowsiness, dizziness, confusion, vision changes, orthostatic hypotension, constipation, runny nose or flu-like symptoms, nausea, vomiting, loss of appetite, or stomach discomfort. Report unresolved constipation or vomiting; chest pain, palpitations, irregular heartbeat; CNS changes (hallucination, loss of memory, seizures, acute headache, nervousness, suicide ideation); painful or difficult urination; stiff neck; increased muscle spasticity, rigidity, or involuntary movements; changes in the appearance of skin moles, skin rash, or other unusual skin changes; or significant worsening of condition.

Dietary Considerations Avoid or limit tyramine-containing foods/beverages (product and/or dose-dependent). Some examples include aged or matured cheese, air-dried or cured meats (including sausages and salamis), fava or broad bean pods, tap/draft beers, Marmite concentrate, sauerkraut, soy sauce and other soybean condiments. Food's freshness is also an important concern; improperly stored or spoiled food can create an environment where tyramine concentrations may increase.

Emsam® 9 mg/24 hours or 12 mg/24 hours: Avoid tyramine-rich foods or beverages beginning the first day of treatment or for 2 weeks after discontinuation or dose reduction to 6 mg/24 hours.
Zelapar®: Do not take with food or liquid.
Some products may contain phenylalanine.

Sertraline (SER tra leen)

Brand Names: U.S. Zoloft®

Index Terms Sertraline Hydrochloride

Pharmacologic Category Antidepressant, Selective Serotonin Reuptake Inhibitor

Medication Safety Issues

Sound-alike/look-alike issues:

Sertraline may be confused with selegiline, Serevent®, Soriatane®

Zoloft® may be confused with Zocor®

Medication Guide Available Yes

Pregnancy Risk Factor C

Lactation Enters breast milk/use caution (AAP rates "of concern"; AAP 2001 update pending)

Breast-Feeding Considerations Sertraline and desmethylsertraline are excreted in breast milk. Infants exposed to sertraline while breast-feeding generally receive a low relative dose and serum concentrations are not detectable in most infants. Adverse reactions have not been reported in nursing infants. Sertraline concentrations in the hindmilk are higher than in foremilk. If the benefits of the mother receiving the sertraline and breast-feeding outweigh the risks, the mother may consider pumping and discarding breast milk with the feeding 7-9 hours after the daily dose to decrease sertraline exposure to the infant. The long-term effects on development and behavior have not been studied. The manufacturer recommends that caution be exercised when administering sertraline to nursing women.

Use Treatment of major depression; obsessive-compulsive disorder (OCD); panic disorder; posttraumatic stress disorder (PTSD); premenstrual dysphoric disorder (PMDD); social anxiety disorder

Unlabeled Use Eating disorders; generalized anxiety disorder (GAD); impulse control disorders; treatment of mild dementia-associated agitation in nonpsychotic patients

Mechanism of Action/Effect Antidepressant with selective inhibitory effects on presynaptic serotonin (5-HT) reuptake and only very weak effects on norepinephrine and dopamine neuronal uptake

Contraindications Hypersensitivity to sertraline or any component of the formulation; use of MAO inhibitors within 14 days; concurrent use of pimozide; concurrent use of sertraline oral concentrate with disulfiram

Warnings/Precautions [U.S. Boxed Warning]: Antidepressants increase the risk of suicidal thinking and behavior in children, adolescents, and young adults (18-24 years of age) with major depressive disorder (MDD) and other psychiatric disorders; consider risk prior to prescribing. Short-term studies did not show an increased risk in patients >24 years of age and showed a decreased risk in patients ≥65 years. Closely monitor patients for clinical worsening, suicidality, or unusual changes in behavior, particularly during the initial 1-2 months of therapy or during periods of dosage adjustments (increases or decreases); the patient's family or caregiver should be instructed to closely observe the patient and communicate condition with healthcare provider. A medication guide concerning the use of antidepressants should be dispensed with each prescription. **Sertraline is not FDA approved for use in children with major depressive disorder (MDD). However, it is approved for the treatment of obsessive-compulsive disorder (OCD) in children ≥6 years of age.**

The possibility of a suicide attempt is inherent in major depression and may persist until remission occurs. Use caution in high-risk patients. Worsening depression and severe abrupt suicidality that are not part of the presenting symptoms may require discontinuation or modification of drug therapy. The patient's family or caregiver should be alerted to monitor patients for the emergence of suicidality and associated behaviors (such as agitation, irritability, hostility, impulsivity, and hypomania) and call healthcare provider.

May worsen psychosis in some patients or precipitate a shift to mania or hypomania in patients with bipolar disorder. Patients presenting with depressive symptoms should be screened for bipolar disorder. Monotherapy in patients with bipolar disorder should be avoided. **Sertraline is not FDA approved for the treatment of bipolar depression.**

Serotonin syndrome and neuroleptic malignant syndrome (NMS)-like reactions have occurred with serotonin/norepinephrine reuptake inhibitors (SNRIs) and selective serotonin reuptake inhibitors (SSRIs) when used alone, and particularly when used in combination with serotonergic agents (eg, triptans) or antidopaminergic agents (eg, antipsychotics). Concurrent use with MAO inhibitors is contraindicated. Has a very low potential to impair cognitive or motor performance. However, caution patients regarding activities requiring alertness until response to sertraline is known. Does not appear to potentiate the effects of alcohol, however, ethanol use is not advised.

Use caution in patients with a previous seizure disorder or condition predisposing to seizures such as brain damage, alcoholism, or concurrent therapy with other drugs which lower the seizure threshold. May increase the risks associated with electroconvulsive therapy. Use with caution in patients with hepatic or renal dysfunction and in elderly patients. May cause hyponatremia/SIADH (elderly at increased risk); volume depletion (diuretics may increase risk). Use with caution in patients with renal insufficiency or other concurrent illness (due to limited experience). Sertraline acts as a mild uricosuric; use with caution in patients at risk of uric acid nephropathy. Use caution with concomitant use of NSAIDs, ASA, or other drugs that affect coagulation; the risk of bleeding may be potentiated. Use with caution in patients where weight loss is undesirable. May cause or exacerbate sexual dysfunction.

Use oral concentrate formulation with caution in patients with latex sensitivity; dropper dispenser contains dry natural rubber. Monitor growth in pediatric patients. Discontinuation symptoms (eg, dysphoric mood, irritability, agitation, confusion, anxiety, insomnia, hypomania) may occur upon abrupt discontinuation. Taper dose when discontinuing therapy.

Drug Interactions

Avoid Concomitant Use

Avoid concomitant use of Sertraline with any of the following: Clopidogrel; Disulfiram; Iobenguane I 123; MAO Inhibitors; Methylene Blue; Pimozide; Tolvaptan; Tryptophan

Decreased Effect

Sertraline may decrease the levels/effects of: Clopidogrel; Iobenguane I 123; Ioflupane I 123

The levels/effects of Sertraline may be decreased by: CarBAMazepine; Cyproheptadine; Darunavir; Efavirenz; Fosphenytoin; NSAID (COX-2 Inhibitor); NSAID (Nonselective); Peginterferon Alfa-2b; Phenytoin; Tocilizumab

Increased Effect/Toxicity

Sertraline may increase the levels/effects of: Alpha-/Beta-Blockers; Anticoagulants; Antidepressants (Serotonin Reuptake Inhibitor/Antagonist); Antiplatelet Agents; Aspirin; Beta-Blockers; Budesonide (Systemic, Oral Inhalation); BusPIRone; CarBAMazepine; CloZAPine; Colchicine; Collagenase (Systemic); CYP2B6 Substrates; CYP2C19 Substrates; CYP2D6 Substrates; CYP3A4 Substrates; Desmopressin; Dextromethorphan; Drotrecogin Alfa (Activated); Eplerenone; Everolimus; Fesoterodine; Fosphenytoin; Galantamine; Halofantrine; Ibritumomab; Ivacaftor; Lithium; Methadone; Methylene Blue; Metoclopramide; NSAID (COX-2 Inhibitor); NSAID (Nonselective); Phenytoin; Pimecrolimus; Pimozide; Ranolazine; RisperiDONE; Rivaroxaban; Salicylates; Salmeterol; Saxagliptin; Serotonin Modulators; Tamoxifen; Thrombolytic Agents; Tolvaptan; Tositumomab and Iodine I 131 Tositumomab; TraMADol; Tricyclic Antidepressants; Vitamin K Antagonists

The levels/effects of Sertraline may be increased by: Abiraterone Acetate; Alcohol (Ethyl); Analgesics (Opioid); Antipsychotics; BusPIRone; Cimetidine; CNS Depressants; Conivaptan; CYP2D6 Inhibitors (Moderate); CYP2D6 Inhibitors (Strong); Dasatinib; Disulfiram; Glucosamine; Herbs (Anticoagulant/Antiplatelet Properties); Linezolid; Macrolide Antibiotics; MAO Inhibitors; Metoclopramide; Omega-3-Acid Ethyl Esters; Pentosan Polysulfate Sodium; Pentoxifylline; Prostacyclin Analogues; TraMADol; Tryptophan; Vitamin E

Nutritional/Ethanol Interactions

Ethanol: May increase CNS depression; monitor for increased effects with coadministration. Caution patients about effects.

Food: Sertraline average peak serum levels may be increased if taken with food.

Herb/Nutraceutical: Avoid valerian, St John's wort, kava kava, gotu kola (may increase CNS depression).

Adverse Reactions

>10%:

Central nervous system: Dizziness, fatigue, headache, insomnia, somnolence
Endocrine & metabolic: Libido decreased
Gastrointestinal: Anorexia, diarrhea, nausea, xerostomia
Genitourinary: Ejaculatory disturbances
Neuromuscular & skeletal: Tremors
Miscellaneous: Diaphoresis

1% to 10%:

Cardiovascular: Chest pain, palpitation
Central nervous system: Agitation, anxiety, hypoesthesia, malaise, nervousness, pain
Dermatologic: Rash
Endocrine & metabolic: Impotence
Gastrointestinal: Appetite increased, constipation, dyspepsia, flatulence, vomiting, weight gain
Neuromuscular & skeletal: Back pain, hypertonia, myalgia, paresthesia, weakness
Ocular: Visual difficulty, abnormal vision
Otic: Tinnitus
Respiratory: Rhinitis
Miscellaneous: Yawning

Additional adverse reactions reported in pediatric patients (frequency >2%): Aggressiveness, epistaxis, hyperkinesia, purpura, sinusitis, urinary incontinence

Pharmacodynamics/Kinetics

Onset of Action Depression: The onset of action is within a week, however, individual response varies greatly and full response may not be seen until 8-12 weeks after initiation of treatment.

Available Dosage Forms

Solution, oral: 20 mg/mL (60 mL)
Zoloft®: 20 mg/mL (60 mL)

Tablet, oral: 25 mg, 50 mg, 100 mg
Zoloft®: 25 mg, 50 mg, 100 mg

General Dosage Range Dosage adjustment recommended in patients with hepatic impairment

Oral:
Children 6-12 years: Initial: 25 mg once daily; Maintenance: 25-200 mg once daily (maximum: 200 mg/day)
Children 13-17 years: Initial: 50 mg once daily; Maintenance: 25-200 mg once daily (maximum: 200 mg/day)
Adults: Initial: 25-50 mg once daily; Maintenance: 50-200 mg once daily (maximum: 200 mg/day)
Elderly: Initial: 25 mg once daily in the morning; Maintenance: 50-100 mg once daily (maximum: 200 mg/day)

Administration

Oral Oral concentrate: Must be diluted before use. Immediately before administration, use the dropper provided to measure the required amount of concentrate; mix with 4 ounces (1/2 cup) of water, ginger ale, lemon/lime soda, lemonade, or orange juice **only**. Do not mix with any other liquids than these. The dose should be taken immediately after mixing; do not mix in advance. A slight haze may appear after mixing; this is normal. **Note:** Use with caution in patients with latex sensitivity; dropper dispenser contains dry natural rubber.

Stability

Storage Tablets and oral solution should be stored at controlled room temperature of 15°C to 30°C (59°F to 86°F).

Nursing Actions

Physical Assessment Assess mental status for worsening of depression, suicide ideation, anxiety, social functioning, mania, or panic attack (especially during initiation of therapy and when dosage is changed). Taper dosage slowly when discontinuing. Pediatric patients: Monitor growth pattern.

Patient Education It may take 2-3 weeks to achieve desired results. Take in the morning to reduce the incidence of insomnia. Avoid alcohol. Maintain adequate hydration unless instructed to restrict fluid intake. You may experience drowsiness, dizziness, lightheadedness, nausea, vomiting, anorexia, dry mouth, postural hypotension, urinary pattern changes, or male sexual dysfunction (reversible). Report persistent insomnia or daytime sedation, agitation, nervousness, fatigue; muscle cramping, tremors, or weakness; chest pain, palpitations, or swelling of extremities; vision changes; ringing in ears; skin rash or irritation; suicide ideation; or worsening of condition.

Sevelamer (se VEL a mer)

Brand Names: U.S. Renagel®; Renvela®

Index Terms Sevelamer Carbonate; Sevelamer Hydrochloride

Pharmacologic Category Phosphate Binder

Medication Safety Issues

Sound-alike/look-alike issues:
Renagel® may be confused with Reglan®, Regonol®, Renal Caps, Renvela®
Renvela® may be confused with Reglan®, Regonol®, Renagel®, Renal Caps
Sevelamer may be confused with Savella®

International issues:
Renagel [U.S., Canada, and multiple international markets] may be confused with Remegel brand name for aluminium hydroxide and magnesium carbonate [Netherlands] and for calcium carbonate [Hungary, Great Britain and Ireland] and with Remegel Wind Relief brand name for calcium carbonate and simethicone [Great Britain]

Pregnancy Risk Factor C

Lactation Excretion in breast milk unknown/use caution (not absorbed systemically but may alter maternal nutrition)

Use Reduction or control of serum phosphorous in patients with chronic kidney disease on hemodialysis

Available Dosage Forms

Powder for suspension, oral:
Renvela®: 0.8 g/packet (90s); 2.4 g/packet (90s)

Tablet, oral:
Renagel®: 400 mg, 800 mg
Renvela®: 800 mg

General Dosage Range Oral: *Adults:* Initial: 800-1600 mg 3 times/day; Maintenance: Up to 2400-14,000 mg/day in 3 divided doses

Administration

Oral Must be administered with meals.
Powder for oral suspension: Mix powder with water prior to administration. The 0.8 g packet should be mixed with 30 mL of water and the 2.4 g packet should be mixed with 60 mL of water (multiple packets may be mixed together using the appropriate amount of water). Stir vigorously to suspend mixture just prior to drinking; powder does not dissolve. Drink within 30 minutes of preparing and resuspend just prior to drinking.
Tablets: Swallow whole; do not crush, chew, or break

Nursing Actions

Physical Assessment Monitor blood pressure; may cause high blood pressure.

Patient Education Take with meals. Do not break or chew tablets. You may experience headache, dizziness, nausea, vomiting, heartburn, diarrhea, itching, or mild neuromuscular pain or stiffness.

Sildenafil (sil DEN a fil)

Brand Names: U.S. Revatio®; Viagra®

Index Terms Sildenafil Citrate; UK92480

Pharmacologic Category Phosphodiesterase-5 Enzyme Inhibitor

Medication Safety Issues

Sound-alike/look-alike issues:
Revatio® may be confused with ReVia®, Revonto™

Sildenafil may be confused with silodosin, tadalafil, vardenafil

Viagra® may be confused with Allegra®, Vaniqa®

Pregnancy Risk Factor B

Lactation Excretion in breast milk unknown/use caution

Use

Revatio®: Treatment of pulmonary arterial hypertension (PAH) (WHO Group I) to improve exercise ability and delay clinical worsening

Viagra®: Treatment of erectile dysfunction (ED)

Unlabeled Use PAH in children; pulmonary hypertension (WHO Group II, III, and IV); persistent pulmonary hypertension after recent left ventricular assist device placement

Mechanism of Action/Effect Sildenafil enhances the effect of nitric oxide by inhibiting phosphodiesterase type 5 (PDE-5), resulting in smooth muscle relaxation. In erectile dysfunction, smooth muscle relaxation results in the inflow of blood into the corpus cavernosum with sexual stimulation. In pulmonary hypertension, smooth muscle relaxation results in pulmonary vasculature; vasodilation reducing pulmonary pressure.

Contraindications Hypersensitivity to sildenafil or any component of the formulation; concurrent use (regularly/intermittently) of organic nitrates in any form (eg, nitroglycerin, isosorbide dinitrate); concurrent use with a protease inhibitor regimen when sildenafil used for pulmonary artery hypertension (eg, Revatio®)

Warnings/Precautions Decreases in blood pressure may occur due to vasodilator effects; use with caution in patients with left ventricular outflow obstruction (aortic stenosis or hypertrophic obstructive cardiomyopathy); may be more sensitive to hypotensive actions. Concurrent use with alpha-adrenergic antagonist therapy or substantial ethanol consumption may cause symptomatic hypotension; patients should be hemodynamically stable prior to initiating therapy at the lowest possible dose. Use with caution in patients with hypotension (<90/50 mm Hg); uncontrolled hypertension (>170/110 mm Hg); life-threatening arrhythmias, stroke or MI within the last 6 months; cardiac failure or coronary artery disease causing unstable angina; safety and efficacy have not been studied in these patients. There is a degree of cardiac risk associated with sexual activity; therefore, physicians should consider the cardiovascular status of their patients prior to initiating any treatment for erectile dysfunction. If pulmonary edema occurs when treating pulmonary arterial hypertension (PAH), consider the possibility of pulmonary veno-occlusive disease (PVOD); continued use is not recommended in patient with PVOD.

Sildenafil should be used with caution in patients with anatomical deformation of the penis (angulation, cavernosal fibrosis, or Peyronie's disease) and in patients who have conditions which may predispose them to priapism (sickle cell anemia, multiple myeloma, leukemia). All patients should be instructed to seek medical attention if erection persists >4 hours.

Vision loss may occur rarely and be a sign of nonarteritic anterior ischemic optic neuropathy (NAION). Risk may be increased with history of vision loss. Other risk factors for NAION include low cup-to-disc ratio ("crowded disc"), coronary artery disease, diabetes, hypertension, hyperlipidemia, smoking, and age >50 years. May cause dose-related impairment of color discrimination. Use caution in patients with retinitis pigmentosa; a minority have genetic disorders of retinal phosphodiesterases (no safety information available). Sudden decrease or loss of hearing has been reported rarely; hearing changes may be accompanied by tinnitus and dizziness. A direct relationship between therapy and vision or hearing loss has not been determined.

The potential underlying causes of erectile dysfunction should be evaluated prior to treatment. The safety and efficacy of sildenafil with other treatments for erectile dysfunction have not been established; use is not recommended. Efficacy with concurrent bosentan therapy has not been evaluated; use with caution. Use with caution in patients taking strong CYP3A4 inhibitors or alpha-blockers. Concomitant use with all forms of nitrates is contraindicated. If nitrate administration is medically necessary, it is not known when nitrates can be safely administered following the use of sildenafil (per manufacturer); the ACC/AHA 2007 guidelines supports administration of nitrates only if 24 hours have elapsed.

Avoid abrupt discontinuation, especially if used as monotherapy in PAH as exacerbation may occur. Use caution in patients with bleeding disorders or with active peptic ulcer disease; safety and efficacy have not been established. Efficacy has not be established for treatment of pulmonary hypertension associated with sickle cell disease. Use with caution in the elderly, or patients with renal or hepatic dysfunction; dose adjustment may be needed.

Drug Interactions

Avoid Concomitant Use

Avoid concomitant use of Sildenafil with any of the following: Amyl Nitrite; Boceprevir; Phosphodiesterase 5 Inhibitors; Pimozide; Telaprevir; Vasodilators (Organic Nitrates)

Decreased Effect

The levels/effects of Sildenafil may be decreased by: Bosentan; CYP3A4 Inducers (Strong); Cyproterone; Deferasirox; Etravirine; Herbs (CYP3A4 Inducers); Peginterferon Alfa-2b; Tocilizumab

Increased Effect/Toxicity

Sildenafil may increase the levels/effects of: Alpha1-Blockers; Amyl Nitrite; Antihypertensives; ARIPiprazole; Bosentan; HMG-CoA Reductase Inhibitors; Phosphodiesterase 5 Inhibitors; Pimozide; Vasodilators (Organic Nitrates)

The levels/effects of Sildenafil may be increased by: Antifungal Agents (Azole Derivatives, Systemic); Boceprevir; CYP3A4 Inhibitors (Moderate); CYP3A4 Inhibitors (Strong); Dasatinib; Erythromycin; Ivacaftor; Protease Inhibitors; Sapropterin; Telaprevir

Nutritional/Ethanol Interactions

Food: Amount and rate of absorption of sildenafil is reduced when taken with a high-fat meal. Serum concentrations/toxicity may be increased with grapefruit juice. Management: Avoid concurrent use of grapefruit juice.

Herb/Nutraceutical: St John's wort may decrease sildenafil levels. Management: Avoid St John's wort.

Adverse Reactions Based upon normal doses for either indication or route. (Adverse effects such as flushing, diarrhea, myalgia, and visual disturbances may be increased with doses >100 mg/24 hours.)

>10%:

Central nervous system: Headache (16% to 46%)

Gastrointestinal: Dyspepsia (7% to 17%; dose related)

2% to 10%:

Cardiovascular: Flushing (10%)

Central nervous system: Insomnia (≤7%), pyrexia (6%), dizziness (2%)

Dermatologic: Erythema (6%), rash (2%)

Gastrointestinal: Diarrhea (3% to 9%), gastritis (≤3%)

Genitourinary: Urinary tract infection (3%)

Hepatic: LFTs increased

Neuromuscular & skeletal: Myalgia (≤7%), paresthesia (≤3%)

Ocular: Abnormal vision (color changes, blurred vision, or increased sensitivity to light 3% to 11%; dose related)

Respiratory: Epistaxis (9% to 13%), dyspnea exacerbated (≤7%), nasal congestion (4%), rhinitis (4%), sinusitis (3%)

Pharmacodynamics/Kinetics

Onset of Action ~60 minutes

Duration of Action 2-4 hours

Available Dosage Forms

Injection, solution:

Revatio®: 0.8 mg/mL (12.5 mL)

Tablet, oral:

Revatio®: 20 mg

Viagra®: 25 mg, 50 mg, 100 mg

General Dosage Range Dosage adjustment recommended in patients with hepatic or renal impairment or on concomitant therapy

I.V.: *Adults:* Revatio®: 10 mg 3 times/day

Oral:

Adults: Revatio®: 20 mg 3 times/day; Viagra®: 25-100 mg once daily

Elderly: Viagra®: Initial: 25 mg

Administration

Oral

Revatio®: Administer tablets without regard to meals at least 4-6 hours apart.

Viagra®: Administer orally 30 minutes to 4 hours before sexual activity.

I.V. Revatio®: Administer injection as an I.V. bolus.

Stability

Storage Store at controlled room temperature of 25°C (77°F); excursions permitted to 15°C to 30°C (59°F to 86°F).

Nursing Actions

Patient Education Sildenafil provides no protection against sexually-transmitted diseases, including HIV. You may experience headache, flushing, or abnormal vision (color changes, blurred or increased sensitivity to light). Report immediately acute allergic reactions, chest pain or palpitations, persistent dizziness, signs of urinary tract infection, skin rash, respiratory difficulty, change in vision, change in hearing or ringing in the ears, or genital swelling. If erection lasts longer than 4 hours, contact prescriber immediately; permanent damage to the penis can occur. If taking for pulmonary arterial hypertension, do not discontinue abruptly.

Dietary Considerations Avoid grapefruit juice.

Silodosin (SI lo doe sin)

Brand Names: U.S. Rapaflo®

Index Terms KMD 3213

Pharmacologic Category Alpha$_1$ Blocker

Medication Safety Issues

Sound-alike/look-alike issues:

Rapaflo® may be confused with Rapamune®

Silodosin may be confused with sildenafil

Pregnancy Risk Factor B

Use Treatment of signs and symptoms of benign prostatic hyperplasia (BPH)

Mechanism of Action/Effect Selectively antagonizes alpha$_{1A}$-adrenoreceptors in the prostate (and bladder) which mediate the dynamic component of urine flow obstruction by regulating smooth muscle tone of the bladder neck and prostate. When given to patients with BPH, blockade of alpha-receptors leads to relaxation of these muscles, resulting in an improvement in urine flow rate and symptoms. Alpha-blockade does not influence the static component of urinary obstruction, which is related to tissue proliferation.

Contraindications Concurrent use with strong CYP3A4 inhibitors (eg, clarithromycin, itraconazole, ketoconazole, ritonavir); severe renal impairment (Cl_{cr} <30 mL/minute); severe hepatic impairment (Child-Pugh class C)

Warnings/Precautions Not intended for use as an antihypertensive drug. May cause significant orthostatic hypotension and syncope, especially with first dose; anticipate a similar effect if therapy is interrupted for a few days, if dosage is rapidly increased, or if another antihypertensive drug (particularly vasodilators) or a PDE-5 inhibitor (eg, sildenafil, tadalafil, vardenafil) is introduced. "First-dose" orthostatic hypotension may occur 4-8 hours after dosing; may be dose related. Patients should be cautioned about performing hazardous tasks when starting new therapy or adjusting dosage upward. Rule out prostatic carcinoma before beginning therapy with silodosin. Intraoperative floppy iris syndrome has been observed in cataract surgery patients who were on or were previously treated with $alpha_1$-blockers; causality has not been established and there appears to be no benefit in discontinuing alpha-blocker therapy prior to surgery. Use with caution in patients with mild-to-moderate hepatic impairment; contraindicated with severe impairment; not studied. Use with caution in patients with moderate renal impairment; dosage adjustment recommended. Contraindicated in patients with severe impairment (Cl_{cr} <30 mL/minute). Not indicated for use in women or children.

Drug Interactions

Avoid Concomitant Use

Avoid concomitant use of Silodosin with any of the following: Alpha1-Blockers; CYP3A4 Inhibitors (Strong); P-glycoprotein/ABCB1 Inhibitors

Decreased Effect

The levels/effects of Silodosin may be decreased by: CYP3A4 Inducers (Strong); Deferasirox; P-glycoprotein/ABCB1 Inducers; Tocilizumab

Increased Effect/Toxicity

Silodosin may increase the levels/effects of: Alpha1-Blockers; Calcium Channel Blockers

The levels/effects of Silodosin may be increased by: Beta-Blockers; CYP3A4 Inhibitors (Moderate); CYP3A4 Inhibitors (Strong); Dasatinib; MAO Inhibitors; P-glycoprotein/ABCB1 Inhibitors; Phosphodiesterase 5 Inhibitors

Nutritional/Ethanol Interactions

Food: AUC decrease by 4% to 49% and C_{max} decreased by ~18% to 43% with moderate calorie/fat meal. Management: Take once daily with a meal.

Herb/Nutraceutical: St John's wort may decrease the levels/effects of silodosin; other herbal medications may have hypotensive properties. There is limited data regarding use with saw palmetto. Management: Avoid St John's wort, black cohosh, California poppy, coleus, golden seal, hawthorn, mistletoe, periwinkle, quinine, and shepherd's purse. Avoid saw palmetto.

Adverse Reactions

>10%: Miscellaneous: Retrograde ejaculation (28%)

1% to 10%:

Cardiovascular: Orthostatic hypotension (3%)

Central nervous system: Dizziness (3%), headache (2%), insomnia (1% to 2%)

Gastrointestinal: Diarrhea (3%), abdominal pain (1% to 2%)

Genitourinary: PSA increased (1% to 2%)

Neuromuscular & skeletal: Weakness (1% to 2%)

Respiratory: Nasal congestion (2%), nasopharyngitis (2%), rhinorrhea (1% to 2%), sinusitis (1% to 2%)

Available Dosage Forms

Capsule, oral:

Rapaflo®: 4 mg, 8 mg

General Dosage Range Dosage adjustment recommended in patients with renal impairment

Oral: *Adults:* Males: 8 mg once daily

Administration

Oral Administer once daily with a meal.

Stability

Storage Store at room temperature of 25°C (77°F); excursions permitted to 15°C to 30°C (59°F to 86°F). Protect from light. Protect from moisture.

Nursing Actions

Physical Assessment Assess potential for interactions or toxicity with other antihypertensives or drugs that may increase hypotensive effect. Monitor symptomatic relief of BPH regularly. Monitor for orthostatic hypotension and syncope when beginning therapy, if therapy is interrupted, or if dose is increased (dose may need to be adjusted). When discontinuing, dose should be tapered and blood pressure monitored closely.

Patient Education Take at the same time each day with a meal. May cause postural hypotension, especially if taken with antihypertensive medications. May cause retrograde ejaculation (consult prescriber).

Dietary Considerations Take with a meal.

Simvastatin (sim va STAT in)

Brand Names: U.S. Zocor®

Pharmacologic Category Antilipemic Agent, HMG-CoA Reductase Inhibitor

Medication Safety Issues

Sound-alike/look-alike issues:

Simvastatin may be confused with atorvastatin, nystatin, pitavastatin

Zocor® may be confused with Cozaar®, Lipitor®, Zoloft®, ZyrTEC®

International issues:

Cardin [Poland] may be confused with Cardem brand name for celiprolol [Spain]; Cardene brand name for nicardipine [U.S., Great Britain, Netherlands]

Pregnancy Risk Factor X

Lactation Excretion in breast milk unknown/contraindicated

Breast-Feeding Considerations Excretion in breast milk is unknown, but would be expected; other medications in this class are excreted in human milk. Breast-feeding is contraindicated.

Use Used with dietary therapy for the following:

Secondary prevention of cardiovascular events in hypercholesterolemic patients with established coronary heart disease (CHD) or at high risk for CHD: To reduce cardiovascular morbidity (myocardial infarction, coronary/noncoronary revascularization procedures) and mortality; to reduce the risk of stroke

Hyperlipidemias: To reduce elevations in total cholesterol (total-C), LDL-C, apolipoprotein B, triglycerides, and VLDL-C, and to increase HDL-C in patients with primary hypercholesterolemia (elevations of 1 or more components are present in Fredrickson type IIa, IIb, III, and IV hyperlipidemias); treatment of homozygous familial hypercholesterolemia

Heterozygous familial hypercholesterolemia (HeFH): In adolescent patients (10-17 years of age, females >1 year postmenarche) with HeFH having LDL-C ≥190 mg/dL **or** LDL-C ≥160 mg/dL with positive family history of premature cardiovascular disease (CVD), or 2 or more CVD risk factors in the adolescent patient

Mechanism of Action/Effect Simvastatin is a derivative of lovastatin that acts by competitively inhibiting 3-hydroxy-3-methylglutaryl-coenzyme A (HMG-CoA) reductase, the enzyme that catalyzes the rate-limiting step in cholesterol biosynthesis; lowers total and LDL-cholesterol with increase in HDL

Contraindications Hypersensitivity to simvastatin or any component of the formulation; active liver disease; unexplained persistent elevations of serum transaminases; concomitant use of strong CYP3A4 inhibitors (eg, clarithromycin, erythromycin, itraconazole, ketoconazole, nefazodone, posaconazole, protease inhibitors [including boceprevir and telaprevir], telithromycin), cyclosporine, danazol, and gemfibrozil; pregnancy; breast-feeding

Warnings/Precautions Secondary causes of hyperlipidemia should be ruled out prior to therapy. Liver enzyme tests should be obtained at baseline and as clinically indicated; routine periodic monitoring of liver enzymes is not necessary. Use with caution in patients who consume large amounts of ethanol or have a history of liver disease; use is contraindicated with active liver disease and with unexplained transaminase elevations. Rhabdomyolysis with acute renal failure has occurred. Risk of rhabdomyolysis is dose-related and increased with high doses (80 mg), concurrent use of lipid-lowering agents which may also cause rhabdomyolysis (other fibrates or niacin doses ≥1 g/day), or moderate-to-strong CYP3A4 inhibitors (eg, amiodarone, grapefruit juice in large quantities, or verapamil), age ≥65 years, female gender, uncontrolled hypothyroidism, and renal dysfunction. In Chinese patients, do not use high-dose simvastatin (80 mg) if concurrently taking niacin ≥1 g/day; may increase risk of myopathy. Concomitant use of simvastatin with some drugs may require cautious use, may not be recommended, may require dosage adjustments, or may be contraindicated. If concurrent use of a contraindicated interacting medication is unavoidable, treatment with simvastatin should be suspended during use or consider the use of an alternative HMG-CoA reductase inhibitor void of CYP3A4 metabolism. Monitor closely if used with other drugs associated with myopathy (eg, colchicine). Increases in Hb A_{1c} and fasting blood glucose have been reported with HMG-CoA reductase inhibitors; however, the benefits of statin therapy far outweigh the risk of dysglycemia. The manufacturer recommends temporary discontinuation for elective major surgery, acute medical or surgical conditions, or in any patient experiencing an acute or serious condition predisposing to renal failure (eg, sepsis, hypotension, trauma, uncontrolled seizures). However, based upon current evidence, HMG-CoA reductase inhibitor therapy should be continued in the perioperative period unless risk outweighs cardioprotective benefit. Use with caution in patients with severe renal impairment; initial dosage adjustment is necessary; monitor closely.

Drug Interactions

Avoid Concomitant Use

Avoid concomitant use of Simvastatin with any of the following: Boceprevir; CYP3A4 Inhibitors (Strong); Erythromycin; Gemfibrozil; Protease Inhibitors; Red Yeast Rice; Telaprevir

Decreased Effect

Simvastatin may decrease the levels/effects of: Lanthanum

The levels/effects of Simvastatin may be decreased by: Antacids; Bosentan; CYP3A4 Inducers (Strong); Deferasirox; Efavirenz; Etravirine; Fosphenytoin; Phenytoin; Rifamycin Derivatives; St Johns Wort; Tocilizumab

Increased Effect/Toxicity

Simvastatin may increase the levels/effects of: ARIPiprazole; DAPTOmycin; Diltiazem; Trabectedin; Vitamin K Antagonists

The levels/effects of Simvastatin may be increased by: Amiodarone; AmLODIPine; Antifungal Agents (Azole Derivatives, Systemic); Boceprevir; Colchicine; CycloSPORINE; CycloSPORINE (Systemic); CYP3A4 Inhibitors (Moderate); CYP3A4 Inhibitors (Strong); Cyproterone; Danazol; Dasatinib; Diltiazem; Dronedarone; Eltrombopag; Erythromycin; Fenofibrate; Fenofibric Acid; Fluconazole; Fusidic Acid; Gemfibrozil; Grapefruit Juice; Green Tea; Imatinib;

Ivacaftor; Macrolide Antibiotics; Niacin; Niacinamide; Protease Inhibitors; QuiNINE; Ranolazine; Red Yeast Rice; Sildenafil; Telaprevir; Ticagrelor; Verapamil

Nutritional/Ethanol Interactions

Ethanol: Excessive ethanol consumption has the potential to cause hepatic effects. Management: Avoid or limit ethanol consumption.

Food: Simvastatin serum concentration may be increased when taken with grapefruit juice. Red yeast rice contains an estimated 2.4 mg lovastatin per 600 mg rice. Management: Avoid concurrent intake of large quantities of grapefruit juice (>1 quart/day).

Herb/Nutraceutical: St John's wort may decrease simvastatin levels. Management: Avoid St John's wort.

Adverse Reactions

1% to 10%:

Cardiovascular: Atrial fibrillation (6%; placebo 5%), edema (3%; placebo 2%)

Central nervous system: Headache (3% to 7%), vertigo (5%)

Dermatologic: Eczema (5%)

Gastrointestinal: Abdominal pain (7%), constipation (2% to 7%), gastritis (5%), nausea (5%)

Hepatic: Transaminases increased (>3 x ULN; 1%)

Neuromuscular & skeletal: CPK increased (>3 x normal; 5%), myalgia (4%)

Respiratory: Upper respiratory infections (9%), bronchitis (7%)

Additional class-related events or case reports (not necessarily reported with simvastatin therapy): Alteration in taste, anorexia, anxiety, bilirubin increased, cataracts, cholestatic jaundice, cirrhosis, decreased libido, depression, erectile dysfunction/impotence, facial paresis, fatty liver, fulminant hepatic necrosis, gynecomastia, hepatoma, hyperbilirubinemia, impaired extraocular muscle movement, increased CPK (>10 x normal), interstitial lung disease, ophthalmoplegia, peripheral nerve palsy, psychic disturbance, renal failure (secondary to rhabdomyolysis), thyroid dysfunction, tremor, vertigo

Pharmacodynamics/Kinetics

Onset of Action >3 days; Peak effect: 2 weeks

Available Dosage Forms

Tablet, oral: 5 mg, 10 mg, 20 mg, 40 mg, 80 mg

Zocor®: 5 mg, 10 mg, 20 mg, 40 mg, 80 mg

General Dosage Range Dosage adjustment recommended in patients with renal impairment or on concomitant therapy

Oral:

Children 10-17 years (females >1 year postmenarche): Initial: 10 mg once daily; Maintenance: 10-40 mg once daily (maximum: 40 mg/day)

Adults: Initial: 10-20 mg once daily; Maintenance: 5-40 mg once daily (maximum: 40 mg/day)

Administration

Oral May be administered without regard to meals. Administer in the evening for maximal efficacy.

Stability

Storage Tablets should be stored in tightly-closed containers at temperatures between 5°C to 30°C (41°F to 86°F).

Nursing Actions

Physical Assessment Assess risk potential for interactions with other prescriptions or herbal products patient may be taking that may increase risk of myopathy or rhabdomyolysis. Assess cholesterol profile prior to treatment and at regular intervals. Assess LFT prior to initiating therapy and recheck when clinically indicated. Teach proper diet and exercise regimen.

Patient Education Take at same time each day, in the evening, with or without food. Follow prescribed cholesterol-lowering diet and exercise regimen. Avoid excessive grapefruit juice (>1 quart/day) and alcohol. You will have periodic blood tests to assess effectiveness. Report unusual muscle cramping or weakness, yellowing of skin or eyes, easy bruising or bleeding, or unusual fatigue.

Dietary Considerations May be taken without regard to meals. Red yeast rice contains an estimated 2.4 mg lovastatin per 600 mg rice.

Sinecatechins (sin e KAT e kins)

Brand Names: U.S. Veregen™

Index Terms Catechins; Green Tea Extract; Kunecatechins; Polyphenols; Polyphenon E

Pharmacologic Category Immunomodulator, Topical; Topical Skin Product

Pregnancy Risk Factor C

Lactation Excretion in breast milk unknown/use caution

Use Treatment of external genital and perianal warts secondary to *Condylomata acuminata*

Available Dosage Forms

Ointment, topical:

Veregen™: 15% (15 g)

General Dosage Range Topical: *Adults:* Apply a thin layer (~0.5 cm strand) 3 times/day

Administration

Topical Wash hands before and after application; apply with fingers, leaving a thin layer of ointment; do not wash ointment off affected area after application. Discontinue treatment if the severity of local skin reactions becomes unacceptable. Do not apply internally; do not apply to open wounds; do not apply occlusive dressing. Sexual contact should be avoided while ointment is on skin. For females requiring tampon use during treatment, tampon should be inserted prior to application of ointment to prevent accidental application of ointment into the vagina. May stain clothing or bedding.

Nursing Actions

Patient Education Apply thin layer of medication; do not wash off. Wash your hands immediately after application. Avoid contact with eyes, nostrils, or mouth. Women using tampons should insert the tampon prior to application so as not to introduce the ointment into the vagina. Avoid exposure to sunlight. Do not apply to open wounds, vagina, or anal area. Avoid sexual contact. Genital warts are sexually transmitted; you may infect your partner. Wash off the ointment before use of a condom or diaphragm; ointment may weaken these forms of birth control. Avoid use of occlusive dressing. You may experience redness, swelling, or itching at the site of application. Report development of open sores or severe reactions.

Sirolimus (sir OH li mus)

Brand Names: U.S. Rapamune®

Index Terms Rapamycin

Pharmacologic Category Immunosuppressant Agent; mTOR Kinase Inhibitor

Medication Safety Issues

Sound-alike/look-alike issues:

Rapamune® may be confused with Rapaflo®

Sirolimus may be confused with everolimus, pimecrolimus, tacrolimus, temsirolimus

Medication Guide Available Yes

Pregnancy Risk Factor C

Lactation Excretion in breast milk unknown/not recommended

Breast-Feeding Considerations Due to the potential for adverse reactions in the breast-fed infant, including possible immunosuppression, breast-feeding is not recommended.

Use Prophylaxis of organ rejection in patients receiving renal transplants

Unlabeled Use Prophylaxis of organ rejection in heart transplant recipients; prevention acute graft-versus-host disease (GVHD) in allogeneic stem cell transplantation; treatment of refractory acute or chronic GVHD; treatment of soft tissue sarcoma (chordoma, angiomyolipoma, or lymphangioleiomyomatosis)

Mechanism of Action/Effect Sirolimus inhibits T-lymphocyte activation and proliferation in response to antigenic and cytokine stimulation and inhibits antibody production (mechanism differs from other immunosuppressants) to inhibit acute rejection of allografts and prolongs graft survival. Sirolimus binds to FKBP-12, an intracellular protein, to form an immunosuppressive complex which inhibits the regulatory kinase, mTOR (mammalian target of rapamycin), which suppresses cytokine mediated T-cell proliferation, halting progression from the G1 to the S phase of the cell cycle.

Contraindications Hypersensitivity to sirolimus or any component of the formulation

Warnings/Precautions Hazardous agent - use appropriate precautions for handling and disposal. **[U.S. Boxed Warning]: Immunosuppressive agents, including sirolimus, increase the risk of infection and may be associated with the development of lymphoma.** Immune suppression may also increase the risk of opportunistic infections (including activation of latent viral infections including BK virus-associated nephropathy), fatal infections, and sepsis. Prophylactic treatment for *Pneumocystis jirovecii* pneumonia (PCP) should be administered for 1 year post-transplant; prophylaxis for cytomegalovirus (CMV) should be taken for 3 months post-transplant in patients at risk for CMV. Progressive multifocal leukoencephalopathy (PML), an opportunistic CNS infection caused by reactivation of the JC virus, has been reported in patients receiving immunosuppressive therapy, including sirolimus. Clinical findings of PML include apathy, ataxia, cognitive deficiency, confusion, and hemiparesis; promptly evaluate any patient presenting with neurological changes; consider decreasing the degree of immunosuppression with consideration to the risk of organ rejection in transplant patients.

[U.S. Boxed Warning]: Sirolimus is not recommended for use in liver or lung transplantation. Bronchial anastomotic dehiscence cases have been reported in lung transplant patients when sirolimus was used as part of an immunosuppressive regimen; most of these reactions were fatal. Studies indicate an association with an increase risk of hepatic artery thrombosis (HAT), graft failure, and increased mortality (with evidence of infection) in liver transplant patients when sirolimus is used in combination with cyclosporine and/or tacrolimus. Most cases of HAT occurred within 30 days of transplant.

In renal transplant patients, *de novo* use without cyclosporine has been associated with higher rates of acute rejection. Sirolimus should be used in combination with cyclosporine (and corticosteroids) initially. Cyclosporine may be withdrawn in low-to-moderate immunologic risk patients after 2-4 months, in conjunction with an increase in sirolimus dosage. In high immunologic risk patients, use in combination with cyclosporine and corticosteroids is recommended for the first year. Safety and efficacy of combination therapy with cyclosporine in high immunologic risk patients has not been studied beyond 12 months of treatment; adjustment of immunosuppressive therapy beyond 12 months should be considered based on clinical judgement. Monitor renal function closely when combined with cyclosporine; consider dosage adjustment or discontinue in patients with increasing serum creatinine.

May increase serum creatinine and decrease GFR. Use caution when used concurrently with medications which may alter renal function. May delay recovery of renal function in patients with delayed allograft function. Increased urinary protein excretion has been observed when converting renal transplant patients from calcineurin inhibitors to sirolimus during maintenance therapy. A higher level of proteinuria prior to sirolimus conversion correlates with a higher degree of proteinuria after conversion. In some patients, proteinuria may reach nephrotic levels; nephrotic syndrome (new onset) has been reported. Increased risk of BK viral-associated nephropathy which may impair renal function and cause graft loss; consider decreasing immunosuppressive burden if evidence of deteriorating renal function.

Use caution with hepatic impairment; a reduction in the maintenance dose is recommended. Has been associated with an increased risk of fluid accumulation and lymphocele; peripheral edema, lymphedema, ascites, and pleural and pericardial effusions (including significant effusions and tamponade) were reported; use with caution in patients in whom fluid accumulation may be poorly tolerated, such as in cardiovascular disease (heart failure or hypertension) and pulmonary disease. Cases of interstitial lung disease (eg, pneumonitis, bronchiolitis obliterans organizing pneumonia [BOOP], pulmonary fibrosis) have been observed; risk may be increased with higher trough levels. Avoid concurrent use of strong CYP3A4 and/or P-glycoprotein (P-gp) inhibitors (eg, clarithromycin, erythromycin, telithromycin, itraconazole, ketoconazole, voriconazole) and strong inducers of CYP3A4 and/or P-gp (eg, rifampin, rifabutin). Concurrent use with a calcineurin inhibitor (cyclosporine, tacrolimus) may increase the risk of calcineurin inhibitor-induced hemolytic uremic syndrome/thrombotic thrombocytopenic purpura/thrombotic microangiopathy (HUS/TTP/TMA).

Hypersensitivity reactions, including anaphylactic/anaphylactoid reactions, angioedema, exfoliative dermatitis, and hypersensitivity vasculitis have been reported. Concurrent use with other drugs known to cause angioedema (eg, ACE inhibitors) may increase risk. Immunosuppressant therapy is associated with an increased risk of skin cancer; limit sun and ultraviolet light exposure; use appropriate sun protection. May increase serum lipids (cholesterol and triglycerides); use with caution in patients with hyperlipidemia. May be associated with wound dehiscence and impaired healing; use caution in the perioperative period. Patients with a body mass index (BMI) >30 kg/m^2 are at increased risk for abnormal wound healing.

Sirolimus tablets and oral solution are not bioequivalent, due to differences in absorption. Clinical equivalence was seen using 2 mg tablet and 2 mg solution. It is not known if higher doses are also clinically equivalent. Monitor sirolimus levels if changes in dosage forms are made. **[U.S. Boxed Warning]: Should only be used by physicians experienced in immunosuppressive therapy and management of transplant patients. Adequate laboratory and supportive medical resources must be readily available.** Sirolimus concentrations are dependent on the assay method (eg, chromatographic and immunoassay) used; assay methods are not interchangeable. Variations in methods to determine sirolimus whole blood concentrations, as well as interlaboratory variations, may result in improper dosage adjustments, which may lead to subtherapeutic or toxic levels. Determine the assay method used to assure consistency (or accommodations if changes occur), and for monitoring purposes, be aware of alterations to assay method or reference range. The manufacturer recommends high performance liquid chromatography (HPLC) as the reference standard to determine sirolimus trough concentrations.

Drug Interactions

Avoid Concomitant Use

Avoid concomitant use of Sirolimus with any of the following: BCG; CloZAPine; Conivaptan; Crizotinib; Natalizumab; Pimecrolimus; Pimozide; Posaconazole; Tacrolimus (Systemic); Tacrolimus (Topical); Vaccines (Live); Voriconazole

Decreased Effect

Sirolimus may decrease the levels/effects of: BCG; Coccidioidin Skin Test; Sipuleucel-T; Tacrolimus; Tacrolimus (Systemic); Vaccines (Inactivated); Vaccines (Live)

The levels/effects of Sirolimus may be decreased by: CYP3A4 Inducers (Strong); Deferasirox; Echinacea; Efavirenz; Fosphenytoin; P-glycoprotein/ABCB1 Inducers; Phenytoin; Rifampin; Tocilizumab

Increased Effect/Toxicity

Sirolimus may increase the levels/effects of: ACE Inhibitors; ARIPiprazole; CloZAPine; CycloSPORINE; CycloSPORINE (Systemic); Hypoglycemic Agents; Leflunomide; Natalizumab; Pimozide; Tacrolimus; Tacrolimus (Systemic); Tacrolimus (Topical); Vaccines (Live)

The levels/effects of Sirolimus may be increased by: Conivaptan; Crizotinib; CycloSPORINE; CycloSPORINE (Systemic); CYP3A4 Inhibitors (Moderate); CYP3A4 Inhibitors (Strong); Dasatinib; Denosumab; Fluconazole; Herbs (Hypoglycemic Properties); Itraconazole; Ketoconazole; Ketoconazole (Systemic); Macrolide Antibiotics; P-glycoprotein/ABCB1 Inhibitors; Pimecrolimus; Posaconazole; Protease Inhibitors; Roflumilast; Tacrolimus; Tacrolimus (Systemic); Tacrolimus (Topical); Telaprevir; Trastuzumab; Voriconazole

Nutritional/Ethanol Interactions

Food: Grapefruit juice may decrease clearance of sirolimus. Ingestion with high-fat meals decreases peak concentrations but increases AUC by 23% to 35%. Management: Avoid grapefruit juice. Take consistently (either with or without food) to minimize variability.

Herb/Nutraceutical: St John's wort may decrease sirolimus levels. Some herbal medications have immunostimulant properties (eg, echinacea). Herbs with hypoglycemic properties may increase the risk of sirolimus-induced hypoglycemia (eg, alfalfa). Management: Avoid St John's wort, cat's claw, and echinacea. Avoid alfalfa, aloe, bilberry, bitter melon, burdock, celery, damiana, fenugreek, garcinia, garlic, ginger, ginseng (American), gymnema, marshmallow, and stinging nettle.

Adverse Reactions Incidence of many adverse effects is dose related.

>20%:

Cardiovascular: Peripheral edema (54% to 58%), hypertension (45% to 49%), edema (18% to 20%)

Central nervous system: Headache (34%), pain (20% to 33%), insomnia (13% to 22%)

Dermatologic: Acne (22%)

Endocrine & metabolic: Hypertriglyceridemia (45% to 57%), hypercholesterolemia (43% to 46%)

Gastrointestinal: Constipation (36% to 38%), abdominal pain (29% to 36%), diarrhea (25% to 36%), nausea (25% to 31%)

Genitourinary: Urinary tract infection (26% to 33%)

Hematologic: Anemia (23% to 33%), thrombocytopenia (14% to 30%)

Neuromuscular & skeletal: Arthralgia (25% to 31%)

Renal: Serum creatinine increased (39% to 40%)

3% to 20%:

Cardiovascular: Atrial fibrillation, CHF, DVT, facial edema, hypervolemia, hypotension, palpitation, peripheral vascular disorder, postural hypotension, syncope, tachycardia, thrombosis, vasodilation

Central nervous system: Anxiety, chills, confusion, depression, dizziness, emotional lability, hypoesthesia, malaise, neuropathy, somnolence

Dermatologic: Rash (10% to 20%), skin carcinoma (up to 3%; includes basal cell carcinoma, squamous cell carcinoma, melanoma), cellulitis, dermal ulcer, dermatitis (fungal), ecchymosis, hirsutism, pruritus, skin hypertrophy, wound healing abnormal

Endocrine & metabolic: Acidosis, Cushing's syndrome, dehydration, diabetes mellitus, glycosuria, hypercalcemia, hyperglycemia, hyperphosphatemia, hypocalcemia, hypoglycemia, hypokalemia, hypomagnesemia, hyponatremia

Gastrointestinal: Abdomen enlarged, anorexia, dysphagia, eructation, esophagitis, flatulence, gastritis, gastroenteritis, gingival hyperplasia, gingivitis, ileus, mouth ulceration, oral moniliasis, stomatitis, weight loss

Genitourinary: Impotence, pelvic pain, scrotal edema, testis disorder

Hematologic: Hemolytic-uremic syndrome, hemorrhage, leukopenia, leukocytosis, polycythemia, TTP

Hepatic: Abnormal liver function tests, alkaline phosphatase increased, LDH increased

Local: Thrombophlebitis

Neuromuscular & skeletal: Arthrosis, bone necrosis, CPK increased, hyper-/hypotonia, leg cramps, myalgia, osteoporosis, paresthesia, tetany

Ocular: Abnormal vision, cataract, conjunctivitis

Otic: Ear pain, otitis media, tinnitus

Renal: Albuminuria, bladder pain, BUN increased, dysuria, hematuria, hydronephrosis, kidney pain, nephropathy (toxic), nocturia, oliguria, pyelonephritis, pyuria, tubular necrosis, urinary frequency, urinary incontinence, urinary retention

Respiratory: Asthma, atelectasis, bronchitis, cough, epistaxis, hypoxia, lung edema, pleural effusion, pneumonia, pulmonary embolism, rhinitis, sinusitis

Miscellaneous: Lymphoproliferative disease/lymphoma (1% to 3%), abscess, diaphoresis, flu-like syndrome, hernia, herpesvirus infection, infection (including opportunistic), lymphadenopathy, lymphocele, peritonitis, sepsis

Available Dosage Forms

Solution, oral:

Rapamune®: 1 mg/mL (60 mL)

Tablet, oral:

Rapamune®: 0.5 mg, 1 mg, 2 mg

General Dosage Range Dosage adjustment recommended in patients with hepatic impairment

Oral:

Children ≥13 years and Adults <40 kg: Low-to-moderate immunologic risk: Loading dose: 3 mg/m² on day 1; Maintenance: 1 mg/m²/day

Children ≥13 years and Adults ≥40 kg: Low-to-moderate immunologic risk: Loading dose: 6 mg on day 1; Maintenance: 2 mg/day (maximum: 40 mg/day)

Adults: High risk: Loading dose: Up to 15 mg on day 1; Maintenance: 5 mg/day (maximum: 40 mg/day)

Administration

Oral Initial dose should be administered as soon as possible after transplant. Sirolimus should be taken 4 hours after oral cyclosporine (Neoral® or Gengraf®). Should be administered consistently (with or without food).

Solution: Mix (by stirring vigorously) with at least 2 ounces of water or orange juice. No other liquids should be used for dilution. Patient should drink diluted solution immediately. The cup should then be refilled with an additional 4 ounces of water or orange juice, stirred vigorously, and the patient should drink the contents at once.

Tablet: Do not crush, split, or chew.

Stability

Storage

Oral solution: Store under refrigeration, 2°C to 8°C (36°F to 46°F). Protect from light. A slight haze may develop in refrigerated solutions, but the quality of the product is not affected. After opening, solution should be used in 1 month. If necessary, may be stored at temperatures up to 25°C (77°F) for ≤15 days after opening. Product may be stored in amber syringe for a maximum of 24 hours (at room temperature or refrigerated). Discard syringe after single use. Solution should be used immediately following dilution.

Tablet: Store at room temperature of 20°C to 25°C (68°F to 77°F). Protect from light.

Nursing Actions

Physical Assessment Monitor blood pressure, weight, and renal function. Assess for signs of fluid retention and infection.

Patient Education Do not mix sirolimus solution with anything other than water or orange juice. Do not crush, split, or chew tablets. May be taken with or without food, but should be taken consistently with regard to food (always on an empty stomach or always with food). Maintain adequate hydration, unless instructed to restrict fluid intake. You will be susceptible to infection. If you have diabetes, monitor glucose levels closely (drug may alter glucose levels). Limit exposure to sunlight by wearing protective clothing or sunscreen. You may experience nausea, vomiting, loss of appetite, constipation, diarrhea, rash, acne, tremor, weight gain, or muscle or back pain. Inform prescriber of unresolved GI problems; respiratory difficulty, cough, or infection; persistent fever; skin rash or irritation; headache, insomnia, anxiety, confusion, or emotional lability; unusual bleeding; changes in voiding pattern or burning, itching, or pain on urination; persistent bone, joint, or muscle cramping, pain or weakness; numbness or tingling of extremities; chest pain, palpitations, or swelling of extremities; weight gain; or hearing or vision changes.

Dietary Considerations Take consistently (with or without food) to minimize variability of absorption.

SitaGLIPtin (sit a GLIP tin)

Brand Names: U.S. Januvia®

Index Terms MK-0431; Sitagliptin Phosphate

Pharmacologic Category Antidiabetic Agent, Dipeptidyl Peptidase IV (DPP-IV) Inhibitor

Medication Safety Issues

Sound-alike/look-alike issues:

Januvia® may be confused with Enjuvia™, Janumet®, Jantoven®

SitaGLIPtin may be confused with saxagliptin, SUMAtriptan

Medication Guide Available Yes

Pregnancy Risk Factor B

Lactation Excretion in breast milk unknown/use caution

Breast-Feeding Considerations It is not known if sitagliptin is excreted in breast milk. The manufacturer recommends that caution be used if administered to breast-feeding women.

Use Management of type 2 diabetes mellitus (noninsulin dependent, NIDDM) as an adjunct to diet and exercise as monotherapy or in combination therapy with other antidiabetic agents

Mechanism of Action/Effect Sitagliptin inhibits dipeptidyl peptidase IV (DPP-IV) enzyme resulting in prolonged active incretin levels. Incretin hormones (eg, glucagon-like peptide-1 [GLP-1] and glucose-dependent insulinotropic polypeptide [GIP]) regulate glucose homeostasis by increasing insulin synthesis and release from pancreatic beta cells and decreasing glucagon secretion from pancreatic alpha cells. Decreased glucagon secretion results in decreased hepatic glucose production. Under normal physiologic circumstances, incretin hormones are released by the intestine throughout the day and levels are increased in response to a meal; incretin hormones are rapidly inactivated by the DPP-IV enzyme.

Contraindications Serious hypersensitivity (eg, anaphylaxis, angioedema) to sitagliptan or any component of the formulation

Warnings/Precautions Avoid use in type 1 diabetes mellitus (insulin dependent, IDDM) and diabetic ketoacidosis (DKA) due to lack of efficacy in these populations. Use caution when used in conjunction with insulin or insulin secretagogues; risk of hypoglycemia is increased. Monitor blood glucose closely; dosage adjustments of insulin or insulin secretagogues may be necessary. Use with caution in patients with moderate-to-severe renal dysfunction and end-stage renal disease (ESRD) requiring hemodialysis or peritoneal dialysis; dosing adjustment required. Safety and efficacy have not been established in severe hepatic dysfunction.

Rare hypersensitivity reactions, including anaphylaxis, angioedema, and/or severe dermatologic reactions (such as Stevens-Johnson syndrome), have been reported in postmarketing surveillance; discontinue if signs/symptoms of hypersensitivity reactions occur. Cases of acute pancreatitis (including hemorrhagic and necrotizing with some fatalities) have been reported with use; monitor for signs/symptoms of pancreatitis. Discontinue use immediately if pancreatitis is suspected and initiate appropriate management. Use with caution in ▶

patients with a history of pancreatitis (not known if this population is at greater risk).

Clinical trials included only a limited number of patients with heart failure (HF). No specific recommendations regarding this population are provided in the approved U.S. labeling (Canadian labeling recommends against use in this population). Diabetes self-management education (DSME) is essential to maximize the effectiveness of therapy.

Drug Interactions

Avoid Concomitant Use There are no known interactions where it is recommended to avoid concomitant use.

Decreased Effect

The levels/effects of SitaGLIPtin may be decreased by: Corticosteroids (Orally Inhaled); Corticosteroids (Systemic); Luteinizing Hormone-Releasing Hormone Analogs; P-glycoprotein/ABCB1 Inducers; Somatropin; Thiazide Diuretics

Increased Effect/Toxicity

SitaGLIPtin may increase the levels/effects of: ACE Inhibitors; Digoxin; Hypoglycemic Agents

The levels/effects of SitaGLIPtin may be increased by: Herbs (Hypoglycemic Properties); Pegvisomant; P-glycoprotein/ABCB1 Inhibitors

Adverse Reactions As reported with monotherapy: 1% to 10%:

Cardiovascular: Peripheral edema (2%)

Endocrine & metabolic: Hypoglycemia (1%)

Gastrointestinal: Diarrhea (4%), constipation (3%), nausea (2%)

Neuromuscular & skeletal: Osteoarthritis (1%)

Respiratory: Nasopharyngitis (5%), pharyngitis (1%), upper respiratory tract infection (viral; 1%)

Available Dosage Forms

Tablet, oral:

Januvia®: 25 mg, 50 mg, 100 mg

General Dosage Range Dosage adjustment recommended in patients with renal impairment

Oral: *Adults:* 100 mg once daily

Administration

Oral May be administered with or without food.

Stability

Storage Store at 20°C to 25°C (68°F to 77°F); excursions permitted to 15°C to 30°C (59°F to 86°F).

Nursing Actions

Physical Assessment With insulin or sulfonylureas, the risk of hypoglycemia may be increased and dosage adjustments may be necessary. Monitor renal function prior to treatment and throughout. Monitor for hypersensitivity reactions and development of pancreatitis. Refer patient to diabetic educator for diabetic education if necessary.

Patient Education This medication will not cure diabetes and may be prescribed in conjunction with another antidiabetic medication. Do not chew or crush tablets. May be taken with or without food. It is important to follow dietary and lifestyle recommendations and glucose monitoring instructions of prescriber or diabetic educator. You will be instructed in signs of hyper-/hypoglycemia; always carry a source of glucose with you in event of hypoglycemia. You may experience mild headache, upper respiratory infection, stuffy or runny nose, sore throat, diarrhea, or constipation when beginning treatment. Notify prescriber of any persistent abdominal pain, anorexia, nausea, or vomiting; or signs of hypersensitivity reaction (swelling of face, lips, or mouth; severe skin rash or eruption; difficulty breathing).

Dietary Considerations May be taken with or without food. Individualized medical nutrition therapy (MNT) based on ADA recommendations is an integral part of therapy.

Sitagliptin and Metformin

(sit a GLIP tin & met FOR min)

Brand Names: U.S. Janumet®; Janumet® XR

Index Terms Metformin and Sitagliptin; Sitagliptin Phosphate and Metformin Hydrochloride

Pharmacologic Category Antidiabetic Agent, Biguanide; Antidiabetic Agent, Dipeptidyl Peptidase IV (DPP-IV) Inhibitor; Hypoglycemic Agent, Oral

Medication Safety Issues

Sound-alike/look-alike issues:

Janumet® may be confused with Jantoven®, Januvia®

Sitagliptin and Metformin may be confused with Linagliptin and Metformin

Sitagliptin and Metformin may be confused with Saxagliptin and Metformin

Medication Guide Available Yes

Pregnancy Risk Factor B

Lactation

Sitagliptin: Excretion in breast milk unknown/use caution

Metformin: Enters breast milk

Use Management of type 2 diabetes mellitus (noninsulin dependent, NIDDM) as an adjunct to diet and exercise in patients not adequately controlled on metformin or sitagliptin monotherapy

Available Dosage Forms

Tablet, oral:

Janumet®: 50/500: Sitagliptin 50 mg and metformin 500 mg; 50/1000: Sitagliptin 50 mg and metformin 1000 mg

Tablet, extended release, oral:

Janumet® XR: 50/500: Sitagliptin 50 mg and metformin 500 mg

Janumet® XR: 50/1000: Sitagliptin 50 mg and metformin 1000 mg

Janumet® XR: 100/1000: Sitagliptin 100 mg and metformin 1000 mg

General Dosage Range Oral: *Adults:*

Immediate release: Sitagliptin 50 mg and metformin 500-1000 mg twice daily (maximum: 100 mg/day [sitagliptin], 2000 mg/day [metformin])

Extended release: Sitagliptin 100 mg and metformin 1000-2000 mg once daily (maximum: 100 mg/day [sitagliptin], 2000 mg/day [metformin])

Administration

Oral Administer with meals, at the same time each day (evening meal preferable for extended release tablets). Swallow extended release tablets whole; do not crush, cut, or chew.

Nursing Actions

Physical Assessment See individual agents.

Patient Education See individual agents.

Sitagliptin and Simvastatin

(sit a GLIP tin & sim va STAT in)

Brand Names: U.S. Juvisync™

Index Terms Simvastatin and Sitagliptin; Sitagliptin Phosphate and Simvastatin

Pharmacologic Category Antidiabetic Agent, Dipeptidyl Peptidase IV (DPP-IV) Inhibitor; Antilipemic Agent, HMG-CoA Reductase Inhibitor

Medication Guide Available Yes

Pregnancy Risk Factor X

Lactation Excretion in breast milk unknown/contraindicated

Use For use when treatment with both sitagliptin and simvastatin is appropriate:

Sitagliptin: Management of type 2 diabetes mellitus (noninsulin dependent, NIDDM) as an adjunct to diet and exercise as monotherapy or in combination therapy with other antidiabetic agents

Simvastatin: Used with dietary therapy for the following:

Secondary prevention of cardiovascular events in hypercholesterolemic patients with established coronary heart disease (CHD) or at high risk for CHD: To reduce cardiovascular morbidity (myocardial infarction, coronary/noncoronary revascularization procedures) and mortality; to reduce the risk of stroke

Hyperlipidemias: To reduce elevations in total cholesterol (total-C), LDL-C, apolipoprotein B, triglycerides, and VLDL-C, and to increase HDL-C in patients with primary hypercholesterolemia (elevations of 1 or more components are present in Fredrickson type IIa, IIb, III, and IV hyperlipidemias); treatment of homozygous familial hypercholesterolemia

Available Dosage Forms Tablet, oral:

Juvisync™ 100/10: Sitagliptin 100 mg and simvastatin 10 mg

Juvisync™ 100/20: Sitagliptin 100 mg and simvastatin 20 mg

Juvisync™ 100/40: Sitagliptin 100 mg and simvastatin 40 mg

General Dosage Range Dosage adjustment recommended in patients on concomitant therapy.

Oral: *Adults:* Initial: Sitagliptin 100 mg and simvastatin 40 mg once daily

Administration

Oral Administer in the evening. Swallow whole; do no crush, split, dissolve, or chew.

Nursing Actions

Physical Assessment See individual agents.

Patient Education See individual agents.

Related Information

Simvastatin *on page 1037*

SitaGLIPtin *on page 1043*

Sodium Bicarbonate

(SOW dee um bye KAR bun ate)

Brand Names: U.S. Brioschi® [OTC]; Neut®

Index Terms Baking Soda; $NaHCO_3$; Sodium Acid Carbonate; Sodium Hydrogen Carbonate

Pharmacologic Category Alkalinizing Agent; Antacid; Electrolyte Supplement, Oral; Electrolyte Supplement, Parenteral

Pregnancy Risk Factor C

Lactation Enters breast milk

Breast-Feeding Considerations Sodium is found in breast milk (IOM, 2004).

Use Management of metabolic acidosis; gastric hyperacidity; as an alkalinization agent for the urine; treatment of hyperkalemia; management of overdose of certain drugs, including tricyclic antidepressants and aspirin

Unlabeled Use Prevention of contrast-induced nephropathy (CIN)

Mechanism of Action/Effect Dissociates to provide bicarbonate ion which neutralizes hydrogen ion concentration and raises blood and urinary pH

Contraindications Alkalosis, hypernatremia, severe pulmonary edema, hypocalcemia, unknown abdominal pain

Warnings/Precautions Rapid administration in neonates and children <2 years of age has led to hypernatremia, decreased CSF pressure and intracranial hemorrhage. **Use of I.V. $NaHCO_3$ should be reserved for documented metabolic acidosis and for hyperkalemia-induced cardiac arrest.** Routine use in cardiac arrest is not recommended. Avoid extravasation, tissue necrosis can occur due to the hypertonicity of $NaHCO_3$. May cause sodium retention especially if renal function is impaired; not to be used in treatment of peptic ulcer; use with caution in patients with HF, edema, cirrhosis, or renal failure. Not the antacid of choice for the elderly because of sodium content and potential for systemic alkalosis.

Drug Interactions

Avoid Concomitant Use There are no known interactions where it is recommended to avoid concomitant use.

Decreased Effect

Sodium Bicarbonate may decrease the levels/effects of: ACE Inhibitors; Anticonvulsants (Hydantoin); Antipsychotic Agents (Phenothiazines); Atazanavir; Bisacodyl; Cefditoren; Cefpodoxime; Cefuroxime; Chloroquine; Corticosteroids (Oral); Dabigatran Etexilate; Dasatinib; Delavirdine; Erlotinib; Flecainide; Gabapentin; HMG-CoA Reductase Inhibitors; Iron Salts; Isoniazid; Itraconazole; Ketoconazole; Ketoconazole (Systemic); Lithium; Mesalamine; Methenamine; PenicillAMINE; Phosphate Supplements; Protease Inhibitors; Rilpivirine; Tetracycline Derivatives; Trientine; Vismodegib

Increased Effect/Toxicity

Sodium Bicarbonate may increase the levels/effects of: Alpha-/Beta-Agonists; Amphetamines; Calcium Polystyrene Sulfonate; Dexmethylphenidate; Flecainide; Memantine; Methylphenidate; QuiNIDine; QuiNINE

The levels/effects of Sodium Bicarbonate may be increased by: AcetaZOLAMIDE

Nutritional/Ethanol Interactions Herb/Nutraceutical: Concurrent doses with iron may decrease iron absorption.

Adverse Reactions Frequency not defined.

Cardiovascular: Cerebral hemorrhage, CHF (aggravated), edema

Central nervous system: Tetany

Gastrointestinal: Belching, flatulence (with oral), gastric distension

Endocrine & metabolic: Hypernatremia, hyperosmolality, hypocalcemia, hypokalemia, increased affinity of hemoglobin for oxygen-reduced pH in myocardial tissue necrosis when extravasated, intracranial acidosis, metabolic alkalosis, milk-alkali syndrome (especially with renal dysfunction)

Respiratory: Pulmonary edema

Pharmacodynamics/Kinetics

Onset of Action Oral: Rapid; I.V.: 15 minutes

Duration of Action Oral: 8-10 minutes; I.V.: 1-2 hours

Available Dosage Forms

Granules for solution, oral:

Brioschi® [OTC]: 2.69 g/capful (120 g, 240 g); 2.69 g/packet (12s)

Injection, solution: 4.2% (10 mL); 8.4% (10 mL, 50 mL, 250 mL, 500 mL)

Neut®: 4% (5 mL)

Injection, solution [preservative free]: 4.2% (5 mL, 10 mL); 7.5% (50 mL); 8.4% (10 mL, 50 mL)

Powder, oral: USP: 100% (120 g, 454 g, 480 g)

Tablet, oral: 325 mg, 650 mg

General Dosage Range

I.V.: *Children and Adults:* Dosage varies greatly depending on indication

Oral:

Children: 1-10 mEq/kg/day as a single dose **or** divided every 4-6 hours

Adults <60 years: 0.5-200 mEq/kg/day in 4-5 divided doses **or** 325 mg to 2 g 1-4 times/day (maximum: 16 g [200 mEq] day)

Adults ≥60 years: 0.5-100 mEq/kg/day in 4-6 divided doses **or** 325 mg to 2 g 1-4 times/day (maximum: 8 g [100 mEq] day)

Administration

Oral Oral product should be administered 1-3 hours after meals.

I.V. Detail Observe for extravasation when giving I.V.

pH: 7.0-8.5

Stability

Reconstitution Prevention of contrast-induced nephropathy (unlabeled use): Remove 154 mL from 1000 mL bag of D_5W; replace with 154 mL of 8.4% sodium bicarbonate; resultant concentration is 154 mEq/L (Merten, 2004); more practically, institutions may remove 150 mL from 1000 mL bag of D_5W and replace with 150 mL of 8.4% sodium bicarbonate; resultant concentration is 150 mEq/L

Storage Store injection at room temperature. Protect from heat and from freezing. Use only clear solutions.

Nursing Actions

Physical Assessment I.V.: Monitor cardiac status, arterial blood gases, and electrolytes. Monitor for CHF. Monitor infusion site for patency (if extravasation occurs, elevate extravasation site and apply warm compresses).

Patient Education Do not use for chronic gastric acidity. Chew tablets thoroughly and follow with a full glass of water, preferably on an empty stomach (2 hours before or after food). Report CNS effects (eg, irritability, confusion), muscle rigidity or tremors, swelling of feet or ankles, respiratory difficulty, chest pain or palpitations, respiratory changes, or tarry stools.

Dietary Considerations Some products may contain sodium. Oral product should be taken 1-3 hours after meals.

Related Information

Compatibility of Drugs *on page 1264*

Management of Drug Extravasations *on page 1269*

Sodium Citrate and Citric Acid

(SOW dee um SIT rate & SI trik AS id)

Brand Names: U.S. Cytra-2; Oracit®; Shohl's Solution (Modified)

Index Terms Bicitra; Citric Acid and Sodium Citrate; Modified Shohl's Solution

Pharmacologic Category Alkalinizing Agent, Oral

Medication Safety Issues

Sound-alike/look-alike issues:

Bicitra may be confused with Polycitra

Pregnancy Risk Factor Not established

Lactation Excretion in breast milk unknown/compatible

Use Treatment of metabolic acidosis; alkalinizing agent in conditions where long-term maintenance of an alkaline urine is desirable

Available Dosage Forms Contains sodium 1 mEq/mL and is equivalent to bicarbonate 1 mEq/mL

Solution, oral: Sodium citrate 500 mg and citric acid 334 mg per 5 mL

Cytra-2: Sodium citrate 500 mg and citric acid 334 mg per 5 mL

Oracit®: Sodium citrate 490 mg and citric acid 640 mg per 5 mL

Shohl's Solution (Modified): Sodium citrate 500 mg and citric acid 300 mg er 5 mL

General Dosage Range Oral:

Infants and Children: 2-3 mEq/kg/day in 3-4 divided doses **or** 5-15 mL after meals and at bedtime

Adults: 10-30 mL after meals and at bedtime

Administration

Oral Administer after meals. Dilute with 30-90 mL of water to enhance taste. Chilling solution prior to dosing helps to enhance palatability.

Nursing Actions

Physical Assessment Assess kidney function prior to treatment. Monitor cardiac status and serum potassium prior to treatment and at regular intervals.

Patient Education Take after meals. Dilute with 1-3 oz of water and follow with additional water; chilling solution prior to taking will help to improve taste. You may experience diarrhea or nausea and vomiting; if severe, contact prescriber. Report CNS changes (eg, irritability, tremors, confusion), swelling of feet or ankles, respiratory difficulty or palpitations, abdominal pain, or tarry stools.

Sodium Polystyrene Sulfonate

(SOW dee um pol ee STYE reen SUL fon ate)

Brand Names: U.S. Kalexate; Kayexalate®; Kionex®; SPS®

Pharmacologic Category Antidote

Medication Safety Issues

Sound-alike/look-alike issues:

Kayexalate® may be confused with Kaopectate®

Sodium polystyrene sulfonate may be confused with calcium polystyrene sulfonate

Administration issues:

Always prescribe either one-time doses or as a specific number of doses (eg, 15 g q6h x 2 doses). Scheduled doses with no dosage limit could be given for days leading to dangerous hypokalemia.

International issues:

Kionex [U.S.] may be confused with Kinex brand name for biperiden [Mexico]

Pregnancy Risk Factor C

Lactation Excretion in breast milk unknown/use caution

Use Treatment of hyperkalemia

Mechanism of Action/Effect Removes potassium by exchanging sodium ions for potassium ions in the intestine (especially the large intestine) before the resin is passed from the body

Contraindications Hypersensitivity to sodium polystyrene sulfonate or any component of the formulation; hypokalemia; obstructive bowel disease; neonates with reduced gut motility (postoperatively or drug-induced); oral administration in neonates

Additional contraindications: Sodium polystyrene sulfonate suspension (**with** sorbitol): Rectal administration in neonates (particularly in premature infants); any postoperative patient until normal bowel function resumes

Warnings/Precautions Intestinal necrosis (including fatalities) and other serious gastrointestinal events (eg, bleeding, ischemic colitis, perforation) have been reported, especially when administered with sorbitol. Increased risk may be associated with a history of intestinal disease or surgery, hypovolemia, prematurity, and renal insufficiency or failure; use with sorbitol is not recommended. Avoid use in any postoperative patient until normal bowel function resumes or in patients at risk for constipation or impaction; discontinue use if constipation occurs. Oral or rectal administration of sorbitol-containing sodium polystyrene sulfonate suspensions is contraindicated in neonates (particularly with prematurity). Use with caution in patients with severe HF, hypertension, or edema; sodium load may exacerbate condition. Effective lowering of serum potassium from sodium polystyrene sulfonate may take hours to days after administration; consider alternative measures (eg, dialysis) or concomitant therapy (eg, I.V. sodium bicarbonate) in situations where rapid correction of severe hyperkalemia is required. Severe hypokalemia may occur; frequent monitoring of serum potassium is recommended within each 24-hour period; ECG monitoring may be appropriate in select patients. In addition to serum potassium-lowering effects, cation-exchange resins may also affect other cation concentrations possibly resulting in decreased serum magnesium and calcium. Large oral doses may cause fecal impaction (especially in elderly).

Concomitant administration of oral sodium polystyrene sulfonate with nonabsorbable cation-donating antacids or laxatives (eg, magnesium hydroxide) may result in systemic alkalosis and may diminish ability to reduce serum potassium concentrations; use with such agents is not recommended. In addition, intestinal obstruction has been reported with concomitant administration of aluminum hydroxide due to concretion formation. Enema will reduce the serum potassium faster than oral administration, but the oral route will result in a greater reduction over several hours. Oral administration in neonates and use in neonates with reduced gut motility (postoperatively or drug-induced) is contraindicated. Oral or rectal administration of sorbitol-containing sodium polystyrene sulfonate suspensions in neonates (particularly with prematurity) is also contraindicated due to propylene glycol content and risk of intestinal necrosis and digestive hemorrhage. Use sodium polystyrene sulfonate (**without** sorbitol) with caution in premature or low-birth-weight infants. Use with caution in children when administering rectally; excessive dosage or inadequate dilution may result in fecal impaction.

Drug Interactions

Avoid Concomitant Use

Avoid concomitant use of Sodium Polystyrene Sulfonate with any of the following: Laxatives; Meloxicam; Sorbitol

Decreased Effect

Sodium Polystyrene Sulfonate may decrease the levels/effects of: Lithium; Thyroid Products

Increased Effect/Toxicity

Sodium Polystyrene Sulfonate may increase the levels/effects of: Aluminum Hydroxide; Digoxin

The levels/effects of Sodium Polystyrene Sulfonate may be increased by: Antacids; Laxatives; Meloxicam; Sorbitol

Nutritional/Ethanol Interactions Food: Some liquids may contain potassium: Management: Do not mix in orange juice or in any fruit juice known to contain potassium.

Adverse Reactions Frequency not defined.

Endocrine & metabolic: Hypernatremia, hypocalcemia, hypokalemia, hypomagnesemia, sodium retention

Gastrointestinal: Anorexia, constipation, diarrhea, fecal impaction, intestinal necrosis (rare), intestinal obstruction (due to concretions in association with aluminum hydroxide), nausea, vomiting

Pharmacodynamics/Kinetics

Onset of Action 2-24 hours

Available Dosage Forms

Powder for suspension, oral/rectal: (454 g)

Kalexate: (454 g)

Kayexalate®: (454 g)

Kionex®: (454 g)

Suspension, oral/rectal:

Kionex®: 15 g/60 mL (60 mL, 480 mL)

SPS®: 15 g/60 mL (60 mL, 120 mL, 473 mL)

General Dosage Range

Oral:

Children: 1 g/kg/dose every 6 hours

Adults: 15 g 1-4 times/day

Rectal:

Children: 1 g/kg/dose every 2-6 hours

Adults: 30-50 g every 6 hours

Administration

Oral Shake suspension well prior to administration. Administer orally (or via NG tube) as a suspension. **Do not mix in orange juice.** Chilling the oral mixture will increase palatability.

Powder for suspension: For each 1 g of the powdered resin, add 3-4 mL of water or syrup (amount of fluid usually ranges from 20-100 mL)

Other Rectal: Enema route is less effective than oral administration. Administer cleansing enema first. Each dose of the powder for suspension should be suspended in 100 mL of aqueous vehicle and administered as a warm emulsion (body temperature). The commercially available suspension should also be warmed to body temperature. During administration, the solution should be agitated gently. Retain enema in colon for at least 30-60 minutes and for several hours, if possible. Once retention time is complete, irrigate colon with a nonsodium-containing solution to remove resin.

Stability

Storage Store at 25°C (77°F); excursions permitted to 15°C to 30°C (59°F to 86°F). Store repackaged product in refrigerator and use within 14 days. Freshly prepared suspensions should be used within 24 hours. Do not heat resin suspension.

Nursing Actions

Physical Assessment Monitor ECG until potassium levels are normal. Monitor bowel function; can cause constipation and/or fecal impaction.

Patient Education You will be monitored for effects of this medication and frequent blood tests may be necessary. Oral: Mix well with a full glass of a chilled liquid (not orange juice or any other juice containing potassium). Avoid use of antacids, laxatives, or preparations containing sorbitol while taking this medication. You may experience nausea, vomiting, or constipation. Report persistent constipation, abdominal pain, or GI distress; chest pain or rapid heartbeat; or mental confusion or muscle weakness.

Dietary Considerations Do **not** mix in orange juice or in any fruit juice known to contain potassium. Some products may contain sodium.

Solifenacin (sol i FEN a sin)

Brand Names: U.S. VESIcare®

Index Terms Solifenacin Succinate; YM905

Pharmacologic Category Anticholinergic Agent

Medication Safety Issues

Sound-alike/look-alike issues:

VESIcare® may be confused with Visicol®

Pregnancy Risk Factor C

Lactation Excretion in breast milk unknown/not recommended

Use Treatment of overactive bladder with symptoms of urinary frequency, urgency, or urge incontinence

Mechanism of Action/Effect Inhibits muscarinic receptors resulting in decreased urinary bladder contraction, increased residual urine volume, and decreased detrusor muscle pressure.

Contraindications Hypersensitivity to solifenacin or any component of the formulation; urinary retention; gastric retention; uncontrolled narrow-angle glaucoma.

Warnings/Precautions Cases of angioedema involving the face, lips, tongue, and/or larynx have been reported. Immediately discontinue if tongue, hypopharynx, or larynx are involved. May cause drowsiness and/or blurred vision, which may impair physical or mental abilities; patients must be cautioned about performing tasks which require mental alertness (eg, operating machinery or driving). Heat prostration may occur in the presence of increased environmental temperature; use caution in hot weather and/or exercise. Use with caution in patients with bladder outflow obstruction, gastrointestinal obstructive disorders, and decreased gastrointestinal motility. Use with caution in patients with a known history of QT prolongation or other risk factors for QT prolongation (eg, concomitant use of medications known to prolong QT interval and/or electrolyte abnormalities); the risk for QT prolongation is dose-related. Use with caution in patients with controlled (treated) narrow-angle glaucoma; use is contraindicated with uncontrolled narrow-angle glaucoma. Dosage adjustment is required for patients with severe renal impairment (Cl_{cr} <30 mL/minute) or moderate (Child-Pugh class B) hepatic impairment; use is not recommended with severe hepatic impairment (Child-Pugh class C). Patients on potent CYP3A4 inhibitors require the lower dose of solifenacin.

Drug Interactions

Avoid Concomitant Use

Avoid concomitant use of Solifenacin with any of the following: Conivaptan

Decreased Effect

Solifenacin may decrease the levels/effects of: Acetylcholinesterase Inhibitors (Central); Secretin

The levels/effects of Solifenacin may be decreased by: Acetylcholinesterase Inhibitors (Central); CYP3A4 Inducers (Strong); Deferasirox; Herbs (CYP3A4 Inducers); Tocilizumab

Increased Effect/Toxicity

Solifenacin may increase the levels/effects of: AbobotulinumtoxinA; Anticholinergics; Cannabinoids; OnabotulinumtoxinA; Potassium Chloride; RimabotulinumtoxinB

The levels/effects of Solifenacin may be increased by: Antifungal Agents (Azole Derivatives, Systemic); Conivaptan; CYP3A4 Inhibitors (Moderate); CYP3A4 Inhibitors (Strong); Dasatinib; Ivacaftor; Pramlintide

Nutritional/Ethanol Interactions

Food: Grapefruit juice may increase the serum level effects of solifenacin.

Herb/Nutraceutical: St John's wort (*Hypericum*) may decrease the levels/effects of solifenacin.

Adverse Reactions

>10%: Gastrointestinal: Xerostomia (11% to 28%; dose-related), constipation (5% to 13%; dose-related)

1% to 10%:

Cardiovascular: Edema (≤1%), hypertension (≤1%)

Central nervous system: Headache (3% to 6%), fatigue (1% to 2%), depression (≤1%)

Gastrointestinal: Dyspepsia (1% to 4%), nausea (2% to 3%), upper abdominal pain (1% to 2%)

Genitourinary: Urinary tract infection (3% to 5%), urinary retention (≤1%)

Ocular: Blurred vision (4% to 5%), dry eyes (≤2%)

Respiratory: Cough (≤1%)

Miscellaneous: Influenza (≤2%)

Available Dosage Forms

Tablet, oral:

VESIcare®: 5 mg, 10 mg

General Dosage Range Dosage adjustment recommended in patients with hepatic or renal impairment and on concomitant therapy

Oral: *Adults:* 5-10 mg/day

Administration

Oral Swallow tablet whole; administer with liquids; may be administered without regard to meals.

Stability

Storage Store at controlled room temperature of 25°C (77°F); excursions permitted to 15°C to 30°C (59°F to 86°F).

Nursing Actions

Physical Assessment Monitor urination pattern.

Patient Education Maintain adequate hydration unless instructed to restrict fluid intake by prescriber. This medication may cause dry mouth. You may be more susceptible to heat prostration due to decreased ability to sweat. Use caution in hot weather. You may experience constipation, nausea, vomiting, blurred vision, and dry eyes. Report difficulty, pain, or burning on urination.

Dietary Considerations May be taken without regard to meals.

Somatropin (soe ma TROE pin)

Brand Names: U.S. Genotropin Miniquick®; Genotropin®; Humatrope®; Norditropin FlexPro®; Norditropin® NordiFlex®; Norditropin® [DSC]; Nutropin AQ Pen®; Nutropin AQ®; Nutropin AQ® NuSpin™; Nutropin®; Omnitrope®; Saizen®; Serostim®; Tev-Tropin®; Zorbtive®

Index Terms Growth Hormone, Human; hGH; Human Growth Hormone

Pharmacologic Category Growth Hormone

Medication Safety Issues

Sound-alike/look-alike issues:

Humatrope® may be confused with homatropine

Somatrem may be confused with somatropin

Somatropin may be confused with homatropine, sumatriptan

Pregnancy Risk Factor B/C (depending upon manufacturer)

Lactation Excretion in breast milk unknown/use caution

Use

Children:

Treatment of growth failure due to inadequate endogenous growth hormone secretion (Genotropin®, Humatrope®, Norditropin®, Nutropin®, Nutropin AQ®, Omnitrope®, Saizen®, Tev-Tropin®)

Treatment of short stature associated with Turner syndrome (Genotropin®, Humatrope®, Norditropin®, Nutropin®, Nutropin AQ®, Omnitrope®)

Treatment of Prader-Willi syndrome (Genotropin®, Omnitrope®)

Treatment of growth failure associated with chronic renal insufficiency (CRI) up until the time of renal transplantation (Nutropin®, Nutropin AQ®)

Treatment of growth failure in children born small for gestational age who fail to manifest catch-up growth by 2 years of age (Genotropin®, Omnitrope®) or by 2-4 years of age (Humatrope®, Norditropin®)

Treatment of idiopathic short stature (nongrowth hormone-deficient short stature) defined by height standard deviation score (SDS) ≤-2.25 and growth rate not likely to attain normal adult height (Genotropin®, Humatrope®, Nutropin®, Nutropin AQ®, Omnitrope®)

Treatment of short stature or growth failure associated with short stature homeobox gene (SHOX) deficiency (Humatrope®)

Treatment of short stature associated with Noonan syndrome (Norditropin®)

Adults:

HIV patients with wasting or cachexia with concomitant antiviral therapy (Serostim®)

Replacement of endogenous growth hormone in patients with adult growth hormone deficiency who meet both of the following criteria (Genotropin®, Humatrope®, Norditropin®, Nutropin®, Nutropin AQ®, Omnitrope®, Saizen®):

Biochemical diagnosis of adult growth hormone deficiency by means of a subnormal response to a standard growth hormone stimulation test (peak growth hormone ≤5 mcg/L). Confirmatory testing may not be required in patients with congenital/genetic growth hormone deficiency or multiple pituitary hormone deficiencies due to organic diseases.

and

Adult-onset: Patients who have adult growth hormone deficiency whether alone or with multiple hormone deficiencies (hypopituitarism) as a result of pituitary disease, hypothalamic disease, surgery, radiation therapy, or trauma

or

Childhood-onset: Patients who were growth hormone deficient during childhood, confirmed as an adult before replacement therapy is initiated

Treatment of short-bowel syndrome (Zorbtive®)

Unlabeled Use Pediatric HIV patients with wasting/cachexia (Serostim®); HIV-associated adipose redistribution syndrome (HARS) (Serostim®)

Mechanism of Action/Effect Human growth hormone assists in growth of linear bone, skeletal muscle, and organs; stimulates erythropoietin which increases red blood cell mass; exerts both insulin-like and diabetogenic effects; enhances transmucosal transport of water, electrolytes, and nutrients across the gut

Contraindications Hypersensitivity to growth hormone or any component of the formulation; growth promotion in pediatric patients with closed epiphyses; progression or recurrence of any underlying intracranial lesion or actively growing intracranial tumor; acute critical illness due to complications following open heart or abdominal surgery; multiple accidental trauma or acute respiratory failure; evidence of active malignancy; active proliferative or severe nonproliferative diabetic retinopathy; use in patients with Prader-Willi syndrome **without** growth hormone deficiency (except Genotropin®) or in patients with Prader-Willi syndrome **with** growth hormone deficiency who are severely obese, have a history of upper airway obstruction or sleep apnea, or have severe respiratory impairment

Warnings/Precautions Initiation of somatropin is contraindicated with acute critical illness due to complications following open heart or abdominal surgery, multiple accidental trauma, or acute respiratory failure; mortality may be increased. The safety of continuing somatropin in patients who develop these illnesses during therapy has not been established; use with caution. Use in contraindicated with active malignancy; monitor patients with pre-existing tumors or growth failure secondary to an intracranial lesion for recurrence or progression of underlying disease; discontinue therapy with evidence of recurrence. An increased risk of second neoplasm has been reported in childhood cancer survivors treated with somatropin; the most common second neoplasms were meningiomas in patients treated with radiation to the head for their first neoplasm. Monitor patients for any malignant transformation of skin lesions.

Somatropin may decrease insulin sensitivity; use with caution in patients with diabetes or with risk factors for impaired glucose tolerance. Adjustment of antidiabetic medications may be necessary. Pancreatitis has been rarely reported; incidence in children (especially girls) with Turner syndrome may be greater than adults. Monitor for hypersensitivity reactions. Patients with hypoadrenalism may require increased dosages of glucocorticoids (especially cortisone acetate and prednisone) due to somatropin-mediated inhibition of 11 beta-hydroxysteroid dehydrogenase type 1; undiagnosed central hypoadrenalism may be unmasked. Excessive glucocorticoid therapy may inhibit the growth promoting effects of somatropin in children; monitor and adjust glucocorticoids carefully. Untreated/undiagnosed hypothyroidism may decrease response to therapy; monitor thyroid function test periodically and initiate/adjust thyroid replacement therapy as needed. Closely monitor other hormonal replacement treatments in patients with hypopituitarism. Obese patients may experience an increased incidence of adverse events when using a weight-based dosing regimen. Intracranial hypertension (IH) with headache, nausea, papilledema, visual changes, and/or vomiting has been reported with somatropin; funduscopic examination prior to initiation of therapy and periodically thereafter is recommended. Treatment should be discontinued in patients who develop papilledema; resuming treatment at a lower dose may be considered once IH-associated signs and symptoms have resolved. Patients with Turner syndrome, chronic renal failure and Prader-Willi syndrome may be at increased risk for IH. Progression of scoliosis may occur in children experiencing rapid growth. Patients with growth hormone deficiency may develop slipped capital epiphyses more frequently, evaluate any child with new onset of a limp or with complaints of hip or knee pain. Patients with Turner syndrome are at increased risk for otitis media and other ear/hearing disorders, cardiovascular disorders (including stroke, aortic aneurysm, hypertension), and thyroid disease, monitor carefully. Fluid retention may occur frequently in adults during use; manifestations of fluid retention (eg, edema, arthralgia, myalgia, nerve compression syndromes/paresthesias) are generally transient and dose dependent. Products may contain benzyl alcohol or m-cresol. When administering to newborns, reconstitute with sterile water or saline for injection. Not for I.V. injection.

Fatalities have been reported in pediatric patients with Prader-Willi syndrome following the use of growth hormone. The reported fatalities occurred in patients with one or more risk factors, including severe obesity, sleep apnea, respiratory impairment, or unidentified respiratory infection; male patients with one or more of these factors may be at greater risk. Treatment interruption is recommended in patients who show signs of upper airway obstruction, including the onset of, or increased, snoring. In addition, evaluation of and/or monitoring for sleep apnea and respiratory infections are recommended.

Patients with HIV infection should be maintained on antiretroviral therapy to prevent the potential increase in viral replication.

Elderly patients may be more sensitive to the actions of somatropin; consider lower starting doses. Safety and efficacy have not been established for the treatment of Noonan syndrome in children with significant cardiac disease. Children with epiphyseal closure who are treated for adult GHD need reassessment of therapy and dose. Administration site rotation is necessary to prevent tissue atrophy.

Drug Interactions

Avoid Concomitant Use There are no known interactions where it is recommended to avoid concomitant use.

Decreased Effect

Somatropin may decrease the levels/effects of: Antidiabetic Agents; Cortisone; PredniSONE

The levels/effects of Somatropin may be decreased by: Estrogen Derivatives

Increased Effect/Toxicity There are no known significant interactions involving an increase in effect.

Adverse Reactions

Growth hormone deficiency: Adverse reactions reported with growth hormone deficiency vary greatly by age. Generally, percentages are less in pediatric patients than adults, and many of the reactions reported in adults are dose related. Percentages reported also vary by product. Below is a listing by age group; events reported more commonly overall are noted with an asterisk (*).

Children: Antibodies development, arthralgia, benign intracranial hypertension, edema, eosinophilia, glycosuria, Hb A_{1c} increased, headache, hematoma, hematuria, hyperglycemia (mild), hypertriglyceridemia, hypoglycemia, hypothyroidism, injection site reaction, intracranial tumor, leg pain, lipoatrophy, leukemia, meningioma, muscle pain, papilledema, pseudotumor cerebri, psoriasis exacerbation, rash, scoliosis progression, seizure, slipped capital femoral epiphysis, weakness

Adults: Acne, ALT increased, AST increased, arthralgia*, back pain, bronchitis, carpal tunnel syndrome, chest pain, cough, depression, diabetes mellitus (type 2), diaphoresis, dizziness, edema*, fatigue, flu-like syndrome*, gastritis, glucose intolerance, glucosuria, headache*, hyperglycemia (mild), hypertension, hypoesthesia, hypothyroidism, infection, insomnia, insulin resistance, joint disorder, leg edema, muscle pain, myalgia*, nausea, pain in extremities, paresthesia*, peripheral edema*, pharyngitis, retinopathy, rhinitis, skeletal pain*, stiffness in extremities, surgical procedure, upper respiratory tract infection, weakness

Additional/postmarketing reactions observed with growth hormone deficiency: Gynecomastia, increased growth of pre-existing nevi, pancreatitis

HARS: Serostim®: Limited to >10%: Edema (peripheral) (19% to 45%), arthralgia (28% to 37%), pain (extremity) (5% to 19%), hypoesthesia (9% to 15%), headache (4% to 14%), blood glucose increased (4% to 14%), paresthesia (11% to 13%), myalgia (3% to 13%)

Idiopathic short stature: Percentages reported using Humatrope® versus placebo: Myalgia (24%), scoliosis (19%), otitis media (16%), arthralgia (11%), arthrosis (11%), hyperlipidemia (8%), gynecomastia (5%), hip pain (3%), hypertension (3%). Additional adverse reactions listed as reported using other products from ISS NCGS Cohort (frequencies <1%): Aggressiveness, benign intracranial hypertension, diabetes, edema, hair loss, headache, injection site reaction

Prader-Willi syndrome: Genotropin® (frequency not defined): Aggressiveness, arthralgia, edema, hair loss, headache, benign intracranial hypertension, myalgia; fatalities associated with use in this population have been reported

Turner syndrome: Percentages reported using Humatrope® compared to untreated patients. Additional adverse reactions reported from other products, frequency not specified: Surgical procedures (45%), otitis media (43%), ear disorders (18%), joint pain, respiratory illness, urinary tract infection

HIV patients with wasting or cachexia: Serostim® (limited to ≥5%): Musculoskeletal disorders (arthralgia, arthrosis, myalgia: 78%), peripheral edema (26%), headache (13%), nausea (9%), paresthesia (8%), edema (6%), gynecomastia (6%), hypoesthesia (5%)

Short-bowel syndrome: Zorbtive® (limited to >10%): Peripheral edema (69% to 81%), facial edema (44% to 50%), arthralgia (31% to 44%), nausea (13% to 31%), injection site pain (up to 31%), flatulence (25%), injection site reaction (19% to 25%), abdominal pain (13% to 25%), vomiting (19%), pain (6% to 19%), chest pain (up to 19%), dehydration (up to 19%), infection (up to 19%), rhinitis (up to 19%), hearing symptoms (13%), dizziness (6% to 13%), rash (6% to 13%), diaphoresis (up to 13%), generalized edema (up to 13%), malaise (up to 13%), moniliasis (up to 13%), myalgia (up to 13%)

SHOX deficiency: Humatrope®: Arthralgia (11%), gynecomastia (8%), excessive cutaneous nevi (7%), scoliosis (4%)

Small for gestational age: Genotropin®, Humatrope® (frequency not defined): Mild, transient hyperglycemia; benign intracranial hypertension (rare); central precocious puberty; jaw prominence (rare); aggravation of pre-existing scoliosis (rare); injection site reactions; progression of pigmented nevi; carpal tunnel syndrome (rare) diabetes mellitus (rare); otitis media; headache; slipped capital femoral epiphysis

Pharmacodynamics/Kinetics

Duration of Action Maintains supraphysiologic levels for 18-20 hours

Available Dosage Forms

Injection, powder for reconstitution:

Genotropin®: 5.8 mg, 13.8 mg
Humatrope®: 5 mg, 6 mg, 12 mg, 24 mg
Nutropin®: 5 mg, 10 mg
Omnitrope®: 5.8 mg
Saizen®: 5 mg, 8.8 mg
Serostim®: 4 mg, 5 mg, 6 mg
Tev-Tropin®: 5 mg
Zorbtive®: 8.8 mg

Injection, powder for reconstitution [preservative free]:

Genotropin Miniquick®: 0.2 mg, 0.4 mg, 0.6 mg, 0.8 mg, 1 mg, 1.2 mg, 1.4 mg, 1.6 mg, 1.8 mg, 2 mg

Injection, solution:

Norditropin FlexPro®: 5 mg/1.5 mL (1.5 mL); 10 mg/1.5 mL (1.5 mL); 15 mg/1.5 mL (1.5 mL)
Norditropin® NordiFlex®: 30 mg/3 mL (3 mL)
Nutropin AQ Pen®: 10 mg/2 mL (2 mL); 20 mg/2 mL (2 mL)
Nutropin AQ®: 10 mg/2 mL (2 mL)
Nutropin AQ® NuSpin™: 5 mg/2 mL (2 mL); 10 mg/2 mL (2 mL); 20 mg/2 mL (2 mL)
Omnitrope®: 5 mg/1.5 mL (1.5 mL); 10 mg/1.5 mL (1.5 mL)

General Dosage Range I.M., SubQ: *Children and Adults:* Dosage varies greatly depending on indication

Administration

I.M. Not all products are approved for I.M. administration. Rotate administration sites to avoid tissue atrophy.

Other Do not shake; administer SubQ or I.M. (not all products are approved for I.M. administration). Rotate administration sites to avoid tissue atrophy. When administering to newborns, do not reconstitute with a diluent that contains benzyl alcohol; sterile water for injection may be used as an alternative. Norditropin® cartridge must be administered using the corresponding color-coded NordiPen® injection pen. Solution in the Omnitrope® cartridges must be administered using the Omnitrope® pen; when installing a new cartridge, prime pen prior to first use. When administering Tev-Tropin®, SubQ injections of solutions >1 mL not recommended.

Stability

Reconstitution

Genotropin®: Reconstitute with diluent provided.

Genotropin MiniQuick®: Reconstitute with diluent provided. Consult the instructions provided with the reconstitution device.

Humatrope®:

Cartridge: Consult HumatroPen™ User Guide for complete instructions for reconstitution. **Dilute with solution provided with cartridges ONLY; do not use diluent provided with vials.**

Vial: 5 mg: Reconstitute with 1.5-5 mL diluent provided. Swirl gently; do not shake.

Nutropin®: Vial:

5 mg: Reconstitute with 1-5 mL bacteriostatic water for injection. Swirl gently, do not shake.

10 mg: Reconstitute with 1-10 mL bacteriostatic water for injection. Swirl gently, do not shake.

Omnitrope® powder: Reconstitute with provided diluent. Swirl gently; do not shake.

Saizen®: Vial:

5 mg: Reconstitute with 1-3 mL bacteriostatic water for injection or sterile water for injection. Gently swirl; do not shake.

8.8 mg: Reconstitute with 2-3 mL bacteriostatic water for injection or sterile water for injection. Gently swirl; do not shake.

Serostim®: Vial: Reconstitute with 0.5-1 mL sterile water for injection.

Tev-Tropin®: Reconstitute with 1-5 mL of diluent provided. Gently swirl; do not shake. May use preservative-free NS for use in newborns.

Zorbtive®: 8.8 mg vial: Reconstitute with 1-2 mL bacteriostatic water for injection. Swirl gently.

Storage

Genotropin®: Store at 2°C to 8°C (36°F to 46°F); do not freeze. Protect from light. Following reconstitution of 5.8 mg and 13.8 mg cartridge, store under refrigeration and use within 21 days.

Genotropin® Miniquick®: Store in refrigerator prior to dispensing, but may be stored ≤25°C (77°F) for up to 3 months after dispensing. Once reconstituted, solution must be refrigerated and used within 24 hours. Discard unused portion.

Humatrope®:

Vial: Before and after reconstitution, store at 2°C to 8°C (36°F to 46°F); do not freeze. When reconstituted with provided diluent or bacteriostatic water for injection, use within 14 days. When reconstituted with sterile water for injection, use within 24 hours and discard unused portion.

Cartridge: Before and after reconstitution, store at 2°C to 8°C (36°F to 46°F); do not freeze. Following reconstitution with provided diluent, stable for 28 days under refrigeration.

Norditropin®: Store at 2°C to 8°C (36°F to 46°F); do not freeze. Avoid direct light.

Cartridge: When refrigerated, must be used within 4 weeks once inserted into pen. Orange cartridges (5 mg/1.5 mL) may also be stored up to 3 weeks at ≤25°C (77°F).

Prefilled pen: When refrigerated, must be used within 4 weeks after initial injection. Orange and blue prefilled pens may also be stored up to 3 weeks at ≤25°C (77°F).

Nutropin®: Before and after reconstitution, store at 2°C to 8°C (36°F to 46°F); do not freeze.

Nutropin® vial: Use reconstituted vials within 14 days. When reconstituted with sterile water for injection, use immediately and discard unused portion.

Nutropin® AQ formulations: Use within 28 days following initial use.

Omnitrope®:

Powder for injection: Prior to reconstitution, store under refrigeration at 2°C to 8°C (36°F to 46°F); do not freeze. Protect from light. Reconstitute with provided diluent. Swirl gently; do not shake. Following reconstitution with the provided diluents, the 5.8 mg vial may be stored under refrigeration for up to 3 weeks. Store vial in carton to protect from light.

Solution: Prior to use, store under refrigeration at 2°C to 8°C (36°F to 46°F). Once the cartridge is loaded into the pen delivery system, store under refrigeration for up to 21 days after first use.

Saizen®: Prior to reconstitution, store at room temperature 15°C to 30°C (59°F to 86°F). Following reconstitution with bacteriostatic water for injection, reconstituted solution should be refrigerated and used within 14 days. When reconstituted with sterile water for injection, use immediately and discard unused portion. The Saizen® easy click cartridge, when reconstituted with the provided bacteriostatic water, should be stored under refrigeration and used within 21 days.

Serostim®: Prior to reconstitution, store at room temperature 15°C to 30°C (59°F to 86°F). When reconstituted with sterile water for injection, use immediately and discard unused portion.

Tev-Tropin®: Prior to reconstitution, store at 2°C to 8°C (36°F to 46°F). Following reconstitution with bacteriostatic NS, solution should be refrigerated and used within 14 days. Some cloudiness may occur; do not use if cloudiness persists after warming to room temperature.

Zorbtive®: Store unopened vials and diluent at room temperature of 15°C to 30°C (59°F to 86°F). Store reconstituted vial under refrigeration at 2°C to 8°C (36°F to 46°F) for up to 14 days; do not freeze.

Nursing Actions

Physical Assessment Instruct patients with diabetes to monitor glucose levels closely. Encourage funduscopic examinations at initiation of therapy and periodically during treatment. Instruct patient in proper use if self-administered (storage, reconstitution, injection techniques, and syringe/needle disposal). Pediatrics: Monitor growth curve; annually determine bone age.

Patient Education This drug can only be administered by injection. If self-administered, you will be instructed by prescriber on proper storage, reconstitution, injection technique, and syringe/needle disposal. Report immediately pain, redness, burning, drainage, or swelling at injection site. If you have diabetes, monitor glucose levels closely. Report immediately swelling of extremities, headache, nausea or vomiting, any rash, sudden change in vision, increased urination, thirst, or weight loss.

Dietary Considerations

Prader-Willi syndrome: All patients should have effective weight control (use is contraindicated in severely-obese patients).

Short-bowel syndrome: Intravenous parenteral nutrition requirements may need reassessment as gastrointestinal absorption improves.

Sorafenib (sor AF e nib)

Brand Names: U.S. NexAVAR®

Index Terms BAY 43-9006; Sorafenib Tosylate

Pharmacologic Category Antineoplastic Agent, Tyrosine Kinase Inhibitor; Vascular Endothelial Growth Factor (VEGF) Inhibitor

Medication Safety Issues

Sound-alike/look-alike issues:

NexAVAR® may be confused with NexIUM®

SORAfenib may be confused with axitinib, gefitinib, imatinib, SUNItinib, vandetanib, vemurafenib

High alert medication:

This medication is in a class the Institute for Safe Medication Practices (ISMP) includes among its list of drug classes which have a heightened risk of causing significant patient harm when used in error.

Pregnancy Risk Factor D

Lactation Excretion in breast milk unknown/not recommended

Breast-Feeding Considerations According to the manufacturer, the decision to continue or discontinue breast-feeding during therapy should take into account the risk of exposure to the infant and the benefits of treatment to the mother.

Use Treatment of advanced renal cell cancer (RCC); treatment of unresectable hepatocellular cancer (HCC)

Unlabeled Use Treatment of advanced thyroid cancer, recurrent or metastatic angiosarcoma, resistant gastrointestinal stromal tumor (GIST)

Mechanism of Action/Effect Prevents tumor growth by inhibiting both tumor cell proliferation and tumor angiogenesis through kinase inhibition

Contraindications Hypersensitivity to sorafenib or any component of the formulation; use in combination with carboplatin and paclitaxel in patients with squamous cell lung cancer

Warnings/Precautions Hazardous agent - use appropriate precautions for handling and disposal. May cause hypertension (generally mild-to-moderate), especially in the first 6 weeks of treatment; monitor; use caution in patients with underlying or poorly-controlled hypertension; consider discontinuing (temporary or permanent) in patients who develop severe or persistent hypertension while on appropriate antihypertensive therapy. May cause cardiac ischemia or infarction; consider discontinuing (temporarily or permanently) in patients who develop these; use in patients with unstable coronary artery disease or recent myocardial infarction has not been studied. QT prolongation has been observed; may increase the risk for ventricular arrhythmia. Avoid use in patients with congenital long QT syndrome; use with caution and monitor closely in patients with heart failure, bradyarrhythmias, concurrent medications know to prolong the QT interval, and electrolyte (calcium, magnesium, potassium) imbalances.

Serious bleeding events may occur (consider permanently discontinuing if serious); monitor PT/INR in patients on warfarin therapy. May complicate wound healing; temporarily withhold treatment for patients undergoing major surgical procedures (the appropriate timing for reinitiation after surgical procedures has not been determined). Gastrointestinal perforation has been reported (rare); monitor patients for signs/symptoms (abdominal pain, constipation, or vomiting); discontinue treatment if gastrointestinal perforation occurs. Avoid concurrent use with strong CYP3A4 inducers (eg, carbamazepine, dexamethasone, phenobarbital, phenytoin, rifampin, St John's wort); may decrease sorafenib levels/effects. Use caution when administering sorafenib with compounds that are metabolized predominantly via UGT1A1 (eg, irinotecan). Use in combination with carboplatin and paclitaxel in patients with squamous cell lung cancer is contraindicated.

Hand-foot skin reaction and rash are the most common adverse events and typically appear within the first 6 weeks of treatment; usually managed with topical treatment, treatment delays, and/or dose reductions. Consider permanently discontinuing with severe or persistent dermatological toxicities. The risk for hand-foot syndrome increased with cumulative doses of sorafenib. The incidence of hand-foot syndrome is also increased in patients treated with sorafenib plus bevacizumab in comparison to those treated with sorafenib monotherapy. Sorafenib levels in patients with mild-to-moderate hepatic impairment (Child-Pugh classes A and B) were similar to levels observed in patients without hepatic impairment; has not been studied in patients with severe hepatic impairment. In a small study of Asian patients with advanced HCC, sorafenib demonstrated efficacy with adequate tolerability in a hepatitis B-endemic area (Yau, 2009). There have been reports of sorafenib-induced hepatitis, including hepatic failure and death.

Drug Interactions

Avoid Concomitant Use

Avoid concomitant use of SORAfenib with any of the following: BCG; CARBOplatin; CloZAPine; CYP3A4 Inducers (Strong); Natalizumab; PACLitaxel; Pimecrolimus; St Johns Wort; Tacrolimus (Topical); Vaccines (Live)

Decreased Effect

SORAfenib may decrease the levels/effects of: BCG; Cardiac Glycosides; Coccidioidin Skin Test; Dacarbazine; Fluorouracil; Fluorouracil (Systemic); Fluorouracil (Topical); Sipuleucel-T; Vaccines (Inactivated); Vaccines (Live); Vitamin K Antagonists

The levels/effects of SORAfenib may be decreased by: CYP3A4 Inducers (Strong); Echinacea; Herbs (CYP3A4 Inducers); Neomycin; St Johns Wort; Tocilizumab

Increased Effect/Toxicity

SORAfenib may increase the levels/effects of: Acetaminophen; CARBOplatin; Carvedilol; CloZAPine; CYP2B6 Substrates; CYP2C8 Substrates; CYP2C9 Substrates; DOCEtaxel; DOXOrubicin; Fluorouracil; Fluorouracil (Systemic); Fluorouracil (Topical); Irinotecan; Leflunomide; Natalizumab; PACLitaxel; Treprostinil; Vaccines (Live); Vitamin K Antagonists; Warfarin

The levels/effects of SORAfenib may be increased by: Acetaminophen; Bevacizumab; CYP3A4 Inhibitors (Strong); Denosumab; Pimecrolimus; Roflumilast; Tacrolimus (Topical); Trastuzumab

Nutritional/Ethanol Interactions

Food: Bioavailability is decreased 29% with a high-fat meal (bioavailability is similar to fasting state when administered with a moderate-fat meal). Management: Administer on an empty stomach 1 hour before or 2 hours after eating.

Herb/Nutraceutical: St John's wort may decrease the levels/effects of sorafenib. Management: Avoid St John's wort.

Adverse Reactions

>10%:

Cardiovascular: Hypertension (9% to 17%; grade 3: 3% to 4%; grade 4: <1%; onset: ~3 weeks)

Central nervous system: Fatigue (37% to 46%), sensory neuropathy (≤13%), pain (11%)

Dermatologic: Rash/desquamation (19% to 40%; grade 3: ≤1%), hand-foot syndrome (21% to 30%; grade 3: 6% to 8%), alopecia (14% to 27%), pruritus (14% to 19%), dry skin (10% to 11%), erythema

Endocrine & metabolic: Hypoalbuminemia (≤59%), hypophosphatemia (35% to 45%; grade 3: 11% to 13%; grade 4: <1%)

Gastrointestinal: Diarrhea (43% to 55%; grade 3: 2% to 10%; grade 4: <1%), lipase increased (40% to 41% [usually transient]), amylase increased (30% to 34% [usually transient]), abdominal pain (11% to 31%), weight loss (10% to 30%), anorexia (16% to 29%), nausea (23% to 24%), vomiting (15% to 16%), constipation (14% to 15%)

Hematologic: Lymphopenia (23% to 47%; grades 3/4: ≤13%), thrombocytopenia (12% to 46%; grades 3/4: 1% to 4%), INR increased (≤42%), neutropenia (≤18%; grades 3/4: ≤5%), hemorrhage (15% to 18%; grade 3: 2% to 3%; grade 4: ≤2%), leukopenia

Hepatic: Liver dysfunction (≤11%; grade 3: 2%; grade 4: 1%)

Neuromuscular & skeletal: Muscle pain, weakness

Respiratory: Dyspnea (≤14%), cough (≤13%)

1% to 10%:

Cardiovascular: Cardiac ischemia/infarction (≤3%), heart failure (2%; congestive), flushing

Central nervous system: Headache (≤10%), depression, fever

Dermatologic: Acne, exfoliative dermatitis

Gastrointestinal: Appetite decreased, dyspepsia, dysphagia, esophageal varices bleeding (2%), glossodynia, mucositis, stomatitis, xerostomia

Genitourinary: Erectile dysfunction

Hematologic: Anemia

Hepatic: Transaminases increased (transient)

Neuromuscular & skeletal: Joint pain (≤10%), arthralgia, myalgia

Renal: Renal failure

Respiratory: Hoarseness

Miscellaneous: Flu-like syndrome

Available Dosage Forms

Tablet, oral:

NexAVAR®: 200 mg

General Dosage Range Dosage adjustments recommended in patients with hepatic or renal impairment, or who develop toxicities

Oral: *Adults:* 400 mg twice daily

Administration

Oral Administer on an empty stomach (1 hour before or 2 hours after eating).

Stability

Storage Store at room temperature of 25°C (77°F); excursions permitted to 15°C and 30°C (59°F and 86°F). Protect from moisture.

Nursing Actions

Physical Assessment Monitor for gastrointestinal perforation (abdominal pain, constipation, vomiting), diarrhea, fatigue, rash, or hand-foot syndrome; dosing adjustments may be necessary.

Patient Education Take on an empty stomach 1 hour before or 2 hours after eating. You may need periodic laboratory tests while taking this medication. Maintain adequate hydration unless instructed to restrict fluid intake. You may experience loss of appetite, nausea, vomiting, diarrhea, or hair loss (may grow back when treatment is discontinued). Report immediately persistent or acute headache, dizziness, or vision changes (monitor blood pressure if recommended by prescriber); chest pain or palpitations; or unusual bleeding. Report unusual skin rash; hand and foot syndrome (redness, tenderness, dryness, peeling, numbness, or tingling of the palms and soles); persistent gastrointestinal upset (diarrhea, constipation, abdominal pain); unusual or persistent cough; bone, joint, or muscle weakness or pain or loss of sensation; or flu-like symptoms.

Dietary Considerations Take without food (1 hour before or 2 hours after eating).

Sorbitol (SOR bi tole)

Pharmacologic Category Genitourinary Irrigant; Laxative, Osmotic

Pregnancy Risk Factor C

Lactation Excretion in breast milk unknown

Use Genitourinary irrigant in transurethral prostatic resection or other transurethral resection or other transurethral surgical procedures; diuretic; humectant; sweetening agent; hyperosmotic laxative; facilitate the passage of sodium polystyrene sulfonate through the intestinal tract

Available Dosage Forms

Solution, genitourinary irrigation [preservative free]: 3% (3000 mL, 5000 mL); 3.3% (2000 mL, 4000 mL)

Solution, oral: 70% (30 mL, 473 mL, 480 mL, 3840 mL)

General Dosage Range

Oral:

Children 2-11 years: 2 mL/kg (70% solution) as a single dose

Children ≥12 years and Adults: 30-150 mL (70% solution) as a single dose

Rectal:

Children 2-11 years: 30-60 mL (25% to 30% solution) as a single dose

Children ≥12 years and Adults: 120 mL (25% to 30% solution) as a single dose

Topical: *Adults:* 3% to 3.3% as a transurethral irrigation

Nursing Actions

Physical Assessment When used as cathartic, determine cause of constipation before use.

Sotalol (SOE ta lole)

Brand Names: U.S. Betapace AF®; Betapace®; Sorine®

Index Terms Sotalol Hydrochloride

Pharmacologic Category Antiarrhythmic Agent, Class II; Antiarrhythmic Agent, Class III; Beta-Adrenergic Blocker, Nonselective

Medication Safety Issues

Sound-alike/look-alike issues:

Sotalol may be confused with Stadol, Sudafed®

Betapace® may be confused with Betapace AF®

Pregnancy Risk Factor B

Lactation Enters breast milk/consider risk:benefit (AAP rates "compatible"; AAP 2001 update pending)

Breast-Feeding Considerations Sotalol is excreted into breast milk in concentrations higher than those found in the maternal serum. Although adverse events in nursing infants have not been observed in case reports, close monitoring for bradycardia, hypotension, respiratory distress, and hypoglycemia is advised. According to the manufacturer, the decision to continue or discontinue breast-feeding during therapy should take into account the risk of exposure to the infant and the benefits of treatment to the mother.

Use Treatment of documented ventricular arrhythmias (ie, sustained ventricular tachycardia), that in the judgment of the physician are life-threatening; maintenance of normal sinus rhythm in patients with symptomatic atrial fibrillation and atrial flutter who are currently in sinus rhythm. Manufacturer states substitutions should not be made for Betapace AF® since Betapace AF® is distributed with a patient package insert specific for atrial fibrillation/flutter.

Injection: Substitution for oral sotalol in those who are unable to take sotalol orally

Unlabeled Use Fetal tachycardia; alternative antiarrhythmic for the treatment of atrial fibrillation in patients with hypertrophic cardiomyopathy (HCM)

Mechanism of Action/Effect

Beta-blocker which contains both beta-adrenoreceptor-blocking (Vaughan Williams Class II) and cardiac action potential duration prolongation (Vaughan Williams Class III) properties

Class II effects: Increased sinus cycle length, slowed heart rate, decreased AV nodal conduction, and increased AV nodal refractoriness

Class III effects: Prolongation of the atrial and ventricular monophasic action potentials, and effective refractory prolongation of atrial muscle, ventricular muscle, and atrioventricular accessory pathways in both the antegrade and retrograde directions

Contraindications Hypersensitivity to sotalol or any component of the formulation; bronchial asthma; sinus bradycardia; second- or third-degree AV block (unless a functioning pacemaker is present); congenital or acquired long QT syndromes; cardiogenic shock; uncontrolled heart failure

Additional contraindications: Betapace AF® and the injectable formulation: Baseline QT_c interval >450 msec; bronchospastic conditions; Cl_{cr} <40 mL/minute; serum potassium <4 mEq/L; sick sinus syndrome

Warnings/Precautions [U.S. Boxed Warning] Manufacturer recommends initiation (or reinitiation) and doses increased in a hospital setting with continuous monitoring and staff familiar with the recognition and treatment of life-threatening arrhythmias. Some experts will initiate therapy on an outpatient basis in a patient without heart disease or bradycardia, who has a baseline uncorrected QT interval <450 msec, and normal serum potassium and magnesium levels; close ECG monitoring during this time is necessary. ACC/AHA guidelines for management of atrial fibrillation also recommend that for outpatient initiation the patient not have risk factors predisposing to drug-induced ventricular proarrhythmia (Fuster, 2006). Dosage should be adjusted gradually with 3 days between dosing increments to achieve steady-state concentrations, and to allow time to monitor QT intervals. **[U.S. Boxed Warning]: Adjust dosing interval based on creatinine clearance to decrease risk of proarrhythmia; QT interval prolongation is directly related to sotalol concentration.** Creatinine clearance must be calculated with dose initiation and dose increases. Use cautiously in the renally-impaired (dosage adjustment required). Betapace AF® and the injectable formulation are contraindicated in patients with Cl_{cr} <40 mL/minute.

[U.S. Boxed Warning]: Sotalol injection: Sotalol can cause life-threatening ventricular tachycardia associated with QT-interval prolongation (ie, torsade de pointes). Do not initiate if baseline QTc interval is >450 msec. If QT_c exceeds 500 msec during therapy, reduce the dose, prolong the infusion duration, or discontinue use. If while on oral sotalol therapy baseline QT_c interval is >500 msec, use I.V. sotalol with particular caution; serious consideration should be given to reducing the dose or discontinuing I.V. sotalol when QT_c exceeds 520 msec. QT_c prolongation is directly related to the concentration of sotalol; reduced creatinine clearance, female gender, and large doses increase the risk of QT_c prolongation and subsequent torsade de pointes. Monitor and adjust dose to prevent QT_c prolongation. Concurrent use with other QT_c-prolonging drugs (including Class I and Class III antiarrhythmics) and use within 3 months of discontinuing amiodarone is generally not recommended. To reduce the chance of excessive QT_c-prolongation, withhold QT_c-prolonging drugs for at least 3 half-lives (or 3 months for amiodarone) before initiating sotalol.

Correct electrolyte imbalances before initiating (especially hypokalemia and hypomagnesemia). Consider pre-existing conditions such as sick sinus syndrome before initiating. Conduction abnormalities can occur particularly sinus bradycardia. Use cautiously within the first 2 weeks post-MI especially in patients with markedly impaired ventricular function (experience limited). Administer cautiously in compensated heart failure and monitor for a worsening of the condition. May precipitate or aggravate symptoms of arterial insufficiency in patients with PVD and Raynaud's disease; use with caution and monitor for progression of arterial obstruction. Bradycardia may be observed more frequently in elderly patients (>65 years of age); dosage reductions may be necessary. Beta-blocker therapy should not be withdrawn abruptly (particularly in patients with CAD), but gradually tapered to avoid acute tachycardia, hypertension, and/or ischemia. Chronic beta-blocker therapy should not be routinely withdrawn prior to major surgery. Use caution with concurrent use of digoxin, verapamil, or diltiazem; bradycardia or heart block can occur. Use with caution in patients receiving inhaled anesthetic agents known to depress myocardial contractility. Use cautiously in diabetics because it can mask prominent hypoglycemic symptoms. Use with caution in patients with bronchospastic disease, myasthenia gravis or psychiatric disease. Adequate alpha-blockade is required prior to use of any beta-blocker for patients with untreated pheochromocytoma. May mask signs of hyperthyroidism (eg, tachycardia); if hyperthyroidism is suspected, carefully manage and monitor; abrupt withdrawal may exacerbate symptoms of hyperthyroidism or precipitate thyroid storm. Use caution with history of severe anaphylaxis to allergens; patients taking beta-blockers may become more sensitive to repeated challenges. Treatment of anaphylaxis (eg, epinephrine) in patients taking beta-blockers may be ineffective or promote undesirable effects.

[U.S. Boxed Warning]: Betapace® should not be substituted for Betapace® AF; Betapace® AF is distributed with an educational insert specifically for patients with atrial fibrillation/flutter.

Drug Interactions

Avoid Concomitant Use

Avoid concomitant use of Sotalol with any of the following: Artemether; Beta2-Agonists; Dronedarone; Floctafenine; Lumefantrine; Methacholine; Nilotinib; Pimozide; QUEtiapine; QuiNINE; Tetrabenazine; Thioridazine; Toremifene; Vandetanib; Vemurafenib; Ziprasidone

Decreased Effect

Sotalol may decrease the levels/effects of: Beta2-Agonists; Theophylline Derivatives

The levels/effects of Sotalol may be decreased by: Barbiturates; Herbs (Hypertensive Properties); Methylphenidate; Nonsteroidal Anti-Inflammatory Agents; Rifamycin Derivatives; Yohimbine

Increased Effect/Toxicity

Sotalol may increase the levels/effects of: Alpha-/Beta-Agonists (Direct-Acting); Alpha1-Blockers; Alpha2-Agonists; Amifostine; Antihypertensives; Antipsychotic Agents (Phenothiazines); Bupivacaine; Cardiac Glycosides; Cholinergic Agonists; ▶

Dronedarone; Fingolimod; Hypotensive Agents; Insulin; Lidocaine; Lidocaine (Systemic); Lidocaine (Topical); Mepivacaine; Methacholine; Midodrine; Pimozide; QTc-Prolonging Agents; QuiNINE; RiTUXimab; Sulfonylureas; Tetrabenazine; Thioridazine; Toremifene; Vandetanib; Vemurafenib; Ziprasidone

The levels/effects of Sotalol may be increased by: Acetylcholinesterase Inhibitors; Alfuzosin; Aminoquinolines (Antimalarial); Amiodarone; Anilidopiperidine Opioids; Antipsychotic Agents (Phenothiazines); Artemether; Calcium Channel Blockers (Dihydropyridine); Calcium Channel Blockers (Nondihydropyridine); Chloroquine; Ciprofloxacin; Ciprofloxacin (Systemic); Diazoxide; Dipyridamole; Disopyramide; Dronedarone; Eribulin; Fingolimod; Floctafenine; Gadobutrol; Herbs (Hypotensive Properties); Indacaterol; Lidocaine (Topical); Lumefantrine; MAO Inhibitors; Nilotinib; Pentoxifylline; Phosphodiesterase 5 Inhibitors; Propafenone; Prostacyclin Analogues; QUEtiapine; QuiNIDine; QuiNINE; Reserpine

Nutritional/Ethanol Interactions

Food: Sotalol peak serum concentrations may be decreased if taken with food.

Herb/Nutraceutical: Avoid ephedra (may worsen arrhythmia).

Adverse Reactions Note: No clinical experience with I.V. sotalol; however, since exposure is similar between I.V. and oral sotalol, adverse reactions are expected to be similar.

>10%:

Cardiovascular: Bradycardia (13% to 16%), chest pain (3% to 16%), palpitation (14%)

Central nervous system: Fatigue (20%), dizziness (20%), lightheadedness (12%)

Neuromuscular & skeletal: Weakness (13%)

Respiratory: Dyspnea (21%)

1% to 10%:

Cardiovascular: Edema (8%), abnormal ECG (7%), hypotension (6%), proarrhythmia (5%), syncope (5%), CHF (5%), torsade de pointes (dose related; 1% to 4%), peripheral vascular disorders (3%), ventricular tachycardia worsened (1%), QT_c interval prolongation (dose related)

Central nervous system: Headache (8%), sleep problems (8%), mental confusion (6%), anxiety (4%), depression (4%)

Dermatologic: Itching/rash (5%)

Endocrine & metabolic: Sexual ability decreased (3%)

Gastrointestinal: Nausea/vomiting (10%), diarrhea (7%), stomach discomfort (3% to 6%), flatulence (2%)

Genitourinary: Impotence (2%)

Hematologic: Bleeding (2%)

Neuromuscular & skeletal: Extremity pain (7%), paresthesia (4%), back pain (3%)

Ocular: Visual problems (5%)

Respiratory: Upper respiratory problems (5% to 8%), asthma (2%)

Pharmacodynamics/Kinetics

Onset of Action Oral: Rapid, 1-2 hours; when administered I.V. for ongoing VT over 5 minutes, onset of action is ~5-10 minutes (Ho, 1994)

Duration of Action 8-16 hours

Available Dosage Forms

Injection, solution [preservative free]: 15 mg/mL (10 mL)

Tablet, oral: 80 mg, 120 mg, 160 mg, 240 mg

Betapace AF®: 80 mg, 120 mg, 160 mg

Betapace®: 80 mg, 120 mg, 160 mg, 240 mg

Sorine®: 80 mg, 120 mg, 160 mg, 240 mg

General Dosage Range Dosage adjustment recommended in patients with renal impairment or who develop toxicities

I.V.: *Adults:* Initial: 75 mg twice daily; Maintenance: 75-150 mg twice daily (maximum: 300 mg/day)

Oral:

Children ≤2 years: Dosage should be adjusted (decreased) by plotting of the child's age on a logarithmic scale; **Note:** Refer to manufacturer's package labeling

Children >2 years: Initial: 90 mg/m²/day in 3 divided doses; Maintenance: 90-180 mg/m²/day in 3 divided doses (maximum: 180 mg/m²/day)

Adults: Initial: 80 mg twice daily; Maintenance: 240-320 mg/day in 2-3 divided doses (maximum: 320 mg/day)

Administration

Oral Administer without regard to meals.

I.V.

Substitution for oral: Administer over 5 hours.

Hemodynamically stable monomorphic VT: Administer I.V. push over 5 minutes; use with caution due to increased risk of adverse events (eg, bradycardia, hypotension, torsade de pointes) (ACLS, 2010)

Stability

Storage Store at 25°C (77°F); excursions permitted to 15°C to 30°C (59°F to 86°F). To prepare sotalol infusion, see manufacturer's prescribing information.

Nursing Actions

Physical Assessment Monitor laboratory tests, blood pressure, and heart rate prior to and following first dose and with any change in dosage. Monitor cardiac and pulmonary status. Advise patients with diabetes to monitor glucose levels closely; beta-blockers may alter glucose tolerance. Should not be stopped abruptly; dose should be tapered gradually when discontinuing. Teach patient hypotension precautions.

Patient Education Take pulse daily (prior to medication) and follow prescriber's instruction about holding of medication. If you have diabetes, monitor serum sugar closely; drug may alter glucose tolerance or mask signs of hypoglycemia.

May cause fatigue, dizziness, lightheadedness, postural hypotension, alteration in sexual performance (reversible), nausea, vomiting, or diarrhea. Report immediately any chest pain, palpitations, irregular heartbeat; swelling of extremities, weight gain, respiratory difficulty, new cough, or unusual fatigue; persistent nausea, vomiting, or diarrhea; or unusual muscle weakness.

Dietary Considerations May be taken without regard to meals.

Spinosad (SPIN oh sad)

Brand Names: U.S. Natroba™

Index Terms NatrOVA

Pharmacologic Category Antiparasitic Agent, Topical; Pediculocide

Pregnancy Risk Factor B

Lactation Use caution

Use Topical treatment of head lice (*Pediculosis capitis*) infestation in adults and children ≥4 years of age

Unlabeled Use Topical treatment of head lice (*Pediculosis capitis*) infestation in children ≥6 months and <4 years of age

Available Dosage Forms

Suspension, topical:

Natroba™: 0.9% (120 mL)

General Dosage Range Topical: *Children ≥4 years old and Adults:* Apply sufficient amount to cover dry scalp and hair; may repeat in 7 days

Administration

Topical Topical suspension. For external use only. Shake bottle well. Apply to dry scalp and rub gently until the scalp is thoroughly moistened, then apply to dry hair; completely covering scalp and hair. Leave on for 10 minutes (start timing treatment after the scalp and hair have been completely covered). The hair should then be rinsed thoroughly with warm water. Shampoo may be used immediately after the product is completely rinsed off. If live lice are seen 7 days after the first treatment, repeat with second application. Avoid contact with the eyes. Nit combing is not required, although a fine-tooth comb may be used to remove treated lice and nits.

Spinosad should be a portion of a whole lice removal program, which should include washing or dry cleaning all clothing, hats, bedding and towels recently worn or used by the patient and washing combs, brushes and hair accessories in hot water.

Spironolactone (speer on oh LAK tone)

Brand Names: U.S. Aldactone®

Pharmacologic Category Diuretic, Potassium-Sparing; Selective Aldosterone Blocker

Medication Safety Issues

Sound-alike/look-alike issues:

Aldactone® may be confused with Aldactazide®

International issues:

Aldactone: Brand name for spironolactone [U.S., Canada, multiple international markets], but also the brand name for potassium canrenoate [Austria, Czech Republic, Germany, Hungary, Poland]

Pregnancy Risk Factor C

Lactation Enters breast milk/not recommended (AAP rates "compatible"; AAP 2001 update pending)

Breast-Feeding Considerations The active metabolite of spironolactone has been found in breast milk. Effects to humans are not known; however, this metabolite was found to be carcinogenic in rats. The manufacturer recommends discontinuing spironolactone or using an alternative method of feeding.

Use Management of edema associated with excessive aldosterone excretion; hypertension; primary hyperaldosteronism; hypokalemia; cirrhosis of liver accompanied by edema or ascites; nephrotic syndrome; severe heart failure (NYHA class III-IV) to increase survival and reduce hospitalization when added to standard therapy

Unlabeled Use Female acne (adjunctive therapy); hirsutism; hypertension (pediatric); diuretic (pediatric)

Mechanism of Action/Effect Competes with aldosterone for receptor sites in the distal renal tubules, increasing sodium chloride and water excretion while conserving potassium and hydrogen ions; may block the effect of aldosterone on arteriolar smooth muscle as well

Contraindications Anuria; acute renal insufficiency; significant impairment of renal excretory function; hyperkalemia

Warnings/Precautions Monitor serum potassium closely in patients being treated for heart failure. Avoid potassium supplements, potassium-containing salt substitutes, a diet rich in potassium, or other drugs that can cause hyperkalemia. Excess amounts can lead to profound diuresis with fluid and electrolyte loss; close medical supervision and dose evaluation are required. Watch for and correct electrolyte disturbances; adjust dose to avoid dehydration. In cirrhosis, avoid electrolyte and acid/base imbalances that might lead to hepatic encephalopathy. Gynecomastia is related to dose and duration of therapy. Discontinue use prior to adrenal vein catheterization. When evaluating a heart failure patient for spironolactone treatment, creatinine should be ≤2.5 mg/dL in men or ≤2 mg/dL in women and potassium <5 mEq/L. Discontinue or interrupt therapy if serum potassium >5 mEq/L or serum creatinine >4 mg/dL. **[U.S. Boxed Warning]: Shown to be a tumorigen in chronic toxicity animal studies. Avoid unnecessary use.**

Drug Interactions

Avoid Concomitant Use

Avoid concomitant use of Spironolactone with any of the following: CycloSPORINE; CycloSPORINE (Systemic); Tacrolimus; Tacrolimus (Systemic)

Decreased Effect

Spironolactone may decrease the levels/effects of: Alpha-/Beta-Agonists; Cardiac Glycosides; Mitotane; QuiNIDine

The levels/effects of Spironolactone may be decreased by: Herbs (Hypertensive Properties); Methylphenidate; Nonsteroidal Anti-Inflammatory Agents; Yohimbine

Increased Effect/Toxicity

Spironolactone may increase the levels/effects of: ACE Inhibitors; Amifostine; Ammonium Chloride; Antihypertensives; Cardiac Glycosides; CycloSPORINE; CycloSPORINE (Systemic); Digoxin; Hypotensive Agents; Neuromuscular-Blocking Agents (Nondepolarizing); RiTUXimab; Sodium Phosphates; Tacrolimus; Tacrolimus (Systemic)

The levels/effects of Spironolactone may be increased by: Alfuzosin; Angiotensin II Receptor Blockers; Diazoxide; Drospirenone; Eplerenone; Herbs (Hypotensive Properties); MAO Inhibitors; Nitrofurantoin; Nonsteroidal Anti-Inflammatory Agents; Pentoxifylline; Phosphodiesterase 5 Inhibitors; Potassium Salts; Prostacyclin Analogues; Tolvaptan; Trimethoprim

Nutritional/Ethanol Interactions

Ethanol: Increases risk of orthostasis.

Food: Food increases absorption.

Herb/Nutraceutical: Avoid natural licorice (due to mineralocorticoid activity)

Adverse Reactions Frequency not defined.

Cardiovascular: Vasculitis

Central nervous system: Ataxia, confusion, drowsiness, fever, headache, lethargy

Dermatologic: Drug rash with eosinophilia and systemic symptoms (DRESS), maculopapular or erythematous cutaneous eruptions, Stevens-Johnson syndrome, toxic epidermal necrolysis, urticaria

Endocrine & metabolic: Amenorrhea, gynecomastia, hyperkalemia, impotence, irregular menses, postmenopausal bleeding

Gastrointestinal: Cramps, diarrhea, gastritis, gastric bleeding, nausea, ulceration, vomiting

Hematologic: Agranulocytosis

Hepatic: Cholestatic/hepatocellular toxicity

Renal: BUN increased, renal dysfunction, renal failure

Miscellaneous: Anaphylactic reaction, breast cancer

Pharmacodynamics/Kinetics

Duration of Action 2-3 days

Available Dosage Forms

Tablet, oral: 25 mg, 50 mg, 100 mg

Aldactone®: 25 mg, 50 mg, 100 mg

General Dosage Range Dosage adjustment recommended in patients with renal impairment

Oral:

Adults: 12.5-400 mg/day in 1-2 divided doses

Elderly: Initial: 25-50 mg/day in 1-2 divided doses

Stability

Storage Store below 25°C (77°F).

Nursing Actions

Physical Assessment Diuretic effect may be delayed 2-3 days. Monitor serum electrolytes on a regular basis during therapy. Assess fluid status and monitor for CNS changes (drowsiness, headache, confusion), rash, gynecomastia, and hyperkalemia during therapy.

Patient Education Take with meals. Avoid any potassium supplements (vitamin/mineral products), potassium-containing salt substitutes, natural licorice, or extra dietary intake of potassium. Weigh yourself weekly and report weight loss. May cause dizziness, drowsiness, confusion, headache, nausea, vomiting, dry mouth, or gynecomastia. Report mental confusion; clumsiness; persistent fatigue, chills, numbness, or muscle weakness in hands, feet, or face; acute persistent diarrhea; chest pain, rapid heartbeat, or palpitations; excessive thirst; respiratory difficulty; or inability to achieve erection in males.

Dietary Considerations Should be taken with food to decrease gastrointestinal irritation and to increase absorption. Excessive potassium intake (eg, salt substitutes, low-salt foods, bananas, nuts) should be avoided.

Stavudine (STAV yoo deen)

Brand Names: U.S. Zerit®

Index Terms d4T

Pharmacologic Category Antiretroviral Agent, Reverse Transcriptase Inhibitor (Nucleoside)

Medication Safety Issues

Sound-alike/look-alike issues:

Zerit® may be confused with Zestril®, Ziac®, ZyrTEC®

Medication Guide Available Yes

Pregnancy Risk Factor C

Lactation Excretion in breast milk unknown/contraindicated

Breast-Feeding Considerations Maternal or infant antiretroviral therapy does not completely eliminate the risk of postnatal HIV transmission. In addition, multiclass-resistant virus has been detected in breast-feeding infants despite maternal therapy. Therefore, in the United States, where formula is accessible, affordable, safe, and sustainable, and the risk of infant mortality due to diarrhea and respiratory infections is low, complete avoidance of breast-feeding by HIV-infected women is recommended to decrease potential transmission of HIV (DHHS [perinatal], 2011).

Use Treatment of HIV infection in combination with other antiretroviral agents

Mechanism of Action/Effect Inhibits reverse transcriptase of the human immunodeficiency virus (HIV)

Contraindications Hypersensitivity to stavudine or any component of the formulation

Warnings/Precautions Use with caution in patients who demonstrate previous hypersensitivity to zidovudine, didanosine, zalcitabine, pre-existing bone marrow suppression, renal insufficiency (dosage adjustment recommended), hepatic impairment, or peripheral neuropathy. Peripheral neuropathy may be a treatment-limiting side effect; consider permanent discontinuation. Zidovudine should not be used in combination with stavudine. **[U.S. Boxed Warning]: Lactic acidosis and severe hepatomegaly with steatosis have been reported with stavudine use, including fatal cases;** combination therapy with didanosine may increase risk; use with caution in patients with risk factors for liver disease (although acidosis has occurred in patients without known risk factors, risk may be increased with female gender, obesity, pregnancy, or prolonged exposure). Suspend treatment in any patient who develops clinical or laboratory findings suggestive of lactic acidosis or hepatotoxicity. Mortality of 50% associated in some case series, notably with serum lactate >10 mmol/L (DHHS, 2011). Severe motor weakness (resembling Guillain-Barré syndrome) has been reported (including fatal cases, usually in association with lactic acidosis); manufacturer recommends discontinuation if motor weakness develops (with or without lactic acidosis). May cause redistribution of fat (eg, buffalo hump, peripheral wasting with increased abdominal girth, cushingoid appearance). Patients may develop immune reconstitution syndrome resulting in the occurrence of an inflammatory response to an indolent or residual opportunistic infection; further evaluation and treatment may be required. **[U.S. Boxed Warning]: Pancreatitis (including some fatal cases) has occurred during combination therapy with didanosine.** Suspend stavudine and didanosine combination therapy, and any other agents toxic to the pancreas, in patients with suspected pancreatitis. If pancreatitis diagnosis confirmed, use extreme caution if reinitiating stavudine; monitor closely and do not use didanosine in regimen. Use with caution in combination with interferon alfa with or without ribavirin in HIV/HBV coinfected patients; monitor closely for hepatic decompensation, anemia, or neutropenia; dose reduction or discontinuation of interferon and/or ribavirin may be required if toxicity evident. Combination therapy with didanosine or hydroxyurea may increase risk of hepatotoxicity, pancreatitis, or severe peripheral neuropathy; avoid stavudine or hydroxyurea combination.

Drug Interactions

Avoid Concomitant Use

Avoid concomitant use of Stavudine with any of the following: Hydroxyurea; Zidovudine

Decreased Effect

The levels/effects of Stavudine may be decreased by: DOXOrubicin; DOXOrubicin (Liposomal); Zidovudine

Increased Effect/Toxicity

Stavudine may increase the levels/effects of: Didanosine; Hydroxyurea

The levels/effects of Stavudine may be increased by: Hydroxyurea; Ribavirin

Adverse Reactions Adverse reactions reported below represent experience with combination therapy with other nucleoside analogues and protease inhibitors.

>10%:

Central nervous system: Headache (25% to 46%)

Dermatologic: Rash (18% to 30%)

Gastrointestinal: Nausea (43% to 53%; less than comparator group), vomiting (18% to 30%; less than comparator group), diarrhea (34% to 45%)

Hepatic: Hyperbilirubinemia (65% to 68%; grade 3/4: 7% to 16%), AST increased (42% to 53%; grade 3/4: 5% to 7%), ALT increased (40% to 50%; grade 3/4: 6% to 8%), GGT increased (15% to 28%; grade 3/4: 2% to 5%)

Neuromuscular & skeletal: Peripheral neuropathy (8% to 21%)

Miscellaneous: Amylase increased (21% to 31%; grade 3/4: 4% to 8%), lipase increased (~27%; grade 3/4: 5% to 6%)

Available Dosage Forms

Capsule, oral: 15 mg, 20 mg, 30 mg, 40 mg

Zerit®: 15 mg, 20 mg, 30 mg, 40 mg

Powder for solution, oral:

Zerit®: 1 mg/mL (200 mL)

General Dosage Range Dosage adjustment recommended in patients with renal impairment.

Oral:

Newborns (Birth to 13 days): 0.5 mg/kg every 12 hours

Children ≥14 days and <30 kg: 1 mg/kg every 12 hours

Children and Adults 30-59 kg: 30 mg every 12 hours

Children and Adults ≥60 kg: 40 mg every 12 hours

Administration

Oral May be administered without regard to meals. Oral solution should be shaken vigorously prior to use.

Stability

Reconstitution Reconstitute powder for oral suspension with 202 mL of purified water as specified on the bottle. Shake vigorously until suspended. Final suspension will be 1 mg/mL (200 mL).

Storage Capsules and powder for reconstitution may be stored at controlled room temperature of 25°C (77°F). Reconstituted oral solution should be stored in refrigerator at 2°C to 8°C (36°F to 46°F) and is stable for 30 days.

Nursing Actions

Physical Assessment Allergy history should be assessed prior to beginning treatment. Monitor patient closely for peripheral neuropathy, lactic acidosis, hepatomegaly, and motor weakness; may require suspension of therapy. Teach patient proper timing of multiple medications.

Patient Education This drug will not cure HIV, nor has it been found to reduce transmission of HIV; use appropriate precautions to prevent spread to other persons. This drug is prescribed as one part of a multidrug combination; take exactly as directed, for full course of therapy. Maintain adequate hydration unless advised by prescriber to restrict fluids. Frequent blood tests may be required. May cause dizziness, weakness, nausea, or vomiting. Report immediately any tingling, pain, or loss of sensation in hands or feet; alterations in urinary pattern; swelling of extremities; or weight gain. If you are instructed to stop the medication, do not restart without specific instruction by your prescriber.

Dietary Considerations May be taken without regard to meals. Some products may contain sucrose.

Streptozocin (strep toe ZOE sin)

Brand Names: U.S. Zanosar®

Pharmacologic Category Antineoplastic Agent, Alkylating Agent

Medication Safety Issues

Sound-alike/look-alike issues:

Streptozocin may be confused with streptomycin

High alert medication:

The Institute for Safe Medication Practices (ISMP) includes this medication among its list of drugs which have a heightened risk of causing significant patient harm when used in error.

Pregnancy Risk Factor D

Lactation Enters breast milk/contraindicated

Use Treatment of metastatic islet cell carcinoma of the pancreas

Unlabeled Use Treatment of adrenal tumors

Available Dosage Forms

Injection, powder for reconstitution:

Zanosar®: 1 g

General Dosage Range Dosage adjustment recommended in patients with renal impairment

I.V.: *Children and Adults:* 1-1.5 g/m^2 weekly for 6 weeks followed by a 4-week rest period **or** 0.5-1 g/m^2 for 5 consecutive days as combination therapy followed by a 4- to 6-week rest period

Administration

I.V. Administer as short (30-60 minutes) or 6-hour infusion; may be given by rapid I.V. push

I.V. Detail pH: 3.5-4.5

Nursing Actions

Physical Assessment Antiemetic should be administered prior to therapy (emetic potential 100%). Infusion site should be monitored closely to prevent extravasation. Monitor for nephrotoxicity (I & O, edema, hematuria, BUN), hepatotoxicity (jaundice, fatigue, LFTs), hypoglycemia, and diarrhea (dehydration) on a regular basis. Caution patients with diabetes to monitor glucose levels closely (may precipitate hypoglycemia).

Patient Education This drug can only be given I.V.; report immediately any redness, swelling, pain, or burning at infusion site. Maintain adequate hydration unless instructed to restrict fluid intake. You will be more sensitive to infection. If you have diabetes, monitor glucose levels closely; may cause hypoglycemia. May cause nausea and vomiting; nervousness, dizziness, confusion, or lethargy; or loss of body hair (reversible when treatment is finished). Report unusual back pain, change in urinary pattern; persistent fever, chills, or sore throat; unusual bleeding; blood in urine, vomitus, or stool; chest pain, palpitations, or respiratory difficulty; or swelling of feet or lower legs.

Related Information

Management of Drug Extravasations *on page 1269*

Succinylcholine (suks in il KOE leen)

Brand Names: U.S. Anectine®; Quelicin®

Index Terms Succinylcholine Chloride; Suxamethonium Chloride

Pharmacologic Category Neuromuscular Blocker Agent, Depolarizing

Medication Safety Issues

High alert medication:

The Institute for Safe Medication Practices (ISMP) includes this medication among its list of drugs which have a heightened risk of causing significant patient harm when used in error.

Other safety concerns:

United States Pharmacopeia (USP) 2006: The Interdisciplinary Safe Medication Use Expert Committee of the USP has recommended the following:

- Hospitals, clinics, and other practice sites should institute special safeguards in the storage, labeling, and use of these agents and should include these safeguards in staff orientation and competency training.

- Healthcare professionals should be on high alert (especially vigilant) whenever a neuromuscular-blocking agent (NMBA) is stocked, ordered, prepared, or administered.

International issues:

Quelicin [U.S., Brazil, Canada, Indonesia] may be confused with Keflin brand name for cefalotin [Argentina, Brazil, Mexico, Netherlands, Norway]

Pregnancy Risk Factor C

Lactation Excretion in breast milk unknown/use caution

Use To facilitate both rapid sequence and routine endotracheal intubation and to relax skeletal muscles during surgery

Note: Does not relieve pain or produce sedation

Unlabeled Use To reduce the intensity of muscle contractions of electroconvulsive therapy (ECT)

Available Dosage Forms

Injection, solution:

Anectine®: 20 mg/mL (10 mL)

Quelicin®: 20 mg/mL (10 mL)

Injection, solution [preservative free]:

Quelicin®: 100 mg/mL (10 mL)

General Dosage Range Dosage adjustment recommended in patients with renal or hepatic impairment

I.M.: *Children and Adults:* Up to 3-4 mg/kg (maximum: 150 mg total dose)

I.V.:

Smaller Children: Intermittent: Initial: 2 mg/kg/dose; Maintenance: 0.3-0.6 mg/kg/dose every 5-10 minutes as needed

Older Children and Adolescents: Intermittent: Initial: 1 mg/kg/dose; Maintenance: 0.3-0.6 mg/kg every 5-10 minutes as needed

Adults: Intubation: 0.6 mg/kg (range: 0.3-1.1 mg/kg); Rapid sequence intubation: 1-1.5 mg/kg

Administration

I.M. I.M. injections should be made deeply, preferably high into deltoid muscle. Use only when I.V. access is not available.

I.V. May be given by rapid I.V. injection without further dilution.

I.V. Detail pH: 3.0-4.5

Nursing Actions

Physical Assessment Ventilatory support must be instituted and maintained until adequate respiratory muscle function and/or airway protection are assured. This drug is not an anesthetic or analgesic; pain must be treated with appropriate analgesic agents. Continuous monitoring of vital signs, cardiac status, respiratory status, and degree of neuromuscular block (objective assessment with external nerve stimulator) is mandatory during infusion and until full muscle tone has returned. Safety precautions regarding ventilation must be maintained until full muscle tone has returned. Safety precautions regarding ventilation must be maintained until full muscle tone has returned.

Patient Education Patient will usually be unconscious prior to administration. Reassurance of constant monitoring and emotional support to reduce fear and anxiety should precede and follow administration. Following return of muscle tone, do not attempt to change position or rise from bed without assistance. Report immediately any skin rash or hives, pounding heartbeat, respiratory difficulty, or muscle tremors.

Sucralfate (soo KRAL fate)

Brand Names: U.S. Carafate®

Index Terms Aluminum Sucrose Sulfate, Basic

Pharmacologic Category Gastrointestinal Agent, Miscellaneous

Medication Safety Issues

Sound-alike/look-alike issues:

Sucralfate may be confused with salsalate

Carafate® may be confused with Cafergot®

Pregnancy Risk Factor B

Lactation Excretion in breast milk unknown/use caution

Use Short-term (≤8 weeks) management of duodenal ulcers; maintenance therapy for duodenal ulcers

Unlabeled Use Gastric ulcers; suspension may be used topically for treatment of stomatitis due to cancer chemotherapy and other causes of esophageal and gastric erosions; GERD, esophagitis; treatment of NSAID mucosal damage; prevention of stress ulcers; postsclerotherapy for esophageal variceal bleeding

Available Dosage Forms

Suspension, oral: 1 g/10 mL (10 mL)

Carafate®: 1 g/10 mL (420 mL)

Tablet, oral: 1 g

Carafate®: 1 g

General Dosage Range Oral: *Adults:* 1 g 2-4 times/day

Administration

Oral Tablet may be broken or dissolved in water before ingestion. Administer with water on an empty stomach.

Nursing Actions

Physical Assessment Teach patient proper timing of other medications. May cause constipation.

Patient Education Take recommended dose with water on an empty stomach, 1 hour before or 2 hours after meals. Take any other medications at least 2 hours before taking sucralfate. May cause constipation. If constipation persists, consult prescriber for stool softener.

SulfADIAZINE (sul fa DYE a zeen)

Pharmacologic Category Antibiotic, Sulfonamide Derivative

Medication Safety Issues

Sound-alike/look-alike issues:

SulfADIAZINE may be confused with sulfaSALAzine, sulfiSOXAZOLE

Pregnancy Risk Factor C

Lactation Enters breast milk/contraindicated

Use Treatment of the following conditions (per product labeling): Chancroid, trachoma, inclusion conjunctivitis, nocardiosis, urinary tract infections, toxoplasmosis encephalitis, malaria, meningococcal meningitis, acute otitis media, rheumatic fever (prophylaxis), meningitis (adjunctive)

Refer to current guidelines for appropriate use.

Available Dosage Forms

Tablet, oral: 500 mg

General Dosage Range Oral:

Children >2 months: Initial: 75 mg/kg; Maintenance: 150 mg/kg/day (maximum: 6 g/24 hours)

Children <30 kg and Adults <30 kg: 0.5 g/day (rheumatic fever prophylaxis)

Children ≥30 kg and Adults ≥30 kg: 1 g/day (rheumatic fever prophylaxis)

Adults: 2-4 g/day in divided doses

Administration

Oral Administer with at least 8 ounces of water and around-the-clock to promote less variation in peak and trough serum levels. Oral sodium bicarbonate may be used to alkalinize the urine of patients unable to maintain adequate fluid intake (in order to prevent crystalluria, azotemia, oliguria) (Lerner, 1996).

Nursing Actions

Physical Assessment Allergy history should be assessed prior to starting therapy (sulfonamides). Monitor for rash, photosensitivity, gastrointestinal disturbance (nausea, vomiting, anorexia), anemia, jaundice, and hematuria. Have patient call prescriber immediately if any signs of rash.

Patient Education Inform prescriber of any allergies you have. Take as directed at regular intervals around-the-clock. Take on an empty stomach, 1 hour before or 2 hours after meals with full glass of water. Maintain adequate hydration to prevent kidney damage, unless instructed to restrict fluid intake. May cause dizziness, headache, photosensitivity, nausea, vomiting, or loss of appetite. Notify prescriber of red, blistered, or swollen skin or red or purple patches under the skin; decreased urine or trouble urinating; persistent nausea; vomiting; diarrhea; opportunistic infection (sore throat, fever, vaginal itching or discharge, unusual bruising or bleeding, fatigue); dark urine; yellow skin or eyes; seizures; hallucinations; joint pain; persistent headache; abdominal pain; or respiratory difficulty.

Sulfamethoxazole and Trimethoprim

(sul fa meth OKS a zole & trye METH oh prim)

Brand Names: U.S. Bactrim™; Bactrim™ DS; Septra® DS

Index Terms Co-Trimoxazole; SMX-TMP; SMZ-TMP; Sulfatrim; TMP-SMX; TMP-SMZ; Trimethoprim and Sulfamethoxazole

Pharmacologic Category Antibiotic, Miscellaneous; Antibiotic, Sulfonamide Derivative

Medication Safety Issues

Sound-alike/look-alike issues:

Bactrim™ may be confused with bacitracin, Bactine®, Bactroban®

Co-trimoxazole may be confused with clotrimazole

Septra® may be confused with Ceptaz, Sectral®

Septra® DS may be confused with Semprex®-D

Pregnancy Risk Factor C

Lactation Enters breast milk/contraindicated (AAP rates "compatible"; AAP 2001 update pending)

Use

Oral treatment of urinary tract infections due to *E. coli*, *Klebsiella* and *Enterobacter* sp, *M. morganii*, *P. mirabilis* and *P. vulgaris*; acute otitis media in children; acute exacerbations of chronic bronchitis in adults due to susceptible strains of *H. influenzae* or *S. pneumoniae*; treatment and prophylaxis of *Pneumocystis jirovecii* pneumonia (PCP); traveler's diarrhea due to enterotoxigenic *E. coli*; treatment of enteritis caused by *Shigella flexneri* or *Shigella sonnei*

I.V. treatment of severe or complicated infections when oral therapy is not feasible, for documented PCP, empiric treatment of PCP in immune compromised patients; treatment of documented or suspected shigellosis, typhoid fever, or other infections caused by susceptible bacteria

Unlabeled Use Cholera and *Salmonella*-type infections and nocardiosis; chronic prostatitis; as prophylaxis in neutropenic patients with *P. jirovecii* infections, in leukemia patients, and in patients following renal transplantation, to decrease incidence of PCP; treatment of *Cyclospora* infection, typhoid fever, *Nocardia asteroides* infection; prophylaxis against urinary tract infection; alternative treatment for MRSA infections

Available Dosage Forms The 5:1 ratio (SMX:TMP) remains constant in all dosage forms.

Injection, solution: Sulfamethoxazole 80 mg and trimethoprim 16 mg per mL (5 mL, 10 mL, 30 mL)

Suspension, oral: Sulfamethoxazole 200 mg and trimethoprim 40 mg per 5 mL

Tablet: Sulfamethoxazole 400 mg and trimethoprim 80 mg

Bactrim™: Sulfamethoxazole 400 mg and trimethoprim 80 mg

Tablet, double-strength: Sulfamethoxazole 800 mg and trimethoprim 160 mg

Bactrim™ DS, Septra® DS: Sulfamethoxazole 800 mg and trimethoprim 160 mg

General Dosage Range Dosage adjustment recommended in patients with renal impairment

I.V.: *Children >2 months and Adults:* 8-20 mg TMP/kg/day divided every 6-12 hours

Oral:

Children >2 months: 6-20 mg TMP/kg/day divided every 6-12 hours **or** 150 mg TMP/m^2/day in divided doses every 12-24 hours for 3-7 days/week (maximum: sulfamethoxazole 1600 mg/day; trimethoprim 320 mg/day)

Adults: 1 or 2 double-strength tablets (sulfamethoxazole 800-1600 mg; trimethoprim 160-320 mg) every 12-24 hours **or** 15-20 mg TMP/kg/day in 3-4 divided doses

Administration

Oral Administer without regard to meals. Administer with at least 8 ounces of water.

I.V. Infuse over 60-90 minutes, must dilute well before giving (ie, 1:15 to 1:25, which equates to 5 mL of drug solution diluted in 75-125 mL base solution).

I.V. Detail Not for I.M. injection. Administer around-the-clock every 6-12 hours.

pH: 10

Nursing Actions

Physical Assessment Perform culture and sensitivity tests prior to initiating therapy.

Patient Education Maintain adequate hydration unless instructed to restrict fluid intake. May cause nausea, vomiting, or GI upset. Report skin rash, severe GI upset or diarrhea, dark urine, yellow skin or eyes, or unusual bleeding or bruising. May cause photosensitivity reactions; avoid sun, sunlamps, and tanning beds. Use sunscreen and wear clothing and eyewear that protects you from the sun.

Related Information

Trimethoprim *on page 1152*

Sulfasalazine (sul fa SAL a zeen)

Brand Names: U.S. Azulfidine EN-tabs®; Azulfidine®

Index Terms Salicylazosulfapyridine

Pharmacologic Category 5-Aminosalicylic Acid Derivative

Medication Safety Issues

Sound-alike/look-alike issues:

SulfaSALAzine may be confused with salsalate, sulfADIAZINE, sulfiSOXAZOLE

Azulfidine® may be confused with Augmentin®, azaTHIOprine

Pregnancy Risk Factor B

Lactation Enters breast milk/use caution (AAP recommends use "with caution"; AAP 2001 update pending)

Use Treatment of mild-to-moderate ulcerative colitis or as adjunctive therapy in severe ulcerative colitis; enteric coated tablets are also used for rheumatoid arthritis (including juvenile idiopathic arthritis [JIA]) in patients who inadequately respond to analgesics and NSAIDs

Unlabeled Use Ankylosing spondylitis, Crohn's disease, psoriasis, psoriatic arthritis

Available Dosage Forms

Tablet, oral: 500 mg

Azulfidine®: 500 mg

Tablet, delayed release, enteric coated, oral: 500 mg

Azulfidine EN-tabs®: 500 mg

General Dosage Range Oral:

Delayed release:

Children ≥6 years: Initial: 1/4 to 1/3 of expected maintenance dose; Maintenance: 30-50 mg/kg/day in 2 divided doses (maximum: 2 g/day)

Adults: Initial: 0.5-1 g/day; Maintenance: 2 g/day in 2 divided doses (maximum: 3 g/day)

Immediate release:

Children ≥6 years: Initial: 40-60 mg/kg/day in 3-6 divided doses; Maintenance: 30 mg/kg/day in 4 divided doses

Adults: Initial: 3-4 g/day in evenly divided doses at ≤8-hour intervals; Maintenance: 2 g/day in divided doses at ≤8-hour intervals

Administration

Oral GI intolerance is common during the first few days of therapy (give with meals). Do not crush enteric coated tablets.

Nursing Actions

Physical Assessment Allergy history should be assessed prior to starting therapy (sulfa drugs, salicylates). Monitor for photosensitivity, gastrointestinal disturbance [nausea, vomiting, anorexia], anemia, jaundice, or hematuria. Caution patients with diabetes to monitor glucose levels closely; may cause altered effect of oral hypoglycemic agents.

Patient Education Take with food, at regular intervals. Do not crush, chew, or dissolve coated tablets. Maintain adequate hydration to prevent kidney damage, unless instructed to restrict fluid intake. May cause dizziness, headache, nausea, vomiting, or loss of appetite. Report rash; persistent nausea, vomiting, diarrhea, or GI pain; opportunistic infection (sore throat, fever, vaginal itching or discharge, unusual bruising or bleeding, fatigue); blood in urine or change in urinary pattern; swelling of face, lips, or tongue; or tightness in chest, bad cough, or blue skin color.

Sulindac (SUL in dak)

Brand Names: U.S. Clinoril®

Pharmacologic Category Nonsteroidal Anti-inflammatory Drug (NSAID), Oral

Medication Safety Issues

Sound-alike/look-alike issues:

Clinoril® may be confused with Cleocin®, Clozaril®

Medication Guide Available Yes

Pregnancy Risk Factor C

Lactation Excretion in breast milk unknown/not recommended

Breast-Feeding Considerations It is not known if sulindac is excreted into breast milk. Breast-feeding is not recommended by the manufacturer.

Use Management of inflammatory diseases including osteoarthritis, rheumatoid arthritis, acute gouty arthritis, ankylosing spondylitis, acute painful shoulder (bursitis/tendonitis)

Unlabeled Use Management of preterm labor

Mechanism of Action/Effect Reversibly inhibits cyclooxygenase-1 and 2 (COX-1 and 2) enzymes, which results in decreased formation of prostaglandin precursors; has antipyretic, analgesic, and anti-inflammatory properties

Contraindications Hypersensitivity or allergic-type reactions to sulindac, aspirin, other NSAIDs, or any component of the formulation; perioperative pain in the setting of coronary artery bypass graft (CABG) surgery

Warnings/Precautions [U.S. Boxed Warning]: NSAIDs are associated with an increased risk of adverse cardiovascular thrombotic events, including MI and stroke. Use caution with fluid retention. Avoid use in heart failure. Concurrent administration of ibuprofen, and potentially other nonselective NSAIDs, may interfere with aspirin's cardioprotective effect. May cause new-onset hypertension or worsening of existing hypertension. NSAID use may compromise existing renal function; dose-dependent decreases in prostaglandin synthesis may result from NSAID use, reducing renal blood flow which may cause renal decompensation. NSAID use may increase the risk for hyperkalemia. Patients with impaired renal function, dehydration, heart failure, liver dysfunction, those taking diuretics, and ACE inhibitors, and the elderly are at greater risk of renal toxicity and hyperkalemia. Rehydrate patient before starting therapy; monitor renal function closely. Not recommended for use in patients with advanced renal disease. Long-term NSAID use may result in renal papillary necrosis. Use caution in patients with renal lithiasis; sulindac metabolites have been reported as components of renal stones. Maintain adequate hydration in patients with a history of renal stones. Use with caution in patients with decreased hepatic function. May require dosage adjustment in hepatic dysfunction; sulfide and sulfone metabolites may accumulate. The elderly are at increased risk for adverse effects. **[U.S. Boxed Warning]: Use is contraindicated for treatment of perioperative pain in the setting of coronary artery bypass graft (CABG) surgery.** Risk of MI and stroke may be increased with use following CABG surgery.

[U.S. Boxed Warning]: NSAIDs may increase risk of gastrointestinal irritation, inflammation, ulceration, bleeding, and perforation. Use the lowest effective dose for the shortest duration of time, consistent with individual patient goals, to reduce risk of cardiovascular or GI adverse events. When used concomitantly with ≤325 mg of aspirin, a substantial increase in the risk of gastrointestinal complications (eg, ulcer) occurs; concomitant gastroprotective therapy (eg, proton pump inhibitors) is recommended (Bhatt, 2008). Pancreatitis has been reported; discontinue with suspected pancreatitis.

NSAIDS may cause drowsiness, dizziness, blurred vision and other neurologic effects which may impair physical or mental abilities; patients must be cautioned about performing tasks which require mental alertness (eg, operating machinery or driving). Discontinue use with blurred or diminished vision and perform ophthalmologic exam. Monitor vision with long-term therapy.

Platelet adhesion and aggregation may be decreased, may prolong bleeding time; patients with coagulation disorders or who are receiving anticoagulants should be monitored closely. Anemia may occur; patients on long-term NSAID therapy should be monitored for anemia. Rarely, NSAID use may cause severe blood dyscrasias (eg, agranulocytosis, aplastic anemia, thrombocytopenia). NSAIDs may cause serious skin adverse events including exfoliative dermatitis, Stevens-Johnson syndrome (SJS) and toxic epidermal necrolysis (TEN); discontinue use at first sign of skin rash or hypersensitivity. Anaphylactoid reactions may occur. Do not use in patients who experience bronchospasm, asthma, rhinitis, or urticaria with NSAID or aspirin therapy. Use caution in other forms of asthma. May increase the risk of aseptic meningitis, especially in patients with systemic lupus erythematosus (SLE) and mixed connective tissue disorders.

Withhold for at least 4-6 half-lives prior to surgical or dental procedures.

Drug Interactions

Avoid Concomitant Use

Avoid concomitant use of Sulindac with any of the following: Floctafenine; Ketorolac; Ketorolac (Nasal); Ketorolac (Systemic)

Decreased Effect

Sulindac may decrease the levels/effects of: ACE Inhibitors; Aliskiren; Angiotensin II Receptor Blockers; Antiplatelet Agents; Beta-Blockers; Eplerenone; HydrALAZINE; Loop Diuretics; Potassium-Sparing Diuretics; Salicylates; Selective Serotonin Reuptake Inhibitors; Thiazide Diuretics

The levels/effects of Sulindac may be decreased by: Bile Acid Sequestrants; Nonsteroidal Anti-Inflammatory Agents; Salicylates

Increased Effect/Toxicity

Sulindac may increase the levels/effects of: Aliskiren; Aminoglycosides; Anticoagulants; Antiplatelet Agents; Bisphosphonate Derivatives; Collagenase (Systemic); CycloSPORINE; CycloSPORINE (Systemic); Deferasirox; Desmopressin; Digoxin; Drotrecogin Alfa (Activated); Eplerenone; Haloperidol; Ibritumomab; Methotrexate; Nonsteroidal Anti-Inflammatory Agents; PEMEtrexed; Porfimer; Potassium-Sparing Diuretics; PRALAtrexate; Quinolone Antibiotics; Rivaroxaban; Salicylates; Thrombolytic Agents; Tositumomab and Iodine I 131 Tositumomab; Vancomycin; Vitamin K Antagonists

The levels/effects of Sulindac may be increased by: ACE Inhibitors; Angiotensin II Receptor Blockers; Antidepressants (Tricyclic, Tertiary Amine); Corticosteroids (Systemic); CycloSPORINE; CycloSPORINE (Systemic); Dasatinib; Dimethyl Sulfoxide; Floctafenine; Glucosamine; Herbs (Anticoagulant/Antiplatelet Properties); Ketorolac; Ketorolac (Nasal); Ketorolac (Systemic); Nonsteroidal Anti-Inflammatory Agents; Omega-3-Acid Ethyl Esters; Pentosan Polysulfate Sodium; Pentoxifylline; Probenecid; Prostacyclin Analogues; Selective Serotonin Reuptake Inhibitors; Serotonin/Norepinephrine Reuptake Inhibitors; Sodium Phosphates; Treprostinil; Vitamin E

Nutritional/Ethanol Interactions

Ethanol: Avoid ethanol (may enhance gastric mucosal irritation).

Herb/Nutraceutical: Avoid alfalfa, anise, bilberry, bladderwrack, bromelain, cat's claw, celery, chamomile, coleus, cordyceps, dong quai, evening primrose, fenugreek, feverfew, garlic, ginger, ginkgo biloba, ginseng (American, Panax, Siberian), grapeseed, green tea, guggul, horse chestnut seed, horseradish, licorice, prickly ash, red clover, reishi, SAMe (S-adenosylmethionine), sweet clover, turmeric, white willow (all have additional antiplatelet activity).

Adverse Reactions 1% to 10%:

Cardiovascular: Edema (1% to 3%)

Central nervous system: Dizziness (3% to 9%), headache (3% to 9%), nervousness (1% to 3%)

Dermatologic: Rash (3% to 9%), pruritus (1% to 3%)

Gastrointestinal: GI pain (10%), constipation (3% to 9%), diarrhea (3% to 9%), dyspepsia (3% to 9%), nausea (3% to 9%), abdominal cramps (1% to 3%), anorexia (1% to 3%), flatulence (1% to 3%), vomiting (1% to 3%)

Otic: Tinnitus (1% to 3%)

Available Dosage Forms

Tablet, oral: 150 mg, 200 mg

Clinoril®: 200 mg

General Dosage Range Dosage adjustment recommended in patients with hepatic impairment

Oral: *Adults:* 150-200 mg twice daily (maximum: 400 mg/day)

Administration

Oral Should be administered with food or milk.

Stability

Storage Store at room temperature of 15°C to 30°C (59°F to 86°F).

Nursing Actions

Physical Assessment Monitor blood pressure at the beginning of therapy and periodically during use. Monitor for adverse GI and respiratory response, hepatotoxicity, and ototoxicity at beginning of therapy and periodically throughout. Schedule ophthalmic evaluations for patients who develop eye complaints during long-term NSAID therapy.

Patient Education Take with food or milk to reduce GI distress. Do not use alcohol. Regularly scheduled ophthalmic exams are advised with long-term use of NSAIDs. You may experience dizziness, nervousness, headache, nausea, vomiting, heartburn, or constipation; GI bleeding, ulceration, or perforation can occur with or without pain; discontinue medication and contact prescriber if persistent abdominal pain, cramping, or blood in stool occurs. Report respiratory difficulty; chest pain; bruising or bleeding; blood in urine, stool, mouth, or vomitus; unusual fatigue; skin rash; or ringing in ears.

Dietary Considerations Drug may cause GI upset, bleeding, ulceration, perforation; take with food or milk to minimize GI upset.

SUMAtriptan (soo ma TRIP tan)

Brand Names: U.S. Alsuma™; Imitrex®; Sumavel™ DosePro™

Index Terms Sumatriptan Succinate

Pharmacologic Category Antimigraine Agent; Serotonin 5-$HT_{1B, 1D}$ Receptor Agonist

Medication Safety Issues

Sound-alike/look-alike issues:

SUMAtriptan may be confused with saxagliptin, sitaGLIPtin, somatropin, ZOLMitriptan

Pregnancy Risk Factor C

Lactation Enters breast milk/use caution (AAP rates "compatible"; AAP 2001 update pending)

Breast-Feeding Considerations The amount of sumatriptan an infant would be exposed to following breast-feeding is considered to be small (although the mean milk-to-plasma ratio is ~4.9, weight adjusted doses estimates suggest breastfed infants receive 3.5% of a maternal dose). Expressing and discarding the milk for 8-12 hours after a single dose is suggested to reduce the amount present even further. The half-life of sumatriptan in breast milk is 2.22 hours.

Use

Intranasal, Oral, SubQ: Acute treatment of migraine with or without aura

SubQ: Acute treatment of cluster headache episodes

Mechanism of Action/Effect Selective agonist for serotonin receptor in cranial arteries; causes vasoconstriction and relief of migraine

Contraindications Hypersensitivity to sumatriptan or any component of the formulation; patients with ischemic heart disease or signs or symptoms of ischemic heart disease (including Prinzmetal's angina, angina pectoris, myocardial infarction, silent myocardial ischemia); cerebrovascular syndromes (including strokes, transient ischemic attacks); peripheral vascular disease (including ischemic bowel disease); uncontrolled hypertension; use within 24 hours of ergotamine derivatives; use within 24 hours of another 5-HT_1 agonist; concurrent administration or within 2 weeks of discontinuing an MAO type A inhibitors (oral and nasal sumatriptan only; see Warnings/Precautions); management of hemiplegic or basilar migraine; severe hepatic impairment (oral and nasal sumatriptan, and injectable Imitrex® only); not for I.V. administration

Warnings/Precautions Sumatriptan is only indicated for the acute treatment of migraine or cluster headache (product dependent); not indicated for migraine prophylaxis, or for the treatment of hemiplegic or basilar migraine. If a patient does not respond to the first dose, the diagnosis of migraine or cluster headache should be reconsidered; rule out underlying neurologic disease in patients with atypical headache and in patients with no prior history of migraine or cluster headache. Cardiac events (coronary artery vasospasm, transient ischemia, myocardial infarction, ventricular tachycardia/fibrillation, cardiac arrest and death), cerebral/subarachnoid hemorrhage, and stroke have been reported with 5-HT_1 agonist administration. Patients who experience sensations of chest pain/pressure/tightness or symptoms suggestive of angina following dosing should be evaluated for coronary artery disease or Prinzmetal's angina before receiving additional doses; if dosing is resumed and similar symptoms recur, monitor with ECG. Do not give to patients with risk factors for CAD until a cardiovascular evaluation has been performed; if evaluation is satisfactory, the healthcare provider should administer the first dose (consider ECG monitoring) and cardiovascular status should be periodically evaluated.

Significant elevation in blood pressure, including hypertensive crisis, has also been reported on rare occasions in patients with and without a history of hypertension; use is contraindicated in patients with uncontrolled hypertension. Vasospasm-related reactions have been reported other than coronary artery vasospasm. Peripheral vascular ischemia and colonic ischemia with abdominal pain and bloody diarrhea have occurred. Transient and permanent blindness and significant partial vision loss have been very rarely reported. Use with caution in patients with a history of seizure disorder or in patients with a lowered seizure threshold. Use the oral formulation with caution (and with dosage limitations) in patients with hepatic impairment where treatment is necessary and advisable. Presystemic clearance of orally administered sumatriptan is reduced in hepatic impairment, leading to increased plasma concentrations; dosage reduction of the oral product is recommended. Non-oral routes of administration (nasal, subcutaneous formulations) do not undergo similar hepatic first-pass metabolism and are not expected to result in significantly altered pharmacokinetics in patients with hepatic impairment. Use of the oral, nasal, or Imitrex® injectable is contraindicated in severe hepatic impairment.

Symptoms of agitation, confusion, hallucinations, hyper-reflexia, myoclonus, shivering, and tachycardia (serotonin syndrome) may occur with concomitant proserotonergic drugs (ie, SSRIs/SNRIs or triptans) or agents which reduce sumatriptan's metabolism. Concurrent use of serotonin precursors (eg, tryptophan) is not recommended. If concomitant administration with SSRIs is warranted, monitor closely, especially at initiation and with dose increases. Concurrent use with an MAO inhibitor may result in increased sumatriptan concentrations and increased risk for dose-related adverse effects (eg, serotonin syndrome); use with oral or nasal sumatriptan is contraindicated. Although generally not recommended, if concomitant use of MAO inhibitors with injectable sumatriptan is deemed necessary, careful monitoring and appropriate dosage adjustments are required. I.V. administration is contraindicated due to the potential to cause coronary vasospasm. Not recommended for use in elderly patients; older adults are at a higher risk for coronary artery disease and may be more likely to have reduced hepatic function.

Drug Interactions

Avoid Concomitant Use

Avoid concomitant use of SUMAtriptan with any of the following: Ergot Derivatives; MAO Inhibitors

Decreased Effect There are no known significant interactions involving a decrease in effect.

Increased Effect/Toxicity

SUMAtriptan may increase the levels/effects of: Ergot Derivatives; Metoclopramide; Serotonin Modulators

The levels/effects of SUMAtriptan may be increased by: Antipsychotics; Ergot Derivatives; MAO Inhibitors

Adverse Reactions

Injection:

>10%:

Central nervous system: Dizziness (12%), warm/hot sensation (11%)

Local: Injection site reaction (≤86%; includes bleeding, bruising, edema, and erythema)

Neuromuscular & skeletal: Paresthesia (5% to 14%)

1% to 10%:

Cardiovascular: Chest discomfort/tightness/pressure (2% to 5%)

Central nervous system: Burning sensation (7%), feeling of heaviness (7%), flushing (7%), pressure sensation (7%), feeling of tightness (5%), drowsiness (3%), feeling strange (2%), headache (2%), tight feeling in head (2%), anxiety (1%), cold sensation (1%), malaise/fatigue (1%)

Gastrointestinal: Nausea/vomiting (4%), abdominal discomfort (1%), dysphagia (1%)

Neuromuscular & skeletal: Neck pain/stiffness (5%), numbness (5%), weakness (5%), jaw discomfort (2%), myalgia (2%), muscle cramps (1%)

Ocular: Vision alterations (1%)

Respiratory: Throat discomfort (3%), nasal disorder/discomfort (2%), bronchospasm (1%)

Miscellaneous: Diaphoresis (2%)

Nasal spray:

>10%: Gastrointestinal: Bad taste (13% to 24%), nausea (11% to 13%), vomiting (11% to 13%)

1% to 10%:

Central nervous system: Dizziness (1% to 2%)

Respiratory: Nasal disorder/discomfort (2% to 4%), throat discomfort (1% to 2%)

Tablet:

1% to 10%:

Cardiovascular: Chest pain/tightness/heaviness/pressure (1% to 2%), palpitation (1%), syncope (1%)

Central nervous system: Burning (1%), dizziness (>1%), drowsiness (>1%), malaise/fatigue (2% to 3%), headache (>1%), nonspecified pain (1% to 2%, placebo 1%), vertigo (<1% to 2%), migraine (>1%), sleepiness (>1%)

Gastrointestinal: Diarrhea (1%), nausea (>1%), vomiting (>1%), hyposalivation (>1%)

Hematologic: Hemolytic anemia (1%)

Neuromuscular & skeletal: Neck, throat, and jaw pain/tightness/pressure (2% to 3%), paresthesia (3% to 5%), myalgia (1%), numbness (1%)

Otic: Ear hemorrhage (1%), hearing loss (1%), sensitivity to noise (1%), tinnitus (1%)

Renal: Hematuria (1%)

Respiratory: Allergic rhinitis (1%), dyspnea (1%), nasal inflammation (1%), nose/throat hemorrhage (1%), sinusitis (1%), upper respiratory inflammation (1%)

Miscellaneous: Hypersensitivity reactions (1%), nonspecified pressure/tightness/heaviness (1% to 3%, placebo 2%); warm/cold sensation (2% to 3%, placebo 2%)

Pharmacodynamics/Kinetics

Onset of Action Oral: ~30 minutes; Nasal: ~15-30 minutes; SubQ: ~10 minutes

Available Dosage Forms

Injection, solution: 4 mg/0.5 mL (0.5 mL); 6 mg/0.5 mL (0.5 mL)

Alsuma™: 6 mg/0.5 mL (0.5 mL)

Imitrex®: 4 mg/0.5 mL (0.5 mL); 6 mg/0.5 mL (0.5 mL)

Sumavel™ DosePro™: 6 mg/0.5 mL (0.5 mL)

Injection, solution [preservative free]: 6 mg/0.5 mL (0.5 mL)

Solution, intranasal: 5 mg/0.1 mL (6s); 20 mg/0.1 mL (6s)

Imitrex®: 5 mg/0.1 mL (6s); 20 mg/0.1 mL (6s)

Tablet, oral: 25 mg, 50 mg, 100 mg

Imitrex®: 25 mg, 50 mg, 100 mg

General Dosage Range Dosage adjustment recommended for oral route in patients with hepatic impairment

Intranasal: *Adults:* 5-20 mg in one nostril as a single dose (may divide dose into both nostrils); may repeat after 2 hours (maximum: 40 mg/day)

Oral: *Adults:* 25-100 mg as a single dose; may repeat after 2 hours (maximum: 200 mg/day)

SubQ: *Adults:* Initial: Up to 6 mg; may repeat if needed ≥1 hour after initial dose (maximum: Two 6 mg injections per 24-hour period)

Administration

Oral Should be administered as soon as symptoms appear.

Other Should be administered as soon as symptoms appear.

Intranasal: Each nasal spray unit is preloaded with 1 dose; **do not** test the spray unit before use; remove unit from plastic pack when ready to use; while sitting down, gently blow nose to clear nasal passages; keep head upright and close one nostril gently with index finger; hold container with other hand, with thumb supporting bottom and index and middle fingers on either side of nozzle; insert nozzle into nostril about 1/2 inch; close mouth; take a breath through nose while releasing spray into nostril by pressing firmly on blue plunger; remove nozzle from nostril; keep head level for 10-20 seconds and gently breathe in through nose and out through mouth; **do not breathe deeply**

SubQ: Not for I.M. or I.V. use. Needle penetrates 1/4 inch of skin; use in areas of the body with adequate skin and subcutaneous thickness. Alsuma™ is a prefilled single-use autoinjector device.

Needleless administration (Sumavel™ DosePro™): Administer to the abdomen (>2 inches from the navel) or thigh; not for I.M. or I.V. administration. Do not administer to other areas of the body (eg, arm). Device is for single use only, discard after use; do not use if the tip of the device is tilted or broken.

Stability

Storage

Alsuma™: Store at 25°C (77°F); excursions permitted between 15°C and 30°C (59°F and 86°F); do not refrigerate. Protect from light.

Imitrex® injectable, tablet, nasal spray: Store at 2°C to 30°C (36°F to 86°F). Protect from light.

Sumavel™ DosePro™: Store at 20°C to 25°C (68°F to 77°F); excursions permitted between 15°C and 30°C (59°F and 86°F); do not freeze.

Nursing Actions

Physical Assessment For use only with a clear diagnosis of acute migraine or cluster headaches (not for prophylaxis). Cardiovascular status should be evaluated prior to initiating medication and periodically thereafter. Evaluate carefully for use-related cautions (eg, history of, current, or risk factors for coronary heart disease; hepatic impairment; or seizure history). Monitor for hypertension, cardiac event, cerebrovascular event, dizziness, tingling, drowsiness, myalgia, vision alternation, nausea, and vomiting. With SubQ, teach patient appropriate injection technique and syringe/needle disposal.

Patient Education Take at first sign of migraine attack. This drug is to be used to reduce your migraine, not to prevent or reduce the number of attacks. If using injection formulation, follow instructions for injection and disposal of needle and syringe. May cause flushing, nausea, or vomiting. Report immediately any chest tightness, pain, or pressure; pressure or tight feeling in head; balance change; muscle weakness on one side of the body; sudden eyesight change; or very nervous and excitable feeling.

Sumatriptan and Naproxen

(soo ma TRIP tan & na PROKS en)

Brand Names: U.S. Treximet™

Index Terms Naproxen and Sumatriptan; Naproxen Sodium and Sumatriptan; Naproxen Sodium and Sumatriptan Succinate; Sumatriptan Succinate and Naproxen; Sumatriptan Succinate and Naproxen Sodium

Pharmacologic Category Antimigraine Agent; Nonsteroidal Anti-inflammatory Drug (NSAID), Oral; Serotonin 5-$HT_{1B, 1D}$ Receptor Agonist

Medication Safety Issues

Sound-alike/look-alike issues:

Naproxen may be confused with Natacyn®, Nebcin, neomycin, niacin

SUMAtriptan may be confused with somatropin, ZOLMitriptan

Treximet™ may be confused with Trexall™

Medication Guide Available Yes

Pregnancy Risk Factor C

Lactation Enters breast milk/not recommended

Use Acute treatment of migraine with or without aura

Available Dosage Forms

Tablet:

Treximet™ 85/500: Sumatriptan 85 mg and naproxen sodium 500 mg

General Dosage Range Oral: *Adults:* 1 tablet (sumatriptan 85 mg and naproxen 500 mg); may repeat in 2 hours if needed (maximum: 2 tablets/24 hours)

Administration

Oral May be administered with or without food. Swallow tablet whole; tablet should not be divided, crushed, or chewed.

Nursing Actions

Physical Assessment See individual agents.

Patient Education See individual agents.

Tacrolimus (Systemic) (ta KROE li mus)

Brand Names: U.S. Hecoria™; Prograf®

Index Terms FK506

Pharmacologic Category Calcineurin Inhibitor; Immunosuppressant Agent

Medication Safety Issues

Sound-alike/look-alike issues:

Prograf® may be confused with Gengraf®, PROzac®

Tacrolimus may be confused with everolimus, pimecrolimus, sirolimus, temsirolimus

Medication Guide Available Yes

Pregnancy Risk Factor C

Lactation Enters breast milk/not recommended

Breast-Feeding Considerations Concentrations of tacrolimus in breast milk are lower than that of the maternal serum. The low bioavailability of tacrolimus following oral absorption may also decrease the amount of exposure to a nursing infant.

Use

Prograf®:

U.S. labeling: Prevention of organ rejection in heart, kidney, or liver transplant recipients

Canadian labeling: Prevention of organ rejection in heart, kidney, or liver transplant recipients; treatment of refractory rejection in kidney or liver transplant recipients; treatment of active rheumatoid arthritis in adult patients nonresponsive to disease-modifying antirheumatic drug (DMARD) therapy or when DMARD therapy is inappropriate

Advagraf® (Canadian availability; not available in U.S.): Prevention of organ rejection in kidney transplant recipients

Unlabeled Use Prevention of organ rejection in lung, small bowel transplant recipients; prevention and treatment of graft-versus-host disease (GVHD) in allogenic hematopoietic stem cell transplantation

Mechanism of Action/Effect Suppresses cellular immunity (inhibits T-lymphocyte activation)

Contraindications Hypersensitivity to tacrolimus or any component of the formulation

Warnings/Precautions Hazardous agent - use appropriate precautions for handling and disposal. **[U.S. Boxed Warning]: Risk of developing infections (including bacterial, viral [including CMV], fungal, and protozoal infections [including opportunistic infections]) is increased.** Latent viral infections may be activated, including BK virus (associated with polyoma virus-associated nephropathy [PVAN]) and JC virus (associated with progressive multifocal leukoencephalopathy [PML]); may result in serious adverse effects. The risk of CMV disease is increased for patients who are CMV-seronegative prior to transplant and receive a graft from a CMV-seropositive donor. Consider reduction in immunosuppression if PVAN, PML, CMV viremia and/or CMV disease occurs. **[U.S. Boxed Warning]: Immunosuppressive therapy may result in the development of lymphoma and other malignancies (predominantly skin malignancies)**. The risk for new-onset diabetes and insulin-dependent post-transplant diabetes mellitus (PTDM) is increased with tacrolimus use after transplantation, including in patients without pretransplant history of diabetes mellitus; insulin dependence may be reversible; increased risk in African-American and Hispanic kidney transplant patients. Nephrotoxicity has has been reported, especially with higher doses; to avoid excess nephrotoxicity do not administer simultaneously with other nephrotoxic drugs (eg sirolimus, cyclosporine). Neurotoxicity may occur especially when used in high doses; tremor headache, coma and delirium have been reported and are associated with serum concentrations. Seizures may also occur. Posterior reversible encephalopathy syndrome (PRES) may also occur; symptoms (altered mental status, headache, hypertension, seizures, and visual disturbances) are reversible with dose reduction or discontinuation of therapy; stabilize blood pressure and reduce dose with suspected or confirmed PRES diagnosis.

Pure red cell aplasia (PRCA) has been reported in patients receiving tacrolimus. Use with caution in patients with risk factors for PRCA including parvovirus B19 infection, underlying disease, or use of concomitant medications associated with PRCA (eg, mycophenolate). Discontinuation of therapy should be considered with diagnosis of PRCA. Monitoring of serum concentrations (trough for oral therapy) is essential to prevent organ rejection and reduce drug-related toxicity. A period of ≥24 hours should elapse between discontinuation of cyclosporine and the initiation of tacrolimus. Delay initiation further with persistently elevated tacrolimus/cyclosporine levels. Use caution in renal or hepatic dysfunction, dosing adjustments may be required. Delay initiation of therapy in kidney transplant patients if postoperative oliguria occurs; begin therapy no sooner than 6 hours and within 24 hours post-transplant, but may be delayed until renal function has recovered. Use may be associated with the development of hypertension (common); hyperkalemia has been reported; avoid use of potassium-sparing diuretics. Myocardial hypertrophy has been reported (rare). Concurrent use with strong CYP3A4 inhibitors (eg, ritonavir, ketoconazole, itraconazole, voriconazole, clarithromycin) or inducers (eg, rifampin, rifabutin) is not recommended without close monitoring of tacrolimus trough concentrations.

Each mL of injection contains polyoxyl 60 hydrogenated castor oil (HCO-60) (200 mg) and dehydrated alcohol USP 80% v/v. Anaphylaxis has been reported with the injection, use should be reserved for those patients not able to take oral medications. Patients should not be immunized with live vaccines during or shortly after treatment and should avoid close contact with recently vaccinated (live vaccine) individuals. Oral formulations contain lactose; the Canadian labeling does not recommend use of these products in patients who may be lactose intolerant (eg, Lapp lactase deficiency, glucose-galactose malabsorption, galactose intolerance). **[U.S. Boxed Warning]: Should be administered under the supervision of a physician experienced in immunosuppressive therapy and organ transplantation in a facility appropriate for monitoring and managing therapy.**

Drug Interactions

Avoid Concomitant Use

Avoid concomitant use of Tacrolimus (Systemic) with any of the following: Artemether; BCG; Conivaptan; Crizotinib; CycloSPORINE (Systemic); Dronedarone; Eplerenone; Grapefruit Juice; Lumefantrine; Natalizumab; Nilotinib; Pimecrolimus; Pimozide; Potassium-Sparing Diuretics; QUEtiapine; QuiNINE; Silodosin; Sirolimus; Tacrolimus (Topical); Temsirolimus; Tetrabenazine; Thioridazine; Topotecan; Toremifene; Vaccines (Live); Vandetanib; Vemurafenib; Ziprasidone

Decreased Effect

Tacrolimus (Systemic) may decrease the levels/effects of: BCG; Coccidioidin Skin Test; Sipuleucel-T; Vaccines (Inactivated); Vaccines (Live)

The levels/effects of Tacrolimus (Systemic) may be decreased by: Caspofungin; Cinacalcet; CYP3A4 Inducers (Strong); Deferasirox; Echinacea; Efavirenz; Fosphenytoin; P-glycoprotein/ABCB1 Inducers; Phenytoin; Rifamycin Derivatives; Sirolimus; St Johns Wort; Temsirolimus; Tocilizumab

Increased Effect/Toxicity

Tacrolimus (Systemic) may increase the levels/effects of: ARIPiprazole; Colchicine; CycloSPORINE (Systemic); Dabigatran Etexilate; Dronedarone; Everolimus; Fosphenytoin; Leflunomide; ▶

Natalizumab; P-glycoprotein/ABCB1 Substrates; Phenytoin; Pimozide; Prucalopride; QTc-Prolonging Agents; QuiNINE; Rivaroxaban; Silodosin; Sirolimus; Temsirolimus; Tetrabenazine; Thioridazine; Topotecan; Toremifene; Vaccines (Live); Vandetanib; Vemurafenib; Ziprasidone

The levels/effects of Tacrolimus (Systemic) may be increased by: Alfuzosin; Antidepressants (Serotonin Reuptake Inhibitor/Antagonist); Artemether; Calcium Channel Blockers (Dihydropyridine); Calcium Channel Blockers (Nondihydropyridine); Chloramphenicol; Chloroquine; Ciprofloxacin; Ciprofloxacin (Systemic); Clotrimazole; Clotrimazole (Oral); Conivaptan; Crizotinib; CycloSPORINE (Systemic); CYP3A4 Inhibitors (Moderate); CYP3A4 Inhibitors (Strong); Danazol; Denosumab; Eplerenone; Fluconazole; Gadobutrol; Grapefruit Juice; Indacaterol; Itraconazole; Ketoconazole; Ketoconazole (Systemic); Lumefantrine; Macrolide Antibiotics; MetroNIDAZOLE; MetroNIDAZOLE (Systemic); Nilotinib; P-glycoprotein/ABCB1 Inhibitors; Pimecrolimus; Posaconazole; Potassium-Sparing Diuretics; Protease Inhibitors; Proton Pump Inhibitors; QUEtiapine; QuiNINE; Ranolazine; Roflumilast; Sirolimus; Tacrolimus (Topical); Telaprevir; Temsirolimus; Trastuzumab; Voriconazole

Nutritional/Ethanol Interactions

Food: Food decreases rate and extent of absorption. High-fat meals have most pronounced effect (37% decrease in AUC, 77% decrease in C_{max}). Grapefruit juice, a CYP3A4 inhibitor, may increase serum level and/or toxicity of tacrolimus. Management: Administer with or without food, but be consistent. Avoid concurrent use of grapefruit juice.

Herb/Nutraceutical: St John's wort may reduce tacrolimus serum concentrations. Management: Avoid St John's wort.

Adverse Reactions As reported for kidney, liver, and heart transplantation:

≥15%:

Cardiovascular: Hypertension (13% to 62%), edema (peripheral 11% to 36%), chest pain (19%), edema (18%), pericardial effusion (heart transplant 15%)

Central nervous system: Headache (24% to 64%), insomnia (30% to 64%), pain (24% to 63%), fever (19% to 48%), postprocedural pain (kidney transplant 29%), dizziness (19%)

Dermatologic: Pruritus (15% to 36%), rash (10% to 24%)

Endocrine & metabolic: New-onset diabetes after transplant (75% kidney transplant), hypophosphatemia (28% to 49%), hypomagnesemia (16% to 48%), hyperglycemia (21% to 47%), hyperkalemia (13% to 45%), hyperlipemia (10% to 31%), hypokalemia (13% to 29%), diabetes mellitus (24% to 26%), post-transplant diabetes mellitus (heart transplant 13% to 22%; kidney transplant 20%; liver transplant 11% to 18%)

Gastrointestinal: Diarrhea (25% to 72%), abdominal pain (29% to 59%), nausea (32% to 46%), constipation (23% to 36%), anorexia (7% to 34%), vomiting (14% to 29%), dyspepsia (18% to 28%)

Genitourinary: Urinary tract infection (16% to 34%)

Hematologic: Anemia (5% to 50%), leukopenia (13% to 48%), leukocytosis (8% to 32%), thrombocytopenia (14% to 24%)

Hepatic: Liver function tests abnormal (6% to 36%), ascites (7% to 27%)

Local: Incision site complication (kidney transplant 28%)

Neuromuscular & skeletal: Tremor (15% to 56%; heart transplant 15%), weakness (11% to 52%), paresthesia (17% to 40%), back pain (17% to 30%), arthralgia (25%)

Renal: Abnormal kidney function (36% to 56%), creatinine increased (23% to 45%), BUN increased (12% to 30%), oliguria (18% to 19%)

Respiratory: Atelectasis (5% to 28%), pleural effusion (30% to 36%), dyspnea (5% to 29%), cough increased (18%), bronchitis (17%)

Miscellaneous: Infection (24% to 45%), CMV infection (heart transplant 32%), graft dysfunction (kidney transplant 24%)

<15%:

Cardiovascular: Abnormal ECG (QRS or ST segment abnormal), arrhythmia, atrial fibrillation, atrial flutter, bradycardia, cardiopulmonary failure, deep thrombophlebitis, heart failure, heart rate decreased, hemorrhage, hemorrhagic stroke, hypervolemia, hypotension, peripheral vascular disorder, phlebitis, postural hypotension, syncope, tachycardia, thrombosis, vasodilation

Central nervous system: Abnormal dreams, abnormal thinking, agitation, amnesia, anxiety, chills, confusion, depression, emotional lability, encephalopathy, flaccid paralysis, hallucinations, mood elevated, nervousness, psychosis, quadriparesis, seizure, somnolence, vertigo

Dermatologic: Acne, alopecia, bruising, cellulitis, exfoliative dermatitis, fungal dermatitis, hirsutism, photosensitivity reaction, skin discoloration, skin disorder, skin neoplasm, skin ulcer, wound healing impaired

Endocrine & metabolic: Acidosis, alkalosis, bicarbonate decreased, Cushing's syndrome, dehydration, gout, hypercholesterolemia, hyper-/hypocalcemia, hyponatremia, hyperphosphatemia, hyperuricemia, hypoproteinemia, serum iron decreased

Gastrointestinal: Appetite increased, cramps, duodenitis, dysphagia, enlarged abdomen, esophagitis (including ulcerative), flatulence, gastritis, gastroesophagitis, GI perforation/hemorrhage, ileus, oral moniliasis, pancreatic pseudocyst, rectal disorder, stomatitis, weight gain

Genitourinary: Bladder spasm, cystitis, dysuria, nocturia, urge incontinence, urinary frequency, urinary incontinence, urinary retention, vaginitis

Hematologic: Coagulation disorder, decreased prothrombin, hypochromic anemia, polycythemia

Hepatic: Alkaline phosphatase increased, bilirubinemia, cholangitis, cholestatic jaundice, GGT increased, hepatitis (including granulomatous), jaundice, LDH increased, liver damage

Local: Phlebitis

Neuromuscular & skeletal: Hypertonia, incoordination, joint disorder, leg cramps, monoparesis, myalgia, myasthenia, myoclonus, nerve compression, neuropathy, osteoporosis, quadriparesis

Ocular: Abnormal vision, amblyopia

Otic: Ear pain, otitis media, tinnitus

Renal: Acute renal failure, albuminuria, BK nephropathy, hematuria, hydronephrosis, renal tubular necrosis, toxic nephropathy

Respiratory: Asthma, emphysema, lung disorder, lung function decreased, pharyngitis, pneumonia, pneumothorax, pulmonary edema, respiratory disorder, rhinitis, sinusitis, voice alteration

Miscellaneous: Abscess, abnormal healing, allergic reaction, crying, diaphoresis, flu-like syndrome, generalized spasm, hernia, herpes simplex, hiccups, peritonitis, sepsis, writing impaired

Available Dosage Forms

Capsule, oral: 0.5 mg, 1 mg, 5 mg

Hecoria™: 0.5 mg, 1 mg, 5 mg

Prograf®: 0.5 mg, 1 mg, 5 mg

Injection, solution:

Prograf®: 5 mg/mL (1 mL)

General Dosage Range

I.V.:

Children: 0.03-0.05 mg/kg/day as a continuous infusion

Adults: 0.01-0.05 mg/kg/day as a continuous infusion

Oral:

Children: 0.15-0.2 mg/kg/day in divided doses every 12 hours

Adults: 0.075-0.2 mg/kg/day in divided doses every 12 hours

Administration

Oral Administer with or without food; be consistent with timing and composition of meals if GI intolerance occurs and administration with food becomes necessary (per manufacturer). If dosed once daily, administer in the morning. If dosed twice daily, doses should be 12 hours apart. If the morning and evening doses differ, the larger dose (differences are never >0.5-1 mg) should be given in the morning. If dosed 3 times/day, separate doses by 8 hours.

Advagraf®: Canadian labeling recommends that missed doses may be taken up to 14 hours after scheduled time; if >14 hours, resume at next regularly scheduled time.

I.V. If I.V. administration is necessary, administer by continuous infusion only. Do not use PVC tubing when administering diluted solutions. Tacrolimus is usually intended to be administered as a continuous infusion over 24 hours.

I.V. Detail Do not mix with solutions with a pH ≥9 (eg, acyclovir or ganciclovir) due to chemical degradation of tacrolimus (use different ports in multilumen lines). Do not alter dose with concurrent T-tube clamping. Adsorption of the drug to PVC tubing may become clinically significant with low concentrations.

Stability

Reconstitution Dilute with 5% dextrose injection or 0.9% sodium chloride injection to a final concentration between 0.004 mg/mL and 0.02 mg/mL.

Storage

Injection: Prior to dilution, store at 5°C to 25°C (41°F to 77°F). Following dilution, stable for 24 hours in D_5W or NS in glass or polyethylene containers.

Capsules: Store at room temperature of 25°C (77°F); excursions permitted to 15°C to 30°C (59°F to 86°F).

Nursing Actions

Physical Assessment Monitor blood pressure frequently; can cause hypertension. Patients with diabetes should monitor glucose levels closely (this medication may alter glucose levels). Monitor for signs of opportunistic infection (eg, persistent fever, malaise, sore throat, unusual bleeding or bruising).

Patient Education Take on an empty stomach. Maintain adequate hydration during entire course of therapy, unless instructed to restrict fluid intake. You will be susceptible to infection. If you have diabetes, monitor glucose levels closely (drug may alter glucose levels). You may experience nausea, vomiting, or diarrhea. Report chest pain, severe headache, respiratory difficulty, unresolved GI effects, fatigue, chills, fever, unhealed sores, white plaques in mouth, pain on urination or change in urinary patterns, or rash.

Dietary Considerations Capsule: Administer with or without food; be consistent with timing and composition of meals, food decreases bioavailability. Avoid grapefruit juice.

Tacrolimus (Topical) (ta KROE li mus)

Brand Names: U.S. Protopic®

Pharmacologic Category Calcineurin Inhibitor; Topical Skin Product

Medication Safety Issues

Sound-alike/look-alike issues:

Tacrolimus may be confused with everolimus, pimecrolimus, sirolimus, temsirolimus

Medication Guide Available Yes

Pregnancy Risk Factor C

Lactation Enters breast milk/not recommended

Use Moderate-to-severe atopic dermatitis in immunocompetent patients not responsive to conventional therapy or when conventional therapy is not appropriate

Canadian labeling: Additional use (not in U.S. labeling): Maintenance therapy to prevent flares and extend flare-free intervals in patients with moderate-to-severe atopic dermatitis who are responsive to initial therapy and experiencing ≥5 flares per year

Available Dosage Forms

Ointment, topical:

Protopic®: 0.03% (30 g, 60 g, 100 g); 0.1% (30 g, 60 g, 100 g)

General Dosage Range Topical:

Children ≥2-15 years: Apply thin layer of 0.03% to affected area twice daily

Children >15 years and Adults: Apply thin layer of 0.03% or 0.1% to affected area twice daily

Administration

Topical Do not use with occlusive dressings. Burning at the application site is most common in first few days; improves as atopic dermatitis improves. Limit application to involved areas. Continue as long as signs and symptoms persist; discontinue if resolution occurs; re-evaluate if symptoms persist >6 weeks.

Nursing Actions

Physical Assessment Monitor for signs of opportunistic infection.

Patient Education Before applying, wash area gently and thoroughly. Apply in thin film to affected area. Do not cover skin with bandages. Wash hands only if not treating skin on the hands. Protect skin from sunlight or exposure to UV light.

Tadalafil (tah DA la fil)

Brand Names: U.S. Adcirca®; Cialis®

Index Terms GF196960

Pharmacologic Category Phosphodiesterase-5 Enzyme Inhibitor

Medication Safety Issues

Sound-alike/look-alike issues:

Tadalafil may be confused with sildenafil, vardenafil

Adcirca® may be confused with Advair® Diskus®, Advair® HFA, Advicor®

Pregnancy Risk Factor B

Lactation Excretion in breast milk unknown/use caution

Use

Adcirca®: Treatment of pulmonary arterial hypertension (PAH) (WHO Group I) to improve exercise ability

Cialis®: Treatment of erectile dysfunction (ED); treatment of signs and symptoms of benign prostatic hyperplasia (BPH)

Mechanism of Action/Effect

BPH: Exact mechanism unknown; effects likely due to PDE-5 mediated reduction and/or relaxation of prostate and bladder tissues, nerves and muscles

Erectile dysfunction: Tadalafil enhances the effect of nitric oxide (NO) by inhibiting phosphodiesterase type 5 (PDE-5), which is responsible for degradation of cGMP in the corpus cavernosum; when sexual stimulation causes local release of NO, inhibition of PDE-5 by tadalafil causes increased levels of cGMP in the corpus cavernosum, resulting in smooth muscle relaxation and inflow of blood to the corpus cavernosum. At recommended doses, it has no effect in the absence of sexual stimulation.

PAH: Inhibits phosphodiesterase type 5 (PDE-5) in smooth muscle of pulmonary vasculature where PDE-5 is responsible for the degradation of cyclic guanosine monophosphate (cGMP). Increased cGMP concentration results in pulmonary vasculature relaxation; vasodilation in the pulmonary bed and the systemic circulation (to a lesser degree) may occur.

Contraindications Known serious hypersensitivity to tadalafil or any component of the formulation; concurrent use (regularly/intermittently) of organic nitrates in any form (eg, nitroglycerin, isosorbide dinitrate)

Warnings/Precautions There is a degree of cardiac risk associated with sexual activity; therefore, physicians should consider the cardiovascular status of their patients prior to initiation. Use is not recommended in patients with hypotension (<90/50 mm Hg), uncontrolled hypertension (>170/100 mm Hg), NYHA class II-IV heart failure within the last 6 months, uncontrolled arrhythmias, stroke within the last 6 months, MI within the last 3 months, unstable angina or angina during sexual intercourse; safety and efficacy have not been evaluated in these patients. Safety and efficacy in PAH have not been evaluated in patients with clinically significant aortic and/or mitral valve disease, life-threatening arrhythmias, hypotension (<90/50 mm Hg), uncontrolled hypertension, significant left ventricular dysfunction, pericardial constriction, restrictive or congestive cardiomyopathy, symptomatic coronary artery disease. Use caution in patients with left ventricular outflow obstruction (eg, aortic stenosis, hypertrophic obstructive cardiomyopathy); may be more sensitive to vasodilator effects.

Patients experiencing anginal chest pain after tadalafil administration should seek immediate medical attention. Concomitant use (regularly/intermittently) with all forms of nitrates is contraindicated. When used for BPH, erectile dysfunction, or PAH and nitrate administration is medically necessary following use, at least 48 hours should elapse after the tadalafil dose and nitrate administration. When used for PAH, per the manufacturer, nitrate may be administered within 48 hours of tadalafil. For both situations, administration of nitrates should only be done under close medical supervision with hemodynamic monitoring.

Concurrent use with alpha-adrenergic antagonist therapy or substantial alcohol consumption may cause symptomatic hypotension; patients should be hemodynamically stable prior to initiating tadalafil therapy at the lowest possible dose. When used for BPH or erectile dysfunction, use caution in patients receiving strong CYP3A4 inhibitors. When used for PAH, avoid use in patients taking strong CYP3A4 inducers/inhibitors. Use in patients receiving or about to receive ritonavir requires dosage adjustment or interruption of therapy, respectively. Canadian labeling does not recommend use of tadalafil in patients with PAH who are also receiving protease inhibitors.

Pulmonary vasodilators may exacerbate the cardiovascular status in patients with pulmonary veno-occlusive disease (PVOD); use is not recommended. In patients with unrecognized PVOD, signs of pulmonary edema should prompt investigation into this diagnosis. Use with caution in patients with mild-to-moderate hepatic impairment; dosage adjustment/limitation is needed. Use is not recommended in patients with severe hepatic impairment or cirrhosis. Use with caution in patients with renal impairment; dosage adjustment/limitation is needed. Safety and efficacy with other tadalafil brands or other PDE-5 inhibitors (ie, sildenafil and vardenafil) have not been established. Patients should be informed not to take with other tadalafil brands or other PDE-5 inhibitors. Use caution in patients with bleeding disorders or peptic ulcer disease due to effect on platelets (bleeding).

When used to treat BPH or erectile dysfunction, potential underlying causes of BPH or erectile dysfunction should be evaluated prior to treatment. Use with caution in patients with anatomical deformation of the penis (angulation, cavernosal fibrosis, or Peyronie's disease), or who have conditions which may predispose them to priapism (sickle cell anemia, multiple myeloma, leukemia). Instruct patients to seek immediate medical attention if erection persists >4 hours. Safety and efficacy with other tadalafil brands or other PDE-5 inhibitors (ie, sildenafil and vardenafil) have not been established. Patients should be informed not to take with other tadalafil brands or other PDE-5 inhibitors.

The safety and efficacy of tadalafil with other treatments for erectile dysfunction have not been studied and are, therefore, not recommended as combination therapy.

Rare cases of nonarteritic anterior ischemic optic neuropathy (NAION) have been reported; risk may be increased with history of vision loss or NAION in one eye. Other risk factors for NAION include heart disease, diabetes, hypertension, smoking, age >50 years, or history of certain eye problems. Sudden decrease or loss of hearing has been reported rarely; hearing changes may be accompanied by tinnitus and dizziness. A direct relationship between therapy and vision or hearing loss has not been determined. Instruct patients to seek medical assistance for sudden loss of vision in one or both eyes, sudden decrease in hearing, or sudden loss of hearing.

Patients with genetic retinal disorders (eg, retinitis pigmentosa) were not evaluated in clinical trials; use is not recommended. Use with caution in the elderly.

Drug Interactions

Avoid Concomitant Use

Avoid concomitant use of Tadalafil with any of the following: Amyl Nitrite; Boceprevir; Phosphodiesterase 5 Inhibitors; Telaprevir; Vasodilators (Organic Nitrates)

Decreased Effect

The levels/effects of Tadalafil may be decreased by: Bosentan; CYP3A4 Inducers (Strong); Etravirine; Tocilizumab

Increased Effect/Toxicity

Tadalafil may increase the levels/effects of: Alpha1-Blockers; Amyl Nitrite; Antihypertensives; Bosentan; Phosphodiesterase 5 Inhibitors; Vasodilators (Organic Nitrates)

The levels/effects of Tadalafil may be increased by: Antifungal Agents (Azole Derivatives, Systemic); Boceprevir; CYP3A4 Inhibitors (Moderate); CYP3A4 Inhibitors (Strong); Dasatinib; Ivacaftor; Ritonavir; Sapropterin; Telaprevir

Nutritional/Ethanol Interactions

Ethanol: Substantial consumption of ethanol may increase the risk of hypotension and orthostasis. Lower ethanol consumption has not been associated with significant changes in blood pressure or increase in orthostatic symptoms. Management: Avoid or limit ethanol consumption.

Food: Rate and extent of absorption are not affected by food. Grapefruit juice may increase serum levels/toxicity of tadalafil. Management: Use of grapefruit juice should be limited or avoided.

Herb/Nutraceutical: St John's wort may decrease the levels/effectiveness of tadalafil. Management: Avoid or use caution with concomitant use.

Adverse Reactions Based upon usual doses for either indication. For erectile dysfunction, similar adverse events are reported with once-daily versus intermittent dosing, but are generally lower than with doses used intermittently.

>10%:

Cardiovascular: Flushing (1% to 13%; dose related)

Central nervous system: Headache (3% to 42%; dose related)

Gastrointestinal: Dyspepsia (1% to 13%), nausea (10% to 11%)

Neuromuscular & skeletal: Myalgia (1% to 14%; dose related), back pain (2% to 12%), extremity pain (1% to 11%)

Respiratory: Respiratory tract infection (3% to 13%), nasopharyngitis (2% to 13%)

2% to 10%:

Cardiovascular: Hypertension (1% to 3%)

Gastrointestinal: Gastroenteritis (viral; 3% to 5%), GERD (1% to 3%), abdominal pain (1% to 2%), diarrhea (1% to 2%)

Genitourinary: Urinary tract infection (≤2%)

Respiratory: Nasal congestion (≤9%), cough (2% to 4%), bronchitis (≤2%)

Miscellaneous: Flu-like syndrome (2% to 5%)

Pharmacodynamics/Kinetics

Onset of Action Within 1 hour

Peak effect: Pulmonary artery vasodilation: 75-90 minutes (Ghofrani, 2004)

Duration of Action Erectile dysfunction: Up to 36 hours

Available Dosage Forms

Tablet, oral:

Adcirca®: 20 mg

Cialis®: 2.5 mg, 5 mg, 10 mg, 20 mg

General Dosage Range Dosage adjustment recommended in patient with hepatic or renal impairment or on concomitant therapy

Oral: *Adults:* Benign prostatic hyperplasia: 5 mg once daily; Erectile dysfunction: As-needed dosing: 5-20 mg prior to anticipated sexual activity as a single dose (maximum: 1 dose/day); Once-daily dosing: 2.5-5 mg once daily; Pulmonary arterial hypertension: 40 mg once daily

Administration

Oral May be administered with or without food.

Adcirca®: Administer daily dose all at once; dividing doses throughout the day is not advised.

Cialis®: When used on an as-needed basis, should be taken at least 30 minutes prior to sexual activity. When used on a once-daily basis, should be taken at the same time each day, without regard to timing of sexual activity.

Stability

Storage Store at 25°C (77°F); excursions permitted to 15°C to 30°C (59°F to 86°F).

Nursing Actions

Physical Assessment Monitor for postural hypotension.

Patient Education Take at the same time daily. Avoid taking with grapefruit juice. Change positions slowly. Avoid substantial consumption of alcohol. This drug provides no protection against sexually-transmitted diseases, including HIV. You may experience headache, fatigue, dizziness, blurred vision, or back or limb pain. Report immediately chest pain, palpitations, respiratory difficulty, unusual dizziness, change in vision, change in hearing or ringing in the ears, signs of urinary tract infection, skin rash, genital swelling or priapism, or erection lasting >4 hours.

Dietary Considerations May be taken with or without food.

Tafluprost (TA floo prost)

Index Terms Zioptan™

Pharmacologic Category Ophthalmic Agent, Antiglaucoma; Prostaglandin, Ophthalmic

Pregnancy Risk Factor C

Lactation Excretion in breast milk unknown/use caution

Use Reduction of intraocular pressure (IOP) in patients with open-angle glaucoma or ocular hypertension

Product Availability Zioptan™ (preservative free ophthalmic solution): FDA approved February 2012; availability is expected in March 2012. Consult prescribing information for additional information.

Available Dosage Forms

Solution, ophthalmic [drops], preservative free:

Zioptan™: 0.0015%

General Dosage Range Ophthalmic: *Adults:* One drop in the affected eye(s) once daily

Administration

Other For ophthalmic use only. Wash hands before use. Avoid touching the tip of the single-use container to eye or other surfaces. Each single-use container has adequate solution to treat both eyes (if applicable); discard immediately after use. If more than one topical ophthalmic drug is being used, administer the drugs at least 5 minutes apart.

Nursing Actions

Physical Assessment Monitor for blurred vision, burning and stinging, conjunctival hyperemia, foreign body sensation, itching, increased pigmentation of the iris, and punctate epithelial keratopathy.

Patient Education For use in eyes only. Iris color may change because of an increase of the brown pigment. Iris pigmentation changes may be more noticeable in patients with green-brown, blue/gray-brown, or yellow-brown irides. If any ocular reaction develops, particularly conjunctivitis and lid reactions, immediately notify prescriber. If more than one topical ophthalmic drug is being used, administer the drugs at least 5 minutes apart. Do not let tip of applicator touch eye; do not contaminate tip of applicator (may cause eye infection, eye damage, or vision loss).

Tamoxifen (ta MOKS i fen)

Index Terms ICI-46474; Nolvadex; Tamoxifen Citras; Tamoxifen Citrate

Pharmacologic Category Antineoplastic Agent, Estrogen Receptor Antagonist; Selective Estrogen Receptor Modulator (SERM)

Medication Safety Issues

Sound-alike/look-alike issues:

Tamoxifen may be confused with pentoxifylline, Tambocor™, tamsulosin, temazepam

Medication Guide Available Yes

Pregnancy Risk Factor D

Lactation Excretion in breast milk unknown/not recommended

Breast-Feeding Considerations It is not known if tamoxifen is excreted in breast milk, however, it has been shown to inhibit lactation. Due to the potential for adverse reactions, women taking tamoxifen should not breast-feed.

Use Treatment of metastatic (female and male) breast cancer; adjuvant treatment of breast cancer after primary treatment with surgery and radiation; reduce risk of invasive breast cancer in women with ductal carcinoma *in situ* (DCIS) after surgery and radiation; reduce the incidence of breast cancer in women at high risk

Unlabeled Use Treatment of mastalgia, gynecomastia, ovarian cancer, endometrial cancer, uterine sarcoma, and desmoid tumors; risk reduction in women with Paget's disease of the breast (with DCIS or without associated cancer); induction of ovulation; treatment of precocious puberty in females, secondary to McCune-Albright syndrome

Mechanism of Action/Effect Competitively binds to estrogen receptors on tumors and other tissue targets, producing a nuclear complex that decreases DNA synthesis and inhibits estrogen effects; nonsteroidal agent with potent antiestrogenic properties which compete with estrogen for binding sites in breast and other tissues; cells accumulate in the G_0 and G_1 phases; therefore, tamoxifen is cytostatic rather than cytocidal.

Contraindications Hypersensitivity to tamoxifen or any component of the formulation; concurrent warfarin therapy or history of deep vein thrombosis or pulmonary embolism (when tamoxifen is used for cancer risk reduction in women at high risk for breast cancer and in women with DCIS)

Warnings/Precautions Hazardous agent - use appropriate precautions for handling and disposal. **[U.S. Boxed Warning]: Serious and life-threatening events (including stroke, pulmonary emboli, and uterine malignancy) have occurred at an incidence greater than placebo during use for breast cancer risk reduction in women at high-risk for breast cancer and in women with DCIS;** these events are rare, but require consideration in risk:benefit evaluation. An increased incidence of thromboembolic events, including DVT and pulmonary embolism, has been associated with use for breast cancer; risk is increased with concomitant chemotherapy; use with caution in individuals with a history of thromboembolic events. Thrombocytopenia and/or leukopenia may occur; neutropenia and pancytopenia have been reported rarely. Although the relationship to tamoxifen therapy is uncertain, rare hemorrhagic episodes have occurred in patients with significant thrombocytopenia. Use with caution in patients with hyperlipidemias; infrequent postmarketing cases of hyperlipidemias have been reported. Decreased visual acuity, retinal vein thrombosis, retinopathy, corneal changes, color perception changes, and increased incidence of cataracts (and the need for cataract surgery), have been reported. Hypercalcemia has occurred in patients with bone metastasis, usually within a few weeks of therapy initiation; institute appropriate hypercalcemia management; discontinue if severe. Local disease flare and increased bone and tumor pain may occur in patients with metastatic breast cancer; may be associated with (good) tumor response.

Tamoxifen is associated with a high potential for drug interactions, including CYP- and Pgp-mediated interactions. Decreased efficacy and an increased risk of breast cancer recurrence has been reported with concurrent moderate or strong CYP2D6 inhibitors (Aubert, 2009; Dezentje, 2009). Concomitant use with select SSRIs may result in decreased tamoxifen efficacy. Strong CYP2D6 inhibitors (eg, fluoxetine, paroxetine) and moderate CYP2D6 inhibitors (eg, sertraline) are reported to interfere with transformation to the active metabolite endoxifen. Weak CYP2D6 inhibitors (eg, venlafaxine, citalopram) have minimal effect on the conversion to endoxifen (Jin, 2005; NCCN Breast Cancer Risk Reduction Guidelines v.2.2010); escitalopram is also a weak CYP2D6 inhibitor. Lower plasma concentrations of endoxifen (active metabolite) have been observed in patients associated with reduced CYP2D6 activity (Jin, 2005) and may be associated with reduced efficacy. In a retrospective analysis of breast cancer patients taking tamoxifen and SSRIs, concomitant use of paroxetine and tamoxifen was associated with an increased risk of death due to breast cancer (Kelly, 2010).

Tamoxifen use may be associated with changes in bone mineral density (BMD) and the effects may be dependent upon menstrual status. In postmenopausal women, tamoxifen use is associated with a protective effect on bone mineral density (BMD), preventing loss of BMD which lasts over the 5-year treatment period. In premenopausal women, a decline (from baseline) in BMD mineral density has been observed in women who continued to menstruate; may be associated with an increased risk of fractures. Liver abnormalities such as cholestasis, fatty liver, hepatitis, and hepatic necrosis have occurred. Hepatocellular carcinomas have been reported in some studies; relationship to treatment is unclear. Tamoxifen is associated with an increased incidence of uterine or endometrial cancers. Endometrial hyperplasia, polyps, endometriosis, uterine fibroids, and ovarian cysts have occurred. Monitor and promptly evaluate any report of abnormal vaginal bleeding. Amenorrhea and menstrual irregularities have been reported with tamoxifen use.

Drug Interactions

Avoid Concomitant Use

Avoid concomitant use of Tamoxifen with any of the following: Conivaptan; CYP2D6 Inhibitors (Strong); Pimozide; Silodosin; Topotecan; Vitamin K Antagonists

Decreased Effect

Tamoxifen may decrease the levels/effects of: Anastrozole; Letrozole

The levels/effects of Tamoxifen may be decreased by: Aminoglutethimide; CYP2C9 Inducers (Strong); CYP3A4 Inducers (Strong); Cyproterone; Deferasirox; Herbs (CYP3A4 Inducers); Peginterferon Alfa-2b; Rifamycin Derivatives; Tocilizumab

Increased Effect/Toxicity

Tamoxifen may increase the levels/effects of: ARIPiprazole; Colchicine; CYP2C8 Substrates; Dabigatran Etexilate; Everolimus; P-glycoprotein/ABCB1 Substrates; Pimozide; Prucalopride; Rivaroxaban; Silodosin; Topotecan; Vitamin K Antagonists

The levels/effects of Tamoxifen may be increased by: Abiraterone Acetate; Conivaptan; CYP2C9 Inhibitors (Moderate); CYP2C9 Inhibitors (Strong); CYP2D6 Inhibitors (Moderate); CYP2D6 Inhibitors (Strong); CYP3A4 Inhibitors (Moderate); CYP3A4 Inhibitors (Strong); Darunavir; Dasatinib; Ivacaftor

Nutritional/Ethanol Interactions

Food: Grapefruit juice may decrease the metabolism of tamoxifen. Management: Avoid grapefruit juice.

Herb/Nutraceutical: Black cohosh and dong quai have estrogenic properties. St John's wort may decrease levels/effects of tamoxifen. Management: Avoid black cohosh and dong quai in estrogen-dependent tumors. Avoid St John's wort.

Adverse Reactions

>10%:

Cardiovascular: Vasodilation (41%), flushing (33%), hypertension (11%), peripheral edema (11%)

Central nervous system: Mood changes (12% to 18%), pain (3% to 16%), depression (2% to 12%)

Dermatologic: Skin changes (6% to 19%), rash (13%)

Endocrine & metabolic: Hot flashes (3% to 80%), fluid retention (32%), altered menses (13% to 25%), amenorrhea (16%)

Gastrointestinal: Nausea (5% to 26%), weight loss (23%), vomiting (12%)

Genitourinary: Vaginal discharge (13% to 55%), vaginal bleeding (2% to 23%)

Neuromuscular & skeletal: Weakness (18%), arthritis (14%), arthralgia (11%)

Respiratory: Pharyngitis (14%)

Miscellaneous: Lymphedema (11%)

1% to 10%:

Cardiovascular: Chest pain (5%), venous thrombotic events (5%), edema (4%), cardiovascular ischemia (3%), angina (2%), deep venous thrombus (≤2%), MI (1%)

Central nervous system: Insomnia (9%), dizziness (8%), headache (8%), anxiety (6%), fatigue (4%)

Dermatologic: Alopecia (≤5%)

Endocrine & metabolic: Oligomenorrhea (9%), breast pain (6%), menstrual disorder (6%), breast neoplasm (5%), hypercholesterolemia (4%)

Gastrointestinal: Abdominal pain (9%), weight gain (9%), constipation (4% to 8%), diarrhea (7%), dyspepsia (6%), throat irritation (oral solution 5%), abdominal cramps (1%), anorexia (1%)

Genitourinary: Urinary tract infection (10%), leukorrhea (9%), vaginal hemorrhage (6%), vaginitis (5%), vulvovaginitis (5%), ovarian cyst (3%)

Hematologic: Thrombocytopenia (≤10%), anemia (5%)

Hepatic: AST increased (5%), serum bilirubin increased (2%)

Neuromuscular & skeletal: Back pain (10%), bone pain (6% to 10%), osteoporosis (7%), fracture (7%), arthrosis (5%), joint disorder (5%), myalgia (5%), paresthesia (5%), musculoskeletal pain (3%)

Ocular: Cataract (7%)

Renal: Serum creatinine increased (≤2%)

Respiratory: Cough (4% to 9%), dyspnea (8%), bronchitis (5%), sinusitis (5%)

Miscellaneous: Infection/sepsis (≤9%), diaphoresis (6%), flu-like syndrome (6%), cyst (5%), neoplasm (5%), allergic reaction (3%)

Available Dosage Forms

Tablet, oral: 10 mg, 20 mg

General Dosage Range Oral: *Adults:* 20-40 mg/day

Administration

Oral Administer with or without food.

Stability

Storage Store at room temperature of 20°C to 25°C (68°F to 77°F). Protect from light.

Nursing Actions

Physical Assessment Evaluate for use-related precautions prior to beginning therapy. Monitor for thromboembolism, flushing, fluid retention, hot flashes, vaginal bleeding or discharge, constipation, rash, or mood changes. Teach patient importance of periodic ophthalmic evaluations and annual gynecological exams and mammograms with long-term use.

Patient Education You should schedule an annual ophthalmic examination, gynecological exam, and mammogram if this medication is used long-term. You may experience hot flashes, hair loss, or loss of libido (these will subside when treatment is completed). May cause nausea, vomiting, and increased blood pressure. Notify prescriber if menstrual irregularities, vaginal bleeding, or intolerable hot flashes occur. Report unusual bleeding or bruising, severe weakness or unusual fatigue, CNS changes (depression, mood changes), persistent bone changes, changes in strength on one side of the body, chest pain or pressure, swelling or pain in calves, respiratory difficulty, or vision changes.

Dietary Considerations May be taken with or without food. Avoid grapefruit and grapefruit juice.

Tamsulosin (tam SOO loe sin)

Brand Names: U.S. Flomax®

Index Terms Tamsulosin Hydrochloride

Pharmacologic Category Alpha$_1$ Blocker

Medication Safety Issues

Sound-alike/look-alike issues:

Flomax® may be confused with Flonase®, Flovent®, Foltx®, Fosamax®

Tamsulosin may be confused with tacrolimus, tamoxifen, terazosin

International issues:

Flomax [U.S., Canada, and multiple international markets] may be confused with Flomox brand name for cefcapene [Japan]; Volmax brand name for salbutamol [multiple international markets]

Flomax: Brand name for tamsulosin [U.S., Canada, and multiple international markets], but also the brand name for morniflumate [Italy]

Pregnancy Risk Factor B

Use Treatment of signs and symptoms of benign prostatic hyperplasia (BPH)

Unlabeled Use Symptomatic treatment of bladder outlet obstruction or dysfunction; facilitation of expulsion of ureteral stones

Mechanism of Action/Effect Antagonizes alpha$_{1A}$-adrenoreceptors in the prostate which mediate the dynamic component of urine flow obstruction by regulating smooth muscle tone of the bladder neck and prostate. When given to patients with BPH, blockade of alpha-receptors leads to relaxation of these muscles, resulting in an improvement in urine flow rate and symptoms. Alpha-blockade does not influence the static component of urinary obstruction, which is related to tissue proliferation.

Contraindications Hypersensitivity to tamsulosin or any component of the formulation

Warnings/Precautions Not intended for use as an antihypertensive drug. May cause significant orthostatic hypotension and syncope, especially with first dose; anticipate a similar effect if therapy is interrupted for a few days, if dosage is rapidly increased, or if another antihypertensive drug (particularly vasodilators) or a PDE-5 inhibitor (eg, sildenafil, tadalafil, vardenafil) is introduced. "First-dose" orthostatic hypotension may occur 4-8 hours after dosing; may be dose related. Patients should be cautioned about performing hazardous tasks when starting new therapy or adjusting dosage upward. Discontinue if symptoms of angina occur or worsen. Rule out prostatic carcinoma before beginning therapy with tamsulosin. Intraoperative floppy iris syndrome has been observed in cataract surgery patients who were on or were previously treated with alpha$_1$-blockers; causality has not been established and there appears to be no benefit in discontinuing alpha-blocker therapy prior to surgery; instruct patients to inform ophthalmologist of tamsulosin use when considering eye surgery. Priapism has been associated with use (rarely). Rarely, patients with a sulfa allergy have also developed an allergic reaction to tamsulosin; avoid use when previous reaction has been severe.

Drug Interactions

Avoid Concomitant Use

Avoid concomitant use of Tamsulosin with any of the following: Alpha1-Blockers; CYP3A4 Inhibitors (Strong)

Decreased Effect

The levels/effects of Tamsulosin may be decreased by: CYP3A4 Inducers (Strong); Deferasirox; Herbs (CYP3A4 Inducers); Peginterferon Alfa-2b; Tocilizumab

Increased Effect/Toxicity

Tamsulosin may increase the levels/effects of: Alpha1-Blockers; Calcium Channel Blockers

The levels/effects of Tamsulosin may be increased by: Beta-Blockers; CYP3A4 Inhibitors (Moderate); CYP3A4 Inhibitors (Strong); Dasatinib; Ivacaftor; MAO Inhibitors; Phosphodiesterase 5 Inhibitors

Nutritional/Ethanol Interactions

Food: Fasting increases bioavailability by 30% and peak concentration 40% to 70%. Management: Administer 30 minutes after the same meal each day.

Herb/Nutraceutical: St John's wort may decrease the levels/effects of tamsulosin. Some herbal medications have hypotensive properties or may increase the hypotensive effect of tamsulosin. Limited information is available regarding combination with saw palmetto. Management: Avoid St John's wort, black cohosh, California poppy, coleus, golden seal, hawthorn, mistletoe, periwinkle, quinine, and shepherd's purse. Avoid saw palmetto.

Adverse Reactions

>10%:

Cardiovascular: Orthostatic hypotension (6% to 19%)

Central nervous system: Headache (19% to 21%), dizziness (15% to 17%)

Genitourinary: Abnormal ejaculation (8% to 18%)

Respiratory: Rhinitis (13% to 18%)

Miscellaneous: Infection (9% to 11%)

1% to 10%:

Cardiovascular: Chest pain (4%)

Central nervous system: Somnolence (3% to 4%), insomnia (1% to 2%), vertigo (≤1%)

Endocrine & metabolic: Libido decreased (1% to 2%)

Gastrointestinal: Diarrhea (4% to 6%), nausea (3% to 4%), gum pain, toothache

Neuromuscular & skeletal: Weakness (8% to 9%), back pain (7% to 8%)

Ocular: Blurred vision (≤2%)

Respiratory: Pharyngitis (5% to 6%), cough (3% to 5%), sinusitis (2% to 4%)

Available Dosage Forms

Capsule, oral: 0.4 mg

Flomax®: 0.4 mg

Tablet, oral: 0.4 mg

General Dosage Range Oral: *Adults:* Initial: 0.4 mg once daily; Maintenance: 0.4-0.8 mg once daily

Administration

Oral Administer 30 minutes after the same meal each day. Capsules should be swallowed whole; do not crush, chew, or open.

Stability

Storage Store at room temperature of 25°C (77°F); excursions permitted to 15°C to 30°C (59°F to 86°F).

Nursing Actions

Physical Assessment Assess blood pressure and monitor for hypotension, dizziness, somnolence, and impotence at beginning of therapy and on a regular basis.

Patient Education May cause dizziness with first doses; may cause postural hypotension, ejaculatory disturbance (reversible, may resolve with continued use of drug), headache, or rhinitis. Report palpitations or rapid heartbeat, chest pain, severe dizziness or passing out, or erection that lasts more than 4 hours.

Dietary Considerations Take once daily, 30 minutes after the same meal each day.

Tapentadol (ta PEN ta dol)

Brand Names: U.S. Nucynta®; Nucynta® ER

Index Terms CG5503; Tapentadol Hydrochloride

Pharmacologic Category Analgesic, Opioid

Medication Safety Issues

Sound-alike/look-alike issues:

Tapentadol may be confused with traMADol

Medication Guide Available Yes

Pregnancy Risk Factor C

Lactation Excretion in breast milk unknown/not recommended

Breast-Feeding Considerations Limited information available on the excretion of tapentadol in human milk; however, data suggests it may be excreted in human milk. The possibility of sedation or respiratory depression in the nursing infant should be considered.

Use

Immediate release formulation: Relief of moderate-to-severe acute pain

Long acting formulation: Relief of moderate-to-severe chronic pain when continuous, around-the-clock analgesia is necessary for an extended period of time

Mechanism of Action/Effect Binds to μ-opiate receptors in the CNS causing inhibition of ascending pain pathways, altering the perception of and response to pain; also inhibits the reuptake of norepinephrine, which also modifies the ascending pain pathway

Contraindications Hypersensitivity to tapentadol or any component of the formulation; impaired pulmonary function (severe respiratory depression, acute or severe asthma or hypercapnia) in unmonitored settings or in absence of resuscitative equipment or ventilatory support; paralytic ileus; use of MAO inhibitors within 14 days

Canadian labeling: Additional contraindications (not in U.S. labeling): Hypersensitivity to opioids; any disease/condition that affects bowel transit (eg, ileus of any type, strictures); severe renal impairment (Cl_{cr} <30 mL/minute); severe hepatic impairment (Child-Pugh class C); mild, intermittent, or short-duration pain that can be managed with alternative pain medication; management of perioperative pain; acute alcoholism, delirium tremens, and seizure disorders; severe CNS depression, increased cerebrospinal or intracranial pressure or head injury; pregnancy; breast-feeding; use during labor/delivery

Warnings/Precautions Extended release tablets: **[U.S. Boxed Warning]: Use of alcohol or alcohol-containing medications should be avoided;** concomitant use with alcohol may increase tapentadol systemic exposure which may lead to possible fatal overdose. **[U.S. Boxed warning]: NOT intended for use as an as-needed analgesic; NOT intended for the management of acute or postoperative pain;** approved for the treatment of chronic pain only (not an as-needed basis). **[U.S. Boxed Warning]: Extended-release tablets must be swallowed whole and should NOT be**

split, crushed, broken, chewed or dissolved. [U.S. Boxed Warning]: Healthcare provider should be alert to problems of abuse, misuse, and diversion. May cause severe hypotension; use with caution in patients with risk factors (eg. hypovolemia, concomitant use of other hypotensive agents).

Use with caution in patients with respiratory disease or respiratory compromise (eg, asthma, chronic obstructive pulmonary disease [COPD], cor pulmonale, sleep apnea, severe obesity, kyphoscoliosis, hypoxia, hypercapnia); critical respiratory depression may occur, even at therapeutic dosages. May cause CNS depression, which may impair physical or mental abilities; patients must be cautioned about performing tasks which require mental alertness (eg, operating machinery or driving). Use with caution in patients with CNS depression or coma. Effects may be potentiated when used with other sedative drugs or ethanol. Use with caution in patients with adrenal insufficiency, hypothyroidism or prostatic hyperplasia/urinary stricture.

Serotonin syndrome (SS) may occur with serotonin/norepinephrine reuptake inhibitors (SNRIs), including tapentadol. Signs of SS may include agitation, tachycardia, hyperthermia, nausea, and vomiting. Avoid use with serotonergic agents such as TCAs, triptans, venlafaxine, trazodone, lithium, sibutramine, meperidine, dextromethorphan, St John's wort, SNRIs, and SSRIs; concomitant use has been associated with the development of serotonin syndrome. Contraindicated with MAO inhibitor use within 14 days.

Use caution in patients with biliary tract dysfunction or acute pancreatitis; opioids may cause spasm of the sphincter of Oddi. Opioid use may obscure diagnosis or clinical course of patients with acute abdominal conditions. Use with extreme caution in patients with head injury, intracranial lesions, or elevated intracranial pressure (ICP); exaggerated elevation of ICP may occur. Serum concentrations are increased in hepatic impairment; use with caution in patients with moderate hepatic impairment (dosage adjustment required). Not recommended for use in severe hepatic impairment (not studied). Use with caution in patients with mild-to-moderate renal impairment (no dosage adjustment recommended). Not recommended for use in severe renal impairment (not studied). Use caution in patients with a history of seizures or conditions predisposing patients to seizures; patients with a history of seizures were excluded in clinical trials of tapentadol. Tramadol, an analgesic with similar pharmacologic properties to tapentadol, has been associated with seizures, particularly in patients with predisposing factors.

Prolonged use increases risk of abuse, addiction, and withdrawal symptoms. An opioid-containing regimen should be tailored to each patient's needs with respect to degree of tolerance for opioids (naïve versus chronic user), age, weight, and medical condition. Healthcare provider should be alert to problems of abuse, misuse, and diversion. Abrupt discontinuation may lead to withdrawal symptoms. Symptoms may be decreased by tapering prior to discontinuation. Use opioids with caution in elderly; consider decreasing initial dose. Use caution in debilitated patients; there is a greater potential for critical respiratory depression, even at therapeutic dosages.

During dosage adjustments, the Canadian labeling recommends that immediate release tramadol may be used as rescue medication (maximum dose: 400 mg/day) and that fentanyl should not be used as rescue medication.

Drug Interactions

Avoid Concomitant Use

Avoid concomitant use of Tapentadol with any of the following: Alcohol (Ethyl); MAO Inhibitors

Decreased Effect

Tapentadol may decrease the levels/effects of: Pegvisomant

The levels/effects of Tapentadol may be decreased by: Ammonium Chloride; Mixed Agonist / Antagonist Opioids; Peginterferon Alfa-2b

Increased Effect/Toxicity

Tapentadol may increase the levels/effects of: Alvimopan; CNS Depressants; Desmopressin; MAO Inhibitors; Metoclopramide; Selective Serotonin Reuptake Inhibitors; Serotonin Modulators; Thiazide Diuretics

The levels/effects of Tapentadol may be increased by: Alcohol (Ethyl); Amphetamines; Antipsychotic Agents (Phenothiazines); Antipsychotics; HydrOXYzine; Succinylcholine

Nutritional/Ethanol Interactions

Ethanol: May increase CNS depression; monitor for increased effects with coadministration. Caution patients about effects. Bioavailability of extended release tablets may be increased by alcohol; combined use should be avoided.

Food: When administered after a high fat/calorie meal, the AUC and C_{max} increased by 25% and 16%, respectively; may administer without regard to meals.

Herb/Nutraceutical: Avoid St John's wort (may increase CNS depression and risk of serotonin syndrome).

Adverse Reactions

Immediate release;

>10%:

Central nervous system: Dizziness (24%), somnolence (15%)

Gastrointestinal: Nausea (30%), vomiting (18%), constipation (8%)

≤1% to 10%:

Central nervous system: Fatigue (3%), insomnia (2%), anxiety (1%), confusion (1%), dreams abnormal (1%), lethargy (1%), attention disturbances (<1%), headache (<1%)

Dermatologic: Pruritus (3% to 5%), hyperhidrosis (3%), rash (1%)

Endocrine & metabolic: Hot flushes (1%)

Gastrointestinal: Xerostomia (4%), appetite decreased (2%), dyspepsia (2%)

Genitourinary: Urinary tract infection (1%)

Neuromuscular & skeletal: Arthralgia (1%), tremor (1%)

Respiratory: Nasopharyngitis (1%), upper respiratory tract infection (1%), dyspnea (<1%)

Extended release:

>10%:

Central nervous system: Dizziness (17%), headache (15%), somnolence (12%)

Gastrointestinal: Nausea (21%), constipation (17%), vomiting (8%)

1% to 10%:

Central nervous system: Fatigue (9%), insomnia (4%), anxiety (2%), lethargy (2%), vertigo (2%), attention disturbances (1%), chills (1%), depression/depressed mood (1%)

Dermatologic: Hyperhidrosis (5%), pruritus (5%), rash (1%)

Endocrine & metabolic: Hot flushes (2%)

Gastrointestinal: Xerostomia (7%), dyspepsia (3%), appetite decreased (2%)

Genitourinary: Erectile dysfunction (1%)

Neuromuscular & skeletal: Weakness (2%), tremor (1%)

Ocular: Vision blurred (1%)

Respiratory: Dyspnea (1%)

Controlled Substance C-II

Available Dosage Forms

Tablet, oral:

Nucynta®: 50 mg, 75 mg, 100 mg

Tablet, extended release, oral:

Nucynta® ER: 50 mg, 100 mg, 150 mg, 200 mg, 250 mg

General Dosage Range Dosage adjustment recommended in patients with hepatic impairment

Oral:

Immediate release: *Adults:* 50-100 mg every 4-6 hours as needed (maximum: 700 mg/day on day 1; 600 mg/day subsequent days)

Extended release: *Adults:* 50-250 mg twice daily (maximum: 500 mg/day)

Administration

Oral Administer orally with or without food. Long acting formulations must be swallowed whole and should **not** be split, crushed, broken, chewed, or dissolved.

Stability

Storage Store at room temperature up to 25°C (77°F); excursions permitted to 15°C to 30°C (59°F to 86°F). Protect from moisture.

Nursing Actions

Physical Assessment Monitor respiratory and CNS status. Assess patient's physical and/or psychological dependence. For inpatients, implement safety measures (eg, side rails up, call light within reach, instructions to call for assistance). Discontinue slowly after prolonged use. If case of overdose, call Poison Help at 1-800-222-1222.

Patient Education May cause physical and/or psychological dependence. While using this medication, do not use alcohol and other prescription or OTC medications (especially sedatives, tranquilizers, antihistamines, or pain medications) without consulting prescriber. Maintain adequate hydration, unless instructed to restrict fluid intake. May cause itching, hypotension, dizziness, drowsiness, impaired coordination, or blurred vision; loss of appetite, dry mouth, nausea, or vomiting; or constipation. Report dizziness, changes in mental status, skin rash, or shortness of breath. Do not crush, chew, or break extended release tablets. Overdose symptoms include vomiting, shallow breathing, and slowed heart rate. If overdose or symptoms of overdose occur, call Poison Help at 1-800-222-1222. Do not suddenly stop this medication. Keep this medicine in a secure place.

Dietary Considerations May be taken without regard to meals.

Tazarotene (taz AR oh teen)

Brand Names: U.S. Avage®; Tazorac®

Pharmacologic Category Acne Products; Keratolytic Agent; Topical Skin Product, Acne

Pregnancy Risk Factor X

Lactation Excretion in breast milk unknown/use caution

Use Topical treatment of facial acne vulgaris; topical treatment of stable plaque psoriasis; mitigation (palliation) of facial skin wrinkling, facial mottled hyper-/hypopigmentation, and benign facial lentigines

Available Dosage Forms

Cream, topical:

Avage®: 0.1% (30 g)

Tazorac®: 0.05% (30 g, 60 g); 0.1% (30 g, 60 g)

Gel, topical:

Tazorac®: 0.05% (30 g, 100 g); 0.1% (30 g, 100 g)

General Dosage Range Topical: *Children ≥12 years and Adults:* Apply a pea-sized amount or thin film **or** 2 mg/cm^2 once daily

Administration

Topical Do not apply to eczematous or sunburned skin; avoid eyes and mouth

Acne: Apply in evening after gently cleansing and drying face; apply enough to cover entire affected area.

Palliation of fine facial wrinkles, facial mottled hyper-/hypopigmentation, benign facial lentigines: Apply to clean dry face at bedtime; lightly cover entire face including eyelids if desired. Emollients or moisturizers may be applied before or after; if applied before tazarotene, ensure cream or lotion has absorbed into the skin and has dried completely.

Psoriasis: Apply in evening. If a bath or shower is taken prior to application, dry the skin before applying. If emollients are used, apply them at least 1 hour prior to application. Unaffected skin may be more susceptible to irritation, avoid application to these areas.

Nursing Actions

Physical Assessment Assess for accumulated photosensitivity.

Patient Education This medication is for external use only; avoid using near eyes or mouth. Severe skin reactions may occur. Avoid any other skin products (including cosmetics or personal products that may contain medications, alcohols, or irritants) that are not approved by your prescriber. May cause photosensitivity, which will cause severe rash or burning (use sunblock SPF 15 or higher, wear protective clothing and eyewear, and avoid direct sunlight, sunlamps, or tanning beds). Report redness or discoloration, irritation, burning, stinging, excessive dryness, or worsening of condition.

Application: Wash affected area gently and completely dry before applying medication. Apply a thin layer to cover affected area. Wash off any medication that gets on unaffected skin areas and wash hands thoroughly after application.

Tegaserod (teg a SER od)

Brand Names: U.S. Zelnorm®

Index Terms HTF919; Tegaserod Maleate

Pharmacologic Category Serotonin 5-HT_4 Receptor Agonist

Pregnancy Risk Factor B

Lactation Excretion in breast milk unknown/not recommended

Use Emergency treatment of irritable bowel syndrome with constipation (IBS-C) and chronic idiopathic constipation (CIC) in women (<55 years of age) in which no alternative therapy exists

Available Dosage Forms

Tablet, oral:

Zelnorm®: 2 mg, 6 mg

General Dosage Range Oral: *Adults (females <55 years of age):* 6 mg twice daily

Administration

Oral Administer 30 minutes before meals.

Nursing Actions

Physical Assessment For emergency use only under FDA emergency investigational new drug process. Monitor for cardiac event, clinically-significant diarrhea (hypovolemia, hypotension, syncope), and ischemic colitis (rectal bleeding, bloody diarrhea, abdominal pain) frequently when beginning therapy and at regular intervals during treatment.

Patient Education Take on an empty stomach, 30 minutes before meals. Effectiveness of treatment will need to be evaluated by prescriber; maintain contact/appointment schedule as directed. May cause headache, dizziness, nausea, flatulence, or diarrhea. Stop taking Zelnorm® and contact prescriber immediately with any new or sudden worsening abdominal pain or rectal bleeding, or severe or bloody diarrhea. Seek emergency medical care immediately if you experience severe chest pain, shortness of breath, dizziness, sudden onset of weakness, or difficulty walking or talking.

Telaprevir (tel A pre vir)

Brand Names: U.S. Incivek™

Index Terms LY570310; MP-424; MP424; VRT111950; VX-950; VX950

Pharmacologic Category Antiviral Agent; Protease Inhibitor

Medication Guide Available Yes

Pregnancy Risk Factor B / X (in combination with ribavirin)

Lactation Excretion in breast milk unknown/not recommended

Breast-Feeding Considerations It is not known if telaprevir or ribavirin are excreted into breast milk. The manufacturer recommends that breast feeding be discontinued prior to the initiation of treatment.

Use Treatment of genotype 1 chronic hepatitis C (in combination with peginterferon alfa and ribavirin) in adult patients with compensated liver disease (including cirrhosis) who are treatment naive or who have received previous interferon-based treatment, including null or partial responders, and treatment relapsers.

Mechanism of Action/Effect Inhibits viral protein synthesis; direct-acting antiviral against the hepatitis C virus

Contraindications Hypersensitivity to telaprevir or any component of the formulation; pregnancy; male partners of pregnant women

Coadministration with CYP 3A4 highly dependent substrates (alfuzosin, atorvastatin, cisapride, ergot derivatives, lovastatin, midazolam [oral], pimozide, sildenafil/tadalafil [when used for treatment of pulmonary arterial hypertension], simvastatin, triazolam), or strong CYP 3A4 inducers (rifampin, St John's wort)

Canadian labeling: Additional contraindications (not in U.S. labeling): Coadministration with amiodarone, eletriptan, flecainide, propafenone, quinidine, terfenadine, vardenafil

Also refer to Peginterferon Alfa and Ribavirin monographs for individual product contraindications.

Warnings/Precautions Avoid pregnancy in female patients and female partners of male patients, during therapy, and for at least 6 months after treatment; two forms of nonhormonal contraception should be used. Safety and efficacy have not been established in patients who have uncompensated cirrhosis, received organ transplants, or been coinfected with hepatitis B or HIV, or who have failed to respond to other NS3/4A inhibitors. Monotherapy is not effective for chronic hepatitis C infection.

Anemia has been reported with peginterferon alfa and ribavirin; addition of telaprevir is associated with further hemoglobin decreases. Low hemoglobin levels were measured during the first 4 weeks of treatment, and the lowest at the end of telaprevir treatment (week 12). Dose modifications of ribavirin were needed more often in patients also taking telaprevir. Assess complete blood count (CBC) pretreatment and at weeks 2, 4, 8, and 12, and when clinically indicated. May require ribavirin dose reduction, interruption or discontinuation of treatment. Do not reduce telaprevir dose. If ribavirin is discontinued, telaprevir must also be discontinued. Do not restart telaprevir if ribavirin therapy is reinitiated. Mild-to-severe skin reactions, including DRESS (drug rash with eosinophilia with systemic symptoms [fever, facial edema, hepatitis or nephritis with or without eosinophilia]) and Stevens-Johnson syndrome (SJS) have been reported; discontinue telaprevir combination therapy immediately if patient develops DRESS or SJS. Severe rashes (other than DRESS, SJS) are generalized, bullous, vesicular or ulcerative; may also have an eczematous appearance. Discontinue telaprevir (may continue peginterferon alfa and ribavirin) for severe rash or for mild-to-moderate rash that progresses or leads to systemic involvement; if no improvement in rash within 1 week of stopping telaprevir, interruption or discontinuation of peginterferon alfa and/or ribavirin should be considered (or sooner if clinically indicated). May use oral antihistamines/topical corticosteroids for rash treatment; do not use systemic corticosteroids. Do not restart telaprevir if discontinued due to any rash severity. High potential for CYP3A-mediated interactions. Hormonal contraceptives may not be effective in patients taking telaprevir or for two weeks after discontinuing therapy. Not recommended in moderate or severe hepatic impairment (Child-Pugh class B or C) or decompensated hepatic disease.

Drug Interactions

Avoid Concomitant Use

Avoid concomitant use of Telaprevir with any of the following: Alfuzosin; Atorvastatin; Axitinib; CarBAMazepine; Cisapride; Conivaptan; Crizotinib; Darunavir; Dronedarone; Eplerenone; Ergot Derivatives; Everolimus; Fluticasone (Oral Inhalation); Fosamprenavir; Fosphenytoin; Halofantrine; Lapatinib; Lopinavir; Lovastatin; Lurasidone; Midazolam; Nilotinib; Nisoldipine; PHENobarbital; Phenytoin; Pimozide; Ranolazine; Rifabutin; Rifampin; Rivaroxaban; RomiDEPsin; Salmeterol; Sildenafil; Silodosin; Simvastatin; St Johns Wort; Tadalafil; Tamsulosin; Ticagrelor; Tolvaptan; Topotecan; Toremifene; Triazolam

Decreased Effect

Telaprevir may decrease the levels/effects of: Contraceptives (Estrogens); Contraceptives (Progestins); Darunavir; Efavirenz; Escitalopram; Fosamprenavir; Fosphenytoin; Methadone; PHENobarbital; Phenytoin; Prasugrel; Ticagrelor; Voriconazole; Warfarin; Zolpidem

The levels/effects of Telaprevir may be decreased by: Atazanavir; Bosentan; CarBAMazepine; Corticosteroids; Corticosteroids (Systemic); CYP3A4 Inducers (Strong); Darunavir; Deferasirox; Efavirenz; Fosamprenavir; Fosphenytoin; Lopinavir; P-glycoprotein/ABCB1 Inducers; PHENobarbital; Phenytoin; Rifabutin; Rifampin; Ritonavir; St Johns Wort; Tocilizumab

Increased Effect/Toxicity

Telaprevir may increase the levels/effects of: Alfuzosin; Almotriptan; Alosetron; ALPRAZolam; Amiodarone; ARIPiprazole; Atazanavir; Atorvastatin; Axitinib; Bepridil [Off Market]; Bortezomib; Bosentan; Brentuximab Vedotin; Brinzolamide; Budesonide (Nasal); Budesonide (Systemic, Oral Inhalation); CarBAMazepine; Ciclesonide; Cisapride; Clarithromycin; Colchicine; Conivaptan; Corticosteroids; Corticosteroids (Orally Inhaled); Corticosteroids (Systemic); Crizotinib; CycloSPORINE; CycloSPORINE (Systemic); CYP3A4 Substrates; Dabigatran Etexilate; Desipramine; Dienogest; Digoxin; Dronedarone; Dutasteride; Eplerenone; Ergot Derivatives; Erythromycin; Everolimus; FentaNYL; Fesoterodine; Flecainide; Fluticasone (Nasal); Fluticasone (Oral Inhalation); Fosphenytoin; GuanFACINE; Halofantrine; Iloperidone; Itraconazole; Ivacaftor; Ixabepilone; Ketoconazole; Ketoconazole (Systemic); Lapatinib; Lidocaine; Lidocaine (Systemic); Lovastatin; Lumefantrine; Lurasidone; Maraviroc; MethylPREDNISolone; Midazolam; Nilotinib; Nisoldipine; Paricalcitol; Pazopanib; P-glycoprotein/ABCB1 Substrates; PHENobarbital; Phenytoin; Pimecrolimus; Pimozide; Posaconazole; Propafenone; Prucalopride; QuiNIDine; Ranolazine; Rifabutin; Rivaroxaban; RomiDEPsin; Ruxolitinib; Salmeterol; Saxagliptin; Sildenafil; Silodosin; Simvastatin; Sirolimus; SORAfenib; Tacrolimus; Tacrolimus (Systemic); Tadalafil; Tamsulosin; Telithromycin; Tenofovir; Ticagrelor; Tolterodine; Tolvaptan; Topotecan; Toremifene; TraZODone;

Triazolam; Vardenafil; Vemurafenib; Vilazodone; Voriconazole; Warfarin; Zuclopenthixol

The levels/effects of Telaprevir may be increased by: Clarithromycin; CYP3A4 Inhibitors (Moderate); CYP3A4 Inhibitors (Strong); Dasatinib; Erythromycin; Itraconazole; Ketoconazole; Ketoconazole (Systemic); P-glycoprotein/ABCB1 Inhibitors; Posaconazole; Ritonavir; Telithromycin; Voriconazole

Available Dosage Forms

Tablet, oral:

Incivek™: 375 mg

General Dosage Range Oral: Adults: 750 mg 3 times/day

Administration

Oral Administer with a meal (not low fat). Doses should be taken approximately every 7-9 hours. Administer concurrently with peginterferon alfa and ribavirin.

Stability

Storage Store at 25°C (77°F); excursions permitted to 15°C to 30°C (59°F to 86°F). Keep container tightly closed. Opened bottle must be used within 28 days.

Nursing Actions

Physical Assessment This drug is typically not indicated for use alone; it must be taken along with peginterferon alfa-2a and ribavirin. These drugs are known to cause birth defects so there must be a negative pregnancy test prior to treatment and two forms of birth control must be used for 6 months after treatment. Do not use with moderate-to-severe liver damage. Instruct patient that medication must be taken with food. There is no renal impairment with this drug, so monitoring renal function is not necessary.

Patient Education Instruct patient to inform prescriber if they have a history of hepatitis B, anemia, or gout. Since this drug is to be given with peginterferon alfa-2a and ribavirin, instruct patients on the fact that these drugs cause birth defects. It is important to use two forms of birth control while on treatment and have a pregnancy test prior to beginning treatment. Dietary counseling may be needed, as this drug is to be taken with food to increase its absorption. Side effects include nausea, vomiting, diarrhea, and rash. Notify prescriber if rash worsens or if mouth sores or ulcers develop along with fever. Due to taking multiple drugs together, the potential for anemia worsens; instruct patient to monitor for symptoms of fatigue, shortness of breath, or rapid heartbeat.

Dietary Considerations Take with a meal (not low fat).

Telbivudine (tel BI vyoo deen)

Brand Names: U.S. Tyzeka®

Index Terms L-Deoxythymidine; LdT

Pharmacologic Category Antiretroviral Agent, Reverse Transcriptase Inhibitor (Nucleoside)

Medication Guide Available Yes

Pregnancy Risk Factor B

Lactation Excretion in breast milk unknown/not recommended

Use Treatment of chronic hepatitis B with evidence of viral replication and either persistent transaminase elevations or histologically-active disease

Mechanism of Action/Effect Telbivudine, a synthetic thymidine nucleoside analogue (L-enantiomer of thymidine), is intracellularly phosphorylated to the active triphosphate form, which competes with the natural substrate, thymidine 5'-triphosphate, to inhibit hepatitis B viral DNA polymerase; enzyme inhibition blocks reverse transcriptase activity thereby reducing viral DNA replication.

Contraindications There are no contraindications in the manufacturers labeling.

Warnings/Precautions [U.S. Boxed Warnings]: Cases of lactic acidosis and severe hepatomegaly with steatosis, some fatal, have been reported with the use of nucleoside analogues. Severe, acute exacerbation of hepatitis B may occur upon discontinuation. Monitor liver function several months after stopping treatment; reinitiation of antihepatitis B therapy may be required. Myopathy (eg, unexplained muscle aches and/or muscle weakness in conjunction with increases serum creatine kinase) has been reported with telbivudine initiation after several weeks to months; therapy should be interrupted if myopathy suspected and discontinued if diagnosed. Patients taking concomitant medications associated with myopathy should be monitored closely. Concomitant use with peginterferon alfa-2a has been associated with an increased risk of peripheral neuropathy; interrupt therapy for suspected peripheral neuropathy and discontinue if confirmed. Use caution in patients with renal impairment or patients receiving concomitant therapy which may reduce renal function; dosage adjustment required (Cl_{cr} <50 mL/minute). Monitor renal function before and during treatment in liver transplant patients receiving concurrent therapy of cyclosporine or tacrolimus; telbivudine may need to be adjusted. Safety and efficacy in liver transplant patients have not been established.

Not recommended as first-line therapy of chronic HBV due to high rate of resistance; use may be appropriate in short-term treatment of acute HBV (Lok, 2009). Cross-resistance among other antivirals for hepatitis B may occur; use caution in patients failing previous therapy with lamivudine. Telbivudine does not exhibit any clinically-relevant activity against human immunodeficiency virus (HIV type 1). Safety and efficacy have not been studied in patients coinfected with HIV, hepatitis C virus (HCV), or hepatitis D virus (HDV).

Drug Interactions

Avoid Concomitant Use

Avoid concomitant use of Telbivudine with any of the following: Interferon Alfa-2b; Peginterferon Alfa-2a; Peginterferon Alfa-2b

Decreased Effect There are no known significant interactions involving a decrease in effect.

Increased Effect/Toxicity

The levels/effects of Telbivudine may be increased by: Interferon Alfa-2b; Peginterferon Alfa-2a; Peginterferon Alfa-2b

Nutritional/Ethanol Interactions

Ethanol: Should be avoided in hepatitis B infection due to potential hepatic toxicity.

Food: Does not have a significant effect on telbivudine absorption.

Adverse Reactions

>10%:

Central nervous system: Fatigue (13%), headache (10%)

Neuromuscular & skeletal: CPK increased (79%; grades 3/4: 13%)

1% to 10%:

Central nervous system: Dizziness (4%), fever (4%), insomnia (3%)

Dermatologic: Rash (4%), pruritus (2%)

Endocrine & metabolic: Lipase increased (grades 3/4: 2%)

Gastrointestinal: Abdominal pain (3% to 6%), diarrhea (6%), nausea (5%), abdominal distension (3%), dyspepsia (3%)

Hematologic: Neutropenia (grades 3/4: 2%)

Hepatic: ALT increased (grades 3/4: 5% to 7%), AST increased (grades 3/4: 6%)

Neuromuscular & skeletal: Arthralgia (4%), back pain (4%), myalgia (3%)

Respiratory: Cough (6%), pharyngolaryngeal pain (5%)

Product Availability Tyzeka® oral solution: FDA approved April 2009; anticipated availability is currently undetermined

Available Dosage Forms

Tablet, oral:

Tyzeka®: 600 mg

General Dosage Range Dosage adjustment recommended in patients with renal impairment

Oral: *Children ≥16 years and Adults:* 600 mg once daily

Administration

Oral May be administered without regard to food.

Stability

Storage Store at 25°C (77°F); excursions permitted to 15°C to 30°C (59°F to 86°F).

Nursing Actions

Physical Assessment Monitor for peripheral neuropathy or myopathy (may be necessary to discontinue drug), gastrointestinal effects (pain or vomiting), or upper respiratory infection. Monitor closely for several months following discontinuation for possible clinical exacerbations.

Patient Education This medication does not stop you from spreading HBV to others; consult prescriber about safe sex practices and do not share needles or personal items that may have blood or body fluids on them. Take as directed with or without food. Avoid alcohol (may increase potential for liver damage). Maintain adequate hydration unless instructed to restrict fluid intake. Frequent blood tests may be required. May cause dizziness, fatigue, headache, muscle pain, or rash. Report immediately any signs of lactic acidosis (eg, persistent lethargy or fatigue, unusual muscle pain or weakness, cold feeling [especially in arms and legs], rapid or irregular heart beat, or difficulty breathing); liver toxicity (eg, yellowing of eyes or skin, pale stool and dark urine); or upper respiratory infection.

Dietary Considerations May be taken without regard to food.

Telithromycin (tel ith roe MYE sin)

Brand Names: U.S. Ketek®

Index Terms HMR 3647

Pharmacologic Category Antibiotic, Ketolide

Medication Safety Issues

Sound-alike/look-alike issues:

Telithromycin may be confused with telavancin

Medication Guide Available Yes

Pregnancy Risk Factor C

Lactation Excretion in breast milk unknown/use caution

Breast-Feeding Considerations It is not known if telithromycin is excreted in breast milk. The manufacturer recommends caution if using telithromycin in a breast-feeding woman.

Use Treatment of community-acquired pneumonia (mild-to-moderate) caused by susceptible strains of *Streptococcus pneumoniae* (including multidrug-resistant isolates), *Haemophilus influenzae*, *Chlamydophila pneumoniae*, *Moraxella catarrhalis*, and *Mycoplasma pneumoniae*

Mechanism of Action/Effect Inhibits bacterial protein synthesis by binding to two sites on the 50S ribosomal subunit.

Contraindications Hypersensitivity to telithromycin, macrolide antibiotics, or any component of the formulation; myasthenia gravis; history of hepatitis and/or jaundice associated with telithromycin or other macrolide antibiotic use; concurrent use of cisapride or pimozide

Warnings/Precautions Acute hepatic failure and severe liver injury, including hepatitis and hepatic necrosis (leading to some fatalities) have been reported, in some cases after only a few doses; if signs/symptoms of hepatitis or liver damage occur, discontinue therapy and initiate liver function tests. **[U.S. Boxed Warning]: Life-threatening (including fatal) respiratory failure has occurred in patients with myasthenia gravis;** use in these patients is contraindicated. May prolong QT_c interval, leading to a risk of ventricular arrhythmias; closely-related antibiotics have been associated with malignant ventricular arrhythmias and torsade de pointes. Avoid in patients with prolongation of QTc interval due to congenital causes, history of long QT syndrome, uncorrected electrolyte disturbances (hypokalemia or hypomagnesemia), significant bradycardia (<50 bpm), or concurrent therapy with QT_c-prolonging drugs (eg, class Ia and class III antiarrhythmics). Avoid use in patients with a prior history of confirmed cardiogenic syncope or ventricular arrhythmias while receiving macrolide antibiotics or other QT_c-prolonging drugs. May cause severe visual disturbances (eg, changes in accommodation ability, diplopia, blurred vision). May cause loss of consciousness (possibly vagal-related); caution patients that these events may interfere with ability to operate machinery or drive, and to use caution until effects are known. Use caution in renal impairment; severe impairment (Cl_{cr} <30 mL/minute) requires dosage adjustment. Pseudomembranous colitis has been reported. Safety and efficacy not established in pediatric patients <13 years of age per Canadian approved labeling and <18 years of age per U.S. approved labeling.

Drug Interactions

Avoid Concomitant Use

Avoid concomitant use of Telithromycin with any of the following: Alfuzosin; Artemether; Axitinib; BCG; Cisapride; Conivaptan; Crizotinib; Disopyramide; Dronedarone; Eplerenone; Everolimus; Fluticasone (Oral Inhalation); Halofantrine; Lapatinib; Lovastatin; Lumefantrine; Lurasidone; Nilotinib; Nisoldipine; Pimozide; QUEtiapine; QuiNINE; Ranolazine; Rivaroxaban; RomiDEPsin; Salmeterol; Silodosin; Simvastatin; Tamsulosin; Terfenadine; Tetrabenazine; Thioridazine; Ticagrelor; Tolvaptan; Toremifene; Vandetanib; Vemurafenib; Ziprasidone

Decreased Effect

Telithromycin may decrease the levels/effects of: BCG; Clopidogrel; Prasugrel; Ticagrelor; Typhoid Vaccine

The levels/effects of Telithromycin may be decreased by: CYP3A4 Inducers (Strong); Cyproterone; Deferasirox; Etravirine; Herbs (CYP3A4 Inducers); Tocilizumab

Increased Effect/Toxicity

Telithromycin may increase the levels/effects of: Alfentanil; Alfuzosin; Almotriptan; Alosetron; Antifungal Agents (Azole Derivatives, Systemic); Antineoplastic Agents (Vinca Alkaloids); ARIPiprazole; Axitinib; Benzodiazepines (metabolized by oxidation); Bortezomib; Brentuximab Vedotin; Brinzolamide; Budesonide (Nasal); Budesonide (Systemic, Oral Inhalation); BusPIRone; Calcium Channel Blockers; CarBAMazepine; Cardiac Glycosides; Ciclesonide; Cilostazol; Cisapride; CloZAPine; Colchicine; Conivaptan; Corticosteroids (Orally Inhaled); Corticosteroids (Systemic); Crizotinib; CycloSPORINE; CycloSPORINE (Systemic); CYP3A4 Substrates; Dienogest; Disopyramide; Dronedarone; Dutasteride; Eletriptan; Eplerenone; Ergot Derivatives; Everolimus; FentaNYL; Fesoterodine; Fluticasone (Nasal); Fluticasone (Oral Inhalation); GuanFACINE; Halofantrine; HMG-CoA Reductase Inhibitors; Iloperidone; Ivacaftor; Ixabepilone; Lapatinib; Lovastatin; Lumefantrine; Lurasidone; Maraviroc; MethylPREDNISolone; Nilotinib; Nisoldipine; Paricalcitol; Pazopanib; Pimecrolimus; Pimozide; Propafenone; QTc-Prolonging Agents; QuiNIDine; QuiNINE; Ranolazine; Repaglinide; Rifamycin Derivatives; Rivaroxaban; RomiDEPsin; Ruxolitinib; Salmeterol; Saxagliptin; Selective Serotonin Reuptake Inhibitors; Sildenafil; Silodosin; Simvastatin; Sirolimus; SORAfenib; Tacrolimus; Tacrolimus (Systemic); Tacrolimus (Topical); Tadalafil; Tamsulosin; Telaprevir; Temsirolimus; Terfenadine; Tetrabenazine; Thioridazine; Ticagrelor; Tolterodine; Tolvaptan; Toremifene; Vandetanib; Vardenafil; Vemurafenib; Verapamil; Vilazodone; Vitamin K Antagonists; Ziprasidone; Zopiclone; Zuclopenthixol

The levels/effects of Telithromycin may be increased by: Alfuzosin; Antifungal Agents (Azole Derivatives, Systemic); Artemether; Chloroquine; Ciprofloxacin; Ciprofloxacin (Systemic); CYP3A4 Inhibitors (Moderate); CYP3A4 Inhibitors (Strong); Gadobutrol; Indacaterol; Lumefantrine; Nilotinib; QUEtiapine; QuiNINE; Telaprevir

Nutritional/Ethanol Interactions Herb/nutraceutical: St John's wort: May decrease the levels/effects of telithromycin.

Adverse Reactions

>10%: Gastrointestinal: Diarrhea (10% to 11%)

2% to 10%:

- Central nervous system: Headache (2% to 6%), dizziness (3% to 4%)
- Gastrointestinal: Nausea (7% to 8%), vomiting (2% to 3%), loose stools (2%), dysgeusia (2%)

≥0.2% to <2%:

- Central nervous system: Fatigue, insomnia, somnolence, vertigo
- Dermatologic: Rash
- Gastrointestinal: Abdominal distension, abdominal pain, anorexia, constipation, dyspepsia, flatulence, gastritis, gastroenteritis, GI upset, glossitis, stomatitis, watery stools, xerostomia
- Genitourinary: Vaginal candidiasis
- Hematologic: Platelets increased
- Hepatic: Transaminases increased
- Ocular: Blurred vision, accommodation delayed, diplopia
- Miscellaneous: Candidiasis, diaphoresis increased

Available Dosage Forms

Tablet, oral:

Ketek®: 300 mg, 400 mg

General Dosage Range Dosage adjustment recommended in patients with renal impairment

Oral: *Adults:* 800 mg once daily

Administration

Oral May be administered with or without food.

Stability

Storage Store at 15°C to 30°C (59°F to 86°F).

Nursing Actions

Physical Assessment Culture and sensitivity report and previous allergy history should be assessed prior to therapy. Monitor LFTs. Monitor for jaundice, gastrointestinal disturbance (nausea, vomiting, diarrhea), CNS (vertigo, insomnia), rash, opportunistic infection, QT prolongation, and arrhythmias. Teach patient to report any signs of jaundice or hepatic impairment.

Patient Education Take with or without food. May cause headache, dizziness, insomnia, blurred vision, difficulty focusing, nausea, vomiting, loss of appetite, diarrhea, or watery stools (consult prescriber if persistent). If you experience visual difficulties, loss of consciousness (fainting), dark urine, pale stool, or yellowing of skin or eyes, contact prescriber immediately before taking another dose. Report chest pain, palpitations, or irregular heart beat; flushing or facial swelling; CNS disturbance (dizziness, headache, anxiety, abnormal dreams, tremor); unusual muscle weakness; skin rash; or vaginal itching, burning, or discharge.

Dietary Considerations May be taken with or without food.

Telmisartan (tel mi SAR tan)

Brand Names: U.S. Micardis®

Pharmacologic Category Angiotensin II Receptor Blocker

Pregnancy Risk Factor D

Lactation Excretion in breast milk unknown/not recommended

Use Treatment of hypertension (may be used alone or in combination with other antihypertensive agents); cardiovascular risk reduction in patients ≥55 years of age unable to take ACE inhibitors and who are at high risk of major cardiovascular events (eg, MI, stroke, death)

Mechanism of Action/Effect Telmisartan, a nonpeptide angiotensin receptor antagonist, binds to the AT1 angiotensin II receptor thereby blocking the vasoconstriction and the aldosterone secreting effects of angiotensin II.

Contraindications Hypersensitivity to telmisartan or any component of the formulation.

Canadian labeling: Additional contraindications: Second and third trimesters of pregnancy; breast-feeding; fructose intolerance

Warnings/Precautions [U.S. Boxed Warning]: Drugs that act on the renin-angiotensin system can cause injury and death to the developing fetus. Discontinue as soon as possible once pregnancy is detected. May cause hyperkalemia; avoid potassium supplementation unless specifically required by healthcare provider. Avoid use or use a smaller dose in patients who are volume depleted; correct depletion first. May be associated with deterioration of renal function and/or increases in serum creatinine, particularly in patients with low renal blood flow (eg, renal artery stenosis, heart failure) whose glomerular filtration rate (GFR) is dependent on efferent arteriolar vasoconstriction by angiotensin II. Use with caution in unstented unilateral/bilateral renal artery stenosis. When unstented bilateral renal artery stenosis is present, use is generally avoided due to the elevated risk of deterioration in renal function unless possible benefits outweigh risks. Use with caution with preexisting renal insufficiency; significant aortic/mitral stenosis. Concurrent use of ACE inhibitors may increase the risk of clinically-significant adverse events (eg, renal dysfunction, hyperkalemia). Concurrent use with ramipril is not recommended. Use with caution in patients who have biliary obstructive disorders or hepatic dysfunction. Product contains sorbitol. The Canadian labeling (not in U.S. labeling) contraindicates use in fructose intolerant patients.

Drug Interactions

Avoid Concomitant Use There are no known interactions where it is recommended to avoid concomitant use.

Decreased Effect

The levels/effects of Telmisartan may be decreased by: Herbs (Hypertensive Properties); Methylphenidate; Nonsteroidal Anti-Inflammatory Agents; Yohimbine

Increased Effect/Toxicity

Telmisartan may increase the levels/effects of: ACE Inhibitors; Amifostine; Antihypertensives; Cardiac Glycosides; Hypotensive Agents; Lithium; Nonsteroidal Anti-Inflammatory Agents; Potassium-Sparing Diuretics; Ramipril; RiTUXimab; Sodium Phosphates

The levels/effects of Telmisartan may be increased by: Alfuzosin; Diazoxide; Eplerenone; Herbs (Hypotensive Properties); MAO Inhibitors; Pentoxifylline; Phosphodiesterase 5 Inhibitors; Potassium Salts; Prostacyclin Analogues; Tolvaptan; Trimethoprim

Nutritional/Ethanol Interactions Herb/Nutraceutical: Some herbal medications may have hypertensive or hypotensive properties; others may increase or decrease the antihypertensive effect of telmisartan. Management: Avoid bayberry, blue cohosh, cayenne, ephedra, ginger, ginseng (American), kola, licorice, and yohimbe. Avoid black cohosh, California poppy, coleus, golden seal, hawthorn, mistletoe, periwinkle, quinine, and shepherd's purse.

Adverse Reactions May be associated with worsening of renal function in patients dependent on renin-angiotensin-aldosterone system.

1% to 10%:

Cardiovascular: Intermittent claudication (7%; placebo 6%), chest pain (≥1%), hypertension (≥1%), peripheral edema (≥1%)

Central nervous system: Dizziness (≥1%), fatigue (≥1%), headache (≥1%), pain (≥1%)

Dermatologic: Skin ulcer (3%; placebo 2%)

Gastrointestinal: Diarrhea (3%), abdominal pain (≥1%), dyspepsia (≥1%), nausea (≥1%)

Genitourinary: Urinary tract infection (≥1%)

Neuromuscular & skeletal: Back pain (3%), myalgia (≥1%)

Respiratory: Upper respiratory infection (7%), sinusitis (3%), cough (≥1%), pharyngitis (1%)

Pharmacodynamics/Kinetics

Onset of Action 1-2 hours; Peak effect: 0.5-1 hours

Duration of Action Up to 24 hours

Available Dosage Forms

Tablet, oral:

Micardis®: 20 mg, 40 mg, 80 mg

General Dosage Range Oral:

Adults: Initial: 40-80 mg once daily; Maintenance: 20-80 mg/day once daily

Elderly: Initial: 20-80 mg once daily

Administration

Oral May be administered without regard to meals.

Stability

Storage Store at 25°C (77°F); excursions between 15°C to 30°C (59°F to 86°F) permitted. Protect from moisture and do not remove from blister pack until immediately before use.

Nursing Actions

Physical Assessment Assess potential for interactions with other pharmacological agents and herbal products (eg, increased risk of hyperkalemia or increased hypotensive effects). Monitor for hypotension, diarrhea, URI, and cough on a regular basis during therapy. Teach patient need for regular blood pressure monitoring.

Patient Education Monitor blood pressure on a regular basis at same time of day, as advised by prescriber. This drug does not eliminate need for diet or exercise regimen as recommended by prescriber. May cause dizziness, fainting, lightheadedness, or postural hypotension. Report unusual weight gain and swelling of ankles, hands, face, lips, throat, or tongue; persistent fatigue; dry cough or respiratory difficulty; palpitations or chest pain; CNS changes; GI disturbances; muscle or bone pain, cramping, or tremors; change in urinary pattern; or changes in hearing or vision.

Dietary Considerations May be taken without regard to meals. Product contains sorbitol.

Telmisartan and Amlodipine

(tel mi SAR tan & am LOE di peen)

Brand Names: U.S. Twynsta®

Index Terms Amlodipine and Telmisartan; Amlodipine Besylate and Telmisartan

Pharmacologic Category Angiotensin II Receptor Blocker; Antianginal Agent; Calcium Channel Blocker; Calcium Channel Blocker, Dihydropyridine

Pregnancy Risk Factor C (1st trimester); D (2nd and 3rd trimesters)

Lactation Excretion in breast milk unknown/not recommended

Use Treatment of hypertension, including initial treatment in patients who will require multiple antihypertensives for adequate control

Available Dosage Forms

Tablet, oral:

Twynsta® 40/5: Telmisartan 40 mg and amlodipine 5 mg; Twynsta® 40/10: telmisartan 40 mg and amlodipine 10 mg; Twynsta® 80/5: telmisartan 80 mg and amlodipine 5 mg; Twynsta® 80/10: telmisartan 80 mg and amlodipine10 mg

General Dosage Range Oral: *Adults:* Amlodipine 5-10 mg and telmisartan 40-80 mg once daily (maximum: 10 mg/day [amlodipine]; 80 mg/day [telmisartan])

Administration

Oral May be administered without regard to meals.

Nursing Actions

Physical Assessment See individual agents.

Patient Education See individual agents.

Related Information

AmLODIPine *on page 65*

Telmisartan *on page 1088*

Telmisartan and Hydrochlorothiazide

(tel mi SAR tan & hye droe klor oh THYE a zide)

Brand Names: U.S. Micardis® HCT

Index Terms Hydrochlorothiazide and Telmisartan

Pharmacologic Category Angiotensin II Receptor Blocker; Diuretic, Thiazide

Pregnancy Risk Factor D

Lactation Enters breast milk/not recommended

Use Treatment of hypertension; combination product should not be used for initial therapy

Available Dosage Forms

Tablet, oral:

Micardis® HCT: 40/12.5: Telmisartan 40 mg and hydrochlorothiazide 12.5 mg; 80/12.5: Telmisartan 80 mg and hydrochlorothiazide 12.5 mg; 80/25: Telmisartan 80 mg and hydrochlorothiazide 25 mg

General Dosage Range Oral: *Adults:* Initial: Telmisartan 80 mg and hydrochlorothiazide 12.5-25 mg once daily; Maintenance: Telmisartan 80-160 mg and hydrochlorothiazide 12.5-25 mg once daily

Administration

Oral May be administered without regard to meals.

Nursing Actions

Physical Assessment See individual agents.

Patient Education See individual agents.

Related Information

Hydrochlorothiazide *on page 570*
Telmisartan *on page 1088*

Temazepam (te MAZ e pam)

Brand Names: U.S. Restoril™

Pharmacologic Category Benzodiazepine

Medication Safety Issues

Sound-alike/look-alike issues:

Temazepam may be confused with flurazepam, LORazepam, tamoxifen

Restoril™ may be confused with Resotran™, RisperDAL®, Vistaril®, Zestril®

BEERS Criteria medication:

This drug may be inappropriate for use in geriatric patients (high severity risk).

Medication Guide Available Yes

Pregnancy Risk Factor X

Lactation Enters breast milk/use caution (AAP rates "of concern"; AAP 2001 update pending)

Use Short-term treatment of insomnia

Unlabeled Use Treatment of anxiety

Controlled Substance C-IV

Available Dosage Forms

Capsule, oral: 7.5 mg, 15 mg, 22.5 mg, 30 mg
Restoril™: 7.5 mg, 15 mg, 22.5 mg, 30 mg

General Dosage Range Oral:
Adults: 7.5-30 mg at bedtime
Elderly: Initial: 7.5 mg at bedtime

Nursing Actions

Physical Assessment For short-term use. Assess for history of addiction; long-term use can result in dependence, abuse, or tolerance. For inpatient use, institute safety measures (side rails, night light, call bell, assistance with ambulation) to prevent falls. For outpatients, monitor for CNS depression at beginning of therapy and periodically throughout.

Patient Education Drug may cause physical and/or psychological dependence. May take with food to decrease GI upset. While using this medication, do not use alcohol. Maintain adequate hydration unless instructed to restrict fluid intake. You may experience drowsiness, dizziness, lightheadedness, blurred vision, dry mouth, or GI discomfort. Report CNS changes (confusion, depression, increased sedation, excitation, headache, abnormal thinking, insomnia, or nightmares, memory impairment, impaired coordination), respiratory difficulty, persistent dizziness, alterations in normal gait, vision changes, or ineffectiveness of medication.

Temozolomide (te moe ZOE loe mide)

Brand Names: U.S. Temodar®

Index Terms SCH 52365; TMZ

Pharmacologic Category Antineoplastic Agent, Alkylating Agent (Triazene)

Medication Safety Issues

Sound-alike/look-alike issues:

Temodar® may be confused with Tambocor™

Temozolomide may be confused with temsirolimus

High alert medication:

This medication is in a class the Institute for Safe Medication Practices (ISMP) includes among its list of drug classes which have a heightened risk of causing significant patient harm when used in error.

Pregnancy Risk Factor D

Lactation Excretion in breast milk unknown/not recommended

Use Treatment of newly-diagnosed glioblastoma multiforme (initially in combination with radiotherapy, then as maintenance treatment); treatment of refractory anaplastic astrocytoma

Canadian labeling (not an approved indication in the U.S.): Treatment of recurrent or progressive glioblastoma multiforme

Unlabeled Use Treatment of recurrent glioblastoma multiforme, low-grade astrocytoma, low-grade oligodendroglioma, anaplastic oligodendroglioma, metastatic CNS lesions, refractory primary CNS lymphoma, advanced or metastatic melanoma, cutaneous T-cell lymphomas (mycosis fungoides [MF] and Sézary syndrome [SS]), advanced neuroendocrine tumors (carcinoid or islet cell), Ewing's sarcoma (recurrent or progressive), soft tissue sarcomas (extremity/retroperitoneal/intra-abdominal or hemangiopericytoma/solitary fibrous tumor), treatment of pediatric neuroblastoma

Available Dosage Forms

Capsule, oral:
Temodar®: 5 mg, 20 mg, 100 mg, 140 mg, 180 mg, 250 mg

Injection, powder for reconstitution:
Temodar®: 100 mg

General Dosage Range Dosage adjustment recommended in patients who develop toxicities.

I.V., Oral: *Adults:* Dosage varies greatly depending on indication

Administration

Oral Swallow capsules whole with a glass of water. Absorption is affected by food. Administer consistently either with food or without food (was administered in studies under fasting and non-fasting conditions). May administer on an empty stomach or at bedtime to reduce nausea and vomiting. Standard antiemetics may be administered if needed. Do not repeat dose if vomiting occurs after dose is administered; wait until the next scheduled dose. Do not open or chew capsules; avoid contact with skin if capsules are accidentally opened or damaged.

I.V. Infuse over 90 minutes. Flush line before and after administration. May be administered through the same I.V. line as sodium chloride 0.9%; do not administer other medications through the same I.V. line.

Nursing Actions

Physical Assessment Monitor for convulsions, fatigue, impaired coordination, ataxia, gastrointestinal disturbance (nausea, vomiting, constipation), myelosuppression, rash, opportunistic infection, vision disturbance, and cough on a regular basis.

Patient Education If administered I.V., report immediately any swelling, pain, or burning at infusion site. May cause headache, dizziness, confusion, fatigue, anxiety, insomnia, impaired coordination, nausea, vomiting, loss of appetite, constipation, or diarrhea. Report chest pain or palpitations; acute headache; unusual swelling of legs or feet; visual disturbances; unresolved GI problems; itching or burning on urination or vaginal discharge; acute joint, back, bone, or muscle pain or unusual weakness; difficulty breathing; cough; or signs of respiratory infection.

Oral: Take always with food or always without food; taking at bedtime may reduce nausea or vomiting. Swallow whole with 8 ounces of water. Do not open, crush, or chew capsules; if capsule is accidentally broken, do not inhale powder (wash hands thoroughly if powder gets on skin).

Temsirolimus (tem sir OH li mus)

Brand Names: U.S. Torisel®

Index Terms CCI-779

Pharmacologic Category Antineoplastic Agent, mTOR Kinase Inhibitor

Medication Safety Issues

Sound-alike/look-alike issues:

Temsirolimus may be confused with everolimus, sirolimus, tacrolimus, temozolomide, tesamorelin

High alert medication:

This medication is in a class the Institute for Safe Medication Practices (ISMP) includes among its list of drug classes which have a heightened risk of causing significant patient harm when used in error.

Administration issues:

Temsirolimus requires a two-step dilution process prior to administration. The medication is supplied in a vial containing a total amount of 30 mg in a total volume of 1.2 mL (25 mg/mL). The vial must initially be diluted to 10 mg/mL (with provided 1.8 mL of diluent), then the intended dose should be withdrawn from the 10 mg/mL diluted vial (ie, 2.5 mL for a 25 mg dose) and further diluted for infusion in 250 mL sodium chloride 0.9%. Errors have occurred due to improper preparation.

Temsirolimus, for the treatment of advanced renal cell cancer, is a flat dose (25 mg if no dosage reductions) and is not based on body surface area (BSA).

Pregnancy Risk Factor D

Lactation Excretion in breast milk unknown/not recommended

Use Treatment of advanced renal cell cancer (RCC)

Available Dosage Forms

Injection, solution:

Torisel®: 25 mg/mL (1.2 mL)

General Dosage Range Dosage adjustment recommended in patients with hepatic impairment, on concomitant therapy, or who develop toxicities

I.V.: *Adults:* 25 mg once weekly

Administration

I.V. Infuse over 30-60 minutes via an infusion pump (preferred). Use polyethylene-lined non-DEHP administration tubing. Administer through an inline polyethersulfone filter ≤5 micron; if set does not contain an inline filter, a polyethersulfone end filter (0.2-5 micron) should be added (do not use both an inline and an end filter). Premedicate with an H_1 antagonist (eg, diphenhydramine 25-50 mg I.V.) ~30 minutes prior to infusion. Monitor during infusion; interrupt infusion for hypersensitivity/infusion reaction; monitor for 30-60 minutes; may reinitiate at a reduced infusion rate (over 60 minutes) with discretion, 30 minutes after administration of a histamine H_1 antagonist and/or a histamine H_2 antagonist (eg, famotidine or ranitidine). Administration should be completed within 6 hours of admixture.

Nursing Actions

Physical Assessment Administer premedication as ordered prior to infusion. Monitor patient closely for anaphylaxis, dyspnea, flushing, and chest pain during and following each infusion; medication/equipment for treating reactions should be readily available. Monitor for altered glucose control (hyper-/hypoglycemia), opportunistic infection, interstitial lung disease (dyspnea, cough, hypoxia, fever, worsening respiratory condition), bowel perforation (abdominal pain, blood in stool), and renal failure at each infusion and throughout therapy; notify prescriber of serious adverse reactions.

Patient Education This medication can only be administered by infusion; you will be closely monitored during infusion. Report immediately unusual back or abdominal pain; acute headache; difficulty breathing or chest pain; difficulty swallowing; itching or rash; or redness, swelling, or pain at infusion site. Maintain adequate nutrition and hydration between treatments, unless instructed to restrict fluid intake. You will be required to have regularly scheduled laboratory tests while on this medication. You will be more susceptible to infection. If you have diabetes, you will be instructed to check your glucose levels closely and notify prescriber of significant changes, excessive thirst, or frequency of urination. This medication can affect glucose control and diabetic medications may need to be adjusted. You may experience headache, insomnia, loss of appetite, nausea, dry mouth, taste changes, rash, or dry skin. Report immediately changes in respiratory status (difficulty breathing, dyspnea, unusual cough, or fever), abdominal pain or blood in stool, signs or symptoms of any urinary tract infection (difficulty urinating, burning on urination, or perineal itching), or unusual infection or delayed wound healing.

Tenecteplase (ten EK te plase)

Brand Names: U.S. TNKase®

Pharmacologic Category Thrombolytic Agent

Medication Safety Issues

Sound-alike/look-alike issues:

TNKase® may be confused with Activase®, t-PA

TNK (occasional abbreviation for TNKase®) is an error-prone abbreviation (mistaken as TPA)

High alert medication:

The Institute for Safe Medication Practices (ISMP) includes this medication (I.V.) among its list of drugs which have a heightened risk of causing significant patient harm when used in error.

Pregnancy Risk Factor C

Lactation Use caution

Use Thrombolytic agent used in the management of ST-elevation myocardial infarction (STEMI) for the lysis of thrombi in the coronary vasculature to restore perfusion and reduce mortality.

Recommended criteria for treatment: STEMI: Chest pain ≥20 minutes duration, onset of chest pain within 12 hours of treatment (or within prior 12-24 hours in patients with continuing ischemic symptoms), and S-T segment elevation >0.1 mV in at least two contiguous precordial leads or two adjacent limb leads on ECG or new or presumably new left bundle branch block (LBBB)

Unlabeled Use Acute MI - combination regimen of tenecteplase (unlabeled dose), abciximab, and heparin (unlabeled dose)

Mechanism of Action/Effect Initiates fibrinolysis by binding to fibrin and converting plasminogen to plasmin.

Contraindications Hypersensitivity to tenecteplase or any component of the formulation; active internal bleeding; history of stroke; intracranial/intraspinal surgery or trauma within 2 months; intracranial neoplasm; arteriovenous malformation or aneurysm; bleeding diathesis; severe uncontrolled hypertension

Warnings/Precautions Stop antiplatelet agents and heparin if serious bleeding occurs. Avoid I.M. injections and nonessential handling of the patient for a few hours after administration. Monitor for bleeding complications. Venipunctures should be performed carefully and only when necessary. If arterial puncture is necessary, then use an upper extremity that can be easily compressed manually. For the following conditions, the risk of bleeding is higher with use of tenecteplase and should be weighed against the benefits: Recent major surgery, cerebrovascular disease, recent GI or GU bleed, recent trauma, uncontrolled hypertension (systolic BP ≥180 mm Hg and/or diastolic BP ≥110 mm Hg), suspected left heart thrombus, acute pericarditis, subacute bacterial endocarditis, hemostatic defects, severe hepatic dysfunction, pregnancy, hemorrhagic diabetic retinopathy or other hemorrhagic ophthalmic conditions, septic thrombophlebitis or occluded arteriovenous cannula at seriously infected site, advanced age, anticoagulants, recent administration of GP IIb/IIIa inhibitors. Coronary thrombolysis may result in reperfusion arrhythmias. Caution with readministration of tenecteplase. Safety and efficacy have not been established in pediatric patients. Cholesterol embolism has rarely been reported.

Drug Interactions

Avoid Concomitant Use There are no known interactions where it is recommended to avoid concomitant use.

Decreased Effect

The levels/effects of Tenecteplase may be decreased by: Aprotinin

Increased Effect/Toxicity

Tenecteplase may increase the levels/effects of: Anticoagulants; Drotrecogin Alfa (Activated)

The levels/effects of Tenecteplase may be increased by: Antiplatelet Agents; Herbs (Anticoagulant/Antiplatelet Properties); Nonsteroidal Anti-Inflammatory Agents; Salicylates

Adverse Reactions As with all drugs which may affect hemostasis, bleeding is the major adverse effect associated with tenecteplase. Hemorrhage may occur at virtually any site. Risk is dependent on multiple variables, including the dosage administered, concurrent use of multiple agents which alter hemostasis, and patient predisposition. Rapid lysis of coronary artery thrombi by thrombolytic agents may be associated with reperfusion-related arterial and/or ventricular arrhythmia. The incidence of stroke and bleeding increase in patients >65 years.

>10%:

Hematologic: Bleeding (22% minor: ASSENT-2 trial)

Local: Hematoma (12% minor)

1% to 10%:

Central nervous system: Stroke (2%)

Gastrointestinal: GI hemorrhage (1% major, 2% minor), epistaxis (2% minor)
Genitourinary: GU bleeding (4% minor)
Hematologic: Bleeding (5% major: ASSENT-2 trial)
Local: Bleeding at catheter puncture site (4% minor), hematoma (2% major)
Respiratory: Pharyngeal bleeding (3% minor)

Additional cardiovascular events associated with use in MI: Cardiogenic shock, arrhythmia, AV block, pulmonary edema, heart failure, cardiac arrest, recurrent myocardial ischemia, myocardial reinfarction, myocardial rupture, cardiac tamponade, pericarditis, pericardial effusion, mitral regurgitation, thrombosis, embolism, electromechanical dissociation, hypotension, fever, nausea, vomiting

Available Dosage Forms

Injection, powder for reconstitution:
TNKase®: 50 mg

General Dosage Range I.V.:
Adults <60 kg: 30 mg as a single dose
Adults ≥60 to <70 kg: 35 mg as a single dose
Adults ≥70 to <80 kg: 40 mg as a single dose
Adults ≥80 to <90 kg: 45 mg as a single dose
Adults ≥90 kg: 50 mg as a single dose

Administration

I.V. Tenecteplase should be reconstituted using the supplied 10 mL syringe with TwinPak™ Dual Cannula Device and 10 mL SWFI. Do not shake when reconstituting. Slight foaming is normal; will dissipate if left standing for several minutes. Any unused solution should be discarded. The reconstituted solution is 5 mg/mL. Dextrose-containing lines must be flushed with a saline solution before and after administration. Check frequently for signs of bleeding. Avoid I.M. injections and nonessential handling of patient.

Stability

Reconstitution Tenecteplase should be reconstituted using the supplied 10 mL syringe with TwinPak™ Dual Cannula Device and 10 mL sterile water for injection.

Storage Store at room temperature not to exceed 30°C (86°F) or under refrigeration 2°C to 8°C (36°F to 46°F). If reconstituted and not used immediately, store in refrigerator and use within 8 hours.

Nursing Actions

Physical Assessment Monitor patient closely for bleeding during and following treatment. Monitor infusion site, neurological status (eg, intracranial hemorrhage), vital signs, and ECG (reperfusion arrhythmias). Arrhythmias may occur; antiarrhythmic drugs should be immediately available. Maintain bedrest and bleeding precautions. Avoid I.M. injections, venipuncture (unless absolutely necessary), and nonessential handling of the patient. If arterial puncture is necessary, an upper extremity vessel that can be manually compressed should be used.

Patient Education This medication is only administered by infusion; you will be monitored closely during and after treatment. Immediately report burning, pain, redness, swelling, or oozing at infusion site. Following infusion you will have a tendency to bleed easily; use caution to prevent injury and follow instructions for strict bedrest to reduce the risk of injury. If bleeding does occur, report immediately and apply pressure to bleeding spot until bleeding stops completely. Report unusual pain (acute headache, joint pain, chest pain); unusual bruising or bleeding; blood in urine, stool, or vomitus; bleeding gums; vision changes; or respiratory difficulty.

Tenofovir (te NOE fo veer)

Brand Names: U.S. Viread®

Index Terms PMPA; TDF; Tenofovir Disoproxil Fumarate

Pharmacologic Category Antiretroviral Agent, Reverse Transcriptase Inhibitor (Nucleotide)

Pregnancy Risk Factor B

Lactation Enters breast milk/contraindicated

Breast-Feeding Considerations Maternal or infant antiretroviral therapy does not completely eliminate the risk of postnatal HIV transmission. In addition, multiclass-resistant virus has been detected in breast-feeding infants despite maternal therapy. Therefore, in the United States, where formula is accessible, affordable, safe, and sustainable, and the risk of infant mortality due to diarrhea and respiratory infections is low, complete avoidance of breast-feeding by HIV-infected women is recommended to decrease potential transmission of HIV (DHHS [perinatal], 2011).

Use Management of HIV infections in combination with at least two other antiretroviral agents; treatment of chronic hepatitis B virus (HBV) in patients with compensated or decompensated liver disease

Mechanism of Action/Effect Tenofovir blocks replication of HIV virus by inhibiting the reverse transcriptase enzyme. It is chemically similar to adenosine 5'-monophosphate (a nucleotide), which is required to form DNA. Tenofovir inhibits replication of HBV by inhibiting HBV polymerase.

Contraindications There are no contraindications listed within the FDA-approved labeling.

Warnings/Precautions [U.S Boxed Warning]: Lactic acidosis and severe hepatomegaly with steatosis have been reported with tenofovir and other nucleoside analogues, including fatal cases; use with caution in patients with risk factors for liver disease (risk may be increased in obese patients or prolonged exposure) and suspend treatment in any patient who develops clinical or laboratory findings suggestive of lactic acidosis (transaminase elevation may/may not accompany hepatomegaly and steatosis). May cause redistribution of fat (eg, buffalo hump, peripheral wasting with increased abdominal girth, cushingoid appearance). Immune reconstitution syndrome may develop resulting in the occurrence of an inflammatory response to an indolent or residual opportunistic infection during initial treatment or activation of autoimmune disorders (eg, Graves' disease, polymyositis, Guillain-Barré syndrome) later in therapy; further evaluation and treatment may be required. Use caution in hepatic impairment; no dosage adjustment is required; limited studies indicate the pharmacokinetics of tenofovir are not altered in hepatic dysfunction. Limited data supporting treatment of chronic hepatitis B in patients with decompensated liver disease; observe for increased adverse reactions, including renal dysfunction.

May cause osteomalacia; increased biochemical markers of bone metabolism, serum parathyroid hormone levels, and 1,25 vitamin D levels have been noted with tenofovir use. A 5% to 7% loss of bone mineral density (BMD) has been reported in some patients. BMD monitoring should be considered in patients with a history of bone fracture or risk factors for osteopenia or bone loss. Bone effects in tenofovir-treated HIV children and adolescents were similar to adults; long-term bone health and fracture risk unknown.

Do not use as monotherapy in treatment of HIV. Treatment of HIV in patients with unrecognized/untreated HBV may lead to rapid HBV resistance. Patients should be tested for presence of chronic hepatitis B infection prior to initiation of therapy.

Use caution in renal impairment. Calculate creatinine clearance prior to initiation of therapy and monitor renal function (including recalculation of creatinine clearance and serum phosphorus) during therapy. Dosage adjustment required in patients with Cl_{cr} <50 mL/minute. May cause acute renal failure or Fanconi syndrome; use caution with other nephrotoxic agents (especially those which compete for active tubular secretion), patients with low body weight, or concurrent medications which increase tenofovir levels. Use caution in the elderly; dosage adjustment based on renal function may be required.

[U.S. Boxed Warning]: If treating HBV, acute exacerbation of hepatitis B may occur upon discontinuation. Monitor liver function closely for several months after discontinuing treatment; reinitiation of antihepatitis B therapy may be required. Treatment of HBV in patients with unrecognized/untreated HIV may lead to HIV resistance; patients should be tested for presence of HIV infection prior to initiating therapy. Do not use as monotherapy in treatment of HIV. Treatment of HIV in patients with unrecognized/untreated HBV may lead to rapid HBV resistance. Patients should be tested for presence of chronic hepatitis B prior to initiation of therapy. Use with caution in patients taking strong CYP3A4 inhibitors, moderate or strong CYP3A4 inducers and major CYP3A4 substrates (see Drug Interactions); consider alternative agents that avoid or lessen the potential for CYP-mediated interactions. Do not use concurrently with adefovir or tenofovir combination products.

Drug Interactions

Avoid Concomitant Use

Avoid concomitant use of Tenofovir with any of the following: Adefovir; Didanosine

Decreased Effect

Tenofovir may decrease the levels/effects of: Atazanavir; Didanosine; Protease Inhibitors

The levels/effects of Tenofovir may be decreased by: Adefovir

Increased Effect/Toxicity

Tenofovir may increase the levels/effects of: Adefovir; Didanosine; Ganciclovir-Valganciclovir

The levels/effects of Tenofovir may be increased by: Acyclovir-Valacyclovir; Adefovir; Atazanavir; Ganciclovir-Valganciclovir; Lopinavir; Protease Inhibitors; Telaprevir

Nutritional/Ethanol Interactions Food: Fatty meals may increase the bioavailability of tenofovir. Tenofovir may be taken with or without food.

Adverse Reactions Frequencies listed are treatment-emergent adverse effects noted at higher frequency than in the placebo group or comparator group. Only adverse events from treatment-naive studies which varied significantly were noted (eg, rash event). Patients treated for chronic hepatitis B had similar reactions and frequencies.

>10%:

Central nervous system: Insomnia (3% to 4%; decompensated liver disease 18%), pain (7% to 13%), dizziness (3%; treatment naive 8%; decompensated liver disease 13%), depression (4% to 8%; treatment naive 9% to 11%), fever (2% to 4%; treatment naive 8%; decompensated liver disease 11%)

Dermatologic: Rash event (includes maculopapular, pustular, or vesiculobullous rash, pruritus or urticaria 5% to 7%; treatment naive 18%)

Endocrine & metabolic: Triglycerides increased (grades 3/4: 11%; treatment naive 4%)

Gastrointestinal: Abdominal pain (4% to 7%; decompensated liver disease 22%), nausea (8% to 11%; decompensated liver disease 20%), diarrhea (11% to 16%), vomiting (4% to 7%; decompensated liver disease 13%)

Neuromuscular & skeletal: Creatine kinase increased (9% to 12%), weakness (7% to 11%)

1% to 10%:

Cardiovascular: Chest pain (3%)

Central nervous system: Fatigue (9%), headache (5% to 8%), anxiety (6%)

Endocrine & metabolic: Hyperglycemia (grades 3/4: 3%)

Gastrointestinal: Serum amylase increased (grades 3/4: 4% to 7%; treatment naive 8% to 9%), anorexia (3% to 4%), dyspepsia (3% to 4%), flatulence (3% to 4%), weight loss (2% to 4%)

Genitourinary: Hematuria (grades 3/4: 3% to 7%)

Hematologic: Neutropenia (1% to 3%)

Hepatic: Transaminases increased (2% to 5%), alkaline phosphatase increased (1%)

Neuromuscular & skeletal: Back pain (3% to 4%; treatment naive 9%), peripheral neuropathy (3% to 5%), myalgia (3% to 4%)

Renal: Serum creatinine increased (decompensated liver disease 9%), renal failure (decompensated liver disease 7%), glycosuria (grades 3/4: 3%)

Respiratory: Upper respiratory tract infection (8%), sinusitis (8%), nasopharyngitis (5%), pneumonia (2% to 3%; treatment naive 5%)

Miscellaneous: Diaphoresis (3%)

Product Availability Viread® oral powder formulation and 150 mg, 200 mg, 250 mg tablets: FDA approved January 2012; availability expected in February 2012.

Available Dosage Forms

Powder, oral:

Viread®: 40 mg/g (60 g)

Tablet, oral:

Viread®: 150 mg, 200 mg, 250 mg, 300 mg

General Dosage Range Dosage adjustment recommended in patients with renal impairment

Oral:

Children ≥2 years and Adolescents: 8 mg/kg once daily (maximum: 300 mg once daily)

Adults: 300 mg once daily

Administration

Oral Tablets may be administered without regard to meals. Powder should be mixed with 2-4 ounces of soft food (applesauce, baby food, yogurt) and swallowed immediately (avoids bitter taste); do not mix in liquid (powder may float on top of the liquid even after stirring). Measure powder using only the supplied dosing scoop.

Stability

Storage Store at 25°C (77°F); excursions permitted to 15°C to 30°C (59°F to 86°F).

Nursing Actions

Physical Assessment Allergy history should be assessed prior to beginning treatment. Monitor for lactic acidosis, elevated transaminases, osteomalacia, nausea, vomiting, diarrhea, neutropenia, myalgia, and peripheral neuropathy on a regular basis. Teach patient drugs that should not be used concurrently.

Patient Education This drug will not cure HIV, nor has it been found to reduce transmission of HIV; use appropriate precautions to prevent spread to other people. When used to treat HIV, this drug will be prescribed as one part of a multidrug combination; take exactly as directed for full course of therapy. You may be susceptible to infection because of your underlying disease. Regular monitoring of effectiveness of therapy will be necessary. Tablets can be taken at any time; powder must be mixed with soft food, not in a drink. May cause headache, nausea, vomiting, diarrhea, or weak bones with long-term use. Report immediately any trouble breathing, severe dizziness or passing out, rapid pulse, severe abdominal pain; severe nausea, vomiting, or diarrhea; severe muscle pain or weakness, dark urine, yellow skin or eyes, feeling unusually tired or weak, feeling cold, or signs of infection (burning on urination, perineal itching, white plaques in mouth, unhealed sores, persistent sore throat, or cough). If you are instructed to stop the medication, do not restart without specific instruction by your prescriber.

Dietary Considerations Consider calcium and vitamin D supplementation in patients with history of bone fracture or osteopenia.

Terazosin (ter AY zoe sin)

Index Terms Hytrin

Pharmacologic Category Alpha$_1$ Blocker

Pregnancy Risk Factor C

Lactation Excretion in breast milk unknown/use caution

Use Management of mild-to-moderate hypertension; alone or in combination with other agents such as diuretics or beta-blockers; benign prostate hyperplasia (BPH)

Unlabeled Use Pediatric hypertension

Available Dosage Forms

Capsule, oral: 1 mg, 2 mg, 5 mg, 10 mg

General Dosage Range Dosage adjustment recommended in patients on concomitant therapy

Oral: *Adults:* Initial: 1 mg at bedtime; Maintenance: 1-20 mg once daily (maximum: 20 mg/day)

Administration

Oral Administered without regard to meals at the same time each day.

Nursing Actions

Physical Assessment Monitor blood pressure and for hypotension, dizziness, somnolence, and impotence at beginning of therapy and on a regular basis. When discontinuing, dose should be tapered and blood pressure monitored closely.

Patient Education Take at the same time each day. Follow recommended diet and exercise program. May cause drowsiness, dizziness, postural hypotension, nausea, or sexual dysfunction (reversible, may resolve with continued use). Report altered CNS status (eg, fatigue, lethargy, confusion, nervousness); sudden weight gain; unusual or persistent swelling of ankles, feet, or extremities; palpitations or rapid heartbeat; respiratory difficulty; or muscle weakness.

Terbinafine (Systemic) (TER bin a feen)

Brand Names: U.S. LamISIL®; Terbinex™

Index Terms Terbinafine Hydrochloride

Pharmacologic Category Antifungal Agent, Oral

Medication Safety Issues

Sound-alike/look-alike issues:

Terbinafine may be confused with terbutaline

LamISIL® may be confused with LaMICtal®, Lomotil®

Pregnancy Risk Factor B

Lactation Enters breast milk/not recommended

Breast-Feeding Considerations Terbinafine is found in breast milk following oral administration. The milk/plasma ratio is 7:1.

Use Active against most strains of *Trichophyton mentagrophytes*, *Trichophyton rubrum*; may be effective for infections of *Microsporum gypseum* and *M. nanum*, *Trichophyton verrucosum*, *Epidermophyton floccosum*, *Candida albicans*, and *Scopulariopsis brevicaulis*

Onychomycosis of the toenail or fingernail due to susceptible dermatophytes; treatment of tinea capitis

Mechanism of Action/Effect Synthetic allylamine derivative which inhibits squalene epoxidase, a key enzyme in sterol biosynthesis in fungi. This results in a deficiency in ergosterol within the fungal cell wall and results in fungal cell death.

Contraindications Hypersensitivity to terbinafine or any component of the formulation

Warnings/Precautions While rare, the following complications have been reported and may require discontinuation of therapy: Changes in the ocular lens and retina, pancytopenia, neutropenia, Stevens-Johnson syndrome, toxic epidermal necrolysis. Precipitation or exacerbation of cutaneous or systemic lupus erythematosus has been observed; discontinue if signs and/or symptoms develop. Rare cases of hepatic failure, including fatal cases, have been reported following treatment of onychomycosis. Not recommended for use in patients with active or chronic liver disease. Discontinue if symptoms or signs of hepatobiliary dysfunction or cholestatic hepatitis develop. Products are not recommended for use with pre-existing liver or renal disease (Cl_{cr} ≤50 mL/minute). Use caution in patients sensitive to allylamine antifungals (eg, naftifine, butenafine); cross sensitivity to terbinafine may exist.

Drug Interactions

Avoid Concomitant Use

Avoid concomitant use of Terbinafine (Systemic) with any of the following: Axitinib; Pimozide; Tamoxifen; Thioridazine

Decreased Effect

Terbinafine (Systemic) may decrease the levels/effects of: ARIPiprazole; Axitinib; Codeine; CycloSPORINE; Iloperidone; Saccharomyces boulardii; Saxagliptin; TraMADol

The levels/effects of Terbinafine (Systemic) may be decreased by: Cyproterone; Rifamycin Derivatives; Tocilizumab

Increased Effect/Toxicity

Terbinafine (Systemic) may increase the levels/effects of: ARIPiprazole; Atomoxetine; CYP2D6 Substrates; Fesoterodine; Iloperidone; Nebivolol; Pimozide; Propafenone; Tamoxifen; Tetrabenazine; Thioridazine; Tricyclic Antidepressants

The levels/effects of Terbinafine (Systemic) may be increased by: Conivaptan

Adverse Reactions Adverse events listed for tablets unless otherwise specified. Granules were studied in patients 4-12 years of age.

>10%: Central nervous system: Headache (13%; granules 7%)

1% to 10%:

Central nervous system: Fever (granules 7%)

Dermatologic: Rash (6%; granules 2%), pruritus (3%; granules 1%), urticaria (1%)

Gastrointestinal: Diarrhea (6%; granules 3%), vomiting (<1%; granules 5%), dyspepsia (4%), nausea (3%; granules 2%), taste disturbance (3%), abdominal pain (2%; granules 2% to 4%), toothache (granules 1%)

Hepatic: Liver enzyme abnormalities (3%)

Respiratory: Nasopharyngitis (granules 10%), cough (granules 6%), nasal congestion (granules 2%), pharyngeal pain (granules 2%), rhinorrhea (granules 2%)

Available Dosage Forms

Granules, oral:

LamISIL®: 125 mg/packet (14s, 42s); 187.5 mg/packet (14s, 42s)

Tablet, oral: 250 mg

LamISIL®: 250 mg

Terbinex™: 250 mg

General Dosage Range

Oral granules: *Children ≥4 years:*

<25 kg: 125 mg once daily for 6 weeks

25-35 kg: 187.5 mg once daily for 6 weeks

>35 kg: 250 mg once daily for 6 weeks

Oral tablet: *Adults:* 250-500 mg daily in 1-2 divided doses

Administration

Oral Tablets may be administered without regard to meals. Granules should be sprinkled on a spoonful of nonacidic food (eg, mashed potatoes); swallow granules without chewing.

Stability

Storage

Granules: Store at controlled room temperature of 15°C to 30°C (59°F to 86°F).

Tablet: Store below 25°C (77°F). Protect from light.

Nursing Actions

Physical Assessment Use with caution in presence of hepatic or renal impairment.

Patient Education Take at same time of day, with or without regard to meals. Granules may be sprinkled on a spoonful of nonacidic food; swallow granules without chewing. It is important to take full prescription, even if symptoms appear resolved; may take several months for full treatment (inadequate treatment may result in reinfection). May cause altered taste (normal); nausea, vomiting, or abdominal pain; or diarrhea. Report unusual fatigue; persistent gastrointestinal upset; nasal congestion, runny nose, sore throat, or unusual cough; skin rash or blistering; or dark urine/pale stool.

Terbutaline (ter BYOO ta leen)

Index Terms Brethaire [DSC]; Brethine; Bricanyl [DSC]

Pharmacologic Category Beta$_2$ Agonist

Medication Safety Issues

Sound-alike/look-alike issues:

Brethine may be confused with Methergine®

Terbutaline may be confused with terbinafine, TOLBUTamide

Terbutaline and methylergonovine parenteral dosage forms look similar. Due to their contrasting indications, use care when administering these agents.

Pregnancy Risk Factor C

Lactation Enters breast milk/compatible

Use Bronchodilator in reversible airway obstruction and bronchial asthma

Unlabeled Use Injection: Tocolytic agent (short-term [≤72 hours] prevention or management of preterm labor

Available Dosage Forms

Injection, solution: 1 mg/mL (1 mL)

Tablet, oral: 2.5 mg, 5 mg

General Dosage Range Dosage adjustment recommended in patients with renal impairment

Oral:

Children 12-15 years: 2.5 mg every 6 hours 3 times/day (maximum: 7.5 mg/day)

Children >15 years and Adults: 2.5-5 mg every 6 hours 3 times/day (maximum: 15 mg/day)

SubQ:

Children <12 years: 0.005-0.01 mg/kg/dose to a maximum of 0.4 mg/dose; may repeat in 15-20 minutes

Children ≥12 years and Adults: 0.25 mg/dose; may repeat in 15-30 minutes (maximum: 0.5 mg/4-hour period)

Administration

Oral Administer around-the-clock to promote less variation in peak and trough serum levels.

I.V. Use infusion pump.

I.V. Detail pH: 3-5 (adjusted)

Nursing Actions

Physical Assessment Respiratory use: Monitor for cardiac and CNS changes at beginning of therapy and periodically throughout. For inpatient care, monitor vital signs and lung sounds prior to and periodically during therapy. **Preterm labor use: Inpatient:** Monitor maternal vital signs; respiratory, fluid, cardiac, and electrolyte status; frequency, duration, and intensity of contractions; and fetal heart rate.

Patient Education You may experience nervousness, dizziness, fatigue, dry mouth, and stomach upset. Report unresolved GI upset; dizziness or fatigue; vision changes; sudden weight gain; swelling of extremities; chest pain, rapid heartbeat, or palpitations; insomnia, nervousness, or hyperactivity; muscle cramping, tremors, or pain; or rash.

Terconazole (ter KONE a zole)

Brand Names: U.S. Terazol® 3; Terazol® 7

Index Terms Triaconazole

Pharmacologic Category Antifungal Agent, Vaginal

Medication Safety Issues

Sound-alike/look-alike issues:

Terconazole may be confused with tioconazole

International issues:

Terazol [U.S., Canada] may be confused with Theradol brand name for tramadol [Netherlands]

Pregnancy Risk Factor C

Lactation Excretion in breast milk unknown/not recommended

Use Local treatment of vulvovaginal candidiasis

Available Dosage Forms

Cream, vaginal: 0.4% (45 g); 0.8% (20 g)

Terazol® 7: 0.4% (45 g)

Terazol® 3: 0.8% (20 g)

Suppository, vaginal: 80 mg (3s)

Terazol® 3: 80 mg (3s)

General Dosage Range Intravaginal: *Adults:* Insert 1 applicatorful or suppository at bedtime

Administration

Other Intravaginal:

Vaginal cream: Use applicator provided by manufacturer. Insertion should be as far as possible into the vagina without causing discomfort. Wash applicator after each use; allow to dry thoroughly before putting back together.

Vaginal suppository: Remove foil package prior to use. Insertion should be as far as possible into the vagina without causing discomfort. If the provided applicator is used for insertion, wash and dry thoroughly prior to additional use.

Nursing Actions

Patient Education Sexual partner may experience irritation; best to refrain from intercourse during period of treatment. Suppositories may cause breakdown of rubber/latex products such as diaphragms; avoid concurrent use. Report persistent vaginal burning, itching, irritation, or rash.

Teriparatide (ter i PAR a tide)

Brand Names: U.S. Forteo®

Index Terms Parathyroid Hormone (1-34); Recombinant Human Parathyroid Hormone (1-34); rhPTH(1-34)

Pharmacologic Category Parathyroid Hormone Analog

Medication Guide Available Yes

Pregnancy Risk Factor C

Lactation Excretion in breast milk unknown/not recommended

Breast-Feeding Considerations Indicated for use in postmenopausal women. Studies have not been conducted to determine excretion in breast milk. Not recommended for use in breast-feeding women.

Use Treatment of osteoporosis in postmenopausal women at high risk of fracture; treatment of primary or hypogonadal osteoporosis in men at high risk of fracture; treatment of glucocorticoid-induced osteoporosis in men and women at high risk for fracture

Mechanism of Action/Effect An analog of parathyroid hormone, teriparatide stimulates osteoblast function, increases gastrointestinal calcium absorption, and increases renal tubular reabsorption of calcium. Treatment with teriparatide increases bone mineral density, bone mass, and strength. In postmenopausal women, it has been shown to decrease osteoporosis-related fractures.

Contraindications Hypersensitivity to teriparatide or any component of the formulation

Canadian labeling: Additional contraindications (not in U.S. labeling): Pre-existing hypercalcemia; severe renal impairment; metabolic bone diseases other than primary osteoporosis (including hyperparathyroidism and Paget's disease of the bone); unexplained elevations of alkaline phosphatase; prior external beam or implant radiation therapy involving the skeleton; bone metastases or history of skeletal malignancies; pregnancy; breast-feeding mothers; pediatric patients or young adults with open epiphysis

Warnings/Precautions [U.S. Boxed Warning]: In animal studies, teriparatide has been associated with an increase in osteosarcoma; risk was dependent on both dose and duration. Avoid use in patients with an increased risk of osteosarcoma (including Paget's disease, prior radiation, unexplained elevation of alkaline phosphatase, or in patients with open epiphyses). Do not use in patients with a history of skeletal metastases, hyperparathyroidism, or pre-existing hypercalcemia. Not for use in patients with metabolic bone disease other than osteoporosis. Use caution in patients with active or recent urolithiasis. Use caution in patients at risk of orthostasis (including concurrent antihypertensive therapy), or in patients who may not tolerate transient hypotension (cardiovascular or cerebrovascular disease). Use caution in patients with cardiac, renal or hepatic impairment (limited data available concerning safety and efficacy). Use in severe renal impairment is contraindicated in the Canadian labeling. Use of teriparatide for longer than 2 years is not recommended. Not approved for use in pediatric patients.

Drug Interactions

Avoid Concomitant Use There are no known interactions where it is recommended to avoid concomitant use.

Decreased Effect There are no known significant interactions involving a decrease in effect.

Increased Effect/Toxicity There are no known significant interactions involving an increase in effect.

Nutritional/Ethanol Interactions

Ethanol: Excessive intake may increase risk of osteoporosis.

Herb/Nutraceutical: Ensure adequate calcium and vitamin D intake.

Adverse Reactions

>10%: Endocrine & metabolic: Hypercalcemia (transient increases noted 4-6 hours postdose [women 11%; men 6%])

1% to 10%:

Cardiovascular: Orthostatic hypotension (5%; transient), chest pain (3%), syncope (3%)

Central nervous system: Dizziness (8%), insomnia (4% to 5%), anxiety (≤4%), depression (4%), vertigo (4%)

Dermatologic: Rash (5%)

Endocrine & metabolic: Hyperuricemia (3%)

Gastrointestinal: Nausea (9% to 14%), gastritis (≤7%), dyspepsia (5%), vomiting (3%)

Neuromuscular & skeletal: Arthralgia (10%), weakness (9%), leg cramps (3%)

Respiratory: Rhinitis (10%), pharyngitis (6%), dyspnea (4% to 6%), pneumonia (4% to 6%)

Miscellaneous: Antibodies to teriparatide (3% of women in long-term treatment; hypersensitivity reactions or decreased efficacy were not associated in preclinical trials), herpes zoster (≤3%)

Available Dosage Forms

Injection, solution:

Forteo®: 250 mcg/mL (2.4 mL)

General Dosage Range

SubQ: *Adults:* 20 mcg once daily

Administration

Other Administer by subcutaneous injection into the thigh or abdominal wall. Initial administration should occur under circumstances in which the patient may sit or lie down, in the event of orthostasis. **Note:** The 3 mL prefilled pen (Canadian availability; not available in U.S.) must be primed prior to each dose.

Stability

Storage Store at 2°C to 8°C (36°F to 46°F); do not freeze. Protect from light. Discard pen 28 days after first injection. Do not use if solution is cloudy, colored, or contains solid particles.

Nursing Actions

Physical Assessment Initial administration should occur where patient may sit or lie down, in the event of orthostasis. Monitor for chest pain, hypotension, nausea, vomiting, arthralgia, leg cramps, and dyspnea. Teach patient proper administration and disposal and proper diet with adequate calcium and vitamin D.

Patient Education Rotate injection sites in thigh or abdominal wall. Sit when administering to reduce possibility of falling or injury. Avoid excess alcohol (may increase risk of osteoporosis) and follow dietary instructions of prescriber. May cause dizziness; nausea, vomiting, or upset stomach; or muscle or skeletal pain, weakness, or cramping. Report chest pain or palpitations or respiratory difficulty.

Tesamorelin (tes a moe REL in)

Brand Names: U.S. Egrifta™

Index Terms Tesamorelin Acetate; TH9507

Pharmacologic Category Growth Hormone Releasing Factor

Medication Safety Issues

Sound-alike/look-alike issues:

Tesamorelin may be confused with temsirolimus

Pregnancy Risk Factor X

Lactation Excretion in breast milk unknown/not recommended

Use Reduction of excess abdominal fat in HIV-infected patients with lipodystrophy

Available Dosage Forms

Injection, powder for reconstitution:

Egrifta™: 1 mg

General Dosage Range SubQ: *Adults:* 2 mg once daily

Administration

Other SubQ: The abdomen is the preferred site of administration; site should be rotated within the abdomen. Avoid injection into scar tissue, bruises, or the navel. The reconstituted solution should be visually inspected for particulate matter and discoloration; do not administer if solution is not clear, colorless and free of particulate matter. **Note:** Syringes and needles are single-use only and should not be shared between patients.

Testosterone (tes TOS ter one)

Brand Names: U.S. Androderm®; AndroGel®; Axiron®; Delatestryl®; Depo®-Testosterone; First®-Testosterone; First®-Testosterone MC; Fortesta™; Striant®; Testim®; Testopel®

Index Terms Axiron®; Testosterone Cypionate; Testosterone Enanthate

Pharmacologic Category Androgen

Medication Safety Issues

Sound-alike/look-alike issues:

Testosterone may be confused with testolactone

Testoderm may be confused with Estraderm®

AndroGel® 1% may be confused with AndroGel® 1.62%

Other safety concerns:

Transdermal patch may contain conducting metal (eg, aluminum); remove patch prior to MRI.

Medication Guide Available Yes

Pregnancy Risk Factor X

Lactation Enters breast milk/contraindicated

Breast-Feeding Considerations High levels of endogenous maternal testosterone, such as those caused by certain ovarian cysts, suppress milk production. Maternal serum testosterone levels generally fall following pregnancy and return to normal once breast-feeding is stopped. The amount of testosterone present in breast milk or the effect to the nursing infant following maternal supplementation is not known. Some products are contraindicated while breast-feeding. Females who are nursing should avoid skin-to-skin contact to areas where testosterone has been applied topically on another person.

Use

Injection: Androgen replacement therapy in the treatment of delayed male puberty; male hypogonadism (primary or hypogonadotropic); inoperable metastatic female breast cancer (enanthate only)

Pellet: Androgen replacement therapy in the treatment of delayed male puberty; male hypogonadism (primary or hypogonadotropic)

Buccal system, topical gel, topical solution, transdermal system: Male hypogonadism (primary or hypogonadotropic)

Capsule (not available in U.S.): Conditions associated with a deficiency or absence of endogenous testosterone

Unlabeled Use Androgen deficiency in men with AIDS wasting; postmenopausal women (short-term use in select cases)

Mechanism of Action/Effect Principal endogenous androgen responsible for promoting the growth and development of the male sex organs and maintaining secondary sex characteristics in androgen-deficient males

Contraindications Hypersensitivity to testosterone or any component of the formulation; males with known or suspected carcinoma of the breast or prostate; specific products are contraindicated in women

Depo®-Testosterone: Also contraindicated in serious hepatic, renal, or cardiac disease

Warnings/Precautions When used to treat delayed male puberty, perform radiographic examination of the hand and wrist every 6 months to determine the rate of bone maturation. May cause hypercalcemia in patients with prolonged immobilization or cancer. May accelerate bone maturation without producing compensating gain in linear growth. Has both androgenic and anabolic activity, the anabolic action may enhance hypoglycemia. May alter serum cholesterol; use caution with history of MI or coronary artery disease. Use caution in elderly patients or patients with other demographic factors which may increase the risk of prostatic carcinoma; careful monitoring is required. Urethral obstruction may develop in patients with BPH; treatment should be discontinued if this should occur (use lower dose if restarted). Withhold treatment pending urological evaluation in patients with palpable prostate nodule or induration, PSA >4 ng/mL, or PSA >3 ng/mL in men at high risk of prostate cancer (Bhasin, 2010). Use with caution in patients with conditions influenced by edema (eg, cardiovascular disease, migraine, seizure disorder, renal or hepatic impairment) or medications that enhance edema formation (eg, corticosteroids); testosterone may cause fluid retention. May cause gynecomastia. Large doses may suppress spermatogenesis. During treatment for metastatic breast cancer, women should be monitored for signs of virilization; discontinue if mild virilization is present to prevent irreversible symptoms.

Prolonged use of high doses of androgens has been associated with serious hepatic effects (peliosis hepatis, hepatic neoplasms, cholestatic hepatitis, jaundice). May potentiate sleep apnea in some male patients (obesity or chronic lung disease). May increase hematocrit requiring dose adjustment or discontinuation; monitor.

[U.S. Boxed Warning]: Virilization in children has been reported following contact with unwashed or unclothed application sites of men using topical testosterone. Patients should strictly adhere to instructions for use in order to prevent secondary exposure. Virilization of female sexual partners has also been reported with male use of topical testosterone. Symptoms of virilization generally regress following removal of exposure; however, in some children, enlarged genitalia and bone age did not fully return to age appropriate normal. Signs of inappropriate virilization in women or children following secondary exposure to topical testosterone should be brought to the attention of a healthcare provider. Axiron® and Fortesta™ are not interchangeable with other topical testosterone products; AndroGel® 1% and AndroGel® 1.62% are not interchangeable. Transdermal patch may contain conducting metal (eg, aluminum); remove patch prior to MRI. Gels, solution, transdermal, and buccal system have not been evaluated in males <18 years of age; safety and efficacy of injection have not been established in males <12 years of age. Some testosterone products may be chemically synthesized from soy. Some products may contain benzyl alcohol. Use of Axiron® in males with BMI >35 kg/m^2 has not been established.

Drug Interactions

Avoid Concomitant Use There are no known interactions where it is recommended to avoid concomitant use.

Decreased Effect

The levels/effects of Testosterone may be decreased by: Tocilizumab

Increased Effect/Toxicity

Testosterone may increase the levels/effects of: CycloSPORINE; CycloSPORINE (Systemic); Vitamin K Antagonists

The levels/effects of Testosterone may be increased by: Conivaptan

Nutritional/Ethanol Interactions Herb/Nutraceutical: St John's wort may decrease testosterone levels.

Adverse Reactions Frequency not always defined.

Cardiovascular: Deep venous thrombosis, edema, hypertension, vasodilation

Central nervous system: Abnormal dreams, aggressive behavior, anger, amnesia, anxiety, blood pressure increased/decreased, chills, depression, dizziness, emotional lability, excitation, fatigue, headache, hostility, insomnia, malaise, memory loss, mood swings, nervousness, seizure, sleep apnea, sleeplessness

Dermatologic: Acne, alopecia, contact dermatitis, dry skin, erythema, folliculitis, hair discoloration, hirsutism (increase in pubic hair growth), pruritus, rash, seborrhea

Endocrine & metabolic: Breast pain/soreness, gonadotropin secretion decreased, growth acceleration, gynecomastia, hot flashes, hypercalcemia, hyperchloremia, hypercholesterolemia, hyper-/hypoglycemia, hyper-/hypokalemia, hyperlipidemia, hypernatremia, inorganic phosphate retention, libido changes, menstrual problems (including amenorrhea), virilism, water retention

Gastrointestinal: Appetite increased, diarrhea, gastroesophageal reflux, GI bleeding, GI irritation, nausea, taste disorder, vomiting, weight gain

Following buccal administration (most common): Bitter taste, gum edema, gum or mouth irritation, gum pain, gum tenderness, taste perversion

Genitourinary: Bladder irritability, impotence, oligospermia, penile erections (spontaneous), priapism, prostatic carcinoma, prostatic hyperplasia, prostatitis, PSA increased, testicular atrophy, urination impaired

Hepatic: Bilirubin increased, cholestatic hepatitis, cholestatic jaundice, hepatic dysfunction, hepatic necrosis, hepatocellular neoplasms, liver function test changes, peliosis hepatis
Hematologic: Anemia, bleeding, hematocrit/hemoglobin increased, leukopenia, polycythemia, suppression of clotting factors
Local: Application site reaction (gel, solution), injection site inflammation/pain
Transdermal system: Pruritus at application site (17% to 37%), burn-like blisters under system (12%), erythema at application site (≤7%), vesicles at application site (6%), allergic contact dermatitis to system (4%), burning at application site (3%), induration at application site (3%), exfoliation at application site (<3%)
Neuromuscular & skeletal: Back pain, hemarthrosis, hyperkinesias, paresthesia, weakness
Ocular: Lacrimation increased
Renal: Creatinine increased, hematuria, polyuria
Respiratory: Dyspnea, nasopharyngitis
Miscellaneous: Anaphylactoid reactions, diaphoresis, hypersensitivity reactions, smell disorder

Pharmacodynamics/Kinetics

Duration of Action Route and ester dependent; I.M.: Cypionate and enanthate esters have longest duration, ≤2-4 weeks; gel: 24-48 hours

Controlled Substance C-III

Available Dosage Forms

Cream, topical:
First®-Testosterone MC: 2% (60 g)

Gel, topical:
AndroGel®: 1% [5 g gel/packet] (30s); 1% [2.5 g gel/packet] (30s); 1% [1.25 g gel/actuation] (75 g); 1.62% [1.25 g gel/actuation] (75 g)
Fortesta™: 10 mg/actuation (60 g)
Testim®: 1% [5 g gel/tube] (30s)

Implant, subcutaneous:
Testopel®: 75 mg (10s, 24s, 100s)

Injection, oil: 100 mg/mL (10 mL); 200 mg/mL (1 mL, 5 mL, 10 mL)
Delatestryl®: 200 mg/mL (5 mL)
Depo®-Testosterone: 100 mg/mL (10 mL); 200 mg/mL (1 mL, 10 mL)

Mucoadhesive, for buccal application:
Striant®: 30 mg (60s)

Ointment, topical:
First®-Testosterone: 2% (60 g)

Patch, transdermal:
Androderm®: 2 mg/24 hours (60s); 4 mg/24 hours (30s)

Powder, for prescription compounding: USP: 100% (5 g, 25 g)

Solution, topical:
Axiron®: 30 mg/actuation (110 mL)

General Dosage Range

Buccal: *Adults (males):* 30 mg every 12 hours

I.M.: *Adolescents and Adults (males):* 50-400 mg every 2-4 weeks

SubQ: *Adolescents and Adults (males):* 150-450 mg every 3-6 months

Transdermal: *Adults (males):* Androderm®: Apply 2-7.5 mg/day; AndroGel® 1%, Testim®: 5-10 g (50-100 mg testosterone) applied once daily (maximum: 10 g/day); AndroGel® 1.62%: Apply 20.25-81 mg/day; Axiron®: Apply 30-120 mg/day; Fortesta™: Apply 10-70 mg/day

Administration

Oral

Oral, buccal application (Striant®): One mucoadhesive for buccal application (buccal system) should be applied to a comfortable area above the incisor tooth. Apply flat side of system to gum. Rotate to alternate sides of mouth with each application. Hold buccal system firmly in place for 30 seconds to ensure adhesion. The buccal system should adhere to gum for 12 hours. If the buccal system falls out, replace with a new system. If the system falls out within 4 hours of next dose, the new buccal system should remain in place until the time of the following scheduled dose. System will soften and mold to shape of gum as it absorbs moisture from mouth. Do not chew or swallow the buccal system. The buccal system will not dissolve; gently remove by sliding downwards from gum; avoid scratching gum.

Oral, capsule (Andriol®; not available in the U.S.): Should be administered with meals. Should be swallowed whole; do not crush or chew.

I.M. Warm injection to room temperature and shaking vial will help redissolve crystals that have formed after storage. Administer by deep I.M. injection into the upper outer quadrant of the gluteus maximus.

Other

Transdermal patch (Androderm®): Apply patch to clean, dry area of skin on the back, abdomen, upper arms, or thigh. Do not apply to bony areas or parts of the body that are subject to prolonged pressure while sleeping or sitting. **Do not apply to the scrotum.** Avoid showering, washing the site, or swimming for 3 hours after application. Following patch removal, mild skin irritation may be treated with OTC hydrocortisone cream. A small amount of triamcinolone acetonide 0.1% cream may be applied under the system to decrease irritation; do not use ointment. Patch should be applied nightly. Rotate administration sites, allowing 7 days between applying to the same site.

Topical gel and solution: Apply to clean, dry, intact skin. Application sites should be allowed to dry for a few minutes prior to dressing. Hands should be washed with soap and water after application. **Do not apply testosterone gel or solution to the genitals.** Alcohol-based gels and solutions are flammable; avoid fire or smoking until dry. Testosterone may be transferred to another person following skin-to-skin contact with the application site. Strict adherence to application instructions is needed in order to decrease secondary exposure. Thoroughly wash hands after application and cover application site with clothing (ie, shirt) once gel or solution has dried, or clean application site thoroughly with soap and water prior to contact in order to minimize transfer. In addition to skin-to-skin contact, secondary exposure has also been reported following exposure to secondary items (eg, towel, shirt, sheets). If secondary exposure occurs, the other person should thoroughly wash the skin with soap and water as soon as possible.

AndroGel® 1%, AndroGel® 1.62%, Testim®: Apply (preferably in the morning) to clean, dry, intact skin of the shoulder and upper arms. AndroGel® 1% may also be applied to the abdomen; do not apply AndroGel® 1.62% or Testim® to the abdomen. Area of application should be limited to what will be covered by a short sleeve t-shirt. Apply at the same time each day. Upon opening the packet(s), the entire contents should be squeezed into the palm of the hand and immediately applied to the application site(s). Alternatively, a portion may be squeezed onto palm of hand and applied, repeating the process until entire packet has been applied. Application site should not be washed for ≥2 hours following application of AndroGel® 1.62% or Testim®, or >5 hours for AndroGel® 1%.

AndroGel® 1% multidose pump: Prime pump 3 times (and discard this portion of product) prior to initial use. Each actuation delivers 1.25 g of gel (4 actuations = 5 g; 6 actuations = 7.5 g; 8 actuations = 10 g); each actuation may be applied individually or all at the same time.

AndroGel® 1.62% multidose pump: Prime pump 3 times (and discard this portion of product) prior to initial use. Each actuation delivers 20.25 mg of gel (2 actuations = 40.5 mg; 3 actuations = 60.75 mg; 4 actuations = 81 mg); each actuation may be applied individually or all at the same time.

Axiron®: Apply using the applicator to the axilla at the same time each morning. Do not apply to other parts of the body (eg, abdomen, genitals, shoulders, upper arms). Avoid washing the site or swimming for 2 hours after application. Prior to first use, prime the applicator pump by depressing it 3 times (discard this portion of the product). After priming, position the nozzle over the applicator cup and depress pump fully one time; ensure liquid enters cup. Each pump actuation delivers testosterone 30 mg. No more than 30 mg (one pump) should be added to the cup at one time. The total dose should be divided between axilla (example, 30 mg/day: apply to one axilla only; 60 mg/day: apply 30 mg to each axilla; 90 mg/day: apply 30 mg to each axilla, allow to dry, then apply an additional 30 mg to one axilla; etc). To apply dose, keep applicator upright and wipe into the axilla; if solution runs or drips, use cup to wipe. Do not rub into skin with fingers or hand. If more than one 30 mg dose is needed, repeat process. Apply roll-on or stick antiperspirants or deodorants prior to testosterone. Once application site is dry, cover with clothing. After use, rinse applicator under running water and pat dry with a tissue. The application site and dose of this product are not interchangeable with other topical testosterone products.

Fortesta™: Apply to skin of front and inner thighs. Do not apply to other parts of the body. Use one finger to rub gel evenly onto skin of each thigh. Avoid showering, washing the site, or swimming for 2 hours after application. Prior to first dose, prime the pump by holding canister upright and fully depressing the pump 8 times (discard this portion of the product). Each pump actuation delivers testosterone 10 mg. The total dose should be divided between thighs (example, 10 mg/day: apply 10 mg to one thigh only; 20 mg/day: apply 10 mg to each thigh; 30 mg/day: apply 20 mg to one thigh and 10 mg to the other thigh; etc). Once application site is dry, cover with clothing. The application site and dose of this product are not interchangeable with other topical testosterone products.

Stability

Storage

Androderm®: Store at room temperature. Do not store outside of pouch. Excessive heat may cause system to burst.

AndroGel® 1%, AndroGel® 1.62%, Axiron®, Delatestryl®, Striant®, Testim®: Store at room temperature.

Depo® Testosterone: Store at room temperature. Protect from light.

Fortesta™: Store at room temperature; do not freeze

Testopel®: Store in a cool location.

Nursing Actions

Physical Assessment Instruct patients to apply to clean, dry skin and that area should be covered with clothing to prevent transmission.

Patient Education Instruct patient that this drug is not to be used by women except in rare situations. Drug can cause male-like features in females or children, such as changes in sex drive, increased body hair, acne, aggressive behavior, or irregular periods. It should be applied to clean, dry skin and then covered with clothing. No swimming or showering should be allowed up to ≥2 hours (product-dependent) after topical application. Inform patients that testosterone may lower blood sugars and that symptoms of hypoglycemia, such as shaking, hunger, blurred vision, or rapid heartbeat, should be monitored. Inform prescriber if patient has history of diabetes or liver or kidney disease. Serious side effects which need to be reported include problems with urination, ankle swelling, nausea or stomach pains, or frequent or prolonged erections.

Dietary Considerations Testosterone USP may be synthesized from soy. Food and beverages have not been found to interfere with buccal system; ensure system is in place following eating, drinking, or brushing teeth.

Tetrabenazine (tet ra BEN a zeen)

Brand Names: U.S. Xenazine®

Pharmacologic Category Central Monoamine-Depleting Agent

Medication Guide Available Yes

Pregnancy Risk Factor C

Lactation Excretion in breast milk unknown/not recommended

Use Treatment of chorea associated with Huntington's disease

Canadian labeling: Treatment of hyperkinetic movement disorders, including Huntington's chorea, hemiballismus, senile chorea, Tourette syndrome, and tardive dyskinesia

Available Dosage Forms

Tablet, oral:

Xenazine®: 12.5 mg, 25 mg

General Dosage Range Dosage adjustment recommended in patients on concomitant therapy or who develop toxicities

Oral: *Adults:* 12.5 mg once daily; Maintenance: 25-100 mg/day in 2-3 divided doses

Administration

Oral May administer without regard to meals.

Nursing Actions

Physical Assessment Monitor psychiatric status and for CNS changes at beginning of therapy, with any dose change, and at frequent intervals during therapy.

Patient Education May cause dizziness, headache, sedation, nausea, or vomiting. Report immediately any signs of CNS changes (mood changes, increased irritability or anxiety, depression, suicide ideation) or difficulty breathing.

Tetracycline (tet ra SYE kleen)

Index Terms Achromycin; TCN; Tetracycline Hydrochloride

Pharmacologic Category Antibiotic, Tetracycline Derivative

Medication Safety Issues

Sound-alike/look-alike issues:

Tetracycline may be confused with tetradecyl sulfate

Achromycin may be confused with actinomycin, Adriamycin®

Pregnancy Risk Factor D

Lactation Enters breast milk/not recommended (AAP rates "compatible"; AAP 2001 update pending)

Use Treatment of susceptible bacterial infections of both gram-positive and gram-negative organisms; also infections due to *Mycoplasma*, *Chlamydia*, and *Rickettsia*; indicated for acne, exacerbations of chronic bronchitis, and treatment of gonorrhea and syphilis in patients who are allergic to penicillin; as part of a multidrug regimen for *H. pylori* eradication to reduce the risk of duodenal ulcer recurrence

Unlabeled Use Treatment of periodontitis associated with presence of *Actinobacillus actinomycetemcomitans* (AA)

Available Dosage Forms

Capsule, oral: 250 mg, 500 mg

General Dosage Range Dosage adjustment recommended in patients with renal impairment

Oral:

Children >8 years: 25-50 mg/kg/day divided every 6 hours

Adults: 250-500 mg 2-4 times/day

Administration

Oral Oral should be given on an empty stomach (ie, 1 hour prior to, or 2 hours after meals) to increase total absorption. Administer at least 1-2 hours prior to, or 4 hours after antacid because aluminum and magnesium cations may chelate with tetracycline and reduce its total absorption. Administer around-the-clock to promote less variation in peak and trough serum levels.

Nursing Actions

Physical Assessment Results of culture and sensitivity tests and patient's allergy history should be assessed prior to beginning therapy. Monitor for nausea, diarrhea, pericarditis, photosensitivity, rash, opportunistic infection, and hypersensitivity.

Patient Education Preferable to take on an empty stomach, 1 hour before or 2 hours after meals. Avoid antacids, iron, or dairy products within 2 hours of taking tetracycline. You may experience photosensitivity, dizziness, lightheadedness, or nausea/vomiting. Report rash or intense itching; yellowing of skin or eyes; fever or chills; watery, bloody, or foul-smelling stool; vaginal itching or discharge; excessive thirst or urination; acute headache; unresolved or persistent diarrhea; respiratory difficulty; if condition does not improve; or worsening of condition. Do not take antidiarrheal medication unless instructed by prescriber.

Thalidomide (tha LI doe mide)

Brand Names: U.S. Thalomid®

Pharmacologic Category Angiogenesis Inhibitor; Immunomodulator, Systemic; Tumor Necrosis Factor (TNF) Blocking Agent

Medication Safety Issues

Sound-alike/look-alike issues:

Thalidomide may be confused with flutamide, lenalidomide

Thalomid® may be confused with thiamine

High alert medication:

This medication is in a class the Institute for Safe Medication Practices (ISMP) includes among its list of drugs which have a heightened risk of causing significant patient harm when used in error.

International issues:

Thalomid [U.S., Canada] may be confused with Thilomide brand name for lodoxamide [Greece, Turkey]

Medication Guide Available Yes

Pregnancy Risk Factor X

Lactation Excretion in breast milk unknown/not recommended

Use Treatment of newly-diagnosed multiple myeloma; treatment and maintenance of cutaneous manifestations of erythema nodosum leprosum (ENL)

Unlabeled Use Treatment of refractory Crohn's disease; treatment of chronic graft-versus-host disease (GVHD) in hematopoietic stem cell transplantation; AIDS-related aphthous stomatitis; Waldenström's macroglobulinemia; maintenance therapy of multiple myeloma (following autologous stem cell transplant)

Available Dosage Forms

Capsule, oral:

Thalomid®: 50 mg, 100 mg, 150 mg, 200 mg

General Dosage Range Dosage adjustment recommended in patients who develop toxicities

Oral: *Children ≥12 years and Adults:* Initial: 100-300 mg once daily (maximum: 400 mg/day)

Administration

Oral Administer orally with water, preferably at bedtime once daily on an empty stomach, at least 1 hour after the evening meal. Doses >400 mg/day may be given in 2-3 divided doses. For missed doses, if <12 hours patient may receive dose; if >12 hours wait till next dose due.

Avoid extensive handling of capsules; capsules should remain in blister pack until ingestion. If exposed to the powder content from broken capsules or body fluids from patients receiving thalidomide, the exposed area should be washed with soap and water.

Nursing Actions

Physical Assessment Patient must be capable of complying with STEPS® program. Instruct patient on risks of pregnancy, appropriate contraceptive measures, and necessity for frequent pregnancy testing (schedule pregnancy testing at time of dispensing and give patient schedule in writing). Monitor for signs of fluid retention, weight gain, and hypotension. Monitor closely for signs of neuropathy (ie, numbness, tingling, and pain in extremities), CNS depression, and altered blood counts.

Patient Education You will be given oral and written instructions about the necessity of using two methods of contraception and the necessity of keeping return visits for pregnancy testing. Do not donate blood while taking this medicine. Male patients should not donate sperm. Avoid extensive handling of capsules; capsules should remain in blister pack until ingestion. If exposed to the powder content from broken capsules or body fluids from patients receiving thalidomide, the exposed area should be washed with soap and water. Avoid alcohol. You may experience postural hypotension, sleepiness, dizziness, fatigue, fever, headaches, lack of concentration, nausea or vomiting or loss of appetite, constipation or diarrhea, oral thrush (frequent mouth care is necessary), or sexual dysfunction (reversible). Report any of the above if persistent or severe. Report chest pain or palpitations or swelling of extremities; respiratory difficulty; back, neck, muscle pain, muscle weakness, or stiffness; numbness or pain in extremities; significant weight loss or gain; skin rash or eruptions; or increased nervousness, anxiety, confusion, or insomnia.

Theophylline (thee OFF i lin)

Brand Names: U.S. Elixophyllin® Elixir; Theo-24®

Index Terms Theophylline Anhydrous

Pharmacologic Category Theophylline Derivative

Pregnancy Risk Factor C

Lactation Enters breast milk/compatible (AAP rates "compatible"; AAP 2001 update pending)

Use Treatment of symptoms and reversible airway obstruction due to chronic asthma, or other chronic lung diseases

Note: The Global Initiative for Asthma Guidelines (2009) and the National Heart, Lung and Blood Institute Guidelines (2007) do not recommend oral theophylline as a long-term control medication for asthma in children ≤5 years of age; use has been shown to be effective as an add-on (but not preferred) agent in older children and adults with severe asthma treated with inhaled or oral glucocorticoids. The guidelines do not recommend theophylline for the treatment of exacerbations of asthma.

The Global Initiative for Chronic Obstructive Lung Disease Guidelines (2009) suggest that while higher doses of slow release formulations of theophylline have been proven to be effective for use in COPD, it is not a preferred agent due to its potential for toxicity.

Available Dosage Forms

Capsule, extended release, oral:

Theo-24®: 100 mg, 200 mg, 300 mg, 400 mg

Infusion, premixed in D_5W: 400 mg (100 mL, 250 mL, 500 mL, 1000 mL); 800 mg (250 mL, 500 mL, 1000 mL)

Solution, oral: 80 mg/15 mL (15 mL, 473 mL)

Elixophyllin® Elixir: 80 mg/15 mL (473 mL)

Tablet, extended release, oral: 100 mg, 200 mg, 300 mg, 400 mg, 450 mg, 600 mg

General Dosage Range

I.V.:

Infants 6-52 weeks: mg/kg/hour = (0.008) (age in weeks) + 0.21

Children 1-9 years: 0.8 mg/kg/hour

Children 9-12 years and Adolescents 12-16 years (cigarette or marijuana smokers): 0.7 mg/kg/hour

Adolescents 12-16 years (nonsmokers): 0.5 mg/kg/hour; maximum 900 mg/day unless serum levels indicate need for larger dose

Adults 16-60 years (otherwise healthy, nonsmokers): 0.4 mg/kg/hour; maximum 900 mg/day unless serum levels indicate need for larger dose

Adults >60 years: 0.3 mg/kg/hour; maximum 400 mg/day unless serum levels indicate need for larger dose

Oral solution:

Full-term Infants and Infants <26 weeks: Total daily dose (mg) = [(0.2 x age in weeks) +5] x (weight in kg); divide dose into 3 equal amounts and administer at 8-hour intervals

Full-term Infants and Infants ≥26 weeks and <52 weeks: Total daily dose (mg) = [(0.2 x age in weeks) +5] x (weight in kg); divide dose into 4 equal amounts and administer at 6-hour intervals

Children ≥1 year and <45 kg: Initial: 10-14 mg/kg/day in divided doses (maximum dose: 300 mg/day); titrate to maintenance dose: 20 mg/kg/day in divided doses every 4-6 hours (maximum dose: 600 mg/day)

Children >45 kg and Adults: Initial: 300 mg/day in divided doses; titrate to maintenance dose: 600 mg/day in divided doses every 6-8 hours

Oral extended release formulations:

Children ≥1 year and <45 kg: Initial: 10-14 mg/kg once daily (maximum dose: 300 mg/day); titrate to maintenance dose: 20 mg/kg once daily (maximum dose: 600 mg/day)

Children >45 kg and Adults: 300-600 mg once daily

Administration

Oral Long-acting preparations should be taken with a full glass of water, swallowed whole, or cut in half if scored. Do **not** crush. Extended release capsule forms may be opened and the contents sprinkled on soft foods; do **not** chew beads.

I.V. Administer loading dose over 30 minutes; follow with a continuous infusion as appropriate.

I.V. Detail pH: 4.3

Nursing Actions

Physical Assessment Evaluate effectiveness of therapy (prevention of bronchospasm). Monitor for cardiac and CNS changes at beginning of therapy and periodically throughout.

Patient Education Preferable to take on empty stomach, 1 hour before or 2 hours after meals, with a full glass of water. Do not chew or crush sustained release forms; capsules may be opened and contents sprinkled on soft food (do not chew beads). Avoid dietary stimulants (eg, caffeine, tea, colas, or chocolate). You may experience nausea, vomiting, or loss of appetite. Report acute insomnia or restlessness, chest pain or rapid heartbeat, emotional lability or agitation, muscle tremors or cramping, acute headache, persistent and repetitive vomiting, abdominal pain and cramping, blackened stool, or worsening of respiratory condition.

Related Information

Peak and Trough Guidelines *on page 1276*

Thiamine (THYE a min)

Index Terms Aneurine Hydrochloride; Thiamin; Thiamine Hydrochloride; Thiaminium Chloride Hydrochloride; Vitamin B_1

Pharmacologic Category Vitamin, Water Soluble

Medication Safety Issues

Sound-alike/look-alike issues:

Thiamine may be confused with Tenormin®, Thalomid®, Thorazine

International issues:

Doxal [Brazil] may be confused with Doxil brand name for doxorubicin [U.S.]

Doxal: Brand name for pyridoxine/thiamine [Brazil], but also the brand name for doxepin [Finland]

Pregnancy Risk Factor A

Lactation Enters breast milk/use caution (AAP rates "compatible"; AAP 2001 update pending)

Use Treatment of thiamine deficiency including beriberi, Wernicke's encephalopathy, Korsakoff's syndrome, neuritis associated with pregnancy, or in alcoholic patients; dietary supplement

Available Dosage Forms

Injection, solution: 100 mg/mL (2 mL)

Tablet, oral: 50 mg, 100 mg, 250 mg, 500 mg

General Dosage Range

I.M., I.V.:

Children: 10-25 mg/dose daily (thiamine deficiency)

Adults: 5-30 mg/dose 3 times/day (thiamine deficiency) **or** 50-250 mg/day (Wernicke's encephalopathy)

Oral:

Infants: 0.2-0.3 mg/day (adequate intake)

Children: 0.5-1.4 mg/day (recommended daily intake) **or** 5-50 mg/day (thiamine deficiency)

Adults: 1.1-1.4 mg/day (recommended daily intake) **or** 5-30 mg/day in 1-3 divided doses (thiamine deficiency)

Administration

I.M. Parenteral form may be administered I.M.

I.V. Parenteral form may be administered by I.V. injection. Various rates of administration have been reported. Local injection reactions may be minimized by slow administration (~30 minutes) into larger, more proximal veins. Thiamine should be administered prior to parenteral glucose solutions to prevent precipitation of acute symptoms of thiamine deficiency in the poorly nourished.

I.V. Detail pH: 2.5-4.5

Nursing Actions

Physical Assessment If self-administered, teach patient appropriate injection technique and needle disposal. Provide patient appropriate dietary instruction. Be alert to the potential for hypersensitivity reaction, especially if given I.V.

Patient Education Follow dietary instructions. Report shortness of breath, itching, or rash.

Thioguanine (thye oh GWAH neen)

Brand Names: U.S. Tabloid®

Index Terms 2-Amino-6-Mercaptopurine; 6-TG (error-prone abbreviation); 6-Thioguanine (error-prone abbreviation); TG; Tioguanine

Pharmacologic Category Antineoplastic Agent, Antimetabolite (Purine Analog)

Medication Safety Issues

Sound-alike/look-alike issues:

Thioguanine may be confused with thiotepa

High alert medication:

This medication is in a class the Institute for Safe Medication Practices (ISMP) includes among its list of drug classes which have a heightened risk of causing significant patient harm when used in error.

Other safety concerns:

6-thioguanine and 6-TG are error-prone abbreviations (associated with sixfold overdoses of thioguanine)

International issues:

Lanvis [Canada and multiple international markets] may be confused with Lantus brand name for insulin glargine [U.S., Canada, and multiple international markets]

Pregnancy Risk Factor D

Lactation Excretion in breast milk unknown/not recommended

Use Treatment of acute myelogenous (nonlymphocytic) leukemia (AML)

Unlabeled Use Treatment of pediatric acute lymphoblastic leukemia (ALL)

Available Dosage Forms

Tablet, oral:

Tabloid®: 40 mg

Administration

Oral For oral use; total daily dose can be given at one time.

Nursing Actions

Physical Assessment Monitor for myelosuppression, nausea, vomiting, anorexia, malaise, and hepatotoxicity weekly when beginning therapy, then monthly. Teach patient necessity for contraception and importance of adequate hydration.

Patient Education Maintain adequate hydration, unless instructed to restrict fluid intake. You may be required to have regularly scheduled laboratory testing to evaluate response to this medication. May cause nausea, vomiting, loss of appetite, weakness or lethargy, or mouth sores. You will be more susceptible to infection. Report signs or symptoms of infection (eg, fever, chills, sore throat, burning urination, fatigue); bleeding or easy bruising; dark urine, light-colored stool, or yellowing of skin or eyes; unresolved mouth sores, nausea, or vomiting; weight gain; or swelling of abdomen.

Thioridazine (thye oh RID a zeen)

Index Terms Mellaril; Thioridazine Hydrochloride

Pharmacologic Category Antipsychotic Agent, Typical, Phenothiazine

Medication Safety Issues

Sound-alike/look-alike issues:

Thioridazine may be confused with thiothixene, Thorazine

Mellaril may be confused with Elavil, Mebaral®

BEERS Criteria medication:

This drug may be inappropriate for use in geriatric patients (high severity risk).

Pregnancy Risk Factor C

Use Management of schizophrenic patients who fail to respond adequately to treatment with other antipsychotic drugs, either because of insufficient effectiveness or the inability to achieve an effective dose due to intolerable adverse effects from those medications

Unlabeled Use Behavior problems (children); severe psychoses (children); schizophrenia/psychoses (children); depressive disorders/dementia (children and adults); behavioral symptoms associated with dementia (elderly); psychosis/agitation related to Alzheimer's dementia

Available Dosage Forms

Tablet, oral: 10 mg, 25 mg, 50 mg, 100 mg

General Dosage Range Oral:

Children >2-12 years: 0.5-3 mg/kg/day in 2-3 divided doses **or** 10-25 mg 2-3 times/day (maximum: 3 mg/kg/day)

Children >12 years and Adults: Initial: 50-100 mg 3 times/day; Maintenance: 150-800 mg/day in 2-4 divided doses (maximum: 800 mg/day) **or** Initial: 25 mg 3 times/day; Maintenance: 20-200 mg/day

Elderly: Initial: 10-25 mg 1-2 times/day; Maintenance: 10-400 mg/day in 1-2 divided doses (maximum: 400 mg/day)

Administration

Oral Do not take antacid within 2 hours of taking drug.

Nursing Actions

Physical Assessment Monitor for excess sedation, extrapyramidal symptoms, tardive dyskinesia, and CNS changes. Monitor level of sedation.

Patient Education May be taken with food. Avoid alcohol. Maintain adequate hydration unless instructed to restrict fluid intake. You may experience excess drowsiness, lightheadedness, dizziness, blurred vision, nausea, vomiting, dry mouth, constipation, urinary retention, ejaculatory dysfunction (reversible), decreased perspiration, or photosensitivity. Report persistent CNS effects (eg, trembling fingers, altered gait or balance, excessive sedation, seizures, unusual movements, anxiety, confusion); chest pain, palpitations, or rapid heartbeat; severe dizziness; unresolved urinary retention; altered menstrual pattern; change in libido; swelling or pain in breasts (male or female); vision changes; skin rash or changes in color of skin (gray-blue); or worsening of condition.

Thiotepa (thye oh TEP a)

Index Terms TESPA; Thiophosphoramide; Thioplex; Triethylenethiophosphoramide; TSPA

Pharmacologic Category Antineoplastic Agent, Alkylating Agent

Medication Safety Issues

Sound-alike/look-alike issues:

Thiotepa may be confused with thioguanine

High alert medication:

This medication is in a class the Institute for Safe Medication Practices (ISMP) includes among its list of drugs which have a heightened risk of causing significant patient harm when used in error.

Administration issues:

Intrathecal medication safety: The American Society of Clinical Oncology (ASCO)/Oncology Nursing Society (ONS) chemotherapy administration safety standards (Jacobson, 2009) encourage the following safety measures for intrathecal chemotherapy:

- Intrathecal medication should not be prepared during the preparation of any other agents
- After preparation, store in an isolated location or container clearly marked with a label identifying as "intrathecal" use only
- Delivery to the patient should only be with other medications intended for administration into the central nervous system

Pregnancy Risk Factor D

Lactation Excretion in breast milk unknown/not recommended

Use Treatment of superficial papillary bladder cancer; palliative treatment of adenocarcinoma of breast or ovary; controlling intracavitary effusions caused by metastatic tumors

Unlabeled Use Intrathecal treatment of leptomeningeal metastases

Available Dosage Forms

Injection, powder for reconstitution: 15 mg

General Dosage Range Dosage adjustment recommended in patients who develop toxicities

I.V.: *Adults:* 0.3-0.4 mg/kg every 1-4 weeks

Intracavitary: *Adults:* 0.6-0.8 mg/kg

Intravesical: *Adults:* 60 mg retained for 2 hours once weekly for 4 weeks

Administration

I.V. Administer as a rapid injection. Infusion times may be longer for high-dose (unlabeled use) treatment; refer to specific protocols.

I.V. Detail pH: 5.5-7.5

Other Intravesical instillation: Instill directly into the bladder and retain for 2 hours; patient should be repositioned every 15-30 minutes for maximal exposure.

Nursing Actions

Physical Assessment Monitor laboratory tests regularly during treatment and for at least 3 weeks following treatment. Monitor for myelosuppression, leukopenia, dysuria, bleeding, and infection. Teach patient importance of adequate hydration.

Patient Education Do not take any aspirin or aspirin-containing products during therapy unless approved by prescriber. If administered by infusion, report immediately any redness, pain, swelling, or burning at infusion site. You will require regular blood tests to assess response to therapy. Maintain adequate hydration to prevent kidney damage, unless instructed to restrict fluid intake. You may have increased sensitivity to infection. May cause mild nausea, vomiting, or loss of appetite; rash; hair loss; or change in skin color (usually reversible after discontinuing treatment). Report any changes in urinary pattern or blood in your urine, unusual bleeding or bruising, persistent fever or chills, sore throat, sores in mouth or vagina, blackened stool, unusual or persistent weakness, difficulty swallowing, or respiratory difficulty.

Related Information

Management of Drug Extravasations *on page 1269*

Thiothixene (thye oh THIKS een)

Brand Names: U.S. Navane® [DSC]

Index Terms Tiotixene

Pharmacologic Category Antipsychotic Agent, Typical

Medication Safety Issues

Sound-alike/look-alike issues:

Thiothixene may be confused with FLUoxetine, thioridazine

Navane® may be confused with Norvasc®, Nubain

Use Management of schizophrenia

Unlabeled Use Psychotic disorders (children); rapid tranquilization of the agitated patient (children); nonpsychotic patient, dementia behavior (elderly); psychosis/agitation related to Alzheimer's dementia

Available Dosage Forms

Capsule, oral: 1 mg, 2 mg, 5 mg, 10 mg

General Dosage Range Oral: *Adults:* Initial: 6-10 mg/day in 2-3 divided doses; Maintenance: 20-60 mg/day in 2-3 divided doses (maximum: 60 mg/day)

Nursing Actions

Physical Assessment Review ophthalmic exam at beginning of therapy and periodically throughout. Monitor for excess sedation, extrapyramidal symptoms, tardive dyskinesia, and CNS changes.

Patient Education Capsules may be taken with food. Avoid alcohol. Maintain adequate hydration unless instructed to restrict fluid intake. You may experience excess drowsiness, lightheadedness, dizziness, blurred vision, nausea, vomiting, constipation, postural hypotension, urinary retention, ejaculatory dysfunction (reversible), decreased perspiration, or photosensitivity. Report persistent CNS effects (eg, trembling fingers, altered gait or balance, excessive sedation, seizures, unusual movements, anxiety, abnormal thoughts, confusion, personality changes); chest pain, palpitations, or rapid heartbeat; severe dizziness; unresolved urinary retention or changes in urinary pattern; altered menstrual pattern; change in libido; swelling or pain in breasts (male or female); vision changes; skin rash, irritation, or changes in color of skin (gray-blue); or worsening of condition.

Thyroid, Desiccated (THYE roid DES i kay tid)

Brand Names: U.S. Armour® Thyroid; Nature-Throid™; Westhroid™

Index Terms Desiccated Thyroid; Levothyroxine and Liothyronine; Tetraiodothyronine and Triiodothyronine; Thyroid Extract; Thyroid USP

Pharmacologic Category Thyroid Product

Medication Safety Issues

BEERS Criteria medication:

This drug may be inappropriate for use in geriatric patients (high severity risk).

Pregnancy Risk Factor A

Lactation Enters breast milk/use caution

Use Replacement or supplemental therapy in hypothyroidism; pituitary TSH suppressants (thyroid nodules, thyroiditis, multinodular goiter, thyroid cancer)

Available Dosage Forms

Tablet, oral:

Armour® Thyroid: 15 mg, 30 mg, 60 mg, 90 mg, 120 mg, 180 mg, 240 mg, 300 mg

Nature-Throid™: 16.25 mg, 32.5 mg, 65 mg, 130 mg, 195 mg

Westhroid™: 32.5 mg, 65 mg, 130 mg

General Dosage Range Oral:

Children 0-6 months: 15-30 mg/day **or** 4.8-6 mg/kg/day

Children 6-12 months: 30-45 mg/day **or** 3.6-4.8 mg/kg/day

Children 1-5 years: 45-60 mg/day **or** 3-3.6 mg/kg/day

Children 6-12 years: 60-90 mg/day **or** 2.4-3 mg/kg/day

Children >12 years: >90 mg/day **or** 1.2-1.8 mg/kg/day

Adults: Initial: 15-30 mg/day; Maintenance: 60-120 mg/day

Administration

Oral Administer on an empty stomach. Take in the morning before breakfast.

Nursing Actions

Physical Assessment Ineffective for weight reduction. Monitor for hyperthyroidism (weight loss, nervousness, sweating, tachycardia, insomnia, heat intolerance, palpitations, vomiting, psychosis, fever, seizures, angina, arrhythmias). Caution patients with diabetes to monitor glucose levels closely (may increase need for oral hypoglycemics or insulin).

Patient Education Thyroid replacement therapy is generally for life. Take in the morning before breakfast. Do not take antacids or iron preparations within 8 hours of thyroid medication. If you have diabetes, monitor glucose levels closely (may increase need for oral hypoglycemics or insulin). Report chest pain, rapid heart rate, palpitations, heat intolerance, excessive sweating, increased nervousness, agitation, or lethargy.

TiaGABine (tye AG a been)

Brand Names: U.S. Gabitril®

Index Terms Tiagabine Hydrochloride

Pharmacologic Category Anticonvulsant, Miscellaneous

Medication Safety Issues

Sound-alike/look-alike issues:

TiaGABine may be confused with tiZANidine

Medication Guide Available Yes

Pregnancy Risk Factor C

Lactation Enters breast milk/not recommended

Use Adjunctive therapy in adults and children ≥12 years of age in the treatment of partial seizures

Mechanism of Action/Effect The exact mechanism by which tiagabine exerts antiseizure activity is not definitively known; however, *in vitro* experiments demonstrate that it enhances the activity of gamma aminobutyric acid (GABA), the major neuroinhibitory transmitter in the nervous system; it is thought that binding to the GABA uptake carrier inhibits the uptake of GABA into presynaptic neurons, allowing an increased amount of GABA to be available to postsynaptic neurons; based on *in vitro* studies, tiagabine does not inhibit the uptake of dopamine, norepinephrine, serotonin, glutamate, or choline

Contraindications Hypersensitivity to tiagabine or any component of the formulation

Warnings/Precautions Antiepileptics are associated with an increased risk of suicidal behavior/thoughts with use (regardless of indication); patients should be monitored for signs/symptoms of depression, suicidal tendencies, and other unusual behavior changes during therapy and instructed to inform their healthcare provider immediately if symptoms occur. New-onset seizures and status epilepticus have been associated with tiagabine use when taken for unlabeled indications. Often these seizures have occurred shortly after the initiation of treatment or shortly after a dosage increase. Seizures have also occurred with very low doses or after several months of therapy. In most cases, patients were using concomitant medications (eg, antidepressants, antipsychotics, stimulants, narcotics). In these instances, the discontinuation of tiagabine, followed by an evaluation for an underlying seizure disorder, is suggested. Use for unapproved indications, however, has not been proven to be safe or effective and is not recommended. When tiagabine is used as an adjunct in partial seizures (an FDA-approved indication), it should not be abruptly discontinued because of the possibility of increasing seizure frequency, unless safety concerns require a more rapid withdrawal. Rarely, nonconvulsive status epilepticus has been reported following abrupt discontinuation or dosage reduction.

Use with caution in patients with hepatic impairment. Experience in patients not receiving enzyme-inducing drugs has been limited; caution should be used in treating any patient who is not receiving one of these medications (decreased dose and slower titration may be required). Weakness, sedation, and confusion may occur with tiagabine use. Patients must be cautioned about performing tasks which require mental alertness (eg, operating machinery or driving). Effects with other sedative drugs or ethanol may be potentiated. May cause serious rash, including Stevens-Johnson syndrome.

Drug Interactions

Avoid Concomitant Use

Avoid concomitant use of TiaGABine with any of the following: Conivaptan

Decreased Effect

The levels/effects of TiaGABine may be decreased by: CYP3A4 Inducers (Strong); Deferasirox; Herbs (CYP3A4 Inducers); Ketorolac; Ketorolac (Nasal); Ketorolac (Systemic); Mefloquine; Tocilizumab

Increased Effect/Toxicity

TiaGABine may increase the levels/effects of: Alcohol (Ethyl); CNS Depressants; Methotrimeprazine; Selective Serotonin Reuptake Inhibitors

The levels/effects of TiaGABine may be increased by: Conivaptan; CYP3A4 Inhibitors (Moderate); CYP3A4 Inhibitors (Strong); Dasatinib; Droperidol; HydrOXYzine; Ivacaftor; Methotrimeprazine

Nutritional/Ethanol Interactions

Ethanol: May increase CNS depression; monitor for increased effects with coadministration. Caution patients about effects.

Food: Food reduces the rate but not the extent of absorption.

Herb/Nutraceutical: St John's wort may decrease tiagabine levels. Avoid valerian, St John's wort, kava kava, gotu kola (may increase CNS depression).

Adverse Reactions

>10%:

Central nervous system: Concentration decreased, dizziness, nervousness, somnolence

Gastrointestinal: Nausea

Neuromuscular & skeletal: Weakness, tremor

1% to 10%:

Cardiovascular: Chest pain, edema, hypertension, palpitation, peripheral edema, syncope, tachycardia, vasodilation

Central nervous system: Agitation, ataxia, chills, confusion, difficulty with memory, confusion, depersonalization, depression, euphoria, hallucination, hostility, insomnia, malaise, migraine, paranoid reaction, personality disorder, speech disorder

Dermatologic: Alopecia, bruising, dry skin, pruritus, rash

Gastrointestinal: Abdominal pain, diarrhea, gingivitis, increased appetite, mouth ulceration, stomatitis, vomiting, weight gain/loss

Neuromuscular & skeletal: Abnormal gait, arthralgia, dysarthria, hyper-/hypokinesia, hyper-/hypotonia, myasthenia, myalgia, myoclonus, neck pain, paresthesia, reflexes decreased, stupor, twitching, vertigo

Ocular: Abnormal vision, amblyopia, nystagmus

Otic: Ear pain, hearing impairment, otitis media, tinnitus

Respiratory: Bronchitis, cough, dyspnea, epistaxis, pneumonia

Miscellaneous: Allergic reaction, cyst, diaphoresis, flu-like syndrome, lymphadenopathy

Available Dosage Forms

Tablet, oral:

Gabitril®: 2 mg, 4 mg, 12 mg, 16 mg

General Dosage Range Dosage adjustment recommended in patients on concomitant therapy

Oral:

Children 12-18 years: Initial: 4 mg once daily; Maintenance: 8-32 mg/day in 2-4 divided doses

Adults: Initial: 4 mg once daily; Maintenance: 8-56 mg/day in 2-4 divided doses

Nursing Actions

Physical Assessment Monitor therapeutic response (seizure activity, type, duration) at beginning of therapy and throughout. Use and teach seizure/safety precautions.

Patient Education While using this medication, do not use alcohol. Maintain adequate hydration unless instructed to restrict fluid intake. You may experience drowsiness, dizziness, disturbed concentration, blurred vision, nausea, vomiting, or loss of appetite. Wear identification of epileptic status and medications. Report behavioral or CNS changes, suicide ideation, or depression; skin rash; muscle cramping, weakness, tremors, changes in gait; vision difficulties; persistent GI distress (cramping, pain, vomiting); chest pain, irregular heartbeat, or palpitations; cough or respiratory difficulty; or worsening of seizure activity or loss of seizure control.

Dietary Considerations Take with food.

Ticagrelor (tye KA grel or)

Brand Names: U.S. Brilinta™

Index Terms AZD6140

Pharmacologic Category Antiplatelet Agent; Antiplatelet Agent, Cyclopentyltriazolopyrimidine

Medication Guide Available Yes

Pregnancy Risk Factor C

Breast-Feeding Considerations Excretion into breast milk is unknown; use is not recommended.

Use Used in conjunction with aspirin for secondary prevention of thrombotic events in patients with unstable angina, non-ST-elevation myocardial infarction (NSTEMI), or ST-elevation myocardial infarction (STEMI) managed medically or with percutaneous coronary intervention (PCI) and/or coronary artery bypass graft (CABG)

Mechanism of Action/Effect Reversibly and noncompetitively blocks ADP-mediated platelet aggregation; recovery of platelet function is likely to depend on serum concentrations of ticagrelor and its active metabolite.

Contraindications Active pathological bleeding (eg, peptic ulcer or intracranial hemorrhage); history of intracranial hemorrhage; hepatic impairment

Canadian labeling: Additional contraindications (not in U.S. labeling): Hypersensitivity to ticagrelor or any component of the formulation; moderate hepatic impairment; concomitant use of strong CYP3A4 inhibitors (eg, ketoconazole, clarithromycin, ritonavir, atazanavir, nefazodone)

Warnings/Precautions [U.S. Boxed Warning]: Ticagrelor increases the risk of bleeding including significant and sometimes fatal bleeding. Use is contraindicated in patients with active pathological bleeding and presence or history of intracranial hemorrhage. Additional risk factors for bleeding include propensity to bleed (eg, recent trauma or surgery, recent or recurrent GI bleeding, active PUD, moderate-to-severe hepatic impairment), CABG or other surgical procedure, concomitant use of medications that increase risk of bleeding (eg, warfarin, NSAIDs), and advanced age. Bleeding should be suspected if patient becomes hypotensive after undergoing recent coronary angiography, PCI, CABG, or other surgical procedure even if overt signs of bleeding do not exist. **Where possible, manage bleeding without discontinuing ticagrelor as the risk of cardiovascular events is increased upon discontinuation.** If discontinuation of ticagrelor is necessary, resume as soon as possible after the bleeding source is identified and controlled. Hemostatic benefits of platelet transfusions are not known; may inhibit transfused platelets. Premature discontinuation of therapy may increase the risk of cardiac events (eg, stent thrombosis with subsequent fatal or nonfatal MI). Duration of therapy, in general, is determined by the type of stent placed (bare metal or drug eluting) and whether an ACS event was ongoing at the time of placement. Use with caution in patients who are at an increased risk of bradycardia (eg, second- or third-degree AV block, sick sinus syndrome) or taking other bradycardic-inducing agents (eg, beta blockers, nondihydropyridine calcium channel blockers). Ventricular pauses ≥3 seconds were noted more frequently with ticagrelor than with clopidogrel in a substudy of the Platelet Inhibition and Patient Outcomes (PLATO) trial. Dyspnea (often mild-to-moderate and transient) was observed more frequently in patients receiving ticagrelor than clopidogrel during clinical trials. Ticagrelor-related dyspnea does not require specific treatment nor does it warrant therapy interruption (Canadian labeling recommends discontinuing therapy in patients unable to tolerate ticagrelor related dyspnea0.

[U.S. Boxed Warning]: Maintenance doses of aspirin greater than 100 mg/day reduce the efficacy of ticagrelor and should be avoided. Use of higher maintenance doses of aspirin (ie, >100 mg/day) was associated with relatively unfavorable outcomes for ticagrelor versus clopidogrel in the PLATO trial (Gaglia, 2011; Wallentin, 2009). Canadian labeling recommends a maximum maintenance aspirin dose of 150 mg/day.

[U.S. Boxed Warning]: Avoid initiation of ticagrelor when urgent CABG surgery is planned; when possible discontinue use at least 5 days before any surgery. Discontinue 5 days before elective surgery (except in patients with cardiac stents that have not completed their full course of dual antiplatelet therapy; patient-specific situations need to be discussed with cardiologist). When urgent CABG is necessary, the ACCF/AHA CABG guidelines recommend discontinuation for at least 24 hours prior to surgery (Hillis, 2011).

Use is contraindicated in patients with severe hepatic impairment (Canadian labeling also contraindicates use in moderate-to-severe hepatic impairment). Use with caution in patients with renal impairment, a history of hyperuricemia or gouty arthritis. Canadian labeling does not recommend use in patients with uric acid nephropathy. Avoid concomitant use with strong CYP3A4 inhibitors (eg, ketoconazole, ritonavir, nefazodone) or strong CYP3A4 inducers (eg, rifampin, carbamazepine, dexamethasone, phenobarbital, phenytoin). Canadian labeling contraindicates use with strong CYP3A4 inhibitors.

Drug Interactions

Avoid Concomitant Use

Avoid concomitant use of Ticagrelor with any of the following: CYP3A4 Inducers (Strong); CYP3A4 Inhibitors (Strong)

Decreased Effect

The levels/effects of Ticagrelor may be decreased by: Aspirin; CYP3A4 Inducers (Strong); CYP3A4 Inhibitors (Strong); Deferasirox; Herbs (CYP3A4 Inducers); Nonsteroidal Anti-Inflammatory Agents; Tocilizumab

Increased Effect/Toxicity

Ticagrelor may increase the levels/effects of: Anticoagulants; Antiplatelet Agents; ARIPiprazole; Carvedilol; Collagenase (Systemic); CYP2C9 Substrates; Digoxin; Drotrecogin Alfa (Activated); Ibritumomab; Lovastatin; Rivaroxaban; Salicylates; Simvastatin; Thrombolytic Agents; Tositumomab and Iodine I 131 Tositumomab

The levels/effects of Ticagrelor may be increased by: Aspirin; CYP3A4 Inhibitors (Strong); Dasatinib; Glucosamine; Herbs (Anticoagulant/Antiplatelet Properties); Nonsteroidal Anti-Inflammatory Agents; Omega-3-Acid Ethyl Esters; Pentosan Polysulfate Sodium; Pentoxifylline; Prostacyclin Analogues; Vitamin E

Adverse Reactions Note: As with all drugs which may affect hemostasis, bleeding is associated with ticagrelor. Hemorrhage may occur at virtually any site. Risk is dependent on multiple variables, including the concurrent use of multiple agents which alter hemostasis and patient susceptibility.

Frequencies as reported in PLATO trial versus clopidogrel:

>10%: Respiratory: Dyspnea (≤14%)

1% to 10%:

Cardiovascular: Ventricular pauses (6%; 2% after 1 month of therapy), atrial fibrillation (4%), hypertension (4%), angina (3%), hypotension (3%), bradycardia (1% to 3%), cardiac failure (2%), peripheral edema (2%), ventricular tachycardia (2%), palpitation (1%), syncope (1%), ventricular extrasystoles (1%), ventricular fibrillation (1%)

Central nervous system: Headache (7%), dizziness (5%), fatigue (3%), fever (3%), anxiety (2%), insomnia (2%), vertigo (2%), depression (1%)

Dermatologic: Bruising (2% to 4%), rash (2%), pruritus (1%), subcutaneous or dermal bleeding

Endocrine & metabolic: Hypokalemia (2%), diabetes mellitus (1%), dyslipidemia (1%), hypercholesterolemia (1%)

Gastrointestinal: Diarrhea (4%), nausea (4%), vomiting (3%), abdominal pain (2%), constipation (2%), dyspepsia (2%), GI hemorrhage

Genitourinary: Urinary tract infection (2%), urinary tract bleeding

Hematologic: Major bleeding (12%; composite of major fatal/life threatening and other major bleeding events), minor bleeding (~5%), anemia (2%), hematoma (2%), postprocedural hemorrhage (2%)

Local: Puncture site hematoma (2%)

Neuromuscular & skeletal: Back pain (4%), noncardiac chest pain (4%), extremity pain (2%), arthralgia (2%), musculoskeletal pain (2%), weakness (2%), myalgia (1%)

Renal: Creatinine increased (7%; mechanism undetermined), hematuria (2%), renal failure (1%)

Respiratory: Epistaxis (6%), cough (5%), nasopharyngitis (2%), bronchitis (1%), pneumonia (1%)

Pharmacodynamics/Kinetics

Onset of Action Inhibition of platelet aggregation (IPA): 180 mg loading dose: ~41% within 30 minutes (similar to clopidogrel 600 mg at 8 hours); Peak effect: Time to maximal IPA: 180 mg loading dose: IPA ~88% at 2 hours post administration

Duration of Action IPA: 180 mg loading dose: 87% to 89% maintained from 2-8 hours; 24 hours after the last maintenance dose, IPA is 58% (similar to maintenance clopidogrel)

Time after discontinuation when IPA is 30%: ~56 hours; IPA 10%: ~110 hours (Gurbel, 2009). Mean IPA observed with ticagrelor at 3 days post-discontinuation was comparable to that observed with clopidogrel at 5 days post discontinuation.

Available Dosage Forms

Tablet, oral:

Brilinta™: 90 mg

General Dosage Range Oral: *Adults:* Loading dose: 180 mg; Maintenance: 90 mg twice daily

Administration

Oral May be administered without regard to meals. Missed doses should be taken at their next regularly scheduled time.

Stability

Storage Store in the original container at 25°C (77°F); excursions permitted to 15°C to 30°C (59°F to 86°F).

Nursing Actions

Physical Assessment

Not to be used in patients with significant active bleeding. Drug should be held prior to surgery except with stent patients; discuss with cardiologist. Shortness of breath can occur early in therapy; treatment is not required but healthcare provider needs to be notified to ensure that there is not another cause of symptom. Other serious side effects include allergic reactions and bleeding.

Patient Education Patients need to be aware of bleeding risks and inform physician of any blood in urine, stool, or sputum. Side effects that are more common include back pain, cough, diarrhea, nausea, fatigue, and headache. Serious side effects that require immediate medical attention include chest tightness or chest pain, shortness of breath, or bleeding.

Dietary Considerations May be taken without regard to meals.

Ticarcillin and Clavulanate Potassium

(tye kar SIL in & klav yoo LAN ate poe TASS ee um)

Brand Names: U.S. Timentin®

Index Terms Ticarcillin and Clavulanic Acid

Pharmacologic Category Antibiotic, Penicillin

Pregnancy Risk Factor B

Lactation Enters breast milk/use caution

Use Treatment of lower respiratory tract, urinary tract, skin and skin structures, bone and joint, gynecologic (endometritis) and intra-abdominal (peritonitis) infections, and septicemia caused by susceptible organisms. Clavulanate expands activity of ticarcillin to include beta-lactamase producing strains of *S. aureus, H. influenzae, Bacteroides* species, and some other gram-negative bacilli

Available Dosage Forms

Infusion [premixed, frozen]:

Timentin®: Ticarcillin 3 g and clavulanic acid 0.1 g (100 mL)

Injection, powder for reconstitution:

Timentin®: Ticarcillin 3 g and clavulanic acid 0.1 g (3.1 g, 31 g)

General Dosage Range Dosage adjustment recommended in patients with hepatic or renal impairment

I.V.:

Children and Adults <60 kg: 200-300 mg of ticarcillin component/kg/day in divided doses every 4-6 hours

Children ≥60 kg and Adults: 3.1 g (ticarcillin 3 g plus clavulanic acid 0.1 g) every 4-6 hours (maximum: 24 g of ticarcillin component/day)

Administration

I.V. Infuse over 30 minutes.

Some penicillins (eg, carbenicillin, ticarcillin, and piperacillin) have been shown to inactivate aminoglycosides *in vitro*. This has been observed to a greater extent with tobramycin and gentamicin, while amikacin has shown greater stability against inactivation. Concurrent use of these agents may pose a risk of reduced antibacterial efficacy *in vivo*, particularly in the setting of profound renal impairment. However, definitive clinical evidence is lacking. If combination penicillin/aminoglycoside therapy is desired in a patient with renal dysfunction, separation of doses (if feasible), and routine monitoring of aminoglycoside levels, CBC, and clinical response should be considered.

I.V. Detail pH: 5.5-7.5

Tigecycline (tye ge SYE kleen)

Brand Names: U.S. Tygacil®

Index Terms GAR-936

Pharmacologic Category Antibiotic, Glycylcycline

Pregnancy Risk Factor D

Lactation Excretion in breast milk unknown/use caution

Use Treatment of complicated skin and skin structure infections caused by susceptible organisms, including methicillin-resistant *Staphylococcus aureus* and vancomycin-sensitive *Enterococcus faecalis*; complicated intra-abdominal infections (cIAI); community-acquired pneumonia

Available Dosage Forms

Injection, powder for reconstitution:

Tygacil®: 50 mg

General Dosage Range Dosage adjustment recommended in patients with hepatic impairment

I.V.: *Adults:* Initial: 100 mg as a single dose; Maintenance: 50 mg every 12 hours

Administration

I.V. Infuse over 30-60 minutes through dedicated line or via Y-site

Nursing Actions

Physical Assessment Culture and sensitivity tests should be assessed prior to beginning therapy. May cause life-threatening anaphylaxis/anaphylactoid reactions. Monitor for nausea, vomiting, diarrhea, headache, rash, anemia, dyspnea, and opportunistic infection.

Patient Education This medication is only administered intravenously. Report immediately any burning, pain, or swelling at infusion site; difficulty breathing or swallowing; chest pain; or chills. Report gastrointestinal upset (nausea, vomiting, diarrhea, constipation, stomach pain), headache or dizziness, changes in respirations, increased sweating, or rash.

Tiludronate (tye LOO droe nate)

Brand Names: U.S. Skelid®

Index Terms Tiludronate Disodium

Pharmacologic Category Bisphosphonate Derivative

Pregnancy Risk Factor C

Lactation Excretion in breast milk unknown/use caution

Use Treatment of Paget's disease of the bone (osteitis deformans) in patients who have a level of serum alkaline phosphatase (SAP) at least twice the upper limit of normal, or who are symptomatic, or who are at risk for future complications of their disease

Available Dosage Forms

Tablet, oral:

Skelid®: 200 mg

General Dosage Range Oral: *Adults:* 400 mg once daily

Administration

Oral Administer as a single oral dose, take with 6-8 oz of plain water. Should not be taken with beverages containing minerals (eg, mineral water), food, or with other medications (may reduce absorption). Do not take within 2 hours of food. Take calcium or mineral supplements at least 2 hours before or after tiludronate. Take aluminum- or magnesium-containing antacids at least 2 hours after taking tiludronate. Patients should be instructed to stay upright (not to lie down) for at least 30 minutes and until after first food of the day (to reduce esophageal irritation).

Nursing Actions

Physical Assessment Monitor blood pressure at the beginning of therapy and periodically during use. Patients at risk for osteonecrosis of the jaw (eg, chemotherapy, corticosteroids, poor oral hygiene) should have dental exams; necessary preventive dentistry should be done before beginning bisphosphonate therapy. Teach patient appropriate administration of medication (eg, timing with food, supplements, and other medications). Instruct patient in lifestyle and dietary changes.

Patient Education In order to be effective, this medication must be taken with a full glass of water (6-8 oz) at least 2 hours before or 2 hours after food. Do not take aspirin, antacids, or vitamin-mineral supplements containing calcium, magnesium, or aluminum within 2 hours of this medication. Consult prescriber to determine recommended lifestyle changes (eg, decreased smoking, decreased alcohol intake, dietary supplements). Certain dental procedures should be avoided if possible while you are taking this medication. Notify prescriber at once if experiencing any difficulty swallowing, pain when swallowing, or severe or persistent heartburn. You may experience mild/temporary skin rash, abdominal pain, or constipation. Report persistent muscle or bone pain or pain in the mouth, jaw, or teeth.

Timolol (Ophthalmic) (TIM oh lol)

Brand Names: U.S. Betimol®; Istalol®; Timolol GFS; Timoptic-XE®; Timoptic®; Timoptic® in OcuDose®

Index Terms Timolol Hemihydrate; Timolol Maleate

Pharmacologic Category Beta Blocker, Nonselective; Ophthalmic Agent, Antiglaucoma

Medication Safety Issues

Sound-alike/look-alike issues:

Timolol may be confused with atenolol, Tylenol®

Timoptic® may be confused with Betoptic S®, Talacen, Viroptic®

Other safety concerns:

Bottle cap color change: Timoptic®: Both the 0.25% and 0.5% strengths are now packaged in bottles with yellow caps; previously, the color of the cap on the product corresponded to different strengths.

International issues:

Betimol [U.S.] may be confused with Betanol brand name for metipranolol [Monaco]

Pregnancy Risk Factor C

Lactation Enters breast milk/ consider risk:benefit (AAP rates "compatible"; AAP 2001 update pending)

Use Treatment of elevated intraocular pressure such as glaucoma or ocular hypertension

Available Dosage Forms

Gel forming solution, ophthalmic: 0.25% (5 mL); 0.5% (5 mL)

Timolol GFS: 0.25% (5 mL); 0.5% (5 mL)

Timoptic-XE®: 0.25% (5 mL); 0.5% (5 mL)

Solution, ophthalmic: 0.25% (5 mL, 10 mL, 15 mL); 0.5% (5 mL, 10 mL, 15 mL)

Betimol®: 0.25% (5 mL); 0.5% (5 mL, 10 mL, 15 mL)

Istalol®: 0.5% (2.5 mL, 5 mL)

Timoptic®: 0.25% (5 mL); 0.5% (5 mL, 10 mL)

Solution, ophthalmic [preservative free]:

Timoptic® in OcuDose®: 0.25% (0.2 mL); 0.5% (0.2 mL)

General Dosage Range Ophthalmic:

Gel-forming solution: *Children and Adults:* Instill 1 drop (0.25% or 0.5%) once daily

Solution: *Children and Adults:* Initial: Instill 1 drop (0.25%) twice daily; Maintenance: Instill 1 drop (0.25% or 0.5%) 1-2 times daily (maximum: 2 drops/day [0.5%])

Administration

Other Ophthalmic: Administer other topically-applied ophthalmic medications at least 10 minutes before Timoptic-XE®; wash hands before use; invert closed bottle and shake once before use; remove cap carefully so that tip does not touch anything; hold bottle between thumb and index finger; use index finger of other hand to pull down the lower eyelid to form a pocket for the eye drop and tilt head back; place the dispenser tip close to the eye and gently squeeze the bottle to administer 1 drop; remove pressure after a single drop has been released; **do not allow the dispenser tip to touch the eye**; replace cap and store bottle in an upright position in a clean area; do **not** enlarge hole of dispenser; do **not** wash tip with water, soap, or any other cleaner. Some solutions contain benzalkonium chloride; wait at least 10 minutes after instilling solution before inserting soft contact lenses.

Nursing Actions

Patient Education Wash hands before using. Do not let tip of applicator touch eye; do not contaminate tip of applicator (may cause eye infection, eye damage, or vision loss). Tilt head back and look upward. Gently pull down lower lid and put drop(s) inside lower eyelid at inner corner. Close eye and roll eyeball in all directions. Do not blink for 1/2 minute. Apply gentle pressure to inner corner of eye for 30 seconds. Wipe away excess from skin around eye. Do not use any other eye preparation for at least 10 minutes. Temporary stinging or blurred vision may occur. Remove contact lenses prior to administration. Lenses may be reinserted 15 minutes following administration. Report persistent eye pain, irritation, double vision, vision changes, slow heart rate, dizziness, worsening of condition, or lack of improvement.

Tinidazole (tye NI da zole)

Brand Names: U.S. Tindamax®

Pharmacologic Category Amebicide; Antibiotic, Miscellaneous; Antiprotozoal, Nitroimidazole

Pregnancy Risk Factor C

Lactation Enters breast milk/contraindicated (AAP rates "of concern"; AAP 2001 update pending)

Breast-Feeding Considerations Tinidazole is excreted into breast milk in concentrations similar to those in the maternal serum and can be detected for up to 72 hours after administration. Tinidazole is contraindicated in nursing mothers unless breast-feeding is interrupted during therapy and for 3 days after the last dose.

Use Treatment of trichomoniasis caused by *T. vaginalis*; treatment of giardiasis caused by *G. duodenalis* (*G. lamblia*); treatment of intestinal amebiasis and amebic liver abscess caused by *E. histolytica*; treatment of bacterial vaginosis caused by *Bacteroides* spp, *Gardnerella vaginalis*, and *Prevotella* spp in nonpregnant females

Mechanism of Action/Effect After diffusing into the organism, it is proposed that tinidazole causes cytotoxicity by damaging DNA and preventing further DNA synthesis.

Contraindications Hypersensitivity to tinidazole, nitroimidazole derivatives (including metronidazole), or any component of the formulation; pregnancy (1st trimester); breast-feeding

Warnings/Precautions Use caution with CNS diseases; seizures and peripheral neuropathy have been reported with tinidazole and other nitroimidazole derivatives. **[U.S. Boxed Warning]: Carcinogenicity has been observed with another nitroimidazole derivative (metronidazole) in animal studies;** use should be reserved for approved indications only. Use caution with current or history of blood dyscrasias or hepatic impairment. When used for amebiasis, not indicated for the treatment of asymptomatic cyst passage. Prolonged use may result in fungal or bacterial superinfection, including *C. difficile*-associated diarrhea (CDAD), pseudomembranous colitis, and/or vaginal candidiasis. CDAD has been observed >2 months postantibiotic treatment. Safety and efficacy have not been established in children ≤3 years of age.

Drug Interactions

Avoid Concomitant Use There are no known interactions where it is recommended to avoid concomitant use.

Decreased Effect Specific interaction studies have not been conducted. Refer to Metronidazole (Systemic) monograph on page 771.

Increased Effect/Toxicity Specific interaction studies have not been conducted. Refer to Metronidazole (Systemic) monograph on page 771.

Nutritional/Ethanol Interactions

Ethanol: The manufacturer recommends to avoid all ethanol or any ethanol-containing drugs (may cause disulfiram-like reaction characterized by flushing, headache, nausea, vomiting, sweating or tachycardia) during and for at least 3 days after completion of treatment.

Food: Peak antibiotic serum concentration lowered and delayed, but total drug absorbed not affected.

Adverse Reactions

1% to 10%:

Central nervous system: Fatigue/malaise (1% to 2%), dizziness (≤1%), headache (≤1%)

Endocrine & metabolic: Menorrhagia (>2%)

Gastrointestinal: Metallic/bitter taste (4% to 6%), nausea (3% to 5%), anorexia (2% to 3%), appetite decreased (>2%), flatulence (>2%), dyspepsia/cramps/epigastric discomfort (1% to 2%), vomiting (1% to 2%), constipation (≤1%)

Genitourinary: *Candida* vaginitis (5%), painful urination (>2%), pelvic pain (>2%), urine abnormality (>2%), vaginal odor (>2%), vulvovaginal discomfort (>2%)

Neuromuscular & skeletal: Weakness (1% to 2%)

Renal: Urinary tract infection (>2%)
Respiratory: Upper respiratory tract infection (>2%)

Frequency not defined:
Cardiovascular: Flushing, palpitation
Central nervous system: Ataxia, coma (rare), confusion (rare), depression (rare), drowsiness, fever, giddiness, insomnia, seizure, vertigo
Dermatologic: Angioedema, pruritus, rash, urticaria
Gastrointestinal: Abdominal pain, diarrhea, furry tongue (rare), oral candidiasis, salivation, stomatitis, thirst, tongue discoloration, xerostomia
Genitourinary: Urine darkened, vaginal discharge increased
Hematologic: Leukopenia (transient), neutropenia (transient), thrombocytopenia (reversible; rare)
Hepatic: Transaminases increased
Neuromuscular & skeletal: Arthralgia, arthritis, myalgia, peripheral neuropathy (transient, includes numbness and paresthesia)
Respiratory: Bronchospasm (rare), dyspnea (rare), pharyngitis (rare)
Miscellaneous: Burning sensation, *Candida* overgrowth, diaphoresis

Available Dosage Forms

Tablet, oral:
Tindamax®: 250 mg, 500 mg

General Dosage Range Oral:
Children >3 years: 50 mg/kg/day (maximum: 2 g/day)
Adults: 1-2 g/day

Administration

Oral Administer with food.

Stability

Storage Store at controlled room temperature of 15°C to 30°C (59°F to 86°F). Protect from light.

Nursing Actions

Patient Education Avoid all alcohol while taking this medication and for 3 days following completion; may cause unpleasant reaction (flushing, nausea, vomiting, sweating, headache, rapid heart beat). Refrain from sexual intercourse or use contraceptive if being treated for trichomoniasis. May cause headache, drowsiness or dizziness; mild gastrointestinal disturbance (nausea, vomiting, constipation, diarrhea, metallic/bitter taste, abdominal discomfort). Report severe fatigue or weakness, chest pain or palpitations, swelling of lips or mouth, or lack of improvement or worsening of condition.

Dietary Considerations Take with food. The manufacturer recommends that ethanol be avoided during treatment and for 3 days after therapy is complete.

Tinzaparin (tin ZA pa rin)

Brand Names: U.S. Innohep® [DSC]
Index Terms Tinzaparin Sodium
Pharmacologic Category Low Molecular Weight Heparin

Medication Safety Issues

High alert medication:
The Institute for Safe Medication Practices (ISMP) includes this medication among its list of drug classes which have a heightened risk of causing significant patient harm when used in error.

National Patient Safety Goals:
The Joint Commission (TJC) requires healthcare organizations that provide anticoagulant therapy to have a process in place to reduce the risk of anticoagulant-associated patient harm. Patients receiving anticoagulants should receive individualized care through a defined process that includes standardized ordering, dispensing, administration, monitoring and education. This does not apply to routine short-term use of anticoagulants for prevention of venous thromboembolism when the expectation is that the patient's laboratory values will remain within or close to normal values (NPSG.03.05.01).

Pregnancy Risk Factor B

Lactation Excretion in breast milk unknown/use caution

Use Treatment of acute symptomatic deep vein thrombosis, with or without pulmonary embolism, in conjunction with warfarin sodium

Unlabeled Use Prophylaxis of deep vein thrombosis following hip or knee replacement surgery, and general surgery

Mechanism of Action/Effect Standard heparin consists of components with molecular weights ranging from 4000-30,000 daltons with a mean of 16,000 daltons. Heparin acts as an anticoagulant by enhancing the inhibition rate of clotting proteases by antithrombin III, impairing normal hemostasis and inhibition of factor Xa. Low molecular weight heparins have a small effect on the activated partial thromboplastin time and strongly inhibit factor Xa. The primary inhibitory activity of tinzaparin is through antithrombin. Tinzaparin is derived from porcine heparin that undergoes controlled enzymatic depolymerization. The average molecular weight of tinzaparin ranges between 5500 and 7500 daltons which is distributed as <2000 daltons (<10%), 2000-8000 daltons (60% to 72%), and >8000 daltons (22% to 36%). The anti-Xa activity is approximately 100 int. units/mg.

Contraindications Hypersensitivity to tinzaparin sodium, heparin, or any component of the formulation; active major bleeding; heparin-induced thrombocytopenia (current or history of)

Warnings/Precautions **[U.S. Boxed Warning]: Spinal or epidural hematomas, including subsequent paralysis, may occur with recent or anticipated neuraxial anesthesia (epidural or spinal) or spinal puncture in patients anticoagulated with LMWH or heparinoids.** Consider risk versus benefit prior to spinal procedures; risk is increased by the use of concomitant agents which may alter hemostasis, the use of indwelling epidural catheters for analgesia, a history of spinal deformity or spinal surgery, as well as traumatic or repeated epidural or spinal punctures. Patient should be observed closely for signs and symptoms of neurological impairment. Not to be used interchangeably (unit for unit) with heparin or any other low molecular weight heparins.

Monitor patient closely for signs or symptoms of bleeding. Certain patients are at increased risk of bleeding. Risk factors include bacterial endocarditis; congenital or acquired bleeding disorders; active ulcerative or angiodysplastic GI diseases; severe uncontrolled hypertension; history of hemorrhagic stroke; use shortly after brain, spinal, or ophthalmologic surgery; patients treated concomitantly with platelet inhibitors; recent GI bleeding; thrombocytopenia or platelet defects; severe liver disease; hypertensive or diabetic retinopathy; or in patients undergoing invasive procedures. Monitor platelet count closely. Rare cases of thrombocytopenia have occurred. Manufacturer recommends discontinuation of therapy if platelets are <100,000/mm^3. Rare cases of thrombocytopenia with thrombosis have occurred.

Reduced tinzaparin clearance was observed in patients with moderate-to-severe renal impairment; use with caution or avoid use in patients with renal insufficiency. The 2008 *Chest* guidelines recommend that patients with Cl_{cr} <30 mL/minute be treated with unfractionated heparin instead of LMWH (Hirsh, 2008). Use with caution in the elderly (delayed elimination may occur). Use in patients ≥70 years of age with renal insufficiency (Cl_{cr} ≤30 mL/minute or ≥75 years of age and Cl_{cr} ≤60 mL/minute) has been associated with an increased risk of death compared to use of unfractionated heparin; consider alternative treatments in these patients.

Heparin can cause hyperkalemia by suppressing aldosterone production; similar reactions could occur with LMWHs. Monitor for hyperkalemia which most commonly occurs in patients with risk factors for the development of hyperkalemia (eg, renal dysfunction, concomitant use of potassium-sparing diuretics or potassium supplements, hematoma in body tissues). For subcutaneous use only; do not administer intramuscularly or intravenously. Clinical experience is limited in patients with BMI >40 kg/m^2. Derived from porcine intestinal mucosa. Contains benzyl alcohol and sodium metabisulfite.

Drug Interactions

Avoid Concomitant Use

Avoid concomitant use of Tinzaparin with any of the following: Rivaroxaban

Decreased Effect There are no known significant interactions involving a decrease in effect.

Increased Effect/Toxicity

Tinzaparin may increase the levels/effects of: Anticoagulants; Collagenase (Systemic); Deferasirox; Drotrecogin Alfa (Activated); Ibritumomab; Rivaroxaban; Tositumomab and Iodine I 131 Tositumomab

The levels/effects of Tinzaparin may be increased by: 5-ASA Derivatives; Antiplatelet Agents; Dasatinib; Herbs (Anticoagulant/Antiplatelet Properties); Nonsteroidal Anti-Inflammatory Agents; Pentosan Polysulfate Sodium; Pentoxifylline; Prostacyclin Analogues; Salicylates; Thrombolytic Agents

Adverse Reactions As with all anticoagulants, bleeding is the major adverse effect of tinzaparin. Hemorrhage may occur at virtually any site. Risk is dependent on multiple variables.

>10%:

Hepatic: ALT increased (13%)

Local: Injection site hematoma (16%)

1% to 10%:

Cardiovascular: Angina pectoris, chest pain (2%), hyper-/hypotension, tachycardia

Central nervous system: Confusion, dizziness, fever (2%), headache (2%), insomnia, pain (2%)

Dermatologic: Bullous eruption, pruritus, rash (1%), skin disorder

Gastrointestinal: Constipation (1%), dyspepsia, flatulence, nausea (2%), nonspecified gastrointestinal disorder, vomiting (1%)

Genitourinary: Dysuria, urinary retention, urinary tract infection (4%)

Hematologic: Anemia, hematoma, hemorrhage (2%), thrombocytopenia (1%)

Hepatic: AST increased (9%)

Local: Thrombophlebitis (deep)

Neuromuscular & skeletal: Back pain (2%)

Renal: Hematuria (1%)

Respiratory: Dyspnea (1%), epistaxis (2%), pneumonia, pulmonary embolism (2%), respiratory disorder

Miscellaneous: Impaired healing, infection, unclassified reactions

Pharmacodynamics/Kinetics

Onset of Action 2-3 hours

General Dosage Range SubQ: *Adults:* 175 anti-Xa int. units/kg of body weight once daily

Administration

Other Patient should be lying down or sitting. Administer by deep SubQ injection, alternating between the left and right anterolateral and left and right posterolateral abdominal wall. Vary site daily. The entire needle should be introduced into the skin fold formed by the thumb and forefinger. Hold the skin fold until injection is complete. To minimize bruising, do not rub the injection site.

Stability

Storage Store at 15°C to 30°C (59°F to 86°F).

Nursing Actions

Physical Assessment Monitor for bleeding, rash, and confusion on a regular basis throughout therapy. Observe and teach bleeding precautions. If self-administered, teach patient appropriate injection technique and syringe/needle disposal.

Patient Education This drug can only be administered by injection; if self-administered, inject exactly as directed and follow instructions for syringe disposal. Report excessive bruising, swelling, or redness at injection site. You may have a tendency to bleed easily while taking this drug. Report immediately any unusual bleeding or bruising (eg, mouth, nose, blood in urine or stool), severe headache or confusion, dizziness, or skin rash.

Tioconazole (tye oh KONE a zole)

Brand Names: U.S. 1-Day™ [OTC]; Vagistat®-1 [OTC]

Pharmacologic Category Antifungal Agent, Vaginal

Medication Safety Issues

Sound-alike/look-alike issues:

Tioconazole may be confused with terconazole

Pregnancy Risk Factor C

Lactation Excretion in breast milk unknown/not recommended

Use Local treatment of vulvovaginal candidiasis

Available Dosage Forms For available OTC formulations, consult specific product labeling.

General Dosage Range Intravaginal: *Adults:* Insert 1 applicatorful prior to bedtime, as a single dose

Nursing Actions

Patient Education Consult with prescriber if treating a vaginal yeast infection for the first time. Insert high into the vagina. Refrain from intercourse during treatment. May interact with condoms and vaginal contraceptive diaphragms (ie, weaken latex); do not rely on these products for 3 days following treatment. Do not use tampons, douches, spermicides, or other vaginal products during treatment. Although product is used for a single day, relief from symptoms usually takes longer than 1 day. Report persistent (>3 days) vaginal burning, irritation, or discharge.

Tiotropium (ty oh TRO pee um)

Brand Names: U.S. Spiriva® HandiHaler®

Index Terms Tiotropium Bromide Monohydrate

Pharmacologic Category Anticholinergic Agent

Medication Safety Issues

Sound-alike/look-alike issues:

Spiriva® may be confused with Inspra™, Serevent®

Tiotropium may be confused with ipratropium

Administration issues:

Spiriva® capsules for inhalation are for administration via HandiHaler® device and are **not** for oral use

Pregnancy Risk Factor C

Lactation Excretion in breast milk unknown/use caution

Use Maintenance treatment of bronchospasm associated with COPD (including bronchitis and emphysema); reduction of COPD exacerbations

Mechanism of Action/Effect Blocks the action of acetylcholine at parasympathetic sites in bronchial smooth muscle causing bronchodilation

Contraindications Hypersensitivity to tiotropium or ipratropium, or any component of the formulation (contains lactose)

Warnings/Precautions Rarely, paradoxical bronchospasm may occur with use of inhaled bronchodilating agents; discontinue use and consider other therapy if bronchospasm occurs.

Not indicated for the initial (rescue) treatment of acute episodes of bronchospasm. Use with caution in patients with myasthenia gravis, narrow-angle glaucoma, prostatic hyperplasia, moderate-severe renal impairment (Cl_{cr} ≤50 mL/minute), or bladder neck obstruction; avoid inadvertent instillation of powder into the eyes. Immediate hypersensitivity reactions may occur; discontinue immediately if signs/symptoms occur. Use with caution in patients with a history of hypersensitivity to atropine.

The contents of Spiriva® capsules are for inhalation only via the HandiHaler® device. There have been reports of incorrect administration (swallowing of the capsules). Capsule for oral inhalation contains lactose; use with caution in patients with severe milk protein allergy.

Drug Interactions

Avoid Concomitant Use There are no known interactions where it is recommended to avoid concomitant use.

Decreased Effect

Tiotropium may decrease the levels/effects of: Acetylcholinesterase Inhibitors (Central); Secretin

The levels/effects of Tiotropium may be decreased by: Acetylcholinesterase Inhibitors (Central); Peginterferon Alfa-2b; Tocilizumab

Increased Effect/Toxicity

Tiotropium may increase the levels/effects of: AbobotulinumtoxinA; Anticholinergics; Cannabinoids; OnabotulinumtoxinA; Potassium Chloride; RimabotulinumtoxinB

The levels/effects of Tiotropium may be increased by: Conivaptan; Pramlintide

Adverse Reactions

>10%:

Gastrointestinal: Xerostomia (5% to 16%)

Respiratory: Upper respiratory tract infection (41%), pharyngitis (9% to 13%), sinusitis (7% to 11%)

1% to 10%:

Cardiovascular: Chest pain (1% to 7%), edema (dependent, 5%)

Central nervous system: Headache (6%), insomnia (4%), depression (1% to 4%), dysphonia (1% to 3%)

Dermatologic: Rash (4%)

Endocrine & metabolic: Hypercholesterolemia (1% to 3%), hyperglycemia (1% to 3%)

Gastrointestinal: Dyspepsia (6%), abdominal pain (5%), constipation (4% to 5%), vomiting (4%), gastroesophageal reflux (1% to 3%), stomatitis (including ulcerative; 1% to 3%)

Genitourinary: Urinary tract infection (7%)

Neuromuscular & skeletal: Arthralgia (4%), myalgia (4%), arthritis (≥3%), leg pain (1% to 3%), paresthesia (1% to 3%), skeletal pain (1% to 3%)

Ocular: Cataract (1% to 3%)

Respiratory: Rhinitis (6%), epistaxis (4%), cough (≥3%), laryngitis (1% to 3%)

Miscellaneous: Infection (4%), moniliasis (4%), flu-like syndrome (≥3%), allergic reaction (1% to 3%), herpes zoster (1% to 3%)

Available Dosage Forms

Powder, for oral inhalation:

Spiriva® HandiHaler®: 18 mcg/capsule (5s, 30s, 90s)

General Dosage Range Inhalation: *Adults:* Contents of 1 capsule (18 mcg) once daily

Administration

Oral For oral inhalation only. Capsule should not be swallowed.

Inhalation Administer once daily at the same time each day. Remove capsule from foil blister immediately before use. Capsule should not be swallowed. Place capsule in the capsule-chamber in the base of the HandiHaler® Inhaler. Must only use the HandiHaler® Inhaler. Close mouthpiece until a click is heard, leaving dustcap open. Exhale fully. Do not exhale into inhaler. Tilt head slightly back and inhale (rapidly, steadily and deeply); the capsule vibration may be heard within the device. Hold breath as long as possible. If any powder remains in capsule, exhale and inhale again. Repeat until capsule is empty. Throw away empty capsule; do not leave in inhaler. Do not use a spacer with the HandiHaler® Inhaler. Do not use HandiHaler® device for other medications. Always keep capsules and inhaler dry.

Delivery of dose: Instruct patient to place mouthpiece gently between teeth, closing lips around inhaler. Instruct patient to inhale deeply and hold breath for 5-10 seconds. The amount of drug delivered is small, and the individual will not sense the medication as it is inhaled. Remove mouthpiece prior to exhalation. Patient should not breathe out through the mouthpiece.

Stability

Storage Store at 25°C (77°F); excursions permitted to 15°C to 30°C (59°F to 86°F). Avoid excessive temperatures and moisture. Do not store capsules in HandiHaler® device. Capsules should be stored in the blister pack and only removed immediately before use. Once protective foil is peeled back and/or removed the capsule should be used immediately; if capsule is not used immediately it should be discarded.

Nursing Actions

Physical Assessment Monitor pulmonary tests prior to and periodically during therapy.

Patient Education Use inhaler and medication as instructed - once daily, at same time each day. Do not use as an acute "rescue" bronchodilator. Capsules are not to be swallowed. May cause nausea or vomiting, dry mouth, hyperglycemia (if you have diabetes, monitor serum glucose closely), or muscle or skeletal pain. Report swelling of face, mouth, or tongue; skin rash; chest pain or palpitations; persistent gastrointestinal effects; muscle or skeletal pain or weakness; change in vision; numbness or weakness of extremities; slurred speech; or respiratory changes, sore throat, or flu-like symptoms.

Administration of HandiHaler® Inhaler: Remove capsule from blister pack immediately before using. Place capsule in capsule chamber in the base of inhaler. Close mouthpiece until a click is heard, leaving dustcap open. Exhale fully (do not exhale into inhaler). Place mouthpiece gently between teeth, closing lips around inhaler. Tilt head back slightly and inhale once rapidly, steadily, and deeply (the capsule vibration may be heard within the inhaler, but you will not sense the medication as it is inhaled.) Hold breath as long as possible. Remove inhaler from mouth before exhaling. If any powder remains in capsule, repeat inhalation again. Throw away empty capsule. Do not store capsule in inhaler and always keep inhaler and capsules dry.

Tipranavir (tip RA na veer)

Brand Names: U.S. Aptivus®

Index Terms PNU-140690E; TPV

Pharmacologic Category Antiretroviral Agent, Protease Inhibitor

Pregnancy Risk Factor C

Lactation Excretion in breast milk unknown/contraindicated

Breast-Feeding Considerations Maternal or infant antiretroviral therapy does not completely eliminate the risk of postnatal HIV transmission.

In addition, multiclass-resistant virus has been detected in breast-feeding infants despite maternal therapy. Therefore, in the United States, where formula is accessible, affordable, safe, and sustainable, and the risk of infant mortality due to diarrhea and respiratory infections is low, complete avoidance of breast-feeding by HIV-infected women is recommended to decrease potential transmission of HIV (DHHS [perinatal], 2011).

Use Treatment of HIV-1 infections in combination with ritonavir and other antiretroviral agents; limited to highly treatment-experienced or multiprotease inhibitor-resistant patients.

Mechanism of Action/Effect Blocks the site of HIV-1 protease activity, resulting in the formation of immature, noninfectious viral particles.

Contraindications Concurrent therapy of tipranavir/ritonavir with alfuzosin, amiodarone, bepridil, cisapride, ergot derivatives (eg, dihydroergotamine, ergonovine, ergotamine, methylergonovine), flecainide, lovastatin, midazolam (oral), pimozide, propafenone, quinidine, rifampin, sildenafil (for pulmonary arterial hypertension [eg, Revatio®]), simvastatin, St John's wort, and triazolam; moderate-to-severe hepatic impairment (Child-Pugh class B or C)

Warnings/Precautions Coadministration with ritonavir is required. **[U.S. Boxed Warning]: In combination with ritonavir, may cause hepatitis (including fatalities) and/or exacerbate pre-existing hepatic dysfunction (causal relationship not established); patients with chronic hepatitis B or C are at increased risk.** Monitor patients closely; discontinue use if signs or symptoms of toxicity occur or if asymptomatic AST/ALT elevations >10 times upper limit of normal or AST/ALT elevations >5-10 times upper limit of normal concurrently with total bilirubin >2.5 times the upper limit of normal occur. Use with caution in patients with mild hepatic impairment; contraindicated in moderate-to-severe impairment. May be associated with fat redistribution (buffalo hump, increased abdominal girth, breast engorgement, facial atrophy). Use caution in hemophilia. May increase cholesterol and/or triglycerides; hypertriglyceridemia may increase risk of pancreatitis. May cause hyperglycemia. Use with caution in patients with sulfonamide allergy. Protease inhibitors have been associated with a variety of hypersensitivity events (some severe), including rash, anaphylaxis (rare), angioedema, bronchospasm, erythema multiforme, and/or Stevens-Johnson syndrome (rare). It is generally recommended to discontinue treatment if severe rash or moderate symptoms accompanied by other systemic symptoms occur. Immune reconstitution syndrome, including inflammatory responses to indolent infections, has been associated with antiretroviral therapy; additional evaluation and treatment may be required.

[U.S. Boxed Warning]: Tipranavir in combination with ritonavir has been associated with rare reports of fatal and nonfatal intracranial hemorrhage; causal relationship not established. Events often occurred in patients with medical conditions (eg, CNS lesions, head trauma, recent neurosurgery, coagulopathy, alcohol abuse) or concurrent therapy which may have influenced these events. Tipranavir may inhibit platelet aggregation. Use with caution in patients who may be at risk for increased bleeding (trauma, surgery or other medical conditions) or in patients receiving concurrent medications which may increase the risk of bleeding, including antiplatelet agents and anticoagulants.

Use with caution in patients taking strong CYP3A4 inhibitors and moderate CYP3A4 inducers. Concomitant use with selected major CYP3A4 substrates and strong CYP3A4 inducers is contraindicated (see Drug Interactions); consider alternative agents that avoid or lessen the potential for CYP-mediated interactions. Do not coadminister colchicine in patient with renal or hepatic impairment; avoid concurrent use with salmeterol. Coadministration with anticoagulants or antiplatelet agents may increase the risk of bleeding. Women receiving estrogen (as hormonal contraception or replacement therapy) have an increased incidence of rash. Alternative forms of contraception may be needed. Do not coadminister with etravirine. Oral solution formulation contains vitamin E; additional vitamin E supplements should be avoided. Safety and efficacy have not been established in children <2 years of age.

Drug Interactions

Avoid Concomitant Use

Avoid concomitant use of Tipranavir with any of the following: Alfuzosin; Amiodarone; Bepridil [Off Market]; Cisapride; Dabigatran Etexilate; Ergot Derivatives; Etravirine; Flecainide; Lovastatin; Midazolam; Pimozide; Propafenone; QuiNIDine; Rifampin; Simvastatin; St Johns Wort; Tamoxifen; Thioridazine; Triazolam

Decreased Effect

Tipranavir may decrease the levels/effects of: Abacavir; Boceprevir; Clarithromycin; Codeine; Contraceptives (Estrogens); Dabigatran Etexilate; Delavirdine; Didanosine; Divalproex; Estrogen Derivatives; Etravirine; Fosphenytoin; Iloperidone; Linagliptin; Meperidine; Methadone; P-glycoprotein/ABCB1 Substrates; PHENobarbital; Phenytoin; Proton Pump Inhibitors; Raltegravir; Theophylline Derivatives; TraMADol; Valproic Acid; Zidovudine

The levels/effects of Tipranavir may be decreased by: Antacids; Boceprevir; CarBAMazepine; CYP3A4 Inducers (Strong); Deferasirox; Efavirenz; Fosphenytoin; Garlic; PHENobarbital; Phenytoin; Rifampin; St Johns Wort; Tenofovir; Tocilizumab

Increased Effect/Toxicity Note: Listed interactions include interactions resulting from coadministration with ritonavir. Refer to Ritonavir monograph on page 1003 for additional interaction concerns. The serum concentrations of tipranavir may be increased by ritonavir. This combination is recommended to enhance the effect ("boost") tipranavir.

Tipranavir/ritonavir may increase the levels/effects of CYP3A4 substrates. Tipranavir/ritonavir may increase the toxicity of benzodiazepines; concurrent use of midazolam and triazolam is specifically contraindicated. Tipranavir may increase serum concentrations of cisapride, increasing the risk of malignant arrhythmias; use is contraindicated. Toxicity of pimozide is significantly increased by tipranavir/ritonavir; concurrent use is contraindicated. Tipranavir/ritonavir may increase serum concentrations/toxicity of several antiarrhythmic agents; contraindicated with amiodarone, flecainide, propafenone, and quinidine (use extreme caution with lidocaine). Tipranavir/ritonavir may also increase serum concentrations/effects of calcium channel blockers and immunosuppressants (cyclosporine, sirolimus, tacrolimus).

Serum concentrations of HMG-CoA reductase inhibitors (atorvastatin, cerivastatin, lovastatin, simvastatin) may be increased by tipranavir/ritonavir, increasing the risk of myopathy/rhabdomyolysis. Lovastatin and simvastatin are not recommended. Use lowest possible dose of atorvastatin. Fluvastatin and pravastatin may be safer alternatives. Serum concentrations of rifabutin may be increased by tipranavir/ritonavir; dosage adjustment of rifabutin is required.

The toxicity of ergot alkaloids (dihydroergotamine, ergotamine, ergonovine, methylergonovine) is increased by tipranavir; concurrent use is contraindicated. Effects of hypoglycemic agents may be altered by tipranavir/ritonavir. Concurrent therapy with tipranavir may increase serum concentrations of normeperidine, and decrease serum concentrations of meperidine. The serum concentrations of sildenafil, tadalafil, and vardenafil may be increased by tipranavir/ritonavir; dose adjustment and limitations related to ritonavir coadministration must be recognized.

Concurrent use of disulfiram with tipranavir oral solution is contraindicated due to risk of adverse reaction (due to alcohol content of formulation). Clarithromycin may increase serum concentrations of tipranavir. Tipranavir/ritonavir may increase serum concentrations of clarithromycin. Use with caution and adjust dose of clarithromycin during concurrent therapy in renally impaired patients.

Nutritional/Ethanol Interactions

Ethanol: Capsules contain dehydrated alcohol 7% w/w (0.1 g per capsule)

Herb/Nutraceutical: St John's wort may decrease the levels/effects of tipranavir/ritonavir. Vitamin E (high dose) may increase the risk of bleeding. Garlic may decrease the serum concentration of tipranavir. Management: Avoid St John's wort; concurrent use is contraindicated. Avoid vitamin E supplementation. Garlic supplementation is not recommended.

Adverse Reactions

>10%:

Dermatologic: Rash (children 21%; adults 3% to 10%)

Endocrine & metabolic: Hypertriglyceridemia (>400 mg/dL: 61%), hypercholesterolemia (>300 mg/dL: 22%)

Gastrointestinal: Diarrhea (15%)

Hepatic: Transaminases increased (>2.5 x ULN: 26% to 32%; grade 3/4: 10% to 20%)

Neuromuscular & skeletal: CPK increased (grade 3/4: children 11%)

2% to 10%:

Central nervous system: Fever (6% to 8%), fatigue (6%), headache (5%)

Endocrine & metabolic: Dehydration (2%)

Gastrointestinal: Nausea (5% to 9%), amylase increased (grade 3: 6% to 8%), vomiting (6%), abdominal pain (4%), diarrhea (children 4%), weight loss (3%)

Hematologic: Bleeding (children 8%), WBC decreased (grades 3: 5%), anemia (3%), neutropenia (2%)

Hepatic: ALT increased (2%, grades 3/4: 10%), AST increased (grades 3/4: 6%), GGT increased (2%)

Neuromuscular & skeletal: Myalgia (2%)

Respiratory: Cough (children 6%), dyspnea (2%), epistaxis (children 4%)

Available Dosage Forms

Capsule, soft gelatin, oral:

Aptivus®: 250 mg

Solution, oral:

Aptivus®: 100 mg/mL (95 mL)

General Dosage Range Dosage adjustment recommended in patients on concomitant therapy

Oral:

Children ≥2 years: 12-14 mg/kg or 290-375 mg/m² (maximum: 500 mg/dose) twice daily

Adults: 500 mg twice daily

Administration

Oral Coadministration with ritonavir is required. Administer with ritonavir capsules or solution without regard to meals; administer with ritonavir tablets with meals.

Stability

Storage

Capsule: Prior to opening bottle, store under refrigeration at 2°C to 8°C (36°F to 46°F). After bottle is opened, may be stored at controlled room temperature of 25°C (77°F) for up to 60 days.

Oral solution: Store at 15°C to 30°C (59°F to 86°F). After bottle is open, use within 60 days. Do not refrigerate or freeze oral solution.

Nursing Actions

Physical Assessment Monitor for adherence to regimen. Monitor for gastrointestinal disturbance (nausea, vomiting, diarrhea) that can lead to dehydration and weight loss, hyperlipidemia, redistribution of body fat, and rash. Caution patients to monitor glucose levels closely; may alter effects of hypoglycemic agents or cause hyperglycemia. Teach patient proper timing of multiple medications. Instruct patient on glucose testing.

Patient Education This is not a cure for HIV, nor has it been found to reduce transmission of HIV; use appropriate precautions to prevent spread to other persons. Maintain adequate hydration, unless instructed to restrict fluid intake. Frequent blood tests may be required. You may be advised to check your glucose levels; this drug can cause exacerbation or new-onset diabetes. May cause body changes due to redistribution of body fat, facial atrophy, or breast enlargement (normal effects of drug). May cause dizziness, insomnia, abnormal thinking, nausea, vomiting, taste perversion, muscle weakness, headache, or insomnia. Inform prescriber if you experience muscle numbness or tingling; unresolved persistent vomiting, diarrhea, or abdominal pain; respiratory difficulty or chest pain; unusual skin rash; or change in color of stool or urine.

Dietary Considerations Capsule contains dehydrated ethanol. Oral solution formulation contains vitamin E; additional vitamin E supplements should be avoided.

Tirofiban (tye roe FYE ban)

Brand Names: U.S. Aggrastat®

Index Terms MK383; Tirofiban Hydrochloride

Pharmacologic Category Antiplatelet Agent, Glycoprotein IIb/IIIa Inhibitor

Medication Safety Issues

Sound-alike/look-alike issues:

Aggrastat® may be confused with Aggrenox®, argatroban

High alert medication:

The Institute for Safe Medication Practices (ISMP) includes this medication among its list of drugs which have a heightened risk of causing significant patient harm when used in error.

Pregnancy Risk Factor B

Lactation Excretion in breast milk unknown/contraindicated

Use Treatment of acute coronary syndrome (ie, unstable angina/non-ST-elevation myocardial infarction [UA/NSTEMI]) in combination with heparin

Unlabeled Use To support PCI (administered at the time of PCI) for ST-elevation myocardial infarction (STEMI), UA/NSTEMI, and stable ischemic heart disease (ie, elective PCI)

Mechanism of Action/Effect A reversible antagonist of fibrinogen binding to the GP IIb/IIIa receptor, the major platelet surface receptor involved in platelet aggregation. Platelet aggregation inhibition is reversible following cessation of the infusion.

Contraindications Hypersensitivity to tirofiban or any component of the formulation; active internal bleeding or a history of bleeding diathesis within the previous 30 days; history of intracranial hemorrhage, intracranial neoplasm, arteriovenous malformation, or aneurysm; history of thrombocytopenia following prior exposure; history of CVA within 30 days or any history of hemorrhagic stroke; major surgical procedure or severe physical trauma within the previous month; history, symptoms, or findings suggestive of aortic dissection; severe hypertension (systolic BP >180 mm Hg and/or diastolic BP >110 mm Hg); concomitant use of another parenteral GP IIb/IIIa inhibitor; acute pericarditis

Warnings/Precautions Bleeding is the most common complication encountered during this therapy; most major bleeding occurs at the arterial access site for cardiac catheterization. Caution in patients with platelets <150,000/mm^3; patients with hemorrhagic retinopathy; chronic dialysis patients; when used in combination with other drugs impacting on coagulation. Prior to pulling the sheath, heparin should be discontinued for 3-4 hours and ACT <180 seconds or aPTT <45 seconds. Use standard compression techniques after sheath removal. Watch the site closely afterwards for further bleeding. Sheath hemostasis should be achieved at least 4 hours before hospital discharge. Other trauma and vascular punctures should be minimized. Avoid obtaining vascular access through a noncompressible site (eg, subclavian or jugular vein). Discontinue at least 2-4 hours prior to coronary artery bypass graft surgery (Hillis, 2011). Patients with severe renal insufficiency require dosage reduction.

Drug Interactions

Avoid Concomitant Use There are no known interactions where it is recommended to avoid concomitant use.

Decreased Effect

The levels/effects of Tirofiban may be decreased by: Nonsteroidal Anti-Inflammatory Agents

Increased Effect/Toxicity

Tirofiban may increase the levels/effects of: Anticoagulants; Antiplatelet Agents; Collagenase (Systemic); Drotrecogin Alfa (Activated); Ibritumomab; Rivaroxaban; Salicylates; Thrombolytic Agents; Tositumomab and Iodine I 131 Tositumomab

The levels/effects of Tirofiban may be increased by: Dasatinib; Glucosamine; Herbs (Anticoagulant/Antiplatelet Properties); Nonsteroidal Anti-Inflammatory Agents; Omega-3-Acid Ethyl Esters; Pentosan Polysulfate Sodium; Pentoxifylline; Prostacyclin Analogues; Vitamin E

Adverse Reactions Bleeding is the major drug-related adverse effect. Patients received background treatment with aspirin and heparin. Major bleeding was reported in 1.4% to 2.2%; minor bleeding in 10.5% to 12%; transfusion was required in 4% to 4.3%.

>1% (nonbleeding adverse events):

Cardiovascular: Coronary artery dissection (5%), bradycardia (4%), edema (2%)

Central nervous system: Dizziness (3%), vasovagal reaction (2%), fever (>1%), headache (>1%)

Gastrointestinal: Nausea (>1%)

Genitourinary: Pelvic pain (6%)

Hematologic: Thrombocytopenia: <90,000/mm^3 (1.5%), <50,000/mm^3 (0.3%)

Neuromuscular & skeletal: Leg pain (3%)

Miscellaneous: Diaphoresis (2%)

Available Dosage Forms

Infusion, premixed in NS [preservative free]:

Aggrastat®: 50 mcg/mL (250 mL)

General Dosage Range Dosage adjustment recommended in patients with renal impairment

I.V.: *Adults:* Initial: 0.4 mcg/kg/minute for 30 minutes; Maintenance infusion: 0.1 mcg/kg/minute

Administration

I.V. For unstable angina/non-ST-elevation MI (UA/NSTEMI), infuse loading dose over 30 minutes, followed by continuous infusion. When used during percutaneous coronary intervention (PCI), may administer loading dose over 3 minutes, followed by continuous infusion. Tirofiban injection must be diluted to a concentration of 50 mcg/mL (premixed solution does not require dilution). Unused solution should be discarded.

I.V. Detail Intended for intravenous delivery using sterile equipment and technique. Do not add other drugs or remove solution directly from the bag with a syringe. Do not use plastic containers in series connections. Such use can result in air embolism by drawing air from the first container if it is empty of solution. Discard any unused solution. May be administered through the same catheter as heparin, lidocaine, dopamine, potassium chloride, and famotidine.

Stability

Storage Store at 25°C (77°F); do not freeze. Protect from light during storage.

Nursing Actions

Physical Assessment Monitor vital signs prior to, during, and after therapy. Assess infusion insertion site during and after therapy (every 15 minutes or as institutional policy). Monitor closely for bleeding (eg, CNS changes; blood in urine, stool, or vomitus; unusual bruising or bleeding). Monitor closely for signs of unusual or excessive bleeding.

Patient Education This medication can only be administered I.V. You will have a tendency to bleed easily during administration of this medication. If bleeding occurs, apply pressure to bleeding spot until bleeding stops completely. Report unusual bruising or bleeding (eg, blood in urine, stool, or vomitus; bleeding gums; vaginal bleeding; nosebleeds); unusual and persistent fever; dizziness or vision changes; back, leg, or pelvic pain; or persistent nausea or vomiting.

TiZANidine (tye ZAN i deen)

Brand Names: U.S. Zanaflex Capsules®; Zanaflex®

Index Terms Sirdalud®

Pharmacologic Category Alpha$_2$-Adrenergic Agonist

Medication Safety Issues

Sound-alike/look-alike issues:

TiZANidine may be confused with tiaGABine

Zanaflex® may be confused with Xiaflex®

Other safety concerns:

Zanaflex® capsules and Zanaflex® tablets (or generic tizanidine tablets) are not interchangeable

Pregnancy Risk Factor C

Lactation Excretion in breast milk unknown

Breast-Feeding Considerations Excretion in breast milk is unknown, but expected due to lipid solubility.

Use Skeletal muscle relaxant used for treatment of muscle spasticity

Unlabeled Use Tension headaches, low back pain, and trigeminal neuralgia

Mechanism of Action/Effect Acts within CNS at the level of the spinal cord to reduce excitation of motor neurons, resulting in muscle relaxation

Contraindications Hypersensitivity to tizanidine or any component of the formulation; concomitant therapy with ciprofloxacin or fluvoxamine (potent CYP1A2 inhibitors)

Warnings/Precautions Significant hypotension (possibly with bradycardia or orthostatic hypotension) and sedation may occur; use caution in patients with cardiac disease or those at risk for severe hypotensive or sedative effects. Should not be used with other alpha$_2$-adrenergic agonists.

Avoid concomitant administration with CYP1A2 inhibitors; increased tizanidine levels/effects (severe hypotension and sedation) may occur. These effects may also be increased with concomitant administration with other CNS depressants and/or antihypertensives; use caution. Elderly patients are at risk due to decreased clearance, particulary in elderly patients with renal insufficiency (Cl_{cr} <25 mL/minute) compared to healthy elderly subjects; this may lead to an increased risk of adverse effects and/or a longer duration of effects. Use caution in any patient with renal impairment; reduced initial doses recommended in patient with Cl_{cr} <25 mL/minute. Use with extreme caution or avoid in hepatic impairment due to extensive hepatic metabolism and potential hepatotoxicity; AST/ALT elevations (≥2 times baseline) and rarely hepatic failure have occurred; monitoring recommended.

Use has been associated with visual hallucinations or delusions, generally in first 6 weeks of therapy; use caution in patients with psychiatric disorders. Withdrawal resulting in rebound hypertension, tachycardia, and hypertonia may occur upon discontinuation; doses should be decreased slowly, particularly in patients receiving high doses for prolonged periods. Pharmacokinetics and bioequivalence between capsules and tablets altered by nonfasting vs fasting conditions. Limited data exists for chronic use of single doses >8 mg and multiple doses >24 mg/day.

Drug Interactions

Avoid Concomitant Use

Avoid concomitant use of TiZANidine with any of the following: Ciprofloxacin; Ciprofloxacin (Systemic); FluvoxaMINE; Iobenguane I 123

Decreased Effect

TiZANidine may decrease the levels/effects of: Iobenguane I 123

The levels/effects of TiZANidine may be decreased by: Antidepressants (Alpha2-Antagonist); Cyproterone; Serotonin/Norepinephrine Reuptake Inhibitors; Tricyclic Antidepressants

Increased Effect/Toxicity

TiZANidine may increase the levels/effects of: ACE Inhibitors; Alcohol (Ethyl); CNS Depressants; Hypotensive Agents; Lisinopril; Methotrimeprazine; Selective Serotonin Reuptake Inhibitors

The levels/effects of TiZANidine may be increased by: Abiraterone Acetate; Beta-Blockers; Ciprofloxacin; Ciprofloxacin (Systemic); Contraceptives (Estrogens); CYP1A2 Inhibitors (Moderate); CYP1A2 Inhibitors (Strong); Deferasirox; Droperidol; FluvoxaMINE; HydrOXYzine; MAO Inhibitors; Methotrimeprazine

Nutritional/Ethanol Interactions

Ethanol: May increase CNS depression; monitor for increased effects with coadministration. Caution patients about effects.

Food: The tablet and capsule dosage forms are not bioequivalent when administered with food. Food increases both the time to peak concentration and the extent of absorption for both the tablet and capsule. However, maximal concentrations of tizanidine achieved when administered with food were increased by 30% for the tablet, but decreased by 20% for the capsule. Under fed conditions, the capsule is approximately 80% bioavailable relative to the tablet.

Herb/Nutraceutical: Avoid valerian, St John's wort, kava kava, gotu kola (may increase CNS depression). Avoid black cohosh, California poppy, coleus, golden seal, hawthorn, mistletoe, periwinkle, quinine, shepherd's purse (may increase hypotensive effects).

Adverse Reactions Frequency percentages below reported during multiple-dose studies, unless specified otherwise.

>10%:

Cardiovascular: Hypotension (single-dose study with doses ≥8 mg: 16% to 33%)

Central nervous system: Somnolence (48%), dizziness (16%)

Gastrointestinal: Xerostomia (49%)

Neuromuscular & skeletal: Weakness (41%)

1% to 10%:

Cardiovascular: Bradycardia (single-dose study with doses ≥8 mg: 2% to 10%)

Central nervous system: Nervousness (3%), speech disorder (3%), visual hallucinations/delusions (3%; generally occurring in first 6 weeks of therapy), anxiety (1%), depression (1%), fever (1%)

Dermatologic: Rash (1%), skin ulcer (1%)

Gastrointestinal: Constipation (4%), vomiting (3%), abdominal pain (1%), diarrhea (1%), dyspepsia (1%)

Genitourinary: UTI (10%), urinary frequency (3%)

Hepatic: Liver enzymes increased (3% to 5%)

Neuromuscular & skeletal: Dyskinesia (3%), back pain (1%), myasthenia (1%), paresthesia (1%)

Ocular: Blurred vision (3%)

Respiratory: Pharyngitis (3%), rhinitis (3%)

Miscellaneous: Infection (6%), flu-like syndrome (3%), diaphoresis (1%)

Pharmacodynamics/Kinetics

Duration of Action 3-6 hours

Available Dosage Forms

Capsule, oral: 2 mg, 4 mg, 6 mg

Zanaflex Capsules®: 2 mg, 4 mg, 6 mg

Tablet, oral: 2 mg, 4 mg

Zanaflex®: 4 mg

General Dosage Range Oral: *Adults:* Initial: 2-4 mg 3 times/day; Maintenance: 6-36 mg/day in 3 divided doses (maximum: 36 mg/day)

Administration

Oral Capsules may be opened and contents sprinkled on food; however, extent of absorption is increased up to 20% relative to administration of the capsule under fasted conditions.

Stability

Storage Store at 25°C (77°F); excursions permitted to 15°C to 30°C (59°F to 86°F).

Nursing Actions

Physical Assessment May cause hypotension; monitor blood pressure periodically. Do not discontinue medication abruptly; can cause hypertension and tachycardia.

Patient Education If you miss a dose, take the missed dose as soon as possible if it is within an hour or so of the regular time. If not within an hour or so, skip the missed dose and go back to your regular dosing schedule. Do not double doses. Avoid alcohol. May cause dizziness, nervousness, insomnia, daytime drowsiness, postural hypotension, nausea, vomiting, dry mouth, mouth sores, or upset stomach. Report persistent dizziness or GI symptoms, chest pain or palpitations, CNS disturbances (delusions, confusion), muscle weakness or tremors, rash, or respiratory difficulty.

Dietary Considerations Administration with food compared to administration in the fasting state results in clinically-significant differences in absorption and other pharmacokinetic parameters. Patients should be consistent and should not switch administration of the tablets or the capsules between the fasting and nonfasting state. In addition, switching between the capsules and the tablets in the fed state will also result in significant differences. Opening capsule contents to sprinkle on applesauce compared to swallowing intact capsules whole will also result in significant absorption differences. Patients should be consistent with regards to administration.

Tobramycin (Systemic, Oral Inhalation) (toe bra MYE sin)

Brand Names: U.S. TOBI®

Index Terms Tobramycin Sulfate

Pharmacologic Category Antibiotic, Aminoglycoside

Medication Safety Issues

Sound-alike/look-alike issues:

Tobramycin may be confused with Trobicin®, vancomycin

International issues:

Nebcin [Multiple international markets] may be confused with Naprosyn brand name for naproxen [U.S., Canada, and multiple international markets]; Nubain brand name for nalbuphine [Multiple international markets]

High alert medication:

The Institute for Safe Medication Practices (ISMP) includes this medication (intrathecal administration) among its list of drug classes which have a heightened risk of causing significant patient harm when used in error.

Pregnancy Risk Factor D

Lactation Enters breast milk/not recommended

Breast-Feeding Considerations Tobramycin is excreted into breast milk and breast-feeding is not recommended by the manufacturer; however, tobramycin is not well absorbed when taken orally. This limited oral absorption may minimize exposure to the nursing infant. Nondose-related effects could include modification of bowel flora.

Use Treatment of documented or suspected infections caused by susceptible gram-negative bacilli, including *Pseudomonas aeruginosa*. Tobramycin solution for inhalation and powder for inhalation (Canadian availability; not available in the U.S.) are indicated for the management of cystic fibrosis patients (>6 years of age) with *Pseudomonas aeruginosa*.

Mechanism of Action/Effect Interferes with bacterial protein synthesis, resulting in a defective bacteriocidal cell membrane

Contraindications Hypersensitivity to tobramycin, other aminoglycosides, or any component of the formulation; pregnancy

Warnings/Precautions [U.S. Boxed Warning]: Aminoglycosides may cause neurotoxicity and/or nephrotoxicity; usual risk factors include pre-existing renal impairment, concomitant neuro-/nephrotoxic medications, advanced age, and dehydration. Ototoxicity may be directly proportional to the amount of drug given and the duration of treatment; tinnitus or vertigo are indications of vestibular injury and impending hearing loss; renal damage is usually reversible. May cause neuromuscular blockade and respiratory paralysis, especially when given soon after anesthesia or muscle relaxants.

Not intended for long-term therapy due to toxic hazards associated with extended administration; use caution in pre-existing renal insufficiency, vestibular or cochlear impairment, myasthenia gravis, hypocalcemia, and conditions which depress neuromuscular transmission. Dosage modification required in patients with impaired renal function. Prolonged use may result in fungal or bacterial superinfection, including *C. difficile*-associated diarrhea (CDAD) and pseudomembranous colitis; CDAD has been observed >2 months postantibiotic treatment. Solution may contain sodium metabisulfate; use caution in patients with sulfite allergy.

Drug Interactions

Avoid Concomitant Use

Avoid concomitant use of Tobramycin (Systemic, Oral Inhalation) with any of the following: BCG; Gallium Nitrate

Decreased Effect

Tobramycin (Systemic, Oral Inhalation) may decrease the levels/effects of: BCG; Typhoid Vaccine

The levels/effects of Tobramycin (Systemic, Oral Inhalation) may be decreased by: Penicillins

Increased Effect/Toxicity

Tobramycin (Systemic, Oral Inhalation) may increase the levels/effects of: AbobotulinumtoxinA; Bisphosphonate Derivatives; CARBOplatin; Colistimethate; CycloSPORINE; CycloSPORINE (Systemic); Gallium Nitrate; Neuromuscular-Blocking Agents; OnabotulinumtoxinA; RimabotulinumtoxinB

The levels/effects of Tobramycin (Systemic, Oral Inhalation) may be increased by: Amphotericin B; Capreomycin; Cephalosporins (2nd Generation); Cephalosporins (3rd Generation); Cephalosporins (4th Generation); CISplatin; Loop Diuretics; Nonsteroidal Anti-Inflammatory Agents; Vancomycin

Adverse Reactions

Injection: Frequency not defined:

Central nervous system: Confusion, disorientation, dizziness, fever, headache, lethargy, vertigo

Dermatologic: Exfoliative dermatitis, itching, rash, urticaria

Endocrine & metabolic: Serum calcium, magnesium, potassium, and/or sodium decreased

Gastrointestinal: Diarrhea, nausea, vomiting

Hematologic: Anemia, eosinophilia, granulocytopenia, leukocytosis, leukopenia, thrombocytopenia

Hepatic: ALT increased, AST increased, bilirubin increased, LDH increased

Local: Pain at the injection site

Otic: Hearing loss, tinnitus, ototoxicity (auditory), ototoxicity (vestibular), roaring in the ears

Renal: BUN increased, cylindruria, serum creatinine increased, oliguria, proteinuria

Inhalation (as reported for solution for inhalation unless otherwise noted):

>10%:

Gastrointestinal: Sputum discoloration (21%)

Respiratory: Cough (22% [powder for inhalation]), voice alteration (13%)

1% to 10%:

Cardiovascular: Chest discomfort (3% [powder for inhalation])

Central nervous system: Malaise (6%), pyrexia (1% [powder for inhalation])

Gastrointestinal: Abnormal taste (5% [powder for inhalation]), xerostomia (2% [powder for inhalation])

Otic: Tinnitus (3%)

Respiratory: Dyspnea (4% [powder for inhalation]), oropharyngeal pain (4% [powder for inhalation]), throat irritation (3% [powder for inhalation]), FEV decreased (2% [powder for inhalation]), pulmonary function decreased (2% [powder for inhalation]), bronchospasm (1% [powder for inhalation]), upper respiratory tract infection (1% [powder for inhalation])

Available Dosage Forms

Infusion, premixed in NS: 80 mg (100 mL)

Injection, powder for reconstitution: 1.2 g

Injection, solution: 10 mg/mL (2 mL, 8 mL); 40 mg/mL (2 mL, 30 mL, 50 mL)

Solution, for nebulization [preservative free]: TOBI®: 300 mg/5 mL (56s)

General Dosage Range Dosage adjustment recommended for the I.M. and I.V. routes in patients with renal impairment

I.M.:

Infants and Children <5 years: 2.5 mg/kg every 8 hours

Children ≥5 years: 2-3.3 mg/kg every 6-8 hours

Adults: 1-2.5 mg/kg every 8-12 hours (1 mg/kg used for synergy) **or** 4-7 mg/kg/day as a single daily dose

Elderly: 1.5-5 mg/kg/day in 1-2 divided doses

I.V.:

Infants and Children <5 years: 2.5 mg/kg every 8 hours

Children ≥5 years: 2-3.3 mg/kg every 6-8 hours

Adults: 1-2.5 mg/kg every 8-12 hours (1 mg/kg/dose used for synergy) **or** 4-7 mg/kg/day as a single daily dose

Elderly: 1.5-5 mg/kg/day in 1-2 divided doses **or** 5-7 mg/kg given every 24, 36, or 48 hours based on Cl_{cr}

Inhalation: *Children ≥6 years and Adults:* 300 mg every 12 hours [TOBI®]

Administration

I.V. Infuse over 30-60 minutes.

Some penicillins (eg, carbenicillin, ticarcillin, and piperacillin) have been shown to inactivate aminoglycosides *in vitro*. This has been observed to a greater extent with tobramycin and gentamicin, while amikacin has shown greater stability against inactivation. Concurrent use of these agents may pose a risk of reduced antibacterial efficacy *in vivo*, particularly in the setting of profound renal impairment. However, definitive clinical evidence is lacking. If combination penicillin/aminoglycoside therapy is desired in a patient with renal dysfunction, separation of doses (if feasible), and routine monitoring of aminoglycoside levels, CBC, and clinical response should be considered.

I.V. Detail Flush with saline before and after administration. **Incompatible** with heparin.

pH: 3.0-6.5 (injection, adjusted); 6-8 (reconstituted solution from powder)

Inhalation

TOBI®: To be inhaled over ~15 minutes using a handheld nebulizer (PARI-LC PLUS™). If multiple different nebulizer treatments are required, administer bronchodilator first, followed by chest physiotherapy, any other nebulized medications, and then TOBI® last. Do not mix with other nebulizer medications.

TOBI® Podhaler® (Canadian availability; not available in the U.S.): Capsules should be administered by oral inhalation via Podhaler® device following manufacturer recommendations for use and handling. Capsules should not be swallowed. Patients requiring bronchodilator therapy should administer the bronchodilator 15-90 minutes prior to TOBI® Podhaler®. The sequence of chest physiotherapy and additional inhaled therapies is at the discretion of the healthcare provider however TOBI® Podhaler® should always be administered last.

Stability

Reconstitution Dilute in 50-100 mL NS, D_5W for I.V. infusion.

Storage

Injection: Stable at room temperature both as the clear, colorless solution and as the dry powder. Reconstituted solutions remain stable for 24 hours at room temperature and 96 hours when refrigerated.

Powder, for inhalation (TOBI® Podhaler®) [Canadian availability; not available in the U.S.]): Store in original package at 15°C to 30°C (59°F to 86°F). Protect from moisture.

Solution, for inhalation (TOBI®): Store under refrigeration at 2°C to 8°C (36°F to 46°F). May be stored in foil pouch at room temperature of 25°C (77°F) for up to 28 days. Avoid intense light. Solution may darken over time; however, do not use if cloudy or contains particles.

Nursing Actions

Physical Assessment Assess patient's hearing level before, during, and following therapy; report changes to prescriber immediately. Monitor for neurotoxicity (vertigo, ataxia) and opportunistic infection (fever, mouth and vaginal sores or plaques) at beginning of therapy and throughout.

Patient Education Maintain adequate hydration unless instructed to restrict fluid intake. Report decreased urine output, swelling of extremities, respiratory difficulty, vaginal itching or discharge, rash, diarrhea, oral thrush, dizziness, change in hearing acuity or ringing in ears, or worsening of condition.

Dietary Considerations May require supplementation of calcium, magnesium, potassium.

Related Information

Peak and Trough Guidelines *on page 1276*

Tolcapone (TOLE ka pone)

Brand Names: U.S. Tasmar®

Pharmacologic Category Anti-Parkinson's Agent, COMT Inhibitor

Pregnancy Risk Factor C

Lactation Excretion in breast milk unknown/not recommended

Use Adjunct to levodopa and carbidopa for the treatment of signs and symptoms of idiopathic Parkinson's disease in patients with motor fluctuations not responsive to other therapies

Mechanism of Action/Effect Tolcapone is a selective and reversible inhibitor of catechol-o-methyltransferase (COMT) which leads to more sustained blood levels of levodopa.

Contraindications Hypersensitivity to tolcapone or any component of the formulation; history of liver disease or tolcapone-induced hepatocellular injury; nontraumatic rhabdomyolysis or hyperpyrexia and confusion

Warnings/Precautions [U.S. Boxed Warning]: Due to reports of fatal liver injury associated with use of this drug, the manufacturer is advising that tolcapone be reserved for patients who are experiencing inadequate symptom control or who are not appropriate candidates for other available treatments. Patients must provide written consent acknowledging the risks of hepatic injury. Liver disease should be excluded prior to initiation; laboratory monitoring is recommended. Discontinue if signs and/or symptoms of hepatic injury are noted (eg, transaminases >2 times upper limit of normal) or if clinical improvement is not evident after 3 weeks of therapy. Use with caution in patients with pre-existing dyskinesias; exacerbation of pre-existing dyskinesia and severe rhabdomyolysis has been reported. Levodopa dosage reduction may be required, particularly in patients with levodopa dosages >600 mg daily or with moderate-to-severe dyskinesia prior to initiation.

May cause orthostatic hypotension and syncope; Parkinson's disease patients appear to have an impaired capacity to respond to a postural challenge; use with caution in patients at risk of hypotension (such as those receiving antihypertensive drugs) or where transient hypotensive episodes would be poorly tolerated (cardiovascular disease or cerebrovascular disease). Parkinson's patients being treated with dopaminergic agonists ordinarily require careful monitoring for signs and symptoms of postural hypotension, especially during dose escalation, and should be informed of this risk. May cause hallucinations, which may improve with reduction in levodopa therapy. Use with caution in patients with lower gastrointestinal disease or an increased risk of dehydration; tolcapone has been associated with delayed development of diarrhea (onset after 2-12 weeks).

Tolcapone, in conjunction with other drug therapy that alters brain biogenic amine concentrations (eg, MAO inhibitors, SSRIs), has been associated with a syndrome resembling neuroleptic malignant syndrome (hyperpyrexia and confusion - some fatal) on abrupt withdrawal or dosage reduction. Concomitant use of tolcapone and nonselective MAO inhibitors should be avoided. Selegiline is a selective MAO type B inhibitor (when given orally at ≤10 mg/day) and can be taken with tolcapone. Dopaminergic agents have been associated with compulsive behaviors and/or loss of impulse control, which has manifested as pathological gambling, libido increases (hypersexuality), and/or binge eating. Causality has not been established, and controversy exists as to whether this phenomenon is related to the underlying disease, prior behaviors/addictions and/or drug therapy. Dose reduction or discontinuation of therapy has been reported to reverse these behaviors in some, but not all cases. Risk for melanoma development is increased in Parkinson's disease patients; drug causation or factors contributing to risk have not been established. Patients should be monitored closely and periodic skin examinations should be performed. Dopaminergic agents from the ergot class have also been associated with fibrotic complications, such as retroperitoneal fibrosis, pulmonary infiltrates or effusion and pleural thickening. It is unknown whether non-ergot, pro-dopaminergic agents like tolcapone confer this risk. Use caution in patients with hepatic impairment or severe renal impairment.

Drug Interactions

Avoid Concomitant Use There are no known interactions where it is recommended to avoid concomitant use.

Decreased Effect There are no known significant interactions involving a decrease in effect.

Increased Effect/Toxicity

Tolcapone may increase the levels/effects of: Alcohol (Ethyl); CNS Depressants; COMT Substrates; MAO Inhibitors; Methotrimeprazine; Selective Serotonin Reuptake Inhibitors

The levels/effects of Tolcapone may be increased by: Droperidol; HydrOXYzine; MAO Inhibitors; Methotrimeprazine

Nutritional/Ethanol Interactions

Ethanol: May increase CNS depression; monitor for increased effects with coadministration. Caution patients about effects.

Food: Tolcapone, taken with food within 1 hour before or 2 hours after the dose, decreases bioavailability by 10% to 20%.

Avoid valerian, St John's wort, kava kava, gotu kola (may increase CNS depression).

Adverse Reactions

>10%:

Cardiovascular: Orthostatic hypotension (17%)

Central nervous system: Somnolence (14% to 32%), sleep disorder (24% to 25%), hallucinations (8% to 24%), excessive dreaming (16% to 21%), dizziness (6% to 13%), headache (10% to 11%), confusion (10% to 11%)

Gastrointestinal: Nausea (28% to 50%), diarrhea (16% to 34%; approximately 3% to 4% severe), anorexia (19% to 23%)

Neuromuscular & skeletal: Dyskinesia (42% to 51%), dystonia (19% to 22%), muscle cramps (17% to 18%)

1% to 10%:

Cardiovascular: Syncope (4% to 5%), chest pain (1% to 3%), hypotension (2%), palpitation

Central nervous system: Fatigue (3% to 7%), loss of balance (2% to 3%), agitation (1%), euphoria (1%), hyperactivity (1%), malaise (1%), panic reaction (1%), irritability (1%), mental deficiency (1%), fever (1%), depression, hypoesthesia, tremor, speech disorder, vertigo, emotional lability, hyperkinesia

Dermatologic: Alopecia (1%), bleeding (1%), tumor (1%), rash

Gastrointestinal: Vomiting (8% to 10%), constipation (6% to 8%), xerostomia (5% to 6%), abdominal pain (5% to 6%), dyspepsia (3% to 4%), flatulence (2% to 4%)

Genitourinary: UTI (5%), hematuria (4% to 5%), urine discoloration (2% to 3%), urination disorder (1% to 2%), uterine tumor (1%), incontinence, impotence

Hepatic: Transaminases increased (1% to 3%; 3 times ULN, usually with first 6 months of therapy)

Neuromuscular & skeletal: Paresthesia (1% to 3%), hyper-/hypokinesia (1% to 3%), arthritis (1% to 2%), neck pain (2%), stiffness (2%), myalgia, rhabdomyolysis

Ocular: Cataract (1%), eye inflammation (1%)

Otic: Tinnitus

Respiratory: Upper respiratory infection (5% to 7%), dyspnea (3%), sinus congestion (1% to 2%), bronchitis, pharyngitis

Miscellaneous: Diaphoresis (4% to 7%), influenza (3% to 4%), burning (1% to 2%), flank pain, injury, infection

Available Dosage Forms

Tablet, oral:

Tasmar®: 100 mg

General Dosage Range Oral: *Adults:* Initial: 100 mg 3 times/day; Maintenance: 100-200 mg 3 times/day

Administration

Oral May be administered without regard to meals. In clinical studies, the first dose of the day was administered with carbidopa/levodopa, and the subsequent doses were administered 6 hours and 12 hours later.

Stability

Storage Store at 20°C to 25°C (68°F to 77°F).

Nursing Actions

Physical Assessment May exacerbate the adverse effects of levodopa, including levodopa toxicity. Assess therapeutic response (eg, mental status and involuntary movements). Monitor for CNS depression. Monitor blood pressure.

Patient Education May be prescribed in conjunction with levodopa/carbidopa. Therapeutic effects may take several weeks or months to achieve and you may need frequent monitoring during first weeks of therapy. Best to take 2 hours before or after a meal; however, may be taken with meals if GI upset occurs. Take at the same time each day. Maintain adequate hydration unless instructed to restrict fluid intake. Do not use alcohol and prescription or OTC sedatives or CNS depressants without consulting prescriber. Urine or perspiration may appear darker. You may experience drowsiness, dizziness, confusion, vision changes, orthostatic hypotension, increased susceptibility to heat stroke, decreased perspiration, constipation, dry skin or nasal passages, nausea, vomiting, loss of appetite, or stomach discomfort. Report unresolved constipation or vomiting; chest pain or irregular heartbeat; respiratory difficulty; acute headache or dizziness; CNS changes (hallucination, loss of memory, nervousness, etc); painful or difficult urination; unusual muscle cramping or pain; yellowing of skin or eyes; easy bruising or bleeding; dry, colored stools; abdominal pain or blood in stool; increased muscle spasticity, rigidity, or involuntary movements; skin rash, persistent itching, changes in the appearance of skin moles, or other unusual skin changes; or significant worsening of condition.

Dietary Considerations May be taken without regard to meals.

Tolterodine (tole TER oh deen)

Brand Names: U.S. Detrol®; Detrol® LA

Index Terms Tolterodine Tartrate

Pharmacologic Category Anticholinergic Agent

Medication Safety Issues

Sound-alike/look-alike issues:

Tolterodine may be confused with fesoterodine

Detrol® may be confused with Ditropan

Pregnancy Risk Factor C

Lactation Excretion in breast milk unknown/not recommended

Use Treatment of patients with an overactive bladder with symptoms of urinary frequency, urgency, or urge incontinence

Mechanism of Action/Effect Antagonizes muscarinic receptors of the urinary bladder resulting in decreased bladder pressure and contraction.

Contraindications Hypersensitivity to tolterodine or fesoterodine (both are metabolized to 5-hydroxymethyl tolterodine) or any component of the formulation; urinary retention; gastric retention; uncontrolled narrow-angle glaucoma

Warnings/Precautions Cases of angioedema have been reported with oral tolterodine; some cases have occurred after a single dose. Discontinue immediately if develops. May cause drowsiness and/or blurred vision, which may impair physical or mental abilities; patients must be cautioned about performing tasks which require mental alertness (eg, operating machinery or driving). Use with caution in patients with bladder flow obstruction, may increase the risk of urinary retention. Use with caution in patients with gastrointestinal obstructive disorders (ie, pyloric stenosis), may increase the risk of gastric retention. Use with caution in patients with myasthenia gravis and controlled (treated) narrow-angle glaucoma; metabolized in the liver and excreted in the urine and feces, dosage adjustment is required for patients with renal or hepatic impairment. Tolterodine has been associated with QT_c prolongation at high (supratherapeutic) doses. The manufacturer recommends caution in patients with congenital prolonged QT or in patients receiving concurrent therapy with QT_c-prolonging drugs (class Ia or III antiarrhythmics). However, the mean change in QT_c even at supratherapeutic dosages was less than 15 msec. Individuals who are CYP2D6 poor metabolizers or in the presence of inhibitors of CYP2D6 and CYP3A4 may be more likely to exhibit prolongation. Dosage adjustment is recommended in patients receiving CYP3A4 inhibitors (a lower dose of tolterodine is recommended).

Drug Interactions

Avoid Concomitant Use There are no known interactions where it is recommended to avoid concomitant use.

Decreased Effect

Tolterodine may decrease the levels/effects of: Acetylcholinesterase Inhibitors (Central); Secretin

The levels/effects of Tolterodine may be decreased by: Acetylcholinesterase Inhibitors (Central); CYP3A4 Inducers (Strong); Deferasirox; Herbs (CYP3A4 Inducers); Peginterferon Alfa-2b; Tocilizumab

Increased Effect/Toxicity

Tolterodine may increase the levels/effects of: AbobotulinumtoxinA; Anticholinergics; Cannabinoids; OnabotulinumtoxinA; Potassium Chloride; RimabotulinumtoxinB; Warfarin

The levels/effects of Tolterodine may be increased by: Abiraterone Acetate; Antifungal Agents (Azole Derivatives, Systemic); CYP2D6 Inhibitors (Moderate); CYP2D6 Inhibitors (Strong); CYP3A4 Inhibitors (Moderate); CYP3A4 Inhibitors (Strong); Dasatinib; Fluconazole; Ivacaftor; Pramlintide; VinBLAStine

Nutritional/Ethanol Interactions
Food: Increases bioavailability (~53% increase) of tolterodine tablets (dose adjustment not necessary); does not affect the pharmacokinetics of tolterodine extended release capsules. As a CYP3A4 inhibitor, grapefruit juice may increase the serum level and/or toxicity of tolterodine, but unlikely secondary to high oral bioavailability.
Herb/Nutraceutical: St John's wort (*Hypericum*) appears to induce CYP3A enzymes.

Adverse Reactions As reported with immediate release tablet, unless otherwise specified
>10%: Gastrointestinal: Dry mouth (35%; extended release capsules 23%)
1% to 10%:
Cardiovascular: Chest pain (2%)
Central nervous system: Headache (7%; extended release capsules 6%), somnolence (3%; extended release capsules 3%), fatigue (4%; extended release capsules 2%), dizziness (5%; extended release capsules 2%), anxiety (extended release capsules 1%)
Dermatologic: Dry skin (1%)
Gastrointestinal: Abdominal pain (5%; extended release capsules 4%), constipation (7%; extended release capsules 6%), dyspepsia (4%; extended release capsules 3%), diarrhea (4%), weight gain (1%)
Genitourinary: Dysuria (2%; extended release capsules 1%)
Neuromuscular & skeletal: Arthralgia (2%)
Ocular: Abnormal vision (2%; extended release capsules 1%), dry eyes (3%; extended release capsules 3%)
Respiratory: Bronchitis (2%), sinusitis (extended release capsules 2%)
Miscellaneous: Flu-like syndrome (3%), infection (1%)

Available Dosage Forms
Capsule, extended release, oral:
Detrol® LA: 2 mg, 4 mg
Tablet, oral:
Detrol®: 1 mg, 2 mg

General Dosage Range Dosage adjustment recommended in patients with hepatic or renal impairment and on concomitant therapy
Oral: *Adults:* Extended release: 2-4 mg once daily; Immediate release: 1-2 mg twice daily

Administration
Oral Extended release capsule: Swallow whole; do not crush, chew, or open

Stability
Storage Store at 25°C (77°F); excursions permitted to 15°C to 30°C (59°F to 86°F). Protect from light.

Nursing Actions
Patient Education Take as directed. Do not break, crush, or chew extended release medication. May cause headache, dry mouth, dizziness, nervousness, sleepiness, abdominal discomfort, diarrhea, constipation, nausea, or vomiting. Report back pain, muscle spasms, alteration in gait, or numbness of extremities; unresolved or persistent constipation, diarrhea, or vomiting; or symptoms of upper respiratory infection or flu. Report immediately any chest pain or palpitations, difficulty urinating, or pain on urination.

Tolvaptan (tol VAP tan)

Brand Names: U.S. Samsca™
Index Terms OPC-41061
Pharmacologic Category Vasopressin Antagonist
Medication Guide Available Yes
Pregnancy Risk Factor C
Lactation Excretion in breast milk unknown/not recommended
Use Treatment of clinically significant hypervolemic or euvolemic hyponatremia (associated with heart failure, cirrhosis, or SIADH) with either a serum sodium <125 mEq/L or less marked hyponatremia that is symptomatic and resistant to fluid restriction
Mechanism of Action/Effect Tolvaptan blocks the antidiuretic action of arginine vasopressin in the kidney, leading to the excretion of free water without loss of serum sodium.
Contraindications Hypovolemic hyponatremia; urgent need to raise serum sodium acutely; use in patients unable to sense or appropriately respond to thirst; anuria; concurrent use with strong CYP3A inhibitors (eg, ketoconazole, itraconazole, ritonavir, indinavir, nelfinavir, saquinavir, nefazodone, telithromycin, clarithromycin)

Canadian labeling: Additional contraindications (not in U.S. labeling): Hypersensitivity to tolvaptan or any component of the formulation

Warnings/Precautions [U.S. Boxed Warning]: Tolvaptan should be initiated and reinitiated in patients only in a hospital where serum sodium can be closely monitored. Too rapid correction of hyponatremia (ie, >12 mEq/L/24 hours) can cause osmotic demyelination resulting in dysarthria, mutism, dysphagia, lethargy, affective changes, spastic quadriparesis, seizures, coma, and death. In susceptible patients (including those with severe malnutrition, alcoholism, or advanced liver disease), slower rates of correction may be advisable. Patients with SIADH or very low baseline serum sodium concentrations may be at greater risk of overly-rapid correction.

Interrupt or discontinue therapy in patients who develop medically significant signs or symptoms of hypovolemia. Patients should ingest fluids in response to thirst. Gastrointestinal bleeding can occur in patients with cirrhosis; use only if the need to treat outweighs the risk. Reductions in extracellular fluid volumes may cause hyperkalemia. Patients with a pretreatment serum potassium >5 mEq/L should be monitored after initiation of therapy.

Use in patients with creatinine clearance <10 mL/minute has not been studied. Do not use in anuric patients. Use with hypertonic saline is not recommended. Use contraindicated in patients taking strong CYP3A inhibitors; avoid use in patients taking moderate CYP3A4 inhibitors. If possible, avoid use with CYP3A4 inducers; if administered with CYP3A4 inducers, dose increases may be necessary. Dose reductions may be necessary if administered with P-gp inhibitors. Consider alternative agents that avoid or lessen the potential for CYP- or P-gp mediated interactions. Patients receiving medications known to increase potassium should be monitored for hyperkalemia.

Monitor closely for rate of serum sodium increase and neurological status; rapid serum sodium correction (>12 mEq/L/24 hours) can lead to permanent neurological damage. Discontinue use if rate of serum sodium increase is undesirable; fluid restriction during the first 24 hours of sodium correction can increase the risk of overly-rapid correction and should generally be avoided; not intended for urgent correction of serum sodium to prevent or treat serious neurologic symptoms; it has not been demonstrated that raising serum sodium with tolvaptan provides a symptomatic benefit.

Drug Interactions

Avoid Concomitant Use

Avoid concomitant use of Tolvaptan with any of the following: CYP3A4 Inducers (Strong); CYP3A4 Inhibitors (Moderate); CYP3A4 Inhibitors (Strong); Pimozide; Sodium Chloride

Decreased Effect

The levels/effects of Tolvaptan may be decreased by: CYP3A4 Inducers (Strong); Deferasirox; P-glycoprotein/ABCB1 Inducers; Tocilizumab

Increased Effect/Toxicity

Tolvaptan may increase the levels/effects of: ACE Inhibitors; Angiotensin II Receptor Blockers; ARIPiprazole; Digoxin; Pimozide; Potassium-Sparing Diuretics

The levels/effects of Tolvaptan may be increased by: CYP3A4 Inhibitors (Moderate); CYP3A4 Inhibitors (Strong); Dasatinib; P-glycoprotein/ABCB1 Inhibitors; Sodium Chloride

Nutritional/Ethanol Interactions

Food: Tolvaptan exposure may be doubled when taken with grapefruit juice. Management: Avoid grapefruit juice.

Herb/Nutraceutical: St John's wort may decrease tolvaptan serum concentrations. Management: Avoid St John's wort.

Adverse Reactions

>10%:

Gastrointestinal: Nausea (21%), xerostomia (7% to 13%)

Renal: Pollakiuria (4% to 11%), polyuria (4% to 11%)

Miscellaneous: Thirst (12% to 16%)

2% to 10%:

Central nervous system: Pyrexia (4%)

Endocrine & metabolic: Hyperglycemia (6%)

Gastrointestinal: Constipation (7%), anorexia (4%)

Neuromuscular & skeletal: Weakness (9%)

Pharmacodynamics/Kinetics

Onset of Action 2-4 hour; Peak effect: 4-8 hours

Duration of Action 60% peak serum sodium elevation is retained at 24 hours; urinary excretion of free water is no longer elevated

Available Dosage Forms

Tablet, oral:

Samsca™: 15 mg, 30 mg

General Dosage Range Oral: *Adults:* 15-60 mg once daily

Administration

Oral Treatment should be initiated or reinitiated in a hospital. May be administered without regards to meals.

Stability

Storage Store at 25°C (77°F); excursions permitted between 15°C and 30°C (59°F and 86°F).

Nursing Actions

Physical Assessment Therapy should be initiated (or reinitiated) in hospital. Monitor serum sodium and neurological status at beginning of therapy and on a regular basis throughout. Teach patient importance of adequate fluid intake.

Patient Education May be taken with or without food. Do not drink grapefruit juice while being treated; may cause dangerous increase in levels of tolvaptan. Follow directions for fluid intake. Report vomiting or diarrhea or if you cannot drink normally, dizziness, unusual weakness, or change in thinking.

Dietary Considerations May be taken without regards to meals. Avoid grapefruit juice.

Topiramate (toe PYRE a mate)

Brand Names: U.S. Topamax®

Pharmacologic Category Anticonvulsant, Miscellaneous

Medication Safety Issues

Sound-alike/look-alike issues:

Topamax® may be confused with Sporanox®, TEGretol®, TEGretol®-XR, Toprol-XL®

Medication Guide Available Yes

Pregnancy Risk Factor D

Lactation Enters breast milk/use caution

Breast-Feeding Considerations Based on limited data, topiramate was found in breast milk. Infant plasma concentrations of topiramate have been reported as 10% to 20% of the maternal plasma concentration.

Use Monotherapy or adjunctive therapy for partial onset seizures and primary generalized tonic-clonic seizures; adjunctive treatment of seizures associated with Lennox-Gastaut syndrome; prophylaxis of migraine headache

Unlabeled Use Diabetic neuropathy, infantile spasms, neuropathic pain; prophylaxis of cluster headache

Mechanism of Action/Effect Anticonvulsant activity may be due to a combination of potential mechanisms: Blocks neuronal voltage-dependent sodium channels, enhances GABA(A) activity, antagonizes AMPA/kainate glutamate receptors, and weakly inhibits carbonic anhydrase.

Contraindications There are no contraindications listed in the manufacturers' labeling.

Canadian labeling (not in U.S. labeling): Hypersensitivity to topiramate or any component of the formulation or container; pregnancy and women in childbearing years not using effective contraception (migraine prophylaxis only)

Warnings/Precautions Antiepileptics are associated with an increased risk of suicidal behavior/thoughts with use (regardless of indication); patients should be monitored for signs/symptoms of depression, suicidal tendencies, and other unusual behavior changes during therapy and instructed to inform their healthcare provider immediately if symptoms occur. Use with caution in patients with hepatic, respiratory, or renal impairment. Topiramate may decrease serum bicarbonate concentrations (up to 67% of patients); treatment-emergent metabolic acidosis is less common. Risk may be increased in patients with a predisposing condition (organ dysfunction, ketogenic diet, or concurrent treatment with other drugs which may cause acidosis). Metabolic acidosis may occur at dosages as low as 50 mg/day. Monitor serum bicarbonate as well as potential complications of chronic acidosis (nephrolithiasis, osteomalacia, and reduced growth rates in children). Kidney stones have been reported in both children and adults; the risk of kidney stones is about 2-4 times that of the untreated population; the risk of this event may be reduced by increasing fluid intake.

Cognitive dysfunction, psychiatric disturbances (mood disorders), and sedation (somnolence or fatigue) may occur with topiramate use; incidence may be related to rapid titration and higher doses. Patients must be cautioned about performing tasks which require mental alertness (eg, operating machinery or driving). Topiramate may also cause paresthesia, dizziness, and ataxia. Topiramate has been associated with acute myopia and secondary angle-closure glaucoma in adults and children, typically within 1 month of initiation; discontinue in patients with acute onset of decreased visual acuity or ocular pain. Hyperammonemia with or without encephalopathy may occur with or without concomitant valproate administration; valproic acid dose-dependency was observed in limited pediatric studies; use with caution in patients with inborn errors of metabolism or decreased hepatic mitochondrial activity. Hypothermia (core body temperature <35°C [95°F]) has been reported with concomitant use of topiramate and valproic acid; may occur with or without associated hyperammonemia and may develop after topiramate initiation or dosage increase; discontinuation of topiramate or valproic acid may be necessary. Topiramate may be associated (rarely) with severe oligohydrosis and hyperthermia, most frequently in children; use caution and monitor closely during strenuous exercise, during exposure to high environmental temperature, or in patients receiving receiving other carbonic anhydrase inhibitors and drugs with anticholinergic activity. Concurrent use of topiramate and hydrochlorothiazide may increase the risk for hypokalemia; monitor potassium closely.

Avoid abrupt withdrawal of topiramate therapy, it should be withdrawn/tapered slowly to minimize the potential of increased seizure frequency. Doses were also gradually withdrawn in migraine prophylaxis studies. Effects with other sedative drugs or ethanol may be potentiated. Safety and efficacy have not been established in children <2 years of age for treatment of seizures. In pediatric patients, weight loss may occur most often early in therapy; in clinical trials of at least 1 year, the majority of patients with weight loss had a resumption of weight gain within the study period. Safety and efficacy have not been established in children for migraine prophylaxis.

Drug Interactions

Avoid Concomitant Use

Avoid concomitant use of Topiramate with any of the following: Axitinib; Carbonic Anhydrase Inhibitors

Decreased Effect

Topiramate may decrease the levels/effects of: ARIPiprazole; Axitinib; Contraceptives (Estrogens); Contraceptives (Progestins); Lithium; Methenamine; Primidone; Saxagliptin

The levels/effects of Topiramate may be decreased by: CarBAMazepine; Fosphenytoin; Ketorolac; Ketorolac (Nasal); Ketorolac (Systemic); Mefloquine; Phenytoin

Increased Effect/Toxicity

Topiramate may increase the levels/effects of: Alcohol (Ethyl); Alpha-/Beta-Agonists; Amphetamines; Anticonvulsants (Barbiturate); Anticonvulsants (Hydantoin); CarBAMazepine; Carbonic Anhydrase Inhibitors; CNS Depressants; Flecainide; Fosphenytoin; Lithium; Memantine; MetFORMIN; Methotrimeprazine; Phenytoin; Primidone; QuiNIDine; Selective Serotonin Reuptake Inhibitors; Valproic Acid

The levels/effects of Topiramate may be increased by: Divalproex; Droperidol; HydrOXYzine; Methotrimeprazine; Salicylates; Thiazide Diuretics

Nutritional/Ethanol Interactions

Ethanol: May increase CNS depression; monitor for increased effects with coadministration. Caution patients about effects.

Food: Ketogenic diet may increase the possibility of acidosis and/or kidney stones.

Herb/Nutraceutical: Avoid evening primrose (seizure threshold decreased).

Adverse Reactions Adverse events are reported for placebo-controlled trials of adjunctive therapy in adult and pediatric patients. Unless otherwise noted, the percentages refer to incidence in epilepsy trials. **Note:** A wide range of dosages were studied; incidence of adverse events was frequently lower in the pediatric population studied.

>10%:

Central nervous system: Somnolence (15% to 29%), dizziness (4% to 25%; dose dependent), fatigue (9% to 16%; dose-dependent), nervousness (9% to 18%), ataxia (6% to 16%), psychomotor slowing (3% to 13%; dose dependent), speech problems (2% to 13%), memory difficulties (2% to 12%), behavior problems (children 11%), confusion (4% to 11%)

Endocrine & metabolic: Serum bicarbonate decreased (dose related: 7% to 67%; marked reductions [to <17 mEq/L] 1% to 11%)

Gastrointestinal: Anorexia (4% to 24%; dose dependent), nausea (6% to 10%; migraine trial: 9% to 14%)

Neuromuscular & skeletal: Paresthesia (1% to 11%; migraine trial: 35% to 51%)

Ocular: Abnormal vision (2% to 13%)

Respiratory: Upper respiratory infection (migraine trial: 12% to 14%)

Miscellaneous: Injury (14%)

1% to 10%:

Cardiovascular: Chest pain (2% to 4%), edema (2%), hypertension (1% to 2%), bradycardia (1%), pallor (1%), syncope (1%)

Central nervous system: Difficulty concentrating (5% to 10%), aggressive reactions (2% to 9%), depression (5% to 9%; dose dependent, insomnia (4% to 8%), mood problems (≤6%), abnormal coordination (4%), agitation (3%), cognitive problems (3%), emotional lability (3%), anxiety (2% to 3%; dose dependent), hypoesthesia (2%; migraine trial: 6% to 8%), stupor (2%), vertigo (2%), fever (migraine trial: 1% to 2%), apathy (1%), hallucination (1%), neurosis (1%), psychosis (1%), seizure (1%), suicide attempt (1%)

Dermatologic: Pruritus (migraine trial: 2% to 4%), skin disorder (2% to 3%), alopecia (2%), dermatitis (2%), hypertrichosis (2%), rash erythematous (1% to 2%), eczema (1%), seborrhea (1%), skin discoloration (1%)

Endocrine & metabolic: Breast pain (4%), hot flashes (1% to 2%), libido decreased (<1% to 2%), menstrual irregularities (1% to 2%), hypoglycemia (1%), metabolic acidosis (hyperchloremia, nonanion gap)

Gastrointestinal: Weight loss (4% to 9%), dyspepsia (2% to 7%), abdominal pain (5% to 6%), salivation increased (6%), constipation (4% to 5%), gastroenteritis (2% to 3%), vomiting (migraine trial: 1% to 3%), diarrhea (2%; migraine trial: 9% to 11%), dysgeusia (2%; migraine trial: 8% to 15%), xerostomia (2%), loss of taste (migraine trial: ≤2%), appetite increased (1%), dysphagia (1%), fecal incontinence (1%), flatulence (1%), GERD (1%), gingivitis (1%), glossitis (1%), gum hyperplasia (1%), weight gain (1%)

Genitourinary: Incontinence (2% to 4%), UTI (2%), premature ejaculation (migraine trial: ≤3%), cystitis (2%), leukorrhea (2%), impotence (1%), nocturia (1%)

Hematologic: Purpura (8%), leukopenia (2%), anemia (1%), hematoma (1%), prothrombin time increased (1%), thrombocytopenia (1%)

Neuromuscular & skeletal: Tremor (3% to 9%), gait abnormal (3% to 8%), arthralgia (migraine trial: 1% to 7%), weakness (6%), hyperkinesia (5%), back pain (1% to 5%), involuntary muscle contractions (2%; migraine trial: 2% to 4%), leg cramps (2%), leg pain (2%), myalgia (2%), hyporeflexia (2%), rigors (1%), skeletal pain (1%)

Ocular: Diplopia (1% to 10%), nystagmus (10%), conjunctivitis (1%), lacrimation abnormal (1%), myopia (1%)

Otic: Hearing decreased (2%), tinnitus (2%), otitis media (migraine trial: 1% to 2%)

Renal: Hematuria (2%), renal calculus (migraine trial ≤2%)

Respiratory: Rhinitis (4% to 7%), pharyngitis (6%), sinusitis (5%; migraine trial: 6% to 10%), pneumonia (5%), epistaxis (2% to 4%), cough (migraine trial: 2% to 4%), bronchitis (migraine trial: 3%), dyspnea (migraine trial: 1% to 3%)

Miscellaneous: Viral infection (2% to 7%: migraine trial: 3% to 4%), flu-like syndrome (3%), allergy (2%), infection (2%), thirst (2%), body odor (1%), diaphoresis (1%), moniliasis (1%)

Available Dosage Forms

Capsule, sprinkle, oral: 15 mg, 25 mg

Topamax®: 15 mg, 25 mg

Tablet, oral: 25 mg, 50 mg, 100 mg, 200 mg

Topamax®: 25 mg, 50 mg, 100 mg, 200 mg

General Dosage Range Dosage adjustment recommended in patients with renal impairment

Oral:

Children 2-9 years: Initial: 25 mg once daily **or** 1-3 mg/kg/day; Maintenance: 150-400 mg/day in 2 divided doses **or** 5-9 mg/kg/day in 2 divided doses

Children 10-16 years: Initial: 25 mg once or twice daily **or** 1-3 mg/kg/day; Maintenance: 5-9 mg/kg/day in 2 divided doses **or** 25-200 mg twice daily

Children ≥17 years: Initial: 25 mg once or twice daily; Maintenance: 100-200 mg twice daily

Adults: Initial: 25-50 mg/day in 1-2 divided doses; Maintenance: 50-200 mg twice daily

Administration

Oral May be administered without regard to meals

Capsule sprinkles: May be swallowed whole or opened to sprinkle the contents on a small amount (~1 teaspoon) of soft food (drug/food mixture should not be chewed; swallow immediately).

Tablet: Because of bitter taste, tablets should not be broken or chewed.

Stability

Storage Store at room temperature of 15°C to 30°C (59°F to 86°F). Protect from moisture.

Nursing Actions

Physical Assessment Monitor therapeutic response (seizure activity, force, type, duration) at beginning of therapy and throughout. Use and teach seizure/safety precautions. May cause weight loss; monitor weight periodically.

Patient Education While using this medication, do not use alcohol. Maintain adequate hydration, unless instructed to restrict fluid intake, to prevent the development of kidney stones and dehydration. You may be at risk for decreased sweating and increased body temperature, especially in hot weather. You may experience drowsiness, dizziness, disturbed concentration, memory changes, blurred vision, mouth sores, nausea, vomiting, or loss of appetite. Wear identification of epileptic status and medications. Report behavioral or CNS changes, suicide ideation, depression, skin rash, muscle cramping, numbness in extremities, weakness, tremors, changes in gait, chest pain, irregular heartbeat, palpitations, hearing loss, cough, respiratory difficulty, or worsening of seizure activity or loss of seizure control. Seek immediate medical evaluation if you experience sudden vision changes, periorbital pain, flank pain, or blood in urine.

Topotecan (toe poe TEE kan)

Brand Names: U.S. Hycamtin®

Index Terms Hycamptamine; SKF 104864; SKF 104864-A; Topotecan Hydrochloride

Pharmacologic Category Antineoplastic Agent, Camptothecin; Antineoplastic Agent, Natural Source (Plant) Derivative; Antineoplastic Agent, Topoisomerase I Inhibitor

Medication Safety Issues

Sound-alike/look-alike issues:

Hycamtin® may be confused with Mycamine®

Topotecan may be confused with irinotecan

High alert medication:

This medication is in a class the Institute for Safe Medication Practices (ISMP) includes among its list of drug classes which have a heightened risk of causing significant patient harm when used in error.

Pregnancy Risk Factor D

Lactation Excretion in breast milk unknown/contraindicated

Breast-Feeding Considerations Breast-feeding should be discontinued in women who are receiving topotecan.

Use Treatment of metastatic ovarian cancer, relapsed or refractory small cell lung cancer, recurrent or resistant (stage IVB) cervical cancer (in combination with cisplatin)

Unlabeled Use Treatment of central nervous system lesions (metastatic from lung cancer), central nervous system lymphoma (primary), Ewing's sarcoma, rhabdomyosarcoma (pediatrics), neuroblastoma (pediatrics)

Mechanism of Action/Effect Binds to topoisomerase I and stabilizes the cleavable complex so that religation of the cleaved DNA strand cannot occur. This results in the accumulation of cleavable complexes and single-strand DNA breaks. Topotecan acts in S phase of the cell cycle.

Contraindications Hypersensitivity to topotecan or any component of the formulation; severe bone marrow depression; pregnancy; breast-feeding

Canadian labeling: Additional contraindications (not in U.S. labeling): Severe renal impairment (Cl_{cr} <20 mL/minute)

Warnings/Precautions Hazardous agent - use appropriate precautions for handling and disposal. **[U.S. Boxed Warning]: May cause neutropenia, which may be severe or lead to infection or fatalities. Monitor blood counts frequently. Do NOT administer to patients with baseline neutrophils <1500/mm^3 and platelets <100,000/mm^3.** The dose-limiting toxicity is bone marrow suppression (primarily neutropenia); may also cause thrombocytopenia and anemia. Neutropenia is not cumulative overtime. In a clinical study comparing I.V. to oral topotecan, G-CSF support was administered in a higher percentage of patients receiving oral topotecan (Eckerd, 2007). Topotecan-induced neutropenia may lead to neutropenic colitis (including fatalities); should be considered in patients presenting with neutropenia, fever and abdominal pain.

Diarrhea has been reported with oral topotecan; may be severe (requiring hospitalization); incidence may be higher in the elderly; educate patients on early recognition and proper management, including diet changes, increase in fluid intake, antidiarrheals, and antibiotics. Interstitial lung disease (ILD) (with fatalities) has been reported; discontinue use in patients with confirmed ILD; risk factors for ILD include a history of ILD, pulmonary fibrosis, lung cancer, thoracic radiation, and the use of colony-stimulating factors or medication with pulmonary toxicity; monitor pulmonary symptoms (cough, fever, dyspnea, and/or hypoxia) and discontinue if ILD is diagnosed. Use caution in renal impairment; may require dose adjustment (use in severe renal impairment is contraindicated in the Canadian labeling).

Drug Interactions

Avoid Concomitant Use

Avoid concomitant use of Topotecan with any of the following: BCG; CloZAPine; Natalizumab; P-glycoprotein/ABCB1 Inhibitors; Pimecrolimus; Tacrolimus (Topical); Vaccines (Live)

Decreased Effect

Topotecan may decrease the levels/effects of: BCG; Coccidioidin Skin Test; Sipuleucel-T; Vaccines (Inactivated); Vaccines (Live)

The levels/effects of Topotecan may be decreased by: Echinacea

Increased Effect/Toxicity

Topotecan may increase the levels/effects of: CloZAPine; Leflunomide; Natalizumab; Vaccines (Live)

The levels/effects of Topotecan may be increased by: BCRP/ABCG2 Inhibitors; Denosumab; Filgrastim; P-glycoprotein/ABCB1 Inhibitors; Pimecrolimus; Platinum Derivatives; Roflumilast; Tacrolimus (Topical); Trastuzumab

Nutritional/Ethanol Interactions Ethanol: Avoid ethanol (due to GI irritation).

Adverse Reactions

>10%:

Central nervous system: Fatigue (6% to 29%), fever (5% to 28%), pain (5% to 23%), headache (18%)

Dermatologic: Alopecia (10% to 49%), rash (16%)

Gastrointestinal: Nausea (8% to 64%), vomiting (10% to 45%), diarrhea (6% to 32%; Oral: grade 3: 4%; grade 4: ≤1%; onset: 9 days), constipation (5% to 29%), abdominal pain (5% to 22%), anorexia (7% to 19%), stomatitis (18%)

Hematologic: Anemia (89% to 98%; grade 4: 7% to 37%; nadir: 15 days), neutropenia (83% to 97%; grade 4: 32% to 80%; nadir 12-15 days; duration: 7 days), leukopenia (86% to 97%; grade 4: 15% to 32%), thrombocytopenia (69% to 81%; grade 4: 6% to 27%; nadir: 15 days; duration: 3-5 days), neutropenic fever/sepsis (2% to 43%)

Neuromuscular & skeletal: Weakness (3% to 25%)

Respiratory: Dyspnea (6% to 22%), cough (15%)

1% to 10%:

Gastrointestinal: Obstruction (5%)

Hepatic: Liver enzymes increased (transient; 8%; grades 3/4: 4%), bilirubin increased (grades 3/4: <2%)

Neuromuscular & skeletal: Paresthesia (7%)

Respiratory: Pneumonia (8%)

Miscellaneous: Sepsis (grades 3/4: 5%)

Available Dosage Forms

Capsule, oral:

Hycamtin®: 0.25 mg, 1 mg

Injection, powder for reconstitution: 4 mg

Hycamtin®: 4 mg

Injection, solution: 1 mg/mL (4 mL)

General Dosage Range Dosage adjustment recommended in patients with renal impairment or who develop toxicities

Oral: *Adults:* 2.3 mg/m^2/day for 5 days; repeated every 21 days

I.V.: *Adults:* IVPB: 1.5 mg/m^2/day for 5 days; repeated every 21 days **or** 0.75 mg/m^2/day for 3 days; repeated every 21 days

Administration

Oral Administer without regard to meals. Swallow whole; do not crush, chew, or divide capsule. If vomiting occurs after dose, do not take replacement dose.

I.V. Administer IVPB over 30 minutes. For combination chemotherapy with cisplatin, administer pretreatment hydration.

Stability

Reconstitution Reconstitute lyophilized powder with 4 mL SWFI. Further dilute in 50-100 mL D_5W or NS for infusion.

Storage

I.V.:

Solution for injection: Store intact vials at 2°C to 8°C (36°F to 45°F). Protect from light. Single-use vials should be discarded after initial vial entry; solutions for infusion are stable for 24 hours at room temperature after diluted.

Lyophilized powder: Store intact vials at room temperature of 20°C to 25°C (68°F to 77°F). Protect from light. Reconstituted solution is stable for up to 28 days at room temperature of 20°C to 25°C (68°F to 77°F), although the manufacturer recommends use immediately after reconstitution. Further dilute in 50-100 mL D_5W or NS. This solution is stable for 24 hours at room temperature (manufacturer recommendation) or up to 7 days under refrigeration (Craig, 1997).

Oral: Store at 2°C to 8°C (36°F to 46°F). Protect from light.

Nursing Actions

Physical Assessment Evaluate renal function (I & O, edema) and monitor for signs of myelosuppression, gastrointestinal disturbance (nausea, vomiting, diarrhea, pain), and dyspnea prior to each infusion and on a regular basis with oral formulation.

Patient Education If this drug is administered by intravenous infusion, report immediately any burning, pain, redness, or swelling at infusion site; sudden chest pain; difficulty breathing or swallowing; or chills. Oral form may be taken with or without food. Swallow whole; do not crush, chew, or divide capsule. If vomiting occurs after dose, do not take replacement dose; take next dose at scheduled time. Maintain adequate hydration (3-4 L/day of fluids) unless instructed to restrict fluid intake during therapy. Maintain good oral hygiene. You will be more susceptible to infection. May cause nausea, vomiting, diarrhea, or hair loss (will regrow after treatment is completed). Report unresolved diarrhea, nausea, vomiting, or unusual abdominal pain; alterations in urinary pattern (increased or decreased); opportunistic infection (fever, chills, unusual bruising or bleeding, fatigue, purulent vaginal discharge, unhealed mouth sores); chest pain; respiratory difficulty; or unexplained weakness or fatigue.

Dietary Considerations May be taken without regard to meals.

Related Information

Management of Drug Extravasations *on page 1269*

Toremifene (tore EM i feen)

Brand Names: U.S. Fareston®

Index Terms FC1157a; Toremifene Citrate

Pharmacologic Category Antineoplastic Agent, Estrogen Receptor Antagonist; Selective Estrogen Receptor Modulator (SERM)

Pregnancy Risk Factor D

Lactation Excretion in breast milk unknown/not recommended

Use Treatment of metastatic breast cancer in postmenopausal women with estrogen receptor positive or estrogen receptor status unknown

Unlabeled Use Treatment of soft tissue sarcoma (desmoid tumors)

Available Dosage Forms

Tablet, oral:

Fareston®: 60 mg

General Dosage Range Oral: *Adults:* 60 mg once daily

Administration

Oral Administer orally, as a single daily dose, with or without food.

Nursing Actions

Physical Assessment Monitor for thromboembolism, MI, edema, hypercalcemia, endometriosis, nausea, vomiting, and vision changes.

Patient Education Take without regard to food. You may experience an initial "flare" of this disease (eg, increased bone pain and hot flashes), which will subside with continued use. May cause nausea, vomiting, loss of appetite, or dizziness. Report vomiting that occurs immediately after taking medication; chest pain, palpitations, or swollen extremities; vaginal bleeding, hot flashes, or excessive perspiration; chest pain, unusual coughing, or respiratory difficulty; or any vision changes or dry eyes.

Torsemide (TORE se mide)

Brand Names: U.S. Demadex®

Pharmacologic Category Diuretic, Loop

Medication Safety Issues

Sound-alike/look-alike issues:

Torsemide may be confused with furosemide

Demadex® may be confused with Denorex®

Pregnancy Risk Factor B

Lactation Excretion in breast milk unknown/use caution

Use Management of edema associated with heart failure and hepatic or renal disease (including chronic renal failure); treatment of hypertension

Mechanism of Action/Effect Inhibits reabsorption of sodium and chloride in the ascending loop of Henle and distal renal tubule, interfering with the chloride-binding cotransport system, thus causing increased excretion of water, sodium, chloride, magnesium, and calcium; does not alter GFR, renal plasma flow, or acid-base balance

Contraindications Hypersensitivity to torsemide, any component of the formulation, or any sulfonylurea; anuria

Warnings/Precautions Loop diuretics are potent diuretics; excess amounts can lead to profound diuresis with fluid and electrolyte loss; close medical supervision and dose evaluation are required. Potassium supplementation and/or use of potassium-sparing diuretics may be necessary to prevent hypokalemia. Use with caution in patients with cirrhosis; avoid sudden changes in fluid and electrolyte balance and acid/base status which may lead to hepatic encephalopathy. Administration with an aldosterone antagonist or potassium-sparing diuretic may provide additional diuretic efficacy and maintain normokalemia. Coadministration of antihypertensives may increase the risk of hypotension.

Monitor fluid status and renal function in an attempt to prevent oliguria, azotemia, and reversible increases in BUN and creatinine; close medical supervision of aggressive diuresis required. Ototoxicity has been demonstrated following oral administration of torsemide and following rapid I.V. administration of other loop diuretics. Other possible risk factors may include use in renal impairment, excessive doses, and concurrent use of other ototoxins (eg, aminoglycosides).

Chemical similarities are present among sulfonamides, sulfonylureas, carbonic anhydrase inhibitors, thiazides, and loop diuretics (except ethacrynic acid). Use in patients with sulfonylurea allergy is specifically contraindicated in product labeling; a risk of cross-reaction exists in patients with allergy to any of these compounds; avoid use when previous reaction has been severe. Discontinue if signs of hypersensitivity are noted.

Drug Interactions

Avoid Concomitant Use There are no known interactions where it is recommended to avoid concomitant use.

Decreased Effect

Torsemide may decrease the levels/effects of: Lithium; Neuromuscular-Blocking Agents

The levels/effects of Torsemide may be decreased by: Bile Acid Sequestrants; CYP2C9 Inducers (Strong); Fosphenytoin; Herbs (Hypertensive Properties); Methotrexate; Methylphenidate; Nonsteroidal Anti-Inflammatory Agents; Peginterferon Alfa-2b; Phenytoin; Probenecid; Salicylates; Yohimbine

Increased Effect/Toxicity

Torsemide may increase the levels/effects of: ACE Inhibitors; Allopurinol; Amifostine; Aminoglycosides; Antihypertensives; Cardiac Glycosides; CISplatin; Dofetilide; Hypotensive Agents; Lithium; Methotrexate; Neuromuscular-Blocking Agents; RisperiDONE; RiTUXimab; Salicylates; Sodium Phosphates; Warfarin

The levels/effects of Torsemide may be increased by: Alfuzosin; Beta2-Agonists; Corticosteroids (Orally Inhaled); Corticosteroids (Systemic); CycloSPORINE (Systemic); CYP2C9 Inhibitors (Moderate); CYP2C9 Inhibitors (Strong); Diazoxide; Eltrombopag; Herbs (Hypotensive Properties); Licorice; MAO Inhibitors; Methotrexate; Pentoxifylline; Phosphodiesterase 5 Inhibitors; Probenecid; Prostacyclin Analogues

Nutritional/Ethanol Interactions Herb/Nutraceutical: Avoid herbs with *hypertensive* properties (bayberry, blue cohosh, cayenne, ephedra, ginger, ginseng [American], kola, licorice); may diminish the antihypertensive effect of torsemide. Avoid herbs with *hypotensive* properties (black cohosh, California poppy, coleus, golden seal, hawthorn, mistletoe, periwinkle, quinine, shepherd's purse); may enhance the hypotensive effect of torsemide.

Adverse Reactions

1% to 10%:

Cardiovascular: ECG abnormality (2%), chest pain (1%)

Central nervous system: Nervousness (1%)

Gastrointestinal: Constipation (2%), diarrhea (2%), dyspepsia (2%), nausea (2%), sore throat (2%)

Genitourinary: Excessive urination (7%)

Neuromuscular & skeletal: Arthralgia (2%), myalgia (2%), weakness (2%)

Respiratory: Rhinitis (3%), cough (2%)

Pharmacodynamics/Kinetics

Onset of Action Diuresis: Oral: Within 1 hour; Peak effect: Diuresis: Oral: 1-2 hours; Antihypertensive: Oral: 4-6 weeks (up to 12 weeks)

Duration of Action Diuresis: Oral: ~6-8 hours

Available Dosage Forms

Injection, solution: 10 mg/mL (2 mL, 5 mL)

Tablet, oral: 5 mg, 10 mg, 20 mg, 100 mg

Demadex®: 5 mg, 10 mg, 20 mg, 100 mg

General Dosage Range

I.V.: *Adults:* 10-200 mg once daily

Oral: *Adults:* 5-200 mg once daily (maximum: 200 mg/day)

Administration

Oral Administer without regard to meals; patients may be switched from the I.V. form to the oral (and vice-versa) with no change in dose.

I.V. Administer over ≥2 minutes; reserve I.V. administration for situations which require rapid onset of action.

I.V. Detail pH: >8.3

Stability

Storage

I.V.: Store at 15°C to 30°C (59°F to 86°F). If torsemide is to be administered via continuous infusion, stability has been demonstrated through 24 hours at room temperature in plastic containers for the following fluids and concentrations:

200 mg torsemide (10 mg/mL) added to 250 mL D_5W, 250 mL NS or 500 mL 0.45% sodium chloride

50 mg torsemide (10 mg/mL) added to 500 mL D_5W, 500 mL NS, or 500 mL 0.45% sodium chloride

Tablets: Store at 15°C to 30°C (59°F to 86°F).

Nursing Actions

Physical Assessment Assess for allergy to sulfonylurea before beginning therapy. Monitor for dehydration, electrolyte imbalance, and postural hypotension on a regular basis during therapy.

Patient Education Take with food or milk (to reduce GI distress), early in the day. If taken twice daily, take last dose in early afternoon in order to avoid sleep disturbance and achieve maximum therapeutic effect. Include potassium-rich foods in daily diet. Do not take potassium supplements without consulting prescriber. Weigh yourself each day when beginning therapy and weekly on long-term therapy; report unusual or unanticipated weight gain or loss. May cause transient drowsiness, blurred vision, dizziness, or constipation. Report unusual weight gain or loss, swelling of ankles and hands, persistent fatigue, weakness, fatigue, dizziness, vomiting, cramps, change in hearing, or chest pain or palpitations.

Dietary Considerations May be taken without regard to meals; however, food slows the rate and reduces the extent of absorption and may reduce diuretic efficacy (Bard, 2004). May require increased intake of potassium-rich foods.

TraMADol (TRA ma dole)

Brand Names: U.S. ConZip™; Rybix™ ODT; Ryzolt™; Ultram®; Ultram® ER

Index Terms Tramadol Hydrochloride

Pharmacologic Category Analgesic, Opioid

Medication Safety Issues

Sound-alike/look-alike issues:

TraMADol may be confused with tapentadol, Toradol®, Trandate®, traZODone, Voltaren®

Ultram® may be confused with Ultane®, Ultracet®, Voltaren®

International issues:

Theradol [Netherlands] may be confused with Foradil brand name for formoterol [U.S., Canada, and multiple international markets], Terazol brand name for terconazole [U.S. and Canada], and Toradol brand name for ketorolac [Canada and multiple international markets]

Trexol [Mexico] may be confused with Trexall brand name for methotrexate [U.S.]; Truxal brand name for chlorprothixene [multiple international markets]

Pregnancy Risk Factor C

Lactation Enters breast milk/not recommended

Breast-Feeding Considerations Sixteen hours following a single 100 mg I.V. dose, the amount of tramadol found in breast milk was 0.1% of the maternal dose. Use is not recommended by the manufacturer for postdelivery analgesia in nursing mothers.

Use Relief of moderate to moderately-severe pain

Extended release formulations are indicated for patients requiring around-the-clock management of moderate to moderately-severe pain for an extended period of time

Mechanism of Action/Effect Tramadol and its active metabolite (M1) binds to μ-opiate receptors in the CNS causing inhibition of ascending pain pathways, altering the perception of and response to pain; also inhibits the reuptake of norepinephrine and serotonin, which also modifies the ascending pain pathway

Contraindications Hypersensitivity to tramadol, opioids, or any component of the formulation

Additional contraindications for Ultram®, Rybix™ ODT, and Ultram® ER: Any situation where opioids are contraindicated, including acute intoxication with alcohol, hypnotics, centrally-acting analgesics, opioids, or psychotropic drugs

Additional contraindications for ConZip™, Ryzolt™: Severe/acute bronchial asthma, hypercapnia, or significant respiratory depression in the absence of appropriately monitored setting and/or resuscitative equipment

Canadian product labeling:

Tramadol is contraindicated during or within 14 days following MAO inhibitor therapy

Extended release formulations (Ralivia™ ER [CAN], Tridural™[CAN], and Zytram® XL [CAN]): Additional contraindications: Severe (Cl_{cr} <30 mL/minute) renal dysfunction, severe (Child-Pugh class C) hepatic dysfunction

Warnings/Precautions Rare but serious anaphylactoid reactions (including fatalities) often following initial dosing have been reported. Pruritus, hives, bronchospasm, angioedema, toxic epidermal necrolysis (TEN) and Stevens-Johnson syndrome also have been reported with use. Previous anaphylactoid reactions to opioids may increase risks for similar reactions to tramadol. Caution patients to swallow extended release tablets whole. Rapid release and absorption of tramadol from extended release tablets that are broken, crushed, or chewed may lead to a potentially lethal overdose. May cause CNS depression, which may impair physical or mental abilities; patients must be cautioned about performing tasks which require mental alertness (eg, operating machinery or driving). May cause CNS depression and/or respiratory depression, particularly when combined with other CNS depressants. Use with caution and reduce dosage when administered to patients receiving other CNS depressants. An increased risk of seizures may occur in patients receiving serotonin reuptake inhibitors (SSRIs or anorectics), tricyclic antidepressants or other cyclic compounds (including cyclobenzaprine, promethazine), neuroleptics, drugs which may lower seizure threshold, or drugs which impair metabolism of tramadol (ie, CYP2D6 and 3A4 inhibitors). Patients with a history of seizures, or with a risk of seizures (head trauma, metabolic disorders, CNS infection, or malignancy, or during ethanol/drug withdrawal) are also at increased risk. Avoid use, if possible, with serotonergic agents such as TCAs, MAO inhibitors (use with extreme caution; contraindicated in Canadian product labeling), triptans, venlafaxine, trazodone, lithium, sibutramine, meperidine, dextromethorphan, St John's wort, SNRIs, and SSRIs; use caution with drugs which impair metabolism of tramadol (ie, CYP2D6 and 3A4 inhibitors); concomitant may increase the risk of serotonin syndrome.

Elderly (particularly >75 years of age), debilitated patients and patients with chronic respiratory disorders may be at greater risk of adverse events. Use with caution in patients with increased intracranial pressure or head injury. Avoid use in patients who are suicidal or addiction prone; use with caution in patients taking tranquilizers and/or antidepressants, or those with an emotional disturbance including depression. Healthcare provider should be alert to problems of abuse, misuse, and diversion. Use caution in heavy alcohol users. Use caution in treatment of acute abdominal conditions; may mask pain. Use tramadol with caution and reduce dosage in patients with liver disease or renal dysfunction. Avoid using extended release tablets in severe hepatic impairment. Do not use Ryzolt™ in any degree of hepatic impairment. Tolerance or drug dependence may result from extended use (withdrawal symptoms have been reported); abrupt discontinuation should be avoided. Tapering of dose at the time of ▶

discontinuation limits the risk of withdrawal symptoms. Some products may contain phenylalanine.

Drug Interactions

Avoid Concomitant Use

Avoid concomitant use of TraMADol with any of the following: Conivaptan

Decreased Effect

TraMADol may decrease the levels/effects of: Pegvisomant

The levels/effects of TraMADol may be decreased by: Ammonium Chloride; CYP2D6 Inhibitors (Moderate); CYP2D6 Inhibitors (Strong); CYP3A4 Inducers (Strong); Deferasirox; Mixed Agonist / Antagonist Opioids; Tocilizumab

Increased Effect/Toxicity

TraMADol may increase the levels/effects of: Alcohol (Ethyl); Alvimopan; CNS Depressants; Desmopressin; MAO Inhibitors; Metoclopramide; Selective Serotonin Reuptake Inhibitors; Serotonin Modulators; Thiazide Diuretics; Vitamin K Antagonists

The levels/effects of TraMADol may be increased by: Amphetamines; Antipsychotic Agents (Phenothiazines); Antipsychotics; Conivaptan; CYP3A4 Inhibitors (Moderate); CYP3A4 Inhibitors (Strong); Dasatinib; HydrOXYzine; Ivacaftor; Selective Serotonin Reuptake Inhibitors; Succinylcholine; Tricyclic Antidepressants

Nutritional/Ethanol Interactions

Ethanol: May increase CNS depression; monitor for increased effects with coadministration. Caution patients about effects.

Food:

Immediate release tablet: Rate and extent of absorption were not significantly affected.

Extended release:

ConZip™: Rate and extent of absorption were unaffected.

Ryzolt™: Increased C_{max}; no effect on AUC.

Ultram® ER: High-fat meal reduced C_{max} and AUC, and increased T_{max} by 3 hours.

Orally disintegrating tablet: Food delays the time to peak serum concentration by 30 minutes; extent of absorption was not significantly affected.

Herb/Nutraceutical: Avoid valerian, St John's wort, kava kava, gotu kola (may increase CNS depression).

Adverse Reactions

>10%:

Cardiovascular: Flushing (8% to 16%)

Central nervous system: Dizziness (10% to 33%), headache (4% to 32%), somnolence (7% to 25%), insomnia (2% to 11%)

Dermatologic: Pruritus (3% to 12%)

Gastrointestinal: Constipation (9% to 46%), nausea (15% to 40%), vomiting (5% to 17%), dyspepsia (1% to 13%)

Neuromuscular & skeletal: Weakness (4% to 12%)

1% to 10%:

Cardiovascular: Postural hypotension (2% to 5%), chest pain (1% to <5%), hypertension (1% to <5%), peripheral edema (1% to <5%), vasodilation (1% to <5%)

Central nervous system: Agitation (1% to <5%), anxiety (1% to <5%), apathy (1% to <5%), chills (1% to <5%), confusion (1% to <5%), coordination impaired (1% to <5%), depersonalization (1% to <5%), depression (1% to <5%), euphoria (1% to <5%), fever (1% to <5%), hypoesthesia (1% to <5%), lethargy (1% to <5%), nervousness (1% to <5%), pain (1% to <5%), pyrexia (1% to <5%), restlessness (1% to <5%), malaise (<1% to <5%), fatigue (2%), vertigo (2%)

Dermatologic: Dermatitis (1% to <5%), rash (1% to <5%)

Endocrine & metabolic: Hot flashes (2% to 9%), hyperglycemia (1% to <5%), menopausal symptoms (1% to <5%)

Gastrointestinal: Diarrhea (5% to 10%), xerostomia (3% to 13%), anorexia (1% to 6%), abdominal pain (1% to <5%), appetite decreased (1% to <5%), weight loss (1% to <5%), flatulence (<1% to <5%)

Genitourinary: Pelvic pain (1% to <5%), prostatic disorder (1% to <5%), urine abnormalities (1% to <5%), urinary tract infection (1% to <5%), urinary frequency (<1% to <5%), urinary retention (<1% to <5%)

Neuromuscular & skeletal: Arthralgia (1% to 5%), back pain (1% to <5%), creatine phosphokinase increased (1% to <5%), myalgia (1% to <5%), hypertonia (1% to <5%), neck pain (1% to <5%), rigors (1% to <5%), paresthesia (1% to <5%), tremor (1% to <5%)

Ocular: Blurred vision (1% to <5%), miosis (1% to <5%)

Respiratory: Bronchitis (1% to <5%), congestion (nasal/sinus) (1% to <5%), cough (1% to <5%), dyspnea (1% to <5%), nasopharyngitis (1% to <5%), pharyngitis (1% to <5%), rhinitis (1% to <5%), rhinorrhea (1% to <5%), sinusitis (1% to <5%), sneezing (1% to <5%), sore throat (1% to <5%), upper respiratory infection (1% to <5%)

Miscellaneous: Diaphoresis (2% to 9%), flu-like syndrome (1% to < 5%), withdrawal syndrome (1% to <5%), shivering (<1% to <5%)

A withdrawal syndrome may include anxiety, diarrhea, hallucinations (rare), nausea, pain, piloerection, rigors, sweating, and tremor. Uncommon discontinuation symptoms may include severe anxiety, panic attacks, or paresthesia.

Pharmacodynamics/Kinetics

Onset of Action Immediate release: ~1 hour

Duration of Action 9 hours

Available Dosage Forms

Capsule, variable release, oral:

ConZip™: 100 mg [25 mg (immediate release) and 75 mg (extended release)]

ConZip™: 200 mg [50 mg (immediate release) and 150 mg (extended release)]
ConZip™: 300 mg [50 mg (immediate release) and 250 mg (extended release)]

Tablet, oral: 50 mg
Ultram®: 50 mg

Tablet, extended release, oral: 100 mg, 200 mg, 300 mg
Ryzolt™: 100 mg, 200 mg, 300 mg
Ultram® ER: 100 mg, 200 mg, 300 mg

Tablet, orally disintegrating, oral:
Rybix™ ODT: 50 mg

General Dosage Range Dosage adjustment recommended in patients with hepatic or renal impairment

Oral:
Immediate release:
Children ≥17 years: 50-100 mg every 4-6 hours (maximum: 400 mg/day)
Adults: 50-100 mg every 4-6 hours (maximum: 400 mg/day)
Elderly >75 years: Maximum: 300 mg/day
Extended release: *Adults:* 100-300 once daily (maximum: 300 mg/day)

Administration

Oral
Immediate release: Administer without regard to meals.
Extended release: Swallow whole; do not crush, chew, or split.
ConZip™, Zytram® XL (Canadian labeling, not available in U.S.): May administer without regard to meals.
Ultram® ER, Ralivia™ ER (Canadian labeling, not available in U.S.), Tridural™ (Canadian labeling, not available in U.S.): May administer without regard to meals, but administer in a consistent manner of either with or without meals.
Orally-disintegrating tablet: Remove from foil blister by peeling back (do not push tablet through the foil). Place tablet on tongue and allow to dissolve (may take ~1 minute); water is not needed, but may be administered with water. Do not chew, break, or split tablet.

Stability

Storage Store at 25°C (77°F); excursions permitted to 15°C to 30°C (59°F to 86°F).

Nursing Actions

Physical Assessment Assess patient's physical and/or psychological dependence. Discontinue slowly after prolonged use.

Patient Education Extended release tablet must be swallowed whole; do not break, chew, or crush. May cause physical and/or psychological dependence. While using this medication, do not use alcohol and other prescription or OTC medications (especially pain medications, sedatives, antihistamines, or cough preparations) without consulting prescriber. Maintain adequate hydration, unless instructed to restrict fluid intake. You may experience headache, drowsiness, dizziness, dry mouth, or blurred vision; nausea, vomiting, or loss of appetite; insomnia; or constipation. Report severe unresolved constipation, respiratory difficulty or shortness of breath, excessive sedation or increased insomnia and restlessness, rash or hives, seizures, muscle weakness or tremors, or chest pain or palpitations.

Dietary Considerations Some products may contain phenylalanine.

Trandolapril (tran DOE la pril)

Brand Names: U.S. Mavik®

Pharmacologic Category Angiotensin-Converting Enzyme (ACE) Inhibitor

Pregnancy Risk Factor D

Lactation Excretion in breast milk unknown/not recommended

Breast-Feeding Considerations It is not known if trandolapril is excreted in breast milk. Breast-feeding is not recommended by the manufacturer.

Use Treatment of hypertension alone or in combination with other antihypertensive agents; treatment of heart failure (HF) or left ventricular (LV) dysfunction after myocardial infarction (MI)

Unlabeled Use To delay the progression of nephropathy and reduce risks of cardiovascular events in hypertensive patients with type 1 or 2 diabetes mellitus

Mechanism of Action/Effect Competitive inhibitor of angiotensin-converting enzyme (ACE); prevents conversion of angiotensin I to angiotensin II, a potent vasoconstrictor; results in lower levels of angiotensin II which causes an increase in plasma renin activity and a reduction in aldosterone secretion

Contraindications Hypersensitivity to trandolapril or any component of the formulation; history of angioedema related to previous treatment with an ACE inhibitor; patients with idiopathic or hereditary angioedema

Warnings/Precautions Anaphylactic reactions may occur rarely with ACE inhibitors. At any time during treatment (especially following first dose) angioedema may occur rarely with ACE inhibitors; it may involve the head and neck (potentially compromising the airway) or the intestine (presenting with abdominal pain). African-Americans and patients with idiopathic or hereditary angioedema may be at an increased risk. Prolonged frequent monitoring may be required especially if tongue, glottis, or larynx are involved as they are associated with airway obstruction. Patients with a history of airway surgery may have a higher risk of airway obstruction. Aggressive early and appropriate management is critical. Use in patients with previous angioedema associated with ACE inhibitor therapy is contraindicated. Severe anaphylactoid reactions may be seen during hemodialysis (eg, CVVHD) with high-flux dialysis membranes (eg, AN69). Rare cases of anaphylactoid reactions have been reported in patients undergoing sensitization treatment with hymenoptera (bee, wasp) venom while receiving ACE inhibitors.

Symptomatic hypotension with or without syncope can occur with ACE inhibitors (usually with the first several doses); effects are most often observed in volume-depleted patients; correct volume depletion prior to initiation; close monitoring of patient is required especially with initial dosing and dosing increases; blood pressure must be lowered at a rate appropriate for the patient's clinical condition. Initiation of therapy in patients with ischemic heart disease or cerebrovascular disease warrants close observation due to the potential consequences posed by falling blood pressure (eg, MI, stroke). Use with caution in hypertrophic cardiomyopathy with outflow tract obstruction, severe aortic stenosis, or before, during, or immediately after major surgery. **[U.S. Boxed Warning]: Drugs that act on the renin-angiotensin system can cause injury and death to the developing fetus. Discontinue as soon as possible once pregnancy is detected.**

Hyperkalemia may occur with ACE inhibitors; risk factors include renal dysfunction, diabetes mellitus, concomitant use of potassium-sparing diuretics, potassium supplements, and/or potassium-containing salts. Use cautiously, if at all, with these agents and monitor potassium closely. Cough may occur with ACE inhibitors. Other causes of cough should be considered (eg, pulmonary congestion in patients with heart failure) and excluded prior to discontinuation.

Dosage adjustment needed in severe renal dysfunction (Cl_{cr} <30 mL/minute) or hepatic cirrhosis. May be associated with deterioration of renal function and/or increases in serum creatinine, particularly in patients with low renal blood flow (eg, renal artery stenosis, heart failure) whose glomerular filtration rate (GFR) is dependent on efferent arteriolar vasoconstriction by angiotensin II; deterioration may result in oliguria, acute renal failure, and progressive azotemia. Small increases in serum creatinine may occur following initiation; consider discontinuation only in patients with progressive and/or significant deterioration in renal function. Use with caution in patients with unstented unilateral/bilateral renal artery stenosis. When unstented bilateral renal artery stenosis is present, use is generally avoided due to the elevated risk of deterioration in renal function unless possible benefits outweigh risks. Concurrent use of angiotensin receptor blockers may increase the risk of clinically-significant adverse events (eg, renal dysfunction, hyperkalemia).

Rare toxicities associated with ACE inhibitors include cholestatic jaundice (which may progress to fulminant hepatic necrosis), agranulocytosis, neutropenia, or leukopenia with myeloid hypoplasia. Patients with collagen vascular diseases (especially with concomitant renal impairment) or renal impairment alone may be at increased risk for hematologic toxicity; periodically monitor CBC with differential in these patients.

Drug Interactions

Avoid Concomitant Use There are no known interactions where it is recommended to avoid concomitant use.

Decreased Effect

The levels/effects of Trandolapril may be decreased by: Antacids; Aprotinin; Herbs (Hypertensive Properties); Icatibant; Lanthanum; Methylphenidate; Nonsteroidal Anti-Inflammatory Agents; Salicylates; Yohimbine

Increased Effect/Toxicity

Trandolapril may increase the levels/effects of: Allopurinol; Amifostine; Antihypertensives; AzaTHIOprine; CycloSPORINE; CycloSPORINE (Systemic); Ferric Gluconate; Gold Sodium Thiomalate; Hypotensive Agents; Iron Dextran Complex; Lithium; Nonsteroidal Anti-Inflammatory Agents; RiTUXimab; Sodium Phosphates

The levels/effects of Trandolapril may be increased by: Alfuzosin; Angiotensin II Receptor Blockers; Diazoxide; DPP-IV Inhibitors; Eplerenone; Everolimus; Herbs (Hypotensive Properties); Loop Diuretics; MAO Inhibitors; Pentoxifylline; Phosphodiesterase 5 Inhibitors; Potassium Salts; Potassium-Sparing Diuretics; Prostacyclin Analogues; Sirolimus; Temsirolimus; Thiazide Diuretics; TiZANidine; Tolvaptan; Trimethoprim

Nutritional/Ethanol Interactions Herb/Nutraceutical: Some herbal medications may worsen hypertension (eg, licorice); others may increase the antihypertensive effects of trandolapril (eg, shepherd's purse). Management: Avoid bayberry, blue cohosh, cayenne, ephedra, ginger, ginseng (American), kola, licorice, and yohimbe. Avoid black cohosh, California poppy, coleus, golden seal, hawthorn, mistletoe, periwinkle, quinine, and shepherd's purse.

Adverse Reactions Note: Frequency ranges include data from hypertension and heart failure trials. Higher rates of adverse reactions have generally been noted in patients with CHF. However, the frequency of adverse effects associated with placebo is also increased in this population.

>1%:

Cardiovascular: Hypotension (<1% to 11%), syncope (6%), bradycardia (<1% to 5%), cardiogenic shock (4%), intermittent claudication (4%)

Central nervous system: Dizziness (1% to 23%), stroke (3%)

Endocrine & metabolic: Uric acid increased (15%), hyperkalemia (5%), hypocalcemia (5%)
Gastrointestinal: Gastritis (4%), diarrhea (1%)
Neuromuscular & skeletal: Myalgia (5%), weakness (3%)
Renal: BUN increased (9%), serum creatinine increased (1% to 5%)
Respiratory: Cough (2% to 35%)

Worsening of renal function may occur in patients with bilateral renal artery stenosis or hypovolemia. In addition, a syndrome which may include fever, myalgia, arthralgia, interstitial nephritis, vasculitis, rash, eosinophilia and positive ANA, and elevated ESR has been reported with ACE inhibitors. Eosinophilic pneumonitis has also been reported with other ACE inhibitors.

Pharmacodynamics/Kinetics

Onset of Action 1-2 hours; Peak effect: Reduction in blood pressure: 6 hours

Duration of Action Prolonged; 72 hours after single dose

Available Dosage Forms

Tablet, oral: 1 mg, 2 mg, 4 mg
Mavik®: 1 mg, 2 mg, 4 mg

General Dosage Range Dosage adjustment recommended in patients with hepatic or renal impairment

Oral: *Adults:* Initial: 1-2 mg once daily; Maintenance: 1-4 mg once daily

Stability

Storage Store at controlled room temperature of 20°C to 25°C (68°F to 77°F).

Nursing Actions

Physical Assessment Assess potential for interactions with other pharmacological agents or herbal products that may impact fluid balance or cardiac status. Monitor for hypovolemia, angioedema, and postural hypotension with first doses and on a regular basis during therapy.

Patient Education Take first dose at bedtime. This drug does not eliminate need for diet or exercise regimen as recommended by prescriber. May cause dizziness, fainting, lightheadedness, postural hypotension, or diarrhea. Report immediately any swelling of face, mouth, lips, tongue or throat; or respiratory difficulty. Report chest pain or palpitations, swelling of extremities, skin rash, or unusual cough.

Trandolapril and Verapamil

(tran DOE la pril & ver AP a mil)

Brand Names: U.S. Tarka®

Index Terms Verapamil and Trandolapril

Pharmacologic Category Angiotensin-Converting Enzyme (ACE) Inhibitor; Calcium Channel Blocker

Pregnancy Risk Factor D

Lactation Enters breast milk/contraindicated

Use Treatment of hypertension; however, not indicated for initial treatment of hypertension

Available Dosage Forms

Tablet, variable release: Trandolapril 2 mg [immediate release] and verapamil 180 mg [sustained release]; Trandolapril 2 mg [immediate release] and verapamil 240 mg [sustained release]; Trandolapril 4 mg [immediate release] and verapamil 240 mg [sustained release]

Tarka®:
1/240: Trandolapril 1 mg [immediate release] and verapamil 240 mg [sustained release]
2/180: Trandolapril 2 mg [immediate release] and verapamil 180 mg [sustained release]
2/240: Trandolapril 2 mg [immediate release] and verapamil 240 mg [sustained release]
4/240: Trandolapril 4 mg [immediate release] and verapamil 240 mg [sustained release]

General Dosage Range Dosage adjustment recommended in patients with hepatic or renal impairment

Oral: *Adults:* Trandolapril 1-4 mg and verapamil 180-240 mg once daily

Nursing Actions

Physical Assessment See individual agents.

Patient Education See individual agents.

Related Information

Trandolapril *on page 1139*
Verapamil *on page 1173*

Tranylcypromine

(tran il SIP roe meen)

Brand Names: U.S. Parnate®

Index Terms Transamine Sulphate; Tranylcypromine Sulfate

Pharmacologic Category Antidepressant, Monoamine Oxidase Inhibitor

Medication Guide Available Yes

Lactation Enters breast milk/not recommended

Use Treatment of major depressive episode without melancholia

Available Dosage Forms

Tablet, oral: 10 mg
Parnate®: 10 mg

General Dosage Range Oral: *Adults:* 10-30 mg twice daily (maximum: 60 mg/day)

Nursing Actions

Physical Assessment Monitor therapeutic response (eg, mental status, mood, affect, suicide ideation) at beginning of therapy and periodically throughout. Monitor blood pressure. Observe for clinical worsening, suicidality, or unusual behavior changes, especially during the initial few months of therapy or during dosage changes.

Patient Education It may take 2-3 weeks to achieve desired results. Take in the morning to reduce the incidence of insomnia. Avoid alcohol, caffeine, and other prescription or OTC medications not approved by prescriber. Avoid tyramine-containing foods; see prescriber for complete list of foods to be avoided. Maintain adequate hydration unless instructed to restrict fluid intake. If you have diabetes, monitor blood glucose closely at the beginning of therapy. May cause hypoglycemia. You may experience drowsiness, dizziness, blurred vision, anorexia, dry mouth, constipation, diarrhea, orthostatic hypotension, or altered sexual ability (reversible). Report persistent excessive sedation; muscle cramping, tremors, weakness, or change in gait; chest pain, palpitations, rapid heartbeat, or swelling of extremities; vision changes; suicide ideation; or worsening of condition.

Trastuzumab (tras TU zoo mab)

Brand Names: U.S. Herceptin®

Index Terms anti-c-erB-2; anti-ERB-2; MOAB HER2; rhuMAb HER2

Pharmacologic Category Antineoplastic Agent, Monoclonal Antibody; Monoclonal Antibody

Medication Safety Issues

High alert medication:

This medication is in a class the Institute for Safe Medication Practices (ISMP) includes among its list of drug classes which have a heightened risk of causing significant patient harm when used in error.

Pregnancy Risk Factor D

Lactation Excretion in breast milk unknown/not recommended

Breast-Feeding Considerations It is not known whether trastuzumab is secreted in human milk. Because many immunoglobulins are secreted in milk, and the potential for serious adverse reactions in the nursing infant exists, patients should discontinue nursing during treatment; the extended half-life should be considered for decisions regarding breast-feeding after therapy completion.

Use Treatment (adjuvant) of HER-2 overexpressing breast cancer; treatment of HER-2 overexpressing metastatic breast cancer; treatment of HER-2 overexpressing metastatic gastric or gastroesophageal junction adenocarcinoma (in patients who have not received prior treatment)

Mechanism of Action/Effect Trastuzumab is a monoclonal antibody which binds to the extracellular domain of the human epidermal growth factor receptor 2 protein (HER-2). It mediates antibody-dependent cellular cytotoxicity by inhibiting proliferation of cells which overexpress HER-2 protein.

Contraindications There are no contraindications listed within the manufacturer's labeling.

Canadian labeling: Hypersensitivity to trastuzumab, Chinese hamster ovary (CHO) cell proteins, or any component of the formulation

Warnings/Precautions Hazardous agent - use appropriate precautions for handling and disposal. **[U.S. Boxed Warning]: Trastuzumab is associated with symptomatic and asymptomatic reductions in left ventricular ejection fraction (LVEF) and heart failure (HF); the incidence is highest in patients receiving trastuzumab with an anthracycline-containing chemotherapy regimen. Evaluate LVEF in all patients prior to and during treatment; discontinue for cardiomyopathy.** Extreme caution should be used in patients with pre-existing cardiac disease or dysfunction. Prior or concurrent exposure to anthracyclines or radiation therapy significantly increases the risk of cardiomyopathy; other potential risk factors include advanced age, high or low body mass index, smoking, diabetes, and hyper/hypothyroidism. Discontinuation should be strongly considered in patients who develop a clinically significant reduction in LVEF during therapy; treatment with HF medications (eg, ACE inhibitors, beta-blockers) should be initiated. Withhold treatment for ≥16% decrease from pretreatment levels or LVEF below normal limits and ≥10% decrease from baseline. Cardiomyopathy due to trastuzumab is generally reversible over a period of 1-3 months after discontinuation. Trastuzumab is also associated with arrhythmias, hypertension, mural thrombus formation, stroke, and even cardiac death.

[U.S. Boxed Warning]: Serious adverse events, including hypersensitivity reaction (anaphylaxis), infusion reactions (including fatalities), and pulmonary events (including acute respiratory distress syndrome [ARDS]) have been associated with trastuzumab. Discontinue for anaphylaxis, angioedema, ARDS or interstitial pneumonitis. Most of these events occur with the first infusion; pulmonary events may occur during or within 24 hours of the first infusion; delayed reactions have occurred. Interrupt infusion for dyspnea or significant hypotension; monitor until symptoms resolve. Infusion reactions may consist of fever and chills, and may also include nausea, vomiting, pain, headache dizziness, dyspnea, hypotension, rash and weakness. Retreatment of patients who experienced severe hypersensitivity reactions has been attempted (with premedication). Some patients tolerated retreatment, while others experienced a second severe reaction. When used in combination with myelosuppressive chemotherapy, trastuzumab may increase the incidence of neutropenia (moderate-to-severe) and febrile neutropenia; the incidence of anemia may be higher when trastuzumab is added to chemotherapy. Rare cases of nephrotic syndrome with evidence of glomerulopathy have been reported, with an onset of 4-18 months from trastuzumab initiation; complications may include volume overload and HF. The incidence of renal impairment was increased in metastatic gastric cancer patients when trastuzumab is added to chemotherapy.

May cause serious pulmonary toxicity (dyspnea, hypoxia, interstitial pneumonitis, pulmonary infiltrates, pleural effusion, noncardiogenic pulmonary edema, pulmonary insufficiency, acute respiratory distress syndrome, and/or pulmonary fibrosis); use caution in patients with pre-existing pulmonary disease or patients with extensive pulmonary tumor involvement. **[U.S. Boxed Warning]: Trastuzumab exposure during pregnancy may result in oligohydramnios and oligohydramnios sequence (pulmonary hypoplasia, skeletal malformations and neonatal death).** Effective contraception is recommended during and for 6 months after treatment for women of childbearing potential.

Drug Interactions

Avoid Concomitant Use

Avoid concomitant use of Trastuzumab with any of the following: Belimumab

Decreased Effect

Trastuzumab may decrease the levels/effects of: PACLitaxel

Increased Effect/Toxicity

Trastuzumab may increase the levels/effects of: Antineoplastic Agents (Anthracycline, Systemic); Belimumab; Immunosuppressants

The levels/effects of Trastuzumab may be increased by: Abciximab; PACLitaxel

Adverse Reactions Note: Percentages reported with single-agent therapy.

>10%:

Cardiovascular: LVEF decreased (4% to 22%)

Central nervous system: Pain (47%), fever (6% to 36%), chills (5% to 32%), headache (10% to 26%), insomnia (14%), dizziness (4% to 13%)

Dermatologic: Rash (4% to 18%)

Gastrointestinal: Nausea (6% to 33%), diarrhea (7% to 25%), vomiting (4% to 23%), abdominal pain (2% to 22%), anorexia (14%)

Neuromuscular & skeletal: Weakness (4% to 42%), back pain (5% to 22%)

Respiratory: Cough (5% to 26%), dyspnea (3% to 22%), rhinitis (2% to 14%), pharyngitis (12%)

Miscellaneous: Infusion reaction (21% to 40%, chills and fever most common; severe: 1%), infection (20%)

1% to 10%:

Cardiovascular: Peripheral edema (5% to 10%), edema (8%), HF (2% to 7%; severe: <1%), tachycardia (5%), hypertension (4%), arrhythmia (3%), palpitation (3%)

Central nervous system: Depression (6%)

Dermatologic: Acne (2%), nail disorder (2%), pruritus (2%)

Gastrointestinal: Constipation (2%), dyspepsia (2%)

Genitourinary: Urinary tract infection (3% to 5%)

Hematologic: Anemia (4%), leukopenia (3%)

Neuromuscular & skeletal: Paresthesia (2% to 9%), bone pain (3% to 7%), arthralgia (6% to 8%), myalgia (4%), muscle spasm (3%), peripheral neuritis (2%), neuropathy (1%)

Respiratory: Sinusitis (2% to 9%), nasopharyngitis (8%), upper respiratory infection (3%), epistaxis (2%), pharyngolaryngeal pain (2%)

Miscellaneous: Flu-like syndrome (2% to 10%), accidental injury (6%), influenza (4%), allergic reaction (3%), herpes simplex (2%)

Available Dosage Forms

Injection, powder for reconstitution:

Herceptin®: 440 mg

General Dosage Range Dosage adjustment recommended in patients who develop toxicities

I.V.: *Adults:* Loading dose: 4 mg/kg; Maintenance: 2 mg/kg once weekly **or** Loading dose: 8 mg/kg; Maintenance: 6 mg/kg every 3 weeks

Administration

I.V. Administered by I.V. infusion; loading doses are infused over 90 minutes; maintenance doses may be infused over 30 minutes if tolerated. Do not administer with D_5W. **Do not administer I.V. push or by rapid bolus.** Treatment with acetaminophen, diphenhydramine, and/or meperidine is usually effective for managing infusion-related events.

I.V. Detail Observe patients closely during the infusion for fever, chills, or other infusion-related symptoms. Treatment with acetaminophen, diphenhydramine, and/or meperidine is usually effective for managing infusion-related events.

pH: 6

Stability

Reconstitution Reconstitute each vial with 20 mL of bacteriostatic sterile water for injection to a concentration of 21 mg/mL. Swirl gently; do not shake. Allow vial to rest for ~5 minutes. If the patient has a known hypersensitivity to benzyl alcohol, trastuzumab may be reconstituted with sterile water for injection without preservatives, which must be used immediately. Further dilute the appropriate volume for the trastuzumab dose in 250 mL NS prior to administration. Gently invert bag to mix.

Storage Prior to reconstitution, store intact vials under refrigeration at 2°C to 8°C (36°F to 46°F). Following reconstitution with bacteriostatic SWFI, the solution in the vial is stable refrigerated for 28 days from the date of reconstitution; do not freeze. Solutions reconstituted with sterile water for injection without preservatives must be used immediately. The solution diluted in 250 mL NS for infusion is stable for 24 hours refrigerated; do not freeze.

Nursing Actions

Physical Assessment Assess for signs of infusion reaction during infusion. If patient is pregnant, monitor amniotic fluid volume. Evaluate cardiac and respiratory function and vital signs. Monitor for arrhythmias, difficulty breathing, peripheral edema, and sudden weight gain.

Patient Education This medication can only be administered by infusion. Report immediately any respiratory difficulty, chills, fever, headache, backache, nausea, or vomiting. You will be susceptible to infection. You may experience dizziness, weakness, nausea, vomiting, diarrhea, headache, or back or joint pain. Report persistent GI effects; sore throat, runny nose, or respiratory difficulty; chest pain, irregular heartbeat, palpitations, swelling of extremities, or unusual weight gain; muscle or joint weakness, numbness, or pain; skin rash or irritation; itching or pain on urination; unhealed sores, white plaques in mouth or genital area, or unusual bruising or bleeding.

Travelers' Diarrhea and Cholera Vaccine

(TRAV uh lerz dahy uh REE uh & KOL er uh vak SEEN)

Index Terms *Vibrio cholera* and Enterotoxigenic *Escherichia coli Vaccine*; Cholera and Traveler's Diarrhea Vaccine; Cholera Vaccine; Enterotoxigenic *Escherichia coli* and *Vibrio cholera* Vaccine; Oral Cholera Vaccine; Traveller's Diarrhea Vaccine and Cholera

Pharmacologic Category Vaccine

Use Protection against travelers' diarrhea and/or cholera in adults and children ≥2 years of age who will be visiting areas where there is a risk of contracting travelers' diarrhea caused by enterotoxigenic *E. coli* (ETEC) or cholera caused by *V. cholerae* O1 (classical and El Tor biotypes; Inaba and Ogawa serotypes)

Product Availability Not available in U.S.

General Dosage Range Oral:

Children 2-6 years: Cholera: Primary immunization: 3 doses given at intervals of ≥1 week

Children ≥2 years: ETEC: Primary immunization: 2 doses given at intervals of ≥1 week

Children >6 years: Cholera: Primary immunization: 2 doses given at intervals of ≥1 week

Adults: Cholera: Primary immunization: 2 doses given at intervals of ≥1 week; ETEC: Primary immunization: 2 doses given at intervals of ≥1 week

Administration

Oral For oral use only; do no administer I.M., I.V., or SubQ. Oral administration of other medications, vaccines, and consumption of food should be avoided 1 hour before and 1 hour following vaccine administration.

Administration with other vaccines (manufacturer recommendations): *Typhoid vaccine, oral:* Separate by at least 8 hours

Acetaminophen may be used when needed to provide comfort; however, routine prophylactic administration of acetaminophen to prevent fever due to vaccine use is not recommended. There is evidence of a decreased immune response to some vaccines associated with acetaminophen administration; the clinical significance of this reduction in immune response has not been established.

Nursing Actions

Physical Assessment Patient history of prior exposure to cholera vaccine should be assessed prior to treatment. Instruct patient about safe eating and drinking practices. All serious adverse reactions must be reported to the U.S. DHHS. U.S. federal law also requires entry into the patient's medical record. Instruct patient about anaphylactic treatment that should be available during use.

Patient Education Emergency treatment for anaphylactic reaction should be available during use. Granules must be dissolved in a glass with water (do not use juice, milk, or other beverages). Contact healthcare provider if you develop severe belly pain, diarrhea, or rash. May cause mild transient abdominal pain or diarrhea.

Travoprost (TRA voe prost)

Brand Names: U.S. Travatan Z®

Pharmacologic Category Ophthalmic Agent, Antiglaucoma; Prostaglandin, Ophthalmic

Medication Safety Issues

Sound-alike/look-alike issues:

Travatan® may be confused with Xalatan®

Pregnancy Risk Factor C

Lactation Excretion in breast milk unknown/use caution

Use Reduction of elevated intraocular pressure in patients with open-angle glaucoma or ocular hypertension who are intolerant of the other IOP-lowering medications or insufficiently responsive (failed to achieve target IOP determined after multiple measurements over time) to another IOP-lowering medication

Available Dosage Forms

Solution, ophthalmic:

Travatan Z®: 0.004% (2.5 mL, 5 mL)

General Dosage Range Ophthalmic: *Adults:* Instill 1 drop into affected eye(s) once daily

Administration

Other May be used with other eye drops to lower intraocular pressure. If using more than one ophthalmic product, wait at least 5 minutes in between application of each medication.

Nursing Actions

Patient Education For use in eyes only. Wash hands before instilling. Sit or lie down to instill. Open eye, look at ceiling, and instill prescribed amount of solution. Apply gentle pressure to inner corner of eye. Do not let tip of applicator touch eye; do not contaminate tip of applicator (may cause eye infection, eye damage, or vision loss). May cause permanent changes in eye color, eyelid, and eyelashes. May also increase the length and/or number of eyelashes. Changes may occur slowly (months to years). May be used with other eye drops to lower intraocular pressure. If using more than one eye drop medicine, wait at least 5 minutes in between application of each medication. Notify prescriber if conjunctivitis or eyelid reactions occur with use of this product.

TraZODone (TRAZ oh done)

Brand Names: U.S. Oleptro™

Index Terms Desyrel; Trazodone Hydrochloride

Pharmacologic Category Antidepressant, Serotonin Reuptake Inhibitor/Antagonist

Medication Safety Issues

Sound-alike/look-alike issues:

Desyrel may be confused with deferoxamine, Demerol®, Delsym®, Zestril®

TraZODone may be confused with traMADol, ziprasidone

International issues:

Desyrel [Canada, Turkey] may be confused with Deseril brand name for methysergide [Australia, Belgium, Great Britain, Netherlands]

Medication Guide Available Yes

Pregnancy Risk Factor C

Lactation Enters breast milk/use caution (AAP rates "of concern"; AAP 2001 update pending)

Use Treatment of major depressive disorder

Unlabeled Use Potential augmenting agent for antidepressants, hypnotic

Available Dosage Forms

Tablet, oral: 50 mg, 100 mg, 150 mg, 300 mg

Tablet, extended release, oral:

Oleptro™: 150 mg, 300 mg

General Dosage Range Oral:

Adults: Immediate release: Initial: 150 mg/day in 3 divided doses; Maintenance: 150-600 mg/day in 3 divided doses; Extended-release: Initial: 150 mg once daily; Maximum dose: 375 mg/day

Elderly: Immediate release: Initial: 25-50 mg at bedtime; Maintenance: 25-150 mg/day at bedtime

Administration

Oral

Immediate release tablet: Dosing after meals may decrease lightheadedness and postural hypotension

Extended release tablet: Take on an empty stomach; swallow whole or as a half tablet without food. Tablet may be broken along the score line, but do not crush or chew.

Nursing Actions

Physical Assessment Monitor therapeutic response (eg, mental status, mood, affect, suicide ideation) at beginning of therapy and periodically throughout.

Patient Education It may take 2-4 weeks to achieve desired results. Take immediate release tablet after meals. Extended release tablet should be taken on an empty stomach. Do not crush or chew tablet. Avoid excessive alcohol. Maintain adequate hydration unless instructed to restrict fluid intake. You may experience drowsiness, lightheadedness, dizziness, postural hypotension, nausea, dry mouth, constipation, or diarrhea. Report persistent dizziness or headache; muscle cramping, tremors, or altered gait; blurred vision or eye pain; chest pain or irregular heartbeat; suicide ideation; or worsening of condition. Report prolonged or inappropriate erections.

Treprostinil (tre PROST in il)

Brand Names: U.S. Remodulin®; Tyvaso™

Index Terms Treprostinil Sodium

Pharmacologic Category Prostacyclin; Prostaglandin; Vasodilator

Pregnancy Risk Factor B

Lactation Excretion in breast milk unknown/use caution

Use

Injection: Treatment of pulmonary arterial hypertension (PAH) (WHO Group I) in patients with NYHA Class II-IV symptoms to decrease exercise-associated symptoms; to diminish clinical deterioration when transitioning from epoprostenol (I.V.)

Inhalation: Treatment of pulmonary arterial hypertension (PAH) (WHO Group I) in patients with NYHA Class III symptoms to improve exercise ability. **Note:** Nearly all controlled clinical trial experience has been with concomitant bosentan or sildenafil.

Mechanism of Action/Effect Treprostinil is a direct vasodilator of both pulmonary and systemic arterial vascular beds.

Contraindications There are no contraindications listed in the FDA-approved labeling.

Warnings/Precautions May produce symptomatic hypotension; use with caution in patients with low systemic arterial blood pressure. Abrupt withdrawal/large dosage reductions may worsen symptoms of PAH. If a SubQ or I.V. infusion is restarted within a few hours of discontinuation, the same dose rate may be used. Interruptions for longer periods may require retitration. Regardless of administration route (inhalation, I.V., or SubQ), treatment interruptions should be avoided. Immediate access to medication, back-up inhalation device, or pump and infusion sets is essential to prevent treatment interruptions. Chronic continuous I.V. infusion of treprostinil via a chronic indwelling central venous catheter has been associated with serious blood stream infections. This method of administration should be reserved for patients who are intolerant of the SubQ route or in whom the benefit outweighs the potential risks. Treprostinil should only be used by clinicians experienced in the treatment of PAH. Prior to initiation, patients should be carefully evaluated for ability to administer treprostinil, either as an I.V./SubQ infusion or inhalation, and care for the infusion system/inhalation device. Initiation of infusion must occur in a setting where adequate personnel and equipment necessary for hemodynamic monitoring and emergency treatment is available. Use with caution in patients with hepatic impairment; dose reduction is recommended for the initial dose (I.V./SubQ) in patients with mild-to-moderate hepatic insufficiency; titrate dose slowly in patients with hepatic insufficiency; has not been studied in severe hepatic impairment. Has not been studied in renal impairment; use with caution in renal impairment; titrate dose slowly in patients with renal insufficiency. Use with caution in patients ≥65 years of age. Inhalation: Safety and efficacy have not been established in patients with underlying pulmonary disease (eg, asthma, COPD). Patients with acute pulmonary infections should be monitored closely for exacerbation or reduced efficacy. Treprostinil inhibits platelet aggregation, increasing the risk of bleeding; use with caution in patients receiving concurrent anticoagulant/antiplatelet therapy.

Drug Interactions

Avoid Concomitant Use There are no known interactions where it is recommended to avoid concomitant use.

Decreased Effect

The levels/effects of Treprostinil may be decreased by: CYP2C8 Inducers (Strong)

Increased Effect/Toxicity

Treprostinil may increase the levels/effects of: Anticoagulants; Antihypertensives; Antiplatelet Agents; Nonsteroidal Anti-Inflammatory Agents; Salicylates

The levels/effects of Treprostinil may be increased by: CYP2C8 Inhibitors (Strong)

Adverse Reactions

>10%:

Cardiovascular: Flushing (11%; inhalation: 15%)

Central nervous system: Headache (27% to 41%)

Dermatologic: Rash (14%)

Gastrointestinal: Diarrhea (25%), nausea (19% to 22%)

Local: Infusion site pain (SubQ: 85%; may improve after several months of therapy), infusion site reaction (SubQ: 83%)

Neuromuscular & skeletal: Jaw pain (13%)

Respiratory: Cough (inhalation: 54%), throat irritation/pharyngolaryngeal pain (inhalation: 25%)

1% to 10%:

Cardiovascular: Edema (9%), syncope (inhalation: 6%), hypotension (4%)

Central nervous system: Dizziness (9%)

Dermatologic: Pruritus (8%)

Respiratory: Epistaxis (inhalation), hemoptysis, pneumonia, wheezing (inhalation)

Available Dosage Forms

Injection, solution:

Remodulin®: 1 mg/mL (20 mL); 2.5 mg/mL (20 mL); 5 mg/mL (20 mL); 10 mg/mL (20 mL)

Solution, for oral inhalation:

Tyvaso™: 0.6 mg/mL (2.9 mL)

General Dosage Range Dosage adjustment recommended for the I.V. infusion and SubQ routes in patients with hepatic impairment

Inhalation: *Adults:* Initial: 18 mcg (or 3 inhalations) every 4 hours 4 times/day; Maintenance: Maximum dose: 54 mcg (or 9 inhalations) 4 times/day

I.V. Infusion, SubQ: *Adults:* Initial: 0.625-1.25 ng/kg/minute; Maintenance: 1.25-40 ng/kg/minute

Administration

I.V. Avoid abrupt withdrawal (including interruptions in delivery) or rapid large dosage reductions. Immediate access to a back-up pump, infusion sets, and medication is essential to prevent treatment interruptions.

I.V. infusion: I.V. use is recommended when SubQ infusion is not tolerated or when the benefit outweighs the potential risks of an indwelling central venous catheter. Solution must be diluted in SWFI, NS, or Flolan® sterile diluent prior to use and administered by continuous infusion using a central indwelling catheter and infusion pump. The ambulatory infusion pump should be small and lightweight; have occlusion/no delivery, low battery, programming error, and motor malfunction alarms; have ± 6% accuracy of the programmed rate; and be positive pressure driven. The reservoir should be made of polyvinyl chloride, polypropylene, or glass. Peripheral infusion may be used temporarily until central line is established.

I.V. Detail pH 6-7.2

Other Avoid abrupt withdrawal (including interruptions in delivery) or rapid large dosage reductions. Immediate access to medication, a back-up inhalation device, or pump and infusion sets is essential to prevent treatment interruptions.

Inhalation: Do not mix with other medications. For inhalation only via the Tyvaso™ Inhalation System; consists of the Optineb-ir Model ON-100/7 (an ultrasonic, pulsed-delivery device) and accessories. Prior to the first treatment session of each day, transfer the entire contents of one ampule into the medicine chamber; one ampule contains sufficient volume of medication for all 4 treatment sessions in a single day. Between each session, the device should be capped and stored upright with the remaining medication inside. At the end of each day, the medicine chamber and any remaining medication must be discarded. Avoid contact of solution with eyes or skin; wash hands after handling.

SubQ infusion (preferred): Administer undiluted via continuous SubQ infusion using an appropriately-designed infusion pump. The ambulatory infusion pump should be small and lightweight; be able to adjust infusion rates in ~0.002 mL/hour increments; have occlusion/no delivery, low battery, programming error, and motor malfunction alarms; have ± 6% accuracy of the programmed rate; and be positive pressure driven. The reservoir should be made of polyvinyl chloride, polypropylene, or glass. Infusion site reactions may be helped by moving the infusion site every 3 days, local application of topical hot and cold packs, topical or oral analgesics. Injection site pain and erythema may improve after several months of treprostinil therapy.

Stability

Reconstitution Injection solution: For SubQ infusion, **product should not be diluted prior to use**. For I.V. infusion, dilute in SWFI, NS, or Flolan® sterile diluent to a final volume of either 50 mL or 100 mL (dependent on system reservoir and calculated dose).

Storage

Injection solution: Store vials at 25°C (77°F); excursions permitted to 15°C to 30°C (59°F to 86°F). Contents of a vial should not be used past 30 days after initial needle access into the vial. Stability for up to 48 hours at 37°C has been shown for I.V. infusion concentrations as low as 4000 ng/mL.

Solution for inhalation: Store ampules in foil packs at 25°C (77°F); excursions permitted to 15°C to 30°C (59°F to 89°F). Protect from light. Once foil pack is opened, ampules should be used within 7 days. Following transfer of solution to inhalation device, solution should remain in device for no more than 24 hours; discard unused portion.

Nursing Actions

Physical Assessment To be used only by clinicians experienced in the diagnosis and treatment of PAH. Initiation of therapy must be performed in a monitored setting. Therapy may be needed long-term; patient's ability to prepare, administer, and care for necessary equipment should be carefully assessed. Evaluate effectiveness of therapy (improved pulmonary function and quality of life). Teach patient/caregiver how to care for equipment and monitor for any malfunction. Instruct patient/caregiver to monitor vital signs on regular basis.

Patient Education Therapy will probably be long-term. You will be taught how to store and prepare medication and how to care for and monitor the equipment; follow these directions completely. Notify contact person immediately with any problems or questions with equipment. You will be required to monitor your blood pressure and heart rate at regular intervals. You may experience mild headache, nervousness, dizziness, nausea, vomiting, diarrhea, or muscular pain. Report immediately any signs or symptoms of increased dizziness, acute or severe headache, increased difficulty breathing, fever or chills, unusual bleeding or bruising, or chest pain or palpitations. If administering through an I.V., notify healthcare provider if site is increasingly painful, red, or has pus forming.

Tretinoin (Topical) (TRET i noyn TOP i kal)

Brand Names: U.S. Atralin™; Avita®; Refissa™; Renova®; Retin-A Micro®; Retin-A®; Tretin-X™

Index Terms *trans*-Retinoic Acid; Retinoic Acid; Vitamin A Acid

Pharmacologic Category Acne Products; Retinoic Acid Derivative; Topical Skin Product, Acne

Medication Safety Issues

Sound-alike/look-alike issues:

Tretinoin may be confused with ISOtretinoin, Tenormin®, triamcinolone, trientine

International issues:

Renova [U.S., Canada] may be confused with Remov brand name for nimesulide [Italy]

Pregnancy Risk Factor C

Lactation Enters breast milk/compatible

Use Treatment of acne vulgaris; photodamaged skin; palliation of fine wrinkles, mottled hyperpigmentation, and tactile roughness of facial skin as part of a comprehensive skin care and sun avoidance program

Unlabeled Use Some skin cancers

Available Dosage Forms

Cream, topical: 0.025% (20 g, 45 g); 0.05% (20 g, 45 g); 0.1% (20 g, 45 g)

Avita®: 0.025% (20 g, 45 g)

Refissa™: 0.05% (40 g)

Renova®: 0.02% (40 g, 44 g, 60 g)

Retin-A®: 0.025% (20 g, 45 g); 0.05% (20 g, 45 g); 0.1% (20 g, 45 g)

Tretin-X™: 0.025% (35 g); 0.0375% (35 g); 0.05% (35 g); 0.1% (35 g)

Gel, topical: 0.01% (15 g, 45 g); 0.025% (15 g, 45 g)

Atralin™: 0.05% (45 g)

Avita®: 0.025% (20 g, 45 g)

Retin-A Micro®: 0.04% (20 g, 45 g, 50 g); 0.1% (20 g, 45 g, 50 g)

Retin-A®: 0.01% (15 g, 45 g); 0.025% (15 g, 45 g)

Tretin-X™: 0.01% (35 g); 0.025% (35 g)

General Dosage Range Topical: *Children >12 years and Adults:* Apply once daily **or** every other day

Administration

Topical Palliation of fine wrinkles, mottled hyperpigmentation, and tactile roughness of facial skin: Cream: Prior to application, gently wash face with a mild soap. Pat dry. Wait 20-30 minutes to apply cream. Avoid eyes, ears, nostrils, and mouth.

Nursing Actions

Patient Education For once-daily use, do not overuse. Thoroughly wash hands before applying. Wash area to be treated at least 30 minutes before applying. Do not wash face more frequently than 2-3 times a day. Do not apply to areas near your mouth, eyes, corners of your nose, or open sores. Avoid using topical preparations that contain alcohol or harsh chemicals during treatment. It may take several weeks before the full benefit of the medication is seen. You may experience increased sensitivity to sunlight; protect skin with sunblock (minimum SPF 15), wear protective clothing, and avoid direct sunlight. Stop treatment and inform prescriber if rash, skin irritation, redness, scaling, or excessive dryness occurs. When used for hyperpigmentation and tactile redness of facial skin, wrinkles will not be eliminated. Must be used in combination with a comprehensive skin care program.

Triamcinolone (Systemic)

(trye am SIN oh lone)

Brand Names: U.S. Aristospan®; Kenalog®-10; Kenalog®-40

Index Terms Triamcinolone Acetonide, Parenteral; Triamcinolone Hexacetonide

Pharmacologic Category Corticosteroid, Systemic

Medication Safety Issues

Sound-alike/look-alike issues:

Kenalog® may be confused with Ketalar®

Other safety concerns:

TAC (occasional abbreviation for triamcinolone) is an error-prone abbreviation (mistaken as tetracaine-adrenaline-cocaine)

Pregnancy Risk Factor C

Lactation Excretion in breast milk unknown/use caution

Breast-Feeding Considerations Corticosteroids are excreted in human milk; information specific to triamcinolone has not been located.

Use

Intra-articular (soft tissue): Acute gouty arthritis, acute/subacute bursitis, acute tenosynovitis, epicondylitis, rheumatoid arthritis, synovitis of osteoarthritis

Intralesional: Alopecia areata, discoid lupus erythematosus, keloids, granuloma annulare lesions (localized hypertrophic, infiltrated, or inflammatory), lichen planus plaques, lichen simplex chronicus plaques, psoriatic plaques, necrobiosis lipoidica diabeticorum, cystic tumors of aponeurosis or tendon (ganglia)

Systemic: Adrenocortical insufficiency, dermatologic diseases, endocrine disorders, gastrointestinal diseases, hematologic and neoplastic disorders, nervous system disorders, nephrotic syndrome, rheumatic disorders, allergic states, respiratory diseases, systemic lupus erythematosus (SLE), and other diseases requiring anti-inflammatory or immunosuppressive effects

Mechanism of Action/Effect Decreases inflammation by suppression of migration of polymorphonuclear leukocytes and reversal of increased capillary permeability; suppresses the immune system by reducing activity and volume of the lymphatic system; suppresses adrenal function at high doses

Contraindications Hypersensitivity to triamcinolone or any component of the formulation; systemic fungal infections; cerebral malaria; idiopathic thrombocytopenic purpura (I.M. injection)

Warnings/Precautions May cause hypercorticism or suppression of hypothalamic-pituitary-adrenal (HPA) axis, particularly in younger children or in patients receiving high doses for prolonged periods. HPA axis suppression may lead to adrenal crisis. Withdrawal and discontinuation of a corticosteroid should be done slowly and carefully.

Acute myopathy has been reported with high-dose corticosteroids, usually in patients with neuromuscular transmission disorders; may involve ocular and/or respiratory muscles; monitor creatine kinase; recovery may be delayed. Corticosteroid use may cause psychiatric disturbances, including depression, euphoria, insomnia, mood swings, and personality changes. Pre-existing psychiatric conditions may be exacerbated by corticosteroid use. Prolonged use of corticosteroids may also increase the incidence of secondary infection, mask acute infection (including fungal infections), prolong or exacerbate viral infections, or limit response to vaccines. Exposure to chickenpox should be avoided; corticosteroids should not be used to treat ocular herpes simplex. Corticosteroids should not be used for cerebral malaria or viral hepatitis. Close observation is required in patients with latent tuberculosis and/or TB reactivity; restrict use in active TB (only in conjunction with antituberculosis treatment). Use with caution in patients with threadworm infection; may cause serious hyperinfection. Prolonged treatment with corticosteroids has been associated with the development of Kaposi's sarcoma (case reports); if noted, discontinuation of therapy should be considered. Avoid use in head injury patients.

Use with caution in patients with thyroid disease, hepatic impairment, renal impairment, cardiovascular disease, diabetes, myasthenia gravis, patients at risk for osteoporosis, patients at risk for seizures, or GI diseases (diverticulitis, peptic ulcer, ulcerative colitis) due to perforation risk. Avoid use in head injury patients. Use caution following acute MI (corticosteroids have been associated with myocardial rupture). Because of the risk of adverse effects, systemic corticosteroids should be used cautiously in the elderly in the smallest possible effective dose for the shortest duration. Patients should not be immunized with live, viral vaccines while receiving immunosuppressive doses of corticosteroids. The ability to respond to dead viral vaccines is unknown.

Withdraw therapy with gradual tapering of dose. There have been reports of systemic corticosteroid withdrawal symptoms (eg, joint/muscle pain, lassitude, depression) when withdrawing oral inhalation therapy. Injection suspension contains benzyl alcohol; benzyl alcohol has been associated with the "gasping syndrome" in neonates and low-birth-weight infants. Administer products only via recommended route (depending on product used). Do **not** administer any triamcinolone product via the epidural or intrathecal route; serious adverse events, including fatalities, have been reported.

Drug Interactions

Avoid Concomitant Use

Avoid concomitant use of Triamcinolone (Systemic) with any of the following: Aldesleukin; BCG; Natalizumab; Pimecrolimus; Tacrolimus (Topical)

Decreased Effect

Triamcinolone (Systemic) may decrease the levels/effects of: Aldesleukin; Antidiabetic Agents; BCG; Calcitriol; Coccidioidin Skin Test; Corticorelin; Isoniazid; Salicylates; Sipuleucel-T; Telaprevir; Vaccines (Inactivated)

The levels/effects of Triamcinolone (Systemic) may be decreased by: Aminoglutethimide; Barbiturates; Echinacea; Mitotane; Primidone; Rifamycin Derivatives

Increased Effect/Toxicity

Triamcinolone (Systemic) may increase the levels/effects of: Acetylcholinesterase Inhibitors; Amphotericin B; Deferasirox; Leflunomide; Loop Diuretics; Natalizumab; NSAID (COX-2 Inhibitor); NSAID (Nonselective); Thiazide Diuretics; Vaccines (Live); Warfarin

The levels/effects of Triamcinolone (Systemic) may be increased by: Antifungal Agents (Azole Derivatives, Systemic); Aprepitant; Calcium Channel Blockers (Nondihydropyridine); Denosumab; Estrogen Derivatives; Fluconazole; Fosaprepitant; Indacaterol; Macrolide Antibiotics; Neuromuscular-Blocking Agents (Nondepolarizing); Pimecrolimus; Quinolone Antibiotics; Roflumilast; Salicylates; Tacrolimus (Topical); Telaprevir; Trastuzumab

Adverse Reactions Frequency not defined; reactions reported with corticosteroid therapy in general:

Cardiovascular: Arrhythmia, bradycardia, cardiac arrest, cardiac enlargement, CHF, circulatory collapse, edema, hypertension, hypertrophic cardiomyopathy (premature infants), myocardial rupture (following recent MI), syncope, tachycardia, thromboembolism, vasculitis

Central nervous system: Arachnoiditis (I.T.), depression, emotional instability, euphoria, headache, insomnia, intracranial pressure increased, malaise, meningitis (I.T.), mood changes, neuritis, neuropathy, personality change, pseudotumor cerebri (with discontinuation), seizure, spinal cord infarction, stroke, vertigo

Dermatologic: Abscess (sterile), acne, allergic dermatitis, angioedema, atrophy (cutaneous/subcutaneous), bruising, dry skin, erythema, hair thinning, hirsutism, hyper-/hypopigmentation, hypertrichosis, impaired wound healing, lupus erythematosus-like lesions, petechiae, purpura, rash, skin test suppression, striae, thin skin

Endocrine & metabolic: Carbohydrate intolerance, Cushingoid state, diabetes mellitus, fluid retention, glucose intolerance, growth suppression (children), hypokalemia, hypokalemic alkalosis, menstrual irregularities, negative nitrogen balance, sodium retention, sperm motility altered

Gastrointestinal: Abdominal distention, appetite increased, GI hemorrhage, GI perforation, nausea, pancreatitis, peptic ulcer, ulcerative esophagitis, weight gain

Hepatic: Hepatomegaly, liver function tests increased

Local: Thrombophlebitis

Neuromuscular & skeletal: Aseptic necrosis of femoral and humeral heads, calcinosis, Charcot-like arthropathy, fractures, joint tissue damage, muscle mass loss, myopathy, osteoporosis, parasthesia, paraplegia, quadriplegia, tendon rupture, vertebral compression fractures, weakness

Ocular: Cataracts, cortical blindness, exophthalmos, glaucoma, ocular pressure increased, papilledema

Renal: Glycosuria

Respiratory: Pulmonary edema

Miscellaneous: Abnormal fat deposits, anaphylactoid reaction, anaphylaxis, diaphoresis, hiccups, infection, moon face

Available Dosage Forms

Injection, suspension:

Aristospan®: 5 mg/mL (5 mL); 20 mg/mL (1 mL, 5 mL)

Kenalog®-10: 10 mg/mL (5 mL)

Kenalog®-40: 40 mg/mL (1 mL, 5 mL, 10 mL)

General Dosage Range

I.M.:

Children 6-12 years: Acetonide: Initial: 40 mg; Range: 2.5-100 mg/day

Children >12 years: Acetonide: Initial: 60 mg; Range: 2.5-100 mg/day

Adults: Acetonide: Initial: 60 mg; Range: 2.5-100 mg/day, may repeat with 20-100 mg when symptoms recur; Multiple sclerosis: 160 mg/day for 1 week, then 64 mg every other day

Intra-articular: *Adults:* Acetonide: 2.5-80 mg; Hexacetonide: 2-20 mg

Intradermal: *Adults:* Acetonide: 1 mg/site

Intralesional: *Adults:* Acetonide: 1-30 mg (usually 1 mg/injection site); Hexacetonide: Up to 0.5 mg/sq inch

Intrasynovial: *Adults:* Acetonide: 5-40 mg

Tendon Sheath: *Adults:* Acetonide: 2.5-10 mg

Administration

I.M. Shake well before use to ensure suspension is uniform. Inspect visually to ensure no clumping; administer immediately after withdrawal so settling does not occur in the syringe. Do **not** administer any product I.V. or via the epidural or intrathecal route

Kenalog®-40 injection: For intra-articular, soft tissue or I.M. administration. When administered I.M., inject deep into the gluteal muscle using a minimum needle length of 1½ inches for adults. Obese patients may require a longer needle. Alternate sites for subsequent injections.

Other Shake well before use to ensure suspension is uniform. Inspect visually to ensure no clumping; administer immediately after withdrawal so settling does not occur in the syringe. Do **not** administer any product I.V. or via the epidural or intrathecal route.

Aristospan® (20 mg/mL concentration): For intra-articular and soft tissue administration only; a ≥23-gauge needle is preferred.

Aristospan® (5 mg/mL concentration): For intralesional or sublesional administration only; a ≥23-gauge needle is preferred.

Kenalog®-10 injection: For intra-articular or intralesional administration only. When administered intralesionally, inject directly into the lesion (ie, intradermally or subcutaneously). Tuberculin syringes with a 23- to 25-gauge needle are preferable for intralesional injections.

Kenalog®-40 injection: May administer intra-articularly or into soft tissue.

Stability

Reconstitution Hexacetonide injectable suspension: Avoid diluents containing parabens, phenol, or other preservatives (may cause flocculation). Suspension for intralesional use may be diluted with D_5NS, D_{10}NS, NS, or SWFI to a 1:1, 1:2, or 1:4 concentration. Solutions for intra-articular use, may be diluted with lidocaine 1% or 2%.

Storage Injection, suspension:

Acetonide injectable suspension: Kenalog®: Store at 20°C to 25°C (68°F to 77°F); avoid freezing. Protect from light.

Hexacetonide injectable suspension: Store at 20°C to 25°C (68°F to 77°F); avoid freezing. Protect from light. Diluted suspension stable up to 1 week.

Nursing Actions

Physical Assessment Patients with diabetes should monitor glucose levels closely (corticosteroids may alter glucose levels). When used for >10-14 days, do not discontinue abruptly; decrease dosage incrementally.

Patient Education Avoid alcohol. If you have diabetes, monitor glucose levels closely (antidiabetic medication may need to be adjusted). Inform prescriber if you are experiencing greater than normal levels of stress (medication may need adjustment). You may be more susceptible to infection. Report promptly excessive nervousness or sleep disturbances, any signs of infection (sore throat, unhealed injuries), excessive growth of body hair or loss of skin color, vision changes, weight gain, swelling of face or extremities, muscle weakness, change in color of stools (black or tarry) or persistent abdominal pain, or worsening of condition or failure to improve.

Dietary Considerations Ensure adequate intake of calcium and vitamins (or consider supplementation) in patients on medium-to-high doses of systemic corticosteroids.

Triamcinolone (Nasal) (trye am SIN oh lone)

Brand Names: U.S. Nasacort® AQ

Index Terms Triamcinolone acetonide

Pharmacologic Category Corticosteroid, Nasal

Medication Safety Issues

Sound-alike/look-alike issues:

Nasacort® may be confused with NasalCrom®

Other safety concerns:

TAC (occasional abbreviation for triamcinolone) is an error-prone abbreviation (mistaken as tetracaine-adrenaline-cocaine)

Pregnancy Risk Factor C

Lactation Excretion in breast milk unknown/use caution

Use Management of seasonal and perennial allergic rhinitis

Available Dosage Forms

Suspension, intranasal: 55 mcg/inhalation (16.5 g)

Nasacort® AQ: 55 mcg/inhalation (16.5 g)

General Dosage Range Inhalation:

Nasal inhaler:

Children 6-11 years: 220 mcg/day as 2 sprays in each nostril once daily

Children ≥12 years and Adults: 220-440 mcg/day as 2-4 sprays in each nostril 1-4 times/day

Nasal spray:

Children 2-5 years: 110 mcg/day as 1 spray in each nostril once daily (maximum: 110 mcg/day)

Children 6-11 years: Initial: 110 mcg/day as 1 spray in each nostril once daily; Maintenance: 110-220 mcg/day as 1-2 sprays in each nostril

Children ≥12 years and Adults: 110-220 mcg/day as 1-2 sprays in each nostril once daily

Administration

Inhalation Shake well prior to use. Gently blow nose to clear nostrils.

Nasacort® AQ: Prime prior to first use, by shaking contents well and releasing 5 sprays into the air. If product is not used for more than 2 weeks, reprime with 1 spray.

Nursing Actions

Patient Education Do not use if you have a nasal infection, nasal injury, or recent nasal surgery. Report unusual cough or spasm; persistent nasal bleeding, burning, or irritation; or worsening of condition.

Triamcinolone (Topical) (trye am SIN oh lone)

Brand Names: U.S. Kenalog®; Oralone®; Pediaderm™ TA; Trianex™; Triderm®; Zytopic™

Pharmacologic Category Corticosteroid, Topical

Medication Safety Issues

Sound-alike/look-alike issues:

Kenalog® may be confused with Ketalar®

Other safety concerns:

TAC (occasional abbreviation for triamcinolone) is an error-prone abbreviation (mistaken as tetracaine-adrenaline-cocaine)

Pregnancy Risk Factor C

Lactation Excretion in breast milk unknown/use caution

Use

Oral topical: Adjunctive treatment and temporary relief of symptoms associated with oral inflammatory lesions and ulcerative lesions resulting from trauma

Topical: Inflammatory dermatoses responsive to steroids

Available Dosage Forms

Aerosol, spray, topical:

Kenalog®: 0.2 mg/2-second spray (63 g, 100 g)

Cream, topical: 0.025% (15 g, 80 g, 454 g); 0.1% (15 g, 30 g, 80 g, 454 g, 2240 g, 2270 g); 0.5% (15 g)

Pediaderm™ TA: 0.1% (30 g)

Triderm®: 0.1% (30 g, 85 g)

Zytopic™: 0.1% (85 g)

Lotion, topical: 0.025% (60 mL); 0.1% (60 mL)

Ointment, topical: 0.025% (15 g, 80 g, 454 g); 0.05% (430 g); 0.1% (15 g, 80 g, 454 g); 0.5% (15 g)

Trianex™: 0.05% (17 g, 85 g)

Paste, oral topical: 0.1% (5 g)

Oralone®: 0.1% (5 g)

General Dosage Range Topical: *Adults:* Cream, ointment: Apply thin film to affected areas 2-4 times/day; Oral: Press a small dab (about 1/4") to the lesion until a thin film develops; Spray: Apply to affected area 3-4 times/day

Administration

Topical

Oral topical: Apply small dab to lesion until a thin film develops; do not rub in. Apply at bedtime or after meals if applications are needed throughout the day.

Topical:

Ointment: Apply a thin film sparingly. Do not use on open skin or wounds. Do not occlude area unless directed; if using occluding dressing, monitor for infection.

Spray: Avoid eyes and do not inhale if spraying near face. Occlusive dressing may be used if instructed; monitor for infection.

Nursing Actions

Patient Education Report promptly any signs of infection. For external use only. Not for eyes or mucous membranes or open wounds. Apply in very thin layer. Avoid prolonged or excessive use around sensitive tissues, genital, or rectal areas. Inform prescriber if condition worsens (swelling, redness, irritation, pain, open sores) or fails to improve.

Triazolam (trye AY zoe lam)

Brand Names: U.S. Halcion®

Pharmacologic Category Benzodiazepine

Medication Safety Issues

Sound-alike/look-alike issues:

Triazolam may be confused with alPRAZolam

Halcion® may be confused with halcinonide, Haldol®

BEERS Criteria medication:

This drug may be inappropriate for use in geriatric patients (high severity risk).

Medication Guide Available Yes

Pregnancy Risk Factor X

Lactation Excretion in breast milk unknown/not recommended

Use Short-term treatment of insomnia

Unlabeled Use Treatment of anxiety before dental procedures

Controlled Substance C-IV

Available Dosage Forms

Tablet, oral: 0.125 mg, 0.25 mg

Halcion®: 0.25 mg

General Dosage Range Dosage adjustment recommended in patients with hepatic impairment

Oral:

Adults: 0.125-0.25 mg at bedtime (maximum: 0.5 mg/day)

Elderly: Initial: 0.125 mg at bedtime (maximum: 0.25 mg/day)

Administration

Oral May take with food. Tablet may be crushed or swallowed whole. Onset of action is rapid, patient should be in bed when taking medication.

Nursing Actions

Physical Assessment Assess for history of addiction; long-term use can result in dependence, abuse, or tolerance. For inpatient use, institute safety measures to prevent falls.

Patient Education Drug may cause physical and/or psychological dependence. Do not use alcohol. Avoid grapefruit juice. Maintain adequate hydration unless instructed to restrict fluid intake. You may experience drowsiness, lightheadedness, impaired coordination, dizziness, blurred vision, nausea, vomiting, dry mouth, constipation, or photosensitivity. Report persistent CNS effects (eg, memory impairment; confusion; depression; increased sedation; excitation; headache; agitation; insomnia or nightmares; dizziness; fatigue; impaired coordination; changes in personality, behavior, or cognition) or worsening of condition.

Trihexyphenidyl (trye heks ee FEN i dil)

Index Terms Artane; Benzhexol Hydrochloride; Trihexyphenidyl Hydrochloride

Pharmacologic Category Anti-Parkinson's Agent, Anticholinergic; Anticholinergic Agent

Medication Safety Issues

Sound-alike/look-alike issues:

Trihexyphenidyl may be confused with trifluoperazine

Pregnancy Risk Factor C

Lactation Excretion in breast milk unknown/use caution

Use Adjunctive treatment of Parkinson's disease; treatment of drug-induced extrapyramidal symptoms

Available Dosage Forms

Elixir, oral: 2 mg/5 mL (473 mL)

Tablet, oral: 2 mg, 5 mg

General Dosage Range Oral: *Adults:* Initial: 1 mg/day; Maintenance: 3-15 mg/day in 3-4 divided doses

Administration

Oral May be administered before or after meals; tolerated best if given in 3 daily doses and with food. High doses (>10 mg/day) may be divided into 4 doses, at meal times and at bedtime.

Nursing Actions

Physical Assessment Monitor renal function. Monitor for Parkinsonian symptoms and anticholinergic syndrome (dry mouth and mucous membranes, constipation, epigastric distress, CNS disturbances, paralytic ileus).

Patient Education Take with meals if GI upset occurs. Maintain adequate hydration unless instructed to restrict fluid intake; void before taking medication. Do not use alcohol. You may experience drowsiness, confusion, vision changes, increased susceptibility to heat stroke, decreased perspiration, constipation, or dry skin or nasal passages. Report unresolved constipation, chest pain or palpitations, respiratory difficulty, CNS changes (hallucination, loss of memory, nervousness, etc), painful or difficult urination, increased muscle spasticity or rigidity, skin rash, or significant worsening of condition.

Trimethobenzamide (trye meth oh BEN za mide)

Brand Names: U.S. Tigan®

Index Terms Trimethobenzamide Hydrochloride

Pharmacologic Category Antiemetic

Medication Safety Issues

Sound-alike/look-alike issues:

Tigan® may be confused with Tiazac®, Ticlid

Trimethobenzamide may be confused with metoclopramide, trimethoprim

BEERS Criteria medication:

This drug may be inappropriate for use in geriatric patients (high severity risk).

Lactation Excretion in breast milk unknown

Use Treatment of postoperative nausea and vomiting; treatment of nausea associated with gastroenteritis

Available Dosage Forms

Capsule, oral: 300 mg

Tigan®: 300 mg

Injection, solution:

Tigan®: 100 mg/mL (20 mL)

Injection, solution [preservative free]:

Tigan®: 100 mg/mL (2 mL)

General Dosage Range

I.M.: *Adults:* 200 mg 3-4 times/day **or** 200 mg as a single dose, repeat 1 hour later

Oral: *Children >40 kg and Adults:* 300 mg 3-4 times/day

Administration

Oral Capsule: Administer capsule orally without regard to meals.

I.M. Injection: Administer I.M. only. Inject deep into upper outer quadrant of gluteal muscle.

I.V. Injection: Not for I.V. administration.

I.V. Detail pH: 5

Nursing Actions

Physical Assessment Monitor for hypovolemia, angioedema, and postural hypotension. If self-administered injection, teach patient appropriate injection technique and syringe disposal.

Patient Education If using injection formulation, follow directions for injection and disposal of syringe. May cause drowsiness, blurred vision, or diarrhea. Report chest pain or palpitations, persistent dizziness or blurred vision, or CNS changes (disorientation, depression, confusion).

Trimethoprim (trye METH oh prim)

Brand Names: U.S. Primsol®

Index Terms TMP

Pharmacologic Category Antibiotic, Miscellaneous

Pregnancy Risk Factor C

Lactation Enters breast milk/use caution

Breast-Feeding Considerations Trimethoprim is excreted in breast milk. The manufacturer recommends caution while using trimethoprim in a breast-feeding woman because trimethoprim may interfere with folic acid metabolism. Nondose-related effects could include modification of bowel flora. Also see the sulfamethoxazole and trimethoprim monograph for additional information.

Use Treatment of urinary tract infections due to susceptible strains of *E. coli*, *P. mirabilis*, *K. pneumoniae*, *Enterobacter* spp and coagulase-negative *Staphylococcus* including *S. saprophyticus*; acute otitis media due to susceptible strains of *S. pneumoniae* and *H. influenzae* in children

Unlabeled Use Alternative agent for *Pneumocystis jirovecii* pneumonia (in combination with dapsone)

Mechanism of Action/Effect Inhibits folic acid reduction to tetrahydrofolate, and thereby inhibits microbial growth

Contraindications Hypersensitivity to trimethoprim or any component of the formulation; megaloblastic anemia due to folate deficiency

Warnings/Precautions Use with caution in patients with impaired renal or hepatic function or with possible folate deficiency. Prolonged use may result in fungal or bacterial superinfection, including *C. difficile*-associated diarrhea (CDAD) and pseudomembranous colitis; CDAD has been observed >2 months postantibiotic treatment.

Drug Interactions

Avoid Concomitant Use

Avoid concomitant use of Trimethoprim with any of the following: BCG; Dofetilide

Decreased Effect

Trimethoprim may decrease the levels/effects of: BCG; Typhoid Vaccine

The levels/effects of Trimethoprim may be decreased by: CYP2C9 Inducers (Strong); CYP3A4 Inducers (Strong); Deferasirox; Herbs (CYP3A4 Inducers); Leucovorin Calcium-Levoleucovorin; Peginterferon Alfa-2b; Tocilizumab

Increased Effect/Toxicity

Trimethoprim may increase the levels/effects of: ACE Inhibitors; Amantadine; Angiotensin II Receptor Blockers; Antidiabetic Agents (Thiazolidinedione); AzaTHIOprine; Carvedilol; CYP2C8 Substrates; CYP2C9 Substrates; Dapsone; Dapsone (Systemic); Dapsone (Topical); Dofetilide; Eplerenone; Fosphenytoin; LamiVUDine; Memantine; Mercaptopurine; Methotrexate; Phenytoin; PRALAtrexate; Procainamide; Repaglinide; Spironolactone; Varenicline

The levels/effects of Trimethoprim may be increased by: Amantadine; Conivaptan; CYP2C9 Inhibitors (Moderate); CYP2C9 Inhibitors (Strong); Dapsone; Dapsone (Systemic); Memantine

Adverse Reactions Frequency not defined.

Central nervous system: Aseptic meningitis (rare), fever

Dermatologic: Maculopapular rash (3% to 7% at 200 mg/day; incidence higher with larger daily doses), erythema multiforme (rare), exfoliative dermatitis (rare), pruritus (common), phototoxic skin eruptions, Stevens-Johnson syndrome (rare), toxic epidermal necrolysis (rare)

Endocrine & metabolic: Hyperkalemia, hyponatremia

Gastrointestinal: Epigastric distress, glossitis, nausea, vomiting

Hematologic: Leukopenia, megaloblastic anemia, methemoglobinemia, neutropenia, thrombocytopenia

Hepatic: Cholestatic jaundice (rare), liver enzymes increased

Renal: BUN and creatinine increased

Miscellaneous: Anaphylaxis, hypersensitivity reactions

Available Dosage Forms

Solution, oral:

Primsol®: 50 mg (base)/5 mL (473 mL)

Tablet, oral: 100 mg

General Dosage Range Dosage adjustment recommended in patients with renal impairment

Oral:

Children ≥2 months: 4-12 mg/kg/day in divided doses every 12 hours

Adults: 100 mg once daily **or** 100 mg every 12 hours **or** 200 mg every 24 hours; up to 15mg/kg/day

Administration

Oral Administer with milk or food.

Stability

Storage

Solution: Store between 15°C to 25°C (59°F to 77°F). Protect from light.

Tablets: Store at 20°C to 25°C (68°F to 77°F). Protect from light.

Nursing Actions

Physical Assessment Culture and sensitivity should be assessed prior to initiating therapy.

Patient Education Maintain adequate hydration unless instructed to restrict fluid intake. May cause nausea, vomiting, or GI upset. Report skin rash, redness, or irritation; feelings of acute fatigue or weakness; or unusual bleeding or bruising.

Dietary Considerations May cause folic acid deficiency, supplements may be needed. Should be taken with milk or food.

Trimipramine (trye MI pra meen)

Brand Names: U.S. Surmontil®

Index Terms Trimipramine Maleate

Pharmacologic Category Antidepressant, Tricyclic (Tertiary Amine)

Medication Safety Issues

Sound-alike/look-alike issues:

Trimipramine may be confused with triamterene

Medication Guide Available Yes

Pregnancy Risk Factor C

Use Treatment of depression

Available Dosage Forms

Capsule, oral:

Surmontil®: 25 mg, 50 mg, 100 mg

General Dosage Range
Oral:
Adolescents: Initial: 50 mg/day (maximum: 100 mg/day)
Adults: 50-200 mg at bedtime (maximum: 200 mg/day [outpatient] or 300 mg/day [inpatient])
Elderly: 50-100 mg at bedtime (maximum: 100 mg/day)

Nursing Actions
Physical Assessment Monitor therapeutic response (eg, mental status, mood, affect, suicide ideation).
Patient Education It may take 2-3 weeks to achieve desired results. Take at bedtime. Avoid alcohol. Maintain adequate hydration unless instructed to restrict fluid intake. You may experience drowsiness, lightheadedness, dizziness, blurred vision, nausea, altered taste, dry mouth, constipation, diarrhea, increased appetite, postural hypotension, urinary retention, or sexual dysfunction (reversible). Report persistent CNS effects (eg, insomnia, restlessness, fatigue, anxiety, impaired cognitive function, seizures, suicide ideation); muscle cramping or tremors; chest pain, palpitations, rapid heartbeat, swelling of extremities, or severe dizziness; unresolved urinary retention; vision changes or eye pain; yellowing of eyes or skin; pale stools/dark urine; suicide ideation; or worsening of condition.

Triptorelin (trip toe REL in)

Brand Names: U.S. Trelstar®
Index Terms AY-25650; CL-118,532; D-Trp(6)-LHRH; Detryptoreline; Triptorelin Pamoate; Tryptoreline
Pharmacologic Category Gonadotropin Releasing Hormone Agonist
Pregnancy Risk Factor X
Lactation Excretion in breast milk unknown/not recommended
Use Palliative treatment of advanced prostate cancer
Unlabeled Use Treatment of endometriosis, *in vitro* fertilization, precocious puberty, uterine sarcoma
Available Dosage Forms
Injection, powder for reconstitution:
Trelstar®: 3.75 mg, 11.25 mg, 22.5 mg
General Dosage Range I.M.: *Adults:* 3.75 mg once every 4 weeks **or** 11.25 mg once every 12 weeks **or** 22.5 mg once every 24 weeks
Administration
I.M. Administer by I.M. injection into the buttock; alternate injection sites. Administer immediately after reconstitution.
Nursing Actions
Physical Assessment Hypersensitivity reactions, including angioedema, anaphylaxis, and anaphylactic shock, have rarely occurred; discontinue if severe reaction occurs.
Patient Education This medication can only be administered by injection. If you have diabetes, monitor blood sugar closely; may alter blood glucose levels. Report swelling, pain, or burning at injection site. May cause disease flare (increased bone pain), blood in urine, urinary retention during early treatment (usually resolves within 1 week), impotence, or hot flashes. Report any persistent adverse GI upset; chest pain, rapid heartbeat, or palpations; numbness in extremities; acute headache; or alterations in urinary pattern. Report immediately sudden headache, severe vomiting, visual or mental status change, and cardiovascular collapse.

Ulipristal (ue li PRIS tal)

Brand Names: U.S. ella®
Index Terms CDB-2914; Ulipristal Acetate
Pharmacologic Category Contraceptive; Progestin Receptor Modulator
Medication Safety Issues
Sound-alike/look-alike issues:
Ulipristal may be confused with ursodiol
Pregnancy Risk Factor X
Lactation Excretion unknown/not recommended
Use Emergency contraception following unprotected intercourse or possible contraceptive failure
Available Dosage Forms
Tablet, oral:
ella®: 30 mg
General Dosage Range Oral: *Adults:* 1 tablet (30 mg) as a single dose
Administration
Oral Administer with or without food at anytime during menstrual cycle. If vomiting occurs within 3 hours of administration, consider repeating dose.

Ursodiol (ur soe DYE ol)

Brand Names: U.S. Actigall®; Urso 250®; Urso Forte®
Index Terms Ursodeoxycholic Acid
Pharmacologic Category Gallstone Dissolution Agent
Medication Safety Issues
Sound-alike/look-alike issues:
Ursodiol may be confused with ulipristal
Pregnancy Risk Factor B
Lactation Excretion in breast milk unknown/use caution
Use
Actigall®: Gallbladder stone dissolution; prevention of gallstones in obese patients experiencing rapid weight loss
Urso®, Urso Forte®: Primary biliary cirrhosis

Available Dosage Forms

Capsule, oral: 300 mg

Actigall®: 300 mg

Tablet, oral: 250 mg, 500 mg

Urso 250®: 250 mg

Urso Forte®: 500 mg

General Dosage Range Oral: *Adults:* 8-15 mg/kg/day in 2-4 divided doses **or** 300 mg twice daily

Administration

Oral Do not administer with aluminum-based antacids. If aluminum-based antacids are needed, administer 2 hours after ursodiol. Urso Forte® can be split into halves for appropriate dosage; do not chew. Urso® and Urso Forte® should be taken with food.

Nursing Actions

Patient Education Take with food. Drug will need to be taken for 1-3 months after stone is dissolved; stones may recur. Report any persistent nausea, vomiting, abdominal pain, or yellowing of skin or eyes.

ValACYclovir (val ay SYE kloe veer)

Brand Names: U.S. Valtrex®

Index Terms Valacyclovir Hydrochloride

Pharmacologic Category Antiviral Agent; Antiviral Agent, Oral

Medication Safety Issues

Sound-alike/look-alike issues:

Valtrex® may be confused with Keflex®, Valcyte®, Zovirax®

ValACYclovir may be confused with acyclovir, valGANciclovir, vancomycin

Pregnancy Risk Factor B

Lactation Enters breast milk/use caution

Breast-Feeding Considerations Peak concentrations in breast milk range from 0.5-2.3 times the corresponding maternal acyclovir serum concentration. This is expected to provide a nursing infant with a dose of acyclovir equivalent to ~0.6 mg/kg/day following ingestion of valacyclovir 500 mg twice daily by the mother. Use with caution while breast-feeding.

Use Treatment of herpes zoster (shingles) in immunocompetent patients; treatment of first-episode and recurrent genital herpes; suppression of recurrent genital herpes and reduction of heterosexual transmission of genital herpes in immunocompetent patients; suppression of genital herpes in HIV-infected individuals; treatment of herpes labialis (cold sores); chickenpox in immunocompetent children

Unlabeled Use Prophylaxis of cancer-related HSV, VZV, and CMV infections; treatment of cancer-related HSV, VZV infection

Mechanism of Action/Effect Valacyclovir is rapidly converted to acyclovir before it exerts its antiviral activity against HSV-1, HSV-2, or VZV. Inhibits viral DNA synthesis and replication.

Contraindications Hypersensitivity to valacyclovir, acyclovir, or any component of the formulation

Warnings/Precautions Thrombotic thrombocytopenic purpura/hemolytic uremic syndrome has occurred in immunocompromised patients (at doses of 8 g/day). Safety and efficacy have not been established for treatment/suppression of recurrent genital herpes or disseminated herpes in patients with profound immunosuppression (eg, advanced HIV with CD4 <100 cells/mm^3). CNS adverse effects (including agitation, hallucinations, confusion, delirium, seizures, and encephalopathy) have been reported. Use caution in patients with renal impairment, the elderly, and/or those receiving nephrotoxic agents. Acute renal failure has been observed in patients with renal dysfunction; dose adjustment may be required. Decreased precipitation in renal tubules may occur leading to urinary precipitation; adequately hydrate patient. For cold sores, treatment should begin at with earliest symptom (tingling, itching, burning). For genital herpes, treatment should begin as soon as possible after the first signs and symptoms (within 72 hours of onset of first diagnosis or within 24 hours of onset of recurrent episodes). For herpes zoster, treatment should begin within 72 hours of onset of rash. For chickenpox, treatment should begin with earliest sign or symptom. Use with caution in the elderly; CNS effects have been reported. Safety and efficacy have not been established in patients <2 years of age.

Drug Interactions

Avoid Concomitant Use

Avoid concomitant use of ValACYclovir with any of the following: Zoster Vaccine

Decreased Effect

ValACYclovir may decrease the levels/effects of: Zoster Vaccine

Increased Effect/Toxicity

ValACYclovir may increase the levels/effects of: Mycophenolate; Tenofovir; Zidovudine

The levels/effects of ValACYclovir may be increased by: Mycophenolate

Adverse Reactions

>10%:

Central nervous system: Headache (13% to 38%)

Gastrointestinal: Nausea (5% to 15%), abdominal pain (1% to 11%)

Hematologic: Neutropenia (≤18%)

Hepatic: ALT increased (≤14%), AST increased (2% to 16%)

Respiratory: Nasopharyngitis (≤16%)

1% to 10%:

Central nervous system: Fatigue (≤8%), depression (≤7%), fever (children 4%), dizziness (2% to 4%)

Dermatologic: Rash (≤8%)

Endocrine: Dysmenorrhea (≤1% to 8%), dehydration (children 2%)
Gastrointestinal: Vomiting (<1% to 6%), diarrhea (children 5%; adults <1%)
Hematologic: Thrombocytopenia (≤3%)
Hepatic: Alkaline phosphatase increased (≤4%)
Neuromuscular & skeletal: Arthralgia (<1 to 6%)
Respiratory: Rhinorrhea (children 2%)
Miscellaneous: Herpes simplex (children 2%)

Available Dosage Forms

Caplet, oral: 500 mg, 1 g

Valtrex®: 500 mg, 1 g

Tablet, oral: 500 mg, 1 g

General Dosage Range Dosage adjustment recommended in patients with renal impairment

Oral:

Children 2 to <12 years: 20 mg/kg/dose 3 times/day (maximum: 1 g 3 times/day)

Children ≥12 to <18 years: 2 g every 12 hours for 1 day **or** 20 mg/kg/dose 3 times/day (maximum: 1 g 3 times/day)

Adults: 500 mg to 1 g 1-3 times/day **or** 2 g every 12 hours for 1 day

Administration

Oral If GI upset occurs, administer with meals.

Stability

Storage Store at 15°C to 25°C (59°F to 77°F).

Nursing Actions

Physical Assessment Monitor for CNS changes (dizziness, depression), nausea, vomiting, dysmenorrhea, and arthralgia. Teach patient appropriate timing of treatment.

Patient Education This medication is not a cure for genital herpes; it is not known if it will prevent transmission to others. Use appropriate precautions to prevent spread to other persons. Begin use at first sign of herpes. Maintain adequate hydration, unless instructed to restrict fluid intake. May cause headache, dizziness, nausea, vomiting, or abdominal pain. Immediately report difficulty swallowing or breathing, rash, or hives.

Dietary Considerations May be taken with or without food.

ValGANCIclovir (val gan SYE kloh veer)

Brand Names: U.S. Valcyte®

Index Terms Valganciclovir Hydrochloride

Pharmacologic Category Antiviral Agent

Medication Safety Issues

Sound-alike/look-alike issues:

Valcyte® may be confused with Valium®, Valtrex®

ValGANciclovir may be confused with valACYclovir

Pregnancy Risk Factor C

Lactation Excretion in breast milk unknown/not recommended

Breast-Feeding Considerations HIV-infected mothers are discouraged from breast-feeding to decrease the potential transmission of HIV.

Use Treatment of cytomegalovirus (CMV) retinitis in patients with acquired immunodeficiency syndrome (AIDS); prevention of CMV disease in high-risk patients (donor CMV positive/recipient CMV negative) undergoing kidney, heart, or kidney/pancreas transplantation

Mechanism of Action/Effect Valganciclovir is a prodrug of ganciclovir, and is rapidly metabolized in the body to form ganciclovir. Ganciclovir inhibits the formation of viral DNA within infected cells, blocking reproduction of the virus.

Contraindications Hypersensitivity to valganciclovir, ganciclovir, or any component of the formulation

Warnings/Precautions Hazardous agent - use appropriate precautions for handling and disposal. **[U.S. Boxed Warning]: May cause dose- or therapy-limiting granulocytopenia, anemia, and/or thrombocytopenia;** do not use in patients with an absolute neutrophil count <500/mm^3, platelet count <25,000/mm^3, or hemoglobin <8 g/dL. Uuse with caution in patients with impaired renal function (dose adjustment required). Acute renal failure (ARF) may occur; ensure adequate hydration and use with caution in patients receiving concomitant nephrotoxic agents. Elderly patients with or without pre-existing renal impairment may develop ARF; use with caution and adjust dose as needed. **[U.S. Boxed Warning]: Ganciclovir may be teratogenic, carcinogenic, and cause aspermatogenesis.** Due to its teratogenic potential, contraceptive precautions for female and male patients need to be followed during and for at least 90 days after therapy with the drug. Fertility may be temporarily or permanently impaired in males and females. Due to differences in bioavailability, valganciclovir tablets cannot be substituted for ganciclovir capsules on a one-to-one basis. The preferred dosage form for pediatric patients is the oral solution; however, valganciclovir tablets may used so long as the calculated dose is within 10% of the available tablet strength (450 mg). Not indicated for use in liver transplant patients (higher incidence of tissue-invasive CMV relative to oral ganciclovir was observed in trials). Use of valganciclovir for the treatment of congenital CMV disease has not been evaluated.

Drug Interactions

Avoid Concomitant Use

Avoid concomitant use of ValGANciclovir with any of the following: Imipenem

Decreased Effect There are no known significant interactions involving a decrease in effect.

Increased Effect/Toxicity

ValGANciclovir may increase the levels/effects of: Imipenem; Mycophenolate; Reverse Transcriptase Inhibitors (Nucleoside); Tenofovir

The levels/effects of ValGANciclovir may be increased by: Mycophenolate; Probenecid; Tenofovir

Nutritional/Ethanol Interactions Food: Coadministration with a high-fat meal increased AUC by 30%. Management: Valganciclovir should be taken with meals.

Adverse Reactions

>10%:

Cardiovascular: Hypertension (12% to 18%)

Central nervous system: Fever (9% to 31%), headache (6% to 22%), insomnia (6% to 20%)

Gastrointestinal: Diarrhea (16% to 41%), nausea (8% to 30%), vomiting (3% to 21%), abdominal pain (15%), constipation

Hematologic: Anemia (≤31%), thrombocytopenia (≤22%), neutropenia (3% to 19%)

Neuromuscular & skeletal: Tremor (12% to 28%)

Ocular: Retinal detachment (15%)

Renal: Serum creatinine increased (S_{cr} >1.5-2.5 mg/dL: 12% to 50%; S_{cr} >2.5: 3% to 17%)

Respiratory: Cough, upper respiratory tract infection

5% to 10%: Central nervous system: Peripheral neuropathy (9%), paresthesia (8%)

<5%:

Cardiovascular: Edema, hypotension, peripheral edema

Central nervous system: Agitation, confusion, depression, dizziness, fatigue, hallucination, pain, psychosis, seizure

Dermatologic: Acne, dermatitis, pruritus

Endocrine & metabolic: Dehydration, hyperglycemia, hyper-/hypokalemia, hypocalcemia, hypomagnesemia, hypophosphatemia

Gastrointestinal: Abdominal distention/pain, appetite (decreased), dyspepsia

Genitourinary: Urinary tract infection

Hematologic: Aplastic anemia, bleeding (potentially life-threatening due to thrombocytopenia), bone marrow depression, pancytopenia

Hepatic: Ascites

Neuromuscular & skeletal: Arthralgia, back pain, limb pain, muscle cramps, weakness

Renal: Creatinine clearance (decreased), dysuria, renal impairment

Respiratory: Dyspnea, nasopharyngitis, pharyngitis, pleural effusion, rhinorrhea

Miscellaneous: Allergic reaction, local and systemic infection (including sepsis)

Available Dosage Forms

Powder for solution, oral:

Valcyte®: 50 mg/mL (100 mL)

Tablet, oral:

Valcyte®: 450 mg

General Dosage Range Dosage adjustment recommended in patients with renal impairment

Oral:

Children 4 months to 16 years: Dose (mg) = 7 x body surface area x creatinine clearance once daily

Children >16 years and Adults: 900 mg 1-2 times/day

Administration

Oral Valganciclovir should be taken with meals. The preferred dosage form for pediatric patients is the oral solution; however, valganciclovir tablets may used so long as the calculated dose is within 10% of the available tablet strength (450 mg).

Due to the carcinogenic and mutagenic potential, avoid direct contact with broken or crushed tablets, powder for oral solution, and oral solution. Consideration should be given to handling and disposal according to guidelines issued for antineoplastic drugs. However, there is no consensus on the need for these precautions.

Stability

Reconstitution Oral solution: Prior to dispensing, prepare the oral solution by adding 91 mL of purified water to the bottle; shake well. Discard any unused medication after 49 days. A reconstituted 100 mL bottle will only provide 88 mL of solution for administration.

Storage

Oral solution: Store dry powder at 25°C (77°F); excursions permitted to 15°C to 30°C (59°F to 86°F). Store oral solution under refrigeration at 2°C to 8°C (36°F to 46°F); do not freeze. Discard any unused medication after 49 days.

Tablet: Store at 25°C (77°F); excursions permitted to 15°C to 30°C (59°F to 86°F).

Nursing Actions

Physical Assessment Monitor for peripheral neuropathy, neutropenia, anemia, nephrotoxicity, vomiting, and bloody diarrhea on a regular basis during therapy.

Patient Education This medication is not a cure for CMV retinitis. You will need frequent and regular laboratory tests and ophthalmic exams while taking this medication. Maintain adequate hydration, unless instructed to restrict fluid intake. May cause headache, insomnia, nausea, vomiting, diarrhea, or photosensitivity. Report fever, chills, unusual bleeding or bruising, infection or unhealed sores, white plaques in mouth or vaginal discharge, CNS disturbances (eg, hallucinations, confusion, nightmares), or weakness or loss of feeling in nerves or muscles.

Dietary Considerations Should be taken with meals.

Valproic Acid (val PROE ik AS id)

Brand Names: U.S. Depacon®; Depakene®; Stavzor™

Index Terms 2-Propylpentanoic Acid; 2-Propylvaleric Acid; Dipropylacetic Acid; DPA; Valproate Semisodium; Valproate Sodium

Pharmacologic Category Anticonvulsant, Miscellaneous; Antimanic Agent; Histone Deacetylase Inhibitor

Medication Safety Issues

Sound-alike/look-alike issues:

Depakene® may be confused with Depakote®

Valproate sodium may be confused with vecuronium

Pregnancy Risk Factor D

Lactation Enters breast milk/not recommended (AAP considers "compatible"; AAP 2001 update pending)

Breast-Feeding Considerations Breast milk concentrations of valproic acid have been reported as 1% to 10% of maternal concentration. The weight-adjusted dose to the infant has been calculated to be ~4%.

Use Monotherapy and adjunctive therapy in the treatment of patients with complex partial seizures; monotherapy and adjunctive therapy of simple and complex absence seizures; adjunctive therapy in patients with multiple seizure types that include absence seizures

Stavzor™: Mania associated with bipolar disorder; migraine prophylaxis

Unlabeled Use Status epilepticus, diabetic neuropathy

Mechanism of Action/Effect Causes increased availability of gamma-aminobutyric acid (GABA), an inhibitory neurotransmitter, to brain neurons or may enhance the action of GABA or mimic its action at postsynaptic receptor sites

Contraindications Hypersensitivity to valproic acid, derivatives, or any component of the formulation; hepatic disease or significant impairment; urea cycle disorders

Warnings/Precautions [U.S. Boxed Warning]: Hepatic failure resulting in fatalities has occurred in patients; children <2 years of age are at considerable risk. Other risk factors include organic brain disease, mental retardation with severe seizure disorders, congenital metabolic disorders, and patients on multiple anticonvulsants. Hepatotoxicity has usually been reported within 6 months of therapy initiation. Monitor patients closely for appearance of malaise, weakness, facial edema, anorexia, jaundice, and vomiting; discontinue immediately with signs/symptom of significant or suspected impairment. Liver function tests should be performed at baseline and at regular intervals after initiation of therapy, especially within the first 6 months. Hepatic dysfunction may progress despite discontinuing treatment. Should only be used as monotherapy in children <2 years of age and patients at high risk for hepatotoxicity. Contraindicated with severe impairment.

[U.S. Boxed Warning]: Cases of life-threatening pancreatitis, occurring at the start of therapy or following years of use, have been reported in adults and children. Some cases have been hemorrhagic with rapid progression of initial symptoms to death. Promptly evaluate symptoms of abdominal pain, nausea, vomiting, and/or anorexia; should generally be discontinued if pancreatitis is diagnosed.

[U.S. Boxed Warning]: May cause teratogenic effects such as neural tube defects (eg, spina bifida). Use in women of childbearing potential requires that benefits of use in mother be weighed against the potential risk to fetus, especially when used for conditions not associated with permanent injury or risk of death (eg, migraine).

May cause severe thrombocytopenia, inhibition of platelet aggregation, and bleeding. Tremors may indicate overdosage; use with caution in patients receiving other anticonvulsants. Hypersensitivity reactions affecting multiple organs have been reported in association with valproic acid use; may include dermatologic and/or hematologic changes (eosinophilia, neutropenia, thrombocytopenia) or symptoms of organ dysfunction.

Hyperammonemia and/or encephalopathy, sometimes fatal, have been reported following the initiation of valproic acid therapy and may be present with normal transaminase levels. Ammonia levels should be measured in patients who develop unexplained lethargy and vomiting, changes in mental status, or in patients who present with hypothermia (unintentional drop in core body temperature to <35°C/95°F). Discontinue therapy if ammonia levels are increased and evaluate for possible urea cycle disorder (UCD); contraindicated in patients with UCD. Evaluation of UCD should be considered for the following patients prior to the start of therapy: History of unexplained encephalopathy or coma; encephalopathy associated with protein load; pregnancy or postpartum encephalopathy; unexplained mental retardation; history of elevated plasma ammonia or glutamine; history of cyclical vomiting and lethargy; episodic extreme irritability, ataxia; low BUN or protein avoidance; family history of UCD or unexplained infant deaths (particularly male); or signs or symptoms of UCD (hyperammonemia, encephalopathy, respiratory alkalosis). Hypothermia has been reported with valproic acid therapy; may or may not be associated with hyperammonemia; may also occur with concomitant topiramate therapy.

In vitro studies have suggested valproic acid stimulates the replication of HIV and CMV viruses under experimental conditions. The clinical consequence of this is unknown, but should be considered when monitoring affected patients.

Antiepileptics are associated with an increased risk of suicidal behavior/thoughts with use (regardless of indication); patients should be monitored for signs/symptoms of depression, suicidal tendencies, and other unusual behavior changes during therapy and instructed to inform their healthcare provider immediately if symptoms occur.

Use of Depacon® injection is not recommended for post-traumatic seizure prophylaxis following acute head trauma. Anticonvulsants should not be discontinued abruptly because of the possibility of increasing seizure frequency; valproic acid should be withdrawn gradually to minimize the potential of increased seizure frequency, unless safety concerns require a more rapid withdrawal. Concomitant use with carbapenem antibiotics may reduce valproic acid levels to subtherapeutic levels; monitor levels frequently and consider alternate therapy if levels drop significantly or lack of seizure control occurs. Concomitant use with clonazepam may induce absence status. Patients treated for bipolar disorder should be monitored closely for clinical worsening or suicidality; prescriptions should be written for the smallest quantity consistent with good patient care.

CNS depression may occur with valproic acid use. Patients must be cautioned about performing tasks which require mental alertness (operating machinery or driving). Effects with other sedative drugs or ethanol may be potentiated. Use with caution in the elderly.

Drug Interactions

Avoid Concomitant Use There are no known interactions where it is recommended to avoid concomitant use.

Decreased Effect

Valproic Acid may decrease the levels/effects of: CarBAMazepine; Fosphenytoin; OXcarbazepine; Phenytoin

The levels/effects of Valproic Acid may be decreased by: Barbiturates; CarBAMazepine; Carbapenems; Cyproterone; Ethosuximide; Fosphenytoin; Methylfolate; Phenytoin; Primidone; Protease Inhibitors; Rifampin

Increased Effect/Toxicity

Valproic Acid may increase the levels/effects of: Barbiturates; Ethosuximide; LamoTRIgine; LORazepam; Paliperidone; Primidone; RisperiDONE; Rufinamide; Temozolomide; Tricyclic Antidepressants; Vorinostat; Zidovudine

The levels/effects of Valproic Acid may be increased by: ChlorproMAZINE; Felbamate; GuanFACINE; Salicylates; Topiramate

Nutritional/Ethanol Interactions

Ethanol: Avoid ethanol (may increase CNS depression).

Food: Food may delay but does not affect the extent of absorption. Valproic acid serum concentrations may be decreased if taken with food. Milk has no effect on absorption.

Herb/Nutraceutical: Avoid evening primrose (seizure threshold decreased).

Adverse Reactions

>10%:

Central nervous system: Headache (≤31%), somnolence (≤30%), dizziness (12% to 25%), insomnia (>1% to 15%), nervousness (>1% to 11%), pain (1% to 11%)

Dermatologic: Alopecia (>1% to 24%)

Gastrointestinal: Nausea (15% to 48%), vomiting (7% to 27%), diarrhea (7% to 23%), abdominal pain (7% to 23%), dyspepsia (7% to 23%), anorexia (>1% to 12%)

Hematologic: Thrombocytopenia (1% to 24%; dose related)

Neuromuscular & skeletal: Tremor (≤57%), weakness (6% to 27%)

Ocular: Diplopia (>1% to 16%), amblyopia/blurred vision (≤12%)

Miscellaneous: Infection (≤20%), flu-like syndrome (12%)

1% to 10%:

Cardiovascular: Peripheral edema (>1% to 8%), chest pain (>1% to <5%), edema (>1% to <5%), facial edema (>1% to <5%), hypertension (>1% to <5%), hypotension (>1% to <5%), palpitation (>1% to <5%), postural hypotension (>1% to <5%), tachycardia (>1% to <5%), vasodilation (>1% to <5%), arrhythmia

Central nervous system: Ataxia (>1% to 8%), amnesia (>1% to 7%), emotional lability (>1% to 6%), fever (>1% to 6%), abnormal thinking (≤6%), depression (>1% to 5%), abnormal dreams (>1% to <5%), agitation (>1% to <5%), anxiety (>1% to <5%), catatonia (>1% to <5%), chills (>1% to <5%), confusion (>1% to <5%), coordination abnormal (>1% to <5%), hallucination (>1% to <5%), malaise (>1% to <5%), personality disorder (>1% to <5%), speech disorder (>1% to <5%), tardive dyskinesia (>1% to <5%), vertigo (>1% to <5%), euphoria (1%), hypoesthesia (1%)

Dermatologic: Rash (>1% to 6%), bruising (>1% to 5%), discoid lupus erythematosus (>1% to <5%), dry skin (>1% to <5%), furunculosis (>1% to <5%), petechia (>1% to <5%), pruritus (>1% to <5), seborrhea (>1% to <5%)

Endocrine & metabolic: Amenorrhea (>1% to <5%), dysmenorrhea (>1% to <5%), metrorrhagia (>1% to <5%), hypoproteinemia

Gastrointestinal: Weight gain (4% to 9%), weight loss (6%), appetite increased (≤6%), constipation (>1% to 5%), xerostomia (>1% to 5%), eructation (>1% to <5%), fecal incontinence (>1% to <5%), flatulence (>1% to <5%), gastroenteritis (>1% to <5%), glossitis (>1% to <5%), hematemesis (>1% to <5%), pancreatitis (>1% to <5%), periodontal abscess (>1% to <5%), stomatitis (>1% to <5%), taste perversion (>1% to <5%), dysphagia, gum hemorrhage, mouth ulceration

Genitourinary: Cystitis (>1% to 5%), dysuria (>1% to 5%), urinary frequency (>1% to <5%), urinary incontinence (>1% to <5%), vaginal hemorrhage (>1% to 5%), vaginitis (>1% to <5%)

Hepatic: ALT increased (>1% to <5%), AST increased (>1% to <5%)

Local: Injection site pain (3%), injection site reaction (2%), injection site inflammation (1%)

Neuromuscular & skeletal: Back pain (≤8%), abnormal gait (>1% to <5%), arthralgia (>1% to <5%), arthrosis (>1% to <5%), dysarthria (>1% to <5%), hypertonia (>1% to <5%), hypokinesia (>1% to <5%), leg cramps (>1% to <5%), myalgia (>1% to <5%), myasthenia (>1% to <5%), neck pain (>1% to <5%), neck rigidity (>1% to <5%), paresthesia (>1% to <5%), reflex increased (>1% to <5%), twitching (>1% to <5%)

Ocular: Nystagmus (1% to 8%), dry eyes (>1% to 5%), eye pain (>1% to 5%), abnormal vision (>1% to <5%), conjunctivitis (>1% to <5%)

Otic: Tinnitus (1% to 7%), ear pain (>1% to 5%), deafness (>1% to <5%), otitis media (>1% to <5%)

Respiratory: Pharyngitis (2% to 8%), bronchitis (5%), rhinitis (>1% to 5%), dyspnea (1% to 5%), cough (>1% to <5%), epistaxis (>1% to <5%), pneumonia (>1% to <5%), sinusitis (>1% to <5%)

Miscellaneous: Diaphoresis (1%), hiccups

Available Dosage Forms

Capsule, softgel, oral: 250 mg

Depakene®: 250 mg

Capsule, softgel, delayed release, oral:

Stavzor™: 125 mg, 250 mg, 500 mg

Injection, solution: 100 mg/mL (5 mL)

Injection, solution [preservative free]: 100 mg/mL (5 mL)

Depacon®: 100 mg/mL (5 mL)

Solution, oral: 250 mg/5 mL (5 mL, 473 mL, 480 mL)

Syrup, oral: 250 mg/5 mL (5 mL, 10 mL, 473 mL, 480 mL)

Depakene®: 250 mg/5 mL (473 mL)

General Dosage Range Dosage adjustment recommended in patients with hepatic impairment

I.V.:

Children: Initial: 15 mg/kg/day; Maximum: 60 mg/kg/day

Children ≥10 years and Adults: Initial: 10-15 mg/kg/day; Maximum: 60 mg/kg/day

Oral:

Children: Initial: 15 mg/kg/day; Maximum: 60 mg/kg/day

Children ≥10 years and Adults: Seizures: Initial: 10-15 mg/kg/day; Maximum: 60 mg/kg/day

Children ≥12 years and Adults: Stavzor™: Initial: 250 mg twice daily; Maintenance: Up to 1000 mg/day

Adults: Mania (Stavzor™): Initial: 750 mg/day in divided doses; Maximum recommended dose: 60 mg/kg/day

Administration

Oral Depakene® capsule, Stavzor™: Swallow whole; do not chew.

I.V. Depacon®: Following dilution to final concentration, administer over 60 minutes at a rate ≤20 mg/minute. Alternatively, single doses up to 45 mg/kg have been administered as a rapid infusion over 5-10 minutes (1.5-6 mg/kg/minute).

Stability

Reconstitution Depacon®: Injection should be diluted in 50 mL of a compatible diluent.

Storage

Depakene® solution: Store below 30°C (86°F).

Stavzor™: Store at controlled room temperature of 25°C (77°F).

Depakene® capsule: Store at controlled room temperature of 15°C to 25°C (59°F to 77°F).

Depacon®: Store vial at room temperature of 15°C to 30°C (59°F to 86°F). Stable in D_5W, NS, and LR for at least 24 hours when stored in glass or PVC.

Nursing Actions

Physical Assessment I.V.: Keep patient under observation (vital signs; neurological, cardiac, and respiratory status) and monitor therapeutic response (seizure activity, force, type, duration). Monitor for signs and symptoms of hepatic failure (malaise, weakness, facial edema, anorexia, jaundice, and vomiting), especially when used in children <2 years of age. Monitor for signs and symptoms of pancreatitis (abdominal pain, nausea, vomiting, and/or anorexia). For outpatients, monitor therapeutic effect (seizure activity, frequency, duration). Teach patient seizure safety precautions. Some adverse reactions, including hepatic failure and thrombocytopenia, can occur 3 days to 6 months after beginning therapy.

Patient Education Oral: Do not crush or chew capsule or enteric-coated pill. While using this medication, do not use alcohol. Maintain adequate hydration unless instructed to restrict fluid intake. You may experience nervousness, decreased appetite, insomnia, headache, sleepiness, dizziness, visual changes, and hair loss. Report suicide ideation or depression; alterations in menstrual cycle; abdominal cramps, unresolved diarrhea, vomiting, or constipation; skin rash; tremors; unusual bruising or bleeding; blood in urine, stool, or vomitus; malaise; weakness; facial swelling; yellowing of skin or eyes; persistent abdominal pain; excessive sedation; change in mental status; extreme lethargy; or restlessness.

Dietary Considerations Valproic acid may cause GI upset; take with large amount of water or food to decrease GI upset. May need to split doses to avoid GI upset. Valproate sodium oral solution will generate valproic acid in carbonated beverages and may cause mouth and throat irritation; do not mix valproate sodium oral solution with carbonated beverages.

Related Information

Peak and Trough Guidelines *on page 1276*

Valrubicin (val ROO bi sin)

Brand Names: U.S. Valstar®

Index Terms *N*-trifluoroacetyladriamycin-14-valerate; AD32

Pharmacologic Category Antineoplastic Agent, Anthracycline

Medication Safety Issues

Sound-alike/look-alike issues:

Valrubicin may be confused with DAUNOrubicin, DOXOrubicin, epirubicin, IDArubicin

Valstar® may be confused with valsartan

High alert medication:

The medication is in a class the Institute for Safe Medication Practices (ISMP) includes among its list of drug classes which have a heightened risk of causing significant patient harm when used in error.

Pregnancy Risk Factor C

Lactation Excretion in breast milk unknown/not recommended

Use Intravesical treatment of BCG-refractory bladder carcinoma *in situ*

Available Dosage Forms

Injection, solution [preservative free]:

Valstar®: 40 mg/mL (5 mL)

General Dosage Range Dosage adjustment recommended in patients who develop toxicities

Intravesical: *Adults:* 800 mg once weekly for 6 weeks

Administration

Other Intravesicular bladder instillation: Insert urinary catheter, empty bladder prior to instillation, slowly by gravity flow, instill 800 mg/75 mL (in 0.9% sodium chloride injection), remove catheter. Retain in the bladder for 2 hours, then void. Administer through non-PVC tubing due to the polyoxyl castor oil (Cremophor® EL) diluent. Maintain adequate hydration following treatment. Use appropriate protective gown, goggles, and gloves during administration.

Nursing Actions

Physical Assessment Use caution to prevent inadvertent exposure to this medication. Monitor patient response during and following instillation (genitourinary [frequency, urgency, incontinence, dysuria, bladder spasm or pain, hematuria, urinary tract infection], rash, nausea, vomiting, myalgia, hyperglycemia).

Patient Education This medication will be instilled into your bladder through a catheter. After the catheter is withdrawn, you should not void for two hours (if possible); after 2 hours you should void. It is important that you maintain adequate hydration, unless instructed to restrict fluid intake. If you have diabetes, monitor glucose levels closely (may cause hyperglycemia). Your urine will be red-tinged for the next 24 hours; report promptly if this continues for a longer period. May cause altered urination patterns (increased or decreased frequency or incontinence), bladder pain, pain on urination, or pelvic pain; report if these persist. May cause dizziness, fatigue, nausea, vomiting, or taste disturbance. Report chest pain or palpitations; persistent dizziness; swelling of extremities; persistent nausea, vomiting, diarrhea, or abdominal pain; muscle weakness, pain, or tremors; unusual cough; or respiratory difficulty.

Valsartan (val SAR tan)

Brand Names: U.S. Diovan®

Pharmacologic Category Angiotensin II Receptor Blocker

Medication Safety Issues

Sound-alike/look-alike issues:

Valsartan may be confused with losartan, Valstar®, Valturna®

Diovan® may be confused with Zyban®

International issues:

Diovan [U.S., Canada, and multiple international markets] may be confused with Dianben, a brand name for metformin [Spain]

Pregnancy Risk Factor D

Lactation Excretion in breast milk unknown/not recommended

Breast-Feeding Considerations It is not known if valsartan is found in breast milk; the manufacturer recommends discontinuing the drug or discontinuing nursing based on the importance of the drug to the mother.

Use Alone or in combination with other antihypertensive agents in the treatment of essential hypertension; reduction of cardiovascular mortality in patients with left ventricular dysfunction postmyocardial infarction; treatment of heart failure (NYHA Class II-IV)

Mechanism of Action/Effect Valsartan produces direct antagonism of the angiotensin II (AT2) receptors. Valsartan blocks the vasoconstrictor and aldosterone-secreting effects of angiotensin II. It displaces angiotensin II from the AT1 receptor and produces its blood pressure-lowering effects by antagonizing AT1-induced vasoconstriction, aldosterone release, catecholamine release, arginine vasopressin release, water intake, and hypertrophic responses. This action results in more efficient blockade of the cardiovascular effects of angiotensin II and fewer side effects than the ACE inhibitors.

Contraindications There are no contraindications listed in manufacturer's labeling.

Canadian labeling: Hypersensitivity to valsartan or any component of the formulation

Warnings/Precautions [U.S. Boxed Warning]: Drugs that act on the renin-angiotensin system can cause injury and death to the developing fetus. Discontinue as soon as possible once pregnancy is detected. May cause hyperkalemia; avoid potassium supplementation unless specifically required by healthcare provider. During the initiation of therapy, hypotension may occur, particularly in patients with heart failure or post-MI patients. Use extreme caution with concurrent administration of potassium-sparing diuretics or potassium supplements, in patients with mild-to-moderate hepatic dysfunction (adjust dose), in those who may be sodium/water depleted (eg, on high-dose diuretics), and in the elderly; correct depletion first.

Use caution with unstented unilateral/bilateral renal artery stenosis. When unstented bilateral renal artery stenosis is present, use is generally avoided due to the elevated risk of deterioration in renal function unless possible benefits outweigh risks. Use with caution with preexisting renal insufficiency; significant aortic/mitral stenosis. May be associated with deterioration of renal function and/or increases in serum creatinine, particularly in patients with low renal blood flow (eg, renal artery stenosis, heart failure) whose glomerular filtration rate (GFR) is dependent on efferent arteriolar vasoconstriction by angiotensin II. Use caution in patients with severe renal impairment or significant hepatic dysfunction. Monitor renal function closely in patients with severe heart failure; changes in renal function should be anticipated and dosage adjustments of valsartan or concomitant medications may be needed. Concurrent use of ACE inhibitors may increase the risk of clinically-significant adverse events (eg, renal dysfunction, hyperkalemia). In Canada, use is not approved in patients <18 years of age.

Drug Interactions

Avoid Concomitant Use There are no known interactions where it is recommended to avoid concomitant use.

Decreased Effect

The levels/effects of Valsartan may be decreased by: Herbs (Hypertensive Properties); Methylphenidate; Nonsteroidal Anti-Inflammatory Agents; Yohimbine

Increased Effect/Toxicity

Valsartan may increase the levels/effects of: ACE Inhibitors; Amifostine; Antihypertensives; Hydrochlorothiazide; Hypotensive Agents; Lithium; Nonsteroidal Anti-Inflammatory Agents; Potassium-Sparing Diuretics; RiTUXimab; Sodium Phosphates

The levels/effects of Valsartan may be increased by: Alfuzosin; Diazoxide; Eltrombopag; Eplerenone; Herbs (Hypotensive Properties); Hydrochlorothiazide; MAO Inhibitors; Pentoxifylline; Phosphodiesterase 5 Inhibitors; Potassium Salts; Prostacyclin Analogues; Tolvaptan; Trimethoprim

Nutritional/Ethanol Interactions

Food: Decreases the peak plasma concentration and extent of absorption by 50% and 40%, respectively. Potassium supplements and/or potassium-containing salts may cause or worsen hyperkalemia. Management: Take consistently with regard to food. Consult prescriber before consuming a potassium-rich diet, potassium supplements, or salt substitutes.

Herb/Nutraceutical: Some herbal medications may worsen hypertension (eg, licorice); others may increase the antihypertensive effect of valsartan (eg, shepherd's purse). Management: Avoid bayberry, blue cohosh, cayenne, ephedra, ginger, ginseng (American), kola, licorice, and yohimbe. Avoid black cohosh, California poppy, coleus, golden seal, hawthorn, mistletoe, periwinkle, quinine, and shepherd's purse.

Adverse Reactions

>10%:

Central nervous system: Dizziness (heart failure trials 17%)

Renal: BUN increased >50% (heart failure trials 17%)

1% to 10%:

Cardiovascular: Hypotension (heart failure trials 7%; MI trial 1%), postural hypotension (heart failure trials 2%), syncope (up to >1%)

Central nervous system: Dizziness (hypertension trial 2% to 8%), fatigue (heart failure trials 3%; hypertension trial 2%), postural dizziness (heart failure trials 2%), headache (heart failure trials >1%), vertigo (up to >1%)

Endocrine & metabolic: Serum potassium increased by >20% (4% to 10%), hyperkalemia (heart failure trials 2%)

Gastrointestinal: Diarrhea (heart failure trials 5%), abdominal pain (2%), nausea (heart failure trials >1%), upper abdominal pain (heart failure trials >1%)

Hematologic: Neutropenia (2%)

Neuromuscular & skeletal: Arthralgia (heart failure trials 3%), back pain (up to 3%)

Ocular: Blurred vision (heart failure trials >1%)

Renal: Creatinine doubled (MI trial 4%), creatinine increased >50% (heart failure trials 4%), renal dysfunction (up to >1%)

Respiratory: Cough (1% to 3%)

Miscellaneous: Viral infection (3%)

Pharmacodynamics/Kinetics

Onset of Action ~2 hours

Duration of Action 24 hours

Available Dosage Forms

Tablet, oral:

Diovan®: 40 mg, 80 mg, 160 mg, 320 mg

General Dosage Range Oral:

Children 6-16 years: Initial: 1.3 mg/kg once daily (maximum: 40 mg/day); Maintenance: Up to ≤2.7 mg/kg; 160 mg

Adults: Initial: 20-40 mg twice daily **or** 80-160 mg once daily; Maintenance: 80-160 mg twice daily (maximum: 320 mg/day)

Administration

Oral Administer with or without food.

Stability

Storage Store at 25°C (77°F); excursions permitted to 15°C to 30°C (59°F to 86°F). Protect from moisture.

Nursing Actions

Physical Assessment Assess effectiveness and interactions with other pharmacological agents and herbal products (eg, concurrent use of potassium supplements, ACE inhibitors, potassium-sparing diuretics may increase risk of hyperkalemia). Monitor for changes in renal function, dizziness, cough, headache, nausea, hypotension, and hyperkalemia.

Patient Education This drug does not eliminate need for diet or exercise regimen as recommended by prescriber. May cause dizziness, lightheadedness, postural hypotension, or diarrhea. Report changes in urinary pattern, swelling of extremities, unusual back ache, chest pain or palpitations, unrelenting headache, or unusual cough.

Dietary Considerations Avoid salt substitutes which contain potassium. May be taken with or without food.

Valsartan and Hydrochlorothiazide

(val SAR tan & hye droe klor oh THYE a zide)

Brand Names: U.S. Diovan HCT®

Index Terms Hydrochlorothiazide and Valsartan

Pharmacologic Category Angiotensin II Receptor Blocker; Diuretic, Thiazide

Medication Safety Issues

Sound-alike/look-alike issues:

Diovan® may be confused with Zyban®

Pregnancy Risk Factor D

Lactation Enters breast milk/not recommended

Use Treatment of hypertension

Available Dosage Forms

Tablet:

Diovan HCT®: 80 mg/12.5 mg: Valsartan 80 mg and hydrochlorothiazide 12.5 mg; 160 mg/12.5 mg: Valsartan 160 mg and hydrochlorothiazide 12.5 mg; 160 mg/25 mg: Valsartan 160 mg and hydrochlorothiazide 25 mg; 320 mg/12.5 mg: Valsartan 320 mg and hydrochlorothiazide 12.5 mg; 320 mg/25 mg: Valsartan 320 mg and hydrochlorothiazide 25 mg

General Dosage Range Oral: *Adults:* Valsartan 80-160 mg and hydrochlorothiazide 12.5-25 mg once daily (maximum: 25 mg/day [hydrochlorothiazide]; 320 mg/day [valsartan])

Administration

Oral Administer with or without food.

Nursing Actions

Physical Assessment See individual agents.

Patient Education See individual agents.

Related Information

Hydrochlorothiazide *on page 570*

Valsartan *on page 1161*

Vancomycin (van koe MYE sin)

Brand Names: U.S. Vancocin®

Index Terms Vancomycin Hydrochloride

Pharmacologic Category Glycopeptide

Medication Safety Issues

Sound-alike/look-alike issues:

I.V. vancomycin may be confused with INVanz®

Vancomycin may be confused with clindamycin, gentamicin, tobramycin, valACYclovir, vecuronium, Vibramycin®

High alert medication:

The Institute for Safe Medication Practices (ISMP) includes this medication (intrathecal administration) among its list of drug classes which have a heightened risk of causing significant patient harm when used in error.

Pregnancy Risk Factor B (oral); C (injection)

Lactation Enters breast milk/not recommended

Breast-Feeding Considerations Small amounts of vancomycin are excreted in human milk and use during breast-feeding is not recommended by the manufacturer. If given orally to the mother, the minimal systemic absorption of the dose would limit the amount available to pass into the milk. If given intravenously, the small amount that distributes to the milk would not be expected to cause systemic toxicity due to the lack of GI absorption. Nondose-related effects could include modification of bowel flora.

Use Treatment of patients with infections caused by staphylococcal species and streptococcal species; used orally for staphylococcal enterocolitis or for antibiotic-associated pseudomembranous colitis produced by *C. difficile*

Unlabeled Use Bacterial endophthalmitis; treatment of infections caused by gram-positive organisms in patients who have serious allergies to beta-lactam agents; treatment of beta-lactam resistant gram-positive infections

Mechanism of Action/Effect Inhibits bacterial cell wall synthesis

Contraindications Hypersensitivity to vancomycin or any component of the formulation; avoid in patients with previous severe hearing loss

Warnings/Precautions May cause nephrotoxicity although limited data suggest direct causal relationship; usual risk factors include pre-existing renal impairment, concomitant nephrotoxic medications, advanced age, and dehydration. If multiple sequential (≥2) serum creatinine concentrations demonstrate an increase of 0.5 mg/dL or ≥50% increase from baseline (whichever is greater) in the absence of an alternative explanation, the patient should be identified as having vancomycin-induced nephrotoxicity (Rybak, 2009). Discontinue treatment if signs of nephrotoxicity occur; renal damage is usually reversible. May cause neurotoxicity; usual risk factors include pre-existing renal impairment, concomitant neuro-/nephrotoxic medications, advanced age, and dehydration. Ototoxicity, although rarely associated with monotherapy, is proportional to the amount of drug given and the duration of treatment. Tinnitus or vertigo may be indications of vestibular injury and impending bilateral irreversible damage. Discontinue treatment if signs of ototoxicity occur. Prolonged therapy (>1 week) or total doses exceeding 25 g may increase the risk of neutropenia; prompt reversal of neutropenia is expected after discontinuation of therapy. Prolonged use may result in fungal or bacterial superinfection, including *C. difficile*-associated diarrhea (CDAD) and pseudomembranous colitis; CDAD has been observed >2 months post-antibiotic treatment. Use with caution in patients with renal impairment or those receiving other nephrotoxic or ototoxic drugs; dosage modification required in patients with impaired renal function (especially elderly). Rapid I.V. administration may result in hypotension, flushing, erythema, urticaria, and/or pruritus. Oral vancomycin is only indicated for the treatment of pseudomembranous colitis due to *C. difficile* and enterocolitis due to *S. aureus* and is not effective for systemic infections; parenteral vancomycin is not effective for the treatment of colitis due to *C. difficile* and enterocolitis due to *S. aureus*. **Note:** The Infectious Disease Society of America (IDSA) recommends the use of oral metronidazole for initial treatment of mild-to-moderate *C. difficile* infection and the use of oral vancomycin for initial treatment of severe *C. difficile* infection (Cohen, 2010).

Drug Interactions

Avoid Concomitant Use

Avoid concomitant use of Vancomycin with any of the following: BCG; Gallium Nitrate

Decreased Effect

Vancomycin may decrease the levels/effects of: BCG; Typhoid Vaccine

The levels/effects of Vancomycin may be decreased by: Bile Acid Sequestrants

Increased Effect/Toxicity

Vancomycin may increase the levels/effects of: Aminoglycosides; Colistimethate; Gallium Nitrate; Neuromuscular-Blocking Agents

The levels/effects of Vancomycin may be increased by: Nonsteroidal Anti-Inflammatory Agents

Adverse Reactions

Oral:

>10%: Gastrointestinal: Bitter taste, nausea, vomiting

1% to 10%:

Central nervous system: Chills, drug fever

Hematologic: Eosinophilia

Parenteral:

>10%:

Cardiovascular: Hypotension accompanied by flushing

Dermatologic: Erythematous rash on face and upper body (red neck or red man syndrome - infusion rate related)

1% to 10%:

Central nervous system: Chills, drug fever

Dermatologic: Rash

Hematologic: Eosinophilia, reversible neutropenia

Local: Phlebitis

Available Dosage Forms

Capsule, oral:

Vancocin®: 125 mg, 250 mg

Infusion, premixed iso-osmotic dextrose solution: 500 mg (100 mL); 750 mg (150 mL); 1 g (200 mL)

Injection, powder for reconstitution: 500 mg, 750 mg, 1 g, 5 g, 10 g

General Dosage Range Dosage adjustment recommended in patients with renal impairment

I.V.:

Infants >1 month: 40-60 mg/kg/day in divided doses every 6 hours

Children: 40-60 mg/kg/day in divided doses every 6 hours **or** 20 mg/kg as a single dose

Adults: 30-60 mg/kg/day in divided doses every 6-12 hours **or** 500-750 mg every 6 hours **or** 1 g as a single dose

Intracatheter, intraventricular: *Children and Adults:* 2-5 mg/mL instilled into catheter port with a volume sufficient to fill the catheter (2-5 mL)

Intrathecal: *Children and Adults:* 5-20 mg/day

Oral:

Children: 40 mg/kg/day in 3-4 divided doses (maximum: 2000 mg/day)

Adults: 500-2000 mg/day in 3-4 divided doses (maximum: 2000 mg/day)

Administration

Oral May be administered with food. If patient cannot swallow capsules, the powder for injection (not premixed solution) may be diluted in 30 mL of water for oral administration; flavoring may be added to improve taste. The unflavored, diluted solution may also be administered via nasogastric tube.

I.M. Do not administer I.M.

I.V. Administer vancomycin with a final concentration not to exceed 5 mg/mL by I.V. intermittent infusion over at least 60 minutes (recommended infusion period of ≥30 minutes for every 500 mg administered).

Red man syndrome may occur if the infusion is too rapid. It is not an allergic reaction, but may be characterized by hypotension and/or a maculopapular rash appearing on the face, neck, trunk, and/or upper extremities. If this should occur, slow the infusion rate to over 1½ to 2 hours and increase the dilution volume. Reactions are often treated with antihistamines and steroids.

Extravasation treatment: Monitor I.V. site closely; extravasation will cause serious injury with possible necrosis and tissue sloughing. Rotate infusion site frequently.

I.V. Detail

pH: 3.9 (in distilled water or sodium chloride 0.9%); 2.5-4.5 (5% solution in water)

Other

Intrathecal (unlabeled route): Vancomycin is available as a powder for injection and may be diluted to 1-5 mg/mL concentration in preservative-free 0.9% sodium chloride for intrathecal administration.

Intravitreal (unlabeled use): May be administered by intravitreal injection.

Rectal (unlabeled route): May be administered as a retention enema per rectum (Cohen, 2010).

Stability

Reconstitution Reconstitute vials with 20 mL of SWFI for each 1 g of vancomycin (10 mL/500 mg vial; 20 mL/1 g vial; 100 mL/5 g vial; 200 mL/10 g vial). The reconstituted solution must be further diluted with at least 100 mL of a compatible diluent per 500 mg of vancomycin prior to parenteral administration.

Intrathecal (unlabeled route): Vancomycin is available as a powder for injection and may be diluted to 1-5 mg/mL concentration in preservative free 0.9% sodium chloride for administration into the CSF.

Storage Reconstituted 500 mg and 1 g vials are stable for at either room temperature or under refrigeration for 14 days. **Note:** Vials contain no bacteriostatic agent. Solutions diluted for administration in either D_5W or NS are stable under refrigeration for 14 days or at room temperature for 7 days.

Nursing Actions

Physical Assessment Culture and sensitivity tests and patient's allergy history should be evaluated prior to first dose. Use caution with renal impairment. Premedication with antihistamines may prevent or minimize "red man" reaction. Monitor infusion site closely to prevent extravasation. Monitor for hypotension, rash, neutropenia, nausea, vomiting, and auditory changes on a regular basis during therapy.

Patient Education If administered by infusion, report immediately any chills; pain, swelling, or redness at infusion site; or respiratory difficulty. May cause nausea, vomiting, or GI upset. Report rash or hives, chills or fever, persistent GI disturbances, opportunistic infection (sore throat, chills, fever, burning, itching on urination, vaginal discharge, white plaques in mouth), respiratory difficulty, any change in urine output, chest pain or palpitations, changes in hearing or feeling of fullness in ears, or worsening of condition.

Dietary Considerations May be taken with food.

Related Information

Compatibility of Drugs *on page 1264*

Peak and Trough Guidelines *on page 1276*

Vandetanib (van DET a nib)

Brand Names: U.S. Caprelsa®

Index Terms AZD6474; Zactima; ZD6474; Zictifa

Pharmacologic Category Antineoplastic Agent, Tyrosine Kinase Inhibitor; Epidermal Growth Factor Receptor (EGFR) Inhibitor; Vascular Endothelial Growth Factor (VEGF) Inhibitor

Medication Safety Issues

Sound-alike/look-alike issues:

Vandetanib may be confused with axitinib, dasatinib, erlotinib, gefitinib, imatinib, lapatinib, nilotinib, pazopanib, SORAfenib, SUNItinib, vemurafenib, vismodegib

High alert medication:

This medication is in a class the Institute for Safe Medication Practices (ISMP) includes among its list of drug classes which have a heightened risk of causing significant patient harm when used in error.

Medication Guide Available Yes

Pregnancy Risk Factor D

Lactation Excretion in breast milk unknown/not recommended

Use Treatment of metastatic or unresectable locally advanced medullary thyroid cancer (symptomatic or progressive)

Available Dosage Forms

Tablet, oral: 100 mg, 300 mg

Caprelsa®: 100 mg, 300 mg

Administration

Oral May be administered with or without food. Missed doses should be omitted if within 12 hours of the next scheduled dose. Do not crush tablet. If unable to swallow tablet whole or if nasogastric or gastrostomy tube administration is necessary, disperse one tablet in 2 ounces of water (noncarbonated only) and stir for 10 minutes to disperse (will not dissolve completely) and administer immediately. Rinse residue in glass with additional 4 ounces of water (noncarbonated only) and administer. Use appropriate handling precautions (hazardous agent).

Vardenafil (var DEN a fil)

Brand Names: U.S. Levitra®; Staxyn™

Index Terms Vardenafil Hydrochloride

Pharmacologic Category Phosphodiesterase-5 Enzyme Inhibitor

Medication Safety Issues

Sound-alike/look-alike issues:

Vardenafil may be confused with sildenafil, tadalafil

Levitra® may be confused with Kaletra®, Lexiva®

Pregnancy Risk Factor B

Lactation Excretion in breast milk unknown/not indicated for use in women.

Use Treatment of erectile dysfunction (ED)

Mechanism of Action/Effect Vardenafil enhances the effect of nitric oxide by inhibiting phosphodiesterase type 5 (PDE-5), resulting in smooth muscle relaxation and inflow of blood into the corpus cavernosum with sexual stimulation.

Contraindications Hypersensitivity to vardenafil or any component of the formulation; concurrent (regular or intermittent) use of organic nitrates in any form (eg, nitroglycerin, isosorbide dinitrate)

Warnings/Precautions There is a degree of cardiac risk associated with sexual activity; therefore, physicians may wish to consider the patient's cardiovascular status prior to initiating any treatment for erectile dysfunction. Use caution in patients with anatomical deformation of the penis (angulation, cavernosal fibrosis, or Peyronie's disease) and in patients who have conditions which may predispose them to priapism (sickle cell anemia, multiple myeloma, leukemia). Instruct patients to seek immediate medical attention if erection persists >4 hours.

Use is not recommended in patients with hypotension (<90/50 mm Hg); uncontrolled hypertension (>170/100 mm Hg); unstable angina or angina during intercourse; life-threatening arrhythmias, stroke, or MI within the last 6 months; cardiac failure or coronary artery disease causing unstable angina. Safety and efficacy have not been studied in these patients. Use caution in patients with left ventricular outflow obstruction (eg, aortic stenosis). Use caution with alpha-blockers, effective CYP3A4 inhibitors, the elderly, or those with hepatic impairment (Child-Pugh class B); dosage adjustment is needed.

Rare cases of nonarteritic ischemic optic neuropathy (NAION) have been reported; risk may be increased with history of vision loss. Other risk factors for NAION include heart disease, diabetes, hypertension, smoking, age >50 years, or history of certain eye problems. Sudden decrease or loss of hearing has been reported rarely; hearing changes may be accompanied by tinnitus and dizziness.

Safety and efficacy have not been studied in patients with the following conditions, therefore, use in these patients is not recommended at this time: Congenital QT prolongation, patients taking medications known to prolong the QT interval (avoid use in patients taking Class Ia or III antiarrhythmics); severe hepatic impairment (Child-Pugh class C); end-stage renal disease requiring dialysis; retinitis pigmentosa or other degenerative retinal disorders. The safety and efficacy of vardenafil with other treatments for erectile dysfunction have not been studied and are not recommended as combination therapy. Concomitant use with all forms of nitrates is contraindicated. If nitrate administration is medically necessary, it is not known when nitrates can be safely administered following the use of vardenafil; the ACC/AHA 2007 guidelines support administration of nitrates only if 24 hours have elapsed. Potential underlying causes of erectile dysfunction should be evaluated prior to treatment. Some products may contain phylalanine. Some products may contain sorbitol; do not use in patients with fructose intolerance.

Drug Interactions

Avoid Concomitant Use

Avoid concomitant use of Vardenafil with any of the following: Amyl Nitrite; Phosphodiesterase 5 Inhibitors; Vasodilators (Organic Nitrates)

Decreased Effect

The levels/effects of Vardenafil may be decreased by: Bosentan; Etravirine; Tocilizumab

Increased Effect/Toxicity

Vardenafil may increase the levels/effects of: Alpha1-Blockers; Amyl Nitrite; Antihypertensives; Bosentan; Phosphodiesterase 5 Inhibitors; Vasodilators (Organic Nitrates)

The levels/effects of Vardenafil may be increased by: Antifungal Agents (Azole Derivatives, Systemic); Boceprevir; Clarithromycin; CYP3A4 Inhibitors (Moderate); CYP3A4 Inhibitors (Strong); Dasatinib; Erythromycin; Ivacaftor; Protease Inhibitors; Sapropterin; Telaprevir

Nutritional/Ethanol Interactions Food: High-fat meals decrease maximum serum concentration 18% to 50%. Serum concentrations/toxicity may be increased with grapefruit juice. Management: Do not take with a high-fat meal. Avoid grapefruit juice.

Adverse Reactions

>10%:

Cardiovascular: Flushing (8% to 11%)

Central nervous system: Headache (14% to 15%)

2% to 10%:

Central nervous system: Dizziness (2%)

Gastrointestinal: Dyspepsia (3% to 4%), nausea (2%)

Neuromuscular & skeletal: Back pain (2%), CPK increased (2%)

Respiratory: Rhinitis (9%), nasal congestion (3%), sinusitis (3%)

Miscellaneous: Flu-like syndrome (3%)

Pharmacodynamics/Kinetics

Onset of Action ~60 minutes

Available Dosage Forms

Tablet, oral:

Levitra®: 2.5 mg, 5 mg, 10 mg, 20 mg

Tablet, orally disintegrating, oral:

Staxyn™: 10 mg

General Dosage Range Dosage adjustment recommended in patients with hepatic impairment or on concomitant therapy

Oral:

Adults: Film-coated tablet (Levitra®): 2.5-20 mg as a single dose (maximum: 1 dose/day); Oral disintegrating tablet (Staxyn™): 10 mg as a single dose (maximum: 10 mg/day)

Elderly ≥65 years: 2.5-5 mg as a single dose (maximum: 1 dose/day)

Administration

Oral May be administered with or without food, 60 minutes prior to sexual activity.

Oral disintegrating tablet should not be removed from blister pack until administered. Using dry hands, place immediately on tongue. Tablet will dissolve within seconds; do not take with liquid. Do not crush, split, or chew.

Stability

Storage Store at controlled room temperature of 25°C (77°F); excursions permitted to 15°C to 25°C (59°F to 86°F). Keep oral disintegrating tablets sealed in blisterpack until ready to use.

Nursing Actions

Patient Education Use 60 minutes prior to sexual activity. Avoid taking with high-fat meals. This medication does not provide protection against sexually-transmitted diseases, including HIV. You may experience headache, flushing, or blurred vision. Report immediately chest pain, acute head pain, respiratory difficulty, change in vision (seeing a blue tinge to objects or having difficulty telling the difference between the colors blue and green), change in hearing or ringing in the ears, allergic response (eg, chills, fever, respiratory difficulty, rash), genital swelling, or erection lasting >4 hours. Orally disintegrating tablet: Place on tongue; avoid drinking liquids while administering tablet. Do not crush or chew.

Dietary Considerations May take with or without food. Avoid grapefruit juice. Some products may contain phenylalanine. Some products may contain sorbitol; do not use in patients with fructose intolerance.

Varenicline (var e NI kleen)

Brand Names: U.S. Chantix®

Index Terms Varenicline Tartrate

Pharmacologic Category Partial Nicotine Agonist; Smoking Cessation Aid

Medication Guide Available Yes

Pregnancy Risk Factor C

Lactation Excretion in breast milk unknown/not recommended

Use Treatment to aid in smoking cessation

Mechanism of Action/Effect Decreases nicotine dependence, craving, and withdrawal

Contraindications Known history of serious hypersensitivity or skin reactions to varenicline

Warnings/Precautions [U.S. Boxed Warning]: Serious neuropsychiatric events (including depression, suicidal thoughts, and suicide) have been reported with use; some cases may have been complicated by symptoms of nicotine withdrawal following smoking cessation. Smoking cessation (with or without treatment) is associated with nicotine withdrawal symptoms and the exacerbation of underlying psychiatric illness; however, some of the behavioral disturbances were reported in treated patients who continued to smoke. Neuropsychiatric symptoms (eg, mood disturbances, psychosis, hostility) have occurred in patients with and without pre-existing psychiatric disease; many cases resolved following therapy discontinuation although in some cases, symptoms persisted. Ethanol consumption may increase the risk of psychiatric adverse events. Monitor all patients for behavioral changes and psychiatric symptoms (eg, agitation, depression, suicidal behavior, suicidal ideation); inform patients to discontinue treatment and contact their healthcare provider immediately if they experience any behavioral and/or mood changes. **[U.S. Boxed Warning]: Before prescribing, the risks of serious neuropsychiatric events must be weighed against the immediate and long term benefits of smoking abstinence for each patient.**

Hypersensitivity reactions (including angioedema) and rare cases of serious skin reactions (including Stevens-Johnson syndrome and erythema multiforme) have been reported. Patients should be instructed to discontinue use and contact healthcare provider if signs/symptoms occur. Treatment may increase risk of cardiovascular events (eg, angina pectoris, nonfatal MI, nonfatal stroke, need for coronary revascularization, new diagnosis of or treatment for PVD). Varenicline was not studied in patients with unstable cardiovascular disease or in patients experiencing recent events (<2 months) prior to treatment. Dose-dependent nausea may occur; both transient and persistent nausea has been reported. Dosage reduction may be considered for intolerable nausea. May cause sedation, which may impair physical or mental abilities; patients must be cautioned about performing tasks which require mental alertness (eg, operating machinery or driving).

Use caution in renal dysfunction; dosage adjustment required. Safety and efficacy of varenicline with other smoking cessation therapies have not been established; increased adverse events when used concurrently with nicotine replacement therapy.

Drug Interactions

Avoid Concomitant Use There are no known interactions where it is recommended to avoid concomitant use.

Decreased Effect There are no known significant interactions involving a decrease in effect.

Increased Effect/Toxicity
The levels/effects of Varenicline may be increased by: Alcohol (Ethyl); H2-Antagonists; Quinolone Antibiotics; Trimethoprim

Nutritional/Ethanol Interactions Ethanol: May increase the risk of psychiatric adverse events. Caution patients about the potential effects of ethanol consumption during therapy.

Adverse Reactions

>10%:

Central nervous system: Insomnia (18% to 19%), headache (15% to 19%), abnormal dreams (9% to 13%)

Gastrointestinal: Nausea (16% to 40%; dose related)

1% to 10%:

Central nervous system: Malaise (≤7%), sleep disorder (≤5%), somnolence (3%), nightmares (1% to 2%), lethargy (1% to 2%)

Dermatologic: Rash (≤3%)

Gastrointestinal: Flatulence (6% to 9%), constipation (5% to 8%), abnormal taste (5% to 8%), abdominal pain (≤7%), xerostomia (≤6%), dyspepsia (5%), vomiting (≤5%), appetite increased (3% to 4%), anorexia (≤2%), gastroesophageal reflux (1%)

Respiratory: Upper respiratory tract disorder (5% to 7%), dyspnea (≤2%), rhinorrhea (≤1%)

Available Dosage Forms

Combination package, oral:
Chantix®: Tablet: 0.5 mg (11s) [white tablets] and Tablet: 1 mg (42s) [light blue tablets]

Tablet, oral:
Chantix®: 0.5 mg, 1 mg

General Dosage Range Dosage adjustment recommended in patients with renal impairment or who develop toxicities

Oral: *Adults:* Days 1-3: 0.5 mg once daily; Days 4-7: 0.5 mg twice daily; Maintenance (≥Day 8): 1 mg twice daily

Administration

Oral Administer with food and a full glass of water.

Stability

Storage Store at 25°C (77°F); excursions permitted to 15°C to 30°C (59°F to 86°F).

Nursing Actions

Physical Assessment Provide educational materials and counseling to support an attempt at quitting smoking. Carefully instruct patient in appropriate titration of doses. Monitor for behavioral and emotional changes, such as hostility, agitation, and suicide ideation. Monitor other medications patient is taking for potential need for dose adjustment after quitting smoking.

Patient Education Start medication 1 week prior to quit date designated. Take after eating, with a full glass of water. You may experience nausea, vomiting, constipation, headaches, problems sleeping, or unusual dreams. Report depression, suicide ideation, or emotional/behavioral changes to prescriber.

Dietary Considerations Should be given with food and a full glass of water to decrease gastric upset.

Varicella Virus Vaccine

(var i SEL a VYE rus vak SEEN)

Brand Names: U.S. Varivax®

Index Terms Chickenpox Vaccine; VAR; Varicella-Zoster Virus (VZV) Vaccine (Varicella); VZV Vaccine (Varicella)

Pharmacologic Category Vaccine, Live (Viral)

Medication Safety Issues

Sound-alike/look-alike issues:

Varicella virus vaccine has been given in error (instead of the indicated varicella immune globulin) to pregnant women exposed to varicella.

Other safety concerns:

Both varicella vaccine and zoster vaccine are live, attenuated strains of varicella-zoster virus. Their indications, dosing, and composition are distinct. Varicella is indicated in children to prevent chickenpox, while zoster vaccine is indicated in older individuals to prevent reactivation of the virus which causes shingles. Zoster vaccine is **not** a substitute for varicella vaccine and should not be used in children.

Pregnancy Risk Factor C

Lactation Excretion in breast milk unknown/use caution

Use Immunization against varicella in children ≥12 months of age and adults

The ACIP recommends vaccination for all children, adolescents, and adults who do not have evidence of immunity. Vaccination is especially important for:

- Healthcare personnel
- Persons with close contact to those at high risk for severe disease
- Persons living or working in environments where transmission is likely (teachers, childcare workers, residents and staff of institutional settings)
- Persons in environments where transmission has been reported
- Nonpregnant women of childbearing age
- Adolescents and adults in households with children
- International travelers

Postexposure prophylaxis: Vaccination within 3 days (possibly 5 days) after exposure to rash is effective in preventing illness or modifying severity of disease

Available Dosage Forms

Injection, powder for reconstitution [preservative free]:

Varivax®: 1350 PFU

General Dosage Range SubQ:

Children 12 months to 12 years: 0.5 mL as a single dose; may repeat in ≥3 months

Children ≥13 years and Adults: 2 doses of 0.5 mL separated by 4-8 weeks

Administration

I.M. SubQ administration is recommended; however, doses inadvertently given I.M. have resulted in similar seroconversion.

I.V. Do not administer I.V.

Other For SubQ injection only; inject in the outer aspect of upper arm. Administer immediately following reconstitution.

Simultaneous administration of vaccines helps ensure the patients will be fully vaccinated by the appropriate age. Simultaneous administration of vaccines is defined as administering >1 vaccine on the same day at different anatomic sites. The use of licensed combination vaccines is generally preferred over separate injections of the equivalent components. Separate vaccines should not be combined in the same syringe unless indicated by product specific labeling. Separate needles and syringes should be used for each injection. The ACIP prefers each dose of a specific vaccine in a series come from the same manufacturer when possible. Adolescents and adults should be vaccinated while seated or lying down. In general, preterm infants should be vaccinated at the same chronological age as full-term infants (CDC, 2011).

Antipyretics have not been shown to prevent febrile seizures. Antipyretics may be used to treat fever or discomfort following vaccination (CDC, 2011). One study reported that routine prophylactic administration of acetaminophen to prevent fever prior to vaccination decreased the immune response of some vaccines; the clinical significance of this reduction in immune response has not been established (Prymula, 2009).

Nursing Actions

Physical Assessment U.S. federal law requires entry into the patient's medical record.

Related Information

Immunization Administration Recommendations *on page 1243*

Immunization Recommendations *on page 1248*

Vasopressin (vay soe PRES in)

Brand Names: U.S. Pitressin®

Index Terms 8-Arginine Vasopressin; ADH; Antidiuretic Hormone; AVP

Pharmacologic Category Antidiuretic Hormone Analog; Hormone, Posterior Pituitary

Medication Safety Issues

Administration issues:

Use care when prescribing and/or administering vasopressin solutions. Close attention should be given to concentration of solution, route of administration, dose, and rate of administration (units/minute, units/kg/minute, units/kg/hour).

Pregnancy Risk Factor C

Lactation Enters breast milk/use caution

Use Treatment of central diabetes insipidus; differential diagnosis of diabetes insipidus

Unlabeled Use ACLS guidelines: Pulseless arrest (ventricular tachycardia [VT]/ventricular fibrillation [VF], asystole/pulseless electrical activity [PEA]); cardiac arrest secondary to anaphylaxis (unresponsive to epinephrine)

Adjunct in the treatment of GI hemorrhage and esophageal varices; adjunct in the treatment of vasodilatory shock (septic shock); donor management in brain-dead patients (hormone replacement therapy)

Available Dosage Forms

Injection, solution: 20 units/mL (0.5 mL, 1 mL, 10 mL)

Pitressin®: 20 units/mL (1 mL)

General Dosage Range I.M., SubQ:

Children: 2.5-10 units 2-4 times/day as needed

Adults: 5-10 units 2-4 times/day as needed

Administration

I.V. Usual concentration: 100 units in 500 mL D_5W. **Note:** In one clinical trial with lower dosing (eg, 0.0005 units/kg/hour) in pediatric patients, a more dilute solution (eg, 20 units in 500 mL D_5W) was employed (Wise-Faberowski, 2004).

Vasodilatory shock: Administration through a central catheter is recommended.

I.V. Detail Use extreme caution to avoid extravasation because of risk of necrosis and gangrene. In treatment of varices, infusions are often supplemented with nitroglycerin infusions to minimize cardiac effects.

Topical Topical administration on nasal mucosa: Administer injectable vasopressin on cotton plugs, as nasal spray, or by dropper. Should not be inhaled.

Other Endotracheal: If no I.V./I.O. access may give endotracheally. ACLS guidelines do not recommend a specific endotracheal dose; however, may be given endotracheally using the same I.V. dose (ACLS, 2010; Wenzel, 1997). Mix with 5-10 mL of water or normal saline, and administer down the endotracheal tube.

Nursing Actions

Physical Assessment I.V. requires use of infusion pump and close monitoring to prevent extravasation (may cause severe necrosis and gangrene). Monitor cardiac status, blood pressure, CNS status, fluid balance, and for signs or symptoms of water intoxication or intranasal irritation.

Patient Education This drug will usually be administered by infusion or injection and you will be closely monitored. Report immediately any chest pain or palpitations; difficulty breathing; abdominal cramping; or redness, swelling, pain, or burning at infusion/injection site. May cause dizziness or drowsiness. Report persistent nausea, vomiting, or abdominal cramps; tremor, acute headache, or dizziness; chest pain or irregular heartbeat; respiratory difficulty or excessive perspiration; or CNS changes (confusion, drowsiness).

Related Information

Management of Drug Extravasations *on page 1269*

Vecuronium (vek ue ROE nee um)

Index Terms Norcuron; ORG NC 45

Pharmacologic Category Neuromuscular Blocker Agent, Nondepolarizing

Medication Safety Issues

Sound-alike/look-alike issues:

Vecuronium may be confused with valproate sodium, vancomycin

Norcuron® may be confused with Narcan®

High alert medication:

The Institute for Safe Medication Practices (ISMP) includes this medication among its list of drugs which have a heightened risk of causing significant patient harm when used in error.

Other safety concerns:

United States Pharmacopeia (USP) 2006: The Interdisciplinary Safe Medication Use Expert Committee of the USP has recommended the following:

- Hospitals, clinics, and other practice sites should institute special safeguards in the storage, labeling, and use of these agents and should include these safeguards in staff orientation and competency training.
- Healthcare professionals should be on high alert (especially vigilant) whenever a neuromuscular-blocking agent (NMBA) is stocked, ordered, prepared, or administered.

Pregnancy Risk Factor C

Lactation Excretion in breast milk unknown/use caution

Use To facilitate endotracheal intubation and to relax skeletal muscles during surgery; to facilitate mechanical ventilation in ICU patients; does not relieve pain or produce sedation

Available Dosage Forms

Injection, powder for reconstitution: 10 mg, 20 mg

General Dosage Range Dosage adjustment recommended in patients with hepatic impairment

I.V.: *Children ≥1 year and Adults:* Initial: 0.04-0.1 mg/kg; Maintenance: 0.01-0.015 mg/kg every 12-15 minutes **or** 0.8-1.2 mcg/kg/minute as a continuous infusion

Administration

I.V. Concentration of 1 mg/mL may be administered by rapid I.V. injection. May further dilute reconstituted vial to 0.1-0.2 mg/mL in a compatible solution for I.V. infusion. Concentration of 1 mg/mL may be used for I.V. infusion in fluid-restricted patients.

I.V. Detail pH: 4

Nursing Actions

Physical Assessment Ventilatory support must be instituted and maintained until adequate respiratory muscle function and/or airway protection are assured. This drug is not an anesthetic or analgesic; pain must be treated with other agents. Continuous monitoring of vital signs, cardiac status, respiratory status, and degree of neuromuscular block (objective assessment with peripheral external nerve stimulator) is mandatory during infusion and until full muscle tone has returned. It may take longer for return of muscle tone in obese or elderly patients or patients with renal or hepatic disease, dehydration, electrolyte imbalance, or severe acid/base imbalance.

Long-term use: Monitor level of neuromuscular blockade, skeletal muscle movement, and respiratory effort. Reposition patient and provide appropriate skin care, mouth care, and care of patient's eyes every 2-3 hours while sedated. Provide appropriate emotional and sensory support (auditory and environmental).

Patient Education Patient will usually be unconscious prior to administration. Reassurance of constant monitoring and emotional support to reduce fear and anxiety should precede and follow administration. Following return of muscle tone, do not attempt to change position or rise from bed without assistance.

Vemurafenib (vem ue RAF e nib)

Brand Names: U.S. Zelboraf™

Index Terms BRAF(V600E) Kinase Inhibitor RO5185426; PLX4032; RG7204; RO5185426

Pharmacologic Category Antineoplastic Agent, BRAF Kinase Inhibitor

Medication Safety Issues

Sound-alike/look-alike issues:

Vemurafenib may be confused with axitinib, SORAfenib, vandetanib, vismodegib

High alert medication:

This medication is in a class the Institute for Safe Medication Practices (ISMP) includes among its list of drug classes which have a heightened risk of causing significant patient harm when used in error.

Medication Guide Available Yes

Pregnancy Risk Factor D

Lactation Excretion in breast milk unknown/not recommended

Use Treatment of unresectable or metastatic melanoma in patients with a BRAF^{V600E} mutation (as detected by an FDA-approved test)

Note: Not recommended in patients with wild-type BRAF melanoma

Available Dosage Forms

Tablet, oral:

Zelboraf™: 240 mg

General Dosage Range Dosage adjustment recommended in patients who develop toxicities.

Oral: *Adults:* 960 mg twice daily

Administration

Oral Doses should be administered orally in the morning and evening, ~12 hours apart. Swallow whole with a glass of water; do not crush or chew. May be taken with or without a meal. If a dose is missed, may be taken up to 4 hours prior to the next scheduled dose to maintain a twice daily schedule; both doses should **not** be taken at the same time.

Nursing Actions

Physical Assessment Cardiac assessment is required periodically, focusing on arrhythmia development. Electrolyte (potassium, magnesium, calcium) and ECG monitoring (QT interval) is required. This drug causes photosensitivity reactions; educate the patient on proper sun protection. Monitor skin closely for reactions or development of any skin lesions. Report these to the doctor for further evaluation. Monitor for ocular toxicity: Blurred vision, pain, tearing, or irritation.

Patient Education Medication is taken twice a day, with or without food and separated by ~12 hours. Pills should be taken whole, not broken or crushed. It is important to maintain a twice-a-day schedule. Photosensitivity instructions include avoiding sun exposure, using lip balm, and wearing protective clothing. Common side effects include arthralgias, fatigue, rash, upset stomach, and alopecia. Side effects which need immediate attention include dizziness, fast heartbeat, white patches on eyes, and new or worsening skin lesions. Instruct patients that because of potential side effects, they will need frequent evaluations of their skin, eyes, and heart, including ECGs and electrolytes.

Venlafaxine (ven la FAX een)

Brand Names: U.S. Effexor XR®; Effexor®

Pharmacologic Category Antidepressant, Serotonin/Norepinephrine Reuptake Inhibitor

Medication Safety Issues

Sound-alike/look-alike issues:

Effexor® may be confused with Effexor XR®

Medication Guide Available Yes

Pregnancy Risk Factor C

Lactation Enters breast milk/not recommended

Breast-Feeding Considerations Venlafaxine and ODV are found in breast milk and the serum of nursing infants. Adverse events have not been observed; however, it is recommended to monitor the infant for adverse events if the decision to breast-feed has been made. The long-term effects on neurobehavior have not been studied, thus one should prescribe venlafaxine to a mother who is breast-feeding only when the benefits outweigh the potential risks. The manufacturer does not recommend breast-feeding during therapy.

Use Treatment of major depressive disorder, generalized anxiety disorder (GAD), social anxiety disorder (social phobia), panic disorder

Unlabeled Use Obsessive-compulsive disorder (OCD); hot flashes; neuropathic pain (including diabetic neuropathy); attention-deficit/hyperactivity disorder (ADHD); post-traumatic stress disorder (PTSD)

Mechanism of Action/Effect Venlafaxine and its active metabolite, o-desmethylvenlafaxine (ODV), inhibit the reuptake of both norepinephrine and serotonin (SNRI); improves symptoms of depression.

Contraindications Hypersensitivity to venlafaxine or any component of the formulation; use of MAO inhibitors within 14 days; should not initiate MAO inhibitor within 7 days of discontinuing venlafaxine

Warnings/Precautions [U.S. Boxed Warning]: Antidepressants increase the risk of suicidal thinking and behavior in children, adolescents, and young adults (18-24 years of age) with major depressive disorder (MDD) and other psychiatric disorders; consider risk prior to prescribing. Short-term studies did not show an increased risk in patients >24 years of age and showed a decreased risk in patients ≥65 years. Closely monitor for clinical worsening, suicidality, or unusual changes in behavior; the patient's family or caregiver should be instructed to closely observe the patient and communicate condition with healthcare provider. Reduced growth rate has been observed with venlafaxine therapy in children. A medication guide should be dispensed with each prescription. **Venlafaxine is not FDA approved for use in children.**

The possibility of a suicide attempt is inherent in major depression and may persist until remission occurs. Monitor for worsening of depression or suicidality, especially during initiation of therapy (generally first 1-2 months) or with dose increases or decreases. Use caution in high-risk patients. Worsening depression and severe abrupt suicidality that are not part of the presenting symptoms may require discontinuation or modification of drug therapy. The patient's family or caregiver should be alerted to monitor patients for the emergence of suicidality and associated behaviors (such as agitation, irritability, hostility, impulsivity, and hypomania) and call healthcare provider.

May worsen psychosis in some patients or precipitate a shift to mania or hypomania in patients with bipolar disorder. Patients presenting with depressive symptoms should be screened for bipolar disorder. Monotherapy in patients with bipolar disorder should be avoided. **Venlafaxine is not FDA approved for the treatment of bipolar depression.**

Serotonin syndrome and neuroleptic malignant syndrome (NMS)-like reactions have occurred with serotonin/norepinephrine reuptake inhibitors (SNRIs) and selective serotonin reuptake inhibitors (SSRIs) when used alone, and particularly when used in combination with serotonergic agents (eg, triptans) or antidopaminergic agents (eg, antipsychotics). Concurrent use with MAO inhibitors is contraindicated. May cause sustained increase in blood pressure or tachycardia; dose related and increases are generally modest (12-15 mm Hg diastolic). Control pre-existing hypertension prior to initiation of venlafaxine. Use caution in patients with recent history of MI, unstable heart disease, or hyperthyroidism; may cause increase in anxiety, nervousness, insomnia; may cause weight loss (use with caution in patients where weight loss is undesirable); may cause increases in serum cholesterol. Use caution with hepatic or renal impairment; dosage adjustments recommended. May cause hyponatremia/SIADH (elderly at increased risk); volume depletion (diuretics may increase risk).

May impair platelet aggregation resulting in increased risk of bleeding events, particularly if used concomitantly with aspirin or NSAIDs. Bleeding related to SSRI or SNRI use has been reported to range from relatively minor bruising and epistaxis to life-threatening hemorrhage. Interstitial lung disease and eosinophilic pneumonia have been rarely reported; may present as progressive dyspnea, cough, and/or chest pain. Prompt evaluation and possible discontinuation of therapy may be necessary. Venlafaxine may increase the risks associated with electroconvulsive therapy. Use cautiously in patients with a history of seizures. The risks of cognitive or motor impairment, as well as the potential for anticholinergic effects are very low. May cause or exacerbate sexual dysfunction.

Abrupt discontinuation or dosage reduction after extended (≥6 weeks) therapy may lead to agitation, dysphoria, nervousness, anxiety, and other symptoms. When discontinuing therapy, dosage should be tapered gradually over at least a 2-week period. If intolerable symptoms occur following a decrease in dosage or upon discontinuation of therapy, then resuming the previous dose with a more gradual taper should be considered. Use caution in patients with increased intraocular pressure or at risk of acute narrow-angle glaucoma.

Drug Interactions

Avoid Concomitant Use

Avoid concomitant use of Venlafaxine with any of the following: Conivaptan; Iobenguane I 123; MAO Inhibitors; Methylene Blue

Decreased Effect

Venlafaxine may decrease the levels/effects of: Alpha2-Agonists; Indinavir; Iobenguane I 123; Ioflupane I 123

The levels/effects of Venlafaxine may be decreased by: CYP3A4 Inducers (Strong); Deferasirox; Peginterferon Alfa-2b; Tocilizumab

Increased Effect/Toxicity

Venlafaxine may increase the levels/effects of: Alpha-/Beta-Agonists; Aspirin; Methylene Blue; Metoclopramide; NSAID (Nonselective); Serotonin Modulators; TraZODone; Vitamin K Antagonists

The levels/effects of Venlafaxine may be increased by: Abiraterone Acetate; Alcohol (Ethyl); Antipsychotics; Conivaptan; CYP2D6 Inhibitors (Moderate); CYP2D6 Inhibitors (Strong); CYP3A4 Inhibitors (Moderate); CYP3A4 Inhibitors (Strong); Darunavir; Dasatinib; Ivacaftor; Linezolid; MAO Inhibitors; Metoclopramide; Propafenone; Voriconazole

Nutritional/Ethanol Interactions

Ethanol: May increase CNS depression; monitor for increased effects with coadministration. Caution patients about effects.

Herb/Nutraceutical: Avoid valerian, St John's wort, SAMe, kava kava, tryptophan (may increase risk of serotonin syndrome and/or excessive sedation).

Adverse Reactions Note: Actual frequency may be dependent upon formulation and/or indication

>10%:

Central nervous system: Headache (25% to 38%), somnolence (12% to 26%), dizziness (11% to 24%), insomnia (15% to 24%), nervousness (6% to 21%), anxiety (2% to 11%),

Gastrointestinal: Nausea (21% to 58%), xerostomia (12% to 22%), anorexia (8% to 17%), constipation (8% to 15%)

Genitourinary: Abnormal ejaculation/orgasm (2% to 19%)

Neuromuscular & skeletal: Weakness (8% to 19%)

Miscellaneous: Diaphoresis (7% to 19%)

1% to 10%:

Cardiovascular: Vasodilation (2% to 6%), hypertension (dose related; 3% in patients receiving <100 mg/day, up to 13% in patients receiving >300 mg/day), palpitation (3%), tachycardia (2%), chest pain (2%), postural hypotension (1%), edema

Central nervous system: Yawning (3% to 8%), abnormal dreams (3% to 7%), chills (2% to 7%), agitation (2% to 5%), confusion (2%), abnormal thinking (2%), depersonalization (1%), depression (1% to 3%), fever, migraine, amnesia, hypoesthesia, vertigo

Dermatologic: Rash (3%), pruritus (1%), bruising

Endocrine & metabolic: Libido decreased (2% to 8%), hypercholesterolemia (5%), triglycerides increased

Gastrointestinal: Abdominal pain (8%), diarrhea (8%), vomiting (3% to 8%), dyspepsia (5% to 7%), weight loss (1% to 6%), flatulence (3% to 4%), taste perversion (2%), appetite increased, belching, weight gain

Genitourinary: Impotence (4% to 6%), urinary frequency (3%), urination impaired (2%), urinary retention (1%), metrorrhagia, prostatic disorder, vaginitis

Neuromuscular & skeletal: Tremor (1% to 10%), hypertonia (3%), paresthesia (2% to 3%), twitching (1% to 3%), arthralgia, neck pain, trismus

Ocular: Accommodation abnormal (6% to 9%), abnormal or blurred vision (4% to 6%), mydriasis (2%)

Otic: Tinnitus (2%)

Renal: Albuminuria

Respiratory: Pharyngitis (7%), sinusitis (2%), bronchitis, cough increased, dyspnea

Miscellaneous: Infection (6%), flu-like syndrome (2%), trauma (2%)

Available Dosage Forms

Capsule, extended release, oral: 37.5 mg, 75 mg, 150 mg

Effexor XR®: 37.5 mg, 75 mg, 150 mg

Tablet, oral: 25 mg, 37.5 mg, 50 mg, 75 mg, 100 mg

Effexor®: 50 mg

Tablet, extended release, oral: 37.5 mg, 75 mg, 150 mg, 225 mg

General Dosage Range Dosage adjustment recommended in patients with hepatic or renal impairment

Oral:

Extended release: *Adults:* Initial: 37.5-75 mg/day once daily; Maintenance: 75-225 mg/day once daily (recommended maximum: 225 mg/day)

Immediate release: *Adults:* Initial: 75 mg/day in 2-3 divided doses; Maintenance: 75-375 mg/day in 2-3 divided doses (recommended maximum: 375 mg/day)

Administration

Oral Administer with food.

Extended-release formulations: Swallow capsule or tablet whole; do not crush or chew. Contents of capsule may be sprinkled on a spoonful of applesauce and swallowed immediately without chewing; followed with a glass of water to ensure complete swallowing of the pellets.

Stability

Storage Store at controlled room temperature of 20°C to 25°C (68°F to 77°F).

Nursing Actions

Physical Assessment Monitor blood pressure and weight/height at beginning of therapy and periodically throughout. Observe for clinical worsening, suicide ideation, or unusual behavior changes, especially during the initial few months of therapy or during dosage changes. Taper dosage when discontinuing.

Patient Education It may take 2-3 weeks to achieve desired results. Take with food. Extended release capsules should be swallowed whole; do not crush or chew. Alternatively, contents may be emptied onto a spoonful of applesauce and swallowed without chewing. Avoid alcohol. Maintain adequate hydration unless instructed to restrict fluid intake. You may experience excess drowsiness or insomnia, lightheadedness, dizziness, blurred vision, headache, nausea, vomiting, anorexia, altered taste, dry mouth, constipation, diarrhea, postural hypotension, urinary retention, or sexual dysfunction (reversible). Report persistent CNS effects (eg, insomnia, restlessness, fatigue, anxiety, abnormal thoughts, suicide ideation, confusion, personality changes, impaired cognitive function), muscle cramping or tremors, chest pain, palpitations, rapid heartbeat, swelling of extremities, severe dizziness, unresolved urinary retention, vision changes or eye pain, hearing changes or ringing in ears, skin rash or irritation, or worsening of condition.

Dietary Considerations Should be taken with food.

Verapamil (ver AP a mil)

Brand Names: U.S. Calan®; Calan® SR; Covera-HS®; Isoptin® SR; Verelan®; Verelan® PM

Index Terms Iproveratril Hydrochloride; Verapamil Hydrochloride

Pharmacologic Category Antianginal Agent; Antiarrhythmic Agent, Class IV; Calcium Channel Blocker; Calcium Channel Blocker, Nondihydropyridine

Medication Safety Issues

Sound-alike/look-alike issues:

Calan® may be confused with Colace®, diltiazem

Covera-HS® may be confused with Provera®

Isoptin® may be confused with Isopto® Tears

Verelan® may be confused with Voltaren®

High alert medication:

The Institute for Safe Medication Practices (ISMP) includes this medication (I.V. formulation) among its list of drug classes which have a heightened risk of causing significant patient harm when used in error.

Administration issues:

Significant differences exist between oral and I.V. dosing. Use caution when converting from one route of administration to another.

International issues:

Dilacor [Brazil] may be confused with Dilacor XR brand name for diltiazem [U.S.]

Pregnancy Risk Factor C

Lactation Enters breast milk/not recommended (AAP considers "compatible"; AAP 2001 update pending)

Breast-Feeding Considerations Crosses into breast milk; manufacturer recommends to discontinue breast-feeding while taking verapamil.

Use

Oral: Treatment of hypertension; angina pectoris (vasospastic, chronic stable, unstable) (Calan®, Covera-HS®); supraventricular tachyarrhythmia (PSVT, atrial fibrillation/flutter [rate control])

I.V.: Supraventricular tachyarrhythmia (PSVT, atrial fibrillation/flutter [rate control])

Unlabeled Use Migraine; hypertrophic cardiomyopathy; bipolar disorder (manic manifestations)

Mechanism of Action/Effect Produces relaxation of coronary vascular smooth muscle and coronary vasodilation. Increases myocardial oxygen delivery in patients with vasospastic (Prinzmetal's) angina. Slows automaticity and conduction of AV node.

Contraindications Hypersensitivity to verapamil or any component of the formulation; severe left ventricular dysfunction; hypotension (systolic pressure <90 mm Hg) or cardiogenic shock; sick sinus syndrome (except in patients with a functioning artificial ventricular pacemaker); second- or third-degree AV block (except in patients with a functioning artificial ventricular pacemaker); atrial flutter or fibrillation and an accessory bypass tract (Wolff-Parkinson-White [WPW] syndrome, Lown-Ganong-Levine syndrome)

I.V.: Additional contraindications include concurrent use of I.V. beta-blocking agents; ventricular tachycardia

Warnings/Precautions Avoid use in heart failure; can exacerbate condition; use is contraindicated in severe left ventricular dysfunction. Symptomatic hypotension with or without syncope can rarely occur; blood pressure must be lowered at a rate appropriate for the patient's clinical condition. Rare increases in hepatic enzymes can be observed. Can cause first-degree AV block or sinus bradycardia; use is contraindicated in patients with sick sinus syndrome, second- or third-degree AV block (except in patients with a functioning artificial pacemaker), or an accessory bypass tract (eg, WPW syndrome). Other conduction abnormalities are rare. Considered contraindicated in patients with wide complex tachycardias unless known to be supraventricular in origin; severe hypotension likely to occur upon administration (ACLS, 2010). Use caution when using verapamil together with a beta-blocker. Administration of I.V. verapamil and an I.V. beta-blocker within a few hours of each other may result in asystole and should be avoided; simultaneous administration is contraindicated. Use with other agents known to reduce SA node function and/or AV nodal conduction (eg, digoxin) or reduce sympathetic outflow (eg, clonidine) may increase the risk of serious bradycardia. Verapamil significantly increases digoxin serum concentrations; adjust digoxin dose. Use with caution in patients with hypertrophic cardiomyopathy with outflow tract obstruction (especially those with resting outflow obstruction and severe limiting symptoms); may be used in patients who cannot tolerate beta-blockade.

Decreased neuromuscular transmission has been reported with verapamil; use with caution in patients with attenuated neuromuscular transmission (Duchenne's muscular dystrophy, myasthenia gravis); dosage reduction may be required. Use with caution in renal impairment; monitor hemodynamics and possibly ECG if severe impairment, particularly if concomitant hepatic impairment. Use with caution in patients with hepatic impairment; dosage reduction may be required; monitor hemodynamics and possibly ECG if severe impairment. May prolong recovery from nondepolarizing neuromuscular-blocking agents. Use Covera-HS® (extended-release delivery system) with caution in patients with severe GI narrowing. In patients with extremely short GI transit times (eg, <7 hours), dosage adjustment may be required; inadequate pharmacokinetic data. I.V. use for SVT for is not recommended in infants; use with caution in children as myocardial depression/hypotension may occur.

Drug Interactions

Avoid Concomitant Use

Avoid concomitant use of Verapamil with any of the following: Conivaptan; Disopyramide; Dofetilide; Pimozide; Silodosin; Topotecan

Decreased Effect

Verapamil may decrease the levels/effects of: Clopidogrel

The levels/effects of Verapamil may be decreased by: Barbiturates; Calcium Salts; CarBAMazepine; CYP3A4 Inducers (Strong); Cyproterone; Deferasirox; Herbs (Hypertensive Properties); Methylphenidate; Nafcillin; P-glycoprotein/ABCB1 Inducers; Rifamycin Derivatives; Tocilizumab; Yohimbine

Increased Effect/Toxicity

Verapamil may increase the levels/effects of: Alcohol (Ethyl); Aliskiren; Amifostine; Amiodarone; Antihypertensives; ARIPiprazole;

Atorvastatin; Benzodiazepines (metabolized by oxidation); Beta-Blockers; Budesonide (Systemic, Oral Inhalation); BusPIRone; Calcium Channel Blockers (Dihydropyridine); CarBAMazepine; Cardiac Glycosides; Colchicine; Corticosteroids (Systemic); CycloSPORINE; CycloSPORINE (Systemic); CYP3A4 Substrates; Dabigatran Etexilate; Disopyramide; Dofetilide; Dronedarone; Eletriptan; Eplerenone; Everolimus; Fexofenadine; Fingolimod; Flecainide; Fosphenytoin; Halofantrine; Hypotensive Agents; Lithium; Lovastatin; Lurasidone; Magnesium Salts; Midodrine; Neuromuscular-Blocking Agents (Nondepolarizing); Nitroprusside; P-glycoprotein/ABCB1 Substrates; Phenytoin; Pimecrolimus; Pimozide; Propafenone; Prucalopride; QuiNIDine; Ranolazine; Red Yeast Rice; RisperiDONE; RiTUXimab; Rivaroxaban; Salicylates; Salmeterol; Silodosin; Simvastatin; Tacrolimus; Tacrolimus (Systemic); Tacrolimus (Topical); Topotecan; Vilazodone; Zuclopenthixol

The levels/effects of Verapamil may be increased by: Alpha1-Blockers; Anilidopiperidine Opioids; Antifungal Agents (Azole Derivatives, Systemic); Atorvastatin; Calcium Channel Blockers (Dihydropyridine); Cimetidine; Conivaptan; CycloSPORINE; CycloSPORINE (Systemic); CYP3A4 Inhibitors (Moderate); CYP3A4 Inhibitors (Strong); Dasatinib; Diazoxide; Dronedarone; Fluconazole; Grapefruit Juice; Herbs (Hypotensive Properties); Macrolide Antibiotics; Magnesium Salts; MAO Inhibitors; Pentoxifylline; P-glycoprotein/ABCB1 Inhibitors; Phosphodiesterase 5 Inhibitors; Prostacyclin Analogues; Protease Inhibitors; QuiNIDine; Telithromycin

Nutritional/Ethanol Interactions

Ethanol: Ethanol may increase ethanol levels. Management: Avoid or limit ethanol.

Food: Grapefruit juice may increase the serum concentration of verapamil. Management: Avoid grapefruit juice or use with caution and monitor for effects. Calan® SR and Isoptin® SR products should be taken with food or milk; other formulations may be administered without regard to meals.

Herb/Nutraceutical: St John's wort may decrease levels of verapamil. Some herbal medications have hypertensive properties (eg, licorice); others may increase or decrease the antihypertensive effect of verapamil. Management: Avoid St John's wort, bayberry, blue cohosh, cayenne, ephedra, ginger, ginseng (American), kola, licorice, and yohimbe. Avoid black cohosh, California poppy, coleus, golden seal, hawthorn, mistletoe, periwinkle, quinine, and shepherd's purse.

Adverse Reactions

>10%:

Central nervous system: Headache (1% to 12%)

Gastrointestinal: Gingival hyperplasia (≤19%), constipation (7% to 12%)

1% to 10%:

Cardiovascular: Peripheral edema (1% to 4%), hypotension (3%), CHF/pulmonary edema (2%), AV block (1% to 2%), bradycardia (HR <50 bpm: 1%), flushing (1%)

Central nervous system: Fatigue (2% to 5%), dizziness (1% to 5%), lethargy (3%), pain (2%), sleep disturbance (1%)

Dermatologic: Rash (1% to 2%)

Gastrointestinal: Dyspepsia (3%), nausea (1% to 3%), diarrhea (2%)

Hepatic: Liver enzymes increased (1%)

Neuromuscular & skeletal: Myalgia (1%), paresthesia (1%)

Respiratory: Dyspnea (1%)

Miscellaneous: Flu-like syndrome (4%)

Pharmacodynamics/Kinetics

Onset of Action Oral (immediate release tablets): Peak effect: 1-2 hours; I.V.: Peak effect: 1-5 minutes

Duration of Action Oral: Immediate release tablets: 6-8 hours; I.V.: 10-20 minutes

Available Dosage Forms

Caplet, sustained release, oral:
Calan® SR: 120 mg, 180 mg, 240 mg

Capsule, extended release, oral: 120 mg, 180 mg, 240 mg

Capsule, extended release, controlled onset, oral: 100 mg, 200 mg, 300 mg
Verelan® PM: 100 mg, 200 mg, 300 mg

Capsule, sustained release, oral: 120 mg, 180 mg, 240 mg, 360 mg
Verelan®: 120 mg, 180 mg, 240 mg, 360 mg

Injection, solution: 2.5 mg/mL (2 mL, 4 mL)

Tablet, oral: 40 mg, 80 mg, 120 mg
Calan®: 80 mg, 120 mg

Tablet, extended release, oral: 120 mg, 180 mg, 240 mg

Tablet, extended release, controlled onset, oral:
Covera-HS®: 180 mg, 240 mg

Tablet, sustained release, oral: 240 mg
Isoptin® SR: 120 mg, 180 mg

General Dosage Range

I.V.:

Children 1-15 years: 0.1-0.3 mg/kg/dose (maximum: 5 mg/dose); may repeat dose (maximum for second dose: 10 mg)

Adults: Initial dose: 2.5-5 mg; Second dose: 5-10 mg (maximum: 20-30 mg total dose)

Oral:

Extended release:

Adults: 180-480 mg once daily

Elderly: Initial: 100-180 mg once daily

Immediate release: *Adults:* Initial: 80-120 mg 3 times/day; Maintenance: 80-480 mg/day in 2-4 divided doses (maximum: 480 mg/day)

Sustained release:

Adults: 120-480 mg/day in 1-2 divided doses (maximum: 480 mg/day)

Elderly: Initial: 120 mg/day once daily; Maintenance: 120-360 mg/day in 1-2 divided doses

Administration

Oral Do not crush or chew sustained or extended release products.

Calan® SR, Isoptin® SR: Administer with food.

Verelan®, Verelan® PM: Capsules may be opened and the contents sprinkled on 1 tablespoonful of applesauce, then swallowed immediately without chewing. Do not subdivide contents of capsules.

I.V. Administer over 2 minutes (over 3 minutes in older patients [ACLS, 2010])

I.V. Detail pH: 4-6.5

Stability

Storage Store at controlled room temperature of 15°C to 30°C (59°F to 86°F). Protect from light.

Nursing Actions

Physical Assessment I.V. requires use of infusion pump and continuous cardiac and hemodynamic monitoring. Monitor gums for gingival hyperplasia. Encourage good oral hygiene. Refer to dentist if indicated. Monitor cardiac status when beginning therapy, when titrating dosage, and periodically throughout.

Patient Education Oral: Do not crush or chew sustained or extended release forms. Avoid grapefruit juice; avoid (or limit) alcohol and caffeine. Maintain good oral hygiene to avoid gum disease. You may experience dizziness or lightheadedness, nausea, vomiting, constipation, or diarrhea. Report chest pain, palpitations, or irregular heartbeat; unusual cough, respiratory difficulty, or swelling of extremities (feet/ankles); muscle tremors or weakness; confusion or acute lethargy; or skin irritation or rash. **Pregnancy precaution:** Inform prescriber if you are or intend to become pregnant.

Dietary Considerations Calan® SR and Isoptin® SR products may be taken with food or milk, other formulations may be administered without regard to meals; sprinkling contents of Verelan® or Verelan® PM capsule onto applesauce does not affect oral absorption.

Vilazodone (vil AZ oh done)

Brand Names: U.S. Viibryd™

Index Terms EMD 68843; SB659746-A; Vilazodone Hydrochloride

Pharmacologic Category Antidepressant, Selective Serotonin Reuptake Inhibitor/5-HT_{1A} Receptor Partial Agonist

Medication Guide Available Yes

Pregnancy Risk Factor C

Lactation Excretion in breast milk unknown/consider risk:benefit

Use Treatment of major depressive disorder

Mechanism of Action/Effect Vilazodone inhibits CNS neuron serotonin uptake; minimal or no effect on reuptake of norepinephrine or dopamine. It also binds selectively with high affinity to 5-HT_{1A} receptors and is a 5-HT_{1A} receptor partial agonist. 5-HT_{1A} receptor activity may be altered in depression and anxiety.

Contraindications Concomitant use with MAO inhibitors or within 2 weeks of discontinuing MAO inhibitors

Warnings/Precautions [U.S. Boxed Warning]: Antidepressants increase the risk of suicidal thinking and behavior in children, adolescents, and young adults (18-24 years of age) with major depressive disorder (MDD) and other psychiatric disorders; consider risk prior to prescribing. Short-term studies did not show an increased risk in patients >24 years of age and showed a decreased risk in patients ≥65 years. Closely monitor patients for clinical worsening, suicidality, or unusual changes in behavior, particularly during the initial 1-2 months of therapy or during periods of dosage adjustments (increases or decreases); the patient's family or caregiver should be instructed to closely observe the patient and communicate condition with healthcare provider. A medication guide concerning the use of antidepressants should be dispensed with each prescription. **Vilazodone is not FDA approved for use in children.**

The possibility of a suicide attempt is inherent in major depression and may persist until remission occurs. Use caution in high-risk patients. Worsening depression and severe abrupt suicidality that are not part of the presenting symptoms may require discontinuation or modification of drug therapy. The patient's family or caregiver should be alerted to monitor patients for the emergence of suicidality and associated behaviors (such as agitation, irritability, hostility, impulsivity, and hypomania) and call healthcare provider.

May worsen psychosis in some patients or precipitate a shift to mania or hypomania in patients with bipolar disorder. Patients presenting with depressive symptoms should be screened for bipolar disorder. Monotherapy in patients with bipolar disorder should be avoided. **Vilazodone is not FDA approved for the treatment of bipolar depression.**

Serotonin syndrome and neuroleptic malignant syndrome (NMS)-like reactions have occurred with serotonin/norepinephrine reuptake inhibitors (SNRIs) and selective serotonin reuptake inhibitors (SSRIs) when used alone, and particularly when used in combination with serotonergic agents (eg, triptans) or antidopaminergic agents (eg, antipsychotics). Concurrent use or use within 2 weeks of discontinuing MAO inhibitors is contraindicated. In addition, allow at least 14 days after stopping vilazodone before starting an MAO inhibitor. High potential for interaction with concomitant medications (see Drug Interactions); monitor closely for toxicity or adverse effects. Dose reductions are recommended with concomitant use of strong or moderate CYP3A4 inhibitors. May increase the risks associated with electroconvulsive therapy. Has a low potential to impair cognitive or motor performance; caution operating hazardous machinery or driving.

Use with caution in patients with hepatic impairment, seizure disorder, in elderly patients, or on concomitant CNS depressants. Use caution with concomitant use of aspirin, NSAIDs, warfarin, or other drugs that affect coagulation; the risk of bleeding may be potentiated. May cause hyponatremia/SIADH (elderly at increased risk); volume depletion and diuretics may increase risk. May cause or exacerbate sexual dysfunction. Upon discontinuation of vilazodone therapy, gradually taper dose. If intolerable symptoms occur following a decrease in dosage or upon discontinuation of therapy, consider resuming the previous dose with a more gradual taper.

Drug Interactions

Avoid Concomitant Use

Avoid concomitant use of Vilazodone with any of the following: Iobenguane I 123; MAO Inhibitors; Methylene Blue; Pimozide; Tryptophan

Decreased Effect

Vilazodone may decrease the levels/effects of: Iobenguane I 123; Ioflupane I 123

The levels/effects of Vilazodone may be decreased by: CarBAMazepine; CYP3A4 Inducers (Strong); Cyproheptadine; Deferasirox; NSAID (COX-2 Inhibitor); NSAID (Nonselective); Peginterferon Alfa-2b; Tocilizumab

Increased Effect/Toxicity

Vilazodone may increase the levels/effects of: Alpha-/Beta-Blockers; Anticoagulants; Antidepressants (Serotonin Reuptake Inhibitor/Antagonist); Antiplatelet Agents; Aspirin; Benzodiazepines (metabolized by oxidation); Beta-Blockers; BusPIRone; CarBAMazepine; CloZAPine; Collagenase (Systemic); CYP2D6 Substrates; Desmopressin; Dextromethorphan; Drotrecogin Alfa (Activated); Fesoterodine; Galantamine; Ibritumomab; Lithium; Methadone; Methylene Blue; Metoclopramide; Mexiletine; NSAID (COX-2 Inhibitor); NSAID (Nonselective); Pimozide; RisperiDONE; Rivaroxaban; Salicylates; Serotonin Modulators; Tamoxifen; Thrombolytic Agents; Tositumomab and Iodine I 131 Tositumomab; TraMADol; Tricyclic Antidepressants; Vitamin K Antagonists

The levels/effects of Vilazodone may be increased by: Alcohol (Ethyl); Analgesics (Opioid); Antipsychotics; BusPIRone; Cimetidine; CNS Depressants; CYP3A4 Inhibitors (Moderate); CYP3A4 Inhibitors (Strong); Dasatinib; Glucosamine; Herbs (Anticoagulant/Antiplatelet Properties); Linezolid; Macrolide Antibiotics; MAO Inhibitors; Metoclopramide; Omega-3-Acid Ethyl Esters; Pentosan Polysulfate Sodium; Pentoxifylline; Propafenone; Prostacyclin Analogues; TraMADol; Tryptophan; Vitamin E

Nutritional/Ethanol Interactions

Ethanol: Ethanol may increase CNS depression. Management: Avoid or limit use and monitor for increased effects.

Food: Management: Take with food.

Adverse Reactions

>10%:

Gastrointestinal: Diarrhea (28%), nausea (23%)

1% to 10%:

Cardiovascular: Palpitation (2%)

Central nervous system: Dizziness (9%), insomnia (6%), dreams abnormal (4%), fatigue (4%), restlessness (3%), somnolence (3%), migraine (≥1%), sedation (≥1%)

Dermatologic: Hyperhidrosis (≥1%)

Endocrine & metabolic: Libido decreased (3% to 5%), orgasm abnormal (2% to 4%), sexual dysfunction (≤2%)

Gastrointestinal: Xerostomia (8%), vomiting (5%), dyspepsia (3%), flatulence (3%), gastroenteritis (3%), appetite increased (2%), appetite decreased (≥1%)

Genitourinary: Ejaculation delayed (2%), erectile dysfunction (2%)

Neuromuscular & skeletal: Arthralgia (3%), paresthesia (3%), jittery (2%), tremor (2%)

Ocular: Blurred vision (≥1%), dry eyes (≥1%)

Miscellaneous: Night sweats (≥1%)

Available Dosage Forms

Tablet, oral:

Viibryd™: 10 mg, 20 mg, 40 mg

General Dosage Range Dosage adjustment recommended in patients on concomitant therapy

Oral: *Adults:* 10-40 mg once daily

Administration

Oral Administer with food.

Stability

Storage Store at 25°C (77°F); excursions permitted to 15°C to 30°C (50°F to 86°F).

Dietary Considerations Take with food.

VinBLAStine (vin BLAS teen)

Index Terms Velban; Vinblastine Sulfate; Vincaleukoblastine; VLB

Pharmacologic Category Antineoplastic Agent, Natural Source (Plant) Derivative; Antineoplastic Agent, Vinca Alkaloid

Medication Safety Issues

Sound-alike/look-alike issues:

VinBLAStine may be confused with vinCRIStine, vinorelbine

High alert medication:

The Institute for Safe Medication Practices (ISMP) includes this medication among its list of drug classes which have a heightened risk of causing significant patient harm when used in error.

Administration issues:

Must be dispensed in overwrap which bears the statement **"Do not remove covering until the moment of injection. Fatal if given intrathecally. For I.V. use only."** Syringes should be labeled: **"Fatal if given intrathecally. For I.V. use only."**

Pregnancy Risk Factor D

Lactation Excretion in breast milk unknown/not recommended

Breast-Feeding Considerations Due to the potential for serious adverse reactions in the nursing infant, breast-feeding is not recommended.

Use Treatment of Hodgkin's and non-Hodgkin's lymphoma; testicular cancer; breast cancer; mycosis fungoides; Kaposi's sarcoma; histiocytosis (Letterer-Siwe disease); choriocarcinoma

Unlabeled Use Treatment of bladder cancer, melanoma, nonsmall cell lung cancer (NSCLC), ovarian cancer, soft tissue sarcoma (desmoid tumors)

Mechanism of Action/Effect Vinblastine arrests cell cycle growth in metaphase. Also inhibits RNA synthesis and amino acid metabolism resulting in inhibition of metabolic pathways and cell growth.

Contraindications Significant granulocytopenia; presence of bacterial infection; I.T. administration is contraindicated (may result in death)

Warnings/Precautions Hazardous agent - use appropriate precautions for handling and disposal. **[U.S. Boxed Warning]: For I.V. use only. Intrathecal administration may result in death.** Must be dispensed in overwrap which bears the statement **"Do not remove covering until the moment of injection. Fatal if given intrathecally. For I.V. use only." [U.S. Boxed Warning]: Vinblastine is a moderate vesicant; avoid extravasation. Individuals administering should be experienced in vinblastine administration;** assure proper needle or catheter placement prior to administration. Leukopenia is common; granulocytopenia may be severe with higher doses. Leukopenia may be more pronounced in cachectic patients and patients with skin ulceration. Thrombocytopenia and anemia may occur rarely.

Use with caution in patients with hepatic impairment; toxicity may be increased; may require dosage modification. Neurotoxicity is rare at clinical doses; may occur with high doses (symptoms are similar to vincristine toxicity, including peripheral neuropathy, loss of deep tendon reflexes, headache, weakness, urinary retention, and GI symptoms). May rarely cause disabling neurotoxicity (usually reversible). Itraconazole may decrease the metabolism of vinblastine via CYP3A4 inhibition and may increase the effects of vinblastine via P-glycoprotein effects; severe myelosuppression and neurotoxicity may occur. Acute shortness of breath and severe bronchospasm have been reported, most often in association with concurrent administration of mitomycin; may occur within minutes to several hours following vinblastine administration or up to 14 days following mitomycin administration; use caution in patients with pre-existing pulmonary disease. Use with caution in patients with ischemic heart disease. **[U.S. Boxed Warning]: Should be administered under the supervision of an experienced cancer chemotherapy physician.** Some dosage forms may contain benzyl alcohol which has been associated with "gasping syndrome" in neonates.

Drug Interactions

Avoid Concomitant Use

Avoid concomitant use of VinBLAStine with any of the following: BCG; CloZAPine; Conivaptan; Dabigatran Etexilate; Natalizumab; Pimecrolimus; Pimozide; Tacrolimus (Topical); Vaccines (Live)

Decreased Effect

VinBLAStine may decrease the levels/effects of: BCG; Coccidioidin Skin Test; Dabigatran Etexilate; Linagliptin; P-glycoprotein/ABCB1 Substrates; Sipuleucel-T; Vaccines (Inactivated); Vaccines (Live)

The levels/effects of VinBLAStine may be decreased by: CYP3A4 Inducers (Strong); Deferasirox; Echinacea; Peginterferon Alfa-2b; P-glycoprotein/ABCB1 Inducers; Tocilizumab

Increased Effect/Toxicity

VinBLAStine may increase the levels/effects of: ARIPiprazole; CloZAPine; Leflunomide; MitoMYcin; Natalizumab; Pimozide; Tolterodine; Vaccines (Live)

The levels/effects of VinBLAStine may be increased by: Conivaptan; CYP3A4 Inhibitors (Moderate); CYP3A4 Inhibitors (Strong); Dasatinib; Denosumab; Itraconazole; Lopinavir; Macrolide Antibiotics; MAO Inhibitors; P-glycoprotein/ABCB1 Inhibitors; Pimecrolimus; Posaconazole; Ritonavir; Roflumilast; Tacrolimus (Topical); Trastuzumab; Voriconazole

Nutritional/Ethanol Interactions Herb/Nutraceutical: Avoid St John's wort (may decrease vinblastine levels). Avoid black cohosh, dong quai in estrogen-dependent tumors.

Adverse Reactions Frequency not defined.

Common:

Cardiovascular: Hypertension

Central nervous system: Malaise

Dermatologic: Alopecia

Gastrointestinal: Constipation

Hematologic: Myelosuppression, leukopenia/granulocytopenia (nadir: 5-10 days; recovery: 7-14 days; dose-limiting toxicity)

Neuromuscular & skeletal: Bone pain, jaw pain, tumor pain

Less common:

Cardiovascular: Angina, cerebrovascular accident, coronary ischemia, ECG abnormalities, limb ischemia, MI, myocardial ischemia, Raynaud's phenomenon

Central nervous system: Depression, dizziness, headache, neurotoxicity (duration: >24 hours), seizure, vertigo

Dermatologic: Dermatitis, photosensitivity (rare), rash, skin blistering

Endocrine & metabolic: Aspermia, hyperuricemia, SIADH

Gastrointestinal: Abdominal pain, anorexia, diarrhea, gastrointestinal bleeding, hemorrhagic enterocolitis, ileus, metallic taste, nausea (mild), paralytic ileus, rectal bleeding, stomatitis, toxic megacolon, vomiting (mild)

Genitourinary: Urinary retention

Hematologic: Anemia, thrombocytopenia (recovery within a few days), thrombotic thrombocytopenic purpura

Local: Cellulitis (with extravasation), irritation, phlebitis (with extravasation), radiation recall

Neuromuscular & skeletal: Deep tendon reflex loss, myalgia, paresthesia, peripheral neuritis, weakness

Ocular: Nystagmus

Otic: Auditory damage, deafness, vestibular damage

Renal: Hemolytic uremic syndrome

Respiratory: Bronchospasm, dyspnea, pharyngitis

Available Dosage Forms

Injection, powder for reconstitution: 10 mg

Injection, solution: 1 mg/mL (10 mL)

General Dosage Range Dosage adjustment recommended in patients with hepatic impairment

I.V.:

Children: Initial dose: 3-6.5 mg/m^2 every 7 days as needed

Adults: Initial: 3.7 mg/m^2; adjust dose every 7 days; Second dose: 5.5 mg/m^2; Third dose: 7.4 mg/m^2; Fourth dose: 9.25 mg/m^2; Fifth dose: 11.1 mg/m^2; Usual range: 5.5-7.4 mg/m^2 every 7 days; Maximum dose: 18.5 mg/m^2

Administration

I.V. Vesicant. **Fatal if given intrathecally.** For I.V. administration only, usually as a slow (2-3 minutes) push, or a bolus (5-15 minutes) infusion; the manufacturer recommends an undiluted 1-minute infusion to prevent venous irritation/extravasation. Prolonged administration times and/or increased administration volumes may the risk of vein irritation and extravasation. Assure proper needle or catheter placement prior to administration.

I.V. Detail pH: 3.5-5.0

Stability

Reconstitution Reconstitute lyophilized powder to a concentration of 1 mg/mL with NS or bacteriostatic NS. For infusion, may dilute in 50 mL NS or D_5W; dilution in larger volumes (≥100 mL) of I.V. fluids is not recommended. Use appropriate precautions for handling and disposal.

Storage Note: Must be dispensed in overwrap which bears the statement "Do not remove covering until the moment of injection. Fatal if given intrathecally. For I.V. use only." Syringes should be labeled: "Fatal if given intrathecally. For I.V. use only."

Store intact vials under refrigeration at 2°C to 8°C (36°F to 46°F). Protect from light. Solutions reconstituted in bacteriostatic NS are stable for 28 days under refrigeration.

Nursing Actions

Physical Assessment Premedication with antiemetic is advisable. Monitor infusion site closely to prevent extravasation (vesicant will cause tissue damage and necrosis). Assess renal function. Monitor for SIADH, bone marrow suppression, leukopenia, hypertension, gastrointestinal disturbance, myalgia, depression, and paresthesia throughout therapy.

Patient Education This medication can only be administered by infusion; report immediately any redness, swelling, burning, or pain at infusion site; sudden difficulty breathing; swelling; chest pain; or chills. Maintain adequate nutrition and hydration, unless instructed to restrict fluid intake. You will be more susceptible to infection. May cause hair loss (will grow back after therapy), nausea or vomiting (request antiemetic), photosensitivity, feelings of extreme weakness or lethargy, or mouth sores. Report persistent constipation or abdominal pain, numbness or tingling in fingers or toes, weakness or pain in muscles or jaw, signs of infection (eg, fever, chills, sore throat, burning urination, fatigue), unusual bleeding (eg, tarry stools, easy bruising, blood in stool, urine, or mouth), unresolved mouth sores, skin rash or itching, or respiratory difficulty.

Related Information

Management of Drug Extravasations *on page 1269*

VinCRIStine (vin KRIS teen)

Brand Names: U.S. Vincasar PFS®

Index Terms Leurocristine Sulfate; Oncovin; Vincristine Sulfate

Pharmacologic Category Antineoplastic Agent, Natural Source (Plant) Derivative; Antineoplastic Agent, Vinca Alkaloid

Medication Safety Issues

Sound-alike/look-alike issues:

VinCRIStine may be confused with vinBLAStine, vinorelbine

Oncovin may be confused with Ancobon®

High alert medication:

This medication is in a class the Institute for Safe Medication Practices (ISMP) includes among its list of drug classes which have a heightened risk of causing significant patient harm when used in error.

Administration issues:

For I.V. use only. Fatal if administered by other routes. To prevent fatal inadvertent intrathecal injection, it is recommended that vincristine doses be dispensed in a small minibag. Vincristine should **NOT** be prepared during the preparation of any intrathecal medications. After preparation, store vincristine in a location **away** from the separate storage location recommended for intrathecal medications. Vincristine should **NOT** be delivered to the patient at the same time with any medications intended for central nervous system administration.

Pregnancy Risk Factor D

Lactation Excretion in breast milk unknown/not recommended

Breast-Feeding Considerations Due to the potential for serious adverse reactions in the nursing infant, breast-feeding is not recommended.

Use Treatment of acute lymphocytic leukemia (ALL), Hodgkin's lymphoma, non-Hodgkin's lymphomas, Wilms' tumor, neuroblastoma, rhabdomyosarcoma

Unlabeled Use Treatment of multiple myeloma, chronic lymphocytic leukemia (CLL), brain tumors, small cell lung cancer, ovarian germ cell tumors

Mechanism of Action/Effect Binds to microtubular protein of the mitotic spindle causing metaphase arrest; cell-cycle phase specific in the M and S phases

Contraindications Patients with demyelinating form of Charcot-Marie-Tooth syndrome

Warnings/Precautions Hazardous agent - use appropriate precautions for handling and disposal; avoid eye contamination.

[U.S. Boxed Warning]: For I.V. administration only; intrathecal administration has uniformly caused severe neurologic damage and/or death; vincristine should never be administered by this route. Vincristine should **NOT** be prepared during the preparation of any intrathecal medications. After preparation, store vincristine in a location **away** from the separate storage location recommended for intrathecal medications. Vincristine should **NOT** be delivered to the patient with any medications intended for central nervous system administration.

[U.S. Boxed Warning]: Vincristine is a vesicant; avoid extravasation. (Individuals administering should be experienced in vincristine administration.) Check for proper needle placement; if extravasation occurs, discontinue vincristine infusion and initiate appropriate extravasation management.

Neurotoxicity, including alterations in mental status such as depression, confusion, or insomnia may occur; neurologic effects are dose-limiting (may require dosage reduction) and may be additive with those of other neurotoxic agents and spinal cord irradiation. Use with caution in patients with preexisting neuromuscular disease and/or with concomitant neurotoxic agents. Constipation, paralytic ileus, intestinal necrosis and/or perforation may occur; constipation may present as upper colon impaction with an empty rectum (may require flat film of abdomen for diagnosis); generally responds to high enemas and laxatives. All patients should be on a prophylactic bowel management regimen.

Use with caution in patients receiving concurrent therapy which alters CYP3A4 activity, may require therapy alterations. Acute shortness of breath and severe bronchospasm have been reported with vinca alkaloids, usually when used in combination with mitomycin-C. Onset may be several minutes to hours after vincristine administration and up to 2 weeks after mitomycin-C. Progressive dyspnea may occur. Permanently discontinue vincristine in this situation.

Use with caution in patients with hepatic impairment; dosage modification required. May be associated with hepatic sinusoidal obstruction syndrome (SOS; formerly called veno-occlusive disease), increased risk in children <3 years of age; use with caution in hepatobiliary dysfunction. Monitor for signs or symptoms of hepatic SOS, including bilirubin >1.4 mg/dL, unexplained weight gain, ascites, hepatomegaly, or unexplained right upper quadrant pain (Arndt, 2004). Acute uric acid nephropathy has been reported with vincristine. Use with caution in the elderly.

Drug Interactions

Avoid Concomitant Use

Avoid concomitant use of VinCRIStine with any of the following: BCG; Conivaptan; Natalizumab; Pimecrolimus; Pimozide; Tacrolimus (Topical); Vaccines (Live)

Decreased Effect

VinCRIStine may decrease the levels/effects of: BCG; Cardiac Glycosides; Coccidioidin Skin Test; Sipuleucel-T; Vaccines (Inactivated); Vaccines (Live); Vitamin K Antagonists

The levels/effects of VinCRIStine may be decreased by: CYP3A4 Inducers (Strong); Deferasirox; Echinacea; P-glycoprotein/ABCB1 Inducers; Tocilizumab

Increased Effect/Toxicity

VinCRIStine may increase the levels/effects of: ARIPiprazole; Leflunomide; MitoMYcin; Natalizumab; Pimozide; Vaccines (Live); Vitamin K Antagonists

The levels/effects of VinCRIStine may be increased by: Conivaptan; CYP3A4 Inhibitors (Moderate); CYP3A4 Inhibitors (Strong); Dasatinib; Denosumab; Itraconazole; Lopinavir; Macrolide Antibiotics; MAO Inhibitors; NIFEdipine; P-glycoprotein/ABCB1 Inhibitors; Pimecrolimus; Posaconazole; Ritonavir; Roflumilast; Tacrolimus (Topical); Teniposide; Trastuzumab; Voriconazole

Nutritional/Ethanol Interactions Herb/Nutraceutical: St John's wort may decrease vincristine levels.

Adverse Reactions Frequency not defined.

Cardiovascular: Edema, hyper-/hypotension, MI, myocardial ischemia

Central nervous system: Ataxia, coma, cranial nerve dysfunction (auditory damage, extraocular muscle impairment, laryngeal muscle impairment, paralysis, paresis, vestibular damage, vocal cord paralysis), dizziness, fever, headache, neurotoxicity, neuropathic pain (common), seizure, vertigo

Dermatologic toxicity: Alopecia (common), rash

Endocrine & metabolic: Hyperuricemia, parotid pain, SIADH (rare)

Gastrointestinal: Abdominal cramps, abdominal pain, anorexia, constipation (common), diarrhea, intestinal necrosis, intestinal perforation, nausea, oral ulcers, paralytic ileus, vomiting, weight loss

Genitourinary: Bladder atony, dysuria, polyuria, urinary retention

Hematologic: Anemia (mild), leukopenia (mild), thrombocytopenia (mild), thrombotic thrombocytopenic purpura

Hepatic: Sinusoidal obstruction (SOS; veno-occlusive liver disease)

Local: Phlebitis, tissue irritation/necrosis (if infiltrated)

Neuromuscular & skeletal: Back pain, bone pain, deep tendon reflex loss, difficulty walking, foot drop, gait changes, jaw pain, limb pain, motor difficulties, muscle wasting, myalgia, paralysis, paresthesia, peripheral neuropathy (common), sensorimotor dysfunction, sensory loss

Ocular: Cortical blindness (transient), nystagmus, optic atrophy with blindness

Otic: Deafness

Renal: Acute uric acid nephropathy, hemolytic uremic syndrome

Respiratory: Bronchospasm, dyspnea, pharyngeal pain

Miscellaneous: Allergic reactions (rare), anaphylaxis (rare), hypersensitivity (rare)

Available Dosage Forms

Injection, solution [preservative free]: 1 mg/mL (1 mL, 2 mL)

Vincasar PFS®: 1 mg/mL (1 mL, 2 mL)

General Dosage Range Dosage adjustment recommended in patients with hepatic impairment

I.V.:

Children ≤10 kg: 0.05 mg/kg once weekly (maximum: 2 mg/dose)

Children >10 kg: 1.5-2 mg/m²/dose (maximum: 2 mg/dose)

Adults: 1.4 mg/m²/dose (maximum: 2 mg/dose)

Administration

I.V. Vesicant; avoid extravasation. **For I.V. administration only. FATAL IF GIVEN INTRATHECALLY.** Vincristine should **NOT** be delivered to the patient at the same time with any medications intended for central nervous system administration.

Usually administered as short 5-10 minute infusion (preferred); may also be administered as a slow (1 minute) push or by a 24-hour continuous infusions (depending on the protocol)

I.V. Detail pH: 3.5-5.5

Stability

Reconstitution Use appropriate precautions for handling and disposal. Solutions for I.V. infusion may be mixed in NS or D_5W. **Note:** In order to prevent inadvertent intrathecal administration the World Health Organization (WHO) and the Institute for Safe Medical Practices (ISMP) recommend dispensing vincristine in a minibag (rather than a syringe). Vincristine should **NOT** be prepared during the preparation of any intrathecal medications. If dispensing vincristine in a syringe, it must be packaged in the manufacturer-provided overwrap which bears the statement **"Do not remove covering until the moment of injection. For intravenous use only. Fatal if given intrathecally."**

Storage Store intact vials under refrigeration. May be stable for up to 30 days at room temperature. Protect from light.

I.V. solution: Diluted in 25-50 mL NS or D_5W, stable for 7 days under refrigeration, or 2 days at room temperature. In ambulatory pumps, solution is stable for 7 days at room temperature. After preparation, store vincristine in a location away from the separate storage location recommended for intrathecal medications.

Nursing Actions

Physical Assessment Premedication with antiemetic is advisable. May cause severe constipation, paralytic ileus, intestinal obstruction, necrosis, and/or perforation. Monitor infusion site closely to prevent extravasation (vesicant will cause tissue damage and necrosis). Assess hepatic function, CNS status (motor difficulties, seizure, depression), neuromuscular status (myalgia, peripheral neuropathy, cramping), and photophobia throughout therapy.

Patient Education This medication can only be administered by infusion; report immediately any redness, swelling, burning, or pain at infusion site. Maintain adequate nutrition and hydration, unless instructed to restrict fluid intake. You will be more susceptible to infection. May cause postural hypotension, hair loss (will grow back after therapy), nausea or vomiting (request antiemetic if persistent), photosensitivity, feelings of extreme weakness or lethargy, or mouth sores. Report persistent gastrointestinal changes (eg, constipation, abdominal cramps, bloating); numbness, tingling, or pain in legs, fingers, or toes; signs of infection (eg, fever, chills, sore throat, burning urination, fatigue); unusual bleeding (eg, tarry stools, easy bruising, blood in stool, urine, or mouth); unresolved mouth sores; skin rash or itching; or respiratory difficulty.

Related Information

Management of Drug Extravasations *on page 1269*

Vinorelbine (vi NOR el been)

Brand Names: U.S. Navelbine®

Index Terms Dihydroxydeoxynorvinkaleukoblastine; Vinorelbine Tartrate

Pharmacologic Category Antineoplastic Agent, Natural Source (Plant) Derivative; Antineoplastic Agent, Vinca Alkaloid

Medication Safety Issues

Sound-alike/look-alike issues:

Vinorelbine may be confused with vinBLAStine, vinCRIStine

High alert medication:

This medication is in a class the Institute for Safe Medication Practices (ISMP) includes among its list of drug classes which have a heightened risk of causing significant patient harm when used in error.

Administration issues:

Vinorelbine is intended **for I.V. use only**: Inadvertent intrathecal administration of other vinca alkaloids has resulted in death. Syringes containing vinorelbine should be labeled **"For I.V. use only. Fatal if given intrathecally."** Vinorelbine should **NOT** be prepared during the preparation of any intrathecal medications. After preparation, store vinorelbine in a location **away** from the separate storage location recommended for intrathecal medications.

Pregnancy Risk Factor D

Lactation Excretion in breast milk unknown/not recommended

Breast-Feeding Considerations Due to the potential for serious adverse reactions in the nursing infant, breast-feeding is not recommended.

Use Treatment of nonsmall cell lung cancer (NSCLC)

Unlabeled Use Treatment of breast cancer (metastatic), cervical cancer, ovarian cancer, malignant pleural mesothelioma, and soft tissue sarcoma

Mechanism of Action/Effect Mitotic inhibition that causes metaphase arrest in neoplastic cells

Contraindications Pretreatment granulocyte counts <1000/mm^3

Warnings/Precautions Hazardous agent - use appropriate precautions for handling and disposal. **[U.S. Boxed Warning]: For I.V. use only; do not administer intrathecally;** intrathecal administration may result in death. **[U.S. Boxed Warning]: Avoid extravasation;** infiltration may cause irritation, thrombophlebitis and/or local tissue necrosis. **[U.S. Boxed Warning]: Severe granulocytopenia may occur with treatment;** granulocytopenia is a dose-limiting toxicity; granulocyte counts should be ≥1000/mm^3 prior to treatment initiation; monitor closely for infections and/or fever; may require dosage adjustment. The incidence of granulocytopenia is significantly higher when given in combination with cisplatin when compared to single-agent vinorelbine. Use with caution in patients with compromised marrow reserve due to prior chemotherapy therapy or prior radiation therapy.

Fatal cases of interstitial pulmonary changes and ARDS have been reported (with single-agent therapy); promptly evaluate changes in baseline pulmonary symptoms or any new onset pulmonary symptoms. Acute shortness of breath and severe bronchospasm have been reported rarely; usually associated with the concurrent administration of mitomycin.

Vinorelbine should **NOT** be prepared during the preparation of any intrathecal medications. After preparation, store vinorelbine in a location **away** from the separate storage location recommended for intrathecal medications. Dosage modification required in patients with impaired hepatic function and neurotoxicity; use with caution. May cause new onset or worsening of pre-existing neuropathy; use with caution in patients with neuropathy. May cause severe constipation (grade 3-4), paralytic ileus, intestinal obstruction, necrosis, and/or perforation. May have radiosensitizing effects with prior or concurrent radiation therapy; radiation recall reactions may occur in patients who have received prior radiation therapy. Avoid eye contamination (exposure may cause severe irritation). **[U.S. Boxed Warning]: Should be administered under the supervision of an experienced cancer chemotherapy physician.**

Drug Interactions

Avoid Concomitant Use

Avoid concomitant use of Vinorelbine with any of the following: BCG; CloZAPine; Conivaptan; Natalizumab; Pimecrolimus; Pimozide; Tacrolimus (Topical); Vaccines (Live)

Decreased Effect

Vinorelbine may decrease the levels/effects of: BCG; Coccidioidin Skin Test; Sipuleucel-T; Vaccines (Inactivated); Vaccines (Live)

The levels/effects of Vinorelbine may be decreased by: CYP3A4 Inducers (Strong);

Deferasirox; Echinacea; Herbs (CYP3A4 Inducers); Peginterferon Alfa-2b; Tocilizumab

Increased Effect/Toxicity

Vinorelbine may increase the levels/effects of: ARIPiprazole; CloZAPine; Leflunomide; MitoMYcin; Natalizumab; Pimozide; Vaccines (Live)

The levels/effects of Vinorelbine may be increased by: CISplatin; Conivaptan; CYP3A4 Inhibitors (Moderate); CYP3A4 Inhibitors (Strong); Dasatinib; Denosumab; Gefitinib; Itraconazole; Ivacaftor; Macrolide Antibiotics; PACLitaxel; PACLitaxel (Protein Bound); Pimecrolimus; Posaconazole; Roflumilast; Tacrolimus (Topical); Trastuzumab; Voriconazole

Nutritional/Ethanol Interactions Herb/Nutraceutical: Avoid St John's wort (may decrease vinorelbine levels).

Adverse Reactions Note: Reported with single-agent therapy.

>10%:

Central nervous system: Fatigue (27%)

Dermatologic: Alopecia (12% to 30%)

Gastrointestinal: Nausea (31% to 44%; grade 3: 1% to 2%), constipation (35%; grade 3: 3%), vomiting (20% to 31%; grade 3: 1% to 2%), diarrhea (12% to 17%)

Hematologic: Leukopenia (83% to 92%; grade 4: 6% to 15%), granulocytopenia (90%; grade 4: 36%; nadir: 7-10 days; recovery 14-21 days; dose-limiting), neutropenia (85%; grade 4: 28%), anemia (83%; grades 3/4: 9%)

Hepatic: AST increased (67%; grade 3: 5%; grade 4: 1%), total bilirubin increased (5% to 13%; grade 3: 4%; grade 4: 3%)

Local: Injection site reaction (22% to 28%; includes erythema, vein discoloration), injection site pain (16%)

Neuromuscular & skeletal: Weakness (36%), peripheral neuropathy (25%; grade 3: 1%; grade 4: <1%)

Renal: Creatinine increased (13%)

1% to 10%:

Cardiovascular: Chest pain (5%)

Dermatologic: Rash (<5%)

Gastrointestinal: Paralytic ileus (1%)

Hematologic: Neutropenic fever/sepsis (8%; grade 4: 4%), thrombocytopenia (3% to 5%; grades 3/4: 1%)

Local: Phlebitis (7% to 10%)

Neuromuscular & skeletal: Loss of deep tendon reflexes (<5%), myalgia (<5%), arthralgia (<5%), jaw pain (<5%)

Otic: Ototoxicity (≤1%)

Respiratory: Dyspnea (7%)

Available Dosage Forms

Injection, solution [preservative free]: 10 mg/mL (1 mL, 5 mL)

Navelbine®: 10 mg/mL (1 mL, 5 mL)

General Dosage Range Dosage adjustment recommended in patients with hepatic impairment or who develop toxicities

I.V.: *Adults:* 25-30 mg/m^2/dose every 7 days

Administration

I.V. FATAL IF GIVEN INTRATHECALLY. Administer as a direct intravenous push or rapid bolus, over 6-10 minutes (up to 30 minutes). Longer infusions may increase the risk of pain and phlebitis. Intravenous doses should be followed by at least 75-125 mL of saline or D_5W to reduce the incidence of phlebitis and inflammation. Assure proper needle or catheter position prior to administration.

I.V. Detail Do not administer in an extremity with poor circulation or repeatedly into the same vein. pH: 3.5 (injection)

Stability

Reconstitution Dilute in D_5W or NS to a final concentration of 1.5-3 mg/mL (for syringe) or 0.5-2 mg/mL (for I.V. bag). Vinorelbine should **NOT** be prepared during the preparation of any intrathecal medications.

Storage Store intact vials under refrigeration at 2°C to 8°C (36°F to 46°F); do not freeze. Protect from light. Intact vials are stable at room temperature of 25°C (77°F) for up to 72 hours. Dilutions in D_5W or NS are stable for 24 hours at room temperature. After preparation, store vinorelbine in a location **away** from the separate storage location recommended for intrathecal medications.

Nursing Actions

Physical Assessment For intravenous use only; fatal if given intrathecally. Premedication with antiemetic is advisable. May cause severe constipation, paralytic ileus, intestinal obstruction, necrosis, and/or perforation. Monitor infusion site closely to prevent extravasation; may cause tissue damage and necrosis. Monitor for peripheral neuropathy. Assess pulmonary status and liver function prior to each infusion and throughout therapy.

Patient Education This medication can only be administered by infusion; report immediately any redness, swelling, burning, or pain at infusion site. Maintain adequate hydration and nutrition. You will be more susceptible to infection. May cause hair loss (will grow back after therapy), nausea or vomiting (request antiemetic if persistent), feelings of weakness or lethargy, or mouth sores. Report persistent constipation or abdominal pain; numbness or tingling in fingers or toes; weakness, numbness, or pain in muscles or extremities; signs of infection (eg, fever, chills, sore throat, burning urination, fatigue); unusual bleeding (eg, tarry stools; easy bruising; blood in stool, urine, or mouth); unresolved mouth sores; skin rash or itching; or respiratory difficulty.

Related Information

Management of Drug Extravasations *on page 1269*

Vismodegib (vis moe DEG ib)

Brand Names: U.S. Erivedge™

Index Terms GDC-0449; Hedgehog Antagonist GDC-0449

Pharmacologic Category Antineoplastic Agent, Hedgehog Pathway Inhibitor

Medication Safety Issues

Sound-alike/look-alike issues:

Vismodegib may be confused with vandetanib, vemurafenib

High alert medication:

This medication is in a class the Institute for Safe Medication Practices (ISMP) includes among its list of drug classes which have a heightened risk of causing significant patient harm when used in error.

Medication Guide Available Yes

Pregnancy Risk Factor D

Lactation Excretion in breast milk unknown/not recommended

Use Treatment of metastatic basal cell carcinoma, or locally-advanced basal cell carcinoma that has recurred following surgery or in patients who are not candidates for surgery, and not candidates for radiation therapy

Available Dosage Forms

Capsule, oral:

Erivedge™: 150 mg

General Dosage Range Oral: *Adults:* 150 mg once daily

Administration

Oral May be taken with or without food. Swallow capsules whole; do not open or crush. If a dose is missed, do not make up; resume dosing with the next scheduled dose.

Nursing Actions

Physical Assessment Re-enforce risk of birth defects in women of childbearing age and men using the drug who may be intimate with women of childbearing age or who are pregnant; discuss need for reliable birth control.

Patient Education Take with or without food; educate appropriate patients about birth control needs and duration of precautions even after treatment completion. Common side effects include fatigue, hair loss, abnormal taste, nausea, diarrhea, weight loss, and muscle spasm. Have patient call prescriber immediately for severe nausea, vomiting, or diarrhea; if pregnancy occurs; or if male and significant other gets a rash.

Voriconazole (vor i KOE na zole)

Brand Names: U.S. VFEND®

Index Terms UK109496

Pharmacologic Category Antifungal Agent, Oral; Antifungal Agent, Parenteral

Pregnancy Risk Factor D

Lactation Excretion in breast milk unknown/not recommended

Breast-Feeding Considerations Excretion in breast milk has not been investigated; avoid breast-feeding until additional data are available.

Use Treatment of invasive aspergillosis; treatment of esophageal candidiasis; treatment of candidemia (in non-neutropenic patients); treatment of disseminated *Candida* infections of the skin and viscera; treatment of serious fungal infections caused by *Scedosporium apiospermum* and *Fusarium* spp (including *Fusarium solani*) in patients intolerant of, or refractory to, other therapy

Unlabeled Use Fungal infection prophylaxis in intermediate or high risk neutropenic cancer patients with myelodysplastic syndrome (MDS) or acute myelogenous leukemia (AML), neutropenic allogeneic hematopoietic stem cell recipients, and patients with significant graft-versus-host disease; empiric antifungal therapy (second-line) for persistent neutropenic fever

Mechanism of Action/Effect Interferes with fungal cytochrome P450 activity (selectively inhibits 14-alpha-lanosterol demethylation), decreasing ergosterol synthesis (principal sterol in fungal cell membrane) and inhibiting fungal cell membrane formation.

Contraindications Hypersensitivity to voriconazole or any component of the formulation (cross-reaction with other azole antifungal agents may occur but has not been established, use caution); coadministration of CYP3A4 substrates which may lead to QT_c prolongation (cisapride, pimozide, or quinidine); coadministration with barbiturates (long acting), carbamazepine, efavirenz (with standard [eg, not adjusted] voriconazole and efavirenz doses), ergot derivatives, rifampin, rifabutin, ritonavir (≥800 mg/day), sirolimus, St John's wort

Warnings/Precautions Visual changes, including blurred vision, changes in visual acuity, color perception, and photophobia, are commonly associated with treatment; postmarketing cases of optic neuritis and papilledema (lasting >1 month) have also been reported. Patients should be warned to avoid tasks which depend on vision, including operating machinery or driving. Changes are reversible on discontinuation following brief exposure/treatment regimens (≤28 days).

Serious hepatic reactions (including hepatitis, cholestasis, and fulminant hepatic failure) have occurred during treatment, primarily in patients with serious concomitant medical conditions. However, hepatotoxicity has occurred in patients with no identifiable risk factors. Use caution in patients with pre-existing hepatic impairment (dose adjustment or discontinuation may be required).

Voriconazole tablets contain lactose; avoid administration in hereditary galactose intolerance, Lapp lactase deficiency, or glucose-galactose malabsorption. Suspension contains sucrose; use caution with fructose intolerance, sucrase-isomaltase deficiency, or glucose-galactose malabsorption. Avoid/limit use of intravenous formulation in patients with renal impairment; intravenous formulation contains excipient cyclodextrin (sulfobutyl ether beta-cyclodextrin), which may accumulate in renal insufficiency. Acute renal failure has been observed in severely ill patients; use with caution in patients receiving concomitant nephrotoxic medications. Anaphylactoid-type infusion-related reactions may occur with intravenous dosing. Consider discontinuation of infusion if reaction is severe.

Use caution in patients taking strong cytochrome P450 inducers, CYP2C9 inhibitors, and major 3A4 substrates (see Drug Interactions); consider alternative agents that avoid or lessen the potential for CYP-mediated interactions. QT interval prolongation has been associated with voriconazole use; rare cases of arrhythmia (including torsade de pointes), cardiac arrest, and sudden death have been reported, usually in seriously ill patients with comorbidities and/or risk factors (eg, prior cardiotoxic chemotherapy, cardiomyopathy, electrolyte imbalance, or concomitant QT_c-prolonging drugs). Use with caution in these patient populations; correct electrolyte abnormalities (eg, hypokalemia, hypomagnesemia, hypocalcemia) prior to initiating therapy. Do not infuse concomitantly with blood products or short-term concentrated electrolyte solutions, even if the two infusions are running in separate intravenous lines (or cannulas).

Rare cases of malignancy (melanoma, squamous cell carcinoma) have been reported in patients (mostly immunocompromised) with prior onset of severe photosensitivity reactions and exposure to long-term voriconazole therapy. Other serious exfoliative cutaneous reactions, including Stevens-Johnson syndrome, have also been reported. Patient should avoid strong, direct exposure to sunlight; may cause photosensitivity, especially with long-term use. Discontinue use in patients who develop an exfoliative cutaneous reaction or a skin lesion consistent with squamous cell carcinoma or melanoma. Periodic total body skin examinations should be performed, particularly with prolonged use.

Monitor pancreatic function in patients (children and adults) at risk for acute pancreatitis (eg, recent chemotherapy or hematopoietic stem cell transplantation); there have been postmarketing reports of pancreatitis in children.

Drug Interactions

Avoid Concomitant Use

Avoid concomitant use of Voriconazole with any of the following: Alfuzosin; Artemether; Axitinib; Barbiturates; CarBAMazepine; Cisapride; Conivaptan; Crizotinib; Darunavir; Dofetilide; Dronedarone; Eplerenone; Ergot Derivatives; Everolimus; Fluconazole; Fluticasone (Oral Inhalation); Halofantrine; Lapatinib; Lopinavir; Lovastatin; Lumefantrine; Lurasidone; Nilotinib; Nisoldipine; Pimozide; QUEtiapine; QuiNIDine; QuiNINE; Ranolazine; Rifamycin Derivatives; Ritonavir; Rivaroxaban; RomiDEPsin; Salmeterol; Silodosin; Simvastatin; Sirolimus; St Johns Wort; Tamsulosin; Tetrabenazine; Thioridazine; Ticagrelor; Tolvaptan; Toremifene; Vandetanib; Vemurafenib; Ziprasidone

Decreased Effect

Voriconazole may decrease the levels/effects of: Amphotericin B; Prasugrel; Saccharomyces boulardii; Ticagrelor

The levels/effects of Voriconazole may be decreased by: Barbiturates; CarBAMazepine; CYP2C19 Inducers (Strong); CYP2C9 Inducers (Strong); Darunavir; Didanosine; Etravirine; Fosphenytoin; Lopinavir; Peginterferon Alfa-2b; Phenytoin; Reverse Transcriptase Inhibitors (Non-Nucleoside); Rifamycin Derivatives; Ritonavir; St Johns Wort; Sucralfate; Telaprevir; Tocilizumab

Increased Effect/Toxicity

Voriconazole may increase the levels/effects of: Alfentanil; Alfuzosin; Almotriptan; Alosetron; Antineoplastic Agents (Vinca Alkaloids); Aprepitant; ARIPiprazole; Axitinib; Benzodiazepines (metabolized by oxidation); Boceprevir; Bortezomib; Bosentan; Brentuximab Vedotin; Brinzolamide; Budesonide (Nasal); Budesonide (Systemic, Oral Inhalation); BusPIRone; Busulfan; Calcium Channel Blockers; CarBAMazepine; Carvedilol; Ciclesonide; Cilostazol; Cinacalcet; Cisapride; Colchicine; Conivaptan; Contraceptives (Estrogens); Contraceptives (Progestins); Corticosteroids (Orally Inhaled); Corticosteroids (Systemic); Crizotinib; CycloSPORINE; CycloSPORINE (Systemic); CYP2C9 Substrates; CYP3A4 Substrates; Diclofenac; Diclofenac (Systemic); Diclofenac (Topical); Dienogest; DOCEtaxel; Dofetilide; Dronedarone; Dutasteride; Eletriptan; Eplerenone; Ergot Derivatives; Erlotinib; Eszopiclone; Etravirine; Everolimus; FentaNYL; Fesoterodine; Fluticasone (Nasal); Fluticasone (Oral Inhalation); Fosaprepitant; Fosphenytoin; Gefitinib; GuanFACINE; Halofantrine; HMG-CoA Reductase Inhibitors; Ibuprofen; Iloperidone; Imatinib; Irinotecan; Ivacaftor; Ixabepilone; Lapatinib; Losartan; Lovastatin; Lumefantrine; Lurasidone; Macrolide Antibiotics; Maraviroc; Meloxicam; Methadone; MethylPREDNISolone; Nilotinib; Nisoldipine; OxyCODONE; Paricalcitol; Pazopanib; Phenytoin; Phosphodiesterase 5 Inhibitors; Pimecrolimus; Pimozide; Propafenone; Protease Inhibitors; QTc-Prolonging Agents; QuiNIDine; QuiNINE; Ramelteon; Ranolazine; Repaglinide; Reverse Transcriptase Inhibitors (Non-Nucleoside); Rifamycin

Derivatives; Rivaroxaban; RomiDEPsin; Ruxolitinib; Salmeterol; Saxagliptin; Sildenafil; Silodosin; Simvastatin; Sirolimus; Solifenacin; SORAfenib; Sulfonylureas; SUNItinib; Tacrolimus; Tacrolimus (Systemic); Tacrolimus (Topical); Tadalafil; Tamsulosin; Telaprevir; Tetrabenazine; Thioridazine; Ticagrelor; Tolterodine; Tolvaptan; Toremifene; Vandetanib; Vardenafil; Vemurafenib; Venlafaxine; Vilazodone; Vitamin K Antagonists; Ziprasidone; Zolpidem; Zuclopenthixol

The levels/effects of Voriconazole may be increased by: Alfuzosin; Artemether; Boceprevir; Chloramphenicol; Chloroquine; Ciprofloxacin; Ciprofloxacin (Systemic); Contraceptives (Estrogens); Contraceptives (Progestins); CYP2C19 Inhibitors (Moderate); CYP2C19 Inhibitors (Strong); CYP2C9 Inhibitors (Moderate); CYP2C9 Inhibitors (Strong); Etravirine; Fluconazole; Gadobutrol; Grapefruit Juice; Indacaterol; Lumefantrine; Macrolide Antibiotics; Nilotinib; Protease Inhibitors; Proton Pump Inhibitors; QUEtiapine; QuiNINE; Telaprevir

Nutritional/Ethanol Interactions

Food: Food may decrease voriconazole absorption. Grapefruit juice may decrease voriconazole levels. Management: Oral voriconazole should be taken 1 hour before or 1 hour after a meal. Avoid grapefruit juice. Maintain adequate hydration unless instructed to restrict fluid intake.

Herb/Nutraceutical: St John's wort may decrease voriconazole levels. Management: Concurrent use of St John's wort with voriconazole is contraindicated.

Adverse Reactions

>10%:

Central nervous system: Hallucinations (4% to 12%; auditory and/or visual and likely serum concentration-dependent)

Ocular: Visual changes (dose related; photophobia, color changes, increased or decreased visual acuity, or blurred vision occur in ~21%)

Renal: Creatinine increased (1% to 21%)

2% to 10%:

Cardiovascular: Tachycardia (≤2%)

Central nervous system: Fever (≤6%), chills (≤4%), headache (≤3%)

Dermatologic: Rash (≤7%)

Endocrine & metabolic: Hypokalemia (≤2%)

Gastrointestinal: Nausea (1% to 5%), vomiting (1% to 4%)

Hepatic: Alkaline phosphatase increased (4% to 5%), AST increased (2% to 4%), ALT increased (2% to 3%), cholestatic jaundice (1% to 2%)

Ocular: Photophobia (2% to 3%)

Available Dosage Forms

Injection, powder for reconstitution:

VFEND®: 200 mg

Powder for suspension, oral:

VFEND®: 40 mg/mL (70 mL)

Tablet, oral: 50 mg, 200 mg

VFEND®: 50 mg, 200 mg

General Dosage Range Dosage adjustment recommended in patients with hepatic impairment

I.V.: *Children ≥12 years and Adults:* Initial: 6 mg/kg every 12 hours for 2 doses; Maintenance: 3-4 mg/kg every 12 hours

Oral: *Children ≥12 years and Adults:* 100-300 mg every 12 hours

Administration

Oral Administer 1 hour before or 1 hour after a meal.

I.V. Infuse over 1-2 hours (rate not to exceed 3 mg/kg/hour). Do not infuse concomitantly into same line or cannula with other drug infusions, including TPN.

Stability

Reconstitution

Powder for injection: Reconstitute 200 mg vial with 19 mL of sterile water for injection (use of automated syringe is not recommended). Resultant solution (20 mL) has a concentration of 10 mg/mL. Prior to infusion, must dilute to 0.5-5 mg/mL with NS, LR, D_5WLR, D_5W1/2NS, D_5W, D_5W with KCl 20 mEq, 1/2NS, or D_5WNS. Do not dilute with 4.2% sodium bicarbonate infusion.

Powder for oral suspension: Add 46 mL of water to the bottle to make 40 mg/mL suspension. Discard unused portion after 14 days.

Storage

Powder for injection: Store at 15°C to 30°C (59°F to 86°F). Reconstituted solutions are stable for up to 24 hours under refrigeration at 2°C to 8°C (36°F to 46°F).

Powder for oral suspension: Store at 2°C to 8°C (36°F to 46°F). Reconstituted oral suspension may be stored at 15°C to 30°C (59°F to 86°F).

Tablets: Store at 15°C to 30°C (59°F to 86°F).

Nursing Actions

Physical Assessment Allergy history should be assessed prior to beginning therapy. Monitor for vision changes (photophobia, changed visual acuity, blurred vision), hepatic toxicity (increased liver enzymes, jaundice), tachycardia, and dermatologic reactions (can be severe; periodic total body examinations should be performed).

Patient Education Maintain adequate hydration unless instructed to restrict fluid intake. Avoid direct exposure to strong sunlight. You may experience headache, dizziness, blurred vision, photophobia, changes in visual acuity (vision changes are reversible shortly after treatment is completed or discontinued), nausea, vomiting, or abdominal pain. Report immediately any change in vision. Report unusual tiredness, flu-like feelings, skin rash or itching, dark urine, light colored stool, yellowing of skin or eyes, fever, chest pain, or rapid heartbeat.

I.V.: You will be monitored during intravenous administration; report immediately any pain, swelling, or redness at infusion site; difficulty breathing or swallowing; back pain; or itching.

Oral: Preferable to take on empty stomach 1 hour before or 1 hour after a meal.

Dietary Considerations Oral: Should be taken 1 hour before or 1 hour after a meal. Voriconazole tablets contain lactose; avoid administration in hereditary galactose intolerance, Lapp lactase deficiency, or glucose-galactose malabsorption. Suspension contains sucrose; use caution with fructose intolerance, sucrose-isomaltase deficiency, or glucose-galactose malabsorption.

Vorinostat (vor IN oh stat)

Brand Names: U.S. Zolinza®

Index Terms SAHA; Suberoylanilide Hydroxamic Acid

Pharmacologic Category Antineoplastic Agent, Histone Deacetylase Inhibitor

Medication Safety Issues

Sound-alike/look-alike issues:

Vorinostat may be confused with Votrient™

High alert medication:

This medication is in a class the Institute for Safe Medication Practices (ISMP) includes among its list of drug classes which have a heightened risk of causing significant patient harm when used in error.

Pregnancy Risk Factor D

Lactation Excretion in breast milk unknown/not recommended

Breast-Feeding Considerations According to the manufacturer, the decision to continue or discontinue breast-feeding during therapy should take into account the risk of exposure to the infant and the benefits of treatment to the mother.

Use Treatment of progressive, persistent, or recurrent cutaneous T-cell lymphoma (CTCL)

Mechanism of Action/Effect Histone deacetylase inhibitor; causes termination of cell growth leading to cell death

Contraindications Severe hepatic impairment.

Canadian labeling: Hypersensitivity to vorinostat or any component of the formulation; severe hepatic impairment (total bilirubin ≥3 times ULN)

Warnings/Precautions Hazardous agent - use appropriate precautions for handling and disposal. Pulmonary embolism and deep vein thrombosis (DVT) have been reported; monitor. Use caution in patients with a history of thrombotic events. Dose-related thrombocytopenia and/or anemia may occur; may require dosage adjustments or discontinuation. QT_c prolongation has been observed; baseline and periodic ECGs were done in clinical trials (Duvic, 2007; Olsen, 2007). Correct electrolyte abnormalities prior to treatment and monitor and correct potassium, calcium, and magnesium levels during therapy. Use caution in patients with a history of QT_c prolongation or with medications known to prolong the QT interval. May cause hyperglycemia; monitor and use with caution in diabetics; may require diet and/or therapy modifications. Nausea, vomiting, and diarrhea may occur; antiemetics and antidiarrheals may be required; control pre-existing nausea and vomiting prior to treatment initiation; replace fluids and electrolytes to avoid dehydration. May cause dizziness or fatigue; caution patients about performing tasks which require mental alertness (eg, operating machinery or driving). Use with caution in patients with mild-to-moderate hepatic impairment (elimination is predominantly hepatic); contraindicated in severe hepatic impairment. In the Canadian labeling, use is also not recommended in patients with moderate hepatic impairment (total bilirubin 1.5-3 times ULN).

Drug Interactions

Avoid Concomitant Use

Avoid concomitant use of Vorinostat with any of the following: Artemether; CloZAPine; Dronedarone; Lumefantrine; Nilotinib; Pimozide; QUEtiapine; QuiNINE; Tetrabenazine; Thioridazine; Toremifene; Vandetanib; Vemurafenib; Ziprasidone

Decreased Effect There are no known significant interactions involving a decrease in effect.

Increased Effect/Toxicity

Vorinostat may increase the levels/effects of: CloZAPine; Dronedarone; Pimozide; QTc-Prolonging Agents; QuiNINE; Tetrabenazine; Thioridazine; Toremifene; Vandetanib; Vemurafenib; Vitamin K Antagonists; Ziprasidone

The levels/effects of Vorinostat may be increased by: Alfuzosin; Artemether; Chloroquine; Ciprofloxacin; Ciprofloxacin (Systemic); Divalproex; Gadobutrol; Indacaterol; Lumefantrine; Nilotinib; QUEtiapine; QuiNINE; Valproic Acid

Adverse Reactions

>10%:

Cardiovascular: Peripheral edema (13%)

Central nervous system: Fatigue (52%), chills (16%), dizziness (15%), headache (12%), fever (11%)

Dermatologic: Alopecia (19%), pruritus (12%)

Endocrine & metabolic: Hyperglycemia (8% to 69%; grade 3: 5%), dehydration (1% to 16%)

Gastrointestinal: Diarrhea (52%), nausea (41%), taste alteration (28%), anorexia (24%), weight loss (21%), xerostomia (16%), constipation (15%), vomiting (15%), appetite decreased (14%)

Hematologic: Thrombocytopenia (26%; grades 3/4: 6%), anemia (14%; grades 3/4: 2%)

Neuromuscular & skeletal: Muscle spasm (20%)

Renal: Proteinuria (51%), creatinine increased (16% to 47%)

Respiratory: Cough (11%), upper respiratory infection (11%)

1% to 10%:

Cardiovascular: QT_c prolongation (3% to 4%)

Dermatologic: Squamous cell carcinoma (4%)

Respiratory: Pulmonary embolism (5%)

Available Dosage Forms

Capsule, oral:

Zolinza®: 100 mg

General Dosage Range Dosage adjustment recommended in patients who develop toxicities

Oral: *Adults:* 400 mg once daily

Administration

Oral Administer with food. Do not open, crush, or chew capsules. Maintain adequate hydration (≥2 L/day fluids) during treatment.

Stability

Storage Store at 20°C to 25°C (68°F to 77°F); excursions permitted to 15°C to 30°C (59°F to 86°F).

Nursing Actions

Physical Assessment Caution patients with diabetes to monitor serum glucose closely. Teach patient correct use and proper handling of capsules.

Patient Education Take with food. Do not open, chew, or crush capsules. If capsule is accidentally opened or crushed, do not touch the capsules or powder. If powder gets on your skin, wash well with water. If you have diabetes, you should monitor your glucose levels closely and report immediately if your blood sugar is higher than normal. Maintain adequate nutrition and hydration, unless instructed to restrict fluid intake. You may experience dry mouth, taste changes, diarrhea, nausea, vomiting, loss of hair (may grow back after treatment is discontinued), dizziness, or headache. Report persistent diarrhea; chest pain or palpitations; upper respiratory infection or difficulty breathing; muscle pain, tremors, weakness, or spasms; swelling in foot, ankle, or leg; or rash or itching.

Dietary Considerations Take with food.

Warfarin (WAR far in)

Brand Names: U.S. Coumadin®; Jantoven®

Index Terms Warfarin Sodium

Pharmacologic Category Anticoagulant, Coumarin Derivative; Vitamin K Antagonist

Medication Safety Issues

Sound-alike/look-alike issues:

Coumadin® may be confused with Avandia®, Cardura®, Compazine, Kemadrin

Jantoven® may be confused with Janumet®, Januvia®

High alert medication:

The Institute for Safe Medication Practices (ISMP) includes this medication among its list of drugs which have a heightened risk of causing significant patient harm when used in error.

National Patient Safety Goals:

The Joint Commission on Accreditation of Healthcare Organizations requires healthcare organizations that provide anticoagulant therapy to have a process in place to reduce the risk of anticoagulant-associated patient harm. Patients receiving anticoagulants should receive individualized care through a defined process that includes standardized ordering, dispensing, administration, monitoring and education. This does not apply to routine short-term use of anticoagulants for prevention of venous thromboembolism when the expectation is that the patient's laboratory values will remain within or close to normal values (NPSG.03.05.01).

Medication Guide Available Yes

Pregnancy Risk Factor D (women with mechanical heart valves)/X (other indications)

Lactation Does not enter breast milk/use caution (AAP rates "compatible"; AAP 2001 update pending)

Breast-Feeding Considerations Breast-feeding women may be treated with warfarin. Based on limited data, warfarin does not pass into breast milk. Women who are breast-feeding should be carefully monitored to avoid excessive anticoagulation. ACCP guidelines recommend continuation of warfarin in lactating women who wish to breastfeed their infants (Bates, 2008). Monitor nursing infants for bruising or bleeding (per manufacturer).

Use Prophylaxis and treatment of thromboembolic disorders (eg, venous, pulmonary) and embolic complications arising from atrial fibrillation or cardiac valve replacement; adjunct to reduce risk of systemic embolism (eg, recurrent MI, stroke) after myocardial infarction

Unlabeled Use Prevention of recurrent transient ischemic attacks

Mechanism of Action/Effect Interferes with hepatic synthesis of vitamin K-dependent coagulation factors (II, VII, IX, X)

Contraindications Hypersensitivity to warfarin or any component of the formulation; hemorrhagic tendencies (eg, patients bleeding from the GI, respiratory, or GU tract; cerebral aneurysm; cerebrovascular hemorrhage; dissecting aortic aneurysm; spinal puncture and other diagnostic or therapeutic procedures with potential for significant bleeding; history of bleeding diathesis); recent or potential surgery of the eye or CNS; major regional lumbar block anesthesia or traumatic surgery resulting in large, open surfaces; blood dyscrasias; severe uncontrolled or malignant hypertension; pericarditis or pericardial effusion; bacterial endocarditis; unsupervised patients with conditions associated with a high potential for noncompliance; eclampsia/pre-eclampsia, threatened abortion, pregnancy (except in women with mechanical heart valves at high risk for thromboembolism)

Warnings/Precautions Hazardous agent - use appropriate precautions for handling and disposal. Use care in the selection of patients appropriate for this treatment. Ensure patient cooperation especially from the alcoholic, illicit drug user, demented, or psychotic patient; ability to comply with routine laboratory monitoring is essential. Use with caution in trauma, acute infection, moderate-severe renal insufficiency, prolonged dietary insufficiencies, moderate-severe hypertension, polycythemia vera, vasculitis, open wound, active TB, any disruption in normal GI flora, history of PUD, anaphylactic disorders, indwelling catheters, severe diabetes, and menstruating and postpartum women. Use with caution in patients with thyroid disease; warfarin responsiveness may increase (Ansell, 2008). Use with caution in protein C deficiency. Use with caution in patients with heparin-induced thrombocytopenia and DVT. Warfarin monotherapy is contraindicated in the initial treatment of active HIT. Reduced liver function, regardless of etiology, may impair synthesis of coagulation factors leading to increased warfarin sensitivity.

[U.S. Boxed Warning]: May cause major or fatal bleeding. Risk factors for bleeding include high intensity anticoagulation (INR >4), age (>65 years), variable INRs, history of GI bleeding, hypertension, cerebrovascular disease, serious heart disease, anemia, malignancy, trauma, renal insufficiency, drug-drug interactions, long duration of therapy, or known genetic deficiency in CYP2C9 activity. Patient must be instructed to report bleeding, accidents, or falls. Unrecognized bleeding sites (eg, colon cancer) may be uncovered by anticoagulation. Patient must also report any new or discontinued medications, herbal or alternative products used, or significant changes in smoking or dietary habits. Necrosis or gangrene of the skin and other tissue can occur, usually in conjunction with protein C or S deficiency. Consider alternative therapies if anticoagulation is necessary. Warfarin therapy may release atheromatous plaque emboli; symptoms depend on site of embolization, most commonly kidneys, pancreas, liver, and spleen. In some cases may lead to necrosis or death. "Purple toes syndrome," due to cholesterol microembolization, may rarely occur. The elderly may be more sensitive to anticoagulant therapy.

Presence of the CYP2C9*2 or *3 allele and/or polymorphism of the vitamin K oxidoreductase (VKORC1) gene may increase the risk of bleeding. Lower doses may be required in these patients; genetic testing may help determine appropriate dosing.

Drug Interactions

Avoid Concomitant Use

Avoid concomitant use of Warfarin with any of the following: Rivaroxaban; Tamoxifen

Decreased Effect

The levels/effects of Warfarin may be decreased by: Aminoglutethimide; Antineoplastic Agents; Antithyroid Agents; Aprepitant; AzaTHIOprine; Barbiturates; Bile Acid Sequestrants; Boceprevir; Bosentan; CarBAMazepine; Coenzyme Q-10; Contraceptives (Estrogens); Contraceptives (Progestins); CYP2C9 Inducers (Strong); Cyproterone; Darunavir; Dicloxacillin; Efavirenz; Fosaprepitant; Ginseng (American); Glutethimide; Green Tea; Griseofulvin; Lopinavir; Mercaptopurine; Nafcillin; Nelfinavir; Peginterferon Alfa-2b; Phytonadione; Rifamycin Derivatives; Ritonavir; St Johns Wort; Sucralfate; Telaprevir; Tocilizumab

Increased Effect/Toxicity

Warfarin may increase the levels/effects of: Anticoagulants; Collagenase (Systemic); Deferasirox; Drotrecogin Alfa (Activated); Ethotoin; Fosphenytoin; Phenytoin; Rivaroxaban

The levels/effects of Warfarin may be increased by: Acetaminophen; Allopurinol; Amiodarone; Androgens; Antineoplastic Agents; Antiplatelet Agents; Atazanavir; Bicalutamide; Boceprevir; Capecitabine; Cephalosporins; Chloral Hydrate; Chloramphenicol; Cimetidine; Clopidogrel; Corticosteroids (Systemic); Cranberry; CYP2C9 Inhibitors (Moderate); CYP2C9 Inhibitors (Strong); Desvenlafaxine; Dexmethylphenidate; Disulfiram; Dronedarone; Efavirenz; Erythromycin (Ophthalmic); Esomeprazole; Ethacrynic Acid; Ethotoin; Etoposide; Exenatide; Fenofibrate; Fenofibric Acid; Fenugreek; Fibric Acid Derivatives; Fluconazole; Fluorouracil; Fluorouracil (Systemic); Fluorouracil (Topical); Fosamprenavir; Fosphenytoin; Gefitinib; Ginkgo Biloba; Glucagon; Green Tea; Herbs (Anticoagulant/Antiplatelet Properties); HMG-CoA Reductase Inhibitors; Ifosfamide; Imatinib; Itraconazole; Ivermectin; Ketoconazole; Ketoconazole (Systemic); Lansoprazole; Leflunomide; Macrolide Antibiotics; Methylphenidate; MetroNIDAZOLE; MetroNIDAZOLE (Systemic); Miconazole (Oral); Miconazole (Topical); Milnacipran; Mirtazapine; Nelfinavir; Neomycin; NSAID (COX-2 Inhibitor); NSAID (Nonselective); Omega-3-Acid Ethyl Esters; Omeprazole; Orlistat; Penicillins; Pentosan Polysulfate Sodium; Pentoxifylline; Phenytoin; Posaconazole; Propafenone; Prostacyclin Analogues; QuiNIDine; QuiNINE; Quinolone Antibiotics; Ranitidine; RomiDEPsin; Salicylates; Saquinavir; Selective Serotonin Reuptake Inhibitors; Sitaxentan; SORAfenib; Sulfinpyrazone [Off Market]; Sulfonamide Derivatives; Tamoxifen; Telaprevir; Tetracycline Derivatives; Thrombolytic Agents; Thyroid Products; Tigecycline; Tolterodine; Toremifene; Torsemide; TraMADol; Tricyclic Antidepressants; Venlafaxine; Vitamin E; Voriconazole; Vorinostat; Zafirlukast; Zileuton

Nutritional/Ethanol Interactions

Ethanol: Acute ethanol ingestion (binge drinking) decreases the metabolism of warfarin and increases PT/INR. Chronic daily ethanol use increases the metabolism of warfarin and decreases PT/INR. Management: Avoid ethanol.

Food: The anticoagulant effects of warfarin may be decreased if taken with foods rich in vitamin K. Vitamin E may increase warfarin effect. Cranberry juice may increase warfarin effect. Management: Maintain a consistent diet; consult prescriber before making changes in diet. Take warfarin at the same time each day.

Herb/Nutraceutical: Some herbal medications (eg, St John's wort) may decrease warfarin levels and effects; many others can add additional antiplatelet activity to warfarin therapy. Management: Avoid ginseng (American), coenzyme Q_{10}, and St John's wort. Avoid cranberry, fenugreek, ginkgo biloba, glucosamine, alfalfa, anise, bilberry, bladderwrack, bromelain, cat's claw, celery, chamomile, coleus, cordyceps, dong quai, evening primrose oil, fenugreek, feverfew, garlic, ginger, ginkgo biloba, ginseng (Panax), ginseng (Siberian), grapeseed, green tea, guggul, horse chestnut seed, horseradish, licorice, omega-3-acids, prickly ash, red clover, reishi, SAMe (s-adenosylmethionine), sweet clover, turmeric, and white willow.

Adverse Reactions Bleeding is the major adverse effect of warfarin. Hemorrhage may occur at virtually any site. Risk is dependent on multiple variables, including the intensity of anticoagulation and patient susceptibility.

Cardiovascular: Vasculitis

Central nervous system: Signs/symptoms of bleeding (eg, dizziness, fatigue, fever, headache, lethargy, malaise, pain)

Dermatologic: Alopecia, bullous eruptions, dermatitis, rash, pruritus, urticaria

Gastrointestinal: Abdominal pain, diarrhea, flatulence, gastrointestinal bleeding, nausea, taste disturbance, vomiting

Genitourinary: Hematuria

Hematologic: Anemia, retroperitoneal hematoma, unrecognized bleeding sites (eg, colon cancer) may be uncovered by anticoagulation

Hepatic: Hepatitis (including cholestatic hepatitis), transaminases increased

Neuromuscular & skeletal: Osteoporosis (potential association with long-term use), paralysis, paresthesia, weakness

Respiratory: Respiratory tract bleeding, tracheobronchial calcification

Miscellaneous: Anaphylactic reaction, hypersensitivity/allergic reactions, skin necrosis, gangrene, "purple toes" syndrome

Pharmacodynamics/Kinetics

Onset of Action Anticoagulation: Oral: 24-72 hours; Peak effect: Full therapeutic effect: 5-7 days; INR may increase in 36-72 hours

Duration of Action 2-5 days

Available Dosage Forms

Injection, powder for reconstitution:

Coumadin®: 5 mg

Tablet, oral: 1 mg, 2 mg, 2.5 mg, 3 mg, 4 mg, 5 mg, 6 mg, 7.5 mg, 10 mg

Coumadin®: 1 mg, 2 mg, 2.5 mg, 3 mg, 4 mg, 5 mg, 6 mg, 7.5 mg, 10 mg

Jantoven®: 1 mg, 2 mg, 2.5 mg, 3 mg, 4 mg, 5 mg, 6 mg, 7.5 mg, 10 mg

General Dosage Range

I.V.: *Adults:* 2-5 mg once daily

Oral:

Adults: Initial: 2-5 mg daily for 2 days; Maintenance: 2-10 mg daily

Elderly: Initial: ≤5 mg/day; Maintenance: 2-5 mg/day

Administration

Oral Administer with or without food. Take at the same time each day.

I.V. Administer as a slow bolus injection over 1-2 minutes. Avoid all I.M. injections.

I.V. Detail pH: 8.1-8.3

Stability

Reconstitution Reconstitute with 2.7 mL of sterile water (yields 2 mg/mL solution).

Storage

Injection: Prior to reconstitution, store at 15°C to 30°C (59°F to 86°F). Following reconstitution with 2.7 mL of sterile water (yields 2 mg/mL solution), stable for 4 hours at 15°C to 30°C (59°F to 86°F). Protect from light.

Tablet: Store at 15°C to 30°C (59°F to 86°F). Protect from light.

Nursing Actions

Physical Assessment Assess potential for interactions with other prescriptions, OTC medications, or herbal products patient may be taking that may affect coagulation or platelet aggregation. Monitor for bleeding from any site, rash, urticaria, gastrointestinal upset, abdominal pain, diarrhea, or hypersensitivity reaction.

Patient Education If dose is missed, take as soon as possible; do not double dose. Laboratory tests will be required. Follow prescriber's recommended diet and activity. Avoid excessive alcohol. Do not make major changes in your dietary intake of vitamin K (green vegetables). You will have a tendency to bleed easily while taking this drug. Report unusual bleeding or bruising, skin rash or irritation, unusual fever, persistent nausea or GI upset, pain in joints or back, swelling or pain at injection site, or unhealed wounds.

Dietary Considerations Foods high in vitamin K (eg, beef liver, pork liver, green tea, and leafy green vegetables) inhibit anticoagulant effect. Do not change dietary habits once stabilized on warfarin therapy. A balanced diet with a consistent intake of vitamin K is essential. Avoid large amounts of alfalfa, asparagus, broccoli, Brussels sprouts, cabbage, cauliflower, green teas, kale, lettuce, spinach, turnip greens, and watercress; decreased efficacy of warfarin. It is recommended that the diet contain a CONSISTENT vitamin K content of 70-140 mcg/day. Check with healthcare provider before changing diet.

Related Information

Peak and Trough Guidelines *on page 1276*

Zafirlukast (za FIR loo kast)

Brand Names: U.S. Accolate®

Index Terms ICI-204,219

Pharmacologic Category Leukotriene-Receptor Antagonist

Medication Safety Issues

Sound-alike/look-alike issues:

Accolate® may be confused with Accupril®, Accutane®, Aclovate®

Pregnancy Risk Factor B

Lactation Enters breast milk/contraindicated

Breast-Feeding Considerations The manufacturer does not recommend breast-feeding due to tumorigenicity observed in animal studies.

Use Prophylaxis and chronic treatment of asthma in adults and children ≥5 years of age

Mechanism of Action/Effect Leukotrienes are inflammatory mediators of asthma. Zafirlukast blocks leukotriene receptors and is able to reduce bronchoconstriction and inflammatory cell infiltration.

Contraindications Hypersensitivity to zafirlukast or any component of the formulation; hepatic impairment

Warnings/Precautions Zafirlukast is not FDA approved for use in the reversal of bronchospasm in acute asthma attacks, including status asthmaticus. Therapy with zafirlukast can be continued during acute exacerbations of asthma.

Hepatic adverse events (including hepatitis, hyperbilirubinemia, and hepatic failure) have been reported; female patients may be at greater risk. Discontinue immediately if liver dysfunction is suspected. Periodic testing of liver function may be considered (early detection is generally believed to improve the likelihood of recovery). If hepatic dysfunction is suspected (due to clinical signs/symptoms), liver function tests should be measured immediately. Do not resume or restart if hepatic function studies are consistent with dysfunction. Use caution in patients with alcoholic cirrhosis; clearance is reduced. Postmarketing reports of behavioral changes (ie, depression, insomnia) have been noted. Monitor INR closely with concomitant warfarin use. Rare cases of eosinophilic vasculitis (Churg-Strauss) have been reported in patients receiving zafirlukast (usually, but not always, associated with reduction in concurrent steroid dosage). No causal relationship established. Monitor for eosinophilic vasculitis, rash, pulmonary symptoms, cardiac symptoms, or neuropathy.

An increased proportion of zafirlukast patients >55 years of age reported infections as compared to placebo-treated patients. These infections were mostly mild or moderate in intensity and predominantly affected the respiratory tract. Infections occurred equally in both sexes, were dose-proportional to total milligrams of zafirlukast exposure, and were associated with coadministration of inhaled corticosteroids.

Drug Interactions

Avoid Concomitant Use

Avoid concomitant use of Zafirlukast with any of the following: Pimozide

Decreased Effect

The levels/effects of Zafirlukast may be decreased by: CYP2C9 Inducers (Strong); Erythromycin; Erythromycin (Systemic); Peginterferon Alfa-2b; Theophylline Derivatives

Increased Effect/Toxicity

Zafirlukast may increase the levels/effects of: ARIPiprazole; Carvedilol; CYP2C9 Substrates; Pimozide; Theophylline Derivatives; Vitamin K Antagonists

The levels/effects of Zafirlukast may be increased by: CYP2C9 Inhibitors (Moderate); CYP2C9 Inhibitors (Strong)

Nutritional/Ethanol Interactions Food: Food decreases bioavailability of zafirlukast by 40%. Management: Take on an empty stomach 1 hour before or 2 hours after meals.

Adverse Reactions

>10%: Central nervous system: Headache (13%)

1% to 10%:

Central nervous system: Dizziness (2%), pain (2%), fever (2%)

Gastrointestinal: Nausea (3%), diarrhea (3%), abdominal pain (2%), vomiting (2%), dyspepsia (1%)

Hepatic: ALT increased (2%)

Neuromuscular & skeletal: Back pain (2%), myalgia (2%), weakness (2%)

Miscellaneous: Infection (4%)

Available Dosage Forms

Tablet, oral: 10 mg, 20 mg

Accolate®: 10 mg, 20 mg

General Dosage Range Oral:

Children 5-11 years: 10 mg twice daily

Children ≥12 years and Adults: 20 mg twice daily

Administration

Oral Administer 1 hour before or 2 hours after meals.

Stability

Storage Store tablets at controlled room temperature of 20°C to 25°C (68°F to 77°F). Protect from light and moisture; dispense in original airtight container.

Nursing Actions

Physical Assessment Not for use in acute asthma attack. Monitor for liver dysfunction.

Patient Education Do not use during acute bronchospasm. Take regularly as prescribed, even during symptom-free periods. This medication should be taken on an empty stomach, 1 hour before or 2 hours after meals. Do not stop taking other antiasthmatic medications unless instructed by prescriber. You may experience headache, drowsiness, dizziness, blurred vision, gastric upset, nausea, or vomiting. Report persistent CNS or GI symptoms; muscle or back pain; weakness, fever, or chills; yellowing of skin or eyes; dark urine or pale stool; or skin rash. Contact prescriber immediately if experiencing right upper abdominal pain; nausea; fatigue; itching; flu-like symptoms; swelling of the eyes, face, neck, or throat; anorexia; or worsening of condition.

Dietary Considerations Should be taken on an empty stomach (1 hour before or 2 hours after meals).

Zaleplon (ZAL e plon)

Brand Names: U.S. Sonata®

Pharmacologic Category Hypnotic, Nonbenzodiazepine

Medication Safety Issues

Sound-alike/look-alike issues:

Sonata® may be confused with Soriatane®

Zaleplon may be confused with Zelapar®, Zemplar®, zolpidem, ZyPREXA® Zydis®

Medication Guide Available Yes

Pregnancy Risk Factor C

Lactation Enters breast milk/not recommended

Use Short-term (7-10 days) treatment of insomnia (has been demonstrated to be effective for up to 5 weeks in controlled trial)

Mechanism of Action/Effect Zaleplon is unrelated to benzodiazepines, barbiturates, or other hypnotics. However, it interacts with the benzodiazepine GABA receptor complex. Nonclinical studies have shown that it binds selectively to the brain omega-1 receptor situated on the alpha subunit of the GABA-A receptor complex.

Contraindications Hypersensitivity to zaleplon or any component of the formulation

Warnings/Precautions Symptomatic treatment of insomnia should be initiated only after careful evaluation of potential causes of sleep disturbance. Failure of sleep disturbance to resolve after 7-10 days may indicate psychiatric and/or medical illness.

Use with caution in patients with depression, particularly if suicidal risk may be present. Use with caution in patients with a history of drug dependence. Abrupt discontinuance may lead to withdrawal symptoms. Hypnotics/sedatives have been associated with abnormal thinking and behavior changes including decreased inhibition, aggression, bizarre behavior, agitation, hallucinations, and depersonalization. These changes may occur unpredictably and may indicate previously unrecognized psychiatric disorders; evaluate appropriately. May impair physical and mental capabilities. Patients must be cautioned about performing tasks which require mental alertness (operating machinery or driving). Amnesia can occur. Use with caution in patients receiving other CNS depressants or psychoactive medications. Effects with other sedative drugs or ethanol may be potentiated. Postmarketing studies have indicated that the use of hypnotic/sedative agents for sleep has been associated with hypersensitivity reactions including anaphylaxis as well as angioedema. An increased risk for hazardous sleep-related activities such as sleep-driving, cooking and eating food, and making phone calls while asleep have been noted.

Use with caution in the elderly, those with compromised respiratory function, or hepatic impairment (dosage adjustment recommended in mild-to-moderate hepatic impairment; avoid use in severe impairment). Because of the rapid onset of action, zaleplon should be administered immediately prior to bedtime or after the patient has gone to bed and is having difficulty falling asleep. Capsules contain tartrazine (FDC yellow #5); avoid in patients with sensitivity (caution in patients with asthma).

Drug Interactions

Avoid Concomitant Use There are no known interactions where it is recommended to avoid concomitant use.

Decreased Effect

The levels/effects of Zaleplon may be decreased by: Flumazenil; Rifamycin Derivatives; Tocilizumab

Increased Effect/Toxicity

Zaleplon may increase the levels/effects of: Alcohol (Ethyl); CNS Depressants; Methotrimeprazine; Selective Serotonin Reuptake Inhibitors

The levels/effects of Zaleplon may be increased by: Cimetidine; Conivaptan; Droperidol; HydrOXYzine; Methotrimeprazine

Nutritional/Ethanol Interactions

Ethanol: Ethanol may increase CNS depression. Management: Avoid or limit use of ethanol and monitor for increased effects.

Food: High-fat meals prolong absorption; delay T_{max} by 2 hours, and reduce C_{max} by 35%. Management: Avoid taking after a high-fat meal.

Herb/Nutraceutical: St John's wort may decrease zaleplon levels. Some herbal medications may increase CNS depression. Management: Avoid St John's wort, valerian, kava kava, and gotu kola.

Adverse Reactions

>10%: Central nervous system: Headache (30% to 42%)

1% to 10%:

Cardiovascular: Chest pain (≥1%), peripheral edema (≤1%)

Central nervous system: Dizziness (7% to 9%), somnolence (5% to 6%), amnesia (2% to 4%), depersonalization (<1% to 2%), hypoesthesia (<1% to 2%), malaise (<1% to 2%), abnormal thinking (≥1%), anxiety (≥1%), depression (≥1%), fever (≥1%), migraine (≥1%), nervousness (≥1%), confusion (≤1%), hallucination (≤1%), vertigo (≤1%)

Dermatologic: Pruritus (≥1%), rash (≥1%), photosensitivity reaction (≤1%)

Endocrine & metabolic: Dysmenorrhea (3% to 4%)

Gastrointestinal: Nausea (6% to 8%), abdominal pain (6%), anorexia (<1% to 2%), constipation (≥1%), dyspepsia (≥1%), taste perversion (≥1%), xerostomia (≥1%), colitis (up to 1%)

Neuromuscular & skeletal: Weakness (5% to 7%), paresthesia (3%), tremor (2%), arthralgia (≥1%), arthritis (≥1%), back pain (≥1%), myalgia (≥1%), hypertonia (1%)

Ocular: Eye pain (3% to 4%), abnormal vision (<1% to 2%), conjunctivitis (≥1%)

Otic: Hyperacusis (1% to 2%), ear pain (≤1%)

Respiratory: Bronchitis (≥1%), epistaxis (≤1%)

Miscellaneous: Parosmia (<1% to 2%)

Pharmacodynamics/Kinetics

Onset of Action Rapid

Controlled Substance C-IV

Available Dosage Forms

Capsule, oral: 5 mg, 10 mg

Sonata®: 5 mg, 10 mg

General Dosage Range Dosage adjustment recommended in patients with hepatic impairment

Oral:

Adults: 5-20 mg at bedtime

Elderly: 5 mg at bedtime (maximum: 10 mg/day)

Administration

Oral Administer immediately before bedtime or when the patient is in bed and cannot fall asleep.

Stability

Storage Store at controlled room temperature of 20°C to 25°C (68°F to 77°F). Protect from light.

Nursing Actions

Physical Assessment Assess for history of addiction (long-term use may result in dependence, abuse, or tolerance). For inpatient use, institute safety measures to prevent falls.

Patient Education Take immediately before bedtime, or when you cannot fall asleep. May be habit forming. Avoid alcohol. You may experience drowsiness, dizziness, or lightheadedness. Discontinue drug and report any severe CNS disturbances (hallucinations, anxiety, persistent sleepiness or lethargy, impaired coordination, amnesia); skin rash; vision changes; respiratory difficulty; or unusual swelling, especially on face or neck.

Dietary Considerations Avoid taking with or after a heavy, high-fat meal; reduces absorption.

Zanamivir (za NA mi veer)

Brand Names: U.S. Relenza®

Pharmacologic Category Antiviral Agent; Neuraminidase Inhibitor

Medication Safety Issues

Sound-alike/look-alike issues:

Relenza® may be confused with Albenza®, Aplenzin™

Pregnancy Risk Factor C

Lactation Excretion in breast milk unknown/use caution

Breast-Feeding Considerations It is not known if zanamivir is found in human milk and the manufacturer recommends that caution be exercised when administering zanamivir to nursing women. According to the CDC, breast-feeding while taking zanamivir can be continued. The CDC recommends that women infected with the influenza virus follow general precautions (eg, frequent hand washing) to decrease viral transmission to the child. Mothers with influenza-like illnesses at delivery should consider avoiding close contact with the infant until they have received 48 hours of antiviral medication, fever has resolved, and cough and secretions can be controlled. These measures may help decrease (but not eliminate) the risk of transmitting influenza to the newborn. During this time, breast milk can be expressed and bottle-fed to the infant by another person who is well. Protective measures, such as wearing a face mask, changing into a clean gown or clothing, and strict hand hygiene should be continued by the mother for ≥7 days after the onset of symptoms or until symptom-free for 24 hours. Infant care should be performed by a noninfected person when possible (consult current CDC guidelines). Influenza may cause serious illness in postpartum women and prompt evaluation for febrile respiratory illnesses is recommended.

Use Treatment of uncomplicated acute illness due to influenza virus A and B in patients who have been symptomatic for no more than 2 days; prophylaxis against influenza virus A and B

The Advisory Committee on Immunization Practices (ACIP) recommends that **treatment** be considered for the following:

- Persons with severe, complicated or progressive illness
- Hospitalized persons

- Persons at higher risk for influenza complications:
  - Children <2 years of age (highest risk in children <6 months of age)
  - Adults ≥65 years of age
  - Persons with chronic disorders of the pulmonary (including asthma) or cardiovascular systems (except hypertension)
  - Persons with chronic metabolic diseases (including diabetes mellitus), hepatic disease, renal dysfunction, hematologic disorders (including sickle cell disease), or immunosuppression (including immunosuppression caused by medications or HIV)
  - Persons with neurologic/neuromuscular conditions (including conditions such as spinal cord injuries, seizure disorders, cerebral palsy, stroke, mental retardation, moderate to severe developmental delay, or muscular dystrophy) which may compromise respiratory function, the handling of respiratory secretions, or that can increase the risk of aspiration
  - Pregnant or postpartum women (≤2 weeks after delivery)
  - Persons <19 years of age on long-term aspirin therapy
  - American Indians and Alaskan Natives
  - Persons who are morbidly obese (BMI ≥40)
  - Residents of nursing homes or other chronic care facilities
- Use may also be considered for previously healthy, nonhigh-risk outpatients with confirmed or suspected influenza based on clinical judgment when treatment can be started within 48 hours of illness onset.

The ACIP recommends that **prophylaxis** be considered for the following:

- Postexposure prophylaxis may be considered for family or close contacts of suspected or confirmed cases, who are at higher risk of influenza complications, and who have not been vaccinated against the circulating strain at the time of the exposure.
- Postexposure prophylaxis may be considered for unvaccinated healthcare workers who had occupational exposure without protective equipment.
- Pre-exposure prophylaxis should only be used for persons at very high risk of influenza complications who cannot be otherwise protected at times of high risk for exposure.
- Prophylaxis should also be administered to all eligible residents of institutions that house patients at high risk when needed to control outbreaks.

Mechanism of Action/Effect Zanamivir inhibits influenza virus neuraminidase enzymes, potentially altering virus particle aggregation and release.

Contraindications Hypersensitivity to zanamivir or any component of the formulation (contains milk proteins)

Warnings/Precautions Allergic-like reactions, including anaphylaxis, oropharyngeal edema, and serious skin rashes have been reported. Rare occurrences of neuropsychiatric events (including confusion, delirium, hallucinations, and/or self-injury) have been reported from postmarketing surveillance; direct causation is difficult to establish (influenza infection may also be associated with behavioral and neurologic changes). Patients must be instructed in the use of the delivery system. Antiviral treatment should begin within 48 hours of symptom onset. However, the CDC recommends that treatment may still be beneficial and should be started in hospitalized patients with severe, complicated or progressive illness if >48 hours. Nonhospitalized persons who are not at high risk for developing severe or complicated illness and who have a mild disease are not likely to benefit if treatment is started >48 hours after symptom onset. Nonhospitalized persons who are already beginning to recover do not need treatment. Effectiveness has not been established in patients with significant underlying medical conditions or for prophylaxis of influenza in nursing home patients (per manufacturer). The CDC recommends zanamivir to be used to control institutional outbreaks of influenza when circulating strains are suspected of being resistant to oseltamivir (refer to current guidelines). Not recommended for use in patients with underlying respiratory disease, such as asthma or COPD, due to lack of efficacy and risk of serious adverse effects. Bronchospasm, decreased lung function, and other serious adverse reactions, including those with fatal outcomes, have been reported in patients with and without airway disease; discontinue with bronchospasm or signs of decreased lung function. For a patient with an underlying airway disease where a medical decision has been made to use zanamivir, a fast-acting bronchodilator should be made available, and used prior to each dose. Not a substitute for annual flu vaccination; has not been shown to reduce risk of transmission of influenza to others. Consider primary or concomitant bacterial infections. Powder for oral inhalation contains lactose; use contraindicated in patients allergic to milk proteins. The inhalation powder should only be administered via inhalation using the provided Diskhaler® delivery device. The commercially available formulation is **not** intended to be solubilized or administered via any nebulizer/ mechanical ventilator; inappropriate administration has resulted in death. Safety and efficacy of repeated courses or use with hepatic impairment or severe renal impairment have not been established. Indicated for children ≥5 years of age (for influenza prophylaxis) and children ≥7 years of age (for influenza treatment); children ages 5-6 years may have inadequate inhalation (via Diskhaler®) for the treatment of influenza.

Drug Interactions

Avoid Concomitant Use There are no known interactions where it is recommended to avoid concomitant use.

Decreased Effect

Zanamivir may decrease the levels/effects of: Influenza Virus Vaccine (Live/Attenuated)

Increased Effect/Toxicity There are no known significant interactions involving an increase in effect.

Adverse Reactions Most adverse reactions occurred at a frequency which was less than or equal to the control (lactose vehicle).

>10%:

Central nervous system: Headache (prophylaxis 13% to 24%; treatment 2%)

Gastrointestinal: Throat/tonsil discomfort/pain (prophylaxis 8% to 19%)

Respiratory: Nasal signs and symptoms (prophylaxis 12% to 20%; treatment 2%), cough (prophylaxis 7% to 17%; treatment ≤2%)

Miscellaneous: Viral infection (prophylaxis 3% to 13%)

1% to 10%:

Central nervous system: Fever/chills (prophylaxis 5% to 9%; treatment <1.5%), fatigue (prophylaxis 5% to 8%; treatment <1.5%), malaise (prophylaxis 5% to 8%; treatment <1.5%), dizziness (treatment 1% to 2%)

Dermatologic: Urticaria (treatment <1.5%)

Gastrointestinal: Anorexia/appetite decreased (prophylaxis 2% to 4%), appetite increased (prophylaxis 2% to 4%), nausea (prophylaxis 1% to 2%; treatment ≤3%), diarrhea (prophylaxis 2%; treatment 2% to 3%), vomiting (prophylaxis 1% to 2%; treatment 1% to 2%), abdominal pain (treatment <1.5%)

Neuromuscular & skeletal: Muscle pain (prophylaxis 3% to 8%), musculoskeletal pain (prophylaxis 6%), arthralgia/articular rheumatism (prophylaxis 2%), arthralgia (treatment <1.5%), myalgia (treatment <1.5%)

Respiratory: Infection (ear/nose/throat; prophylaxis 2%; treatment 1% to 5%), sinusitis (treatment 3%), bronchitis (treatment 2%), nasal inflammation (prophylaxis 1%)

Available Dosage Forms

Powder, for oral inhalation:

Relenza®: 5 mg/blister (20s)

General Dosage Range Oral inhalation:

Children ≥5 years: Prophylaxis: 10 mg once daily

Children ≥7 years: Treatment: 10 mg twice daily

Adolescents and Adults: Prophylaxis: 10 mg once to twice daily; Treatment: 10 mg twice daily

Administration

Inhalation Must be used with Diskhaler® delivery device. The foil blister disk containing zanamivir inhalation powder should not be manipulated, solubilized, or administered via a nebulizer. Patients who are scheduled to use an inhaled bronchodilator should use their bronchodilator prior to zanamivir. With the exception of the initial dose when used for treatment, administer at the same time each day.

Stability

Storage Store at 25°C (77°F); excursions permitted to 15°C to 30°C (59°F to 86°F). Do not puncture blister until taking a dose using the Diskhaler®.

Nursing Actions

Physical Assessment Recommendations for antiviral susceptibility and effectiveness may change. Validate with the CDC recommendations for use prior to prescribing. Therapy for treatment must be started within 48 hours of first influenza symptoms. Monitor for change in behavior.

Patient Education This is not a substitute for the influenza vaccine. If you have asthma or COPD you may be at risk for bronchospasm; see prescriber for appropriate bronchodilator before using zanamivir. Stop using this medication and contact your prescriber if you experience shortness of breath, increased wheezing, or other signs of bronchospasm. You may experience dizziness, headache, sore throat, or nasal congestion. Report unresolved diarrhea, vomiting, or nausea; fever or muscle pain; or change in behavior, including hallucinations, confusion, delirium, or seizures.

Ziconotide (zi KOE no tide)

Brand Names: U.S. Prialt®

Pharmacologic Category Analgesic, Nonopioid; Calcium Channel Blocker, N-Type

Medication Safety Issues

High alert medication:

The Institute for Safe Medication Practices (ISMP) includes this medication among its list of drugs which have a heightened risk of causing significant patient harm when used in error.

Pregnancy Risk Factor C

Lactation Excretion in breast milk unknown/not recommended

Breast-Feeding Considerations The manufacturer recommends discontinuing breast-feeding or discontinuing ziconotide.

Use Management of severe chronic pain in patients requiring intrathecal (I.T.) therapy and who are intolerant or refractory to other therapies

Mechanism of Action/Effect Ziconotide selectively binds to N-type voltage-sensitive calcium channels located on the nociceptive afferent nerves of the dorsal horn in the spinal cord. This binding is thought to block N-type calcium channels, leading to a blockade of excitatory neurotransmitter release and reducing sensitivity to painful stimuli.

Contraindications Hypersensitivity to ziconotide or any component of the formulation; history of psychosis; I.V. administration

I.T. administration is contraindicated in patients with infection at the injection site, uncontrolled bleeding, or spinal canal obstruction that impairs CSF circulation

Warnings/Precautions [U.S Boxed Warning]: Severe psychiatric symptoms and neurological impairment have been reported; interrupt or discontinue therapy if cognitive impairment, hallucinations, mood changes, or changes in consciousness occur. May cause or worsen depression and/or risk of suicide. Cognitive impairment may appear gradually during treatment and is generally reversible after discontinuation (may take up to 2 weeks for cognitive effects to reverse). Use caution in the elderly; may experience a higher incidence of confusion. Patients should be instructed to use caution in performing tasks which require alertness (eg, operating machinery or driving). May have additive effects with opiates or other CNS-depressant medications; may potentiate opioid-induced decreased GI motility; does not interact with opioid receptors or potentiate opiate-induced respiratory depression. Will not prevent or relieve symptoms associated with opiate withdrawal and opiates should not be abruptly discontinued. Unlike opioids, ziconotide therapy can be interrupted abruptly or discontinued without evidence of withdrawal.

Meningitis may occur with use of I.T. pumps; monitor for signs and symptoms of meningitis; treatment of meningitis may require removal of system and discontinuation of intrathecal therapy. Elevated serum creatine kinase can occur, particularly during the first 2 months of therapy; consider dose reduction or discontinuing if combined with new neuromuscular symptoms (myalgias, myasthenia, muscle cramps, weakness) or reduction in physical activity. Safety and efficacy have not been established with renal or hepatic dysfunction, or in pediatric patients. Should not be used in combination with intrathecal opiates.

Drug Interactions

Avoid Concomitant Use There are no known interactions where it is recommended to avoid concomitant use.

Decreased Effect There are no known significant interactions involving a decrease in effect.

Increased Effect/Toxicity

Ziconotide may increase the levels/effects of: Alcohol (Ethyl); CNS Depressants; Methotrimeprazine; Selective Serotonin Reuptake Inhibitors

The levels/effects of Ziconotide may be increased by: Droperidol; HydrOXYzine; Methotrimeprazine

Nutritional/Ethanol Interactions Ethanol: May increase CNS depression; monitor for increased effects with coadministration. Caution patients about effects.

Adverse Reactions

>10%:

Central nervous system: Dizziness (46%), confusion (15% to 33%), memory impairment (7% to 22%), somnolence (17%), ataxia (14%), speech disorder (14%), headache (13%), aphasia (12%), hallucination (12%; including auditory and visual)

Gastrointestinal: Nausea (40%), diarrhea (18%), vomiting (16%)

Neuromuscular & skeletal: Creatine kinase increased (40%; ≥3 times ULN: 11%), weakness (18%), gait disturbances (14%)

Ocular: Blurred vision (12%)

2% to 10%:

Cardiovascular: Hypotension, peripheral edema, postural hypotension

Central nervous system: Abnormal thinking (8%), amnesia (8%), anxiety (8%), vertigo (7%), insomnia (6%), fever (5%), paranoid reaction (3%), delirium (2%), hostility (2%), stupor (2%), agitation, attention disturbance, balance impaired, burning sensation, coordination abnormal, depression, disorientation, fatigue, fever, hypoesthesia, irritability, lethargy, mental impairment, mood disorder, nervousness, pain, sedation

Dermatologic: Pruritus (7%)

Gastrointestinal: Anorexia (6%), taste perversion (5%), abdominal pain, appetite decreased, constipation, xerostomia

Genitourinary: Urinary retention (9%), dysuria, urinary hesitance

Neuromuscular & skeletal: Dysarthria (7%), paresthesia (7%), rigors (7%), tremor (7%), muscle spasm (6%), limb pain (5%), areflexia, muscle cramp, muscle weakness, myalgia

Ocular: Nystagmus (8%), diplopia, visual disturbance

Respiratory: Sinusitis (5%)

Miscellaneous: Diaphoresis (5%)

Available Dosage Forms

Injection, solution [preservative free]:

Prialt®: 25 mcg/mL (20 mL); 100 mcg/mL (1 mL, 5 mL)

General Dosage Range Dosage adjustment recommended in patients who develop toxicities

I.T.: *Adults:* Initial dose: ≤2.4 mcg/day (0.1 mcg/hour); Maintenance range: 2.4-19.2 mcg/day (0.1-0.8 mcg/hour) (maximum: 19.2 mcg/day [0.8 mcg/hour])

Administration

I.V. Not for I.V. administration

Other Not for I.V. administration. **For I.T. administration only** using Medtronic SynchroMed® EL, SynchroMed® II Infusion System, or CADD-Micro® ambulatory infusion pump.

Medtronic SynchroMed® EL or SynchroMed® II Infusion Systems:

Naive pump priming (first time use with ziconotide): Use 2 mL of undiluted ziconotide 25 mcg/mL solution to rinse the internal surfaces of the pump; repeat twice for a total of 3 rinses

Initial pump fill: Use only undiluted 25 mcg/mL solution and fill pump after priming. Following the initial fill only, adsorption on internal device surfaces will occur, requiring the use of the undiluted solution and refill within 14 days.

Pump refills: Contents should be emptied prior to refill. Subsequent pump refills should occur at least every 40 days if using diluted solution or at least every 84 days if using undiluted solution.

CADD-Micro® ambulatory infusion pump: Refer to manufacturers' manual for initial fill and refill instructions

pH: 4-5

Stability

Reconstitution Preservative free NS should be used when dilution is needed.

CADD-Micro® ambulatory infusion pump: Initial fill: Dilute to final concentration of 5 mcg/mL.

Medtronic SynchroMed® EL or SynchroMed® II infusion system: Prior to initial fill, rinse internal pump surfaces with 2 mL ziconotide (25 mcg/mL), repeat twice. Only the 25 mcg/mL concentration (undiluted) should be used for initial pump fill.

Storage Prior to use, store vials at 2°C to 8°C (36°F to 46°F). Once diluted, may be stored at 2°C to 8°C (36°F to 46°F) for 24 hours; refrigerate during transit. Do not freeze. Protect from light.

When using the Medtronic SynchroMed® EL or SynchroMed® II Infusion System, solutions expire as follows:

25 mcg/mL: Undiluted:

Initial fill: Use within 14 days.

Refill: Use within 84 days.

100 mcg/mL:

Undiluted: Refill: Use within 84 days.

Diluted: Refill: Use within 40 days.

Nursing Actions

Physical Assessment This medication is given intrathecally via pump. Monitor for changes in behavior, cognitive impairment, hallucinations, or changes in mood or consciousness.

Patient Education Do not use alcohol. You may experience dizziness, sleepiness, or lightheadedness; nausea or vomiting; constipation; diarrhea; or loss of appetite. Report chest pain, swelling of extremities, muscle weakness and poor coordination, hallucinations, confusion, or extreme weakness.

Zidovudine (zye DOE vyoo deen)

Brand Names: U.S. Retrovir®

Index Terms Azidothymidine; AZT (error-prone abbreviation); Compound S; ZDV

Pharmacologic Category Antiretroviral Agent, Reverse Transcriptase Inhibitor (Nucleoside)

Medication Safety Issues

Sound-alike/look-alike issues:

Azidothymidine may be confused with azaTHIOprine, aztreonam

Retrovir® may be confused with acyclovir, ritonavir

Other safety concerns:

AZT is an error-prone abbreviation (mistaken as azathioprine, aztreonam)

Pregnancy Risk Factor C

Lactation Enters breast milk/contraindicated

Breast-Feeding Considerations Maternal or infant antiretroviral therapy does not completely eliminate the risk of postnatal HIV transmission. In addition, multiclass-resistant virus has been detected in breast-feeding infants despite maternal therapy. Therefore, in the United States, where formula is accessible, affordable, safe, and sustainable, and the risk of infant mortality due to diarrhea and respiratory infections is low, complete avoidance of breast-feeding by HIV-infected women is recommended to decrease potential transmission of HIV (DHHS [perinatal], 2011).

Use Treatment of HIV infection in combination with at least two other antiretroviral agents; prevention of maternal/fetal HIV transmission as monotherapy

Unlabeled Use Postexposure prophylaxis for HIV exposure as part of a multidrug regimen

Mechanism of Action/Effect Zidovudine is a thymidine analog which interferes with the HIV virus that results in inhibition of viral replication.

Contraindications Life-threatening hypersensitivity to zidovudine or any component of the formulation

Warnings/Precautions Hazardous agent - use appropriate precautions for handling and disposal. **[U.S. Boxed Warning]: Often associated with hematologic toxicity including granulocytopenia, severe anemia requiring transfusions, or (rarely) pancytopenia.** Use with caution in patients with bone marrow compromise (granulocytes <1000 cells/mm^3 or hemoglobin <9.5 mg/dL); dosage adjustment may be required in patients who develop anemia or neutropenia. **[U.S. Boxed Warning]: Lactic acidosis and severe hepatomegaly with steatosis have been reported, including fatal cases;** use with caution in patients with risk factors for liver disease (risk may be increased in obese patients or prolonged exposure) and suspend treatment with zidovudine in any patient who develops clinical or laboratory findings suggestive of lactic acidosis (transaminase elevation may/may not accompany hepatomegaly and steatosis). Use caution in combination with interferon alfa with or without ribavirin in HIV/HBV coinfected patients; monitor closely for hepatic decompensation, anemia, or neutropenia; dose reduction or discontinuation of interferon and/or ribavirin may be required if toxicity evident.

[U.S. Boxed Warning]: Prolonged use has been associated with symptomatic myopathy and myositis. May cause redistribution of fat (eg, buffalo hump, peripheral wasting with increased abdominal girth, cushingoid appearance). Immune reconstitution syndrome may develop resulting in the occurrence of an inflammatory response to an indolent or residual opportunistic infection; further evaluation and treatment may be required. Reduce dose in patients with severe renal impairment. Do not administer with combination products that contain zidovudine as one of their components (eg, COMBIVIR® [lamivudine and zidovudine] or TRIZIVIR® [abacavir sulfate, lamivudine, and zidovudine]).

Drug Interactions

Avoid Concomitant Use

Avoid concomitant use of Zidovudine with any of the following: CloZAPine; Stavudine

Decreased Effect

Zidovudine may decrease the levels/effects of: Stavudine

The levels/effects of Zidovudine may be decreased by: Clarithromycin; DOXOrubicin; DOXOrubicin (Liposomal); Protease Inhibitors; Rifamycin Derivatives; Tocilizumab

Increased Effect/Toxicity

Zidovudine may increase the levels/effects of: CloZAPine; Ribavirin

The levels/effects of Zidovudine may be increased by: Acyclovir-Valacyclovir; Clarithromycin; Conivaptan; Divalproex; DOXOrubicin; DOXOrubicin (Liposomal); Fluconazole; Ganciclovir-Valganciclovir; Interferons; Methadone; Probenecid; Ribavirin; Valproic Acid

Adverse Reactions As reported in adult patients with asymptomatic HIV infection. Frequency and severity may increase with advanced disease.

>10%:

Central nervous system: Headache (63%), malaise (53%)

Gastrointestinal: Nausea (51%), anorexia (20%), vomiting (17%)

1% to 10%:

Gastrointestinal: Constipation (6%)

Hematologic: Granulocytopenia (2%; onset 6-8 weeks), anemia (1%; onset 2-4 weeks)

Hepatic: Transaminases increased (1% to 3%)

Neuromuscular & skeletal: Weakness (9%)

Frequency not defined:

Cardiovascular: Cardiomyopathy, chest pain, syncope, vasculitis

Central nervous system: Anxiety, chills, confusion, depression, dizziness, fatigue, insomnia, loss of mental acuity, mania, seizure, somnolence, vertigo

Dermatologic: Pruritus, rash, skin/nail pigmentation changes, Stevens-Johnson syndrome, toxic epidermal necrolysis, urticaria

Endocrine & metabolic: Body fat redistribution, diabetes, dyslipidemias, gynecomastia, insulin resistance

Gastrointestinal: Abdominal cramps, abdominal pain, dyspepsia, dysphagia, flatulence, mouth ulcer, oral mucosa pigmentation, pancreatitis, taste perversion

Genitourinary: Urinary frequency, urinary hesitancy

Hematologic: Aplastic anemia, hemolytic anemia, leukopenia, lymphadenopathy, pancytopenia with marrow hypoplasia, pure red cell aplasia

Hepatic: Hepatitis, hepatomegaly with steatosis, hyperbilirubinemia, jaundice, lactic acidosis

Neuromuscular & skeletal: Arthralgia, back pain, CPK increased, LDH increased, musculoskeletal pain, myalgia, neuropathy, muscle spasm, myopathy, myositis, paresthesia, rhabdomyolysis, tremor

Ocular: Amblyopia, macular edema, photophobia

Otic: Hearing loss

Respiratory: Cough, dyspnea, rhinitis, sinusitis

Miscellaneous: Allergic reactions, anaphylaxis, angioedema, diaphoresis, flu-like syndrome, immune reconstitution syndrome

Available Dosage Forms

Capsule, oral: 100 mg

Retrovir®: 100 mg

Injection, solution [preservative free]:

Retrovir®: 10 mg/mL (20 mL)

Syrup, oral: 50 mg/5 mL (240 mL)

Retrovir®: 50 mg/5 mL (240 mL)

Tablet, oral: 300 mg

Retrovir®: 300 mg

General Dosage Range Dosage adjustment recommended in patients with renal impairment or who develop toxicities

I.V.:

Infants <30 weeks gestation at birth: 1.5 mg/kg/dose every 12 hours; at 4 weeks of age advance to 1.5 mg/kg/dose every 8 hours

Infants ≥30 weeks and <35 weeks gestation at birth: 2 mg/kg/dose every 12 hours; at 2 weeks of age, advance to 1.5 mg/kg/dose every 8 hours

Infants (full term): 1.5 mg/kg/dose every 6 hours

Children 6 weeks to <12 years: 120 mg/m²/dose every 6 hours **or** 20 mg/m²/hour as a continuous infusion

Children ≥12 years and Adults: 1 mg/kg/dose every 4 hours around-the-clock **or** 2 mg/kg bolus followed by 1 mg/kg/hour continuous infusion

Oral:

Infants <30 weeks gestation at birth: 2 mg/kg/dose every 12 hours; at 4 weeks of age advance to 2 mg/kg/dose every 8 hours

Infants ≥30 weeks and <35 weeks gestation at birth: 2 mg/kg/dose every 12 hours; at 2 weeks of age, advance to 2 mg/kg/dose every 8 hours

Infants (full term): 4 mg/kg/dose twice daily

Children 4 weeks to <18 years: 240 mg/m^2 every 12 hours (maximum 300 mg every 12 hours) **or** 160 mg/m^2/dose every 8 hours (maximum: 200 mg every 8 hours)

4 to <9 kg: 12 mg/kg/dose twice daily **or** 8 mg/kg/dose 3 times/day

≥9 to <30 kg: 9 mg/kg/dose twice daily **or** 6 mg/kg/dose 3 times/day

≥30 kg and Adults: 300 mg twice daily **or** 200 mg 3 times/day

Administration

Oral Administer around-the-clock to promote less variation in peak and trough serum levels. Oral zidovudine may be administered without regard to meals.

I.M. Do not give I.M.

I.V. Avoid rapid infusion or bolus injection

Neonates: Infuse over 30 minutes

Adults: Infuse loading dose over 1 hour, followed by continuous infusion

I.V. Detail pH: 5.5

Stability

Reconstitution Solution for injection should be diluted with D_5W to a concentration ≤4 mg/mL. Attempt to administer diluted solution within 8 hours if stored at room temperature or 24 hours if refrigerated to minimize potential for microbial-contaminated solutions ≥≥(vials are single-use and do not contain preservative).

Storage

I.V.: Store undiluted vials at 15°C to 25°C (59°F to 77°F). Protect from light. When diluted, solution is physically and chemically stable for 24 hours at room temperature and 48 hours if refrigerated.

Tablets, capsules, syrup: Store at 15°C to 25°C (59°F to 77°F). Protect capsules from moisture.

Nursing Actions

Physical Assessment Allergy history should be assessed prior to beginning treatment. Monitor for lactic acidosis (elevated transaminases), anemia, neutropenia, hepatic decompensation, gastrointestinal disturbance (nausea, vomiting, diarrhea), myalgia, and peripheral neuropathy. Teach patient proper timing of multiple medications.

Patient Education This drug will not cure HIV, nor has it been found to reduce transmission of HIV; use appropriate precautions to prevent spread to other persons. This drug is prescribed as one part of a multidrug combination; take exactly as directed for full course of therapy. Maintain adequate hydration unless advised by prescriber to restrict fluids. Avoid alcohol. Frequent blood tests may be required. May cause body changes due to redistribution of body fat, facial atrophy, or breast enlargement (normal effects of drug). May cause headache, dizziness, weakness, nausea, vomiting, mouth sores, constipation, CNS changes (anxiety, chills, confusion, depression, loss of mental acuity, or seizures - contact prescriber), or back or muscle pain. Report excessive fatigue, easy bruising or bleeding, change in urinary pattern, dark urine or light stool, chest pain or palpitations, rash or skin sores, muscle or bone pain, or tremor. Stop drug and report immediately symptoms of hypersensitivity/allergic reaction (eg, swelling of lips, face, mouth, or throat; rash; difficulty breathing or chest tightness; excessive sweating; numbness or loss of sensation). Do not restart without specific instruction by your prescriber.

Dietary Considerations May be taken without regard to meals.

Zileuton (zye LOO ton)

Brand Names: U.S. Zyflo CR®; Zyflo®

Pharmacologic Category 5-Lipoxygenase Inhibitor

Pregnancy Risk Factor C

Lactation Excretion in breast milk unknown/not recommended

Breast-Feeding Considerations Due to the potential tumorigenicity of zileuton in animal studies, the manufacturer does not recommend breast-feeding.

Use Prophylaxis and chronic treatment of asthma

Mechanism of Action/Effect Inhibits leukotriene formation which contributes to inflammation, edema, mucous secretion, and bronchoconstriction in the airway of the asthmatic.

Contraindications Hypersensitivity to zileuton or any component of the formulation; active liver disease or transaminase elevations ≥3 times ULN

Warnings/Precautions Not appropriate or indicated for the reversal of bronchospasm in acute asthma attacks, including status asthmaticus; therapy may be continued during acute asthma exacerbations. Hepatic adverse effects have been reported (elevated transaminase levels); females >65 years and patients with pre-existing elevated transaminases may be at greater risk. Serum ALT should be monitored. Discontinue zileuton and follow transaminases until normal if patients develop clinical signs/symptoms of liver dysfunction or with transaminase levels >5 times ULN (use caution with history of liver disease and/or in those patients who consume substantial quantities of ethanol). Postmarketing reports of behavioral changes and sleep disorders have been noted.

Drug Interactions

Avoid Concomitant Use

Avoid concomitant use of Zileuton with any of the following: Pimozide

Decreased Effect

The levels/effects of Zileuton may be decreased by: Cyproterone; Tocilizumab

Increased Effect/Toxicity

Zileuton may increase the levels/effects of: Pimozide; Propranolol; Theophylline; Warfarin

The levels/effects of Zileuton may be increased by: Conivaptan

Nutritional/Ethanol Interactions
Ethanol: Avoid ethanol (may increase CNS depression; may increase risk of hepatic toxicity).
Food: Zyflo CR®: Improved absorption when administered with food.
Herb/Nutraceutical: St John's wort may decrease zileuton levels.

Adverse Reactions
>10%: Central nervous system: Headache (23% to 25%)
1% to 10%:
Cardiovascular: Chest pain
Central nervous system: Pain (8%), dizziness, fever, insomnia, malaise, nervousness, somnolence
Dermatologic: Pruritus, rash
Gastrointestinal: Dyspepsia (8%), diarrhea (5%), nausea (5% to 6%), abdominal pain (5%), constipation, flatulence, vomiting
Genitourinary: Urinary tract infection, vaginitis
Hematologic: Leukopenia (1% to 3%)
Hepatic: ALT increased (≥3 x ULN: 2% to 5%), hepatotoxicity
Neuromuscular & skeletal: Myalgia (7%), weakness (4%), arthralgia, hypertonia, neck pain/rigidity
Ocular: Conjunctivitis
Respiratory: Upper respiratory tract infection (9%), sinusitis (7%), pharyngolaryngeal pain (5%)
Miscellaneous: Hypersensitivity reactions, lymphadenopathy

Available Dosage Forms
Tablet, oral:
Zyflo®: 600 mg [scored]
Tablet, extended release, oral:
Zyflo CR®: 600 mg

General Dosage Range Oral:
Extended release: *Children ≥12 years and Adults:* 1200 mg twice daily
Immediate release: *Children ≥12 years and Adults:* 600 mg 4 times/day

Administration
Oral
Immediate release: Administer without regard to meals.
Extended release: Do not crush, cut, or chew tablet; administer within 1 hour after morning and evening meals.

Stability
Storage Store tablets at 20°C to 25°C (68°F to 77°F). Protect from light.

Nursing Actions
Physical Assessment Not for use to relieve acute asthmatic attacks. Monitor vital signs and lung sounds prior to and periodically during therapy.
Patient Education This medication is not for an acute asthmatic attack. Do not stop other asthma medication. Avoid alcohol. You may experience mild headache, belly pain, nausea, vomiting, or diarrhea. Report skin rash; flu-like symptoms; severe nausea, vomiting, or diarrhea; inability to eat; itching; jaundice or dark urine; or worsening of asthmatic condition.

Dietary Considerations
Immediate release: Take without regard to meals.
Extended release: Take with food.

Ziprasidone (zi PRAS i done)

Brand Names: U.S. Geodon®
Index Terms Zeldox; Ziprasidone Hydrochloride; Ziprasidone Mesylate
Pharmacologic Category Antipsychotic Agent, Atypical

Medication Safety Issues
Sound-alike/look-alike issues:
Ziprasidone may be confused with TraZODone

Pregnancy Risk Factor C
Lactation Excretion in breast milk unknown/not recommended
Use Treatment of schizophrenia; treatment of acute manic or mixed episodes associated with bipolar disorder with or without psychosis; maintenance treatment of bipolar disorder as an adjunct to lithium or valproate; acute agitation in patients with schizophrenia
Unlabeled Use Tourette's syndrome; psychosis/agitation related to Alzheimer's dementia
Mechanism of Action/Effect Ziprasidone is a benzylisothiazolylpiperazine antipsychotic which blocks a number of CNS receptors, including dopamine, serotonin, alpha$_1$ adrenergic, and histamine receptors. Also inhibits reuptake of serotonin and epinephrine. Results in improvement in positive and negative symptoms of schizophrenia.
Contraindications Hypersensitivity to ziprasidone or any component of the formulation; history of (or current) prolonged QT; congenital long QT syndrome; recent myocardial infarction; uncompensated heart failure; concurrent use of other QT$_c$-prolonging agents including arsenic trioxide, chlorpromazine, class Ia antiarrhythmics (eg, disopyramide, quinidine, procainamide), class III antiarrhythmics (eg, amiodarone, dofetilide, ibutilide, sotalol), dolasetron, droperidol, gatifloxacin, levomethadyl, mefloquine, mesoridazine, moxifloxacin, pentamidine, pimozide, probucol, tacrolimus, and thioridazine
Warnings/Precautions [U.S. Boxed Warning]: Elderly patients with dementia-related behavioral disorders treated with antipsychotics are at an increased risk of death compared to placebo. Most deaths appeared to be either cardiovascular (eg, heart failure, sudden death) or infectious (eg, pneumonia) in nature. Ziprasidone is not approved for the treatment of dementia-related psychosis.

May result in QT_c prolongation (dose related), which has been associated with the development of malignant ventricular arrhythmias (torsade de pointes) and sudden death. Note contraindications related to this effect. Observed prolongation was greater than with other atypical antipsychotic agents (risperidone, olanzapine, quetiapine), but less than with thioridazine. Correct electrolyte disturbances, especially hypokalemia or hypomagnesemia, prior to use and throughout therapy. Use caution in patients with bradycardia. Discontinue in patients found to have persistent QT_c intervals >500 msec. Patients with symptoms of dizziness, palpitations, or syncope should receive further cardiac evaluation. May cause orthostatic hypotension. Use is contraindicated in patients with recent acute myocardial infarction (MI), QT prolongation, or uncompensated heart failure. Avoid use in patients with a history of cardiac arrhythmias; use with caution in patients with history of MI or unstable heart disease.

Leukopenia, neutropenia, and agranulocytosis (sometimes fatal) have been reported in clinical trials and postmarketing reports with antipsychotic use; presence of risk factors (eg, pre-existing low WBC or history of drug-induced leuko-/neutropenia) should prompt periodic blood count assessment. Discontinue therapy at first signs of blood dyscrasias or if absolute neutrophil count <1000/mm^3.

May cause extrapyramidal symptoms (EPS). Risk of dystonia (and probably other EPS) may be greater with increased doses, use of conventional antipsychotics, males, and younger patients. Impaired core body temperature regulation may occur; caution with strenuous exercise, heat exposure, dehydration, and concomitant medication possessing anticholinergic effects; not reported in premarketing trials of ziprasidone. Antipsychotic use may also be associated with neuroleptic malignant syndrome (NMS). Use with caution in patients at risk of seizures.

Atypical antipsychotics have been associated with development of hyperglycemia. There is limited documentation with ziprasidone and specific risk associated with this agent is not known. Use caution in patients with diabetes or other disorders of glucose regulation; monitor for worsening of glucose control. May increase prolactin levels; clinical significance of hyperprolactinemia in patients with breast cancer or other prolactin-dependent tumors is unknown.

Cognitive and/or motor impairment (sedation) is common with ziprasidone. Use with caution in disorders where CNS depression is a feature. Use with caution in Parkinson's disease. Antipsychotic use has been associated with esophageal dysmotility and aspiration; use with caution in patients at risk of pneumonia (ie, Alzheimer's disease). Use caution in hepatic impairment. Ziprasidone has been associated with a fairly high incidence of rash (5%). Significant weight gain has been observed with antipsychotic therapy; incidence varies with product. Monitor waist circumference and BMI. Rare cases of priapism have been reported. Use the intramuscular formulation with caution in patients with renal impairment; formulation contains cyclodextrin, an excipient which may accumulate in renal insufficiency.

The possibility of a suicide attempt is inherent in psychotic illness or bipolar disorder; use caution in high-risk patients during initiation of therapy. Prescriptions should be written for the smallest quantity consistent with good patient care.

Drug Interactions

Avoid Concomitant Use

Avoid concomitant use of Ziprasidone with any of the following: Artemether; Dronedarone; Lumefantrine; Metoclopramide; Nilotinib; Pimozide; QTc-Prolonging Agents; QUEtiapine; QuiNINE; Tetrabenazine; Thioridazine; Toremifene; Vandetanib; Vemurafenib

Decreased Effect

Ziprasidone may decrease the levels/effects of: Amphetamines; Anti-Parkinson's Agents (Dopamine Agonist); Quinagolide

The levels/effects of Ziprasidone may be decreased by: CarBAMazepine; Cyproterone; Lithium formulations; Tocilizumab

Increased Effect/Toxicity

Ziprasidone may increase the levels/effects of: Alcohol (Ethyl); ARIPiprazole; CNS Depressants; Dronedarone; Methylphenidate; Pimozide; QTc-Prolonging Agents; QuiNINE; Serotonin Modulators; Tetrabenazine; Thioridazine; Toremifene; Vandetanib; Vemurafenib

The levels/effects of Ziprasidone may be increased by: Acetylcholinesterase Inhibitors (Central); Alfuzosin; Antifungal Agents (Azole Derivatives, Systemic); Artemether; Chloroquine; Ciprofloxacin; Ciprofloxacin (Systemic); Conivaptan; Gadobutrol; HydrOXYzine; Indacaterol; Lithium formulations; Lumefantrine; Methylphenidate; Metoclopramide; Nilotinib; QTc-Prolonging Agents; QUEtiapine; QuiNINE; Tetrabenazine

Nutritional/Ethanol Interactions

Ethanol: May increase CNS depression; monitor for increased effects with coadministration. Caution patients about effects.

Food: Administration with food increases serum levels twofold. Grapefruit juice may increase serum concentration of ziprasidone.

Herb/Nutraceutical: St John's wort may decrease serum levels of ziprasidone, due to a potential effect on CYP3A4. This has not been specifically studied. Avoid kava kava, chamomile (may increase CNS depression).

Adverse Reactions Note: Although minor QT_c prolongation (mean: 10 msec at 160 mg/day) may occur more frequently (incidence not specified), clinically-relevant prolongation (>500 msec) was rare (0.06%) and less than placebo (0.23%).

>10%:

Central nervous system: Extrapyramidal symptoms (2% to 31%), somnolence (8% to 31%), headache (3% to 18%), dizziness (3% to 16%)

Gastrointestinal: Nausea (4% to 12%)

1% to 10%:

Cardiovascular: Postural hypotension (5%), chest pain (3%), hypertension (2% to 3%), tachycardia (2%), bradycardia (≤2%), facial edema (1%), vasodilation (≤1%), orthostatic hypotension

Central nervous system: Akathisia (2% to 10%), anxiety (2% to 5%), insomnia (3%), agitation (2%), speech disorder (2%), personality disorder (2%), akinesia (≥1%), amnesia (≥1%), ataxia (≥1%), confusion (≥1%), coordination abnormal (≥1%), delirium (≥1%), dystonia (≥1%), hostility (≥1%), oculogyric crisis (≥1%), vertigo (≥1%), chills (1%), fever (1%), hypothermia (1%), psychosis (1%)

Dermatologic: Rash (4% to 5%), fungal dermatitis (2%)

Endocrine & metabolic: Dysmenorrhea (2%)

Gastrointestinal: Weight gain (6% to 10%), constipation (2% to 9%), dyspepsia (1% to 8%), diarrhea (3% to 5%), vomiting (3% to 5%), xerostomia (1% to 5%), salivation increased (4%), tongue edema (≤3%), anorexia (2%), abdominal pain (≤2%), dysphagia (≤2%), rectal hemorrhage (≤2%), buccoglossal syndrome (≥1%)

Genitourinary: Priapism (1%)

Local: Injection site pain (7% to 9%)

Neuromuscular & skeletal: Weakness (2% to 6%), hypoesthesia (2%), myalgia (2%), paresthesia (2%), abnormal gait (≥1%), choreoathetosis (≥1%), dysarthria (≥1%), dyskinesia (≥1%), hyper-/hypokinesia (≥1%), hypotonia (≥1%), neuropathy (≥1%), tremor (≥1%), twitching (≥1%), back pain (1%), cogwheel rigidity (1%), hypertonia (1%)

Ocular: Vision abnormal (3% to 6%), diplopia (≥1%)

Respiratory: Infection (8%), rhinitis (1% to 4%), cough (3%), pharyngitis (3%), dyspnea (2%)

Miscellaneous: Diaphoresis (2%), furunculosis (2%), withdrawal syndrome (≥1%), flank pain (1%), flu-like syndrome (1%), photosensitivity reaction (1%),

Available Dosage Forms

Capsule, oral: 20 mg, 40 mg, 60 mg, 80 mg

Geodon®: 20 mg, 40 mg, 60 mg, 80 mg

Injection, powder for reconstitution:

Geodon®: 20 mg

General Dosage Range

I.M.: *Adults:* 10 mg every 2 hours **or** 20 mg every 4 hours (maximum: 40 mg/day)

Oral: *Adults:* Initial: 20-40 mg twice daily; Maintenance: 20-80 mg twice daily (maximum: 200 mg/day)

Administration

Oral Administer with food.

I.M. Injection: For I.M. administration only.

Stability

Reconstitution Each vial should be reconstituted with 1.2 mL SWFI. Shake vigorously; will form a pale, pink solution containing 20 mg/mL ziprasidone.

Storage

Capsule: Store at 25°C (77°F); excursion permitted to 15°C to 30°C (59°F to 86°F).

Vials for injection: Store at 25°C (77°F); excursion permitted to 15°C to 30°C (59°F to 86°F). Protect from light. Following reconstitution, injection may be stored at room temperature up to 24 hours or under refrigeration for up to 7 days. Protect from light.

Nursing Actions

Physical Assessment Monitor weight prior to initiating therapy and at least monthly.

Patient Education It may take 2-3 weeks to achieve desired results. Avoid alcohol. Maintain adequate hydration. If you have diabetes, you may experience increased blood sugars; monitor closely. You may experience drowsiness, lightheadedness, impaired coordination, dizziness, or blurred vision; dry mouth, nausea, or GI upset; postural hypotension; urinary retention; or constipation. Report persistent CNS effects (eg, trembling, altered gait or balance, excessive sedation, seizures, unusual muscle or skeletal movements, excessive anxiety, hallucinations, nightmares, suicide ideation, confusion), swelling or pain in breasts (male or female), altered menstrual pattern, sexual dysfunction, alteration in urinary pattern, vision changes, rash, respiratory difficulty, or chest pain or palpitations.

Dietary Considerations Take with food.

Zoledronic Acid (zoe le DRON ik AS id)

Brand Names: U.S. Reclast®; Zometa®

Index Terms CGP-42446; Zol 446; Zoledronate

Pharmacologic Category Antidote; Bisphosphonate Derivative

Medication Safety Issues

Sound-alike/look-alike issues:

Zometa® may be confused with Zofran®, Zoladex®

Other safety concerns:

Duplicate therapy issues: Reclast® and Aclasta® contain zoledronic acid, which is the same ingredient contained in Zometa®; patients receiving Zometa® should not be treated with Reclast® or Aclasta®

Medication Guide Available Yes

Pregnancy Risk Factor D

Lactation Excretion in breast milk unknown/not recommended

Breast-Feeding Considerations Because it binds to bone long term, zoledronic acid use is not recommended in nursing women.

Use

Oncology-related uses: Treatment of hypercalcemia of malignancy (albumin-corrected serum calcium >12 mg/dL); treatment of multiple myeloma; treatment of bone metastases of solid tumors

Nononcology uses: Treatment of Paget's disease of bone; treatment of osteoporosis in postmenopausal women (to reduce the incidence of fractures or to reduce the incidence of new clinical fractures in patients with low-trauma hip fracture); prevention of osteoporosis in postmenopausal women, treatment of osteoporosis in men (to increase bone mass); treatment and prevention of glucocorticoid-induced osteoporosis (in patients initiating or continuing prednisone ≥7.5 mg/day [or equivalent] and expected to remain on glucocorticoids for at least 12 months)

Unlabeled Use Prevention of bone loss associated with aromatase inhibitor therapy in postmenopausal women with breast cancer; prevention of bone loss associated with androgen deprivation therapy in prostate cancer

Mechanism of Action/Effect A bisphosphonate which inhibits bone resorption via actions on osteoclasts or on osteoclast precursors; inhibits osteoclastic activity and skeletal calcium release induced by tumors. Decreases serum calcium and phosphorus, and increases their elimination. In osteoporosis, zoledronic acid inhibits osteoclast-mediated resorption, therefore reducing bone turnover.

Contraindications Hypersensitivity to zoledronic acid or any component of the formulation; hypocalcemia (Reclast®); in patients with a creatinine clearance (Cl_{cr}) <35 mL/minute and in patients with evidence of acute renal impairment due to an increased risk of renal failure (Reclast®)

Canadian labeling: Hypersensitivity to other bisphosphonates. Aclasta® is also contraindicated with uncorrected hypocalcemia at the time of infusion and in pregnancy and breast-feeding.

Warnings/Precautions Osteonecrosis of the jaw (ONJ) has been reported in patients receiving bisphosphonates. Risk factors include invasive dental procedures (eg, tooth extraction, dental implants, boney surgery); a diagnosis of cancer, with concomitant chemotherapy, radiotherapy, or corticosteroids; poor oral hygiene, ill-fitting dentures; and comorbid disorders (anemia, coagulopathy, infection, pre-existing dental disease). Most reported cases occurred after I.V. bisphosphonate therapy; however, cases have been reported following oral therapy. A dental exam and preventative dentistry should be performed prior to placing patients with risk factors on chronic bisphosphonate therapy. The manufacturer's labeling states that there are no data to suggest whether discontinuing bisphosphonates in patients requiring invasive dental procedures reduces the risk of ONJ. However, other experts suggest that there is no evidence that discontinuing therapy reduces the risk of developing ONJ (Assael, 2009). The benefit/risk must be assessed by the treating physician and/or dentist/surgeon prior to any invasive dental procedure. Patients developing ONJ while on bisphosphonates should receive care by an oral surgeon.

Atypical, low energy, or low trauma femur fractures have been reported in patients receiving bisphosphonates for treatment/prevention of osteoporosis. The fractures include subtrochanteric femur (bone just below the hip joint) and diaphyseal femur (long segment of the thigh bone). Some patients experience prodromal pain weeks or months before the fracture occurs. It is unclear if bisphosphonate therapy is the cause for these fractures; atypical femur fractures have also been reported in patients not taking bisphosphonates, and in patients receiving glucocorticoids. Patients receiving long-term (>3-5 years) bisphosphonate therapy may be at an increased risk. Patients presenting with thigh or groin pain with a history of receiving bisphosphonates should be evaluated for femur fracture. Consider interrupting bisphosphonate therapy in patients who develop a femoral shaft fracture; assess for fracture in the contralateral limb.

Infrequently, severe (and occasionally debilitating) musculoskeletal (bone, joint, and/or muscle) pain have been reported during bisphosphonate treatment. The onset of pain ranged from a single day to several months. Consider discontinuing therapy in patients who experience severe symptoms; symptoms usually resolve upon discontinuation. Some patients experienced recurrence when rechallenged with same drug or another bisphosphonate; avoid use in patients with a history of these symptoms in association with bisphosphonate therapy.

May cause a significant risk of hypocalcemia in patients with Paget's disease, in whom the pretreatment rate of bone turnover may be greatly elevated. Hypocalcemia must be corrected before initiation of therapy in patients with Paget's disease and osteoporosis. Ensure adequate calcium and vitamin D intake during therapy. Use caution in patients with disturbances of calcium and mineral metabolism (eg, hypoparathyroidism, thyroid/parathyroid, surgery, malabsorption syndromes, excision of small intestine).

Reclast®: Use is contraindicated in patients with Cl_{cr} <35 mL/minute and in patients with evidence of acute renal impairment due to an increased risk of renal failure. Re-evaluate the need for continued therapy for the treatment of osteoporosis periodically; the optimal duration of treatment has not yet been determined.

Zometa®: Use caution in mild-to-moderate renal dysfunction; dosage adjustment required. In cancer patients, renal toxicity has been reported with doses >4 mg or infusions administered over 15 minutes. Risk factors for renal deterioration include pre-existing renal insufficiency and repeated doses of zoledronic acid and other bisphosphonates. Dehydration and the use of other nephrotoxic drugs which may contribute to renal deterioration should be identified and managed. Use is not recommended in patients with severe renal impairment (serum creatinine >3 mg/dL or Cl_{cr} <30 mL/minute) and bone metastases (limited data); use in patients with hypercalcemia of malignancy and severe renal impairment (serum creatinine >4.5 mg/dL for hypercalcemia of malignancy) should only be done if the benefits outweigh the risks. Renal function should be assessed prior to treatment; if decreased after treatment, additional treatments should be withheld until renal function returns to within 10% of baseline. Diuretics should not be used before correcting hypovolemia. Renal deterioration, resulting in renal failure and dialysis has occurred in patients treated with zoledronic acid after single and multiple infusions at recommended doses of 4 mg over 15 minutes.

Aclasta® [CAN; not available in U.S.]: Use is not recommended in patients with Cl_{cr} <30 mL/minute.

According to the American Society of Clinical Oncology (ASCO) guidelines for bisphosphonates in multiple myeloma, treatment with zoledronic acid is not recommended for asymptomatic (smoldering) or indolent myeloma or with solitary plasmacytoma (Kyle, 2007). The National Comprehensive Cancer Network® (NCCN) multiple myeloma guidelines (v.1.2011) also do not recommend the use of bisphosphonates in stage 1 or smoldering disease, unless part of a clinical trial.

Adequate hydration is required during treatment (urine output ~2 L/day); avoid overhydration, especially in patients with heart failure. Pre-existing renal compromise, severe dehydration, and concurrent use with diuretics or other nephrotoxic drugs may increase the risk for renal impairment. Single and multiple infusions in patients with both normal and impaired renal function have been associated with renal deterioration, resulting in renal failure and dialysis or death (rare). Patients with underlying moderate-to-severe renal impairment, increased age, concurrent use of nephrotoxic or diuretic medications, or severe dehydration prior to or after zoledronic acid administration may have an increased risk of acute renal impairment or renal failure. Others with increased risk include patients with renal impairment or dehydration secondary to fever, sepsis, gastrointestinal losses, or diuretic use. If history or physical exam suggests dehydration, treatment should not be given until the patient is normovolemic. Creatinine clearance (using actual body weight) should be calculated with the Cockcroft-Gault formula prior to each administration. Transient increases in serum creatinine may be more pronounced in patients with impaired renal function; consider monitoring creatinine clearance in at-risk patients taking other renally-eliminated drugs.

Use caution in patients with aspirin-sensitive asthma (may cause bronchoconstriction) and the elderly. Rare cases of urticaria and angioedema and very rare cases of anaphylactic reactions/shock have been reported. Women of childbearing age should be advised against becoming pregnant. Not approved for use in children. Do not administer Zometa® and Reclast® to the same patient for different indications.

Drug Interactions

Avoid Concomitant Use There are no known interactions where it is recommended to avoid concomitant use.

Decreased Effect

The levels/effects of Zoledronic Acid may be decreased by: Proton Pump Inhibitors

Increased Effect/Toxicity

Zoledronic Acid may increase the levels/effects of: Deferasirox; Phosphate Supplements

The levels/effects of Zoledronic Acid may be increased by: Aminoglycosides; Nonsteroidal Anti-Inflammatory Agents; Thalidomide

Adverse Reactions Note: An acute reaction (eg, arthralgia, fever, flu-like symptoms, myalgia) may occur within the first 3 days following infusion in up to 44% of patients; usually resolves within 3-4 days of onset, although may take up to 14 days to resolve. The incidence may be decreased with acetaminophen (prior to infusion and for 72 hours postinfusion).

Zometa®:

>10%:

Cardiovascular: Leg edema (5% to 21%), hypotension (11%)

Central nervous system: Fatigue (39%), fever (32% to 44%), headache (5% to 19%), dizziness (18%), insomnia (15% to 16%), anxiety (11% to 14%), depression (14%), agitation (13%), confusion (7% to 13%), hypoesthesia (12%)

Dermatologic: Alopecia (12%), dermatitis (11%)

Endocrine & metabolic: Dehydration (5% to 14%), hypophosphatemia (13%), hypokalemia (12%), hypomagnesemia (11%)

Gastrointestinal: Nausea (29% to 46%), vomiting (14% to 32%), constipation (27% to 31%), diarrhea (17% to 24%), anorexia (9% to 22%), abdominal pain (14% to 16%), weight loss (16%), appetite decreased (13%)

Genitourinary: Urinary tract infection (12% to 14%)

Hematologic: Anemia (22% to 33%), neutropenia (12%)

Neuromuscular & skeletal: Bone pain (55%), weakness (5% to 24%), myalgia (23%), arthralgia (5% to 21%), back pain (15%), paresthesia (15%), limb pain (14%), skeletal pain (12%), rigors (11%)

Renal: Renal deterioration (8% to 17%; up to 40% in patients with abnormal baseline creatinine)

Respiratory: Dyspnea (22% to 27%), cough (12% to 22%)

Miscellaneous: Cancer progression (16% to 20%), moniliasis (12%)

1% to 10%:

Cardiovascular: Chest pain (5% to 10%)

Central nervous system: Somnolence (5% to 10%)

Endocrine & metabolic: Hypocalcemia (5% to 10%; grades 3/4: ≤1%), hypermagnesemia (grade 3: 2%)

Gastrointestinal: Dysphagia (5% to 10%), dyspepsia (10%), mucositis (5% to 10%), stomatitis (8%), sore throat (8%)

Hematologic: Granulocytopenia (5% to 10%), pancytopenia (5% to 10%), thrombocytopenia (5% to 10%)

Renal: Serum creatinine increased (grades 3/4: ≤2%)

Respiratory: Upper respiratory tract infection (10%)

Miscellaneous: Infection (nonspecific; 5% to 10%)

Reclast®:

>10%:

Cardiovascular: Hypertension (5% to 13%)

Central nervous system: Pain (2% to 24%), fever (9% to 22%), headache (4% to 20%), chills (2% to 18%), fatigue (2% to 18%)

Endocrine & metabolic: Hypocalcemia (≤3%; Paget's disease 21%)

Gastrointestinal: Nausea (5% to 18%)

Neuromuscular & skeletal: Arthralgia (9% to 27%), myalgia (5% to 23%), back pain (4% to 18%), limb pain (3% to 16%), musculoskeletal pain (≤12%)

Miscellaneous: Acute phase reaction (4% to 25%), flu-like syndrome (1% to 11%)

1% to 10%:

Cardiovascular: Chest pain (1% to 8%), peripheral edema (3% to 6%), atrial fibrillation (1% to 3%), palpitation (≤3%)

Central nervous system: Dizziness (2% to 9%), malaise (1% to 7%), hypoesthesia (≤6%), lethargy (3% to 5%), vertigo (1% to 4%), hyperthermia (≤2%)

Dermatologic: Rash (2% to 3%), hyperhidrosis (≤3%)

Gastrointestinal: Abdominal pain (1% to 9%), diarrhea (5% to 8%), vomiting (2% to 8%), constipation (6% to 7%), dyspepsia (2% to 7%), abdominal discomfort/distension (1% to 2%), anorexia (1% to 2%)

Neuromuscular & skeletal: Bone pain (3% to 9%), arthritis (2% to 9%), rigors (8%), shoulder pain (≤7%), neck pain (1% to 7%), weakness (2% to 6%), muscle spasm (2% to 6%), stiffness (1% to 5%), jaw pain (2% to 4%), joint swelling (≤3%), paresthesia (2%)

Ocular: Eye pain (≤2%)

Renal: Serum creatinine increased (2%)

Respiratory: Dyspnea (5% to 7%)

Miscellaneous: C-reactive protein increased (≤5%)

Available Dosage Forms

Infusion, premixed:

Reclast®: 5 mg (100 mL)

Zometa®: 4 mg (100 mL)

Injection, solution:

Zometa®: 4 mg/5 mL (5 mL)

General Dosage Range Dosage adjustment recommended in patients with renal impairment or who develop toxicities

I.V.: *Adults:*

Zometa®: 4 mg as a single dose or every 3-4 weeks

Reclast®: 5 mg as a single dose, once a year or every 2 years

Administration

I.V. Infuse over at least 15 minutes. Flush I.V. line with 10 mL NS flush following infusion. Infuse in a line separate from other medications. Patients should be appropriately hydrated prior to treatment.

Reclast®, Zometa®: If refrigerated, allow to reach room temperature prior to administration. Acetaminophen after administration may reduce the incidence of acute reaction (eg, arthralgia, fever, flu-like symptoms, myalgia).

I.V. Detail

Zometa®: pH: ~2

Reclast®, Aclasta® [CAN]: pH 6-7 (infusion)

Stability

Reconstitution

Zometa® concentrate vials: Further dilute in 100 mL NS or D_5W prior to administration.

Zometa® ready-to use bottles: No further preparation necessary. If reduced doses are necessary for patients with renal impairment, withdraw the appropriate volume of solution and replace with an equal amount of NS or D_5W.

Storage

Aclasta® [CAN]: Store at room temperature of 15°C to 30°C (59°F to 86°F).

Reclast®: Store at room temperature of 25°C (77°F); excursions permitted to 15°C to 30°C (59°F to 86°F). After opening, stable for 24 hours at 2°C to 8°C (36°F to 46°F).

Zometa®: Store concentrate vials and ready-to-use bottles at 25°C (77°F); excursions permitted to 15°C to 30°C (59°F to 86°F). Diluted solutions for infusion which are not used immediately after preparation should be refrigerated at 2°C to 8°C (36°F to 46°F). Infusion of solution must be completed within 24 hours of preparation. The ready-to-use bottles are for single use only; if any preparation is necessary (preparing reduced dosage for patients with renal impairment), the prepared, diluted solution may be refrigerated at 2°C to 8°C (36°F to 46°F) if not used immediately. Infusion of solution must be completed within 24 hours of preparation. The previously withdrawn volume from the ready-to-use solution should be discarded; do not store or reuse.

Nursing Actions

Physical Assessment Assess kidney function prior to administration. Decision to administer medication may change if patient has severe renal dysfunction. A thorough oral exam should be done prior to initiating any therapy. Patients need to be instructed on maintaining good oral hygiene throughout treatment. It is important to know that if a patient is undergoing chemotherapy, radiation therapy, or a combination of both, they are at a higher risk for osteonecrosis of the jaw.

Patient Education Patients should be aware that a dental exam and any needed dental work should be completed before starting this medication. Patients need to understand the importance of good oral hygiene throughout treatment, especially if they are receiving chemotherapy, radiation therapy, or both.

Dietary Considerations

Multiple myeloma or metastatic bone lesions from solid tumors: Take daily calcium supplement (500 mg) and daily multivitamin (with 400 int. units vitamin D).

Osteoporosis: Ensure adequate calcium and vitamin D supplementation; general requirements are calcium 1200 mg/day and vitamin D 800-1000 int. units/day.

Paget's disease: Take elemental calcium 1500 mg/day (750 mg twice daily or 500 mg 3 times/day) and vitamin D 800 units/day, particularly during the first 2 weeks after administration.

Zolmitriptan (zohl mi TRIP tan)

Brand Names: U.S. Zomig-ZMT®; Zomig®

Index Terms 311C90

Pharmacologic Category Antimigraine Agent; Serotonin 5-$HT_{1B, 1D}$ Receptor Agonist

Medication Safety Issues

Sound-alike/look-alike issues:

ZOLMitriptan may be confused with SUMAtriptan

Pregnancy Risk Factor C

Lactation Excretion in breast milk unknown/use caution

Use Acute treatment of migraine with or without aura

Mechanism of Action/Effect Selective agonist for serotonin receptor in cranial arteries; causes vasoconstriction and relief of migraine

Contraindications Hypersensitivity to zolmitriptan or any component of the formulation; ischemic heart disease or vasospastic coronary artery disease, including Prinzmetal's angina; signs or symptoms of ischemic heart disease; uncontrolled hypertension; symptomatic Wolff-Parkinson-White syndrome or arrhythmias associated with other cardiac accessory conduction pathway disorders; use with ergotamine derivatives (within 24 hours of); use within 24 hours of another 5-HT_1 agonist; concurrent administration or within 2 weeks of discontinuing an MAO inhibitor; management of hemiplegic or basilar migraine

Nasal spray: Additional contraindications with nasal spray: Cerebrovascular syndromes (eg, stroke, TIA); peripheral vascular disease (including ischemic bowel disease)

Warnings/Precautions Zolmitriptan is indicated only in patient populations with a clear diagnosis of migraine. Not for prophylactic treatment of migraine headaches. Cardiac events (coronary artery vasospasm, transient ischemia, myocardial infarction, ventricular tachycardia/fibrillation, cardiac arrest, and death) have been reported with 5-HT_1 agonist administration. Patients who experience sensations of chest pain/pressure/tightness or symptoms suggestive of angina following dosing should be evaluated for coronary artery disease or Prinzmetal's angina before receiving additional doses; if dosing is resumed and similar symptoms recur, monitor with ECG. Should not be given to patients who have risk factors for CAD (eg, hypertension, hypercholesterolemia, smoker, obesity, diabetes, strong family history of CAD, menopause, male >40 years of age) without adequate cardiac evaluation. Patients with suspected CAD should have cardiovascular evaluation to rule out CAD before considering zolmitriptan's use; if cardiovascular evaluation negative, first dose would be safest if given in the healthcare provider's office (consider ECG monitoring). Periodic evaluation of those without cardiovascular disease, but with continued risk factors, should be done. Significant elevation in blood pressure, including hypertensive crisis, has also been reported on rare occasions in patients with and without a history of hypertension. Vasospasm-related reactions have been reported other than coronary artery vasospasm. Peripheral vascular ischemia and colonic ischemia with abdominal pain and bloody diarrhea have occurred. Cerebral/subarachnoid hemorrhage and stroke have been reported with 5-HT_1 agonist administration; nasal spray contraindicated in patients with cerebrovascular syndromes. Rarely, partial vision loss and blindness (transient and permanent) have been reported with 5-HT_1 agonists. Use with caution in patients with hepatic impairment. Zomig-ZMT™ tablets contain phenylalanine. Symptoms of agitation, confusion, hallucinations, hyper-reflexia, myoclonus, shivering, and tachycardia (serotonin syndrome) may occur with concomitant proserotonergic drugs (eg, SSRIs/SNRIs or triptans) or agents which reduce zolmitriptan's metabolism. Concurrent use of serotonin precursors (eg, tryptophan) is not recommended.

Drug Interactions

Avoid Concomitant Use

Avoid concomitant use of ZOLMitriptan with any of the following: Ergot Derivatives; MAO Inhibitors

Decreased Effect

The levels/effects of ZOLMitriptan may be decreased by: Cyproterone

Increased Effect/Toxicity

ZOLMitriptan may increase the levels/effects of: Ergot Derivatives; Metoclopramide; Serotonin Modulators

The levels/effects of ZOLMitriptan may be increased by: Antipsychotics; Cimetidine; Ergot Derivatives; MAO Inhibitors; Propranolol

Nutritional/Ethanol Interactions Ethanol: Limit use (may have additive CNS toxicity).

Adverse Reactions Percentages noted from oral preparations.

1% to 10%:

Cardiovascular: Chest pain (2% to 4%), palpitation (up to 2%)

Central nervous system: Dizziness (6% to 10%), somnolence (5% to 8%), pain (2% to 3%), vertigo (≤2%)

Gastrointestinal: Nausea (4% to 9%), xerostomia (3% to 5%), dyspepsia (1% to 3%), dysphagia (≤2%)

Neuromuscular & skeletal: Paresthesia (5% to 9%), weakness (3% to 9%), warm/cold sensation (5% to 7%), hypoesthesia (1% to 2%), myalgia (1% to 2%), myasthenia (up to 2%)

Miscellaneous: Neck/throat/jaw pain (4% to 10%), diaphoresis (up to 3%), allergic reaction (up to 1%)

Pharmacodynamics/Kinetics

Onset of Action 0.5-1 hour

Available Dosage Forms

Solution, intranasal:

Zomig®: 5 mg/0.1 mL (0.1 mL)

Tablet, oral:

Zomig®: 2.5 mg, 5 mg

Tablet, orally disintegrating, oral:

Zomig-ZMT®: 2.5 mg, 5 mg

General Dosage Range Dosage adjustment recommended in patients with hepatic impairment

Nasal inhalation: *Adults:* 1 spray (5 mg) at the onset of migraine headache; may repeat in 2 hours if no relief (maximum: 10 mg/24 hours)

Oral: *Adults:* 1.25-2.5 mg at the onset of migraine headache; may repeat in 2 hours if no relief (maximum: 10 mg/24 hours)

Administration

Oral Administer as soon as migraine headache starts. Tablets may be broken. Orally-disintegrating tablets: Must be taken whole; do not break, crush or chew. Place on tongue and allow to dissolve. Administration with liquid is not required

Other Nasal spray: Administer as soon as migraine headache starts. Blow nose gently prior to use. After removing protective cap, instill device into nostril. Block opposite nostril; breathe in gently through nose while pressing plunger of spray device. One dose (5 mg) is equal to 1 spray in 1 nostril.

Stability

Storage Store at 20°C to 25°C (68°F to 77°F). Protect from light and moisture.

Nursing Actions

Physical Assessment For use only with a clear diagnosis of migraine headaches. Monitor for hypertension, cardiac events, chest pain, nausea, dizziness, paresthesia, myalgia, and pain. Teach patient proper use (treatment of acute migraine).

Patient Education This drug is to be used to reduce your migraine, not to prevent or reduce the number of attacks. Remove orally-disintegrating tablet from blister package just before using, place on tongue, and allow to dissolve. Do not crush, break, or chew. Regular tablet may be broken in half for use. Do not remove protective cap from nasal spray until ready to use. If first dose brings relief, second dose may be taken anytime after 2 hours if migraine returns. If you have no relief with first dose, do not take a second dose without consulting prescriber. Do not exceed 10 mg in 24 hours. May cause dizziness, drowsiness, or dry mouth. Report immediately any chest pain, heart throbbing, or tightness in throat; swelling of eyelids, face, or lips; skin rash or hives; easy bruising; blood in urine, stool, or vomitus; pain or itching with urination; or pain, warmth, or numbness in extremities.

Dietary Considerations Some products may contain phenylalanine.

Zolpidem (zole PI dem)

Brand Names: U.S. Ambien CR®; Ambien®; Edluar™; Zolpimist®

Index Terms Intermezzo®; Zolpidem Tartrate

Pharmacologic Category Hypnotic, Nonbenzodiazepine

Medication Safety Issues

Sound-alike/look-alike issues:

Ambien® may be confused with Abilify®, Ativan®, Ambi 10®

Sublinox™ may be confused with Suboxone®

Zolpidem may be confused with lorazepam, zaleplon

International issues:

Ambien [U.S., Argentina, Israel] may be confused with Amyben brand name for amiodarone [Great Britain]

Medication Guide Available Yes

Pregnancy Risk Factor C

Lactation Enters breast milk/use caution (AAP rates "compatible"; AAP 2001 update pending)

Use

Ambien®, Edluar™, Zolpimist®: Short-term treatment of insomnia (with difficulty of sleep onset)

Ambien CR®: Treatment of insomnia (with difficulty of sleep onset and/or sleep maintenance)

Sublinox™ (Canadian availability; not available in U.S.): Short-term treatment of insomnia (with difficulty of sleep onset, frequent awakenings, and/or early awakenings)

Mechanism of Action/Effect Zolpidem is structurally dissimilar to benzodiazepines but enhances the activity of γ-aminobutyric acid (GABA) resulting in increased sedation. Zolpidem exhibits minimal anxiolytic, myorelaxant, and anticonvulsant properties.

Contraindications Hypersensitivity to zolpidem or any component of the formulation

Canadian labeling: Additional contraindications (not in U.S. labeling): Significant obstructive sleep apnea syndrome and acute and/or severe impairment of respiratory function; myasthenia gravis; severe hepatic impairment; personal or family history of sleepwalking

Warnings/Precautions Should be used only after evaluation of potential causes of sleep disturbance. Failure of sleep disturbance to resolve after 7-10 days may indicate psychiatric or medical illness. Hypnotics/sedatives have been associated with abnormal thinking and behavior changes including decreased inhibition, aggression, bizarre behavior, agitation, hallucinations, and depersonalization. These changes may occur unpredictably and may indicate previously unrecognized psychiatric disorders; evaluate appropriately. Sedative/hypnotics may produce withdrawal symptoms following abrupt discontinuation. Use with caution in patients with depression; worsening of depression, including suicide or suicidal ideation has been reported with the use of hypnotics. Intentional overdose may be an issue in this population. The minimum dose that will effectively treat the individual patient should be used. Prescriptions should be written for the smallest quantity consistent with good patient care. Causes CNS depression, which may impair physical and mental capabilities. Zolpidem should only be administered when the patient is able to stay in bed a full night (7-8 hours) before being active again. Effects with other sedative drugs or ethanol may be potentiated. Canadian labeling does not recommend concomitant use with alcohol.

Use caution in patients with myasthenia gravis (contraindicated in the Canadian labeling). Avoid use in patients with sleep apnea or a history of sedative-hypnotic abuse. Postmarketing studies have indicated that the use of hypnotic/sedative agents for sleep has been associated with hypersensitivity reactions including anaphylaxis as well as angioedema. An increased risk for hazardous sleep-related activities such as sleep-driving; cooking and eating food, and making phone calls while asleep have also been noted; amnesia may also occur. Discontinue treatment in patients who report any sleep-related episodes. Canadian labeling recommends avoiding use in patients with disorders (eg, restless legs syndrome, periodic limb movement disorder, sleep apnea) that may disrupt sleep and cause frequent awakenings, potentially increasing the risk of complex sleep-related behaviors.

Use caution with respiratory disease (Canadian labeling contraindicates use with acute and/or severe impairment of respiratory function). Use caution with hepatic impairment (Canadian labeling contraindicates use in severe impairment); dose adjustment required. Because of the rapid onset of action, administer immediately prior to bedtime or after the patient has gone to bed and is having difficulty falling asleep.

Use caution in the elderly; dose adjustment recommended. Closely monitor elderly or debilitated patients for impaired cognitive or motor performance. When studied for the unapproved use of insomnia associated with ADHD in children, a higher incidence (~7%) of hallucinations was reported. In addition, sleep latency did not decrease compared to placebo. Zolpidem is **not** FDA- or Health Canada-approved for use in pediatric patients.

Drug Interactions

Avoid Concomitant Use

Avoid concomitant use of Zolpidem with any of the following: Conivaptan

Decreased Effect

The levels/effects of Zolpidem may be decreased by: CarBAMazepine; CYP3A4 Inducers (Strong); Cyproterone; Deferasirox; Flumazenil; Herbs (CYP3A4 Inducers); Peginterferon Alfa-2b; Rifamycin Derivatives; Telaprevir; Tocilizumab

Increased Effect/Toxicity

Zolpidem may increase the levels/effects of: Alcohol (Ethyl); CarBAMazepine; CNS Depressants; Methotrimeprazine; Selective Serotonin Reuptake Inhibitors

The levels/effects of Zolpidem may be increased by: Antifungal Agents (Azole Derivatives, Systemic); Conivaptan; CYP3A4 Inhibitors (Moderate); CYP3A4 Inhibitors (Strong); Dasatinib; Droperidol; HydrOXYzine; Ivacaftor; Methotrimeprazine

Nutritional/Ethanol Interactions

Ethanol: May enhance the adverse/toxic effects of zolpidem. Management: Avoid use of ethanol.

Food: Maximum plasma concentration and bioavailability are decreased with food; time to peak plasma concentration is increased; half-life remains unchanged. Grapefruit juice may decrease the metabolism of zolpidem. Management: Avoid grapefruit juice.

Herb/Nutraceutical: St John's wort may decrease the levels/effects of zolpidem. Some herbal medications should be avoided due to the risk of increased CNS depression. Management: Avoid concomitant use of St John's wort. Avoid valerian, kava kava, and gotu kola.

Adverse Reactions Actual frequency may be dosage form, dose, and/or age dependent

>10%: Central nervous system: Headache (7% to 19%), somnolence (6% to 15%), dizziness (1% to 12%)

1% to 10%:

Cardiovascular: Blood pressure increased, chest discomfort/pain, palpitation

Central nervous system: Abnormal dreams, anxiety, apathy, amnesia, ataxia, attention disturbance, body temperature increased, burning sensation, confusion, depersonalization, depression, disinhibition, disorientation, drowsiness, drugged feeling, euphoria, fatigue, fever, hallucinations, hypoesthesia, insomnia, lethargy, lightheadedness, memory disorder, mood swings, sleep disorder, stress

Dermatologic: Rash, urticaria, wrinkling

Endocrine & metabolic: Menorrhagia

Gastrointestinal: Abdominal discomfort, abdominal pain, abdominal tenderness, appetite disorder, constipation, diarrhea, dyspepsia, flatulence, gastroenteritis, gastroesophageal reflux, hiccup, nausea, vomiting, xerostomia

Genitourinary: Urinary tract infection, vulvovaginal dryness

Neuromuscular & skeletal: Arthralgia, back pain, balance disorder, involuntary muscle contractions, myalgia, neck pain, paresthesia, psychomotor retardation, tremor, weakness

Ocular: Asthenopia, blurred vision, depth perception altered, diplopia, red eye, visual disturbance

Otic: Labyrinthitis, tinnitus, vertigo

Renal: Dysuria

Respiratory: Pharyngitis, sinusitis, throat irritation, upper respiratory tract infection

Miscellaneous: Allergy, binge eating, flu-like syndrome

Pharmacodynamics/Kinetics

Onset of Action Immediate release: 30 minutes

Duration of Action Immediate release: 6-8 hours

Product Availability

Intermezzo® sublingual tablets: FDA approved November 2011; availability anticipated second quarter 2012

Intermezzo® sublingual tablets are indicated for as needed treatment of insomnia when middle-of-the-night awakening is followed by difficulty returning to sleep with ≥4 hours of expected sleep time remaining.

Controlled Substance C-IV

Available Dosage Forms

Solution, oral:

Zolpimist®: 5 mg/actuation (8.2 g)

Tablet, oral: 5 mg, 10 mg

Ambien®: 5 mg, 10 mg

Tablet, sublingual:

Edluar™: 5 mg, 10 mg

Tablet, extended release, oral: 6.25 mg, 12.5 mg

Ambien CR®: 6.25 mg, 12.5 mg

General Dosage Range Dosage adjustment recommended in patients with hepatic impairment.

Oral:

Immediate release tablet, spray, sublingual tablet:

Adults: 10 mg immediately before bedtime

Elderly: 5 mg immediately before bedtime

Extended release tablet:

Adults: 12.5 mg immediately before bedtime

Elderly: 6.25 mg immediately before bedtime

Administration

Oral Ingest immediately before bedtime due to rapid onset of action.

Ambien CR® tablets should be swallowed whole; do not divide, crush, or chew.

Edluar™ or Sublinox™ (Canadian availability; not available in U.S.) sublingual tablets should be placed under the tongue and allowed to disintegrate; do not swallow or administer with water. Do not administer with or immediately after a meal.

Zolpimist® oral spray should be sprayed directly into the mouth over the tongue. Prior to initial use, pump should be primed by spraying 5 times. If pump is not used for at least 14 days, re-prime pump with 1 spray.

Stability

Storage

Ambien®, Edluar™: Store at 20°C to 25°C (68°F to 77°F). Protect sublingual tablets from light and moisture.

Ambien CR®: Store at 15°C to 25°C (59°F to 77°F); limited excursions permitted up to 30°C (86°F).

Zolpimist®: Store at 25°C (77°F); do not freeze. Avoid prolonged exposure to temperatures >30°C (86°F).

Sublinox™ (Canadian availability; not available in U.S.): Store at 15°C to 30°C (59°F to 86°F); protect from light and moisture.

Nursing Actions

Physical Assessment For short-term use. Assess for history of addiction; long-term use can result in dependence, abuse, or tolerance; behaviors that patient has no memory of performing after taking (driving, preparing food, or eating); periodically evaluate need for continued use. Monitor for CNS depression. For inpatient use, institute safety measures to prevent falls.

Patient Education Take immediately before going to bed. Spray mist into mouth over tongue. Only use this medication if you can get a full night's sleep (at least 7-8 hours). Drug may cause physical and/or psychological dependence. While using this medication, do not use alcohol. Avoid grapefruit or grapefruit juice when taking this medication. Do not drive or operate machinery after taking this medication. Report CNS changes (confusion, memory problems, depression, excitation, headache, abnormal thinking or behavior, nightmares); or respiratory difficulty. Report episodes of "sleep driving" or other complex behaviors, such as driving a vehicle, preparing food, or other activities which you have no memory of performing.

Dietary Considerations For faster sleep onset, do not administer with (or immediately after) a meal.

Zonisamide (zoe NIS a mide)

Brand Names: U.S. Zonegran®

Pharmacologic Category Anticonvulsant, Miscellaneous

Medication Safety Issues

Sound-alike/look-alike issues:

Zonegran® may be confused with SINEquan®

Zonisamide may be confused with lacosamide

Medication Guide Available Yes

Pregnancy Risk Factor C

Lactation Excreted into breast milk /not recommended

Breast-Feeding Considerations Zonisamide is excreted into breast milk in concentrations similar to those in the maternal plasma and has been detected in the plasma of a nursing infant. According to the manufacturer, the decision to continue or discontinue breast-feeding during therapy should take into account the risk of exposure to the infant and the benefits of treatment to the mother.

Use Adjunct treatment of partial seizures in children >16 years of age and adults with epilepsy

Unlabeled Use Bipolar disorder

Mechanism of Action/Effect The exact mechanism of action is not known. May stabilize neuronal membranes and suppress neuronal hypersynchronization through action at sodium and calcium channels. Does not affect GABA activity.

Contraindications Hypersensitivity to zonisamide, sulfonamides, or any component of the formulation

Warnings/Precautions Hazardous agent - use appropriate precautions for handling and disposal. Rare, but potentially fatal sulfonamide reactions have occurred following the use of zonisamide. These reactions include Stevens-Johnson syndrome, fulminant hepatic necrosis, agranulocytosis, aplastic anemia, and toxic epidermal necrolysis, usually appearing within 2-16 weeks of drug initiation. Discontinue zonisamide if rash develops. Chemical similarities are present among sulfonamides, sulfonylureas, carbonic anhydrase inhibitors, thiazides, and loop diuretics (except ethacrynic acid). Use in patients with sulfonamide allergy is specifically contraindicated in product labeling, however, a risk of cross-reaction exists in patients with allergy to any of these compounds; avoid use when previous reaction has been severe. Use may be associated with the development of metabolic acidosis (generally dose-dependent) in certain patients; predisposing conditions/therapies include renal disease, severe respiratory disease, diarrhea, surgery, ketogenic diet, and other medications. Pediatric patients may also be at an increased risk for and may have more severe metabolic acidosis. Serum bicarbonate should be monitored in all patients prior to and during use; if metabolic acidosis occurs, consider decreasing the dose or tapering the dose to discontinue. If use continued despite acidosis, alkali treatment should be considered. Untreated metabolic acidosis may increase the risk of developing nephrolithiasis, nephrocalcinosis, osteomalacia (or rickets in children), or osteoporosis; pediatric patients may also have decreased growth rates.

Pooled analysis of trials involving various antiepileptics (regardless of indication) showed an increased risk of suicidal thoughts/behavior (incidence rate: 0.43% treated patients compared to 0.24% of patients receiving placebo); risk observed as early as 1 week after initiation and continued through duration of trials (most trials ≤24 weeks). Monitor all patients for notable changes in behavior that might indicate suicidal thoughts or depression; notify healthcare provider immediately if symptoms occur.

Discontinue zonisamide in patients who develop acute renal failure or a significant sustained increase in creatinine/BUN concentration. Kidney stones have been reported. Do not use in patients with renal impairment (GFR <50 mL/minute); use with caution in patients with hepatic impairment.

Significant CNS effects include psychiatric symptoms, psychomotor slowing, and fatigue or somnolence. Fatigue and somnolence occur within the first month of treatment, most commonly at doses of 300-500 mg/day. Effects with other sedative drugs or ethanol may be potentiated. May cause sedation, which may impair physical or mental abilities; patients must be cautioned about performing tasks which require mental alertness (eg, operating machinery or driving). Abrupt withdrawal may precipitate seizures; discontinue or reduce doses gradually.

Safety and efficacy in children <16 years of age has not been established. Decreased sweating (oligohydrosis) and hyperthermia requiring hospitalization have been reported in children. Pediatric patients may also be at an increased risk and may have more severe metabolic acidosis.

Drug Interactions

Avoid Concomitant Use

Avoid concomitant use of Zonisamide with any of the following: Carbonic Anhydrase Inhibitors; Conivaptan

Decreased Effect

Zonisamide may decrease the levels/effects of: Lithium; Methenamine; Primidone

The levels/effects of Zonisamide may be decreased by: CYP3A4 Inducers (Strong); Deferasirox; Fosphenytoin; Herbs (CYP3A4 Inducers); Ketorolac; Ketorolac (Nasal); Ketorolac (Systemic); Mefloquine; PHENobarbital; Phenytoin; Tocilizumab

Increased Effect/Toxicity

Zonisamide may increase the levels/effects of: Alcohol (Ethyl); Alpha-/Beta-Agonists; Amphetamines; Anticonvulsants (Barbiturate); Anticonvulsants (Hydantoin); CarBAMazepine; Carbonic Anhydrase Inhibitors; CNS Depressants; Flecainide; Memantine; MetFORMIN; Methotrimeprazine; Primidone; QuiNIDine; Selective Serotonin Reuptake Inhibitors

The levels/effects of Zonisamide may be increased by: Conivaptan; CYP3A4 Inhibitors (Moderate); CYP3A4 Inhibitors (Strong); Dasatinib; Droperidol; HydrOXYzine; Ivacaftor; Methotrimeprazine; Salicylates

Nutritional/Ethanol Interactions

Ethanol: May increase CNS depression; monitor for increased effects with coadministration. Caution patients about effects.

Food: Food delays time to maximum concentration, but does not affect bioavailability.

Adverse Reactions Adjunctive therapy: Frequencies noted in patients receiving other anticonvulsants:

>10%:

Central nervous system: Somnolence (17%), dizziness (13%)

Gastrointestinal: Anorexia (13%)

1% to 10%:

Central nervous system: Headache (10%), agitation/irritability (9%), fatigue (8%), tiredness (7%), ataxia (6%), confusion (6%), concentration decreased (6%), memory impairment (6%), depression (6%), insomnia (6%), speech disorders (5%), mental slowing (4%), anxiety (3%), nervousness (2%), schizophrenic/schizophreniform behavior (2%), difficulty in verbal expression (2%), status epilepticus (1%), seizure (1%), hyperesthesia (1%), incoordination (1%)

Dermatologic: Rash (3%), bruising (2%), pruritus (1%)

Gastrointestinal: Nausea (9%), abdominal pain (6%), diarrhea (5%), dyspepsia (3%), weight loss (3%), constipation (2%), taste perversion (2%), xerostomia (2%), vomiting (1%)

Neuromuscular & skeletal: Paresthesia (4%), abnormal gait (1%), tremor (1%), weakness (1%)

Ocular: Diplopia (6%), nystagmus (4%), amblyopia (1%)

Otic: Tinnitus (1%)

Renal: Kidney stones (4%, children 3% to 8%)

Respiratory: Rhinitis (2%), pharyngitis (1%), increased cough (1%)

Miscellaneous: Flu-like syndrome (4%) accidental injury (1%)

Available Dosage Forms

Capsule, oral: 25 mg, 50 mg, 100 mg

Zonegran®: 25 mg, 100 mg

General Dosage Range Oral: *Children >16 years and Adults:* Initial: 100 mg/day; Maintenance: 100-600 mg/day (maximum: 600 mg/day)

Administration

Oral Capsules should be swallowed whole. Dose may be administered once or twice daily. Doses of 300 mg/day and higher are associated with increased side effects. Steady-state levels are reached in 14 days.

Stability

Storage Store at controlled room temperature 25°C (77°F). Protect from moisture and light.

Nursing Actions

Physical Assessment Observe and teach seizure precautions.

Patient Education Take at the same time each day, with or without food. Do not chew, crush, or open capsules; swallow whole. Maintain adequate hydration unless instructed to restrict fluid intake. While using this medication, avoid alcohol. Wear/carry identification of epileptic status and medications. You may experience drowsiness, dizziness, blurred vision, nausea, vomiting, constipation, dry mouth, or loss of appetite. Report CNS changes (changes in speech patterns, mentation changes, suicide ideation, depression, changes in cognition or memory, unusual thought patterns, coordination difficulties, or excessive drowsiness); extreme fatigue, loss of appetite, or hyperventilation; respiratory difficulty or tightening of the throat; swelling of mouth, lips, or tongue; muscle cramping, weakness, or pain; rash or skin irritations; unusual bruising or bleeding (mouth, urine, stool); fever, sore throat, or sores in your mouth; swelling of extremities; sudden back pain, pain on urination, or dark/bloody urine (signs of kidney stones); or change in seizure type or frequency.

Dietary Considerations May be taken without regard to meals.

Zoster Vaccine (ZOS ter vak SEEN)

Brand Names: U.S. Zostavax®

Index Terms Shingles Vaccine; Varicella-Zoster (VZV) Vaccine (Zoster); VZV Vaccine (Zoster); ZOS

Pharmacologic Category Vaccine, Live (Viral)

Medication Safety Issues

Administration issues:

Both varicella vaccine and zoster vaccine are live, attenuated strains of varicella-zoster virus. Their indications, dosing, and composition are distinct. Varicella vaccine is indicated for the prevention of chickenpox, while zoster vaccine is indicated in older individuals to prevent reactivation of the virus which causes shingles. Zoster vaccine is **not** a substitute for varicella vaccine and should not be used in children.

Lactation Excretion in breast milk unknown/use caution

Use Prevention of herpes zoster (shingles) in patients ≥50 years of age

The Advisory Committee on Immunization Practices (ACIP) recommends routine vaccination of all patients ≥60 years of age, including:

- Patients who report a previous episode of zoster.
- Patients with chronic medical conditions (eg, chronic renal failure, diabetes mellitus, rheumatoid arthritis, chronic pulmonary disease) unless those conditions are contraindications.
- Residents of nursing homes and other long-term care facilities ≥60 years of age, without contraindications.

Although not specifically recommended for their profession, healthcare providers within the recommended age group should also receive the zoster vaccine (CDC, 61[4], 2012)

Available Dosage Forms

Injection, powder for reconstitution [preservative free]:

Zostavax®: 19,400 PFU

General Dosage Range SubQ: *Adults ≥50 years:* 0.65 mL as a single dose

Administration

I.M. Not for I.M. administration

I.V. Not for I.V. administration

Other Inject immediately after reconstitution. Inject SubQ into the deltoid region of the upper arm, if possible. In persons anticipating immunosuppression, give at least 14 days to 1 month prior to starting immunosuppressant.

Administration with chronic use of acyclovir, famciclovir, or valacyclovir: Discontinue ≥24 hours before administration of zoster vaccine. Do not use for ≥14 days after vaccination.

Simultaneous administration of vaccines helps ensure the patients will be fully vaccinated by the appropriate age. Simultaneous administration of vaccines is defined as administering >1 vaccine on the same day at different anatomic sites. Separate vaccines should not be combined in the same syringe unless indicated by product specific labeling. Separate needles and syringes should be used for each injection. The ACIP prefers each dose of a specific vaccine in a series come from the same manufacturer when possible. Adolescents and adults should be vaccinated while seated or lying down (CDC, 2011).

Antipyretics have not been shown to prevent febrile seizures. Antipyretics may be used to treat fever or discomfort following vaccination (CDC, 2011). One study reported that routine prophylactic administration of acetaminophen to prevent fever prior to vaccination decreased the immune response of some vaccines; the clinical significance of this reduction in immune response has not been established (Prymula, 2009).

Nursing Actions

Physical Assessment Not for use in patients <50 years of age or in the treatment of active zoster outbreak. Treatment for anaphylactic/anaphylactoid reaction should be immediately available. U.S. federal law requires entry into the patient's medical record.

Patient Education This vaccine is not a treatment for shingles, but may help prevent the occurrence of shingles or reduce the pain if shingles develops despite the vaccination. Avoid other vaccinations for 2 months following this vaccine unless approved by prescriber. Avoid close and/or prolonged contact with highly susceptible individuals (newborns, pregnant women, immunocompromised persons) for six weeks following vaccination; there is a rare risk of transmitting the vaccine virus to those who have not had chickenpox. Notify prescriber immediately of any acute reaction to vaccination (eg, difficulty breathing, chest pain, acute headache, rash, or difficulty swallowing). May cause mild fever and some irritation or swelling at injection site; consult prescriber if excessive or persisting. U.S. federal law requires entry into the patient's medical record.

Related Information

Immunization Administration Recommendations *on page 1243*

Immunization Recommendations *on page 1248*

Zucapsaicin (zu kap SAY sin)

Pharmacologic Category Analgesic, Topical; Topical Skin Product; Transient Receptor Potential Vanilloid 1 (TRPV1) Agonist

Lactation Excretion in human breast milk is unknown/use caution

Use In conjunction with an oral NSAID or COX-2 inhibitor for short-term (≤3 months) treatment of severe pain associated with osteoarthritis of the knee that is not controlled by NSAID or COX-2 inhibitor monotherapy

Product Availability Not available in the U.S.

General Dosage Range Topical: *Adults:* Apply a pea-sized amount to each of 3 different locations around affected knee 3 times/day (minimum interval between applications: 4 hours) (maximum: 3 applications/day)

Administration

Topical For external use only on intact skin; do not apply to broken or irritated skin. Gently rub into affected knee until no residue is left on skin. Do not cover treated area with occlusive dressing. Wash hands thoroughly after application. Avoid taking a hot bath or shower immediately before or after administration (may cause burning sensation). Avoid contact with eyes, lips, and genital area. Avoid concomitant application of other topical medications to treated areas.

APPENDIX TABLE OF CONTENTS

ABBREVIATIONS, ACRONYMS, AND SYMBOLS

Abbreviations Which May Be Used in This Reference

Abbreviation	Meaning
½NS	0.45% sodium chloride
5-HT	5-hydroxytryptamine
AAP	American Academy of Pediatrics
AAPC	antibiotic-associated pseudomembranous colitis
ABG	arterial blood gases
ABMT	autologous bone marrow transplant
ABW	adjusted body weight
AACT	American Academy of Clinical Toxicology
ACC	American College of Cardiology
ACE	angiotensin-converting enzyme
ACLS	advanced cardiac life support
ACOG	American College of Obstetricians and Gynecologists
ACTH	adrenocorticotrophic hormone
ADH	antidiuretic hormone
ADHD	attention-deficit/hyperactivity disorder
ADI	adequate daily intake
ADLs	activities of daily living
AED	antiepileptic drug
AHA	American Heart Association
AHCPR	Agency for Health Care Policy and Research
AIDS	acquired immunodeficiency syndrome
AIMS	Abnormal Involuntary Movement Scale
ALL	acute lymphoblastic leukemia
ALS	amyotrophic lateral sclerosis
ALT	alanine aminotransferase (formerly called SGPT)
AMA	American Medical Association
AML	acute myeloblastic leukemia
ANA	antinuclear antibodies
ANC	absolute neutrophil count
ANLL	acute nonlymphoblastic leukemia
aPTT	activated partial thromboplastin time
ARB	angiotensin receptor blocker
ARDS	acute respiratory distress syndrome
ASA-PS	American Society of Anesthesiologists – Physical Status P1: Normal, healthy patient P2: Patient having mild systemic disease P3: Patient having severe systemic disease P4: Patient having severe systemic disease which is a constant threat to life P5: Moribund patient; not expected to survive without the procedure P6: Patient declared brain-dead; organs being removed for donor purposes
AST	aspartate aminotransferase (formerly called SGOT)
ATP	adenosine triphosphate
AUC	area under the curve (area under the serum concentration-time curve)
A-V	atrial-ventricular
BDI	Beck Depression Inventory
BEC	blood ethanol concentration
BLS	basic life support
BMI	body mass index
BMT	bone marrow transplant
BP	blood pressure
BPD	bronchopulmonary disease or dysplasia
BPH	benign prostatic hyperplasia
BPRS	Brief Psychiatric Rating Scale
BSA	body surface area
BUN	blood urea nitrogen

Abbreviations Which May Be Used in This Reference *(continued)*

Abbreviation	Meaning
CABG	coronary artery bypass graft
CAD	coronary artery disease
CADD	computer ambulatory drug delivery
cAMP	cyclic adenosine monophosphate
CAN	Canadian
CAPD	continuous ambulatory peritoneal dialysis
CAS	chemical abstract service
CBC	complete blood count
CBT	cognitive behavioral therapy
Cl_{cr}	creatinine clearance
CDC	Centers for Disease Control and Prevention
CF	cystic fibrosis
CFC	chlorofluorocarbons
CGI	Clinical Global Impression
CHD	coronary heart disease
CHF	congestive heart failure; chronic heart failure
CI	cardiac index
CIE	chemotherapy-induced emesis
C-II	schedule two controlled substance
C-III	schedule three controlled substance
C-IV	schedule four controlled substance
C-V	schedule five controlled substance
CIV	continuous I.V. infusion
Cl_{cr}	creatinine clearance
CLL	chronic lymphocytic leukemia
C_{max}	maximum plasma concentration
C_{min}	minimum plasma concentration
CML	chronic myelogenous leukemia
CMV	cytomegalovirus
CNS	central nervous system or coagulase negative staphylococcus
COLD	chronic obstructive lung disease
COPD	chronic obstructive pulmonary disease
COX	cyclooxygenase
CPK	creatine phosphokinase
CPR	cardiopulmonary resuscitation
CRF	chronic renal failure
CRP	C-reactive protein
CRRT	continuous renal replacement therapy
CSF	cerebrospinal fluid
CSII	continuous subcutaneous insulin infusion
CT	computed tomography
CVA	cerebrovascular accident
CVP	central venous pressure
CVVH	continuous venovenous hemofiltration
CVVHD	continuous venovenous hemodialysis
CVVHDF	continuous venovenous hemodiafiltration
CYP	cytochrome
$D_5/^1/_4NS$	dextrose 5% in sodium chloride 0.2%
$D_5/^1/_2NS$	dextrose 5% in sodium chloride 0.45%
D_5/LR	dextrose 5% in lactated Ringer's
D_5/NS	dextrose 5% in sodium chloride 0.9%
D_5W	dextrose 5% in water
$D_{10}W$	dextrose 10% in water
DBP	diastolic blood pressure
DEHP	di(3-ethylhexyl)phthalate
DIC	disseminated intravascular coagulation
DL_{co}	pulmonary diffusion capacity for carbon monoxide

Abbreviations Which May Be Used in This Reference *(continued)*

Abbreviation	Meaning
DM	diabetes mellitus
DMARD	disease modifying antirheumatic drug
DNA	deoxyribonucleic acid
DSC	discontinued
DSM-IV	Diagnostic and Statistical Manual
DVT	deep vein thrombosis
EBV	Epstein-Barr virus
ECG	electrocardiogram
ECHO	echocardiogram
ECMO	extracorporeal membrane oxygenation
ECT	electroconvulsive therapy
ED	emergency department
EEG	electroencephalogram
EF	ejection fraction
EG	ethylene glycol
EGA	estimated gestational age
EIA	enzyme immunoassay
ELBW	extremely low birth weight
ELISA	enzyme-linked immunosorbent assay
EPS	extrapyramidal side effects
ESR	erythrocyte sedimentation rate
ESRD	end stage renal disease
E.T.	endotracheal
EtOH	alcohol
FDA	Food and Drug Administration (United States)
FEV_1	forced expiratory volume exhaled after 1 second
FSH	follicle-stimulating hormone
FTT	failure to thrive
FVC	forced vital capacity
G-6-PD	glucose-6-phosphate dehydrogenase
GA	gestational age
GABA	gamma-aminobutyric acid
GAD	generalized anxiety disorder
GE	gastroesophageal
GERD	gastroesophageal reflux disease
GFR	glomerular filtration rate
GGT	gamma-glutamyltransferase
GI	gastrointestinal
GU	genitourinary
GVHD	graft versus host disease
HAM-A	Hamilton Anxiety Scale
HAM-D	Hamilton Depression Scale
Hct	hematocrit
HDL-C	high density lipoprotein cholesterol
HF	heart failure
HFA	hydrofluoroalkane
HFSA	Heart Failure Society of America
Hgb	hemoglobin
HIV	human immunodeficiency virus
HMG-CoA	3-hydroxy-3-methylglutaryl-coenzyme A
HOCM	hypertrophic obstructive cardiomyopathy
HPA	hypothalamic-pituitary-adrenal
HPLC	high performance liquid chromatography
HSV	herpes simplex virus
HTN	hypertension
HUS	hemolytic uremic syndrome
IBD	inflammatory bowel disease

Abbreviations Which May Be Used in This Reference *(continued)*

Abbreviation	Meaning
IBS	irritable bowel syndrome
IBW	ideal body weight
ICD	implantable cardioverter defibrillator
ICH	intracranial hemorrhage
ICP	intracranial pressure
IDDM	insulin-dependent diabetes mellitus
IDSA	Infectious Diseases Society of America
IgG	immune globulin G
IHSS	idiopathic hypertrophic subaortic stenosis
I.M.	intramuscular
ILCOR	International Liaison Committee on Resuscitation
INR	international normalized ration
Int. unit	international unit
I.O.	intraosseous
I & O	input and output
IOP	intraocular pressure
IQ	intelligence quotient
I.T.	intrathecal
ITP	idiopathic thrombocytopenic purpura
IUGR	intrauterine growth retardation
I.V.	intravenous
IVH	intraventricular hemorrhage
IVP	intravenous push
IVPB	intravenous piggyback
JIA	juvenile idiopathic arthritis
JNC	Joint National Committee
JRA	juvenile rheumatoid arthritis
kg	kilogram
KIU	kallikrein inhibitor unit
KOH	potassium hydroxide
LAMM	L-α-acetyl methadol
LDH	lactate dehydrogenase
LDL-C	low density lipoprotein cholesterol
LE	lupus erythematosus
LFT	liver function test
LGA	large for gestational age
LH	luteinizing hormone
LP	lumbar posture
LR	lactated Ringer's
LV	left ventricular
LVEF	left ventricular ejection fraction
LVH	left ventricular hypertrophy
MAC	*Mycobacterium avium* complex
MADRS	Montgomery Asbery Depression Rating Scale
MAO	monoamine oxidase
MAOIs	monamine oxidase inhibitors
MAP	mean arterial pressure
MDD	major depressive disorder
MDRD	modification of diet in renal disease
MDRSP	multidrug resistant *streptococcus pneumoniae*
MI	myocardial infarction
MMSE	mini mental status examination
MOPP	mustargen (mechlorethamine), Oncovin® (vincristine), procarbazine, and prednisone
M/P	milk to plasma ratio
MPS I	mucopolysaccharidosis I
MRHD	maximum recommended human dose
MRI	magnetic resonance imaging

Abbreviations Which May Be Used in This Reference *(continued)*

Abbreviation	Meaning
MRSA	methicillin-resistant *Staphylococcus aureus*
MUGA	multiple gated acquisition scan
NAEPP	National Asthma Education and Prevention Program
NAS	neonatal abstinence syndrome
NCI	National Cancer Institute
ND	nasoduodenal
NF	National Formulary
NFD	Nephrogenic fibrosing dermopathy
NG	nasogastric
NIDDM	noninsulin-dependent diabetes mellitus
NIH	National Institute of Health
NKA	no known allergies
NKDA	No known drug allergies
NMDA	n-methyl-d-aspartate
NMS	neuroleptic malignant syndrome
NNRTI	non-nucleoside reverse transcriptase inhibitor
NRTI	nucleoside reverse transcriptase inhibitor
NS	normal saline (0.9% sodium chloride)
NSAID	nonsteroidal anti-inflammatory drug
NSF	nephrogenic systemic fibrosis
NSTEMI	Non-ST-elevation myocardial infarction
NYHA	New York Heart Association
OA	osteoarthritis
OCD	obsessive-compulsive disorder
OHSS	ovarian hyperstimulation syndrome
O.R.	operating room
OTC	over-the-counter (nonprescription)
PABA	para-aminobenzoic acid
PACTG	Pediatric AIDS Clinical Trials Group
PALS	pediatric advanced life support
PAT	paroxysmal atrial tachycardia
PCA	patient-controlled analgesia
PCP	*Pneumocystis jiroveci* pneumonia (also called *Pneumocystis carinii* pneumonia)
PCWP	pulmonary capillary wedge pressure
PD	Parkinson's disease; peritoneal dialysis
PDA	patent ductus arteriosus
PDE-5	phosphodiesterase-5
PE	pulmonary embolism
PEG tube	percutaneous endoscopic gastrostomy tube
P-gp	P-glycoprotein
PHN	post-herpetic neuralgia
PICU	Pediatric Intensive Care Unit
PID	pelvic inflammatory disease
PIP	peak inspiratory pressure
PMA	postmenstrual age
PMDD	premenstrual dysphoric disorder
PNA	postnatal age
PONV	postoperative nausea and vomiting
PPHN	persistent pulmonary hypertension of the neonate
PPN	peripheral parenteral nutrition
PROM	premature rupture of membranes
PSVT	paroxysmal supraventricular tachycardia
PT	prothrombin time
PTH	parathyroid hormone
PTSD	post-traumatic stress disorder
PTT	partial thromboplastin time
PUD	peptic ulcer disease

Abbreviations Which May Be Used in This Reference *(continued)*

Abbreviation	Meaning
PVC	premature ventricular contraction
PVD	peripheral vascular disease
PVR	peripheral vascular resistance
QT_c	corrected QT interval
QT_c-F	corrected QT interval by Fredricia's formula
RA	rheumatoid arthritis
RAP	right arterial pressure
RDA	recommended daily allowance
REM	rapid eye movement
REMS	risk evaluation and mitigation strategies
RIA	radioimmunoassay
RNA	ribonucleic acid
RPLS	reversible posterior leukoencephalopathy syndrome
RSV	respiratory syncytial virus
SA	sinoatrial
SAD	seasonal affective disorder
SAH	subarachnoid hemorrhage
SBE	subacute bacterial endocarditis
SBP	systolic blood pressure
S_{cr}	serum creatinine
SERM	selective estrogen receptor modulator
SGA	small for gestational age
SGOT	serum glutamic oxaloacetic aminotransferase
SGPT	serum glutamic pyruvate transaminase
SI	International System of Units or Systeme international d'Unites
SIADH	syndrome of inappropriate antidiuretic hormone secretion
SLE	systemic lupus erythematosus
SLEDD	sustained low-efficiency daily diafiltration
SNRI	serotonin norepinephrine reuptake inhibitor
SSKI	saturated solution of potassium iodide
SSRIs	selective serotonin reuptake inhibitors
STD	sexually transmitted disease
STEM I	ST-elevation myocardial infarction
SVR	systemic vascular resistance
SVT	supraventricular tachycardia
SWFI	sterile water for injection
SWI	sterile water for injection
$T_{1/2}$	half-life
T_3	triiodothyronine
T_4	thyroxine
TB	tuberculosis
TC	total cholesterol
TCA	tricyclic antidepressant
TD	tardive dyskinesia
TG	triglyceride
TIA	transient ischemic attack
TIBC	total iron binding capacity
TMA	thrombotic microangiopathy
T_{max}	time to maximum observed concentration, plasma
TNF	tumor necrosis factor
TPN	total parenteral nutrition
TSH	thyroid stimulating hormone
TT	thrombin time
TTP	thrombotic thrombocytopenic purpura
UA	urine analysis
UC	ulcerative colitis
ULN	upper limits of normal

Abbreviations Which May Be Used in This Reference *(continued)*

Abbreviation	Meaning
URI	upper respiratory infection
USAN	United States Adopted Names
USP	United States Pharmacopeia
UTI	urinary tract infection
UV	ultraviolet
V_d	volume of distribution
V_{dss}	volume of distribution at steady-state
VEGF	vascular endothelial growth factor
VF	ventricular fibrillation
VLBW	very low birth weight
VMA	vanillylmandelic acid
VT	ventricular tachycardia
VTE	venous thromboembolism
vWD	von Willebrand disease
VZV	varicella zoster virus
WHO	World Health Organization
w/v	weight for volume
w/w	weight for weight
YBOC	Yale Brown Obsessive-Compulsive Scale
YMRS	Young Mania Rating Scale

Common Weights, Measures, or Apothecary Abbreviations

Abbreviation	Meaning
<[1]	less than
>[1]	greater than
≤	less than or equal to
≥	greater than or equal to
ac	before meals or food
ad	to, up to
ad lib	at pleasure
AM	morning
AMA	against medical advice
amp	ampul
amt	amount
aq	water
aq. dest.	distilled water
ASAP	as soon as possible
a.u.[1]	each ear
bid	twice daily
bm	bowel movement
C	Celsius, centigrade
cal	calorie
cap	capsule
cc[1]	cubic centimeter
cm	centimeter
comp	compound
cont	continue
d	day
d/c[1]	discharge
dil	dilute
disp	dispense
div	divide
dtd	give of such a dose
Dx	diagnosis
elix, el	elixir

Common Weights, Measures, or Apothecary Abbreviations *(continued)*

Abbreviation	Meaning
emp	as directed
et	and
ex aq	in water
F	Fahrenheit
f, ft	make, let be made
g	gram
gr	grain
gtt	a drop
h	hour
hs[1]	at bedtime
kcal	kilocalorie
kg	kilogram
L	liter
liq	a liquor, solution
M	molar
mcg	microgram
m. dict	as directed
mEq	milliequivalent
mg	milligram
microL	microliter
min	minute
mL	milliliter
mm	millimeter
mM	millimole
mm Hg	millimeters of mercury
mo	month
mOsm	milliosmoles
ng	nanogram
nmol	nanomole
no.	number
noc	in the night
non rep	do not repeat, no refills
NPO	nothing by mouth
NV	nausea and vomiting
O, Oct	a pint
o.d.[1]	right eye
o.l.	left eye
o.s.[1]	left eye
o.u.[1]	each eye
pc, post cib	after meals
PM	afternoon or evening
P.O.	by mouth
P.R.	rectally
prn	as needed
pulv	a powder
q	every
qad	every other day
qd[1,2]	every day, daily
qh	every hour
qid	four times a day
qod[1,2]	every other day
qs	a sufficient quantity
qs ad	a sufficient quantity to make
Rx	take, a recipe
S.L.	sublingual
stat	at once, immediately
SubQ	subcutaneous

Common Weights, Measures, or Apothecary Abbreviations *(continued)*

Abbreviation	Meaning
supp	suppository
syr	syrup
tab	tablet
tal	such
tid	three times a day
tr, tinct	tincture
trit	triturate
tsp	teaspoon
u.d.	as directed
ung	ointment
v.o.	verbal order
w.a.	while awake
x3	3 times
x4	4 times
y	year

[1]ISMP error-prone abbreviation

[2]JCAHO Do Not Use list

Additional abbreviations used and defined within a specific monograph or text piece may only apply to that text.

REFERENCES

The Institute for Safe Medication Practices (ISMP) list of Error-Prone Abbreviations, Symbols, and Dose Designations. Available at http://www.ismp.org/Tools/errorproneabbreviations.pdf

The Joint Commission Official "Do Not Use" list. Available at http://www.jointcommission.org/assets/1/18/Official_Do_Not_Use_List_6_111.PDF

APOTHECARY/METRIC EQUIVALENTS

Approximate Liquid Measures

Basic equivalent: 1 fluid ounce = 30 mL

Examples:

1 gallon	=	3800 mL
1 quart	=	960 mL
1 pint	=	480 mL
8 fluid oz	=	240 mL
4 fluid oz	=	120 mL

1 gallon	=	128 fluid ounces
1 quart	=	32 fluid ounces
1 pint	=	16 fluid ounces
15 minims	=	1 mL
10 minims	=	0.6 mL

Approximate Household Equivalents

1 teaspoonful	=	5 mL
1 tablespoonful	=	15 mL

Weights

Basic equivalents:

1 oz	=	30 g
15 gr	=	1 g

Examples:

4 oz	=	120 g
2 oz	=	60 g
10 gr	=	600 mg
7 1/2 gr	=	500 mg
16 oz	=	1 lb

1 gr	=	60 mg
1/100 gr	=	600 mcg
1/150 gr	=	400 mcg
1/200 gr	=	300 mcg

Metric Conversions

Basic equivalents:

1 g	=	1000 mg
1 mg	=	1000 mcg

Examples:

5 g	=	5000 mg
0.5 g	=	500 mg
0.05 g	=	50 mg

5 mg	=	5000 mcg
0.5 mg	=	500 mcg
0.05 mg	=	50 mcg

Exact Equivalents

1 g	=	15.43 gr
1 mL	=	16.23 minims
1 minim	=	0.06 mL
1 gr	=	64.8 mg
1 pint (pt)	=	473.2 mL
1 oz	=	28.35 g
1 lb	=	453.6 g
1 kg	=	2.2 lb
1 qt	=	946.4 mL

0.1 mg	=	1/600 gr
0.12 mg	=	1/500 gr
0.15 mg	=	1/400 gr
0.2 mg	=	1/300 gr
0.3 mg	=	1/200 gr
0.4 mg	=	1/150 gr
0.5 mg	=	1/120 gr
0.6 mg	=	1/100 gr
0.8 mg	=	1/80 gr
1 mg	=	1/65 gr

Solids[1]

1/4 grain	=	15 mg
1/2 grain	=	30 mg
1 grain	=	60 mg

1 1/2 grains	=	90 mg
5 grains	=	300 mg
10 grains	=	600 mg

[1]Use exact equivalents for compounding and calculations requiring a high degree of accuracy.

AVERAGE WEIGHTS AND SURFACE AREAS

Average Height, Weight, and Surface Area by Age and Gender

Age	Girls			Boys		
	Height (cm)	Weight (kg)	BSA (m^2)	Height (cm)	Weight (kg)	BSA (m^2)
Birth	49.5	3.4	0.22	50	3.6	0.22
3 mo	59	5.6	0.3	61	6	0.32
6 mo	65	7.2	0.36	67	7.9	0.38
9 mo	70	8.3	0.4	72	9.3	0.43
12 mo	74.5	9.5	0.44	75.5	10.3	0.46
15 mo	77	10.3	0.47	79	11.1	0.49
18 mo	80	11	0.49	82	11.7	0.52
21 mo	83	11.6	0.52	85	12.2	0.54
2 y	86	12	0.54	87.5	12.6	0.55
2.5 y	91	13	0.57	92	13.5	0.59
3 y	94.5	13.8	0.6	96	14.3	0.62
3.5 y	97	15	0.64	98	15	0.64
4 y	101	16	0.67	102	16	0.67
4.5 y	104	17	0.7	105	17	0.7
5 y	107.5	18	0.73	109	18.5	0.75
6 y	115	20	0.80	115	21	0.82
7 y	121.5	23	0.88	122	23	0.88
8 y	127.5	25.5	0.95	127.5	26	0.96
9 y	133	29	1.04	133.5	28.5	1.03
10 y	138	33	1.12	138.5	32	1.1
11 y	144	37	1.22	143.5	36	1.2
12 y	151	41.5	1.32	149	40.5	1.29
13 y	157	46	1.42	156	45.5	1.4
14 y	160.5	49.5	1.49	163.5	51	1.52
15 y	162	52	1.53	170	56	1.63
16 y	162.5	54	1.56	173.5	61	1.71
17 y	163	55	1.58	175	64.5	1.77
Adult[1]	163.5	58	1.62	177	83.5	2.03

Data extracted from the CDC growth charts based on the 50th percentile height and weight for a given age[2]

Body surface area calculation[3]: Square root of [(Ht x Wt) / 3600]

[1]McDowell MA, Fryar CD, Hirsch R, et al, "Anthropometric Reference Data for Children and Adults: U.S. Population, 1999-2002," *Adv Data*, 2005, (361):1-5.

[2]Centers for Disease Control and Prevention, "2000 CDC Growth Charts: United States". Available at http://www.cdc.gov/growthcharts. Accessed November 16, 2007.

[3]Mosteller RD, "Simplified Calculation of Body-Surface Area," *N Engl J Med*, 1987, 317(17):1098.

BODY SURFACE AREA OF ADULTS AND CHILDREN

Calculating Body Surface Area in Children

In a child of average size, find weight and corresponding surface area on the boxed scale to the left or use the nomogram to the right. Lay a straightedge on the correct height and weight points for the child, then read the intersecting point on the surface area scale. (**Note:** 2.2 lb = 1 kg)

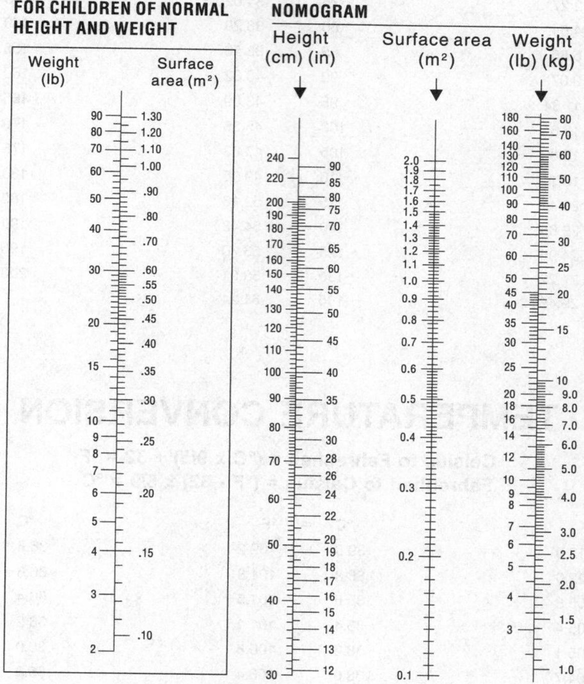

BODY SURFACE AREA FORMULA
(Adult and Pediatric)

$$BSA (m^2) = \sqrt{\frac{Ht (in) \times Wt (lb)}{3131}} \text{ or, in metric: } BSA (m^2) = \sqrt{\frac{Ht (cm) \times Wt (kg)}{3600}}$$

References

Lam TK and Leung DT, "More on Simplified Calculation of Body Surface Area," *N Engl J Med*, 1988, 318(17):1130 (Letter).

Mosteller RD, "Simplified Calculation of Body Surface Area", *N Engl J Med*, 1987, 317(17):1098 (Letter).

POUNDS/KILOGRAMS CONVERSION

1 pound = 0.45359 kilograms
1 kilogram = 2.2 pounds

lb	=	kg	lb	=	kg	lb	=	kg
1		0.45	70		31.75	140		63.50
5		2.27	75		34.02	145		65.77
10		4.54	80		36.29	150		68.04
15		6.80	85		38.56	155		70.31
20		9.07	90		40.82	160		72.58
25		11.34	95		43.09	165		74.84
30		13.61	100		45.36	170		77.11
35		15.88	105		47.63	175		79.38
40		18.14	110		49.90	180		81.65
45		20.41	115		52.16	185		83.92
50		22.68	120		54.43	190		86.18
55		24.95	125		56.70	195		88.45
60		27.22	130		58.91	200		90.72
65		29.48	135		61.24			

TEMPERATURE CONVERSION

Celsius to Fahrenheit = (°C x 9/5) + 32 = °F
Fahrenheit to Celsius = (°F - 32) x 5/9 = °C

°C	=	°F	°C	=	°F	°C	=	°F
100.0		212.0	39.0		102.2	36.8		98.2
50.0		122.0	38.8		101.8	36.6		97.9
41.0		105.8	38.6		101.5	36.4		97.5
40.8		105.4	38.4		101.1	36.2		97.2
40.6		105.1	38.2		100.8	36.0		96.8
40.4		104.7	38.0		100.4	35.8		96.4
40.2		104.4	37.8		100.1	35.6		96.1
40.0		104.0	37.6		99.7	35.4		95.7
39.8		103.6	37.4		99.3	35.2		95.4
39.6		103.3	37.2		99.0	35.0		95.0
39.4		102.9	37.0		98.6	0		32.0
39.2		102.6						

REFERENCE VALUES FOR ADULTS

CHEMISTRY

Test	Values	Remarks
Serum/Plasma		
Acetone	Negative	
Albumin	3.2-5 g/dL	
Alcohol, ethyl	Negative	
Aldolase	1.2-7.6 IU/L	
Ammonia	20-70 mcg/dL	Specimen to be placed on ice as soon as collected.
Amylase	30-110 units/L	
Bilirubin, direct	0-0.3 mg/dL	
Bilirubin, total	0.1-1.2 mg/dL	
Calcium	8.6-10.3 mg/dL	
Calcium, ionized	2.24-2.46 mEq/L	
Chloride	95-108 mEq/L	
Cholesterol, total	≤200 mg/dL	Fasted blood required – normal value affected by dietary habits. This reference range is for a general adult population.
HDL cholesterol	40-60 mg/dL	Fasted blood required – normal value affected by dietary habits.
LDL cholesterol	<160 mg/dL	If triglyceride is >400 mg/dL, LDL cannot be calculated accurately (Friedewald equation). Target LDL-C depends on patient's risk factors.
CO_2	23-30 mEq/L	
Creatine kinase (CK) isoenzymes		
CK-BB	0%	
CK-MB (cardiac)	0%-3.9%	
CK-MM (muscle)	96%-100%	
CK-MB levels must be both ≥4% and 10 IU/L to meet diagnostic criteria for CK-MB positive result consistent with myocardial injury.		
Creatine phosphokinase (CPK)	8-150 IU/L	
Creatinine	0.5-1.4 mg/dL	
Ferritin	13-300 ng/mL	
Folate	3.6-20 ng/dL	
GGT (gamma-glutamyltranspeptidase)		
male	11-63 IU/L	
female	8-35 IU/L	
GLDH	To be determined	
Glucose (preprandial)	<115 mg/dL	Goals different for diabetics.
Glucose, fasting	60-110 mg/dL	Goals different for diabetics.
Glucose, nonfasting (2-h postprandial)	<120 mg/dL	Goals different for diabetics.
Hemoglobin A_{1c}	<8	
Hemoglobin, plasma free	<2.5 mg/100 mL	
Hemoglobin, total glycosolated (Hb A_1)	4%-8%	
Iron	65-150 mcg/dL	
Iron binding capacity, total (TIBC)	250-420 mcg/dL	
Lactic acid	0.7-2.1 mEq/L	Specimen to be kept on ice and sent to lab as soon as possible.
Lactate dehydrogenase (LDH)	56-194 IU/L	

CHEMISTRY *(continued)*

Test	Values	Remarks
Lactate dehydrogenase (LDH) isoenzymes		
LD_1	20%-34%	
LD_2	29%-41%	
LD_3	15%-25%	
LD_4	1%-12%	
LD_5	1%-15%	
Flipped LD_1/LD_2 ratios (>1 may be consistent with myocardial injury) particularly when considered in combination with a recent CK-MB positive result.		
Lipase	23-208 units/L	
Magnesium	1.6-2.5 mg/dL	Increased by slight hemolysis.
Osmolality	289-308 mOsm/kg	
Phosphatase, alkaline		
adults 25-60 y	33-131 IU/L	
adults ≥61 y	51-153 IU/L	
infancy-adolescence	Values range up to 3-5 times higher than adults	
Phosphate, inorganic	2.8-4.2 mg/dL	
Potassium	3.5-5.2 mEq/L	Increased by slight hemolysis.
Prealbumin	>15 mg/dL	
Protein, total	6.5-7.9 g/dL	
AST	<35 IU/L (20-48)	
ALT (10-35)	<35 IU/L	
Sodium	134-149 mEq/L	
Thyroid stimulating hormone (TSH)		
adults ≤20 y	0.7-6.4 mIU/L	
21-54 y	0.4-4.2 mIU/L	
55-87 y	0.5-8.9 mIU/L	
Transferrin	>200 mg/dL	
Triglycerides	45-155 mg/dL	Fasted blood required.
Troponin I	<1.5 ng/mL	
Urea nitrogen (BUN)	7-20 mg/dL	
Uric acid		
male	2-8 mg/dL	
female	2-7.5 mg/dL	
Cerebrospinal Fluid		
Glucose	50-70 mg/dL	
Protein	15-45 mg/dL	CSF obtained by lumbar puncture.
Note: Bloody specimen gives erroneously high value due to contamination with blood proteins		
Urine (24-hour specimen is required for all these tests unless specified)		
Amylase	32-641 units/L	The value is in units/L and **not** calculated for total volume.
Amylase, fluid (random samples)		Interpretation of value left for physician, depends on the nature of fluid.
Calcium	Depends upon dietary intake	
Creatine		
male	150 mg/24 h	Higher value on children and during pregnancy.
female	250 mg/24 h	
Creatinine	1000-2000 mg/24 h	
Creatinine clearance (endogenous)		
male	85-125 mL/min	A blood sample must accompany urine specimen.
female	75-115 mL/min	

CHEMISTRY *(continued)*

Test	Values	Remarks
Glucose	1 g/24 h	
5-hydroxyindoleacetic acid	2-8 mg/24 h	
Iron	0.15 mg/24 h	Acid washed container required.
Magnesium	146-209 mg/24 h	
Osmolality	500-800 mOsm/kg	With normal fluid intake.
Oxalate	10-40 mg/24 h	
Phosphate	400-1300 mg/24 h	
Potassium	25-120 mEq/24 h	Varies with diet; the interpretation of urine electrolytes and osmolality should be left for the physician.
Sodium	40-220 mEq/24 h	
Porphobilinogen, qualitative	Negative	
Porphyrins, qualitative	Negative	
Proteins	0.05-0.1 g/24 h	
Salicylate	Negative	
Urea clearance	60-95 mL/min	A blood sample must accompany specimen.
Urea N	10-40 g/24 h	Dependent on protein intake.
Uric acid	250-750 mg/24 h	Dependent on diet and therapy.
Urobilinogen	0.5-3.5 mg/24 h	For qualitative determination on random urine, send sample to urinalysis section in Hematology Lab.
Xylose absorption test		
children	16%-33% of ingested xylose	
Feces		
Fat, 3-day collection	<5 g/d	Value depends on fat intake of 100 g/d for 3 days preceding and during collection.
Gastric Acidity		
Acidity, total, 12 h	10-60 mEq/L	Titrated at pH 7.

Blood Gases

	Arterial	Capillary	Venous
pH	7.35-7.45	7.35-7.45	7.32-7.42
pCO_2 (mm Hg)	35-45	35-45	38-52
pO_2 (mm Hg)	70-100	60-80	24-48
HCO_3 (mEq/L)	19-25	19-25	19-25
TCO_2 (mEq/L)	19-29	19-29	23-33
O_2 saturation (%)	90-95	90-95	40-70
Base excess (mEq/L)	-5 to +5	-5 to +5	-5 to +5

HEMATOLOGY

Complete Blood Count

Age	Hgb (g/dL)	Hct (%)	RBC (mill/mm^3)	RDW
0-3 d	15.0-20.0	45-61	4.0-5.9	<18
1-2 wk	12.5-18.5	39-57	3.6-5.5	<17
1-6 mo	10.0-13.0	29-42	3.1-4.3	<16.5
7 mo to 2 y	10.5-13.0	33-38	3.7-4.9	<16
2-5 y	11.5-13.0	34-39	3.9-5.0	<15
5-8 y	11.5-14.5	35-42	4.0-4.9	<15
13-18 y	12.0-15.2	36-47	4.5-5.1	<14.5
Adult male	13.5-16.5	41-50	4.5-5.5	<14.5
Adult female	12.0-15.0	36-44	4.0-4.9	<14.5

Age	MCV (fL)	MCH (pg)	MCHC (%)	Plts (x 10^3/mm^3)
0-3 d	95-115	31-37	29-37	250-450
1-2 wk	86-110	28-36	28-38	250-450
1-6 mo	74-96	25-35	30-36	300-700
7 mo to 2 y	70-84	23-30	31-37	250-600
2-5 y	75-87	24-30	31-37	250-550
5-8 y	77-95	25-33	31-37	250-550
13-18 y	78-96	25-35	31-37	150-450
Adult male	80-100	26-34	31-37	150-450
Adult female	80-100	26-34	31-37	150-450

WBC and Differential

Age	WBC (x 10^3/mm^3)	Segs	Bands	Lymphs	Monos
0-3 d	9.0-35.0	32-62	<18	19-29	5-7
1-2 wk	5.0-20.0	14-34	<14	36-45	6-10
1-6 mo	6.0-17.5	13-33	<12	41-71	4-7
7 mo to 2 y	6.0-17.0	15-35	<11	45-76	3-6
2-5 y	5.5-15.5	23-45	<11	35-65	3-6
5-8 y	5.0-14.5	32-54	<11	28-48	3-6
13-18 y	4.5-13.0	34-64	<11	25-45	3-6
Adults	4.5-11.0	35-66	<11	24-44	3-6

Age	Eosinophils	Basophils	Atypical Lymphs	No. of NRBCs
0-3 d	0-2	0-1	0-8	0-2
1-2 wk	0-2	0-1	0-8	0
1-6 mo	0-3	0-1	0-8	0
7 mo to 2 y	0-3	0-1	0-8	0
2-5 y	0-3	0-1	0-8	0
5-8 y	0-3	0-1	0-8	0
13-18 y	0-3	0-1	0-8	0
Adults	0-3	0-1	0-8	0

Segs = segmented neutrophils.

Bands = band neutrophils.

Lymphs = lymphocytes.

Monos = monocytes.

Erythrocyte Sedimentation Rates and Reticulocyte Counts

Sedimentation rate, Westergren	Children	0-20 mm/h
	Adult male	0-15 mm/h
	Adult female	0-20 mm/h
Sedimentation rate, Wintrobe	Children	0-13 mm/h
	Adult male	0-10 mm/h
	Adult female	0-15 mm/h
Reticulocyte count	Newborns	2%-6%
	1-6 mo	0%-2.8%
	Adults	0.5%-1.5%

REFERENCE VALUES FOR CHILDREN

		Normal Values
CHEMISTRY		
Albumin	0-1 y	2-4 g/dL
	1 y to adult	3.5-5.5 g/dL
Ammonia	Newborns	90-150 mcg/dL
	Children	40-120 mcg/dL
	Adults	18-54 mcg/dL
Amylase	Newborns	0-60 units/L
	Adults	30-110 units/L
Bilirubin, conjugated, direct	Newborns	<1.5 mg/dL
	1 mo to adult	0-0.5 mg/dL
Bilirubin, total	0-3 d	2-10 mg/dL
	1 mo to adult	0-1.5 mg/dL
Bilirubin, unconjugated, indirect		0.6-10.5 mg/dL
Calcium	Newborns	7-12 mg/dL
	0-2 y	8.8-11.2 mg/dL
	2 y to adult	9-11 mg/dL
Calcium, ionized, whole blood		4.4-5.4 mg/dL
Carbon dioxide, total		23-33 mEq/L
Chloride		95-105 mEq/L
Cholesterol	Newborns	45-170 mg/dL
	0-1 y	65-175 mg/dL
	1-20 y	120-230 mg/dL
Creatinine	0-1 y	≤0.6 mg/dL
	1 y to adult	0.5-1.5 mg/dL
Glucose	Newborns	30-90 mg/dL
	0-2 y	60-105 mg/dL
	Children to Adults	70-110 mg/dL
Iron	Newborns	110-270 mcg/dL
	Infants	30-70 mcg/dL
	Children	55-120 mcg/dL
	Adults	70-180 mcg/dL
Iron binding	Newborns	59-175 mcg/dL
	Infants	100-400 mcg/dL
	Adults	250-400 mcg/dL
Lactic acid, lactate		2-20 mg/dL
Lead, whole blood		<10 mcg/dL
Lipase	Children	20-140 units/L
	Adults	0-190 units/L
Magnesium		1.5-2.5 mEq/L
Osmolality, serum		275-296 mOsm/kg
Osmolality, urine		50-1400 mOsm/kg

(continued)

		Normal Values
Phosphorus	Newborns	4.2-9 mg/dL
	6 wk to 19 mo	3.8-6.7 mg/dL
	19 mo to 3 y	2.9-5.9 mg/dL
	3-15 y	3.6-5.6 mg/dL
	>15 y	2.5-5 mg/dL
Potassium, plasma	Newborns	4.5-7.2 mEq/L
	2 d to 3 mo	4-6.2 mEq/L
	3 mo to 1 y	3.7-5.6 mEq/L
	1-16 y	3.5-5 mEq/L
Protein, total	0-2 y	4.2-7.4 g/dL
	>2 y	6-8 g/dL
Sodium		136-145 mEq/L
Triglycerides	Infants	0-171 mg/dL
	Children	20-130 mg/dL
	Adults	30-200 mg/dL
Urea nitrogen, blood	0-2 y	4-15 mg/dL
	2 y to Adult	5-20 mg/dL
Uric acid	Male	3-7 mg/dL
	Female	2-6 mg/dL
ENZYMES		
Alanine aminotransferase (ALT)	0-2 mo	8-78 units/L
	>2 mo	8-36 units/L
Alkaline phosphatase (ALKP)	Newborns	60-130 units/L
	0-16 y	85-400 units/L
	>16 y	30-115 units/L
Aspartate aminotransferase (AST)	Infants	18-74 units/L
	Children	15-46 units/L
	Adults	5-35 units/L
Creatine kinase (CK)	Infants	20-200 units/L
	Children	10-90 units/L
	Adult male	0-206 units/L
	Adult female	0-175 units/L
Lactate dehydrogenase (LDH)	Newborns	290-501 units/L
	1 mo to 2 y	110-144 units/L
	>16 y	60-170 units/L

Blood Gases

	Arterial	Capillary	Venous
pH	7.35-7.45	7.35-7.45	7.32-7.42
pCO_2 (mm Hg)	35-45	35-45	38-52
pO_2 (mm Hg)	70-100	60-80	24-48
HCO_3 (mEq/L)	19-25	19-25	19-25
TCO_2 (mEq/L)	19-29	19-29	23-33
O_2 saturation (%)	90-95	90-95	40-70
Base excess (mEq/L)	-5 to +5	-5 to +5	-5 to +5

Thyroid Function Tests

Test	Age	Normal Values
T_4 (thyroxine)	1-7 d	10.1-20.9 mcg/dL
	8-14 d	9.8-16.6 mcg/dL
	1 mo to 1 y	5.5-16 mcg/dL
	>1 y	4-12 mcg/dL
FTI	1-3 d	9.3-26.6
	1-4 wk	7.6-20.8
	1-4 mo	7.4-17.9
	4-12 mo	5.1-14.5
	1-6 y	5.7-13.3
	>6 y	4.8-14
T_3 by RIA	Newborns	100-470 ng/dL
	1-5 y	100-260 ng/dL
	5-10 y	90-240 ng/dL
	10 y to Adult	70-210 ng/dL
T_3 uptake		35%-45%
TSH	Cord	3-22 µIU/mL
	1-3 d	<40 µIU/mL
	3-7 d	<25 µIU/mL
	>7 d	0-10 µIU/mL

DIAGNOSTICS AND SURGICAL AIDS

Agent	Use
Arginine (R-Gene® 10)	Pituitary function test (growth hormone)
Atopiclair® (multiple ingredients)	Manage and relieve symptoms of dermatoses, including atopic dermatitis and allergic contact dermatitis; helps to relieve dry, waxy skin by maintaining a moist skin environment
Candida albicans (Monilia) (Candin®)	Screen for the detection of nonresponsiveness to antigens in immunocompromised individuals
Cellulose (oxidized regenerated) (Surgicel®)	Hemostatic; temporary packing for the control of capillary, venous, or small arterial hemorrhage
Chondroitin sulfate – sodium hyaluronate (DisCoVisc®; Viscoat®)	Ophthalmic surgical aid in the anterior segment during cataract extraction and intraocular lens implantation
Collagen hemostat (Avitene®; EndoAvitene®; Helistat®; Helitene®; Instat™; SyringeAvitene™)	Adjunct to hemostasis when control of bleeding by ligature is ineffective or impractical
Corticorelin (Acthrel®)	Diagnostic test used in adrenocorticotropic hormone (ACTH)-dependent Cushing's syndrome to differentiate between pituitary and ectopic production of ACTH
Corticotropin (H.P. Acthar® Gel)	Acute exacerbations of multiple sclerosis; diagnostic aid in adrenocortical insufficiency, severe muscle weakness in myasthenia gravis Cosyntropin is preferred over corticotropin for diagnostic test of adrenocortical insufficiency (cosyntropin is less allergenic and test is shorter in duration)
Cosyntropin (Cortrosyn®)	Diagnostic test to differentiate primary adrenal from secondary (pituitary) adrenocortical insufficiency
Cyclopentolate (AK-Pentolate™; Cyclogyl®; Cylate™)	Diagnostic procedures requiring mydriasis and cycloplegia
Cyclopentolate and phenylephrine (Cyclomydril®)	Induce mydriasis greater than that produced with cyclopentolate HCl alone
Fluorescein (AK-Fluor®; Angiofluor™; Angiofluor™ Lite; Fluorescite®; Fluorets®; Ful-Glo®)	Injection: Diagnostic aid in ophthalmic angiography and angioscopy Topical: To stain the anterior segment of the eye for procedures (such as fitting contact lenses), disclosing corneal injury, and in applanation tonometry
Fluorescein and benoxinate (EyeFlur; Fluress®; Flurox™)	For use in ophthalmic procedures when a topical disclosing agent is needed along with an anesthetic
Gelatin, absorbable (Gelfilm®; Gelfoam®)	Adjunct to provide hemostasis in surgery; used in open prostatic surgery
Hydroxyamphetamine and tropicamide (Paremyd®)	Short-term pupil dilation for diagnostic procedures and exams
Hydroxypropyl methylcellulose (Cellugel®; GenTeal® Mild; GenTeal®; Gonak™; Goniosoft™; Isopto® Tears; Tearisol®; Tears Again® MC)	Relief of burning and minor irritation due to dry eyes; diagnostic agent in gonioscopic examination
Indocyanine green (IC-Green™)	Determine hepatic function, cardiac output, and liver blood flow; ophthalmic angiography
Isosulfan Blue (Lymphazurin™)	Adjunct to lymphography for visualization of the lymphatic system; sentinel node identification
Methacholine (Provocholine®)	Diagnosis of bronchial airway hyperactivity
Metyrapone (Metopirone®)	Diagnostic test for hypothalamic-pituitary ACTH function
MimyX® (multiple ingredients)	Manage and relieve the symptoms of dermatoses, including atopic dermatitis, allergic contact dermatitis, and radiation dermatitis; used to maintain a moist wound and skin environment; restores the natural components of the stratum corneum; re-establishes barrier function of the outer layers of the epidermis
Perflutren Protein Type A (Optison™)	Opacification of left ventricular chamber and improvement of delineation of the left ventricular endocardial border in patients with suboptimal echocardiograms
Proparacaine (Alcaine®; Ophthetic®; Parcaine™)	Anesthesia for tonometry, gonioscopy; suture removal from cornea; removal of corneal foreign body; cataract extraction, glaucoma surgery; short operative procedure involving the cornea and conjunctiva
Proparacaine and fluorescein (Flucaine®)	Anesthesia for tonometry, gonioscopy; suture removal from cornea; removal of corneal foreign body; cataract extraction, glaucoma surgery
Regadenoson (Lexiscan®)	Radionuclide myocardial perfusion imaging (MPI) in patients unable to undergo adequate exercise stress testing
Secretin (ChiRhoStim™)	Secretin-stimulation testing to aid in diagnosis of pancreatic exocrine dysfunction; diagnosis of gastrinoma (Zollinger-Ellison syndrome); facilitation of endoscopic retrograde cholangiopancreatography (ERCP) visualization

(continued)

Agent	Use
Sincalide (Kinevac®)	Postevacuation cholecystography; gallbladder bile sampling; stimulate pancreatic secretion for analysis; accelerate the transit of barium through the small bowel
Thrombin (topical) (Evithrom™; Recothrom™; Thrombi-Gel®; Thrombi-Pad®; Thrombin-JMI®)	Hemostasis whenever minor bleeding from capillaries and small venules is accessible Thrombi-Gel®; Thrombi-Pad®: Temporary control as trauma dressing for moderate-to-severe bleeding wounds; control of surface bleeding from vascular access sites and percutaneous catheter/tubes
Thyrotropin Alfa (Thyrogen®)	As an adjunctive diagnostic tool for serum thyroglobulin (Tg) testing; adjunctive treatment for radioiodine ablation of thyroid tissue remnants after total or near-total thyroidectomy in patients with well-differentiated thyroid cancer without evidence of metastatic disease Potential clinical uses include: Patients with an undetectable Tg on thyroid hormone suppressive therapy to exclude the diagnosis of residual or recurrent thyroid cancer, patients requiring serum Tg testing and radioiodine imaging who are unwilling to undergo thyroid hormone withdrawal testing and whose treating physician believes that use of a less sensitive test is justified, patients who are either unable to mount an adequate endogenous TSH response to thyroid hormone withdrawal or in whom withdrawal is medically contraindicated, and patients without evidence of metastatic disease to ablate thyroid remnants (in combination with radioiodine [I^{131}]) following near-total thyroidectomy.
Trichophyton skin test	Assess cell-mediated immunity
Tropicamide (Mydral™; Mydriacyl®; Tropicacyl®)	Short-acting mydriatic used in diagnostic procedures, as well as preoperatively and postoperatively; treatment of some cases of acute iritis, iridocyclitis, and keratitis

HERBAL AND NUTRITIONAL PRODUCTS

HERBS AND COMMON NATURAL AGENTS

The authors have chosen to include this list of natural products and proposed medical claims. However, due to limited scientific investigation to support these claims, this list is not intended to imply that these claims have been scientifically proven.

Proposed Treatments

Herb	Treatment
Agrimony	Digestive disorders
Alfalfa	High cholesterol; menopause
Allspice	General health
Aloe vera	Healing agent; minor bites and stings; constipation
Alpha-lipoic acid	Glaucoma; neuropathies
Androstenedione	Increased strength and muscle mass
Anise (seed)	Prevent gas
Astragalus	Enhance energy reserves; immune system modulation; adjunctive treatment for cancer
Barberry (bark)	Halitosis
Bayberry (bark)	Relieve and prevent varicose veins
Bay (leaf)	Relieves cramps
Bee pollen	Renewal of enzymes, hormones, vitamins, amino acids, and others
Bergamot	Calming effect
Bifidobacterium bifidum (bifidus)	Gastrointestinal microflora recolonization (anaerobic)
Bilberry (leaf)	Increases night vision; reduces eye fatigue; antioxidant; circulation
Birch (bark)	Urinary problems; used for rheumatism
Blackberry (leaf)	Diarrhea
Black cohosh	Relieves menstrual cramps; menopause
Blueberry (leaf)	Diarrhea
Blue cohosh	Regulate menstrual flow
Blue flag	Skin diseases and constipation
Boldo (leaf)	Stimulates digestion; gallstones
Boneset	Colds and flu
Bromelain	Digestive enzyme
Buchu (leaf)	Diuretic
Buckthorn (bark)	Expels worms; laxative
Burdock (leaf and root)	Eczema
Butternut	Works well for constipation
Calendula	Mending and healing of cuts or wounds topically; burns
Capsicum (cayenne)	Normalizes blood pressure; circulation; arthritis; neuralgia pain
Caraway (seed)	Aids digestion
Cascara sagrada	Remedies for chronic constipation
Catnip	Calming effect in children
Cat's claw	Asthma; cancer
Celery	Blood pressure; diuretic
Centaury	Stimulates the salivary gland
Chamomile	Headache; colic; minor bites and stings; anxiety/tension
Chaste tree	Acne; menopause
Chickweed	Rich in vitamin C and minerals (calcium, magnesium, and potassium); diuretic; thyroid stimulant
Chicory (root)	Effective in disorders of the kidneys, liver, and urinary canal

Proposed Treatments *(continued)*

Herb	Treatment
Chondroitin	Osteoarthritis
Cinnamon (bark)	Prevents infection and indigestion; helps break down fats during digestion
Cleavers	Kidney and bladder disorders; useful in obstructions of the urinary organ
Cloves	General medicinal
Coenzyme Q_{10}	Cardiovascular disorders (angina, heart failure, hypertension)
Coriander (seed)	Stomach tonic
Cranberry	Urinary tract health; bladder infections; cystitis
Cubeb (berry)	Chronic bladder trouble; increases flow of urine
Damiana (leaf)	Sexual impotency
Dandelion (leaf)	Diuretic; appetite stimulation; liver conditions
Dandelion (root)	Detoxify poisons in the liver; beneficial in lowering blood pressure
Dehydroepiandrosterone (DHEA)	Improvement in energy, muscle mass, mood, memory
Devil's claw	Arthritis; back pain
Dill weed	Digestive health
Dong quai (root)	Menopause and PMS symptoms; anemia
Echinacea (root)	Colds and viruses; immune modulating
Eucalyptus (leaf)	Mucolytic
Elder	Antiviral; boils and skin ulcers; cough
Elecampane (root)	Cough with mucus
Evening primrose	Arthritis; diabetes; eczema
Eyebright (*Euphrasia officinalis*)	Eye-related inflammatory conditions
Fennel (seed)	Remedies for gas and acid stomach
Fenugreek (seed)	Allergies; coughs; digestion; emphysema; headaches; migraines; intestinal inflammation; ulcers; lungs; mucous membranes; and sore throat
Feverfew	Migraines
Fish oil	Hypercholesterolemia; cardiovascular health
Flax seed	Cardiovascular health
Garlic (bulb)	Lowers blood cholesterol; anti-infective; protective against cancer
Gentian	Digestive health
Ginger (root)	Antiemetic; arthritis
Ginkgo biloba	Improves blood circulation to the brain; dementia; impotence
Ginseng, Siberian (root)	Resistance against stress; slows the aging process; fatigue
Glucosamine	Osteoarthritis
Goldenseal	Digestive disorders
Gota kola	"Memory herb"; nerve tonic; wound healing
Gravelroot (queen of the meadow)	Remedy for stones in the kidney and bladder
Green tea	Antioxidant
Hawthorn	Cardiotonic; hypertension; circulatory problems
Hibiscus (flower)	Diuretic
Hops (flower)	Insomnia; used to decrease the desire for alcohol
Horehound	Acute or chronic sore throat and coughs
Horsetail (shavegrass)	Rich in minerals, especially silica; used to develop strong fingernails and hair, good for split ends; diuretic
Hydrangea (root)	Backaches
Juniper (berry)	Diuretic; arthritis; bladder infections; cystitis
Kava (root)	Calm nervousness; anxiety; pain
Kelp	High contents of natural plant iodine, for proper function of the thyroid; high levels of natural calcium, potassium, and magnesium
Lactobacillus acidophilus	Gastrointestinal microflora recolonization (anaerobic)
Lavender (oil)	Wound healing; decrease scarring (topical)

Proposed Treatments *(continued)*

Herb	Treatment
Lecithin	Break up cholesterol; prevent arteriosclerosis
Licorice (root)	Expectorant; used in peptic ulceration; adrenal exhaustion; canker sores
Lobelia	Cough
Ma huang (ephedra)	Asthma
Malva (flower)	Soothes inflammation in the mouth and throat; helpful for earaches
Marjoram	Beneficial for a sour stomach or loss of appetite
Marshmallow (leaf)	Demulcent
Milk thistle	Liver detoxifier; antioxidant; diuretic
Motherwort	Hypertension; regulate blood circulation
Mugwort	Used for rheumatism and gout
Mullein (leaf)	High in iron, magnesium, and potassium; sinuses; relieves swollen joints; soothing bronchial tissue
Mustard (seed)	General medicinal
Myrrh (gum)	Removes bad breath; sinus problems
Nettle (leaf)	Dandruff; antihistaminic qualities; allergies; asthma; hay fever
Nettle (root)	Used in benign prostatic hyperplasia (BPH); arthritis
Nutmeg	Gas
Oregano (leaf)	Settles the stomach after meals; helps treat colds
Oregon grape (root)	Gallbladder problems
Papaya (leaf)	Digestive stimulant; contains the enzyme papain
Paprika (sweet)	Stimulates the appetite and gastric secretions
Passion (flower)	Mild sedative
Pau d'arco	Protects immune system; antifungal
Peppermint (leaf)	Excellent for headaches; digestive stimulation; indigestion; colic
Poppy seed blue	Excellent in the making of breads and desserts
Prickly ash (bark)	Increases circulation
Psyllium (seed)	Lubricant to the intestinal tract
Red clover	Phytoestrogenic properties
Red raspberry (leaf)	Decreases menstrual bleeding; childbirth; diarrhea
Red yeast rice	Lowers cholesterol levels
Rhubarb (root)	Powerful laxative
Rose hips	High content of vitamin C
SAMe (S-adenosyl methionine)	Depression
Sassafras oil	Mild counterirritant on skin (eg, insect bites)
Saw palmetto (berry)	Benign prostatic hyperplasia (BPH)
Schisandra	Increasing the body's ability to adapt to stresses from chemical, physical, psychological, and environmental sources
Scullcap	Anxiety and tension
Seawrack (bladderwrack)	Combat obesity; contains iodine
Senna (leaf)	Laxative
Shepherd's purse	Female reproductive health
Sheep sorrel	Diuretic
Slippery elm (bark)	Normalize bowel movement; beneficial for hemorrhoids and constipation
Solomon's seal (root)	Poultice for bruises
Spikenard	Skin ailments such as acne, pimples, blackheads, rashes, and general skin problems
Star anise	Promotes appetite and relieves flatulence
St John's wort	Depression; neuralgia pain
Summer savory (leaf)	Diarrhea, upset stomach, and sore throat
Tea tree oil	Antifungal, antibacterial; dental and oral health (mouthwash); burns, cuts, scrapes, insect bites, dandruff; acne

Proposed Treatments *(continued)*

Herb	Treatment
Thyme (leaf)	Ulcers (peptic); cough; antifungal
Tumeric	Arthritis; liver detoxifier
Uva-ursi (leaf)	Diuretic; used in urinary tract health; bladder infections; cystitis
Valerian (root)	Insomnia; anxiety and tension; neuralgia pain
Vanadium	Diabetes mellitus
Vervain	Remedy for fevers
White oak (bark)	Strong astringent
White willow	Arthritis; back pain; migraines
Wild alum (root)	Powerful astringent; used as rinse for sores in mouth and bleeding gums
Wild cherry	Cough suppressant
Wild Oregon grape (root)	Chronic skin disease
Wild yam (root)	Menopause
Wintergreen (leaf)	Valuable for colic and gas in the bowels
Witch hazel (bark and leaf)	Hemorrhoids
Wormwood	Antiparasitic
Yarrow (root)	Fevers; hemorrhoid
Yellow dock (root)	Good in all skin problems
Yerba santa	Bronchial congestion
Yohimbe	Natural aphrodisiac
Yucca (root)	Reduces inflammation of the joints

IMMUNIZATION ADMINISTRATION RECOMMENDATIONS

The following tables are taken from the General Recommendations on Immunization, 2011:

- Guidelines for Spacing of Live and Inactivated Antigens
- Guidelines for Administering Antibody-Containing Products and Vaccines
- Recommended Intervals Between Administration of Antibody-Containing Products and Measles- or Varicella-Containing Vaccine, by Product and Indication for Vaccination
- Vaccination of persons with Primary and Secondary Immunodeficiencies
- Needle length and Injection Site of I.M. injections

Guidelines for Spacing of Live and Inactivated Antigens

Antigen Combination	Recommended Minimum Interval Between Doses
Two or more inactivated[1]	May be administered simultaneously or at any interval between doses
Inactivated and live	May be administered simultaneously or at any interval between doses
Two or more live injectable[2]	28 days minimum interval, if not administered simultaneously

[1]Certain experts suggest a 28-day interval between tetanus toxoid, reduced diphtheria toxoid, and reduced acellular pertussis (Tdap) vaccine and tetravalent meningococcal conjugate vaccine if they are not administered simultaneously.

[2]Live oral vaccines (eg, Ty21a typhoid vaccine and rotavirus vaccine) may be administered simultaneously or at any interval before or after inactivated or live injectable vaccines.

Adapted from American Academy of Pediatrics, "Pertussis," In: Pickering LK, Baker CJ, Kimberlin DW, et al, eds, *Red Book*: 2009 Report of the Committee on Infectious Diseases, 28th ed, Elk Grove Village, IL: American Academy of Pediatrics, 2009, 22.

Guidelines for Administering Antibody-Containing Products[1] and Vaccines

Simultaneous Administration (during the same office visit)

Products Administered	Recommended Minimum Interval Between Doses
Antibody-containing products and inactivated antigen	Can be administered simultaneously at different anatomic sites or at any time interval between doses.
Antibody-containing products and live antigen	Should **not** be administered simultaneously.[2] If simultaneous administration of measles-containing vaccine or varicella vaccine is unavoidable, administer at different sites and revaccinate or test for seroconversion after the recommended interval.

Nonsimultaneous Administration

Products Administered: Administered first	Products Administered: Administered second	Recommended Minimum Interval Between Doses
Antibody-containing products	Inactivated antigen	No interval necessary
Inactivated antigen	Antibody-containing products	No interval necessary
Antibody-containing products	Live antigen	Dose-related[2,3]
Live antigen	Antibody-containing products	2 weeks[2]

[1]Blood products containing substantial amounts of immune globulin include intramuscular and intravenous immune globulin, specific hyperimmune globulin (eg, hepatitis B immune globulin, tetanus immune globulin, varicella zoster immune globulin, and rabies immune globulin), whole blood, packed red blood cells, plasma, and platelet products.

[2]Yellow fever vaccine, rotavirus vaccine, oral Ty21a typhoid vaccine, live-attenuated influenza vaccine, and zoster vaccine are exceptions to these recommendations. These live-attenuated vaccines can be administered at any time before, after, or simultaneously with an antibody-containing product.

[3]The duration of interference of antibody-containing products with the immune response to the measles component of measles-containing vaccine, and possibly varicella vaccine, is dose-related.

Recommended Intervals Between Administration of Antibody-Containing Products and Measles- or Varicella-Containing Vaccine, by Product and Indication for Vaccination

Product/Indication	Dose (mg IgG/kg) and Route[1]	Recommended Interval Before Measles- or Varicella-Containing Vaccine[2] Administration (mo)
Tetanus IG	I.M.: 250 units (10 mg IgG/kg)	3
Hepatitis A IG		
Contact prophylaxis	I.M.: 0.02 mL/kg (3.3 mg IgG/kg)	3
International travel	I.M.: 0.06 mL/kg (10 mg IgG/kg)	3
Hepatitis B IG	I.M.: 0.06 mL/kg (10 mg IgG/kg)	3
Rabies IG	I.M.: 20 int. units/kg (22 mg IgG/kg)	4
Varicella IG	I.M.: 125 units/10 kg (60-200 mg IgG/kg) (maximum: 625 units)	5
Measles prophylaxis IG		
Standard (ie, nonimmunocompromised) contact	I.M.: 0.25 mL/kg (40 mg IgG/kg)	5
Immunocompromised contact	I.M.: 0.50 mL/kg (80 mg IgG/kg)	6
Blood transfusion		
Red blood cells (RBCs), washed	I.V.: 10 mL/kg (negligible IgG/kg)	None
RBCs, adenine-saline added	I.V.: 10 mL/kg (10 mg IgG/kg)	3
Packed RBCs (hematocrit 65%)[3]	I.V.: 10 mL/kg (60 mg IgG/kg)	6
Whole blood cells (hematocrit 35% to 50%)[3]	I.V.: 10 mL/kg (80-100 mg IgG/kg)	6
Plasma/platelet products	I.V.: 10 mL/kg (160 mg IgG/kg)	7
Cytomegalovirus intravenous immune globulin (IGIV)	150 mg/kg maximum	6
IGIV		
Replacement therapy for immune deficiencies[4]	I.V.: 300-400 mg/kg[4]	8
Immune thrombocytopenic purpura treatment	I.V.: 400 mg/kg	8
Postexposure varicella prophylaxis[5]	I.V.: 400 mg/kg	8
Immune thrombocytopenic purpura treatment	I.V.: 1000 mg/kg	10
Kawasaki disease	I.V.: 2 g/kg	11
Monoclonal antibody to respiratory syncytial virus F protein (Synagis® [Medimmune])[6]	I.M.: 15 mg/kg	None

HIV = human immunodeficiency virus, IG = immune globulin, IgG = immune globulin G, IGIV = intravenous immune globulin, mg IgG/kg = milligrams of immune globulin G per kilogram of body weight, I.M. = intramuscular, I.V. = intravenous, RBCs = red blood cells

[1]This table is not intended for determining the correct indications and dosages for using antibody-containing products. Unvaccinated persons might not be fully protected against measles during the entire recommended interval, and additional doses of IG or measles vaccine might be indicated after measles exposure. Concentrations of measles antibody in an IG preparation can vary by manufacturer's lot. Rates of antibody clearance after receipt of an IG preparation also might vary. Recommended intervals are extrapolated from an estimated half-life of 30 days for passively acquired antibody and an observed interference with the immune response to measles vaccine for 5 months after a dose of 80 mg IgG/kg.

[2]Does not include zoster vaccine. Zoster vaccine may be given with antibody-containing blood products.

[3]Assumes a serum IgG concentration of 16 mg/mL

[4]Measles and varicella vaccinations are recommended for children with asymptomatic or mildly symptomatic HIV infection but are contraindicated for persons with severe immunosuppression from HIV or any other immunosuppressive disorder.

[5]The investigational product VariZIG™, similar to licensed varicella-zoster IG (VZIG), is a purified human IG preparation made from plasma containing high levels of anti-varicella antibodies (IgG). The interval between VariZIG™ and varicella vaccine (Var or MMRV) is 5 months.

[6]Contains antibody only to respiratory syncytial virus

Vaccination of Persons With Primary and Secondary Immunodeficiencies

Category	Specific Immunodeficiency	Contraindicated Vaccines[1]	Risk-Specific Recommended Vaccines[1]	Effectiveness and Comments
Primary				
B-lymphocyte (humoral)	Severe antibody deficiencies (eg, X-linked agammaglobulinemia and common variable immunodeficiency)	Oral poliovirus (OPV)[2] Smallpox Live-attenuated influenza vaccine (LAIV) BCG Ty21a (live oral typhoid) Yellow fever	Pneumococcal Consider measles and varicella vaccination	The effectiveness of any vaccine is uncertain if it depends only on the humoral response (eg, PPSV or MPSV4) IGIV interferes with the immune response to measles vaccine and possibly varicella vaccine
	Less severe antibody deficiencies (eg, selective IgA deficiency and IgG subclass deficiency)	OPV[2] BCG Yellow Fever Other live-vaccines appear to be safe	Pneumococcal	All vaccines likely effective; immune response may be attenuated
T-lymphocyte (cell-mediated and humoral)	Complete defects (eg, severe combined immunodeficiency [SCID] disease, complete DiGeorge syndrome)	All live vaccines[3,4,5]	Pneumococcal	Vaccines might be ineffective
	Partial defects (eg, most patients with DiGeorge syndrome, Wiskott-Aldrich syndrome, ataxia-telangiectasia)	All live vaccines[3,4,5]	Pneumococcal Meningococcal Hib (if not administered in infancy)	Effectiveness of any vaccine depends on degree of immune suppression
Complement	Persistent complement, properdin, or factor B deficiency	None	Pneumococcal Meningococcal	All routine vaccines likely effective
Phagocytic function	Chronic granulomatous disease, leukocyte adhesion defect, and myeloperoxidase deficiency	Live bacterial vaccines[3]	Pneumococcal[6]	All inactivated vaccines safe and likely effective; live viral vaccines likely safe and effective

Vaccination of Persons With Primary and Secondary Immunodeficiencies *continued*

Category	Specific Immunodeficiency	Contraindicated Vaccines[1]	Risk-Specific Recommended Vaccines[1]	Effectiveness and Comments
Secondary				
	HIV/AIDS	OPV[2] Smallpox BCG LAIV Withhold MMR and varicella in severely immunocompromised persons Yellow fever vaccine might have a contraindication or a precaution depending on clinical parameters of immune function[9]	Pneumococcal Consider Hib (if not administered in infancy) and meningococcal vaccination.	MMR, varicella, rotavirus, and all inactivated vaccines, including inactivated influenza, might be effective.[7]
	Malignant neoplasm, transplantation, immunosuppressive or radiation therapy	Live viral and bacterial, depending on immune status[3,4]	Pneumococcal	Effectiveness of any vaccine depends on degree of immune suppression
	Asplenia	None	Pneumococcal Meningococcal Hib (if not administered in infancy)	All routine vaccines likely effective
	Chronic renal disease	LAIV	Pneumococcal Hepatitis B[8]	All routine vaccines likely effective

AIDS = acquired immunodeficiency syndrome; BCG = bacille Calmette-Guerin; Hib = *Haemophilus influenzae* type b; HIV = human immunodeficiency virus; IG = immunoglobulin; IGIV = immune globulin intravenous; LAIV = live, attenuated influenza vaccine; MMR = measles, mumps, and rubella; MPSV4 = quadrivalent meningococcal polysaccharide vaccine; OPV = oral poliovirus vaccine (live); PPSV = pneumococcal polysaccharide vaccine; TIV = trivalent inactivated influenza vaccine

[1]Other vaccines that are universally or routinely recommended should be administered if not contraindicated.

[2]OPV is no longer available in the United States.

[3]Live bacterial vaccines: BCG and oral Ty21a *Salmonella typhi* vaccine

[4]Live viral vaccines: MMR, MMRV, OPV, LAIV, yellow fever, zoster, rotavirus, varicella, and vaccinia (smallpox). Smallpox vaccine is not recommended for children or the general public.

[5]Regarding T-lymphocyte immunodeficiency as a contraindication for rotavirus vaccine, data exist only for severe combined immunodeficiency.

[6]Pneumococcal vaccine is not indicated for children with chronic granulomatous disease beyond age-based universal recommendations for PCV. Children with chronic granulomatous disease are not at increased risk for pneumococcal disease.

[7]HIV-infected children should receive IG after exposure to measles and may receive varicella and measles vaccine if $CD4^+$ lymphocyte count is ≥15%.

[8]Indicated based on the risk from dialysis-based bloodborne transmission

[9]Symptomatic HIV infection or $CD4^+$ T-lymphocyte count of <200/mm^3 or <15% of total lymphocytes for children aged <6 years is a containdication to yellow fever vaccine administration. Asymptomatic HIV infection with $CD4^+$ T-lymphocyte count of 200-499/mm^3 for persons aged ≥6 years or 15% to 24% of total lymphocytes for children aged <6 years is a precaution for yellow fever vaccine administration. Details of yellow fever vaccine recommendations are available from the CDC. (CDC, "Yellow Fever Vaccine: Recommendations of the Advisory Committee on Immunization Practices [ACIP]," *MMWR Recomm Rep*, 2010, 59[No. RR-7].)

Adapted from American Academy of Pediatrics, "Passive Immunization," In: Pickering LK, Baker CJ, Kimberline DW, et al, eds, *Red Book*: 2009 Report of the Committee on Infectious Diseases, 28th ed, Elk Grove Village, IL: American Academy of Pediatrics, 2009, 74-5.

Needle Length and Injection Site of I.M. for Children Aged ≤18 years (by age) and Adults Aged ≥19 years (by sex and weight)

Age Group	Needle Length	Injection Site
Children (birth to 18 y)		
Neonates[1]	5/8" (16 mm)[2]	Anterolateral thigh
Infant 1-12 mo	1" (25 mm)	Anterolateral thigh
Toddler 1-2 y	1-1¼" (25-32 mm)	Anterolateral thigh[3]
	5/8[2]-1" (16-25 mm)	Deltoid muscle of the arm
Children 3-18 y	5/8[2]-1" (16-25 mm)	Deltoid muscle of the arm[3]
	1-1¼" (25-32 mm)	Anterolateral thigh
Adults ≥19 y		
Men and women <60 kg (130 lb)	1" (25 mm)[4]	Deltoid muscle of the arm
Men and women 60-70 kg (130-152 lb)	1" (25 mm)	
Men 70-118 kg (152-260 lb)	1-1½" (25-38 mm)	
Women 70-90 kg (152-200 lb)		
Men >118 kg (260 lb)	1½" (38 mm)	
Women >90 kg (200 lb)		

I.M. = intramuscular

[1]First 28 days of life

[2]If skin is stretched tightly and subcutaneous tissues are not bunched

[3]Preferred site

[4]Some experts recommend a 5/8" needle for men and women who weigh <60 kg.

Adapted from Poland GA, Borrud A, Jacobsen RM, et al, "Determination of Deltoid Fat Pad Thickness: Implications for Needle Length in Adult Immunization," *JAMA*, 1997, 277:1709-11.

RECOMMENDATIONS FOR TRAVELERS

The Centers for Disease Control and Prevention (CDC) also provides guidance to assist travelers and their healthcare providers in deciding the vaccines, medications, and other measures necessary to prevent illness and injury during international travel. Available at http://wwwnc.cdc.gov/travel

REFERENCE

Centers for Disease Control, "Recommendations of the Advisory Committee on Immunization Practices (ACIP): General Recommendations on Immunization," *MMWR Recomm Rep*, 2011, 60(2):1-61.

IMMUNIZATION RECOMMENDATIONS

Recommended immunization schedule for persons aged 0 through 6 years — United States, 2012
For those who fall behind or start late, see the catch-up schedule

Vaccine ▼ Age ▶	Birth	1 month	2 months	4 months	6 months	9 months	12 months	15 months	18 months	19–23 months	2–3 years	4–6 years
Hepatitis B[1]	HepB	HepB			HepB							
Rotavirus[2]			RV	RV	RV[2]							
Diphtheria, tetanus, pertussis[3]			DTaP	DTaP	DTaP		See footnote[3]	DTaP				DTaP
***Haemophilus influenzae* type b**[4]			Hib	Hib	Hib[4]		Hib					
Pneumococcal[5]			PCV	PCV	PCV		PCV				PPSV	
Inactivated poliovirus[6]			IPV	IPV	IPV							IPV
Influenza[7]					Influenza (yearly)							
Measles, mumps, rubella[8]							MMR		See footnote[8]			MMR
Varicella[9]							VAR		See footnote[9]			VAR
Hepatitis A[10]							Dose 1[10]				HepA series	
Meningococcal[11]						MCV4 — See footnote[11]						

Range of recommended ages for all children

Range of recommended ages for certain high-risk groups

Range of recommended ages for all children and certain high-risk groups

This schedule includes recommendations in effect as of December 23, 2011. Any dose not administered at the recommended age should be administered at a subsequent visit, when indicated and feasible. The use of a combination vaccine generally is preferred over separate injections of its equivalent component vaccines. Vaccination providers should consult the relevant Advisory Committee on Immunization Practices (ACIP) statement for detailed recommendations: **http://www.cdc.gov/vaccines/pubs/acip-list.htm**. Clinically significant adverse events that follow vaccination should be reported to the Vaccine Adverse Event Reporting System (VAERS) at http://www.vaers.hhs.gov or by telephone, **(800) 822-7967**.

Footnotes to Recommended Immunization Schedule for Persons 0-6 Years of Age

[1]**Hepatitis B vaccine (HepB)** *(Minimum age: Birth)*

At birth:

- Administer monovalent HepB vaccine to all newborns before hospital discharge.
- For infants born to hepatitis B surface antigen (HB_sAg)-positive mothers, administer HepB vaccine and 0.5 mL of hepatitis B immune globulin (HBIG) within 12 hours of birth. These infants should be tested for HB_sAg and antibody to HB_sAg (anti-HBs) 1-2 months after completion of at least 3 doses of the HepB series, at 9-18 months of age (generally at the next well-child visit).
- If mother's HB_sAg status is unknown, within 12 hours of birth, administer HepB vaccine for infants weighing ≥2,000 grams and HepB vaccine plus HBIG for infants weighing <2,000 grams. Determine mother's HB_sAg status as soon as possible and, if she is HB_sAg-positive, administer HBIG for infants weighing ≥2,000 grams (no later than 1 week of age).

Doses after the birth dose:

- The second dose should be administered at 1 or 2 months of age. Monovalent HepB vaccine should be used for doses administered before 6 weeks of age.
- Administration of a total of 4 doses of HepB to infants is permissible when a combination vaccine containing HepB is administered after the birth dose.
- Infants who did not receive a birth dose should receive 3 doses of a HepB-containing vaccine starting as soon as feasible.

- The minimum interval between dose 1 and 2 is 4 weeks, and between dose 2 and 3 is 8 weeks. The final (third or fourth) dose in the HepB vaccine series should be administered no earlier than 24 weeks of age and ≥16 weeks after the first dose.

[2]**Rotavirus vaccine (RV)** *(Minimum age: 6 weeks for both RV-1 [Rotarix®] and RV-5 [RotaTeq®])*

- The maximum age for the first dose in the series is 14 weeks, 6 days; and 8 months, 0 days for the final dose in the series. Vaccination should not be initiated for infants ≥15 weeks, 0 days of age.
- If RV-1 (Rotarix®)is administered at 2 and 4 months of age, a dose at 6 months of age is not indicated.

[3]**Diphtheria and tetanus toxoids and acellular pertussis vaccine (DTaP)** *(Minimum age: 6 weeks)*

- The fourth dose may be administered as early as 12 months of age, provided ≥6 months have elapsed since the third dose.

[4] ***Haemophilus influenzae* type b conjugate vaccine (Hib)** *(Minimum age: 6 weeks)*

- If PRP-OMP (PedvaxHIB® or ComVax® [HepB-Hib]) is administered at 2 and 4 months of age, a dose at 6 months of age is not indicated.
- Hiberix® should only be used for the booster (final) dose in children 12 months to 4 years of age.

[5]**Pneumococcal vaccine** *(Minimum age: 6 weeks for pneumococcal conjugate vaccine [PCV]; 2 years for pneumococcal polysaccharide vaccine [PPSV])*

- Administer 1 dose of PCV to all healthy children 24-59 months of age who are not completely vaccinated for their age.
- For children who have received an age-appropriate series of 7-valent PCV (PCV7), a single supplemental dose of 13-valent PCV (PCV13) is recommended for:
  - All children 14-59 months of age
  - Children 60-71 months of age with underlying medical conditions
- Administer PPSV ≥8 weeks after last dose of PCV to children ≥2 years of age with certain underlying medical conditions, including a cochlear implant. See *MMWR*, 2010, 59(No. RR-11), available at http://www.cdc.gov/mmwr/pdf/rr/rr5911.pdf.

[6]**Inactivated poliovirus vaccine (IPV)** *(Minimum age: 6 weeks)*

- If ≥4 doses are administered prior to 4 years of age, an additional dose should be administered at 4-6 years of age.
- The final dose in the series should be administered on or after the fourth birthday and ≥6 months after the previous dose.

[7]**Influenza vaccines** *(Minimum age: 6 months for trivalent inactivated influenza vaccine [TIV]; 2 years for live, attenuated influenza vaccine [LAIV])*

- For most healthy children ≥2 years of age, either LAIV or TIV may be used. However, LAIV should not be administered to some children, including children with asthma, children 2-4 years of age who had wheezing in the past 12 months, or children who have any other underlying medical conditions that predispose them to influenza complications. For all other contraindications to use of LAIV, see *MMWR*, 2010, 59(No. RR-8), available at http://www.cdc.gov/mmwr/pdf/rr/rr5908.pdf.
- For children 6 months to 8 years of age:
  - For the 2011-12 season, administer 2 doses (separated by ≥4 weeks) to those who did not receive ≥1 dose of the 2010-11 vaccine. Those who received ≥1 dose of the 2010-11 vaccine require 1 dose for the 2011-12 season.
  - For the 2012-13 season, follow dosing guidelines in the 2012 ACIP influenze vaccine recommendations.

[8]**Measles, mumps, and rubella vaccine (MMR)** *(Minimum age: 12 months)*

- The second dose may be administered before 4 years of age, provided ≥4 weeks have elapsed since the first dose.
- Administer MMR vaccine to infants 6-11 months of age who are traveling internationally. These children should be revaccinated with 2 doses of MMR vaccine, the first at 12-15 months of age and ≥4 weeks after the previous dose, and second at 4-6 years of age.

[9]**Varicella vaccine (VAR)** *(Minimum age: 12 months)*

- The second dose may be administered before 4 years of age, provided ≥3 months have elapsed since the first dose.

- For children 12 months to 12 years of age, the recommended minimum interval between doses is 3 months. However, if the second dose was administered ≥4 weeks after the first dose, it can be accepted as valid.

[10]**Hepatitis A vaccine (HepA)** *(Minimum age: 12 months)*

- Administer the second (final) dose 6-18 months after the first dose.
- Unvaccinated children ≥24 months of age at high risk should be vaccinated. See *MMWR*, 2006, 55(No. RR-7), available at http://www.cdc.gov/mmwr/pdf/rr/rr5507.pdf.
- A 2-dose HepA vaccine series is recommended for anyone ≥24 months of age, previously unvaccined, for whom immunity against hepatitis A virus infection is desired.

[11]**Meningococcal conjugate vaccines, quadrivalent (MCV4)** *(Minimum age: 9 months for Menactra® [MCV4-D]; 2 years for Menveo® [MCV4-CRM])*

- For children 9-23 months of age with persistent complement component deficiency, who are residents of or travelers to countries with hyperendemic or epidemic disease, or who are present during outbreaks caused by a vaccine serogroup, administer 2 primary doses of MCV4-D, ideally at 9-12 months of age or ≥8 weeks apart.
- For children ≥24 months of age with persistent complement component deficiency who have not been previously vaccinated or with anatomic/functional asplenia, administer 2 primary doses of either MCV4 ≥8 weeks apart.
- For children with anatomic/functional asplenia, if MCV4-D (Menactra®) is used, administer at a minimum age of 2 years and ≥4 weeks after completion of all PCV doses.
- See *MMWR*, 2011, 60:72-6, available at http://www.cdc.gov/mmwr/pdf/wk/mm6003.pdf; Vaccines for Children Program resolution No. 6/11-1, available at http://www.cdc.gov/vaccines/programs/vfc/downloads/resolutions/06-11mening-mcv.pdf; and *MMWR*, 2011, 60:1391-2, available at http://www.cdc.gov/mmwr/pdf/wk/mm6040.pdf, for further guidance, including revaccination guidelines.

The recommended immunization schedules for persons 0-18 years of age are approved by the Advisory Committee on Immunization Practices (**http://www.cdc.gov/vaccines/recs/acip**), the American Academy of Pediatrics (**http://www.aap.org**), and the American Academy of Family Physicians (**http://www.aafp.org**).

Recommended immunization schedule for persons aged 7 through 18 years — United States, 2012
For those who fall behind or start late, see the catch-up schedule

Vaccine ▼ / Age ▶	7–10 years	11–12 years	13–18 years
Tetanus, diphtheria, pertussis[1]	1 dose (if indicated)	1 dose	1 dose (if indicated)
Human papillomavirus[2]	*See footnote*[2]	3 doses	Complete 3-dose series
Meningococcal[3]	See footnote[3]	Dose 1	Booster at age 16 years
Influenza[4]	Influenza (yearly)		
Pneumococcal[5]	See footnote[5]		
Hepatitis A[6]	Complete 2-dose series		
Hepatitis B[7]	Complete 3-dose series		
Inactivated poliovirus[8]	Complete 3-dose series		
Measles, mumps, rubella[9]	Complete 2-dose series		
Varicella[10]	Complete 2-dose series		

Legend: Range of recommended ages for all children; Range of recommended ages for catch-up immunization; Range of recommended ages for certain high-risk groups

This schedule includes recommendations in effect as of December 23, 2011. Any dose not administered at the recommended age should be administered at a subsequent visit, when indicated and feasible. The use of a combination vaccine generally is preferred over separate injections of its equivalent component vaccines. Vaccination providers should consult the relevant Advisory Committee on Immunization Practices (ACIP) statement for detailed recommendations, available at **http://www.cdc.gov/vaccines/pubs/acip-list.htm**. Clinically significant adverse events that follow vaccination should be reported to the Vaccine Adverse Event Reporting System (VAERS) at **http://www.vaers.hhs.gov** or by telephone, **(800) 822-7967**.

Footnotes to Recommended Immunization Schedule for Persons 7-18 Years of Age

[1]**Tetanus and diphtheria toxoids and acellular pertussis vaccine (Tdap)** *(Minimum age: 10 years for Boostrix® and 11 years for Adacel®)*

- Persons 11-18 years of age who have not received Tdap should receive a dose, followed by tetanus and diphtheria toxoids (Td) booster doses, every 10 years thereafter.
- Tdap vaccine should be substituted for a single dose of Td in the catch-up series for children 7-10 years of age. Refer to the catch-up schedule if additional doses of tetanus and diphtheria toxoid–containing vaccine are needed.
- Tdap vaccine can be administered regardless of the interval since the last tetanus and diphtheria toxoid–containing vaccine.

[2]**Human papillomavirus vaccine (HPV) (HPV4 [Gardasil®] and HPV2 [Cervarix®])** *(Minimum age: 9 years)*

- Either HPV4 or HPV2 is recommended in a 3-dose series for females 11-12 years of age. HPV4 is recommended in a 3-dose series for males 11-12 years of age.
- The vaccine series can be started beginning at 9 years of age.
- Administer the second dose 1-2 months after the first dose and the third dose 6 months after the first dose (≥24 weeks after the first dose).
- See *MMWR*, 2010, 59:626-32, available at http://www.cdc.gov/mmwr/pdf/wk/mm5920.pdf.

[3]**Meningococcal conjugate vaccines, quadrivalent (MCV4)**

- Administer MCV4 at 11-12 years of age, with a booster dose at 16 years of age.
- Administer MCV4 at 13-18 years of age if patient is not previously vaccinated.
- If the first dose is administered at 13-15 years of age, a booster dose should be administered at 16-18 years of age with a minimum interval of ≥8 weeks after the preceding dose.
- If the first dose is administered at ≥16 years of age, a booster dose is not needed.
- Administer 2 primary doses ≥8 weeks apart to previously unvaccinated persons with persistent complement component deficiency or anatomic/functional asplenia, and 1 dose every 5 years thereafter.
- Adolescents 11-18 years of age with human immunodeficiency virus (HIV) infection should receive a 2-dose primary series of MCV4, ≥8 weeks apart.
- See *MMWR*, 2011, 60:72-6, available at http://www.cdc.gov/mmwr/pdf/wk/mm6003.pdf, and Vaccines for Children Program resolution No. 6/11-1, available at http://www.cdc.gov/vaccines/programs/vfc/downloads/resolutions/06-11mening-mcv.pdf, for further guidelines.

[4]**Influenza vaccines (trivalent inactivated influenza vaccine [TIV] and live, attenuated influenza vaccine [LAIV])**

- For most healthy, nonpregnant persons, either LAIV or TIV may be used, except LAIV should not be used for some persons, including those with asthma or any other underlying medical conditions that predispose them to influenza complications. For all other contraindications to use of LAIV, see *MMWR*, 2010, 59(No. RR-8), available at http://www.cdc.gov/mmwr/pdf/rr/rr5908.pdf.
- Administer 1 dose to persons ≥9 years of age.
- For children 6 months to 8 years of age:
  - For the 2011-12 season, administer 2 doses (separated by ≥4 weeks) to those who did not receive ≥1 dose of the 2010-11 vaccine. Those who received ≥1 dose of the 2010-11 vaccine require 1 dose for the 2011-12 season.
  - For the 2012-13 season, follow dosing guidelines in the 2012 ACIP influenza vaccine recommendations.

[5]Pneumococcal vaccines (pneumococcal conjugate vaccine [PCV] and pneumococcal polysaccharide vaccine [PPSV])

- A single dose of PCV may be administered to children 6-18 years of age who have anatomic/functional asplenia, HIV infection or other immunocompromising condition, cochlear implant, or cerebral spinal fluid leak. See *MMWR*, 2010, 59(No. RR-11), available at http://www.cdc.gov/mmwr/pdf/rr/rr5911.pdf.
- Administer PPSV ≥8 weeks after the last dose of PCV to children ≥2 years of age with certain underlying medical conditions, including a cochlear implant. A single revaccination should be administered after 5 years to children with anatomic/functional asplenia or an immunocompromising condition.

[6]Hepatitis A vaccine (HepA)

- HepA vaccine is recommended for children >23 months of age who live in areas where vaccination programs target older children, who are at increased risk of infection, or for whom immunity against hepatitis A infection is desired. See *MMWR*, 2006, 55(No. RR-7), available at http://www.cdc.gov/mmwr/pdf/rr/rr5507.pdf.
- Administer 2 doses ≥6 months apart to unvaccinated persons.

[7]Hepatitis B vaccine (HepB)

- Administer the 3-dose series to those not previously vaccinated.
- For those with incomplete vaccination, see the **Catch-up Immunization Schedule**.
- A 2-dose series (doses separated by ≥4 months) of adult formulation Recombivax HB® is licensed for use in children 11-15 years of age.

[8]Inactivated poliovirus vaccine (IPV)

- The final dose in the series should be administered ≥6 months after the previous dose.
- If both OPV and IPV were administered as part of a series, a total of 4 doses should be administered, regardless of the child's current age.
- IPV is not routinely recommended for U.S. residents ≥18 years of age.

[9]Measles, mumps, and rubella vaccine (MMR)

- The minimum interval between the 2 doses of MMR vaccine is 4 weeks.

[10]Varicella vaccine (VAR)

- For persons without evidence of immunity, administer 2 doses if not previously vaccinated or the second dose if only 1 dose has been administered. See *MMWR*, 2007, 56(RR-4), available at http://www.cdc.gov/mmwr/pdf/rr/rr5604.pdf.
- For persons 7-12 years of age, the recommended minimum interval between doses is 3 months. However, if the second dose was administered ≥4 weeks after the first dose, it can be accepted as valid.
- For persons ≥13 years of age, the minimum interval between doses is 4 weeks.

This schedule is approved by the Advisory Committee on Immunization Practices (**http://www.cdc.gov/vaccines/recs/acip**), the American Academy of Pediatrics (**http://www.aap.org**), and the American Academy of Family Physicians (**http://www.aafp.org**).

REFERENCE

Centers for Disease Control and Prevention (CDC), "Recommended Immunization Schedules for Persons Aged 0-18 Years – United States, 2012," *MMWR Recomm Rep*, 2012, 61(5). Available at http://www.cdc.gov/mmwr/PDF/wk/mm6105-Immunization.pdf

Catch-up Immunization Schedule for Persons 4 Months to 18 Years of Age Who Start Late or Who Are >1 Month Behind – United States, 2012

This table provides catch-up schedules and minimum intervals between doses for children whose vaccinations have been delayed. A vaccine series does not need to be restarted, regardless of the time that has elapsed between doses. Use the section appropriate for the child's age.

Vaccine	Minimum Age for Dose 1	Minimum Interval Between Doses			
		Dose 1 to Dose 2	Dose 2 to Dose 3	Dose 3 to Dose 4	Dose 4 to Dose 5
Catch-up Schedule for Persons 4 Months to 6 Years of Age					
Hepatitis B	Birth	**4 weeks**	**8 weeks** and ≥16 weeks after first dose; minimum age for final dose is 24 weeks		
Rotavirus[1]	6 weeks	**4 weeks**	**4 weeks**[1]		
Diphtheria, tetanus, pertussis[2]	6 weeks	**4 weeks**	**4 weeks**	**6 months**	**6 months**[2]
Haemophilus influenzae type b[3]	6 weeks	**4 weeks** if first dose administered at <12 months of age **8 weeks** (as final dose) if first dose administered at 12-14 months of age **No further doses needed** if first dose administered at ≥15 months of age	**4 weeks**[3] if currently <12 months of age **8 weeks** (as final dose)[3] if currently ≥12 months of age and first dose administered at <12 months of age and second dose administered at <15 months of age **No further doses needed** if previous dose administered at ≥15 months of age	**8 weeks** (as final dose) This dose only necessary for children 12-59 months of age who received 3 doses before 12 months of age	
Pneumococcal[4]	6 weeks	**4 weeks** if first dose administered at <12 months of age **8 weeks** (as final dose for healthy children) if first dose administered at ≥12 months of age or currently 24-59 months of age **No further doses needed** for healthy children if first dose administered at ≥24 months of age	**4 weeks** if currently <12 months of age **8 weeks** (as final dose for healthy children) if currently ≥12 months of age **No further doses needed** for healthy children if previous dose administered at ≥24 months of age	**8 weeks** (as final dose) This dose only necessary for children 12-59 months of age who received 3 doses before 12 months of age or for high-risk children who received 3 doses at any age	
Inactivated poliovirus[5]	6 weeks	**4 weeks**	**4 weeks**	**6 months**[5] minimum 4 years of age for final dose	
Meningococcal[6]	9 months	**8 weeks**[6]			
Measles, mumps, rubella[7]	12 months	**4 weeks**			
Varicella[8]	12 months	**3 months**			
Hepatitis A	12 months	**6 months**			
Catch-up Schedule for Persons 7-18 Years of Age					
Tetanus, diphtheria/ tetanus, diphtheria, pertussis[9]	7 years[9]	**4 weeks**	**4 weeks** if first dose administered at <12 months of age **6 months** if first dose administered at ≥12 months of age	**6 months** if first dose administered at <12 months of age	
Human papillomavirus[10]	9 years	Routine dosing intervals are recommended[10]			
Hepatitis A	12 months	**6 months**			
Hepatitis B	Birth	**4 weeks**	**8 weeks** (and ≥16 weeks after first dose)		

(continued)

Vaccine	Minimum Age for Dose 1	Minimum Interval Between Doses			
		Dose 1 to Dose 2	Dose 2 to Dose 3	Dose 3 to Dose 4	Dose 4 to Dose 5
Inactivated poliovirus[5]	6 weeks	**4 weeks**	**4 weeks**[5]	**6 months**[5]	
Meningococcal[6]	9 months	**8 weeks**[6]			
Measles, mumps, rubella[7]	12 months	**4 weeks**			
Varicella[8]	12 months	**3 months** if person is <13 years of age **4 weeks** if person is ≥13 years of age			

Footnotes to Catch-up Immunization Schedule Table

[1]Rotavirus vaccines (RV-1 [Rotarix®] and RV-5 [RotaTeq®])

- The maximum age for the first dose is 14 weeks 6 days, and 8 months 0 days for the final dose in the series. Vaccination should not be initiated for infants ≥15 weeks 0 days of age.
- If RV-1 was administered for the first and second doses, a third dose is not indicated.

[2]Diphtheria and tetanus toxoids and acellular pertussis vaccine (DTaP)

- The fifth dose is not necessary if the fourth dose was administered at ≥4 years of age.

[3] *Haemophilus influenzae* type b conjugate vaccine (Hib)

- Hib vaccine should be considered for unvaccinated persons ≥5 years of age who have sickle cell disease, leukemia, human immunodeficiency virus (HIV) infection, or anatomic/functional asplenia.
- If the first 2 doses were PRP-OMP (PedvaxHIB® or ComVax®) and were administered at ≤11 months of age, the third (and final) dose should be administered at 12-15 months of age and ≥8 weeks after the second dose.
- If first dose was administered at 7-11 months of age, administer second dose ≥4 weeks later and a final dose at 12-15 months of age.

[4]Pneumococcal vaccine *(Minimum age: 6 weeks for pneumococcal conjugate vaccine [PCV]; 2 years for pneumococcal polysaccharide vaccine [PPSV])*

- For children 24-71 months of age with underlying medical conditions, administer 1 dose of PCV if 3 doses of PCV were received previously, or administer 2 doses of PCV ≥8 weeks apart if <3 doses of PCV were received previously.
- A single dose of PCV may be administered to certain children 6-18 years of age with underlying medical conditions. See age-specific schedules for details.
- Administer PPSV to children ≥2 years of age with certain underlying medical conditions. See *MMWR*, 2010, 59(No. RR-11), available at http://www.cdc.gov/mmwr/pdf/rr/rr5911.pdf

[5]Inactivated poliovirus vaccine (IPV)

- A fourth dose is not necessary if the third dose was administered at ≥4 years of age and ≥6 months after the previous dose.
- In the first 6 months of life, minimum age and minimum intervals are only recommended if the person is at risk for imminent exposure to circulating poliovirus (ie, travel to a polio-endemic region or during an outbreak).
- IPV is not routinely recommended for U.S. residents ≥18 years of age.

[6]Meningococcal conjugate vaccines, quadrivalent (MCV4) *(Minimum age: 9 months for Menactra® [MCV4-D]; 2 years for Menveo® [MCV4-CRM])*

- See **Recommended Immunization Schedule for Persons 0-6 Years of Age** and **Recommended Immunization Schedule for Persons 7-18 Years of Age**, for further guidance.

[7]Measles, mumps, and rubella vaccine (MMR)

- Administer the second dose routinely at 4-6 years of age.

[8]Varicella vaccine (VAR)

- Administer the second dose routinely at 4-6 years of age. If the second dose was administered ≥4 weeks after the first dose, it can be accepted as valid.

[9]**Tetanus and diphtheria toxoids vaccine (Td) and tetanus and diphtheria toxoids and acellular pertussis vaccine (Tdap)**

- For children 7-10 years of age who are not fully immunized with the childhood DTaP vaccine series, Tdap vaccine should be substituted for a single dose of Td vaccine in the catch-up series; if additional doses are needed, use Td vaccine. For these children, an adolescent Tdap vaccine dose should not be given.
- An inadvertent dose of DTaP vaccine administered to children 7-10 years of age can count as part of the catch-up series. This dose can count as the adolescent Tdap dose, or the child can later receive a Tdap booster dose at 11-12 years of age.

[10]**Human papillomavirus (HPV) vaccines (HPV4 [Gardasil®] and HPV2 [Cervarix®])**

- Administer the vaccine series to females (either HPV2 or HPV4) and males (HPV4) at 13-18 years of age if not previously vaccinated.
- Use recommended routine dosing intervals for series catch-up; see **Recommended Immunization Schedule for Persons 7-18 Years of Age**.

Clinically significant adverse events that follow vaccination should be reported to the Vaccine Adverse Event Reporting System (VAERS) online (http://www.vaers.hhs.gov) or by telephone, (800) 822-7967. Suspected cases of vaccine-preventable diseases should be reported to the state or local health departments. Additional information, including precautions and contraindications for immunization, is available from CDC online (http://www.cdc.gov/vaccines) or by telephone, (800) CDC-INFO (800-232-4636).

Recommended adult immunization schedule, by vaccine and age group[1] — United States, 2012

VACCINE ▼ AGE GROUP ▶	19–21 years	22–26 years	27–49 years	50–59 years	60–64 years	≥65 years
Influenza[2,*]			1 dose annually			
Tetanus, diphtheria, pertussis (Td/Tdap)[3,*]		Substitute 1-time dose of Tdap for Td booster; then boost with Td every 10 years				Td/Tdap[3]
Varicella[4,*]			2 doses			
Human papillomavirus (HPV)[5,*] Female	3 doses					
Human papillomavirus (HPV)[5,*] Male	3 doses					
Zoster[6]					1 dose	
Measles, mumps, rubella (MMR)[7,*]	1 or 2 doses			1 dose		
Pneumococcal (polysaccharide)[8,9]			1 or 2 doses			1 dose
Meningococcal[10,*]			1 or more doses			
Hepatitis A[11,*]			2 doses			
Hepatitis B[12,*]			3 doses			

*Covered by the Vaccine Injury Compensation Program

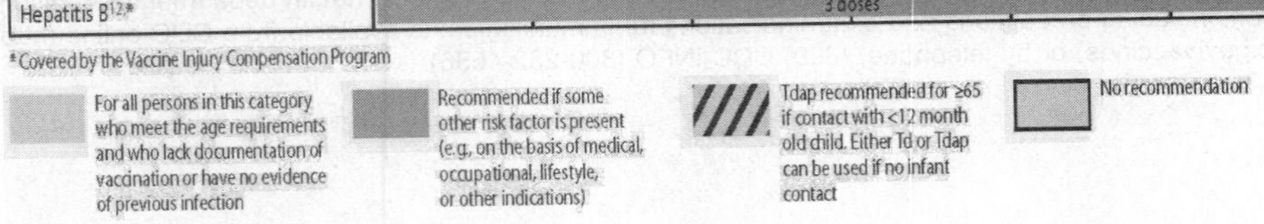

Vaccines that might be indicated for adults, based on medical and other indications[1] — United States, 2012

VACCINE ▼ INDICATION ▶	Pregnancy	Immunocompromising conditions (excluding human immunodeficiency virus [HIV])[4,6,7,14]	HIV infection[4,7,13,14] CD4+ T lymphocyte count: <200 cells/μL	HIV infection CD4+ T lymphocyte count: ≥200 cells/μL	Men who have sex with men (MSM)	Heart disease, chronic lung disease, chronic alcoholism	Asplenia[13] (including elective splenectomy and persistent complement component deficiencies)	Chronic liver disease	Diabetes, kidney failure, end-stage renal disease, receipt of hemodialysis	Health-care personnel
Influenza[2,*]		1 dose TIV annually			1 dose TIV or LAIV annually		1 dose TIV annually			1 dose TIV or LAIV annually
Tetanus, diphtheria, pertussis (Td/Tdap)[3,*]				Substitute 1-time dose of Tdap for Td booster; then boost with Td every 10 years						
Varicella[4,*]		Contraindicated					2 doses			
Human papillomavirus (HPV)[5,*] Female		3 doses through age 26 years					3 doses through age 26 years			
Human papillomavirus (HPV)[5,*] Male		3 doses through age 26 years					3 doses through age 21 years			
Zoster[6]		Contraindicated					1 dose			
Measles, mumps, rubella[7,*]		Contraindicated					1 or 2 doses			
Pneumococcal (polysaccharide)[8,9]					1 or 2 doses					
Meningococcal[10,*]					1 or more doses					
Hepatitis A[11,*]					2 doses					
Hepatitis B[12,*]					3 doses					

*Covered by the Vaccine Injury Compensation Program

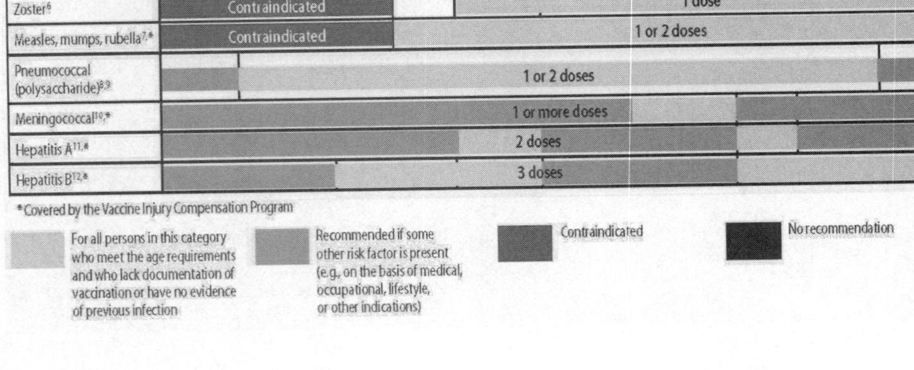

Footnotes to Recommended Adult Immunization Schedule

[1]Additional information

- Advisory Committee on Immunization Practices (ACIP) vaccine recommendations and additional information are available at http://www.cdc.gov/vaccines/pubs/acip-list.htm.
- Information on travel vaccine requirements and recommendations (eg, for hepatitis A and B, meningococcal, and other vaccines) are available at http://wwwnc.cdc.gov/travel/page/vaccinations.htm.

[2]Influenza vaccine

- Annual vaccination against influenza is recommended for all persons ≥6 months of age.
- Persons ≥6 months of age, including pregnant women, can receive the trivalent inactivated vaccine (TIV).
- Healthy, nonpregnant adults <50 years of age without high-risk medical conditions can receive either intranasally administered live, attenuated influenza vaccine (LAIV) (FluMist®) or TIV. Healthcare personnel who care for severely immunocompromised persons (ie, those who require care in a protected environment) should receive TIV, rather than LAIV. Other persons should receive TIV.
- The intramuscularly or intradermally administered TIV are options for adults 18-64 years of age.
- Adults ≥65 years of age can receive the standard-dose TIV or the high-dose TIV (Fluzone® High Dose).

[3]Tetanus, diphtheria, and acellular pertussis vaccine (Td/Tdap)

- Administer a one-time dose of Tdap to adults <65 years of age who have not received Tdap previously or for whom vaccine status is unknown to replace one of the 10-year Td boosters.
- Tdap is specifically recommended for the following persons:
  - Pregnant women >20 weeks gestation
  - Adults, regardless of age, who are close contacts of infants <12 months of age (eg, parents, grandparents, or child-care providers), and
  - Healthcare personnel
- Tdap can be administered regardless of interval since the most recent tetanus or diphtheria-containing vaccine.
- Pregnant women not vaccinated during pregnancy should receive Tdap immediately postpartum.
- Adults ≥65 years of age may receive Tdap.
- Adults with unknown or incomplete history of completing a 3-dose primary vaccination series with Td-containing vaccines should begin or complete a primary vaccination series. Tdap should be substituted for a single dose of Td in the vaccination series, with Tdap preferred as the first dose.
- For unvaccinated adults, administer the first 2 doses ≥4 weeks apart and the third dose 6-12 months after the second.
- If incompletely vaccinated (ie, less than 3 doses), administer remaining doses. Refer to the ACIP statement for recommendations for administering Td/Tdap as prophylaxis in wound management (see footnote 1).

[4]Varicella vaccine

- All adults without evidence of immunity to varicella should receive 2 doses of single-antigen varicella vaccine or a second dose if they have received only 1 dose.
- Special consideration should be given to those who:
  - Have close contact with persons at high risk for severe disease (eg, healthcare personnel and family contacts of persons with immunocompromising conditions), or
  - Are at high risk for exposure or transmission (eg, teachers; child-care employees; residents and staff members of institutional settings, including correctional institutions; college students; military personnel; adolescents and adults living in households with children; nonpregnant women of childbearing age; international travelers)
- Pregnant women should be assessed for evidence of varicella immunity. Women who do not have evidence of immunity should receive the first dose of varicella vaccine upon completion or termination of pregnancy and before discharge from the healthcare facility. The second dose should be administered 4-8 weeks after the first dose.

- Evidence of immunity to varicella in adults includes any of the following:
  - Documentation of 2 doses of varicella vaccine ≥4 weeks apart
  - U.S.-born before 1980 (although for healthcare personnel and pregnant women, birth before 1980 should not be considered evidence of immunity)
  - History of varicella based on diagnosis or verification of varicella by a healthcare provider (for a patient reporting a history of or having an atypical case, a mild case, or both, healthcare providers should seek either an epidemiologic link with a typical varicella case or to a laboratory-confirmed case or evidence of laboratory confirmation if it was performed at the time of acute disease)
  - History of herpes zoster based on diagnosis or verification of herpes zoster by a healthcare provider, or
  - Laboratory evidence of immunity or laboratory confirmation of disease

[5]Human papillomavirus vaccine (HPV)

- Two vaccines are licensed for use in females, bivalent HPV vaccine (HPV2) and quadrivalent HPV vaccine (HPV4), and one HPV vaccine for use in males (HPV4).
- For females, either HPV4 or HPV2 is recommended in a 3-dose series for routine vaccination at 11 or 12 years of age, and for those 13-26 years of age, if not previously vaccinated.
- For males, HPV4 is recommended in a 3-dose series for routine vaccination at 11 or 12 years of age, and for those 13-21 years of age, if not previously vaccinated. Males 22-26 years of age may be vaccinated.
- HPV vaccines are not live vaccines and can be administered to persons who are immunocompromised as a result of infection (including HIV infection), disease, or medications. Vaccine is recommended for immunocompromised persons through 26 years of age who did not get any or all doses when they were younger. The immune response and vaccine efficacy might be less than that in immunocompetent persons.
- Men who have sex with men (MSM) might especially benefit from vaccination to prevent condyloma and anal cancer. HPV4 is recommended for MSM through 26 years of age who did not get any or all doses when they were younger.
- Ideally, vaccine should be administered before potential exposure to HPV through sexual activity; however, persons who are sexually active should still be vaccinated consistent with age-based recommendations. HPV vaccine can be administered to persons with a history of genital warts, abnormal Papanicolaou test, or positive HPV DNA test.
- A complete series for either HPV4 or HPV2 consists of 3 doses. The second dose should be administered 1–2 months after the first dose; the third dose should be administered 6 months after the first dose (≥24 weeks after the first dose).
- Although HPV vaccination is not specifically recommended for healthcare personnel (HCP) based on their occupation, HCP should receive the HPV vaccine if they are in the recommended age group.

[6]Zoster vaccine

- A single dose of zoster vaccine is recommended for adults ≥60 years of age, regardless of whether they report a prior episode of herpes zoster. Although the vaccine is licensed by the Food and Drug Administration (FDA) for use among and can be administered to persons ≥50 years of age, ACIP recommendes that vaccination begin at 60 years of age.
- Persons with chronic medical conditions may be vaccinated, unless their condition constitutes a contraindication, such as pregnancy or severe immunodeficiency.
- Although zoster vaccination is not specifically recommended for healthcare personnel (HCP), HCP should receive the vaccine if they are in the recommended age group.

[7]Measles, mumps, rubella vaccine (MMR)

- Adults born before 1957 generally are considered immune to measles and mumps. All adults born in 1957 or later should have documentation of ≥1 dose of MMR vaccine, unless they have a medical contraindication to the vaccine, laboratory evidence of immunity to each of the three diseases, or documentation of provider-diagnosed measles or mumps disease. For rubella, documentation of provider-diagnosed disease is not considered acceptable evidence of immunity.

- *Measles component:*
  - A routine second dose of MMR vaccine, administered a minimum of 28 days after the first dose, is recommended for adults who:
    - Are students in postsecondary educational institutions
    - Work in a healthcare facility, or
    - Plan to travel internationally
  - Persons who received inactivated (killed) measles vaccine or measles vaccine of unknown type during 1963–1967 should be revaccinated with 2 doses of MMR vaccine.
- *Mumps component:*
  - A routine second dose of MMR vaccine, administered a minimum of 28 days after the first dose, is recommended for adults who:
    - Are students in postsecondary educational institutions
    - Work in a healthcare facility, or
    - Plan to travel internationally
  - Persons vaccinated before 1979 with either killed mumps vaccine or mumps vaccine of unknown type who are at high risk for mumps infection (eg, persons who are working in a healthcare facility) should be considered for revaccination with 2 doses of MMR vaccine.
- *Rubella component:* For women of childbearing age, regardless of birth year, rubella immunity should be determined. If there is no evidence of immunity, women who are not pregnant should be vaccinated. Pregnant women who do not have evidence of immunity should receive MMR vaccine upon completion or termination of pregnancy and before discharge from the healthcare facility.
- *Healthcare personnel born before 1957:* For unvaccinated healthcare personnel born before 1957 who lack laboratory evidence of measles, mumps, and/or rubella immunity or laboratory confirmation of disease, healthcare facilities should consider routinely vaccinating personnel with 2 doses of MMR vaccine at the appropriate interval for measles and mumps or 1 dose of MMR vaccine for rubella.

[8]Pneumococcal polysaccharide vaccine (PPSV)

- Vaccinate all persons with the following indications:
  - ≥65 years of age without a history of PPSV vaccination
  - Adults <65 years of age with chronic lung disease (including chronic obstructive pulmonary disease, emphysema, and asthma), chronic cardiovascular diseases, diabetes mellitus, chronic liver diseases (including cirrhosis), alcoholism, cochlear implants, cerebrospinal fluid leaks, immunocompromising conditions, and functional or anatomic asplenia (eg, sickle cell disease and other hemoglobinophathies, congenital or acquired asplenia, splenic dysfunction, or splenectomy [if elective splenectomy is planned, vaccinate ≥2 weeks before surgery])
  - Residents of nursing homes or long-term care facilities, and
  - Adults who smoke cigarettes
- Persons with asymptomatic or symptomatic HIV infection should be vaccinated as soon as possible after their diagonosis.
- When cancer chemotherapy or other immunosuppressive therapy is being considered, the interval between vaccination and initiation of immunosuppresive therapy should be ≥2 weeks. Vaccination during chemotherapy or radiation therapy should be avoided.
- Routine use of PPSV is not recommended for American Indians/Alaska Natives or other persons <65 years of age, unless they have underlying medical conditions that are PPSV indications. However, public health authorities may consider recommending PPSV for American Indians/Alaska Natives who are living in areas where the risk for invasive pneumococcal disease is increased.

[9]Revaccination with PPSV

- One-time revaccination 5 years after the first dose is recommended for persons 19-64 years of age with chronic renal failure or nephrotic syndrome, functional or anatomic asplenia (eg, sickle cell disease or splenectomy), and for persons with immunocompromising conditions.

- Persons who received PPSV before 65 years of age for any indication should receive another dose of the vaccine at ≥65 years of age if ≥5 years have passed since their previous dose.
- No further doses are needed for persons vaccinated with PPSV ≥65 years of age.

[10]Meningococcal vaccine

- Administer 2 doses of meningococcal conjugate vaccine quadrivalent (MCV4) ≥2 months apart to adults with functional asplenia or persistent complement component deficiencies.
- HIV-infected persons who are vaccinated should also receive 2 doses.
- Administer a single dose of meningococcal vaccine to microbiologists routinely exposed to isolates of *Neisseria meningitidis*, military recruits, and persons who travel to or live in countries in which meningococcal disease is hyperendemic or epidemic.
- First-year college students ≤21 years of age who are living in residence halls should be vaccinated if they have not received a dose on or after their 16th birthday.
- MCV4 is preferred for adults with any of the preceding indications who are ≤55 years of age; meningococcal polysaccharide vaccine (MPSV4) is preferred for adults ≥56 years of age.
- Revaccination with MCV4 every 5 years is recommended for adults previously vaccinated with MCV4 or MPSV4 who remain at increased risk for infection (eg, adults with anatomic or functional asplenia or persistent complement component deficiencies).

[11]Hepatitis A vaccine

- Vaccinate any person seeking protection from hepatitis A virus (HAV) infection and persons with any of the following indications:
  - Men who have sex with men and persons who use injection drugs
  - Persons working with HAV-infected primates or with HAV in a research laboratory setting
  - Persons with chronic liver disease and persons who receive clotting factor concentrates
  - Persons traveling to or working in countries that have high or intermediate endemicity of hepatitis A, and
  - Unvaccinated persons who anticipate close personal contatct (eg, household or regular babysitting) with an international adoptee during the first 60 days after arrival in the United States from a country with high or intermediate endemicity (see footnote 1 for more information on travel recommendations). The first dose of the 2-dose hepatitis A vaccine series should be administered as soon as adoption is planned, ideally 2 or more weeks before the arrival of the adoptee.
- Single-antigen vaccine formulations should be administered in a 2-dose schedule at either 0 and 6-12 months (Havrix®), or 0 and 6-18 months (VAQTA®). If the combined hepatitis A and hepatitis B vaccine (Twinrix®) is used, administer 3 doses at 0, 1, and 6 months; alternatively, a 4-dose schedule may be used, administered on days 0, 7, and 21-30, followed by a booster dose at month 12.

[12]Hepatitis B vaccine

- Vaccinate persons with any of the following indications and any person seeking protection from hepatitis B virus (HBV) infection:
  - Sexually active persons who are not in a long-term, mutually monogamous relationship (eg, persons with more than one sex partner during the previous 6 months); persons seeking evaluation or treatment for a sexually transmitted disease (STD); current or recent injection-drug users; and men who have sex with men.
  - Healthcare personnel and public-safety workers who are exposed to blood or other potentially infectious body fluids.
  - Persons with diabetes <60 years of age as soon as feasible after diagnosis; persons with diabetes who are ≥60 years of age at the discretion of the treating clinician, based on increased need for assisted blood glucose monitoring in long-term care facilities, likelihood of acquiring hepatitis B infection, its complications, or chronic sequelae, and likelihood of immune response to vaccination
  - Persons with end-stage renal disease, including patients receiving hemodialysis; persons with HIV infection; and persons with chronic liver disease

- Household contacts and sex partners of persons with chronic HBV infection; clients and staff members of institutions for persons with developmental disabilities; and international travelers to countries with high or intermediate prevalence of chronic HBV infection; and
- All adults in the following settings: STD treatment facilities, HIV testing and treatment facilities, facilities providing drug-abuse treatment and prevention services, healthcare settings targeting services to injection-drug users or men who have sex with men, correctional facilities, end-stage renal disease programs and facilities for chronic hemodialysis patients, and institutions and nonresidential daycare facilities for persons with developmental disabilities

- Administer missing doses to complete a 3-dose series of hepatitis B vaccine to those persons not vaccinated or not completely vaccinated. The second dose should be administered 1 month after the first dose; the third dose should be given ≥2 months after the second dose (and ≥4 months after the first dose). If the combined hepatitis A and hepatitis B vaccine (Twinrix®) is used, give 3 doses at 0, 1, and 6 months; alternatively, a 4-dose Twinrix® schedule, administered on days 0, 7, and 21-30, followed by a booster dose at month 12, may be used.
- Adult patients receiving hemodialysis or with other immunocompromising conditions should receive 1 dose of 40 μg/mL (Recombivax HB®), administered on a 3-dose schedule, or 2 doses of 20 μg/mL (Engerix-B®), administered simultaneously on a 4-dose schedule at 0, 1, 2, and 6 months.

[13]Selected conditions for which *Haemophilus influenzae* type b (Hib) vaccine may be used

- One dose of Hib vaccine should be considered for persons who have sickle cell disease, leukemia, or HIV infection, or who have anatomic or functional asplenia if they have not previously received Hib vaccine.

[14]Immunocompromising conditions

- Inactivated vaccines generally are acceptable (eg, pneumococcal, meningococcal, influenza [inactivated influenza vaccine]) and live vaccines generally are avoided in persons with immune deficiencies or immunocompromising conditions. Information on specific conditions is available at http://www.cdc.gov/vaccines/pubs/acip-list.htm.

REFERENCE

"Recommended Adult Immunization Schedule – United States, 2012," *MMWR Recomm Rep*, 2012, 61(4):Q1-5. Available at http://www.cdc.gov/mmwr/pdf/rr/rr6002.pdf

These schedules indicate the recommended age groups and medical indications for which administration of currently licensed vaccines is commonly indicated for adults ≥19 years of age, as of January 1, 2011. For all vaccines being recommended on the adult immunization schedule, a vaccine series does not need to be restarted, regardless of the time that has elapsed between doses. Licensed combination vaccines may be used whenever any components of the combination are indicated and when the vaccine's other components are not contraindicated. For detailed recommendations on all vaccines, including those used primarily for travelers or that are issued during the year, consult the manufacturers' package inserts and the complete statements from the Advisory Committee on Immunization Practices (http://www.cdc.gov/vaccines/pubs/acip-list.htm).

Report all clinically significant postvaccination reactions to the Vaccine Adverse Event Reporting System (VAERS). Reporting forms and instructions on filing a VAERS report are available at http://www.vaers.hhs.gov or by telephone, (800) 822-7967.

Information on how to file a Vaccine Injury Compensation Program claim is available at http://www.hrsa.gov/vaccinecompensation or by telephone, (800) 338-2382. Information about filing a claim for vaccine injury is available through the U.S. Court of Federal Claims, 717 Madison Place, N.W., Washington, D.C. 20005; telephone, (202) 357-6400.

Additional information about the vaccines in this schedule, extent of available data, and contraindications for vaccination also is available at http://www.cdc.gov/vaccines or from the CDC-INFO Contact Center at (800) CDC-INFO (800-232-4636) in English and Spanish, 8 a.m. to 8 p.m., Monday through Friday, excluding holidays.

Use of trade names and commercial sources is for identification only and does not imply endorsement by the U.S. Department of Health and Human Services.

U.S. Department of Health and Human Services • Centers for Disease Control and Prevention

VACCINE INJURY TABLE

The Vaccine Injury Table makes it easier for some people to get compensation. The table lists and explains injuries/conditions that are presumed to be caused by vaccines. It also lists time periods in which the first symptom of these injuries/conditions must occur after receiving the vaccine. If the first symptom of these injuries/conditions occurs within the listed time periods, it is presumed that the vaccine was the cause of the injury or condition unless another cause is found. For example, if the patient received the tetanus vaccines and had a severe allergic reaction (anaphylaxis) within 4 hours after receiving the vaccine, then it is presumed that the tetanus vaccine caused the injury if no other cause is found.

If the injury/condition is not on the table or if the injury/condition did not occur within the time period on the table, it must be proven that the vaccine caused the injury/condition. Such proof must be based on medical records or opinion, which may include expert witness testimony.

Vaccine Injury Table[1]

Vaccine		Illness, Disability, Injury, or Condition Covered	Time Period for First Symptom or Manifestation of Onset or of Significant Aggravation After Vaccine Administration
Vaccines containing tetanus toxoid (eg, DTaP, DTP, DT, Td, TT)	A.	Anaphylaxis or anaphylactic shock	4 hours
	B.	Brachial neuritis	2-28 days
	C.	Any acute complication or sequela (including death) of above events	Not applicable
Vaccines containing whole cell pertussis bacteria, extracted or partial cell pertussis bacteria, or specific pertussis antigen(s) (eg, DTP, DTaP, P, DTP-Hib)	A.	Anaphylaxis or anaphylactic shock	4 hours
	B.	Encephalopathy (or encephalitis)	72 hours
	C.	Any acute complication or sequela (including death) of above events	Not applicable
Measles, mumps, and rubella vaccine or any of its components (eg, MMR, MR, M, R)	A.	Anaphylaxis or anaphylactic shock	4 hours
	B.	Encephalopathy (or encephalitis)	5-15 days
	C.	Any acute complication or sequela (including death) of above events	Not applicable
Vaccines containing rubella virus (eg, MMR, MR, R)	A.	Chronic arthritis	7-42 days
	B.	Any acute complication or sequela (including death) of above events	Not applicable
Vaccines containing measles virus (eg, MMR, MR, M)	A.	Thrombocytopenic purpura	7-30 days
	B.	Vaccine-strain measles viral infection in an immunodeficient recipient	6 months
	C.	Any acute complication or sequela (including death) of above events	Not applicable
Vaccines containing polio live virus (OPV)	A.	Paralytic polio	
		• In a nonimmunodeficient recipient	30 days
		• In an immunodeficient recipient	6 months
		• In a vaccine-associated community case	Not applicable
	B.	Vaccine-strain polio viral infection	
		• In a nonimmunodeficient recipient	30 days
		• In an immunodeficient recipient	6 months
		• In a vaccine-associated community case	Not applicable
	C.	Any acute complication or sequela (including death) of above events	Not applicable
Vaccines containing polio inactivated (eg, IPV)	A.	Anaphylaxis or anaphylactic shock	4 hours
	B.	Any acute complication or sequela (including death) of above events	Not applicable
Hepatitis B vaccines	A.	Anaphylaxis or anaphylactic shock	4 hours
	B.	Any acute complication or sequela (including death) of above events	Not applicable
Hemophilus influenzae type b polysaccharide conjugate vaccines	A.	No condition specified	Not applicable
Varicella vaccine	A.	No condition specified	Not applicable
Rotavirus vaccine	A.	No condition specified	Not applicable
Pneumococcal conjugate vaccines	A.	No condition specified	Not applicable
Hepatitis A vaccines	A.	No condition specified	Not applicable
Trivalent influenza vaccines	A.	No condition specified	Not applicable
Meningococcal vaccines	A.	No condition specified	Not applicable

Vaccine Injury Table[1] *(continued)*

Vaccine		Illness, Disability, Injury, or Condition Covered	Time Period for First Symptom or Manifestation of Onset or of Significant Aggravation After Vaccine Administration
Human papillomavirus (HPV) vaccines	A.	No condition specified	Not applicable
Any new vaccine recommended by the Centers for Disease Control and Prevention for routine administration to children, after publication by Secretary, HHS of a notice of coverage	A.	No condition specified	Not applicable

[1]Effective date: July 22, 2011

COMPATIBILITY OF DRUGS

Drug Compatibility Guide

KEY
C = Compatible
X = Incompatible
Ø = Conflicting Reports
Blank = No information

	azithromycin	butorphanol	calcium gluconate	cefazolin	ciprofloxacin	cisatracurium	clindamycin	dobutamine	dopamine	drotrecogin alfa	fentanyl	fluconazole	furosemide	heparin	lansoprazole	levofloxacin	lorazepam	magnesium
azithromycin	■				X		X				X		X			X		
butorphanol		■				C									X			
calcium gluconate			■		C	C					C	X		C	X			
cefazolin				■		Ø					C	C		C	X			C
ciprofloxacin	X		C		■	C		C	C	X			X	X	X		C	X
cisatracurium		C	C	Ø	C	■	C	C	C	C	C	C	Ø	Ø			C	C
clindamycin	X					C	■			X	C	X		C	X	C		C
dobutamine					C	C		■		X	C	C		Ø	X	C		
dopamine					C	C			■	X	C	C		C	X	C		
drotrecogin alfa					X	C	X	X	X	■		C	X	X		X		X
fentanyl	X		C	C		C	C	C	C		■		C	C	C	C	C	
fluconazole			X	C		C	X	C	C	C		■	X	C	C		C	
furosemide	X				X	Ø				X	C	X	■	C	X	X	C	
heparin			C	C	X	Ø	C	Ø	C	X	C	C	C	■	C	X	C	C
lansoprazole		X	X	X	X		X	X	X		C	C	X	C	■	X	X	X
levofloxacin	X						C	C	C	X	C		X	X	X	■	C	
lorazepam					C	C					C	C	C	C	X	C	■	
magnesium				C	X	C	C			X				C	X			■
methylprednisolone					X	Ø								Ø	X			
metronidazole					C	C			Ø	X	C	C		C	X	C	C	C
midazolam			C	C	C	C	C	Ø	C	X	C	C	X	C	X			
morphine	X			C		C	C		C			C	X	C	X	C		C
nesiritide								C	C		C		X	X				
nitroglycerin						C				C	C	C	X	Ø	X	X		
nitroprusside						Ø				X				C		X		
norepinephrine						C			C	X				C				
pantoprazole			X	X	X		X	Ø	X		X	X	X	X		X	X	Ø
piperacillin & tazobactam																		
potassium chloride	X		C		C	C			C	C	C		C		X		C	C
potassium phosphate					X					X					X			
prochlorperazine			Ø			C						C		C	X			
promethazine					C	C						C	X	C	X			
propofol		C	C	C	C		C	C	C		Ø	C	C	C			Ø	C
ranitidine				C	C	C		C	C	X		C		C	X		C	
sodium bicarbonate					Ø	Ø					C			C	X	C		
vancomycin				Ø		C				X	C	C		Ø	X	C	C	C

Note: Because the compatibility of two or more drugs in solution depends on several variables such as the solution itself, drug concentration and the method of mixing (bottle, syringe, or Y-site), this table is intended to be used solely as a guide to general drug compatibilities. Before mixing any drugs, the healthcare professional should ascertain if a potential incompatibility exists by referring to an appropriate information source.

Drug Compatibility Guide

KEY

C = Compatible
X = Incompatible
Ø = Conflicting Reports
Blank = No information

	methylprednisolone	metronidazole	midazolam	morphine	nesiritide	nitroglycerin	nitroprusside	norepinephrine	pantoprazole	piperacillin & tazobactam	potassium chloride	potassium phosphate	prochlorperazine	promethazine	propofol	ranitidine	sodium bicarbonate	vancomycin
azithromycin				X							X							
butorphanol															C			
calcium gluconate			C						X		C		Ø		C			
cefazolin			C	C					X						C	C		Ø
ciprofloxacin	X	C	C						X		C	X		C	C	C	Ø	
cisatracurium	Ø	C	C	C		C	Ø	C			C		C	C		C	Ø	C
clindamycin			C	C					X						C			
dobutamine			Ø		C				Ø						C	C		
dopamine		Ø	C	C	C			C	X		C				C	C		
drotrecogin alfa		X	X			C	X	X			C	X				X		X
fentanyl		C	C		C	C			X		C				Ø		C	C
fluconazole		C	C	C		C			X				C	C	C	C		C
furosemide			X	X	X	X			X		C			X	C			
heparin	Ø	C	C	C	X	Ø	C	C	X				C	C	C	C	C	Ø
lansoprazole	X	X	X	X		X					X	X	X	X		X	X	X
levofloxacin		C		C		X	X		X								C	C
lorazepam		C							X		C				Ø	C		C
magnesium		C		C					Ø		C				C			C
methylprednisolone	■	C	X	C					X		X				X			
metronidazole	C	■	C	C					X									
midazolam	X	C	■	C		C	C	C	X		Ø				C	C	X	C
morphine	C	C	C	■	C		C	C	X		C				C			C
nesiritide				C	■	C	C	C										
nitroglycerin			C		C	■			X						C	C		
nitroprusside			C	C	C		■		X									
norepinephrine			C	C	C			■	X		C				C			
pantoprazole	X	X	X	X		X	X	X	■	X	C	X	X		X	X	X	C
piperacillin & tazobactam									X	■								
potassium chloride	X		Ø	C				C	C		■		C	C	C		C	
potassium phosphate									X			■						
prochlorperazine									X		C		■		C			
promethazine											C			■				
propofol	X		X	C		C		C	X		C		C		■	C	C	C
ranitidine			C			C			X						C	■		
sodium bicarbonate			X						X		C				C		■	
vancomycin			C	C					C						C			■

Chart created using the King Guide to Parental Admixtures, available through Lexi-Drugs Online www.lexi.com.

LATEX ALLERGY

The incidence of clinically significant latex allergy is increasing. This increase has been suggested to be due in part to the implementation of universal precautions by the CDC in 1987 secondary to the AIDS epidemic. **Because of the increased incidence of latex allergy, all patients need a complete history, including risk factor evaluation and previous evidence of clinical signs and symptoms suggesting contact dermatitis or urticaria.** For example, patients should be questioned about the presence of swelling or itching of the hands or other areas after contact with rubber gloves, condoms, diaphragms, toys, or other rubber products and about itching or swelling of the lips or mouth after dental exams, blowing up balloons, or after eating bananas, chestnuts, and avocados.

It is important today for healthcare institutions to have a comprehensive plan (including a perioperative component) in place for dealing with latex-allergic patients and healthcare personnel. In cardiovascular medicine, the high proportion of procedures and imaging modalities heightens exposure to latex allergens, usually related to rubber gloves. This is a potentially life-threatening problem, both for the patient and healthcare personnel, in situations such as the cardiac catheterization laboratory. Some institutions have avoided use of latex products throughout the hospital environment.

HYPERSENSITIVITY REACTIONS CAUSED BY LATEX

Latex-containing products can produce type I and type IV hypersensitivity reactions.

The type I (IgE-mediated) hypersensitivity reaction is the true "allergic" reaction seen with latex products. Proteins found in the latex promote the production of an antibody of the IgE class which attaches to basophils and mast cells. When the antigen (protein) is encountered again, histamine and other physiologically active mediators are released from mast cells and basophils. The clinical manifestations can include single or multiple system involvement, be mild or severe, ranging from itching to edema, and from mild hypotension to shock. It has been estimated that 10% of the true anaphylactic reactions during anesthesia are due to latex allergy. These reactions are usually seen 5-30 minutes after induction of anesthesia and start of surgery. Seventy-nine percent of of type I patients previously had type IV symptoms.

In the type IV (delayed type) reaction, a contact dermatitis is seen. The preservatives, stabilizers, accelerators, and antioxidants used in the latex manufacturing process serve as the antigens for T-cell lymphocytes. The dermatitis produced can be uncomfortable, but is not life-threatening and usually occurs over a 24-hour period; limited to site of contact. Not all patients with type IV symptoms will progress to type I reactivity.

ROUTES OF EXPOSURE TO LATEX PROTEINS

It is important to consider the route of exposure of the latex protein in allergic patients as this can be a determinant of the type of reaction produced. The following table summarizes major routes of exposure.

Type of Exposure	Reaction
Direct skin contact	Localized or generalized urticaria
Mucous membrane	Rhinitis, conjunctivitis, stomatitis, angioedema; severe anaphylactic reactions and death reported
Inhalation of airborne starch-protein particles	Wheezing, bronchospasm, reduced lung compliance, episodes of desaturation and/or severe hypoxemia
Intravascular absorption of water soluble latex particles from surgical gloves	Sudden tachycardia, severe hypotension, cardiorespiratory collapse

HIGH-RISK PATIENTS

Several groups have been identified as "high-risk" for allergic reactions to latex. Special consideration should be given these individuals.

Patients having multiple surgical procedures (eg, spina bifida patients/patients with congenital urologic abnormalities). A 30% to 70% incidence of latex allergy has been reported for spina bifida patients. These patients are routinely exposed to latex-containing urinary catheters.

Healthcare providers. Latex sensitivity may be as high as 17%. Approximately 70% of adverse events reported to FDA regarding latex involve healthcare workers.

Workers with occupational exposure to natural rubber latex (eg, hairdressers, greenhouse workers, latex manufacturers).

Patients with a history of atopy, hay fever, rhinitis, asthma, or eczema. Atopy is one of the significant predisposing risk factors for latex allergy.

Patients with a history of food allergy to tropical fruits (eg, avocado, kiwi, bananas), chestnuts, stone fruits, and additional specific foods. These plants contain several proteins similar/identical to those found in latex.

Individuals with severe or anaphylactic responses to latex should consider having an Epi-Pen® available at all times, and having a Medic-Alert® bracelet to alert healthcare workers to the potential for life-threatening allergic reactions.

TREATMENT OF ANAPHYLACTIC REACTION

Management of an anaphylactic reaction which is thought to be due to latex allergy must be immediate. Initial therapy should consist of the following.

- Stop administration of offending agent.
- Remove all latex products (switch to nonlatex gloves and latex-free intravenous tubing). Latex-free precautions must accompany the patient throughout the perioperative and hospital stay (PACU, ICU, general floor, and discharge unit).
- Discontinue all antibiotic and blood administration.
- Maintain airway with 100% oxygen.
- Intubate the trachea (as indicated).
- Intravascular volume expansion with crystalloid or colloid.
- Epinephrine administration (see Epinephrine (Systemic, Oral Inhalation) on page 397).
- Discontinue all anesthetic agents if appropriate.
- Consider use of Military Anti-Shock Trousers (MAST).
- Display prominent signs to identify latex allergy.
- When appropriate, administer antihistamines (eg, diphenhydramine), corticosteroids (eg, hydrocortisone), catecholamine infusions (eg, norepinephrine), inhaled bronchodilators (eg, albuterol) for bronchospasm, and sodium bicarbonate (guided by arterial blood gas results). Patients should be admitted to the ICU for 24 hours following an anaphylactic reaction because of the possibility of recurrent "late-phase" reactions. To confirm a latex allergy, RAST or AlaSTAT test may be performed.
- Details of any allergic reaction should be clearly documented in the patient's chart and reported to FDA MedWatch program.
- Contact dermatitis and type IV reactions:
  - Avoid irritating skin cleansers.
  - Topical corticosteroids can be applied locally.

PERIOPERATIVE MANAGEMENT OF A LATEX ALLERGIC PATIENT

No evidence exists to demonstrate that prophylaxis before surgery prevents latex-induced anaphylactic reactions. In spite of this, prophylaxis has been used in patients with a positive history of allergy. One suggested regimen uses diphenhydramine P.O. or I.V. every 6 hours at 13, 7, and 1 hours before surgery; prednisone P.O. every 6 hours at 13, 7, and 1 hours before surgery (hydrocortisone I.V. may be substituted); and ranitidine P.O. or I.V. every 12 hours at 13 and 1 hours before surgery. This regimen is continued for 12 hours after surgery.

The key to the hospital management of the latex-allergic patient is to provide a latex-free environment. To accomplish this, the following actions should be taken.

- Substitute all items with nonlatex alternatives when possible; if there is a question concerning the latex content of a product, the manufacturer should be called.
- Gloves made of neoprene or other polymers should be used.
- Latex-based adhesives should be eliminated.
- Stopcocks should be used for drug administration instead of injection ports on I.V. tubing.
- Syringes not containing rubber tips on the plunger should be used.

- Drug products in glass ampuls should be used whenever possible; if a vial must be used, utilize a vial stopper remover so the stopper does not have to be punctured or puncture only once.

- To reduce exposure to aerosolized glove powder which is a known carrier of latex proteins, schedule the surgery as the first case of the day. Some institutions have reserved an O.R. suite for latex-allergic patients.

TESTING FOR LATEX ALLERGY

Testing for latex allergy is recommended for high-risk patients. Both *in vitro* and *in vivo* tests are available as seen in the following table.

Test	Type	Description
Skin prick (SPT)	*in vivo*	Sensitive method to confirm IgE-mediated latex hypersensitivity; correlates well with clinical presence of allergy; high sensitivity (100%), high specificity (99%)
Patch	*in vivo*	Test for type IV hypersensitivity reaction; test performed with 1 inch square of rubber glove; skin observed for contact dermatitis after 48 hours
Radioallergosorbent (RAST)	*in vitro*	Performed on the serum of patients with natural latex as the antigen; used to detect and quantify allergen specific IgE in patient's serum; positive RAST response correlates strongly with *in vivo* allergic response; sensitivity 67% to 82%
Enzymeallergosorbent (EAST)	*in vitro*	Enzyme-linked immunometric assay used to measure latex-specific IgE antibodies; can be false negatives

REFERENCES AND RECOMMENDED READING

Dakin MJ and Yentis SM, "Latex Allergy: A Strategy for Management," *Anaesthesia*, 1998, 53(8):774-81.

Hancock DL, "Latex Allergy. Prevention and Treatment," *Anesthesiol Rev*, 1994, 21(5):153-63.

Katz JD, Holzman RS, Brown RH, et al, "Natural Rubber Latex Allergy: Considerations for Anesthesiologists," American Society of Anesthesiologists (ASA), 2005. Available at http://ecommerce.asahq.org/publicationsAndServices/latexallergy.pdf. Accessed December 6, 2007.

Senst BL and Johnson RA, "Latex Allergy," *Am J Health Syst Pharm*, 1997, 54(9):1071-5.

Steelman VM, "Latex Allergy Precautions. A Research-Based Protocol," *Nurs Clin North Am*, 1995, 30(3):475-93.

Sussman G and Gold M, "Guidelines for the Management of Latex Allergies and Safe Latex Use in Health Care Facilities." Available at http://www.acaai.org/public/physicians/latex.htm

MANAGEMENT OF DRUG EXTRAVASATIONS

Vesicant: An agent that has the potential to cause blistering, severe tissue injury, or tissue necrosis when extravasated.

Irritant: An agent that causes aching, tightness, and phlebitis with or without inflammation, but does not typically cause tissue necrosis. Irritants can cause necrosis if the extravasation is severe or left untreated.

Extravasation: Unintentional leakage (or instillation) of fluid out of a blood vessel into surrounding tissue.

Flare: Local, nonpainful, possibly allergic reaction often accompanied by reddening along the vein.

A potential complication of drug therapy is extravasation caused by leakage of the drug solution or instillation out of the vein. A variety of symptoms, including erythema, ulceration, pain, tissue sloughing, and necrosis, is possible. This problem is not unique to antineoplastic therapy; a variety of drugs have been reported to cause tissue damage if extravasated. See table.

Vesicant Agents

Antineoplastic Agents	Nonantineoplastic Agents
Amsacrine[1]	Acyclovir (>7 mg/mL)
CISplatin (≥0.5 mg/mL)	Aminophylline
DACTINomycin	Calcium chloride (>10%)
DAUNOrubicin	Calcium gluconate
DOXOrubicin	Calcium gluceptate[1]
Epirubicin	ChlordiazePOXIDE
IDArubicin	Contrast media
Mechlorethamine	Crystalline amino acids (4.25%)
MitoMYcin	Dantrolene
MitoXANtrone	Dextrose (>10%)
Oxaliplatin	Diazepam
Streptozocin	Digoxin
Trabectedin[1]	DOPamine
VinBLAStine	EPINEPHrine
VinCRIStine	Esmolol
Vindesine[1]	HydrOXYzine
Vinorelbine	Mannitol (>5%)
	Nafcillin
	Nitroglycerin
	Norepinephrine
	Phenylephrine
	Phenytoin
	Potassium acetate (>2 mEq/mL)
	Potassium chloride (>2 mEq/mL)
	Promethazine
	Propylene glycol
	Sodium bicarbonate (≥8.4%)
	Sodium chloride (>1%)
	Sodium thiopental
	Tromethamine
	Vasopressin

[1]Not commercially available in the U.S.

Antineoplastic Agents Associated With Irritation or Occasional Extravasation Reactions

Arsenic Trioxide	Etoposide
Bendamustine	Floxuridine
Bleomycin	Fluorouracil
Bortezomib	Gemcitabine
Busulfan	Ibritumomab
CARBOplatin	Ifosfamide
Carmustine	Irinotecan
CISplatin (<0.5 mg/mL)	Melphalan
Cladribine	PACLitaxel
Cyclophosphamide	PACLitaxel (Protein Bound)
Dacarbazine	Teniposide
DAUNOrubicin Citrate (Liposomal)	Thiotepa
DOCEtaxel	Topotecan
DOXOrubicin (Liposomal)	

The actual incidence of drug extravasations is unknown. Some of the uncertainty stems from varying definitions of incidence. Incidence rates have been reported based on total number of drug doses administered, number of vesicant doses administered, number of treatments, number of patients treated with vesicants, and total number of patients treated. Most estimates place the incidence of extravasations with cytotoxic agents to be in the range of 1% to 7%.

MANAGEMENT OF DRUG EXTRAVASATIONS

The best management for extravasation is prevention, education, and close monitoring. Although it is not possible to prevent all accidents, a few simple precautions can minimize the risk to the patient. The vein used should be a large, intact vessel with good blood flow. Veins in the forearm (ie, basilic, cephalic, and median antebrachial) are usually good options for peripheral infusions. To minimize the risk of dislodging the catheter, veins in the hands, dorsum of the foot, and any joint space (eg, antecubital) should be avoided. It is also important to remember to not administer chemotherapy distal to a recent venipuncture.

A frequently recommended precaution against drug extravasation is the use of a central venous catheter. Use of a central line has several advantages, including high patient satisfaction, reliable venous access, high flow rates, and rapid dilution of the drug. Many institutions encourage or require use of a vascular access device for administration of vesicant agents. Despite their benefit, central lines are not an absolute solution. Vascular access devices are subject to a number of complications. Misplacement/migration of the catheter or improper placement of the needle in accessing injection ports, and cuts, punctures, infections, or rupture of the catheter itself have all been reported.

Education of both the patient and practitioner is imperative. Educate the patient to immediately report any signs of pain, itching, tingling, burning, redness, or discomfort, all of which could be signs of extravasation. Ensure the healthcare team is informed of the risks and management strategies for both prevention and treatment of extravasations.

The nurse administering the chemotherapy agents needs to monitor the patient and I.V. site frequently. Prior to drug administration, the patency of the I.V. line should be verified. The line should be flushed with 5-10 mL of a saline or dextrose solution (depending on compatibility) and the drug(s) infused through the side of a free-flowing I.V. line over 2-5 minutes. If an extravasation occurs, it is important to monitor the site closely at 24 hours, 1 week, 2 weeks, and as necessary for any signs and symptoms of extravasation.

When a drug extravasation does occur, a number of immediate actions are recommended.

1. **Stop the infusion.** At the first suspicion of extravasation, the drug infusion and I.V. fluids should be stopped.
2. **Do NOT remove the catheter/needle.** The I.V. tubing should be disconnected, but the catheter/needle should not be removed. It should be left in place to facilitate aspiration of fluid from the extravasation site and, if appropriate, administration of an antidote.
3. **Aspirate fluid.** To the extent possible, the extravasated drug solution should be removed from the subcutaneous tissues. It is important to avoid any friction or pressure to the area.
4. **Do NOT flush the line.** Flooding the infiltration site with saline or dextrose in an attempt to dilute the drug solution is not recommended.
5. **Remove the catheter/needle.** If an antidote is not going to be injected into the extravasation site, the catheter/needle should be removed. If an antidote is to be injected into the area, it should be injected through the catheter to ensure delivery of the antidote to the extravasation site. When this has been accomplished, the catheter should then be removed.
6. In addition, the affected extremity should be elevated, marked, and photographed if possible. Documentation of the event and follow-up is also highly recommended.

Two issues for which there is less consensus are the application of heat or cold and the use of various antidotes. A variety of recommendations exists for each of these concerns; however, there is no consensus concerning the proper approach.

Cold: Intermittent cooling of the area of extravasation results in vasoconstriction, potentially restricting the spread of the drug and decreasing the pain and inflammation in the area. Application of cold is usually recommended as immediate treatment for most drug extravasations, except the vinca alkaloids and epipodophyllotoxins (eg, etoposide).

Heat: Application of heat results in a localized vasodilation and increased blood flow. Increased circulation is believed to facilitate removal of the drug from the area of extravasation. Heat is generally recommended for treatment for vinca alkaloid and epipodophyllotoxin extravasations. Most data are from animal studies with relatively few human case reports. Animal models indicate application of heat exacerbates the damage from anthracycline extravasations.

For some agents, such as cisplatin, epipodophyllotoxins, mechlorethamine, and paclitaxel, there are conflicting recommendations. Some reports recommend application of cold; others recommend heat. At least one report suggests neither cold nor heat is effective for paclitaxel extravasations.

EXTRAVASATION-SPECIFIC ANTIDOTES

A very wide variety of agents have been reported as possible antidotes for extravasated drugs, with no consensus on their proper use. For a number of reasons, evaluation of the various reports is difficult.

Agents Used as Antidotes

Dexrazoxane	Sodium thiosulfate
Hyaluronidase	Dimethyl sulfoxide

Dexrazoxane: Dexrazoxane, a derivative of EDTA, is an intracellular chelating agent used as a cardioprotective agent in patients receiving anthracycline therapy. It is believed that the cardioprotective effect of dexrazoxane is a result of chelating iron following intracellular hydrolysis. Dexrazoxane is not an effective chelator itself but is hydrolyzed intracellularly to an open-ring chelator form, which complexes with iron, other heavy metals, and doxorubicin complexes to inhibit the generation of free radicals. It has been postulated that dexrazoxane's chelating effect and its ability to stabilize topoisomerase II may be useful in preventing tissue damage from anthracycline extravasations.

Dexrazoxane was FDA-approved in 2007 for the treatment of anthracycline-induced extravasations. Approval was based on two clinical trials, including a total of 80 patients with anthracycline extravasations. Dexrazoxane was administered as 3 I.V. infusions over 1-2 hours through a different venous access location: 1000 mg/m^2 within 6 hours, 1000 mg/m^2 after 24 hours, and 500 mg/m^2 after 48 hours of the actual extravasation up to a maximum total dose of 2000 mg on days 1 and 2 and 1000 mg on day 3, respectively. Although localized cooling was permitted (except within 15 minutes of dexrazoxane infusion) in the trials, the number of patients in which this was used was not reported. Fifty-four of the 80 patients were evaluable. The primary endpoint was rate of surgical resection and necrosis. One patient (2%) required surgery and two patients (4%) developed tissue necrosis. Seventy-one percent of the patients were able to maintain chemotherapy appointments on schedule. Treatment has been associated with neutropenia, leukopenia, and thrombocytopenia. Hematological and liver function tests should be monitored. Other common yet reversible adverse events include nausea and vomiting, diarrhea, stomatitis, and infusion site burning. The proportion of toxicities that were attributable to dexrazoxane or as a result of primary antineoplastic therapy was not clear. Prior to administering dexrazoxane, discontinue DMSO as studies suggest the single agent is more effective than when used in combinations with DMSO.

Hyaluronidase: Hyaluronidase is an enzyme that destroys hyaluronic acid, an essential component of connective tissue. This results in increased permeability of the tissue, facilitating diffusion and absorption of fluids. It is postulated that increasing the diffusion of extravasated fluids results in more rapid absorption, thereby limiting tissue damage. In individual case reports, hyaluronidase has been reported effective in preventing tissue damage from a wide variety of agents, including vinca alkaloids, epipodophyllotoxins, and taxanes. The recommended total dose is 1 mL (150 units) administered as 5 separate 0.2 mL SubQ injections via a 24-gauge or smaller needle. It is recommended to use a new syringe for each injection site.

Sodium thiosulfate: Sodium thiosulfate (1/6 molar) has been recommended for treatment of mechlorethamine, dacarbazine, and cisplatin extravasations. Sodium thiosulfate provides a substrate for alkylation by mechlorethamine, preventing the alkylation and subsequent destruction in subcutaneous tissue. The use of sodium thiosulfate to treat mechlorethamine extravasations is based almost exclusively on *in vitro* and animal data. A single case report of successful sodium thiosulfate treatment of an accidental intramuscular mechlorethamine injection has been published. Thus far, no reports of sodium thiosulfate treatment of mechlorethamine infiltrations have been published.

Preparation of a 1/6 molar solution of sodium thiosulfate:

- Dilute 4 mL of a sodium thiosulfate 10% solution into a syringe with 6 mL of sterile water for injection, resulting in 10 mL of 1/6 molar solution

  or

- Dilute 1.6 mL of a sodium thiosulfate 25% solution with 8.4 mL of sterile water for injection, resulting in 10 mL of 1/6 molar solution

Inject 1-5 mL of the 1/6 molar sodium thiosulfate solution subcutaneously around the edge of the extravasation site using a tuberculin syringe. The dose of sodium thiosulfate depends on the amount of drug extravasated. For mechlorethamine, administer 2 mL of sodium thiosulfate 1/6 molar for every estimated 1 mg of mechlorethamine extravasated. For a cisplatin extravasation, it is recommended to inject 2 mL of sodium thiosulfate for each estimated 100 mg of cisplatin extravasated. It is recommended to use a new syringe for each injection site.

Dimethyl sulfoxide (DMSO): A number of case reports and small clinical trials have suggested that the application of DMSO is an effective treatment for chemotherapy extravasations. It is believed DMSO's protective effect is due to its ability to act as a free radical scavenger. DMSO may be considered as a treatment option for extravasations due to anthracyclines, mitomycin C, and actinomycin D. The optimal dose and duration is unknown. Common doses are to apply 1.5 mL of 50% DMSO topically with a saturated gauze pad every 6 hours for 7-14 days. Gently paint DMSO solution onto an area twice the size of the extravasation. Allow the site to dry. Do not cover with a dressing, as severe blistering may result. During application, DMSO may cause mild local burning, blistering, erythema, and itching.

There are a number of limitations for the use of DMSO. Results in animal models have been equivocal, with some reports indicating DMSO is beneficial and some showing little or no effect. Clinical reports of its use are extremely difficult to interpret due to variations in DMSO concentration (50% to 99%), number of applications/day, duration of therapy, inclusion of nonvesicants in studies, and concomitant treatments. A number of different treatments, including cold, steroids, vitamin E, and sodium bicarbonate, have been used in conjunction with DMSO. Also, most reports that suggest DMSO is effective in preventing tissue damage used DMSO concentrations >90%, which is not available for clinical use in the United States. The product is only commercially available in the United States at a concentration 50% (vol/vol) solution in water; however, higher concentrations may be purchased at health food stores. And lastly, the only FDA-approved indication is symptomatic relief interstitial cystitis (intravesicular administration). Based on these limitations, many institutions, ONS, and the prescribing information do not include DMSO as a treatment option for anthracycline extravasations.

Accepted Treatment Regimens for Specific Drug Extravasations

Medication Extravasated	Treatment	Dose	Route	Duration	Preparation	Administration	Concomitant Therapy
Anthracycline (DAUNOrubicin, DOXOrubicin, epirubicin, IDArubicin)	Children <18 years: Dimethyl sulfoxide[1]	90% to 99% every 6-8 hours	Topical	7-14 days	N/A	Topical; apply to area twice the size of the extravasation; do not cover with dressing	Cold[2]
	Adults: Dexrazoxane	1000 mg/m^2 500 mg/m^2	I.V.	Days 1 and 2 Day 3	1000 mL NS	I.V. (in a large vein remote from extravasation) over 1-2 hours	Cold[2,4] **Note:** Withhold cooling for 15 min before dexrazoxane infusion; may reinstitute cooling 15 minutes after infusion complete
MitoMYcin	Dimethyl sulfoxide[1]	90% to 99% every 6-8 hours	Topical	7-14 days	N/A	Topical	Cold[2]
Aminophylline, calcium salts, nafcillin, phenytoin, potassium	Hyaluronidase	150-900 units (total)	I.V., SubQ	One time	Reconstitute with 1 mL NS[6]	1-6 mL into I.V. line of extravasated solution (if still accessed) or SubQ; typical dose of 1 mL per each mL extravasated or 5 injections (0.2 mL) SubQ into area of extravasation in a clockwise manner	Use of either heat or cold therapy has not been determined
Epipodophyllotoxins (eg, etoposide, teniposide)[5], Vinca alkaloids (eg, vinBLAStine, vinCRIStine, vinorelbine)	Hyaluronidase	150-900 units (total)	I.V., SubQ	One time	Reconstitute with 1 mL NS[6]	1-6 mL into I.V. line of extravasated solution (if still accessed) or SubQ; typical dose of 1 mL per each mL extravasated or 5 injections (0.2 mL) SubQ into area of extravasation in a clockwise manner	Heat[3]
Amino acid solutions, contrast media[4], dextrose, mannitol	Hyaluronidase	150-900 units (total)	I.V., SubQ	One time	Reconstitute with 1 mL NS[6]	1-6 mL into I.V. line of extravasated solution (if still accessed) or SubQ; typical dose of 1 mL per each mL extravasated or 5 injections (0.2 mL) SubQ into area of extravasation in a clockwise manner	Cold[2]
Docetaxel, paclitaxel							Cold[2]
Mechlorethamine, CISplatin	Sodium thiosulfate	¹/₆M	I.V., SubQ	One time	Mix 4 mL of 10% sodium thiosulfate with 6 mL sterile water	Mechlorethamine: Inject 2 mL for each 1 mg of mechlorethamine; Cisplatin: Inject locally 2 mL for each 100 mL of cisplatin infiltrated (cisplatin >20 mL and >0.5 mg/mL)	Cold[2]

Accepted Treatment Regimens for Specific Drug Extravasations *continued*

Medication Extravasated	Treatment	Dose	Route	Duration	Preparation	Administration	Concomitant Therapy
Vasopressors (DOPamine, EPINEPHrine, norepinephrine, phenylephrine)	Phentolamine	5 mg	SubQ	1 day	Mix 5 mg with 9 mL NS	Inject small amounts(s) of solution into area of extravasation. Blanching should reverse immediately; if blanching should recur, additional injections may be needed.	None
	or						
	Terbutaline **Note:** Phentolamine is the preferred antidote for these extravasations; terbutaline has been used during phentolamine shortage	1 mg	SubQ	One time	Larger extravasations: Mix 1 mg in 10 mL NS Smaller extravasations (eg, accidental epinephrine autoinjection into digit): Mix 1 mg in 1 mL NS	Inject small amounts(s) of solution into area of extravasation. Blanching should reverse immediately; if blanching should recur, additional injections may be needed.	None

N/A = not applicable, I.V. = intravenous, SubQ = subcutaneous, I.D. = intradermal

[1]DMSO concentration >50% are not available for human use in the U.S.

[2] **Cold therapy:** Mechlorethamine: Apply ice for 6-12 hours (after sodium thiosulfate); for most other antineoplastic agents (when cold is recommended): Apply cold pack for 15 minutes at least 4 times/day for 24 hours. For all other (nonantineoplastic) agents: Apply cold pack for 15 minutes 4 times/day for 3-4 days.

[3] **Heat therapy:** For vinca alkaloids and epipodophyllotoxins: Apply warm pack for 15-20 minutes at least 4 times/day for 1-2 days.

[4]Large extravasations only

[5]In some instances (eg, small extravasations or diluted solution), the use of hyaluronidase for epipodophyllotoxin extravasation may not be necessary.

[6] **Hyaluronidase:** Some institutions utilize a 1:10 dilution in infants and children; prepare by mixing 0.1 mL of 150 units/mL solution with 0.9 mL NS in 1 mL syringe to make final concentration = 15 units/mL

SELECTED READINGS

Bellin MF, Jakobsen JA, Tomassin I, et al, "Contrast Medium Extravasation Injury: Guidelines for Prevention and Management," *Eur Radiol*, 2002, 12(11):2807-12.

Bertelli G, "Prevention and Management of Extravasation of Cytotoxic Drugs," *Drug Saf*, 1995, 12(4):245-55.

Boyle DM and Engelking C, "Vesicant Extravasation: Myths and Realities," *Oncol Nurs Forum*, 1995, 22(1):57-67.

Doellman D, Hadaway L, Bowe-Geddes LA, et al, "Infiltration and Extravasation: Update on Prevention and Management," *J Infus Nurs*, 2009, 32(4):203-11.

Dorr RT, "Antidotes to Vesicant Chemotherapy Extravasations," *Blood Rev*, 1990, 4(1):41-60.

Dorr RT, Soble M, and Alberts DS, "Efficacy of Sodium Thiosulfate as a Local Antidote to Mechlorethamine Skin Toxicity in the Mouse," *Cancer Chemother Pharmacol*, 1988, 22(4):299-302.

Ener RA, Meglathery SB, and Styler M, "Extravasation of Systemic Hemato-Oncological Therapies," *Ann Oncol*, 2004, 15(6):858-62.

Hadaway L, "Infiltration and Extravasation," *Am J Nurs*, 2007, 107(8):64-72.

Kurul S, Saip P, and Aydin T, "Totally Implantable Venous-Access Ports: Local Problems and Extravasation Injury," *Lancet Oncol*, 2002, 3(11):684-92.

Larson DL, "Alterations in Wound Healing Secondary to Infusion Injury," *Clin Plast Surg*, 1990, 17(3):509-17.

Larson DL, "Treatment of Tissue Extravasation by Antitumor Agents," *Cancer*, 1982, 49(9):1796-9.

Larson DL, "What Is the Appropriate Management of Tissue Extravasation by Antitumor Agents?" *Plast Reconstr Surg*, 1985, 75 (3):397-405.

MacCara ME, "Extravasation: A Hazard of Intravenous Therapy," *Drug Intell Clin Pharm*, 1983, 17(10):713-7.

Mouridsen HT, Langer SW, Buter J, et al, "Treatment of Anthracycline Extravasation With Savene (Dexrazoxane): Results From Two Prospective Clinical Multicentre Studies," *Ann Oncol*, 2007, 18(3):546-50.

Perry MC, "Extravasation," *The Chemotherapy Source Book*, 4th ed, Philadelphia, PA, 2008.

Polovich M, Whitford JN and Olsen M, *Chemotherapy and Biotherapy Guidelines and Reccomendations for Practice*, 3rd ed, Pittsburgh, PA: Oncology Nursing Society, 2009.

Schrijvers DL, "Extravasation: A Dreaded Complication of Chemotherapy," *Ann Oncol*, 2003, 14 Suppl 3:iii26-30.

Schulmeister L and Camp-Sorrell D, "Chemotherapy Extravasation From Implanted Ports," *Oncol Nurs Forum*, 2000, 27(3):531-8.

Schulmeister L, "Preventing and Managing Vesicant Chemotherapy Extravasations," *J Support Oncol*, 2010, 8(5):212-5.

Stier PA, Bogner MP, Webster K, et al, "Use of Subcutaneous Terbutaline to Reverse Peripheral Ischemia," *Am J Emerg Med*, 1999, 17 (1):91-4.

Wang CL, Cohan RH, Ellis JH, et al, "Frequency, Management, and Outcome of Extravasation of Nonionic Iodinated Contrast Medium in 69,657 Intravenous Injections," *Radiology*, 2007, 243(1):80-7.

PEAK AND TROUGH GUIDELINES

Drug	When to Sample	Therapeutic Levels*	Usual Half-Life	Steady State (Ideal Sampling Time)	Potentially Toxic Levels*
Antibiotics					
Gentamicin Tobramycin	30 min after 30 min infusion Trough: <0.5 h before next dose	Peak: 4-10 mcg/mL Trough: <2.0 mcg/mL	2 h	15 h	Peak: >12 mcg/mL Trough: >2 mcg/mL
Amikacin		Peak: 20-35 mcg/mL Trough: <8 mcg/mL			Peak: >35 mcg/mL Trough: >8 mcg/mL
Vancomycin	Peak: 1 h after 1 h infusion Trough: <0.5 h before next dose	Peak: 30-40 mcg/mL Trough: ≥10-20 mcg/mL depending upon severity/type of infection	6-8 h	24 h	Peak: >80 mcg/mL
Anticonvulsants					
CarBAMazepine	Trough: Just before next oral dose In combination with other anticonvulsants	4-12 mcg/mL 4-8 mcg/mL	15-20 h	7-12 d	>12 mcg/mL
Ethosuximide	Trough: Just before next oral dose	40-100 mcg/mL	30-60 h	10-13 d	>100 mcg/mL
PHENobarbital	Trough: Just before next dose	15-40 mcg/mL	40-120 h	20 d	>40 mcg/mL
Phenytoin Free phenytoin	Trough: Just before next dose Draw at same time as total level.	10-20 mcg/mL 1-2 mcg/mL	Concentration dependent	5-14 d	>20 mcg/mL
Primidone	Trough: Just before next dose (**Note:** Primidone is metabolized to phenobarb, order levels separately.)	5-12 mcg/mL	10-12 h	5 d	>12 mcg/mL
Valproic acid	Trough: Just before next dose	Seizures: 50-100 mcg/mL Mania: 85-125 mcg/mL	5-20 h	4 d	>150 mcg/mL
Bronchodilators					
Aminophylline (I.V.)	18-24 h after starting or changing a maintenance dose; given as a constant infusion	5-15 mcg/mL	Nonsmoking adult: 8 h Children and smoking adults: 4 h	2 d	>20 mcg/mL
Theophylline (P.O.)	Peak levels: Not recommended Trough level: Just before next dose				
Cardiovascular Agents					
Digoxin	Trough: Just before next dose (levels drawn earlier than 6 h after a dose will be artificially elevated)	0.5-2 ng/mL	36 h	5 d	>2 ng/mL
Lidocaine	Steady-state levels are usually achieved after 6-12 h	1.2-5.0 mcg/mL	1.5 h	5-10 h	>6 mcg/mL
Procainamide	Trough: Just before next oral dose I.V.: 6-12 h after infusion started Combined procainamide plus NAPA	4-10 mcg/mL NAPA: 6-10 h 5-30 mcg/mL	Procain: 2.7-5 h >30 (NAPA + procain)	20 h	>10 mcg/mL
QuiNIDine	Trough: Just before next oral dose	2-5 mcg/mL	6 h	24 h	>10 mcg/mL
Warfarin	Same time of day each draw	See Warfarin monograph.	42 h	5-7 d	See Warfarin monograph.

continued

Drug	When to Sample	Therapeutic Levels*	Usual Half-Life	Steady State (Ideal Sampling Time)	Potentially Toxic Levels*
Other Agents					
Amitriptyline plus nortriptyline	Trough: Just before next dose	120-250 ng/mL		4-80 d	
CycloSPORINE		Months post-transplant: Plasma: 50-150 ng/mL Whole blood: 150-450 ng/mL		Variable	
Desipramine		50-300 ng/mL	12-54 h	3-11 d	
Imipramine plus desipramine		150-300 ng/mL	9-24 h	2-5 d	
Lithium		0.6-1.2 mEq/mL (acute)	18-20 h	2-7 d	>1.5 mEq/mL
Nortriptyline		50-140 ng/mL		4-19 d	

*Due to methodology differences, reference ranges may vary from laboratory to laboratory; check with the laboratory service used for their appropriate levels.

ORAL MEDICATIONS THAT SHOULD NOT BE CRUSHED OR ALTERED

There are a variety of reasons for crushing tablets or capsule contents prior to administering to the patient. Patients may have nasogastric tubes which do not permit the administration of tablets or capsules, an oral solution for a particular medication may not be available from the manufacturer or readily prepared by pharmacy, patients may have difficulty swallowing capsules or tablets, or mixing of powdered medication with food or drink may make the drug more palatable.

Generally, medications which should not be crushed fall into one of the following categories:

- **Extended Release Products:** The formulation of some tablets is specialized as to allow the medication within it to be slowly released into the body. This may be accomplished by centering the drug within the core of the tablet, with a subsequent shedding of multiple layers around the core. Wax melts in the GI tract, releasing drug contained within the wax matrix (eg, OxyCONTIN®). Capsules may contain beads which have multiple layers which are slowly dissolved with time.

  Common Abbreviations for Extended Release Products

CD	Controlled dose
CR	Controlled release
CRT	Controlled release tablet
LA	Long-acting
SR	Sustained release
TR	Timed release
TD	Time delay
SA	Sustained action
XL	Extended release
XR	Extended release

- **Medications Which Are Irritating to the Stomach:** Tablets which are irritating to the stomach may be enteric-coated which delays release of the drug until the time when it reaches the small intestine. Enteric-coated aspirin is an example of this.
- **Foul-Tasting Medication:** Some drugs are quite unpleasant to taste so the manufacturer coats the tablet in a sugar coating to increase its palatability. By crushing the tablet, this sugar coating is lost and the patient tastes the unpleasant tasting medication.
- **Sublingual Medication:** Medication intended for use under the tongue should not be crushed. While it appears to be obvious, it is not always easy to determine if a medication is to be used sublingually. Sublingual medications should indicate on the package that they are intended for sublingual use.
- **Effervescent Tablets:** These are tablets which, when dropped into a liquid, quickly dissolve to yield a solution. Many effervescent tablets, when crushed, lose their ability to quickly dissolve.
- **Potentially Hazardous Substances:** Certain drugs, including antineoplastic agents, hormonal agents, some antivirals, some bioengineered agents, and other miscellaneous drugs, are considered potentially hazardous when used in humans based on their characteristics. Examples of these characteristics include carcinogenicity, teratogenicity, reproductive toxicity, organ toxicity at low doses, or genotoxicity. Exposure to these substances can result in adverse effects and should be avoided. Crushing or breaking a tablet or opening a capsule of a potentially hazardous substance may increase the risk of exposure to the substance through skin contact, inhalation, or accidental ingestion. The extent of exposure, potency, and toxicity of the hazardous substance determines the health risk. Institutions have policies and procedures to follow when handling any potentially hazardous substance. **Note:** All potentially hazardous substances may not be represented in this table. Refer to institution-specific guidelines for precautions to observe when handling hazardous substances.

RECOMMENDATIONS

1. It is not advisable to crush certain medications.
2. Consult individual monographs prior to crushing capsule or tablet.
3. If crushing a tablet or capsule is contraindicated, consult with your pharmacist to determine whether an oral solution exists or can be compounded.

Drug Product	Dosage Form	Dosage Reasons/Comments
Accutane®	Capsule	Mucous membrane irritant; teratogenic potential
Aciphex®	Tablet	Slow release
Actiq®	Lozenge	Slow release. This lollipop delivery system requires the patient to dissolve it slowly.
Actoplus Met® XR	Tablet	Slow release
Actonel®	Tablet	Irritant. Chewed, crushed, or sucked tablets may cause oropharyngeal irritation.
Adalat® CC	Tablet	Slow release
Adderall XR®	Capsule	Slow release[1]
Adenovirus (Types 4, 7) Vaccine	Tablet	Teratogenic potential; enteric-coated; do not disrupt tablet to avoid releasing live adenovirus in upper respiratory tract
Advicor®	Tablet	Slow release
AeroHist Plus™	Tablet	Slow release[8]
Afeditab® CR	Tablet	Slow release
Afinitor®	Tablet	Mucous membrane irritant; teratogenic potential; potentially hazardous substance[10]
Aggrenox®	Capsule	Slow release. Capsule may be opened; contents include an aspirin tablet that may be chewed and dipyridamole pellets that may be sprinkled on applesauce.
Alavert™ Allergy Sinus 12 Hour	Tablet	Slow release
Allegra-D®	Tablet	Slow release
Alophen®	Tablet	Enteric-coated
ALPRAZolam ER	Tablet	Slow release
Altoprev®	Tablet	Slow release
Ambien CR®	Tablet	Slow release
Amitiza®	Capsule	Slow release
Amnesteem®	Capsule	Mucous membrane irritant; teratogenic potential
Ampyra™	Tablet	Slow release
Amrix®	Capsule	Slow release
Aplenzin™	Tablet	Slow release
Apriso™	Capsule	Slow release[1]
Aptivus®	Capsule	Taste. Oil emulsion within spheres
Aricept® 23 mg	Tablet	Film-coated; chewing or crushing may increase rate of absorption
Arava®	Tablet	Teratogenic potential; hazardous substance[10]
Arthrotec®	Tablet	Enteric-coated
Asacol®	Tablet	Slow release
Ascriptin® A/D	Tablet	Enteric-coated
Atelvia™	Tablet	Slow release; tablet coating is an important part of the delayed release
Augmentin XR®	Tablet	Slow release[2, 8]
AVINza™	Capsule	Slow release[1] (applesauce)
Avodart®	Capsule	Capsule should not be handled by pregnant women due to teratogenic potential[9]; hazardous substance[10]
Azulfidine® EN-tabs®	Tablet	Enteric-coated

(continued)

Drug Product	Dosage Form	Dosage Reasons/Comments
Bayer® Aspirin EC	Caplet	Enteric-coated
Bayer® Aspirin, Low Adult 81 mg	Tablet	Enteric-coated
Bayer® Aspirin, Regular Strength 325 mg	Caplet	Enteric-coated
Biaxin® XL	Tablet	Slow release
Biltricide®	Tablet	Taste[8]
Biohist LA	Tablet	Slow release[8]
Bisa-Lax	Tablet	Enteric-coacted[3]
Bisac-Evac™	Tablet	Enteric-coated[3]
Bisacodyl	Tablet	Enteric-coated[3]
Boniva®	Tablet	Irritant. Chewed, crushed, or sucked tablets may cause oropharyngeal irritation.
Bontril® Slow-Release	Capsule	Slow release
Bromfed®	Capsule	Slow release
Bromfed®-PD	Capsule	Slow release
Budeprion SR®, Budeprion XL®	Tablet	Slow release
Buproban®	Tablet	Slow release
BuPROPion SR	Tablet	Slow release
Campral®	Tablet	Enteric-coated; slow release
Calan® SR	Tablet	Slow release[8]
Caprelsa®	Tablet	Teratogenic potential; hazardous substance[10]
Carbatrol®	Capsule	Slow release[1]
Cardene® SR	Capsule	Slow release
Cardizem®	Tablet	Not described as slow release but releases drug over 3 hours.
Cardizem® CD	Capsule	Slow release
Cardizem® LA	Tablet	Slow release
Cardura® XL	Tablet	Slow release
Cartia® XT	Capsule	Slow release
Casodex®	Tablet	Teratogenic potential; hazardous substance[10]
CeeNU®	Capsule	Teratogenic potential; hazardous substance[10]
Cefaclor extended release	Tablet	Slow release
Ceftin®	Tablet	Taste[2]. Use suspension for children.
Cefuroxime	Tablet	Taste[2]. Use suspension for children.
CellCept®	Capsule, tablet	Teratogenic potential; hazardous substance[10]
Charcoal Plus®	Tablet	Enteric-coated
Chlor-Trimeton® 12-Hour	Tablet	Slow release[2]
Cipro® XR	Tablet	Slow release
Claravis™	Capsule	Mucous membrane irritant; teratogenic potential
Claritin-D® 12-Hour	Tablet	Slow release
Claritin-D® 24-Hour	Tablet	Slow release
Colace®	Capsule	Taste[5]
Colestid®	Tablet	Slow release
Commit®	Lozenge	Integrity compromised by chewing or crushing.
Concerta®	Tablet	Slow release
ConZip™	Capsule	Extended release; tablet disruption may cause overdose
Coreg CR®	Capsule	Slow release[1]
Cotazym-S®	Capsule	Enteric-coated[1]
Covera-HS®	Tablet	Slow release
Creon®	Capsule	Slow release[1]

(continued)

Drug Product	Dosage Form	Dosage Reasons/Comments
Crixivan®	Capsule	Taste. Capsule may be opened and mixed with fruit puree (eg, banana).
Cymbalta®	Capsule	Enteric-coated
Cytoxan®	Tablet	Drug may be crushed, but manufacturer recommends using injection; hazardous substance[10]
Depakene®	Capsule	Slow release; mucous membrane irritant[2]
Depakote®	Tablet	Slow release
Depakote® ER	Tablet	Slow release
Detrol® LA	Capsule	Slow release
Dexedrine® Spansule®	Capsule	Slow release
Dexilant™	Capsule	Slow release[1]
Diamox® Sequels®	Capsule	Slow release
Dilacor® XR	Capsule	Slow release
Dilatrate-SR®	Capsule	Slow release
Dilt-CD	Capsule	Slow release
Dilt-XR	Capsule	Slow release
Diltia XT®	Capsule	Slow release
Ditropan® XL	Tablet	Slow release
Divalproex ER	Tablet	Slow release
Donnatal® Extentab®	Tablet	Slow release[2]
Doxidan®	Tablet	Enteric-coated[3]
Drisdol®	Capsule	Liquid filled[4]
Drixoral®	Tablet	Slow release
Droxia®	Capsule	May be opened; wear gloves to handle; hazardous substance[10]
Drysec	Tablet	Slow release[8]
Dulcolax®	Capsule	Liquid-filled
Dulcolax®	Tablet	Enteric-coated[3]
DynaCirc® CR	Tablet	Slow release
Easprin®	Tablet	Enteric-coated
EC-Naprosyn®	Tablet	Enteric-coated
Ecotrin® Adult Low Strength	Tablet	Enteric-coated
Ecotrin® Maximum Strength	Tablet	Enteric-coated
Ecotrin® Regular Strength	Tablet	Enteric-coated
Ed A-Hist™	Tablet	Slow release[2]
E.E.S.® 400	Tablet	Enteric-coated[2]
Effer-K™	Tablet	Effervescent tablet[6]
Effervescent Potassium	Tablet	Effervescent tablet[6]
Effexor® XR	Capsule	Slow release
Embeda™	Capsule	Slow release; can open capsule and sprinkle on applesauce; do not give via NG tube
E-Mycin®	Tablet	Enteric-coated
Enablex®	Tablet	Slow release
Entocort® EC	Capsule	Enteric-coated[1]
Equetro®	Capsule	Slow release[1]
Ergomar®	Tablet	Sublingual form[7]
Ery-Tab®	Tablet	Enteric-coated
Erythromycin Stearate	Tablet	Enteric-coated
Erythromycin Base	Tablet	Enteric-coated
Erythromycin Delayed-Release	Capsule	Enteric-coated pellets[1]

(continued)

Drug Product	Dosage Form	Dosage Reasons/Comments
Etoposide	Capsule	Hazardous substance[10]
Evista®	Tablet	Taste; teratogenic potential; hazardous substance[10]
Eviredge™	Capsule	Teratogenic potential[10]
Exalgo™	Tablet	Slow release; breaking, chewing, crushing, or dissolving before ingestion increases the risk of overdose
ExeFen-PD	Tablet	Slow release[8]
Fareston®	Tablet	Teratogenic potential; hazardous substance[10]
Feen-A-Mint®	Tablet	Enteric-coated[3]
Feldene®	Capsule	Mucous membrane irritant
Fentora®	Tablet	Buccal tablet
Feosol®	Tablet	Enteric-coated[2]
Feratab®	Tablet	Enteric-coated[2]
Fergon®	Tablet	Enteric-coated
Fero-Grad 500®	Tablet	Slow release
Ferro-Sequels®	Tablet	Slow release
Flagyl ER®	Tablet	Slow release
Flomax®	Capsule	Slow release
Focalin® XR	Capsule	Slow release[1]
Fosamax®	Tablet	Mucous membrane irritant
Fosamax Plus D™	Tablet	Mucous membrane irritant
Gengraf®	Capsule	Teratogenic potential; hazardous substance[10]
Gleevec®	Tablet	Taste[8]. May be dissolved in water or apple juice; hazardous substance[10]
GlipiZIDE ER	Tablet	Slow release
Glucophage® XR	Tablet	Slow release
Glucotrol® XL	Tablet	Slow release
Glumetza™	Tablet	Slow release
Gralise™	Tablet	Slow release
Guaifenex® GP	Tablet	Slow release[8]
Guaifenex® PSE	Tablet	Slow release[8]
Guaimax-D®	Tablet	Slow release[8]
Halfprin®	Tablet	Enteric coated
Hexalen®	Capsule	Teratogenic potential; hazardous substance[10]
Horizant™	Tablet	Slow release
Hycamtin®	Capsule	Teratogenic potential; hazardous substance[10]
Hydrea®	Capsule	Can be opened and mixed with water; wear gloves to handle; hazardous substance[10]
Imdur®	Tablet	Slow release[8]
Inderal® LA	Capsule	Slow release
Indocin® SR	Capsule	Slow release[1,2]
Inlyta®	Tablet	Teratogenic potential; hazardous substance[10]
InnoPran XL®	Capsule	Slow release
Intelence™	Tablet	Tablet should be swallowed whole and not crushed; tablet may be dispersed in water
Intuniv™	Tablet	Slow release
Invega®	Tablet	Slow release
Ionamin®	Capsule	Slow release
Isochron™	Tablet	Slow release
Isoptin® SR	Tablet	Slow release[8]
Isordil® Sublingual	Tablet	Sublingual form[7]

(continued)

Drug Product	Dosage Form	Dosage Reasons/Comments
Isosorbide Dinitrate Sublingual	Tablet	Sublingual form[7]
Isosorbide SR	Tablet	Slow release
Jalyn®	Capsule	Capsule should not be handled by pregnant women due to teratogenic potential[9]; hazardous substance[10]
Janumet®	Tablet	Slow release
Kadian®	Capsule	Slow release[1]. Do not give via NG tubes.
Kaletra®	Tablet	Film coated
Kaon-Cl®	Tablet	Slow release[2]
Kapidex™	Capsule	Slow release[1]
Kapvay™	Tablet	Slow release
K-Dur®	Tablet	Slow release
Keppra®	Tablet	Taste[2]
Keppra® XR	Tablet	Slow release
Ketek®	Tablet	Slow release
Klor-Con®	Tablet	Slow release[2]
Klor-Con® M	Tablet	Slow release[2]; some strengths are scored
Klotrix®	Tablet	Slow release[2]
K-Lyte®	Tablet	Effervescent tablet[6]
K-Lyte/Cl®	Tablet	Effervescent tablet[6]
K-Lyte DS®	Tablet	Effervescent tablet[6]
Kombiglyze™ XR	Tablet	Slow release; tablet matrix may remain in stool
K-Tab®	Tablet	Slow release[2]
LaMICtal® XR™	Tablet	Slow release
Lescol® XL	Tablet	Slow release
Letairis®	Tablet	Film coated
Leukeran®	Tablet	Teratogenic potential; hazardous substance[10]
Levbid®	Tablet	Slow release[8]
Levsinex® Timecaps®	Capsule	Slow release
Lexxel®	Tablet	Slow release
Lialda™	Tablet	Delayed release, enteric coated
Lipram 4500	Capsule	Enteric-coated[1]
Lipram-PN	Capsule	Slow release[1]
Lipram-UL	Capsule	Slow release[1]
Liquibid-D®	Tablet	Slow release
Lithobid®	Tablet	Slow release
Lodrane® 24	Capsule	Slow release
Lodrane® 24D	Capsule	Slow release
LoHist 12D	Tablet	Slow release
Lovaza®	Capsule	Contents of capsule may erode walls of styrofoam or plastic materials
Luvox® CR	Capsule	Slow release
Lysodren®	Tablet	Hazardous substance[10]
Mag-Tab® SR	Tablet	Slow release
Matulane®	Capsule	Teratogenic potential; hazardous substance[10]
Maxifed DMX ER	Tablet	Slow release[8]
Maxifed-G®	Tablet	Slow release
Maxiphen DM	Tablet	Slow release[8]
Medent-DM	Tablet	Slow release
Mestinon® Timespan®	Tablet	Slow release[2]
Metadate® CD	Capsule	Slow release[1]

ORAL MEDICATIONS THAT SHOULD NOT BE CRUSHED OR ALTERED

(continued)

Drug Product	Dosage Form	Dosage Reasons/Comments
Metadate® ER	Tablet	Slow release
Methylin® ER	Tablet	Slow release
Metoprolol ER	Tablet	Slow release
MicroK® Extencaps	Capsule	Slow release[1,2]
Minocin	Capsule	Slow release
Morphine sulfate extended-release	Tablet	Slow release
Motrin®	Tablet	Taste[5]
Moxatag™	Tablet	Slow release
MS Contin®	Tablet	Slow release[2]
Mucinex®	Tablet	Slow release
Mucinex® DM	Tablet	Slow release[2]
Myfortic®	Tablet	Slow release; teratogenic potential; hazardous substance[10]
Namenda® XR	Capsule	Slow release[1]
Naprelan®	Tablet	Slow release
Neoral®	Capsule	Teratogenic potential; hazardous substance[10]
NexIUM®	Capsule	Slow release[1]
Niaspan®	Tablet	Slow release
Nicotinic Acid	Capsule, Tablet	Slow release[8]
Nifediac® CC	Tablet	Slow release
Nifedical® XL	Tablet	Slow release
NIFEdipine ER	Tablet	Slow release
Nitrostat®	Tablet	Sublingual route[7]
Norflex™	Tablet	Slow release
Norpace® CR	Capsule	Slow release
Norvir®	Tablet	Crushing tablets has resulted in decreased bioavailability of drug[2]
Nucynta® ER	Tablet	Slow release; tablet disruption may cause a potentially fatal overdose
Oforta™	Tablet	Teratogenic potential; hazardous substance[10]
Oleptro™	Tablet	Slow release[8]
Opana® ER	Tablet	Slow release; tablet disruption may cause a potentially fatal overdose
Oracea™	Capsule	Slow release
Oramorph SR®	Tablet	Slow release[2]
Orphenadrine citrate ER	Tablet	Slow release
OxyCONTIN®	Tablet	Slow release; surrounded by wax matrix; tablet disruption may cause a potentially fatal overdose
Pancrease MT®	Capsule	Enteric-coated[1]
Pancreaze™	Capsule	Enteric-coated[1]
Pancrelipase™	Capsule	Enteric-coated[1]
Paxil CR®	Tablet	Slow release
Pentasa®	Capsule	Slow release
Plendil®	Tablet	Slow release
Pradaxa®	Capsule	Bioavailability increases by 75% when the pellets are taken without the capsule shell
Prevacid®	Capsule	Slow release[1]
Prevacid®	Suspension	Slow release. Contains enteric-coated granules. Not for use in NG tubes.
Prevacid® SoluTab™	Tablet	Orally disintegrating. Do not swallow; dissolve in water only and dispense via dosing syringe or NG tube.
PriLOSEC®	Capsule	Slow release

(continued)

Drug Product	Dosage Form	Dosage Reasons/Comments
PriLOSEC OTC™	Tablet	Slow release
Pristiq®	Tablet	Slow release
Procardia XL®	Tablet	Slow release
Propecia®	Tablet	Women who are, or may become, pregnant should not handle crushed or broken tablets due to teratogenic potential[9]; hazardous substance[10]
Proquin® XR	Tablet	Slow release
Proscar®	Tablet	Women who are, or may become, pregnant should not handle crushed or broken tablets due to teratogenic potential[9]; hazardous substance[10]
Protonix®	Tablet	Slow release
PROzac® Weekly™	Capsule	Enteric coated
Purinethol®	Tablet	Teratogenic potential[9]; hazardous substance[10]
QuiNIDine ER	Tablet	Slow release[8]; enteric-coated
Ralix	Tablet	Slow release
Ranexa®	Tablet	Slow release
Rapamune®	Tablet	Taste; hazardous substance[10]
Razadyne™ ER	Capsule	Slow release
Renagel®	Tablet	Expands in liquid if broken/crushed.
Renvela	Tablet	Enteric-coated
Requip® XL™	Tablet	Slow release
Rescon®	Tablet	Slow release
Rescon-Jr	Tablet	Slow release
Rescriptor®	Tablet	If unable to swallow, may dissolve 100 mg tablets in water and drink; 200 mg tablets must be swallowed whole
Revlimid®	Capsule	Teratogenic potential; hazardous substance[10]; healthcare workers should avoid contact with capsule contents/body fluids
RisperDAL® M-Tab	Tablet	Orally disintegrating. Do not chew or break tablet; after dissolving under tongue, tablet may be swallowed
Ritalin® LA	Capsule	Slow release[1]
Ritalin-SR®	Tablet	Slow release
R-Tanna	Tablet	Slow release[2]
Rybix™ ODT	Tablet	Orally disintegrating. Do not chew, break, or split tablet; after dissolving on the tongue, may swallow.
Rythmol® SR	Capsule	Slow release
Ryzolt™	Tablet	Slow release; tablet disruption may cause overdose
SandIMMUNE®	Capsule	Teratogenic potential; hazardous substance[10]
Saphris®	Tablet	Sublingual form[7]
Sensipar®	Tablet	Tablets are not scored and cutting may cause inaccurate dosage
SEROquel® XR	Tablet	Slow release
Sinemet® CR	Tablet	Slow release
SINUvent® PE	Tablet	Slow release[8]
Slo-Niacin®	Tablet	Slow release[8]
Slow-Mag®	Tablet	Slow release
Solodyn®	Tablet	Slow release
Somnote®	Capsule	Liquid filled
Sotret®	Capsule	Mucous membrane irritant; teratogenic potential
Sprycel®	Tablet	Film coated. Active ingredients are surrounded by a wax matrix to prevent healthcare exposure. Women who are, or may become pregnant, should not handle crushed or broken tablets; teratogenic potential; hazardous substance[10]

ORAL MEDICATIONS THAT SHOULD NOT BE CRUSHED OR ALTERED

(continued)

Drug Product	Dosage Form	Dosage Reasons/Comments
Stavzor™	Capsule	Slow release
Strattera®	Capsule	Capsule contents can cause ocular irritation.
Sudafed® 12-Hour	Capsule	Slow release[2]
Sudafed® 24-Hour	Capsule	Slow release[2]
Sulfazine EC	Tablet	Delayed release, enteric coated
Sular®	Tablet	Slow release
Sustiva®	Tablet	Tablets should not be broken (capsules should be used if dosage adjustment needed)
Symax® Duotab	Tablet	Slow release
Symax® SR	Tablet	Slow release
Syprine®	Capsule	Potential risk of contact dermatitis
Tabloid®	Tablet	Teratogenic potential; hazardous substance[10]
Tamoxifen®	Tablet	Teratogenic potential; hazardous substance[10]
Tasigna®	Capsule	Potentially hazardous substance[10]; altering capsule may lead to high blood levels, increasing the risk of toxicity
Taztia XT®	Capsule	Slow release[1]
TEGretol®-XR	Tablet	Slow release
Temodar®	Capsule	Teratogenic potential; hazardous substance[10]. **Note:** If capsules are accidentally opened or damaged, rigorous precautions should be taken to avoid inhalation or contact of contents with the skin or mucous membranes.
Tessalon®	Capsule	Swallow whole; pharmacologic action may cause choking if chewed or opened and swallowed.
Thalomid®	Capsule	Teratogenic potential; hazardous substance[10]
Theo-24®	Tablet	Slow release[2]
Theochron™	Tablet	Slow release[2]
Tiazac®	Capsule	Slow release[1]
Topamax®	Capsule	Taste[1]
Topamax®	Tablet	Taste
Toprol XL®	Tablet	Slow release[8]
Touro® CC/CC-LD	Caplet	Slow release[2,8]
Touro® DM®	Tablet	Slow release[2]
Touro LA®	Caplet	Slow release
Toviaz™	Tablet	Slow release
Tracleer®	Tablet	Teratogenic potential; hazardous substance[9,10]
TRENtal®	Tablet	Slow release
Treximet™	Tablet	Unique formulation enhances rapid drug absorption
Tylenol® Arthritis Pain	Caplet	Slow release
Tylenol® 8 Hour	Caplet	Slow release
Ultram® ER	Tablet	Slow release. Tablet disruption my cause a potentially fatal overdose.
Ultrase®	Capsule	Enteric-coated[1]
Ultrase® MT	Capsule	Enteric-coated[1]
Uniphyl®	Tablet	Slow release
Urocit®-K	Tablet	Wax-coated
Uroxatral®	Tablet	Slow release
Valcyte®	Tablet	Irritant potential; teratogenic potential; hazardous substance[10]
Verapamil SR	Tablet	Slow release[8]
Verelan®	Capsule	Slow release[1]
Verelan® PM	Capsule	Slow release[1]
Vesanoid®	Capsule	Teratogenic potential; hazardous substance[10]

(continued)

Drug Product	Dosage Form	Dosage Reasons/Comments
VESIcare®	Tablet	Enteric-coated
Videx® EC	Capsule	Slow release
Vimovo™	Tablet	Slow release
Viramune® XR™	Tablet	Slow release[2]
Voltaren®-XR	Tablet	Slow release
VoSpire ER®	Tablet	Slow release
Votrient™	Tablet	Crushing significantly increases AUC and T_{max}
Wellbutrin SR®	Tablet	Slow release
Wellbutrin XL™	Tablet	Slow release
Xalkori®	Capsule	Teratogenic potential; hazardous substance[10]
Xanax XR®	Tablet	Slow release
Xeloda®	Tablet	Teratogenic potential; hazardous substance[10].
Zegerid OTC™	Capsule	Slow release
Zelboraf™	Tablet	Teratogenic potential; hazardous substance[10]
ZENPEP®	Capsule	Slow release[1]
Zolinza®	Capsule	Irritant; avoid contact with skin or mucous membranes; use gloves to handle; teratogenic potential; hazardous substance[10]
Zomig-ZMT®	Tablet	Sublingual form[7]
ZORprin®	Tablet	Slow release
Zortress®	Tablet	Mucous membrane irritant; teratogenic potential; potentially hazardous substance[10]
Zyban®	Tablet	Slow release
Zyflo CR®	Tablet	Slow release
ZyrTEC-D® Allergy & Congestion	Tablet	Slow release
Zytiga™	Tablet	Teratogenic potential; hazardous substance[10]

[1]Capsule may be opened and the contents taken without crushing or chewing; soft food, such as applesauce or pudding, may facilitate administration; contents may generally be administered via nasogastric tube using an appropriate fluid, provided entire contents are washed down the tube.

[2]Liquid dosage forms of the product are available; however, dose, frequency of administration, and manufacturers may differ from that of the solid dosage form.

[3]Antacids and/or milk may prematurely dissolve the coating of the tablet.

[4]Capsule may be opened and the liquid contents removed for administration.

[5]The taste of this product in a liquid form would likely be unacceptable to the patient; administration via nasogastric tube should be acceptable.

[6]Effervescent tablets must be dissolved in the amount of diluent recommended by the manufacturer.

[7]Tablets are made to disintegrate under (or on) the tongue.

[8]Tablet is scored and may be broken in half without affecting release characteristics.

[9]Prescribing information recommends that women who are, or may become, pregnant should not handle medication, especially if crushed or broken; avoid direct contact.

[10]Potentially hazardous or hazardous substance; refer to institution-specific guidelines for precautions to observe when handling this substance.

REFERENCES

Mitchell JF, "Oral Dosage Forms That Should Not Be Crushed." Available at http://www.ismp.org/tools/DoNotCrush.pdf. Accessed November 11, 2011.

National Institute for Occupational Safety and Health, "NIOSH List of Antineoplastic and Other Hazardous Drugs in Healthcare Settings 2010." Available at http://www.cdc.gov/niosh/docs/2010-167. Accessed September 20, 2010.

VITAMIN K CONTENT IN SELECTED FOODS

The following list describes the relative amounts of vitamin K in foods generally considered high in vitamin K. This is a partial listing of foods with estimated portions. For more complete information, refer to the USDA National Nutrient Database for Standard Reference, Release 23, at http://www.ars.usda.gov/SP2UserFiles/Place/12354500/Data/SR23/nutrlist/sr23w430.pdf.

Foods	Portion Size	Vitamin K Content (mcg)
Kale	1 cup	1062-1147
Collards	1 cup	836-1059
Beet greens	1 cup	697
Dandelion greens	1 cup	579
Turnip greens	1 cup	529-851
Mustard greens	1 cup	419
Brussels sprouts	1 cup	219-300
Onions	1 cup	207
Parsley	10 sprigs	164
Noodles	1 cup	162
Spinach	1 cup	145-1027
Asparagus	1 cup	144
Lettuce	1 head	130-167
Endive	1 cup	116
Broccoli	1 cup	90-220
Okra	1 cup	64
Peas	1 cup	63
Cabbage	1 cup	53-163
Cucumber	1 large	49
Asparagus	4 spears	48
Oil, canola	1 Tbsp	10
Oil, olive, salad, or cooking	1 Tbsp	8

ALPHABETICAL INDEX

Horizant™ *see* Gabapentin Enacarbil ... 529

Oxecta™ *see* OxyCODONE 870

Notes

Notes

Notes

Notes

Notes

Notes

Notes

Notes

Notes

Notes

Notes

Notes

Notes

Notes

Notes

Notes

Notes

Notes

Notes

Notes

Notes

Notes

Other Products Offered by Lexicomp

Anesthesiology & Critical Care Drug Handbook

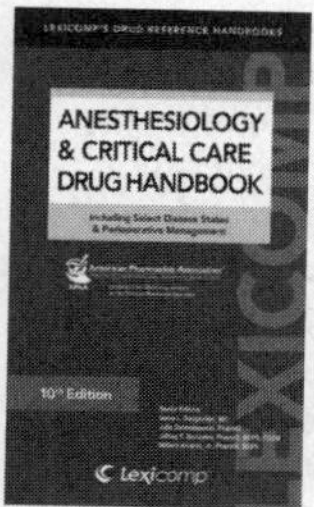

Designed for anesthesiologists, critical care practitioners, and all healthcare professionals involved in the treatment of surgical or ICU patients.

Includes: Comprehensive drug information to ensure appropriate clinical management of patients; Intensivist and Anesthesiologist perspective; Over 2000 medications most commonly used in the preoperative and critical care setting; Special Topics/Issues addressing frequently encountered patient conditions.

Drug Information Handbook

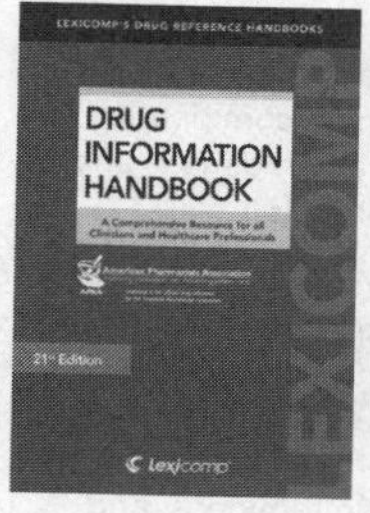

This easy-to-use drug reference is for the pharmacist, physician, or other healthcare professional requiring fast access to comprehensive drug information.

Over 1450 drug monographs are detailed with up to 37 fields of information per monograph. A valuable appendix offers charts and reviews of special topics such as guidelines for treatment and therapy recommendations. A pharmacologic category index is also provided.

Drug Information Handbook with International Trade Names Index

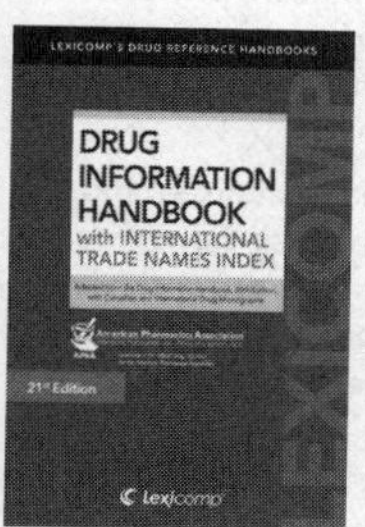

The *Drug Information Handbook with International Trade Names Index* includes the content of our *Drug Information Handbook*, plus international drug monographs for use worldwide! This easy-to-use reference is complied especially for the pharmacist, physician, or other healthcare professional seeking quick access to comprehensive drug information.

Drug Information Handbook for Advanced Practice Nursing

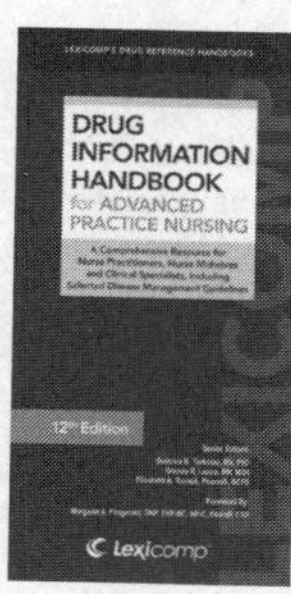

Designed to assist the advanced practice nurse with prescribing, monitoring and educating patients.

Includes: Over 4800 generic and brand names cross-referenced by page number; Generic drug names and cross-references highlighted in RED; Labeled and Investigational indications; Adult, Geriatric, and Pediatric dosing; and up to 60 fields of information per monograph, including Patient Education and Physical Assessment.

Other Products Offered by Lexicomp

Drug Information Handbook for Oncology

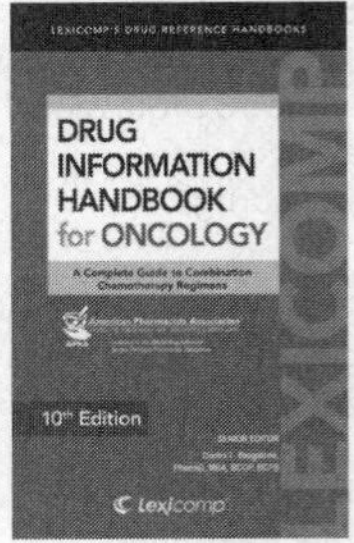

Designed for oncology professionals requiring information on combination chemotherapy regimens and dosing protocols.

Includes: Monographs containing warnings, adverse reaction profiles, drug interactions, dosing for specific indications, vesicant, emetic potential, combination regimens, and more; where applicable, a special Combination Chemotherapy field links to specific oncology monographs; Special Topics such as Cancer Treatment Related Complications, Bone Marrow Transplantation, and Drug Development.

Drug Information Handbook for Psychiatry

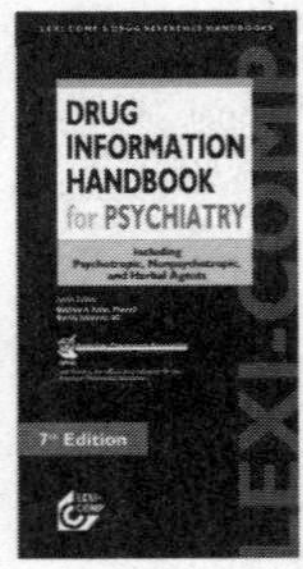

Designed for any healthcare professional requiring quick access to comprehensive drug information as it relates to mental health issues.

Includes: Drug monographs for psychotropic, nonpsychotropic, and herbal medications; Special fields such as Mental Health Comment (useful clinical pearls), Medication Safety Issues, Effects on Mental Status, and Effects on Psychiatric Treatment.

Geriatric Dosage Handbook

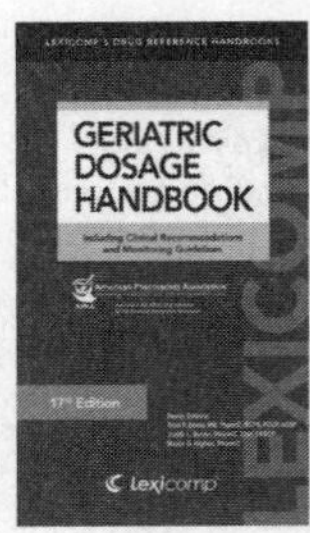

Designed for healthcare professionals managing geriatric patients.

Includes: Complete adult and geriatric dosing; Special geriatric considerations; Up to 41 key fields of information in each monograph, including Medication Safety Issues; Extensive information on drug interactions, as well as dosing for patients with renal/hepatic impairment.

Pharmacogenomics Handbook

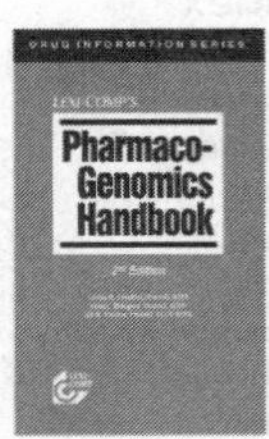

Ideal for any healthcare professional or student wishing to gain insight into the emerging field of pharmacogenomics.

Includes: Information concerning key genetic variations that may influence drug disposition and/or sensitivity; brief introductions to fundamental concepts in genetics and genomics. A foundation for all clinicians who will be called on to integrate rapidly-expanding genomics knowledge into the management of drug therapy.

To order, call Customer Service at 1-866-397-3433 or visit www.lexi.com.
Outside of the U.S., call +1-330-650-6506 or visit www.lexi.com.

Other Products Offered by Lexicomp

Pediatric Dosage Handbook

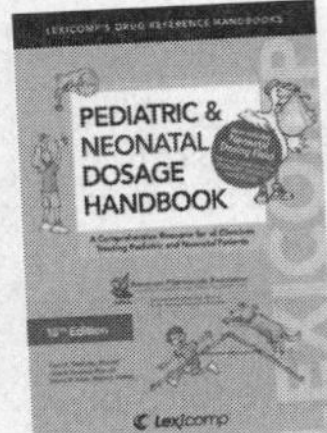

This book is desigrd for healthcare professionals requirg quick access to comprehensive pdiatric drug information. Each mograph contains multiple fiel of content, including usual dosagby age group, indication,ancoute of administration. Drug inractions, adverse reactions, xteporaneous preparations, pharmacynamics/ pharmacokinetic data, d medication safet issues e covered.

Also available:
Manual de Preripción ediátrica (Spanish versi

Pediatric Dosage Handbook with International Trade Names Index

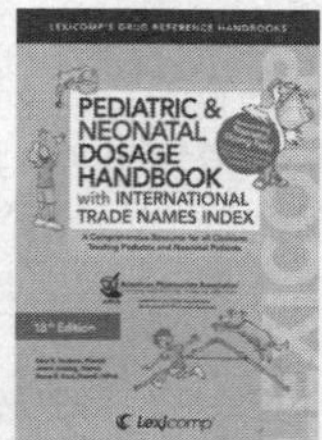

The *Pediatric Dosage Handbook with International Trade Names Index* is the trusted pediatric drug resource of medical professionals worldwide. The International Edition contains all the content of Lexi-Comp's *Pediatric Dosage Handbook*, plus an International Trade Names Index including trade names from over 100 countries.

Rating Scales for MerHealth

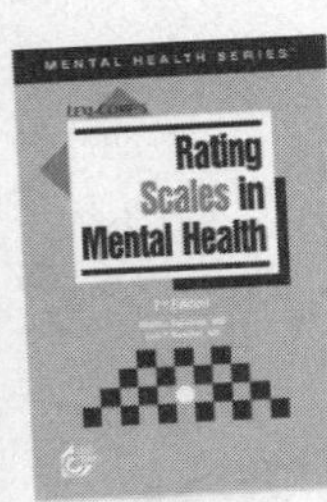

Ideal icians as well as admirors, this book provi overview of over 100 mended rating scalmental assessment.

IncRating scales for co s such as General Anxiety, Somily Functioning, Eating D s, and Sleep Disorders; aph format covering such s Overview of Scale, Applications, Psychometric ies, and References.

, call Customer Service at 1-866-397-3433 or visit www.lexi.com.
tside of the U.S., call +1-330-650-6506 or visit www.lexi.com.

Other Products Offered by Lexicomp

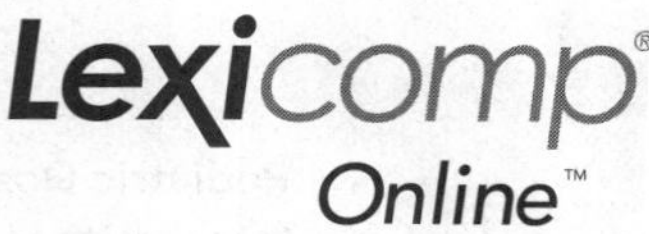

Nine of the top 10 hospitals in U.S. News & World Report's 211-12 Honor Roll ranking utilize Lexicomp's clinical databases and technology. These includeohns Hopkins, Massachusetts General, Mayo Clinic, Cleveland Clinic and others.

Lexicomp Online™ integrates industry-leading databases adenhanced searching technology to bring you time-sensitive clinical information at the poino'-care. Our easy-to-use interface and concise information eliminate the need to navigate thoug multiple pages or make unnecessary mouse clicks.

Lexicomp Online includes multiple databases and moduls coving the following topic areas:

- Core drug information with specialty fields
- Pediatrics and Geriatrics
- Interaction Analysis
- Pharmacogenomics
- Infectious Diseases
- Laboratory Tests and Diagnostic Procedures
- Natural Products
- Patient Education
- Drug Identification
- Calculations
- I.V. Compatibility: *King® Guide to Parenteral Admixtures®*
- Toxicology

Register for a FREE 45-day trial

Visit www.lexi.com/institutions

Academic and Institutional licenses available.

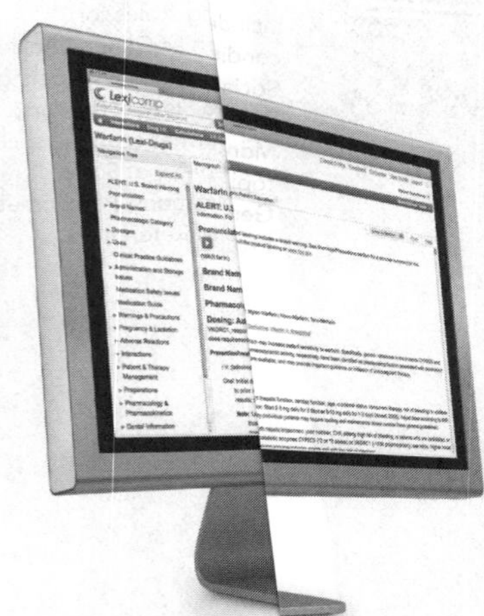

To order, call Customer Service at 1-866-397-3433 or visit w om.
Outside of the U.S., call +1-330-650-6506 or visit www.l

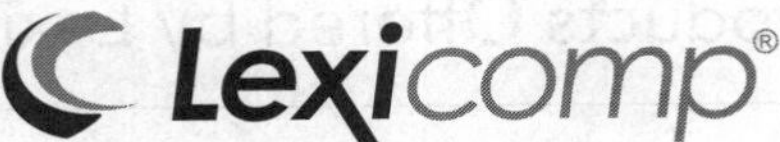

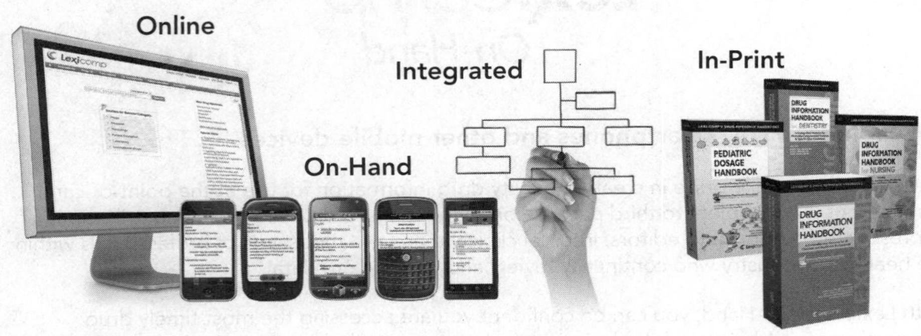

The Lexicomp Knowledge Solution™

The Lexicomp Knowledge Solution provides expert clinical decision support across four platforms, equipping your entire facility with the most trusted drug and clinical information available. Accessible In-Print, Online, On-Hand and Integrated within your HIS system, the Knowledge Solution is your single source for the point-of-care answers you need, when and where you need them. Contact Lexicomp to discuss how we can customize the Knowledge Solution to best serve your facility.

Lexicomp Online™ is the only hospital-wide drug information solution offering access to two levels of information. Lexicomp provides clear, concise, point-of-care knowledge, while AHFS® content allows you to dig deeper, should you need a more in-depth and authoritative research solution.

Lexicomp On-Hand™ is the most versatile and comprehensive drug information software available. Simply point, click and access Lexicomp's continually updated content, available on numerous mobile device platforms.

Lexicomp Integrated™ supplies the tools and content needed when integrating data into your HIS system. Drug interaction, allergy, duplicate therapy and dose range checking content provides a core clinical decision framework to improve decision making and ultimately influence positive patient outcomes.

Lexicomp In-Print™ offers a variety of handbooks designed for point-of-care use. For over 30 years, our handbooks have delivered the most trusted content in the industry. Choose from multiple titles, each focusing on a specific knowledge area.

For more information on the Lexicomp Knowledge Solution, visit our web site at www.lexi.com or call 1-800-837-5394.